THE Foundations OF Chinese Medicine

evolve

You've just purchased more than a textbook!

Evolve Student Resources for *Maciocia, The Foundations of Chinese Medicine, Third Edition*, include the following:

- Presents a new way of relating each pattern to a precursor and a consequence
- Introduces a unique and inventive new way of learning patterns (syndromes) to help you memorize them
- Contains a series of learning tools to help you remember patterns and point combinations
- A series of case studies give details of patient symptoms with a self-assessment option so that you can give your own diagnosis and check the suggested diagnosis

- Includes learning activities so that you can check and test your knowledge
- Contains over 600 MCQs to help you consolidate learning and prepare for exams
- Presents over 500 true/false questions you revise
- More than 800 short questions practise writing and learning by reading

Activate the complete learning experience with NEW text by registering at

https://evolve.elsevier.com/maciocia/foundations

REGISTER TODAY!

You can now purchase Elsevier products on Evolve!
Go to evolve.elsevier.com/html/shop-promo.html to search and browse for products.

For Elsevier
Content Strategist: *Alison Taylor*
Content Development Specialist: *Martin Mellor Publishing Services Ltd*
Project Manager: *Andrew Riley*
Designer/Design Direction: *Miles Hitchen*
Illustration Manager: *Ceil Nuyianes*

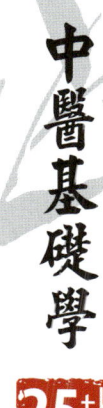

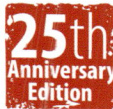

THE
Foundations
OF Chinese Medicine

THIRD EDITION

A Comprehensive Text

Giovanni Maciocia C.Ac. (Nanjing)

Acupuncturist and Medical Herbalist
Visiting Associate Professor at the Nanjing University of Traditional Chinese Medicine

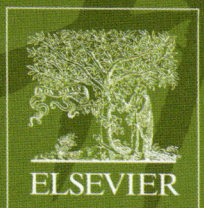

ELSEVIER

Edinburgh   London   New York   Oxford   Philadelphia   St Louis   Sydney   Toronto   2015

ELSEVIER

© 2015 Elsevier Ltd. All rights reserved.

No part of this publication may be reproduced or transmitted in any form or by any means, electronic or mechanical, including photocopying, recording, or any information storage and retrieval system, without permission in writing from the publisher. Details on how to seek permission, further information about the Publisher's permissions policies and our arrangements with organizations such as the Copyright Clearance Center and the Copyright Licensing Agency, can be found at our website: www.elsevier.com/permissions.

This book and the individual contributions contained in it are protected under copyright by the Publisher (other than as may be noted herein).

First edition 1989
Second edition 2005
Third edition 2015

ISBN (9780702052163)

British Library Cataloguing in Publication Data
A catalogue record for this book is available from the British Library

Library of Congress Cataloging in Publication Data
A catalog record for this book is available from the Library of Congress

Notices
Knowledge and best practice in this field are constantly changing. As new research and experience broaden our understanding, changes in research methods, professional practices, or medical treatment may become necessary.

Practitioners and researchers must always rely on their own experience and knowledge in evaluating and using any information, methods, compounds, or experiments described herein. In using such information or methods they should be mindful of their own safety and the safety of others, including parties for whom they have a professional responsibility.

With respect to any drug or pharmaceutical products identified, readers are advised to check the most current information provided (i) on procedures featured or (ii) by the manufacturer of each product to be administered, to verify the recommended dose or formula, the method and duration of administration, and contraindications. It is the responsibility of practitioners, relying on their own experience and knowledge of their patients, to make diagnoses, to determine dosages and the best treatment for each individual patient, and to take all appropriate safety precautions.

To the fullest extent of the law, neither the Publisher nor the authors, contributors, or editors, assume any liability for any injury and/or damage to persons or property as a matter of products liability, negligence or otherwise, or from any use or operation of any methods, products, instructions, or ideas contained in the material herein.

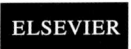 your source for books, journals and multimedia in the health sciences
www.elsevierhealth.com

The publisher's policy is to use **paper manufactured from sustainable forests**

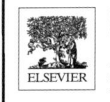 Working together to grow libraries in developing countries

www.elsevier.com • www.bookaid.org

Printed in China

Contents

Preface *xv*
Acknowledgements *xix*
Note on the translation of Chinese terms *xxi*

PART 1
GENERAL THEORY *1*
INTRODUCTION *2*

CHAPTER 1 Yin–Yang *3*

Historical Development *4*
Nature of the Yin–Yang Concept *4*
Application of Yin–Yang to Medicine *9*
Application of the Four Principles of Yin–Yang to Medicine *11*

CHAPTER 2 The Five Elements *19*

The Five Elements in Nature *20*
The Five Elements in Chinese Medicine *26*

CHAPTER 3 The Vital Substances *43*

The Concept of Qi in Chinese Philosophy *43*
The Concept of Qi in Chinese Medicine *45*

CHAPTER 4 The Transformations of Qi *75*

The Original Qi as the Motive Force for the Transformation of Qi *75*
The Fire of the Gate of Life as the Warmth for the Transformation of Qi *76*
The Dynamics and Physiology of the Transformation of Qi *78*
The Triple Burner's Transformation of Qi *87*
Pathology of Qi Transformation *89*

PART 2
THE FUNCTIONS OF THE INTERNAL ORGANS *93*

SECTION 1
THE FUNCTIONS OF THE YIN ORGANS *95*
INTRODUCTION *96*

CHAPTER 5 The Functions of the Internal Organs – Introduction *97*

The Internal Organs and the Vital Substances *98*
The Internal Organs and the Tissues *98*
The Internal Organs and the Sense Organs *98*
The Internal Organs and the Emotions *99*
The Internal Organs and the Spiritual Aspects *100*
The Internal Organs and Climates *101*
The External Manifestations of the Internal Organs *101*
The Internal Organs and the Fluids *101*
The Internal Organs and the Odours *102*
The Internal Organs and the Colours *102*
The Internal Organs and the Tastes *103*
The Internal Organs and the Sounds *103*
Yin (*Zang*) and Yang (*Fu*) Organs *103*

CHAPTER 6 The Functions of the Heart *107*

Functions of the Heart *107*
Other Heart Relationships *114*
Dreams *115*
Sayings *115*

CHAPTER 7 The Functions of the Liver *117*

Functions of the Liver *118*
Other Liver Relationships *125*
Dreams *126*
Sayings *126*

CHAPTER 8 The Functions of the Lungs *129*

The Functions of the Lungs *130*
Other Lung Relationships *140*
Dreams *141*
Sayings *141*

CHAPTER 9 The Functions of the Spleen *143*

The Functions of the Spleen *144*
Other Spleen Relationships *151*
Dreams *151*
Sayings *151*

CHAPTER 10 The Functions of the Kidneys *155*

The functions of the Kidneys *157*
Other Kidney relationships *165*
Dreams *165*
Sayings *165*

CHAPTER 11 The Functions of the Pericardium 169

The Pericardium as an organ 169
The Pericardium as a channel 170
The Pericardium and the Mind-Spirit 171
Relationship between the Pericardium and
the Minister Fire 171
Relationship between the Pericardium and the Uterus 172

CHAPTER 12 Yin Organ Interrelationships 175

Heart and Lungs 175
Heart and Liver 176
Heart and Kidneys 177
Liver and Lungs 179
Liver and Spleen 181
Liver and Kidneys 181
Spleen and Lungs 182
Spleen and Kidneys 183
Lungs and Kidneys 183
Spleen and Heart 184

SECTION 2
THE FUNCTIONS OF THE YANG ORGANS 189
INTRODUCTION 190

CHAPTER 13 The Functions of the Stomach 193

The Stomach Controls Receiving 193
The Stomach Controls The 'Rotting and Ripening'
Of Food 194
The Stomach Controls the Transportation of Food
Essences 194
The Stomach Controls the Descending of Qi 196
The Stomach is the Origin of Fluids 197
Other Aspects of the Stomach 197

CHAPTER 14 The Functions of the Small Intestine 201

The Small Intestine Controls Receiving and Transforming 201
The Small Intestine Separates Fluids 202
Other Aspects of the Small Intestine 202

CHAPTER 15 The Functions of the Large Intestine 205

The Large Intestine Controls Passage and
Conduction 205
The Large Intestine Transforms Stools and
Reabsorbs Fluids 206
Other Aspects of the Large Intestine 206

CHAPTER 16 Functions of the Gall Bladder 209

The Gall Bladder Stores and Excretes Bile 209
The Gall Bladder Controls Decisiveness 210
The Gall Bladder Controls the Sinews 211
Other Aspects of the Gall Bladder 211

CHAPTER 17 The Functions of the Bladder 215

The Bladder Removes Water by Qi Transformation 215
Other Aspects of the Bladder 216

CHAPTER 18 The Functions of the Triple Burner 219

Functions of the Triple Burner 219
Four Views of the Triple Burner 223
Other Aspects of the Triple Burner 229

SECTION 3
THE FUNCTIONS OF THE SIX EXTRAORDINARY YANG ORGANS 233
INTRODUCTION 234

CHAPTER 19 The Functions of the Six Extraordinary Yang Organs (the Four Seas) 235

The Uterus 235
The Brain 240
Marrow 241
The Bones 242
The Blood Vessels 243
The Gall Bladder 243
The Four Seas 243

PART 3
THE CAUSES OF DISEASE 247
INTRODUCTION 248

CHAPTER 20 Internal Causes of Disease 251

Anger 259
Joy 261
Sadness 261
Worry 263
Pensiveness 264
Fear 264
Shock 265

CHAPTER 21 External Causes of Disease 267

Climate as a Cause of Disease 268
Bacteria and Viruses in Relation to 'Wind' 269
Historical Background 270
Climatic Factors as Patterns of Disharmony 271
Artificial 'Climates' as Causes of Disease 272
Pathology and Clinical Manifestations of Exterior Pathogenic
Factors 272
Aversion to Cold and Fever 274
Symptoms and Signs of Exterior Pathogenic Factors
Patterns 276
Consequences of Invasion of Exterior Pathogenic Factors 277

CHAPTER 22 Miscellaneous Causes of Disease 279

Weak Constitution 279
Overwork 283

Excessive Physical Work (and Lack of Exercise) *284*
Excessive Sexual Activity *285*
Diet *290*
Trauma *292*
Parasites and Poisons *292*
Wrong Treatment *293*
Medicinal Drugs *293*
Drugs *294*

PART 4
DIAGNOSIS *297*
INTRODUCTION *298*

CHAPTER 23 Diagnosis by Observation *301*

Introduction *301*
Spirit *306*
Body *307*
Demeanour and Body Movements *313*
Head and Face *313*
Eyes *317*
Nose *318*
Ears *319*
Mouth and Lips *319*
Teeth and Gums *319*
Throat *320*
Limbs *321*
Skin *324*
Tongue *324*
Channels *331*

CHAPTER 24 Diagnosis by Interrogation *335*

Nature of Diagnosis by Interrogation *337*
Nature of 'Symptoms' in Chinese Medicine *337*
The Art of Interrogation: Asking the Right Questions *338*
Terminology Problems in Interrogation *338*
Procedure for Interrogation *339*
Identification of Patterns and Interrogation *339*
Tongue and Pulse Diagnosis: Integration with Interrogation *340*
The 10 Traditional Questions *340*
Three New Questions for Western Patients *341*
The 16 Questions *342*

CHAPTER 25 Diagnosis by Palpation *373*

Pulse Diagnosis *374*
Palpating the Skin *389*
Palpating the Limbs *390*
Palpating the Chest *392*
Palpating the Abdomen *394*
Palpating Points *394*

CHAPTER 26 Diagnosis by Hearing and Smelling *397*

Diagnosis by Hearing *397*
Diagnosis by Smelling *399*

PART 5
PATHOLOGY *401*
INTRODUCTION *402*

CHAPTER 27 The Pathology of Full and Empty Conditions *403*

Introduction *403*
Nature of 'Pathogenic Factor' in Chinese Medicine *403*
Full Conditions *411*
Empty Conditions *411*
Full/Empty Conditions *412*
Interaction Between Pathogenic Factors and Upright Qi *415*

CHAPTER 28 The Pathology of Yin–Yang Imbalance *419*

Imbalance of Yin and Yang *419*
Yin–Yang Imbalance and Heat–Cold Patterns *420*
Transformation and Interaction between Yin and Yang *420*
Excess of Yang *421*
Deficiency of Yang *421*
Excess of Yin *422*
Deficiency of Yin *422*
Principles of Treatment *423*

CHAPTER 29 Pathology of the Qi Mechanism *425*

Pathology of the Ascending/Descending of Qi *426*
Pathology of the Entering/Exiting of Qi *432*

PART 6
IDENTIFICATION OF PATTERNS *439*
INTRODUCTION *440*

SECTION 1
IDENTIFICATION OF PATTERNS ACCORDING TO THE EIGHT PRINCIPLES AND QI–BLOOD–BODY FLUIDS *447*
INTRODUCTION *448*

CHAPTER 30 Identification of Patterns according to the Eight Principles *451*

Exterior–Interior *453*
Hot–Cold *455*
Combined Hot and Cold *460*
Full–Empty *461*
Yin–Yang *465*

CHAPTER 31 Identification of Patterns according to Qi–Blood–Body Fluids *469*

Qi Pattern Identification *470*
Blood Pattern Identification *471*
Body Fluid Pattern Identification *476*

SECTION 2
IDENTIFICATION OF PATTERNS ACCORDING TO THE INTERNAL ORGANS 483
INTRODUCTION 484

CHAPTER 32 Heart Patterns 489

General aetiology 490
Deficiency Patterns 491
Excess Patterns 500
Deficiency–Excess Patterns 510
Combined Patterns 513

CHAPTER 33 Pericardium Patterns 515

The pericardium in invasions of exterior pathogenic factors 515
The pericardium as the 'house' of the mind 518
The pericardium as the 'centre of the thorax' 524

CHAPTER 34 Liver Patterns 529

General Aetiology 530
Full Patterns 532
Empty Patterns 548
Full/Empty Patterns 552
Combined Patterns 559

CHAPTER 35 Lung Patterns 571

General Aetiology 572
Empty Patterns 573
Full Patterns: Exterior 579
Full Patterns: Interior 584
Combined Patterns 594

CHAPTER 36 Spleen Patterns 597

General Aetiology 598
Empty Patterns 599
Full Patterns 608
Combined Patterns 612

CHAPTER 37 Kidney Patterns 621

General Aetiology 623
Empty Patterns 625
Empty/Full Patterns 635
Combined Patterns 640

CHAPTER 38 Stomach Patterns 651

General Aetiology 653
Empty Patterns 655
Full Patterns 660
Combined Patterns 672

CHAPTER 39 Small Intestine Patterns 677

General Aetiology 677
Full Patterns 678
Empty Pattern 684

CHAPTER 40 Large Intestine Patterns 687

General Aetiology 687
Full Patterns 688
Empty Patterns 697

CHAPTER 41 Gall Bladder Patterns 703

General Aetiology 703
Full Patterns 704
Empty Patterns 708
Combined Patterns 710

CHAPTER 42 Bladder Patterns 713

General Aetiology 713
Full Patterns 714
Empty Patterns 718

SECTION 3
IDENTIFICATION OF PATTERNS ACCORDING TO PATHOGENIC FACTORS 723
INTRODUCTION 724

CHAPTER 43 Identification of Patterns According to Pathogenic Factors 725

Wind 727
Cold 732
Summer-Heat 736
Dampness 737
Dryness 743
Fire 745

CHAPTER 44 Identification of Patterns According to the Six Stages 751

Greater Yang Stage 753
Channel Patterns 754
Organ Patterns 756
Bright Yang Stage 757
Lesser Yang (*Shao Yang*) Stage 759
Greater Yin (*Tai Yin*) Stage 760
Lesser Yin (*Shao Yin*) Stage 761
Terminal Yin (*Jue Yin*) Stage 762

CHAPTER 45 Identification of Patterns According to the Four Levels 765

Defensive Qi (*Wei*) Level 770
Qi Level 773

Nutritive Qi (*Ying*) Level 775
Blood Level 776
Latent Heat 779
Relationships between the Four Levels, Six Stages and Three Burners 781

CHAPTER 46 Identification of Patterns According to the Three Burners 787

Upper Burner 787
Middle Burner 789
Lower Burner 790

SECTION 4 793
IDENTIFICATION OF PATTERNS ACCORDING TO THE 12 CHANNELS, EIGHT EXTRAORDINARY VESSELS AND FIVE ELEMENTS 793
INTRODUCTION 794

CHAPTER 47 Identification of Patterns According to the 12 Channels 795

CHAPTER 48 Identification of Patterns According to the Eight Extraordinary Vessels 807

Governing Vessel (*Du Mai*) 807
Directing Vessel (*Ren Mai*) 808
Penetrating Vessel (*Chong Mai*) 809
Combined Directing and Penetrating Vessel Patterns 810
Girdle Vessel (*Dai Mai*) 815
Yin Stepping Vessel (*Yin Qiao Mai*) 816
Yang Stepping Vessel (*Yang Qiao Mai*) 817
Yin Linking Vessel (*Yin Wei Mai*) 817
Yang Linking Vessel (*Yang Wei Mai*) 818

CHAPTER 49 Identification of Patterns According to the Five Elements 821

Generating Sequence Patterns 821
Overacting Sequence Patterns 822
Insulting Sequence Patterns 823

PART 7
THE ACUPUNCTURE POINTS 825
INTRODUCTION 826

SECTION 1
CATEGORIES OF POINTS 827
INTRODUCTION 828

CHAPTER 50 The Five Transporting Points (*Shu* Points) 829

Energetic Actions of the Five Transporting Points 832
Actions of the Five Transporting Points From the Classics 834
Summary 839

CHAPTER 51 The Functions of Specific Categories of Points 845

Source (*Yuan*) Points 845
Connecting (*Luo*) Points 848
Back Transporting (*Shu*) Points 853
Front Collecting (*Mu*) Points 857
Accumulation (*Xi*) Points 858
Gathering (*Hui*) Points 859
Points of the Four Seas 859
Window of Heaven Points 860
12 Heavenly Star Points of Ma Dan Yang 862
Sun Si Miao's 13 Ghost Points 862
Points of the Eye System (*Mu Xi*) 863
Five Command Points 864

CHAPTER 52 The Eight Extraordinary Vessels – Introduction 867

Introduction 868
Functions of the Extraordinary Vessels 868
Energetic dynamics of the extraordinary vessels 874
Clinical Use of the Extraordinary Vessels 880

CHAPTER 53 The Eight Extraordinary Vessels 889

Governing Vessel (*Du Mai*) 892
Directing Vessel (*Ren Mai*) 897
Penetrating Vessel (*Chong Mai*) 902
Girdle Vessel (*Dai Mai*) 918
Yin Stepping Vessel (*Yin Qiao Mai*) 922
Yang Stepping Vessel (*Yang Qiao Mai*) 925
Combined Yin and Yang Stepping Vessel Pathology 929
Yin Linking Vessel (*Yin Wei Mai*) 931
Yang Linking Vessel (*Yang Wei Mai*) 934
Combined Yin and Yang Linking Vessel Pathology 936

SECTION 2
THE FUNCTIONS OF THE POINTS 941
INTRODUCTION 942

CHAPTER 54 Lung Channel 949

LU-1 Zhongfu *Central Palace* 949
LU-2 Yunmen *Cloud Door* 950
LU-3 Tianfu *Heavenly Palace* 951
LU-5 Chize *Foot Marsh* 952
LU-6 Kongzui *Convergence Hole* 953
LU-7 Lieque *Branching Cleft* 954
LU-8 Jingqu *River [Point] Ditch* 956
LU-9 Taiyuan *Supreme Abyss* 956
LU-10 Yuji *Fish Border* 957
LU-11 Shaoshang *Lesser Metal* 958

CHAPTER 55 Large Intestine Channel 961

L.I.-1 Shangyang *Metal Yang* 962
L.I.-2 Erjian *Second Interval* 962

L.I.-3 Sanjian *Third Interval* 963
L.I.-4 Hegu *Enclosed Valley* 963
L.I.-5 Yangxi *Yang Stream* 964
L.I.-6 Pianli *Lateral Passage* 965
L.I.-7 Wenliu *Warm Gathering* 965
L.I.-10 Shousanli *Arm Three Miles* 966
L.I.-11 Quchi *Pool on Bend* 967
L.I.-12 Zhouliao *Elbow Crevice* 968
L.I.-14 Binao *Upper Arm* 968
L.I.-15 Jianyu *Shoulder Bone* 968
L.I.-16 Jugu *Great Bone* 969
L.I.-17 Tianding *Heaven's Tripod* 969
L.I.-18 Futu *Support the Protuberance* 969
L.I.-20 Yingxiang *Welcome Fragrance* 970

CHAPTER 56 Stomach Channel 973

ST-1 Chengqi *Containing Tears* 974
ST-2 Sibai *Four Whites* 974
ST-3 Juliao *Great Crevice* 975
ST-4 Dicang *Earth Granary* 975
ST-6 Jiache *Jaw Chariot* 976
ST-7 Xiaguan *Lower Gate* 976
ST-8 Touwei *Head Corner* 977
ST-9 Renying *Person's Welcome* 977
ST-12 Quepen *Empty Basin* 978
ST-18 Rugen *Breast Root* 978
ST-19 Burong *Full* 979
ST-20 Chengman *Supporting Fullness* 979
ST-21 Liangmen *Beam Door* 979
ST-22 Guanmen *Pass Gate* 980
ST-25 Tianshu *Heavenly Pivot* 980
ST-27 Daju *Big Greatness* 981
ST-28 Shuidao *Water Passages* 982
ST-29 Guilai *Return* 982
ST-30 Qichong *Penetrating Qi* 983
ST-31 Biguan *Thigh Gate* 984
ST-32 Futu *Crouching Rabbit* 984
ST-34 Liangqiu *Beam Mound* 985
ST-35 Dubi *Calf Nose* 985
ST-36 Zusanli *Three Miles of the Foot* 985
ST-37 Shangjuxu *Upper Great Emptiness* 987
ST-38 Tiaokou *Narrow Opening* 987
ST-39 Xiajuxu *Lower Great Emptiness* 988
ST-40 Fenglong *Abundant Bulge* 988
ST-41 Jiexi *Dispersing Stream* 989
ST-42 Chongyang *Penetrating Yang* 990
ST-43 Xiangu *Sinking Valley* 990
ST-44 Neiting *Inner Courtyard* 991
ST-45 Lidui *Sick Mouth* 991

CHAPTER 57 Spleen Channel 995

SP-1 Yinbai *Hidden White* 995
SP-2 Dadu *Big Capital* 996
SP-3 Taibai *Supreme White* 997
SP-4 Gongsun *Minute Connecting Channels* 998
SP-5 Shangqiu *Metal Mound* 999

SP-6 Sanyinjiao *Three Yin Meeting* 1000
SP-8 Diji *Earth Pivot* 1001
SP-9 Yinlingquan *Yin Mound Spring* 1002
SP-10 Xuehai *Sea of Blood* 1003
SP-12 Chongmen *Penetrating Door* 1004
SP-15 Daheng *Big Horizontal Stroke* 1004
SP-21 Dabao *General Control* 1005

CHAPTER 58 Heart Channel 1007

HE-1 Jiquan *Supreme Spring* 1007
HE-3 Shaohai *Lesser-Yin Sea* 1008
HE-4 Lingdao *Spirit Path* 1008
HE-5 Tongli *Inner Communication* 1009
HE-6 Yinxi *Yin Crevice* 1010
HE-7 Shenmen *Mind Door* 1010
HE-8 Shaofu *Lesser-Yin Mansion* 1012
HE-9 Shaochong *Lesser-Yin Penetrating* 1013

CHAPTER 59 Small Intestine Channel 1015

S.I.-1 Shaoze *Lesser Marsh* 1016
S.I.-2 Qiangu *Front Valley* 1016
S.I.-3 Houxi *Back Stream* 1017
S.I.-4 Wangu *Wrist Bone* 1018
S.I.-5 Yanggu *Yang Valley* 1019
S.I.-6 Yanglao *Nourishing the Elderly* 1019
S.I.-7 Zhizheng *Branch to Heart Channel* 1020
S.I.-8 Xiaohai *Small Intestine Sea* 1020
S.I.-9 Jianzhen *Upright Shoulder* 1021
S.I.-10 Naoshu *Humerus Transporting Point* 1021
S.I.-11 Tianzong *Heavenly Attribution* 1021
S.I.-12 Bingfeng *Watching Wind* 1022
S.I.-13 Quyuan *Bent Wall* 1022
S.I.-14 Jianwaishu *Transporting Point of the Outside of the Shoulder* 1023
S.I.-15 Jianzhongshu *Transporting Point of the Centre of the Shoulder* 1023
S.I.-16 Tianchuang *Heavenly Window* 1024
S.I.-17 Tianrong *Heavenly Appearance* 1024
S.I.-18 Quanliao *Zygoma Crevice* 1025
S.I.-19 Tinggong *Listening Palace* 1025

CHAPTER 60 Bladder Channel 1027

BL-1 Jingming *Eye Brightness* 1027
BL-2 Zanzhu (or Cuanzhu) *Gathered Bamboo* 1029
BL-5 Wuchu *Five Places* 1029
BL-7 Tongtian *Penetrating Heaven* 1029
BL-9 Yuzhen *Jade Pillow* 1030
BL-10 Tianzhu *Heaven Pillar* 1030
BL-11 Dazhu *Big Shuttle* 1031
Fengmen BL-12 *Wind Door* 1033
BL-13 Feishu *Lung Back Transporting Point* 1034
BL-14 Jueyinshu *Terminal Yin Back Transporting Point* 1035
BL-15 Xinshu *Heart Back Transporting Point* 1035
BL-16 Dushu *Governing Vessel Back Transporting Point* 1036

BL-17 Geshu *Diaphragm Back Transporting Point* 1036
BL-18 Ganshu *Liver Back Transporting Point* 1037
BL-19 Danshu *Gall Bladder Back Transporting Point* 1038
BL-20 Pishu *Spleen Back Transporting Point* 1039
BL-21 Weishu *Stomach Back Transporting Point* 1039
BL-22 Sanjiaoshu *Triple Burner Back Transporting Point* 1040
BL-23 Shenshu *Kidney Back Transporting Point* 1041
BL-24 Qihaishu *Sea of Qi Back Transporting Point* 1043
BL-25 Dachangshu *Large Intestine Back Transporting Point* 1043
BL-26 Guanyuanshu *Origin Gate Back Transporting Point* 1044
BL-27 Xiaochangshu *Small Intestine Back Transporting Point* 1044
BL-28 Pangguangshu *Bladder Back Transporting Point* 1045
BL-30 Baihuanshu *White Ring Transporting Point* 1045
BL-32 Ciliao *Second Crevice* 1046
BL-36 Chengfu *Receiving Support* 1046
BL-37 Yinmen *Huge Gate* 1047
BL-39 Weiyang *Supporting Yang* 1047
BL-40 Weizhong *Supporting Middle* 1047
BL-42 Pohu *Door of the Corporeal Soul* 1048
BL-43 Gaohuangshu (or Gaohuang) *Transporting Point of Gaohuang* 1049
BL-44 Shentang *Mind Hall* 1050
BL-47 Hunmen *Door of the Ethereal Soul* 1050
BL-49 Yishe *Intellect Abode* 1051
BL-51 Huangmen *Door of Gaohuang* 1052
BL-52 Zhishi *Room of Will-Power* 1052
BL-53 Baohuang *Bladder Vitals* 1053
BL-54 Zhibian *Lowermost Edge* 1054
BL-57 Chengshan *Supporting Mountain* 1055
BL-58 Feiyang *Flying Up* 1055
BL-59 Fuyang *Instep Yang* 1056
BL-60 Kunlun *Kunlun (Mountains)* 1056
BL-62 Shenmai *Ninth Channel* 1057
BL-63 Jinmen *Golden Door* 1058
BL-64 Jinggu *Capital Bone* 1058
BL-65 Shugu *Binding Bone* 1059
BL-66 Tonggu *Passing Valley* 1059
BL-67 Zhiyin *Reaching Yin* 1060

CHAPTER 61 Kidney Channel 1063

KI-1 Yongquan *Bubbling Spring* 1063
KI-2 Rangu *Blazing Valley* 1064
KI-3 Taixi *Greater Stream* 1065
KI-4 Dazhong *Big Bell* 1066
KI-5 Shuiquan *Water Spring* 1066
KI-6 Zhaohai *Shining Sea* 1067
KI-7 Fuliu *Returning Current* 1068
KI-8 Jiaoxin *Meeting the Spleen Channel* 1068
KI-9 Zhubin *Guest House* 1069
KI-10 Yingu *Yin Valley* 1069
KI-11 Henggu *Pubic Bone* 1070
KI-12 Dahe *Big Glory* 1070
KI-13 Qixue *Qi Hole* 1071

KI-14 Siman *Four Fullnesses* 1072
KI-16 Huangshu *Transporting Point of 'Huang'* 1073
KI-17 Shangqu *Bent Metal* 1073
KI-21 Youmen *Door of Darkness* 1074
KI-23 Shenfeng *Mind Seal* 1075
KI-24 Lingxu *Spirit Burial Ground* 1075
KI-25 Shencang *Mind Storage* 1075
KI-27 Shufu *Transporting Point Mansion* 1076

CHAPTER 62 Pericardium Channel 1079

P-1 Tianchi *Heavenly Pool* 1079
P-3 Quze *Marsh on Bend* 1080
P-4 Ximen *Cleft Door* 1081
P-5 Jianshi *Intermediary* 1081
P-6 Neiguan *Inner Gate* 1082
P-7 Daling *Great Hill* 1083
P-8 Laogong *Labour Palace* 1084
P-9 Zhongchong *Centre Rush* 1085

CHAPTER 63 Triple Burner Channel 1087

T.B.-1 Guanchong *Penetrating the Gate* 1088
T.B.-2 Yemen *Fluid Door* 1089
T.B.-3 Zhongzhu *Middle Islet* 1089
T.B.-4 Yangchi *Yang Pond* 1090
T.B.-5 Waiguan *Outer Gate* 1091
T.B.-6 Zhigou *Branching Ditch* 1092
T.B.-7 Huizong *Converging Channels* 1093
T.B.-8 Sanyangluo *Connecting Three Yang* 1093
T.B.-10 Tianjing *Heavenly Well* 1094
T.B.-13 Naohui *Shoulder Convergence* 1094
T.B.-14 Jianliao *Shoulder Crevice* 1095
T.B.-15 Tianliao *Heavenly Crevice* 1095
T.B.-16 Tianyou *Window of Heaven* 1096
T.B.-17 Yifeng *Wind Screen* 1096
T.B.-21 Ermen *Ear Door* 1096
T.B.-23 Sizhukong *Silk Bamboo Hole* 1097

CHAPTER 64 Gall Bladder Channel 1099

G.B.-1 Tongziliao *Pupil Crevice* 1100
G.B.-2 Tinghui *Hearing Convergence* 1100
G.B.-4 Hanyan *Jaw Serenity* 1101
G.B.-5 Xuanlu *Hanging Skull* 1101
G.B.-6 Xuanli *Deviation From Hanging Skull* 1101
G.B.-8 Shuaigu *Leading Valley* 1102
G.B.-9 Tianchong *Penetrating Heaven* 1102
G.B.-11 Touqiaoyin *(Head) Yin Orifices* 1103
G.B.-12 Wangu *Whole Bone* 1103
G.B.-13 Benshen *Mind Root* 1104
G.B.-14 Yangbai *Yang White* 1105
G.B.-15 Linqi *Falling Tears* 1105
G.B.-17 Zhengying *Top Convergence* 1106
G.B.-18 Chengling *Spirit Receiver* 1106
G.B.-19 Naokong *Brain Cavity* 1106
G.B.-20 Fengchi *Wind Pool* 1107
G.B.-21 Jianjing *Shoulder Well* 1108

G.B.-22 Yuanye *Axilla Abyss* 1109
G.B.-24 Riyue *Sun and Moon* 1109
G.B.-25 Jingmen *Capital Door* 1110
G.B.-26 Daimai *Girdle Vessel* 1110
G.B.-29 Juliao *Squatting Crevice* 1110
G.B.-30 Huantiao *Jumping Circle* 1111
G.B.-31 Fengshi *Wind Market* 1112
G.B.-33 Xiyangguan *Knee Yang Gate* 1112
G.B.-34 Yanglingquan *Yang Hill Spring* 1112
G.B.-35 Yangjiao *Yang Crossing* 1113
G.B.-36 Waiqiu *Outer Mound* 1113
G.B.-37 Guangming *Brightness* 1114
G.B.-38 Yangfu *Yang Aid* 1114
G.B.-39 Xuanzhong *Hanging Bell* 1115
G.B.-40 Qiuxu *Mound Ruins* 1115
G.B.-41 Zulinqi *(Foot) Falling Tears* 1116
G.B.-43 Xiaxi *Stream Insertion* 1116
G.B.-44 Zuqiaoyin *(Foot) Yin Orifice* 1117

CHAPTER 65 Liver Channel 1119

LIV-1 Dadun *Big Mound* 1120
LIV-2 Xingjian *Temporary in-Between* 1120
LIV-3 Taichong *Bigger Penetrating* 1121
LIV-4 Zhongfeng *Middle Seal* 1123
LIV-5 Ligou *Gourd Ditch* 1123
LIV-6 Zhongdu *Middle Capital* 1124
LIV-7 Xiguan *Knee Gate* 1124
LIV-8 Ququan *Spring on Bend* 1124
LIV-13 Zhangmen *Completion Gate* 1125
LIV-14 Qimen *Cyclic Gate* 1125

CHAPTER 66 Directing Vessel (Ren Mai) 1129

REN-1 Huiyin *Meeting of Yin* 1129
REN-2 Qugu *Curved Bone* 1130
REN-3 Zhongji *Middle Pole* 1131
REN-4 Guanyuan *Gate to the Original Qi* 1132
REN-5 Shimen *Stone Door* 1133
REN-6 Qihai *Sea of Qi* 1134
REN-7 Yinjiao *Yin Crossing* 1135
REN-8 Shenque *Spirit Palace* 1136
REN-9 Shuifen *Water Separation* 1138
REN-10 Xiawan *Lower Epigastrium* 1138
REN-11 Jianli *Building Mile* 1139
REN-12 Zhongwan *Middle of Epigastrium* 1139
REN-13 Shangwan *Upper Epigastrium* 1140
REN-14 Juque *Great Palace* 1141
REN-15 Jiuwei *Dove Tail* 1142
REN-17 Shanzhong (or Tanzhong) *Middle of Chest* 1143
REN-22 Tiantu *Heaven Projection* 1144
REN-23 Lianquan *Corner Spring* 1144
REN-24 Chengjiang *Saliva Receiver* 1144

CHAPTER 67 Governing Vessel 1147

Du-1 Changqiang *Long Strength* 1148
Du-2 Yaoshu *Transporting Point of Lower Back* 1148
Du-3 Yaoyangguan *Lumbar Yang Gate* 1148
Du-4 Mingmen *Gate of Life* 1149
Du-8 Jinsuo *Tendon Spasm* 1150
Du-9 Zhiyang *Reaching Yang* 1151
Du-11 Shendao *Mind Way* 1151
Du-12 Shenzhu *Body Pillar* 1151
Du-13 Taodao *Kiln Way* 1152
Du-14 Dazhui *Big Vertebra* 1152
Du-15 Yamen *Door to Dumbness* 1153
Du-16 Fengfu *Wind Palace* 1154
Du-17 Naohu *Brain Window* 1154
Du-19 Houding *Posterior Vertex* 1155
Du-20 Baihui *Hundred Meetings* 1155
Du-23 Shangxing *Upper Star* 1156
Du-24 Shenting *Mind Courtyard* 1156
Du-26 Renzhong *Middle of Person* 1157

CHAPTER 68 Extra Points 1159

Sishencong *Four Mind Alertness* 1159
Yintang *Seal Hall* 1159
Taiyang *Greater Yang* 1160
Yuyao *Fish Spine* 1160
Bitong *Free Nose Passages* 1161
Jingzhong *Middle of Periods* 1161
Qimen *Door of Qi* 1161
Zigong *Palace of Child* 1162
Tituo *Lift and Support* 1162
Dingchuan *Stopping Asthma* 1162
Jinggong *Palace of Essence* 1163
Huatuojiaji *Hua Tuo Back Filling Points* 1163
Shiqizhuixia *Below the 17Th Vertebra* 1164
Jianneiling *Inner Shoulder Mound* 1164
Baxie *Eight Pathogenic Factors* 1165
Sifeng *Four Cracks* 1165
Shixuan *Ten Declarations* 1166
Xiyan *Knee Eyes* 1166
Dannangxue *Gall Bladder Point* 1167
Lanweixue *Appendix Point* 1167
Bafeng *Eight Winds* 1167

PART 8
PRINCIPLES OF TREATMENT 1169
INTRODUCTION 1170

CHAPTER 69 Principles of Treatment 1171

The Root and the Manifestation (*Ben* and *Biao*) 1173
When to Tonify Upright Qi, When to Expel Pathogenic Factors 1178
Differences between Acupuncture and Herbal Therapy in the Application of the Treatment Principle 1184

CHAPTER 70 Principles of Combination of Points 1191

Balancing Distal and Local Points 1195
Balancing Upper and Lower Parts of the Body 1202
Balancing Left and Right 1204

Balancing Yin and Yang *1206*
Balancing Front and Back *1207*

Appendix 1: Prescriptions *1209*
Appendix 2: Glossary of Chinese Terms *1231*

Appendix 3: Chronology of Chinese Dynasties *1241*
Appendix 4: Bibliography *1243*
Appendix 5: The Classics of Chinese Medicine *1249*
Appendix 6: Self-Assesment Answers *1255*
Index *1267*

Preface

It is now 27 years since I started writing the first edition of the 'Foundations of Chinese Medicine': this proved to be very popular with students and it has been adopted as a textbook by many acupuncture colleges all over the world. The present edition is a revision of the second edition published in 2005.

As its name implies, this book is intended to give the foundations of the principles of Chinese medicine: it is therefore only the beginning in the journey of learning this ancient art. There are of course, very many different traditions of Chinese medicine and especially, acupuncture: I hope that this book can provide a 'foundation' from which a practitioner can build and branch out in different directions.

My main sources (indicated in the bibliography) for this book are modern Chinese textbooks and some ancient ones and in particular the Yellow Emperor's Classic of Internal Medicine (Simple Questions *Su Wen* and Spiritual Axis *Ling Shu*) and the Classic of Difficulties (*Nan Jing*). I have tried to present the theory of Chinese medicine from Chinese books but I have also occasionally presented my own experience gleaned from nearly 40 years of practice. Whenever I present my own experience, I precede this with the statement '*in my experience*' or '*in my opinion*'.

It is worth mentioning the main changes made in the second edition:

1. An expanded discussion of the functions of the Pericardium
2. An expanded discussion of the functions and nature of the Triple Burner
3. An expanded discussion of external pathogenic factors both as causes of disease and as patterns
4. An expanded section on Diagnosis
5. A new section on pathology (chapters 27, 28 and 29)
6. A complete revision of the clinical manifestations of the patterns of the Internal Organs with a clearer distinction between Yin deficiency and Empty Heat for each organ and the addition of herbal prescriptions for each pattern
7. An expanded discussion of the Identification of Patterns according to the 6 Stages, 4 Levels and 3 Burners.
8. A greatly expanded discussion of the nature, functions and clinical application of the 8 Extraordinary Vessels
9. The discussion of categories of point not previously discussed, e.g. points of the 4 Seas, Window of Heaven points, 12 Heavenly Star points, Sun Si Miao's Ghost points, points of the Eye System and 5 Command points
10. A complete revision of the functions of the points with a new heading of 'Clinical manifestations' and the addition of some points not previously discussed
11. An expanded discussion of the principles of combination of acupuncture points.

The present revision made the following changes or additions to the 2005 edition:

1. Over 200 new figures throughout the book
2. New self-assessment tests to help students in their studies
3. Case histories with self-assessment tests
4. New diagrams illustrating the precursors and developments of the Internal Organs patterns.
5. New guidelines with figures as to how to learn the patterns of the Internal Organs in a logical, simple way, avoiding mere memorization
6. More clinical notes throughout the text
7. More acupuncture point combinations with analysis of points actions
8. More case histories
9. Location of acupuncture points mentioned

The reader will notice that I do not use the term 'Traditional Chinese Medicine' (TCM) in my books as I personally do not agree with this term. It is a term that came to be used purely by chance when Westerners started attending courses at Chinese colleges, all of which are called 'College of Traditional Chinese Medicine'. In China, Chinese Medicine is simply called '*Zhong Yi*' (which means 'Chinese medicine') to distinguish it from Western medicine (*Xi Yi*).

When the Chinese colleges started running courses for foreigners they coined the term 'Traditional Chinese medicine'. The Chinese colleges did not use the word 'traditional' with the same meaning as most acupuncturist would give it in the West. Unfortunately, the word 'traditional' is often used in the West by followers of particular styles of acupuncture, each claiming to be more 'traditional' or 'classical' than another.

Especially in the context of Chinese medicine, the word 'traditional' can mean anything depending on which tradition one refers to. Is a tradition from the Han dynasty more 'traditional' than one from the Song dynasty because it is older? More importantly, is an innovation introduced post 1949 to be discarded because it is 'marxist-leninist' or 'maoist'?

As the Chinese colleges were called 'College of Traditional Chinese Medicine' and taught courses in 'traditional Chinese medicine', the term TCM began to be used to identify Chinese medicine and acupuncture '*as it is practised and taught in modern China*'.

For me, the main problems with the term 'TCM' are two. Firstly, this term implies that Chinese medicine 'as it is practised and taught in modern China' is rigidly monolithic and uniform and not allowing any diversity. This is simply not the case.

There are as many styles of acupuncture in China as there are provinces, counties and colleges. While a certain 'systematization' is encouraged, diversity is not suppressed. One only needs to walk into a bookshop in China and check the Chinese medicine section: there are always many texts called 'Collection of Experiences of Modern Chinese medicine doctors' (apart from the collections of experiences of ancient doctors). It is wrong to make a judgment on the state of Chinese medicine in modern China purely on the basis of the few textbooks translated into English and on the basis of the curriculum of the courses run for foreigners. That diversity is not suppressed is also evidenced by the reverence demonstrated towards old doctors '*lao zhong yi*'") and the appreciation of their particular styles and theories.

Secondly, the term 'TCM' is difficult to define as a particular style of acupuncture in the West. There is certainly no uniformity of 'TCM' acupuncture among Western practitioners. For example, if TCM is defined as 'Chinese medicine and acupuncture as they are taught and practised in modern China', then I personally do not practise 'TCM' and neither do any of the colleagues I know.

There is an on-going debate as to how much the modern Chinese (post 1949) have changed, excessively 'systematized' or even corrupted Chinese medicine and acupuncture. This is a very wide issue that could actually be the subject of a book in itself. Of course the modern Communist Chinese regime has influenced Chinese medicine, in the same way as any previous dynasty also influenced Chinese medicine. Undoubtedly, there has been a 'systematization' of Chinese medicine which, in my opinion, was dictated more by the need to train vast numbers of doctors of Chinese medicine in the dramatic public health situation of 1950 than by the desire to consciously impose a Marxist orthodoxy onto Chinese medicine. Moreover, some of the 'systematization' actually started before 1949.[i]

The new Communist government was faced with the huge task of delivering healthcare to a population weakened by innumerable infectious diseases, malnutrition, 25 years of civil war and famines: the new Government made the conscious decision to rely on Chinese medicine and raise it to a new level. They had little choice but to do that. Indeed, they did that not through a conviction in the value of Chinese medicine but out of sheer necessity as many millions of peasants relied only on Chinese medicine for their health.

Another important factor that drove such 'systematization' was the necessity to make Chinese medicine appear more 'scientific' so that it would be more readily accepted by the Western-trained Chinese doctors of Western medicine. We should realize that there was a fierce struggle going on in the Chinese Ministry of Public Health in the 1950s between the promoters of Chinese medicine and the 'modernizers'. Again, such need to make Chinese medicine appear more 'scientific' started before 1949. Indeed, it was in the 1930s and at the hand of the Nationalist government (of Chang Kai Shek) that they tried to suppress Chinese medicine entirely.

The systematization that occurred in modern China, therefore, was more the result of a necessity to set up solid colleges with a common syllabus that could train thousands of doctors of Chinese medicine in a rational manner, rather than of a conscious Marxist agenda bent on suppressing divergent views. Any group of persons which decides to set up a college needs to draw up a syllabus that necessarily represents a 'systematization' of a subject and one that necessarily includes certain subjects and excludes others.

That the modern Chinese did not set out to deliberately and systematically to eradicate any classic influence from Chinese medicine is evidenced by two main factors amongst others.

Firstly, the modern Chinese have reprinted all the old classics in simplified characters which makes them easier to study to the new generations and such classics form part of the curriculum of Chinese colleges (all major colleges of Chinese Medicine have a *Nei Jing* department).

Secondly, there are dozens and dozens of modern books collecting the experiences of both ancient and modern famous doctors, one of which has been translated into English and called '*Essentials of Contemporary Chinese Acupuncturists' Clinical Experience*': strangely, very few colleagues seem to have read this interesting book.[ii]

Moreover, some of the 'systematization' of Chinese medicine is welcome. The logical and structured way of teaching the functions and patterns of the internal organs is very helpful in practice. For example, when we study the functions of the internal organs, we do so systematically listing the sense organ, tissue and vital substance influenced by a particular organ. Such systematization is useful as the information from which it is derived is scattered in different chapters of the classics. For example, chapter 9 of the Simple Questions says that the Liver manifests on the nails and controls the sinews, chapter 5 of the Simple Questions and chapter 17 of the Spiritual Axis say that the Liver opens into the eyes, etc.

Of course, the Marxist outlook promoted by the modern Chinese did influence Chinese medicine in eliminating or glossing over aspects of Chinese medicine that do not fit in with a 'scientific', Marxist philosophy. For example, going back to the functions of the internal organs, Chinese books will say that the Liver stores Blood, that it opens into the eyes and that it controls the sinews, but not that it houses the Ethereal Soul (*Hun*) as a Marxist is obviously uncomfortable with the concept of Ethereal Soul. However, there are some modern books that do mention the Ethereal Soul in the context of mental diseases.[iii]

I personally do not see the Marxist influence on Chinese medicine as a big impediment for two main reasons: firstly, we have access to all the classics of Chinese medicine (many of which have been translated into English) and we can therefore restore any of the ancient concepts that the modern Chinese have chosen to overlook.

Secondly, in my opinion, the Marxist influence on Chinese medicine is a thin veneer under which there is a more lasting layer of Neo-Confucianist influence. Indeed, it would be interesting to explore how much the Neo-Confucianist thinkers of the Song and Ming dynasties, changed, systematized or even distorted Chinese medicine: in my opinion, they did so in a more profound and lasting way than the Marxists could ever do.

We tend to think of the *Nei Jing* as our 'bible' dating back to the Han dynasty if not even to the Warring States Period (476-221 BC). In reality, the text we have dates back to 762 AD and to the three revisions that took place during the Song dynasty (960-1279). We should remember that the Song dynasty represented the triumph of Confucianism in every way: that inevitably included medicine. We should not therefore look upon any development before 1949 as 'good' (or 'spiritual') and post-1949 as 'bad'.

In this revision of the second edition, in the chapters dealing with the acupuncture points (chapters 54 to 67) I have added the location of the acupuncture points. The location of the acupuncture points mentioned in the text was added not to replace a good book on acupuncture where there is not only the location but also location guidelines and a figure. The location was added primarily as quick reminder to the reader, saving the time to look the point up in another book. This was done particularly bearing in mind less common points such as, for example, G.B.17 Zhengying.

Finally, another new feature of the book is its association with a website. The website will be designed to reflect the design of the print book and will be easier to navigate than a CD. There will be an image bank of all images and flowcharts from the book and over 1000 self-assessment questions with a mixture of MCQ, True and False, labelling and drag and drop.

Giovanni Maciocia
Santa Barbara

Notes

i   Scheid V 2002 Chinese Medicine in Contemporary China, Duke University Press, Durham, p. 32.

ii Chen Youbang and Deng Liangyue 1989 Essentials of Contemporary Chinese Acupuncturists' Clinical Experiences, Foreign Languages Press, Beijing.

iii Wang Ke Qin 1988 Theory of the Mind in Chinese Medicine (*Zhong Yi Shen Zhu Xue Shuo* 中医神主学说), Ancient Chinese Medical Texts Publishing House, Beijing.

Acknowledgements

My first trip to China, where I attended my first acupuncture course at the Nanjing University of Traditional Chinese Medicine in 1980, was an important milestone in my professional development. My first teacher there was the late Dr Su Xin Ming who played an important role in the development of my acupuncture skills. I am indebted to him for the patient way in which he communicated his skills to me.

I am grateful to Dr Zhou Zhong Ying of the Nanjing University of Chinese Medicine for teaching me his knowledge and skills in diagnosis and herbal medicine. I am indebted to many other teachers and clinical teachers from the Nanjing University of Traditional Chinese Medicine.

I am indebted to the late Dr J.H.F. Shen for communicating his great skills, particularly in the field of aetiology and diagnosis. Dr Shen has been one of the most important persons in my professional development particularly with regard to pulse diagnosis. He truly adapted Chinese medicine to his Western patients but stayed faithful to its roots.

Backed by his considerable teaching and clinical experience, Peter Valaskatgis helped greatly with his constant feedback and his extremely valuable suggestions which enhanced the book.

Dr J.D. Van Buren was my very first teacher more than 40 years ago: from him I learned the importance of diagnosis and especially of pulse diagnosis. I owe him a debt of gratitude for being my first source of inspiration in Chinese medicine.

I am indebted to Jason Smith for his comments, proof-reading, suggestions and support.

Finally, I would like to thank Claire Wilson, Alison Taylor and Barbara Simmons of Elsevier Science for their professionalism and support.

Giovanni Maciocia
Santa Barbara

Note on the translation of Chinese terms

The terminology used in this book generally follows that used in the second edition of *Foundations of Chinese Medicine*, *Obstetrics and Gynaecology in Chinese Medicine*, *Diagnosis in Chinese Medicine*, the second edition of *Practice of Chinese Medicine* and *The Psyche in Chinese Medicine*. As in those books, I have opted for translating all Chinese medical terms with the exception of 'Yin', 'Yang', 'Qi' and '*cun*' (unit of measurement).

I have continued using initial capitals for the terms which are specific to Chinese medicine. For example, 'Blood' indicates one of the vital substances of Chinese medicine, whereas 'blood' denotes the liquid flowing in the blood vessels; e.g. '*In Blood deficiency the menstrual blood may be pale*'. I use initial capitals also for all pulse qualities and for pathological colours and shapes of the tongue body.

This system has served readers of my previous books well. As most teachers (including myself) use Chinese terms when lecturing (e.g. *Yuan Qi* rather than 'Original Qi'), I have given each term in *pinyin* especially when it is introduced for the first time. One change I have introduced in this book (as in the second editions of 'Foundations of Chinese Medicine', 'Practice of Chinese Medicine' and 'The Psyche in Chinese Medicine') is to use the *pinyin* terms more often throughout the text and at least once in each chapter when the Chinese term is first introduced. I have done this to reduce the frequency with which the reader may need to consult the Glossary.

I made the choice of translating all Chinese terms (with the exceptions indicated above) mostly for reasons of style: I believe that a well-written English text reads better than one peppered with Chinese terms in *pinyin*. Leaving Chinese terms in *pinyin* is probably the easiest option but this is not ideal also because a single *pinyin* word can often have more than one meaning; for example, *jing* can mean 'channels', 'periods', 'Essence' or 'shock', while *shen* can mean 'Kidneys', 'Mind' or 'Spirit'.

I am conscious of the fact that there is no such thing as a 'right' translation of a Chinese medicine term and my terminology is not proposed in this spirit; in fact, Chinese medicine terms are essentially impossible to translate. The greatest difficulty in translating Chinese terms is probably that a term has many facets and different meanings in different contexts: thus it would be impossible for one translation to be 'right' in every situation and every context. For example, the term *jue* (厥) has many different meanings; a translation can illustrate only one aspect of a multi-faceted term. In fact, *jue* can mean a state of collapse with unconsciousness; coldness of hands and feet; or a critical situation of retention of urine. In other contexts it has other meanings: e.g. *jue qi* (厥气), a condition of chaotic Qi; *jue xin tong* (厥心痛), a condition of violent chest pain with cold hands; and *jue yin zheng* (厥阴证), the Terminal-Yin pattern within the Six-Stage Identification of Patterns characterized by Heat above and Cold below.

Many sinologists concur that Chinese philosophical terms are essentially impossible to translate and that, the moment we translate them, we distort them with a world-view that is not Chinese. Ames is particularly clear about the intrinsic distortion of Chinese concepts when they are translated. He gives examples of Chinese terms that are distorted when translated, such as *Tian* 天 ('Heaven'), *You-Wu* 有无 ('Being" and 'Non-Being'), *Dao* 道 ('Way'), *Xing* 性 ('human nature'), *Ren* 仁 ('benevolence'), *Li* 理 ('Principle'), *Qi* 气 ('primal substance'), etc.[i]

Ames is particularly forceful in rejecting a single, one-to-one translation of a Chinese term into a Western one in the introduction of his book 'Focusing the Familiar' (a translation of the Confucian text *Zhong Yong*).[ii] Ames says: '*Our Western languages are substance-oriented and are therefore most relevant to the descriptions of a world defined by discreteness, objectivity and permanence. Such languages are ill disposed to describe and interpret a world,* such as that of the Chinese, that is primarily characterized by continuity, process and becoming.'[iii]

Ames then gives some examples of what he considers to be serious mis-translations of Chinese philosophical terms. The important thing is that these are not 'mis-translations' because the terms are 'wrong' but because of the intrinsic difference between Chinese and Western thinking and therefore the inherent inability of Western terms to convey Chinese philosophical ideas.

Ames says: 'For example, 'You' 有 and 'Wu' 無 have often been uncritically rendered as 'Being' and 'Non-Being.' Influential translators, until quite recently, have rendered 'wu xing' 五行 as 'Five Elements'. 'Xing' 性 is still most often translated as 'nature'. All these translations promote the fixed and univocal characterizations of objects or essences emergent from a language rooted in a substantialist perspective [our Western languages].'[iv]

Ames stresses that the use of a 'substances language' (i.e. a Western language) to translate Chinese insights into a world of process and change has led to seriously inappropriate interpretations of the Chinese sensibility. Ames asserts that it is the very difference between Chinese and Western philosophy that makes translation of Chinese terms virtually impossible. He says: 'In the classical traditions of the West, being takes precedence over becoming and thus becoming is ultimately unreal. Whatever becomes is realized by achieving its end – that is, coming into being. In the Chinese world, becoming takes precedence over being. 'Being' is interpreted as a transitory state marked by further transition.'[v]

Ames then says: 'The Chinese world is a phenomenal world of continuity, becoming and change. In such a world there is no final discreteness. Things cannot be understood as objects. Without this notion of objectivity, there can only be the flux of passing circumstances in which things dissolve into the flux and flow. A processive language precludes the assumption that objects serve as references of linguistic expressions. The precise referential language of denotation and description is to be replaced by a language of 'deference' in which meanings both allude to and defer to one another in a shifting field of significance. A referential language [Western language] characterizes an event, object, or state of affairs through an act of naming meant to indicate a particular thing. On the other hand, the language of deference [Chinese] does not employ proper names simply as indicators of particular individuals or things, but invokes hints, suggestions, or allusions to indicate foci in a field of meanings.'[vi]

As an example of this intrinsic impossibility of translating a Chinese philosophical term into a Western language, Ames then cites Steve Owen's reluctance in translating shi 詩 as 'poem'. Owen says: 'If we translate 'shi' as 'poem', it is merely for the sake of convenience. 'Shi' is not a 'poem': 'shi' is not a thing made in the same way one makes a bed, a painting or a shoe. A 'shi' can be worked on, polished and crafted; but that has nothing to do with what a 'shi' fundamentally 'is' … 'Shi' is not the 'object' of its writer: it is the writer, the outside of an inside.'[vii]

Ames gives various translations of Li 礼 (a Confucian concept) as an the example of how a multiplicity of terms may apply to a single Chinese term and how none of them is 'wrong'. He says that Li has been variously translated as 'ritual', 'rites', 'customs', 'etiquette', 'propriety', 'morals', 'rules of proper behaviour' and 'worship'. Ames says: 'Properly contextualized, each of these English terms can render Li on occasion. In classical Chinese, however, the character carries all of these meanings on every occasion of its use.'[viii] This confirms clearly how, by the very translation, we limit a Chinese term that is rich with multiple meanings to a single meaning in Chinese.

Ames says that in classical Chinese philosophical texts, allusive and connotatively rich language is more highly prized than clarity, precision and argumentative rigor. This rather dramatic contrast between Chinese and Western languages with respect to the issue of clarity presents the translator of Chinese philosophical texts with a peculiar burden.

For the Chinese, the opposite of clarity is not confusion, but something like *vagueness*. Vague ideas are really determinable in the sense that a *variety* of meanings are associated with them. Each Chinese term constitutes a field of meanings which may be focused by any of a number of its meanings. Ames says that in the translation of Chinese texts we must avoid what Whitehead called 'the Fallacy of the Perfect Dictionary'. By this, he means the assumption that there exists a complete semantic repository of terms of which we may adequately characterize the variety and depth of our experience and that, ideally, one may seek a one-to-one correspondence between word and meaning.

With this 'fallacy' in mind, Ames and Hall say: 'We challenge the wisdom and accuracy of proposing 'one-to-one' equivalencies in translating terms from one language to another. We introduce the notion of 'linguistic clustering' as an alternative strategy to 'literal translation' that allows us to put the semantic value of a term first by parsing *[describe grammatically] its range of meaning according to context, with the assumption that a range of meaning with a different configuration of emphasis is present on each appearance of the term.*'ix

These ideas could not be more apt to illustrate the problems in translating Chinese medicine terms. Of course we must strive for precision and consistency but to think that there is a one-to-one, 'right' correspondence between a Chinese medicine idea and a Western term is a misunderstanding of the very essence of Chinese medicine.

For example, to say that the only 'right' translation of *Chong Mai* is 'Thoroughfare Vessel' makes us fall into the trap of what Whitehead calls the 'Fallacy of the Perfect Dictionary'. Of course, *Chong Mai* can be translated as 'Thoroughfare Vessel' but that is only one of its meanings and it is absolutely impossible for a single Western term to convey the richness of ideas behind the word *Chong Mai* (which I translate as 'Penetrating Vessel'): to think that we can reduce a rich Chinese medicine idea to a single, one-to-one term in a Western language reveals, in my opinion, a misunderstanding of the very essence of Chinese medicine. Therefore, in the example above, I do not proffer 'Penetrating Vessel' as the only 'correct' translation of *Chong Mai*.

Ames makes this point very forcefully. He says: *'The Fallacy of the Perfect Dictionary is largely a consequence of our analytical bias towards univocity. We would suggest that this bias does not serve us well when approaching Chinese texts. Not only is there the continued possibility of novel experiences requiring appeal to novel terminologies, but also there is seldom, if ever, a simple, one-to-one translation of Chinese terms into Western languages. The allusiveness of the classical Chinese language is hardly conducive to univocal translations. We would contend that, in translating Chinese texts into Western languages, it is most unproductive to seek a single equivalent for a Chinese character. In fact, rather than trying to avoid ambiguity by a dogged use of formally stipulated terms, the translator might have to concede that characters often require a cluster of words to do justice to their range of meanings – all of which are suggested in any given rendering of the character. In fact, any attempt to employ univocal translations of Chinese terms justified by appeal to the criteria of clarity or univocity often reduces philosophical insight to nonsense and poetry to doggerel. Such an approach to translation serves only to numb Western readers to the provocative significance harboured within the richly vague and allusive language of the Chinese texts.'*x

As an example of the multiplicity of meanings of a Chinese term and therefore of the fact that it is perfectly legitimate to translate a single Chinese idea into more than one term according to different contexts, Ames says that he translates the term *zhong* ('centre' or 'central') in the title of the Confucian text sometimes as 'focus', sometimes as 'focusing' and other times as 'equilibrium'. Other times, he even translates it as 'centre' or 'impartiality'. He says strongly: *'The Chinese language is not logocentric. Words do not name essences. Rather, they indicate always-transitory processes and events. It is important therefore to stress the gerundative character of the language. The language of process is vague, allusive and suggestive.'*xi

Rosemont makes the same point with regard to the translation of *Li* (rituals). He says *Li* could be translated as 'customs', 'mores', 'propriety', 'etiquette', 'rites', 'rituals', 'rules of proper behaviour', and 'worship'. He says: *'If we can agree that, appropriately contextualized, each of these English terms can translate Li on occasion, we should conclude that the Chinese graph must have all of these meanings on every occasion of its use, and that selecting only one of them can lead only to the result that 'something is lost in translation'*xii

According to Ames, in the field of philosophy, two terms particularly stand out as being influenced by a Western thinking when translated, i.e. *Tian* 天 ('Heaven') and *Ren* 仁 ('benevolence'). Ames says: *'When we translate Tian as 'Heaven', like it or not, we invoke in the Western reader a notion of transcendent creator Deity, along with the language of soul, sin and afterlife…When we translate Ren as 'benevolence', we psychologize and make altruistic a term which originally had a radically different range of sociological connotations. Being altruistic for example, implies being selfless in the service of others. But this 'self-sacrifice' implicitly entails a notion of 'self' which exists independently of others and that can be surrendered – a notion of self which we believe is alien to the world of the Analects [of Confucius]: indeed, such a reading [of the term 'ren'] transforms what is fundamentally a strategy for self-realization into one of self-abnegation.'*xiii

With regard to Chinese medicine, the term *Xue* 血 ('Blood') is a good example of the above-mentioned problem reported by Ames. When we translate the word *Xue* as 'Blood' we immediately alter its essential character and give it a Western medical connotation; in fact, in Chinese medicine, *Xue* is itself actually a form of Qi and one that is closely bound with Nutritive Qi

(*Ying Qi*). Indeed, the term *mai* 脉 appearing in the 'Yellow Emperor's Classic of Internal Medicine' is often ambiguous as it sometimes clearly refers to the acupuncture channels and other times to the blood vessels.

After highlighting the problems in translating Chinese terms, Ames confirms that a single Chinese term may have different meaning in different contexts. For example, the term *shen* 神 in some cases means 'human spirituality', in others it means 'divinity'.[xiv] As he considers only the philosophical meanings of the word *shen*, we could actually add many others in the context of Chinese medicine, e.g. 'mind', 'spirit', 'lustre' (in the context of diagnosis), 'numinous', 'numinosity'.

Graham says: '*Every Western sinologist knows that there is no exact equivalent in his own language for such a word as ren* 仁 *or de* 德, *and that as long as he thinks of it as synonymous with 'benevolence' or 'virtue' he will impose Western preconceptions on the thought he is studying.*'[xv]

Ames then surveys the options that are presented to a translator and seems to favour simply transliterating the Chinese terms and leave them untranslated in pinyin. He says: '*To some, this approach may appear to be simply the laziest way out of a difficult problem. But 'ritual' has a narrowly circumscribed set of meanings in English, and Li an importantly different and less circumscribed set. Just as no Indological scholar would look for English equivalent for 'karma', 'dharma' and so on, perhaps it is time to do the same for classical Chinese, the homonymity of the language notwithstanding.*'[xvi]

Hall confirms that a single Chinese term may have a plurality of meanings. He says: '*The Chinese have traditionally affirmed as the ground of their intellectual and institutional harmony the recognition of the co-presence of a plurality of significances with which any given term might easily resonate.*'[xvii]

Finally, another sinologist, Yung Sik Kim, discusses the difficulty presented by the plurality of meanings of a single Chinese term. He says: '*I have adopted the policy of sticking to one English translation for a particular Chinese word whenever possible…Of course, exceptions cannot be avoided altogether. I have had to resort to different translations for such characters as 'xin'* 心 *which means both 'heart' and 'mind'; 'tian'* 天, *both 'heaven' and 'sky'.*'[xviii]

In another passage, Yung Sik Kim affirms that transliteration of a Chinese term with a plurality of meanings is the only alternative: '*The term 'li'* 理 *is difficult to define. It is difficult even to translate because there is no single word in Western languages that covers all facets of what 'li' meant to the traditional Chinese mind. The existence of many translations for the term, which often leaves transliteration as the only viable option, bespeaks the difficulty.*'[xix]

An example of a Chinese medicine term which has many different meaning in different context is *zhi* 志. *Zhi can have at lest four different meanings. It can mean 'will-power' (the Zhi of the Kidneys) but, in relation to the Kidneys, it also indicates 'memory'. It may also mean 'emotion' (the 5 emotions are often called wu zhi) or 'mind' (as in the treatment principle an shen ding zhi* 安神定志).

The translation of a Chinese term into a Latin-based term can lead to a distortion of the original Chinese idea. The word *zheng* 政, usually translated as 'government' is a good case in point. The Chinese character takes the word *zheng* 正 as its radical: this word means 'correct'. Not by chance, these two words are cognate, i.e. they share the same sound: to 'govern' means to do what is 'proper' and 'correct'. Indeed, Confucius says exactly that in the Analects: '*Governing effectively is doing what is proper. If you lead by doing what is proper, who would dare do otherwise?*'[xx]

Therefore, the Chinese term for 'government' conveys the Confucian idea that to 'govern' consists in behaving correctly and with integrity thus ensuring social harmony. By contrast, the term 'government' derives from the Latin *gubernare* which means to 'steer, to govern': this implies a totally different concept of a top-down approach in which to 'govern' means not to follow the same ethical code as everybody else, but to 'steer', to 'govern' other people.

Although a diversity of translation of Chinese terms may present its problems, these are easily overcome if an author explains the translation in a glossary and, most importantly, explains the meaning of a given Chinese term in its context (in our case, Chinese medicine).

In my books, I have chosen to translate all Chinese medicine terms rather than using *pinyin* purely for reasons of style as a sentence written half in English and half in *pinyin* is often awkward. Moreover, if we use *pinyin* terms in writing, it could be argued that we should be consistent and use *pinyin* terms for *all* Chinese medicine terms and this would not make for very clear reading. Consider the following sentence: '*To treat Pi-Yang Xu we adopt the zhi fa of bu pi and wen Yang*' ('To treat Spleen-Yang deficiency we adopt the treatment principle of tonifying the Spleen and warming Yang').

Moreover, the problem arises only in the written form as, in my experience, most lecturers in colleges throughout the Western world normally prefer using *pinyin* terms rather than their counterparts in English (or any other Western languages). Thus, a lecturer will refer to Kidney-*Jing* rather than 'Kidney-Essence'. Indeed, when I myself lecture, I generally use the *pinyin* terms rather than their English translation. Again, most lecturers use a pragmatic approach translating some terms into English (such as 'treatment principle' instead of '*zhi fa*') and leaving others in *pinyin* such as '*Yuan Qi*' or '*Chong Mai*'.

When I lecture I always try to give the participants an idea of the meaning of a particular Chinese character and its significance and application in Chinese medicine. Indeed, the use of *pinyin* when lecturing renders Chinese medicine truly international as I can lecture in the Czech Republic and mention *Jing*, *Yang Qiao Mai*, *Wei Qi*, etc., knowing that I will be understood by everyone.

A diversity of translation of Chinese terms may even have a positive aspect as each author may highlight a particular facet of a Chinese term so that diversity actually enriches our understanding of Chinese medicine. If someone translates *Zong Qi* (宗气) as 'Initial Qi', for example, we learn something about that author's view and understanding of *Zong Qi*; the translation cannot be branded as 'wrong' (I translate this term as 'Gathering Qi'). Another example: if someone translates *yang qiao mai* as 'Yang Motility Vessel', the translation captures one aspect of this vessel's nature; again, this could not be defined as wrong (I translate the name of this vessel as 'Yang Stepping Vessel').

Trying to impose a standard, 'right' translation of Chinese medicine terms may lead to suppression of healthy debate; I therefore hope that readers will continue to benefit from the diversity of translation of Chinese medical terms and draw inspiration from the rich heritage of Chinese medicine that it represents.

I firmly believe that the future lies not in trying to establish a rigid, embalmed, fossilized, 'right' terminology based on single, one-to-one translations of Chinese ideas. Indeed, I believe this is a potentially dangerous trend as it would, in my opinion, lead students and practitioners away from the richness of Chinese language and richness of meanings of Chinese medicine ideas. The adoption of a standardized, 'approved' terminology of Chinese medical terms may indeed, in time, divorce students and practitioners from the essence of Chinese medicine. If an 'official', standardized translation of Chinese terms took hold, then students would be less inclined to study the Chinese terms to explore their meaning.

Ames and Hall make the same point: '*Such translations have been 'legitimized' by their gradual insinuation into the standard Chinese-English dictionaries and glosses. By encouraging the uncritical assumption in those who consult these reference works that this formula of translations provides the student with a 'literal' rendering of the terms, these lexicons have become complicit in an entrenched cultural equivocation that we strive to avoid.*'[xxi]

They then further make the point that using a one-to-one translation of Chinese terms ignores the cultural background where they came from: '*Our argument is that it is in fact these formulaic usages that are radical interpretations. To our mind, to consciously or unconsciously transplant a text from its own historical and intellectual soil and replant it in one that has decidedly different philosophical landscape is to take liberties with the text and is radical in the sense it tampers with its very roots.*'[xxii]

As I said above, an 'official', standardized translation of Chinese terms may make students and practitioners less inclined to study the Chinese terms to explore their meaning with their own interpretation. Ames and Hall say: '*Our goal is not to replace one inadequate formula with another. Our translations are intended as no more than suggestive 'placeholders' that refer readers back to this glossary to negotiate their own meaning, and, we hope, to appropriate the Chinese terms for themselves.*'[xxiii]

Moreover, imposing an 'approved' terminology in English betrays an Anglo-centric world view: to be consistent, we should then have an 'approved' terminology in every major language of the world. It seems to me much better to try and understand the spirit and the essence of Chinese medicine by studying its characters and their *clinical* significance and using *pinyin* transliteration whenever appropriate.

Trying to fossilize Chinese medicine terms into an imposed terminology goes against the very essence of the Chinese language which, as Ames says, is not logocentric and in which words do not name essences: rather, they indicate always-transitory processes and events. The language of process is vague, allusive and suggestive.

Because Chinese language is a language of *process*, the question arises also whether practising Chinese medicine actually helps the understanding of Chinese medical terminology: in my opinion, in many cases it does. For example, I feel that clinical experience helps us to understand the nature of the *Chong Mai* (Penetrating Vessel) and therefore helps us to understand the term *Chong* in a 'knowing practice' way (as Farquhar defines it)[xxiv] rather than a theoretical way.

Of course, a translator of Chinese books should strive for precision and consistency, but we must accept that there is a rich multiplicity of meanings for any give idea of Chinese medicine. The *Chong Mai* is a good example of this multiplicity as the term *chong* could be translated as 'throroughfare', 'strategic cross-roads', 'to penetrate', 'to rush', 'to rush upwards', 'to charge', 'activity', 'movement' and 'free passage'. Which of these translations is 'correct'? They are all correct as they all convey an idea of the nature and function of the *Chong Mai*.

I therefore think that the future of teaching Chinese medicine lies not in trying to impose the straight-jacket of a rigid terminology of the rich ideas of Chinese medicine, but in teaching students more and more Chinese characters explaining the richness of meanings associated with them in the context of Chinese medicine. I myself, would not like my own terminology to be 'adopted' as the 'correct' or 'official' one: I would rather see colleges teaching more and more Chinese to their students by illustrating the rich meanings of Chinese medicine terms. As mentioned above, my main motive for translating all terms is purely for reasons of style in an English-language textbook; when I lecture I generally use *pinyin* terms but, most of all, I show the students the Chinese characters and try to convey their meaning in the context of Chinese medicine.

Finally, I would like to explain my continued translation of *Wu Xing* as 'Five Elements'. The term 'Five Elements' has been used by most Western practitioners of Chinese Medicine for a long time (also in French and other European languages). Some authors consider this to be a misunderstanding of the meaning of the Chinese term '*Wu Xing*', perpetuated over the years. '*Wu*' means 'five' and '*Xing*' means 'movement', 'process', 'to go', 'conduct' or 'behaviour'. Most authors therefore think that the word '*Xing*' cannot indicate 'element' as a basic constituent of Nature, as was supposedly intended in ancient Greek philosophy.

This is, in my opinion, only partly true as the elements, as they were conceived by various Greek philosophers over the centuries, were not always considered 'basic constituents' of Nature or 'passive motionless fundamental substances'.[xxv] Some Greek philosophers conceived the elements as dynamic qualities of Nature, in a way similar to Chinese philosophy.

For example, Aristotle gave a definite dynamic interpretation to the four elements and called them 'primary form' (*prota somata*). He said: '*Earth and Fire are opposites also due to the opposition of the respective qualities with which they are revealed to our senses: Fire is hot, Earth is cold. Besides the fundamental opposition of hot and cold, there is another one, i.e. that of dry and wet: hence the four possible combinations of hot-dry [Fire], hot-wet [Air], cold-dry [Earth] and cold-wet [Water] ... the elements can mix with each other and can even transform into one another ... thus Earth, which is cold and dry, can generate Water if wetness replaces dryness.*'[xxvi]

To Aristotle, therefore, the four elements became the four basic qualities of natural phenomena, classified as combinations of four qualities, hot, cold, dry and wet. As is apparent from the above statement, the Aristotelian elements could even transform into one another and generate each other.

This interpretation is very similar to the Chinese one, in which the elements are *qualities* of Nature. Furthermore, it is interesting to note the similarity with the Chinese theory of Yin-Yang: the four Aristotelian elements derive from the interaction of the basic Yin-Yang qualities of cold-hot and dry-wet.

Thus, it is not entirely true to say that the Greek elements were conceived only as the basic constituents of matter, the 'building blocks' of Nature which would make the use of the word 'element' wrong to indicate *xing*. Furthermore, the word 'elements' does not necessarily imply that: it does so only in its modern chemical interpretation.

In conclusion, for the above reasons I have kept the word 'element' as a translation of the Chinese word '*xing*'. According to Wang, the term 'Five Elements' could be translate in a number of ways, e.g. 'agents', 'entities', 'goings', 'conduct', 'doings', 'forces', 'activites', and 'stages of change'.[xxvii]

Recently, the term 'Five Phases' is gaining acceptance but some sinologists disagree with this translation and propose returning to 'Five Elements'. Friedrich and Lackner, for example, suggest restoring the term 'elements'.[xxviii] Graham uses the term 'Five Processes'.[xxix] I would probably agree that 'processes' is the best translation of *Wu Xing*. In fact, the book 'Shang Shu' written during the Western Zhou dynasty (1000-771 BC) said: '*The Five Elements are Water, Fire, Wood, Metal and Earth. Water moistens downwards; Fire flares upwards; Wood can be bent and straightened; Metal can be moulded and can harden; Earth allows sowing, growing and reaping.*'[xxx]

Some sinologists (e.g. Needham and Fung Yu Lan) still use the term 'element'. Fung Yu Lan suggests that a possible translation of *wu xing* could be 'Five Activities' or 'Five Agents'.[xxxi] Although the term 'five phases' has gained some acceptance as a translation of '*wu xing*', I find this term restrictive as it clearly refers to only one aspect of the Five Elements, i.e. phases of a (seasonal) cycle.

A glossary with *pinyin* terms, Chinese characters and English translation appears at the end of the book. I have included both a *Pinyin*-English and an English-*Pinyin* glossary.

Notes

i. Ames R T, Rosemont H 1999 The Analects of Confucius – a Philosophical Translation, Ballantine Books, New York, p. 311.
ii. Ames R T and Hall D L 2001 Focusing the Familiar – A Translation and Philosophical Interpretation of the *Zhong Yong*, University of Hawai'i Press, Honolulu, pp. 6 to 16.
iii. Ibid., p. 6.
iv. Ibid., p. 6.
v. Ibid., p. 10.
vi. Ibid., p. 10.
vii. Ibid., p. 13.
viii. Ibid., p. 69.
ix. Ames R T and Hall D L 2003 Daodejing – 'Making This Life Significant' A Philosophical Translation, Ballantine Books, New York, p. 56.
x. Ibid., p. 16.
xi. Ibid., p. 16.
xii. Bockover M (editor) 1991 Rules, Ritual and Responsibility – Essays Dedicated to Herbert Fingarette, Open Court, La Salle, Illinois, p. 98.
xiii. The Analects of Confucius, p. 312.
xiv. Ibid., p. 313.
xv. Hall D L and Ames R T 1998 Thinking from the Han – Self, Truth and Transcendence in Chinese and Western Culture, State University of New York Press, New York, p. 238.
xvi. The Analects of Confucius, p. 314.
xvii. Thinking from the Han, p. 4.
xviii. Kim Yung Sik 2000 The Natural Philosophy of Chu Hsi, American Philosophical Society, Philadelphia, p. 11.
xix. Ibid., p. 19.
xx. Jones D (editor) 2008 Confucius Now, Open Court, Chicago, p. 19.
xxi. Daodejing – 'Making This Life Significant', p. 55.
xxii. Ibid., pp. 55-6.
xxiii. Ibid., p. 56.
xxiv. Farquhar J 1994 Knowing Practice – The Clinical Encounter of Chinese Medicine, Westview Press, Boulder, USA.
xxv. Needham J 1977 Science and Civilization in China, Vol 2, Cambridge University Press, Cambridge, p. 244.
xxvi. Lamanna E P 1967 *Storia della Filosofia* (History of Philosophy), Vol 1.Le Monnier, Florence, p 220–221.
xxvii. Wang Ai He 1999 Cosmology and Political Culture in Early China, Cambridge University Press, Cambridge, p. 3.
xxviii. Friedrich M and Lackner M, 'Once again: the concept of Wu Xing' in 'Early China' 9-10, pp. 218-9.
xxix. Graham A C 1986 Yin-Yang and the Nature of Correlative Thinking, Institute of East Asian Philosophies, Singapore, p. 42-66 and 70-92.
xxx. *Shang Shu* (c 659 BC) cited in 1980 Practical Chinese Medicine (*Shi Yong Zhong Yi Xue* 实用中医学), Beijing Publishing House, Beijing, p. 32. The book *Shang Shu* is placed by some in the early Zhou dynasty (hence c. 1000 BC), but the prevalent opinion is that is was written sometime between 659 BC and 627 BC.
xxxi. Fung Yu Lan 1966 A Short History of Chinese Philosophy, Free Press, New York, p. 131.

PART 1

General Theory

1

INTRODUCTION

Part 1 will discuss the general theory of Chinese medicine. There are three pillars to the general theory of Chinese medicine:

- The theory of Yin–Yang
- The theory of the Five Elements
- The theory of Qi

The theory of Yin–Yang is very ancient. In the 'Book of Changes' (*Yi Jing, c.*700 BC), Yin and Yang are represented by a broken and unbroken line, respectively. Combinations of the eight Trigrams (made up of three lines) form the 64 hexagrams which represent the myriad phenomena of the Universe.

The theory of Yin–Yang was developed systematically by one of the many schools of thought that arose during the Warring States period (476–221 BC); that is, the 'School of Yin–Yang', whose main representative thinker was Zou Yan (*c.*350–270 BC). The application of Yin–Yang to medicine was developed after this school.

The first recorded reference to the Five Elements (*Wu Xing*) dates back to the Zhou dynasty (*c.*1000–770 BC).[1] The theory of the Five Elements was not applied to Chinese medicine throughout its historical development as its popularity waxed and waned through the centuries. During the Warring States period it became immensely popular and was applied to medicine, astrology, the natural sciences, the calendar, music and even politics. Its popularity was such that most phenomena were classified in fives.

From the Han dynasty onwards, the influence of the theory of the Five Elements in Chinese medicine began to wane. However, this theory remained one of the main pillars of Chinese medicine, cropping up in many aspects of Chinese medicine: for example, the five pathological colours of the face, the five flavours of herbs, the five emotions, the five Yin organs, and many others.

The concept of Qi is absolutely at the core of Chinese medical thinking. The changing nature of Qi between a material substance and an ethereal, subtle force is central to the Chinese medicine view of body and mind as an integrated unit.

The infinite variety of phenomena in the universe is the result of the continuous coming together and dispersion of Qi to form phenomena of various degrees of materialization. This idea of aggregation and dispersion of Qi has been discussed by many Chinese philosophers of all times.

Qi is the very basis of the universe's infinite manifestations of life, including minerals, vegetables and animals (including human beings).

Part 1 comprises the following chapters:
Chapter 1   Yin–Yang
Chapter 2   The Five Elements
Chapter 3   The Vital Substances
Chapter 4   The transformations of Qi.

END NOTES

1. Needham J 1977 Science and Civilization in China, Cambridge University Press, Cambridge, vol. 2, p. 232–242.

PART 1

Yin–Yang 1

> **Key contents**
>
> Nature of Yin–Yang concept
>
> Four aspects of Yin–Yang relationship (opposition, interdependence, mutual consumption, intertransformation)
>
> Application of Yin–Yang to medicine

The concept of Yin–Yang is probably the single most important and distinctive theory of Chinese medicine. It could be said that all Chinese medical physiology, pathology and treatment can, eventually, be reduced to Yin–Yang. The concept of Yin–Yang is extremely simple and yet very profound. One can understand it on a rational level, and yet continually find new expressions of it in clinical practice and, indeed, in life.

The concept of Yin–Yang, together with that of Qi, has permeated Chinese philosophy over the centuries and is radically different from any Western philosophical idea. In general, Western logic is based upon the opposition of contraries, which is the fundamental premise of Aristotelian logic. According to this logic, a pair of contraries (such as 'The table is square' and 'The table is not square') cannot both be true. This approach has dominated Western thought for over 2000 years. The Chinese concept of Yin–Yang is radically different from this system of thought: Yin and Yang represent opposite but complementary qualities. Each thing or phenomenon could be both itself and its contrary. Moreover, Yin contains the seed of Yang, so that Yin can transform into Yang, and vice versa.

A passage from a commentary on Zhuang Zi highlights this thinking about the complementarity of opposites: *'There are no two things under Heaven which do not have the mutual relationship of the "self" and the "other". Both the "self" and the "other" equally desire to act for themselves, thus opposing each other as strongly as East and West. On the other hand, the "self" and the "other"* have at the same time the mutual relationship of lips and teeth ... therefore the action of the "other" on its own behalf at the same time helps the "self". Thus, though mutually opposed, they are incapable of mutual negation.'[1]

The discussion of Yin–Yang will be developed under the following headings:

- Historical development
- Nature of the Yin–Yang concept
  - Yin–Yang as two phases of a cyclical movement
  - Yin–Yang as two states of density of matter
  - Four aspects of Yin–Yang relationship
    - The opposition of Yin and Yang
    - The interdependence of Yin and Yang
    - The mutual consuming of Yin and Yang
    - The intertransformation of Yin and Yang
- Application of Yin–Yang to medicine
  - Yin–Yang and the body structures
    - Back–front
    - Head–body
    - Exterior–Interior
    - Above–below waist
    - Posterior–lateral and anterior–medial surfaces
    - Yang and Yin organs
    - Function–structure of organs
    - Qi–Blood
    - Defensive Qi–Nutritive Qi
- Application of the four principles of Yin–Yang to medicine
  - Opposition of Yin and Yang
    - Fire–Water
    - Heat–Cold
    - Redness–paleness
    - Restless–quiet
    - Dry–wet
    - Hard–soft
    - Excitement–inhibition
    - Rapidity–slowness
    - Substantial–non-substantial
    - Transformation/change–conservation/storage/sustainment

- The interdependence of Yin and Yang
  - Yin and Yang organs
  - Structure and function of the organs
- The mutual consuming of Yin and Yang
  - Balance of Yin and Yang
  - Excess of Yin
  - Excess of Yang
  - Consumption of Yang
  - Consumption of Yin
- Intertransformation of Yin and Yang

HISTORICAL DEVELOPMENT

The earliest reference to Yin and Yang is probably the one in the 'Book of Changes' (*Yi Jing*), dating back to about 700 BC. In this book, Yin and Yang are represented by broken and unbroken lines (Fig. 1.1).

Yin   Yang

Figure 1.1 Yin–Yang diagrams

The combination of broken and unbroken lines in pairs forms four sets of diagrams, representing utmost Yin, utmost Yang and two intermediate stages (Fig. 1.2).

The addition of another line to these four diagrams forms, with varying combinations, the eight trigrams (Fig. 1.3).

Finally, the various combinations of the trigrams gives rise to the 64 hexagrams. These are supposed to symbolize all possible phenomena of the universe, and therefore show how all phenomena ultimately depend on the two poles of Yin and Yang.

The philosophical school that developed the theory of Yin and Yang to its highest degree is called the Yin–Yang School, though Needham calls it the 'Naturalist School'.[2] Many schools of thought arose during the Warring States period (476–221 BC), and the Yin–Yang school was one of them. It dedicated itself to the study of Yin–Yang and the Five Elements and its main exponent was Zou Yan (*c*. 350–270 BC). The school is sometimes also called the Naturalist School because it set out to interpret Nature in a positive way and to use natural laws to man's advantage, not through attempting to control and subdue Nature (as in modern Western science), but by acting in harmony with its laws. This school represents a form of what we might call naturalist science today, and the theories of Yin–Yang and the Five Elements served to interpret natural phenomena, including the human body in health and disease.

The theories of Yin–Yang and the Five Elements, systematically elaborated by the Naturalist School, later became the common heritage of subsequent schools of thought, particularly the Neo-Confucianist schools of the Song, Ming and Qing dynasties. These schools combined most of the elements from the previous schools of thought to form a coherent philosophy of nature, ethics, social order and astrology.[3]

I will discuss Yin–Yang from a general philosophical point of view first, and then from a medical point of view.

NATURE OF THE YIN–YANG CONCEPT

The Chinese characters for 'Yin' and 'Yang' are related to the image of a hill with one side dark and the other sunlit. The characters are:

陰
YIN

阝 represents a 'mound' or 'hill'

 represents a 'cloud'

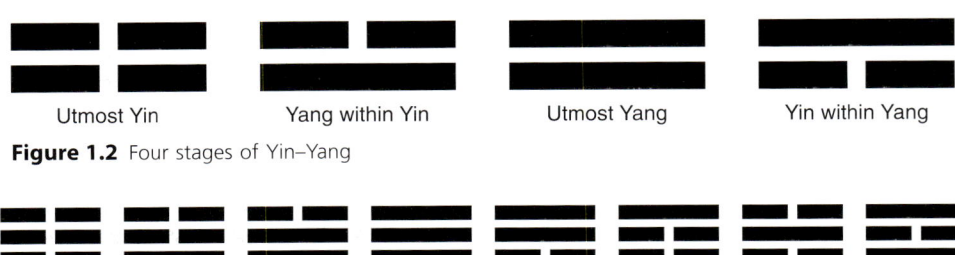

Utmost Yin   Yang within Yin   Utmost Yang   Yin within Yang

Figure 1.2 Four stages of Yin–Yang

The Eight Trigrams

Figure 1.3 The Eight Trigrams

陽
YANG

日 represents the 'sun'
旦 represents the 'sun over the horizon'
勿 represents the 'rays of light'

Thus the character for Yin indicates the shady side of a hill, whilst the character for Yang indicates the sunny side of a hill. By extension, they therefore also indicate 'darkness' and 'light' or 'shady' and 'bright'.

Yin–Yang as two phases of a cyclical movement

The earliest origin of Yin–Yang phenomena must have derived from the peasants' observation of the cyclical alternation of day and night. Thus day corresponds to Yang and night to Yin, and, by extension, activity to Yang and rest to Yin. This led to the first observation of the continuous alternation of every phenomenon between two cyclical poles, one corresponding to light, Sun, brightness and activity (Yang), the other corresponding to darkness, Moon, shade and rest (Yin). From this point of view, Yin and Yang are two stages of a cyclical movement, one constantly changing into the other, such as the day giving way to night and vice versa.

Heaven (where the sun is) is therefore Yang and Earth is Yin. The ancient Chinese farmers conceived Heaven as a round vault, and the Earth as flat. Hence, round is Yang and square is Yin. The Heaven, containing the Sun, Moon and stars on which the Chinese farmers based their calendar, therefore corresponds to time; the Earth, which is parcelled out into fields, corresponds to space.

Because the sun rises in the East and sets in the West, the former is Yang and the latter Yin. If we face South, East will be on the left and West on the right (in the northern hemisphere). In Chinese cosmology, the compass directions were established assuming that one faced South. This was also reflected in imperial ceremonials when 'The Emperor faced South towards his subjects who faced North ... The Emperor thus opened himself to receive the influence of Heaven, Yang and South. South is therefore like Heaven, at the top; North is therefore like Earth, at the bottom ... By facing South, the Emperor identifies his left with East and his right with West.'[4]

Thus, left corresponds to Yang and right to Yin. The 'Simple Questions' relates the correspondence Yang-Left and Yin-Right to physiology. It says: *'East represents Yang ... West represents Yin ... in the West and North there is a deficiency of Heaven, hence the left ear and eyes hear and see better than the right; in the East and South there is a deficiency of Earth, hence the right hand and foot are stronger than the left.'*[5]

The characters for 'left' and 'right' clearly show their relation with Yin and Yang as that for left includes the symbol for work (activity = Yang), and that for right includes a mouth (which eats products of the Earth which is Yin).[6]

左　　右
LEFT　　RIGHT

工 represents 'work'
口 represents 'mouth'

We therefore have the first correspondences:

Yang	Yin
Light	Darkness
Sun	Moon
Brightness	Shade
Activity	Rest
Heaven	Earth
Round	Flat
Time	Space
East	West
South	North
Left	Right

Thus, from this point of view, Yin and Yang are essentially an expression of a duality in time, an alternation of two opposite stages in time. Every phenomenon in the universe alternates through a cyclical movement of peaks and troughs, and the alternation of Yin and Yang is the motive force of its change and development. Day changes into night, summer into winter, growth into decay and vice versa. Thus the development of all phenomena in the universe is the result of the interplay of two opposite stages, symbolized by Yin and Yang, and every phenomenon contains within itself both aspects in different degrees of manifestation. The day belongs to Yang but, after it reaches its peak at midday, the Yin within it gradually begins to unfold and manifest. Thus each phenomenon may belong to a Yang stage or a Yin stage but always contains the seed of the opposite stage within itself. The daily cycle clearly illustrates this (Fig. 1.4).

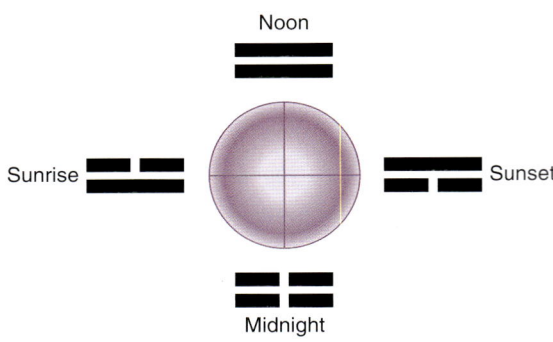

Figure 1.4 Yin–Yang in the daily cycle

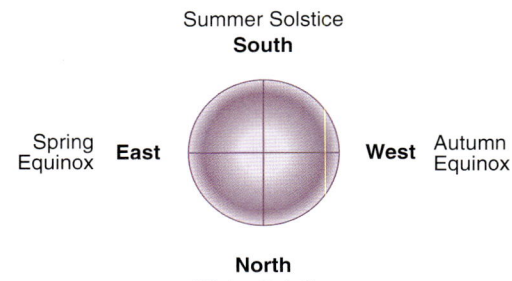

Figure 1.5 Yin–Yang in the seasonal cycle

Exactly the same happens with the yearly cycle and we need only substitute 'spring' for 'dawn', 'summer' for 'noon', 'autumn' for 'dusk' and 'winter' for 'midnight' (Fig. 1.5).

Thus:

> Spring = Yang within Yin = growth of Yang
> Summer = Yang within Yang = maximum Yang
> Autumn = Yin within Yang = growth of Yin
> Winter = Yin within Yin = maximum Yin

The two intermediate stages (dawn–spring and dusk–autumn) do not represent neutral stages in between Yin and Yang: they still pertain primarily to one or the other (i.e. dawn–spring pertains to Yang and dusk–autumn pertains to Yin), so that the cycle can always be narrowed down to a polarity of two stages.

Yin–Yang as two states of density of matter

From a different viewpoint, Yin and Yang stand for two states in the process of change and transformation of all things in the universe. As we have seen above, everything goes through phases of a cycle, and in so doing, its form also changes. For example, the water in lakes and seas heats up during the day and is transformed into vapour. As the air cools down in the evening, vapour condenses into water again.

Matter can acquire different states of density. For example, a table is a dense form of matter and if it is burned, this matter changes into heat and light, less dense forms of matter. From this point of view, Yang symbolizes the more immaterial, rarefied states of matter, whereas Yin symbolizes the more material, dense states of matter. In the above example, the table would represent a dense form of matter that is Yin; the light and heat generated when it is burned represent a less dense form of matter, but matter, nonetheless, that is Yang.

To use the same examples, water in its liquid state pertains to Yin, and the vapour resulting from heat pertains to Yang; similarly wood in its solid state pertains to Yin while the heat and light generated by its burning pertain to Yang.

This duality in the states of condensation of things was often symbolized in ancient China by the duality of 'Heaven' and 'Earth'. 'Heaven' symbolized all rarefied, immaterial, clear and gas-like states of things, whereas 'Earth' symbolized all dense, material, turbid and solid states of things. The 'Simple Questions' in chapter 2 says: '*Heaven is an accumulation of Yang, Earth is an accumulation of Yin.*'[7] Therefore condensation or 'agglomeration' are Yin states of matter while dispersion or evaporation are Yang states of matter.

The important thing to understand is that the two opposite states of condensation or aggregation of things are not independent of each other, but rather change into each other. Yin and Yang symbolize two such opposite states of aggregation of things, the former 'dense' and the latter 'dispersed'. *Lie Zi*, a Daoist text dating from the 5th century BC, said: '*The purer and lighter [elements] tending upwards made the Heaven; the grosser and heavier, tending downwards, made the Earth.*'[8]

In its purest and most rarefied form, Yang is totally immaterial and corresponds to pure energy, and Yin, in its coarsest and densest form, is totally material and corresponds to matter. From this viewpoint, energy and matter are but two states of a continuum, with an infinite possible number of states of aggregation. The 'Simple Questions' in chapter 2 says: '*Yin is quiet, Yang is active. Yang gives life, Yin makes it grow … Yang is transformed into Qi, Yin is transformed into material life.*'[9]

As Yang corresponds to creation and activity, it naturally also corresponds to expansion and it rises. As Yin corresponds to condensation and materialization, it naturally also corresponds to contraction and it descends. Thus we can add a few more qualities to the list of Yin–Yang correspondences:

Yang	Yin
Immaterial	Material
Produces energy	Produces form
Generates	Grows
Non-substantial	Substantial
Energy	Matter
Expansion	Contraction
Rising	Descending
Above	Below
Fire	Water

The relationship and interdependence of Yin–Yang can be represented in the well-known symbol (Fig. 1.6). This symbol is called the 'Supreme Ultimate' (*Tai Ji*) and it represents well the interdependence of Yin and Yang.

The main points of this interdependence are:

- Although they are opposite cyclical stages or opposite states of density of matter, Yin and Yang form a unity and are complementary
- Yang contains the seed of Yin and vice versa. This is represented by the small black and white spots
- Nothing is totally Yin or totally Yang
- Yang changes into Yin and vice versa

Four aspects of Yin–Yang relationship

The main aspects of the Yin–Yang relationship can be summarized into four:

- Opposition of Yin and Yang
- Interdependence of Yin and Yang
- Mutual consuming of Yin and Yang
- Intertransformation of Yin and Yang

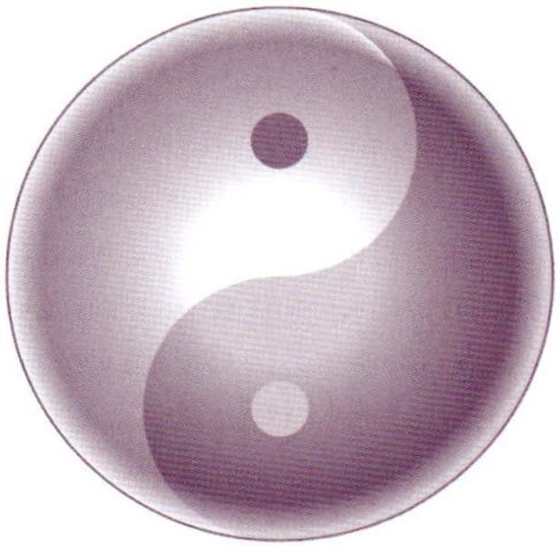

Figure 1.6 Symbol of Yin and Yang

The opposition of Yin and Yang

Yin and Yang are either opposite stages of a cycle or opposite states of aggregation of matter as explained above. Nothing in the natural world escapes this opposition. It is this very inner contradiction that constitutes the motive force of all the changes, development and decay of things.

However, the opposition is relative, not absolute, in so far as nothing is totally Yin or totally Yang. Everything contains the seed of its opposite. Moreover, the opposition of Yin–Yang is relative as the Yin or Yang quality of something is not really intrinsic, but only relative to something else.

Thus, strictly speaking, it is wrong to say that something 'is Yang' or 'is Yin'. Everything only pertains to Yin or Yang in relation to something else. For example, as heat pertains to Yang and cold to Yin, we might say that the climate in Barcelona is Yang in relation to that in Stockholm, but Yin in relation to that in Algiers. To give another example from Chinese dietary principles, vegetables are generally Yin and meat generally Yang. However, within each category there are degrees of Yang or Yin quality: thus, chicken is Yang compared to lettuce but Yin compared to lamb.

Although everything contains Yin and Yang, these are never present in a static 50:50 proportion, but in a dynamic and constantly changing balance. For example, the human body's temperature is nearly constant within a very narrow range. This is not the result of a static situation, but of a dynamic balance of many opposing forces.

The interdependence of Yin and Yang

Although Yin and Yang are opposite, they are also interdependent: one cannot exist without the other. Everything contains opposite forces which are mutually exclusive, but, at the same time, they depend on each other. Day cannot come but after the night and vice versa; there cannot be activity without rest, energy without matter or contraction without expansion.

A passage from chapter 36 of the Daoist classic *Dao De Jing* by Lao Zi illustrates this point well: '*In order to contract, it is necessary first to expand.*'[13]

The mutual consuming of Yin and Yang

Yin and Yang are in a constant state of dynamic balance, which is maintained by a continuous adjustment of their relative levels. When either Yin or Yang is out of balance, they necessarily affect each other and by changing their proportion achieve a new balance.

Besides the normal state of balance of Yin and Yang, there are four possible states of imbalance:

- Preponderance of Yin
- Preponderance of Yang
- Weakness of Yin
- Weakness of Yang

When Yin is preponderant, it induces a decrease of Yang (i.e. the excess of Yin consumes Yang). When Yang is preponderant, it induces a decrease of Yin (i.e. the excess of Yang consumes Yin).

When Yin is weak, Yang is in apparent excess, and when Yang is weak, Yin is in apparent excess. But this is a matter of appearance, as the excess occurs only in relation to the deficient quality, not in absolute.

These four situations can be represented by the diagrams in Figure 1.7. These diagrams will be discussed again in detail when dealing with the application of Yin and Yang to Chinese medicine. Although the diagram of a normal, balanced state of Yin and Yang shows equal proportion of the two qualities, this should not be interpreted literally: the balance is achieved with different dynamic proportions of Yin and Yang.

It is important to see the difference between Preponderance of Yin and Weakness of Yang: these may appear the same, but they are not. It is a question of what is primary and what is secondary. In case of Preponderance of Yin, this is primary and, as a consequence, the excess of Yin consumes the Yang. In case of Weakness of Yang, this is primary and, as a consequence, Yin is in apparent excess. Although it looks as if it is in excess, however, it appears so only relative to the deficiency of Yang. The same applies to Preponderance of Yang and Weakness of Yin.

The intertransformation of Yin and Yang

Yin and Yang are not static, but they actually transform into each other: Yin can change into Yang and vice versa. This change does not happen at random, but only at a certain stage of development of something. Summer changes into winter, day changes into night, life into death, happiness into unhappiness, heat into cold and vice versa. For example, the great euphoria of a drinking spree is quickly followed the next morning by the misery of a hangover.

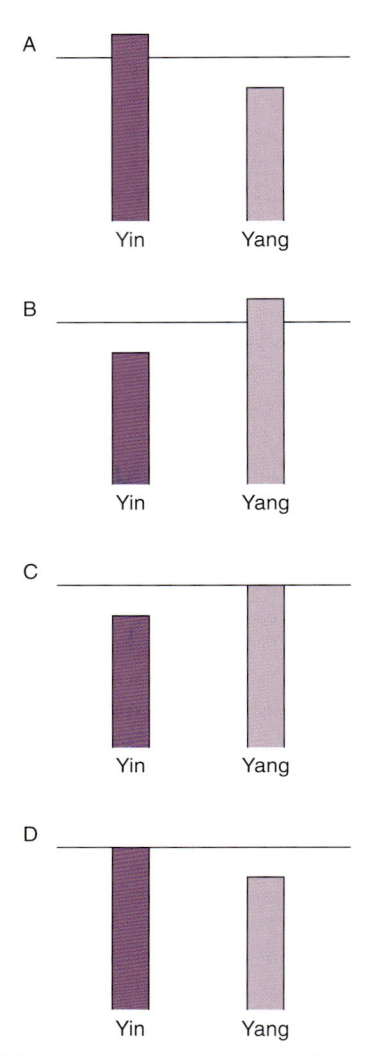

Figure 1.7 Preponderance and weakness of Yin and Yang

There are two conditions for the transformation of Yin into Yang or vice versa. The first concerns internal conditions. Things can change only through internal causes primarily, and external causes secondarily. Change takes place only when the internal conditions are ripe. For example, an egg changes into a chick with the application of heat only because the egg contains within itself the capacity of turning into a chick. Application of heat to a stone will not produce a chick.

The second condition is the time factor. Yin and Yang can transform into each other only at a certain stage of development, when conditions are ripe for the change. In the case of the egg, the chick will hatch only when the time is ripe.

APPLICATION OF YIN–YANG TO MEDICINE

It could be said that the whole of Chinese medicine, its physiology, pathology, diagnosis and treatment, can all be reduced to the basic and fundamental theory of Yin and Yang. Every physiological process and every symptom or sign can be analysed in the light of the Yin–Yang theory.

In treatment, all strategies boil down to four:
1. Tonify Yang
2. Tonify Yin
3. Eliminate excess Yang
4. Eliminate excess Yin

Understanding the application of the theory of Yin–Yang to medicine is therefore of supreme importance in practice: one can say that there is no Chinese medicine without Yin–Yang.

Yin–Yang and the body structures

Every part of the human body is predominantly Yin or Yang in character, and this is important in clinical practice. It must be emphasized, however, that this character is only relative. For example, the chest area is Yang in relation to the abdomen (because it is higher), but Yin in relation to the head.

As a general rule, the following are the characters of various body structures:

Yang	Yin
Superior	Inferior
Exterior	Interior
Posterior–lateral surface	Anterior–medial surface
Back	Front
Function	Structure

More specifically, the Yin–Yang characters of the body structures, organs and energies are as follows (Fig. 1.8):

Yang	Yin
Back	Front (chest-abdomen)
Head	Body
Exterior (skin-muscles)	Interior (organs)
Above the waist	Below the waist
Posterior–lateral surface of limbs	Interior–medial surface of limbs
Yang organs	Yin organs
Function of organs	Structure of organs
Qi	Blood/Body Fluids
Defensive Qi	Nutritive Qi

Each of these will need to be explained in detail.

Back–front

The back is the place where all the Yang channels flow. These carry Yang energy and have the function of protecting the body from exterior pathogenic factors. It is the nature of Yang to be on the Exterior and to protect. It is the nature of Yin to be in the Interior and to nourish. Thus the channels on the back belong to Yang and can be used both to strengthen Yang and therefore our resistance to exterior pathogenic factors, and to eliminate pathogenic factors after these have already invaded the body.

The front (abdomen and chest) is the place where all the Yin channels flow. These carry Yin energy and have the function of nourishing the body. They are often used to tonify Yin.

Head–body

The head is the place where all the Yang channels either end or begin: they therefore all meet and flow into each other on the head. The relation of the head to Yang energy is verified in different ways in practice.

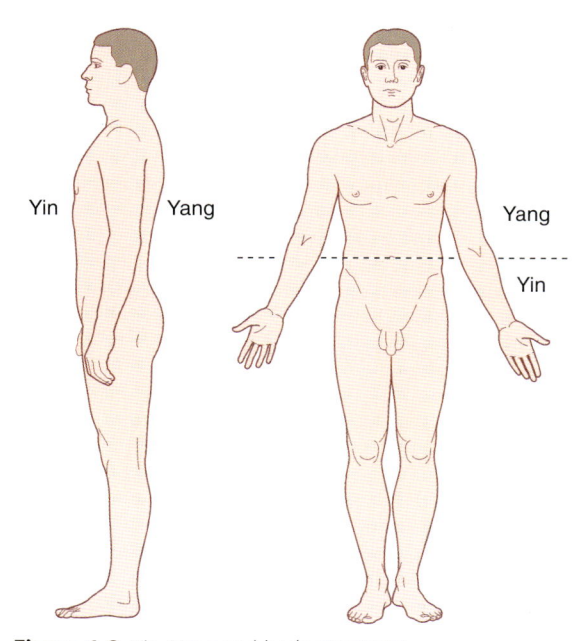

Figure 1.8 Yin–Yang and body structures

First of all, Yang energy tends to rise and, in pathological situations, Heat or Fire will tend to rise. Since the head is the topmost area of the body, Yang energy (be it physiological or pathological) will tend to rise to the head. In pathological circumstances, this will cause red face and red eyes.

The head is also easily affected by Yang pathogenic factors such as Wind and Summer-Heat.

Finally, the head being the convergence place of all the Yang channels, points in this area can be used to raise the Yang energy.

The rest of the body (chest and abdomen) pertains to Yin and is easily affected by Yin pathogenic factors such as Cold and Dampness.

Exterior–Interior

The Exterior of the body includes skin and muscles and pertains to Yang. It has the function of protecting the body from exterior pathogenic factors. The Interior of the body includes the internal organs and it has the function of nourishing the body.

Above–below waist

The area above the waist pertains to Yang and is easily affected by Yang pathogenic factors such as Wind, whereas the area below the waist pertains to Yin and is easily affected by Yin pathogenic factors such as Dampness: this basic general rule is frequently applied in the diagnosis of skin diseases.

Posterior–lateral and anterior–medial surface of limbs

The Yang channels flow on the posterior–lateral surface of limbs, and the Yin channels on the anterior–medial one.

Yang and Yin organs

Some organs pertain to Yang and some to Yin. The Yang organs transform, digest and excrete 'impure' products of food and fluids. The Yin organs store the 'pure' essences, resulting from the process of transformation carried out by the Yang organs. The 'Simple Questions' in chapter 11 says: *'The Five Yin organs store ... and do not excrete ... the 6 Yang organs transform and digest and do not store.'*[10]

Thus the Yang organs, in conformity with the correspondence of Yang to activity, are constantly filling and emptying, transforming, separating and excreting the products of food in order to produce Qi. They are in contact with the exterior as most of the Yang organs (stomach, intestines, bladder) communicate with the exterior, via the mouth, anus or urethra.

The Yin organs, on the contrary, do not transform, digest or excrete, but store the pure essences extracted from food by the Yang organs. In particular they store the Vital Substances: that is, Qi, Blood, Body Fluids and Essence.

Function–structure of organs

Yang corresponds to function and Yin corresponds to structure. We have just said that some organs 'are' Yang and some 'are' Yin. However, in accordance with the principle that nothing is totally Yang or Yin, each organ contains within itself a Yang and a Yin aspect. In particular, the structure of the organ itself and the Blood, Essence or Fluids contained within it, pertain to Yin; they are its Yin aspect.

The functional activity of the organ represents its Yang aspect. The two aspects are of course related and interdependent. For example, the Spleen function of transforming and transporting the essences extracted from food represents its Yang aspect. The Qi extracted in this way from food is then transformed into Blood, which, being Yin, contributes to forming the structure of the Spleen itself. The 'Simple Questions' in chapter 5 says: *'Yang transforms Qi, Yin forms the structure.'*[11] This relationship can be represented with a diagram (Fig. 1.9).

Another good example of function and structure within an organ is that of the Liver. The Liver stores Blood and this represents its Yin aspect and is its structure; on the other hand, the Liver controls the flow of

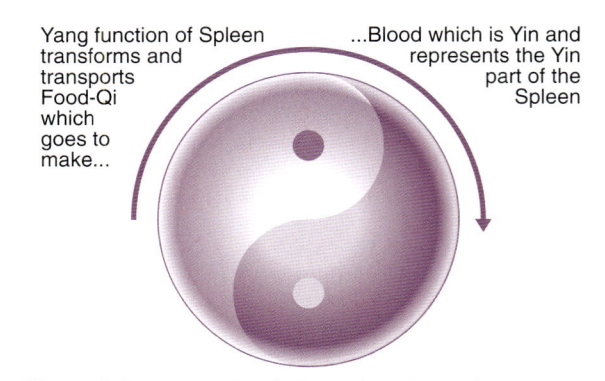

Figure 1.9 Yin–Yang in relation to function and structure

Qi in all parts of the body and this represents its Yang aspect and is its function.

Qi–Blood

Qi is Yang in relation to Blood. Blood, which is a denser and more material form of Qi, is therefore more Yin.

Qi has the role of warming, protecting, transforming and raising, all typically Yang functions. Blood has the role of nourishing and moistening, which are typically Yin functions. The nature and functions of Qi and Blood will be dealt with in detail in chapter 3.

Defensive Qi–Nutritive Qi

Defensive Qi is Yang in relation to Nutritive Qi. Defensive Qi circulates in the skin and muscles (a Yang area) and has the function of protecting and warming the body (a Yang function). Nutritive Qi circulates in the internal organs (a Yin area) and has the function of nourishing the body (a Yin function). Again, the nature and functions of Defensive and Nutritive Qi will be dealt with in detail in chapter 3.

APPLICATION OF THE FOUR PRINCIPLES OF YIN–YANG TO MEDICINE

Let us now discuss in detail the application of the four principles of Yin–Yang interrelationship to Chinese medicine.

Opposition of Yin–Yang

The opposition of Yin–Yang is reflected in medicine in the opposing Yin–Yang structures of the human body, the opposing Yin–Yang character of the organs and, most of all, the opposing symptomatology of Yin and Yang. No matter how complicated, all symptoms and signs in Chinese medicine can be reduced to their elemental, basic character of Yin or Yang.

In order to interpret the character of the clinical manifestations in terms of Yin–Yang, we can refer to certain basic qualities which will guide us in clinical practice. These are:

Yang	Yin
Fire	Water
Heat	Cold
Restless	Quiet
Dry	Wet
Hard	Soft

Excitement	Inhibition
Rapidity	Slowness
Non-substantial	Substantial
Transformation/change	Conservation/storage/sustainment

Fire–Water

This is one of the fundamental dualities of Yin–Yang in Chinese medicine. Although these terms derive from the Five-Element theory, there is an interaction between that and the theory of Yin–Yang.

The balance between Fire and Water in the body is crucial. Fire is essential to all physiological processes: it represents the flame that keeps alive and stokes all metabolic processes. Fire, the physiological Fire, assists the Heart in its function of housing the Mind (*Shen*), it provides the warmth necessary to the Spleen to transform and transport, it stimulates the Small Intestine function of separation, it provides the heat necessary to the Bladder and Lower Burner to transform and excrete fluids and it provides the heat necessary for the Uterus to keep the Blood moving.

If the physiological Fire declines, the Mind will suffer with depression, the Spleen cannot transform and transport, the Small Intestine cannot separate the fluids, the Bladder and Lower Burner cannot excrete the fluids and there will be oedema, and the Uterus turns Cold, which may cause infertility.

This physiological Fire is called the Fire of the Gate of Life (*Ming Men*) and derives from the Kidneys.

> **Clinical note**
>
> The physiological Fire of the body is essential to all physiological processes and to the Mind. Deficiency of the physiological Fire will cause depression. It is stimulated by using moxa on KI-3 Taixi and Du-4 Mingmen.

Water has the function of moistening and cooling during all the body's physiological functions, to balance the warming action of the physiological Fire. The origin of Water is also from the Kidneys.

Thus, the balance between Fire and Water is fundamental to all physiological processes of the body. Fire and Water balance and keep a check on each other in every single physiological process. When Fire gets out of hand and becomes excessive, it has a tendency to flow upwards; hence the manifestations will show on the top part of the body and head, with headaches, red eyes, red face or thirst. When Water become excessive, it has a tendency to flow downwards causing oedema of the legs, excessive urination or incontinence.

Heat–Cold

Excess of Yang is manifested with Heat and excess of Yin is manifested with Cold. For example, a person with excess of Yang will feel hot, and one with excess of Yin will tend to feel always cold. The hot and cold character can also be observed in certain signs themselves. For example, a large single boil that is red and hot to the touch indicates Heat. A lower back area very cold to the touch indicates Cold in the Kidneys.

Redness–paleness

A red complexion indicates excess of Yang (or deficiency of Yin), a pale one excess of Yin (or deficiency of Yang).

Restless–quiet

Restlessness, insomnia, fidgeting or tremors indicate excess of Yang. Quiet behaviour, desire to be immobile or sleepiness indicate excess of Yin.

Dry–wet

Any symptom or sign of dryness such as dry eyes, dry throat, dry skin or dry stools indicates excess of Yang (or deficiency of Yin). Any symptom or sign of excess wetness, such as watery eyes, runny nose, damp pimples on skin or loose stools, indicates excess of Yin (or deficiency of Yang).

Hard–soft

Any lumps, swellings or masses that are hard are usually due to excess of Yang, whereas if they are soft they are due to excess of Yin.

Excitement–inhibition

Whenever a function is in a state of hyperactivity, it indicates an excess of Yang; if it is in a state of hypoactivity, it indicates excess of Yin. For example, a rapid heart rate may indicate excess of Yang of the Heart, whereas a very slow heart rate may indicate excess of Yin of the Heart.

Rapidity–slowness

This shows in two ways: in a person's movements and in the onset of the manifestations.

If a person's movements are rapid, and he or she walks and talks fast, it may indicate an excess of Yang. If a person's movements are slow, and he or she walks and talks slowly, it may indicate an excess of Yin.

If symptoms and signs appear suddenly and change rapidly, they indicate a Yang condition. If they appear gradually and change slowly, they indicate a Yin condition.

Substantial–non-substantial

As explained above, Yang corresponds to a subtle state of aggregation, and Yin corresponds to a dense, coarse state of aggregation. If Yang is normal, things will be kept moving, Qi will flow normally and fluids will be transformed and excreted. If Yang is deficient, Qi stagnates, fluids are not transformed or excreted and therefore Yin will prevail. Thus, Yang keeps things moving and in a state of fluidity or 'non-substantiality'. When Yin prevails, the movement and transformation power of Yang fails, energy condenses into form and it becomes 'substantial'.

For example, if Qi moves normally in the abdomen, the intestine's function of separation and excretion of fluids will be normal. If Yang fails and Qi decreases, the Yang power of moving and transforming is impaired, fluids are not transformed, Blood is not moved, and in time, the stagnation of Qi gives rise to stasis of Blood and then to actual, physical masses or tumours.

Transformation/change–conservation/storage/sustainment

Yin corresponds to conservation and storage: this is reflected in the function of the Yin organs, which store Blood, Body Fluids and Essence and guard them as precious essences. Yang corresponds to transformation and change: this is reflected in the function of the Yang organs, which are constantly filled and emptied and which constantly transform, transport and excrete.

The above are general guidelines, enabling us, through the theory of Yin–Yang, to interpret clinical manifestations. All symptoms and signs can be interpreted in the light of the above guidelines, because all clinical manifestations arise from a separation of Yin and Yang. In health, Yin and Yang are harmoniously blended in a dynamic balance. When Yin and Yang are so balanced, they cannot be identified as separate entities: hence, symptoms and signs do not appear. For example, if Yin and Yang and Qi and Blood are balanced, the face will have a normal, pink, flourishing colour and will be neither too pale nor too red, neither too colourless nor too dark, etc. In other words, nothing can be observed.

If Yin and Yang are out of balance, they become separated; there will be too much of one or the other, and the face will be either too pale (excess of Yin) or too red (excess of Yang). Yin and Yang therefore show themselves when they are out of balance. One can visualize the Yin–Yang Supreme Ultimate symbol (see Fig. 1.6) spinning very fast: in this case the white and the black will not be visible because they cannot be separated by the eye. Similarly, when Yin and Yang are balanced and moving harmoniously, they cannot be separated, they are not visible and symptoms and signs will not arise.

All symptoms and signs can be interpreted in this way, i.e. as a loss of balance of Yin and Yang. Another example: if Yin and Yang are balanced, urine will be of a normal pale-yellow colour and of normal amount. If Yin is in excess, it will be very pale, looking almost like water, and profuse; if Yang is in excess, it will be rather dark and scanty.

All symptoms and signs are ultimately due to an imbalance between Yin and Yang.

Keeping in mind the general principles of the Yin and Yang character of symptoms and signs, we can list the main clinical manifestations as follows:

Yang	Yin
Acute disease	Chronic disease
Rapid onset	Gradual onset
Rapid pathological changes	Lingering disease
Heat	Cold
Restlessness, insomnia	Sleepiness, listlessness
Throws off bedclothes	Likes to be covered
Likes to lie stretched out	Likes to curl up
Hot limbs and body	Cold limbs and body
Red face	Pale face
Likes cold drinks	Likes hot drinks
Loud voice, talks a lot	Weak voice, dislikes talking
Coarse breathing	Shallow, weak breathing
Thirst	No thirst
Scanty-dark urination	Profuse-pale urination
Constipation	Loose stools
Red tongue with yellow coating	Pale tongue
Full pulse	Empty pulse

Finally, following the discussion of the Yin and Yang character of symptoms and signs, it must be emphasized that, although the distinction between Yin and Yang in clinical manifestations is fundamental, it is not detailed enough to be of much clinical use in practice. For example, if the face is too red, it indicates an excess of Yang. However, this conclusion is too general to give any indication as to what the appropriate treatment should be, since the face could, in fact, be red from Full-Heat or Empty-Heat from Yin deficiency (both of which can be classified as 'excess of Yang'). If it was red from Full-Heat, one must further distinguish which organ is mostly involved: it could be red from Liver-Fire, Heart-Fire, Lung-Heat or Stomach-Heat. The treatment would be different in each case.

The theory of Yin–Yang, although fundamental, is thus too general to give concrete guidelines as to the treatment needed. As we will see later, it needs to be integrated with the Eight-Principle and the Internal-Organ pattern theory to be applied to actual clinical situations (see chs 30 to 42). The theory of Yin–Yang is, nevertheless, the necessary foundation for an understanding of symptoms and signs.

The interdependence of Yin and Yang

Yin and Yang are opposite but are also mutually dependent on each other. Yin and Yang cannot exist in isolation, and this is very apparent when considering the body's physiology. All the physiological processes are a result of the opposition and interdependence of Yin and Yang. The functions of the internal organs in Chinese medicine show the interdependence of Yin and Yang very clearly.

Yin and Yang organs

The Yin and Yang organs are very different in their functions, but, at the same time, they depend on each other for the performance of these functions. The Yin organs depend on the Yang ones to produce Qi and Blood from the transformation of food. The Yang organs depend on the Yin ones for their nourishment deriving from Blood and Essence stored by the Yin organs.

Structure and function of the organs

Each organ has a structure represented by the organ itself and the Blood and fluids within it. At the same time, each organ has a certain function which both affects and is affected by its structure. For example, the structure of the Liver is represented by the actual organ and the Blood stored within it. In particular, the Liver has the function of storing Blood. Another function of the Liver is that of ensuring the smooth flow of Qi all over the body. By ensuring the smooth flow of Qi, the Liver also keeps the Blood moving, therefore providing a correct storage of Blood within itself: this is an example of how the Liver function assists the Liver structure. On the other hand, in order to carry out its function, the Liver organ itself needs the nourishment of Blood: this is an example of how the Liver structure assists the Liver function.

Without structure (Yin), the function (Yang) could not perform; without function, the structure would lack transformation and movement.

The 'Simple Questions' in chapter 5 says: *'Yin is in the Interior and is the material foundation of Yang; Yang is on the Exterior and is the manifestation of Yin.'*[12]

The mutual consuming of Yin and Yang

Yin and Yang are in a constant state of change so that when one increases, the other is consumed, to preserve the balance. This can easily be seen in the ebb and flow of night and day. As the day comes to an end, Yang decreases and Yin increases. Exactly the same can be observed in the cycle of seasons. When spring comes, Yin begins to decrease and Yang increases. Beyond the mere preservation of their balance, Yin and Yang also mutually 'consume' each other. When one increases, the other must decrease. For example, if the weather becomes unduly hot (Yang), the water (Yin) in the soil dries up. Thus:

> If Yin is consumed, Yang increases
> If Yang is consumed, Yin increases
> If Yin increases, Yang is consumed
> If Yang increases, Yin is consumed

In the human body, the mutual consuming of Yin and Yang can be seen from a physiological point of view and from a pathological point of view.

From a physiological point of view, the mutual consuming of Yin and Yang is a normal process which keeps the balance of physiological functions. This process can be observed in all physiological processes; for example, in the regulation of sweating, urination, temperature of the body, breathing, etc. In summertime, for instance, the weather is hot (Yang) and we sweat (Yin) more; when the external temperature is very cold (Yin), the body starts trembling (Yang) in an attempt to produce some heat.

From a physiological point of view, the mutual consuming of Yin and Yang can also be observed in the alternation of Yin and Yang in the menstrual cycle. The menstrual cycle can be divided into four phases as follows:

> Phase 1: bleeding phase
> Phase 2: post-menstrual phase (roughly a week after the end of bleeding)
> Phase 3: mid-cycle (roughly a week around ovulation)
> Phase 4: pre-menstrual phase (roughly a week before the period)

In phases 1 and 2, Yang is decreasing and Yin is increasing; i.e. Yin increases and Yang is consumed. In phases 3 and 4, Yang is increasing and Yin decreasing; that is, Yang increases and Yin is consumed (Fig. 1.10). From a Western perspective, the first two phases correspond to the follicular phase and the last two phases to the luteal phase.

From a pathological point of view, Yin or Yang may increase beyond their normal range and lead to consumption of their opposite quality. For example, the

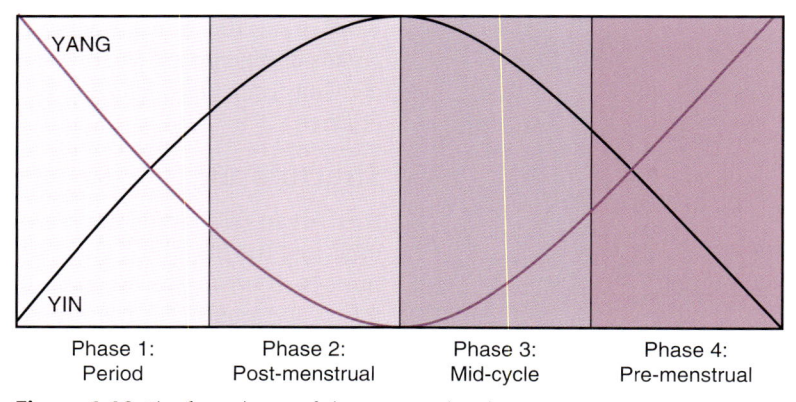

Figure 1.10 The four phases of the menstrual cycle

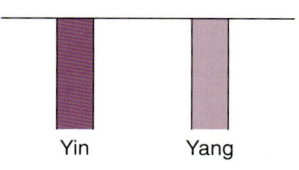

Figure 1.11 Balance of Yin and Yang

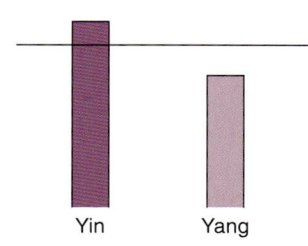

Figure 1.12 Excess of Yin

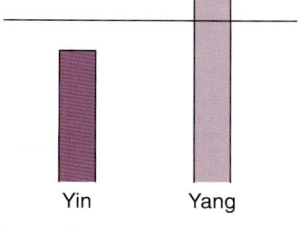

Figure 1.13 Excess of Yang

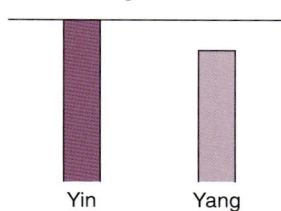

Figure 1.14 Consumption of Yang

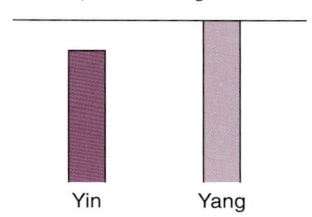

Figure 1.15 Consumption of Yin

temperature may rise (excess of Yang) during an infectious disease. This can lead to dryness and exhaustion of body fluids (consumption of Yin). Although some might still regard this as an attempt by the body to keep the balance between Yin and Yang (the body fluids and temperature), it is not a normal balance, but a pathological balance deriving from an excess of Yang. One might go further and say that the temperature itself was an attempt by the body to fight a pathogenic factor, but this does not change the fact that the rise in temperature represents an excess of Yang, which leads to consumption of Yin.

From a pathological point of view, there can be four different situations of excess of Yin or excess of Yang leading to consumption of Yang or Yin, respectively, or consumption of Yang or consumption of Yin leading to apparent excess of Yin or Yang, respectively. It is important to note that excess of Yang and consumption of Yin are not the same. In excess of Yang, the primary factor is the abnormal increase of Yang, which leads to consumption of Yin. In consumption of Yin, the primary factor is the deficiency of Yin arising spontaneously and leading to an apparent excess of Yang.

Five diagrams will clarify this (Figs 1.11 to 1.15).

Balance of Yin and Yang
(Fig. 1.11)

Excess of Yin
(Fig. 1.12)

An example of this is when excess Cold (interior or exterior) in the body consumes the Yang, especially Spleen-Yang. This is Full-Cold.

Excess of Yang
(Fig. 1.13)

An example of this is when excess Heat (which can be exterior or interior) consumes the body fluids (which pertain to Yin) and leads to dryness. This is Full-Heat.

Consumption of Yang
(Fig. 1.14)

This takes place when the body's Yang energy is spontaneously deficient. The decrease of Yang energy leads to cold, chilliness and other symptoms which, to a certain extent, are similar to those created by excess of Yin. The situation is, however, very different, as in excess of Yin it is the excessive Yin that is the primary aspect and which consumes Yang. In case of consumption of Yang, the decrease of Yang is the primary aspect and the Yin is only apparently in excess. This is called Empty-Cold.

Consumption of Yin
(Fig. 1.15)

This takes place when the body's Yin energies are depleted. The decrease of Yin may lead to symptoms of apparent excess of Yang, such as feelings of heat. Again, this situation is very different from that seen in excess of Yang. In excess of Yang, the excessive Yang is the primary aspect. In case of decrease of Yin, this is the primary aspect, and the Yang is only apparently in excess. This is called Empty-Heat.

The distinction between Empty-Cold and Full-Cold and between Empty-Heat and Full-Heat is all-important in practice: in cases of Emptiness, one needs to tonify, while in cases of Fullness, one needs to expel pathogenic factors (see Box 1.1).

Box 1.1 Mutual consuming of Yin–Yang: Heat and Cold

1. Excess of Yin = Full-Cold
2. Excess of Yang = Full-Heat
3. Consumption of Yang = Empty-Cold
4. Consumption of Yin = Empty-Heat

The intertransformation of Yin and Yang

Although opposite, Yin and Yang can change into one another. This transformation does not take place at random, but is determined by the stage of development and by internal conditions.

First of all, the change takes place when conditions are ripe at a certain point in time. Day cannot turn into night at any time, but only when it has reached its point of exhaustion.

The second condition of change is determined by the internal qualities of any given thing or phenomenon. Wood can turn into coal, but a stone cannot.

The process of transformation of Yin and Yang into each other can be observed in many natural phenomena, such as in the alternation of day and night, the seasons, climate.

The principle of intertransformation of Yin–Yang has many applications in clinical practice. An understanding of this transformation is important for the prevention of disease. If we are aware of how a thing can turn into its opposite, then we can prevent this and achieve a balance which is the essence of Chinese medicine.

For example, excessive work (Yang) without rest induces extreme deficiency (Yin) of the body's energies. Excessive jogging (Yang) induces a very slow (Yin) pulse. Excessive consumption of alcohol creates a pleasant euphoria (Yang) which is quickly followed by a hangover (Yin). Excessive worrying (Yang) depletes (Yin) the energy of the body. Excessive sexual activity (Yang) depletes the Essence (Yin).

Thus, balance in our life, in diet, exercise, work, emotional life and sexual life, is the essence of prevention in Chinese medicine, and an understanding of how Yang can turn into Yin and vice versa can help us to avoid the rapid swings from one to the other which are detrimental to our physical and emotional life. Of course, nothing would be more difficult to achieve in our modern Western societies, which seem to be geared to producing the maximum swing from one extreme to the other.

The transformation of Yin–Yang can also be observed in the pathological changes seen in clinical practice. For example, exterior Cold can invade the body and, after a time, it can easily change into Heat. An Excess condition can easily turn into a Deficiency one. Excessive Heat, for instance, can damage the body fluids and lead to deficiency of fluids. A Deficiency condition can also turn into an Excess one. For example, a deficiency of Spleen-Yang can lead to Excess of Dampness or Phlegm. It is therefore extremely important to be able to discern the transformation of Yin–Yang in clinical practice in order to treat the condition properly.

Learning outcomes

In this chapter you will have learned:
- How to grasp the concept of Yin–Yang
- The classification of phenomena according to Yin–Yang
- The four aspects of Yin–Yang interrelationship
- How to apply the theory of Yin–Yang to Chinese medicine
- How to grasp the concepts of Yin Deficiency, Yang Deficiency, Yin Excess and Yang Excess

Self-assessment questions

1. What do the Chinese characters for Yin and Yang represent?
2. Why do you think left pertains to Yang and right to Yin?
3. Why does round pertain to Yang and square to Yin?
4. How do Yin and Yang relate to the four seasons?
5. You are by a lake on a very hot day and you observe the vapour rising from the surface of the water: how do you interpret this in terms of Yin–Yang?
6. When Yang is preponderant, what happens to Yin?
7. When Yin is deficient, what happens to Yang?

8. Explain the relationship between Liver-Blood and Liver-Qi in terms of Yin–Yang.
9. Mention at least five examples of the opposition of Yin–Yang in symptomatology.
10. Relate Excess of Yin/Yang and Deficiency of Yin/Yang to Heat and Cold (Full or Empty).

See p. 1255 for answers

END NOTES

1. Needham J 1977 Science and Civilization in China, vol. 2, Cambridge University Press, Cambridge, p. 303.
2. Ibid.
3. A deeper discussion of the historical development of the theory of Yin–Yang over the centuries is beyond the scope of this book. The reader is referred to the following works:
   - Fung Yu-Lan 1966 A Short History of Chinese Philosophy, Macmillan, New York.
   - Granet M 1967 La Pensée Chinoise, Albin Michel, Paris.
   - Moore CA 1967 The Chinese Mind, University Press of Hawaii, Honolulu.
   - Needham J 1956 Science and Civilization in China, vol. 2, Cambridge University Press, Cambridge.
   - Wing Tsit Chan 1969 A Source Book in Chinese Philosophy, Princeton University Press, Princeton.
4. Granet M 1967 La Pensée Chinoise, Albin Michel, Paris, p. 367.
5. 1979 The Yellow Emperor's Classic of Internal Medicine – Simple Questions (*Huang Di Nei Jing Su Wen* 黄帝内经素问), People's Health Publishing House, Beijing, p. 44.
6. It is interesting to compare this with the Western cultural attitude to left and right, according to which left is somehow 'bad' and right somehow 'good'. See, for example, certain words such as 'sinister' (etymologically related to 'left'), 'cack-handed' meaning both 'left-handed' and 'clumsy', or 'dexterous' meaning both 'right-handed' and 'skilful'.
7. Simple Questions, p. 31.
8. Science and Civilization in China, vol. 2, p. 41.
9. Simple Questions, p. 31.
10. Ibid., p. 77–78
11. Ibid., p. 32.
12. Ibid., p. 42–43.
13. Lao Zi, Library of Chinese Classics, Foreign Languages Press, Beijing, 1999, p. 73.

BIBLIOGRAPHY AND FURTHER READING

Fung Yu Lan 1966 A Short History of Chinese Philosophy, Free Press, New York
Kaptchuk T 2000 The Web that has no Weaver – Understanding Chinese Medicine, Contemporary Books, Chicago
Moore CA 1967 The Chinese Mind, University Press of Hawaii, Honolulu
Needham J 1977 Science and Civilization in China, vol. 2, Cambridge University Press, Cambridge
Wang Bi 1994 The Classic of Changes (translated by RJ Lynn), Columbia University Press, New York
Wilhelm R 1967 The I Ching, Routledge and Kegan Paul, London
Wing Tsit Chan 1969 A Source Book in Chinese Philosophy, Princeton University Press, Princeton

PART 1

The Five Elements 2

Key contents

The Five Elements in Nature

Nature of the Five Elements

The Five Elements interrelationships

Application of the Five Elements to Chinese medicine

Together with the theory of Yin–Yang, the theory of the Five Elements constitutes the basis of Chinese medical theory. The term 'Five Elements' has been used by most Western practitioners of Chinese medicine for a long time. Some authors consider this to be a misunderstanding of the meaning of the Chinese term '*Wu Xing*', perpetuated over the years. '*Wu*' means 'five' and '*Xing*' means 'movement', 'process', 'to go' or 'conduct, behaviour'. Most authors therefore think that the word '*Xing*' cannot indicate 'element' as a basic constituent of Nature, as was supposedly intended in ancient Greek philosophy.

This is, in my opinion, only partly true. First of all, the elements, as they were conceived by various Greek philosophers over the centuries, were not always considered 'basic constituents' of Nature or 'passive motionless fundamental substances'.[1] Some Greek philosophers thought of the elements as dynamic qualities of Nature, in a way similar to Chinese philosophy.

Greek philosophers used different words to indicate the elements, which proves the lack of a uniform view of them. To Empedocles, they were 'roots' (*rhizomata* ριζωματα), to Plato, 'simple components' (*stoicheia* στοιχεια). Aristotle gave a definite dynamic interpretation to the four elements and called them 'primary form' (*prota somata* πρωτα σωματα). He said: '*Earth and Fire are opposites also due to the opposition of the respective qualities with which they are revealed to our senses: Fire is hot, Earth is cold. Besides the fundamental opposition of hot and cold, there is another one, i.e. that of dry and wet: hence the four possible combinations of hot-dry [Fire], hot-wet [Air], cold-dry [Earth] and cold-wet [Water] … the elements can mix with each other and can even transform into one another … thus Earth, which is cold and dry, can generate Water if wetness replaces dryness.*'[2]

For Aristotle, therefore, the four elements became the four basic qualities of natural phenomena, classified as combinations of four qualities, hot, cold, dry and wet. As is apparent from the above statement, the Aristotelian elements could even transform into one another and generate each other.

This interpretation is very similar to the Chinese one, in which the elements are qualities of Nature. Furthermore, it is interesting to note the similarity with the Chinese theory of Yin–Yang: the four Aristotelian elements derive from the interaction of the basic Yin–Yang qualities of cold-hot and dry-wet.

Thus, it is not entirely true to say that the Greek elements were conceived only as the basic constituents of matter, the 'building blocks' of Nature. Furthermore, the word 'elements' does not necessarily imply that: it does so only in its modern chemical interpretation.

Finally, it is not entirely true either that the Chinese elements were not conceived as basic constituents of matter. Certainly, they are primarily basic qualities of natural phenomena, or movements; however, there are also statements which would seem to imply that the elements are that and basic constituents of Nature as well. For instance: '*When the Qi of the Elements settles, things acquire form.*'[3]

In conclusion, for the above reasons, I have kept the word 'element' as a translation of the Chinese word '*xing*'. Some Sinologists (such as Joseph Needham and Fung Yu Lan) have used the term 'element'. Fung Yu Lan suggested that a possible translation of *wu xing* could be 'Five Activities' or 'Five Agents'.[4] Although the term 'five phases' has gained some acceptance as a translation of '*wu xing*', I find this term restrictive as it

> **Box 2.1 Nature of Five Elements**
>
> - Five basic processes of Nature
> - Five qualities of natural phenomena
> - Five phases of a cycle
> - Five inherent capabilities of change of phenomena

clearly refers to only one aspect of the Five Elements, namely the phases of a (seasonal) cycle.

Therefore, while they are not basic constituents of Nature, the Five Elements, like Yin–Yang, have a multifaceted nature. They can be described as listed in Box 2.1.

The theory of the Five Elements was not applied to Chinese medicine throughout its historical development as its popularity waxed and waned through the centuries. During the Warring States period (see Chinese Chronology, Appendix 3), it became immensely popular and was applied to medicine, astrology, the natural sciences, the calendar, music and even politics. Its popularity was such that most phenomena were classified in fives.

However, critical voices were raised as early as the beginning of the 1st century. The great sceptical philosopher Wang Chong (AD 27–97) criticized the theory of the Five Elements as being too rigid to interpret all natural phenomena correctly. He said: '*The rooster pertains to Metal and the hare to Wood: if Metal really conquers Wood, why is it that roosters do not devour hares?*'[5]

From the Han dynasty onwards, the influence of the theory of the Five Elements in Chinese medicine began to wane. For example, the great Chinese medical classic of the Han dynasty 'Discussion of Cold-induced Diseases', by Zhang Zhong Jing, makes no mention of the Five Elements at all. It was not until the Song dynasty (960–1279) that the theory of the Five Elements regained popularity and was systematically applied to diagnosis, symptomatology and treatment in Chinese medicine.

From the Ming dynasty onwards, the influence of the theory of the Five Elements again decreased as Chinese medicine was dominated by the study of infectious diseases from exterior heat, for the diagnosis and treatment of which the Identification of Patterns according to the Four Levels and Three Burners was used.

For the best critical appraisal of the significance of the Five-Element theory in Chinese medicine see 'The Web that has no Weaver'.[6]

This chapter will be articulated into the following headings:

- The Five Elements in Nature
  - The Five Elements as basic qualities
  - The Five Elements as movements
  - The Five Elements as stages of a seasonal cycle
  - The Five-Element interrelationships
    - The Cosmological sequence
    - The Generating sequence
    - The Controlling sequence
    - The Over-acting sequence
    - The Insulting sequence
  - The Five-Element correspondences
- The Five Elements in Chinese medicine
  - The Five Elements in physiology
    - The Generating and Controlling sequences
    - The Cosmological sequence
    - The system of correspondences in Five-Element physiology
  - The Five Elements in pathology
    - The Over-acting sequence
    - The Insulting sequence
    - The Generating sequence
  - The Five Elements in diagnosis
    - Colours
    - Sounds
    - Smells
    - Emotions
    - Tastes
    - Tissues
    - Sense orifices
    - Climates
  - The Five Elements in acupuncture treatment
    - Treatment according to the various sequences
    - Treatment according to the Five Transporting points
  - The Five Elements in herbal and diet therapy

THE FIVE ELEMENTS IN NATURE

The theory of Five Elements originated at about the same time as that of Yin–Yang. The first references to both Yin–Yang and the Five Elements date back to the Zhou dynasty (about 1000–771 BC).[7]

Some of the earliest references to the Elements do not call them elements at all; instead, an element is a 'seat of government', a 'government repository', a 'mansion' or 'house' (*Fu* 府) or an 'ability, talent, material' (*cai* 柴), and they were at one point considered to be six rather than five. They were in fact called either the 'Five Abilities' or the 'Six Seats of Government'. A book from the Warring States period says: '*Heaven sends the Five Abilities and the people use them.*'[8] And it also says: '*The Six Seats of Government ... are Water, Fire, Metal, Wood, Earth and Grain.*'[9] Thus 'Grain' was considered to be the sixth 'element'.

A Western Han dynasty (206 BC – AD 24) book called the 'Great Transmission of the Valued Book' says: '*Water and Fire provide food, Metal and Wood provide prosperity and the Earth makes provisions.*'[10]

It could be said that the theories of Yin–Yang and of the Five Elements, and their application to medicine, mark the beginning of what one might call 'scientific' medicine and a departure from shamanism. No longer do healers look for a supernatural cause of disease: they now observe Nature and, with a combination of the inductive and deductive methods, they set out to find patterns within it and, by extension, apply these in the interpretation of disease.

> The theory of Yin–Yang and of the Five Elements represented a historical leap in medicine from a view of disease as being caused by evil spirits to a naturalistic view of disease as being caused by lifestyle.

It is therefore not by chance that numbers and numeration are increasingly applied in the interpretation of Nature and the human body: two basic polarities (Yin–Yang), a three-tier cosmological 'structure' (Heaven, Person, Earth), four seasons, Five Elements, six climates in Nature, and five Yin and six Yang organs in the human body. The number 5 and the Five Elements are associated with earthly phenomena, while the number 6 is associated with heavenly phenomena (the six climates). The classification of things in numbers is indicative of an increasingly searching and analytical mode of thought.

Interestingly, more or less the same process was taking place in ancient Greece at roughly the same time, when the Greek theories of the Elements were developed. In his essay 'On the sacred disease', Hippocrates launches an in-depth criticism of the supernatural theory for the aetiology of epilepsy.[11]

The book *Shang Shu*, written during the Western Zhou dynasty (1000–771 BC), said: '*The Five Elements are Water, Fire, Wood, Metal and Earth. Water moistens downwards, Fire flares upwards, Wood can be bent and straightened, Metal can be moulded and can harden, Earth permits sowing, growing and reaping.*'[12] We will return to this statement later as it contains many important concepts on the nature of the Five Elements.

The theory of the Five Elements was developed by the same philosophical school that developed the theory of Yin–Yang, the 'Yin–Yang School', sometimes also called the 'Naturalist School'. The chief exponent of this school was Zou Yan (*c*.350–270 BC). Initially, the theory of the Five Elements had political implications as much as naturalistic ones. The philosophers of this school were highly esteemed, and perhaps somewhat feared, by the ancient Chinese rulers, as they purported to be able to interpret Nature in the light of Yin–Yang and Five Elements and to draw political conclusions from it. For example, a certain ruler was associated with a certain Element and every ceremonial occasion had to conform to that particular Element's colour, season, etc.

Also, these philosophers claimed they could predict the succession of rulers by referring to the various cycles of the Five Elements. Zou Yan said: '*Each of the Five Elements is followed by one it cannot conquer. The dynasty of Shun ruled by the virtue of Earth, the Xia dynasty ruled by the virtue of Wood, the Shang dynasty ruled by the virtue of Metal, and the Zhou dynasty ruled by the virtue of Fire. When some new dynasty is going to arise, heaven exhibits auspicious signs to the people. During the rise of Huang Di [the Yellow Emperor] large earth-worms and large ants appeared. He said: "This indicates that the Element Earth is in the ascendant, so our colour must be yellow, and our affairs must be placed under the sign of Earth." During the rise of Yu the Great, heaven produced plants and trees that did not wither in autumn and winter. He said: "This indicates that the Element Wood is in the ascendant, so our colour must be green, and our affairs must be placed under the signs of Wood."*'[13] One could say that the philosophers of the Naturalist School developed a primitive natural science and occupied a respected social position comparable with that of modern scientists today.

Apart from its political connotation, the theory of the Five Elements has many facets. The three main ones will be discussed as well as the Five-Element interrelationship and correspondences, i.e.:

- Five different qualities of natural phenomena
- Five movements
- Five phases in the cycle of seasons
- Interrelationship among the Five Elements
- Five-Element correspondences

The Five Elements as basic qualities

It is worth repeating here and enlarging the passage from the *Shang Shu*: 'The Five Elements are Water, Fire, Wood, Metal and Earth. Water moistens downwards, Fire flares upwards, Wood can be bent and straightened, Metal can be moulded and can harden, Earth permits sowing, growing and reaping. That which soaks and descends [Water] is salty, that which blazes upwards [Fire] is bitter, that which can be bent and straightened [Wood] is sour, that which can be moulded and become hard [Metal] is pungent, that which permits sowing and reaping [Earth] is sweet.'[14]

This statement clearly shows that the Five Elements symbolize five different inherent qualities and states of natural phenomena. It also relates the tastes (or flavours) to the Five Elements, and it is apparent that the tastes have more to do with an inherent quality of a thing (like its chemical composition in modern terms) than with its actual flavour.

Thus, from this statement, it is apparent that the Five Elements are not five sorts of fundamental matter but five types of processes (Box 2.2). Needham translates these processes in modern terms as follows:

Water: liquidity, fluidity, solution
Fire: heat, combustion
Wood: solidity, workability
Metal: solidity, congelation, mouldability
Earth: nutritivity[15]

The Five Elements as movements

The Five Elements also symbolize five different directions of movement of natural phenomena. Wood represents expansive, outward movement in all directions, Metal represents contractive, inward movement, Water represents downward movement, Fire represents upward movement and Earth represents neutrality or stability (Fig. 2.1).

The very term *xing* (translated as 'Element') means movement: thus, the Five Elements always represented five types of movements rather than fundamental substances. The five movements find important applications in medicine. For example, pathological Fire clearly blazes upwards (causing a red face and feeling of heat), Wood (Liver-Qi) flows freely in every direction, Metal controls the skin which contains the body (contraction), Water (Kidney-Qi) has clearly a downward movement (excretion of impure fluids), and Earth is in the centre and therefore the pivot of reference (Box 2.3).

The Five Elements as stages of a seasonal cycle

Each of the Five Elements represents a season in the yearly cycle. Wood corresponds to spring and is associated with birth, Fire corresponds to summer and is associated with growth, Metal corresponds to autumn and is associated with harvest, Water corresponds to

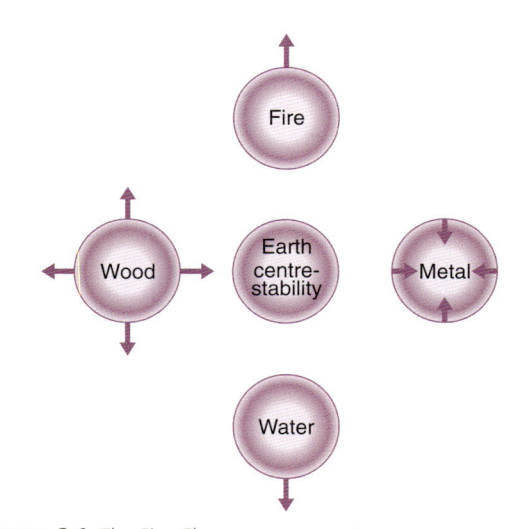

Figure 2.1 The Five-Element movements

Box 2.2 The Five Elements as basic qualities
• Wood: 'can be bent and straightened'
• Fire: 'flares upwards'
• Earth: 'permits sowing, growing and reaping'
• Metal: 'can be moulded and can harden'
• Water: 'moistens downwards'

Box 2.3 The Five Elements as movements
• Wood: expansion
• Fire: upwards
• Earth: centre, point of reference, stability
• Metal: contraction
• Water: downwards

winter and is associated with storage, Earth corresponds to the late season and is associated with transformation.

The position of Earth requires some explanation. Earth does not correspond to any season, as it is the centre, the neutral term of reference around which the seasons and the other elements spin. The 'Classic of Categories' (1624) by Zhang Jie Bin says: *'The Spleen belongs to Earth which pertains to the Centre, its influence manifests for 18 days at the end of each of the four seasons and it does not pertain to any season on its own.'*[16] The 'Discussion of Prescriptions from the Golden Chest' (c.AD 220), by Zhang Zhong Jing, says: *'During the last period of each season, the Spleen is strong enough to resist pathogenic factors.'*[17]

Thus, in the cycle of seasons, the Earth actually corresponds to the late stage of each season. In other words, towards the end of each season, the heavenly energies go back to the Earth for replenishment. Although the Earth element is often associated with 'late summer' or 'Indian summer', it also corresponds to 'late winter', 'late spring' and 'late autumn'.

This could be represented as in Figure 2.2 (see also Box 2.4).

Box 2.4 The Five Elements as seasonal cycles

- Wood: spring
- Fire: summer
- Earth: centre, point of reference, no season
- Metal: autumn
- Water: winter

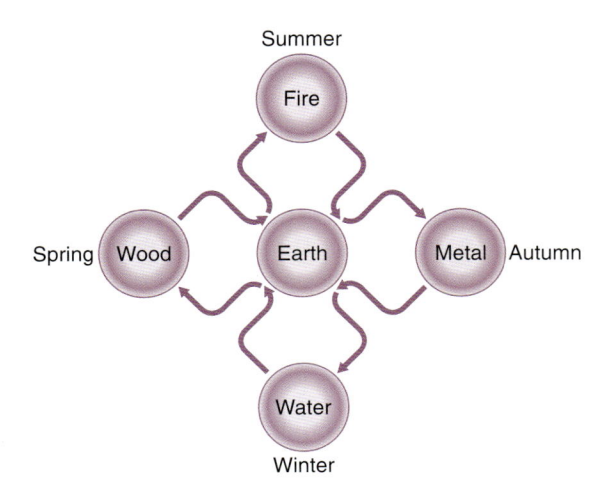

Figure 2.2 The Five-Element seasonal cycle

The Five-Element interrelationships

Essential to the very concept of the Five Elements are the various interactions among them. Different philosophers stressed different relationships among the Five Elements. For example, the main exponent of the Naturalist School, Zou Yan, wrote about only the 'controlling' relationships among the Elements (see below). Thirty-six different arrangements of the Five Elements are mathematically possible. The most common ones are five:

The Cosmological sequence

As was mentioned above, the earliest reference to the Five Elements enumerates them as follows: *'As for the Five Elements, the first is called Water, the second Fire, the third Wood, the fourth Metal and the fifth Earth.'*[18]

The order in which the Elements are enumerated is not a chance one, and is closely related to their numerology. If we assign numbers to each of the Elements in the order in which they are listed, these would be:

1. Water
2. Fire
3. Wood
4. Metal
5. Earth

If we add five to each of these numbers, we get:

6. Water
7. Fire
8. Wood
9. Metal
10. (or 5) Earth

These are the numbers usually associated with the Elements in the list of correspondences (see below). If we arrange the Elements in the above order, they would look like Figure 2.3. In this arrangement Water assumes an important place, as it is the basis, the beginning of the sequence. Bearing in mind the correspondence of the Kidneys to Water, this reflects the important principle of the Kidneys being the foundation of all the other organs.

This sequence also bears out the importance of Earth being the centre, the pivot of reference for all the other Elements. This has important implications in practice which will be discussed shortly.

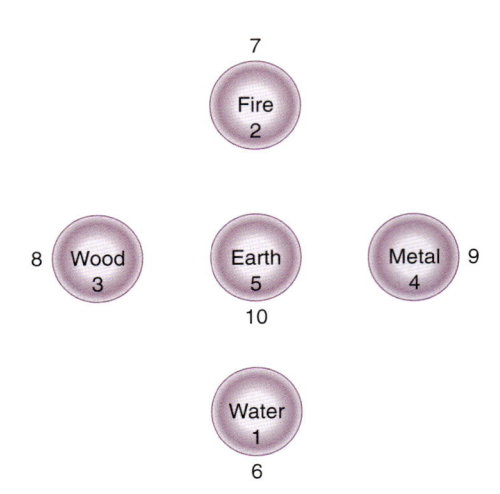

Figure 2.3 The Five-Element numbers

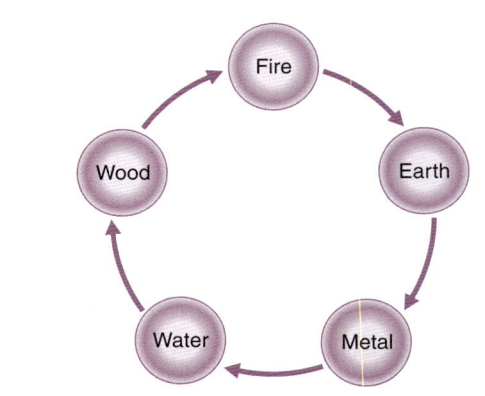

Figure 2.4 The Generating sequence

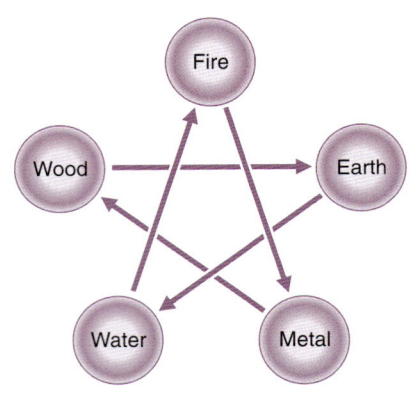

Figure 2.5 The Controlling and Over-acting sequences

The Generating sequence

In this sequence each Element is generated by one and generates another. Thus, Wood generates Fire, Fire generates Earth, Earth generates Metal, Metal generates Water and Water generates Wood; accordingly, Wood, for example, is generated by Water, and it generates Fire, a sequential stage that is sometimes expressed as 'Wood is the Child of Water and the Mother of Fire' (Fig. 2.4).

The Controlling sequence

In this sequence each Element controls another and is controlled by one. Thus, Wood controls Earth, Earth controls Water, Water controls Fire, Fire controls Metal and Metal controls Wood; accordingly, Wood controls Earth, for example, but is controlled by Metal (Fig. 2.5).

The Controlling sequence ensures that a balance is maintained among the Five Elements.

There is also an interrelationship between the Generating and the Controlling sequences. For example, Wood controls Earth, but Earth generates Metal, which controls Wood. Furthermore, on the one hand, Wood controls Earth, but on the other hand, it generates Fire, which, in turn, generates Earth. Thus a self-regulating balance is kept at all times.

The mutual generating and controlling relationships among the Elements is a fine model of the many self-regulating balancing processes to be seen in Nature and in the human body. In Nature, the Five-Element interrelationship and the fine self-regulating balance are clear forerunners of the ideas about ecological balance. Needham cites several interesting examples that clearly illustrate the above principles.[19]

The Over-acting sequence

This follows the same sequence as the Controlling one, but in it, each Element 'over-controls' another, so that it causes it to decrease. This happens when the balance is broken and, under the circumstances, the quantitative relationship among the Elements breaks down, so that, at a particular time, one Element is excessive in relation to another (see Fig. 2.5).

To return to a comparison with natural phenomena, the destructive actions of human beings towards Nature, especially in recent times, provide numerous examples of this sequence.

The Insulting sequence

This sequence is literally called 'insulting' in Chinese. It takes place in the reverse order to the Controlling

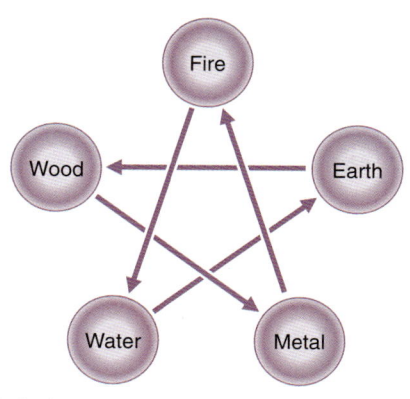

Figure 2.6 The Insulting sequence

sequence. Thus, Wood insults Metal, Metal insults Fire, Fire insults Water, Water insults Earth and Earth insults Wood (Fig. 2.6). This also takes place when the balance is broken.

Thus, the first two sequences deal with the normal balance among the Elements, while the second two (Over-acting and Insulting) deal with the abnormal relationships among the Elements that take place when the balance is broken.

The Five-Element correspondences

The system of correspondences is an important part of the Five-Element theory. This system is typical of the ancient Chinese thought, linking many different phenomena and qualities within the microcosm and macrocosm under the aegis of a certain Element. The ancient Chinese philosophers saw the link among apparently unrelated phenomena as a kind of 'resonance' among them. Various different phenomena would be unified by an indefinable common quality, much as two strings would vibrate in unison.

One of the most typical aspects of Chinese medicine is the common resonance among phenomena in Nature and in the human body. Some of these correspondences are commonly verified and experienced all the time in clinical practice, some may seem far-fetched, but the feeling remains that there is a profound wisdom underlying all of them which is at times unfathomable.

However they were determined, there are many sets of correspondences for each of the Five Elements. The correlation between the Elements and seasons is a very immediate and obvious one, and so is that with the cardinal directions (Fig. 2.7).

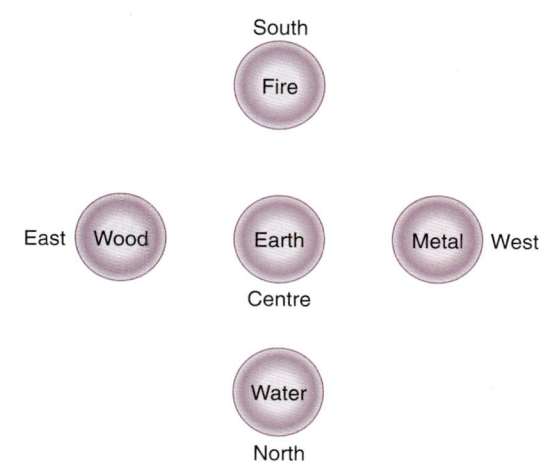

Figure 2.7 The Five Elements and cardinal directions

The main correlations with regard to medicine are found in the 'Simple Questions' chapters 4 and 5.[20]

Some of the main correspondences are as shown in Table 2.1.

These sets of correspondences, especially those related to the human body, show how the organs and their related phenomena form an inseparable and integrated whole. Thus, Wood corresponds to the Liver, eyes, sinews, shouting, green, anger, wheat, spring and birth. All these phenomena are related and all pertain to the Element of Wood. Their application to Chinese medicine will be explained shortly.

Two organs, one Yin, the other Yang, belong to each Element. These are (with the Yin organ listed first):

- Wood: Liver and Gall Bladder
- Fire: Heart and Small Intestine
- Earth: Spleen and Stomach
- Metal: Lungs and Large Intestine
- Water: Kidneys and Bladder

A special mention should be made of the Fire Element. The two organs belonging to Fire are the Heart (Yin) and the Small Intestine (Yang). However, the Fire Element corresponds also to two other organs, namely the Pericardium (Yin) and the Triple Burner (Yang). These two organs together are known as the 'Minister Fire' while the Heart and Small Intestine pertain to the 'Emperor Fire'; this is because the Pericardium and Triple Burner are considered to have the role of serving and protecting the Heart in a way similar to a Prime Minister's (in ancient China) following of the orders of the Emperor. This question will be further discussed in chapters 11 and 18 (Fig. 2.8).

Table 2.1 Some of the main correspondences of the Five Elements

	Wood	Fire	Earth	Metal	Water
Seasons	Spring	Summer	None	Autumn	Winter
Directions	East	South	Centre	West	North
Colours	Green	Red	Yellow	White	Black
Tastes	Sour	Bitter	Sweet	Pungent	Salty
Climates	Wind	Heat	Dampness	Dryness	Cold
Stage of development	Birth	Growth	Transformation	Harvest	Storage
Numbers	8	7	5	9	6
Planets	Jupiter	Mars	Saturn	Venus	Mercury
Yin–Yang	Lesser Yang	Utmost Yang	Centre	Lesser Yin	Utmost Yin
Animals	Fish	Birds	Human	Mammals	Shell-covered
Domestic animals	Sheep	Fowl	Ox	Dog	Pig
Grains	Wheat	Beans	Rice	Hemp	Millet
Yin organs	Liver	Heart	Spleen	Lungs	Kidneys
Yang organs	Gall Bladder	Small Intestine	Stomach	Large Intestine	Bladder
Sense organs	Eyes	Tongue	Mouth	Nose	Ears
Tissues	Sinews	Vessels	Muscles	Skin	Bones
Emotions	Anger	Joy	Pensiveness	Sadness	Fear
Sounds	Shouting	Laughing	Singing	Crying	Groaning

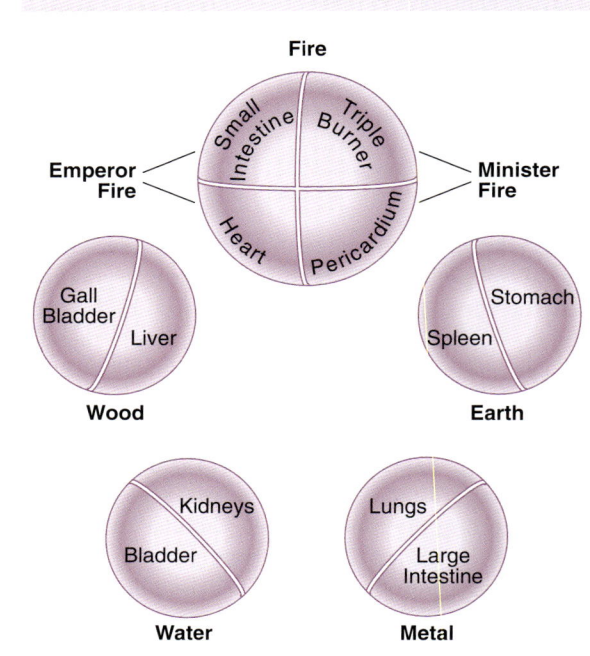

Figure 2.8 The Internal Organs and the Five Elements

THE FIVE ELEMENTS IN CHINESE MEDICINE

The applications of the theory of the Five Elements to Chinese medicine are numerous and very important. We shall explore them in five different areas:

- Physiology
- Pathology
- Diagnosis
- Treatment
- Dietary and herbal therapy

The Five Elements in physiology

The relationships among the Five Elements are like a model of relationships among the internal organs and between them and the various tissues, sense organs, colours, smells, tastes and sounds.

The Generating and Controlling sequences

These provide the basic model of physiological relationships among the internal organs. Just as 'Wood generates Fire and is generated by Water', so we can say that the 'Liver is the mother of the Heart and the child of the Kidneys'. The Generating sequence among the organs is shown in Figure 2.9.

On the other hand, each organ is kept in check by another so that a proper balance among them is kept: this is the Controlling sequence (Fig. 2.10). It is as follows:

- The Liver controls the Spleen
- The Heart controls the Lungs
- The Spleen controls the Kidneys
- The Lungs control the Liver
- The Kidneys control the Heart

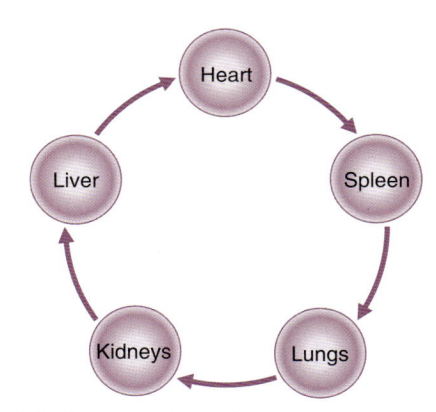

Figure 2.9 The Organ-Generating sequence

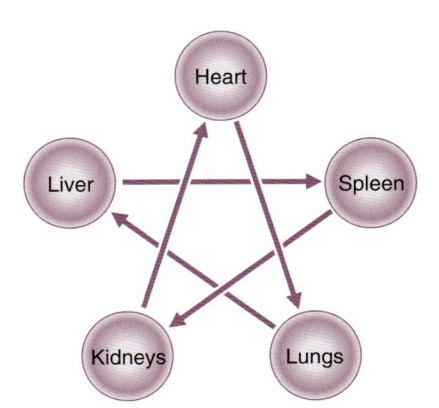

Figure 2.10 The Organ-Controlling and Over-acting sequences

It is very important to remember in practice that the above sequences among the organs are only a Five-Element model of relationships and that, as such, it may suffer from inconsistencies, deficiencies and arbitrariness. Although this model can be extremely useful in clinical practice, one should not lose sight of the actual organ functions and how these interact with each other. In other words, we should not make the mistake of using the Five-Element model in practice in isolation from the actual organ functions which the model itself is trying to represent. There is the danger that one might use the symbols themselves (the Five Elements), and not what they symbolize (the interaction of the internal organs' functions). When properly used, however, the symbols can provide a quick and effective model to refer to in clinical practice and a guideline for diagnosis and treatment.

One could explain all the Five-Element relationships among the organs in terms of organ functions. The organ functions will be discussed in depth in chapters 5 to 18, but it is worth mentioning them at this stage to illustrate how the Five-Element interactions are a model of internal organs' functional relationships. It must be stressed, however, that not all the Five-Element relationships are equally meaningful as a model of organ–function interactions. For example, the generating relationship between Kidneys and Liver has deep implications in practice, that between Heart and Spleen less so.

Furthermore, one should not lose sight of the fact that the Generating and Controlling sequences are only two of the possible models of relationships among the Five Elements. Besides these two, I will discuss a third sequence, the Cosmological sequence, the relationships of which are different from those in the Generating sequence. For example, in the Generating sequence the Heart is the mother of the Spleen, but this relationship has few meaningful applications in practice. In the Cosmological sequence, on the other hand, the Spleen is a supporting organ for the Heart, and this has far more applications in practice as, for instance, the Spleen produces Blood which houses the Mind (*Shen*).

Let us look at some examples of Generating sequence relationships (Fig. 2.11).

The Liver is the mother of the Heart: the Liver stores Blood and Blood houses the Mind. If Liver-Blood is weak, the Heart will suffer; Liver-Blood deficiency often induces Heart-Blood deficiency and they both affect sleep and dreaming.

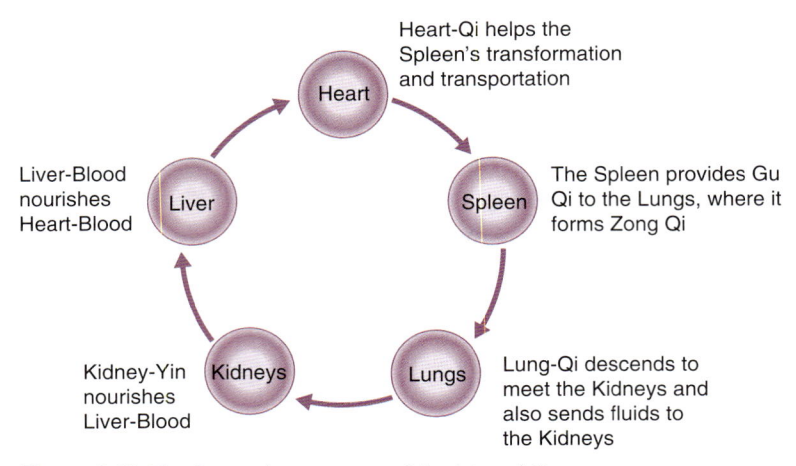

Figure 2.11 The Generating sequence of the Internal Organs

- Heart-Qi helps the Spleen's transformation and transportation
- The Spleen provides Gu Qi to the Lungs, where it forms Zong Qi
- Lung-Qi descends to meet the Kidneys and also sends fluids to the Kidneys
- Kidney-Yin nourishes Liver-Blood
- Liver-Blood nourishes Heart-Blood

The Heart is the mother of the Spleen: Heart-Qi pushes the Blood and thus helps the Spleen function of transportation.

The Spleen is the mother of the Lungs: the Spleen provides Food-Qi to the Lungs, where it interacts with air to form the Gathering Qi. A deficiency of both Spleen- and Lung-Qi is common.

The Lungs are the mother of the Kidneys: Lung-Qi descends to meet Kidney-Qi. The Lungs also send fluids down to the Kidneys.

The Kidneys are the mother of the Liver: Kidney-Yin nourishes Liver-Blood. The Kidneys control the bones and the Liver the sinews: bones and sinews are inseparable.

As for the Controlling sequence, 'controlling' must not be taken literally, as the organs actually support rather than suppress each other's functions along the Controlling sequence. In fact, it will be seen that each organ actually helps the function of the organ it is supposed to 'control'. The following will be a few examples:

The Liver controls the Stomach and Spleen: the Liver, with its free flow of Qi, actually helps the Stomach to rot and ripen food and the Spleen to transform and transport. It is only when the controlling function gets out of hand (in which case it is called 'over-acting') that the Liver can actually interfere with and impair the Stomach and Spleen functions.

The Heart controls the Lungs: Heart and Lungs are closely related as they are both situated in the Upper Burner. The Heart governs Blood and Lungs govern Qi: Qi and Blood mutually assist and nourish each other.

The Spleen controls the Kidneys: both Spleen and Kidneys transform Body Fluids. The Spleen activity in transforming and transporting fluids is essential to the Kidney transformation and excretion of fluids.

The Lungs control the Liver: in this case, unlike the others, there is a certain element of 'control' of the Liver by the Lungs. The Lungs send Qi downwards, whereas the Liver spreads Qi upwards. If Lung-Qi is weak and cannot descend, Liver-Qi may tend to rise too much. This often happens in practice, when a deficiency of the Lungs leads to rising of Liver-Yang or stagnation of Liver-Qi.

The Kidneys control the Heart: Kidneys and Heart actually assist and support each other. A proper communication and interaction between Kidneys and Heart is essential for health. This relationship will be discussed at length shortly, when dealing with the Cosmological sequence.

The Cosmological sequence

This sequence is often overlooked: yet it is very important and meaningful in clinical practice, and in the philosophy of the Five Elements in general.

As was mentioned above, the very first reference to the Five Elements lists them in this order: Water, Fire, Wood, Metal and Earth (see note 12). An assigning of numbers to them would give 1 for Water, 2 for Fire, 3 for Wood, 4 for Metal and 5 for Earth. Adding five to each of these, we would get 6 for Water, 7 for Fire, 8 for Wood, 9 for Metal and 10 (or 5) for Earth. The number to be added is five because five was associated with earthly phenomena in Chinese philosophy whilst

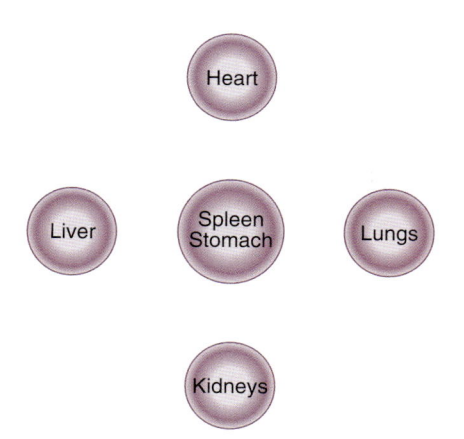

Figure 2.12 The Organ Cosmological sequence

Box 2.5 Five-Element Cosmological sequence

- Water as the foundation
- Axis Kidneys–Heart
- Stomach and Spleen as the centre
- Stomach and Spleen as support for the Heart
- Earth as centre in cycle of seasons
- Axis Essence–Qi–Mind (*Jing–Qi–Shen*)

---

six was associated with heavenly phenomena, and since the Five-Element cosmology describes earthly phenomena, the number five is used. The climates, on the contrary, are heavenly phenomena, and they are classified in six.

The Cosmological sequence can be represented as shown in Figure 2.12 (see also Box 2.5).

This arrangement is significant in clinical practice in many ways:

Water as the foundation

In this sequence, Water is the beginning, the foundation of the other Elements. This corresponds well to the importance of the Kidneys as the foundation of Yin and Yang, the basis for the Yin and Yang of all the other organs. They pertain to Water and store Essence (*Jing*), but also store the Fire of the Gate of Life (*Ming Men*). They are therefore the source of Water and Fire, also called the Original Yin and the Original Yang. From this point of view, Water can be considered the foundation of all the other Elements.

This principle is constantly applied in clinical practice as Kidney-Yin deficiency easily induces a deficiency of Liver-Yin and Heart-Yin, and Kidney-Yang deficiency easily induces a deficiency of Spleen-Yang and Lung-Qi.

Also, the Kidneys store the Essence, which is the material foundation of Qi and Mind.

The relationship between Kidneys and Heart

Kidneys and Heart are related along the vertical axis. There is a direct communication between them, not an indirect one through Wood. This fundamental relationship between Water and Fire is probably the most important and basic balance of the body, as it reflects the basic balance between Yin and Yang.

The Kidneys govern Water and this has to flow upwards to nourish the Heart. The Heart governs Fire and this has to flow downwards to the Kidneys. Thus, far from being a relationship of control or over-action, the relationship between Kidneys and Heart is one of mutual nourishment and assistance.

This relationship also reflects that between Essence and Mind. The Essence is the material basis for the Mind: if Essence is weak, the Mind will necessarily suffer.

If Kidney-Yin is deficient, not enough Yin energy goes through to the Heart: Heart-Yin then becomes deficient and Empty-Heat rises within the Heart. This is a very common situation in clinical practice, particularly in women during the menopause.

The Stomach and Spleen as the centre

From the Cosmological sequence the central role of Stomach and Spleen as a neutral pivot is very apparent. This is also fundamental in clinical practice. The Stomach and Spleen are the Root of the Post-Heaven Qi and the origin of Qi and Blood: they therefore nourish all the other organs and naturally occupy a central place in human physiology. Thus the Cosmological sequence accurately reflects the importance of the Pre-Heaven Qi (in so far as Water is the foundation), and of the Post-Heaven Qi (in so far as Earth is the centre). The arrangement of the Elements in a circle along the Generating cycle does not highlight these two important concepts.

For this reason the tonifying of Stomach and Spleen indirectly tonifies all the other organs. The idea of the Stomach and Spleen being the centre, and therefore the source of tonification of all the other organs, appears throughout the classics, but the most famous and complete exponent of this idea was Li Dong Yuan, who wrote the 'Discussion on Stomach and Spleen' (*Pi Wei Lun*) in 1249.

The Stomach and Spleen as support for the Heart

If we examine the Cosmological sequence diagram, we can see how the Earth is in between Water and Fire and is the support of Fire. Thus Stomach and Spleen are, in practice, the main support for the Heart. In all cases of chronic Heart-Qi or Heart-Blood deficiency, and particularly when the rhythm of the heart is irregular, it is essential to tonify the Stomach. The Spleen also produces Blood on which the Heart depends and which houses the Mind.

The role of Earth in the cycle of seasons

When the Earth is placed in the centre, its role in relation to seasons is apparent. The Earth actually belongs to no season as it is the neutral pivot along which the seasonal cycle unfolds. On the other hand, the Earth does perform the role of replenishment at the end of each season (see Fig. 2.2).

Thus at the end of each season, the energy goes back to the Earth for regeneration. In the human body, this reaffirms the importance of the Stomach and Spleen as the centre. Thus, the Stomach and Spleen might be tonified at the end of each season, particularly at the end of Winter, to regenerate the energy.

The vertical axis as symbol of Essence–Qi–Mind (Jing–Qi–Shen)

The very important vertical axis of Water, Earth and Fire can be seen as a symbol of Essence–Qi–Mind, which is the complex of physical and mental energies in human beings. The Essence belongs to the Kidneys, Qi is derived from Stomach and Spleen and the Mind is housed in the Heart.

The system of correspondences in Five-Element physiology

The system of Five-Element correspondences has wide applications in human physiology. According to this scheme, each Element encompasses numerous phenomena in the universe and the human body which are somehow 'attributed' to that particular Element. Or it could be said that these phenomena 'resonate' at a particular frequency and have particular qualities that respond to a certain Element.

As far as the internal organs are concerned, this theory has points of contact with the theory of the Internal Organs (see ch. 5), in so far as each organ is seen as a sphere of influence which encompasses many functions and phenomena beyond the organ itself. There are, however, some differences between the theory of Five-Element correspondences and that of the Internal Organs. First of all, the theory of Five-Element correspondences encompasses phenomena outside the human body, such as the five planets, the five grains and the five musical notes. Secondly, and most importantly, there are important discrepancies (or differences) between the two theories. For example, the Heart pertains to Fire from the Five-Element point of view, but from the Internal-Organ theory point of view, the Kidneys are the source of physiological Fire in the body. Such discrepancies will be discussed in greater detail shortly. It will be seen that the two concepts are not mutually incompatible.

The system of Five-Element correspondences does, nevertheless, provide a comprehensive and clinically useful model of relationships between the organs and various tissues, sense organs, etc., and also between the organs and various external phenomena such as climates and seasons.

As a way of illustration, we can explore the system of correspondences related to Wood and how they apply in clinical practice.

Season: the season corresponding to Wood is spring. In practice, it is very common for a Liver imbalance to be aggravated in springtime. This is probably because the Liver energy flows upwards and is very active: in springtime, Yang rises and the growing energy is bursting forward and can thus aggravate a Liver imbalance and cause Liver-Qi to rise excessively.

Direction: east winds easily affect the Liver. In practice, some patients suffering from chronic headaches or neck ache sometimes will remark that they get a headache whenever an east wind blows.

Colour: the face colour in Liver imbalances will often be greenish. This is applied in diagnosis.

Taste: a small amount of sour taste in the diet is beneficial to the Liver; and an excess of it is detrimental. Also, an excess of sour taste can damage the Spleen (Over-acting) and be beneficial to the Lungs. This will be discussed in greater detail when dealing with the application of Five-Element theory to diet and herbal therapy.

Climate: wind very clearly affects those who suffer from an imbalance in the Liver, often causing headaches and stiffness in the neck.

Sense organ: the Liver moistens and nourishes the eyes.

Tissue: the Liver also moistens and nourishes sinews.

Emotion: anger is the emotion that is connected to Wood and the Liver. Someone whose Liver energy stagnates or rebels upwards, may be prone to fits of anger.

Sound: related to the above, a person who suffers from a Liver disharmony will be prone to shouting (in anger).

The correspondences for the other Elements apply in the same way. However, it is important to realize that the system of Five-Element correspondences is only one of the theoretical models available, and by no means the only one. Chinese medicine developed over thousands of years and, naturally, different theories arose at different times in its history. Thus, the model presented by the Five-Element system of correspondences may contradict, or complement, that available from other points of view, in exactly the same way that the Generating and Controlling sequences do not represent the only possible relationships among the Five Elements.

Let us look at a few examples of discrepancies or differences between the Five-Element model and other theories of Chinese medicine.

The Heart belongs to Emperor Fire: in Five-Element theory, the Heart belongs to the so-called Emperor Fire and is the most important of all organs, sometimes called the Monarch. But from the point of view of Internal-Organ physiology, one could say that the Kidneys are the 'Emperor' because they are the origin of the Fire of the Gate of Life (*Ming Men*), the source of the Original Yin and the Original Yang and the storehouse of the Essence (*Jing*).

Of course, the Heart does occupy a prominent place among the Internal Organs in so far as it is the organ that houses the Mind (*Shen*): it is really in this sense that the Heart is the 'Emperor'.

Fire pertains to the Heart: this may be true from the Five-Element point of view, but, again, from another point of view, the physiological Fire originates from the Kidney (Yang), and it is the Gate of Life that actually provides Fire to the Heart. This theory started from chapters 36 and 39 of the 'Classic of Difficulties'[21] and later was taken up by many doctors, the most notable of them being Zhao Xian He of the Ming dynasty.

The eyes pertain to Wood (and Liver): although it is true and important in practice that the Liver moistens and nourishes the eyes, it is not the only organ that affects the eyes, and not every eye problem is related to the Liver. For example, Kidney-Yin also moistens the eyes and many chronic eye problems are related to the Kidneys. The Heart also reaches the eye via its Connecting channel. Some acute eye problems such as acute conjunctivitis are often related to no organ but simply due to exterior Wind-Heat. Many other channels are related to the eyes, such as the Lungs, Small Intestine, Gall Bladder and Triple Burner.

The tongue is related to Fire (Heart): this is true, but all the other organs are reflected on the tongue, and this forms the basis of tongue diagnosis.

The ears are related to Water (Kidneys): again, it is true that the Kidney-Essence nourishes the ears, but not every ear problem derives from the Kidneys. For example, acute ear problems, such as acute otitis media, may be due to invasion of exterior Wind-Heat affecting the Gall Bladder channel.

The above are only a few examples of the limitations of the Five-Element model of correspondences. The basic limitation lies in the fact that the Five-Element model of correspondences became a rigid model of relationships between individual parts, and, in the process of fitting everything into a five-fold classification, many assumptions and far-fetched correlations had to be made.

More importantly, the Five-Element model of correspondences sees one-to-one correlations between phenomena; for example, Liver–eyes, Kidney–ears and Spleen–muscles. This may be useful in clinical practice, but the essence of Chinese medicine is to see the whole disharmony and trace the pattern woven by various signs and symptoms. In this way, a one-to-one correlation is no longer valid, as one part could be related to a certain organ in the presence of a certain pattern, but to another organ in the presence of a different pattern. For example, if a woman suffers from blurred vision and, in addition, also has poor memory, scanty periods, numbness and dizziness, we can say that Liver-Blood is not nourishing the eyes: this therefore confirms the relationship between Liver and eye within the Five-Element theory. But if the same woman suffers from dry eyes and glaucoma and, in addition, has lower backache, vertigo, tinnitus and night sweating, we would say that Kidney-Yin is not moistening the eyes: this would therefore be outside the Five-Element model of correspondences.

The Five Elements in pathology

The Five-Element model provides an important and clinically useful pattern of pathological relationships among the internal organs.

In the Five-Element relationships, only two of the possible sequences apply to pathological cases: these are the Over-acting and Insulting sequences. The Generating sequence can also give rise to pathological conditions when it is out of balance.

The essence of the Five-Element relationships is balance: the Generating and Controlling sequences keep a dynamic balance among the Elements. When this balance is upset for a prolonged period of time, disease ensues.

The Over-acting sequence

This occurs when the controlling relationship among the Elements gets out of control and becomes excessive. Similar to the physiological relationships, the Over-acting sequence relationships can be explained in terms of Internal-Organ pathology (Fig. 2.13).

The Liver over-acts on the Stomach and Spleen: if Liver-Qi stagnates, it 'invades' both the Stomach, impairing its function of rotting and ripening, and the Spleen, impairing its function of transforming and transporting. In particular, when Liver-Qi invades the Stomach, it prevents Stomach-Qi from descending, which causes nausea, and it prevents Spleen-Qi from ascending, which causes diarrhoea.

The Heart over-acts on the Lungs: Heart-Fire can dry up the Lung fluids and cause Lung-Yin deficiency.

The Spleen over-acts on the Kidneys: when the Spleen holds Dampness, this can obstruct the Kidney function of transformation and excretion of fluids.

The Lungs over-act on the Liver: if Lung-Qi fails to descend it may impair the physiological rise of Liver-Qi. Also Lung-Heat or Phlegm-Heat may be transmitted to the Liver.

The Kidneys over-act on the Heart: if the Kidneys' fluids accumulate pathologically, they impair the function of the Heart (a pattern called 'Water Overflowing to the Heart').

The insulting sequence

These relationships along the Insulting sequence also occur in pathological conditions (Fig. 2.14).

The Liver insults the Lungs: Liver-Qi can stagnate upwards and obstruct the chest and breathing. Liver-Fire may also obstruct the descending of Lung-Qi and cause asthma.

The Heart insults the Kidneys: Heart-Fire can infuse downwards to the Kidneys and cause Kidney-Yin deficiency.

The Spleen insults the Liver: if the Spleen retains Dampness, this can overflow and impair the free flow of Liver-Qi.

The Lungs insult the Heart: if the Lungs are obstructed by Phlegm, they can impair the circulation of Heart-Qi.

The Kidneys insult the Spleen: if the Kidneys fail to transform fluids, the Spleen will suffer and become obstructed by Dampness.

The Generating sequence

The Generating sequence can also give rise to pathological states when out of balance. There are two possibilities:

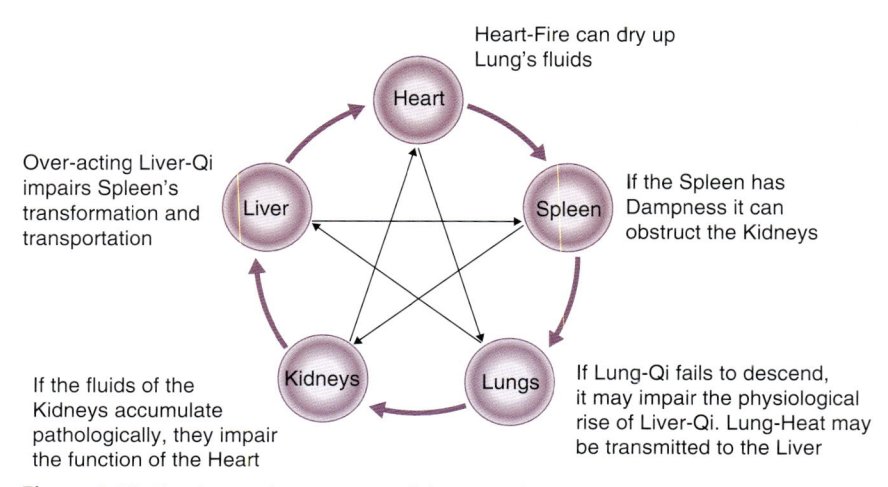

Figure 2.13 The Over-acting sequence of the Internal Organs

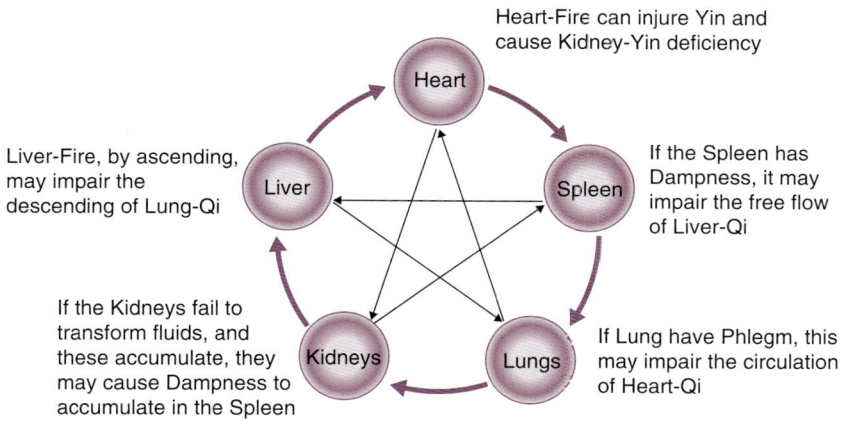

Figure 2.14 The Insulting sequence of the Internal Organs

- Heart-Fire can injure Yin and cause Kidney-Yin deficiency
- If the Spleen has Dampness, it may impair the free flow of Liver-Qi
- If Lung have Phlegm, this may impair the circulation of Heart-Qi
- If the Kidneys fail to transform fluids, and these accumulate, they may cause Dampness to accumulate in the Spleen
- Liver-Fire, by ascending, may impair the descending of Lung-Qi

1. The Mother-Element is not nourishing the Child-Element
2. The Child-Element is taking too much from the Mother-Element

The Liver (Mother) affecting the Heart (Child): this happens when the Liver fails to nourish the Heart. Specifically, when Liver-Blood is deficient, it often affects Heart-Blood, which becomes deficient, and palpitations and insomnia ensue. Another particular way in which Wood affects Fire is in the effect of the Gall Bladder on the Heart. This happens on a psychological level. The Gall Bladder controls the capacity of making decisions, not so much in the sense of being able to distinguish and evaluate what is right and what is wrong, but in the sense of having the courage to act on a decision. Thus, it is said in Chinese medicine that a strong Gall Bladder makes one courageous.

This psychological trait of the Gall Bladder influences the Heart, as the Mind (housed in the Heart) needs the support of decisiveness and courage given by a strong Gall Bladder. In this way, a deficient Gall Bladder can affect the Mind (of the Heart) causing emotional weakness, timidity and lack of assertion.

The Heart (Child) affecting the Liver (Mother): if Heart-Blood is deficient, it can lead to general deficiency of Blood, which will affect the Liver storage of Blood. This causes scanty periods or amenorrhoea.

The Heart (Mother) affecting the Spleen (Child): the Mind of the Heart needs to support the mental faculties and capacity of concentration which belong to the Spleen. Another aspect of this relationship is in Heart-Fire deficient being unable to warm Spleen-Yang and leading to cold feeling and diarrhoea. Ultimately, however, the physiological Fire of the Heart is itself derived from Kidney-Yang.

The Spleen (Child) affecting the Heart (Mother): the Spleen makes Qi and Blood and the Heart needs a strong supply of Blood. If the Spleen does not make enough Blood, the Heart will suffer and palpitations, insomnia, poor memory and slight depression will ensue.

The Spleen (Mother) affecting the Lungs (Child): if the Spleen's function of transformation and transportation of fluids is impaired, Phlegm will be formed. Phlegm often settles in the Lungs and causes breathlessness and asthma.

The Lungs (Child) affecting the Spleen (Mother): the Lungs govern Qi and if Lung-Qi is deficient, Spleen-Qi will be affected, causing tiredness, no appetite and loose stools. In practice, Spleen-Qi and Lung-Qi deficiency often occur together.

The Lungs (Mother) affecting the Kidneys (Child): Lung-Qi normally descends towards the Kidneys which 'hold' it down. Also, the Lungs send fluids down to the Kidneys. Thus, if Lung-Qi is deficient, Qi and fluids cannot descend to the Kidneys, causing breathlessness (Kidney unable to receive Qi) and dryness of the Kidneys.

The Kidneys (Child) affecting the Lungs (Mother): if Kidney-Qi is deficient it will fail to hold Qi down, Qi will rebel upwards and obstruct the Lungs, causing breathlessness.

The Kidneys (Mother) affecting the Liver (Child): Kidney-Yin nourishes Liver-Yin and Liver-Blood. If Kidney-Yin is deficient, Liver-Yin and/or Liver-Blood will become deficient and give rise to tinnitus, dizziness, headaches and irritability. This particular relationship is one of the most important and common in clinical practice.

The Liver (Child) affecting the Kidneys (Mother): Liver-Blood nourishes and replenishes the Kidney-Essence. If Liver-Blood is deficient over a long period of time, it can contribute to deficiency of Kidney-Essence, causing dizziness, tinnitus, poor bone development and sexual weakness.

In conclusion, each Element can be out of balance in four ways (Fig. 2.15):

1. It is in excess and over-acts on another along the over-acting sequence
2. It is in excess and 'draws' excessively from its Mother Element
3. It is deficient and fails to nourish its Child
4. It is deficient and is insulted by another along the insulting sequence

The Five Elements in diagnosis

The Five-Element model of correspondences is extensively used in diagnosis. This is based mostly on the correspondence between Elements and smell, colour, taste and sound. The 'Classic of Difficulties' in chapter 61 says: '*By observation one can distinguish the five colours, thus identifying the disease; by hearing one can distinguish the five sounds, thus identifying the disease; by interrogation one can distinguish the five tastes, thus identifying the disease.*'[22]

The aspects of diagnosis related to the Five Elements discussed are:

- Colours
- Sounds
- Smells
- Emotions
- Tastes
- Tissues
- Sense orifices
- Climates

Colours

Observation of the colours is the most important of all in the Five-Element scheme of diagnosis. The colour of the face is mostly observed and the prevalence of one of the five colours indicates an imbalance in that particular Element, which could be either Deficiency or an Excess.

Thus, a green colour of the face indicates an imbalance in Wood, which could be due to stagnation of Liver-Qi.

A red colour indicates an imbalance in Fire, which could be due to an excess of Heart-Fire.

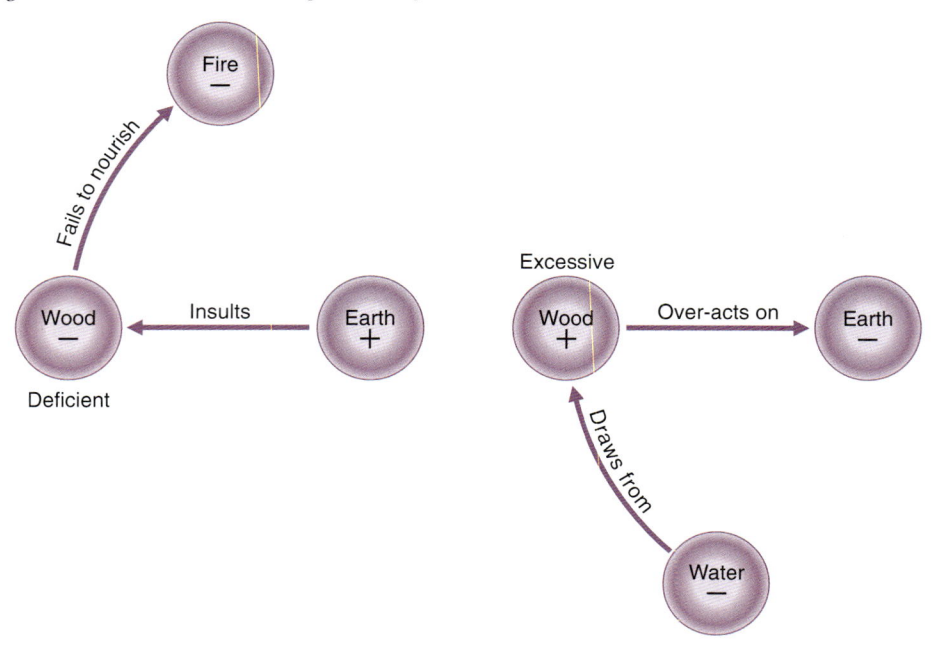

Figure 2.15 Pathology of Generating, Over-acting and Insulting sequences

A yellow, sallow complexion indicates an imbalance in Earth, which could be due to deficiency of Spleen-Qi.

A white colour indicates an imbalance in Metal, which could be due to deficiency of Lung-Qi.

A dark, purplish colour, sometimes greyish, sometimes nearly black, indicates an imbalance in Water, which could be due to Kidney-Yin deficiency.

Sometimes the complexion can show complex interactions between two Elements. For instance, a person may have a very pallid, whitish face with red cheek-bones: this indicates Fire (red cheek-bones) over-acting on Metal (pale-white face). Or one might have a yellow complexion with a greenish tinge around the mouth: this would indicate Wood (green around mouth) over-acting on Earth (yellow complexion).

The face colour does not always accord with the clinical manifestations: in some situations, it may contradict the pattern that they present. In these cases, the face colour usually shows the underlying cause of the imbalance. For example, if a person displays symptoms of Earth deficiency (tiredness, loose stools, no appetite, etc.) and has a greenish colour in the face, it may indicate that the Spleen is weak because the Liver is over-acting on it. Conversely, someone may display symptoms of Wood imbalance (such as gallstones, for instance) and have a yellow complexion. This may indicate that Earth is insulting Wood. If a person has symptoms of Fire imbalance (such as palpitations, a bitter taste, mouth ulcers, and insomnia, indicating Heart-Fire) and the complexion is dark, it may indicate that Water is over-acting on Fire. In the above cases then, the face colour shows the seat of the root imbalance and the clinical manifestations show the resulting pattern.

However, the Five-Element colour correspondences in diagnosis have to be used critically, and they should not be applied mechanically. In interpreting and making deductions from the face colour, one must be very careful to take into account not only the Five-Element theory but also other aspects of Chinese medicine. For example, a yellow complexion indicates an Earth problem from the Five-Element point of view, but it may also indicate retention of Dampness. A dark-blackish complexion indicates a Water problem according to the Five Elements, but it may also indicate stasis of Blood. A white complexion indicates a Metal imbalance from the Five-Element point of view, but it also indicates a Cold condition (which could be of any organ) judged according to the Eight Principles.

According to the Five Elements a green complexion indicates a Wood imbalance, but it also may indicate stasis of Blood or chronic pain. The Five-Element theory tells us that a red complexion indicates a Fire imbalance, but according to the Eight Principles, it may also indicate Heat, which could be in any organ. Diagnosis by observation of the complexion colours is discussed in chapter 23.

As was pointed out before, in Chinese diagnosis it is not always possible to make a direct correlation between two phenomena on a one-to-one basis. What counts is the place of each phenomenon in the whole pattern. For example, if someone has a red face, a bitter taste, insomnia, mouth ulcers and palpitations, this does indicate a problem in the Fire (Heart); but a red face with rapid breathing, yellow mucus and a cough indicates a problem in the Lungs, and a red face with irritability, a bitter taste, headaches and dizziness indicates a problem in the Liver (Box 2.6).

Sounds

The sound and tone of the voice can also be used in diagnosis. If someone tends to shout a lot in anger, it indicates an imbalance in the Wood element. If someone laughs a lot without apparent reason (as sometimes happens when a patient punctuates the interrogation with frequent laughs), it indicates an imbalance in the Fire element.

A singing tone of voice indicates an imbalance in the Earth element. Crying is related to Metal and it often indicates a deficiency of the Lungs (whose emotion is grief). A very thin and weak, often 'weepy' voice also indicates weakness of Lung-Qi. A groaning or husky tone of voice indicates an imbalance in Water (Box 2.7).

Box 2.6 Five-Element colours

- Wood: green
- Fire: red
- Earth: yellow
- Metal: white
- Water: black

Box 2.7 Five-Element sounds

- Wood: shouting
- Fire: laughing
- Earth: singing
- Metal: weeping
- Water: groaning

> **Box 2.8 Five-Element smells**
> - Wood: rancid
> - Fire: scorched
> - Earth: fragrant
> - Metal: rotten
> - Water: putrid

> **Box 2.9 Five-Element emotions**
> - Wood: anger
> - Fire: joy
> - Earth: pensiveness
> - Metal: worry–sorrow–sadness
> - Water: fear

Smells

Smells are also used in diagnosis according to the Five-Element model of correspondences. A rancid smell indicates an imbalance in Wood, often due to stagnation of Heat in the Liver. A burned smell indicates an imbalance in Fire, usually Heart-Fire.

A fragrant, sweetish smell is often associated with Spleen deficiency or Dampness. A rank or rotten smell is often indicative of a Metal imbalance, usually due to chronic retention of Phlegm in the Lungs. A putrid smell is indicative of a Kidney or Bladder imbalance, usually due to retention of Damp-Heat.

Much as colours can be interpreted in other ways than those indicated by the Five-Element model, smells too sometimes do not correspond to this rather rigid system.

For example, a rotten or putrid smell is indicative of Heat of any organ. Also, other types of smells are sometimes described, such as 'leathery', being indicative of Damp-Heat, and 'fishy', being indicative of Damp-Cold (Box 2.8).

Emotions

The relationship between emotions and Elements is important in diagnosis. A person who is prone to outbursts of anger would manifest an imbalance in Wood (usually due to rising of Liver-Yang). The emotion may also be more subdued and less apparent when the anger is repressed.

Joy is the emotion related to Fire and the Heart. Obviously a state of joy is not a harmful emotion. What is meant by 'joy' here, however, is rather a state of excessive or constant excitement which may be typical of some people in our society. An example of the negative effect of excess joy is the migraine attack that can sometimes be triggered not only by bad news but also by sudden good news.

Pensiveness or over-concentration is the 'emotion' related to Earth. Admittedly this is not an 'emotion' in the way we conceive it, but it is nevertheless the mental activity related to the Spleen.[23]

An excessive use of our thinking faculties and over-studying may lead to deficiency of the Spleen.

Grief and sorrow are the emotions related to Metal, and, in practice, there is a direct and common relationship between these emotions and the state of the Lungs. Lung-Qi is very much affected by grief or sadness (and also worry), and these emotions will cause a deficiency of Lung-Qi.

Fear is related to Water and, again, this emotion directly influences the Kidneys and Bladder. A deficiency of the Kidneys often causes anxiety and fears (Box 2.9).

Tastes

The tastes related to the Five Elements are a relatively minor aspect of Chinese diagnosis. They are as follows: sour for Wood, bitter for Fire, sweet for Earth, pungent for Metal and salty for Water.

A sour taste often accompanies Liver disharmonies, a bitter taste is part of the pattern of Heart-Fire, a sweet taste is often indicative of Spleen deficiency, a pungent taste sometimes accompanies Lung disharmonies and a salty taste occasionally is associated with Kidney deficiency.

The taste correspondences also suffer from certain limitations, in the same way as for the colours. For example, a sour taste is more frequently present in Stomach disharmonies, a bitter taste is also more frequently indicative of Liver disharmonies such as Liver-Fire and a sweet taste can also indicate retention of Dampness.

Beside this, there are also other types of taste often described by patients that do not fit into this scheme. For example, a 'flat' taste indicates Spleen deficiency and a 'sticky' taste indicates retention of Dampness. English-speaking patients often report a 'metallic' taste: it would be wrong, in my opinion, to attribute this automatically to the Metal Element as I think it corresponds to what the Chinese call a 'sticky' taste (Box 2.10).

> **Box 2.10 Five-Element tastes**
> - Wood: sour
> - Fire: bitter
> - Earth: sweet
> - Metal: pungent
> - Water: salty

> **Box 2.11 Five-Element tissues**
> - Wood: sinews
> - Fire: blood vessels
> - Earth: muscles
> - Metal: skin
> - Water: bones

Tissues

A pathological state of the tissues can be used in diagnosis as a pointer to disharmony of the relevant Elements. For example, if the tendons are tight and stiff, this indicates a Liver and Gall Bladder or Wood disharmony. A problem with blood vessels points to a Heart or Fire imbalance. A weakness or atrophy of the muscles indicates Spleen or Earth deficiency. The skin is related to Metal and the Lungs, and a Lung weakness is often manifested with spontaneous sweating (the pores being open).

The Kidneys are related to the bones, and bone degenerative diseases which occur in old age, such as osteoporosis, are often due to the decline of Kidney-Essence (Box 2.11).

Sense orifices

Problems with the five senses can also reflect disharmonies in the relevant Elements. For example, blurred vision often reflects Liver deficiency, a problem with the tongue (such as ulcers) can be related to the Heart, problems with the mouth and lips (such as dryness) are often due to Spleen deficiency or Stomach Heat, a problem with dry nostrils or frequent sneezing reflects Lung dryness or deficiency, and a decrease in hearing or chronic tinnitus can be due to Kidney deficiency.

> **Clinical note**
>
> The Back-Transporting points (Back-Shu points) of the Yin organs are used to affect the relevant senses:
> BL-18 Ganshu: sight
> BL-15 Xinshu: tongue
> BL-20 Pishu: taste
> BL-13 Feishu: smell
> Bl-23 Shenshu: hearing

Again, this model of relationships is only partly applicable. For example, there are many eye disorders not related to Wood (as explained above), some tongue pathologies can also be due to Stomach or Kidneys, the lips also manifest the state of Blood, mouth problems can also be due to a Kidney pathology and many ear problems are not due to a Kidney deficiency but to imbalances in other Elements, for example, the Wood Element (Box 2.12).

> **Box 2.12 Five-Element sense organs**
> - Wood: eyes
> - Fire: tongue
> - Earth: mouth and lips
> - Metal: nose
> - Water: ears

Climates

A person's sensitivity to a particular climatic condition often reflects a disharmony in the relevant Element. Thus, a sensitivity to wind often reflects a disharmony in Wood. People with Heart disharmonies often feel much worse in the heat, dampness affects the Spleen, dryness injures the Lungs and cold weakens the Kidneys.

However, this model has limitations too. For example, heat can aggravate a Heat condition of any organ, not just the Heart. Dampness can aggravate a Damp condition not only of the Spleen, but also of Kidneys, Gall Bladder and Bladder. Dryness injures the body fluids not only of the Lungs, but also of Stomach and Kidneys. Cold affects virtually any organ (in particular Stomach, Spleen, Intestines, Lungs, Uterus and Bladder) and not just the Kidneys (Box 2.13).

> **Box 2.13 Five-Element climates**
> - Wood: wind
> - Fire: heat
> - Earth: dampness
> - Metal: dryness
> - Water: cold

The Five Elements in acupuncture treatment

There are several ways in which the theory of the Five Elements is applied in treatment. These could be summarized in two headings:

> 1. Treatment according to the various sequences
> 2. Treatment according to the Five Transporting points

These are not alternative ways of applying the Five-Element theory in treatment, but simply a convenient method of discussing their use, bearing in mind that both are often used at the same time.

Treatment according to the various sequences

When considering a treatment of a certain Element, one should keep in mind the various relationships of that Element with the others along the Generating, Controlling, Over-acting, Insulting and Cosmological sequences.

Let us look, for example, at one Element, Wood; the other four Elements all follow the same general principle.

If there is a Wood disharmony, one must consider first of all if this disharmony may be affected by another Element, and, secondly, whether it is affecting another Element.

For example, if the Liver is deficient and the patient has several signs and symptoms of Liver-Blood deficiency, one should always consider and check whether the Mother Element (Water) is at fault, failing to nourish Wood. On the other hand, we must consider and check whether Wood is deficient from being overacted upon by Metal, or because Fire (the Child) is drawing too much from Wood (the Mother), or even because it is being insulted by Earth. One should also consider and check whether the Liver deficiency is affecting the Child Element, that is, the Heart (Fig. 2.16).

If the Liver is in excess and the patient has symptoms and signs of Liver-Qi stagnation or Liver-Fire, for example, one must check whether this excess is due to deficient Metal failing to control Wood. This often happens in chronic constitutional weakness of the Lungs.

On the other hand, one must check whether the excess in Wood has begun to affect other Elements. For example, when Wood is in excess, it can easily over-act

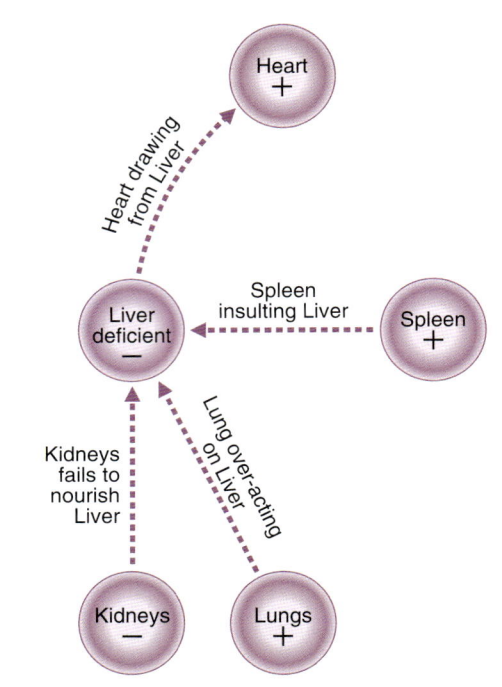

Figure 2.16 Pathological influences between a deficient Liver and other organs

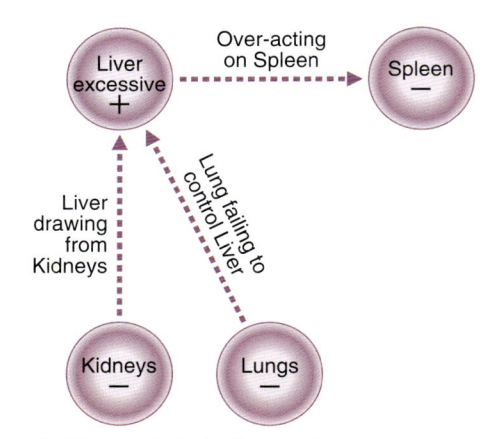

Figure 2.17 Pathological influences between an excessive Liver and other organs

on Earth. This is called 'Wood invading Earth' and is very common in practice. If Wood is in excess, it could also make too much demand on the Mother Element, that is, Water (Fig. 2.17). It is necessary to keep all these relationships in mind when determining the treatment.

Thus, if the Liver is deficient because it is not nourished by its Mother Element, Water, the Kidneys as well as the Liver must be tonified. If the Liver is deficient because it is being over-acted on by Metal, the correct course of action would be to sedate the Lungs. If the Liver is deficient because the Heart (Child) is drawing too much from it, one would have to sedate the Heart. If the Liver is deficient because it is being insulted by the Spleen, treatment demands sedation of the Spleen.

If the Liver deficiency is affecting its Child Element, one would tonify the Heart as well as the Liver.

If the Liver is in excess because Metal is not controlling it, one must tonify Metal (the Lungs), as well as sedating the Liver. If the Liver excess is affecting and depressing Earth, in this case the Spleen requires tonification. If the Liver is in excess and is drawing too much from the Mother Element, one must also tonify the Kidneys.

The 'Classic of Difficulties' says in chapter 77: *'If the Liver is diseased, it can invade the Spleen, one must therefore tonify the Spleen first.'*[24]

Treatment according to the Five Transporting points

This subject will be discussed in detail in chapter 37, and will therefore be dealt with only briefly here.

The Five Transporting points are the points between the fingers and elbows and between the toes and knees: each of the five points is related to an Element, in the order of the Generating sequence, starting with Wood for the Yin channels and Metal for the Yang ones. This principle was established for the first time in the 'Classic of Difficulties' in chapter 64.[25]

In chapter 69 it says: *'In case of Deficiency tonify the Mother, in case of Excess sedate the Child.'*[26]
(Figs 2.18 and 2.19.)

This means that in cases of deficiency of one organ one can choose the point on its channel related to its Mother Element. For example, in a case of deficiency of the Liver channel, one can choose the point on the Liver channel related to its Mother Element, that is, Water: this is LIV-8 Ququan (see Fig. 2.18).

In cases of excess of one organ one can choose the point on its channel related to its Child Element. For example, in a case of excess of the Liver channel, one can choose the point on the Liver channel related to its Child Element, that is, Fire: this is LIV-2 Xingjian (see Fig. 2.19).

Another way of making use of the Five-Element points in treatment is by using them to expel pathogenic factors. Given that Wood corresponds to Wind,

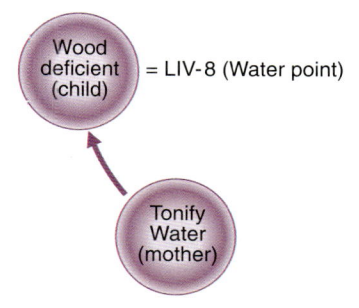

Figure 2.18 Tonify Mother in case of deficiency

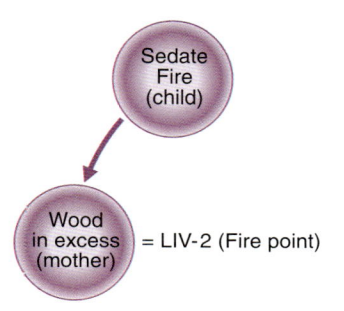

Figure 2.19 Sedate Child in case of excess

Fire to Heat, Earth to Dampness, Metal to Dryness and Water to Cold, one can use (usually sedate) the Element points to expel the relevant pathogenic factor. Thus one would use a Wood point to subdue Wind, a Fire point to clear Heat, an Earth point to resolve Dampness, etc.

The Five Elements in herbal and diet therapy

Diet therapy is a vast subject in Chinese medicine and it will be mentioned only briefly here as it is partly based on the Five-Element model. The principles underlying diet therapy are largely the same as those in herbal therapy, and they will therefore be discussed together.

Each food or herb has a certain taste which is related to one of the Elements. The five tastes are: sour for Wood, bitter for Fire, sweet for Earth, pungent for Metal and salty for Water. Each food or herb is classified as having one of these tastes. The 'taste' of a food or herb is not always related to its actual flavour: for instance, lamb is classified as 'bitter', and so is apple. The 'taste' of a food or herb is therefore more like its intrinsic quality than its actual flavour, although in most cases the two will coincide.

Each of the tastes has a certain effect on the body as described below.

The sour taste generates fluids and Yin. It is astringent and can control perspiration and diarrhoea.

The bitter taste clears Heat, sedates and hardens. It clears Damp-Heat and it subdues rebellious Qi.

The sweet taste tonifies, balances and moderates. It is used to tonify deficiency and to stop pain.

The pungent taste scatters, and is used to expel pathogenic factors.

The salty taste flows downwards, softens hardness and is used to treat constipation and swelling.

When foods or herbs of a certain taste are consumed in excess, the taste will have a negative effect on certain parts of the body.

The sour taste goes to the nerves and, in excess, can upset the Liver, so it should be used sparingly if a person suffers from chronic pain.

The bitter taste goes to the bones, and an excess of it should be avoided in bone diseases.

The sweet taste goes to the muscles and an excess of it can cause weakness in them.

The pungent taste scatters Qi and should be avoided in Qi deficiency.

The salty taste can dry the Blood, and should be avoided in Blood deficiency.

The 'Spiritual Axis' in chapter 56 deals with the effect of the five tastes. It says: *'The sour taste goes to the Liver, the bitter taste goes to the Heart, the sweet taste goes to the Spleen, the pungent taste goes to the Lungs, the salty taste goes to the Kidneys ... if the Liver is diseased one should not eat pungent foods, if the Heart is diseased one should not eat salty foods, if the Spleen is diseased one should not eat sour foods, if the Kidney is diseased one should not eat sweet foods, if the Lung is diseased one should not eat bitter foods.'*[27]

(Fig. 2.20.)

Thus, if an organ is diseased one should avoid the taste related to the Element that controls that organ along the Controlling sequence. For example, the salty taste pertains to Water, Water over-acts on Fire and therefore an excess of salt may injure the Heart (which, interestingly, coincides with the Western view of excessive salt consumption).

Conversely, each organ is nourished by the taste of the Element that it controls. For example, Wood (Liver) controls Earth, sweet is the taste corresponding to Earth; hence foods and herbs with a sweet taste are beneficial to the Liver (Fig. 2.21).

Learning outcomes

In this chapter you will have learned:
- The nature of the Five Elements
- The Five Elements as five basic processes of Nature
- The Five Elements as five qualities of natural phenomena
- The Five Elements as five phases of a cycle
- The Five Elements as five inherent capabilities of change of phenomena
- The concept of Five-Elements interrelationships (Generating, Controlling, Over-acting, Insulting and Cosmological sequences) and how these are applied in Chinese medicine
- How to apply the Five-Element correspondences in diagnosis
- Acupuncture treatment strategies according to the Five Elements

Self-assessment questions

1. In the earliest references, in which order were the Five Elements enumerated and how does this relate to their numerology?
2. Name four aspects of the nature of the Five Elements.
3. What is the Cosmological sequence?
4. Name three Five-Element relationships within the Generating sequence and explain how these relate to the functions of the Internal Organs.
5. Name three Five-Element relationships within the Controlling sequence and explain how these relate to the functions of the Internal Organs.
6. Name three clinical implications of the Cosmological sequence of the Five Elements.
7. Name two relationships within the Over-acting sequence in pathology and how these relate to Internal Organs pathological interactions.

Figure 2.20 Beneficial tastes according to Five-Element sequence

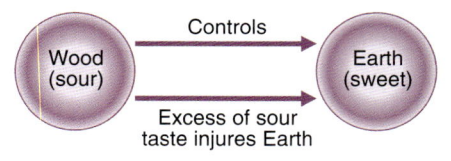

Figure 2.21 Detrimental tastes according to Five-Element sequence

8. Name the five sounds, tastes and emotions corresponding to the Five Elements.
9. What happens if we eat too much salt and how is this explained in the light of the Five Elements?

See p. 1255 for answers

END NOTES

1. Needham J 1977 Science and Civilization in China, vol. 2, Cambridge University Press, Cambridge, p. 244.
2. Lamanna EP 1967 Storia della Filosofia (History of Philosophy), vol. 1, Le Monnier, Florence, p. 220–221.
3. Science and Civilization in China, p. 242.
4. Fung Yu Lan 1966 A Short History of Chinese Philosophy, Free Press, New York, p. 131.
5. Science and Civilization in China, p. 266.
6. Kaptchuk T 1983 The Web that has no Weaver, Congdon and Weed, New York, p. 343–354.
7. Science and Civilization in China, p. 232–242.
8. Gu He Dao 1979 History of Chinese Medicine (*Zhong Guo Yi Xue Shi Lue* 中国医学史略), Shanxi People's Publishing House, Taiyuan, p. 29.
9. History of Chinese Medicine, p. 29.
10. Great Transmission of the Valued Book (*Shang Shu Da Chuan* 尚书大传), cited in History of Chinese Medicine, p. 29.
11. Lloyd G, Chadwick J, Mann W 1983 Hippocratic Writings, Penguin Books, Harmondsworth, p. 237.
12. Shang Shu (*c.*659–627 BC), cited in 1975 Practical Chinese Medicine (*Shi Yong Zhong Yi Xue* 实用中医学), Beijing Publishing House, Beijing, p. 32. The book *Shang Shu* is attributed by some to the early Zhou dynasty (*c.*1000 BC), but the prevalent opinion is that it was written between 659 and 627 BC.
13. Science and Civilization in China, p. 238.
14. Practical Chinese Medicine, p. 32.
15. Science and Civilization in China, p. 243.
16. 1982 Classic of Categories (*Lei Jing* 类经), People's Health Publishing House, Beijing, p. 46 (first published 1624).
17. 1981 Discussion of Prescriptions of the Golden Chest (*Jin Gui Yao Lue Fang Lun* 金匮要略方论), Zhejiang Scientific Publishing House, p. 1 (first published *c.*AD 220).
18. See note 7 above.
19. Science and Civilization in China, vol. 2, p. 258–259.
20. 1979 The Yellow Emperor's Classic of Internal Medicine – Simple Questions (*Huang Ti Nei Jing Su Wen* 黄帝内经素问), People's Health Publishing House, Beijing, p. 22–38 (first published *c.*100 BC).
21. Nanjing College of Traditional Chinese Medicine 1979 A Revised Explanation of the Classic of Difficulties (*Nan Jing Jiao Shi* 难经校释), People's Publishing House, Beijing, p. 90, 95.
22. Classic of Difficulties, p. 134.
23. It is difficult to understand how the Chinese word '*Si*' 思 which is the 'emotion' related to Earth and means 'to think' or 'pensiveness', could be translated as 'sympathy' by some authors.
24. Classic of Difficulties, p. 163.
25. Classic of Difficulties, p. 139.
26. Classic of Difficulties, p. 151.
27. 1981 Spiritual Axis, People's Health Publishing House, Beijing, p. 104 (first compiled *c.*200 BC).

BIBLIOGRAPHY AND FURTHER READING

Beinfield H, Korngold E 1992 Between Heaven and Earth, Ballantine Books, New York
Chan Wing Tsit 1969 A Source Book in Chinese Philosophy, Princeton University Press, Princeton
Fung Yu Lan 1966 A Short History of Chinese Philosophy, Free Press, New York
Kaptchuk T 2000 The Web that has no Weaver – Understanding Chinese Medicine, Contemporary Books, Chicago
Matsumoto K 1993 Five Elements and Ten Stems, Paradigm Publications, Boston
Moore CA 1967 The Chinese Mind, University Press of Hawaii, Honolulu
Needham J 1977 Science and Civilization in China, vol. 2, Cambridge University Press, Cambridge

PART 1

The Vital Substances 3

> **Key contents**
>
> **Origin, nature, function and brief pathology of:**
> *Essence*
> *Qi*
> *Blood*
> *Body Fluids*
> *Mind (Shen)*

Chinese medicine sees the working of the body and mind as the result of the interaction of certain vital substances. These substances manifest in varying degrees of 'substantiality', so that some of them are very rarefied and some totally non-material. All together, they constitute the ancient Chinese view of the body-mind.

In Chinese philosophy and medicine, the body and the mind are not seen as a mechanism (however complex) but as a vortex of Qi in its various manifestations interacting with each other to form an organism. The body and the mind are nothing but forms of Qi. At the basis of all is Qi: all the other vital substances are but manifestations of Qi in varying degrees of materiality, ranging from the completely material, such as Body Fluids, to the totally immaterial, such as the Mind (*Shen*).

The Vital Substances are:

> Qi
> Blood
> Essence (*Jing*)
> Body Fluids
> Mind (*Shen*)

The discussion will be organized under the following headings:

- The concept of Qi in Chinese philosophy
- The concept of Qi in Chinese medicine

- Essence
  - Pre-Heaven Essence
  - Post-Heaven Essence
  - The Kidney-Essence
- Qi
  - Original Qi (*Yuan Qi*)
  - Food-Qi (*Gu Qi*)
  - Gathering Qi (*Zong Qi*)
  - True Qi (*Zhen Qi*)
  - Central Qi (*Zhong Qi*)
  - Upright Qi (*Zheng Qi*)
  - Functions of Qi
  - Direction of Qi movement
  - Pathology of Qi
- Blood
  - Source of Blood
  - Functions of Blood
  - Relation of Blood with internal organs
  - Blood–Qi relationship
  - Blood–Essence relationship
  - Blood pathology
- Body Fluids
  - Source
  - Relations with internal organs
  - Types of Body Fluids
  - Relation between Qi and Body Fluids
  - Relation between Blood and Body Fluids
  - Pathology of body fluids
- Mind (*Shen*)

THE CONCEPT OF QI IN CHINESE PHILOSOPHY

The concept of Qi has occupied Chinese philosophers throughout history, from the beginning of Chinese civilization to our modern times. The character for Qi indicates that it is something which is, at the same time, both material and immaterial.

氣

气 means 'vapour', 'steam', 'gas'

米 means (uncooked) 'rice'

This clearly indicates that Qi can be as rarefied and immaterial as vapour, and as dense and material as rice. It also indicates that Qi is a subtle substance (steam, vapour) deriving from a coarse one (rice) just as steam is produced by cooking rice.

It is very difficult to translate the word 'Qi' and many different translations have been proposed, none of which approximates the essence of Qi exactly. It has variously been translated as 'energy', 'material force', 'matter', 'ether', 'matter-energy', 'vital force', 'life force', 'vital power', 'moving power'. The reason it is so difficult to translate the word 'Qi' correctly lies precisely in its versatile nature whereby Qi can assume different manifestations and be different things in different situations.

The way 'Qi' is translated also depends on the particular viewpoint taken. Most modern physicists would probably agree that 'Qi' may be termed 'energy', since Qi expresses the continuum of matter and energy as it is now understood by modern particle physics. The closeness of the concepts of Qi and energy was highlighted by an article on the nature of Qi written by a professor from the Institute of High Energy Physics of China.[1] According to Needham, 'Qi' also conveys modern scientific ideas of 'aethereal waves' or 'radioactive emanations'.[2]

Most Sinologists generally agree that Qi corresponds to 'matter', although not to matter in a restrictive materialistic sense, as Qi can also assume very rarefied, dispersed, non-material forms. In Chinese philosophy, there is another term to indicate matter in its solid, hard and tangible state, and that is '*Ji*'. Ji is a material form of Qi, but Qi is not always Ji, as it can exist in tenuous and non-perceptible forms. Because of the difficulty in finding an appropriate translation for the term 'Qi', I have chosen to leave it untranslated, as I do for 'Yin' and 'Yang'.

Qi is at the basis of all phenomena in the universe and provides a continuity between coarse, material forms and tenuous, rarefied, non-material energies. It therefore completely side-steps the dilemma that has pervaded Western philosophy from the time of Plato to the present day, that is, the duality and contrast between materialism and idealism. Western philosophy either considered matter as independent of man's perception, or, at the other extreme, considered matter as a mere reflection of ideas. Needham puts this very well: '*both [the macrocosm–microcosm doctrine and organic naturalism] were subject to what I call ... the characteristic European schizophrenia or split-personality. Europeans could only think in terms either of Democritean mechanical materialism or of Platonic theological spiritualism. A deus always had to be found for a machina. Animas, entelechiae, souls, archaei, dance processionally through the history of European thinking.*'[3]

The infinite variety of phenomena in the universe is the result of the continuous coming together and dispersion of Qi to form phenomena of various degrees of materialization. This idea of aggregation and dispersion of Qi has been discussed by many Chinese philosophers of all times.

Qi is the very basis of the universe's infinite manifestations of life, including minerals, vegetables and animals (including human beings). Xun Kuang (c.313–238 BC) said: '*Water and Fire have Qi but not life; plants and trees have life, but not knowledge; birds and animals have knowledge, but no sense of what are rights.*'[4]

Lie Zi, a Daoist text from around 300 BC, said: '*The purer and lighter [elements], tending upwards, made the heaven; the grosser and heavier [elements], tending downwards, made the earth*'.[5]

Thus 'Heaven' and 'Earth' are often used to symbolize two extreme states of utmost rarefaction and dispersion or utmost condensation and aggregation of Qi, respectively (Fig. 3.1).

Huai Nan Zi (c.122 BC), another Daoist text, says: '*Dao originated from Emptiness and Emptiness produced the universe. The universe produced Qi. ... That which was clear and light drifted up to become heaven, and that which was heavy and turbid solidified to form earth.*'[6]

According to these ancient philosophers, life and death themselves are nothing but an aggregation and dispersal of Qi. According to Wang Chong (AD 27–97): '*Qi produces the human body just as water becomes ice. As water freezes into ice, so Qi coagulates to form the human body. When ice melts, it becomes water. When a person dies, he or she becomes spirit [shen] again. It is called spirit, just as melted ice changes its name to water.*'[7] He also said: '*When it came to separation and differentiation, the pure [elements] formed heaven, and the turbid ones formed earth.*'[8]

Zhang Zai (AD 1020–1077) further developed the concept of Qi. He proposed that the Great Void was not

Wang Fu Zhi (1619–1692) reaffirmed the concept of continuity of energy and matter and the condensation of formless Qi into physical shapes. He said: '*Life is not creation from nothing, and death is not complete dispersion and destruction*'.[14] Also: '[*Despite the condensation and dispersion of Qi] its original substance can neither be added nor be lessened.*'[15] Other quotations from his writings further clarify the nature of Qi: '*All that is void and empty is full of Qi which, in its state of condensation and thus visible, is called being, but in its state of dispersion and thus no longer visible, is called non-being.*'[16] '*When dispersing Qi makes the Great Void, only regaining its original misty feature but not perishing; when condensing, it becomes the origin of all beings.*'[17]

In conclusion, we can say that Qi is a continuous form of matter, resulting in physical shape ('*Xing*') when it condenses. *Xing* is a discontinuous form of matter, resulting in Qi when it disperses.

THE CONCEPT OF QI IN CHINESE MEDICINE

All that has been said about Qi so far applies to Chinese medicine. Chinese philosophers and doctors observed the interrelationship between the universe and human beings and considered the human being's Qi as a result of the interaction of the Qi of Heaven and Earth. The 'Simple Questions' in chapter 25 says: '*A human being results from the Qi of Heaven and Earth ... The union of the Qi of Heaven and Earth is called human being.*'[18]

This stresses the interaction between the human being's Qi and natural forces. Chinese medicine emphasizes the relationship between human beings and their environment and takes this into account in determining aetiology, diagnosis and treatment.

Just as Qi is the material substratum of the universe, it is also the material and mental-spiritual substratum of human life. The 'Classic of Difficulties' says: '*Qi is the root of a human being.*'[19]

In particular, two aspects of Qi are especially relevant to medicine:

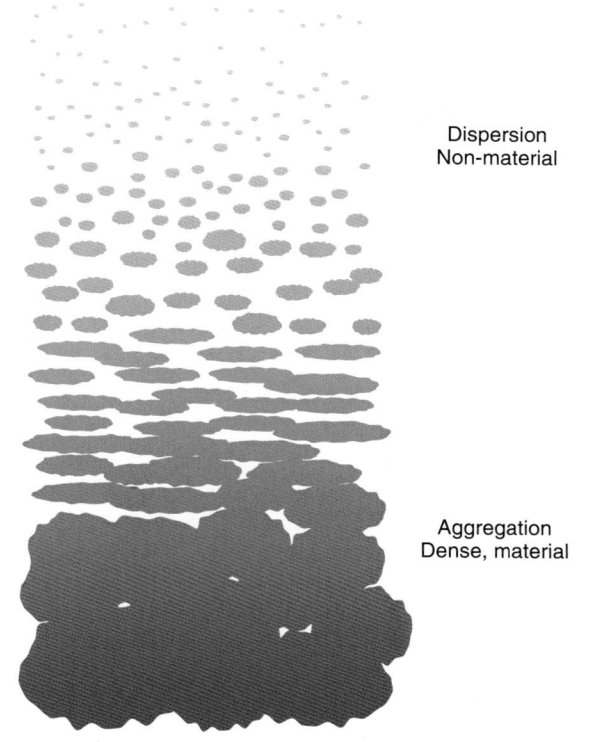

Figure 3.1 Aggregation and dispersion of Qi

mere emptiness, but Qi in its state of continuity. He said the Great Void cannot but consist of Qi. He also further developed the idea of condensation and dissipation of Qi as giving rise to the myriad phenomena in the universe. He affirmed that extreme aggregation of Qi gives rise to actual form, '*Xing*', that is, a material substance. This concept has important applications in Chinese medicine, as we shall see shortly. Zhang Zai said: '*The Great Void consists of Qi. Qi condenses to become the myriad things. Things of necessity disintegrate and return to the Great Void.*'[9] Also: '*If Qi condenses, its visibility becomes effective and physical form appears.*'[10]

Zhang Zai clearly saw the important phenomenon of indestructibility of matter-energy: '*Qi in dispersion is substance, and so is it in condensation.*'[11] Human life, too, is nothing but a condensation of Qi, and death is a dispersal of Qi. He said: '*Every birth is a condensation, every death a dispersal. Birth is not a gain, death not a loss ... when condensed, Qi becomes a living being, when dispersed, it is the substratum of mutations.*'[12]

Zhu Xi (1131–1200) also saw life as a condensation of Qi. He said: '*Qi, condensing, can form beings*'.[13]

1. Qi is in a constant state of flux and in varying states of aggregation. When condensed, Qi gives rise to physical shape; when dispersed, Qi gives rise to subtle forms of energy.
2. Qi is an energy which manifests simultaneously on the physical and emotional-mental-spiritual level.

According to Chinese medicine, there are many different 'types' of Qi affecting our body and mind, ranging from the subtle and rarefied to the very dense and coarse. All the various types of Qi, however, are ultimately one Qi, merely manifesting in different forms.

It is important, therefore, to see the simultaneous universality and particularity of Qi. Whilst ultimately there is only one Qi energy which assumes different forms, in practice it is important to be able to distinguish between the different types of Qi.

Although Qi remains fundamentally the same, it 'puts on different hats' in different places and changes its form according to the place it is in and which of its different functions it is assuming. For example, Nutritive Qi (*Ying Qi*) exists in the Interior of the body. Its function is to nourish, and it is denser than Defensive Qi (*Wei Qi*), which is on the Exterior and protects the body. Derangement of either Defensive or Nutritive Qi will give rise to different clinical manifestations and will require different kinds of treatment. Ultimately, though, they are simply two different manifestations of the same Qi energy (Fig. 3.2).

Poor circulation can result in excessive 'aggregation' or 'condensation' of Qi, which means that Qi becomes pathologically dense, forming lumps, masses or tumours.

The various states of aggregation of Qi also account for its manifestations at a physical and emotional-mental-spiritual level simultaneously. The Blood in the Liver represents a dense, material form of Qi whilst the emotional energy of anger is also a form of Qi, albeit of a more subtle, non-material type.

In Chinese medicine, the term 'Qi' is used in two major ways. Firstly, it indicates the refined energy produced by the internal organs, which has the function of nourishing the body and mind. This refined energy takes several forms depending on its location and function. Gathering Qi (*Zong Qi*), for example, is in the chest and nourishes the Heart and Lungs. Original Qi (*Yuan Qi*) is in the Lower Burner and nourishes the Kidneys.

Two meanings of the term 'Qi':
1. The refined energy produced by the Internal Organs, assuming different forms in different places.
2. The functional activity of an Internal Organ (e.g. Liver-Qi, Lung-Qi).

Secondly, 'Qi' indicates the functional activity of the internal organs. When used in this sense, it does *not* indicate a refined substance as above, but simply the complex of functional activities of any organ. For example, when we speak of Liver-Qi, we do not mean the 'portion' of Qi residing in the Liver, but rather the complex of the Liver's functional activities, that is, ensuring the smooth flow of Qi. In this sense, we can speak of Liver-Qi, Heart-Qi, Lung-Qi, Stomach-Qi, etc.

Essence 精

(Box 3.1)

Box 3.1 Three types of Essence

1. Pre-Heaven Essence
2. Post-Heaven Essence
3. Kidney-Essence

'JING' is usually translated as 'Essence'. The Chinese character for '*jing*' is composed of the character for 'rice' on the left and that for 'clear, refined' on the right, as follows:

米 indicates 'rice' (uncooked)

青 indicates 'clear, refined' when combined with the water radical

Thus the character for 'Essence' gives the idea of something derived from a process of refinement or distillation: it is a distilled, refined essence, extracted from some coarser basis. This process of extraction of a refined essence from a larger, coarser substance implies that the Essence is a rather precious substance to be cherished and guarded.

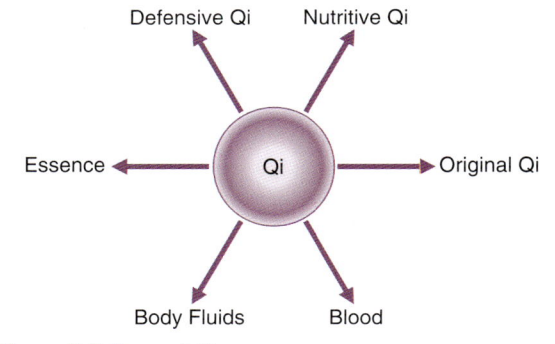

Figure 3.2 Types of Qi

The term 'Essence' occurs in Chinese medicine in three different contexts with slightly different meanings (Box 3.1).

Pre-Heaven Essence

Conception is a blending of the sexual energies of man and woman to form what the ancient Chinese called the 'Pre-Heaven Essence' (in English also known as 'Prenatal Essence') of the newly conceived human being. This Essence nourishes the embryo and fetus during pregnancy and is also dependent on nourishment derived from the mother's Kidneys. The Pre-Heaven Essence is the only kind of essence present in the fetus, as it does not have independent physiological activity.

This Pre-Heaven Essence is what determines each person's basic constitutional make-up, strength and vitality. It is what makes each individual unique.

The Pre-Heaven Essence is closely linked to the Fire of the Gate of Life (*Ming Men*), which is discussed in more detail in chapter 10. Situated in between the Kidneys, the Fire of the Gate of Life is the physiological Fire of the body which provides the warmth that is essential for all the body's physiological processes and for all the internal organs. The Fire of the Gate of Life is already present from birth and, indeed, from conception. The Pre-Heaven Essence is also present from conception and birth but it then 'matures' into the Kidney-Essence (see below) at puberty when it generates menstrual blood and ova in women and sperm in men. Thus, the Fire of the Gate of Life can be said to represent the Yang aspect of the Pre-Heaven Essence, while the Pre-Heaven Essence proper (transforming into Kidney-Essence at puberty) represents the Yin aspect (Fig. 3.3).

The Fire of the Gate of Life accumulates at the point Du-4 Mingmen on the spine at conception, while the Pre-Heaven Essence concentrates at the point Ren-4 Guanyuan, also at conception (Fig. 3.4). This correlates with the Uterus (where menstrual blood is stored) in women and with the Room of Sperm in men.[20] Chapter 36 of the 'Classic of Difficulties' says: '*The Gate of Life is the residence of the Mind and Essence and it is connected to the Original Qi [Yuan Qi]: in men it houses the Sperm; in women the Uterus.*'[21]

Since it is inherited from the parents at conception, the Pre-Heaven Essence can be influenced only with difficulty in the course of adult life. Some say this

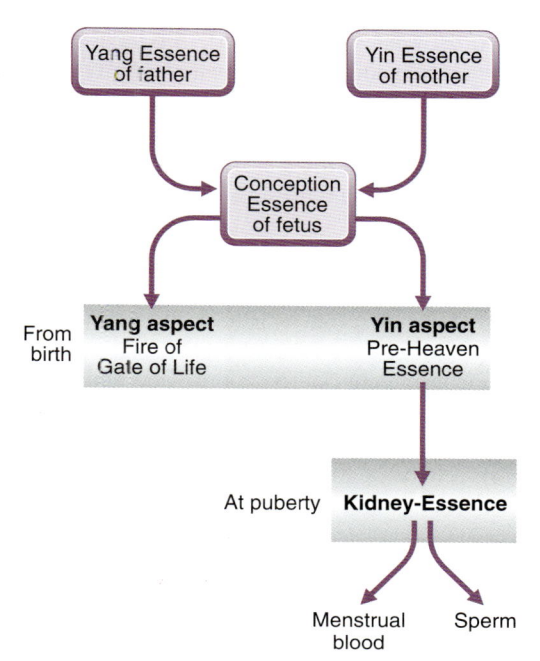

Figure 3.3 Yang and Yin aspects of the Prenatal Essence

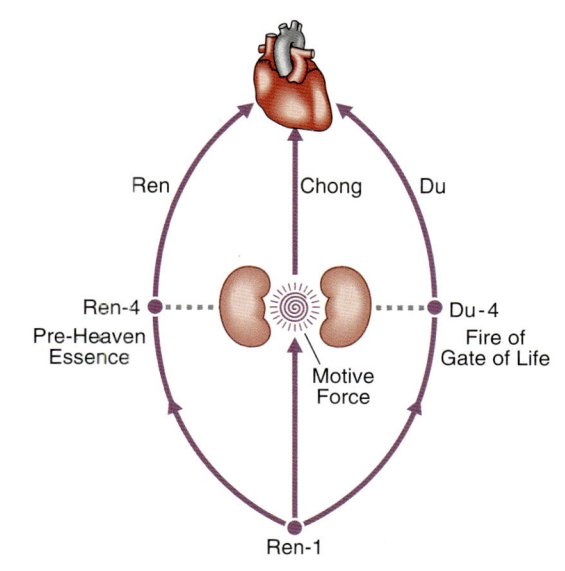

Figure 3.4 The Fire of the Gate of Life and the Pre-Heaven Essence

Essence is 'fixed' in quantity and quality. However, due to its interaction with the Post-Heaven Essence, it can be positively affected, even if not quantitatively increased.[22]

The best way to affect positively one's Pre-Heaven Essence is by striving for balance in one's life activities:

balance between work and rest, restraint in sexual activity and a balanced diet. Any irregularity or excess in these spheres is bound to diminish the Pre-Heaven Essence. A direct way to influence one's Essence positively is through breathing exercises and such exercises as *Tai Ji Quan* and *Qi Gong*.

Post-Heaven Essence

This is the essence that is refined and extracted from food and fluids by the Stomach and Spleen after birth. The newborn baby starts taking nourishment and breathing, its Lungs, Stomach and Spleen start functioning to produce Qi from food, drink and air. The 'Golden Mirror of Medical Collection' says: '*The Pre-Heaven Essence originates from the parents, the Post-Heaven Essence originates from food.*'[23]

The complex of essences refined and extracted from food is collectively known as 'Post-Heaven Essence' (in English also called 'Postnatal Essence'). Because the Stomach and Spleen are responsible for the digestion of food and the transformation and transportation of food essences ultimately leading to the production of Qi, the Post-Heaven Essence is closely related to Stomach and Spleen.

The Post-Heaven Essence is therefore not a specific type of essence, but simply a general term to indicate the essences produced by the Stomach and Spleen after birth, as opposed to the Pre-Heaven Essence which is formed before birth. For this reason, the Stomach and Spleen are also known as the 'Root of the Post-Heaven Essence' and the Kidneys as the 'Root of the Pre-Heaven Essence' (see below).

The Kidney-Essence

Kidney-Essence is a more specific kind of vital substance which plays an extremely important role in human physiology. It derives from both the Pre-Heaven Essence and the Post-Heaven Essence. Like the Pre-Heaven Essence, it is a hereditary energy which determines the person's constitution. Unlike the Pre-Heaven Essence, however, the Kidney Essence interacts with the Post-Heaven Essence and is replenished by it. Kidney Essence therefore partakes of both the Pre-Heaven and the Post-Heaven Essences.

This Essence is stored in the Kidneys, but it also circulates all over the body, particularly in the Eight Extraordinary Vessels (see chapters 52 and 53).

The Kidney-Essence determines growth, reproduction, development, sexual maturation, conception, pregnancy, menopause and ageing.

The following are some differences between Essence and Qi in the human body:

- Essence is primarily derived from the parents before birth, whilst Qi is formed after birth
- Essence is replenished only with difficulty, Qi can easily be replenished on a day-to-day basis
- Essence follows very long cycles of 7 or 8 years, whereas Qi follows briefer cycles, some yearly, some circadian, some even shorter
- Qi moves and changes quickly from moment to moment, whereas the Essence changes only slowly and gradually over long periods of time

The functions of Essence are as follows:

- Growth, reproduction and development
- Basis of Kidney-Qi
- Producer of Marrow
- Basis of constitutional strength
- Basis for the 'Three Treasures' (Essence–Qi–Mind, *Jing–Qi–Shen*)

Growth, reproduction and development

Essence is the organic substance that forms the basis for growth, reproduction and development and ageing. In children, it controls the growth of bones, teeth, hair, normal brain development and sexual maturation. After puberty, it controls the reproductive function and fertility. It forms the basis for successful conception and pregnancy. The natural decline of the Essence during our lifetime leads to the natural decline of sexual energy and fertility. Ageing itself is a process of decline of the Essence.

According to the first chapter of the 'Simple Questions', men's Essence flows in 8-year cycles, and women's Essence in 7-year cycles. '*Tian Gui*' in this passage refers to sperm in men and ova in women. '*The Kidney energy of a girl becomes abundant at the age of 7, her baby teeth are replaced by permanent ones and the hair grows. At the age of 14 the Tian Gui arrives [ovulation and menstruation], the Directing Vessel begins to flow, the Penetrating Vessel is flourishing, the periods come regularly and she can conceive. At the age of 21 the Kidney-Essence peaks, the wisdom teeth come out and growth is at its utmost. At the age of 28, tendons and bones become strong,* the hair grows longest and the body is strong and flourishing. At the age of 35, the Bright Yang channels begin to weaken, the complexion starts to wither and the hair begins to fall. At the age of 42, the three Yang channels are weak, the face darkens and the hair begins to turn grey. At the age of 49, the Directing Vessel is empty, the Penetrating Vessel depleted, the Tian Gui dries up, the Earth Passage [uterus] is not open, so weakness and infertility set in. In a man, at the age of 8 the boy's Kidney energy is abundant, his hair and teeth grow. At the age of 16 his Kidney energy is even more abundant, the Tian Gui arrives, the Essence is luxuriant and flowing, Yin and Yang are harmonized and he can father a child. At the age of 24, the Kidney energy peaks, tendons and bones are strong, the wisdom teeth appear, and growth is at its peak. At the age of 32, tendons and bones are at their strongest, and the muscles are full and strong. At the age of 40, the Kidney is weakened, the hair begins to fall out and the teeth become loose. At the age of 48, Yang Qi is exhausted, the face becomes darker and the hair turns grey. At the age of 56, the Liver energy is weakened, the tendons cannot move, the Tian Gui is dried up, the Kidney becomes weak and the body begins to grow old. At the age of 64, hair and teeth are gone.'[24]

The Essence as basis of Kidney-Qi

There is a close interaction among the various aspects of Kidney energy, that is, Kidney-Essence, Kidney-Yin, Kidney-Yang, Kidney-Qi.

The Essence is fluid-like and naturally has an affinity with Yin; it can therefore be considered as an aspect of Kidney-Yin. In addition, it provides the material basis for Kidney-Yin to produce Kidney-Qi by the heating action of Kidney-Yang. In other words, the Kidneys can be compared to a large cauldron full of water. The fire under the cauldron is provided by Kidney-Yang and the Gate of Life (*Ming Men*, see chapter 10), the water inside the cauldron corresponds to the Kidney-Essence, and the resulting steam (i.e. Qi), corresponds to Kidney-Qi (Fig. 3.5).

Thus, Kidney-Essence is necessary for the transformation of Kidney-Yin into Kidney-Qi through the warming action of Kidney-Yang.

The Essence produces Marrow

The concept of Marrow in Chinese medicine is different from that in Western medicine, and it does not correspond directly to bone marrow.

The Essence produces Marrow, which, in turn, produces bone marrow and fills the spinal cord and the brain. Thus, 'Marrow' is a substance which is the common matrix of the bone marrow, brain and spinal cord: it has no equivalent in Western medicine.

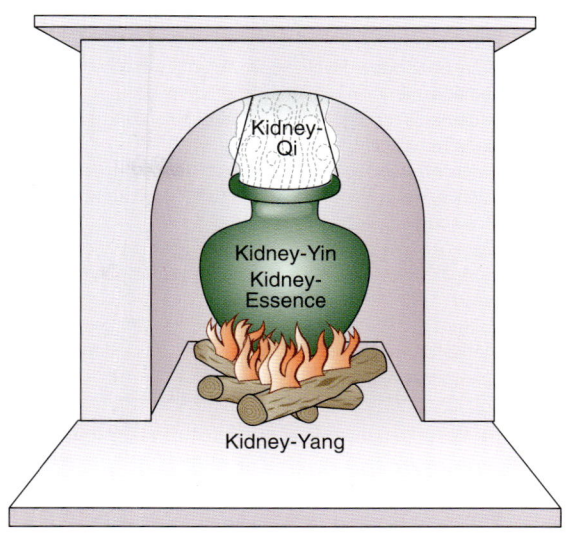

Figure 3.5 Relationship between Kidney-Yin, Kidney-Essence, Kidney-Yang and Kidney-Qi

Essence is therefore extremely important for healthy bone marrow, brain and spinal cord. The 'Spiritual Axis' in chapter 33 says: '*The Brain is the Sea of Marrow*'.[25] Thus, if the Kidney-Essence is weak, the brain may lack nourishment and the person may lack concentration and memory and suffer from dizziness and a feeling of emptiness of the head.

The Essence as the basis of constitutional strength

Finally, the Essence determines our basic constitutional strength and resistance to exterior pathogenic factors. Although the Defensive Qi is mostly responsible for protection from exterior pathogenic factors, it also draws its strength and has its root in the Kidney-Essence. Thus the Kidney-Essence also plays a fundamental role in the protection against exterior pathogenic factors. The 'Simple Questions' in chapter 4 says: '*If the Essence is properly stored [i.e. not dissipated], no exterior febrile diseases will be contracted in the Spring ... if the Essence is not stored in Winter, exterior febrile diseases will be contracted in the Spring.*'[26]

From these four main functions of the Essence, one may deduce the kind of problems that may derive from a deficiency of Essence:

1. *Growth, reproduction and development*: stunted growth in children, poor bone development, infertility, habitual miscarriage, mental retardation in children, bone deterioration in adults, loose teeth and hair falling out or greying prematurely
2. *The Essence as basis for Kidney-Qi*: poor sexual function, impotence, weakness of knees, nocturnal emissions, tinnitus and deafness
3. *The Essence as the basis of Marrow*: poor concentration, poor memory, dizziness, tinnitus and a feeling of emptiness of the head
4. *The Essence as the basis of constitutional strength*: being constantly prone to colds, influenza and other exterior diseases, allergic rhinitis

The Essence as the basis for the 'Three Treasures'

The Essence and Qi are also considered to be the material foundation of the Mind (*Shen*). Essence, Qi and Mind (*Jing, Qi, Shen*) are the three fundamental physical and psychic substances of a human being. For this reason, they are called the 'Three Treasures'.

Essence, Qi and Mind also represent three different states of condensation of Qi, the Essence being the densest, Qi being more rarefied, and the Mind being the most subtle and immaterial. According to Chinese medicine, Essence and Qi are the essential foundation of the Mind. If Essence and Qi are healthy and flourishing, the Mind will be happy and this will lead to a healthy and happy life. If Essence and Qi are both depleted, then the Mind necessarily will suffer.

Thus a healthy Mind depends on the strength of the Essence, which is stored in the Kidneys, and Qi, which is produced by the Stomach and Spleen. In other words, the Mind is dependent on the Pre-Heaven and Post-Heaven Essence.

The triad of Essence, Qi and Mind is often expressed in Chinese medicine as Heaven (the Mind), Person (Qi) and Earth (the Essence), corresponding to the three organs Heart, Stomach/Spleen and Kidneys, respectively.

MIND	HEART	HEAVEN
QI	STOMACH-SPLEEN	PERSON
ESSENCE	KIDNEYS	EARTH

In practice, it is important to make a general assessment of the relative state of these three fundamental substances as the Essence gives an indication of the inherited constitution, Qi gives an indication of the state of Qi produced from day to day, and the Mind gives an indication of the state of the emotional and mental life.

The state of the Essence can to some degree be deduced from the patient's past: a history of serious childhood diseases would indicate a weak constitution. It can also be observed in the pulse: a pulse with a 'Scattered' or 'Leather' (see ch. 25) quality indicates poor and weakened Essence. The tongue can show a weakened Essence if its root has 'no spirit' (see ch. 23).

The state of the Mind can be deduced by observing the 'lustre' of the eyes. Eyes with lustre, that is, with a certain undefinable shine and vitality about them, show a healthy condition of the Mind. Eyes that look dull, as if they have a curtain of mist in front of them, show that the Mind is disturbed. This can frequently be observed in those who have had serious emotional problems for a long period of time, or have had a serious shock, even if this occurred many years previously.

Some Chinese language expressions also show how these concepts are rooted in Chinese culture. '*Jing-shen*' (i.e. Essence-Mind) means 'mind' or 'consciousness', showing the interaction of body and mind; it also means 'vigour', 'vitality', 'drive', all qualities that are present when both the Essence and the Mind are healthy and strong. '*Jing-shen bing*' means 'mental illness'.

The functions of Kidney-Essence are summarized in Box 3.2.

Box 3.2 Functions of Kidney-Essence

1. It determines growth, reproduction and development
2. It is the basis of Kidney-Qi
3. It produces Marrow
4. It is the basis of constitution
5. It is the foundation of the 'Three Treasures' (Essence, Qi, Mind)

Qi 氣

As we have discussed, Qi takes various forms in the body, fulfilling a variety of functions. Let us now discuss the various forms of Qi.

Original Qi (*Yuan Qi*) 原氣

This type of Qi is closely related to the Essence. Indeed, Original Qi is nothing but Essence in the form of Qi; it could be described as Essence transformed into Qi. It is a dynamic and rarefied form of Essence having its origin in the Kidneys. Original Qi is also often said to include the 'Original Yin' (*Yuan Yin*) and 'Original Yang' (*Yuan Yang*): this means that Original Qi is the foundation of all the Yin and Yang energies of the body.

Original Qi, like Essence, relies on nourishment from the Post-Heaven Essence.

Original Qi has many functions:

- It is the Motive Force
- It is the basis of Kidney-Qi
- It facilitates the transformation of Qi
- It is the conduit for the Triple Burner
- It facilitates the transformation of Blood
- It comes out at the Source points

Motive force

Original Qi can be seen as the dynamic motive force that arouses and moves the functional activity of all the organs. It does so because, like the Essence, it is the foundation of vitality and stamina. As a form of Qi, it circulates all over the body, in the channels. It could be said to be the link between Essence, which is more fluid-like and related to slow, long-term cycles and changes, and the day-to-day Qi, which is Qi-like and is related to short-term cycles and changes.

Basis of Kidney-Qi

Original Qi is the basis for Kidney-Qi and is closely related to all the Kidney's functional activities. According to chapter 66 of the 'Classic of Difficulties', Original Qi dwells between the two Kidneys below the umbilicus, at the Gate of Life.[27]

Thus, Original Qi is closely related to the Gate of Life and shares its role of providing the heat necessary to all the body's functional activities.

Facilitates the transformation of Qi

Original Qi acts as the agent of change in the transformation of Gathering Qi (*Zong Qi*) into True Qi (*Zhen Qi*). This is one way in which the Kidneys (where the Original Qi arises from) participate in the production of Qi.

Conduit for the Triple Burner

Chapter 66 of the 'Classic of Difficulties' discusses the connection between the Original Qi (in this chapter called *Dong Qi*, 'Motive Force') and the Triple Burner. It says: '*The Original Qi is the Motive Force [Dong Qi] situated between the two kidneys, it is life-giving and it is the root of the 12 channels. The Triple Burner causes the Original Qi to differentiate [for its different uses around the body]; the Original Qi passes through the Three Burners and then spreads to the 5 Yin and 6 Yang organs and their channels. The places where the Original Qi stays are the Source [Yuan] points.*'[28]

Other authors translate this passage as saying that the Triple Burner is the '*special envoy*' that '*transmits*' the Original Qi.[29] I have adopted Clavey's interpretation of this passage, that is, that the Triple Burner makes the Original Qi separate and differentiate in its different forms in different places around the body.[30] If interpreted in this way, the Triple Burner plays the very important role of allowing the Original Qi to facilitate the transformation of Qi in different places around the body and assume different forms in each place.

Facilitates the transformation of Blood

Original Qi also facilitates the transformation of Food-Qi (*Gu Qi*) into Blood in the Heart (see below). This is one way in which the Kidneys participate in the production of Blood.

Comes out at the Source points

From its origin in between the two Kidneys where the Gate of Life resides, Original Qi passes through the Triple Burner and spreads to the internal organs and channels. The places where the Original Qi stays are the Source (*Yuan*) points (Fig. 3.6).[31]

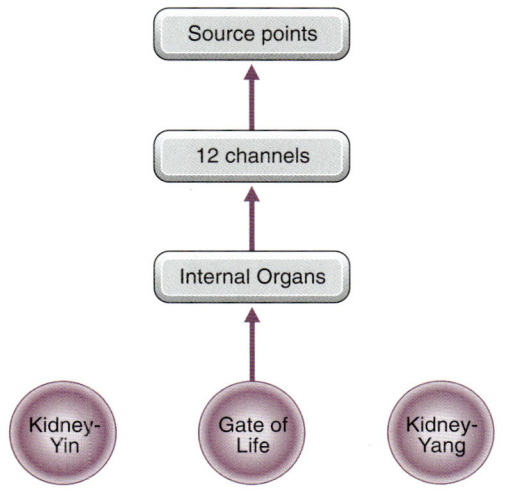

Figure 3.6 Relationship between the Gate of Life, Original Qi and Source points

The following list summarizes the nature of the Original Qi:

- Original Qi is like Essence in 'Qi' form
- It originates between the two Kidneys
- It is derived from the Pre-Heaven Essence
- It is constantly replenished by the Post-Heaven Qi
- It is related to the Gate of Life (*Ming Men*)
- It relies on the transporting function of the Triple Burner to circulate throughout the body
- It circulates in the channels to emerge at the Source points

How can the Original Qi be treated in acupuncture? There are three ways:

1. Needling the Source points (see ch. 51) on the 12 channels
2. Needling and applying moxa to the points on the Directing Vessel below the navel, such as Ren-7 Yinjiao, Ren-6 Qihai, Ren-5 Shimen but especially Ren-4 Guangyuan
3. Needling and applying moxa to the point Du-4 Mingmen, which corresponds to the place from which the Original Qi originates

Clinical note

The Source (*Yuan*) is important to tonify the Internal Organs:
KI-3 Taixi for the Kidneys
LIV-3 Taichong for the Liver
HE-7 Shenmen for the Heart
SP-3 Taibai for the Spleen
LU-9 Taiyuan for the Lungs

Box 3.3 summarizes the functions of Original Qi.

Box 3.3 Functions of Original Qi

1. Is the Motive Force of all physiological activities
2. Is the basis of Kidney-Qi
3. Helps transformation of Gathering Qi (*Zong Qi*) into True Qi (*Zhen Qi*)
4. Helps transformation of Food-Qi (*Gu Qi*) into Blood
5. Comes out at the Source (*Yuan*) points

Food-Qi (*Gu Qi*) 谷 气

'*Gu Qi*', meaning 'Qi of grains' or 'Qi of Food', represents the first stage in the transformation of food into Qi.

Food on entering the Stomach is first 'rotted and ripened', and then is transformed into Food-Qi by the Spleen. This Food-Qi is not yet in a form that the body can use.

From the Middle Burner, Food-Qi rises to the chest and goes to the Lungs where, combining with air, it forms Gathering Qi, called in Chinese '*Zong Qi*' (Fig. 3.7).

From the Middle Burner, Food-Qi also rises to the chest and goes first to the Lungs, and then to the Heart, where it is transformed into Blood. This transformation is helped by Kidney-Qi and Original Qi (Fig. 3.8).

Food-Qi is produced by the Spleen, which has the very important function of transforming and transporting the various products extracted from food.

In so doing, the Spleen has to send the Food-Qi up to the chest: this is one reason why Spleen-Qi ascends. Spleen-Qi normally flows up: if it flows down, the food is not transformed properly and there will be loose stools.

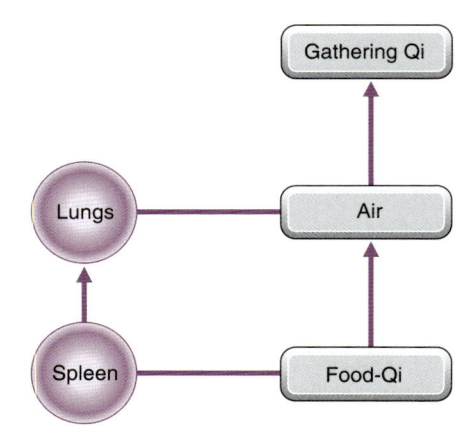

Figure 3.7 Food-Qi and Gathering Qi

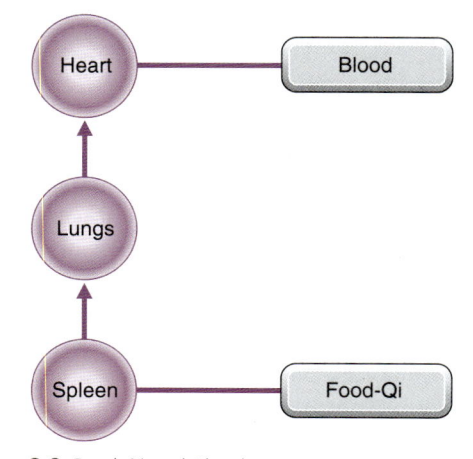

Figure 3.8 Food-Qi and Blood

Although Food-Qi represents the crucial first stage in the transformation of food into Qi, this coarse form of Qi cannot be used by the body as it is: it therefore is the basis for the transformation into more refined forms of Qi.

Since Food-Qi is extracted from food and is the basis for the production of all Qi and Blood, it is easy to see what importance Chinese medicine attributes to the quantity and quality of food eaten. The 'Spiritual Axis' in chapter 56 says: *'If no food is eaten for half a day, Qi is weakened, if no food is eaten for a whole day, Qi is depleted.'*[32] It is apparent from this statement that the ancient Chinese did not believe much in the therapeutic value of fasting!

Clinical note

To tonify Food-Qi (*Gu Qi*) use Ren-12 Zhongwan and ST-36 Zusanli

Food-Qi is summarized in Box 3.4.

Box 3.4 Food-Qi (*Gu Qi*)

- It originates from Stomach and Spleen
- It is the origin of Qi and Blood
- It rises to the chest where, in the Lungs, it combines with air to form Gathering Qi (*Zong Qi*)
- It rises to the chest where, in the Heart, it is transformed into Blood

Gathering Qi (*Zong Qi*) 宗气

This is called in Chinese '*Zong Qi*'. It is probably the type of Qi whose name has had the most translations. The character '*Zong*' 宗 usually means 'ancestor', and for this reason, it is sometimes translated as 'ancestral Qi', a confusing term as some authors use the name 'ancestral Qi' either for the Essence or for the Original Qi. Other authors call it 'genetic Qi', which is also confusing as, of all the types of Qi in the body, the Essence or the Original Qi would best qualify as being a 'genetic' Qi. In the international acupuncture training courses run in China, it is usually called 'Essential Qi'.

I call it 'Gathering Qi', as in the opinion of some authors the character '*Zong*' in this context means to 'gather' or 'collect together' rather than 'ancestor'.[33] I think this translation fits well the function of this type of Qi. The Gathering Qi is also sometimes called 'Chest-Qi' (*Xiong Qi*) or 'Big Qi' (*Da Qi*), or 'Big Qi of the Chest'.

As mentioned before, the Gathering Qi derives from the interaction of Food-Qi with air. The Spleen sends Food-Qi up to the Lungs where, combining with air, it is transformed into Gathering Qi (see Fig. 3.7).

Gathering Qi is a more subtle and refined form of Qi than Food-Qi, and it is usable by the body.

Its main functions are:

- Nourishes Heart and Lungs
- Enhances and promotes the Lung function of controlling Qi and respiration, and the Heart function of governing Blood and blood vessels
- Controls the speech and the strength of the voice
- Affects and promotes blood circulation to extremities

Gathering Qi is closely related to the functions of Heart and Lungs. It assists the Lung and Heart in their functions of controlling Qi and breathing and Blood and blood vessels, respectively. The 'Simple Questions' in chapter 18 says: *'The energy that comes out under the left breast and can be felt under the fingers, is the Gathering Qi.'*[34]

This means that Gathering Qi assists the Heart and Lungs to push Qi and Blood to the limbs, and especially into the hands. The 'Spiritual Axis' in chapter 75 says: *'If the Gathering Qi does not descend, the blood will stagnate in the vessels.'*[35] So if Gathering Qi is weak, the limbs, and especially the hands, will be cold.

Gathering Qi also gathers in the throat and influences speech (which is under the control of the Heart) and the strength of voice (which is under the control of the Lungs). Thus, if Gathering Qi is weak, the speech may be impeded, or the voice may be very weak and fine.

The 'Spiritual Axis' in chapter 71 comments: *'The Gathering Qi accumulates in the chest, rises to the throat, enters the Heart channel and aids breathing.'*[36]

In practice one can gauge the state of Gathering Qi from the health of the Heart and Lungs and from the circulation and voice. A weak voice shows weakness of Gathering Qi and so does poor circulation to the hands.

Being the energy of the chest, Gathering Qi is also affected by emotional problems such as grief and sadness which weaken the Lungs and disperse the energy in the chest. In these cases, both Front positions of left and right (which correspond to Heart and Lungs) of the pulse are very weak or empty.

Finally, Gathering Qi and Original Qi assist each other. Gathering Qi flows downwards to aid the Kidneys, and Original Qi flows upwards to aid breathing. This is another aspect of the relationship of mutual assistance that exists between Lungs and Kidneys.

> **Clinical note**
>
> To tonify Gathering Qi (*Zong Qi*) use Ren-17 Shanzhong and LU-9 Taiyuan

The chest area where Gathering Qi collects is also called the 'Sea of Qi'. This is one of the Four Seas discussed in chapter 33 of the 'Spiritual Axis'. The controlling point for the Sea of Qi (and the Gathering Qi) is Ren-17 Shanzhong. Gathering Qi is also treated via the Heart and Lung channels, and, of course, by breathing exercises (Box 3.5).

Box 3.5 Gathering Qi

- It nourishes Heart and Lungs
- It enhances and promotes the Lung function of controlling Qi and respiration, and the Heart function of governing Blood and blood vessels
- It controls the speech and the strength of voice
- It affects and promotes blood circulation to extremities
- It is coordinated with Original Qi to regulate breathing

True Qi (*Zhen Qi*) 真气

Called in Chinese '*Zhen Qi*', which literally means 'True Qi', this is the last stage of transformation of Qi. Gathering Qi is transformed into True Qi under the catalytic action of Original Qi. True Qi is the final stage in the process of refinement and transformation of Qi; it is the Qi that circulates in the channels and nourishes the organs (Fig. 3.9).

Like Gathering Qi, True Qi also originates eventually from the Lungs; hence the Lung's function of controlling Qi in general.

True Qi assumes two different forms: Nutritive Qi (*Ying Qi*) and Defensive Qi (*Wei Qi*). We cannot therefore discuss the functions of the True Qi without referring to its two different forms. True Qi is summarized in Box 3.6.

Box 3.6 True Qi (*Zhen Qi*)

- Originates from Gathering Qi (*Zong Qi*)
- Originates from the Lungs
- Assumes two forms: Nutritive Qi (*Ying Qi*) and Defensive Qi (*Wei Qi*)

Nutritive Qi (*Ying Qi*) 营气

This is called '*Ying Qi*' in Chinese. It literally means 'Nutritive' or 'Nourishing' Qi. As its name implies, this type of Qi has the function of nourishing the internal organs and the whole body.

Nutritive Qi is closely related to Blood and flows with it in the blood vessels, as well as, of course, in the channels.

The 'Simple Questions' in chapter 43 says: '*Nutritive Qi is extracted from food and water, it regulates the 5 Yin organs, moistens the 6 Yang organs, it enters the blood vessels, it circulates in the channels above and below, is linked with the 5 Yin organs and connects with the 6 Yang organs.*'[37]

This is the Qi that is activated whenever a needle is inserted in an acupuncture point.

The functions of Nutritive Qi are summarized in Box 3.7.

Box 3.7 Nutritive Qi (*Ying Qi*)

- Nourishes the Internal Organs
- Is closely linked to Blood
- Flows in channels and blood vessels

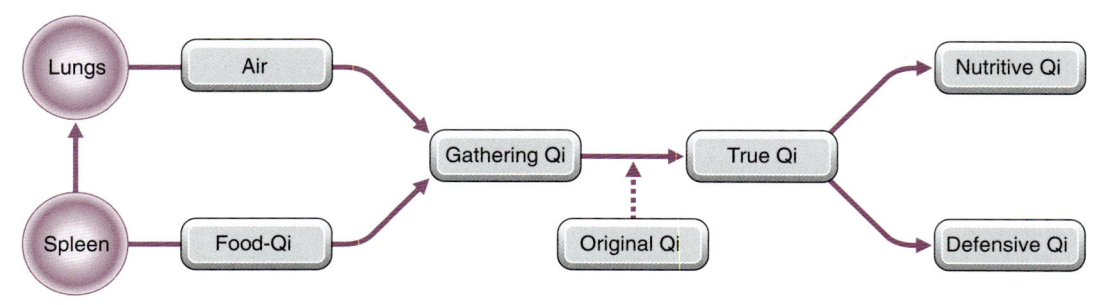

Figure 3.9 The Origin of Qi

Defensive Qi (Wei Qi) 卫气

Defensive Qi is called '*Wei Qi*' in Chinese. 'Wei' means 'to defend' or 'to protect'. Another form assumed by True Qi, when compared with the Nutritive Qi, Defensive Qi is a coarser form of Qi. As it flows on the outer layers of the body, it is Yang in relation to the Nutritive Qi which flows in the inner layers and the internal organs.

The 'Spiritual Axis' in chapter 18 says: '*The human being receives Qi from food: this enters the stomach, is transported to the Lungs [i.e. the Food-Qi] ... it is transformed into Qi, the refined part becomes Nutritive Qi, the coarse part becomes Defensive Qi. Nutritive Qi flows in the blood vessels [and channels], Defensive Qi flows outside the channels.*'[38]

The 'Simple Questions' in chapter 43 says: '*Defensive Qi is derived from the coarse part of food and water, it is slippery in nature, hence it cannot enter the channels. It therefore circulates under the skin, in between the muscles, it vapourizes in between membranes and diffuses over the chest and abdomen.*'[39]

To summarize:

- Nutritive Qi is in the Interior and nourishes
- Defensive Qi is on the Exterior and protects

Nutritive versus Defensive Qi

Nutritive Qi is in the Interior and nourishes, Defensive Qi is on the Exterior and protects.

The main function of Defensive Qi is to protect the body from the attacks of exterior pathogenic factors, such as Wind, Cold, Heat and Dampness. In addition, it warms, moistens and partially nourishes skin and muscles, it adjusts the opening and closing of the pores (and therefore regulates sweating) and (chiefly by so doing) it regulates the body temperature.

The 'Spiritual Axis' in chapter 47 says: '*Defensive Qi warms the muscles, fills up the skin, enters the space between skin and muscles, opens the pores.*'[40]

Being diffused under the skin, Defensive Qi comes under the control of the Lungs. The Lungs regulate the circulation of Defensive Qi to the skin and the opening and closing of the pores. Thus, a weakness of Lung-Qi may lead to a weakness of Defensive Qi. This can make someone prone to frequent colds.

Defensive Qi circulates outside the channels, in the skin and muscles: these are called the Exterior of the body, or also the 'Lung-Defensive Qi Portion'. The Lungs diffuse body fluids to the skin and muscles. These fluids mix with Defensive Qi so that a deficiency of Defensive Qi may cause spontaneous daytime sweating, because if Defensive Qi is weak it fails to hold the fluids in.

This also explains the rationale in promoting sweating when the body is invaded by exterior Wind-Cold. In such cases invading Wind-Cold obstructs the circulation of Defensive Qi in the skin and muscles, blocking the pores and impairing the diffusing function of the Lungs. By restoring the Lung's diffusing function and promoting sweating, the pores will be unblocked, the fluids come out as sweat and, mixed with them, the Wind-Cold is expelled. It is therefore said that the Defensive Qi spreads in the Upper Burner.

However, Defensive Qi also spreads in the Middle and Lower Burner. It spreads in the Middle Burner as it originates from the Food-Qi produced by Stomach and Spleen. On the other hand, the Essence and Original Qi stored in the Kidneys also play a role in the resistance to exterior pathogenic factors, as explained above. Thus, Defensive Qi originates also from the Essence and Original Qi and is transformed from Kidney-Yang. This is another reason why resistance to exterior pathogenic factors is determined by the strength not only of Lung-Qi but also of Kidney-Yang.

To summarize, Defensive Qi has its root in the Lower Burner (Kidneys), it is nourished by the Middle Burner (Stomach and Spleen), and it spreads outwards in the Upper Burner (Lungs). Functions of Defensive Qi are summarized in Box 3.8.

A deficiency of Defensive Qi causes a weakening of the body's defences against exterior pathogenic factors,

---

Box 3.8 Defensive Qi (*Wei Qi*)

- Has its root in the Lower Burner (Kidneys), it is nourished by the Middle Burner (Stomach and Spleen), and it spreads outwards in the Upper Burner (Lungs)
- It is a coarse form of Qi
- It circulates outside the channels in the space between skin and muscles
- It protects the body from invasion of external pathogenic factors
- It warms the muscles
- It is mixed with sweat in the space between skin and muscles and it regulates the opening and closing of pores
- It circulates 50 times in 24 hours: 25 during the day and 25 at night

and the person will be prone to catching cold frequently. The person will always tend to feel easily cold, as the deficient Defensive Qi fails to warm the skin and muscles.

Defensive Qi circulates 50 times in 24 hours: 25 times during the day and 25 times during the night. By day it circulates in the Exterior of the body, and at night it circulates in the Yin organs.[41] In the daytime, it circulates on the Exterior in the Yang superficial channels from the Greater Yang to Lesser Yang to Bright Yang channels. According to the 'Spiritual Axis', it is this very flow of Defensive Qi from the Interior towards the Exterior, emerging at the inner corner of the eye (meeting of Greater Yang Small Intestine and Bladder channels), that opens the eyes and wakes us up in the morning. At night, Defensive Qi flows into the Yin organs, first to the Kidneys, then to Heart, Lung, Liver, Spleen.[42]

As stated above, each 12-hour period is divided into 25 circuits. In the daytime, the Defensive Qi circulates first through Greater Yang, then Lesser Yang, then Bright Yang, and then Yin; it repeats this circuit 25 times. At night it circulates in the same order and again completes 25 circuits (Fig. 3.10).

Clinical note

To tonify the Defensive Qi (*Wei Qi*) use LU-9 Taiyuan and ST-36 Zusanli

Central Qi (*Zhong Qi*) 中 气

'Zhong' means 'middle' or 'centre'. In this case it indicates the Middle Burner. In fact, Central Qi is another way of defining the Qi of Stomach and Spleen, or the Post-Heaven Qi derived from food. It is also another term for the Spleen's function of transformation and transportation. In this sense, Central Qi is also True Qi, but specifically True Qi of the Stomach and Spleen.

The term 'Central Qi' also implies the Spleen's function of raising Qi and the condition of 'sinking' of Spleen-Qi is often referred to as 'deficiency of Central Qi'. Box 3.9 summarizes Central Qi.

Box 3.9 Central Qi (*Zhong Qi*)

Central Qi refers to:
- The True Qi of Stomach and Spleen
- The Spleen's function of transportation and transformation (*yun-hua*)
- The Spleen's function of raising Qi

Upright Qi (*Zheng Qi*) 正 气

The Upright Qi (*Zheng Qi*) is not really another type of Qi, but simply a general term to indicate the various types of Qi that have the function of protecting the body from invasion by exterior pathogenic factors. It should be noted that, although it is the Defensive Qi that circulates on the Exterior of the body to protect it from invasions of external pathogenic factors, the Nutritive Qi and even the Kidney-Essence play a role in the defence from pathogenic factors.

The term 'Upright Qi' is usually used in relation and in contrast to 'pathogenic factor' (*Xie Qi*), and it indicates the body's resistance to exterior diseases. Upright Qi is summarized in Box 3.10.

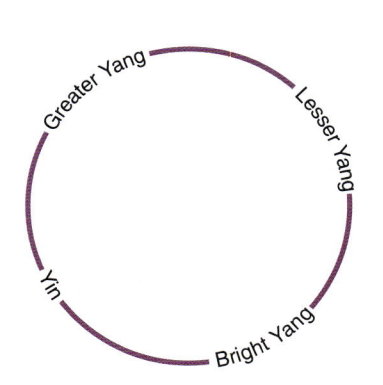

Figure 3.10 Circulation of Defensive Qi

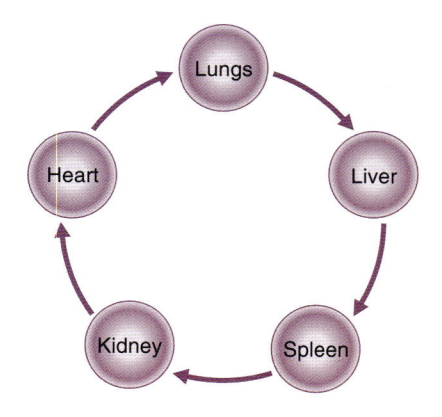

> **Box 3.10 Upright Qi (*Zheng Qi*)**
> - 'Upright Qi' indicates all the types of Qi that play a role in the defence of the body from invasion by external pathogenic factors. These include Defensive Qi, Nutritive Qi and Kidney-Essence
> - 'Upright Qi' (*Zheng Qi*) is contrasted to 'Pathogenic Factor' (*Xie Qi*)

Functions of Qi

Before concluding the discussion of Qi, we need to summarize the basic functions of Qi as observed in clinical practice, irrespective of their various types.

The basic functions of Qi are listed in Box 3.11.

It is worth giving here some examples of these functions of Qi, though these will be clearer after reading chapter 5 on the function of the internal organs (Fig. 3.11).

> **Box 3.11 Functions of Qi**
> - Transforming
> - Transporting
> - Holding
> - Raising
> - Protecting
> - Warming

Transforming

Qi (Yang in nature) is essential for the transformation of food and fluids (Yin in nature) into clear (Yang) and turbid (Yin) parts. This process of transformation is another aspect of the change in the state of aggregation/dispersion of Qi mentioned above. Material, dense forms of matter such as food and fluids need the power of Qi to be transformed into more subtle forms of matter, e.g. food is transformed into Food-Qi which is, in turn, transformed into True Qi.

Examples of transformation of various substances by Qi are: Spleen-Qi transforms food into Food-Qi, Stomach-Qi rots and ripens food, Kidney-Qi transforms fluids, Bladder-Qi transforms urine, Heart-Qi transforms Food-Qi into Blood, Lung-Qi transforms air into True Qi.

Transporting

Transportation, closely linked to transformation, is another essential function of Qi. In the process of transformation of various substances, Qi transports them in and out of various body structures. This transportation movement may be upwards, downwards, inwards or outwards. The ascending/descending and entering/exiting of Qi in the body constitutes what is called the Qi Mechanism (*Qi Ji*).

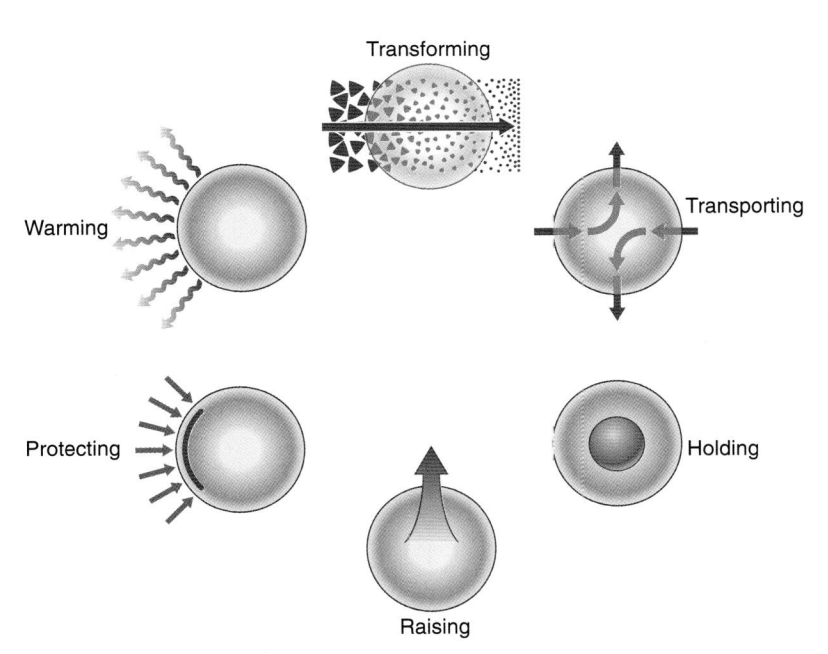

Figure 3.11 Functions of Qi

Examples of Qi transportation are: Spleen-Qi transports Food-Qi, Lung-Qi transports fluids to the skin and diffuses Defensive Qi to the space between skin and muscles, Kidney-Qi transports Qi both upwards to the Lungs and also downwards to the Bladder to transform and excrete fluids, Liver-Qi transports Qi in all directions, Lung-Qi transports Qi downwards.

Holding

'Holding' means that Qi (Yang in nature) holds fluids and Blood (Yin in nature) in their proper places. This is essential so that fluids or blood do not leak out.

Examples of the holding by Qi are: Spleen-Qi holds the Blood in the blood vessels and fluids in the proper spaces, both Spleen-Qi and Kidney-Qi hold Blood in the Uterus vessels, Kidney-Qi and Bladder-Qi hold urine, Lung-Qi holds sweat.

Raising

Qi ensures that the body structures are held in their proper place. If Qi is deficient, particularly in its raising function, it is said to be not only deficient but also 'sinking'.

Examples of raising by Qi are: Spleen-Qi raises the organs in general and Kidney-Qi raises the Uterus.

The raising by Qi refers also to its raising of fluids and Blood and this function is, of course, closely linked to the previous one, i.e. the 'holding' by Qi. In pathological conditions characterized by chronic leakage of mucus or blood (e.g. leukorrhoea and menorrhagia), not only is the holding function of Qi at fault but also its raising function.

Protecting

Qi protects the body from invasion of exterior pathogenic factors. This is primarily (but not exclusively) a function of Defensive Qi. Defensive Qi irrigates the space between the skin and muscles which constitutes the exterior energetic layer of the body. The strength of Defensive Qi in this space determines our resistance to external pathogenic factors such as Wind, Cold and Dampness. Defensive Qi is closely linked to the Lungs which spread it in the space between skin and muscles and therefore Lung-Qi protects the body from exterior pathogenic factors.

However, our overall resistance to external pathogenic factors does not depend only on the strength of Defensive Qi but partly also on that of Nutritive Qi and Kidney-Essence.

Warming

This is a function of Yang-Qi. Warming is an essential role for Qi as all physiological processes depend on 'warmth': this is especially crucial with fluids, as they are Yin in nature and therefore need Yang (warmth) to promote their transformation, transportation and excretion.

The source of Yang and warmth in the body is primarily Kidney-Yang and the Minister Fire. Spleen-Yang also warms the body but it, in turn, derives its warmth primarily from Kidney-Yang.

Direction of Qi movement

The normal physiological functions of the internal organs and the various types of Qi rely on a complex balance not only among the internal organs and between Yin and Yang but also on the direction of movement of Qi.

The 12 internal organs of the body all perform specific functions in relation to the different types of Qi. In order to function properly, the different types of Qi must flow in their appropriate directions.

The complex of different directions of Qi is called 'Ascending-descending and exiting-entering' in the Yellow Emperor's Classic. The 'Simple Questions' in chapter 68 says: *'Without exiting-entering of Qi, there would be no birth, growth, maturity and decline. Without ascending-descending, there would be no birth, growth, transformation, receiving and storage. All organs rely on the ascending-descending and exiting-entering of Qi.'*[43]

The complex of the ascending–descending and entering–exiting of Qi is called the 'Qi Mechanism' (*Qi Ji*). Let us look at some examples of the 'ascending–descending and exiting–entering of Qi' (Fig. 3.12 and Box 3.12).

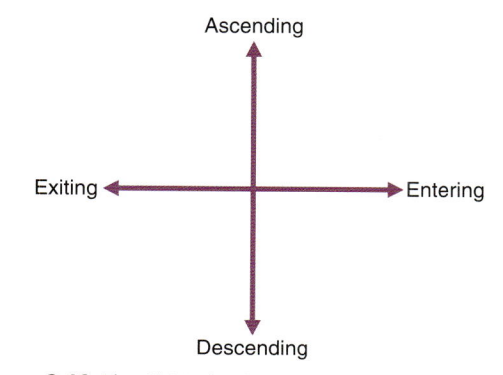

Figure 3.12 The Qi Mechanism

Box 3.12 Qi Mechanism (*Qi Ji*)

- 'Qi Mechanism' indicates the flow of Qi in all organs of the body, all Triple Burner cavities, joints, skin, muscles, diaphragm, Fat Tissue, Membranes
- The movement of Qi in the Qi Mechanism comprises the ascending–descending and entering–exiting of Qi in every part of the body
- The Qi Mechanism is like a vast system of roads and motorways (freeways) where traffic needs to be regulated by one-way streets
- The smooth movement of Qi in the Qi Mechanism relies on the proper ascending and descending of Qi in various organs and structures and also on the entering and exiting of Qi in and out of various structures
- The balance of Yin and Yang is crucial for the smooth movement of Qi, as ascending and exiting are Yang movements while descending and entering are Yin movements
- An excess of Yang will imply excessive ascending and exiting of Qi, while an excess of Yin will imply excessive descending and entering of Qi
- When the Qi Mechanism is disrupted, there will be Qi stagnation or Qi rebellious

and Bladder, it also ascends to diffuse Defensive Qi and sweat to the space between skin and muscles (see chapter 8).

Apart from regulating the ascending and descending, the Lungs also regulate the entering and exiting of Qi in and out of the space between skin and muscles. The entering and exiting of Qi in and out of this space regulates Defensive Qi and sweat and therefore also influences our resistance to external pathogenic factors. If Qi 'exits' too much from this space, the space is too 'open' and external pathogenic factors will enter easily; if Qi 'enters' too much into this space, the space is too 'closed' and when external pathogenic factors penetrate it, the patient will have a high fever.

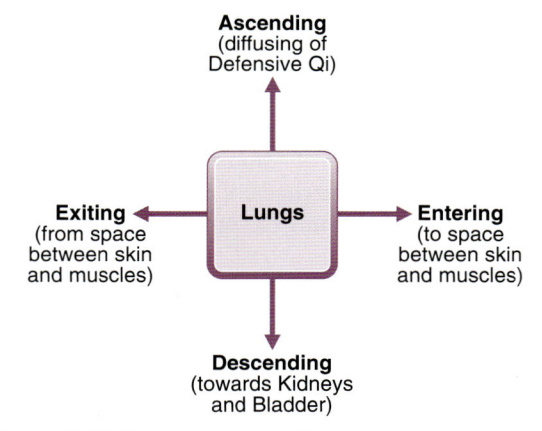

Figure 3.13 Directions of Lung-Qi

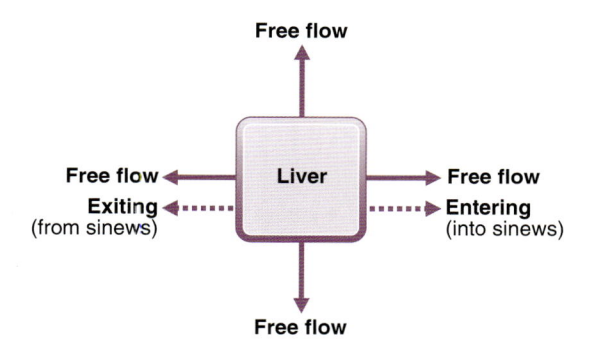

Figure 3.14 Directions of Liver-Qi

Lungs

The Lungs are the uppermost organ and are often compared to a 'lid' or 'canopy'. Their Qi, therefore, naturally descends. Lung-Qi descends towards the Kidneys: when Lung-Qi descends, breathing is normal; when Lung-Qi fails to descend, there is breathlessness or cough. Lung-Qi also descends to communicate with the Bladder and some urinary problems may be due to a Lung pathology, e.g. urinary retention in the elderly due to Lung-Qi deficiency (Fig. 3.13).

However, from some points of view, Lung-Qi also ascends. While Lung-Qi descends towards the Kidneys

Liver

The Liver controls the smooth flow of Qi in all directions. This smooth flow assists all the other organs and it helps them to channel their Qi in the right directions. For example, the smooth flow of Liver-Qi helps Stomach-Qi to descend and Spleen-Qi to ascend; it also helps the Qi of the Intestines and Bladder to descend. Conversely, if Liver-Qi stagnates, it may affect the direction of Qi of other organs, e.g. it may cause Stomach-Qi to ascend and Spleen-Qi to descend (Fig. 3.14).

The Liver has a close relationship with the Lungs. The normal ascending of Liver-Qi is coordinated with the descending of Lung-Qi. In terms of energy, though obviously not of anatomy, the Liver is on the left and the Lungs are on the right: Liver-Qi ascends while Lung-Qi descends. Thus, Lungs and Liver balance each other, in so far as Lung-Qi flows downwards and Liver-Qi flows upwards. This balance is another reflection of the balance existing between Metal and Wood in the Controlling Sequence of the Five Elements (Fig. 3.15).

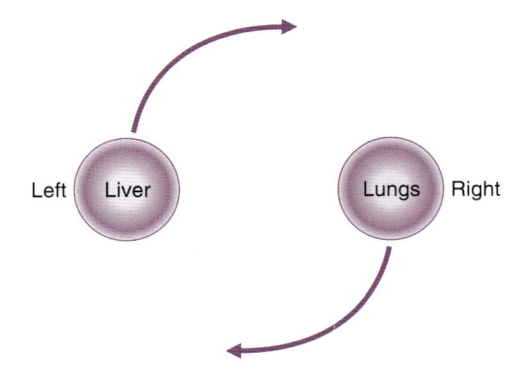

Figure 3.15 Directions of Liver-Qi and Lung-Qi

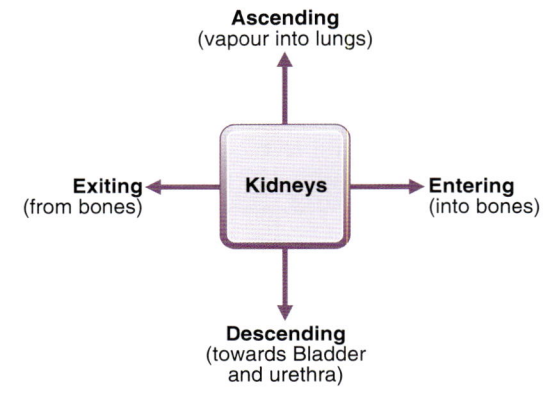

Figure 3.16 Directions of Kidney-Qi

Kidneys

The Kidneys control the transformation of Water, so that the impure fluids flow downwards and the clear part of fluids flows upwards along the spine. Therefore, for certain physiological functions (e.g. urination) Kidney-Qi descends, while for others (in relation to Defensive Qi) Kidney-Qi ascends (Fig. 3.16).

Lungs and Kidneys balance each other, as Lung-Qi descends to the Kidneys, and Kidney-Qi ascends to the Lungs. The Lungs send Qi down, the Kidneys receive Qi. The Lungs control exhalation, Kidneys control inhalation. Lung-Qi flows downwards, whilst Kidney-Qi flows upwards; one's Qi exits, the other's Qi enters (Fig. 3.17). Hence the 'Classic of Difficulties' in chapter 4 says: *'Exhalation is controlled by Lungs and Heart, inhalation is controlled by Kidneys and Liver.'*[44]

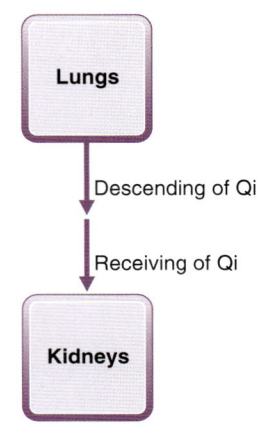

Figure 3.17 Directions of Lung-Qi and Kidney-Qi

The 'Complete Book of [Zhang] Jing Yue' (1634) says: *'The Lungs govern Qi, and the Kidneys are the root of Qi.'*[45]

Spleen–Stomach

The Spleen sends Qi upwards (to Lungs and Heart) and the Stomach sends (impure) Qi downwards. The Spleen controls transformation, the Stomach controls receiving. Hence the ascending of clear Qi and the descending of impure Qi depend on the ascending of Spleen-Qi and the descending of Stomach-Qi. If Spleen-Qi descends, it causes diarrhoea; if Stomach-Qi ascends, it causes nausea, belching or vomiting (Fig. 3.18).

Heart–Kidneys

Heart-Fire flows downwards to meet the Water of the Kidneys, and Kidney-Water rises to meet Heart-Fire. Thus, Heart-Qi descends to meet with Kidney-Qi, which ascends. The communication between Heart and Kidneys is crucial in many physiological processes and especially in the regulation of menstruation (Fig. 3.19).

Thus the normal physiological functioning of the organs depends on the correct direction of Qi flow. A derangement of these different directions can cause various problems. These arise when movement of Qi is impeded, or when the direction of movement is opposite to what it should be, and ascending–descending and exiting–entering are out of balance.

For example, Liver-Qi can stagnate (not flow smoothly in all directions) or it can ascend out of control. Stomach-Qi, as we have seen, can rise instead of descending, Spleen-Qi can descend instead of

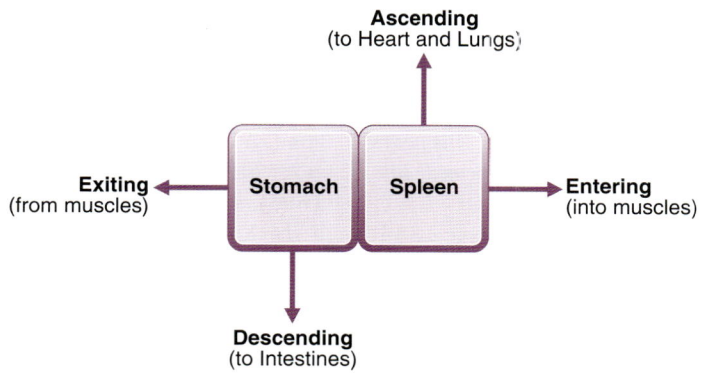

Figure 3.18 Directions of Stomach-Qi and Spleen-Qi

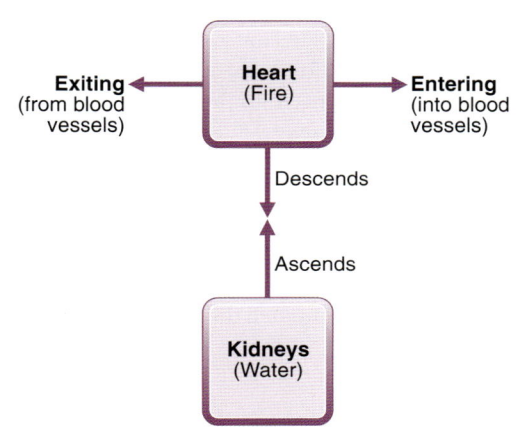

Figure 3.19 Directions of Heart-Qi and Kidney-Qi

ascending, Lung-Qi could fail to descend, Kidney-Qi could fail to receive and ascend, Kidney and Heart could fail to communicate and respond to each other. All these are fairly common pathological occurrences.

Pathology of Qi

Qi pathology can manifest in four different ways as follows:

Qi deficient

Qi can be deficient from various causes, often due to overwork or dietary irregularity. The Qi of Stomach, Spleen, Lungs or Kidneys is especially prone to being deficient.

Qi sinking

If Qi is deficient it can sink, causing prolapse of the organs. This applies mostly to Spleen-Qi and Kidney-Qi.

Qi stagnant

Qi can fail in its movement and stagnate. This applies mostly to Liver-Qi, but also, to a lesser extent, to other organs such as Intestines and Lungs.

Qi rebellious

Qi can flow in the wrong direction: this is called 'rebellious Qi'. Examples are Stomach-Qi failing to descend and flowing upwards, causing nausea or vomiting, or Spleen-Qi failing to ascend and flowing downwards, causing diarrhoea.

All these cases will be discussed in detail in chapter 9. Box 3.13 summarizes Qi pathology.

Box 3.13 Pathology of Qi

1. Qi deficiency
2. Qi sinking
3. Qi stagnation
4. Qi rebellious

Blood 血

The meaning of 'Blood' in Chinese medicine is different from its meaning in Western medicine. In Chinese medicine, Blood is itself a form of Qi, a very dense and material one, but Qi nevertheless. Moreover, Blood is inseparable from Qi itself as Qi infuses life into Blood; without Qi, Blood would be an inert fluid.

Source of Blood

Blood is derived mostly from the Food-Qi produced by the Spleen. The Spleen sends Food-Qi upwards to the Lungs, and through the pushing action of Lung-Qi this is sent to the Heart, where it is transformed into Blood (Fig. 3.20). The 'Spiritual Axis' says in chapter 18: '*The Stomach is in the Middle Burner, it opens onto the Upper Burner, it receives Qi, secretes the dregs, evaporates the fluids transforming them into a refined essence. This pours upwards towards the Lungs and is transformed into Blood.*'[46]

The 'Discussion on Blood' (by Tang Zong Hai, 1884) says: '*Water is transformed into Qi, Fire is transformed into Blood ... How can we say that Fire is transformed into Blood? Blood and Fire are both red in colour, Fire resides in the Heart where it generates Blood, which moistens the whole body. Fire is Yang, and it generates Blood that is Yin.*'[47]

Figure 3.20 illustrates three aspects of the origin of Blood.

1. The Spleen and Stomach are the main source of Blood
2. Lung-Qi plays an important role in pushing Food-Qi to the Heart: this is an example of the general principle that Qi makes Blood move
3. Food-Qi is transformed into Blood in the Heart: this is one aspect of the principle that the Heart governs Blood

According to Chinese medicine there are two other important features in the manufacture of Blood.

One is that the transformation of Food-Qi into Blood is aided by the Original Qi. The other is that the Kidneys store Essence, which produces Marrow: this, in turn, generates bone marrow, which contributes to making Blood. A doctor of the Qing dynasty, Zhang Lu, in his book 'Medical Transmission of the Zhang Family' (1695), says: '*If Qi is not exhausted, it returns essences to the Kidneys to be transformed into Essence; if the Essence is not depleted, it returns Essence to the Liver to be transformed into Blood.*'[48]

From this it is evident that the Kidneys play an important role, as they store Essence and are the source of Original Qi. We can therefore say that Blood is generated by the interaction of the Post-Heaven Qi of the Stomach and Spleen (which are the source of Food-Qi) and the Pre-Heaven Qi (as the Kidneys play a role in its formation). This is illustrated in Figure 3.21. So to nourish Blood, we need to tonify the Spleen and Kidneys.

It seems remarkable that the Chinese account of the blood-forming function of bone marrow, so similar to that given by Western physiology, was formulated during the Qing dynasty before the introduction of Western medicine into China. Lin Pei Qin, a doctor of the Qing dynasty, formulated the theory that 'Liver and

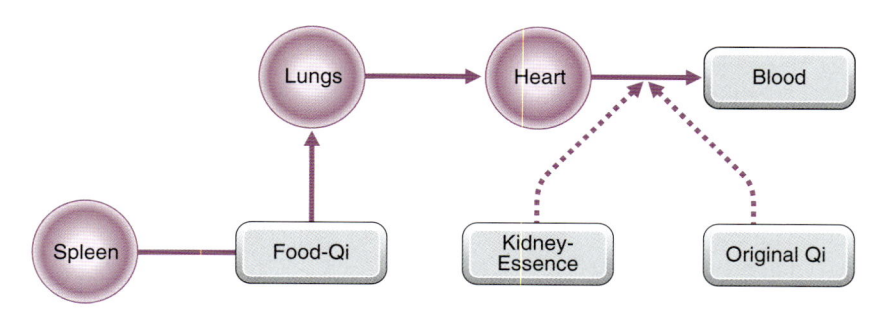

Figure 3.20 Origin of Blood

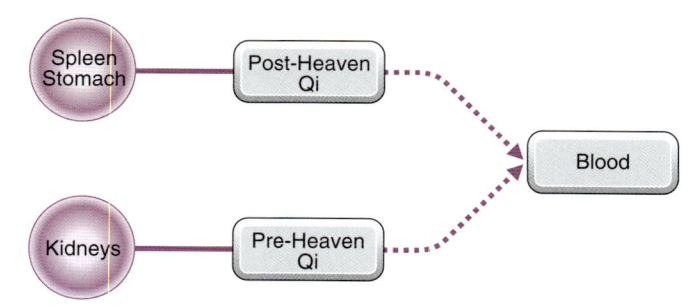

Figure 3.21 Post-Heaven and Pre-Heaven sources of Blood

Kidneys have the same source' and that Blood is transformed from the Kidney-Essence.[49]

Functions of Blood

The main function of Blood is that of nourishing the body. It complements the nourishing action of Qi. Blood is a dense form of Qi and it flows with it all over the body.

Besides providing nourishment, Blood also has a moistening function, which Qi does not have. The Blood ensures that body tissues do not dry out. For example, Liver-Blood moistens eyes and sinews, so that the eyes can see properly and the sinews are flexible and healthy. Liver-Blood also moistens the skin and the hair, ensuring that the skin is not too dry and the hair remains shiny and healthy. Heart-Blood moistens the tongue.

Blood is very important also in another way: it provides the material foundation for the Mind (*Shen*). Blood is part of Yin (as it is dense and fluid-like) and it houses and anchors the Mind. Blood embraces the Mind, providing the harbour within which the Mind can flourish.

The 'Simple Questions' in chapter 26 says: '*Blood is the Mind of a person.*'[50] The 'Spiritual Axis' in chapter 32 says: '*When Blood is harmonized, the Mind has a residence.*'[51]

If the Blood is deficient, the Mind will lack its foundation and so become unhappy or uneasy. This is typically manifested by a 'deficient restlessness' characterized by a vague anxiety, a slight irritability, and a feeling of dissatisfaction. When someone is asleep at night Blood naturally embraces the Mind and the Ethereal Soul, but if Blood is deficient the Mind and Ethereal Soul 'float' and the person cannot sleep or dreams a lot.

Clinical note

To nourish Blood use Ren-4 Guanyuan (especially in women), ST-36 Zusanli, LIV-8 Ququan and SP-6 Sanyinjiao

Blood is summarized in Box 3.14.

Relation of Blood with internal organs

Heart

The Heart governs Blood and the blood vessels, which are responsible for its circulation. As we have seen, the Heart is also the place where the Blood is made through

Box 3.14 Blood

- Originates from Food-Qi (*Gu Qi*) in the Heart under the agency of Original Qi
- The Kidneys contribute to making Blood through Marrow and Kidney-Essence
- Nourishes the body
- Circulates with Nutritive Qi (*Ying Qi*)
- Moistens the body
- Houses the Mind
- Determines menstruation

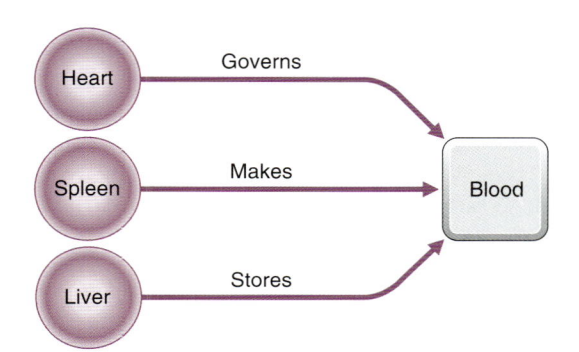

Figure 3.22 Relationship of Heart, Spleen and Liver with Blood

the agency of Heart-Fire. Fire is Yang and it transforms into Yin (Blood). Blood cools down the Fire, preventing it from flaring up excessively. The 'Discussion on Blood' written in 1884 by Tang Zong Hai says: '*Fire is Yang and generates Blood which is Yin. On the other hand, Blood nourishes Fire and makes sure that Fire does not flare up, whilst Blood moistens the lower Burner. It is stored in the Liver, it fills the Sea of Blood and the Penetrating, Directing and Girdle extraordinary vessels, and it warms and nourishes the whole body ... When Blood moistens the Lower Burner and the Sea of Blood, and Heart-Fire follows it down to the umbilicus, then Blood is flourishing and Fire does not flare excessively, so that men are free of disease and women are fertile.*'[52]

From this passage it is apparent that the Heart is essential for the formation of Blood, and that it also has to flow downwards to the Lower Burner to interact with Blood (Fig. 3.22).

Chinese pulse diagnosis confirms that the Heart corresponds to Blood and the Lungs to Qi. Since the Heart is felt on the left side and the Lung on the right, the left side can be taken to reflect the state of Blood, while the right pulse indicates the state of Qi.

Spleen

The Spleen is related to the Blood in two ways. First of all it is the origin of Blood as it produces Food-Qi, which is the basis for the formation of Blood.

Secondly, Spleen-Qi ensures that Blood remains in the blood vessels and does not extravasate. If Spleen-Qi is deficient, Qi cannot hold Blood, and haemorrhages may result.

Liver

The Liver stores Blood: this important function has several meanings. First, from a physiological point of view, when a person is erect and engaged in normal everyday movement, Blood flows to the muscles and sinews. When a person lies down, Blood flows back to the Liver. Wang Ping, a doctor from the Tang dynasty, said: '*When the person is active, Blood circulates in the vessels, when the person rests, Blood goes back to the Liver*'.[53]

When lying down, the Blood regenerates itself in the Liver: hence the importance of having adequate rest (especially lying down), in cases of deficient Liver-Blood.

Second, Blood stored in the Liver has the function of moistening the eyes, which promotes good sight, and moistening the sinews, which promotes flexibility of joints. Chapter 10 of the 'Simple Questions' says: '*Blood goes to the Liver during sleep, so that, when adequately supplied with Blood, the eyes can see, the hands can hold, the fingers can grasp, the feet can walk.*'[54] The 'Spiritual Axis', in chapter 47, says: '*When the Blood is harmonized ... the sinews are strong and the joints supple.*'[55]

Thirdly, a very important aspect of the Liver storage of Blood is in relation to the physiology and pathology of menstruation. The Blood of the Liver supplies the uterus with Blood and is closely related to the Penetrating Vessel (*Chong Mai*). This vessel also supplies the uterus with Blood, but ultimately this supply also is dependent on the provision of Blood from the Liver. Thus Liver-Blood is extremely important for a regular and healthy menstrual function (Fig. 3.23).

The importance of Liver-Blood in women's physiology is partly explained by the close connection existing between Kidneys and Liver. It is said in Chinese medicine that 'Kidneys and Liver have a common origin'. The Kidneys store Essence and the Liver stores Blood. The Kidneys are the mother of the Liver according to the Five Elements, and so Essence and Blood mutually

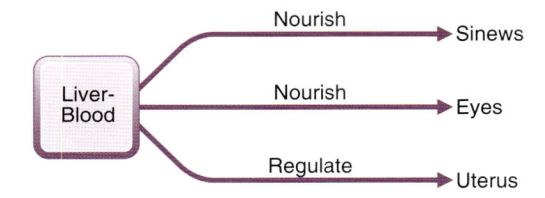

Figure 3.23 Functions of Liver-Blood

influence each other. Essence can be transformed into Blood as mentioned above; on the other hand, Blood also nourishes and replenishes Essence. The Kidney-Essence controls the reproductive function and since it influences Blood, Blood also influences the reproductive function in women. The reason this is more relevant in women than in men is that women's physiology is more dependent on Blood than that of men. For these reasons, it is said that Kidney and Liver have a common origin, and the state of Liver-Blood is extremely important for women's menstrual function.

For example, if Liver-Blood is deficient, this can lead to amenorrhoea or scanty periods; stagnant Liver-Blood can be a cause of painful periods.

Although the storage of Blood by the Liver is essential for a healthy menstrual function, it should be remembered that menstrual blood originates directly from the Kidney-Essence. As mentioned above when discussing the Essence, this matures into *Tian Gui* during puberty (14 years for girls and 16 for boys). Menstrual blood is *Tian Gui* and it is therefore a precious fluid that is a direct manifestation of Kidney-Essence (in the same way that sperm is for men) (Box 3.15).

Lungs

The Lungs affect Blood in several ways. First of all they assist the Spleen in sending Food-Qi to the Heart where it is transformed into Blood.

Besides this, the Lungs control all the channels and blood vessels. This means that the Lungs infuse

---

Box 3.15 *Tian Gui*

Tian Gui is menstrual blood in women and sperm in men. It originates directly from the Kidney-Essence and it matures at puberty. Thus, although part of 'Blood', menstrual blood is a more precious fluid because it derives directly from the Kidney-Essence.

Qi into the blood vessels to assist the pushing action of the Heart. This is another aspect of the relationship between Qi and Blood, which will be discussed in detail below.

Kidneys

As mentioned above, the Kidneys contribute to the production of Blood in two ways: Original Qi assists in the transformation of Food-Qi into Blood, and the Kidney-Essence can also be transformed into Blood.

The implication of this in clinical practice is that, in order to nourish Blood, we need to tonify the Spleen and Kidneys.

Of all the above organs, however, the Heart, Spleen and Liver are the most important ones with relation to Blood. The Heart governs Blood, the Spleen holds Blood in the vessels and the Liver stores Blood.

Blood–Qi relationship

There is a very close relationship between Qi and Blood. Blood is a form of Qi, albeit a very dense one. Qi is Yang if compared with Blood (as it is more subtle), Blood is Yin if compared with Qi (as it is denser).

Qi and Blood are inseparable: Nutritive Qi circulates with Blood in the blood vessels. The close relationship between Qi and Blood is borne out by the fact that the ancient classics seem to use the word *mai* ambiguously, meaning both a 'channel' where Qi flows and also a 'vessel' where Blood flows.

The close relationship between Blood and Qi can be observed in the clinical signs following a serious haemorrhage: often in these cases, after a massive loss of blood, the person develops signs of Qi deficiency, such as sweating, breathlessness and cold limbs. On the other hand, after prolonged and heavy sweating (which depletes Qi), one may develop signs of Blood deficiency, such as pallor, numbness, dizziness and palpitations (Fig. 3.24).

There are four aspects to the Blood–Qi relationship (Fig. 3.25).

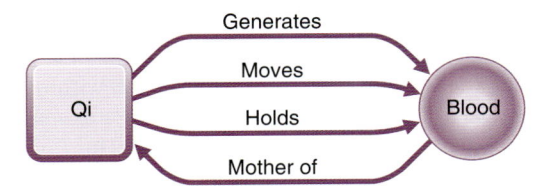

Qi generates Blood

Qi generates Blood in so far as Food-Qi is the basis for Blood, and also Lung-Qi is essential for the production of Blood.

Thus, if Qi is deficient, Blood will eventually also be deficient. In practice, it is often necessary to tonify Qi in order to nourish Blood. This is particularly important in herbal practice, as the herbs to tonify Qi and nourish Blood are in different categories, whereas in acupuncture practice, the difference is not so clear-cut.

Qi moves Blood

Qi is the motive force for Blood. Without Qi, Blood would be an inert substance. Nutritive Qi is very closely related to Blood and flows with it in the blood vessels. Lung-Qi infuses the necessary Qi into the blood vessels.

This relationship between Qi and Blood is often expressed by the saying: '*When Qi moves, Blood follows*', and also '*If Qi stagnates, Blood congeals*'.

If Qi is deficient or stagnant, it cannot push the Blood, which will stagnate.

Qi holds the Blood

Qi holds Blood in the blood vessels, thus preventing haemorrhages. This function belongs primarily to the Spleen. If Spleen-Qi is deficient, Qi cannot hold Blood, and there may be haemorrhages. However, Kidney-Qi also plays an important role in keeping Blood in the Uterus vessels.

The above three aspects of Qi–Blood relationship are often expressed in the saying: '*Qi is the commander of Blood*'.

Blood nourishes Qi

Whereas Blood relies on Qi's generating, pushing and holding actions, Qi, on the other hand, relies on the nutritive function of Blood.

Blood affects Qi in two ways. First of all, Qi relies on Blood for nourishment. Secondly, Blood provides a material and 'dense' basis which prevents Qi from 'floating' and giving rise to symptoms of Empty-Heat.

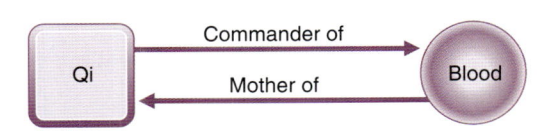

Figure 3.24 Relationship between Qi and Blood

Figure 3.25 Relationship between Qi and Blood

Both these aspects of the Blood–Qi relationship are often expressed in the saying: '*Blood is the mother of Qi*'.

Blood–Essence relationship

Blood and Essence mutually affect each other. Each of them can transform into the other.

As we have already seen, Essence plays an important role in the formation of Blood. On the other hand, Blood continually nourishes and replenishes the Essence.

Blood pathology

There are three basic cases of pathology of Blood:

Blood deficiency

Blood can be deficient when not enough is manufactured. This is mostly caused by a deficiency of Spleen-Qi and Stomach-Qi. However, other organs are also implicated and particularly the Liver and Kidneys.

Blood deficiency manifesting primarily in the menstrual function with scanty periods or amenorrhoea is generally due to a deficiency of the Kidneys and Liver.

Blood Heat

Blood can be hot: this is mostly due to Liver-Heat. As the Liver stores Blood, Liver-Heat or Liver-Fire is transmitted to the Blood, making it 'hot'. In women Blood Heat often causes heavy periods; many skin diseases are due to Blood Heat.

Clinical note

To cool Blood use L.I.-11 Quchi and SP-10 Xuehai

Blood stasis

The Blood can fail to move properly and stagnate. This may be caused by stagnation of Qi (mostly of the Liver), by Heat, or by Cold. All these cases will be discussed in detail in chapter 9. Blood stasis often causes pain.

Clinical note

To invigorate (move) Blood use KI-14 Siman, SP-10 Xuehai and LIV-3 Taichong

Box 3.16 summarizes Blood pathology.

Box 3.16 Blood pathology

1. Blood deficiency
2. Blood Heat
3. Blood stasis

Body Fluids 津 液

Body Fluids are called '*Jin-Ye*' in Chinese. This word is composed of two characters, '*Jin*', meaning 'moist' or 'saliva', and '*Ye*', meaning 'fluid'. '*Jin*' indicates anything that is liquid, while '*Ye*' indicates fluids of living organisms (those found in fruit, for instance). Thus, '*Jin-Ye*' could be translated as 'organic fluids'. I will refer to them as 'Body Fluids'.

Source

Body Fluids originate from our food and drink. These are transformed and separated by the Spleen: some 'clean' fluids then go up from the Spleen to the Lungs, which spread some of them to the skin and send some of them down to the Kidneys; from the Spleen, some 'dirty' fluids go down to the Small Intestine where they are separated again, this time into pure and impure. Following this second separation the pure fluids go to the Bladder and the impure fluids go to the Large Intestine, where some water is re-absorbed. The Bladder further transforms and separates the fluids it receives into pure and impure. The pure fluids flow upwards and go to the Exterior of the body where they form sweat. The impure fluids flow downwards and are transformed into urine.

The Bladder effects this transformation and separation by the power of Qi, which it receives from Kidney-Yang: this function of the Bladder is called 'function of Qi transformation'.

The 'Simple Questions' in chapter 21 says: '*Fluids enter the Stomach and they are separated. A pure part flows upwards from the Spleen to the Lungs, which direct them to the Water Passages and then downwards to the Bladder.*'[56]

The process of formation of Body Fluids is the result of an intricate series of purification processes, each stage further separating the fluids into a pure and impure part. For this reason the Chinese talk of a 'pure within the impure' part and an 'impure within the pure' part. The pure fluids need to be transported upwards, the impure fluids downwards. This correct movement of the pure and the impure fluids depends on the correct ascending/descending and entering/

exiting of Qi and is essential to their proper transformation. Many organs contribute to the transformation, transportation and excretion of Body Fluids but primarily the Lungs, Spleen and Kidneys.

The pure fluids flow upwards to the Lungs, which distribute some to the space under the skin, and some downwards to the Kidneys. For this reason, the Lungs are called the 'Upper Source of Water'. Impure fluids flow downwards to the Small Intestine and the Bladder which carries out its further separation and transformation as described above. The Bladder function of Qi transformation is controlled by Kidney-Yang: hence the Kidneys are called the 'Lower Source of Water' (Fig. 3.26).

Relations with internal organs

Spleen

The Spleen is the most important organ in relation to the physiology and pathology of Body Fluids. It controls the initial transformation and separation into a pure and impure part, as described above. It also controls the crucial direction of moving pure and impure fluids upwards and downwards, respectively, at all stages of Body Fluids production.

For this reason, the Spleen is always treated in any type of disorders of Body Fluids (Fig. 3.27).

Lungs

The Lungs control the diffusing of the pure part of Body Fluids coming from the Spleen to the space under the skin. This is an aspect of the Lung's diffusing function.

They also send some of the fluids down to the Kidneys and Bladder. This is an aspect of the Lung's descending function.

Because of these two functions, the Lungs are said to regulate the 'Water passages'.

Kidneys

The Kidneys are extremely important in the physiology of Body Fluids. First, they vaporize some of the fluids

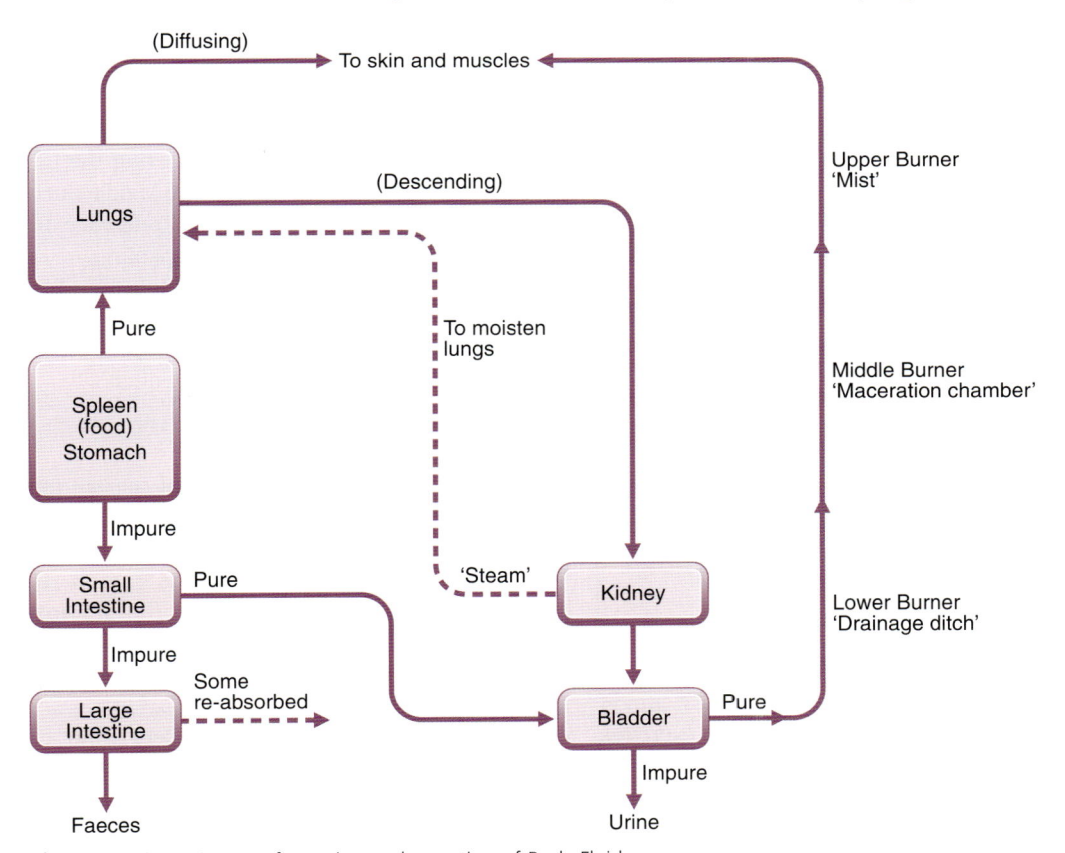

Figure 3.26 Origin, transformation and excretion of Body Fluids

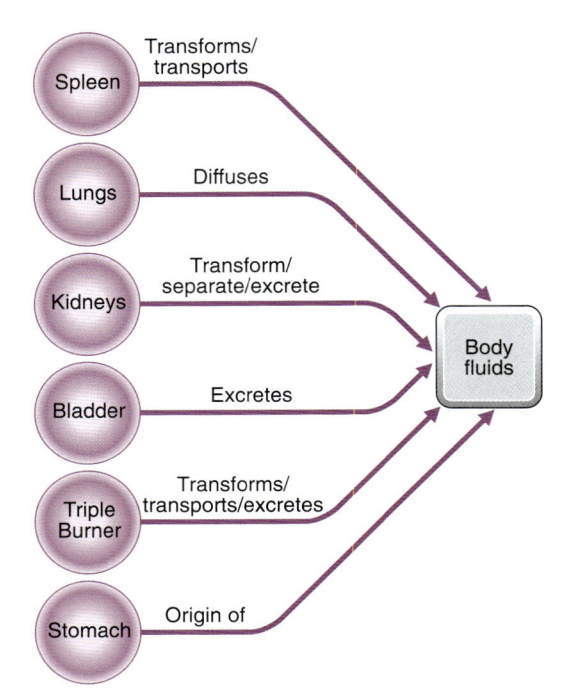

Figure 3.27 Relationship between Internal Organs and Body Fluids

they receive and send them back up to the Lungs, to moisten the Lungs and prevent their getting too dry.

Furthermore, the Kidneys, in particular Kidney-Yang, control many stages of the transformation of fluids. In particular:

- They provide the heat necessary for the Spleen to transform Body Fluids. For this reason, a deficiency of Kidney-Yang nearly always results in a deficiency of Spleen-Yang, with consequent accumulation of fluids
- They assist the Small Intestine in its function of separation of Body Fluids into a pure and impure part
- They provide Qi to the Bladder for its function of Qi transformation
- They assist the Triple Burner transformation and excretion of fluids

For all these reasons, Kidney-Yang is extremely important for the transformation, separation and excretion of fluids.

Small Intestine

The Small Intestine separates the fluids it receives from the Stomach into a 'clean' part which goes to the Bladder for excretion as urine, and a 'dirty' part which goes to the Large Intestine partly for re-absorption and partly for excretion in the stools (see Fig. 14.2).

The Small Intestine function of separating fluids is controlled by the action of Kidney-Yang, which provides the Qi and the heat necessary for this separation to take place.

Bladder

The Bladder separates the fluids it receives into a pure and impure part and it excretes urine by the power of Qi transformation.

Triple Burner

The Triple Burner assists the transformation, transportation and excretion of fluids at all stages. The 'Simple Questions' in chapter 8 says: '*The Triple Burner is the official in charge of irrigation and it controls the water passages.*'[57]

The Upper Burner assists the Spleen in directing the pure fluids upwards, and the Lungs in dispersing them to the space under the skin. For this reason, the Upper Burner is compared with a 'mist'.

The Middle Burner assists the Stomach in its function of churning the fluids and directing the impure part downwards. For this reason, the Middle Burner is compared with a 'muddy pool' (a reference to the Stomach's function of rotting and ripening).

The Lower Burner assists the Small Intestine, Bladder and Kidneys in their functions of transforming, separating and excreting fluids. For this reason, the Lower Burner is compared with a 'drainage ditch'.

Stomach

Even though the Stomach does not appear to play an important role in the transformation of Body Fluids, it nevertheless is the 'source' of Body Fluids. The fluids first enter the Stomach and from there they are transformed and separated by the Spleen. The Stomach likes to be relatively moist, in contrast to the Spleen, which likes dryness and is damaged by too much dampness.

In fact, the Stomach easily suffers from excess dryness, and this can lead to Stomach-Yin deficiency.

For this reason, wet, slippery foods (such as rice or oat porridge) are beneficial to the Stomach, and an excess of very dry foods (such as foods roasted or broiled for a long time) may damage Stomach-Yin.

Types of Body Fluids

There are two types of body fluids:

Fluids in Chinese called *Jin*
Liquids in Chinese called *Ye*

> **Box 3.17 Types of body fluids**
>
> - Fluids (*Jin*): clear, light and watery, they circulate with Defensive Qi in the space between skin and muscles. They moisten skin and muscles
> - Liquids (*Ye*): turbid, heavy and dense, they circulate with Nutritive Qi in the Interior. They moisten brain, spine, bone marrow, joints and sense organs

The 'Spiritual Axis' in chapter 30 says: '*The body fluids that are dispersed in the space between skin and muscles and come out as sweat are the fluids [Jin] ... when food enters the body and Qi is abundant, fluids overflow to the bones, enabling them to bend, irrigating and tonifying the brain and marrow, and moistening the skin; these are called liquids [Ye].*'[58]

Fluids (*Jin*)

The *Jin* fluids are clear, light and thin-watery and they circulate with Defensive Qi on the Exterior (skin and muscles). They move relatively quickly. They are under the control of the Lungs, which spread them to the skin all over the body, and of the Upper Burner, which controls their transformation and movement towards the skin.

Their function is to moisten and in part to nourish skin and muscles. Exuded as sweat, these fluids also manifest as tears, saliva and mucus.

Another important function of the fluids is to become a component of the fluid part of Blood. In other words, these fluids thin the Blood out and prevent its stasis. We discuss this further when dealing with the relation between Blood and fluids.

Liquids (*Ye*)

The *Ye* fluids are more turbid, heavy and dense. They circulate with Nutritive Qi in the Interior. They move relatively slowly. They are under the control of the Spleen and Kidneys for their transformation, and of the Middle and Lower Burner for their movement and excretion. The 'Spiritual Axis' in chapter 36 says: '*The Qi of the Triple Burner goes to the muscles and skin and is transformed into fluids [Jin]. Other body fluids do not move and are transformed into liquids [Ye].*'[59]

Their function is to moisten the joints, spine, brain and bone marrow. They also lubricate the orifices of the sense organs, i.e. eyes, ears, nose and mouth. Box 3.17 summarizes the types of Body Fluids.

Relation between Qi and Body Fluids

Qi and Body Fluids are related in many ways. First of all, Qi transforms and transports fluids. This is an extremely important aspect of the Qi–Body Fluids relationship. Without the transforming and transporting power of Qi, Body Fluids would accumulate, giving rise to disease.

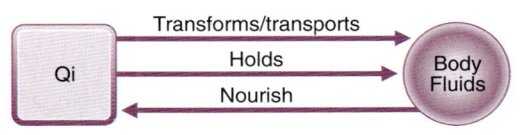

Figure 3.28 Relationship between Qi and Body Fluids

Secondly, Qi also holds in Body Fluids, in the same way as it holds blood. If Qi is deficient, the fluids may leak out, and give rise to urinary incontinence or enuresis (deficiency of Kidney-Qi), spontaneous sweating (deficiency of Lung-Qi) or chronic vaginal discharges (deficiency of Spleen-Qi).

Thirdly, while Qi produces Body Fluids, these, on the other hand, play a minor part in nourishing Qi. A deficiency of the Stomach and Spleen may, in the long run, cause deficiency of fluids (as the Stomach is the origin of fluids). Also, after a significant loss of fluids, such as occurs in profuse sweating, Qi also becomes deficient, and the person may suffer from cold limbs, pallor, dislike of cold, i.e. symptoms of Yang deficiency (Fig. 3.28).

This is because the fluids that form sweat in the space between skin and muscles are blended with Defensive Qi, and profuse sweating also causes a loss of Defensive Qi. Since Defensive Qi pertains to Yang, it is said in Chinese medicine that 'Profuse sweating injures Yang'. Qi may also be consumed by excessive vomiting: hence the saying 'Persistent vomiting certainly depletes Qi'.

On the other hand, if Qi is deficient, fluids may leak out in the form of sweat: hence the saying 'Qi deficiency causes sweating'.

Relationship between Blood and Body Fluids

There is a relationship of mutual nourishment between fluids and Blood. On the one hand, Body Fluids constantly replenish Blood and make it thinner so that it does not coagulate or stagnate. The 'Spiritual Axis' in

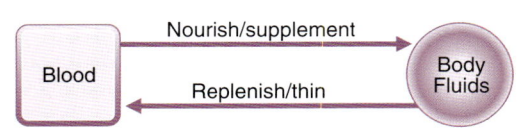

Figure 3.29 Relationship between Blood and Body Fluids

chapter 71 says: '*Nutritive Qi secretes Body Fluids; these enter the blood vessels and are transformed into Blood.*'[60] And also, in chapter 81: '*If Body Fluids are harmonized, they turn red and are transformed into Blood.*'[61]

On the other hand, Blood can also nourish and supplement Body Fluids. Both Blood and Body Fluids pertain to Yin and are somewhat interchangeable. For this reason, if there is a significant loss of Body Fluids over a long period of time, as in chronic spontaneous sweating (or excessive use of saunas), this can lead to deficiency of Blood. Vice versa, if there is a chronic loss of blood, as in menorrhagia, this can lead to deficiency of Body Fluids and dryness (Fig. 3.29).

Because Blood and Body Fluids come from the same source and mutually nourish each other, sweating and bleeding treatment methods are contradictory in practice, and should never be used together. Also, if the patient is bleeding, one should not induce sweating; while if the patient is sweating, bleeding as a treatment method is contraindicated. The 'Spiritual Axis' says in chapter 18: '*If there is profuse bleeding, do not cause sweating; if there is profuse sweating, do not cause bleeding.*'[62] Also, the 'Discussion on Cold-induced Diseases' says: '*In a patient with severe deficiency of Blood, do not cause sweating.*'[63]

Pathology of body fluids

The Body Fluids can be pathologically altered in two different ways:

- Deficiency of Body Fluids
- Accumulation of Body Fluids in the form of oedema, Dampness or Phlegm

These will be dealt with in detail in the chapter on the identification of Qi–Blood–Body Fluids patterns (ch. 31). Box 3.18 summarizes pathology of Body Fluids.

Mind (*Shen*) 神

The Mind (*Shen*) is one of the Vital Substances of the body. As we have seen above, the Vital Substances take

Box 3.18 Pathology of Body Fluids

- Deficiency of Body Fluids (dryness)
- Accumulation of Body Fluids (oedema)

shape in different degrees of aggregation of Qi: the Mind is the most subtle and non-material type of Qi. The word *Shen* is often translated as 'Spirit' in Western acupuncture books and schools; but I prefer to translate *Shen* as 'Mind' since I believe that what we would call 'Spirit' in the West is the complex of all five mental–spiritual aspects of a human being: i.e. the Ethereal Soul (*Hun*) pertaining to the Liver; the Corporeal Soul (*Po*) pertaining to the Lungs; the Intellect (*Yi*) pertaining to the Spleen; the Will-power (*Zhi*) pertaining to the Kidneys; and the Mind (*Shen*) itself.

I translate *Shen* as 'Mind' and use 'Spirit' for the complex of Ethereal Soul (*Hun*), Corporeal Soul (*Po*), Intellect (*Yi*), Will-power (*Zhi*) and Mind (*Shen*) itself

What, then, is the Chinese view of the Mind? As explained above, the Mind, like other Vital Substances, is a form of Qi; in fact, it is Qi's most subtle and non-material type. One of the most important characteristics of Chinese medicine is the close integration of body and mind which is highlighted by the integration of Essence (*Jing*), Qi and Mind, called the 'Three Treasures'.

The Essence is the origin and biological basis of the Mind. The 'Spiritual Axis' in chapter 8 says: '*Life comes about through the Essence; when the two Essences [of mother and father] unite, they form the Mind.*'[64] Zhang Jie Bin says: '*The two Essences, one Yin, one Yang, unite … to form life; the Essences of mother and father unite to form the Mind.*'[65]

Therefore the Mind of a newly conceived being comes from the Pre-Natal Essences of its mother and father. After birth, its Pre-Natal Essence is stored in the Kidneys and this provides the biological foundation for the Mind. The life and Mind of a newly born baby, however, also depend on the nourishment from its own Post-Natal Essence. The 'Spiritual Axis' in chapter 30 says: '*When the Stomach and Intestines are coordinated the 5 Yin organs are peaceful, Blood is harmonized and mental activity is stable. The Mind derives from the refined essence of water and food.*'[66] Thus the Mind draws its basis and nourishment from the Pre-Natal Essence stored in the Kidneys and the Post-Natal Essence produced by the Stomach and Spleen.

Hence the Three Treasures:

```
MIND = HEART
Qi = STOMACH–SPLEEN
ESSENCE = KIDNEYS
```

These Three Treasures represent three different states of condensation of Qi, the Essence being the densest, Qi the more rarefied, and the Mind the most subtle and non-material. The activity of the Mind relies on the Essence and Qi as its fundamental basis. Hence the Essence is said to be the 'foundation of the body and the root of the Mind'. Thus if Essence and Qi are strong and flourishing, the Mind will be happy, balanced and alert. If Essence and Qi are depleted, the Mind will suffer and may become unhappy, depressed, anxious, or clouded. Zhang Jie Bin says: '*If the Essence is strong, Qi flourishes; if Qi flourishes, the Mind is whole.*'[67] However, the state of the Mind also affects Qi and Essence. If the Mind is disturbed by emotional stress, becoming unhappy, depressed, anxious or unstable, it will definitely affect Qi and/or the Essence. In most cases it will affect Qi first since all emotional stress upsets the normal functioning of Qi. Emotional stress will tend to weaken the Essence either when it is combined with overwork and/or excessive sexual activity, or when the Fire generated by long-term emotional tensions injures Yin and Essence.

Of all the organs, the Mind is most closely related to the Heart, which is said to be the Mind's 'residence'. The 'Simple Questions' in chapter 8 says: '*The Heart is the Monarch and it governs the Mind ...*'.[68] The 'Spiritual Axis' in chapter 71 says: '*The Heart is the Monarch of the 5 Yin organs and 6 Yang organs and it is the residence of the Mind.*'[69]

The 'Mind' residing in the Heart is responsible for many different mental activities. Box 3.19 summarizes these.

Of course many of these activities are also carried out by other organs and there is often an overlap between the functions of various organs. For example, although the Mind is mainly responsible for memory, the Spleen and Kidneys also play a role.

Let us now briefly look at the above functions in more detail.

Box 3.19 Functions of the Mind (*Shen*)

- Consciousness
- Thinking
- Memory
- Insight
- Cognition
- Sleep
- Intelligence
- Wisdom
- Ideas
- Affections
- Feelings
- Senses

Consciousness indicates the totality of thoughts and perceptions as well as the state of being conscious. This is the most important of the Mind's characteristics. The Mind residing in the Heart is what makes us conscious as human beings, what gives each of us a sense of being an individual. In psychological terms, we may compare the Mind (*Shen*) with the ego consciousness. The Mind is responsible for the recognition of thoughts, perceptions and feelings. When the Mind is clear, we are conscious; if the Mind is obfuscated or suddenly depleted, we lose consciousness.

Thinking depends on the Mind. If the Mind is strong, thinking will be clear. If the Mind is weak or disturbed, thinking will be slow and dull. The Chinese characters for 'thought' (*yi*), 'to think' (*xiang*) and 'pensiveness' (*si*) all have the character for 'heart' as their radical.

Memory has two different meanings. On the one hand, it indicates the capacity of memorizing data when one is studying or working and, on the other hand, the ability to remember past events. Both of these depend on the Mind and therefore the Heart, although also on the Spleen and Kidneys.

Insight indicates our capacity for self-knowledge and self-recognition. We are subjected to many different emotional stimuli, perceptions, feelings and sensations and all of these are perceived and recognized by the Mind. Insight is lost when the Mind is obstructed by Phlegm, resulting in serious mental illness such as psychosis.

Cognition refers to higher mental processes, memory, language, problem solving, and abstract thinking.

Sleep is dependent on the state of the Mind. If the Mind is calm and balanced, a person sleeps well. If the Mind is restless, the person sleeps badly.

Intelligence also depends on the Heart and the Mind. A strong Heart and Mind will make a person intelligent and bright. A weak Heart and Mind will render a person slow and dull. It should be remembered, however, that the Essence, and therefore heredity, plays a role in determining a person's intelligence.

Wisdom derives from a strong Heart and a healthy Mind. As the Mind is responsible for knowing and perceiving, it also gives us the sagacity to apply this knowledge critically and wisely.

Ideas are another function of the Mind. The Heart and Mind are responsible for our ideas, our projects and the dreams that give our lives purpose. However, the Ethereal Soul also plays an important role in this area.

Affections depend on the Mind as only the Mind (and therefore the Heart) can 'feel' them. I use the term 'affections' to indicate the normal range of affective feelings which all human beings experience; I use the term 'emotions' for affections that, due to being intense and prolonged, become causes of disease. Of course affection and emotions definitely affect all the other organs too, but it is only the Mind that actually recognizes and feels them. For example, anger affects the Liver, but the Liver cannot feel it because it does not house the Mind. Only the Heart can feel it because it houses the Mind, which is responsible for insight. It is for this reason that all emotions eventually affect the Heart (in addition to other specific organs), and it is in this sense that the Heart is the 'emperor' of all the other organs.

Feelings depend on the Mind as it is the Mind that recognizes the stimuli generated by perceptions, touch, taste, pressure, temperature.

Senses and sense organs also rely on the Mind. Each sense is related to a certain organ, i.e. smell to the Lungs, taste to the Spleen and Heart, hearing to the Kidneys and sight to the Liver. However, all senses rely also on the Heart because it is the Mind that ultimately receives the sensory perceptions. The eyes and sight are obviously related to the Liver, especially Liver-Blood, and the Ethereal Soul. However, although the eyes rely on the nourishment from Liver-Blood, blood flows to the eyes through blood vessels which are under the control of the Heart. The 'Simple Questions' says in chapter 10: *'Blood vessels influence the eyes.'*[70] In fact, the 'Simple Questions' also lists excessive use of the eyes as harmful to the blood vessels and Heart. It says in chapter 23: *'Excessive use of the eyes injures Blood [i.e. the Heart].'*[71]

Ren Ying Qiu, in 'Theories of Chinese medicine Doctors', says: *'The Heart governs the Mind ... sight is a manifestation of the activity of the Mind.'*[72] Wang Ken Tang, in 'Standards of Diagnosis and Treatment' (1602) says: *'The eye is an orifice of the Liver ... but a function of the Heart.'*[73] As the Heart influences the eyes, excessive use of the eyes may damage the Heart and therefore the Mind: this explains the damaging effect of excessive TV-watching on the eyes and the Mind in children.

Hearing depends on the Kidneys but the Heart also has an influence on it in so far as it brings Qi and Blood to the ears. The 'Simple Questions', in chapter 4, says: *'The colour of the Southern direction is red, it is related to the Heart which opens into the ears ...'*.[74] Some types of tinnitus are due to Heart-Qi being deficient and not reaching the ears.

The sense of smell is also dependent on the Heart and Mind as well as the Lungs. The 'Simple Questions' in chapter 11 says: *'The five odours enter the nose and are stored by Lungs and Heart; if Lungs and Heart are diseased, the nose cannot smell.'*[75] The 'Classic of Difficulties' in chapter 14 says: *'The nose pertains to the Lungs but its function depends on the Heart.'*

The sense of taste naturally depends on the Heart and Mind as the tongue is an offshoot of the Heart.

The sense of touch is also dependent on the Heart and Mind as this is responsible for the cognition and organization of external stimuli sensations.

To sum up, all sensations of sight, hearing, smell, taste and touch depend on the Mind in much the same way as they depend on the brain in Western medicine.

All senses (sight, hearing, taste, smell, touch) depend on the Heart and the Mind (*Shen*)

Thus if the Heart is strong and the Mind healthy, a person can think clearly, memory is good, consciousness and insight are sharp, the cognition is clear, sleep is sound, intelligence is bright, actions show wisdom, ideas flow easily. If the Heart is affected and the Mind weak or disturbed, a person is unable to think clearly, memory is poor, consciousness is clouded, insight is poor, sleep is restless, intelligence is lacking, actions are unwise and ideas are muddled.

Most of the above functions of the Mind are attributed to the brain in Western medicine. During the course of development of Chinese medicine, too, there have been doctors who attributed mental functions to the brain rather than the Heart: in particular, Sun Si Miao of the Tang dynasty, Zhao You Qin of the Yuan dynasty, Li Shi Zhen of the Ming dynasty and especially Wang Qing Ren of the Qing dynasty.

The Mind is closely related to our affective life because only it can 'feel' affections and feelings. It follows, therefore, that all emotions, besides affecting the relevant organ directly, also affect the Heart and the Mind because it is the latter that 'feels' them. It alone, being responsible for consciousness, affection and feelings, can recognize and feel the effect of emotions. Fei Bo Xiong (1800–1879) put it very clearly when he said: *'The seven emotions injure the 5 Yin organs selectively, but they all affect the Heart. Joy injures the Heart ... Anger injures the Liver, the Liver cannot recognize anger but the Heart can, hence it affects both Liver and Heart. Worry injures the Lungs, the Lungs cannot recognize it but the Heart can, hence it affects both Lungs and Heart. Pensiveness injures the Spleen, the Spleen cannot recognise it but the Heart can, hence it affects both Spleen and Heart.'*[76] Yu Chang in 'Principles of Medical Practice' (1658) says: *'Worry agitates the Heart and has repercussions on the Lungs; pensiveness agitates the Heart and has repercussions on the Spleen; anger agitates the Heart and has repercussions on the Liver; fear agitates the Heart and has repercussions on the Kidneys. Therefore all the five emotions [including joy] affect the Heart.'*[77]

All emotions affect the Heart besides affecting their relevant organ, e.g. anger affects not only the Liver but also the Heart

Chinese writing clearly bears out the idea that all emotions affect the Heart since the characters for all seven emotions are based on the 'heart' radical.

The way that all emotions afflict the Heart also explains why Heart-Fire indicated by a red tip of the tongue is so commonly seen even in emotional problems related to other organs.

Learning outcomes

In this chapter you will have learned:
- The origin, nature and functions of the Pre-Heaven Essence, Post-Heaven Essence and Kidney-Essence
- The origin, nature, functions and brief pathology of Original Qi, Food-Qi, Gathering Qi, True Qi, Nutritive Qi and Defensive Qi
- The functions of Qi in general (transforming, transporting, holding, raising, protecting, warming)
- Directions of Qi movement for each organ
- The origin, nature, functions and brief pathology of Blood
- Relation between Blood and Qi
- Relation between Blood and Essence
- The origin, nature, functions and brief pathology of Body Fluids
- Types of Body Fluids
- Relation between Body Fluids and Blood
- Relation between Body Fluids and Qi
- The functions of the Mind (*Shen*)

Self-assessment questions

1. What does the ancient Chinese character for 'Qi' portray and how does this relate to its nature?
2. List four functions of the Kidney-Essence.
3. What are the Three Treasures and what is their clinical significance?
4. List at least three functions of the Original Qi.
5. Where does Food-Qi derive from?
6. How is Gathering Qi formed?
7. How is True Qi formed?
8. Compare and contrast briefly Nutritive and Defensive Qi.
9. What is the Qi Mechanism?
10. List the physiological direction of Qi movement of Heart, Lungs and Liver.
11. How is Blood formed?
12. Which organs are mostly involved with Blood?
13. What is the relationship between Qi and Blood?
14. Which organs are primarily involved in the transformation, transportation and excretion of Body Fluids?
15. Why is bleeding therapy contraindicated in people who are sweating and sweating therapy contraindicated in people who are bleeding?
16. Why is a red tip of the tongue very common in patients suffering from emotional problems?

See p. 1255 for answers

END NOTES

1. He Zuo Xiu 1968 The Materialistic Theory of Yuan Qi – One of the Brilliant Philosophical Ideas of the Legalist School. Institute of High Energy Physics, Academia Sinica. In: Scientia Sinica, vol. 18, no. 6, Beijing.
2. Needham J 1956 Science and Civilization in China, vol. 2, Cambridge University Press, Cambridge, p. 472.

3. Science and Civilization in China, p. 302.
4. He Zuo Xiu 1968 The Materialistic Theory of Yuan Qi, p. 697.
5. Science and Civilization in China, p. 372.
6. Wing Tsit Chan 1969 A Source Book in Chinese Philosophy, Princeton University Press, Princeton, New Jersey, p. 307.
7. A Source Book in Chinese Philosophy, p. 300.
8. Science and Civilization in China, p. 373.
9. A Source Book in Chinese Philosophy, p. 501.
10. A Source Book in Chinese Philosophy, p. 503.
11. The Materialistic Theory of Yuan Qi, p. 704.
12. Fung Yu Lan 1966 A Short History of Chinese Philosophy, Macmillan, New York, p. 280.
13. Science and Civilization in China, p. 480.
14. Science and Civilization in China, p. 512.
15. The Materialistic Theory of Yuan Qi, p. 704.
16. The Materialistic Theory of Yuan Qi, p. 705.
17. The Materialistic Theory of Yuan Qi, p. 705.
18. 1979 The Yellow Emperor's Classic of Internal Medicine – Simple Questions (*Huang Di Nei Jing Su Wen* 黄帝内经素问). People's Health Publishing House, Beijing, first published c.100 BC, p. 158–159.
19. Nanjing College of Traditional Chinese Medicine 1979 A Revised Explanation of the Classic of Difficulties (*Nan Jing Jiao Shi* 难经校释), People's Health Publishing House, Beijing, first published c.AD 100, p. 17.
20. The 'Room of Sperm' is not an anatomical, physical structure but it simply indicates the Lower *Dan Tian* in a man where sperm was thought to be made by the Kidneys.
21. Classic of Difficulties, p. 90.
22. The ability to enhance the Pre-Heaven Essence in the course of one's lifetime can be compared with the process of adding peat to poor soil in order to 'condition' it. Even though peat does not actually add fertilizing substances to the soil, it increases its fertility by improving the condition and structure of the soil and making the absorption of nutrients by the rootlet system of plants easier. Similarly, even though we cannot quantitatively increase our Pre-Heaven Essence, we can improve the 'soil' of all the body's energies, so that the Pre-Heaven Essence can issue forth and nourish the body more effectively.
23. Wu Qian 1742 The Golden Mirror of Medical Collection, cited in 1981 Syndromes and Treatment of the Internal Organs (*Zang Fu Zheng Zhi* 脏腑证治), Tianjin Scientific Publishing House, Tianjin, p. 34.
24. Simple Questions, p. 4–6.
25. 1981 Spiritual Axis (*Ling Shu Jing* 灵枢经), People's Health Publishing House, Beijing, first published c.100 BC, p. 73.
26. Simple Questions, p. 24.
27. Classic of Difficulties, p. 144.
28. Ibid., p. 144.
29. Unschuld PU 1986 Medicine in China – Nan Ching The Classic of Difficult Issues, University of California Press, Berkeley, USA, p. 561.
30. Clavey S 2002 Fluid Physiology and Pathology in Traditional Chinese Medicine, 2nd edition, Churchill Livingstone, Edinburgh, p. 34–35.
31. Classic of Difficulties, p. 144.
32. Spiritual Axis, p. 104.
33. Dr Chen Jing Hua, personal communication, London, 1986.
34. Simple Questions, p. 111.
35. Spiritual Axis, p. 137.
36. Spiritual Axis, p. 126.
37. Simple Questions, p. 245.
38. Spiritual Axis, p. 51.
39. Simple Questions, p. 245.
40. Spiritual Axis, p. 89.
41. Ibid., p. 139.
42. Ibid., p. 140.
43. Simple Questions, p. 400.
44. Classic of Difficulties, p. 8.
45. Zhang Jing Yue 1634 Complete Book of [Zhang] Jing Yue (*Jing Yue Quan Shu* 景岳全书), cited in Syndromes and Treatment of the Internal Organs, p. 24.
46. Spiritual Axis, p. 52.
47. Tang Zong Hai 1884 Discussion on Blood Patterns (*Xue Zheng Lun* 血证论), edited by Pei Zheng Xue and Yin Xin Min, People's Health Publishing House, 1979, p. 14 and 16.
48. Zhang Lu Medical Transmission of the Zhang Family (*Zhang Shi Yi Tong* 张氏医通), cited in Syndromes and Treatment of the Internal Organs, p. 27.
49. Personal communication from Prof. Meng Jing Chun, Nanjing, 1982. See also Academy of Traditional Chinese Medicine and Guangzhou College of Traditional Chinese Medicine 1980 Concise Dictionary of Chinese Medicine (*Jian Ming Zhong Yi Ci Dian* 简明中医辞典), People's Health Publishing House, Beijing, p. 508.
50. Simple Questions, p. 168.
51. Spiritual Axis, p. 72.
52. Discussion on Blood Patterns, p. 16.
53. Syndromes and Treatment of the Internal Organs, p. 131.
54. Simple Questions, p. 73.
55. Spiritual Axis, p. 89.
56. Simple Questions, p. 139–140.
57. Simple Questions, p. 59.
58. Spiritual Axis, p. 71.
59. Spiritual Axis, p. 76–77.
60. Spiritual Axis, p. 126.
61. Spiritual Axis, p. 153.
62. Spiritual Axis, p. 72.
63. Discussion on Cold-induced Diseases, cited in Syndromes and Treatment of the Internal Organs, p. 41.
64. 1981 Spiritual Axis (*Ling Shu Jing*), People's Health Publishing House, Beijing, first published c.100 BC, p. 23.
65. Zhang Jie Bin 1982 Classic of Categories (*Lei Jing* 类经), People's Health Publishing House, Beijing, p. 49. First published in 1624.
66. Spiritual Axis, p. 71.
67. Classic of Categories, p. 63.
68. 1979 The Yellow Emperor's Classic of Internal Medicine – Simple Questions (*Huang Di Nei Jing Su Wen*), People's Health Publishing House, Beijing, first published c.100 BC, p. 58.
69. Spiritual Axis, p. 128.
70. Simple Questions, p. 72.
71. Ibid., p. 154.
72. Ren Ying Qiu 1985 Theories of Chinese Medicine Doctors cited in Wang Ke Qin 1988 Theory of the Mind in Chinese Medicine (*Zhong Yi Shen Zhu Xue Shuo* 中医神主学说), Ancient Chinese Medical Texts Publishing House, Beijing, p. 22.
73. Wang Ken Tang 1602 Standards of Diagnosis and Treatment (*Zheng Zhi Zhun Sheng*), cited in Theory of the Mind in Chinese Medicine, p.22.
74. Simple Questions, p. 26.
75. Ibid., p. 78.
76. Fei Bo Xiong et al. 1985 Medical Collection from Four Families from Meng He (*Meng He Si Jia Yi Ji* 孟河四家医集), Jiangsu Science Publishing House, p. 40.
77. Principles of Medical Practice, cited in Theory of the Mind in Chinese Medicine, p. 34.

BIBLIOGRAPHY AND FURTHER READING

Clavey S 2002 Fluid Physiology and Pathology in Traditional Chinese Medicine, 2nd edition, Churchill Livingstone, Edinburgh

Kaptchuk T 2000 The Web that has no Weaver – Understanding Chinese Medicine, Contemporary Books, Chicago

Needham J 1977 Science and Civilization in China, vol. 2, Cambridge University Press, Cambridge

PART 1

The Transformations of Qi 4

> **Key contents**
>
> **The Original Qi as the Motive Force for the transformation of Qi**
>
> **The Fire of the Gate of Life as the warmth for the transformation of Qi**
>
> **The dynamics and physiology of transformation of Qi**
> The Qi Mechanism
> - Ascending–descending of Qi
> - Entering–exiting of Qi
>
> The Stomach and Spleen as the 'central axis'
> The Liver and Lungs as the 'outer wheel'
> The Heart and Kidneys as the 'root'
>
> **The Triple Burner's transformation of Qi**
>
> **Pathology of Qi transformation**
> Stomach and Spleen
> Liver and Lungs
> Heart and Kidneys

Human physiology is based on the transformation of Qi. As we have seen, Qi can assume different forms depending on its states of aggregation or dispersal, and it is the motive force of all physiological processes. In the course of its work, Qi assumes many different forms: it is transformed, changed, transported, condensed, dispersed, it enters, exits, rises and descends. All these functional activities of Qi are generally called 'transformation of Qi', as constant transformation and transmutation are the essence of human Qi physiology.

Qi in aggregation forms the material body and is Yin in nature; Qi in dispersal moves and transforms and is Yang in nature. The Yin and Yang aspects of Qi form the basis of human physiology. If Qi is transformed properly, movement, birth, growth and reproduction can take place.

If Qi is flourishing there is health, if it is weak there is disease; if it is balanced there is quietness, if it moves in the wrong direction there is disease. Thus the transformation and proper direction of movement of Qi is the basis for the movement of Blood, the transformation of the Essence, the movement, transformation and excretion of Body Fluids, the digestion of food, the absorption of nourishment, the excretion of waste, the moistening of sinews and bones, the moistening of skin and the resistance to exterior pathogenic factors.

In a broad sense transformation of Qi includes all the various physiological processes and movements of Qi; in a narrow sense, it indicates the transformation of Qi by the Triple Burner.

The discussion of the transformation of Qi will be articulated in the following aspects:

- The Original Qi (*Yuan Qi*) as the Motive Force for the transformation of Qi
- The Fire of the Gate of Life (*Ming Men*) as the warmth for the transformation of Qi
- The dynamics and physiology of transformation of Qi
  - The Qi Mechanism
    - Ascending–descending of Qi
    - Entering–exiting of Qi
  - The Stomach and Spleen as the 'central axis'
  - The Liver and Lungs as the 'outer wheel'
  - The Heart and Kidneys as the 'root'
- The Triple Burner's transformation of Qi
- Pathology of Qi transformation
  - Stomach and Spleen
  - Liver and Lungs
  - Heart and Kidneys

THE ORIGINAL QI AS THE MOTIVE FORCE FOR THE TRANSFORMATION OF QI

The 'Motive Force' is discussed in chapter 66 of the 'Classic of Difficulties'. The Motive Force for the

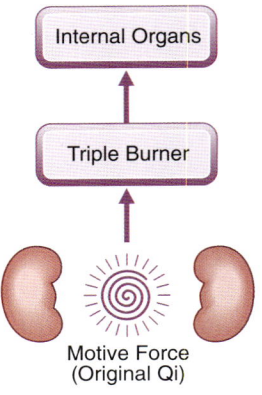

Figure 4.1 Motive force and the Triple Burner

transformation of Qi arises from between the Kidneys and it is another name for the Original Qi (*Yuan Qi*).

As discussed in chapter 3, the Original Qi is related to the Essence and it plays an important role as motive force for transformation in all physiological activities. For example, as discussed in chapter 3, it brings about the transformation of Gathering Qi (*Zong Qi*) into True Qi (*Zhen Qi*), it facilitates the transformation of Food-Qi (*Gu Qi*) into Blood, it is the basis of all Kidney's physiological activities, and so on. Although related to it, Original Qi differs from the Essence (*Jing*) as, compared with it, it is a more rarified form of Qi: indeed, it circulates in the channels and it emerges at the Source points (*Yuan* points).

The Original Qi can be seen as the dynamic motive force that is behind all movement and transformation of Qi in every part of the body. Chapter 66 of the 'Classic of Difficulties' discusses the connection between the Original Qi (in this chapter called *Dong Qi*, 'Motive Force'). It says: '*The Original Qi is the motive force situated between the two kidneys, it is life-giving and it is the root of the 12 channels. The Triple Burner causes the Original Qi to differentiate [for its different uses around the body]; the Original Qi passes through the Three Burners and then spreads to the 5 Yin and 6 Yang organs and their channels. The places where the Original Qi stays are the Source [Yuan] points*'[1] (Figs 4.1 and 4.2).

Other authors translate this passage saying that the Triple Burner is the '*special envoy*' that '*transmits*' the Original Qi.[2] I have adopted Clavey's interpretation of this passage: that is, that the Triple Burner makes the Original Qi separate and differentiate in its different forms in different places around the body.[3] If interpreted in this way, the Triple Burner plays the very

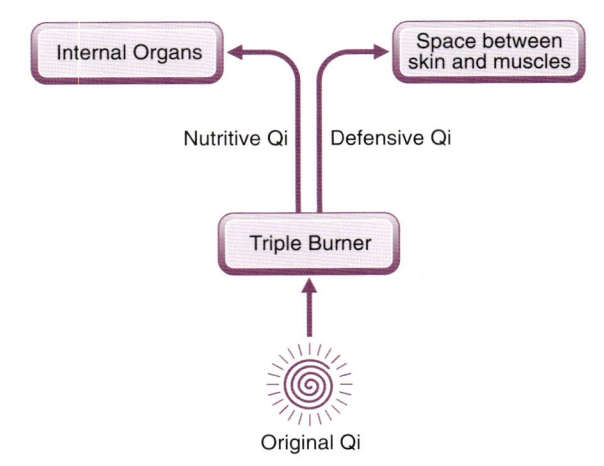

Figure 4.2 Original Qi and the Triple Burner

important role of allowing the Original Qi to facilitate the transformation of Qi in different places around the body assuming different forms in each place.

Clinical note

The Original Qi can be tonified by using KI-3 Taixi with either Du-4 Mingmen or Ren-4 Guanyuan

Box 4.1 summarizes the Original Qi as the motive force for the transformation of Qi.

Box 4.1 The Original Qi (*Yuan Qi*) as the motive force for the transformation of Qi

- Original Qi (*Yuan Qi*) is the Motive Force between the Kidneys (ch. 66 of the 'Classic of Difficulties' (*Nan Jing*))
- Original Qi is the dynamic force driving all movement and transformation of Qi in every part of the body
- The Triple Burner allows the Original Qi emerging from between the kidneys to differentiate in its different forms for its different functions around the body

---

THE FIRE OF THE GATE OF LIFE AS THE WARMTH FOR THE TRANSFORMATION OF QI

The Motive Force between the Kidneys is equivalent to the Original Qi but is also related to the Fire of the Gate of Life (*Ming Men*), itself also called Minister Fire. Zhang Jing Yue (1563–1640) said: '*The Fire of the Gate of Life is the Sea of Essence and Blood, the Stomach and Spleen are the Sea of Food and Water: the two together are*

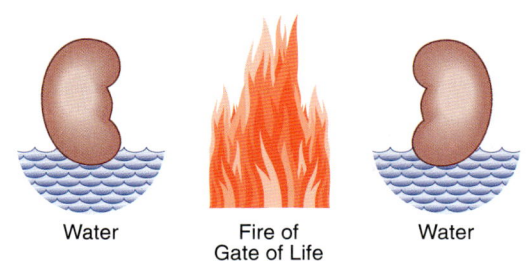

Figure 4.3 Fire of the Gate of Life (*Ming Men*)

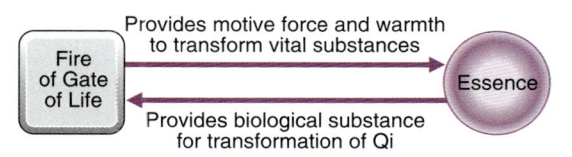

Figure 4.5 Fire of the Gate of Life and the Essence

the root of the 5 Yin and 6 Yang organs. The Gate of Life is the root of the Original Qi'[4] (Fig. 4.3).

The Fire of the Gate of Life, also called the Minister Fire, is the root of Pre-Heaven Qi, the source of Post-Heaven Qi and the foundation for the Original Qi (Fig. 4.4). Thus, the Kidneys are called the 'Root of Pre-Heaven' for two reasons:

1. The Kidneys store the Essence (including the Pre-Heaven and Post-Heaven Essence) which is the fundamental biological substance of life
2. The Kidneys contain the Fire of the Gate of Life which is the motive force that transforms and sets things in motion

Chapter 36 of the 'Classic of Difficulties' says: '*Each of the Yin organs is a single entity; only the kidneys are two, why? The two kidneys are not both kidneys. The left is the kidney [proper] while the right kidney is the Gate of Life (Ming Men). The Gate of Life is the place where the Mind and Spirit and the Essence lodge and the place to which the Original Qi is tied. In men, [the Gate of Life] stores the Essence (sperm); in women, it stores the Uterus*'[5] (Fig. 4.5).

It should be noted here that the present passage reflects the view according to which the right kidney is identified with the Fire of the Gate of Life: therefore the right kidney pertains to Yang and the left to Yin. This view is reflected in pulse diagnosis as the majority of doctors place Kidney-Yang on the right-Rear position and Kidney-Yin on the left-Rear position. However, there is a differing view according to which the Fire of the Gate of Life is placed in between the two kidneys and it is not identified with the right-hand one. The position of the point Du-4 Mingmen (itself meaning 'Gate of Life') would tend to support this view.

The Essence and the Fire of the Gate of Life are another example of Yin–Yang polarity and interdependence. The Fire of the Gate of Life relies on the Essence to provide the basic, fundamental biological substance for all life processes; the Essence relies on the Fire of the Gate of Life to be the motive force and provide the heat that transforms and moves the various physiological substances and that is the basis for the transformation of Qi. Without the Fire of the Gate of Life, the Essence would be a cold, inert substance incapable of nurturing life (see Fig. 4.5; see also Figs 3.3 and 3.4).

The interrelationship between Essence and the Gate of Life is mirrored in the expressions '*Qi is transformed into Essence*' and '*Essence is transformed into Qi.*'[6]

The Fire of the Gate of Life is connected to the Gathering Qi (*Zong Qi*) of the chest: this has the function of assisting the Gate of Life by providing pure Qi from breathing. Gathering Qi has to flow down to the Gate of Life to provide Qi, and the Gate of Life has to flow up to the Lungs to provide heat (Fig. 4.6).

The transformation of Qi relies on warmth as transformation is a Yang process. The Fire of the Gate of Life

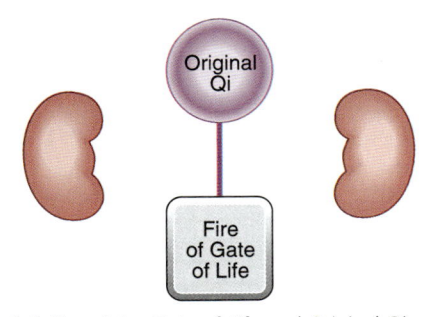

Figure 4.4 Fire of the Gate of Life and Original Qi

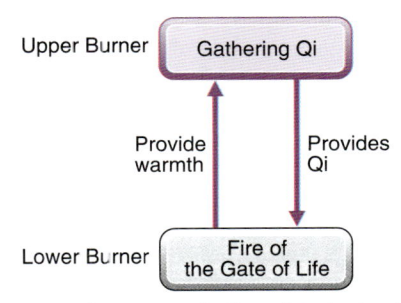

Figure 4.6 Fire of the Gate of Life and Gathering Qi

provides warmth to all the organs for the transformation of Qi in every part of the body. For example, the Fire of the Gate of Life helps Lung-Qi to descend, it helps Spleen-Qi to transform and transport food essences, it helps Bladder-Qi to transform and excrete urine, it assists the Intestines in transporting and transforming, it helps the Heart to house the Mind.

The Fire of the Gate of Life is further discussed in chapter 10 on the functions of the Kidneys.

> **Clinical note**
>
> Direct moxa on Du-4 Mingmen tonifies the Fire of the Gate of Life (*Ming Men*)

Box 4.2 summarizes the Fire of the Gate of Life as the warmth for the transformation of Qi.

Box 4.2 The Fire of the Gate of Life (*Ming Men*) as the warmth for the transformation of Qi

- The Original Qi between the Kidneys is related to the Fire of the Gate of Life (*Ming Men*)
- The Fire of the Gate of Life, also called Minister Fire, is the root of Pre-Heaven Qi, the source of Post-Heaven Qi and the foundation for the Original Qi
- The Essence is Yin and it provides the Fire of the Gate of Life with the biological substance for life
- The Fire of the Gate of Life is Yang and it gives the Essence the necessary warmth for its activation
- The Fire of the Gate of Life provides the warmth necessary to all physiological processes

---

THE DYNAMICS AND PHYSIOLOGY OF THE TRANSFORMATION OF QI

The dynamics and physiology of the transformation of Qi will be differentiated into four areas:

- The Qi Mechanism
  - Ascending–descending of Qi
  - Entering–exiting of Qi
- The Stomach and Spleen as the 'central axis'
- The Liver and Lungs as the 'outer wheel'
- The Heart and Kidneys as the 'root'

The Qi Mechanism

The 'Qi Mechanism' (*Qi Ji*) indicates the complex process of movement of Qi in all parts of the body. The direction of movement of the various types of Qi in various physiological processes is essential to the proper transformation of Qi. The Qi mechanism relies on four fundamental movements of Qi:

- Ascending (a Yang movement)
- Descending (a Yin movement)
- Exiting (a Yang movement)
- Entering (a Yin movement)

Chapter 68 of the 'Simple Questions' says: '*If there is no ascending/descending, there is no birth, growth, maturation and decline. If there is no entering/exiting, there is no birth, growth, transformation, receiving and storage. If the Qi Mechanism functions well there is room for birth and transformation; if the Qi Mechanism is disrupted, there is fragmentation and no birth or transformation.*'[7]

The 'Notes on Reading Medical Books' (*Du Yi Sui Bi*, 1891), by Zhou Xue Hai, says: '*The faculties of seeing, hearing, smelling, tasting and thinking all depend on the smooth ascending/descending and entering/exiting of Qi; if Qi is obstructed [in its ascending/descending and entering/exiting] those faculties are not normal.*'[8]

The ascending–descending and entering–exiting of Qi influences the formation of Qi and Blood at every stage and in every organ. The very production of Qi and Blood relies on the delicate, harmonious balance of ascending–descending and entering–exiting of Qi in every organ, every part of the body, every structure and at every stage. Therefore, any disruption of ascending–descending and/or entering–exiting of Qi may result in a pathology of Qi and/or Blood, which may be a deficiency, a stagnation or a situation of rebellious Qi.

Furthermore, the ascending–descending and entering–exiting of Qi influences the metabolism of fluids: for fluids to be transported, transformed and excreted properly, Qi needs to ascend–descend and enter–exit from body structures in a balanced, regulated way. If the ascending–descending and entering–exiting of Qi is disrupted, this may result in the formation of Dampness, Phlegm or oedema.

The intricate movement of Qi in the Qi Mechanism and its influence on fluid metabolism is closely dependent on the Triple Burner, which is also prone to Qi stagnation. Together with Liver-Qi, the Triple Burner controls the smooth and proper movement of Qi in all three Burners: in the Upper Burner, Qi goes up and enters and is under control of the Lungs; in the Middle

Burner, Qi goes up and down and in and out and is under the control of Stomach and Spleen; in the Lower Burner, Qi mostly descends and exits and is under the control of the Kidneys, Bladder and Intestines.

The Triple Burner assists all the other organs in their functions and, in particular, it makes sure that all passages (of Qi or fluids) are open, that the various types of Qi flow smoothly, that the Original Qi emerges from between the Kidneys and assumes different forms in different places, and that wastes are excreted smoothly (Fig. 4.7).

Ascending–descending of Qi

In certain physiological processes Qi needs to ascend, in others to descend. For example, Spleen-Qi ascends while Stomach-Qi descends: the movement of Qi for each organ has been discussed in chapter 3. Ascending is a Yang movement while descending is a Yin one. For example, the ascending of Spleen-Qi is Yang and, in fact, the Qi of the Spleen fails to ascend when Spleen-Yang of Spleen-Qi is deficient.

The Yang and Yin nature of the ascending and descending processes themselves should not be confused with the descending of Yang and ascending of Yin in another context. The ancient Chinese often identified Yang (which is above) with 'Heaven' and Yin (which is below) with 'Earth'. Heaven pertains to Yang and is above and it therefore descends; Earth pertains to Yin and is below and it therefore ascends.

The 'Simple Questions' in chapter 68 says: *'Descending pertains to Heaven; ascending pertains to Earth. The Qi of Heaven descends flowing to Earth; the Qi of Earth ascends mounting to Heaven.'*[9] This is not in contradiction with the above statement according to which, in the context of transformation of Qi, ascending is a Yang movement and descending a Yin one. Ascending, *as a movement*, is Yang; the fact that Earth (Yin) is below and ascends is not in contradiction with this as Earth is Yin but, when it ascends, that *movement* itself is Yang. In other words, there is Yang (ascending movement) within Yin (Earth, below) and Yin (descending movement) within Yang (Fire) (Fig. 4.8).

- Heaven (Yang) is Above and it descends, but descending is a Yin *movement*.
- Earth (Yin) is Below and it ascends, but ascending is a Yang *movement*.

These various ascendings and descendings of Qi depend on the functions of the internal organs. Each organ has a particular effect on Qi with regard to its ascending or descending. For example, Spleen-Qi

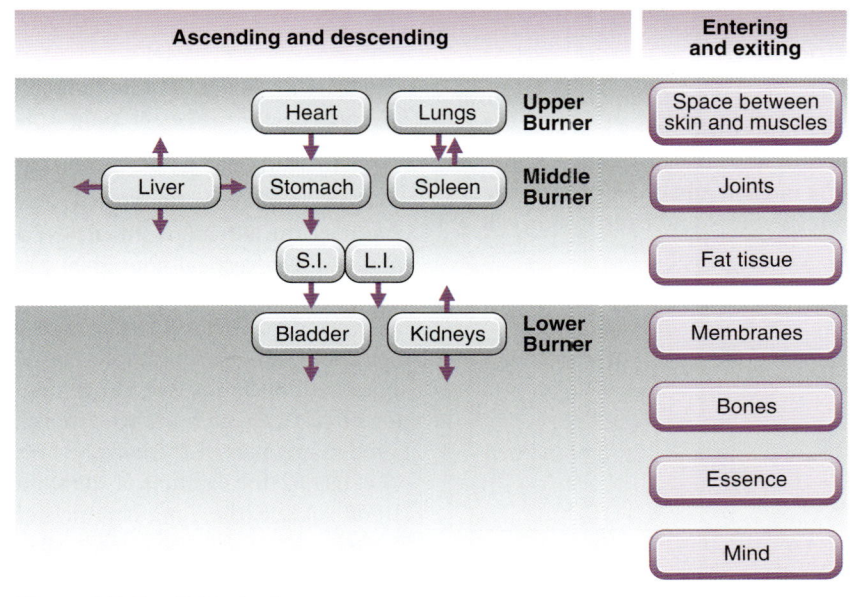

Figure 4.7 The Qi Mechanism

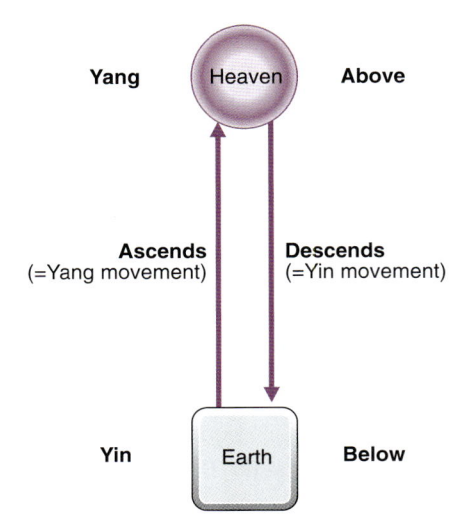

Figure 4.8 Movements of Heaven and Earth

ascends, Lung-Qi descends, Heart-Qi descends, Liver-Qi ascends and extends, Kidney-Qi descends, Stomach-Qi descends, and Bladder, Large and Small Intestine Qi all descend. These movements were described in chapter 3.

The balance of Yin and Yang is crucial for the smooth movement of Qi, as ascending is a Yang movement while descending is a Yin movement. Thus an excess of Yang will imply excessive ascending of Qi (e.g. Liver-Yang rising), while an excess of Yin will imply excessive descending of Qi (Spleen-Qi sinking).

Entering–exiting of Qi

The smooth movement of Qi in the Qi Mechanism relies not only on the proper ascending and descending of Qi in various organs and structures but also on the entering and exiting of Qi in and out of various structures. For example, Qi enters and exits in and out of these structures:

- Channels
- Space between skin and muscles
- Triple Burner cavities
- Joints
- Fat Tissue (*Gao*)
- Membranes (*Huang*)
- Bones
- Mind-Spirit (*Shen*)

Thus, the entering–exiting of Qi provides a horizontal dimension to the movement of Qi, while the ascending–descending of Qi provides a vertical dimension.

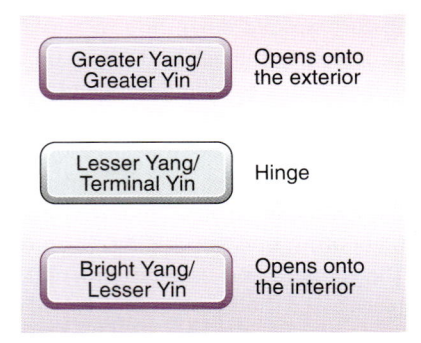

Figure 4.9 Entering and exiting among channels

Channels

The entering–exiting of Qi is also an important aspect of the movement among the three Yang energetic layers of Greater Yang (*Tai Yang*), Lesser Yang (*Shao Yang*) and Bright Yang (*Yang Ming*), and among the three Yin energetic layers of Greater Yin (*Tai Yin*), Terminal Yin (*Jue Yin*) and Lesser Yin (*Shao Yin*).

Within the Yang channels, the Greater Yang is said to 'open onto the Exterior', the Bright Yang 'opens onto the Interior' and the Lesser Yang is the 'hinge' between the two; within the Yin channels, the Greater Yin is said to 'open onto the Exterior', the Lesser Yin 'opens onto the Interior' and the Terminal Yin is the 'hinge' between the two.

In other words, the order of depth is as follows (Fig. 4.9):

	YANG	YIN
Superficial	Greater Yang	Greater Yin
'Hinge'	Lesser Yang	Terminal Yin
Deep	Bright Yang	Lesser Yin

When considering the physiology and pathology of channels, the ascending and descending of Qi is paramount (their 'vertical' movement) but we should not overlook the entering and exiting of Qi (their 'horizontal' movement): by 'horizontal' movement, I mean the movement among the three energetic layers listed above within the Yang or Yin channels. The combination of vertical and horizontal movement of Qi can be found in any part of the body.

Let us take the example of the shoulder area. On the lateral surface, the Yang channels of Small Intestine, Triple Burner and Large Intestine flow from the fingertips to the face: this is the vertical movement of Qi. However, within the shoulder area, there is also a 'horizontal' movement among the Greater Yang (Small

Intestine), Lesser Yang (Triple Burner) and Bright Yang (Large Intestine): this 'horizontal' movement represents the entering and exiting of Qi. The same applies to the Yin channels in the shoulder area (Fig. 4.10).

The entering and exiting of Qi is also controlled by the Corporeal Soul (*Po*), which is in charge of the entering and exiting of the Essence (*Jing*). In other words, the Corporeal Soul and the Essence are closely coordinated and the Corporeal Soul is sometimes described as the 'entering and exiting of the Essence'. For this reason, the Corporeal Soul contributes to all physiological activities.

> The Corporeal Soul (*Po*) is the 'entering and exiting of the Essence'. It brings the Essence into play and regulates all physiological processes

Space between skin and muscles

The space between the skin and muscles is part of the Triple Burner cavities (see below) but may usefully be discussed separately in view of its clinical importance. This space between skin and muscles is one of the body spaces called *Cou Li*. I translate the term *Cou Li* as 'Spaces and Texture' (Fig. 4.11).

The 'space between the skin and muscles' should not be intended in a strict Western anatomical sense, but

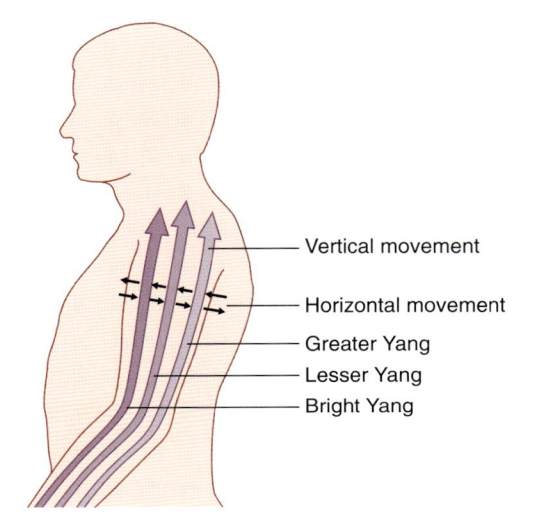

Figure 4.10 Entering and exiting of Qi in shoulder area

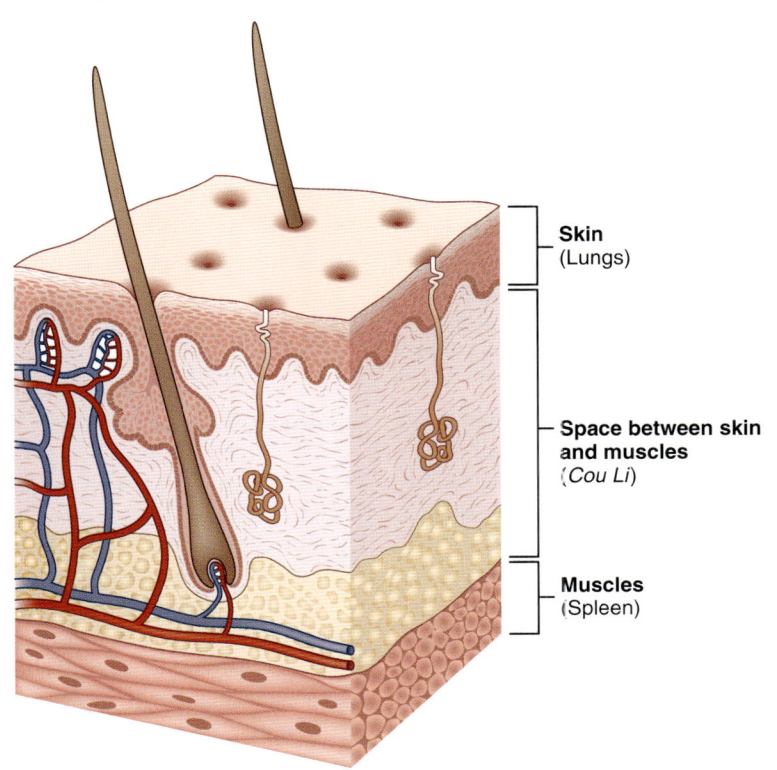

Figure 4.11 Space between skin and muscles (*Cou Li*)

as an energetic layer corresponding to the surface of the body, also called the 'Exterior': this layer is also sometimes called the 'Lung's Defensive Qi portion'. The space between the skin and muscles is the energetic space where the Defensive Qi circulates (to warm and protect the body), where sweat is situated, and where external pathogenic factors first invade the body.

Qi enters into and exits from the space between the skin and muscles, thus regulating the proper circulation of Defensive Qi and the balanced opening and closing of the pores, and therefore regulating sweating. The movement of Qi in and out of the space between skin and muscles relies on Lung-Qi. When the entering and exiting of Qi are properly balanced, Defensive Qi circulates well in the space between the skin and muscles, the pores are regulated, sweating is normal and external pathogenic factors generally will not enter this space (unless they are particularly strong).

Clinical note

LU-7 Lieque, L.I.-4 Hegu and ST-36 Zusanli regulate the *Cou Li* space

Triple Burner cavities

The Triple Burner is discussed in more detail in chapter 18. There are many facets to the nature of the Triple Burner: one of them is that the Triple Burner is a system of body cavities and 'spaces', ranging from the very large to the very small. All these cavities are called *Cou* (as in *Cou Li*, 'Spaces and Texture'). In particular, the Three Burners are the three large cavities of the chest (Upper Burner), the abdomen (Middle Burner) and the pelvis (Lower Burner). The space between the skin and muscles is another example of a Triple Burner cavity (Fig. 4.12).

Together with Liver-Qi, the Triple Burner controls the smooth and proper movement of Qi in all three Burners: in the Upper Burner, Qi mostly ascends and enters and is under control of the Lungs; in the Middle Burner, Qi ascends and descends and enters and exits and is under the control of Stomach and Spleen; in the Lower Burner, Qi mostly descends and exits and is under the control of the Kidneys, Bladder and Intestines. The Triple Burner assists all the other organs in their functions and, in particular, it makes sure that all passages and cavities are open, and that Qi enters into and exits from these cavities in a balanced way.

Figure 4.12 Triple Burner cavities

The Qi of the Triple Burner is prone to stagnate. Stagnation will obstruct the proper entering and exiting of Qi in various spaces of the body, resulting in sensations of distension and pain.

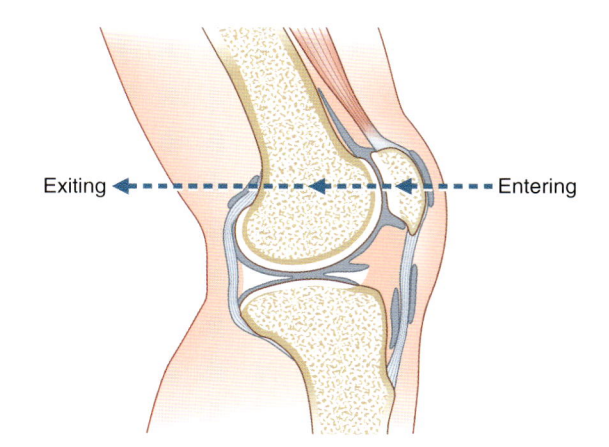

Figure 4.13 Entering and exiting of Qi in joint

Joints

The joint capsules are also spaces or cavities into which Qi enters and from which it exits. The movement of Qi in and out of the joints is controlled primarily by the Liver and Triple Burner in general: however, it obviously also relies on whichever channel traverses a particular joint (Fig. 4.13).

If Qi enters and exits from the joints in a balanced way, the joint will be free of pain and its movement unrestricted. If Qi exits too much, the joint will be rigid and painful, and extension will be difficult; if Qi enters too much, the joint will be weak and achy and adduction will be difficult.

Fat Tissue (Gao)

Fat Tissue is called *Gao* in Chinese. It broadly corresponds to adipose tissue in Western medicine, but it has a slightly different meaning. While from a Western perspective adipose tissue is distributed all over the body, Fat Tissue (*Gao*) in Chinese medicine refers primarily to the adipose tissue in the abdomen (both in men and women) and in the breasts (in women); it also includes the peritoneal membranes that encapsulate the organs (the peritoneal membranes are connective, not adipose, tissue).

The entering and exiting of Qi in and out of the Fat Tissue relies primarily on the Spleen; a balanced entering of Qi into and exiting of Qi from the Fat Tissue will result in normal tissues. Excessive entering of Qi may result in the accumulation of fat and obesity, while excessive exiting of Qi may result in loss of weight.

Membranes (Huang)

'*Huang*' literally means 'membranes' and it refers to membranes that cover the whole body; there is a superficial layer below the skin and an inner layer below that. Membranes have the function of *wrapping* and *anchoring* the organs, muscles and bones and of *connecting* the organs among themselves.

Broadly speaking, Membranes correspond to connective tissues in Western medicine, although not all connective tissues are part of Membranes. In particular, although sinews are a connective tissue, in Chinese medicine they are not Membranes but Sinews (i.e. the tissue of the Liver).

Membranes are found only in the abdomen and they broadly correspond to the fascia (superficial and deep), the peritoneum, mesenterium and omentum. The stroma (i.e. the framework of connective tissue or organs) is also an example of Membranes.

Proper entering and exiting of Qi in and out of the Membranes ensures a smooth circulation of Qi in the abdomen. If there is excessive exiting of Qi, stagnation of Qi in the Membranes will result in abdominal distension and pain; if there is excessive entering of Qi, a deficiency and possibly sinking of Qi will result in a slackening of the Membranes.

Bones

'Bones' in Chinese medicine does not refer purely to the Western anatomical structure of that name, although it does include that. Apart from its anatomical aspect, 'Bones' in Chinese medicine refers also to an energetic layer of the body structures. The body is divided into structures with different energetic layers: in increasing order of depth, they are skin, muscles, sinews, blood vessels and bones. These are controlled by the Lungs, Spleen, Liver, Heart and Kidneys, respectively. Thus, 'Bones' refers also to a deep energetic layer of the body that is influenced by the Kidneys. For example, night sweating is also called 'steaming from the bones' as the nocturnal sweat is deemed to emanate from deep within the bones (as opposed to diurnal sweat that emanates from the space between skin and muscles).

Qi enters and exits from the bones on its way to and from the deep energetic layers of the body. If there is excessive exiting of Qi from the bones there may be night sweating; if there is excessive entering of Qi into the bones there may be a tendency to Blood stasis (Box 4.3).

Mind-Spirit (Shen)

The Mind (*Shen*) is also one of the Vital Substances, albeit the most rarefied and non-substantial of them.[10] As explained in the previous chapter, I translate as 'Mind' the *Shen* of the Heart and as 'Spirit' the whole complex of Ethereal Soul (*Hun*), Corporeal Soul (*Po*), Intellect (*Yi*), Will-Power (*Zhi*) and the Mind (*Shen*) itself.

The entering and exiting of Qi in and out of the Mind must be seen in the context of the coordination between the Mind of the Heart and the Ethereal Soul (*Hun*) of the Liver. Briefly, the Ethereal Soul is a repository of ideas, dreams, projects, aspirations, ideals, inspiration: it provides the Mind with another psychic dimension without which it would be sterile. The Mind, on the other hand, needs to control and integrate all the psychic contents springing from the Ethereal Soul. Sometimes defined as the 'coming and going of the

---

Box 4.3 Five energetic layers

1. Skin = Lungs
2. Muscles = Spleen
3. Sinews = Liver
4. Blood vessels = Heart
5. Bones = Kidneys

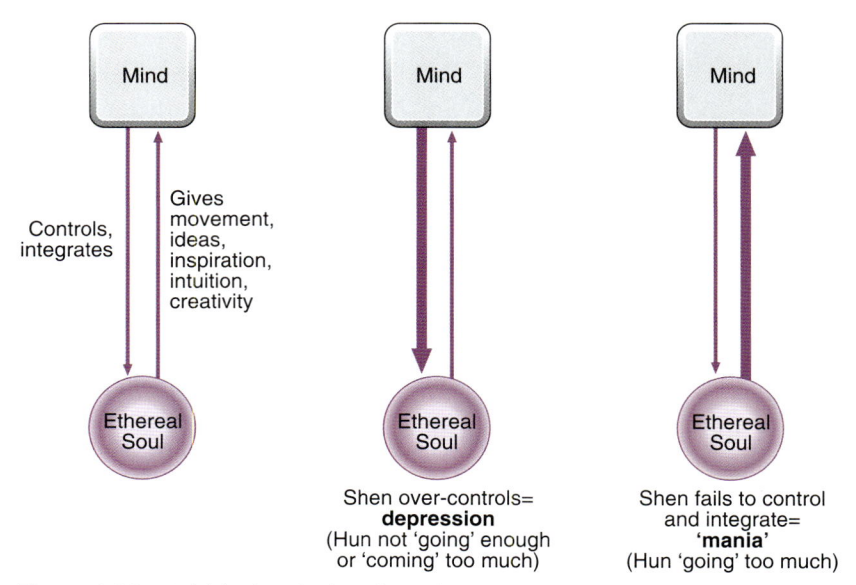

Figure 4.14 Mind (*Shen*) and Ethereal Soul (*Hun*) relationships

Mind', the Ethereal Soul is always searching, dreaming, exploring, making plans, being inspired. Hence, on a psychic level, that constitutes the 'entering and exiting of Qi' (i.e. the 'coming and going') in and out of the Mind (Fig. 4.14).

The pathology of the relationship between the Mind and the Ethereal Soul in relation to entering/exiting of Qi is discussed in chapter 29.

The Ethereal Soul (*Hun*) is the 'coming and going of the Mind (*Shen*)' and is responsible for ideas, aims, projects, ideals, plans, inspiration, life dreams, aspirations

The Stomach and Spleen as the central axis

The movement of Qi of Stomach and Spleen is crucial for most physiological processes. Stomach and Spleen are the 'centre' in more ways than one: physiologically, as they are the source of Qi and Blood and therefore all other organs depend on them for their nourishment; anatomically, as they lie in the Middle Burner at the crossroads of many physiological activities and many different movements of Qi in all directions. The correct functioning of Stomach and Spleen in relation to the direction of movement of Qi is therefore crucial for a proper physiological activity (Figs 4.15 and 4.16).

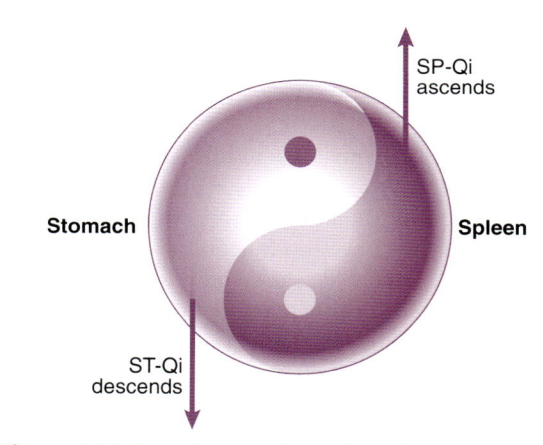

Figure 4.15 Ascending and descending of Stomach and Spleen

Spleen and Stomach complement each other. The Spleen is Yin and its Qi ascends: it transports and transforms (a Yang activity) food essences. The Stomach is Yang and its Qi descends: its functions are to churn food and liquids and provide the source of Body Fluids, all activities which are Yin in nature.

Spleen-Qi ascends to send the essences extracted from food up to the Lungs and Heart where they are

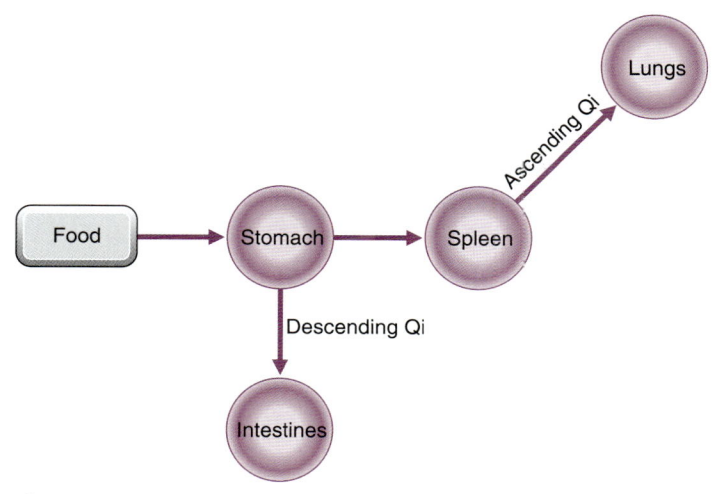

Figure 4.16 Ascending Spleen-Qi and descending Stomach-Qi

transformed into Qi and Blood, respectively. Stomach-Qi descends to send the impure part resulting from the transformation of food down to the Intestines.

Ye Tian Shi (1667–1746) said: 'After food has entered the Stomach, the Spleen transforms and moves it; if Spleen-Qi rises it is healthy. If Stomach-Qi descends there is harmony ... Yang Qi [of the Spleen] moves ... Yin Qi [of the Stomach] is quiet. The Spleen likes dryness, and the Stomach likes moisture.'[11]

Thus the ascending and descending of Spleen-Qi and Stomach-Qi are crucial for the production of Qi and Blood and for the harmonious crossing of Qi in the Middle Burner.

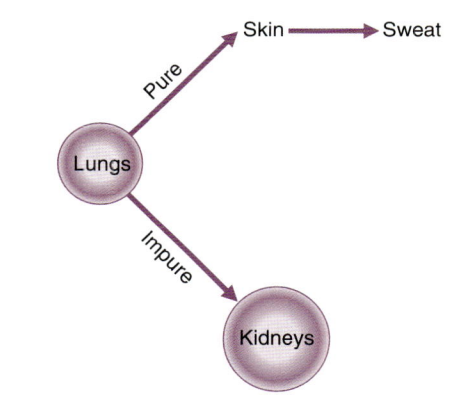

Figure 4.17 Descending of Lung-Qi

Clinical note

Ren-12 Zhongwan is the main point to regulate the ascending and descending of Qi in the Middle Burner

The Liver and Lungs as the outer wheel

The Liver is on the left and its Qi rises, the Lungs are on the right and their Qi descends. Being 'on the left' or 'on the right' should be interpreted not in a strict anatomical sense but in relation to the Five-Element scheme, which places Wood (Liver) on the left and Metal (Lungs) on the right (Figs 4.17 and 4.18).

Ye Tian Shi said: 'The human body mirrors the natural world [so that], the Liver is on the left and its Qi ascends, the Lungs are on the right and their Qi descends. When their ascending and descending are harmonized, Qi can relax and develop ... the Liver makes Qi ascend to the head and the upper orifices; the Lungs make Qi descend to the internal organs and sinews and bones. The two together permit Qi and Blood to flow and extend and the internal organs to be peaceful and balanced.'[12]

The Liver is in the Lower Burner (energetically, not anatomically) and sends Qi upwards, the Lungs are in the Upper Burner and send Qi downwards. The two together ensure the smooth flow of Qi between Upper and Lower Burner and among the internal organs.

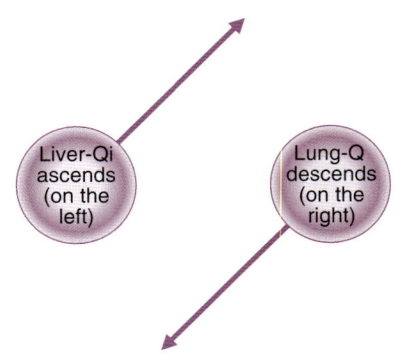

Figure 4.18 Ascending of Liver-Qi and descending of Lung-Qi

The Heart and Kidneys as the root

The Heart houses the Mind and pertains to Fire; the Kidneys store the Essence and pertain to Water. The polarity of Heart and Kidneys is the fundamental polarity between Fire and Water.

The Fire of the Heart descends to the Kidneys to warm them; the Water of the Kidneys rises to the Heart to nourish its Yin aspect.[13] The descending of the Fire of the Heart and the ascending of the Water of the Kidneys keep the fundamental balance between Fire and Water, Yang and Yin, Above and Below. There is a direct connection between Heart and Kidneys and the two have to communicate with each other and be harmonized (Fig. 4.19).

The book 'Wu's Collected Medical Works' (1792) says: *'The Heart pertains to Fire but there is Water within Fire; the Kidneys pertain to Water but there is Fire within Water. Fire governs Water and Heart-Qi descends. Water is the source of Fire and Kidney-Qi ascends. If Water does not ascend, disease ensues: this is due to deficient Kidney-Yang being unable to raise Water upwards. If Fire does not descend, disease ensues: this is due to deficient Heart Yin being unable to lower Fire downwards.'*[14]

Clinical note

Ren-15 Jiuwei and Ren-4 Guanyuan harmonize Heart and Kidneys

We can now summarize these three relationships between Stomach and Spleen, Liver and Lungs and Heart and Kidneys by referring to the Five-Element Cosmological sequence.

We can visualize the Cosmological sequence as a three-dimensional model of the relationships of the internal organs and the movement of Qi in the various directions (Fig. 4.20).

The Heart and Kidneys axis could be seen as an imaginary axis going through the centre of a horizontal wheel; the Stomach and Spleen, as the hub of the wheel; and the Liver and Lungs, as the outer rim of the wheel (Fig. 4.21).

Box 4.4 summarizes the dynamics and physiology of the transformation of Qi.

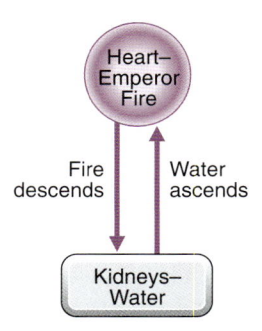

Figure 4.19 Descending of Fire of Heart and ascending of Water of the Kidneys

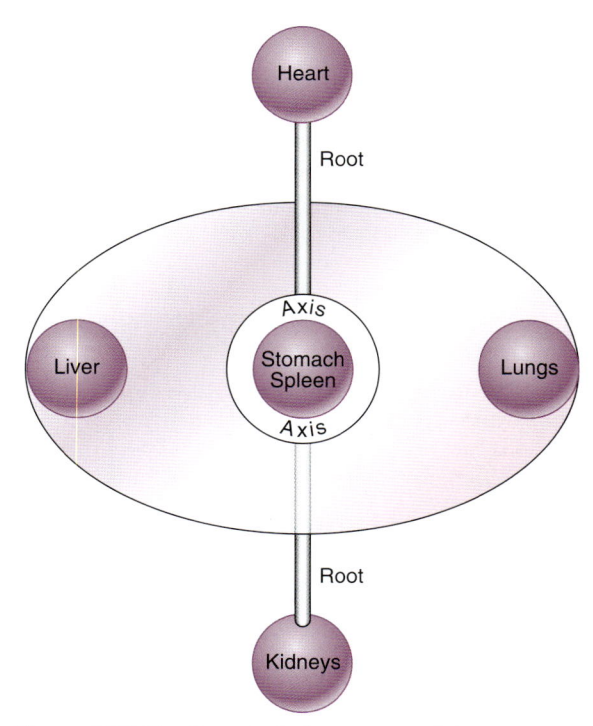

Figure 4.20 The Cosmological sequence and the organ direction of Qi

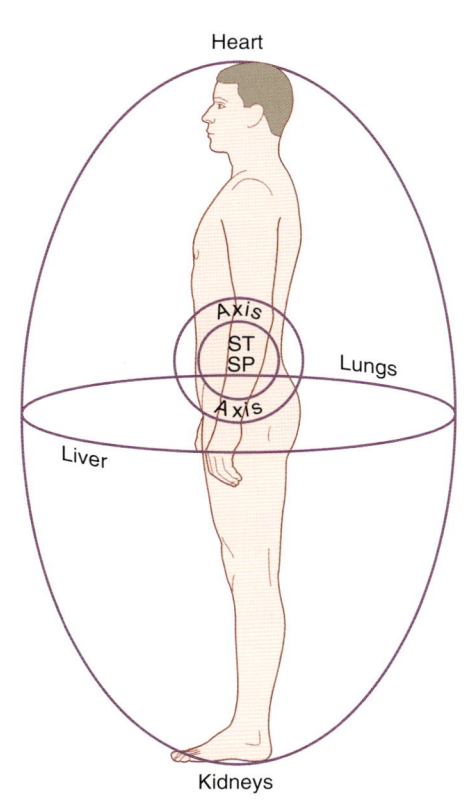

Figure 4.21 The axis, root and outer wheel of the Organs

Box 4.4 Summary box: the dynamics and physiology of the transformation of Qi

1. The Qi Mechanism
   a) 'Qi Mechanism' (*Qi Ji*) indicates the complex process of movement of Qi in all parts of the body
   b) The four basic movements of Qi are: ascending, descending, entering and exiting
2. The Stomach and Spleen as the central axis
   a) The Stomach and Spleen are at the centre of the body's physiology
   b) The ascending of Spleen-Qi and descending of Stomach-Qi are crucial to assist the proper ascending/descending of Qi of all other organs
3. The Liver and Lungs as the outer wheel
   a) Energetically, the 'Liver is on the left and the Lungs on the right'
   b) Liver-Qi ascends and Lung-Qi descends
   c) The coordination between the ascending of Liver-Qi and the descending of Lung-Qi is important to regulate the movement of Qi between the Upper and Lower Burners
4. The Heart and Kidneys as the root
   a) The Fire of the Heart descends towards the Kidneys and the Water of the Kidneys ascends towards the Heart
   b) The coordination between the descending of Heart-Qi and ascending of Kidney-Qi is important to regulate the movement of Qi between the Upper and Lower Burners
   c) The communication between the Heart and Kidneys is important in the gynaecological and sexual spheres

---

THE TRIPLE BURNER'S TRANSFORMATION OF QI

The Triple Burner is one of the six Yang organs. Its nature has been the subject of discussion for centuries and the question of whether it is even an 'organ', as the other five Yang organs are, is debatable. Indeed, one subject of debate has been whether the Triple Burner 'has a form' or not: that is, whether it is an actual organ or just a collective complex of functions.

As far as the transformation of Qi is concerned, the functions of the Triple Burner are expressed in the 'Simple Questions' as 'making things go through' (*tong*) and 'letting out' or 'excrete' (*chu*). In other words, the Triple Burner assists all the other organs in their functions and, in particular, it makes sure that all passages are open, that the various types of Qi flow smoothly and that wastes are excreted properly. This is therefore an essential function in relation to the movement of the various types of Qi and essences in any part of the body. In particular, as the Triple Burner is also a system of body cavities, it also ensures the proper entering and exiting of Qi in and out of such cavities.

Each of the three Burners is in charge of particular functions and particular movements of Qi.

The Upper Burner (which comprises Lungs and Heart) is in charge of diffusing Qi to the skin and muscles: this is a function of Lung-Qi. In particular, it controls the outward movement of Defensive Qi to the skin. From this perspective, the Qi of the Triple Burner ascends as the diffusing action of the Lungs has an outward and ascending movement. However, the Qi of the Triple Burner also descends as Lung-Qi descends. As for entering–exiting, the Qi of the Upper Burner enters and exits from the space between the skin and muscles and in and out of the chest cavity.

The Middle Burner (which comprises Stomach and Spleen) is in charge of digesting food, transforming it and transporting the Food-Qi upwards to Lungs and Heart. In particular, the Middle Burner controls the movement of Nutritive Qi and makes sure that Qi moves in the right directions: that is, Spleen-Qi upwards and Stomach-Qi downwards. As for entering–exiting, the Qi of the Middle Burner goes in and out of the abdominal Membranes.

The Lower Burner (which comprises Liver, Kidneys, Bladder and Intestines) is in charge of the transformation, transportation and excretion of fluids and wastes. Its Qi has a definite downward movement. In particular, the Lower Burner controls the downward movement of the Qi of the Intestines and Bladder. As for entering–exiting, the Qi of the Lower Burner mostly exits but it also enters into the Membranes (Fig. 4.22).

To summarize, the Triple Burner is in charge of the correct direction of movement (both ascending–descending and entering–exiting) of all types of Qi in all parts of the body. If this function of the Triple Burner is impaired, Qi, Blood and Body Fluids do not flow smoothly: they will overflow, passages will be blocked and Qi will stagnate.

The 'Classic of the Secret Transmission', by Hua Tuo (died AD 208), says: *'The Triple Burner ... assembles and directs the 5 Yin and 6 Yang organs, the Nutritive and Defensive Qi and the channels, [it harmonizes] the Qi of interior and exterior, left and right, upper and lower. If the Triple Burner is open, then the interior and exterior, left and right, upper and lower are also open; in this way it regulates and irrigates the body, it harmonizes interior and exterior, left and right, upper and lower.'*[15]

As the Triple Burner, together with Liver-Qi, is in charge of the free flow of Qi in every part of the body, Qi stagnation affects the Triple Burner as well as the Liver and, for this reason, Triple Burner points may be used to relieve stagnation of Qi.

Clinical note

TB-6 Zhigou can be used to relieve Qi stagnation in every part of the body, but especially in the upper part, hypochondrium, flanks and breasts

Clinical note

The Triple Burner's transformation of Qi is stimulated by using points on the Directing Vessel (*Ren Mai*):
- Ren-17 Shanzhong for Upper Burner
- Ren-12 Zhongwan for Middle Burner
- Ren-5 Shimen for Lower Burner

Box 4.5 summarizes the Triple Burner's transformation of Qi.

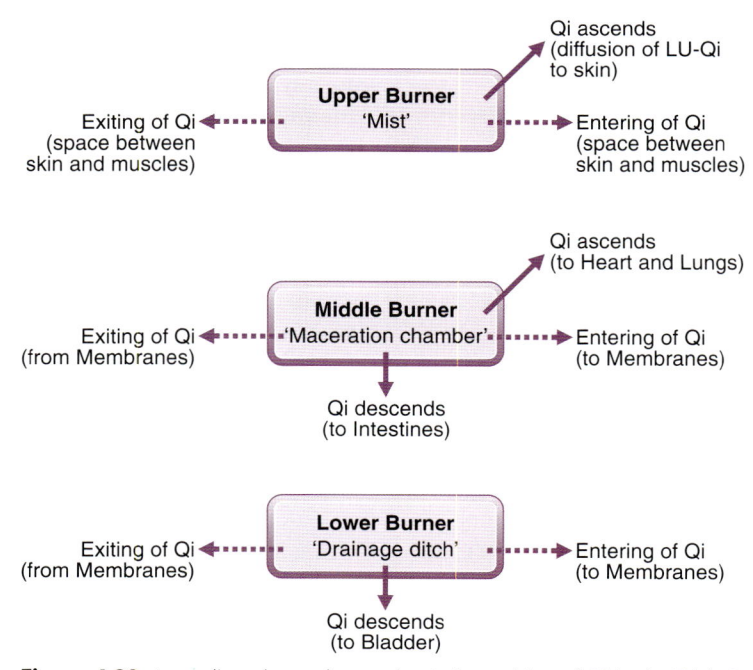

Figure 4.22 Ascending–descending and entering–exiting of Qi in the Triple Burner

> **Box 4.5 Summary box: the Triple Burner's transformation of Qi**
>
> - The Triple Burner is an important organ to promote the transformation of Qi
> - The Triple Burner promotes 'making things go through', 'letting out' and 'excreting'
> - The Triple Burner ensures that all passages of Qi and Water are open
> - The Qi of the Upper Burner generally ascends
> - The Qi of the Middle Burner ascends and descends
> - The Qi of the Lower Burner mostly descends

PATHOLOGY OF QI TRANSFORMATION

The correct direction of movement of the various types of Qi in different situations depends on the internal organs. Each of the internal organs moves its Qi in a particular direction to perform certain functions: thus, the direction of Qi is closely related to a particular internal organ's function. For this reason, any disruption of Qi transformation needs to be viewed in relation to the dysfunction of the internal organs.

Stomach and Spleen

Spleen-Qi normally ascends to Lungs and Heart, in so far as the Spleen directs the pure essences extracted from food upwards to these two organs where they are transformed into Qi and Blood, respectively. If Spleen-Qi does not ascend, the pure essences will not be transported upwards and diarrhoea will ensue.

Apart from diarrhoea, an obvious consequence of Spleen-Qi not rising is that the food essences are not transported to Lungs and Heart and, in the long run, deficiency of Qi and Blood will ensue.

The ascending of Spleen-Qi lifts and keeps the organs in place. If Spleen-Qi sinks, prolapse may ensue. This may involve the stomach, uterus, intestines, kidney, bladder, vagina and rectal veins in the form of haemorrhoids.

Stomach-Qi normally descends to transmit to the Intestines the impure part of food, which is left after the Spleen transformation. If Stomach-Qi does not descend, Qi will escape upwards causing nausea, hiccup, belching and vomiting.

Both Spleen-Qi descending and Stomach-Qi ascending are called 'rebellious' Qi: that is, Qi flowing in the wrong direction. The former is a rebellious Qi of deficient nature (usually called 'sinking Qi'), the latter a rebellious Qi of excess nature. Rebellious Qi is one of the possible pathologies of Qi, in addition to deficiency and stagnation.

> **Clinical note**
>
> The point Du-20 Baihui 'lifts' Spleen-Qi and may be used to correct sinking of Spleen-Qi causing a prolapse; it is normally used with direct moxa cones

Liver and Lungs

Liver-Qi ascends and Lung-Qi descends: if the two are balanced, Qi flows freely and smoothly.

Liver-Qi can, however, fail to ascend and extend, and this becomes a major cause of stagnation of Qi. Stagnation of Liver-Qi may be manifested in many different areas of the body, such as the hypochondrium, epigastrium, abdomen, uterus, throat and head. It may affect the Lungs, impairing the descending of Lung-Qi (manifesting with a feeling of distension of the chest, depression, cough and breathlessness) (Figs 4.23 and 4.24).

The ascending of Liver-Qi can also become 'rebellious' (called 'Liver-Yang rising') and rise to the head causing headaches and irritability: this may also impair the descending of Lung-Qi, causing cough and breathlessness. Liver-Fire may also have the same effect and, in addition, it would cause red eyes.

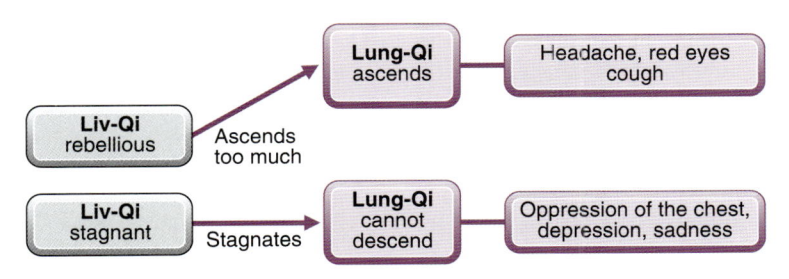

Figure 4.23 Pathology of ascending of Liver-Qi and descending of Lung-Qi

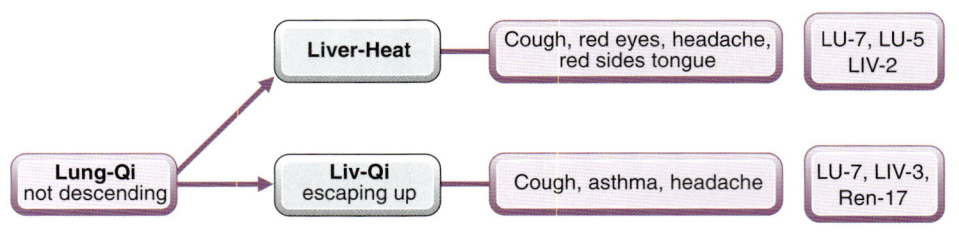

Figure 4.24 Pathology and treatment of ascending of Liver-Qi and descending of Lung-Qi

All the above pathological situations may be described in Five-Element terms as 'Liver insulting the Lungs'.

Descending of Lung-Qi brings Qi and fluids down to the Kidneys and Bladder. If Lung-Qi fails to descend, it will stagnate in the chest and cause cough or asthma. When Lung-Qi fails to descend, it may affect the Liver and the rising of Liver-Yang, which will manifest with cough, breathlessness and headache. The failure of Lung-Qi to descend may also cause Liver-Heat with symptoms of cough, red eyes and headache.

Heart and Kidneys

In health, the Fire of the Heart goes downwards to communicate with the Water of the Kidneys: conversely, the Water of the Kidneys goes upwards to nourish Heart-Yin.

If the Fire of the Heart does not descend to meet the Kidneys, Heart-Heat develops, which can damage Kidney-Yin. If Water is deficient, it cannot rise to meet the Heart, Kidney-Yang is deficient and oedema develops.

This same situation is described by Zhang Jing Yue when he says: '*Fire is the root of Heat, if there is no Water within Fire the Heat becomes excessive and it depletes the Yin which causes the drying and withering of life. Water is the root of Cold, if there is no Fire within the Water, Cold becomes excessive and it injures the Yang which causes things to be lifeless and without Fire.*'[16]

Wang Ping, author of the edition of the 'Yellow Emperor's Classic of Internal Medicine' (AD 762) on which all modern versions are based, says: '*The Heart should not have excessive Heat but enough Yang; the Kidneys should not have excessive Cold but enough Yin.*'[17]

The disharmony between Kidneys and Heart can also be manifested when the Water of the Kidneys, and in particular Kidney-Yin, fails to ascend to cool and nurture Heart-Yin: in this case the lack of nourishment from Kidney-Yin causes an uprising of pathological Fire in the Heart, with such symptoms as insomnia, mental restlessness and anxiety. These symptoms are caused by Empty-Heat of the Heart deriving from Yin deficiency.

Being the root for the ascending and descending of Qi, the axis of Heart and Kidneys affects many other organs. The Liver relies on the nourishment from Kidney-Yin: if Kidney-Yin does not nourish Liver-Yin, Liver-Qi may ascend too much, causing headaches and irritability. The Heart, on the other hand, keeps the Lungs in check, and if Heart-Qi does not descend, Lung-Qi may fail to descend, causing cough or asthma.

The function of Stomach and Spleen is also dependent on the ascending and descending of Heart and Kidney Qi, as these provide the Fire and the Water necessary for the function of digestion, transformation and transportation. He Bo Zhai (1694–?) said: '*The Internal Organs depend on the Stomach and Spleen for their nourishment. After food enters the Stomach, its essence is transported by the Spleen. The ability of the Spleen to transform food depends on the Qi of Fire and Water. If the Fire is in excess, the Stomach and Spleen are too dry; if Water is in excess the Stomach and Spleen are too damp: in both cases they will not be able to transform and disease will ensue.*'[18]

Box 4.6 summarizes the pathology of Qi ascending and descending.

Box 4.6 Summary box: the pathology of Qi ascending and descending

- Failure in the ascending of Spleen-Qi may cause diarrhoea or prolapse of organs
- Failure in descending of Stomach-Qi causes nausea, vomiting, belching, hiccups
- Failure in the ascending and extending of Liver-Qi causes stagnation of Qi manifesting with abdominal distension, irritability and moodiness
- Excessive ascending of Liver-Qi may cause headaches and dizziness
- Failure in the descending of Lung-Qi may cause cough or asthma
- Failure in the descending of Heart-Qi may cause menstrual or sexual problems
- Failure in the ascending of Kidney-Water may cause a feeling of heat and hot flushes

Learning outcomes

In this chapter you will have learned:
- The concept of the 'transformation of Qi' which describes all the functional activities of Qi and their associated physiological processes in the body
- The role of the Original Qi (Yuan Qi) as the dynamic motive force for transformation
- The importance of the Fire of the Gate of Life (Ming Men) in providing the warmth necessary for transformation in every organ and all parts of the body
- The interrelationship of the Essence and the Fire of the Gate of Life, which provide both the fundamental biological substance of life and the motive force and heat necessary for its transformation
- The relationship of the Fire of the Gate of Life and the Gathering Qi of the chest
- The concept of the 'Qi Mechanism' – the process of movement of Qi in all parts of the body
- The importance of harmonious ascending–descending and entering–exiting of Qi for healthy production of Qi and Blood and metabolism of body fluids
- The central role of the Triple Burner in the movement of Qi and fluid metabolism
- The concept of entering–exiting of Qi, which provides a 'horizontal' dimension to the movement of Qi, together with the 'vertical' dimension of ascending–descending of Qi
- The importance of the varying depths of the energetic layers of the six paired Yang and Yin channels when considering the entering–exiting of Qi
- The role of the Corporeal Soul as the 'entering and exiting of the Essence'
- How the entering and exiting of Qi from the space between the skin and muscles regulates sweating
- How Qi enters and exits from the joints, and how this process can become interrupted
- The significance of entering and exiting in and out of the Fat Tissue
- The importance of proper entering and exiting of Qi in and out of the Membranes for a smooth circulation of Qi in the abdomen
- The role of the bones as one of the deepest energetic layers where Qi enters and exits
- The relationship of the Mind and the Ethereal Soul in the entering and exiting of Qi in and out of the Mind
- The role of the Stomach and Spleen as the 'centre'
- The function of the Liver and the Lungs as the 'outer wheel', ensuring the smooth flow of Qi between Upper and Lower Burners and among the internal organs
- The importance of the communication between Heart and Kidneys as the 'root', maintaining the fundamental balance of Fire and Water, Yang and Yin
- The importance of the Triple Burner functions of 'making things go through' and 'letting out' in relation to the transformation of Qi and the harmonious ascending–descending and entering–exiting of Qi in the three Burners
- How disruption of the correct movement of Stomach-Qi and Spleen-Qi produces their associated symptoms
- How the symptoms of deranged Liver-Qi or Lung-Qi relate closely to their functions of ascending–descending and entering–exiting
- The significance of disruption in the ascending and descending of Heart-Qi and Kidney-Qi, which affects many other organs as it is the root of ascending and descending in the body

Self-assessment questions

1. Explain the connection between the Triple Burner and the Original Qi, and the function of this connection in relation to the transformation of Qi.
2. According to chapter 36 of the 'Classic of Difficulties', what is the difference between the two Kidneys?
3. Complete the following: 'The transformation of Qi relies on _____ as transformation is a Yang process.'
4. Summarise the basic movement of Qi in the three burners.
5. Complete the following: 'Heaven (____) is Above and it _____ but _____ is a Yin *movement*. Earth (____) is Below and it _____ but _____ is a Yang *movement*.'
6. List three organs which send Qi downwards.
7. List the Yang channels which traverse the shoulder in order of their depth.
8. Which two organs are associated with the space between the skin and muscles?
9. Which organs control the movement of Qi in and out of the joints?
10. What are the functions of the Membranes?
11. Complete the following: 'The Ethereal Soul is sometimes defined as the '_____ and _____ of the Mind."
12. In which two main ways are the Stomach and Spleen the 'centre'?
13. Energetically speaking, where are the Liver and Lungs positioned, and in which direction does their Qi flow?
14. To which pathology is the Triple Burner especially susceptible?
15. Why, if Lung-Qi fails to descend, might there be symptoms of cough, headache, and red eyes?

See p. 1256 for answers

END NOTES

1. Nanjing College of Traditional Chinese Medicine 1979 A Revised Explanation of the Classic of Difficulties (*Nan Jing Jiao Shi* 难经校释), People's Health Publishing House, Beijing, first published c.AD 100, p. 144.
2. Unschuld PU 1986 Medicine in China – Nan Ching The Classic of Difficult Issues, University of California Press, Berkeley, USA, p. 561.
3. Clavey S 2002 Fluid Physiology and Pathology in Traditional Chinese Medicine, 2nd edition, Churchill Livingstone, Edinburgh, p. 34–35.
4. The Complete Book of Jing Yue, cited in 1981 Syndromes and Treatment of the Internal Organs (*Zang Fu Zheng Zhi* 脏腑证治), Tianjin Scientific Publishing House, Tianjin, p. 48.

5. A Revised Explanation of the Classic of Difficulties, p. 90.
6. 1979 The Yellow Emperor's Classic of Internal Medicine – Simple Questions (*Huang Di Nei Jing Su Wen* 黄帝内经素问), People's Health Publishing House, Beijing, first published *c*.100 BC, ch. 5, p. 33.
7. Ibid., p. 173–174.
8. Cited in Wang Xue Tai 1988 Great Treatise of Chinese Acupuncture (*Zhong Guo Zhen Jiu Da Quan* 中国针灸大全), Henan Science Publishing House, p. 162.
9. Simple Questions, p. 398.
10. Please note that I translate as 'Mind' the *Shen* that resides in the Heart, while as 'Spirit' the complex of the five spiritual aspects of the five Yin organs, i.e. the *Hun* (Ethereal Soul) of the Liver, the *Po* (Corporeal Soul) of the Lungs, the *Yi* (Intellect) of the Spleen, the *Zhi* (Will-power) of the Kidneys and the *Shen* (Mind) of the Heart itself.
11. Cited in Syndromes and Treatment of the Internal Organs, p. 51.
12. Ibid., p. 51.
13. What is described from now on as 'the Fire of the Heart' should not be confused with what will later be described as 'Heart-Fire'. The 'Fire of the Heart' indicates Fire in a Five-Element sense, the normal, physiological Fire to which the Heart pertains, called Emperor Fire. 'Heart-Fire' indicates a pathological condition of the Heart characterized by excess Heat.
14. 1792 Wu's Collected Medical Works, cited in Syndromes and Treatment of the Internal Organs, p. 52.
15. Hua Tuo 1985 The Classic of the Secret Transmission (*Zhong Cang Jing* 中藏经), Jiangsu Scientific Publishing House, Nanjing, originally published *c*.AD 180, p. 39.
16. 1624 The Complete Book of Jing Yue (*Jing Yue Quan Shu*), cited in Syndromes and Treatment of the Internal Organs, p. 52.
17. Wang Ping, cited in Syndromes and Treatment of the Internal Organs, p. 56.
18. He Bo Zhai, cited in Syndromes and Treatment of the Internal Organs, p. 56.

PART 2

The Functions of the Internal Organs

The functions of the Internal Organs (*Zangfu*) form the core of Chinese medical physiology. The general principles of Yin–Yang, the Five Elements and Qi are all at work in the theory of the Internal Organs. For example, we saw in chapter 3 that Qi moves and transforms fluids and that it is primarily Yang Qi that has such a function. When we study the functions of the Internal Organs we see this principle applied to Spleen-Yang and Kidney-Yang and can therefore formulate a theory about the functions of these two aspects of these organs.

The theory of the Internal Organs is often described as the core of Chinese medical theory, because it best represents the Chinese medicine view of the body as an integrated whole. At core, this theory represents a landscape of functional relationships which provide total integration of bodily functions, emotions, mental activities, tissues, sense organs and environmental influences.

There are two types of Internal Organs: Yin (called '*Zang*') and Yang (called '*Fu*') organs. The Chinese name for Internal Organs is simply '*Zangfu*'.

The Internal Organs are functionally related to various vital substances, emotions, tissues, senses: the following are the main aspects of these interrelationships.

The Yin organs store the Vital Substances (Qi, Blood, Essence and Body Fluids). They only store pure, refined substances which they receive from the Yang organs after transformation from food.

The Yang organs, in contrast, do not store but are constantly filled and emptied. They transform and refine food and drink to extract the pure essences which are then stored by the Yin organs. As well as carrying out this process of transformation, the Yang organs also excrete waste products.

There is a close interrelationship between Yin and Yang organs: the two groups of organs are different in function but their difference is only relative. The relationship between Yin and Yang organs is a structural–functional relationship. The Yin organs correspond to structure and store the Vital Substances, while the Yang organs correspond to function.

Part 2 is divided as follows:

SECTION 1 The functions of the Yin organs
- Chapter 5 The functions of the Internal Organs – Introduction
- Chapter 6 The functions of the Heart
- Chapter 7 The functions of the Liver
- Chapter 8 The functions of the Lungs
- Chapter 9 The functions of the Spleen
- Chapter 10 The functions of the Kidneys
- Chapter 11 The functions of the Pericardium
- Chapter 12 Yin organ interrelationships

SECTION 2 The functions of the Yang organs
- Chapter 13 The functions of the Stomach
- Chapter 14 The functions of the Small Intestine
- Chapter 15 The functions of the Large Intestine
- Chapter 16 The functions of the Gall Bladder
- Chapter 17 The functions of the Bladder
- Chapter 18 The functions of the Triple Burner

SECTION 3 The functions of the Six Extraordinary Yang Organs
- Chapter 19 The Uterus, Brain, Marrow, Bones, Blood Vessels, Gall Bladder

---

The Internal Organs and the Vital Substances
The Internal Organs and the tissues
The Internal Organs and the sense organs
The Internal Organs and the emotions
The Internal Organs and the spiritual aspects
The Internal Organs and climates
External manifestations of the Internal Organs
The Internal Organs and the fluids
The Internal Organs and the odours
The Internal Organs and the colours
The Internal Organs and the tastes
The Internal Organs and the sounds

SECTION 1

The functions of the Yin organs

INTRODUCTION

While the theory of the Internal Organs (*Zangfu*) is the core of Chinese physiology and pathology, the Yin organs (*Zang*) are the core of the Internal Organs. In fact, the Yin organs occupy a central place in Chinese physiology and pathology. The Yin organs are called *Zang* in Chinese, which means 'to store': they take this name because they store the precious essences of the body: that is, Blood, Fluids and the Essence itself. In pathology, for example, a deficiency of Yin is more serious and more difficult to treat than a deficiency of Yang.

Also the various correspondences listed in the ancient texts are always referred to the Yin rather than Yang organs (e.g. the correspondence between the Liver, anger, Spring, green, sinews, etc.).

When studying the functions of the Internal Organs, much more space is always dedicated to the Yin than to the Yang organs. This is not because the Yang organs are less 'important' but because many of the functions that we would attribute to the Yang organs in modern medicine are attributed to the Yin organs in Chinese medicine. A good example of this is the digestive system. Many intestinal disorders fall under the pathological umbrella of the Liver and Spleen.

All the ancient text always mentioned the 'five *Zang* and the six *Fu*', the five Yin Organs being the Liver, Heart, Spleen, Lungs and Kidneys, omitting the Pericardium. This is because the Pericardium was included under the sphere of the Heart. Indeed, modern Chinese books dedicate very little space to the functions of the Pericardium when discussing the functions of the Internal Organs and, when discussing the pathology, Pericardium patterns are not even mentioned. The functions and pathology of the Pericardium fall under the sphere of the Heart: hence the ancient texts always mention the 'five *Zang*'.

However, when considering the theory of channels rather than internal organs, the Pericardium is a distinct channel with its own actions, different to those of the Heart channel. For this reason, the ancient texts always mention 11 Internal Organs and 12 channels.

Section 1 of Part 2 comprises the following chapters:

Chapter 5 The functions of the Internal Organs
  – Introduction
Chapter 6 The functions of the Heart
Chapter 7 The functions of the Liver
Chapter 8 The functions of the Lungs
Chapter 9 The functions of the Spleen
Chapter 10 The functions of the Kidneys
Chapter 11 The functions of the Pericardium
Chapter 12 Yin organ interrelationships

For each Yin organ, the following aspects will be discussed:

1. Functions
    a) The type of Qi governed
    b) The tissue it controls
    c) The place where it manifests
    d) The Spiritual Aspect housed
    e) The emotion
    f) The sense organ into which it opens
    g) The fluids it controls
2. Other relationships
    a) Smell
    b) Colour
    c) Taste
    d) Climate
    e) Sound
3. Dreams
4. Sayings

The Functions of the Internal Organs – Introduction

5

Key contents

The Yin and Yang Internal Organs

Correspondences of Internal Organs

The theory of the Internal Organs is often described as the core of Chinese medical theory, because it best represents the Chinese medicine view of the body as an integrated whole. At core, this theory represents a landscape of functional relationships which provide total integration of bodily functions, emotions, mental activities, tissues, sense organs and environmental influences.

When studying the Chinese theory of the Internal Organs, it is best to rid oneself of the Western concept of internal organs entirely. Western medicine sees each organ only in its material–anatomical aspect, whereas Chinese medicine sees each organ as a complex energetic system encompassing its anatomical entity and its mental, emotional and spiritual aspects. As explained in chapter 3, the basis of Chinese medicine is Qi, which assumes different states of aggregation and dispersal. Thus, the aggregation of Qi into dense matter forms the Internal Organs, while the dispersal of Qi in more subtle states forms their emotional, mental and spiritual aspects (Box 5.1).

Each internal organ is therefore not simply an anatomical entity (although also that) but an energetic vortex that manifests in different states of aggregation in many different spheres of life. In fact, each organ is correlated with a particular emotion, tissue, sense organ, mental faculty, colour, climate, taste, smell and more. Throughout this book, organs are described in this way and not in the Western anatomical sense.

The correspondences between the Internal Organs and other manifestations are as follows:

- Vital substances
- Tissues
- Sense organs
- Emotions
- Spiritual aspects
- Climates
- External manifestations
- Fluids
- Odours
- Colours
- Tastes
- Sounds

For example, the Liver is in correspondence with the following:

- Blood
- Sinews
- Eyes
- Anger
- Ethereal Soul
- Wind
- Nails
- Tears
- Rancid
- Green
- Sour
- Shouting

Box 5.1 Internal Organs correspondences

- Vital substances
- Tissues
- Sense organs
- Emotions
- Spiritual aspects
- Climates
- External manifestations
- Fluids
- Odours
- Colours
- Tastes
- Sounds

However, it is often said that Chinese medicine disregards anatomy entirely and only considers the functional relationships: this is not entirely true. While Chinese medicine excels in its acute and detailed observation of complex functional relationships, it does not entirely disregard the study of anatomy. There are many chapters of the 'Yellow Emperor's Classic' and the 'Classic of Difficulties' that describe the anatomy of the internal organs, muscles and bones.[1]

The Internal Organs are functionally related to various vital substances, emotions, tissues and sense organs. It should be pointed out that these functional relationships relate only to the Yin organs. The following are the main aspects of these interrelationships that will be discussed in the following chapters.

- The Internal Organs and the Vital Substances
- The Internal Organs and the tissues
- The Internal Organs and the sense organs
- The Internal Organs and the emotions
- The Internal Organs and the spiritual aspects
- The Internal Organs and climates
- The external manifestations of the Internal Organs
- The Internal Organs and the fluids
- The Internal Organs and the odours
- The Internal Organs and the colours
- The Internal Organs and the tastes
- The Internal Organs and the sounds

THE INTERNAL ORGANS AND THE VITAL SUBSTANCES

One of the main functions of the Internal Organs is to ensure the production, maintenance, replenishment, transformation and movement of the Vital Substances. Each of the Vital Substances, Qi, Blood, Essence, and Body Fluids is related to one or more of the organs, as listed in Box 5.2.

Box 5.2 Internal Organs and Vital Substances

- The Heart governs Blood
- The Liver stores Blood
- The Lungs govern Qi and influence Body Fluids
- The Spleen governs Food-Qi (*Gu Qi*), holds Blood and influences Body Fluids
- The Kidneys store Essence (*Jing*) and influence Body Fluids

---

Clinical note

- As the Liver stores and the Heart governs Blood, tonify Liver and Heart to nourish Blood
- As the Lungs and Spleen govern Qi, tonify Lungs and Spleen to strengthen Qi
- As the Kidneys govern the Essence, strengthen the Kidneys to nourish the Essence

THE INTERNAL ORGANS AND THE TISSUES

Each organ influences one of the tissues of the body: this means that there is a functional relationship between certain tissues and each organ, so that the state of the organ can be deduced by observation of the tissue related to it. For example, the Heart controls the blood vessels, the Liver controls the sinews, the Lungs control the skin, the Spleen controls the muscles, the Kidneys control the bones. Thus, the state of those tissues reflects the state of the corresponding Internal Organs. For example, a weakness and flaccidity of the muscles indicates a deficiency of the Spleen; a tendency to contraction of the sinews indicates a pathology of the Liver; a reduced bone density in old age reflects a deficiency of the Kidneys.

In treatment, treating the Internal Organs will influence their related tissues (Box 5.3).

Box 5.3 Internal Organs and tissues

- Liver – sinews
- Heart – blood vessels
- Spleen – muscles
- Lungs – skin
- Kidneys – bones

THE INTERNAL ORGANS AND THE SENSE ORGANS

Each organ is functionally related to one of the sense organs. This means that the health and acuity of a particular sense organ relies on the nourishment of an internal organ. Thus, the Heart controls the tongue and taste, the Liver controls the eyes and sight, the Lungs control the nose and smell, the Spleen controls the mouth and taste, the Kidneys control the ears and hearing (Box 5.4).

> **Box 5.4 Internal Organs and sense organs**
>
> - Liver – eyes
> - Heart – tongue
> - Spleen – mouth
> - Lungs – nose
> - Kidneys – ears

For example, a loss of taste sensation is usually due to a Spleen deficiency; a decrease in visual acuity is often related to a deficiency of Liver-Blood (but not always), etc.

> **Clinical note**
>
> The Back-Transporting (Back-*Shu*) points of the Yin organs affect the relevant sense organs:
> - BL-13 Feishu (Lungs) for the nose
> - BL-15 Xinshu (Heart) for the tongue and taste
> - BL-18 Ganshu (Liver) for the eyes
> - BL-20 Pishu (Spleen) for the mouth and taste
> - BL-23 Shenshu (Kidneys) for the ears

THE INTERNAL ORGANS AND THE EMOTIONS

This extremely important aspect of the Chinese theory of the Internal Organs illustrates the unity of body and mind in Chinese medicine. The same Qi that is the basis for all the physiological processes is also the basis for emotional and mental processes, since Qi, as we have seen, exists in many different states of aggregation and refinement. Whereas in Western physiology emotional and mental processes are attributed to the brain, in Chinese medicine they are part of the sphere of action of the internal organs. Thus, in Western medicine, the brain and the nervous system are at the top of the mind–body pyramid with the autonomic centres of the brain cortex at the top and the viscera at the bottom (Fig. 5.1); in Chinese medicine, the pyramid is inverted, with the viscera at the top and the mind at the bottom (Fig. 5.2).

The relation between each organ and a particular emotion is mutual: the state of the organ will affect the

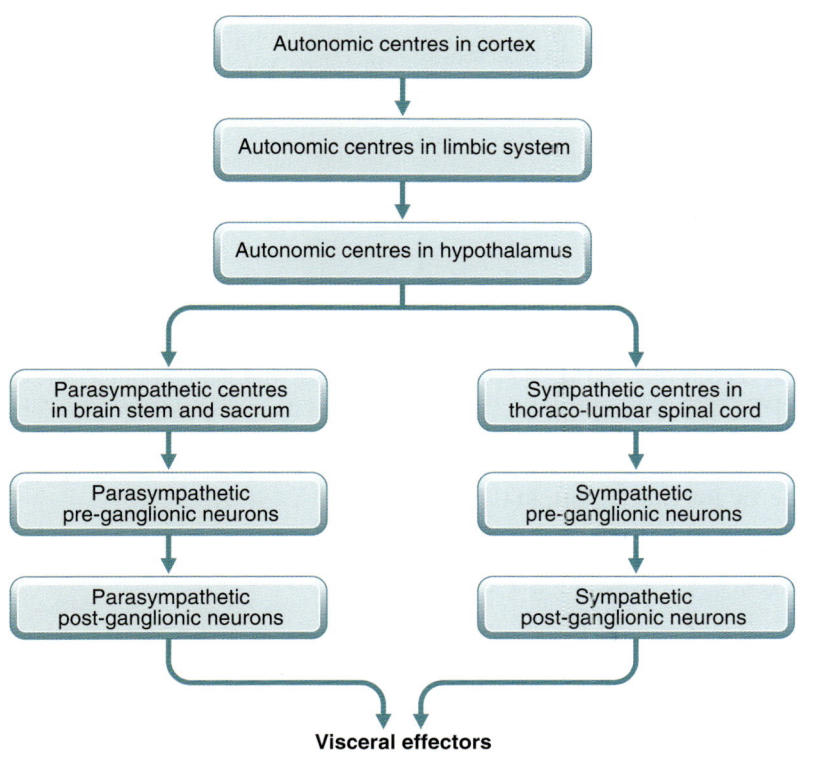

```
Autonomic centres in cortex
          ↓
Autonomic centres in limbic system
          ↓
Autonomic centres in hypothalamus
       ↙        ↘
Parasympathetic centres      Sympathetic centres in
in brain stem and sacrum     thoraco-lumbar spinal cord
       ↓                            ↓
Parasympathetic              Sympathetic
pre-ganglionic neurons       pre-ganglionic neurons
       ↓                            ↓
Parasympathetic              Sympathetic
post-ganglionic neurons      post-ganglionic neurons
       ↘                    ↙
          Visceral effectors
```

Figure 5.1 Mind–body interrelationship in Western medicine

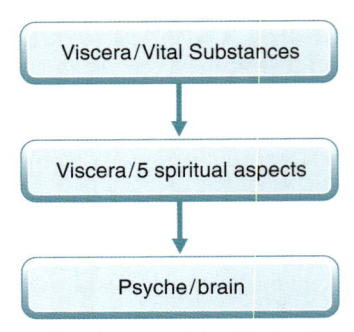

Figure 5.2 Mind–body interrelationship in Chinese medicine

emotions, and emotions will affect the state of the organ. Thus: the Heart relates to joy, the Liver to anger, the Lungs to sadness and worry, the Spleen to thinking and pensiveness and the Kidneys to fear. Thus, for example, a state of persistent anger due to a particular situation in one's life may cause the rising of Liver-Yang; vice versa, if Liver-Yang rises because Liver-Blood is deficient, this may cause the person to become prone to outbursts of anger.

These emotions usually become a cause of imbalance only when they are excessive and prolonged. By treating a specific organ, we can influence the particular emotion related to that organ and help a person to achieve a more balanced emotional state (Box 5.5).

> **Box 5.5 Internal Organs and emotions**
> - Liver – anger
> - Heart – joy
> - Spleen – pensiveness
> - Lungs – worry
> - Kidneys – fear

THE INTERNAL ORGANS AND THE SPIRITUAL ASPECTS

By 'Spiritual Aspects' I refer to the mental–spiritual entities related to the Yin Internal Organs. In Chinese, these are called *Wu Shen* ('Five Shen') or *Wu Zhi* ('Five Zhi').

The five Spiritual Aspects are listed in Box 5.6.

The Ethereal Soul (*Hun*) is a soul that is Yang in nature and that, according to Chinese culture, enters the body three days after birth and is imparted to the baby by the father. After death, the Ethereal Soul survives the body and returns to a world of spirit. The Chinese character for *hun* (Ethereal Soul) confirms its spiritual, non-material nature as it is made up by the radical *gui* which means 'spirit' or 'ghost' and the radical *yun* which means 'clouds'. The Ethereal Soul resides in the Liver and particularly in the Blood and Yin of the Liver where it should be 'anchored': if Liver-Blood is deficient and the Ethereal Soul is not anchored in the Liver, it 'wanders' at night and causes the person to dream a lot. The Ethereal Soul is described as 'the coming and going of the Mind (*Shen*)' and it will be discussed further in chapter 7.

> **Box 5.6 Internal Organs and spiritual aspects**
> - Liver – Ethereal Soul (*Hun*)
> - Heart – Mind (*Shen*)
> - Spleen – Intellect (*Yi*)
> - Lungs – Corporeal Soul (*Po*)
> - Kidneys – Will-power (*Zhi*)

The Ethereal Soul is the 'coming and going of the Mind (*Shen*)'

The Mind (*Shen*) is the consciousness that is responsible for thought, feeling, emotions, perceptions, cognition. The Mind resides in the Heart and it is primarily for this reason that the Heart is called the 'Emperor' in relation to all the other Internal Organs. As the Mind is the consciousness that defines us as individual human beings and is responsible for thinking, willing and feeling, the Heart plays a leading role among the other Internal Organs. I translate *shen* as 'Mind' rather than the more generally used term 'Spirit'. I translate as 'Mind' the Spiritual Aspect of the Heart, that is, the *Shen* which corresponds to consciousness; I translate as 'Spirit' the complex of all five Spiritual Aspects, that is, the Ethereal Soul (*Hun*), the Corporeal Soul (*Po*), the Intellect (*Yi*), the Will-power (*Zhi*) and the Mind itself (*Shen*). The Mind is discussed further in chapter 6.

Remember: I translate *Shen* (of the Heart) as 'Mind' and as 'Spirit', the complex of the Five Spiritual Aspects (*Hun, Po, Yi, Zhi* and *Shen* itself)

The Intellect (*Yi*) is responsible for memory, concentration, thinking, logical thinking, capacity for studying and application. In pathology, the capacity for thinking may become pensiveness, over-thinking, obsessive thinking, fantasizing or brooding. The Intellect resides in the Spleen. The Intellect is discussed further in chapter 9.

The Corporeal Soul (*Po*) is responsible for physical sensations, feelings and generally somatic expressions. It resides in the Lungs and it plays a role in all physiological processes of the body. It is formed at conception (unlike the Ethereal Soul which enters the body after birth), it is Yin in nature (compared to the Ethereal Soul) and, at death, it dies with the body, returning to the Earth (while the Ethereal Soul survives the body and returns to Heaven). The Corporeal Soul is described as the 'entering and exiting of Essence (*Jing*)'. The Corporeal Soul is discussed further in chapter 8.

Clinical note

The outer points on the Bladder channel in the back affect the relevant Spiritual Aspects:
- BL-42 Pohu for the Corporeal Soul
- BL-44 Shentang for the Mind
- BL-47 Hunmen for the Ethereal Soul
- BL-49 Yishe for the Intellect
- BL-52 Zhishi for the Will-power

The Corporeal Soul is the 'entering and exiting of Essence (*Jing*)'

The Will-power (*Zhi*) resides in the Kidneys and it is responsible for will-power, drive, determination, constancy. The Will-power is discussed at greater length in chapter 10.

THE INTERNAL ORGANS AND CLIMATES

Chinese medicine considers that differing climatic conditions influence specific organs. Heat influences the Heart, wind influences the Liver, dryness influences the Lung, dampness influences the Spleen and cold influences the Kidneys.

An excess of these climatic conditions for a prolonged period may adversely affect the relevant organ. Vice versa, a weakness of one of the Internal Organs may render the person prone to attack by its corresponding climate; for example, a Spleen deficiency will make a person prone to invasions of Dampness (Box 5.7).

Box 5.7 Internal Organs and climates
- Liver – wind
- Heart – heat
- Spleen – dampness
- Lungs – dryness
- Kidneys – cold

THE EXTERNAL MANIFESTATIONS OF THE INTERNAL ORGANS

Each internal organ influences a particular part of the body and, conversely, each part of the body reflects the state of a particular organ. The correspondences are as listed in Box 5.8.

Box 5.8 External manifestations of the Internal Organs
- The Heart manifests in the complexion
- The Liver manifests in the nails
- The Lungs manifest in the body hair
- The Spleen manifests on the lips
- The Kidneys manifest in the hair

Thus, for example, the Liver manifests on the nails and therefore the condition of the nails reflects the state of the Liver: brittle nails, for example, indicate deficiency of Liver-Blood. The correspondence between the five Yin organs and five parts of the body is closer for some than for others. In particular, the correspondence between the Liver, Lungs, Spleen and nails, body hair and lips, respectively, is close: that is, the nails will always and only indicate the state of the Liver. The correspondence between the Heart and Kidneys and the complexion and hair, respectively, is less rigid: that is, the appearance of the complexion may indicate the state of any organ and not just of the Heart.

THE INTERNAL ORGANS AND THE FLUIDS

Each Internal Organ is related to a certain body fluids as follows:

- Liver – tears
- Heart – sweat
- Spleen – saliva
- Lungs – snivel
- Kidneys – spittle

By 'tears' is meant mostly the basal and reflex tears of Western medicine (i.e. the tears that lubricate the eye and those that are provoked by a foreign body in the eye, as opposed to tears brought about by emotion). The connection of the Liver with tears is probably the closest and most obvious relationship between an Internal Organ and a fluid. The Liver opens into the eyes, and tears are therefore the fluids naturally related to the Liver. This means that deficiency of Liver-Blood or Liver-Yin may cause dry eyes, while Liver-Yang rising may cause the eyes to water a lot; Damp-Heat in the Liver channel may cause the tears to be sticky and thick.

The Heart influences sweat and this relationship is seen most clearly when a person sweats excessively in response to emotional tension. Sweat is also related to the Lungs and the Lung's influence on the space between skin and muscles where sweat is.

'Saliva' is a translation of the Chinese word '*xian*'. This fluid is described as a thin, watery fluid in the mouth which has the function of moistening the mouth and to aid digestion.

Nasal mucus is naturally related to the Lungs as these open into the nose. By 'nasal mucus' is meant here not the nasal discharge seen in a cold, rhinitis or sinusitis, but the normal mucosal secretion of the lining of the nose.

'Spittle' is a translation of the Chinese word '*tuo*'. This fluid is described as being thick and more turbid than saliva (*xian*). Spittle's function is to lubricate the back of the mouth and throat and it is thought to be an expression of the Kidney-Essence (summarized in Box 5.9).

> **Box 5.9 The Internal Organs and the fluids**
> - Liver – tears
> - Heart – sweat
> - Spleen – saliva
> - Lungs – nasal mucus
> - Kidneys – spittle

THE INTERNAL ORGANS AND THE ODOURS

Each Internal Organ is related to a particular odour as follows:

> - Liver – rancid
> - Heart – scorched
> - Spleen – fragrant, sweetish
> - Lungs – rotten, rank
> - Kidneys – putrid

The rancid odour pertaining to the Liver is like the smell of rancid meat (this is quite common); the scorched smell of the Heart is like that or burnt toast (not common in practice); the fragrant, sweetish smell of the Spleen is like that of a sickly, sweetish perfume; the rotten smell of the Lungs is like that of rotten eggs; the putrid smell of the Kidneys is like that of putrid, stagnant water (a common smell in the elderly).

These odours are body odours that can be smelled as the patient undresses or sometimes even through the clothes and they are used in diagnosis as each odour indicates a pathology of the relevant organ (summarized in Box 5.10).

> **Box 5.10 The Internal Organs and the odours**
> - Liver – rancid
> - Heart – scorched
> - Spleen – fragrant, sweetish
> - Lungs – rotten, rank
> - Kidneys – putrid

THE INTERNAL ORGANS AND THE COLOURS

The colours related to the Internal Organs are as follows:

> - Liver – green
> - Heart – red
> - Spleen – yellow
> - Lungs – white
> - Kidneys – black, dark

The colours of the Internal Organs are observed primarily on the facial complexion and they are an important aspect of diagnosis. Thus, a greenish complexion indicates a Liver pathology such as Liver-Qi stagnation, a red colour on the cheeks may indicate Heart-Fire (but also Heat in other organs), a yellow complexion is typical of a Spleen deficiency or obstruction of the Spleen by Dampness, a white complexion indicates Lung-Qi deficiency (but also a deficiency of Qi or Blood of other organs), and a dark complexion indicates Kidney-Yin deficiency (summarized in Box 5.11).

> **Box 5.11 The Internal Organs and the colours**
>
> - Liver – green
> - Heart – red
> - Spleen – yellow
> - Lungs – white
> - Kidneys – dark, black

THE INTERNAL ORGANS AND THE TASTES

Each Internal Organ is related to a particular taste as follows:

> - Liver – sour
> - Heart – bitter
> - Spleen – sweet
> - Lungs – pungent
> - Kidneys – salty

There are many important implications to the tastes in Chinese medicine. Firstly, a particular taste experienced by a person may indicate a pathology of the relevant organ; for example, a bitter taste often indicates Heart-Fire (although it may also relate to Liver-Fire), while a sweetish taste indicates a Spleen pathology.

Secondly, the tastes are important in Chinese herbal medicine as each herbs is classified as having a particular taste which makes that herb 'enter' the relevant channel (e.g. sour herbs enter the Liver channel). The excess of a particular taste may injure the organ to which it is related and the organ that is over-acted upon (and its relevant tissue): for example, an excessive consumption of herbs with a sour taste may injure the Liver and the also the Spleen and the muscles. On the other hand, each taste is beneficial to the organ that over-acts on the organ related to that particular taste: for example, the sweet taste (related to the Spleen) is beneficial to the Liver.

Thirdly, the tastes are important in Chinese dietary therapy as each food is classified as having a particular taste. The effect of that food on the Internal Organs is the same as that of the herbs mentioned above.

These correspondences are summarized in Box 5.12.

> **Box 5.12 The Internal Organs and the tastes**
>
> - Liver – sour
> - Heart – bitter
> - Spleen – sweet
> - Lungs – pungent
> - Kidneys – salty

THE INTERNAL ORGANS AND THE SOUNDS

Each Internal Organ is related to a sound as follows:

> - Liver – shouting
> - Heart – laughing
> - Spleen – singing
> - Lungs – crying
> - Kidneys – groaning

The sounds refer to the sound and pitch of the voice and are used primarily in diagnosis. Thus, if a person speaks with a very loud, almost shouting voice, it indicates a pathology of the Liver; a person suffering from a Heart pattern may tend to punctuate his or her speech with inappropriate, short bursts of laughter; a melodious, singing tone may indicate a Spleen pathology; a person suffering from Lung deficiency may speak with a tone that is almost as if they were about to burst into tears; a throaty, groaning voice may indicate a Kidney deficiency.

These correspondences are summarized in Box 5.13.

> **Box 5.13 The Internal Organs and the sounds**
>
> - Liver – shouting
> - Heart – laughing
> - Spleen – singing
> - Lungs – crying
> - Kidneys – groaning

YIN (*ZANG*) AND YANG (*FU*) ORGANS

There are two types of Internal Organs: Yin (called '*Zang*') and Yang (called '*Fu*') organs. The Chinese name for Internal Organs is simply '*Zangfu*'.

Both '*Zang*' and '*Fu*' mean 'organ', but an analysis of the Chinese characters can clarify the difference between the two:

ZANG 臟 (simplified: 脏) means organ, viscus

月 this part indicates 'flesh'

藏 this part indicates 'to store'

This indicates that the Yin organs are in charge of storing the vital substances.

FU 腑 also means organ

月 this part indicates 'flesh'

府 this part indicates 'seat of government' or 'administrative centre'

This indicates that the Yang organs are in charge of transforming food and drink to produce Qi and Blood, just as the government in ancient China was considered to be in charge of food distribution.

The 'Simple Questions' in chapter 11 says: *'The 5 Yin organs store Essence and Qi and do not excrete: they can be full but not in excess. The 6 Yang organs transform and digest and do not store: they can be in excess but not full. In fact, after food enters the mouth, the stomach is full and the intestines empty; when the food goes down, the intestines are full and the stomach empty.'*[2]

Thus the Yin organs store the Vital Substances (Qi, Blood, Essence and Body Fluids). They only store pure, refined substances, which they receive from the Yang organs after transformation from food.

Box 5.14 summarizes the functions of the Yin organs.

> **Box 5.14 Yin organs (*Zang*)**
>
> The Yin organs store the Vital Substances: that is, Qi, Blood, Essence and Body Fluids. They store only pure, refined substances which they receive from the Yang organs after transformation from food

The Yang organs, on the contrary, do not store but are constantly filled and emptied. They transform and refine food and drink to extract the pure essences which are then stored by the Yin organs. As well as carrying out this process of transformation, the Yang organs also excrete waste products. The essence of the Yang organs is therefore to 'receive', 'move', 'transform', digest' and 'excrete'. The functions of the Yang organs are often summarized by the two words '*chuan*' and '*xing*', meaning 'to transmit' and 'to move', because they are constantly receiving, transmitting, moving and excreting substances. Perhaps because of this constant moving in and out of substances, the Yang organs are also compared to a government office with a constant coming and going of people, as their name '*Fu*' implies.

The 'Simple Questions' in chapter 9 says: *'The Stomach, Small and Large Intestine, Triple Burner and Bladder are the roots of food storage, they are the residence of Nutritive Qi, they are called containers, they transform waste substances and transmit the incoming and outgoing flavours.'*[3]

Box 5.15 summarizes the functions of the Yang organs.

There is a close interrelationship between Yin and Yang organs: the two groups of organs are different in

> **Box 5.15 Yang organs (*Fu*)**
>
> - The Yang organs do not store
> - They are constantly filled and emptied
> - They transform and refine food and drink to extract the pure essences which are then stored by the Yin organs
> - They excrete waste products
> - The function of the Yang organs is therefore to 'receive', 'move', 'transform', digest and 'excrete'

function but their difference is only relative. The relationship between Yin and Yang organs is a structural–functional relationship. The Yin organs correspond to structure and store the Vital Substances, while the Yang organs correspond to function. Structure and function are interdependent and we can view each Yang organ as the functional aspect of its corresponding Yin organ. For example, one can view the Gall Bladder as the functional aspect of the Liver. Although one Yang and one Yin, the two organs can be seen as a unit, the Liver being the structure and the Gall Bladder its functional expression. This view of the Yin–Yang relationship of the organs is particularly useful in pulse diagnosis where it may be more meaningful to see each pulse position at the superficial level as the function aspect of the relevant Yin organ, rather than considering each of the 12 pulse positions individually and in isolation.

In the Chinese theory of the organs, the Yin organs are the core: they are more important than the Yang organs both in terms of physiology and pathology. The Yin organs are more important because they store all the Vital Substances, while the Yang organs are their functional aspect. For this reason, in what follows, the main focus of attention is on the Yin organs. However, it should be stressed that the priority of the Yin over the Yang organs is not reflected in the theory of the channels: from an acupuncturist's (as opposed to a herbalist's) perspective, all the 14 channels are equally important.

There are 12 organs, six Yin and six Yang:

Yin organs	*Yang organs*	*Element*
Heart	Small Intestine	Emperor Fire
Liver	Gall Bladder	Wood
Lungs	Large Intestine	Metal
Spleen	Stomach	Earth
Kidneys	Bladder	Water
Pericardium	Triple Burner	Minister Fire

For each organ the following aspects will be discussed in detail:

- Its main function or functions
- The tissue it controls
- The sense organ into which it 'opens'
- The part of the body on which it 'manifests'
- The fluid it controls
- Any other function peculiar to each organ

In addition to the above, a few sayings for each organ will be given to illustrate certain other aspects of the organ functions not normally included in the itemized functions.

Learning outcomes

In this chapter you will have learned:

- The nature and functions of the Yin and Yang organs in general
- The essential differences between Yin and Yang organs in general
- The correlation between Internal Organs and Vital Substances, emotions, Spiritual Aspects, tissues, climates, sense organs and external manifestations

Self-assessment questions

1. Which Vital Substance does the Heart 'govern'?
2. Which Vital Substance does the Liver 'store'?
3. A person suffers from rigidity and contraction of the elbow: which tissue is involved and which organ controls that tissue?
4. Which is the sense organ related to the Lungs?
5. Which organs does worry affect primarily?
6. Which type of soul do the Liver and the Lungs 'house'?
7. Which is the climate that affects the Spleen?
8. The nails manifest the state of which organs?
9. Which fluid do the Kidneys control?
10. What odour might you expect to emanate from the body of a patient's suffering from a Heart disharmony?

See p. 1256 for answers

END NOTES

1. 1981 Spiritual Axis (*Ling Shu Jing* 灵枢经), People's Health Publishing House, Beijing, first published *c.*100 BC, chs 10, 13, 14 and 31. Nanjing College of Traditional Chinese Medicine 1979 A Revised Explanation of the Classic of Difficulties (*Nan Jing Jiao Shi* 难经校释). People's Health Publishing House, Beijing, first published *c.*AD 100, chs 41 and 42.
2. 1979 The Yellow Emperor's Classic of Internal Medicine – Simple Questions (*Huang Di Nei Jing Su Wen* 黄帝内经素问), People's Health Publishing House, Beijing, first published *c.*100 BC, p. 77.
3. Ibid., p. 67.

BIBLIOGRAPHY AND FURTHER READING

Kaptchuk T 2000 The Web that has no Weaver – Understanding Chinese Medicine, Contemporary Books, Chicago

SECTION 1   PART 2

The Functions of the Heart 6

Key contents

The functions of the Heart
Governs Blood
Controls the blood vessels
Manifests in the complexion
Houses the Mind (Shen)
Opens into the tongue
Controls sweat

Other Heart relationships
Its smell is scorched
Its colour is red
Its taste is bitter
Its climate is heat
Its sound is laughing

Dreams

Sayings

The Heart is considered to be the most important of all the Internal Organs, sometimes described as the 'ruler', 'emperor' or 'monarch' of the Internal Organs. The 'Simple Questions' in chapter 8 says: '*The Heart is like the Monarch and it governs the Mind (Shen)*.'[1] The 'Spiritual Axis' in chapter 71 says: '*The Heart is the Monarch of the 5 Yin organs and the 6 Yang organs and it is the residence of the Mind (Shen)*.'[2]

The Heart's main functions are to govern Blood and blood vessels and to house the Mind (*Shen*). Its functions can be summarized as follows:

- It governs Blood
- It controls the blood vessels
- It manifests in the complexion
- It houses the Mind (*Shen*)
- It opens into the tongue
- It controls sweat

The discussion of the Heart will be organized under the following headings:

- Functions of the Heart
  - The Heart governs Blood
  - The Heart controls the blood vessels
  - The Heart manifests in the complexion
  - The Heart houses the Mind
  - The Heart is related to joy
  - The Heart opens into the tongue
  - The Heart controls sweat
- Other Heart relationships
  - The smell of the Heart is scorched
  - The colour of the Heart is red
  - The taste of the Heart is bitter
  - The climate of the Heart is heat
  - The sound of the Heart is laughing
- Dreams
- Sayings

FUNCTIONS OF THE HEART

The functions of the Heart discussed are:

- The Heart governs Blood
- The Heart controls the blood vessels
- The Heart manifests in the complexion
- The Heart houses the Mind
- The Heart is related to joy
- The Heart opens into the tongue
- The Heart controls sweat

The Heart governs Blood

The Heart governs Blood in two ways:

1. The transformation of Food-Qi (*Gu Qi*) into Blood takes place in the Heart
2. The Heart s responsible for the circulation of Blood just the same as in Western medicine (although in Chinese medicine, other organs, notably the Lungs, Spleen and Liver, also play a role in the circulation of Blood)

A healthy Heart is essential for a proper supply of blood to all the body tissues. When its function is impaired (i.e. Heart-Blood is deficient), the circulation of Blood is slack and the hands may be cold.

The relationship between Heart and Blood is important in another way as it determines the strength of constitution of an individual.

Although our constitution is primarily related to the Essence (*Jing*) and the Kidney, it is also partly determined by the relative constitutional strength of the Heart and Blood. If the Heart is strong, Blood in ample supply and its circulation good, a person will be full of vigour and have a good constitution. If the Heart is constitutionally weak and Blood deficient, a person will have a poor constitution and lack strength. A constitutional weakness of the Heart is sometimes manifested with a shallow, long crack in the midline of the tongue (Fig. 6.1) and a weak pulse on both the Heart and Kidney positions.

Clinical note

A thin, long, midline crack on the tongue indicates a weak Heart constitution and the tendency to emotional problems.

Heart-Blood also influences menstruation indirectly. Although it is Liver-Blood that is most important for the menstrual function, Heart-Blood also plays a role because the Heart controls the discharge of blood occurring during menstruation; in other words, although it is Liver-Blood that is stored in the Uterus, the Heart controls the downward movement of Qi and Blood that makes menstruation occur.

Heart-Blood plays a role in menstruation.

As explained below, one of the most important functions of Heart-Blood is to 'house' the Mind (*Shen*).

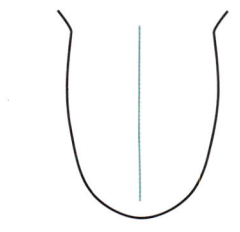

Figure 6.1 Heart crack on the tongue

Box 6.1 The Heart governs Blood

- Food-Qi is transformed into Blood in the Heart
- The Heart controls the circulation of Blood
- Heart-Blood influences menstruation indirectly
- Heart-Blood houses the Mind (*Shen*)

The 'Simple Questions' in chapter 10 says: '*Blood pertains to the Heart.*'[3]

Box 6.1 summarizes these points.

As we will see in the next chapters, three organs influence Blood: the Heart 'governs' Blood, the Liver 'stores' Blood and the Spleen and Kidneys 'make' Blood.

Clinical note

The points that tonify Heart-Blood are Ren-15 Jiuwei, HE-7 Shenmen and BL-15 Xinshu (with moxa cones). The remedy Gui Pi Tang (or *Calm the Shen* in the *Three Treasures*) nourishes Heart-Blood

The Heart controls the blood vessels

As the Heart governs Blood, it naturally also controls the blood vessels (Box 6.2). The state of the Heart's energy is reflected in the state of the blood vessels. Blood vessels depend on the Heart's Qi and Blood. If Heart-Qi is strong, the blood vessels will be in a good state and the pulse will be full and regular. If Heart-Qi is weak, the pulse may be feeble and irregular. The 'Simple Questions' in chapter 44 says: '*The Heart governs the blood vessels.*'[4] If Heart-Blood is abundant, the pulse is full and smooth; if Heart-Blood is deficient, the pulse is Choppy; if Heart-Blood has stasis, the blood vessels feel hard and this may cause arteriosclerosis.

Clinical note

The Heart influences the blood vessels. The elderly often have a very hard pulse, which is often due to arteriosclerosis (hardening of the arteries): this always reflects the state of the Heart (often Heart-Blood stasis)

Box 6.2 The Heart controls the blood vessels

- The Heart influences the state of the blood vessels (e.g. hardening of blood vessels from Heart-Blood stasis)
- The blood vessels identify one of five energetic layers (skin, muscles, sinews, blood vessels, bones)

The 'blood vessels' have also another significance in Chinese medicine in so far as they denote an energetic layer together with skin, muscles, sinews and bones. The energetic layers, in ascending order of depth, are as listed below:

'Blood vessels' refers also to one of five energetic layers:
- Skin (Lungs)
- Muscles (Spleen)
- Sinews (Liver)
- Blood vessels (Heart)
- Bones (Kidneys)

For example, a classification of Painful Obstruction Syndrome (*Bi*) in the 'Yellow Emperor's Classic of Internal Medicine' is based on these five energetic layers with five types of *Bi* (i.e. Skin-*Bi*, Muscles-*Bi*, etc.). The five energetic layers of skin, muscles, sinews, blood vessels and bones are also used in pulse diagnosis as the superficial layer of the pulse reflects skin and muscles (Lungs and Spleen), the middle level sinews and blood vessels (Liver and Heart), and the deep level the bones (Kidneys).

The Heart manifests in the complexion

The Heart governs Blood and blood vessels and distributes Blood all over the body. The state of the Heart and Blood can therefore be reflected in the complexion and particularly the complexion of the face (Box 6.3). If Blood is abundant and the Heart strong, the complexion will be rosy and lustrous. If Blood is deficient, the complexion will be pale or dull white; if Heart-Yang is deficient, the complexion will be bright white. If Blood is stagnant, the complexion will be purplish or dull and dark, and if the Heart has Heat, the complexion will be too red. The 'Simple Questions' in chapter 10 says; '*The Heart ... manifests in the complexion.*'[5]

Of course, the complexion can reflect the state of any organ: for example, red cheeks may indicate Lung-Heat or Liver-Heat.

Box 6.3 The Heart and the complexion
The Heart is reflected in the face complexion: • Dull pale: Heart-Blood deficiency • Bright white: Heart-Yang deficiency • Purplish or dark: Heart-Blood stasis • Red: Heart-Heat.

The Heart houses the Mind

Chinese medicine holds that the Heart is the residence of the Mind (*Shen*).[6] The word *Shen* can have many different meanings and, in Chinese medicine, it is used in at least two different contexts.

Firstly, in a narrow sense, *Shen* indicates the complex of mental faculties which are said to 'reside' in the Heart. In this sense, the *Shen* corresponds to the Mind and is specifically related to the Heart.

Secondly, in a broad sense, *Shen* is used to indicate the whole sphere of mental and spiritual aspects of a human being. In this sense, it is related not only to the Heart but also it encompasses the mental and spiritual phenomena of all the other organs, notably the Yin organs: that is, the Ethereal Soul (*Hun*), Corporeal Soul (*Po*), Intellect (*Yi*), Will-power (*Zhi*) and the Mind (*Shen*) itself.

- In a narrow sense, *Shen* pertains to the Heart (translated as 'Mind')
- In a broad sense, *Shen* pertains to all Yin organs, including *Hun, Po, Yi, Zhi* and *Shen* of the Heart itself (translated as 'Spirit')

The Mind of the Heart

Let us now discuss the nature and functions of the Mind in the first, narrow sense outlined above.

According to Chinese medicine, mental activity and consciousness 'reside' in the Heart. This means that the state of the Heart (and Blood) will affect the mental activities including the emotional state. In particular, five functions are affected by the state of the Heart. These are listed in Box 6.4.

If the Heart is strong and Blood abundant, there will be a normal mental activity, a balanced emotional life, a clear consciousness, a good memory, keen thinking and good sleep. If the Heart is weak and Blood deficient there may be mental–emotional problems

Box 6.4 Five major Heart-Mind functions
• Mental activity (including emotions) • Consciousness • Memory • Thinking • Sleep

(such as depression), poor memory, dull thinking, insomnia or somnolence and in extreme cases, unconsciousness. The 'Simple Questions' in chapter 9 says: *'The Heart ... is in control of the Mind.'*[7] The 'Spiritual Axis' in chapter 71 says: *'The Heart ... is the residence of the Mind.'*[8]

As the Heart controls all mental activities of the Mind and is responsible for insight and cognition, which other organs do not have, this is another reason that it is the 'emperor' of the other internal organs. For this reason, the Heart is also called the 'root of life', as in chapter 9 of the 'Simple Questions': *'The Heart is the root of life and the origin of mental life.'*[9]

The Heart's function of housing the Mind depends on an adequate nourishment from the Blood and, conversely, the Heart's job of governing Blood depends on the Mind. Thus there is a relation of mutual dependence between the function of governing Blood and that of housing the Mind. The Blood is the root of the Mind. This concept is important in practice as Heart-Blood roots the Mind, embraces it and anchors it, so that the Mind will be peaceful and happy. If Heart-Blood is deficient and does not root the Mind, this will result in mental restlessness, depression, anxiety and insomnia. Conversely, mental restlessness, emotional problems and sadness can induce a deficiency of Blood of the Heart causing palpitations, a pale complexion and a weak or irregular pulse. If Heart-Blood has Heat, the person will be restless, agitated and will not sleep well (Fig. 6.2).

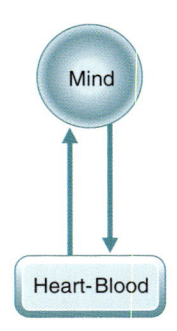

Figure 6.2 Relationship between Heart-Blood and Mind

Apart from the mental activity aspect, the Mind also affects the emotional state. If the Heart is strong, the Mind will also be strong and the person will be happy. If the Heart is weak, the Mind lacks vitality and the person will be sad or depressed or in low spirits. If the Heart is in an excess condition, the Mind will be affected and the person may display symptoms of mental illness, such as manic depression. Of course, this is an oversimplification, as a person's emotional state is related to all the other organs too.

On an emotional level, the state of the Heart determines a person's capacity to form meaningful relationships. A healthy Heart and Mind will positively influence our ability to relate to other people, and conversely, emotional problems due to difficult relationships can weaken the Heart and the Mind.

Clinical note

HE-7 Shenmen and Ren-15 Jiuwei are two of the best points to nourish Heart-Blood when the person is affected by emotional problems and lacks 'joy'

Chinese medicine sees the Mind closely linked to the body. Essence and Qi form the physical basis for the Mind. If the Essence is flourishing and Qi vital, then the Mind will be happy and peaceful. Conversely, if the Essence is weak and Qi deficient, the Mind will suffer. For this reason, the lustre of the eyes shows both the state of Essence and the Mind. Essence, Qi and Mind are called the 'Three Treasures' (see also chapter 3).

The Five Spiritual Aspects

We can now discuss the nature of *Shen* in its second sense, that is, not as the Mind residing in the Heart, but as the whole complex of mental and spiritual aspects of a human being. In this sense, it is related not only to the Heart but also encompasses mental and spiritual aspects related to other organs, and particularly the Yin organs. For this reason, it would be wrong to identify our mental and spiritual life simply with the Heart. All five Yin organs influence emotions, Mind and Spirit in different ways.

Each of the five Yin organs is related to a certain mental–spiritual aspect. These are often called the 'Five Shen' in Chinese:

- The Mind (*Shen*) for the Heart
- The Ethereal Soul (*Hun*) for the Liver
- The Corporeal Soul (*Po*) for the Lungs
- The Will-power (*Zhi*) for the Kidneys
- Intellect (*Yi*) for the Spleen.

> **Box 6.5 Five spiritual aspects**
> - Mind (*Shen*) – Heart
> - Ethereal Soul (*Hun*) – Liver
> - Corporeal Soul (*Po*) – Lungs
> - Intellect (*Yi*) – Spleen
> - Will-power (*Zhi*) – Kidneys

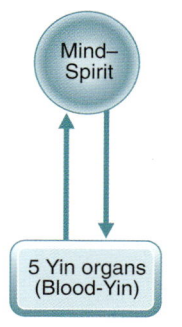

Figure 6.3 Relationship between five Yin organs and Mind-Spirit

The five spiritual aspects are also listed in Box 6.5.

The 'Simple Questions' in chapter 23 says: '*The Heart houses the Mind (Shen), the Lungs house the Corporeal Soul (Po), the Liver houses the Ethereal Soul (Hun), the Spleen houses Intellect (Yi) and the Kidneys house Will Power (Zhi).*'[10] In chapter 9 it says: '*The Heart is the root of life and the origin of the Mind ... the Lungs are the root of Qi and the dwelling of the Corporeal Soul ... the Kidneys are the root of sealed storage [Essence] and the dwelling of Will-Power ... the Liver is the root of harmonization and the residence of the Ethereal Soul.*'[11]

The commentary, based also on passages from the 'Spiritual Axis', adds: '*The Mind is a transformation of Essence and Qi: both Essences [i.e. the Pre-Heaven and Post-Heaven Essences] contribute to forming the Mind. The Corporeal Soul is the assistant of Essence and Qi: it is close to Essence but it moves in and out. The Ethereal Soul complements the Mind and Qi: it is close to the Mind but it comes and goes. Intellect corresponds to memory: it is the memory which depends on the Heart. The Will Power is like a purposeful and focused mind: the Kidneys store Essence ... and through the Will Power they can fulfil our destiny.*'[12]

The complex of these five mental and spiritual phenomena represents the Chinese medical view of body, mind and spirit. Each of these will be discussed in more detail with the functions of their relevant organ. These five aspects together form the 'Spirit', which is also called '*Shen*' or sometimes the '*Five Shen*' in the old classics. The five Yin organs are the residences of '*Shen*' (intended in the broad sense outlined above), that is, the Spirit, and they are sometimes also called the 'Five-*Shen* residences', as in chapter 9 of the 'Simple Questions'.[13]

The five Yin organs are the physiological basis of the Spirit. The indissoluble relationship between them is well known to any acupuncturist. The state of Qi and Blood of each organ can influence the Mind or Spirit and, conversely, alterations of the Mind or Spirit will affect one or more of the internal organs (Fig. 6.3).

The Ethereal Soul (*Hun*) pertaining to the Liver broadly corresponds to our Western concept of 'Soul'. According to ancient Chinese beliefs it enters the body shortly after birth. It is ethereal in nature, as opposed to the Corporeal Soul, which is more physical, and after death it survives the body. The Ethereal Soul can be described as '*that part of the Soul [as opposed to the Corporeal Soul] which at death leaves the body, carrying with it an appearance of physical form.*'[14] This corresponds closely to the ancient Greek views on 'spirit' as being πγευμα (which means 'breath') or 'soul' as being φυκη (which means 'wind or vital breath').

The Corporeal Soul (*Po*) can be defined as '*that part of the Soul [as opposed to the Ethereal Soul] which is indissolubly attached to the body and goes down to Earth with it at death.*'[15] The Corporeal Soul is closely linked to the body and it could be described as the somatic expression of the Soul. As the 'Simple Questions' says in the passage mentioned above, the Corporeal Soul is close to Essence and Qi. The 'Classic of Categories' (1624) says: '*The Corporeal Soul moves and accomplishes things and [when it is active] pain and itching can be felt.*'[16] This passage illustrates just how physical the Corporeal Soul is. It gives us the capacity of sensation, feeling, hearing and sight.

The Will-power (*Zhi*) resides in the Kidneys and is the mental drive that gives us determination and single-mindedness in the pursuit of our goals.

Intellect (*Yi*) resides in the Spleen and corresponds to our capacity for applied thinking, studying, concentrating and memorizing. Although Intellect is said to reside in the Spleen, the Heart also affects thinking and memory, as shown by the passage from the 'Simple Questions' (chapter 23) mentioned above.

> **Clinical note**
>
> The points on the outer Bladder line influence the five spiritual aspects:
> - BL-42 Pohu for the Corporeal Soul
> - BL-44 Shentang for the Mind
> - BL-47 Hunmen for the Ethereal Soul
> - BL-49 Yishe for the Intellect
> - BL-52 Zhishi for the Will-power

Thus, while the *Shen* that resides in the Heart corresponds to the Mind, the *Shen* that indicates the complex of mental and spiritual aspects of a human being more appropriately corresponds to 'Spirit' (Box 6.6).

In some cases, the word *shen* is used in Chinese medical classics to indicate the outward appearance of something. For example, the *shen* of a face indicates an appearance of vitality. A tongue is said to have 'spirit' (*shen*) when it looks vital, bright and flourishing.

Before concluding this section on the relation between the Heart and the Mind, mention should be made of a different viewpoint which emerged during the historical development of Chinese medicine.

Since the Ming dynasty (1368–1644), a few doctors have attributed the functions of intelligence and memory to the brain, not the Heart, as is traditional in Chinese medicine. Li Shi Zhen (1518–1593), the famous herbalist of the Ming dynasty, said: '*The brain is the residence of the Original Mind.*'[17]

Wang Qing Ren, of the early Qing dynasty (1644–1911), dealt at length with the role of the brain in relation to intelligence and memory. He believed that intelligence and memory are functions which depend on the brain rather than the Heart. He said: '*Intelligence and memory reside in the brain. Food generates Qi and Blood ... the clear Essence is transformed into marrow which ascends along the spine to the brain and is called Brain Marrow, or Sea of Marrow.*'[18]

From this it is obvious that, from the Ming dynasty onwards, a new medical theory developed in parallel with the traditional one, whereby the intellectual functions were attributed to the brain rather than the Heart. Significantly, these new theories emerged before the introduction of Western medicine into China.

From the Ming dynasty (1368–1644) onwards, some doctors attributed the 'residence' of the Mind to the brain rather than the Heart.

The Heart is related to joy

Of all the emotions mentioned in Chinese medicine, 'joy' is the most difficult one to explain. Obviously a state of joy is not a cause of disease! Indeed, a normal state of joy is not in itself a cause of disease; on the contrary, it is a beneficial mental state which favours a smooth functioning of the internal organs and their mental faculties. The 'Simple Questions' in chapter 39 says: '*Joy makes the Mind peaceful and relaxed, it benefits the Nutritive and Defensive Qi and it makes Qi relax and slow down.*'[19] On the other hand, in chapter 2, the 'Simple Questions' says: '*The Heart ... controls joy, joy injures the Heart, fear counteracts joy.*'[20]

What is meant by 'joy' as a cause of disease is obviously not a state of healthy contentment but one of excessive excitement and craving which can injure the Heart. This happens to people who live in a state of continuous mental stimulation (however pleasurable) or excessive excitement: in other words, a life of 'hard playing'. I would also define 'excess joy' as 'overstimulation'. Intended in this sense, overstimulation is indeed a cause of disease in patients (e.g. overstimulation from drugs, some medicinal drugs, advertising, consumerism, alcohol, etc.).

'Joy' is also akin to inordinate craving which stirs up the Minister Fire: this flows upwards and overstimulates the Mind.

Joy, in the broad sense indicated above, makes the Heart larger. This leads to excessive stimulation of the Heart, which, in time, may lead to Heart-related

---

Box 6.6 The five spiritual aspects

- **Mind** (*Shen*): resides in the Heart, responsible for consciousness, thinking, affections, memory, sleep
- **Ethereal Soul** (*Hun*): resides in the Liver, responsible for sleep, plans, projects, life aims, 'coming and going of *Shen*'
- **Corporeal Soul** (*Po*): resides in the Lungs, responsible for physiological activities, sensations, sight, hearing, smell, taste, 'entering and exiting of *Jing*'
- **Intellect** (*Yi*): resides in the Spleen, responsible for thinking, memory, concentration
- **Will-power** (*Zhi*): resides in the Kidneys, responsible for will-power, drive, determination

symptoms and signs. These may deviate somewhat from the classical Heart patterns. The main manifestations would be palpitations, overexcitability, insomnia, restlessness, talking a lot and a red tip of the tongue.

Joy may also be marked out as a cause of disease when it is sudden; this happens, for example, on hearing good news unexpectedly. In this situation, 'joy' is akin to shock. Fei Bo Xiong (1800–1879), in 'Medical Collection from Four Families from Meng He', says: '*Joy injures the Heart ... [it causes] Yang Qi to float and the blood vessels to become too open and dilated.*'[21] In these cases of sudden joy and excitement the Heart dilates and slows down and the pulse becomes Slow and slightly Overflowing but Empty. One can understand the effect of sudden joy further if one thinks of situations when a migraine attack is precipitated by the excitement of suddenly hearing good news. Another example of joy as a cause of disease is that of sudden laughter triggering a heart attack; this example also confirms the relationship existing between the Heart and laughter.

Finally, one can also get an idea of joy as an emotion of overexcitement in children, in whom overexcitement usually ends in tears.

The Heart opens into the tongue

The tongue is considered to be the 'offshoot' of the Heart. The Heart controls the colour, form and appearance of the tongue; it is in particular related to the tip of the tongue. It also controls the sense of taste. If the Heart is normal, the tongue will have a normal pale-red colour and the sense of taste will be normal.

If the Heart has Heat, the tongue may be dry and dark red, the tip may be redder and swollen and there may be a bitter taste. If the Heat is severe the tongue may have ulcers that are red and painful. If the Heart is weak and the Blood deficient, the tongue may be pale and thin. The 'Spiritual Axis' in chapter 17 says: '*Heart-Qi communicates with the tongue, if the Heart is normal the tongue can distinguish the five tastes.*'[22]

The condition of the Heart also affects speech and abnormalities may cause stuttering or aphasia. Apart from speech difficulties themselves, the Heart also influences talking and laughing. Often a disharmony of the Heart (whether excess or deficiency) can cause a person to talk incessantly or laugh inappropriately.

Box 6.7 summarizes the relationship between the Heart and the tongue.

Box 6.7 The Heart opens into the tongue

- The Heart influences the tongue itself (e.g. tongue ulcers, tongue soreness)
- The Heart influences the tongue, talking and speech (e.g. talking a lot, speech difficulty, stuttering, aphasia)

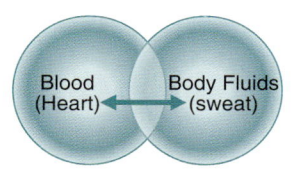

Figure 6.4 Relationship between Blood and Body Fluids

The Heart controls sweat

Blood and Body Fluids have a common origin. Sweat is one of the Body Fluids that come from the space between skin and muscles. As we have seen, Blood and Body Fluids mutually interchange (Fig. 6.4). When Blood is too thick, Body Fluids enter the blood vessels and thin it down. The 'Classic of the Jade Letter of the Golden Shrine' says: '*Body fluids enter the blood vessels and change into Blood.*'[23]

Since the Heart governs Blood and this has a relation of mutual interchange with Body Fluids, of which sweat is part, the Heart is related to sweat. A deficiency of Heart-Qi or Heart-Yang may often cause spontaneous sweating, while a deficiency of Heart-Yin may often cause night sweating and the treatment should be aimed at tonifying Heart-Yang in the former case and Heart-Yin in the latter. On the other hand, excessive sweating, such as happens in hot weather or hot living conditions, may injure Heart-Yang.

Because of the relationship of interchange between Body Fluids and Blood, a patient who is haemorrhaging should not be subjected to sweating, and a patient who is sweating profusely should not have drying herbs, nor should a bleeding technique in acupuncture be used. As the 'Spiritual Axis' in chapter 18 advises: '*Big bleeding, do not cause sweat; big sweat, do not cause bleeding.*'[24]

Furthermore any profuse and continuous sweating in a patient with Heart deficiency should be treated without delay, as a loss of sweat implies loss of Body Fluids, which, in turn, will lead to a deficiency of Blood because of the interchange between Blood and Body Fluids.

Of course, it should be noted that excessive sweating may also be due to organs other than the Heart. In particular, deficiency of Lung-Qi may cause spontaneous sweating. Excess sweating may also be caused by Heat or Damp-Heat, especially of the Stomach. Generally speaking excessive sweating is related to the Heart, especially when it is associated with emotional tension.

Case history

A 45-year-old woman suffered from excessive sweating of the head and chest, which was worse when she was under stress. She had a high-powered job and worked long hours. She suffered from insomnia. Her tongue was red and her pulse was Wiry. I initially attributed the excessive sweating to Stomach-Heat. However, treatment of this pattern did not yield results. I reassessed my diagnosis and came to the conclusion that the sweating derived from Heart-Heat caused by the stress and overwork (the insomnia supported this diagnosis). Treatment of the Heart was successful in reducing sweating. This case history is a good example of excessive sweating due to a Heart disharmony and therefore of the relationship between the Heart and sweat.

OTHER HEART RELATIONSHIPS

The following will be discussed:

- The Heart's smell
- The Heart's colour
- The Heart's taste
- The Heart's climate
- The Heart's sound

The smell of the Heart is scorched

The scorched smell reflects a Heart disharmony and particularly Heart-Fire. The scorched smell is not common in clinical practice and it smells vaguely like burnt toast.

The colour of the Heart is red

A red complexion may indicate a pathology of the Heart and often Heart-Fire as the Heart manifests in the complexion. However, it is important to note that Heat of other organs may also cause a red complexion.

The taste of the Heart is bitter

A bitter taste is often caused by a Heart pattern and particularly Heart-Fire. A bitter taste related to Heart-Fire is often due to intense emotional problems such as frustration, resentment, jealousy or guilt. A bitter taste is frequently related to the Liver as well, and especially Liver-Fire: generally, if the bitter taste is experienced only in the morning after a bad night's sleep, it indicates Heart-Fire; if it is experienced the whole day, it is related to Liver-Fire.

It is interesting to note that in China, the word 'bitter' has clear emotional connotations, as in 'bitter life experiences': for this reason, frequently a Chinese patient complaining of a bitter taste hides some deep emotional scar related to a 'bitter' life experience (a very common occurrence in modern China during the Cultural Revolution).

The climate of the Heart is heat

Each internal organ is affected more by a certain climate. Heat affects the Heart negatively. Although external heat is said not to affect the Heart directly, it affects the Pericardium. For example, in the progression of fevers from external origin, when external heat reaches the Nutritive Qi level, it affects the Pericardium, causing a high fever at night and delirium. It is interesting that, also from the point of view of Western medicine, hot weather affects heart patients adversely.

Heat injures the Heart also because it causes sweating: as sweat is a fluid related to the Heart, excessive sweating may weaken Heart-Yang.

The sound of the Heart is laughing

Laughing is the sound related to the Heart. This relationship manifests in two main ways. Some patients intersperse their talking during the consultation with short bursts of laughter: this often indicates a Heart disharmony which may be both of an Empty (e.g. Heart-Qi deficiency) or a Full nature (e.g. Heart-Fire). On the other hand, people who seem to be very jovial and laugh very loudly may suffer from a Heart disharmony and particularly Heart-Fire.

DREAMS

Since the Heart houses the Mind, it is very closely related to sleep. The Mind should reside in the Heart and if the Heart (particularly Heart-Blood) is strong, a person will fall asleep easily and the sleep will be sound. If the Heart is weak (and especially Heart-Blood), the Mind has no residence and it will 'float' at night causing an inability to fall asleep, disturbed sleep or excessive dreaming. All dreams therefore are, in a way, related to the Heart (as we will see later, they are also related to the Ethereal Soul and the Liver). Certain dreams, however, are more directly indicative of a Heart disharmony.

The 'Simple Questions' in chapter 80 says: *'When the Heart is weak, one dreams of fires; if the dream takes place in summertime, one dreams of volcanic eruptions.'*[25] The 'Spiritual Axis' in chapter 43 says: *'When the Heart is in excess, one dreams of laughing ... when the Heart is deficient, one dreams of mountains, fire and smoke.'*[26]

SAYINGS

- 'The Heart loathes heat'
- 'The Heart controls speech'

'The Heart loathes heat'

Of all the exterior pathogenic factors, Heat is the most pernicious to the Heart. Strictly speaking, Chinese medicine holds that the Heart cannot be invaded by exterior Heat. The Pericardium is closely related to the Heart and can be invaded by exterior Heat, which clouds the 'Heart orifices'. As the Heart houses the Mind, clouding of the Heart orifices can cause coma, delirium or aphasia.

'The Heart controls speech'

The Heart influences speech and this relationship is manifested in different ways. A condition of Heart-Fire (see ch. 32) will cause a person to talk a lot, but sometimes this may also be caused by Heart-Qi deficiency. On the other hand, invasion of the Pericardium by Heat can result in aphasia. Stuttering can be due to a Heart disharmony, as explained above.

Learning outcomes

In this chapter you will have learned:
- The relationship between Heart and Blood
- The relationship between Heart and blood vessels
- The connection between the Heart and the Mind (*Shen*)
- The relationship between the Heart and the complexion
- The relationship between the Heart and sweat
- The relationship between the Heart and the tongue
- An introduction to the nature of the Ethereal Soul (*Hun*), Corporeal Soul (*Po*), Intellect (*Yi*), Mind (*Shen*) and Will-power (*Zhi*)
- Dreams related to the Heart
- Climate detrimental to the Heart
- The taste, colour, sound and smell related to the Heart and their clinical significance

Self-assessment questions

1. In which way does the Heart 'govern' Blood?
2. How does the Heart affect blood vessels?
3. What does a hard blood vessel tell you about the state of the Heart?
4. What does a dull-pale complexion tell you about the state of the Heart?
5. What are the main five functions of the Mind (*Shen*)?
6. Which aspect of the Heart affects sleep?
7. If a patient laughs inappropriately during the consultation, what does that tell you about the Heart?
8. Why do all emotions affect the Heart?
9. How would a deficiency of Heart-Yang affect sweat?

See p. 1256 for answers

END NOTES

1. 1979 The Yellow Emperor's Classic of Internal Medicine – Simple Questions (*Huang Ti Nei Jing Su Wen* 黄帝内经素问), People's Health Publishing House, Beijing, first published *c*.100 BC, p. 58.
2. 1981 Spiritual Axis (*Ling Shu Jing* 灵枢经), People's Health Publishing House, Beijing, first published *c*.100 BC, p. 128.
3. Simple Questions, p. 72.
4. Ibid., p. 246.
5. Ibid., p. 70.
6. I translate the word *Shen* as 'Mind' as its functions, as described in the Chinese medical classics, closely correspond to the mental activities (including emotions) attributed to the 'Mind' in Western psychology. The word *Shen* has many different meanings. In order to obtain a clearer idea of the meaning of this word it is useful to consult pre-1949 dictionaries which are not influenced by a Marxist, materialistic philosophical outlook. The 1912 'Chinese–English Dictionary' by H Giles (Kelly and Walsh Ltd, Shanghai, p. 1194) gives the following possible translations for the word *Shen*: 'Spirits; gods (used by some Protestant sects for "God"); divine; supernatural; mysterious; spiritual (as opposed to material); the soul; the mind; the animal spirits; inspiration; genius; force (as language); expression'. Thus, as it is apparent from the above passage, the translation of *Shen* simply as 'Spirit' (as opposed to the

material body) was influenced by Western Christian missionaries in China during the second half of the 19th century. A Christian philosophical outlook would use the word *Shen* indicating the 'Spirit' (or even 'God') as opposed to the 'body', reflecting a typical Western dualistic attitude to Matter and Spirit which is totally alien to Chinese philosophy. Although the word Shen can have the meaning of 'Spiritual', in Chinese medical classics it was always used to indicate the mental faculties attributed to the Heart, i.e. the Mind. Indeed, the word *Xin* itself (meaning 'Heart') is often used as synonymous with 'Mind' in Chinese medical classics. The problem is not simply semantic as it has repercussions in diagnosis and treatment. Western acupuncture has concentrated entirely on the role of the Heart in mental and spiritual phenomena, based on the idea that 'the Heart houses the Spirit'. This approach is rather partial as, on the one hand, it ignores the role of the Heart for mental faculties, thinking and memory and, on the other hand, it ignores the role of the other Yin organs in the mental–spiritual sphere.

7. Simple Questions, p. 67.
8. Spiritual Axis, p. 128.
9. Simple Questions, p. 67.
10. Simple Questions, p. 153.
11. Ibid., p. 67–68.
12. Ibid., p. 153.
13. Ibid., p. 63.
14. Giles H 1912 Chinese–English Dictionary, Kelly and Walsh, Shanghai, p. 650.
15. Chinese–English Dictionary, p. 1144.
16. Cited in 1980 Concise Dictionary of Chinese Medicine (*Jian Ming Zhong Yi Ci Dian* 简明中医辞典), People's Health Publishing House, Beijing, p. 953.
17. Cited in Wang Xin Hua 1983 Selected Historical Theories in Chinese Medicine (*Zhong Yi Li Dai Yi Lun Xuan* 中医历代医论选), Jiangsu Scientific Publishing House, Jiangsu, p. 31.
18. Correction of the Mistakes of the Medical Forest (*Yi Lin Gai Cuo* 医林改错) by Wang Qing Ren, 1830, cited in Selected Historical Theories in Chinese Medicine, p. 30.
19. Simple Questions, p. 221.
20. Ibid., p. 38.
21. Fei Bo Xiong 1985 Medical Collection from Four Families from Meng He (*Meng He Si Jia Yi Ji* 孟河四家医集), Jiangsu Science Publishing House, Nanjing, p. 40.
22. Spiritual Axis, p. 50.
23. The Classic of the Jade Letter of the Golden Shrine (*Jin Gui Yu Hang Jing* 金匮玉函经), Song Dynasty, cited in 1978 Fundamentals of Chinese Medicine (*Zhong Yi Ji Chu Xue* 中医基础学), Shandong Scientific Publishing House, Jinan, p. 35.
24. Spiritual Axis, p. 52.
25. Simple Questions, p. 569.
26. Spiritual Axis, p. 84–85.

FURTHER READING

Kaptchuk T 2000 The Web that has no Weaver – Understanding Chinese Medicine, Contemporary Books, Chicago

SECTION 1   PART 2

The Functions of the Liver   7

Key contents

The functions of the Liver
It stores Blood
It ensures the smooth flow of Qi
It controls the sinews
It manifests in the nails
It opens into the eyes
It controls tears
It houses the Ethereal Soul
It is affected by anger

Other Liver relationships
Its smell is rancid
Its colour is green
Its taste is sour
Its climate is wind
Its sound is shouting

Dreams

Sayings

The Liver has many important functions, among which are those of storing Blood, ensuring the smooth movement of Qi throughout the body and housing the Ethereal Soul (*Hun*). Liver-Blood is very important for nourishing the sinews, thus allowing physical exercise, and storing Blood for the Uterus, thus ensuring a regular menstruation.

The smooth flow of Liver-Qi is essential to all physiological processes in every organ and every part of the body. On a psychic level, the Ethereal Soul (*Hun*) performs a very important role in our mental and spiritual life by providing the Mind (*Shen*) with inspiration, creativity, life dreams and a sense of direction in life.

The Liver, and in particular Liver-Blood, is also responsible for our capacity for recovering energy and it contributes to the body's resistance to exterior pathogenic factors.

The Liver is often compared to an army general because it is responsible for overall planning of the body's functions by ensuring the smooth flow and proper direction of Qi (see below). While the 'planning' on a physical level is the reflection of the smooth flow of Liver-Qi affecting all organs, on a mental and spiritual level, the Liver influences our capacity for making plans and having a sense of direction in life: this quality depends primarily on the Ethereal Soul. Because of this quality, the Liver is also said to be the origin of courage and resoluteness, if the organ is in a good state of health.[1] However, the quality of courage is also dependent on the state of the Gall Bladder.

The 'Simple Questions' in chapter 8 says: '*The Liver is like an army's general from whom the strategy is derived*'.[2] Owing to this quality, the Liver is also said to influence our capacity to plan our life.

The functions of the Liver are:

- It stores Blood
- It ensures the smooth flow of Qi
- It controls the sinews
- It manifests in the nails
- It opens into the eyes
- It controls tears
- It houses the Ethereal Soul
- It is affected by anger

Other Liver relationships are:

- Its smell is rancid
- Its colour is green
- Its taste is sour
- Its climate is wind
- Its sound is shouting

The discussion of the Liver will be differentiated into the following headings:

- Functions
  - The Liver stores Blood

- The Liver regulates the volume of Blood in the body
- Liver-Blood regulates menstruation
- Liver-Blood moistens eyes and sinews
  - The Liver ensures the smooth flow of Qi
    - Smooth flow of Liver-Qi in relation to emotional state
    - Smooth flow of Liver-Qi assists digestion
    - Smooth flow of Liver-Qi ensures the flow of bile
  - The Liver controls the sinews
  - The Liver manifests in the nails
  - The Liver opens into the eye
  - The Liver controls tears
  - The Liver houses the Ethereal Soul
  - The Liver is affected by anger
- Other Liver relationships
  - The Liver's smell is rancid
  - The Liver's colour is green
  - The Liver's taste is sour
  - The Liver's climate is wind
  - The Liver's sound is shouting
- Dreams
- Sayings

FUNCTIONS OF THE LIVER

The functions of the Liver are discussed under the following headings:

- The Liver stores Blood
  - The Liver regulates the volume of Blood in the body
  - Liver-Blood regulates menstruation
  - Liver-Blood moistens eyes and sinews
- The Liver ensures the smooth flow of Qi
  - Smooth flow of Liver-Qi in relation to emotional state
  - Smooth flow of Liver-Qi assists digestion
  - Smooth flow of Liver-Qi ensures the flow of bile
- The Liver controls the sinews
- The Liver manifests in the nails
- The Liver opens into the eye
- The Liver controls tears
- The Liver houses the Ethereal Soul
- The Liver is affected by anger

The Liver stores Blood

The Liver is the most important organ for storing Blood and, by so doing, it regulates the volume of Blood in the whole body at any one time. The Liver function of storing of Blood has three aspects, as listed in Box 7.1.

Box 7.1 The Liver stores Blood
- It regulates Blood volume in relation to rest and activity
- It regulates menstruation
- It moistens eyes and sinews

The Liver regulates the volume of Blood in the body

The Liver regulates the volume of Blood in the body according to physical activity. When the body is active, Blood flows to the muscles and sinews; when the body is at rest, Blood flows back to the Liver. This is a self-regulating process, depending on physical activity.

The 'Simple Questions' in chapter 62 says: '*The Liver stores Blood*'.[3] In chapter 10 it says: '*When a person lies down Blood returns to the Liver*'.[4] Wang Ping (Tang dynasty) says: '*The Liver stores Blood ... when a person moves, Blood goes to the channels, when at rest it goes to the Liver.*'[5]

When Blood returns to the Liver with the body at rest, it contributes to restoring the person's energy; when it flows to the muscles and sinews during exercise, it nourishes and moistens the muscles and sinews to enable them to perform during exercise (Fig. 7.1).

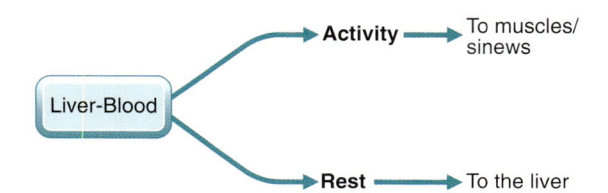

Figure 7.1 Relationship of Liver-Blood to activity and rest

The Liver's job of regulating Blood volume throughout the body has an important influence on a person's level of energy. When the Blood flows to the appropriate places in the body at the appropriate times, it will nourish the necessary tissues, and therefore give us energy. If this regulatory function is impaired, there will be lack of Blood and therefore nourishment where and when it is needed, and the person will become easily tired. The 'Simple Questions' in chapter 10 says: '*When the Liver has enough Blood ... the feet can walk, the hands can hold and the fingers can grasp.*'[6]

Finally, the Liver function of storing and regulating Blood volume also indirectly influences our resistance to external pathogenic factors. If this Liver function is normal, the skin and muscles will be well nourished by Blood and be able to resist attacks of exterior pathogenic factors. If this function is impaired, the skin and muscles will not be irrigated and nourished by Blood at the appropriate times (during exercise), and the body will therefore be more liable to attack by exterior pathogenic factors. There are other more important factors involved in determining the resistance to exterior pathogenic factors, notably the strength of the Defensive Qi and Lung-Qi. However, it is necessary not to overlook the importance of this Liver function in this respect.

> **Clinical note**
>
> To nourish Liver-Blood I use: ST-36 Zusanli, LIV-8 Ququan and SP-6 Sanyinjiao

Liver-Blood plays a role in the body's defence from exterior pathogenic factors

Liver-Blood regulates menstruation

The Liver function of storing Blood has a marked influence on menstruation and is of great relevance in clinical practice (Box 7.2). If the Liver stores Blood normally, menstruation will be normal. If the Blood of the Liver is deficient, there will be amenorrhoea or scanty periods. If the Blood of the Liver is in excess or hot, the periods may be heavy. If the Blood of the Liver is stagnant, the periods will be painful.

> **Box 7.2 Liver-Blood and menstruation**
>
> - Liver-Blood normal: regular and normal menstruation
> - Liver-Blood deficiency: scanty periods or amenorrhoea
> - Liver-Blood stasis: painful periods
> - Liver-Blood Heat: heavy periods

The Liver function of storing Blood is extremely important in women's physiology and pathology. Many gynaecological problems are due to malfunction of Liver-Qi or Liver-Blood. If Liver-Qi is stagnant, this may lead to stasis of Blood of the Liver causing painful periods with premenstrual tension and the menstrual blood will have dark clots.

The Liver storage of Blood also influences the Directing (*Ren Mai*) and Penetrating Vessels (*Chong Mai*), the two extraordinary vessels that are closely related to the uterus. Any malfunction of the Liver will induce an imbalance in these two vessels, affecting menstruation.

> **Clinical note**
>
> To nourish Liver-Blood in women I use: ST-36 Zusanli, LIV-8 Ququan, SP-6 Sanyinjiao and Ren-4 Guanyuan

> **Clinical note**
>
> LIV-3 Taichong is a very important point to regulate menstruation (it also regulates the Penetrating Vessel *Chong Mai*)

Liver-Blood moistens eyes and sinews

The Blood of the Liver also moistens eyes and sinews (Fig. 7.2). The relationship between Liver and eyes is very close (although other organs influence the eyes too). Liver-Blood moistens and 'brightens' the eyes; if Liver-Blood is deficient, the person may suffer from dry eyes and/or blurred vision. If Liver-Blood has Heat, the eyes may become red and painful.

Liver-Blood also moistens and nourishes the sinews (which include tendons, ligaments and cartilages): this is essential for a proper functioning of all joints. If Liver-Blood fails to moisten and nourish the sinews, there will be muscle cramps and contraction of the tendons. If the Liver is affected by Internal Wind, there will be tremor or convulsions (as tremors and convulsions are seen in Chinese medicine as 'shaking of the tendons').

Finally, there is a relationship of reciprocal influence between Blood and Liver: if Blood is abnormal

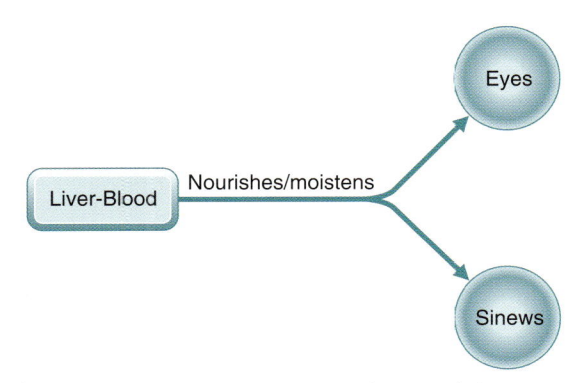

Figure 7.2 Relation between Liver and eyes and sinews

(deficient or hot), it may affect the Liver function. If, on the other hand, the Liver function is abnormal, it may affect the quality of the Blood, causing certain kinds of skin diseases, such as eczema or psoriasis. This last concept has been advanced by Dr J. Shen, who holds that, just as an improper storing medium can spoil food (for instance a dirty container encouraging the growth of bacteria), similarly, an improper Liver function (the storing medium for Blood) can 'spoil' Blood, giving rise to skin diseases.[7]

The Liver ensures the smooth flow of Qi

This is the most important of all the Liver functions and it is central to nearly all Liver disharmonies. The impairment of this function is one of the most common patterns seen in practice. What does it mean that the Liver ensures the 'smooth flow of Qi'? The Chinese words for this function, *shu xie*, literally mean 'to flow' and 'to let out':

疏 *shu* means 'to dredge, disperse, scatter'

泄 *xie* means 'to let out, discharge, release, vent'

When Chinese books explain this function they use such terms as 'disperse', 'extend', 'loosen', 'relax', 'circulate', 'make smooth and free' and 'balance' (literally 'stop extremes'). Thus the Liver ensures the smooth flow of Qi throughout the body, in all organs and in all directions (Fig. 7.3).

This last point is important. As we have seen, every organ's Qi has a normal direction of flow: the Qi of some organs flows downwards (such as that of the Lungs and Stomach), while that of others flows upwards (such as that of the Spleen). The normal direction of movement of Liver-Qi is partially upwards and partially outwards in all directions to ensure the smooth and unimpeded flow of Qi everywhere. For example, the smooth flow of Liver-Qi in the Middle Burner helps Stomach-Qi to descend and Spleen-Qi to ascend. This explains the importance of this function, as it involves all parts of the body and can affect all organs. This movement of Liver-Qi can be related to the character of Wood in terms of the Five Elements, with its expansive movement in all directions.

There are three aspects to this function, as listed in Box 7.3 and described below.

Box 7.3   The smooth flow of Liver-Qi

- Affects emotional state
- Affects digestion
- Affects secretion of bile

Smooth flow of Liver-Qi in relation to the emotional state

The Liver function of ensuring the smooth flow of Qi has a deep influence on the emotional state. Whilst on a physical level the smooth flow of Liver-Qi helps the physiological activities of all organs, on a

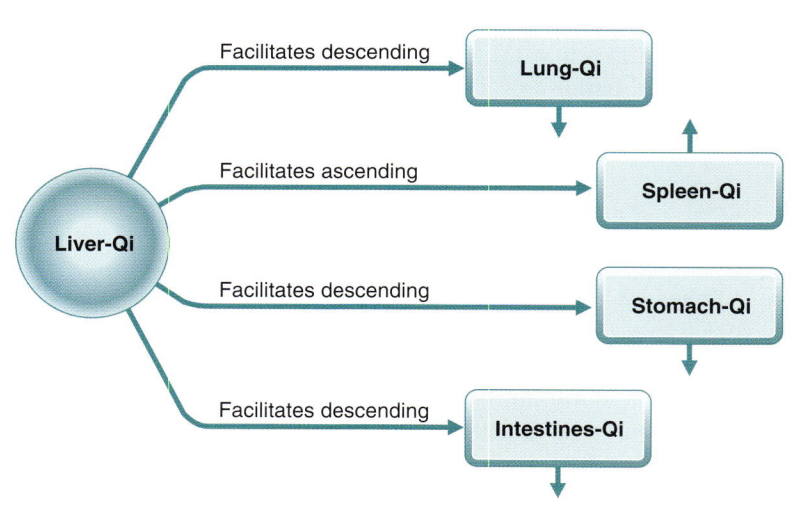

Figure 7.3 Free flow of Liver-Qi in all directions

mental–emotional level, the same smooth flow of Qi ensures a balanced emotional life. This is primarily a function of the Ethereal Soul as the smooth flow of Liver-Qi on a physical level mirrors the smooth 'coming and going of the Ethereal Soul on a psychic level' (see below) and the proper coordination and integration between the Ethereal Soul (*Hun*) and the Mind (*Shen*).

Clinical note

To stimulate the free flow of Liver-Qi in emotional problems I use LIV-3 Taichong

The smooth flow of Liver-Qi is essential for a balanced emotional state

If Liver-Qi flows smoothly, Qi flows normally and the emotional life is happy. If this function is impaired, the circulation of Qi is obstructed, Qi becomes restrained giving rise to emotional frustration, depression or repressed anger, accompanied by such physical symptoms as hypochondrial or abdominal distension, a feeling of oppression in the chest and the sensation of a 'lump' in the throat. In women, it may give rise to premenstrual tension including depression, irritability and distension of the breasts. This is a reciprocal relationship: a restrained Liver function will lead to emotional tension and frustration, and a tense emotional life characterized by frustration or repressed anger will impair the Liver function and lead to a breakdown of the smooth flow of Qi.

The 'Simple Questions' in chapter 3 says: '*Anger makes Qi rise and Blood stagnate in the chest.*'[8]

Smooth flow of Liver-Qi assists digestion

In health, the smooth flow of Liver-Qi assists the Stomach and Spleen digestive function. If Liver-Qi flows smoothly, the Stomach can ripen and rot food and Stomach-Qi can descend; the Spleen can extract Food-Qi and Spleen-Qi can ascend (Fig. 7.4). In disease, if Liver-Qi becomes stagnant or horizontally 'rebellious' it may 'invade' the Stomach preventing the downward movement of Stomach-Qi, resulting in belching, sour regurgitation, nausea or vomiting. If it invades the Spleen, it obstructs the transformation and transportation of food and prevents Spleen-Qi from flowing upwards, resulting in diarrhoea (Fig. 7.5). In Five-Element terms this corresponds to 'Wood overacting on Earth'.

This is a pathological aspect of what is normally a physiological function of Liver-Qi in aiding Stomach and Spleen. The smooth flow of Liver-Qi is all important in ensuring a harmonious movement of Qi in the Middle Burner. Since Stomach-Qi should go down and Spleen-Qi should go up, the Middle Burner is a crossing place of Qi moving in different directions and the Liver makes sure that the Qi of the Stomach and Spleen flow smoothly in the proper directions.

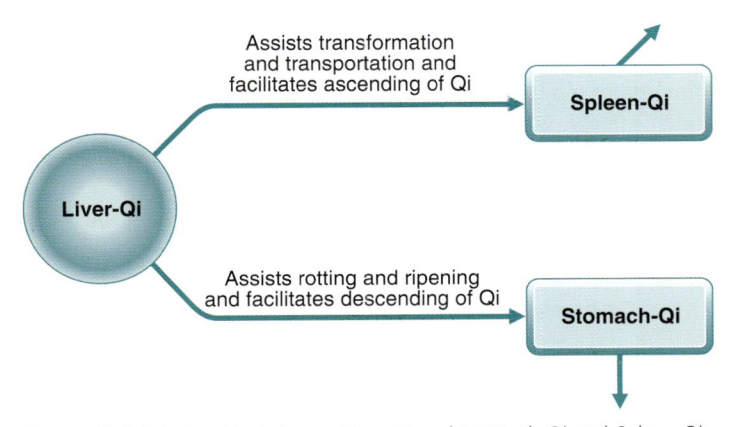

Figure 7.4 Relationship between Liver-Qi and Stomach-Qi and Spleen-Qi

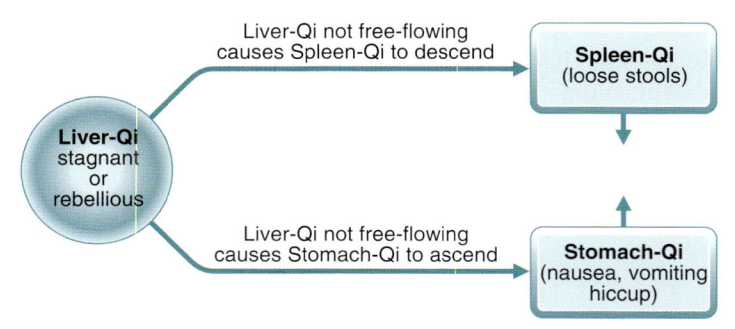

Figure 7.5 Relationship between stagnation of Liver-Qi and Stomach-Qi and Spleen-Qi

> **Clinical note**
>
> To stimulate the free flow of Liver-Qi in digestive problems I use LIV-14 Qimen for the Stomach or LIV-13 Zhangmen for the Spleen, both with Ren-12 Zhongwan.

> **Box 7.4 The Liver nourishes the sinews**
>
> - Liver-Blood normal: supple sinews and tendons, free movement
> - Deficiency of Liver-Blood: cramps, numbness, tingling
> - Liver-Blood stasis: stiffness of sinews, rigidity, pain

The smooth flow of Liver-Qi ensures flow of bile

Finally, the smooth flow of Liver-Qi affects the flow of bile. If Liver-Qi flows smoothly, bile is secreted properly and digestion is good. If Liver-Qi is stagnant, the flow of bile may be obstructed, resulting in bitter taste, belching or jaundice and also in the inability to digest fats.

> **Clinical note**
>
> To stimulate the free flow of Liver-Qi and the flow of bile I use LIV-14 Qimen and G.B.-34 Yanglingquan

The Liver controls the sinews

The state of the sinews (including tendons, cartilages and ligaments of the limbs) affects our capacity for movement and physical activity. The contraction and relaxation of sinews ensures the movement of joints. The sinews' capacity for contraction and relaxation depends on the nourishment and moistening of the Blood from the Liver (Box 7.4). The 'Simple Questions' in chapter 21 says: *'The Qi of food enters the Stomach, the refined essence extracted from food goes to the Liver and the excess Qi from the Liver overflows into the sinews.'*[9] For this reason, the sinews are considered to be an 'extension' of the Liver.

If Liver-Blood is abundant, the sinews will be moistened and nourished, ensuring smooth movement of joints and good muscle action. If Liver-Blood is deficient, the sinews will lack moistening and nourishment which may cause contractions and spasms or impaired extension/flexion, numbness of limbs, tingling, muscle cramps and, if Liver-Wind develops, tremors or convulsions. Tremors are considered to be due to 'shaking of the tendons' and this symptom reflects the presence of Liver-Wind. This is why the 'Simple Questions' in chapter 1 says: *'When Liver-Qi declines, the sinews cannot move.'*[10]

If there is stasis of Liver-Blood, the sinews will lack suppleness and the person may experience stiffness, rigidity and pain of the joints.

The Liver's influence on the sinews has also another meaning, corresponding to certain neurological conditions from a Western medical perspective. For example, if a child contracts an infectious disease such as meningitis manifesting with a high temperature eventually causing convulsions, in Chinese terms this is due to Heat stirring Liver-Wind. The interior Wind of the Liver causes a contraction and tremor of the sinews, which leads to convulsions.

Finally, mention should be made of the fact that most Western books on acupuncture list the 'muscles' as being controlled by the Liver and 'flesh' by the Spleen: I translate *jin* (the tissue controlled by the Liver) as 'sinews' (which includes tendons, ligaments of the limbs and cartilages) and *rou* or *ji rou* (the tissue controlled by the Spleen) as 'muscles'. First of all, it should be noted that *ji rou* indicating 'muscles' refers only to the skeletal muscles in the limbs (and therefore not the cardiac muscle or the smooth muscles). Secondly, obviously there is an overlap in the physiology and pathology of sinews and muscles and therefore between Liver and Spleen. Essentially, a weakness of the limb muscles is related to the Spleen, while cramps, contractions, difficulty in flexion/extension reflect a pathology of the Liver.

> **Box 7.5 The Liver opens into the eyes**
> - Liver-Blood normal: good vision
> - Liver-Blood deficiency: blurred vision, floaters
> - Liver-Yin deficiency: dry, gritty eyes
> - Liver-Blood stasis: painful eyeball
> - Liver-Yang rising: watery eyes
> - Liver-Fire: dry, bloodshot eyes (may also be red, swollen and painful)
> - Liver-Wind: eyeball moving

Clinical note

G.B.-34 Yanglingquan is the Gathering (*Hui*) point for sinews

The Liver manifests in the nails

The nails are considered in Chinese medicine as a 'by-product' of the sinews, and, as such, they are under the influence of Liver-Blood. If Liver-Blood is abundant the nails will be moist and healthy; if Liver-Blood is deficient, the nails will lack nourishment and become ridged, dry, brittle and cracked. If there is stasis of Liver-Blood, the nails will be dark or purple.

The 'Simple Questions' in chapter 10 says: '*The Liver controls the sinews and its flourishing condition manifests on the nails.*'[11] In chapter 9 it says: '*The Liver is a regulatory organ, it is the residence of the Ethereal Soul, it manifests in the nails, controls the sinews.*'[12]

The Liver opens into the eyes

The eye is the sense organ connected to the Liver. It is the nourishment and moistening of Liver-Blood that gives the eyes the capacity to see. If Liver-Blood is abundant, the eyes will be normally moist and the vision will be good. If Liver-Blood is deficient, there may be blurred vision, myopia, 'floaters' in eyes, colour blindness or the eyes may feel dry and gritty.

The 'Simple Questions' in chapter 10 says: '*When the Liver receives Blood the eyes can see.*'[13] The 'Spiritual Axis' in chapter 17 says: '*Liver-Qi extends to the eyes, when the Liver is healthy the eyes can distinguish the five colours.*'[14]

Information about the eye is summarized in Box 7.5.

The 'Spiritual Axis' in chapter 37 says: '*The eye is the sense organ pertaining to the Liver.*'[15] The 'Simple Questions' in chapter 4 says: '*The Liver corresponds to the direction East and the green colour, and it opens into the eye.*'[16]

If the Liver has Heat, the eyes may be bloodshot and feel painful or burning. If the Liver has internal Wind, the eyeball may turn upwards and move involuntarily (nystagmus).

Aside from the Liver, many other Yin and Yang organs affect the eye, in particular the Heart, Kidneys, Lungs, Gall Bladder, Bladder and Small Intestine. The 'Spiritual Axis' in chapter 80 says: '*The Essence from the 5 Yin and 6 Yang organs flows upwards to irrigate the eyes.*'[17]

In particular, the Essence of the Kidneys nourishes the eyes, so that many chronic eye diseases are related to the decline of Kidney-Essence. The Heart is also closely related to the eye. The 'Spiritual Axis' in chapter 80 says: '*The eyes mirror the state of the Heart, which houses the Mind.*'[18]

The 'Simple Questions' in chapter 81 says: '*The Heart concentrates the Essence of the 5 Yin organs and this manifests in the eye.*'[19]

Thus the eyes also reflect the state of the Mind and the Heart. In conclusion, the Kidneys and Heart are the two other Yin organs besides the Liver which are most closely related to the eyes. Heart-Fire can cause pain and redness of the eye and Kidney-Yin deficiency can cause failing eyesight and dryness of the eyes.

Clinical note

The Back-Transporting (Back-Shu) point of the Liver, BL-18 Ganshu, affects the eyes

The Liver is **not** the only organ that affects the eyes

The Liver controls tears

Tears are a fluid related to the Liver. In particular, the basal tears (which lubricate the eyes) and the reflex tears (that occur when a foreign body enters the eye) are related to the Liver (rather than the emotional tears).

Thus, a deficiency of Liver-Blood or Liver-Yin may cause dryness of the eyes, while Liver-Yang rising may cause watery eyes.

The Liver houses the Ethereal Soul

The Ethereal Soul, called *Hun* in Chinese, is the mental–spiritual aspect of the Liver. The 'Simple Questions' in Chapter 9 says: *'The Liver is the residence of the Ethereal Soul.'*[20] The concept of Ethereal Soul is closely linked to the ancient Chinese belief in 'spirits' and 'demons'. According to these beliefs, spirits and demons are spirit-like creatures who preserve a physical appearance and wander in the world of spirit. Some are good and some are evil. In the times prior to the Warring States period (476–221 BC), such spirits were considered to be the main cause of disease. After the Warring States period, naturalistic causes of disease (such as the weather) replaced this belief, which, however, has never really disappeared even to the present day. The character for *Hun* contains the radical *Gui*, which means 'spirit' in the above sense, and the radical *Yun*, for 'cloud'. The combination of these two characters conveys the idea of the nature of the Ethereal Soul: it is like a 'spirit' but it is Yang and ethereal in nature and essentially harmless: that is, it is not one of the evil spirits (hence the presence of the 'cloud' radical).

魂 *Hun*

鬼 *Gui*

云 *Yun*

The Ethereal Soul is thus Yang in nature (as opposed to the Corporeal Soul) and at death survives the body to flow back to a world of subtle, non-material energies.

The Ethereal Soul is said to influence the capacity of planning our life and finding a sense of direction in life. A lack of direction in life and mental confusion could be compared to the wandering of the Ethereal Soul alone in space and time. Thus, if the Liver (in particular Liver-Blood) is flourishing, the Ethereal Soul is firmly rooted and can help us to plan our life with wisdom and vision. If Liver-Blood is weak, the Ethereal Soul is not rooted and cannot give us a sense of direction in life. If Liver-Blood or Liver-Yin is very weak, at times the Ethereal Soul may even leave the body temporarily at night during sleep or just before going to sleep. Those who suffer from severe deficiency of Yin may experience a sensation as if they were floating in the few moments just before falling asleep: this is said to be due to the 'floating' of the Ethereal Soul not rooted in Blood and Yin.

In my experience, the Ethereal Soul is also the source of life dreams, vision, aims, projects, inspiration, creativity, ideas: the Ethereal Soul is described as the '*coming and going of the Mind (Shen)*'. This means that it gives the Mind the necessary other dimension of life: that is, dreams, vision, aims, projects, inspiration, creativity and ideas. Without these, the Mind would be sterile and the person would suffer from depression. On the other hand, the Mind needs to somewhat restrain the 'coming and going' of the Ethereal Soul to keep it under check; it also needs to integrate all the ideas spurting forth from the Ethereal Soul into our psyche in an orderly fashion. The Ethereal Soul is like an 'ocean' of ideas, dreams, projects and inspiration, and the Mind can only cope with one at a time. If the Ethereal Soul brings forth too much material from its 'ocean' without enough control and integration by the Mind, the person's behaviour would become somewhat chaotic and, in extreme cases, positively manic. Figure 7.6 illustrates the relationship between the Mind (*Shen*) and the Ethereal Soul (*Hun*).

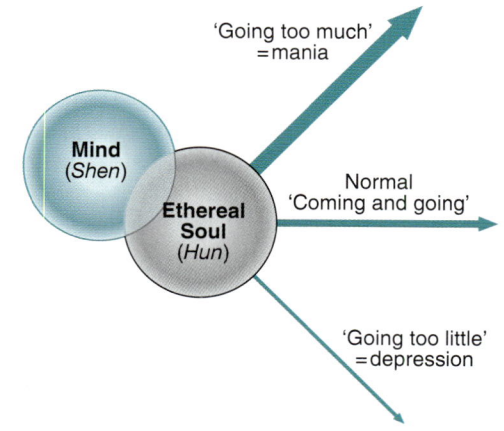

Figure 7.6 Relationship between Mind (*Shen*) and Ethereal Soul (*Hun*)

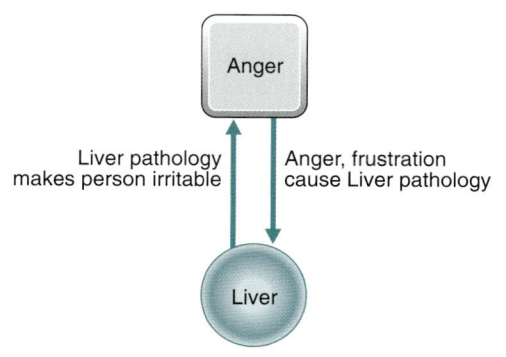

Figure 7.7 Mutual relationship between Liver and anger

The 'Discussion on Blood Diseases' says: *'If Liver-Blood is deficient Fire agitates the Ethereal Soul resulting in nocturnal emissions with dreams.'*[21] This confirms that the Ethereal Soul can become unrooted at night when Blood or Yin are deficient.

A discussion of the nature of the Ethereal Soul is not complete without discussing the Corporeal Soul (*Po*) as the two are but two poles of the same phenomenon. The Corporeal Soul represents a very physical aspect of the Soul, the part of the Soul which is indissolubly linked to the body. At death, it goes back to the Earth. The Chinese concept of 'soul' therefore includes both the Ethereal and Corporeal Soul.

The Liver is affected by anger

Anger is the emotion that is closely related to the Liver. 'Anger' should be intended in a broad sense and includes frustration, resentment, repressed anger and rage.

Anger causes stagnation of Liver-Qi, especially when it is repressed; anger that is vented often causes Liver-Yang rising or Liver-Fire.

As with any other emotion, the relationship between an emotion and the organ is mutual: a state of anger causes a Liver pathology and, vice versa, a Liver pathology may cause the person to become irritable (Fig. 7.7).

OTHER LIVER RELATIONSHIPS

The other Liver relationships discussed are:

- The Liver's smell
- The Liver's colour
- The Liver's taste
- The Liver's climate
- The Liver's sound

Box 7.6 summarizes these relationships.

Box 7.6 Other Liver relationships

- Smell: rancid
- Colour: green
- Taste: sour
- Climate: wind
- Sound: shouting

The Liver's smell is rancid

The smell associated with the Liver is rancidity. This is the smell of rancid meat and it emanates particularly from the axillae. It is a common smell in clinical practice. It indicates Liver pathology, usually with Heat, that is, either Liver-Fire or Damp-Heat in the Liver.

The Liver's colour is green

A Liver pathology such as Liver-Qi stagnation may cause a greenish complexion: the left cheek in particular reflects the state of the Liver.

The green colour's diagnostic significance applies also to other things such as a vaginal discharge: a greenish vaginal discharge indicates Dampness in the Liver channel.

The Liver's taste is sour

If a person experiences a sour taste, it may indicate Liver pathology, and especially one characterized by Heat.

The excessive consumption of foods or herbs with a sour taste (e.g. grapefruit) may injure the Liver, the Spleen and the muscles. On the other hand, the sour taste is beneficial to the Lungs (e.g. the herb Wu Wei Zi *Fructus Schizandrae*, which is a Lung tonic).

Although the taste pertaining to the Liver is the sour one, it should be noted that a bitter taste is very common in Liver-Fire and Damp-Heat in the Liver and Gall Bladder.

The Liver's climate is wind

Wind is the climate related to the Liver. This can be observed in practice in various ways. A patient suffering from a Liver disharmony will often complain of being badly affected by wind (for example causing a migraine) and occasionally patients will even report being adversely affected specifically by an East wind (East is the direction of Wood and of the Liver).

The Liver's sound is shouting

A Liver disharmony, especially an Excess one, will often cause a person to speak with a very loud, almost shouting voice. Shouting is the sound of the Liver also because people shout when they give vent to anger (the emotion of the Liver).

DREAMS

The 'Simple Questions' in chapter 17 says: *'When the Liver is in excess, one dreams of being angry.'*[22]

And in chapter 80 it says: *'When the Liver is deficient, one dreams of very fragrant mushrooms. If the dream takes place in Spring, one dreams of lying under a tree without being able to get up.'*[23]

The 'Spiritual Axis' in chapter 43 says: *'When the Liver is deficient one dreams of forests in the mountains.'*[24]

SAYINGS

There are many saying related to the Liver:

- 'The Liver is a resolute organ'
- 'The Liver influences rising and growth'
- 'The Liver controls planning'
- 'The Liver is a regulating, balancing and harmonizing organ'
- 'The Liver loathes wind'
- 'The Liver can cause convulsions'
- 'The Liver arises from the left side'

'The Liver is a resolute organ'

Just as in disease Liver-Qi easily becomes stagnant and excessive and Liver Yang easily flares upwards causing irritability and anger, in health the same type of energy deriving from the Liver can give a person great creative drive and resoluteness.

For this reason, it is said in Chinese medicine that a healthy Liver function can confer on a person resoluteness, an indomitable spirit and courage. This mental and character quality of a person depends on the state of Liver-Qi and of Gall Bladder-Qi. In fact, the only manifestation of Liver-Qi deficiency (an unusual pattern) is on a character level: that is, timidity, lack or resolve, lack of courage and indecision.

'The Liver influences rising and growth'

In health, Liver-Qi rises upwards and spreads in all directions to promote the smooth flow of Qi in all parts of the body. 'Growth' here should be intended in a symbolical sense as the Liver pertains to Wood and this particular quality is compared to the rising of sap promoting growth in a tree.

In disease, the rising movement of Liver-Qi can get out of control, resulting in a separation of Yin and Yang and the excessive rising of Liver-Yang or Liver-Fire. This causes irritability, outbursts of anger, a red face, dizziness, tinnitus and headaches.

'The Liver controls planning'

This idea is derived from chapter 8 of the 'Simple Questions' already mentioned. The Liver is said to impart to us the capacity to plan our life smoothly and wisely. In disease, a Liver disharmony can manifest with an inability to plan our life and a lack of direction. This function is particularly a function of the Ethereal Soul.

'The Liver is a regulating, balancing and harmonizing organ'

This is a loose translation of an expression that is difficult to translate and that literally means *'The Liver is the root of stopping extremes'*. This expression was first used in chapter 9 of the 'Simple Questions' where it says: *'The Liver has a regulating, balancing function [lit. is the root of stopping extremes], it houses the Ethereal Soul, manifests in the nails.'*[25]

This means that the Liver has an important regulating and balancing activity which is mostly derived from its function of storing Blood and of ensuring the smooth flow of Liver-Qi.

As was mentioned, the Liver regulates the volume of Blood needed by the body according to physical activity. During movement and exercise, the Blood flows to the muscles and sinews; at rest, it flows back to the Liver. By flowing back to the Liver during rest, the Blood helps us to recover energy. Conversely, if the Blood of the Liver is deficient, a person will find it difficult to recover energy by resting.

The smooth flow of Liver-Qi is another manifestation of the regulating and balancing function of the Liver as the smooth flow of its Qi regulates all movements of Qi in every part of the body.

Finally, the regulating and balancing function of the Liver has an important emotional aspect. The Liver, and particularly the Ethereal Soul, is responsible for a balanced emotional life: that is, ensuring that the person is neither overcome by emotions (as happens in an 'emotional' person) nor too indifferent to life's stimuli (as happens in people who are cut off from their feelings).

'The Liver loathes wind'

Windy weather often affects the Liver. Thus the relationship between Liver and 'Wind' concerns not only interior but also exterior Wind. It is not infrequent to hear patients who suffer from a Liver disharmony complaining about headaches and stiffness of the neck appearing after a period of windy weather.

'The Liver can cause convulsions'

Convulsions are a manifestation of interior Wind, which is always related to the Liver. As mentioned above, convulsions are considered to be due to the 'shaking' of the tendons, which are an extension of the Liver.

'The Liver arises from the left side'

Although anatomically situated on the right side, energetically the Liver is on the left (and the Lungs on the right). The Liver is related to the left side of the body in various ways.

Headaches on the left side of the head are said to be related to the Liver, and in particular deficiency of Liver-Blood, while those on the right are said to be related to the Gall Bladder. Of course, this is not always so in practice.

The left side of the tongue reflects more the state of the Liver, while the right side reflects the state of the Gall Bladder.

In pulse diagnosis, of course, the energy of the Liver is felt on the left side.

- An introduction to the relationship between Mind (*Shen*) and Ethereal Soul (*Hun*)
- How anger affects the Liver and how a Liver disharmony affects our moods
- The climate detrimental to the Liver
- The taste, colour, sound and smell related to the Liver and their clinical significance
- Dreams related to the Liver

Self-assessment questions

1. Which are the two main aspects of the Liver's storage of Blood?
2. How does Liver-Blood affect exercise?
3. How does Liver-Blood affect menstruation?
4. Which are the three main aspects of the smooth flow of Liver-Qi?
5. How does the smooth flow of Liver-Qi affect digestion?
6. What is the influence of the smooth flow of Liver-Qi on the emotional state?
7. How does anger affect the Liver?
8. What would be the consequence of an insufficient moistening and nourishment of the sinews by Liver-Blood?
9. What would be the consequence of an insufficient moistening and nourishment of the eyes by Liver-Blood?
10. Describe briefly the characteristics of the Ethereal Soul.
11. Describe briefly the relationship between the Ethereal Soul (*Hun*) and the Mind (*Shen*).

See p. 1256 for answers

END NOTES

1. Beijing College of Traditional Chinese Medicine 1980 Practical Chinese Medicine (*Shi Yong Zhong Yi Xue* 实用中医学), Beijing Publishing House, Beijing, p. 53.
2. 1979 The Yellow Emperor's Classic of Internal Medicine – Simple Questions (*Huang Di Nei Jing Su Wen* 黄帝内经素问), People's Health Publishing House, Beijing, first published c.100 BC, p. 58.
3. Ibid., p. 334.
4. Ibid., p. 73.
5. 1981 Syndromes and Treatment of the Internal Organs (*Zang Fu Zheng Zhi* 脏腑证治), Tianjin Scientific Publishing House, Tianjin, p. 131.
6. Simple Questions, p. 73.
7. Personal communication from Dr JHF Shen.
8. Simple Questions, p. 17.
9. Ibid., p. 139.
10. Ibid., p. 5.
11. Ibid., p. 70.
12. Ibid., p. 68.
13. Ibid., p. 73.
14. 1981 Spiritual Axis (*Ling Shu Jing* 灵枢经), People's Health Publishing House, Beijing, first published c.100 BC, p. 50.
15. Ibid., p. 78.
16. Simple Questions, p. 25.

Learning outcomes

In this chapter you will have learned:
- The clinical significance of the Liver's storage of Blood
- The importance of Liver-Blood in menstruation
- The clinical significance of the smooth flow of Liver-Qi in its three main aspects
- An introduction to the concept of Qi stagnation
- The relationship between Liver and sinews
- The relationship between the Liver and eyes
- The nature and clinical significance of the Ethereal Soul (*Hun*) and its relationship to the Liver

17. Spiritual Axis, p. 151.
18. Ibid., p. 151.
19. Simple Questions, p. 572.
20. Ibid., p. 67.
21. Tang Zong Hai 1979 Discussion on Blood (*Xue Zheng Lun* 血证论), People's Health Publishing House, first published 1884, p. 29.
22. Simple Questions, p. 102.
23. Ibid., p. 569.
24. Spiritual Axis, p. 85.
25. Simple Questions, p. 68.

FURTHER READING

Kaptchuk T 2000 The Web that has no Weaver – Understanding Chinese Medicine, Contemporary Books, Chicago

SECTION 1   PART 2

The Functions of the Lungs   8

Key contents

Functions of the Lungs
They govern Qi and respiration
They control channels and blood vessels
They control the diffusing and descending of Qi
They regulate all physiological activities
They regulate the Water passages
They control the skin and the space between skin and muscles
They manifest in the body hair
They open into the nose
They control nasal mucus
They house the Corporeal Soul
They are affected by worry, sadness and grief

Other Lung relationships
Their smell is rotten
Their colour is white
Their taste is pungent
Their climate is dryness
Their sound is weeping

Dreams

Sayings
'The Lungs control the 100 vessels'
'The Lungs loathe cold'
'The Lungs govern the voice'
'The Lungs are a delicate organ'

'The Simple Questions' in chapter 8 says that *'The Lungs are like a Prime Minister in charge of regulation.'*[1] This statement refers primarily to the part that the Lungs play in aiding the Heart (which is the Emperor) to circulate the Blood.

The functions of the Lungs are:

- They govern Qi and respiration
- They control channels and blood vessels
- They control diffusing and descending of Qi
- They regulate all physiological activities
- They regulate Water passages
- They control skin and hair
- They open into the nose
- They control nasal mucus
- They house the Corporeal Soul (*Po*)

The discussion of the function of the Lungs will be divided into the following headings:

- The functions of the lungs
  - The Lungs govern Qi and respiration
  - The Lungs control channels and blood vessels
  - The Lungs control the diffusing and descending of Qi
  - The Lungs regulate all physiological activities
  - The Lungs regulate Water passages
  - The Lungs control the skin and the space between skin and muscles
  - The Lungs manifest in the body hair
  - The Lungs open into the nose
  - The Lungs control nasal mucus
  - The Lungs house the Corporeal Soul
  - The Lungs are affected by worry, grief and sadness
- Other Lung relationships
  - The smell of the Lungs is rotten
  - The colour of the Lungs is white
  - The taste of the Lungs is pungent
  - The climate of the Lungs is dryness
  - The sound of the Lungs is weeping

The Lungs govern Qi and respiration and in particular are in charge of inhaling air. For this reason, and also because they influence the skin, they are the intermediary organ between the organism and the environment.

They control the blood vessels in that the Qi of the Lungs assists the Heart in controlling blood circulation. They are also said to control the 'Water passages'. This means that they play a vital role in the movement of Body Fluids.

- Dreams
- Sayings
  - 'The Lungs control the 100 vessels'
  - 'The Lungs loathe cold'
  - 'The Lungs govern the voice'
  - 'The Lungs are a delicate organ'

THE FUNCTIONS OF THE LUNGS

The functions of the Lungs discussed are:

- The Lungs govern Qi and respiration
- The Lungs control channels and blood vessels
- The Lungs control diffusing and descending of Qi
- The Lungs regulate all physiological activities
- The Lungs regulate Water passages
- The Lungs control the skin and the space between skin and muscles
- The Lungs manifest in the body hair
- The Lungs open into the nose
- The Lungs control nasal mucus
- The Lungs house the Corporeal Soul
- The Lungs are affected by worry, grief and sadness

The Lungs govern Qi and respiration

This is the most important Lung function since, from the air, the Lungs extract 'clean Qi' for the body, which then combines with Food-Qi coming from the Spleen: the combination of air from the Lungs and Food-Qi from the Spleen forms Gathering Qi (Zong Qi) (see also Fig. 3.7 in chapter 3).

Let us look at the two aspects of this vital work:

1. When we say that the Lungs govern respiration we mean that they inhale 'pure Qi' (air) and exhale 'dirty Qi'. The constant exchange and renewal of Qi performed by the Lungs ensures the proper functioning of all the body's physiological processes that take Qi as their basis. The 'Simple Questions' in chapter 5 says: '*Heavenly Qi goes to the Lung.*'[2] 'Heavenly Qi' here indicates air.

2. The second way in which the Lungs govern Qi is in the actual process of formation of Qi. As we saw in chapter 3, Food-Qi is extracted from food by the Spleen. This is directed to the Lungs where it combines with the inhaled air to form what is called Gathering Qi (*Zong Qi*). Because this process takes place in the chest, the chest is also called 'Sea of Qi' or 'Upper Sea of Qi' (as opposed to the Lower Sea of Qi below the navel). The Gathering Qi is sometimes also called 'Big Qi of the chest' (Fig. 8.1).

After its formation, the Lungs spread Qi all over the body to nourish all tissues and promote all physiological processes.

The 'Spiritual Axis' in chapter 56 says: '*Big Qi gathers together without moving to accumulate in the chest; it is called the Sea of Qi which comes out of the Lungs, goes to the throat and facilitates inhalation and exhalation.*'[3]

Gathering Qi (or Big Qi) resides in the chest and aids the Lung and Heart functions, promoting good circulation to the limbs and controlling the strength of voice. Weak Lung-Qi can therefore cause tiredness, a weak voice and slight breathlessness.

Clinical note

Gathering Qi can be tonified by using Ren-17 Shanzhong

Because of their role in extracting Qi from air, and because they control the skin, the Lungs are the most 'external' of the Yin organs; they are the connection between the body and the outside world. For this reason, the Lungs are easily attacked by exterior pathogenic factors and are sometimes referred to as the

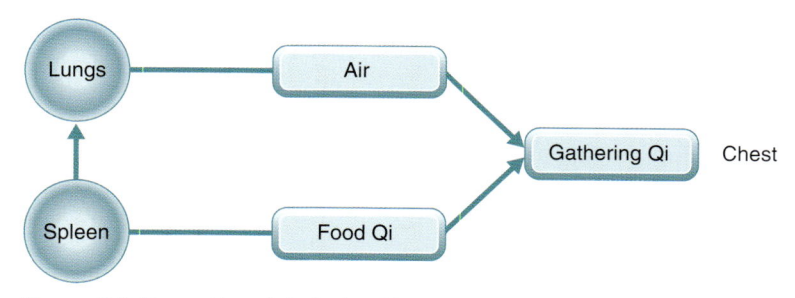

Figure 8.1 The making of Gathering Qi

> **Box 8.1 The lungs govern Qi and respiration**
> - The Lungs inhale 'heavenly Qi', i.e. air
> - The air from the Lungs combines with Food-Qi from the Spleen to form Gathering Qi (*Zong Qi*)
> - The Lungs govern Gathering Qi in the chest

'delicate' organ: that is, delicate and vulnerable to invasion by climatic factors.

This function of the Lungs is summarized in Box 8.1.

The Lungs control channels and blood vessels

As we have seen, the Lungs govern Qi and Qi is essential to aid the Heart to circulate Blood. For this reason, although the Heart controls the blood vessels, the Lungs also play an important part in maintaining the health of blood vessels. In this respect, their scope is somewhat wider than that of the Heart, since the Lungs not only control circulation in the blood vessels themselves but also in all channels. As we have seen in the chapter on Qi, Nutritive Qi is closely related to Blood and the two flow together both in blood vessels and channels. Since the Lungs govern Qi, they control the circulation of Qi in both blood vessels and channels.

It should also be noted that, in the 'Yellow Emperor's Classic of Internal Medicine' the word *mai* ('vessel') is used somewhat ambiguously as, in certain contexts, it clearly refers to channels while in others it refers to blood vessels.

In the 'Yellow Emperor's Classic of Internal Medicine' the word *mai* may mean both 'acupuncture channel' and 'blood vessel'.

If Lung-Qi is strong, the circulation of Qi and Blood will be good and the limbs will be warm. If Lung Qi is weak, Qi will not be able to push the Blood, and the limbs, particularly the hands, will be cold.

This function of the Lungs is summarized in Box 8.2.

> **Box 8.2 The Lungs control channels and blood vessels**
> - As they govern Qi, the Lungs control all (acupuncture) channels
> - As Qi is the commander of Blood and as Nutritive Qi (*Ying Qi*) flows in close contact with Blood, the Lungs also influence all blood vessels

The Lungs control the diffusing and descending of Qi

These two functions are extremely important and essential to grasp in order to understand the Lungs' physiology and pathology.

The diffusing of Qi and fluids

The Lungs have the function of diffusing or spreading Defensive Qi and Body Fluids all over the body to the space between skin and muscles (Fig. 8.2). This is one way in which the Lungs are physiologically related to the skin. The diffusing of Qi ensures that Defensive Qi is equally distributed all over the body under the skin, performing its function of warming the skin and muscles and protecting the body from exterior pathogenic factors.

If Lung-Qi is weak and its diffusing function is impaired, Defensive Qi will not reach the skin and the body will be easily invaded by exterior pathogenic factors. One can have a good idea of what the diffusing function really is by observing what happens when this function is impaired. When a person catches a cold, most of the symptoms and signs are a manifestation of the impairment of the Lungs' diffusing function. The exterior Wind-Cold obstructs the skin, prevents the spreading and diffusing of Defensive Qi and therefore interferes with the Lungs' diffusing function. Qi cannot be diffused and everything feels 'blocked'. That is precisely how one may feel during a heavy cold, with aversion to cold, a headache, sneezing, etc.

The 'Spiritual Axis' in chapter 30 says: *'The Qi of the Upper Burner is in communication with the outside and spreads out, it disseminates the essences of food, it warms the skin, it fills the body and it moistens the hair like irrigation by fog and dew.'*[4]

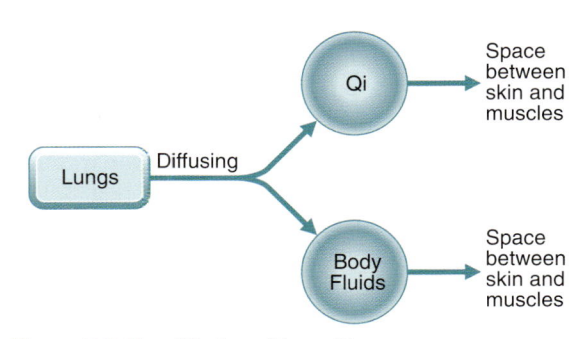

Figure 8.2 The diffusing of Lung-Qi

Besides Qi, the Lungs also diffuse Body Fluids to the skin and to the space between the skin and muscles (*cou li* space) in the form of a fine 'mist'. This is one reason why the Upper Burner is compared to 'Mist'. The fine mist of Body Fluids moistens the skin and regulates the opening and closing of pores and sweating. When this function is normal, the pores open and close normally, and there is a normal, physiological, amount of sweating: in such a case, the space between skin and muscles is said to be well regulated. When this function is impaired, and the condition is one of Excess, the pores become blocked and there is no sweating: in this case, the space between the skin and muscles is said to be too 'tight'. If the condition is one of Deficiency, the pores are over-relaxed and remain open so that there is spontaneous sweating: in such a case, the space between the skin and muscles is said to be too 'loose'.

If the Lung's function of diffusing body fluids is impaired, fluids may accumulate under the skin, causing oedema (usually of the face).

> **Clinical note**
>
> The diffusing of Lung-Qi can be stimulated by LU-7 Lieque

This function of the Lungs is summarized in Box 8.3.

> **Box 8.3 Diffusing of Lung-Qi**
>
> - The Lungs diffuse Qi to the space between skin and muscles (where it forms the Defensive Qi)
> - The Lungs diffuse Body Fluids to the space between skin and muscles (where it forms sweat)

The descending of Qi

Because the Lungs are the uppermost organ in the body, Chinese medical texts often referred to them as the 'lid', or 'magnificent lid'.[5] Because they are the uppermost organ in the body, their Qi must descend. This is what is meant by descending of Qi. As we have seen, Lung-Qi must descend to communicate with the Kidneys and these respond by 'holding' Qi (Fig. 8.3).

If this descending movement of Qi is impaired, Lung-Qi does not flow down and Qi will accumulate in the chest, causing cough, breathlessness and a feeling of oppression of the chest. In some cases, it may affect the function of the Large Intestine. If the Large Intestine does not receive Qi from the Lungs, it will not have the power necessary for defecation (this happens particularly in the elderly). In certain cases, the impairment of the descending of Lung-Qi may also cause retention of urine (again, particularly in old people).

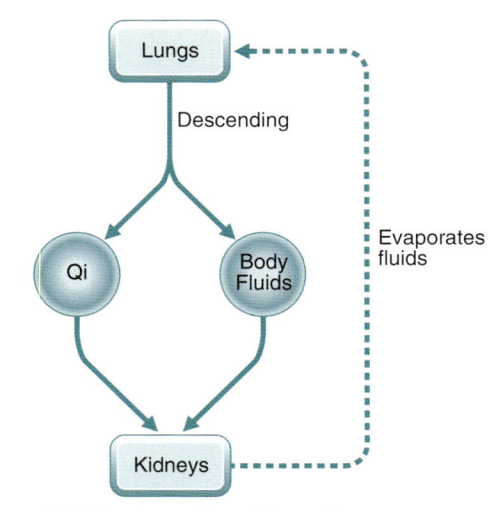

Figure 8.3 The descending of Lung-Qi

The descending function applies not only to Qi but also to Body Fluids, because the Lungs also direct fluids down to the Kidneys and Bladder. The Lungs direct fluids down to the Kidneys where Kidney-Yang evaporates them and sends them back up to the Lungs: these fluids are essential to keep the Lungs moist. The Lungs also send some fluids down to the Bladder where they are excreted as urine. For this reason, some urinary problems, especially in the elderly, may be due to Lung-Qi.

> **Clinical note**
>
> The descending of Lung-Qi can be stimulated by LU-7 Lieque

This function of the Lungs is summarized in Box 8.4.

The role of the Lung's diffusing and descending functions is summarized in Box 8.5.

The Lungs regulate all physiological activities

Chapter 8 of the 'Simple Questions' says: '*The Lungs are like a Prime Minister in charge of regulation.*'[6] This description of the Lungs' function in the 'Simple Questions' should be seen in context and the sentence

Box 8.4 Descending of Lung-Qi

- The Lungs descend Qi to Kidneys (the coordination of Lungs and Kidneys harmonizes breathing)
- The Lungs descend Body Fluids to the Kidneys; they, in turn, evaporate the fluids and send them back up to the Lungs where they moisten the Lungs
- The Lungs descend Body Fluids to the Bladder where they are excreted as urine (for this reason the Lungs influence urination and Lung-Qi deficiency may cause urinary problems)

Box 8.5 The diffusing and descending of the Lungs

- They ensure the proper 'entering and exiting' and 'ascending and descending' of Qi (see ch. 4)
- They ensure the free movement of Qi and regulate breathing
- They regulate the exchange of Qi between the body and the environment
- They ensure that all organs receive the necessary nourishment of Qi, Blood and Body Fluids
- They prevent the fluids from accumulating and stagnating
- They prevent the scattering and exhaustion of Lung-Qi
- They ensure the communication between Lungs and Kidneys

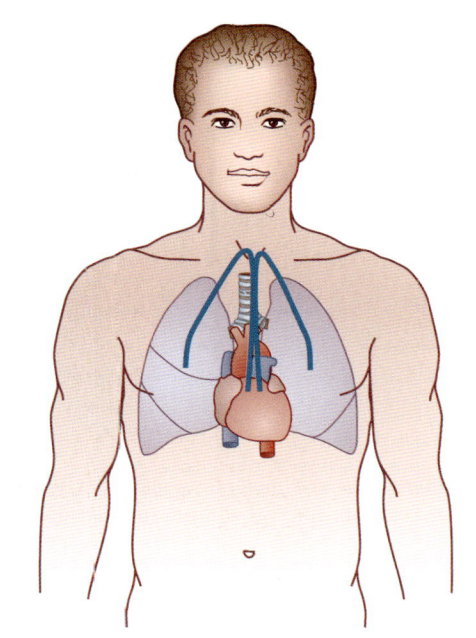

Figure 8.4 Gathering Qi in the chest

preceding the above concerning the function of the Heart says: '*The Heart is like the Emperor, in charge of the Spirit (Shen Ming).*'[7]

Thus, the Heart is compared to an Emperor and the Lungs to a Prime Minister assisting the Emperor.[8] This relationship is an expression of the close relationship between Qi and Blood. The Lungs govern Qi and the Heart governs Blood: Qi is the 'commander of Blood' (it moves Blood) and Blood is the 'mother of Qi'. Qi and Blood assist and depend on each other: hence the comparison of the relationship between the Heart and Lungs to that between an Emperor and his Prime Minister.

Moreover, Heart and Lungs are both in the chest and their relationship is close for other reasons. The Gathering Qi '*Zong Qi*' is a type of Qi and, as such, governed by the Lungs, but it plays an important role in assisting the Heart's functions. The Gathering Qi also plays an important role in the circulation of Blood, which is governed by the Heart. Gathering Qi assists the Heart and Lungs to propel Qi and Blood to the limbs, especially the hands. The 'Spiritual Axis' in chapter 71 comments: '*The Gathering Qi accumulates in the chest, rises to the throat, enters the Heart channel and aids breathing*'[9] (Fig. 8.4).

After saying that the Lungs are like a Prime Minister, the 'Simple Questions' says that the Lungs are in charge of 'regulation'. This means that, just as the Prime Minister regulates all administrative functions, the Lungs help to regulate all physiological activities in every organ and every part of the body, just as the Prime Minister's office controls and directs the administrative functions of all government departments (Fig. 8.5). The Lungs regulate all physiological activities in various ways:

- By governing Qi
- By controlling all channels and blood vessels
- By governing breathing

As Qi is the basis for all physiological activities, the Lungs, by governing Qi, are naturally in charge of all physiological activities. This regulation function is dependent also on the Lungs' action in moving Qi around the body. As the Lungs are the uppermost organ in the body, their Qi naturally descends. In fact, the Lungs are situated at the highest part of the trunk; in the 'Yellow Emperor's Classic of Internal Medicine'

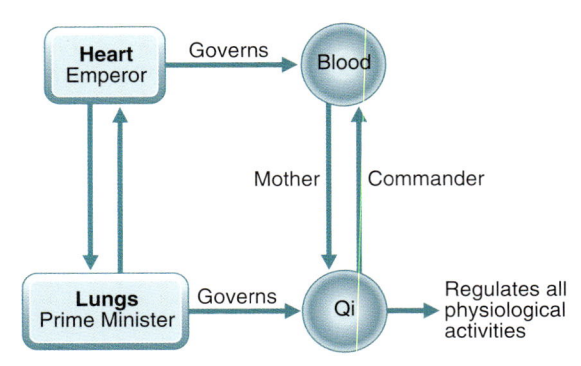

Figure 8.5 Relationship between Heart and Lungs

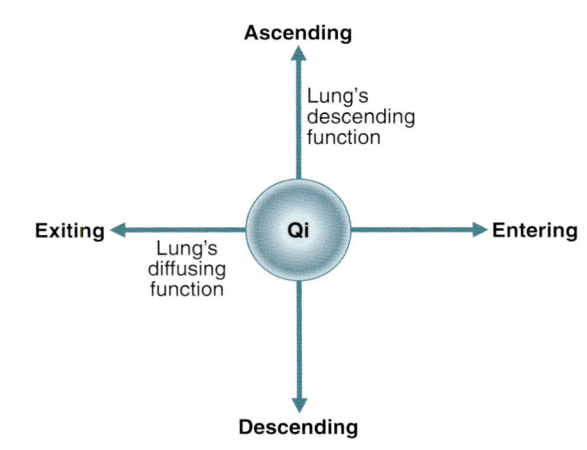

Figure 8.6 Regulation of Qi Mechanism by diffusing and descending of Lung-Qi

they are compared to a '*magnificent lid*'. For this reason, the Lungs regulate the 'ascending and descending' as well as the 'entering and exiting' of Qi of the Qi Mechanism (see ch. 4). They regulate the ascending–descending of Qi through their descending function and the entering–exiting of Qi through their diffusing function.

In turn, the circulation of Qi by the Lungs depends on the Lungs controlling all channels and blood vessels. This is reflected in the expression '*The Lungs rule over the 100 vessels (mai)*.' Note that the word '*mai*' (vessel) is often used in an ambiguous sense in the 'Yellow Emperor's Classic of Internal Medicine' in so far as it sometimes refers to acupuncture channels and sometimes to blood vessels. For this reason I translate that expression by saying that the Lungs govern all channels and blood vessels. Indeed, it is not by chance that we feel the pulse for pulse diagnosis on the radial artery where the Lung channel flows: the pulsation of blood in that blood vessel reflects also the 'pulsation' of Qi.

> **Clinical note**
>
> In Chinese pulse diagnosis, we feel the pulse on the radial artery, a blood vessel. However, it is not by chance that we feel the radial artery where the Lung channel flows. By feeling the radial artery, and due to its connection with the Lung channel, we also get a feel of Qi circulation as the Lungs govern Qi.

As the Lungs govern breathing, this is another way in which they regulate all physiological activities. Through breathing, the Lungs distribute Qi to all tissues in every part of the body and every organ and this naturally plays an important regulating function in all physiological activities. These aspects of the Lungs are summarized in Figure 8.6 and Box 8.6.

> **Box 8.6 The Lungs regulate all physiological activities**
>
> The Lungs regulate all physiological activities by:
> - Governing Qi
> - Controlling breathing
> - Controlling all channels and blood vessels
> - Controlling the ascending–descending and entering–exiting of Qi ('Qi Mechanism')

The Lungs regulate Water passages

After receiving the refined fluids from the Spleen, the Lungs reduce them to a fine mist and 'spray' them throughout the area under the skin and, specifically, the space between skin and muscles (*cou li* space). This process is part of the diffusing function of the Lungs (Fig. 8.7). In health, the fluids are evenly spread all over the body, the opening and closing of the pores is normal and the space between the skin and muscles is properly regulated. If this function is impaired, the fluids may accumulate under the skin and give rise to oedema.

The Lungs also direct fluids down to the Kidneys and Bladder. This process is part of the descending function of the Lungs. The Kidneys receive the fluids and vaporize part of these before sending them back up to the Lungs to keep them moist. The Lungs' job of directing fluids downwards also has an influence on the Bladder

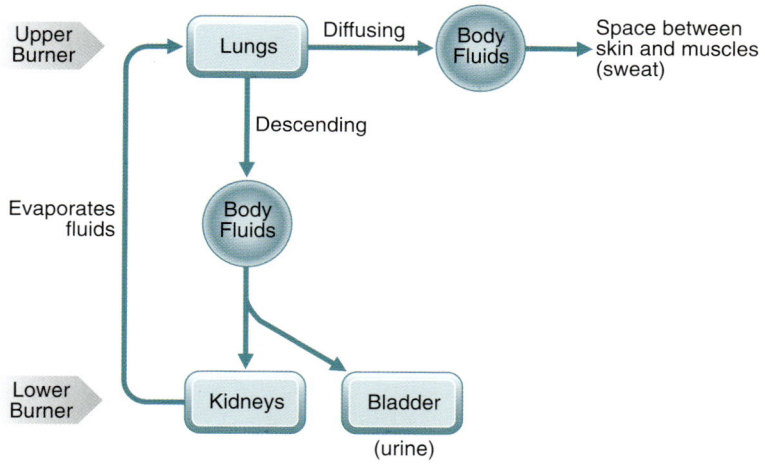

Figure 8.7 The regulation of Water passages by the Lungs

function. If this Lung function is normal, urination will be normal; if it is impaired, there may be urinary retention, especially in old people.

As the Lungs play an important role in the metabolism of fluids in the Upper Burner, they are sometimes called the 'Upper Source of Water'. The 'Simple Questions' in chapter 21 says: *'Fluids enter the Stomach, the refined part is transmitted upward to the Spleen. Spleen-Qi, in turn, spreads it upwards to the Lungs who, regulating the Water passages, send it down to the Bladder.'*[10]

Through its diffusing and descending functions, the Lungs are therefore responsible for the excretion of Body Fluids through sweat (due to the diffusing of fluids in the space between skin and muscles) or urine (due to the connection between Lungs and Bladder).

The Lungs' diffusing and descending of Body Fluids is part of the Upper Burner physiology in fluid metabolism. One of the major functions of the Triple Burner (see ch. 13) is that of transformation, transportation and excretion of fluids. The Triple Burner is a system of body 'cavities', some large and some small. The large cavities are the chest cavity (Upper Burner), abdominal cavity (Middle Burner) and pelvic cavity (Lower Burner). The Triple Burner is in charge of the movement, transformation and excretion of body fluids between these cavities: for this, it relies on a proper ascending–descending and entering–exiting of Qi in all cavities and all organs. The Lungs' activity of regulating Water passages by its diffusing and descending of Qi is part of the Upper Burner's metabolism of fluids.

This function of the Lungs is summarized in Box 8.7.

Box 8.7 The Lungs regulate the Water passages

The Lungs regulate the Water passages by:
- Diffusing Body Fluids to the space between skin and muscles
- Descending Body Fluids to the Kidneys and Bladder

The Lungs control the skin and the space between skin and muscles (*Cou li* space)

This function is closely related to the previous two functions. The Lungs receive fluids from the Spleen and spreads them to the skin and the space between skin and muscles all over the body. This nourishes and moistens the skin. If the Lungs diffuse fluids normally, the skin will have lustre, the opening and closing of the pores is well regulated and sweating will be normal. If this function is impaired, the skin will be deprived of nourishment and moisture, and the skin may be rough and dry (Fig. 8.8).

When Qi and fluids in the space between skin and muscles (*cou li*) are harmonized, the space is properly regulated, sweating is normal and the person has a good resistance to pathogenic factors. In pathology, the space between skin and muscles may be either too 'slack' or 'open', in which case the person sweats abnormally and external pathogenic factors penetrate easily, or too 'tight' or 'closed', in which case there is not enough sweating and, if pathogenic factors do invade the body, the person will usually react strongly with a fever.

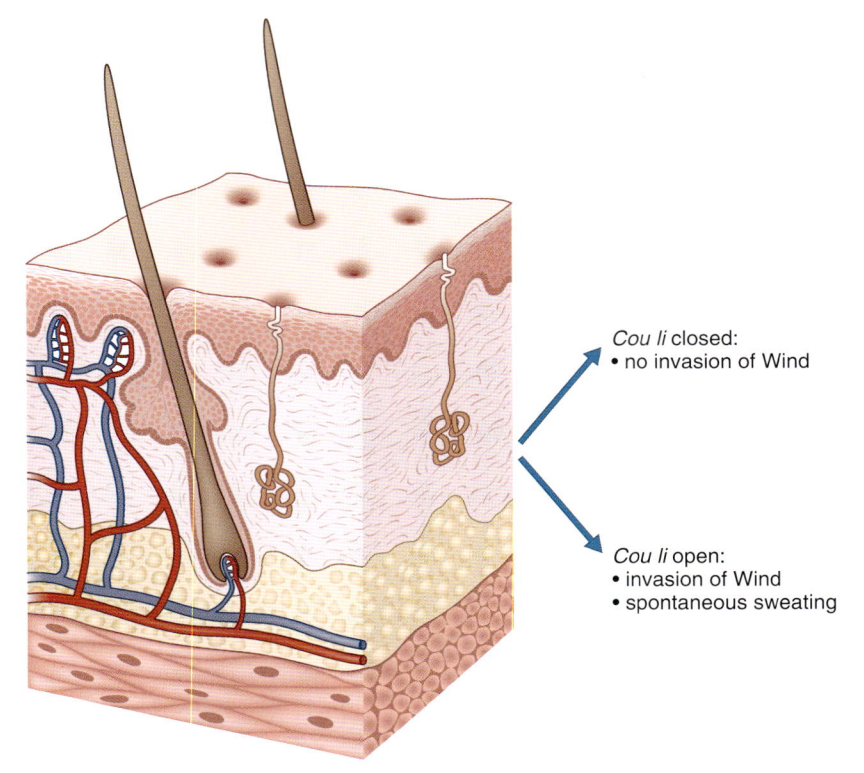

Figure 8.8 The space between skin and muscles (*Cou Li*)

Cou li closed:
- no invasion of Wind

Cou li open:
- invasion of Wind
- spontaneous sweating

> **Clinical note**
>
> The space between skin and muscles (*cou li*)
> - When Qi and fluids in the space between skin and muscles (*cou li*) are harmonized, the space is properly regulated, sweating is normal and the person has a good resistance to pathogenic factors
> - When the space between skin and muscles is too 'open', the person sweats abnormally and external pathogenic factors penetrate easily. To 'tighten' the space, reinforce LU-9 Taiyuan and BL-13 Feishu with direct moxa cones
> - When the space between skin and muscles is too 'closed', there is not enough sweating and, if pathogenic factors do invade the body, the person will usually react strongly with a fever. To 'relax' the space, needle LU-7 Lieque and L.I.-4 Hegu

The Lungs influence Defensive Qi, which flows in the space between skin and muscles. If Lung-Qi is strong, Defensive Qi will be strong and the person will have a good resistance to attack by exterior pathogenic factors. If Lung Qi is weak, the Defensive Qi will also be weak and, because the pores will be open, there may be spontaneous sweating; the person will also be prone to attack by exterior pathogenic factors. When this kind of sweating occurs, a certain amount of Defensive Qi is lost with the sweat. For this reason, the 'Simple Questions' in chapter 3 calls the pores '*doors of Qi*'.[11]

Conversely, if an exterior pathogenic factor does invade the exterior portions of the body, that is, the space between skin and muscles (which can happen even if the Defensive Qi is relatively strong), it will obstruct this space and therefore the circulation of Defensive Qi, which, in turn, will impair the Lung diffusing function, causing aversion to cold, sneezing, etc. (Fig. 8.9).

The 'Simple Questions' in chapter 10 says: '*The Lungs control the skin and manifest on the hair.*'[12] In chapter 9 it says: '*The Lungs are the root of Qi, the residence of the Corporeal Soul (Po), they manifest in the hair, they fill up the skin, they represent Yin within the Yang and pertain to Autumn.*'[13]

This function of the Lungs is summarized in Box 8.8.

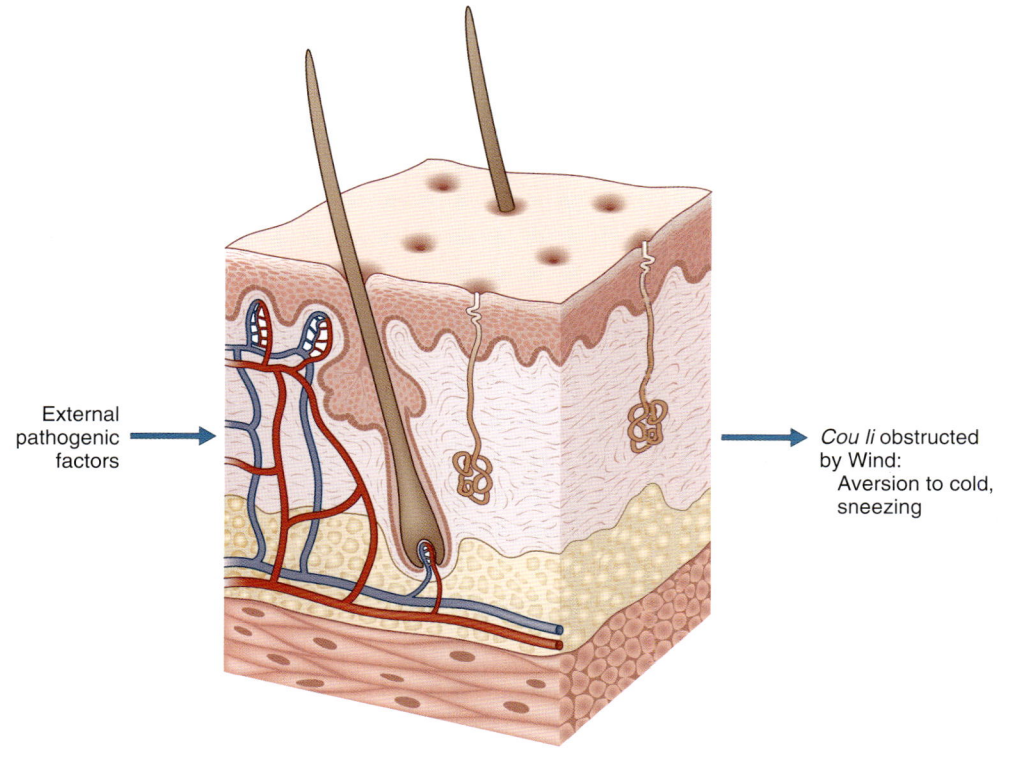

Figure 8.9 Invasion of Wind in the space between the skin and muscles

---

Box 8.8 The Lungs control the skin and the space between skin and muscles (*Cou li*)

- The Lungs diffuse fluids to the skin, giving it lustre
- The Lungs diffuse Qi and fluids to the space between skin and muscles, regulating sweating and providing a normal resistance to pathogenic factors

---

Box 8.9 The Lungs manifest in the body hair

The Lungs diffuse Qi and fluids to the skin and body hair:
- Normal diffusing: hair lustrous
- Abnormal diffusing: brittle and dry hair

The Lungs manifest in the body hair

The Lungs diffuse Defensive Qi and fluids to the skin and hair. Therefore the state of the hair (body hair) reflects the state of the Lungs. The Lungs receive fluids from the Spleen and spread them all over the body to the skin and hair: this nourishes and moistens the body hair.

If the diffusing of Qi and fluids by the Lungs is normal, the hair will be glossy and healthy. If the Lungs do not diffuse Qi and fluids properly, the body hair will lack nourishment and moisture and the hair will have a withered, brittle and dry quality (Fig. 8.10 and Box 8.9.)

The Lungs open into the nose

The nose is the opening of the Lungs, and through it respiration occurs. If Lung-Qi is strong, the nose will be open, breathing will be easy and the sense of smell will be normal. If Lung-Qi is weak, the sense of smell may be weak; if the Lung's Defensive Qi portion is invaded by an exterior pathogenic factor, the nose will be runny, there may be loss of the sense of smell and sneezing; if the Lungs are invaded by Dampness, the nose is blocked; if the Lungs have Heat, there may be bleeding from the nose, loss of the sense of smell and the alae nasi will flap rapidly (as in pneumonia).

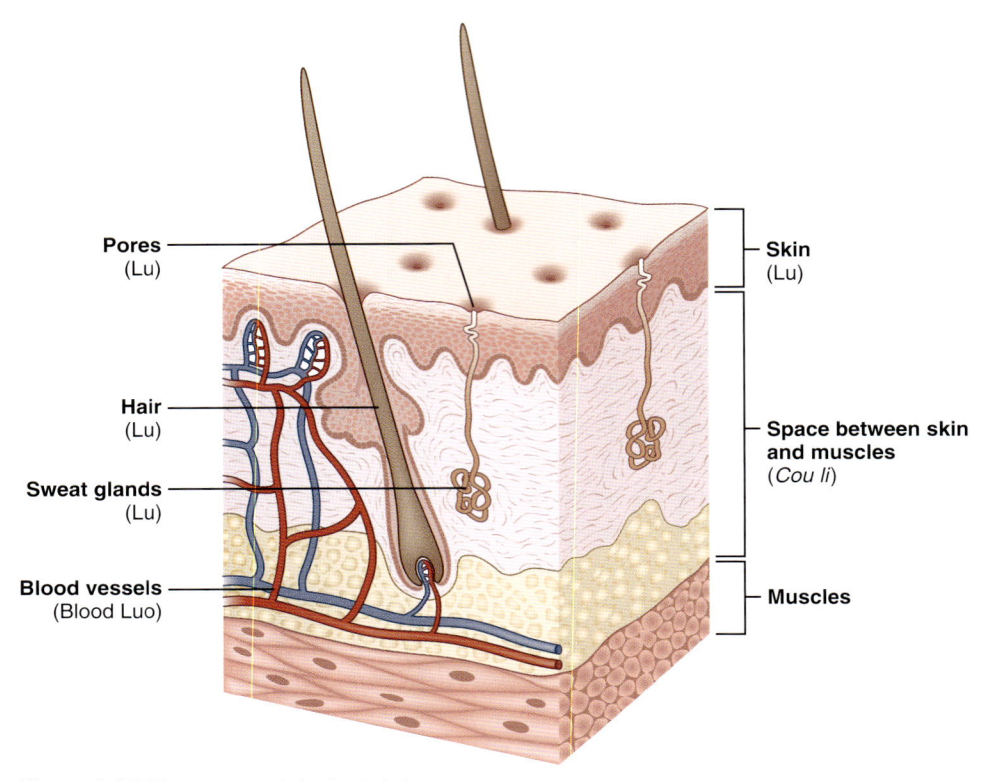

Figure 8.10 The Lungs and the body hair

Clinical note

- Lung-Qi deficient: weak sense of smell (use LU-7 Lieque, L.I.-4 Hegu and extra point Bitong)
- Invasion of Wind: runny nose (use LU-7 Lieque, L.I.-4 Hegu, BL-12 Fengmen and BL-13 Feishu)
- Dampness: blocked nose (use LU-7 Lieque, L.I.-4 Hegu, extra point Bitong and Du-23 Shangxing)
- Lung-Heat: flapping of ala nasi, nosebleed (use LU-5 Chize and L.I.-11 Quchi)

The 'Spiritual Axis' in chapter 17 says: *'The Lungs open into the nose, if the Lung is harmonious, the nose can smell.'*[14]

Finally, it must be remembered that there are also other organs which affect the sense of smell apart from the Lungs, notably the Spleen.

This function of the Lungs is summarized in Box 8.10.

The Lungs control nasal mucus

Of the fluids, the Lungs naturally control nasal mucus and the nose is the orifice pertaining to the Lungs. The

Box 8.10 The Lungs open into the nose

The Lungs open into the nose through which breathing occurs. Ease of breathing through the nose and sense of smell depend on the state of the Lungs

'Simple Questions' says in chapter 23: *'The Lungs control nasal mucus.'*[15] If the diffusing of Qi and fluids by the Lungs is normal, the nose is properly moistened and lubricated by normal mucus secretion, which plays a certain role in the defence from exterior pathogenic factors. If the diffusing and descending of Lung-Qi and fluids is impaired, the nasal secretion may accumulate, causing a nasal discharge or a stuffed nose. If the Lungs are affected by Heat or Phlegm-Heat, the nasal mucus becomes yellow and thick. If the Lungs are affected by dryness, the nasal mucus is insufficient and the nasal mucosa is too dry.

Box 8.11 summarizes this function of the Lungs.

The Lungs house the Corporeal Soul

The Lungs are said to be the residence of the Corporeal Soul (*Po*), which forms the Yin or physical counterpart

Box 8.11 The Lungs control nasal mucus

Nasal mucus is influenced by the Lungs:
- Normal diffusing of Qi and fluids by the Lungs: the nose is properly moistened and lubricated by normal mucus secretion
- Diffusing and descending of Lung-Qi and fluids impaired: nasal secretion accumulates, causing a nasal discharge or a stuffed nose
- Lung-Heat or Phlegm-Heat: thick-yellow nasal mucus
- Dryness in the Lungs: nasal mucus is insufficient and the nasal mucosa is too dry

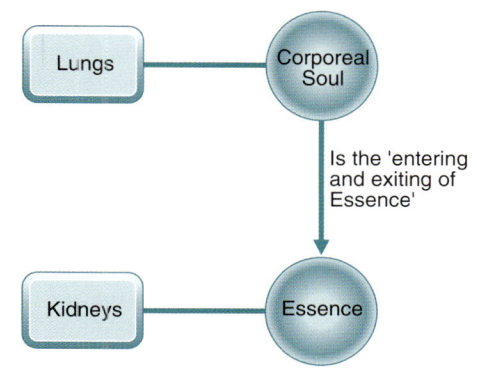

Figure 8.11 The Lungs and the Corporeal Soul

of the Ethereal Soul (*Hun*). Similarly to *Hun*, the Chinese character for *Po* also contains the radical *Gui*, which means 'spirit' or 'demon'.

魄 is the character for *Po*

鬼 is the character for *gui*

白 is the character for 'white'

The Corporeal Soul is the most physical and material part of a human being's soul. It could be said to be the somatic manifestation of the soul. The 'Classic of Categories' (1624) by Zhang Jie Bing says: '*The Corporeal Soul moves and does, ... through it pain and itching can be felt.*'[16]

The Corporeal Soul is Yin compared to the Ethereal Soul (*Hun*) and it is formed at conception (while the Ethereal Soul enters the body 3 days after birth). The Corporeal Soul dies with the body while the Ethereal Soul survives at death. After birth, the newly born baby's whole life revolves around the Corporeal Soul; in those months, the mother's Corporeal Soul nourishes that of the baby.

The Corporeal Soul is closely related to Essence and it could be said to be a manifestation of the Essence in the sphere of sensations and feelings. The Corporeal Soul is called the 'entering and exiting of Essence (*Jing*)'. Essence is the foundation for a healthy body and the Corporeal Soul makes for sharp and clear sensations and movements (Fig. 8.11). Through the Corporeal Soul, the Essence 'enters and exits', which allows it to play a role in all physiological processes.

The relationship between Corporeal Soul and Essence is very important in practice. Firstly, it means that the Essence is not simply the precious constitutional essence that resides in the Kidneys, but it is also an essence that, through the Corporeal Soul, plays a role in all physiological processes.

Secondly, through the Corporeal Soul, the Essence plays a role in defence against exterior pathogenic factors. As we know, Defensive Qi is related to the Lungs: as protection of pathogenic factors is a function of the Defensive Qi, tonifying the Lungs will strengthen Defensive Qi and therefore the resistance to pathogenic factors. However, other factors play a role in protection against pathogenic factors and in the functioning of Defensive Qi; the strength of the Essence is one such factor. The close connection between the Corporeal Soul and the Essence, and especially the fact that the Corporeal Soul makes the Essence 'enter and exit' in all parts of the body, means that the Essence (and therefore the Kidneys) also plays a role in protection from pathogenic factors. In particular, following the Corporeal Soul (and therefore Lung-Qi), the Essence goes to the space between the skin and muscles where it plays a role in protection against exterior pathogenic factors.

Being related to the Lungs, the Corporeal Soul is also closely linked to breathing. The ancient Greeks called the soul ανεμοξ (*anemos*), which means 'wind or vital breath', and the spirit πυεμα (*pneuma,*) which also means 'breath'. The Corporeal Soul, residing in the Lungs, is a direct manifestation of the breath of life. Just as through breathing oxygen enters the blood in Western medicine, in Chinese medicine breathing is a manifestation of the Corporeal Soul which affects all physiological functions.

Sadness and grief constrict the Corporeal Soul, dissolve Lung-Qi and suspend our breathing. The shallow and short breathing of a person who is sad and worried is an expression of the constraint of the Corporeal Soul and Lung-Qi

On an emotional level, the Corporeal Soul is directly affected by emotions of sadness or grief, which constrain its feelings and obstruct its movement. Since the Corporeal Soul resides in the Lungs, such emotions have a powerful and direct effect on breathing, which itself could be seen as the pulsating of the Corporeal Soul.

Sadness and grief constrict the Corporeal Soul, dissolve Lung-Qi and suspend our breathing. The shallow and short breathing of a person who is sad and worried is an example of this. Similarly, the rapid and shallow breathing taking place at the very top of the chest only, almost in the neck, is an expression of the constraint of the Corporeal Soul and Lung-Qi. For this reason, treatment of the Lungs is often very important in emotional problems deriving from depression, sadness, grief, anxiety or bereavement.

This function of the Lungs is summarized in Box 8.12.

Clinical note

The best points to treat the Lungs when the Corporeal Soul is affected by worry, sadness or grief are LU-7 Lieque and BL-42 Pohu

The Lungs are affected by worry, grief and sadness

Worry, grief and sadness affect the Lungs directly. Worry tends to 'knot' Qi, while grief and sadness tend to deplete Qi (Fig. 8.12). The 'knotting' action of worry on Qi may be seen in the shoulder and chest tension

Box 8.12 The Lungs house the Corporeal Soul (*Po*)

- The Corporeal Soul is a 'physical' soul in charge of all physiological processes
- The Corporeal Soul is responsible for feelings and sensations
- The Corporeal Soul is Yin in relation to the Ethereal Soul (*Hun*)
- The Corporeal Soul dies with the body (while the Ethereal Soul survives death)
- The Corporeal Soul is formed at conception
- A newly born baby's life revolves completely around the Corporeal Soul
- The Corporeal Soul is the 'entering and exiting of the Essence'
- Through the Corporeal Soul, the Essence plays a role in all physiological processes
- The Corporeal Soul is affected by worry, sadness and grief

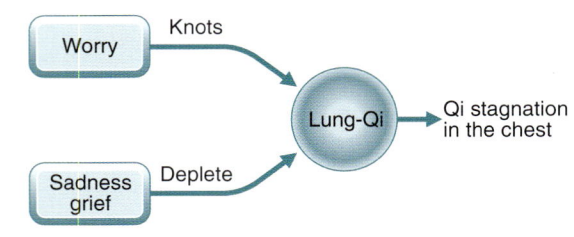

Figure 8.12 Effects of worry, sadness and grief on Lung-Qi

displayed by people who are subject to chronic worry. Qi stagnation in the chest deriving from worry may also affect the breasts in women and it is often at the root of the formation of breast lumps.

Sadness and grief deplete Qi and this can observed in the Lung pulse becoming weak and fine (thin), in the complexion becoming white and in the tone of voice becoming feeble and weepy.

It should be noted that, although sadness and grief deplete Qi in the chest, they also to some extent cause stagnation of Qi in the chest, manifesting with a slight feeling of tightness of the chest and slight breathlessness.

This function of the Lungs is summarized in Box 8.13.

Box 8.13 The Lungs are affected by worry, sadness and grief

- Worry 'knots' Lung-Qi and causes a feeling of tightness of the chest, slight breathlessness and tension of the shoulders. In women, it affects the breasts
- Sadness and grief deplete Lung-Qi and cause a slight breathlessness and tiredness
- All three emotions may lead to Qi stagnation in the chest

OTHER LUNG RELATIONSHIPS

The relationships of the Lungs discussed are:

- The smell of the Lungs
- The colour of the Lungs
- The taste of the Lungs
- The climate of the Lungs
- The sound of the Lungs

The smell of the Lungs is rotten

The smell related to the Lungs is described as 'rotten': this is the smell of purulent sputum in a chest infection of the lungs. This smell can occasionally be smelled also in the absence of a chest infection, particularly when there is Lung-Heat or Phlegm-Heat in the Lungs.

The colour of the Lungs is white

The colour white is associated with the Metal element and the Lungs. In diagnosis, this relationship may be observed, as pale-white cheeks often reflect a deficiency of Lung-Qi.

The taste of the Lungs is pungent

The pungent (including spicy) taste is related to the Lungs. A small amount of pungent (spicy) taste in the diet will gently tonify the Lungs. Please note that the pungent taste is not only the taste of spicy, hot foods such as chilli, curry or cayenne pepper but also the taste of spices such as cinnamon and nutmeg. The pungent taste is often also associated with fragrant herbs (containing volatile oils) such as peppermint: indeed, peppermint will stimulate the diffusing of Lung-Qi.

An excessive consumption of foods with a pungent taste may either weaken Lung-Yin or lead to Lung-Heat; in addition, the excessive consumption of foods with a pungent taste may also injure the Liver (Metal overacting on Wood).

The climate of the Lungs is dryness

An excessively dry climate, such as that found in the desert, injures the Lungs and particularly Lung-Yin. The Lungs need to be kept moist at all times and the 'vapour' released by the heating action of Kidney-Yang rises to the Lungs to keep them moist. Excessive dryness can also be found in certain industrial environments.

The sound of the Lungs is weeping

A person suffering from Lung deficiency may tend to speak with a 'weepy' tone, almost as if that person was about to burst into tears. Apart from the tone of voice, weeping and crying themselves are the sounds related to the Lungs as the Lungs are affected by sadness and grief.

DREAMS

The 'Simple Questions' says in chapter 17: '*When the Lungs are in excess, one dreams of weeping.*'[17] In chapter 80 it says that '*If the Lungs are deficient, one will dream of white objects or about bloody killings. If the dream takes place in the Autumn, one will dream of battles and war.*'[18]

The 'Spiritual Axis' in chapter 43 says: '*When the Lungs are in excess, one will have dreams of worry and fear, or crying and flying ... if the Lungs are deficient one will dream of flying and seeing strange objects made of gold or iron.*'[19]

SAYINGS

The sayings discussed are:

- 'The Lungs control the 100 vessels'
- 'The Lungs loathe cold'
- 'The Lungs govern the voice'
- 'The Lungs are a delicate organ'

'The Lungs govern the 100 vessels'

As the Lungs govern Qi, they have an influence on all channels in so far as they circulate Qi. Given the close relationship between Lungs (governing Qi) and the Heart (governing Blood) and given the close relationship between Qi and Blood ('Qi is the commander of Blood, Blood is the mother of Qi'), the influence of the Lungs naturally extends to the blood vessels. Indeed, it is not by chance that, in Chinese pulse diagnosis, we feel the pulse on the radial artery where the Lung channel flows.

Thus, the above expression, that the Lungs rule over the 100 vessels, refers to both channels and blood vessels.

'The Lungs loathe cold'

The Lungs influence the skin and the Defensive Qi and are easily invaded by exterior pathogenic factors, particularly Wind-Cold.

'The Lungs govern the voice'

The strength, tone and clarity of voice are all dependent on the Lungs. When the Lungs are healthy they are compared to a bell, giving off a clear ringing sound, which is the voice. If the Lungs are weak, the voice may be low, while if the Lungs are obstructed by Phlegm, the voice tone may be muffled.

'The Lungs are a delicate organ'

The Lungs are described as a 'tender' or 'delicate' organs. This is because, of all the internal organs, it is the first one to be invaded by external pathogenic factors: the relative ease with which the Lungs are affected by external pathogenic factors reflects their being 'delicate'.

The propensity to be invaded by external pathogenic factors manifests at two levels. Firstly, the energetic layer corresponding to the 'Exterior' of the body (i.e. the space between the skin and muscles) is under the influence of the Lungs and the Defensive Qi; this is the first energetic layer to be invaded by exterior Wind when we get an upper respiratory infection. Secondly, if the pathogenic factor penetrates into the Interior, it usually affects the Lungs most commonly. In the example given above, if the upper respiratory infection continues, it usually affects the Lungs at the interior level, causing a chest infection.

The Lungs are particularly delicate in children and that is why children are so prone to upper respiratory infections.

Learning outcomes

In this chapter you will have learned:
- The relationship between Qi and the Lungs
- The relationship between the Lungs and both channels and blood vessels
- The clinical significance of the Lungs' position as 'Prime Minister' and of their regulation of all physiological activities
- The clinical significance of the diffusing of Lung-Qi in relation to Qi and fluids
- The clinical significance of the descending of Lung-Qi in relation to Qi and fluids
- The relationship between these two Lung function and the movement of fluids in the Upper Burner
- The clinical significance of the Lungs' regulation of Water passages and how this is related to the diffusing and descending of Qi and fluids by the Lungs
- The relationship between the Lungs and the skin
- The relationship between the Lungs and the space between skin and muscles
- The influence of the Lungs' diffusing of Qi and fluids on the space between skin and muscles
- The influence of the Lungs on the movement of Defensive Qi in the space between skin and muscles
- The influence of the Lungs on sweating in relationship to the space between skin and muscles
- The relationship between the Lungs and the nose and nasal mucus
- The clinical significance of the Corporeal Soul in all physiological activities
- The clinical significance of the relationship between the Corporeal Soul and the Essence
- How worry, sadness and grief affect the Lungs and the Corporeal Soul
- The Lungs' smell, colour, climate and sound
- Dreams related to the Lungs

Self-assessment questions

1. What is the clinical significance of the Lungs governing Qi?
2. Given that the Lungs govern Qi, in which way do they influence the blood vessels (under the control of the Heart and Blood)?
3. Which are the two main aspects of the Lungs' diffusing function?
4. Which are the two main aspects of the Lungs' descending function?
5. How do the dispersing and descending functions of the Lungs help the Qi Mechanism?
6. How do the Lungs regulate all physiological activities?
7. How does the Lungs' regulation of Water passages depend on their diffusing and descending functions?
8. What is the relationship between the Corporeal Soul and the Essence?
9. How do the Lungs influence the space between the skin and muscles?

See p. 1256 for answers

END NOTES

1. 1979 The Yellow Emperor's Classic of Internal Medicine – Simple Questions (*Huang Di Nei Jing Su Wen* 黄帝内经素问), People's Health Publishing House, Beijing, first published *c.*100 BC, p. 58.
2. Ibid., p. 45.
3. 1981 Spiritual Axis (*Ling Shu Jing* 灵枢经), People's Health Publishing House, Beijing, first published *c.*100 BC, p. 104.
4. Ibid., p. 71.
5. Zhao Xian Ke 1687 Medicine Treasure (*Yi Guan*), cited in 1983 Selected Historical Theories in Chinese Medicine (*Zhong Yi Li Dai Yi Lun Xuan* 中医历代医论选), Shandong Scientific Publishing House, Jinan, p. 1.
6. Simple Questions, p. 58.
7. Ibid., p. 58.
8. In order to understand the clinical significance of the Lungs being like a Prime Minister, we should see this statement in the context of the social and political situation of ancient China. In modern Western societies, the Prime Minister has primarily political responsibility and the administration of government is delegated to government departments (or the Civil Service in Britain). In ancient China, society was administered very tightly by a central, pyramidal bureaucracy with the Prime Minister at its apex: the Prime Minister, therefore, was the head of all government departments administering the country. It is in this context that the functions of the Lungs should be seen.
9. Spiritual Axis, p. 126.
10. Simple Questions, p. 139.
11. Ibid., p. 19.
12. Ibid., p. 70.
13. Ibid., p. 67.
14. Spiritual Axis, p. 50.
15. Simple Questions, p. 152.
16. Cited in 1980 Concise Dictionary of Chinese Medicine (*Jian Ming Zhong Yi Ci Dian* 简明中医辞典), People's Health Publishing House, Beijing, p. 953.
17. Simple Questions, p. 102.
18. Ibid., p. 569.
19. Spiritual Axis, p. 85.

FURTHER READING

Kaptchuk T 2000 The Web that has no Weaver – Understanding Chinese Medicine, Contemporary Books, Chicago

SECTION 1 PART 2

The Functions of the Spleen 9

Key contents

Functions of the Spleen
Governs transformation and transportation
Controls the ascending of Qi
Controls Blood
Controls the muscles and the four limbs
Opens into the mouth
Manifests in the lips
Controls saliva
Controls the raising of Qi
Houses the Intellect (Yi)
It is affected by pensiveness

Other Spleen relationships
Its smell is fragrant
Its colour is yellow
Its taste is sweet
Its climate is Dampness
Its sound is singing

Dreams

Sayings
'The Spleen governs the four limbs'
'The Spleen transforms fluids for the Stomach'
'The Spleen is the Root of Post-Heaven Qi'
'The Spleen is the origin of birth and development'
'The Spleen raises the clear (Yang) upwards'
'The Spleen loathes Dampness'
'The Spleen likes dryness'

The Spleen's main function is to assist the Stomach digestion by transporting and transforming food essences, absorbing the nourishment from food and separating the usable from the unusable part of food. The Spleen is the central organ in the production of Qi: from the food and drink ingested, it extracts Food-Qi (*Gu Qi*), which is the basis for the formation of Qi and Blood. In fact, Food-Qi produced by the Spleen combines with air in the Lungs to form the Gathering Qi, which itself is the basis for the formation of True Qi (*Zhen Qi*) (see Figs 3.7, 3.8, 3.9 in ch. 3).

Food-Qi of the Spleen is also the basis for the formation of Blood, which takes place in the Heart (see Fig. 3.8 in ch. 3). Because the Food-Qi extracted by the Spleen is the material basis for the production of Qi and Blood, the Spleen (together with the Stomach) is often called the Root of Post-Heaven Qi.

Since the Spleen is the central organ in the digestive process, it is often referred to as the '*Granary official from whom the five tastes are derived*'.[1]

The Spleen, together with the Stomach, occupies a central place in physiology and pathology, so much so that tonification of the Stomach and Spleen was advocated by one of the four major 'schools of thought' in Chinese medicine. The school of thought, placing the Stomach and Spleen at the centre of physiology and pathology and therefore advocating tonification and regulation of the Stomach and Spleen as the main treatment principle, was started by the celebrated Li Dong Yuan (1180–1251). In his important work 'Discussion on Stomach and Spleen' (*Pi Wei Lun*), Dr Li maintained that injury to the Stomach and Spleen, caused by an irregular diet and overwork, was the origin of numerous diseases. Dr Li also highlighted the influence of the Stomach and Spleen on the Original Qi (*Yuan Qi*): although related to the Kidneys, the Original Qi is replenished by the Stomach and Spleen and a depletion of Stomach and Spleen in chronic diseases involves a decline of the Original Qi. The famous prescription formulated by Dr Li, Bu Zhong Yi Qi Tang, *Tonifying the Centre and Benefiting Qi Decoction*, is aimed at strengthening the Original Qi by tonifying Stomach and Spleen.

The functions of the Spleen are:

- It governs transformation and transportation
- It controls the Blood
- It controls the muscles and the four limbs
- It opens into the mouth and manifests in the lips
- It controls the 'raising of Qi'
- It houses the Intellect (*Yi*)

> **Note on the pancreas**
>
> Chinese medical books never mention the pancreas and some authors think that, functionally, the pancreas is included with the Chinese notion of 'Spleen'. It would seem that many of the Spleen functions affecting digestion could be correlated with the pancreas secretion of digestive enzymes.
>
> One of the few mentions of the pancreas is in chapter 42 of the 'Classic of Difficulties' where it says: *'The spleen weighs 2 pounds and 3 ounces, it is 3 inches wide, 5 inches long and has ½ pound of fatty tissues surrounding it.'*[2] It would appear that the '½ pound of fatty tissue surrounding it' is the pancreas.

The functions of the Spleen are discussed under the following headings:

- The functions of the Spleen
  - The Spleen governs transformation and transportation
    - The Spleen's transformation and transportation of food essences and Qi
    - The Spleen's transformation and transportation of fluids
  - The Spleen controls the ascending of Qi
    - The ascending of Spleen-Qi in relation to Qi, food essences and fluids
    - The ascending of Spleen-Qi in relation to the 'lifting' of organs
  - The Spleen controls Blood
  - The Spleen controls the muscles and the four limbs
  - The Spleen opens into the mouth
  - The Spleen manifests in the lips
  - The Spleen controls saliva
  - The Spleen controls the raising of Qi
  - The Spleen houses the Intellect (*Yi*)
  - The Spleen is affected by pensiveness
- Other Spleen relationships
  - Its smell is fragrant
  - Its colour is yellow
  - Its taste is sweet
  - Its climate is Dampness
  - Its sound is singing
- Dreams
- Sayings
  - 'The Spleen governs the four limbs'
  - 'The Spleen transforms fluids for the Stomach'
  - 'The Spleen is the Root of Post-Heaven Qi'
  - 'The Spleen is the origin of birth and development'
  - 'The Spleen raises the clear (Yang) upwards'
  - 'The Spleen loathes Dampness'
  - 'The Spleen likes dryness'

THE FUNCTIONS OF THE SPLEEN

The functions of the Spleen are discussed under the following headings:

- The Spleen governs transformation and transportation
  - The Spleen's transformation and transportation of food essences and Qi
  - The Spleen's transformation and transportation of fluids
- The Spleen controls the ascending of Qi
  - The ascending of Spleen-Qi in relation to Qi, food essences and fluids
  - The ascending of Spleen-Qi in relation to the 'lifting' of organs
- The Spleen controls Blood
- The Spleen controls the muscles and the four limbs
- The Spleen opens into the mouth
- The Spleen manifests in the lips
- The Spleen controls saliva
- The Spleen controls the raising of Qi
- The Spleen houses the Intellect (*Yi*)
- The Spleen is affected by pensiveness

The Spleen governs transformation and transportation

The Spleen's function of transformation and transportation (*yun hua*) concerns food essences, Qi and fluids.

The Spleen's transformation and transportation of food essences and Qi

The Spleen transforms the ingested food and drink to extract Qi from it: this is called Food-Qi and is the basis for the production of Qi and Blood. Once Food-Qi is formed, the Spleen transports this and some other refined parts of food, called 'food essences', to the various organs and parts of the body.

The 'Simple Questions' in chapter 21 says: *'Food enters the Stomach, the refined part goes to the Liver, the excess goes to the sinews. Food enters the Stomach, the unrefined part goes to the Heart, the excess goes to the blood vessels ... fluids enter the Stomach ... the upper part go to the Spleen, the Spleen transports the refined essence upwards to the Lungs.'*[3] This passage describes the Spleen's role of separating the usable from unusable part of food and directing Food-Qi upwards to the Lungs to combine with air to form Gathering Qi and to the Heart to form Blood (Fig. 9.1; see also Figs 3.7, 3.8 and 3.20 in chapter 3). The various transformations and movements described, 'the refined part to the Liver', 'the unrefined to the Heart' 'the refined upwards to the Lungs', are all under the control of the Spleen.

The Spleen's transformation and transportation of food essences is crucial to the process of digestion and production of Qi and Blood. If this function is normal, the digestion will be good, with good appetite, normal absorption and regular bowel movements. If this function is impaired, there may be poor appetite, bad digestion, abdominal distension and loose stools.

> **Clinical note**
>
> Spleen-Qi deficiency leading to digestive problems is one of the common patterns encountered in practice. ST-36 Zusanli and SP-6 Sanyinjiao are a simple and very effective combination to tonify Spleen-Qi in digestive problems

The Spleen's transformation and transportation of fluids

Apart from governing the movement of the various food essences and Qi, the Spleen also controls the transformation, separation and movement of fluids. The Spleen separates the usable from the unusable part of the fluids ingested; the 'clear' part goes upwards to the Lungs to be distributed to the skin and the space between the skin and muscles, and the 'turbid' part goes downward to the Intestines where it is further separated (Fig. 9.2). If this Spleen function is normal, the transformation and movement of fluids will be normal. If this function is impaired, the fluids will not be transformed or transported properly and may accumulate to form Dampness or Phlegm or cause oedema.

The implication here is that the Spleen must always be treated when there is Dampness, Phlegm or oedema. Moreover, the Spleen is also easily affected by external Dampness, which may impair its function of transformation and transportation.

> **Clinical note**
>
> To stimulate the Spleen's function of transforming fluids one can reinforce Ren-12 Zhongwan, ST-36 Zusanli and BL-20 Pishu and reduce SP-9 Yinlingquan and SP-6 Sanyinjiao

This function of the Spleen is summarized in Box 9.1.

The Spleen controls the ascending of Qi

The Spleen separates the usable from the unusable part of food and directs Food-Qi upwards to the Lungs to combine with air to form Gathering Qi and to the Heart to form Blood (see Fig. 9.1). The various transformations and movements described in the passage from chapter 21 of the 'Simple Questions' quoted above (i.e. 'the refined part to the Liver', 'the unrefined to

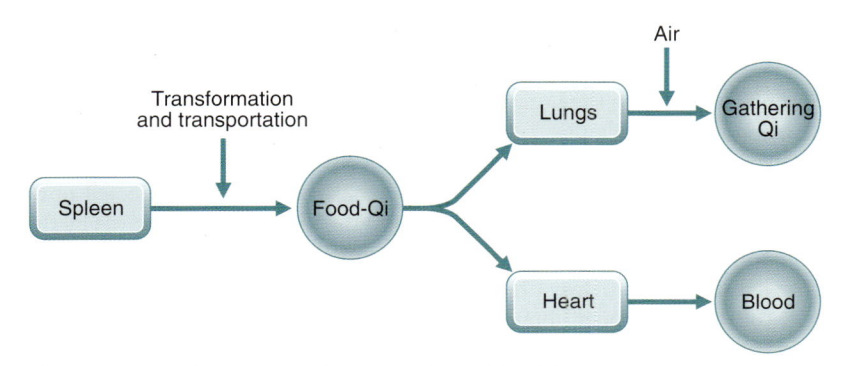

Figure 9.1 Transformation and transportation of the Spleen

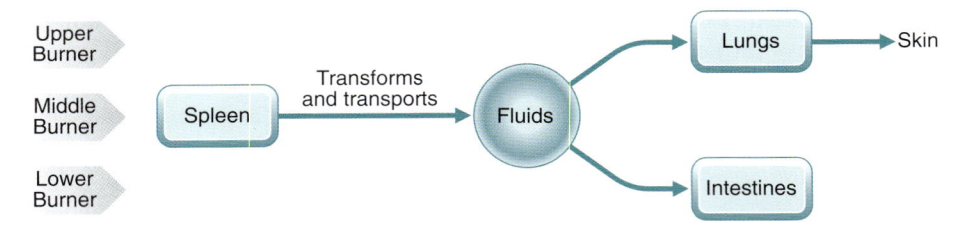

Figure 9.2 Spleen's transformation and transportation of fluids

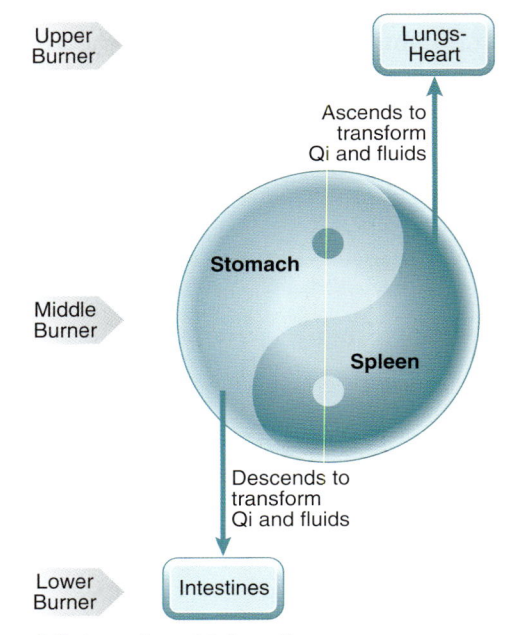

Figure 9.3 Ascending of Spleen-Qi

Box 9.1 The Spleen governs transformation and transportation

- Spleen-Qi transforms and transports food essences and Qi in the process of digestion, leading to the formation of Qi and Blood
- Spleen-Qi transforms and transports fluids

---

the Heart' and 'the refined upwards to the Lungs') are all dependent on the ascending of Spleen-Qi.

The Spleen and the Stomach are at the heart of the Middle Burner, in the centre of the Qi Mechanism described in chapter 4. Being in the centre, the Stomach and Spleen control the movement and direction of Qi in all Burners: they are like a vital motorway (freeway) interlink that is essential to the proper movement, direction and transformation of Qi in all three Burners (Fig. 9.3).

The ascending of Spleen-Qi in relation to Qi, food essences and fluids

The Spleen's function of transformation and transportation is inextricably linked to the ascending of Spleen-Qi. In a specific sense, Spleen-Qi ascends in so far as it transports Qi and food essences to the Lungs where it forms Gathering Qi after combining with air. In Chinese books, the 'ascending' of Spleen-Qi is always linked to the notion of 'clear': that is, the Spleen carries the clear part of food essences and Qi extracted from food upwards to the Upper Burner. Li Dong Yuan said: *'Food enters the Stomach and the Spleen directs the clear essence of food up to the Lungs ... to nourish the whole body.'*[4]

In a general sense, the 'ascending' of Spleen-Qi includes all movements of Spleen-Qi in the process of digestion and not just the upward movement towards the Lungs. In this sense, the ascending of Spleen-Qi is essential for a proper transformation and transportation of food essence, Qi and fluids by the Spleen.

The ascending of Spleen-Qi is coordinated with the descending of Stomach-Qi. Spleen-Qi ascends (to the Lungs and Heart) and Stomach-Qi descends (to the Intestines): the coordination of the ascending of Spleen-Qi and descending of Stomach-Qi is essential for the production of Qi and Blood in the Middle Burner.

Ye Tian Shi (1667–1746), the celebrated specialist in Warm Diseases, said: *'Spleen-Qi goes up, Stomach-Qi goes down'*[5] (see Fig. 9.3).

The coordination between the ascending of Spleen-Qi and the descending of Stomach-Qi is essential for a proper movement of Qi in the body during digestion, so that the clear Qi is directed upwards by the Spleen and the turbid Qi downwards by the Stomach. Qi connects upwards with the Lungs and Heart and downwards with the Intestines, Liver and Kidneys. Only if these ascending and descending movements of Qi are coordinated can the clear Yang ascend to the upper (sense) orifices and the turbid Yin descend to the two lower orifices. If the descending and ascending movements are impaired, the clear Yang does not ascend, refined Qi extracted from food cannot be stored and turbid Qi cannot be excreted.

Such coordination between the ascending Spleen-Qi and descending Stomach-Qi is essential also to the transformation and transportation of fluids: when Spleen-Qi fails to ascend, it may affect the transformation and transportation of fluids in the Middle Burner, leading to the formation of Dampness, Phlegm or oedema.

The ascending of Spleen-Qi in relation to the 'lifting' of organs

The ascending of Spleen-Qi has another important function as it serves to 'lift' the internal organs to keep them in their proper place. The failing of this ascending movement may cause prolapse of an internal organ. This function is described in more detail below.

> **Clinical note**
>
> To stimulate the ascending of Spleen-Qi in relation to lifting of organs, one can use Du-20 Baihui, Ren-12 Zhongwan and Ren-6 Qihai

This function is summarized in Box 9.2.

> **Box 9.2 The Spleen controls the ascending of Qi**
>
> - Spleen-Qi ascends to send Qi, food essences and fluids up to the Lungs
> - The ascending Spleen-Qi 'lifts' the organs, keeping them in place
> - The ascending of Spleen-Qi is coordinated with the descending of Stomach-Qi

The Spleen controls Blood

'Control' in this case has two separate meanings: on the one hand, it means that Spleen-Qi keeps or 'holds' the blood in the vessels; on the other hand, it means that the Spleen plays an important role in the making of Blood. The 'Classic of Difficulties' in chapter 42 says that the '*the Spleen is in charge of holding the Blood together*'.[6] While it is Qi in general that holds the blood in the vessels, it is Spleen-Qi in particular that performs this function. The Spleen's function of keeping the blood in the vessels is also closely linked to the ascending of Spleen-Qi: that is, the failure of

Spleen-Qi to control Blood implies an impairing of the ascending of Spleen-Qi.

If Spleen-Qi is healthy, Blood will circulate normally and stay in the vessels. If Spleen-Qi is deficient and not ascending properly, Blood may spill out of the vessels, resulting in haemorrhage. The failure of the ascending of Spleen-Qi and the failure in controlling Blood normally causes bleeding downwards, for example from the uterus, bladder or intestines (Fig. 9.4).

> **Clinical note**
>
> To stimulate the Spleen's function of holding Blood (stopping bleeding), one can use Ren-12 Zhongwan, ST-36 Zusanli and SP-10 Xuehai

Besides controlling the Blood and preventing haemorrhages, the Spleen also plays an important role in making Blood. In fact, the Spleen extracts Food-Qi from food and this forms Blood in the Heart with the assistance of the Original Qi from the Kidneys. The Spleen is therefore the central, essential organ for the production of both Qi and Blood. This is another reason why it is called the 'Root of Post-Heaven Qi'. In this context, 'Qi' in the expression 'Post-Heaven Qi' should be intended in a broad sense which includes Blood. If we wish to tonify the Blood, therefore, we must always tonify the Spleen.

With reference to the making of Blood, it should be pointed out that the Spleen plays an important role; however, menstrual Blood is different to Blood in other parts of the body. In fact, menstrual Blood is

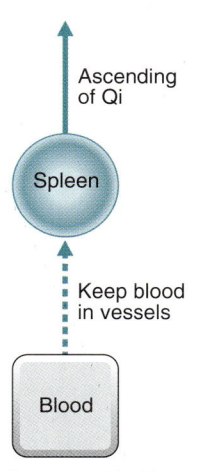

Figure 9.4 Spleen's function of holding Blood

called *Tian Gui* and it derives directly from the Kidney-Essence; the most important organ in the making of menstrual Blood is therefore not the Spleen but the Kidneys.

> Menstrual Blood (called *Tian Gui*) is different to Blood in other parts of the body. Menstrual Blood derives from Kidney-Essence; Blood in the body derives from the Spleen and Kidneys

As the Root of Post-Heaven Qi, the Spleen also plays a role in supplementing and nourishing the Original Qi (*Yuan Qi*). Li Dong Yuan (1180–1251), author of the famous 'Discussion on Stomach and Spleen', says: '*The Original Qi can only be strong if the Spleen and Stomach are not weakened and can nourish it. If the Stomach is weak and food is not transformed, the Stomach and Spleen are weakened, they cannot nourish the Original Qi which becomes empty and disease results.*'[7]

This function is summarized in Box 9.3.

Box 9.3 The Spleen controls blood

- The Spleen 'holds' Blood in the vessels, thus preventing bleeding
- The Spleen makes Blood from Food-Qi

The Spleen controls the muscles and the four limbs

The Spleen extracts Food-Qi from food so as to nourish all tissues in the body. This refined Qi is transported throughout the body by the Spleen. If the Spleen is strong, refined Qi is directed to the muscles, particularly those of the limbs. If Spleen-Qi is weak, the refined Qi cannot be transported to the muscles and the person will feel weary, the muscles will be weak and, in severe cases, may atrophy (Fig. 9.5).

The state of the Spleen is one of the most important factors determining the amount of physical energy a person has. Tiredness is a common complaint and in these cases the Spleen must always be tonified.

> **Clinical note**
>
> A deficiency of Spleen-Qi causing chronic tiredness is one of the most common pathologies encountered in the clinic. ST-36 Zusanli, SP-6 Sanyinjiao, BL-20 Pishu and BL-21 Weishu are an excellent combination for this condition

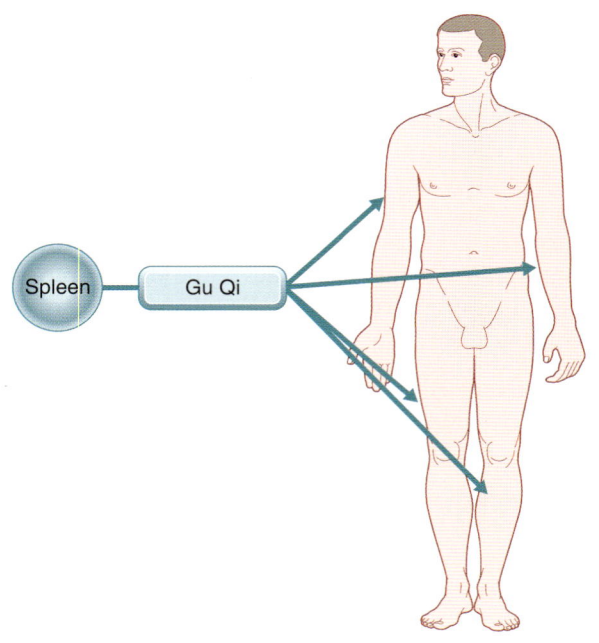

Figure 9.5 The Spleen and the muscles

Box 9.4 The Spleen controls the muscles and the four limbs

The Spleen transports food essences to all the muscles of the body (especially motor muscles) and in particular in the four limbs

The 'Simple Questions' in chapter 44 says: '*The Spleen governs the muscles ... if the Spleen has Heat, there will be thirst, the muscles will be weak and atrophied.*'[8] In chapter 29 it says: '*The four limbs depend on the Stomach for Qi, but Stomach-Qi can only reach the channels through the transmission of the Spleen. If the Spleen is diseased it cannot transport the fluids of the Stomach, with the result that the four limbs cannot receive the Qi of Food.*'[9]

This function is summarized in Box 9.4.

The Spleen opens into the mouth

The action of chewing prepares food for the Spleen to transform and transport its food essences. For this reason the mouth has a functional relationship with the Spleen. When Spleen-Qi is normal, the sense of taste is good and chewing is normal. If Spleen-Qi is abnormal, there may be impairment of the sense of taste, difficulty in chewing and lack of appetite The

'Spiritual Axis' in chapter 17 says: '*Spleen-Qi connects with the mouth, if the Spleen is healthy, the mouth can taste the five grains.*'[10]

This function is summarized in Box 9.5.

Box 9.5 The Spleen opens into the mouth

The Spleen controls the mouth, enabling chewing and taste

The Spleen manifests in the lips

The lips reflect the state of the Spleen; in particular, they reflect the Blood rather than the Qi of the Spleen. When Spleen-Qi and Spleen-Blood are healthy, the lips are rosy and moist. If Spleen-Blood is deficient, the lips are pale; if Spleen-Yin is deficient, the lips are dry; if the Spleen has Heat, the lips will tend to be red and dry and the patient may complain of a sweet taste.

The 'Simple Questions' says in chapter 10 that the '*Spleen controls the muscles and manifests in the lips*'.[11]

This function is summarized in Box 9.6.

Box 9.6 The Spleen manifests in the lips

The Spleen influences the lips. Indeed, the lips are a reliable indicator of the state of the Spleen. When the Spleen is normal, the lips are rosy and moist

---

The Spleen controls saliva

As the Spleen controls the mouth, it naturally controls the secretion of saliva. 'Saliva' is my translation of the Chinese word '*xian*', which is used to describe the fluid related to the Spleen. Saliva's function is to moisten the mouth and to aid digestion by mixing the food with fluids to ease digestion (obviously the ancient Chinese were not aware of the digestive enzymes present in saliva).

Saliva is described in Chinese books as being a 'clear and thin' fluid, in contrast to spittle (of the Kidneys), which is a 'turbid and thick' fluid.

This function is summarized in Box 9.7.

Box 9.7 The Spleen controls saliva

- The Spleen influences saliva, which promotes its digestion
- Saliva is called '*xian*' and is described as a thin and clear fluid (in contrast to *tuo*, the fluid corresponding to the Kidneys, that is thick and turbid and which I translate as 'spittle')

The Spleen controls the raising of Qi

The Spleen produces a 'lifting' effect on the organs: this 'raising' of Qi is also an expression of the ascending of Spleen-Qi. It is this force that makes sure that the internal organs are in their proper place.

If Spleen-Qi is deficient and its 'raising Qi' function weak, there may be prolapse of various organs such as uterus, stomach, kidney, bladder or anus (Fig. 9.6).

Although the raising action of Spleen-Qi is the predominant factor in 'lifting' the organs to keep them in their proper place, the descending of Qi also plays a role in keeping the organs in place. The coordination between the ascending of (clear) Qi (Yang in nature) and the descending of (turbid) Qi (Yin in nature) also plays a role in keeping the organs in place. In some cases, the clear Yang cannot ascend because turbid Yin is not descending: in other words, if turbid Yin does not descend properly, it then stays above, thus preventing the clear Yang from ascending.

The Spleen houses the Intellect

The Spleen is said to be the 'residence' of the Intellect (*Yi*). The Intellect resides in the Spleen and is responsible for applied thinking, studying, memorizing, focusing, concentrating and generating ideas. The Postnatal Qi and Blood are the physiological basis for the Intellect. Thus, if the Spleen is strong, thinking will be clear, memory good and the capacity for concentrating, studying and generating ideas will also be good. If the Spleen is weak, the Intellect will be dull and

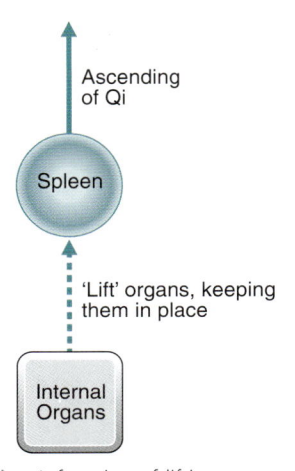

Figure 9.6 Spleen's function of lifting organs

thinking will be slow, memory poor and the capacity for studying, concentrating and focusing will all be weak. Conversely, excessive studying, mental work and concentration for sustained periods can weaken the Spleen.

- The Spleen controls studying, memorizing, concentrating
- The Heart controls memory of distant events
- The Kidneys control memory of recent events

In the sphere of thinking, remembering and memorizing there is considerable overlap between the Intellect (*Yi*) of the Spleen, the Mind (*Shen*) of the Heart, and the Will-power (*Zhi*) of the Kidneys (Fig. 9.7). The Spleen influences our capacity for thinking in the sense of studying, concentrating and memorizing work or schoolwork subjects. The Heart houses the Mind and influences thinking in the sense of being able to think clearly when faced with life problems and it affects long-term memory of past events. The connection and interaction between the Intellect of the Spleen and the Mind of the Heart is very close in the sphere of memory. The 'Spiritual Axis' says in chapter 8: '*The Heart function of recollecting is called Intellect.*'[12]

The Kidneys nourish the brain and influence short-term memory in everyday life. In fact, in old age there is a decline of Kidney-Essence, which fails to nourish the brain. For this reason, many old people often forget recent events (which is due to a Kidney weakness), and yet may be able to remember long-past events (which is dependent on the Heart). As for the Intellect of the Spleen, some people may have an extraordinary memory in their work or study field (which is dependent on the Spleen) and yet be very forgetful in everyday life (which is dependent on the Heart). The memorizing function of the Intellect of the Spleen is so closely related to the Will-power of the Kidneys that the same chapter continues: '*The storing [of data] of the Intellect is called Memory [Zhi].*'[13] It should be noted here that I translate the mental aspect of the Kidneys *Zhi* as 'Will-power', although it also has the meaning of 'memory' or 'mind'. In the above-mentioned quotation, *Zhi* has the meaning of 'memory'.

Box 9.8 The Spleen houses the Intellect (*Yi*)

The Spleen houses the Intellect, which is responsible for memory, concentration and focus

Clinical note

To stimulate the Spleen's memory, one can use Ren-12 Zhongwan, ST-36 Zusanli, BL-20 Pishu and BL-49 Yishe

This function is summarized in Box 9.8.

The Spleen is affected by pensiveness

Pensiveness is very similar to worry in its character and effect. Pensiveness consists in brooding, constantly thinking about certain events or people (even though not worrying), or nostalgic hankering after the past. In extreme cases, pensiveness leads to obsessive thoughts. In a different sense, pensiveness also includes excessive mental work in the process of one's work or study. In a way, pensiveness is nothing but the negative equivalent of the Intellect's capacity for focus and concentration: just as the Intellect allows us to focus and concentrate with a clear mind, when the person is affected by pensiveness, the same mental powers are manifested in a negative way with excessive thinking, brooding, etc.

Pensiveness affects the Spleen and, like worry, it knots Qi; however, worry will tend to knot Qi in the Upper Burner, while pensiveness knots Qi in the Middle Burner. Stagnation of Qi in the Middle Burner will cause poor digestion and a feeling of distension of the epigastrium.

Clinical note

To treat pensiveness, one can use BL-49 Yishe

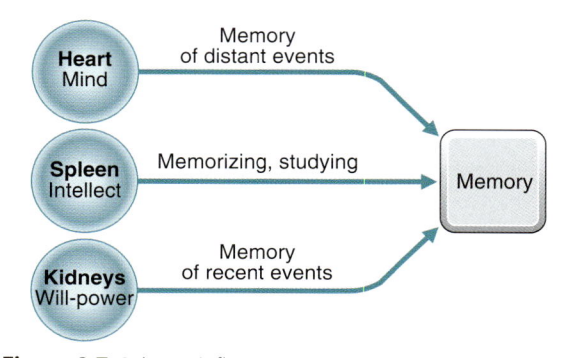

Figure 9.7 Spleen's influence on memory

This is summarized in Box 9.9.

> **Box 9.9 The Spleen is affected by pensiveness**
> - 'Pensiveness' includes thinking too much, brooding, hankering after the past, obsessive thinking
> - A Spleen deficiency may induce pensiveness
> - Pensiveness injures the Spleen

OTHER SPLEEN RELATIONSHIPS

Other Spleen relationships discussed are:

- Its smell is fragrant
- Its colour is yellow
- Its taste is sweet
- Its climate is Dampness
- Its sound is singing

Its smell is fragrant

The body odour related to the Spleen is fragrant, sometimes also described as sweetish (although the sweetish smell is more related to Heat patterns of the Spleen).

The fragrant Spleen smell really is like a perfume but with a faint, sweet, sickly overtone. Such a smell may indicate either a Spleen deficiency or Dampness obstructing the Spleen.

Its colour is yellow

A complexion that is yellow in colour is extremely common. It is usually seen on the cheeks, forehead or chin. A pale, dull-yellow colour indicates Spleen deficiency; a richer, fuller, bright, yellow colour indicates Damp-Heat, while if it is dull it indicates chronic Dampness (without Heat).

Its taste is sweet

A sweet taste in the mouth may indicate Dampness, especially with Heat. As for the taste of foodstuffs, foods with a sweet taste nourish the Spleen if taken in moderation. In excess, they weaken the Spleen as well as the Kidneys.

Its climate is Dampness

External Dampness is a major pathogenic factor as it is very common. Please note that 'external Dampness' denotes not just a damp climate, but also damp living conditions (such as living in a basement with a damp problem in the walls), and also some habits such as wearing a wet swimming suit after swimming or sitting on damp grass.

External Dampness enters the channels of the legs and especially the Spleen, settling in the Lower Burner where it may cause many different problems such as excessive vaginal discharge or urinary problems.

> **Clinical note**
>
> Invasion of external Dampness in the Spleen channel is extremely common. SP-9 Yinlingquan is the best point to drain Dampness from the Lower Burner

Its sound is singing

A 'singing' tone of voice is characteristic of people with a constitutional Spleen deficiency. Singing as a sound related to the Spleen may also be observed in people who have the habit of humming a tune (often an unrecognizable one) while they go about their daily activities.

DREAMS

The 'Simple Questions' in chapter 80 says: '*If the Spleen is deficient, one dreams of being hungry; if the dream takes place in late summer, one dreams of building a house.*'[14]

The 'Spiritual Axis' in chapter 43 says: '*If the Spleen is in excess one dreams of singing and being very heavy ... if the Spleen is deficient one dreams of abysses in mountains and of marshes.*'[15]

SAYINGS

The sayings considered are:

- 'The Spleen governs the four limbs'
- 'The Spleen transforms fluids for the Stomach'
- 'The Spleen is the Root of Post-Heaven Qi'
- 'The Spleen is the origin of birth and development'
- 'The Spleen raises the clear (Yang) upwards'
- 'The Spleen loathes Dampness'
- 'The Spleen likes dryness'

'The Spleen governs the four limbs'

The Spleen distributes food essences to all parts of the body and in particular to the limbs. For this reason, when the Spleen is deficient, the food essences cannot reach the limbs, which will feel cold and weak. One can observe this in practice as often digestive disturbances cause one's limbs to go cold.

'The Spleen transforms fluids for the Stomach'

The Stomach is the origin of fluids in the body and the Spleen transforms and transports them. The Stomach fluids are part of Stomach-Yin, while the activity of fluid transformation and transportation is carried out by Spleen-Yang. It is interesting to note that, although the Stomach is a Yang organ, it is the origin of fluids (Yin), and although the Spleen is a Yin organ, it provides the Yang energy to transport and transform fluids.

'The Spleen is the Root of Post-Heaven Qi'

The Spleen is the origin of Qi and Blood in the body. For this reason, it is called, together with the Stomach, the Root of Post-Heaven Qi: that is, the Qi and Blood produced after birth as opposed to the Pre-Heaven Qi (related to the Kidneys), which nourishes the fetus before birth and which determines our hereditary constitution.

'The Spleen is the origin of birth and development'

This refers to the central role played by the Spleen in nourishing the body and promoting development in so far as the Spleen is the origin of Qi and Blood.

'The Spleen raises the clear (Yang) upwards'

As we have seen, Spleen-Qi ascends: we can see this ascending movement in the ascending of Food-Qi to the Lungs (to make Gathering Qi) and to the Heart (to make Blood). The ascending of Spleen-Qi is also essential to transform and transport fluids.

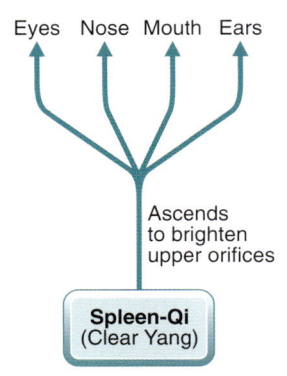

Figure 9.8 Ascending of Spleen's clear Yang to the upper orifices

The ascending of Spleen-Qi implies ascending of clear Qi. In relation to the head, this is often called 'clear Yang': as it rises to the head, clear Yang brightens the upper orifices (eyes, nose, ears and mouth), thus enabling us to see, smell, hear and taste clearly. Therefore, Spleen-Qi flows upwards to carry the clear Yang energies upwards to the head (Fig. 9.8). If Spleen-Qi does not lift the clear Yang towards the head, either because it is deficient or because it is obstructed by Dampness, the clear Yang cannot rise to the head and this results in a dull headache and a feeling of heaviness and muzziness of the head.

'The Spleen loathes Dampness'

Dampness easily obstructs the Spleen, causing a dysfunction of its activity of transformation and transportation. This can cause abdominal fullness, urinary problems or vaginal discharges. In the head, Dampness prevents the rising of Spleen-Qi, causing a dull headache and a feeling of heaviness and muzziness.

'The Spleen likes dryness'

In connection with the transformation of food and digestion, it is said that the Spleen 'likes dryness': this means that the Spleen's activity of transformation and transportation can be easily impaired by the excessive consumption of cold liquids or icy drinks (so common in many Western countries). In contrast, the Stomach 'likes wetness', i.e. foods that are moist and not drying.

Learning outcomes

In this chapter you will have learned:
- The clinical significance of the Spleen's function of transformation and transportation in physiology and pathology
- How the Spleen's transformation and transportation is the basis for the formation of Qi and Blood
- The clinical significance of the ascending of Spleen-Qi in relation to the production of Qi and Blood
- The coordination between the ascending of Spleen-Qi and the descending of Stomach-Qi
- The importance of the Spleen in holding blood in the vessels
- The relationship between the Spleen and muscles of the limbs
- How the Spleen affects energy
- The relationship between the Spleen and the mouth, lips and saliva
- The clinical significance of the Spleen's raising of Qi in relation to prolapse of the internal organs
- The relationships between the Spleen and the Intellect (*Yi*)
- How the Intellect of the Spleen affects memory and how it differs from the Heart's and the Kidneys' influence on memory
- The nature of 'pensiveness' and how it affects the Spleen
- The smell, colour, taste, climate and sound associated with the Spleen
- Dreams reflecting disharmonies of the Spleen
- Sayings relating to the Spleen

Self-assessment questions

1. How does the Spleen's function of transformation and transportation affect the making of Qi and Blood?
2. How does the Spleen's function of transformation and transportation affect the metabolism of fluids?
3. Spleen-Qi ascends to which organ?
4. How does the Spleen coordinate with the Stomach?
5. What is the meaning of the Spleen's 'control' of Blood?
6. How does a feeling of heaviness and muzziness of the head relate to the Spleen and, in particular, to which Spleen function?
7. How does the Spleen affect the muscles and what is the consequence of Spleen-Qi deficiency in this area?
8. What is the consequence of an impairment of the Spleen's raising of Qi?
9. What are the main functions of the Intellect (*Yi*)?
10. What is the nature of pensiveness and how does it affect the Spleen?

See p. 1257 for answers

END NOTES

1. 1979 The Yellow Emperor's Classic of Internal Medicine – Simple Questions (*Huang Di Nei Jing Su Wen* 黄帝内经素问), People's Health Publishing House, Beijing, first published *c.*100 BC, p. 58.
2. Nanjing College of Traditional Chinese Medicine 1979 A Revised Explanation of the Classic of Difficulties (*Nan Jing Jiao Shi* 难经校释), People's Health Publishing House, Beijing, first published *c.*AD 100, p. 99.
3. Simple Questions, p. 139.
4. 1981 Syndromes and Treatment of the Internal Organs (*Zang Fu Zheng Zhi* 脏腑证治), Tianjin Scientific Publishing House, Tianjin, p. 170.
5. Syndromes and Treatment of the Internal Organs, p. 170.
6. A Revised Explanation of the Classic of Difficulties, p. 99.
7. Syndromes and Treatment of the Internal Organs, p. 168.
8. Simple Questions, p. 246.
9. Ibid., p. 180.
10. 1981 Spiritual Axis (*Ling Shu Jing* 灵枢经), People's Health Publishing House, Beijing, first published *c.*100 BC, p. 50.
11. Simple Questions, p. 70.
12. Spiritual Axis, p. 23.
13. Ibid., p. 23.
14. Simple Questions, p. 569.
15. Spiritual Axis, p. 85.

FURTHER READING

Kaptchuk T 2000 The Web that has no Weaver – Understanding Chinese Medicine, Contemporary Books, Chicago

SECTION 1 PART 2

The Functions of the Kidneys 10

> **Key contents**
>
> **Functions of the Kidney**
> *Store the Essence and govern birth, growth, reproduction and development*
> *Produce Marrow, fill up the brain and control bones*
> *Govern Water*
> *Control the reception of Qi*
> *Open into the ears*
> *Manifest in the hair*
> *Control spittle*
> *Control the two lower orifices*
> *House the Will-power (Zhi)*
> *Control the Gate of Life (Minister Fire, Ming Men)*
>
> **Other Kidney relationships**
> *Its smell is putrid*
> *Its colour is black*
> *Its taste is salty*
> *Its climate is cold*
> *Its sound is groaning*
>
> **Dreams**
>
> **Sayings**
> *'The Kidneys control opening and closing'*
> *'The Kidneys control strength and skill'*
> *'The Kidneys are the Root of Pre-Heaven Qi'*
> *'The Kidneys loathe dryness'*
> *'The Kidneys are the Gate of the Stomach'*

The Kidneys are often referred to as the 'Root of Life' or the 'Root of the Pre-Heaven Qi'. This is because they store the Essence (*Jing*), which, in its Pre-Heaven form, is derived from the parents and established at conception; this Essence determines our basic constitution: hence the description of the Kidneys as the 'Root of Life'.

Like every other Yin organ, the Kidneys have a Yin and a Yang aspect. However, these two aspects acquire a different meaning for the Kidneys because they are the foundation of the Yin and Yang for all the other organs. For this reason, Kidney-Yin and Kidney-Yang are also called 'Primary Yin' and 'Primary Yang', respectively. We could look upon Kidney-Yin as the foundation of all the Yin energies of the body, in particular that of the Liver, Heart and Lungs, and Kidney-Yang as the foundation of all the Yang energies of the body, in particular that of the Spleen, Lungs and Heart (Fig. 10.1).

> The Kidneys are the foundation for all the Yin and Yang energies of the body

Kidney-Yin is the fundamental substance for birth, growth and reproduction while Kidney-Yang is the motive force of all physiological processes. Kidney-Yin is the material foundation for Kidney-Yang, and Kidney-Yang represents the physiological activity that transforms Kidney-Yin. In health, these two poles form

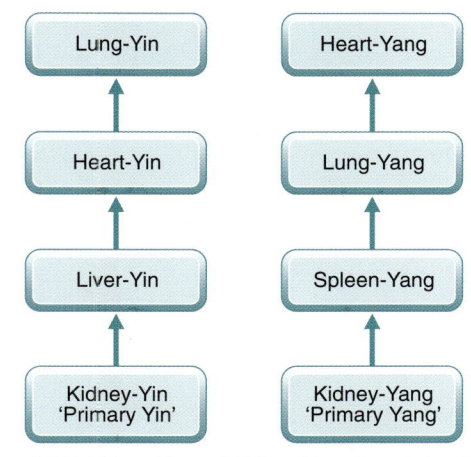

```
  Lung-Yin              Heart-Yang
     ↑                      ↑
  Heart-Yin             Lung-Yang
     ↑                      ↑
  Liver-Yin             Spleen-Yang
     ↑                      ↑
  Kidney-Yin            Kidney-Yang
  'Primary Yin'         'Primary Yang'
```

Figure 10.1 Kidney-Yin and Kidney-Yang foundation for other organs

a unified whole. In disease, however, a separation of Kidney-Yin and Kidney-Yang occurs (Fig. 10.2).

Kidney-Yin and Kidney-Yang have the same root and they rely on each other for their existence. Kidney-Yin provides the material substratum for Kidney-Yang, and Kidney-Yang provides the heat necessary to all the Kidney functions. Because they are fundamentally one and interdependent, deficiency of one necessarily implies deficiency of the other, albeit always in differing proportions.

Kidney-Yin and Kidney-Yang could be likened to an oil lamp, the oil representing Kidney-Yin and the flame representing Kidney-Yang. If the oil (Kidney-Yin) decreases, the flame (Kidney-Yang) will also decrease; if we increase the oil (Kidney-Yin) too much, it may simply smother the flame (Kidney-Yang) (Fig. 10.3). It follows that, in treating Kidney disharmonies, one usually needs to tonify both Kidney-Yin and Kidney-Yang (albeit in differing proportions) to prevent the exhaustion of one of them.

Clinical note

When tonifying the Kidneys with herbal medicine, it is necessary to tonify both Kidney-Yin and Kidney-Yang (although with different emphasis according to condition)

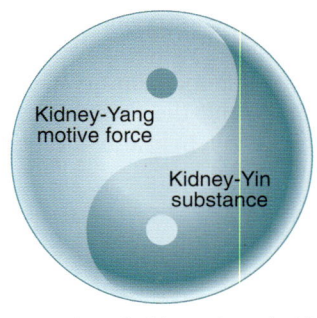

Figure 10.2 Interaction of Kidney-Yin and Kidney-Yang

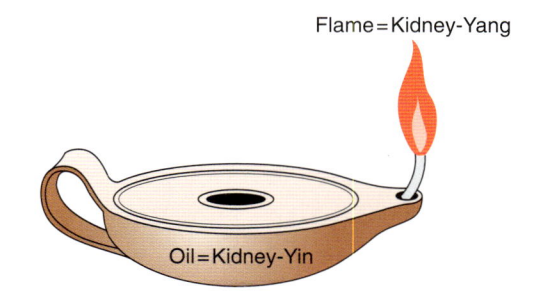

Figure 10.3 Kidney-Yin and Kidney-Yang as oil lamp

A good example of this principle can be seen in the composition of two classic herbal prescriptions to tonify Kidney-Yin and Kidney-Yang. The classic prescription to tonify Kidney-Yin is Liu Wei Di Huang Wan *Six-Flavour Rehmannia Decoction*, while the classic prescription to tonify Kidney-Yang, Jin Gui Shen Qi Wan *Golden Chest Kidney-Qi Decoction*, is nothing but the *Six-Flavour Rehmannia Decoction* with the addition of two hot herbs, namely Fu Zi *Radix lateralis Aconiti Carmichaeli preparata* and Gui Zhi *Ramulus Cinnamomi cassiae*. This shows very clearly that in order to tonify Kidney-Yang, one must also, to a certain extent, tonify Kidney-Yin and vice versa.

The two other important decoctions to tonify Kidney-Yin and Kidney-Yang from Zhang Jie Bin illustrate the same principle. In fact, the formula Zuo Gui Wan *Restoring the Left [Kidney] Pill*, which nourishes Kidney-Yin, contains some Kidney-Yang tonics such as Tu Si Zi *Semen Cuscutae* and Lu Jiao Jiao *Colla Cornu Cervi*, while the formula You Gui Wan *Restoring the Right [Kidney] Decoction*, which tonifies Kidney-Yang, contains some Kidney-Yin tonics such as Gou Qi Zi *Fructus Lycii*.

Clinical note

With acupuncture, the same points (e.g. KI-3 Taixi) can tonify Kidney-Yang or nourish Kidney-Yin. The main difference is in the use of moxa: the same point can tonify Kidney-Yang with moxa or nourish Kidney-Yin without moxa

Therefore, the Kidneys are different from other Yin organs because they are the foundation for all the Yin and Yang energies of the body, and also because they are the origin of Water and Fire in the body. Although according to the Five Elements the Kidneys belong to Water, they are also the source of Fire in the body, which is called the 'Fire of the Gate of Life' (*Ming Men*) or Minister Fire, a physiological Fire (see below) (Fig. 10.4).

The functions of the Kidneys are:

- They store Essence (*Jing*) and govern birth, growth, reproduction and development
- They produce Marrow, fill up the Brain and control bones
- They govern Water
- They control the reception of Qi
- They open into the ears
- They manifest in the hair
- They control the two lower orifices
- They house Will-power
- They control the Gate of Life (*Ming Men*, Minister Fire)

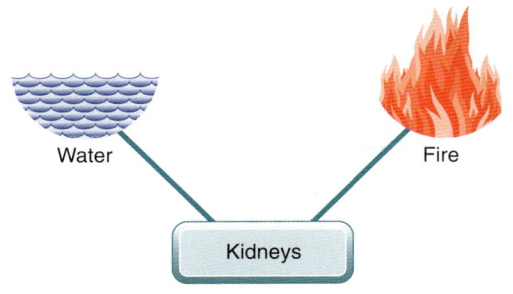

Figure 10.4 The Kidneys as origin of Water and Fire

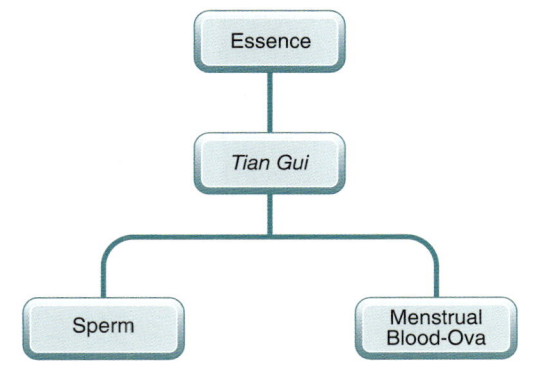

Figure 10.5 The Kidneys and *Tian Gui*

The functions of the Kidneys are discussed under the following headings:

- The functions of the Kidneys
  - The Kidneys store Essence and govern birth, growth, reproduction and development
  - The Kidneys produce Marrow, fill up the Brain and control bones
  - The Kidneys govern Water
  - The Kidneys control the reception of Qi
  - The Kidneys open into the ears
  - The Kidneys manifest in the hair
  - The Kidneys control spittle
  - The Kidneys control the two lower orifices
  - The Kidneys house Will-power
  - The Kidneys control the Gate of Life (*Ming Men*)
- Other Kidney relationships
  - Their smell is putrid
  - Their colour is black
  - Their taste is salty
  - Their climate is cold
  - Their sound is groaning
- Dreams
- Sayings
  - 'The Kidneys control opening and closing'
  - 'The Kidneys control strength and skill'
  - 'The Kidneys are the Root of Pre-Heaven Qi'
  - 'The Kidneys loathe dryness'
  - 'The Kidneys are the Gate of the Stomach'

THE FUNCTIONS OF THE KIDNEYS

The following functions of the Kidneys are discussed:

- Store Essence and govern birth, growth, reproduction and development
- Produce Marrow, fill up the brain and control bones
- Govern Water
- Control the reception of Qi
- Open into the ears
- Manifest in the hair
- Control spittle
- Control the two lower orifices.
- House Will-power
- Control the Gate of Life (*Ming Men* or Minister Fire)

The Kidneys store Essence and govern birth, growth, reproduction and development

As we discussed in chapter 3, the Essence (*Jing*) of the Kidneys is a precious substance which is inherited from the parents but also partly replenished by the Qi extracted from food. The Kidneys' function of storing Essence has two aspects:

1. They store the Pre-Heaven Essence, which is, the inherited Essence that before birth nourishes the fetus and after birth controls growth, sexual maturation, fertility and development. This Essence determines our basic constitution, strength and vitality. It is also the basis of sexual life, and the material foundation for the manufacture of sperm in men and ova and menstrual blood in women. As mentioned before, menstrual Blood (called *Tian Gui*) is different from other types of Blood as it derives directly from the Kidney-Essence (Fig. 10.5). Insufficient Essence may be a cause of infertility, impotence, underdevelopment in children (physical or mental), retarded growth and premature senility.
2. They store the Post-Heaven Essence, which is, the refined essence extracted from food through the transforming power of the Internal Organs.

I shall refer to 'Kidney-Essence' as the Essence that derives from both the Pre-Heaven and Post-Heaven Essence. Like the Pre-Heaven Essence, it is a hereditary energy which determines the person's constitution. Unlike the Pre-Heaven Essence, however, the Kidney-Essence interacts with the Post-Heaven Essence and is replenished by it. Kidney-Essence therefore partakes of both the Pre-Heaven and the Post-Heaven Essence.

This Essence is stored in the Kidneys, but it also circulates all over the body, particularly in the Eight Extraordinary Vessels (see ch. 39) (Fig. 10.6).

The Kidney-Essence determines growth, reproduction, development, sexual maturation, conception, pregnancy, menopause and ageing. The Kidney-Essence also controls the various stages of change in life, i.e. birth, puberty, menopause and death. The Kidney-Essence is essentially in charge of what we would call hormonal changes in Western medicine: that is, the changes occurring at puberty, during pregnancy and after childbirth in women, and during the menopause. Ageing itself is due to a physiological decline of Essence during life. The first chapter of the 'Simple Questions' describes the various stages of life in cycles of 7 years for women and 8 years for men.

The Kidney-Essence provides the material basis for both Kidney-Yin and Kidney-Yang. To put it differently, the Kidney-Essence has a Yin and a Yang aspect. The Yang aspect of the Essence is the Fire of the Gate of Life (*Ming Men*) that is active from conception (see Fig. 3.3 in chapter 3), concentrating at the point Du-4 Mingmen. The Yin aspect of the Kidney-Essence is the Water aspect of the Essence: that is, the sperm in men and the menstrual blood and ova in women. The Yin aspect of the Essence concentrates at the point Ren-4 Guanyuan (Figs 10.7 and 3.4).

Clinical note

- Du-4 Mingmen is the concentration point of the Yang aspect of the Essence, i.e. the Fire of the Gate of Life (*Ming Men*)
- Ren-4 Guanyuan is the concentration point of the Yin aspect of the Essence

As we have seen in chapter 3, the Kidney-Essence is the organic basis for the transformation of Kidney-Yin into Kidney-Qi by the warming and evaporating action of Kidney-Yang (see Fig. 3.5 in chapter 3).

The state of the Essence determines the state of the Kidneys. If Essence is flourishing and abundant, the Kidneys are strong and there will be great vitality, sexual power and fertility. If Essence is weak, the Kidneys are weak and there will be lack of vitality, infertility or sexual weakness.

Box 10.1 summarizes these functions of the Kidneys.

The Kidneys produce Marrow, fill up the brain and control bones

The Kidney's influence on Marrow is also derived from the Essence. Essence is the organic foundation for the production of Marrow. 'Marrow' (*sui*) does not correspond to bone marrow of Western medicine.

Box 10.1 The Kidney-Essence functions

- Governs growth
- Governs reproduction
- Governs development
- Governs sexual maturation
- Determines the 7- and 8-year cycles
- Influences conception
- Supports pregnancy
- Its decline induces menopause
- Determines ageing
- Is the material basis for Kidney-Yin and Kidney-Yang
- It has a Yin aspect (Essence) and a Yang aspect (Minister Fire)
- It is the basis for the transformation of Kidney-Yin into Kidney-Qi under the influence of Kidney-Yang

---

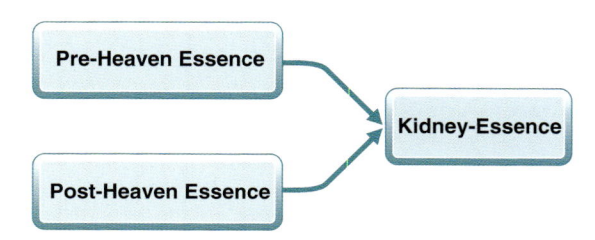

Figure 10.6 The Kidney-Essence and the Pre-Heaven and Post-Heaven Essence

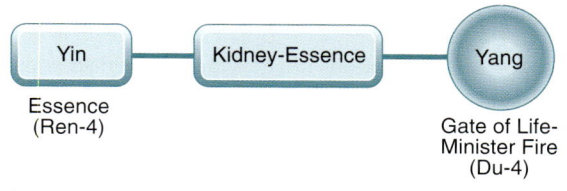

Figure 10.7 Yin and Yang aspects of Kidney-Essence

'Marrow' in Chinese medicine is a substance which is the common matrix of bones, bone marrow, brain and spinal cord (Fig. 10.8). The 'Simple Questions' says in chapter 34: *'The Kidneys pertain to Water and they generate the bones. If the Kidneys are not flourishing the Marrow cannot be filled.'*[1]

The 'Spiritual Axis' says in chapter 36: *'The five flavours and fluids amalgamate to form fat: this irrigates the cavities inside the bones, it tonifies the Brain and the Marrow and flows to the thighs.'*[2] This statement is interesting in its reference to a form of 'fat' formed by food and drink which goes to form bone marrow and the spinal cord and brain. Therefore the bone marrow, spinal cord and brain (all manifestations of 'Marrow') are a dense, material type of Qi which the 'Spiritual Axis' calls 'fat'. Another interesting aspect of the above statement is the reference to the Marrow flowing to the thighs: therefore the ancient Chinese seem to have grasped the fact that long bones contain bone marrow.

The Kidney-Essence produces Marrow, which generates the spinal cord and 'fills up' the brain. The 'Spiritual Axis' in chapter 33 says: *'The Brain is the Sea of Marrow.'*[3] For this reason, in Chinese medicine the brain has a physiological relationship with the Kidneys. If Kidney-Essence is strong, it will nourish the brain and memory, concentration, thinking and sight will all be keen. Chinese medicine holds that 'the Kidneys are the origin of skill and intelligence'. If the brain is not adequately nourished by the Essence, there may be poor memory and concentration, dizziness, dull thinking and poor sight. Brain and spinal cord are also referred to as 'Sea of Marrow' (Fig. 10.9).

> **Clinical note**
>
> The Kidney-Essence nourishes the brain; hence memory depends on the state of the Kidneys. BL-23 Shenshu and Du-20 Baihui can tonify the Kidneys to stimulate memory

The Marrow is also the basis for the formation of bone marrow, which nourishes the bones. Thus the Kidneys also govern the bone marrow and bones. The 'Simple Questions' in chapter 17 says: *'The bones are the Fu [organ] of the Marrow.'*[4] If the Kidney-Essence is strong, the bones will be strong, and the teeth will be firm. If the Kidney-Essence is weak, the bones will be brittle and the teeth loose. A weak Kidney-Essence in children will cause poor bone development, pigeon-chest, etc. The 'Simple Questions' in chapter 44 says: *'Kidneys control the bone marrow … if the Kidneys have Heat, the spine will not be straight, the bones will wither,*

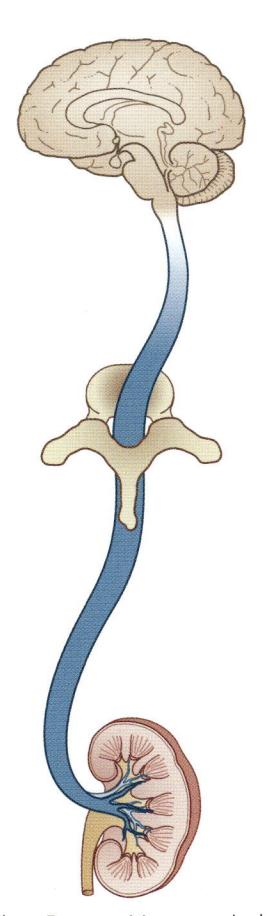

Figure 10.8 Kidney-Essence, Marrow, spinal cord and brain

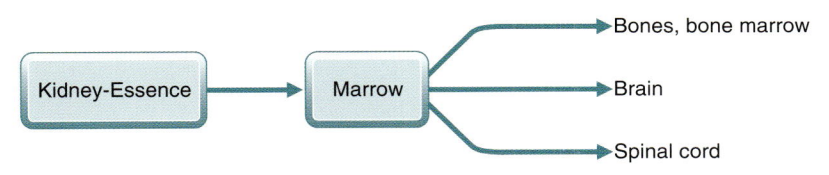

Figure 10.9 Kidney-Essence and Marrow

the marrow will decrease.'⁵ The decline of Kidney-Essence occurring with the menopause in women means that the Essence does not nourish the Marrow and bones so that they become brittle, leading to osteoporosis.

> **Clinical note**
>
> The Kidney-Essence nourishes the bones through Marrow. Osteoporosis is due to the decline of Kidney-Essence. The points BL-23 Shenshu, KI-3 Taixi and BL-11 Dashu can tonify the Kidneys to nourish bones

The Kidney-Essence has also an important influence on vitality and mental vigour. The 'Simple Questions' says in chapter 8: '*The Kidneys are the strong official from whom ingenuity is derived.*'⁶ This means that the Kidneys determine both the physical and mental strength of an individual. They also determine our will-power, as will be explained shortly.

> **Clinical note**
>
> To nourish the Kidney-Essence to tonify the brain, one can use the Governing Vessel, i.e. S.I.-3 Houxi with BL-62 Shenmai plus BL-23 Shenshu, KI-3 Taixi, Du-16 Fengfu and Du-20 Baihui

This function of the Kidneys is summarized in Box 10.2.

The Kidneys govern Water

As we have seen, according to the Five Elements, the Kidneys belong to Water and they govern the transformation and transportation of Body Fluids in many different ways:

- The Kidneys are like a gate that opens and closes in order to control the flow of Body Fluids in the Lower Burner. Under normal physiological conditions there will be a correct balance between Kidney-Yin and Kidney-Yang, resulting in the correct regulation of the opening and closing of the 'gate'. Urination will therefore be normal in quantity and colour. In disease, there is an imbalance between Kidney-Yin and Kidney-Yang, resulting in a malfunctioning of the 'gate' in opening and closing: it will either be too open (deficiency of Kidney-Yang), causing profuse and pale urination, or too closed (deficiency of Kidney-Yin), causing scanty and dark urination
- The Kidneys belong to the Lower Burner, which is sometimes compared to a 'drainage ditch'. The organs of the Lower Burner are particularly concerned with the excretion of impure Body Fluids. The Kidneys have the function of providing Qi for the Bladder to store and transform urine
- The Small Intestine and Large Intestine, also in the Lower Burner, play a part in separating clean from dirty fluids. This intestinal function of separating fluids is also under the control of the Kidneys, in particular Kidney-Yang
- The Kidneys receive fluids from the Lungs, some of which are excreted and some of which are vaporized, in which form they return to the Lungs to keep them moist
- The Spleen plays a very important role in the transformation and transportation of Body Fluids. Kidney-Yang provides the Spleen with the heat it needs to carry out its function of transforming and transporting fluids

This function of the Kidneys is summarized in Box 10.3.

The Kidneys control the reception of Qi

To make use of the clear Qi of the air, the Lungs and Kidneys work together. The Lungs have a descending action on Qi, directing it down to the Kidneys. The Kidneys respond by 'holding' this Qi down. If the Kidneys cannot hold Qi down it 'rebels' upward, creating congestion in the chest, resulting in breathlessness and asthma. This is a very frequent cause of chronic asthma (Fig. 10.10).

> **Box 10.2 The Kidneys produce Marrow, fill up the brain and control bones**
>
> - The Kidney-Essence produces Marrow
> - Marrow is the substance that forms the brain
> - Marrow is also transformed into bone marrow
> - Marrow and bone marrow generate the bones

> **Box 10.3 The Kidneys control Water**
>
> - The Kidneys are the 'gate' that controls urination
> - The Kidneys influence the Lower Burner's excretion of fluids
> - Kidney-Yang influences the Intestines' capacity for transforming and separating fluids
> - The Kidneys receive fluids from the Lungs and they also send vaporized fluids up to the Lungs
> - Kidney-Yang provides heat to the Spleen for the transformation and transportation of fluids

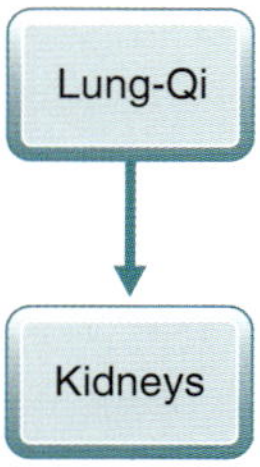

Figure 10.10 The Kidney's reception of Qi

> **Clinical note**
>
> The main points to stimulate the Kidneys' grasping of Qi (from the Lungs) are KI-7 Fuliu, Ren-4 Guanyuan and KI-13 Qixue

This function of the Kidneys is summarized in Box 10.4.

> **Box 10.4 The Kidneys control the reception of Qi**
>
> The Lungs send Qi down to the Kidneys; the Kidneys respond by 'receiving' or 'grasping' Qi to hold it down. If the Kidneys do not receive and hold Qi down, this will escape upwards, causing breathlessness.

The Kidneys open into the ears

The ears rely on the nourishment of the Essence for their proper functioning, and are therefore physiologically related to the Kidneys. The 'Spiritual Axis' in chapter 17 says: *'The Kidneys open into the ears, if the Kidneys are healthy the ears can hear the five sounds.'*[7]

If the Kidneys are weak, hearing may be impaired and there may be tinnitus.

This function of the Kidneys is summarized in Box 10.5.

> **Box 10.5 The Kidneys open into the ears**
>
> The Kidneys nourish the ears: a Kidney deficiency may cause deafness and/or tinnitus

The Kidneys manifest in the hair

The hair relies on the nourishment of the Kidney-Essence to grow. If the Kidney-Essence is abundant, the hair will grow well and will be healthy and glossy. If the Kidney-Essence is weak or is declining, the hair will become thin, brittle, dull-looking and may fall out altogether. The first chapter of the 'Simple Questions' says: *'If the Kidneys are strong, the teeth will be firm and the hair grow well ... if the Kidneys are declining in energy, the hair will fall out and the teeth become loose.'*[8]

The quality and colour of the hair are also related to the state of the Kidney-Essence. If the Kidney-Essence is strong, the hair will be thick and of a good colour. If the Kidney-Essence is weak, the hair will be thin and become grey. The 'Simple Questions' in chapter 10 says: *'The Kidneys control the bones and manifest in the hair.'*[9]

Remember that Liver-Blood also influences the hair and there is therefore an overlap between the Kidneys and the Liver as the organs influencing the state of the hair. Thus, dull, brittle and dry hair may indicate a Kidney deficiency or a Liver-Blood deficiency; however, prematurely grey hair generally indicates a Kidney deficiency.

This function is summarized in Box 10.6.

> **Box 10.6 The Kidneys manifest in the hair**
>
> The Kidneys nourish the hair: thin, brittle, dry, dull, prematurely grey hair may indicate Kidney deficiency (remember that Liver-Blood also influences the hair)

The Kidneys control spittle

'Spittle' is the translation of the word '*tuo*', which modern dictionaries also translate as 'saliva'. I translate *tuo* (of the Kidneys) as 'spittle' to distinguish it from *xian* (of the Spleen), which I translate as 'saliva'.

Spittle is described as a thick fluid in the mouth deriving from the root of the tongue and the back of the throat (whilst saliva is a thin fluids that originates from the mouth itself). Spittle is a fluid that actually moistens the Kidneys and benefits the Kidney-Essence. Indeed, excessive spitting was considered to be detrimental to the Kidney-Essence. For this reason, in many Daoist exercises, the practitioner should roll the tongue around the gums in order to produce spittle which should then be gulped down and mentally directed to the Lower *Dan Tian* (i.e. the area below the umbilicus): this was thought to nourish the Kidney-Essence.

This function of the Kidneys is summarized in Box 10.7.

> **Box 10.7 The Kidneys control spittle**
>
> 'Spittle' is a thick fluid at the back of the tongue and throat. Spittle both derives from Kidney-Essence and nourishes Kidney-Essence

The Kidneys control the two lower orifices

The two lower orifices are the front and the rear lower orifices. The front orifices include the urethra and spermatic duct in men; the rear orifice is the anus. These orifices are functionally related to the Kidneys. The urethra is obviously related to the Kidneys since the Bladder derives the Qi necessary for the transformation of urine from the Kidneys. If the Kidney energy is weak, urine may leak out causing incontinence or enuresis.

The spermatic duct is related to the Kidney as sperm is the outer manifestation of the Kidney-Essence. A deficiency of Kidney-Qi or Kidney-Essence may cause spermatorrhoea or nocturnal emissions. Finally, the anus, although anatomically related to the Large Intestine, is also functionally related to the Kidneys. If Kidney-Qi is weak, there may be diarrhoea or prolapse of the anus.

In conclusion, Kidney-Qi is essential for the normal functioning of all the lower orifices and a deficiency of Kidney-Qi will induce a 'leaking' of each orifice: that is, urinary incontinence, spermatorrhoea and diarrhoea.

This function of the Kidneys is summarized in Box 10.8.

> **Box 10.8 The Kidneys control the two lower orifices**
>
> The Kidneys influence:
> - The urethra (e.g. urethral discharge, urethritis)
> - The spermatic duct (e.g. sperm discharge)
> - The anus (e.g. incontinence of stool)

The Kidneys house Will-power

It is said in Chinese medicine that the Kidneys are the 'residence' of Will power (*Zhi*).[10] The Simple Questions' says in chapter 23: '*The Kidneys house Will Power.*'[11] This means that the Kidneys determine our will-power: this includes also determination, enthusiasm, spirit of initiative and steadfastness.

If the Kidneys are strong, the Will-power will be strong, the Mind will be focused on goals that it sets itself and it will pursue them in a single-minded way. Conversely, if the Kidneys are weak, Will-power will be lacking, the Mind will be easily discouraged and swayed from its aims. Lack of will-power and motivation are often important aspects of mental depression and tonification of the Kidneys will often give very good results.

> **Clinical note**
>
> BL-52 Zhishi can strengthen Will-power

As *Zhi* also has the meaning of 'memory', the Kidneys' housing of *Zhi* also implies that the Kidneys influence memory and recalling.

This function is summarized in Box 10.9.

> **Box 10.9 The Kidneys control Will-power**
>
> - The Kidneys control will-power, determination, single-mindedness, tenacity
> - The Kidneys control memory

The Kidneys control the Gate of Life (*Ming Men*)

A discussion of the Kidney functions would not be complete without reference to the Gate of Life (*Ming Men*). The first discussion of the Gate of Life can be found in the 'Classic of Difficulties', especially in chapters 36 and 39. Chapter 36 says: '*The Kidneys are not really two, as the left Kidney is a Kidney proper and the right Kidney is the Gate of Life [Ming Men]. The Gate of Life is the residence of the Mind [Shen] and is related to the Original Qi [Yuan Qi]: in men it stores Essence [Jing], in women it is connected to the uterus. That is why there is only one Kidney.*'[12]

Chapter 39 says: '*Why does the classic say that there are 5 Yang and 6 Yin organs? The reason is that the Yin organs count as 6 since there are two Kidneys. The left Kidney is the Kidney proper, the right Kidney is the Gate of Life [Ming Men] ... the reason that there are 6 Yang organs is that each of the 5 Yin organs has a corresponding Yang organ, plus an extra one being the Triple Burner.*'[13]

These two passages clearly show that, according to the 'Classic of Difficulties', the Gate of Life corresponds to the right Kidney, and is therefore functionally inseparable from the Kidneys. The 'Pulse Classic' written by

Wang Shu He in the Han dynasty confirms this in assigning the Kidney and Gate of Life to the right Rear (proximal) position on the pulse.

Chen Wu Ze of the Song dynasty wrote: '*The ancients considered the left Kidney as Kidney proper, related to the Bladder, and the right Kidney as the Gate of Life related to the Triple Burner.*'[14] However, for several centuries, up to the Ming dynasty, medical writers seldom discussed the Gate of Life as something separate from the Kidney, and simply referred to it as 'Kidney-Qi' (Fig. 10.11).

With the beginning of the Ming dynasty, the concept of Gate of Life (*Ming Men*) was greatly developed, and ideas on it differed from those expounded in the 'Classic of Difficulties'. During the Ming dynasty, Chinese physicians no longer considered the Gate of Life as part of the right Kidney, but as occupying the place between the two Kidneys. Zhang Jie Bin (1563–1640) said: '*There are two Kidneys ... the Gate of Life is in between them. ... The Gate of Life is the organ of Water and Fire, it is the residence of Yin and Yang, the Sea of Essence and it determines life and death.*'[15] Li Shi Zhen also said that the Gate of Life is in between the two Kidneys (Fig. 10.12).

Before the Ming dynasty the Gate of Life (*Ming Men*) was identified with the right Kidney. After the Ming dynasty, the Gate of Life was thought to be an independent entity residing between the two kidneys

Zhao Xian He was a doctor who discussed the Gate of Life in greatest depth in his book 'Medicine Treasure' (*Yi Gui*) published in 1687. Most of this book deals with physiological and pathological aspects of the Gate of Life. Zhao Xian He also regarded the Gate of Life as being between the two Kidneys (Fig. 10.13).

He wrote that the Gate of Life is the motive force of all functional activities of the body, being the physiological Fire which is essential to life. This Fire is also called 'True Fire' or 'Minister Fire' (in quite a different sense that is sometimes attributed to the Pericardium). The importance of the Fire nature of the Gate of Life is that it provides heat for all our bodily functions and for the Kidney-Essence itself. The Kidneys are unlike any other organ in so far as they are the origin of Water and Fire of the body, the Primary Yin and Primary Yang. The Gate of Life is the embodiment of the Fire within the Kidneys and the Minister Fire is a special type of Fire in that not only it does not extinguish Water, but it can actually produce Water.

In this respect the Gate of Life theory is at variance with the Five-Element theory according to which Fire is derived from the Heart, not from the Gate of Life (i.e. the Kidneys). These theories simply spring from two different perspectives and are both valid. Indeed, the two Fires (of the Heart and Kidneys) are called Emperor and Minister Fire, respectively. However, in clinical practice, the theory that attributes the origin of Fire to the Gate of Life, and hence the Kidneys, is more significant and more widely used when treating pathological conditions deriving from Yang deficiency and weakness of the Minister Fire. For example, when the Spleen- and Kidney-Yang are depleted and the Minister Fire weak and the patient suffers from tiredness, exhaustion, oedema, etc., it is necessary to tonify the Minister Fire of the Kidneys and not the (Emperor) Fire of the Heart.

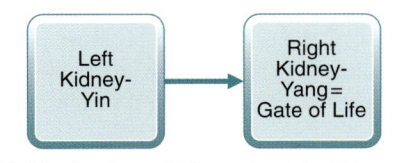

Figure 10.11 The Gate of Life as the right Kidney

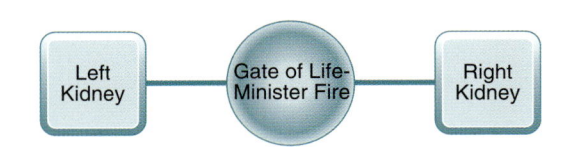

Figure 10.12 The Gate of Life in between the Kidneys

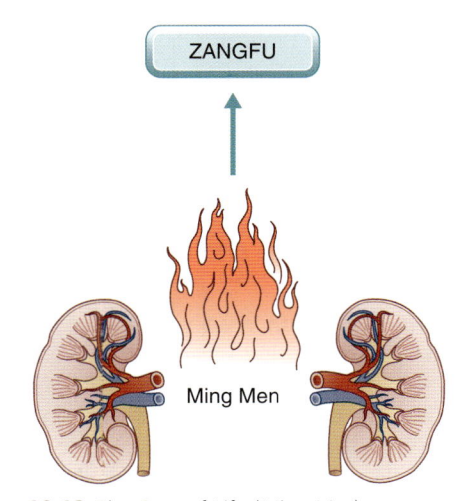

Figure 10.13 The Gate of Life (*Ming Men*)

The main functions of the Gate of Life can be summarized as follows:

It is the Root of the Original Qi (Yuan Qi)

Both the Gate of Life and Original Qi are related to the Kidneys, and are interdependent. Original Qi is a form of dynamically activated Essence which has many functions, among which is that of assisting in the making of Blood. Original Qi relies on heat for its performance and this heat is provided by the Gate of Life. If the Fire of the Gate of Life is deficient, Original Qi will suffer, and will inevitably lead to a general deficiency of Qi and Blood.

It is the source of (physiological) Fire for all the Internal Organs

All the organs rely on the heat provided by the Fire of the Gate of Life to function properly. The Spleen needs its heat to transform and transport food essences, the Stomach needs it to rot and ripen food, the Heart needs it to house the Mind, the Lungs needs it to send Qi downwards and to diffuse Qi, the Liver needs it to ensure the free flow of Qi, the Intestines need it to move food and stools, the Gall Bladder needs it to secrete bile and the Triple Burner needs it to transform and excrete fluids.

If the Fire of the Gate of Life declines, the functional activity of all organs will be impaired, leading to tiredness, mental depression, lack of vitality, negativity and a pronounced feeling of cold.

It warms the Lower Burner and Bladder

The Lower Burner transforms and excretes fluids, with the assistance of the Bladder. The heat of the Gate of Life is essential to transform fluids in the Lower Burner. If the Gate of Life Fire is weak, the Lower Burner and Bladder will lack the Heat necessary to transform fluids: these will therefore accumulate, giving rise to Dampness or oedema.

It warms the Stomach and Spleen to aid digestion

Heat is essential to the Spleen for its functions of transportation, separation and transformation. All this requires heat supplied by the Gate of Life. If the Fire of the Gate of Life is deficient, the Spleen cannot transform and the Stomach cannot digest the food, leading to diarrhoea, tiredness, feelings of cold and cold limbs.

It harmonizes the sexual function and warms the Essence and Uterus

The Fire of the Gate of Life is essential for a healthy sexual function and to warm the Essence and the Uterus. The Fire of the Gate of Life (Minister Fire) could be seen as the Yang aspect of the Essence. Sexual performance, fertility, puberty and menstruation all depend on the Fire of the Gate of Life. If the Fire of the Gate of Life declines, the Essence in men and the Uterus in women will turn cold, causing impotence and sterility in men and lack of sexual desire and infertility in women.

It assists the Kidney function of reception of Qi

The function of reception of Qi depends on Kidney-Yang, which requires the Fire of the Gate of Life for its performance. For Kidney-Yang to function normally, there must be communication between the Gathering Qi (Zong Qi) of the chest and the Original Qi (Yuan Qi) of the lower abdomen, which itself relies on the heat from the Gate of Life for its activity.

If the Fire of the Gate of Life is deficient, the Kidneys' ability to receive Qi will be impaired, causing breathlessness, asthma, a feeling of oppression of the chest and cold hands.

It assists the Heart function of housing the Mind

The Fire of the Gate of Life has to ascend from the Kidneys and communicate with the Heart, to provide it with the heat necessary for its functions. Because of this, the Fire of the Gate of Life assists the Heart in housing the Mind. This means that the Fire of the Gate of Life has a strong influence on the mental state and happiness. If the Fire of the Gate of Life is deficient, the Heart cannot house the Mind, and the person will be depressed, unhappy and lack vitality. Vice versa, if the Minister Fire of the Gate of Life becomes pathological (from emotional problems, for example), it flares upwards, harassing the Heart and Pericardium.

> **Clinical note**
>
> The Fire of the Gate of Life (*Ming Men*) is tonified by using Du-4 Mingmen, Ren-4 Guanyuan and KI-3 Taixi with moxa

These functions are summarized in Box 10.10.

> **Box 10.10 Functions of the Gate of Life**
> - It is the Root of the Original Qi
> - It is the Source of Fire for all the Internal Organs
> - It warms the Lower Burner and Bladder
> - It warms the Stomach and Spleen to aid digestion
> - It harmonizes the sexual function and warms the Essence and Uterus
> - It assists the Kidney reception of Qi
> - It assists the Heart in housing the Mind

OTHER KIDNEY RELATIONSHIPS

The other Kidney relationships discussed are:

- Their smell
- Their colour
- Their taste
- Their climate
- Their sound

Their smell is putrid

The putrid smell is frequent in clinical practice. It is particularly frequent in the elderly and it always indicates a Kidney deficiency. The putrid smell is like the smell of stagnant water.

Their colour is black

The 'black' colour of the Kidneys is not literally black but dark, often somewhat dark-grey. This can be observed on the cheeks or under the eyes, usually indicating Kidney-Yin deficiency. However, a dark-bluish colour may also relate to the Kidneys and it may be observed on the cheeks, indicating Kidney-Yang deficiency.

Their taste is salty

The salty taste is not common and very few patients will report experiencing such a taste. A salty taste indicates a Kidney deficiency, which may be of Yin or Yang.

A small amount of salty taste is beneficial to the Kidneys and especially Kidney-Yin. In fact, some doctors, when prescribing Kidney-Yin tonic tablets, advise patients to take these in the evening with slightly salted hot water. Conversely, an excessive amount of salt in the diet will harm not only the Kidneys but also the Heart (as Water over-acts on Fire along the Controlling Cycle of the Five Elements).

Their climate is cold

External cold injures the Kidneys and particularly Kidney-Yang. External cold affects the Kidneys when it invades the lower back and loins; this is all the more likely to occur in modern women since modern fashion often leaves the lower abdominal area and loins exposed.

Cold in the Kidneys may cause lumbago, abdominal pain, diarrhoea, and painful periods. Cold injures Yang and leads eventually to Kidney-Yang deficiency.

Their sound is groaning

The voice sound related to the Kidneys is groaning: this is a low, deep, somewhat rasping and hoarse sound.[16]

Other Kidney relationships are summarized in Box 10.11.

> **Box 10.11 Other Kidney relationships**
> - Their smell is putrid
> - Their colour is black
> - Their taste is salty
> - Their climate is cold
> - Their sound is groaning

DREAMS

The 'Simple Questions' in chapter 80 says: *'When the Kidneys are weak, one dreams of swimming after a shipwreck; if the dream takes place in winter, one dreams of plunging in water and being scared.'*[17]

The 'Spiritual Axis' in chapter 43 says: *'When the Kidneys are in excess one dreams that the spine is detached from the body ... when they are weak, one dreams of being immersed in water.'*[18]

SAYINGS

The sayings discussed are:

- 'The Kidneys control opening and closing'
- 'The Kidneys control strength and skill'
- 'The Kidneys are the Root of Pre-Heaven Qi'
- 'The Kidneys loathe dryness'
- 'The Kidneys are the Gate of the Stomach'

'The Kidneys control opening and closing'

The Kidneys function like a 'gate' in relation to urination. As was mentioned before, if Kidney-Yang is deficient (i.e. the gate is open), urine will be abundant and clear. If Kidney-Yin is deficient (i.e. the gate is closed), urine will be scanty and dark.

Besides controlling urination, the Kidneys also influence the anus and defecation and if Kidney-Yang is deficient there may be diarrhoea. For this reason, the Kidneys influence the 'opening and closing' of both lower Yin orifices (i.e. the anus and the urethra).

'The Kidneys control strength and skill'

The Kidneys control our capacity for hard work. If the Kidneys are strong, a person can work hard and purposefully for long periods of time. If the Kidneys are weak, a person will lack the strength necessary for long periods of hard work. Conversely, a Kidney disharmony can sometimes drive a person to overwork beyond measure, becoming a 'workaholic'.

Besides strength, the Kidneys also influence our capacity for skilled and delicate activities.

'The Kidneys are the Root of Pre-Heaven Qi'

Just as the Spleen is the Root of Post-Heaven Qi, being the origin of Qi and Blood produced after birth, the Kidneys are the Root of Pre-Heaven Qi because they store the Essence, which is inherited from our parents.

'The Kidneys loathe dryness'

Dry weather or internal Dryness can injure Kidney-Yin. Interior Dryness can be produced by a Stomach deficiency, by profuse and continued loss of fluids (such as occurs in sweating or diarrhoea) or by smoking. According to Chinese medicine, tobacco dries Blood and Essence and it can injure Kidney-Yin.

Although the Kidneys dislike dryness and the Lungs dislike cold, some doctors also say that the Kidneys dislike cold and the Lungs dryness. This view is also valid.

'The Kidneys are the Gate of the Stomach'

The Stomach is the origin of fluids and the Kidneys transform and excrete fluids. If the Kidneys cannot excrete fluids properly, these will stagnate and affect the Stomach. Conversely, a lack of Stomach fluids can lead to Kidney-Yin deficiency.

Box 10.12 lists the sayings about the Kidneys.

Box 10.12 Sayings about the Kidneys

- 'The Kidneys control opening and closing'
- 'The Kidneys control strength and skill'
- 'The Kidneys are the Root of Pre-Heaven Qi'
- 'The Kidneys loathe dryness'
- 'The Kidneys are the Gate of the Stomach'

Learning outcomes

In this chapter you will have learned:
- The significance of the Kidneys as the foundation of Yin and Yang, the origin of Fire and Water in the body
- The unity and interdependence of Kidney-Yin and Kidney-Yang
- The relationship between the Kidney-Essence and Marrow, brain, bones and teeth
- How the Kidneys govern transformation and transportation of Body Fluids
- The role of the Kidneys in controlling reception of Qi
- How the Kidney-Essence nourishes the ears and hair
- The function of the Kidneys in controlling the lower orifices
- The relationship between the Kidneys and the Will-power (*Zhi*)
- The significance of the Kidneys in controlling the Gate of Life
- The smell, colour, taste, climate and sound of the Kidneys
- Dreams reflecting disharmonies of the Kidneys
- Sayings related to the Kidneys

Self-assessment questions

1. Describe Kidney-Yin and Kidney-Yang using the analogy of an oil lamp.
2. Why in herbal medicine is it common to tonify both Kidney-Yin and Kidney-Yang together?
3. List the physiological processes which are governed or influenced by the Kidney-Essence.
4. Describe the development of osteoporosis in older women in terms of Kidney-Essence, Marrow and bones.
5. Give three examples of the Kidneys controlling Water.
6. What would happen if the Kidneys failed to 'grasp' the Qi sent down by the Lungs?
7. Give examples of symptoms which would occur if weak Kidney-Qi failed to control the two lower orifices.
8. If a patient suffers from tiredness, exhaustion, and oedema why might it be necessary to tonify the Kidneys?
9. What are the smell, colour, taste, climate and sound of the Kidneys?
10. How might a state of Interior Dryness arise, and how would it affect the Kidneys?

See p. 1257 for answers

END NOTES

1. 1979 The Yellow Emperor's Classic of Internal Medicine – Simple Questions (*Huang Di Nei Jing Su Wen* 黄帝内经素问), People's Health Publishing House, Beijing, first published *c*.100 BC, p. 198.
2. 1981 Spiritual Axis (*Ling Shu Jing* 灵枢经), People's Health Publishing House, Beijing, first published *c*.100 BC, p. 77.
3. Ibid., p. 73.
4. Simple Questions, p. 100.
5. Ibid., p. 247
6. Ibid., p. 58.
7. Spiritual Axis, p. 50.
8. Simple Questions, p. 4.
9. Ibid., p. 70.
10. Please note that I translate '*Zhi*' as Will-power, but this Chinese word has many different meanings, among which are 'memory', 'aspiration', 'ideal'.
11. Simple Questions, p. 153.
12. A Revised Explanation of the Classic of Difficulties, p. 90.
13. Ibid., p. 95.
14. 1979 Patterns and Treatment of Kidney diseases (*Shen Yu Shen Bing de Zheng Zhi* 肾与肾病的证治), Hebei People's Publishing House, Hebei, p. 2.
15. Ibid., p. 3.
16. The actress Demi Moore, for example, has a groaning voice.
17. Simple Questions, p. 569.
18. Spiritual Axis, p. 85.

FURTHER READING

Kaptchuk T 2000 The Web that has no Weaver – Understanding Chinese Medicine, Contemporary Books, Chicago

SECTION 1　PART 2

The Functions of the Pericardium   11

Key contents

Functions of the Pericardium

The Pericardium as an organ
- It is the membrane wrapping around the Heart
  - Protects the Heart
  - Like the Heart, it governs Blood and houses the Mind
  - Pericardium points can invigorate Blood or cool Blood
  - Pericardium points stimulate or calm the Mind

The Pericardium as a channel
- Sphere of influence is the centre of the thorax
- Exteriorly–interiorly related to the Triple Burner channel

The Pericardium and the Mind-Spirit
- The Pericardium houses the Mind (with the Heart)
- Blood deficiency of the Pericardium will cause depression and slight anxiety
- Blood Heat of the Pericardium will cause anxiety, insomnia and agitation
- Phlegm in the Pericardium will cause mental confusion and, in severe cases, mental illness
- Points on the Pericardium channel are often used to treat emotional problems

Other Pericardium relationships

The Pericardium and the Minister Fire
- From a Five-Element perspective, the Pericardium pertains to the Minister Fire, along with the Triple Burner
- From the perspective of channel relationships, the Pericardium pertains to the Minister Fire along with the Triple Burner
- From the perspective of organs, the Ministerial Fire originates from the Kidneys

The Pericardium is an organ that is not so clearly defined as the other Yin organs. We translate as 'Pericardium' various Chinese terms such as 'Master of the Heart' (*Xin Zhu*), 'Envelope of the Heart' (*Xin Bao*) and 'Connecting Channel of the Envelope of the Heart' (*Xin Bao Luo*). The uncertain nature of the Pericardium derives also from it being linked to the Heart from the point of view of organs (as it is obviously so close to the Heart itself) but to the Triple Burner from the point of view of channels (Fig. 11.1). It is therefore best to discuss the functions and nature of the Pericardium as an organ and as a channel separately.

Names for 'Pericardium'

What we translate as 'Pericardium' takes various names in Chinese:
- 'Master of the Heart' *Xin Zhu*
- 'Envelope of the Heart' *Xin Bao*
- 'Connecting Channel of the Envelope of the Heart' *Xin Bao Luo*

The discussion of the Pericardium will be according to the following topics:

- The Pericardium as an organ
- The Pericardium as a channel
- The Pericardium and the Mind-Spirit
- Relationship between the Pericardium and the Minister Fire
- Relationship between the Pericardium and the Uterus

THE PERICARDIUM AS AN ORGAN

As an organ, the Pericardium is closely related to the Heart. The 'Selected Historical Theories of Chinese Medicine' confirms the nature of the Pericardium as the outer covering of the Heart by saying: 'The

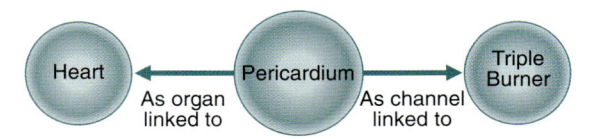

Heart ←— As organ linked to —→ Pericardium ←— As channel linked to —→ Triple Burner

Figure 11.1 Pericardium connections

Pericardium [xin bao luo] is a membrane wrapping around the Heart.'[1]

The traditional view of the Pericardium is that it functions as an external covering of the Heart, protecting it from attacks by exterior pathogenic factors. The 'Spiritual Axis' in chapter 71 says: '*The Heart is the Ruler of the 5 Yin organs and 6 Yang organs, it is the residence of the Mind and it is so tough that no pathogenic factor can take hold in it. If the Heart is attacked by a pathogenic factor, the Mind suffers, which can lead to death. If a pathogenic factor does attack the Heart, it will be deviated to attack the Pericardium instead. For this reason, the Heart has no Stream Transporting point.*'[2] The protective function of the Pericardium in respect of the Heart is mentioned in 'Selected Historical Theories of Chinese Medicine': '*The Triple Burner protects the Internal Organs on the outside and the Pericardium protects the Heart on the outside.*'[3]

The Yellow Emperor's Classic normally only mentions 11 organs: this book (and many other classics) constantly refers to the '5 Zang and 6 Fu', the Pericardium being a mere appendage of the Heart. In fact, the 'Spiritual Axis' in chapter 1 says that the Stream (*Shu*) and Source (*Yuan*) point of the Heart is Daling (Pericardium-7).[4] This is why the 'Spiritual Axis' in chapter 17 quoted above says that '*the Heart has no Stream Transporting point*'.

According to the theory of the Internal Organs, the functions of the Pericardium are more or less identical with those of the Heart: it governs Blood and it houses the Mind. For example, in relation to its function of governing Blood, the Pericardium channel can be used to invigorate Blood with acupuncture and P-6 Neiguan or to cool Blood with P-3 Quze. With regard to the function of housing the Mind, many Pericardium channel points have a powerful influence on the mental and emotional state (see below).

The Pericardium is of secondary importance to the Heart as it displays many of the same functions. In herbal medicine, the Pericardium is usually only referred to in the context of infectious diseases caused by exterior Heat. Such diseases correspond to the Upper Burner stage in the model of Identification of Patterns according to the Three Burners or to the Heat in Pericardium Pattern at the Nutritive Qi level within the Identification of Patterns according to the Four Levels, both characterized by delirium, mental confusion, aphasia and very high temperature, all symptoms of invasion of the Pericardium by extreme Heat. In terms of acupuncture, however, the Pericardium channel has as much importance as the Heart or any other channel (see below).

Box 11.1 summarizes this aspect of the Pericardium.

Box 11.1 The Pericardium as an organ

- Closely related to the Heart
- It is the 'membrane wrapping around the Heart'
- It protects the Heart
- Like the Heart, it governs Blood and houses the Mind
- Pericardium points can invigorate Blood or cool Blood
- Pericardium points stimulate or calm the Mind
- In acute febrile diseases, the Pericardium may be obstructed by Heat manifesting with high fever and delirium

THE PERICARDIUM AS A CHANNEL

Whilst as an organ the Pericardium is the outer covering of the Heart and its functions are the same as those of the Heart, from the point of view of channels, the Pericardium channel is quite distinct from the Heart channel and, on a physical level, has a different sphere of action, influencing the area at the centre of the thorax (Fig. 11.2).

The 'Yellow Emperor's Classic' often refers to the Pericardium as the 'centre of the thorax': hence the important action of P-6 Neiguan on the chest. The Pericardium channel goes to the centre of the thorax and this area, called *Shan Zhong*, is under the influence of the Pericardium. Chapter 35 of the 'Spiritual Axis' says: '*The centre of the thorax [shan zhong] is the palace of the Pericardium [Xin Zhu].*'[5]

Being in the centre of the chest, the Pericardium influences the Gathering Qi (*Zong Qi*) and therefore both Heart and Lungs. The Pericardium in this area acts as the agent of propulsion for the Qi and Blood of both Heart and Lungs and, for this reason, Pericardium

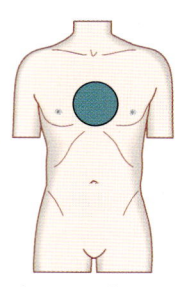

Figure 11.2 Sphere of action of Pericardium channel

patterns are characterized by clinical manifestations along the chest channels, causing tightness, stuffiness, distension, oppression or pain of the chest.

Thus, whilst in terms of organ functions the Pericardium is obviously closely related to the Heart, in terms of channels, it is exteriorly–interiorly related to the Triple Burner channel, the Pericardium being Yin and the Triple Burner Yang.

THE PERICARDIUM AND THE MIND-SPIRIT

The 'Simple Questions' in chapter 8 says: *'The Pericardium is the ambassador and from it joy and happiness derive.'*[6] Like the Heart, the Pericardium houses the Mind and it therefore influences our mental–emotional state deeply. For example, a deficiency of Blood will affect the Pericardium as well as the Heart, making the person depressed and slightly anxious. Heat in the Blood will agitate the Pericardium and make the person agitated and restless. Phlegm obstructing the Pericardium will also obstruct the Mind, causing mental confusion.

The Pericardium's function on the mental–emotional plane is probably the psychic equivalent of the above-mentioned function of the Pericardium in the chest with regard to moving Qi and Blood of Heart and Lungs: just as it does that on a physical level, on a mental–emotional level the Pericardium is responsible for 'movement' towards others (i.e. in relationships). Given that the Pericardium is related to the Liver within the Terminal-Yin channels, this 'movement' is also related to the 'movement' of the Ethereal Soul from the ego towards others in social relationships and familial interactions. For this reason, on a mental–emotional level, the Pericardium is particularly responsible for a healthy interaction with other people in social, love and family relationships.

Indeed, many Pericardium channel points have a deep influence on the mental state and are frequently used in mental–emotional problems. Three good examples are those of P-6 Neiguan, which stimulates the mood and lifts depression, P-7 Daling, which calms the Mind and settles anxiety, and P-5 Jianshi, which resolves Phlegm misting the Mind. In particular, the Pericardium also influences a person's relations with other people, and the points on its channel are often used to treat emotional problems caused by relationship difficulties (e.g. P-7 Daling).

Clinical note

- P-6 Neiguan lifts mood and treats depression
- P-7 Daling calms the Mind
- P-5 Jianshi resolves Phlegm from the Pericardium to treat mental confusion

It could be said that the protective function of the Pericardium in relation to the Heart, mentioned above, is reflected primarily in the mental–emotional sphere where the 'Minister Fire' of the Pericardium protects the 'Emperor Fire' of the Heart.

Box 11.2 summarizes this aspect of the Pericardium.

Box 11.2 The Pericardium and the Mind-Spirit

- The Pericardium houses the Mind (with the Heart)
- Blood deficiency of the Pericardium will cause depression and slight anxiety
- Blood-Heat of the Pericardium will cause anxiety, insomnia and agitation
- Phlegm in the Pericardium will cause mental confusion and, in severe cases, mental illness
- The Pericardium affects emotional problems from relationship problems

RELATIONSHIP BETWEEN THE PERICARDIUM AND THE MINISTER FIRE

Before concluding this section on the Pericardium, mention should be made of the question of the 'Minister Fire'. The prevailing view in the history of Chinese medicine has been that the 'Minister Fire' is the Fire of the Gate of Life (*Ming Men*). As we have seen in the chapter on the Kidneys, this physiological Fire stems from the Kidneys and is essential to the healthy functioning of the body.

Although many doctors such as Zhu Zhen Heng (1281–1358) identified 'Minister Fire' with the Fire of the Gate of Life (and therefore the Kidneys),[7] others, such as Zhang Jie Bin (1563–1640), identified the 'Minister Fire' with such internal organs as the Kidney, Liver, Triple Burner, Gall Bladder and Pericardium.[8] In fact, the Minister Fire is said to go upwards to the Liver, Gall Bladder and Pericardium (in so doing it is compared to the 'Fire Dragon flying to the top of a high mountain') and downwards to the Kidneys (in so doing it is compared to the 'Fire Dragon immersing in the deep sea')[9] (Fig. 11.3).

Thus, purely from a Five-Element perspective, the Pericardium pertains to the Minister Fire (with the Triple Burner) compared to the Emperor Fire of the Heart, while from the perspective of the Internal Organs, the Minister Fire is the Fire of the Gate of Life pertaining to the Kidneys. However, there is a connection between the two views as the Minister Fire does flow up to the Liver, Gall Bladder and Pericardium (Fig. 11.4). In pathology, this has an even greater relevance as the pathological Minister Fire (driven by emotional stress) flares upwards to harass the Pericardium, causing mental restlessness, agitation, anxiety and insomnia.[10]

Box 11.3 summarizes this aspect of the Pericardium.

> **Box 11.3 Pericardium and the Minister Fire**
>
> - Pericardium pertains to Minister Fire with the Triple Burner (in terms of channels)
> - Pericardium pertains to Minister Fire with the Kidneys as Minister Fire originates there
> - The Minister Fire flares upwards to Liver, Gall Bladder and Pericardium and flows downwards to the Kidneys
> - From a Five-Element perspective, the Pericardium pertains to the Minister Fire channels with the Triple Burner
> - From an organ perspective, the Minister Fire originates from the Kidneys
> - Pathological Minister Fire flares upwards to harass the Pericardium

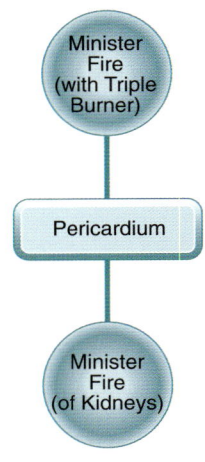

Figure 11.3 Relationship between Pericardium and Minister Fire

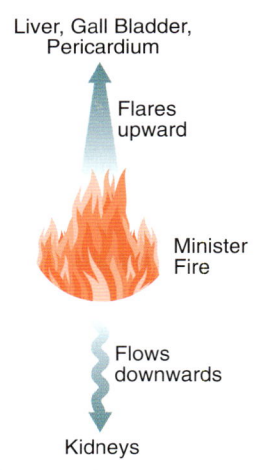

Figure 11.4 Relationship between Minister Fire and Internal Organs

RELATIONSHIP BETWEEN THE PERICARDIUM AND THE UTERUS

The Uterus is related to the Kidneys via a channel called the 'Uterus Channel' (*Bao Luo*) and to the Heart via a vessel called the 'Uterus Vessel' (*Bao Mai*). The latter vessel is, in particular, related to the Pericardium. The 'Selected Historical Theories of Chinese Medicine' says: '*The Pericardium (Xin Bao) is a membrane wrapping the Heart on the outside ... the Uterus connects downwards with the Kidneys and upwards with the Heart where it receives the name of "Luo of the Envelope of the Heart" (Xin Bao Luo).*'[11]

This provides the basis for an interesting observation regarding pulse diagnosis as it might explain the attribution of the right-Rear position to different organs in different systems. Some authors assign the right-Rear position to the Uterus and the Fire of the Gate of Life, while the 'Classic of Difficulties' assigns it to the Pericardium. The connection between the Uterus and the Pericardium might explain why both these systems, as contradictory as they might seem, could be both right.

Given the relationship between the Pericardium and the Uterus, a pathology of the Pericardium may affect menstruation. Thus, a deficiency of Blood of the Pericardium may cause scanty periods or amenorrhoea, Pericardium-Fire might heat the Blood and cause heavy periods, while Blood stasis in the Pericardium might cause painful periods.

As the Pericardium is also the house of the Mind (together with the Heart), its connection with the Uterus also explains the profound influence on emotional problems on the menstrual function in women.

Learning outcomes

In this chapter you will have learned:
- The various Chinese terms which are translated as 'Pericardium', and the reasons why there is uncertainty regarding the nature of the Pericardium
- The role of the Pericardium as an organ, the outer protective covering of the Heart
- The omission of the Pericardium in references from the Yellow Emperor's Classic to the '5 Yin and 6 Yang organs'
- The similarity of the functions of Pericardium and Heart (governing Blood and housing the Mind)
- The importance of the Pericardium channel in acupuncture treatment, compared with its narrower role in herbal medicine to treat febrile diseases
- The sphere of action of the Pericardium channel as the 'centre of the thorax'
- The influence of the Pericardium on the Gathering-Qi and the Heart and Lungs
- The significance of the Pericardium in the mental–emotional sphere, including facilitating healthy interaction with others in social, intimate and family relationships
- The theories concerning the association of the Pericardium and Minister Fire
- The connection between the Pericardium and the Uterus, via the 'Uterus Vessel' (*Bao Mai*), and the implications of this in pulse diagnosis

Self-assessment questions

1. How does the Pericardium function as an external covering of the Heart?
2. According to the theory of the Internal Organs, what are the two primary functions of the Pericardium?
3. What effect can points on the Pericardium channel have on Blood?
4. What effect can points on the Pericardium channel have on the Mind-Spirit?
5. What is the sphere of influence of the Pericardium channel?
6. In terms of channels, which channel is the Pericardium channel interiorly–exteriorly related to?
7. What is the relationship between the Minister Fire and the Pericardium?

See p. 1257 for answers

END NOTES

1. Wang Xin Hua 1983 Selected Historical Theories of Chinese Medicine (*Zhong Yi Li Dai Yi Lun Xuan* 中医历代医论选), Jiangsu Scientific Publishing House, p. 159.
2. 1981 Spiritual Axis (*Ling Shu Jing* 灵枢经), People's Health Publishing House, Beijing, first published *c*.100 BC, p. 128.
3. Selected Historical Theories of Chinese Medicine, p. 154.
4. Spiritual Axis, p. 3.
5. Spiritual Axis, p. 75.
6. Simple Questions, p. 58.
7. Selected Historical Theories of Chinese Medicine, p. 195.
8. Selected Historical Theories of Chinese Medicine, p. 195.
9. Selected Historical Theories of Chinese Medicine, p. 159.
10. There is an intriguing possibility that the *Xin Zhu* (translated as Pericardium) is the same as the Minister Fire. Chapter 18 of the 'Classic of Difficulties' attributes the right-Rear pulse position to the Fire of Lesser Yang (Triple Burner) and of *Xin Zhu*' (Nanjing College of Traditional Chinese Medicine 1979 A Revised Explanation of the Classic of Difficulties (*Nan Jing Jiao Shi* 难经校释), People's Health Publishing House, Beijing, first published *c*.AD 100, p. 45.) '*Xin Zhu*' here has always been translated as 'Pericardium'. Chapter 52 of the 'Simple Questions' says: '*Above the diaphragm, in the middle there are the Father and Mother [i.e. the Heart and Lungs]; beside the 7th node [i.e. the 2nd lumbar vertebra] there is a "Small Fire": if one follows it happiness will result, if one goes against it misery will result*' (1979 The Yellow Emperor's Classic of Internal Medicine – Simple Questions (*Huang Ti Nei Jing Su Wen* 黄帝内经素问), People's Health Publishing House, Beijing, first published *c*.100 BC, p. 276.) The 'Small Fire' in the lumbar region seems to be the Minister Fire of the Kidneys. If we refer to the pulse positions, it is interesting that the 'Classic of Difficulties' places the *Xin Zhu* on the right-Rear position where later doctors usually place the Minister Fire. It is therefore possible that the *Xin Zhu* of chapter 18 of the 'Classic of Difficulties' is the same as the 'Small Heart' (*Xiao Xin*) of chapter 52 of the 'Simple Questions'. This would mean that the Minister Fire has always been the Fire of the Kidneys and that the *Xin Zhu* of chapter 18 of the 'Classic of Difficulties' refers not to the Pericardium but to the Minister Fire of the Kidneys (called 'Small Heart' in chapter 52 of the 'Simple Questions'). This would make sense as the 'Simple Questions' would then refer to the Fire of the Heart above and a Fire of a 'Small Heart' below, i.e. the Minister Fire. If this is true it would at a stroke solve the conundrum as to why the 'Classic of Difficulties' attributes the right-Rear position of the pulse to the Pericardium and most later doctors attribute that position to the Minister Fire of the Kidneys. The fact that that pulse position is also associated with the Triple Burner is not contradictory and it would actually reinforce this apparent contradiction. In fact, the Triple Burner can be neatly assigned to the right-Rear position with the Pericardium as the two *channels* are exteriorly–interiorly related. However, the Triple Burner can also be assigned to the right-Rear position because it is the vehicle through which the Original Qi emerges from the space between the Kidneys (a view found in the 'Classic of Difficulties' itself in chapter 66). In other words, in terms of *channels* the Triple Burner is paired with the Pericardium, but in terms of *organs* it is the organ through which the Original Qi emerges from the space between the Kidneys.
11. Selected Historical Theories of Chinese Medicine, p. 160.

SECTION 1   PART 2

Yin Organ Interrelationships | 12

Key contents

Interrelationships between:

Heart and Lungs
Heart and Liver
Heart and Kidneys
Liver and Lungs
Liver and Spleen
Liver and Kidneys
Spleen and Lungs
Spleen and Kidneys
Lungs and Kidneys
Spleen and Heart

Interrelationship is the essence of Chinese medicine since the body is regarded as an integrated whole. Because of this it is not enough to consider the Yin organs merely on an individual basis. To understand them properly we must consider how they interrelate, since a person's health depends on a proper balance being maintained among the internal organs.

The Interrelationships of the Yin organs will be discussed under the following headings:

- Heart and Lungs
- Heart and Liver
- Heart and Kidneys
  - The mutual assistance of Fire and Water
  - The common root of Mind (*Shen*) and Essence (*Jing*)
  - The interrelationship of Heart and Kidneys in the menstrual cycle
- Liver and Lungs
  - The relationship between Lung-Qi and Liver-Blood
  - The relationship between the descending of Lung-Qi and the ascending of Liver-Qi
- Liver and Spleen
- Liver and Kidneys
- Spleen and Lungs
- Spleen and Kidneys
- Lungs and Kidneys
  - The relationship between Lungs and Kidneys with regard to Qi
  - The relationship between Lungs and Kidneys with regard to fluids
- Spleen and Heart

HEART AND LUNGS

The Heart governs Blood and the Lungs govern Qi: the relationship between Heart and Lungs is thus essentially the relationship between Qi and Blood (Fig. 12.1). Qi and Blood are mutually dependent as Qi is the commander of Blood and Blood is the mother of Qi. As Qi is the commander of Blood, Qi makes Blood circulate and if Qi stagnates (or if it is deficient), Blood stagnates. Blood needs the power of Qi in order to circulate in the blood vessels and Qi can only circulate throughout the body by 'concentrating' in the blood vessels. That is why it is said in Chinese medicine that 'Qi controls warmth' (here 'warmth' means warm nourishment and motive power), and that 'Blood controls immersion' ('immersion' here means the fluids which provide the vehicle for this nourishment and motive power).[1]

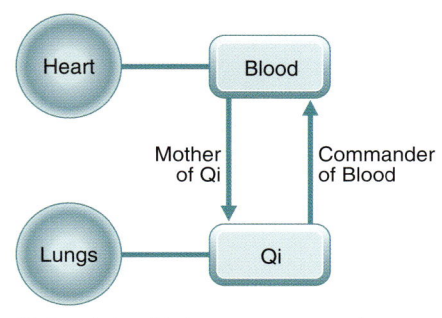

Figure 12.1 Relationship between Heart and Lungs

Blood needs the warmth of Qi to circulate, while Qi needs the 'immersion' (i.e. liquid quality) of Blood as a vehicle to circulate

On the other hand, as Blood is the mother of Qi, Blood nourishes Qi.

The relationship between Qi and Blood in this respect depends on the relationship between Lungs and Heart. Although it is the Heart that drives the Blood through the blood vessels, it relies on the Lungs to provide the Qi for this job. On the other hand, the Lungs rely on Blood from the Heart for nourishment.

Because of this, if Lung-Qi is deficient, it can lead to stagnation of Qi of the Heart, which, in turn, causes stagnation of Blood of the Heart. This manifests with palpitations, pain in the chest and blue lips. Excessive Heart-Fire dries up the Lung fluids, causing a dry cough, dry nose and thirst.

In practice it is common for both Heart- and Lung-Qi to be deficient at the same time as they are so closely related and they are both situated in the chest. Furthermore, Gathering Qi (*Zong Qi*), which collects in the chest, influences both Heart and Lung functions and the circulation of both Qi and Blood. If Gathering Qi is weak, the voice will be weak and the hands will be cold, as Qi and Blood of Lung and Heart will be diminished.

Clinical note

Ren-17 Shanzhong tonifies the Gathering Qi (*Zong Qi*) and both Lungs and Heart

Sadness often depletes both Lung- and Heart-Qi and is manifested with a pulse that is Weak in the Front position of both left and right side.

Clinical note

When sadness affects both Lungs and Heart and the pulse is weak on both Front positions, LU-7 Lieque and HE-7 Shenmen are indicated

Finally, the relationship between Lungs and Heart is seen also in the process leading to Blood. Food-Qi (*Gu Qi*) of the Spleen goes to the Heart to make Blood: however, it ascends to the Heart, through the moving action of Lung-Qi.

Box 12.1 summarizes the interrelationship between the Heart and the Lungs.

Box 12.1 Heart and Lungs

- Heart governs Blood, Lungs govern Qi
- Qi is the commander of Blood, Blood is the mother of Qi
- If Qi circulates well, Blood circulates; if Qi is stagnant, Blood stagnates
- Qi provides warmth to Blood, Blood provides a liquid vehicle for Qi
- Gathering Qi of the chest is influenced by both Lungs and Heart
- Food Qi of the Spleen goes to the Heart to make Blood through the agency of the Lungs

HEART AND LIVER

The interrelationship between Heart and Liver hinges on their roles in respect of Blood. The Heart governs Blood while the Liver stores Blood and regulates its volume: these two activities must be coordinated and harmonized. It is very common for a deficiency of Liver-Blood to cause a deficiency of Heart-Blood as not enough Blood is stored by the Liver to nourish the Heart, causing palpitations and insomnia. In Five-Element terms this situation would be described as the 'Mother not nourishing the Child'.

Clinical note

Liver-Blood deficiency leading to Heart-Blood deficiency is a common cause of postnatal depression. Blood loss from the uterus during childbirth causes Liver-Blood deficiency, which, in turn, induces Heart-Blood deficiency. Deficient Heart-Blood fails to anchor and house the Mind (*Shen*): this causes depression, anxiety, insomnia and palpitations

On the other hand, if Heart-Blood is deficient, this may disrupt the Liver's ability to regulate the Blood and it gives rise to dizziness and excessive dreaming. In Five-Element terms this situation would be described as the 'Child draining the Mother'.

On a mental level, the Heart houses the Mind and influences the mood and spirits of a person, while the Liver is responsible for the smooth flow of Qi. The smooth flow of Qi of the Liver has a deep influence on the emotional state; on an emotional level, the smooth flow of Liver-Qi ensures that the emotions experienced by the patients 'flow' smoothly, that they are not repressed, that they are expressed appropriately, and that they do not take over the person's life: in short, the smooth flow of Liver-Qi on an emotional level ensures that our emotions do not turn into moods to possess us (Fig. 12.2). The Mind (through the Heart) and our emotional state (through the Liver) are interdependent. The Mind controls the emotions in the sense that it recognizes and feels them: this has an influence on the recognition and expression of our emotions in an appropriate way. On the other hand, the Liver, through the smooth flow of its Qi ensures that the emotions flow smoothly and do not affect the Mind in a prolonged way.

A weak Heart and a low Mind may lead to depression and anxiety: this would influence the smooth flow of Liver-Qi and therefore the emotional state. On the other hand, stagnation of Liver-Qi impairs the smooth flow of Qi and constrains the emotions, which may lead to a weakening of the Mind and a lowering of vitality (Fig. 12.3).

Finally, the Heart and Liver are closely linked on a psychological level through the connection between Mind (*Shen*) and Ethereal Soul (*Hun*) (see Fig. 12.3). As described in chapter 7, the Ethereal Soul represents the 'coming and going of the Mind' which means that it gives the Mind 'movement' in the sense of relationships with others, inspiration, vision, capacity for planning, a sense of direction in life, etc. On the other hand, the Mind controls, directs and integrates the psychic material coming from the Ethereal Soul so that this is integrated properly within our psyche (see Fig. 4.14).

Box 12.2 summarizes the interrelationship between the Heart and the Liver.

> **Box 12.2 Heart and Liver**
>
> - The Heart governs Blood, the Liver stores Blood
> - Liver-Blood deficiency often leads to Heart-Blood deficiency
> - The Heart houses the Mind, the Liver houses the Ethereal Soul
> - The Heart (through the Mind) recognizes, controls and integrates emotions; the Liver ensures the smooth flow of emotions
> - The Ethereal Soul (of the Liver) is the 'coming and going' of the Mind (of the Heart)

HEART AND KIDNEYS

The interrelationship of Heart and Kidneys is very important in clinical practice. This relationship has three aspects:

- The mutual assistance of Fire and Water
- The common root of Mind (*Shen*) and Essence (*Jing*)
- The interrelationship of Heart and Kidneys in the menstrual cycle

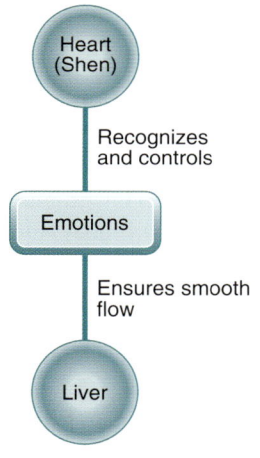

Figure 12.2 Relationship between Heart and Liver with regard to emotions

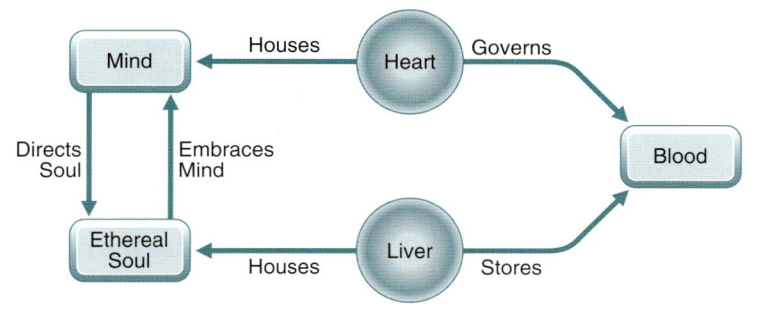

Figure 12.3 Relationship between Mind and Ethereal Soul and emotions

The mutual assistance of Fire and Water

Heart belongs to Fire and is in the Upper Burner: Fire is Yang in nature and corresponds to movement.

The Kidneys belong to Water and are in the Lower Burner: Water is Yin in nature and corresponds to stillness. Heart and Kidneys must be in balance as they represent two fundamental poles of Yang and Yin, Fire and Water. It should be stressed here that although from a Five-Element perspective Fire and Water control each other (i.e. Fire dries up Water and Water douses Fire), in this context, Fire and Water interact with each other and mutually nourish each other. The relationship between Fire and Water highlights the importance of a connection and link between these two Elements and therefore between Heart and Kidneys. In a way, this relationship is similar to that between Lungs and Kidneys: as described in chapter 10, Lung-Qi descends to the Kidneys and the Kidneys respond by 'grabbing' and holding Qi down. Similarly, Heart-Qi descends to the Kidneys, which hold it; likewise, Kidney-Qi ascends to the Heart.

Fire and Water are interdependent and mutually assist each other. In physiology, Fire does not dry up Water and Water does not douse Fire

Heart-Yang descends to warm Kidney-Yin; Kidney-Yin ascends to nourish and cool Heart-Yang. The energy of the Heart and Kidneys is in constant interchange above and below. Chinese medicine refers to this as the 'mutual support of Fire and Water', or the 'mutual support of Heart and Kidneys'.

Clinical note

Ren-15 Jiuwei and Ren-4 Guanyuan promote the communication between Heart and Kidneys

If Kidney-Yang is deficient, the Kidneys cannot transform the fluids, which can overflow towards the top, causing the pattern called 'Water insulting the Heart'. If Kidney-Yin is deficient, it cannot rise to nourish Heart-Yin, which leads to the development of Empty-Heat of the Heart, causing palpitations, mental restlessness, insomnia, red flushed cheekbones, night sweats, and a Red Peeled tongue with a crack in the centre. These two situations are characterized by a loss of contact between Heart and Kidneys.

The common root of Mind (*Shen*) and Essence (*Jing*)

The Heart houses the Mind; the Kidneys store Essence. Mind and Essence have a common root. Essence is the fundamental substance from which the Mind is derived. As we saw in chapter 3, Essence, Qi and Mind represent three different states of condensation of Qi, the Essence being the densest, Qi being more rarefied, and the Mind being the most subtle and immaterial. According to Chinese medicine, Essence and Qi are the essential foundation of the Mind. If Essence and Qi are healthy and flourishing, the Mind will be happy and this will lead to a healthy and happy life. If Essence and Qi are both depleted, then the Mind necessarily will suffer.

Thus a healthy Mind depends on the strength of the Essence, which is stored in the Kidneys. The Pre-Heaven Essence is the foundation of the Mind, while the Post-Heaven Essence provides nourishment for the Mind. An ample supply of Essence is the precondition for a normal activity of the Mind and a vigorous Mind is the precondition for a productive Essence. The relationship between Essence and Mind highlights the Chinese view of the body and mind as an integrated whole, one influencing the other, with both body and mind having a common root in Qi.

If Essence is weak, the Mind will suffer and the person will lack vitality, self-confidence and will-power. If the Mind is perturbed by emotional problems, the Essence will not be directed by the Mind and the person will feel permanently tired and lack motivation (Fig. 12.4).

The relationship between the Mind and Essence reflects also that between the Mind and Will-power (*Zhi*), which is the spiritual aspect of the Kidneys. If the Kidney-Essence is weak, the Will-power will be diminished and this will affect the Mind negatively: the person will be depressed and lacking in vitality, will-power, drive and determination.

The interrelationship of Heart and Kidneys in the menstrual cycle[2]

The interrelationship between Heart and Kidneys is essential for a healthy menstrual cycle. The menstrual

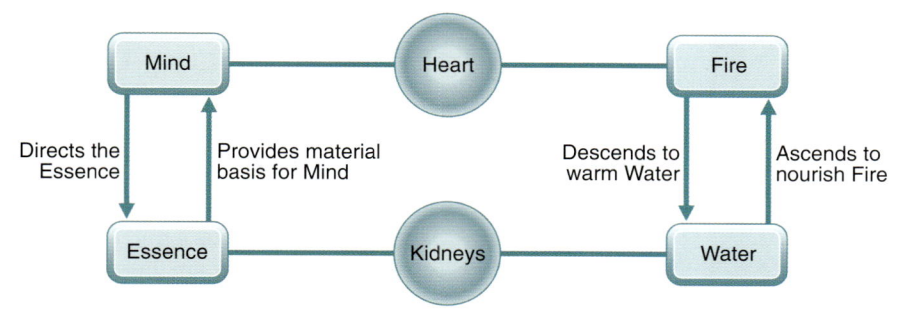

Figure 12.4 Relationship between Mind and Essence

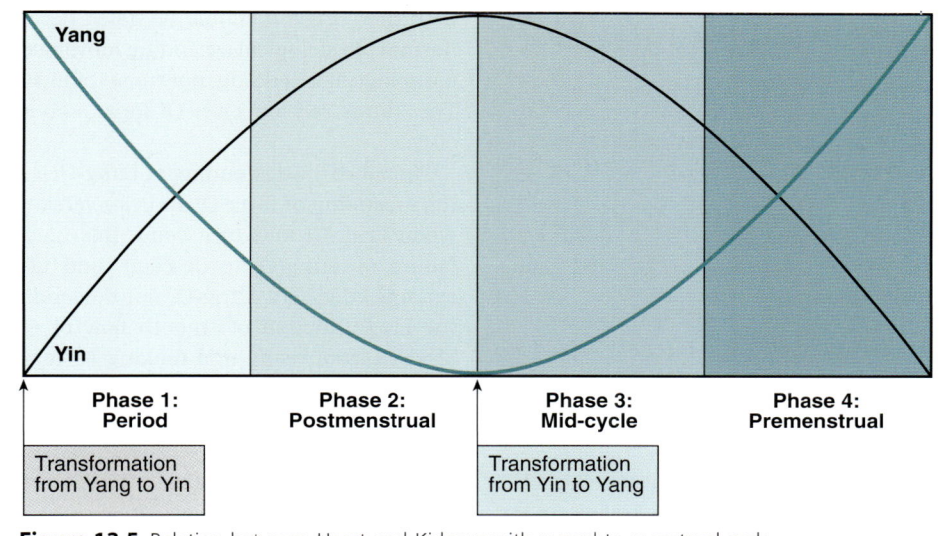

Figure 12.5 Relation between Heart and Kidneys with regard to menstrual cycle

cycle itself is a flow of Kidney-Yin and Kidney-Yang as the Kidneys are the origin of *Tian Gui*, which is the basis for menstrual blood. In the first half of the cycle Yin is growing, reaching a maximum at ovulation; with ovulation, Yin begins to decrease and Yang to increase, reaching a maximum just before the onset of the period. This ebb and flow of Yin and Yang is determined by Kidney-Yin and Kidney-Yang. Thus, the onset of the period marks a rapid change from Yang to Yin (i.e. Yang decreases rapidly), while ovulation marks a rapid change from Yin to Yang (i.e. Yin has reached its maximum). Therefore, the onset of the period and ovulation represent two moments of transformation from Yang to Yin and Yin to Yang, respectively. Whilst the Kidneys provide the material Yin and Yang basis for such ebb and flow, the Heart provides the impetus for the transformation of Yang to Yin and vice versa. Moreover, Heart-Qi and Heart-Blood descend during the period to promote the downwards flow of blood and during ovulation to promote the discharge of the eggs (Fig. 12.5).

Box 12.3 summarizes the interrelationship between the Heart and the Kidneys.

LIVER AND LUNGS

There are two aspects to the relationship between Liver and Lungs:

- The relationship between Lung-Qi and Liver-Blood
- The relationship between the descending of Lung-Qi and the ascending of Liver-Qi

Box 12.3 Heart and Kidneys

- The mutual assistance of Fire and Water
  - The Heart pertains to Fire and is in the Upper Burner; the Kidneys pertain to Water and are in the Lower Burner
  - Fire and Water communicate with each and mutually assist each other
  - Heart-Yang descends to the Kidneys, Kidney-Yin ascends to the Heart
- The common root of Mind and Essence
  - The Heart houses the Mind, the Kidneys house the Essence and Will-power (*Zhi*)
  - The Essence is the basis for a stable and happy Mind; the state of the Mind influences the Essence
  - The Mind of the Heart and the Will-power of the Kidneys mutually affect each other
- The interrelationship of Heart and Kidneys in the menstrual cycle
  - The interrelationship between Heart and Kidneys is essential for a healthy menstrual cycle
  - The Kidneys are the origin of menstrual blood and are the source of the ebb and flow of Yin and Yang in the menstrual cycle
  - The Heart controls the discharge of menstrual blood at menstruation and of eggs at ovulation
  - The Heart controls the transformation of Yang to Yin with the period and of Yin to Yang with ovulation

The relationship between Lung-Qi and Liver-Blood

The relationship between Lungs and Liver reflects the relationship between Qi and Blood. The Lungs govern Qi, the Liver regulates and stores Blood, and the two rely on each other to perform their respective functions. The Liver relies on Lung-Qi to regulate Blood as Lung-Qi drives Blood in the blood vessels; on the other hand, as Blood is the mother of Qi, Liver-Blood provides the moisture and nourishment for Lung-Qi to circulate properly (Fig. 12.6, left).

The relationship between the descending of Lung-Qi and the ascending of Liver-Qi

The relationship between Lung-Qi and Liver-Qi is based on the direction of flow of their respective Qi: Lung-Qi descends while Liver-Qi ascends (Fig 12.6, right). It is said, in fact, that 'the Liver is on the left and its Qi ascends, the Lungs are on the right and their Qi descends' ('left' and 'right' here should not be understood in a Western anatomical sense).

Although Liver-Qi flows in all directions, in this context it ascends to coordinate the movement of Qi with the Lungs. It should be noted here that this is a normal physiological ascending movement and not the pathological ascending movement of Liver-Yang rising. The Lungs rely on Liver-Qi for a smooth movement of Qi.

Therefore the descending of Lung-Qi is dependent on the ascending of Liver-Qi and vice versa. In some cases when Liver-Qi fails to ascend, this may be due to a failure of Lung-Qi to descend, and vice versa. For example, deficient Lung-Qi not descending can affect the Liver function of smooth flow of Qi, preventing Liver-Qi from rising and making it stagnate. In such cases, a person will experience listlessness (from deficiency of Qi), depression (from stagnation of Liver-Qi), cough and hypochondrial pain. This situation corresponds to 'Metal not controlling Wood' from the Five-Element point of view.

On the other hand, if Liver-Qi stagnates in the chest and fails to ascend to the Lungs, it can obstruct the flow of Lung-Qi, impairing the descending of its Qi and causing cough, breathlessness and hypochondrial distension. This situation corresponds to 'Wood insulting Metal' according to the Five Elements (see Figs 12.6 and 3.15).

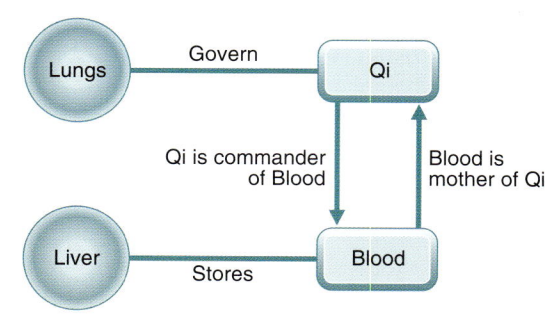

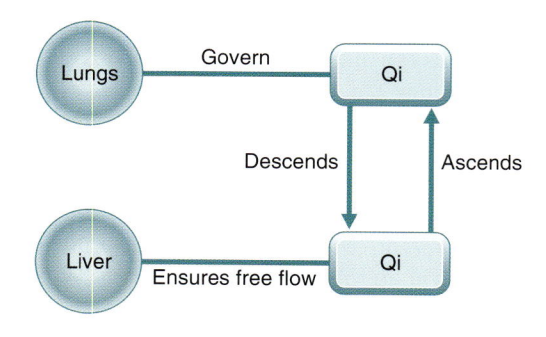

Figure 12.6 Relationship between Liver and Lungs

Box 12.4 summarizes the interrelationship between the Liver and the Lungs.

> **Box 12.4 Liver and Lungs**
>
> - The relationship between Lung-Qi and Liver-Blood
>   - The Lungs govern Qi; the Liver stores Blood
>   - The Liver relies on Lung-Qi to regulate Blood; Lung-Qi relies on the moisture and nourishment of Liver-Blood
> - The relationship between the descending of Lung-Qi and the ascending of Liver-Qi
>   - Lung-Qi descends, Liver-Qi ascends
>   - The descending of Lung-Qi and ascending of Liver-Qi rely on each other
>   - Lung-Qi needs to descend for Liver-Qi to ascend and vice versa

LIVER AND SPLEEN

Liver and Spleen have a very close relationship, disturbances of which frequently occur in clinical practice. Under normal circumstances, Liver-Qi, with its smooth flow, helps the Spleen to transform, separate and transport. Furthermore, Liver-Qi ensures the smooth flow of bile, which also helps digestion. If Liver-Qi is normal, digestion will be good and the Spleen will be aided in the performance of its function. By ensuring the smooth flow of Qi all over the body and in all directions, the Liver ensures that Spleen-Qi flows upwards, the normal direction of Spleen-Qi (Fig. 12.7).

Stagnant Liver-Qi disrupts the Spleen's ability to transform and transport food and fluids and, in particular, the upward flow of Spleen-Qi. This manifests as abdominal distension, hypochondrial pain and loose stools. This situation corresponds to 'Wood overacting on Earth' according to the theory of the Five Elements, and is a common clinical finding.

As usual there is a reciprocal relationship, and the ascending of Spleen-Qi also aids the Liver's smooth flow of Qi. If Spleen-Qi is deficient and its transformation and transportation impaired, food will not be digested properly and will be retained in the Middle Burner, often also with the formation of Dampness. This in turn may affect the circulation of Liver-Qi and impair the smooth flow of Qi in the Middle Burner, causing abdominal distension, hypochondrial pain and irritability. This situation corresponds to 'Earth insulting Wood' according to the theory of the Five Elements (Fig. 12.8).

> **Clinical note**
>
> LIV-14 Qimen harmonizes Liver and Stomach; LIV-13 Zhangmen harmonizes Liver and Spleen

Box 12.5 summarizes the interrelationship between the Liver and the Spleen.

> **Box 12.5 Liver and Spleen**
>
> - The Liver stores Blood; the Spleen makes Blood
> - The free flow of Liver-Qi helps the Spleen's function of transformation and transportation
> - The ascending of Spleen-Qi helps the free flow of Liver-Qi

LIVER AND KIDNEYS

The relationship between Liver and Kidneys, of considerable clinical significance, is based on the mutual exchange between Blood and Essence. Liver-Blood nourishes and replenishes Kidney-Essence, and this in turn contributes to the making of Blood (because the Essence produces bone marrow, which makes Blood). The Kidneys also contribute to making Blood through the action of the Original Qi (ch. 3). This is why it is said that 'Liver and Kidneys have a common origin' and 'Essence and Blood have a common source'. Moreover, Kidney-Yin nourishes Liver-Yin (which includes Liver-Blood), in agreement with the Five-Element theory which states that 'Water nourishes Wood'.

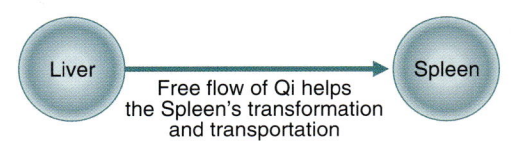

Figure 12.7 Free flow of Liver-Qi influence on Spleen

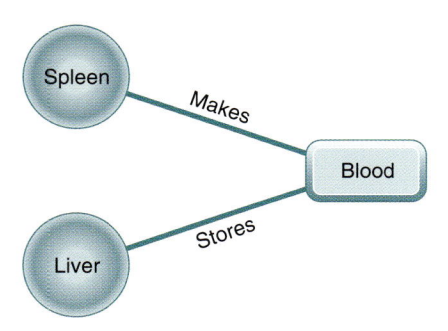

Figure 12.8 Relationship between Liver and Spleen

Deficient Kidney-Essence may lead to deficiency of Blood, with symptoms of dizziness, blurred vision and tinnitus. If Kidney-Yin is deficient it fails to nourish Liver-Yin. Deficient Liver-Yin leads to hyperactivity and rising of Liver-Yang, causing blurred vision, tinnitus, dizziness, irritability, and headaches.

Deficient Liver-Blood may cause weakness of Kidney-Essence, because this will lack the nourishment of Liver-Blood: the result will be deafness, tinnitus and nocturnal emissions (Fig. 12.9).

The relationship between Liver and Kidneys is particularly important in gynaecology. The Liver stores the Blood that supplies the Uterus with Blood, while the Kidneys are the origin of *Tian Gui*, which is the substance from which menstrual blood derives (Fig. 12.10). Therefore, these two organs are of paramount importance for the woman to have a regular and normal menstrual cycle. The Liver and Kidney channels are especially important in gynaecology because they are closely linked with the Directing and Penetrating Vessels (*Ren Mai* and *Chong Mai*).

Box 12.6 summarizes the interrelationship between the Liver and the Kidneys.

Box 12.6 Liver and Kidneys

- The Liver stores Blood and the Kidneys store Essence
- Liver-Blood replenishes the Essence
- The Essence contributes to making Blood, which is stored by the Liver
- The Original Qi of the Kidneys also contributes to making Blood
- In gynaecology, the Kidneys are the origin of *Tian Gui* and menstrual blood, while the Liver provides Blood to the Uterus
- Both Liver and Kidney channels are closely connected to the Directing and Penetrating Vessels (*Ren Mai* and *Chong Mai*)

SPLEEN AND LUNGS

The Spleen and Lungs mutually assist each other in their functions. The Spleen extracts the refined Essence of Food and sends it up to the Lungs where it combines with air to form Gathering Qi (*Zong Qi*). In this way, Spleen-Qi benefits Lung-Qi, as it provides Food-Qi from which Qi is formed. In its turn, the Spleen relies on the descending of Lung-Qi to help in the transformation and transportation of food and Body Fluids (Fig. 12.11). Thus Lung-Qi has an influence on Spleen-Qi. Hence the saying: 'The Spleen is the origin of Qi and the Lungs are the axis of Qi'.

If Spleen-Qi is deficient, then Food-Qi (*Food Qi*) will be deficient and the production of Qi, particularly that of the Lungs, will be impaired. This will result in tiredness, weak limbs, breathlessness and a weak voice. The theory of the Five Elements describes this as 'Earth not producing Metal'.

Another important consequence of Spleen deficiency is that the fluids will not be transformed and may accumulate to form Phlegm, which usually settles in the Lungs, impairing the Lung functions. Hence the

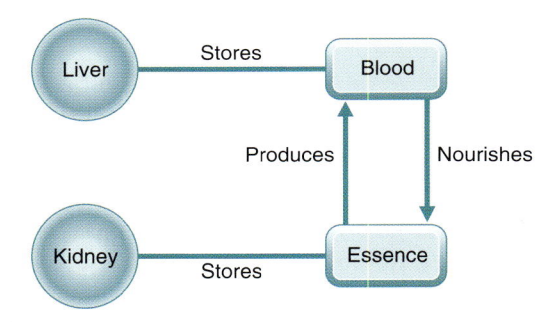

Figure 12.9 Relationship between Liver and Kidneys

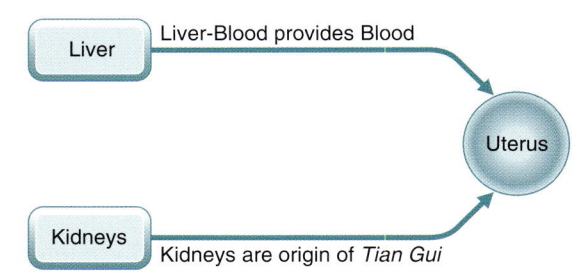

Figure 12.10 Relationship between Liver and Kidneys with regard to menstruation

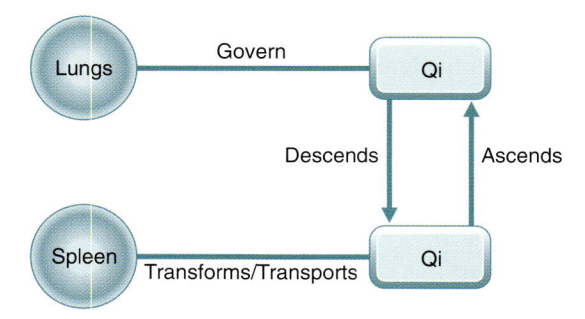

Figure 12.11 Relationship between Spleen and Lungs

saying 'The Spleen is the origin of Phlegm and the Lungs store it'.

If Lung-Qi is weak and its descending impaired, the Spleen cannot transform and transport the fluids, causing oedema.

Box 12.7 summarizes the interrelationship between the Spleen and the Lungs.

> **Box 12.7 Spleen and Lungs**
> - The Spleen makes Qi; the Lungs govern Qi
> - Spleen-Qi ascends, Lung-Qi descends
> - Spleen-Qi transports Food-Qi to the Lungs: hence the Lungs are dependent on ascending of Spleen-Qi
> - The descending of Lung-Qi helps the Spleen's transformation and transportation of food essence
> - Deficiency of Spleen-Qi may lead to Phlegm, which affects the Lungs

SPLEEN AND KIDNEYS

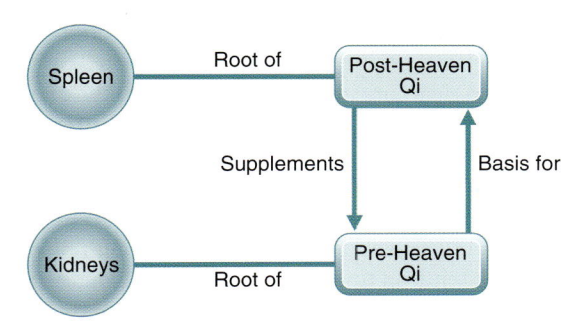

The relationship between Spleen and Kidneys is one of mutual nourishment. The Spleen is the Root of Post-Heaven Qi, while the Kidneys are the Root of Pre-Heaven Qi (Fig. 12.12). As mentioned before, the Post-Heaven and Pre-Heaven Qi mutually support one another. The Post-Heaven Qi continually replenishes the Pre-Heaven Qi with the Qi produced from food, and the Pre-Heaven Qi assists in the production of Qi by providing the heat necessary for digestion and transformation (through the Fire of the Gate of Life).

If Spleen-Qi is deficient, not enough Qi will be produced to replenish Kidney-Essence; this may cause tiredness, lack of appetite, tinnitus, dizziness and lower backache.

If Kidney-Yang is deficient, the Fire of the Gate of Life cannot warm the Spleen in its activity of transformation and transportation, causing diarrhoea and chilliness. This is termed by the Five-Element theory 'Fire not producing Earth'.

The Spleen and Kidney also assist each other in the transformation and transportation of Body Fluids: Kidney-Yang provides the heat necessary to the Spleen in order to transform and transport fluids. Spleen-Qi helps the Kidneys in transforming and excreting fluids. If Spleen-Qi cannot transform and transport the fluids, these may accumulate to form Dampness, which can impair the Kidney function of governing Water, further aggravating the Dampness. On the other hand, if Kidney-Yang is deficient, the Fire of the Gate of Life cannot provide the heat necessary for the Spleen to transform the fluids and this can cause Dampness or oedema, diarrhoea and chilliness.

Box 12.8 summarizes the interrelationship between the Spleen and the Kidneys.

> **Box 12.8 Spleen and Kidneys**
> - The Spleen is the Root of Post-Heaven Qi, the Kidneys are the Root of Pre-Heaven Qi
> - Kidney-Yang provides the heat to the Spleen necessary to transport and transform food essence
> - Spleen-Qi helps the Kidneys' transformation and excretion of fluids

LUNGS AND KIDNEYS

The Lungs and Kidneys are related in many ways. First of all, the Lungs send Qi and fluids down to the Kidneys, and the Kidneys respond by holding the Qi down and evaporating some of the fluids and sending the resulting vapour back up to the Lungs to keep them moist. The relationship between Lungs and Kidneys can therefore be analysed in terms of Qi or fluids:

> - The relationship between Lungs and Kidneys with regard to Qi
> - The relationship between Lungs and Kidneys with regard to fluids

The relationship between Lungs and Kidneys with regard to Qi

In terms of Qi, the Lungs govern Qi and respiration and send Qi down to the Kidneys. The Kidneys respond by holding Qi down. Thus, Lungs and Kidneys must communicate with and respond to each other to achieve

Figure 12.12 Relationship between Spleen and Kidneys

proper breathing. This relationship is also mirrored in the relationship between Gathering Qi in the chest (which pertains to the Lungs) and Original Qi in the lower abdomen (which belongs to the Kidneys). Gathering Qi has to flow down to obtain nourishment from the Original Qi, while this has to flow up to the chest to assist in the production of Qi and Blood. Thus, the Lungs' function of governing Qi and respiration is dependent on the Kidneys' function of reception of Qi and vice versa.

If the Kidneys are weak and their function of reception of Qi is impaired, the Kidneys will fail to hold Qi down and Qi will flow back up to the chest, obstructing the Lungs' descending function and causing breathlessness (more on inhalation), cough and asthma.

Clinical note

The points to stimulate the descending of Lung-Qi to the Kidneys and the Kidneys' grasping of Qi are LU-7 Lieque, Ren-4 Guanyuan and KI-13 Qixue

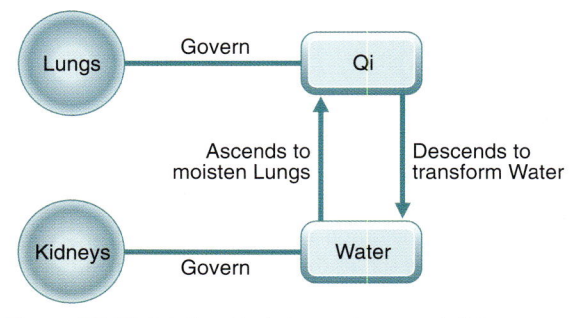

The relationship between Lungs and Kidneys with regard to fluids

In terms of fluids, the Lungs control the Water passages and send fluids down to the Kidneys; the Kidneys respond by evaporating some of the fluids and sending them back up to the Lungs to keep them moist (Fig. 12.13). This is why it is said in Chinese medicine that the 'Kidneys govern Water and the Lungs are the Upper Source of Water'.

If Lung-Qi is deficient, it cannot send fluids downwards and the Lungs cannot communicate with the Kidneys and Bladder, causing incontinence or retention of urine. If Kidney-Yang is deficient and cannot transform and excrete the fluids in the Lower Burner, they may accumulate to cause oedema, which will impair the descending and diffusing of Lung-Qi. Deficiency of Kidney-Yin results in deficiency of fluids in the Lower Burner. The consequence of this is that fluids fail to rise to keep the Lungs moist, thus causing deficiency of Lung-Yin. The symptoms of this are a dry throat at night, a dry cough, night sweating and a feeling of heat in the palms and soles of feet.

Box 12.9 summarizes the interrelationship between the Lungs and the Kidneys.

Box 12.9 Lungs and Kidneys

- Relationship between Lungs and Kidneys with regard to Qi
  - The Lungs send Qi down to the Kidneys, which 'hold' it: this makes breathing normal
  - Gathering Qi of the chest (related to the Lungs) communicates with Original Qi in the abdomen (related to the Kidneys)
- Relationship between Lungs and Kidneys with regard to fluids
  - Lung-Qi sends fluids down to the Kidneys
  - Kidney-Yang evaporates some and sends resulting 'vapour' back up to the Lungs to moisten them

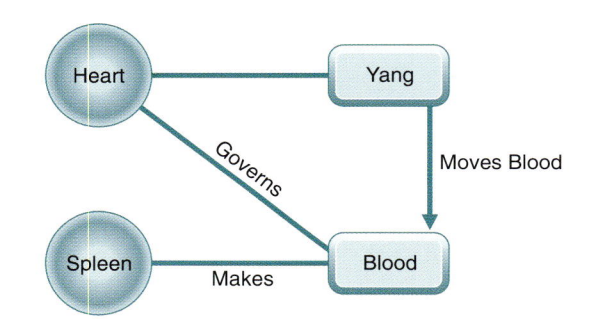

Figure 12.14 Relationship between Spleen and Heart

SPLEEN AND HEART

Spleen and Heart are interrelated because of their connection with Blood. The Spleen makes Blood (because it provides the Essence of Food, which is the basis for Blood) and it is therefore of paramount importance to the Heart, which governs Blood (Fig. 12.14). If Spleen-Qi is deficient and cannot make enough Blood, this will often lead to deficiency of Heart-Blood, with symptoms of dizziness, poor memory, insomnia and palpitations.

Figure 12.13 Relationship between Lungs and Kidneys

Box 12.10 Spleen and Heart

- The Spleen makes Blood; the Heart governs Blood
- Spleen-Qi transports Food-Qi to the Heart where it is transformed into Blood
- Heart-Blood nourishes the Spleen
- The descending of Heart-Qi helps the Spleen's transformation and transportation of food essences

On the other hand, Heart-Yang pushes Blood in the vessels and Heart-Blood nourishes the Spleen. If Heart-Yang is deficient it will fail to push the Blood in the vessels and the Spleen will suffer as it makes and controls Blood.

Box 12.10 summarizes the interrelationship between the Spleen and the Heart.

Learning outcomes

In this section you will have learned:
- Heart and Lungs
  - Heart governs Blood, Lungs govern Qi
  - Qi is the commander of Blood, Blood is the mother of Qi
  - If Qi circulates well, Blood circulates; if Qi is stagnant, Blood stagnates
  - Qi provides warmth to Blood; Blood provides a liquid vehicle for Qi
  - Gathering Qi of the chest is influenced by both Lungs and Heart
  - Food Qi of the Spleen goes to the Heart to make Blood via the agency of the Lungs
- Heart and Liver
  - Heart governs Blood, Liver stores Blood
  - Liver-Blood deficiency often leads to Heart-Blood deficiency
  - The Heart houses the Mind, the Liver houses the Ethereal Soul
  - The Heart (through the Mind) recognizes, controls and integrates emotions; the Liver ensures the smooth flow of emotions
  - The Ethereal Soul (of the Liver) is the 'coming and going' of the Mind (of the Heart)
- Heart and Kidneys
  - The relationship between Fire and Water
  - The interrelationship of the Heart and Kidneys in the menstrual cycle
  - The common root of Mind and Essence
- Liver and Lungs
  - The relationship between Lung-Qi and Liver-Blood
  - The Lungs govern Qi, the Liver stores Blood
  - The Liver relies on Lung-Qi to regulate blood: Lung-Qi relies on the moisture and nourishment of Liver-Blood
  - The relationship between the descending of Lung-Qi and the ascending of Liver-Qi
  - Lung-Qi descends, Liver-Qi ascends
  - The descending of Lung-Qi and Liver-Qi rely on each other: Lung-Qi needs to descend for Liver-Qi to ascend and vice versa
- Liver and Spleen
  - The Liver stores Blood, the Spleen makes Blood
  - The free flow of Liver-Qi helps the Spleen's function of transformation and transportation
  - The ascending of Spleen-Qi helps the free flow of Liver-Qi
- Liver and Kidneys
  - The Liver stores Blood and the Kidneys store Essence
  - Liver-Blood replenishes the Essence
  - The Essence contributes to making Blood, which is stored by the Liver
  - The Original Qi of the Kidneys also contributes to making Blood
  - In gynaecology, the Kidneys are the origin of *Tian Gui* and menstrual blood, while the Liver provides Blood to the Uterus
  - Both Liver and Kidney channels are closely connected to the Directing and Penetrating Vessels (*Ren Mai* and *Chong Mai*)
- Spleen and Lungs
  - The Spleen makes Qi, the Lungs govern Qi
  - Spleen-Qi ascends, Lung-Qi descends
  - Spleen-Qi transports Food-Qi to the Lungs: therefore function of the Lungs is dependent on ascending of Spleen-Qi
  - The descending of Lung-Qi helps the Spleen's transformation and transportation of food essence
  - Deficiency of Spleen-Qi may lead to the formation of Phlegm, which affects the Lungs
- Spleen and Kidneys
  - The Spleen is the root of Post-Heaven Qi; the Kidneys are the root of Pre-Heaven Qi
  - Kidney-Yang provides the heat to the Spleen necessary to transport and transform food essence
  - Spleen-Qi helps the Kidneys' function of the transformation and excretion of fluids
- Lungs and Kidneys
  - Relationship between the Lungs and Kidneys with regard to Qi
    - The Lungs send Qi down to the Kidneys, which 'hold' it: this makes breathing normal
    - Gathering Qi of the chest (related to the Lungs) communicates with Original Qi in the abdomen (related to the Kidneys)
  - Relationship between the Lungs and Kidneys with regard to fluids
    - Lung-Qi sends fluids down to the Kidneys
    - Kidney-Yang evaporates some and sends the resulting 'vapour' back up to the Lungs to moisten them
- Spleen and Heart
  - The Spleen makes Blood, the Heart governs Blood
  - Spleen-Qi transports Food-Qi to the heart where it is transformed into Blood
  - Heart-Blood nourishes the Spleen
  - The descending of Heart-Qi helps the Spleen's transformation and transportation of food essences

Self-assessment questions

Heart and Lungs

1. Which two vital substances do the Heart and Lungs govern? How does this affect the relationship between the two organs?
2. Explain the relationship between Qi and Blood.
3. If Lung-Qi is deficient, what can happen to Heart-Qi?
4. How can the pattern of Excessive Heart Fire affect the Lungs?
5. Why is it common for both Heart- and Lung-Qi to be deficient at the same time?
6. How does Gathering Qi affect the function of the Heart and Lungs?
7. What emotion depletes both Heart- and Lung-Qi?

Heart and Liver

1. Explain the relationship between the Heart and Liver in terms of their action upon Blood.
2. What effect can Liver-Blood deficiency have on the Heart?
3. How may deficient Heart-Blood affect the Liver? What symptoms might this situation give rise to?
4. Which psychological aspects of the person can the Liver and Heart be said to 'house'?
5. Explain how both the Heart and the Liver have an effect upon the emotions and psychological state.

Heart and Kidneys

1. In terms of the theory of the Five Elements, which elements do the Heart and Kidneys correspond to? Explain the relationship of these two elements:
   i. from a Five-Element perspective
   ii. from an organ perspective.
2. Which Heart pattern can develop if Kidney-Yang is deficient?
3. Which Heart pattern can develop if Kidney-Yin is deficient?
4. Explain how the Mind and Essence have a common root.
5. What can happen to the Mind if a person's Essence is weak?
6. What can happen to the Essence if a person's Mind is disturbed by emotional problems? How might this manifest?
7. What is the spiritual aspect of the Kidney organ?
8. Explain how the relationship between the Mind and Essence reflects the relationship between the Mind and the Will-power. (For example, how will the Will-power be affected if the Essence is weak, and vice versa?)
9. Describe what happens to Kidney-Yin and Kidney-Yang during the menstrual cycle.
10. In which two ways does the Heart play a role in the menstrual cycle?

Liver and Lungs

1. The relationship between the Liver and Lungs reflects the relationship between which two vital substances? Explain.
2. How does the Liver rely on Lung-Qi to regulate Blood?
3. How does Liver-Blood affect Lung-Qi?
4. What is the direction of the flow of Lung-Qi and Liver-Qi?
5. Explain how deficient Lung-Qi will affect the Liver function of the smooth flow of Qi. What situation does this correspond to in Five-Element terms?

Liver and Spleen

1. In what two ways does the Liver help the Spleen to transform, separate and transport food and fluids?
2. What is the normal direction of Spleen-Qi?
3. What symptoms can occur if stagnant Liver-Qi disrupts the Spleen's ability to transform food and fluids? What situation does this correspond to in Five-Element terms?
4. How can deficient Spleen-Qi affect Liver-Qi? Which symptoms can this cause? Which Five-Element pattern does this situation correspond to?
5. Explain how both the Liver and Spleen have a relationship with Blood.

Liver and Kidneys

1. Explain how the relationship between the Liver and Kidneys is based on the mutual exchange between Blood and Essence.
2. What is the relationship between Kidney-Yin and Liver-Yin and Blood? Describe this relationship in Five-Element terms.
3. If Liver-Blood is deficient, what can happen to Kidney-Essence? What symptoms an occur in this situation?
4. If Kidney-Yin is deficient, what an happen to Liver-Yin and Liver-Blood? What symptoms can occur in this situation?
5. Explain how both the Liver and Kidneys play a role in ensuring a regular menstrual cycle.
6. Which extraordinary channels are the Liver and Kidney channels closely linked to?

Spleen and Lungs

1. Explain the role played by the Spleen and Lungs in the formation of Gathering Qi.
2. What is the direction of Lung-Qi? How does this direction of Lung-Qi aid the action of Spleen-Qi?
3. If Spleen-Qi is deficient, how can Lung-Qi be affected? In this situation, what symptoms may occur? In Five-Element terms, how is this situation described?
4. Describe the relationship the Spleen and Lungs have with Phlegm.

Spleen and Kidneys

1. The Spleen is the root of Post-Heaven Qi while the Kidneys are the root of Pre-Heaven Qi. How do Post- and Pre-Heaven Qi mutually support each other?
2. How can a deficiency of Spleen-Qi affect Kidney-Essence? What symptoms may occur in this situation?
3. What can happen to Spleen-Qi if Kidney-Yang is deficient? In this situation, what symptoms may occur? In Five-Element terms, how is this situation described?
4. Describe the role played by the Spleen and Kidneys with regards to Body Fluids.

Lungs and Kidneys

1. Explain how the Lungs and Kidneys are related in terms of Qi and fluids.
2. Explain the relationship of Gathering Qi and Original Qi.
3. What happens to the Kidney organ if Lung-Qi is deficient? What symptoms may occur?
4. How will Kidney-Yang deficiency affect the Lungs? What symptoms may occur?
5. How will a deficiency of Kidney-Yin affect the Lungs? What symptoms may occur?

Spleen and Heart

1. Explain the role the Spleen and Heart play with regards to Blood.
2. If Spleen-Qi is deficient and cannot make enough blood, what can happen to the Heart?

See p. 1258 for answers

END NOTES

1. Beijing College of Traditional Chinese Medicine 1980 Practical Chinese Medicine (*Shi Yong Zhong Yi Xue* 实用中医学), Beijing Publishing House, Beijing, p. 51.
2. Although the role of the Kidneys and Heart in regulating the menstrual cycle is recognized in traditional Chinese medicine, the more specific aspects of the influence of the Heart on the discharge of menstrual blood and eggs is modern. This account is based on personal communications from Dr Xia Gui Cheng, former director of the Gynaecology Department of the Affiliated Hospital for Traditional Chinese Medicine in Nanjing.

SECTION 2

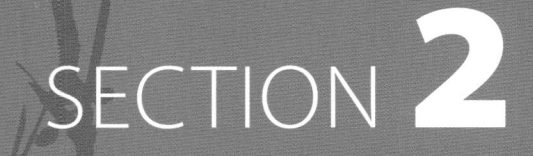

The functions of the Yang organs

INTRODUCTION

The Yang organs are called *Fu* in Chinese. *Fu* can mean 'seat of government', 'administrative centre' or 'palace'. Unlike the Yin organs, which store precious essences, the Yang organs do not store but are constantly filled and emptied. Also, they do not deal with pure substances as the Yin organs do, but with impure ones (e.g. food, impure fluids, urine, stools, etc.).

In the theory of the Internal Organs (*Zangfu*), the physiology and pathology of the Yin organs has predominance over that of the Yang organs. For example, the various Five-Element associations of colours, emotions, odours, sounds, etc., are always associated with their relevant Yin, rather than Yang, organs (e.g. the scorched smell refers to the Heart rather than to the Small Intestine). One reason for this predominance is that many of the functions of the Yang organs are subsumed under those of the Yin organs (not necessarily its coupled organ within Yin–Yang). For example, many of the stomach and intestinal digestive functions fall under the umbrella of the Spleen and Liver. Also, from the Yin–Yang point of view, the Small Intestine is associated with the Heart and the Large Intestine with the Lungs; however, the free flow of Liver-Qi has an important influence on both the Small and Large Intestine and stagnation of Qi in the Intestines is almost always associated with Liver-Qi stagnation. Similarly, the Spleen also exerts an important influence on the Intestines: for example, a condition of Cold in the Intestines causing loose stools and abdominal pain is nearly always associated with Cold in the Spleen.

The six Yang organs include the Triple Burner, which is an entity peculiar to Chinese medicine. Whilst there is some correspondence between, say, the Chinese 'Stomach' and the 'stomach' of modern medicine, the Triple Burner has no equivalent in modern medicine.

It should be stressed that, although from the point of view of organ physiology and pathology the Yin organs are more important than the Yang ones, from the point of view of channels all 12 channels are equally important.

From the point of view of physiology and pathology, the Yin organs are more important than the Yang ones; from the point of view of treatment, all channels, Yin and Yang, are equally important

The functions of the Yang organs will be discussed under the following headings:

1. The Functions of the Stomach

1. Controls 'receiving'
2. Controls the 'rotting and ripening' of food
3. Controls the transportation of food essences
4. Controls the descending of Qi
5. Is the origin of fluids
6. Other aspects:
   a) Mental aspect
   b) Dreams
   c) Relationship with the Spleen

2. The Functions of the Small Intestine

1. Controls receiving and transforming
2. Separates fluids
3. Other aspects
   a) Mental aspect
   b) Dreams
   c) Relationship with the Heart

3. The Functions of the Large Intestine

1. Controls passage and conduction
2. Transforms stools and reabsorbs fluids
3. Other aspects:
   a) Mental aspect
   b) Dreams
   c) Relationship with the Lungs

4. The Functions of the Gall Bladder

1. Stores and excretes bile
2. Controls decisiveness
3. Controls the sinews
4. Other aspects
   a) Mental aspect
   b) Dreams
   c) Relationship with the Liver

5. The Functions of the Bladder

1. Removes Water by Qi transformation
2. Other aspects
   a) Mental aspect
   b) Dreams
   c) Relationship with the Kidneys

6. The Functions of the Triple Burner

1. Functions of the Triple Burner
   a) It mobilizes the Original Qi (*Yuan Qi*)
   b) It controls the transportation and penetration of Qi
   c) It controls the Water Passages and the excretion of fluids
2. Four views of the Triple Burner
   a) The Triple Burner as one the six Yang organs
   b) The Triple Burner as a 'mobilizer of the Original Qi'
   c) The Triple Burner as the three divisions of the body:
      i. the Upper Burner is like a mist
      ii. the Middle Burner is like a maceration chamber
      iii. the Lower Burner is like a ditch
   d) The Triple Burner as body cavities
3. Other aspects
   a) Mental aspect
   b) Dreams
   c) Relationship with the Pericardium

The Functions of the Stomach

SECTION 2　PART 2　13

Key contents

The Stomach controls 'receiving'

The Stomach controls the 'rotting and ripening' of food

The Stomach controls the transportation of food essences

The Stomach controls the descending of Qi

The Stomach is the origin of fluids

Other aspects of the Stomach
Mental aspect
Dreams
Relationship with the Spleen

- Other aspects of the Stomach
  - Mental aspect
  - Dreams
  - Relationship with the Spleen

THE STOMACH CONTROLS RECEIVING

The functions of the Stomach are summarized in Box 13.1.

Box 13.1 Functions of the Stomach

- Controls 'receiving'
- Controls the rotting and ripening of food
- Controls the transportation of food essences
- Controls the descending of Qi
- Is the origin of fluids

The Stomach is the most important of all the Yang organs. Together with the Spleen, it is known as the 'Root of Post-Heaven Qi' because it is the origin of all Qi and Blood produced after birth (as opposed to the Pre-Heaven Qi, which is formed at conception). The 'Simple Questions' says in chapter 8: *'The Spleen and Stomach are the officials in charge of food storage and from whom the 5 flavours are derived.'*[1]

In chapter 11 it says: *'The Stomach is the Sea of water and grains and the great Source of nourishment for the 6 Yang organs. The 5 flavours enter the mouth to be stored in the Stomach for nourishing the 5 Yin organs ... and thus the flavours of the 5 Yin and 6 Yang organs are all derived from the Stomach.'*[2]

The functions of the Stomach and other aspects will be discussed under the following headings:

- The Stomach controls 'receiving'
- The Stomach controls the 'rotting and ripening' of food
- The Stomach controls the transportation of food essences
- The Stomach controls the descending of Qi
- The Stomach is the origin of fluids

Food and drink enter the mouth and then reach the stomach via the pharynx and oesophagus. Therefore the Stomach 'receives' food and drink and keeps them down. 'Receiving' here does not merely indicate the obvious fact that the Stomach receives ingested food and drink but it implies also that the Stomach holds these down too.

Because the Stomach receives food and drink it is called the 'Great Granary' and also the 'Sea of Food and Drink'. Chapter 60 of the 'Spiritual Axis' says: *'Human beings receive Qi from food and food is received by the Stomach: hence the Stomach is the Sea of Qi and Blood and of Food and Drink.'*[3]

The Stomach function of receiving also has a relationship to the appetite: a good, healthy appetite indicates a strong Stomach 'receiving'; a poor appetite indicates a weak Stomach 'receiving'; and the total absence of appetite denotes the complete collapse of the Stomach 'receiving'. Belching, nausea and vomiting also indicate a weak Stomach 'receiving' and Stomach-Qi 'rebelling' upwards.

> **Clinical note**
>
> The best point to stimulate the receiving o the Stomach is Ren-12 Zhongwan

This function of the Stomach is summarized in Box 13.2.

> **Box 13.2 The Stomach controls 'receiving'**
>
> - The Stomach receives food and drink and holds them down
> - 'Receiving' is also related to the appetite
> - The Stomach is called the 'Great Granary' and the 'Sea of Food and Drink'

THE STOMACH CONTROLS THE 'ROTTING AND RIPENING' OF FOOD

The Stomach transforms ingested food and drink by a process of fermentation described as 'rotting and ripening'. The 'Classic of Difficulties' in chapter 31 says: *'The Middle Burner is in the Stomach ... and controls the rotting and ripening of food and drink.'*[4] This activity of the Stomach prepares the ground for the Spleen to separate and extract the refined essence from food. Because of the Stomach function of rotting and ripening, the Middle Burner is often compared to a bubbling cauldron. After transformation in the Stomach, food is passed down to the Small Intestine for further separation and absorption.

The Stomach's role in transforming food means that the Stomach, together with the Spleen, is the origin of Qi and Blood in the body, and for this reason it is called the 'Root of Post-Heaven Qi'.

The 'Simple Questions' in chapter 19 says: *'The 5 Yin organs all derive Qi from the Stomach, and thus the Stomach is the root of the 5 Yin organs.'*[5]

Throughout the development of traditional Chinese medical theory, the Stomach was taken to be the origin of the Qi of the body. 'Stomach-Qi' became synonymous with a good prognosis and life itself, while 'absence of Stomach-Qi' became synonymous with a poor prognosis and death. No matter how serious the disease, if Stomach-Qi is still strong, the prognosis will be good. Hence the saying 'If there is Stomach-Qi there is life, if there is no Stomach-Qi there is death.' It should be noted, however, that, in this context, the expression 'Stomach-Qi' includes Spleen-Qi as well.

Yu Jia Yan (1585–1664) said: *'If Stomach-Qi is strong the 5 Yin organs are healthy, if Stomach-Qi is weak they will decline.'*[6] Zhang Jie Bin said: *'Stomach-Qi is the nourishment of life itself, if the Stomach is strong life will be healthy, if the Stomach is weak, life will be unhealthy.'*[7] He also said: *'The doctor who wants to nourish life has to tonify Stomach and Spleen.'*[8]

It is for the above reasons that tonification of the points ST-36 Zusanli and SP-6 Sanyinjiao is a very simple but powerful treatment to tonify Qi and Blood.

> **Clinical note**
>
> ST-36 Zusanli and SP-6 Sanyinjiao are a simple and very powerful combination to tonify Qi and Blood in general

The tongue coating gives a good idea of the relative strength or weakness of Stomach-Qi. The normal coating derives from the normal functioning of the Stomach and therefore a thin-white coating with root reflects the good state of Stomach-Qi.[9] Indeed, even if the coating is pathological (e.g. yellow and too thick), if it has a root, it indicates that Stomach-Qi is still intact (even though the patient harbours a pathogenic factor, in this case Heat) and that the condition can be treated relatively easily.

A school of thought developed that stressed the importance of 'Preserving Stomach-Qi' as the most important treatment method. The most famous exponent of this school was Li Dong Yuan (1180–1251), author of the celebrated 'Discussion on Stomach and Spleen' (*Pi Wei Lun*).

Box 13.3 summarizes this function of the Stomach.

> **Box 13.3 The Stomach controls the rotting and ripening of food**
>
> - The Stomach macerates food to break it down
> - The Stomach is the origin of Qi and Blood as Food-Qi (*Gu Qi*) is extracted from the Stomach
> - Strong Stomach-Qi indicates good prognosis; weak Stomach-Qi indicates poor prognosis
> - The tongue coating reflects good Stomach-Qi

THE STOMACH CONTROLS THE TRANSPORTATION OF FOOD ESSENCES

The Stomach, together with the Spleen, is responsible for the transportation of food essences to the whole

```
Stomach rotting  →  Food essences  →  Whole body
and ripening
```

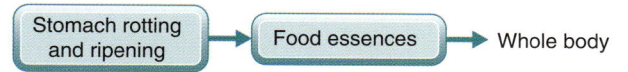

Figure 13.1 Food essences from the Stomach

body, in particular the limbs (Fig. 13.1). From this point of view, the Spleen and Stomach roles are inseparable.

If the Stomach is strong and has enough Qi to extract and transport food essences throughout the body, a person will feel strong and full of energy. If the Stomach is deficient, food essences will be weak too and the Stomach will lack Qi to transport them to the whole body so that the person will feel tired and suffer from weakness of the muscles. A deficiency of both Stomach and Spleen is one of the common conditions encountered in practice: it will make the person tired and the limbs weak (see Fig. 13.1).

Clinical note

A deficiency of Stomach- and Spleen-Qi is one of the most common clinical situations, making the person chronically tired. The best points for this condition are ST-36 Zusanli and SP-6 Sanyinjiao

The Stomach function of transporting food essences also has an influence on the pulse. The 'Simple Questions' in chapter 19 says: *'The Qi of the organs relies on Stomach-Qi to reach the Lung channel.'*[10]

This means that, by transporting food essences to all the organs, Stomach-Qi also ensures that the Qi of the organs reaches the pulse (which, of course, is on the Lung channel). There are certain qualities of a normal pulse that are associated with a good Stomach-Qi. A pulse with good Stomach-Qi is said to be neither weak nor strong, with Yin and Yang perfectly harmonized, having a regular and rather slow beat. A good Stomach-Qi is also said to make the pulse 'soft and gentle': if a pulse feels too rough or hard, it indicates that it lacks Stomach-Qi.

Clinical note

The condition of Stomach-Qi can be diagnosed from:
- Tongue coating: thin white coating with root indicates good Stomach-Qi
- Pulse: a gentle, flowing and relatively soft pulse indicates good Stomach-Qi

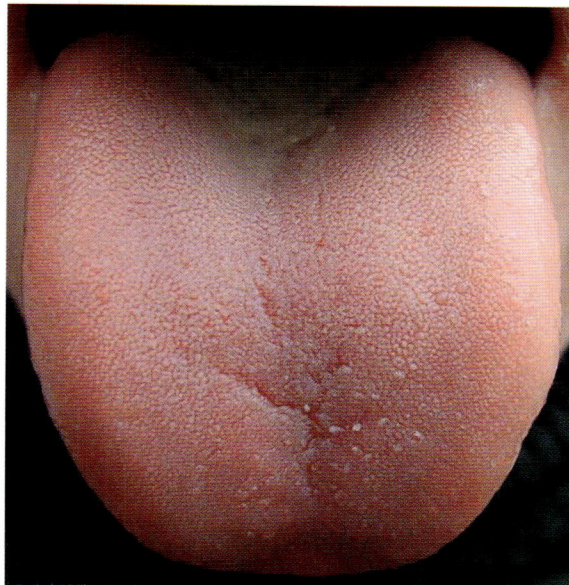

Figure 13.2 Tongue with a normal coating

Finally, in relation to the Stomach function of transporting food essences, the Stomach is very closely related to the tongue coating. This is formed by the 'dirty dampness' that is generated as a by-product of the Stomach activity of rotting and ripening: this dirty dampness subsequently rises up to the tongue to form the coating. A thin white coating therefore indicates that the Stomach is functioning properly. The absence of coating indicates that the Stomach function of digestion is impaired and Stomach-Qi is severely weakened. The colour of the coating also closely reflects Stomach pathology: a thick white coating indicates Cold in the Stomach, while a thick yellow coating indicates Heat.

Figure 13.2 shows a relatively normal coating, Figure 13.3 shows a tongue without coating and Figure 13.4 a tongue with a thick coating.

Box 13.4 summarizes this function of the Stomach.

Box 13.4 The Stomach controls the transportation of food essences

- The Stomach transports food essence all over the body and particularly to the limbs
- If this transportation is impaired, the person will feel tired and the limbs will feel weak
- The Stomach transports the Qi of Food to the pulse
- The Stomach transports some 'dirty dampness' to the tongue, producing a normal tongue coating

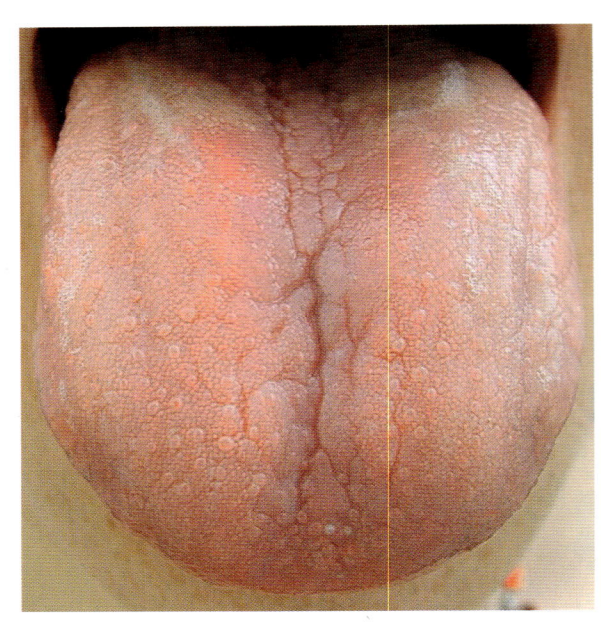

Figure 13.3 Tongue without a coating

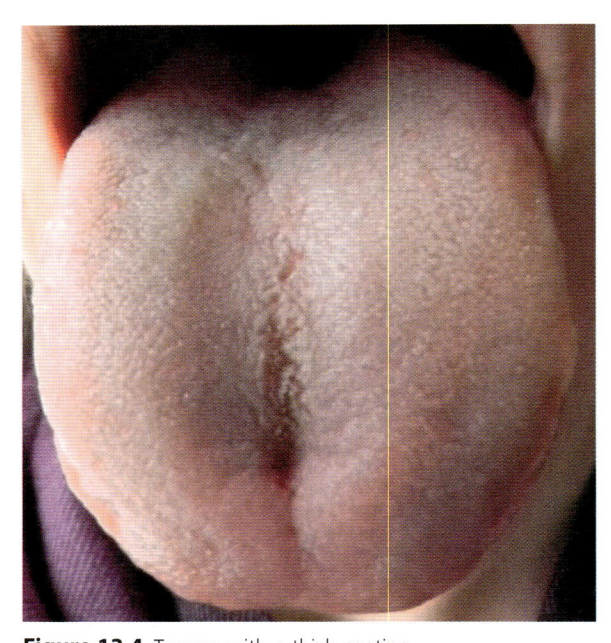

Figure 13.4 Tongue with a thick coating

Clinical note

Whenever I see a tongue completely or partially without coating, I tonify the Stomach, even in the absence of any digestive symptoms. In such a case, I would use Ren-12 Zhongwan, ST-36 Zusanli and SP-6 Sanyinjiao.

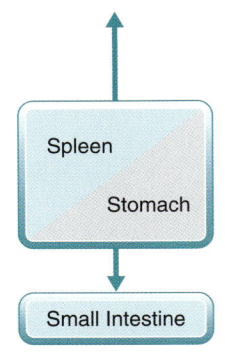

Figure 13.5 The descending of Stomach-Qi

THE STOMACH CONTROLS THE DESCENDING OF QI

The Stomach sends transformed food downwards to the Small Intestine: for this reason in health, Stomach-Qi has a downward movement. If Stomach-Qi descends, digestion will be good and trouble-free. If Stomach-Qi fails to descend, food will stagnate in the stomach, leading to a feeling of fullness and distension, sour regurgitation, belching, hiccup, nausea and vomiting.

Clinical note

The best point to stimulate the descending of Stomach-Qi is Ren-10 Xiawan

However, the descending of Stomach-Qi has a wider meaning than just the descending of Qi from the Stomach to the Small Intestine (Fig. 13.5). The Stomach pertains to Earth, which occupies a central place within the Five Elements. The Stomach and Spleen are the axis of the body (see ch. 4 and Figs 4.17 and 4.18) and the Stomach and Spleen pertain to the Middle Burner. Therefore, for all these reasons, the Stomach and Spleen occupy a very important, strategic central place among the organs and structures and the ascending of Spleen-Qi and descending of Stomach-Qi are crucial for the proper movement of Qi in the Three Burners.

Box 13.5 summarizes this function of the Stomach.

The Liver helps the descending of Stomach-Qi and, under normal conditions, Liver-Qi contributes to the descending of Stomach-Qi and so helps digestion. If Liver-Qi stagnates in the Middle Burner, it can interfere

> **Box 13.5 The Stomach controls the descending of Qi**
>
> - Stomach-Qi descends to transport food dregs to the Small Intestine
> - The Stomach is in the Centre and the descending of its Qi is essential
> - Liver-Qi helps the descending of Stomach-Qi

> **Box 13.6 The Stomach is the origin of fluids**
>
> - The Stomach is the origin of fluids through its process of maceration of food and drink
> - In relation to fluids, the Stomach is the Gate to the Kidneys
> - A deficiency of Stomach fluids is the beginning of a process leading to Yin deficiency

with the descending of Stomach-Qi, giving rise to belching, hiccupping, nausea and vomiting.

THE STOMACH IS THE ORIGIN OF FLUIDS

To rot and ripen food the Stomach needs an abundance of fluids, just as sufficient fluids are needed to extract the vital principles from a herbal decoction or a soup. Furthermore, fluids themselves are derived from the food and drink ingested. The Stomach ensures that the part of food and drink that does not go to make essences of food condenses to form Body Fluids.

The Stomach is thus an important source of fluids in the body, and for this reason it is said that the Stomach 'likes wetness and dislikes dryness'.

If Stomach fluids are abundant, digestion will be good and the sense of taste normal. If Stomach fluids are deficient, a person will be thirsty, the tongue will be dry and cracked and digestion will be poor. One of the main reasons for deficiency of Stomach fluids is eating too late at night.

The Stomach function as origin of fluids is closely related to the Kidneys. The Kidneys are sometimes called the 'Gate of the Stomach', because they transform fluids in the Lower Burner. If this Kidney function is impaired, fluids will stagnate in the Lower Burner and overflow upwards to the Stomach, impairing the digestion.

Moreover, a long-standing deficiency of Stomach fluids will often lead to a deficiency of Kidney-Yin, so that in very chronic cases, deficiency of Stomach-Yin is nearly always associated with deficiency of Kidney-Yin.

The Stomach's role as origin of fluids points to a rather strange anomaly in the theory of the Internal Organs. Although the Spleen is a Yin and the Stomach a Yang organ, in many ways the situation is reversed, the Stomach having many Yin functions and the Spleen many Yang functions (see 'Clinical Note' box).

Furthermore, the Stomach is Yang but its channel is (uniquely) on the front of the body, which is Yin.

Box 13.6 summarizes this function of the body.

> **Clinical note**
>
> **Comparison of stomach and spleen**
>
> - The Stomach (Yang organ) is the origin of fluids, which are Yin
> - The Spleen (Yin organ) has the function of transporting and moving, which is Yang in nature
> - The Spleen is a Yin organ but its Qi ascends (which is a Yang-type movement); the Stomach is a Yang organ but its Qi descends (which is a Yin-type movement)
> - The Spleen is Yin but likes dryness; the Stomach is Yang but likes wetness
> - The Stomach channel is the only Yang channel in the anterior aspect of the body
> - The Stomach often suffers from Yin deficiency, whilst the Spleen seldom suffers from Yin deficiency, but very often from Yang deficiency

OTHER ASPECTS OF THE STOMACH

The other aspects discussed are:

- Mental aspect
- Dreams
- Relationship with the Spleen

Mental aspect

Mention should be made here of the Stomach's influence on the mental state. The Stomach easily suffers from Excess patterns, such as Fire, or Phlegm-Fire. Fire easily agitates the Mind and causes mental symptoms. On a mental level, a condition of Excess of the Stomach can manifest as shutting oneself in the house, closing all doors and windows, wanting to be by oneself, uncontrolled talking or laughing or singing, violent behaviour or taking off of one's clothes. These symptoms described in the ancient classics correspond to what we would today call manic behaviour; however, it is important to note that they may occur in only a mild degree as well.

In less serious cases, Stomach-Fire or Stomach Phlegm-Fire can cause mental confusion, severe anxiety, hypomania and hyperactivity.

Dreams

The 'Spiritual Axis' in chapter 43 says: *'When the Stomach is deficient one dreams of having a large meal.'*[11]

> **Clinical note**
>
> The best point to treat the mental aspect of a Stomach pathology is ST-40 Fenglong

Relationship with the Spleen

According to the Five Elements, Stomach and Spleen belong to the Earth Element, one being Yang and the other Yin. The relationship between these two organs is very close indeed, so much so that they could be considered as two aspects of the same organ system. Indeed, the relationship between the Stomach and Spleen is probably closer than that of any of the other Yin–Yang pairs of organs (Fig. 13.6).

In fact, the Stomach function of rotting and ripening is closely coordinated with the Spleen function of transforming and transporting essences of food. The Spleen function of transporting Food-Qi to the whole body is closely dependent on Stomach-Qi. The Stomach is the origin of fluids and must rely on the Spleen function of transforming and separating the Body Fluids. The coordination and complementarity between Stomach and Spleen may be summarized as follows:

- The Stomach is Yang, the Spleen is Yin
- Stomach-Qi descends, Spleen-Qi ascends
- The Stomach likes wetness and dislikes dryness; the Spleen likes dryness and dislikes wetness
- If the Stomach is too dry, Stomach-Qi cannot descend and food cannot be moved down to the Small Intestine. If the Spleen is too damp, Spleen-Qi cannot ascend and fluids and food cannot be transformed
- The Stomach easily suffers from Excess; the Spleen easily suffers from Deficiency
- The Stomach is prone to Heat, the Spleen to Cold
- The Stomach tends to suffer from deficiency of Yin, the Spleen from deficiency of Yang (although each of them may also suffer from the opposite)

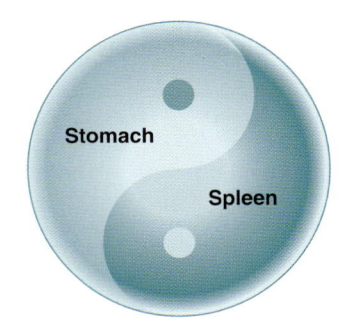

Figure 13.6 Relationship between Stomach and Spleen

Box 13.7 Stomach and Spleen

- The Stomach is Yang, the Spleen is Yin
- Stomach-Qi descends, Spleen-Qi ascends
- The Stomach likes wetness and dislikes dryness; the Spleen likes dryness and dislikes wetness
- If the Stomach is too dry, Stomach-Qi cannot descend and food cannot be moved down to the Small Intestine. If the Spleen is too damp, Spleen-Qi cannot ascend and fluids and food cannot be transformed
- The Stomach easily suffers from Excess, the Spleen from Deficiency
- The Stomach is prone to Heat, the Spleen to Cold
- The Stomach tends to suffer from deficiency of Yin, the Spleen from deficiency of Yang (although each of them may also suffer from the opposite)

The relationship between the Stomach and the Spleen is also summarized in Box 13.7.

> **Learning outcomes**
>
> In this chapter you will have learned:
> - The significance of the Stomach (along with the Spleen) as the 'Root of Post-Heaven Qi'
> - The role of the Stomach in receiving and holding down food and drink
> - The importance of the 'rotting and ripening' of the Stomach in transforming food
> - The relationship between Stomach-Qi and prognosis of disease
> - The role of the Stomach in transporting food essences
> - The manifestation of Stomach-Qi in the pulse and the tongue coating
> - The significance of the descending movement of Stomach-Qi
> - How the Stomach functions as the origin of fluids in the body
> - The influence of Excess patterns of the Stomach on mental state
> - Dreams reflecting disharmonies of the Stomach
> - The closeness of the relationship between Stomach and Spleen

Self-assessment questions

1. Give three symptoms which might indicate that the 'receiving' function of the Stomach had been compromised.
2. Why is the Stomach, together with the Spleen, known as the 'Root of Post-Heaven Qi', with good Stomach-Qi being synonymous with a good prognosis?
3. What kind of tongue coating indicates healthy Stomach Qi?
4. Give two symptoms which might indicate a breakdown in the Stomach's transportation of food essences.
5. What happens if Stomach-Qi fails to descend?
6. Give two examples of the relationship between the Stomach, the Kidneys and Body Fluids.
7. Which two Excess Stomach patterns can cause manic behaviour?
8. Describe the close relationship of the Stomach and Spleen in terms of transformation and transportation of food and fluids.

See p. 1259 for answers

END NOTES

1. 1979 The Yellow Emperor's Classic of Internal Medicine – Simple Questions (*Huang Di Nei Jing Su Wen* 黄帝内经素问), People's Health Publishing House, Beijing, first published *c*.100 BC, p. 58.
2. Simple Questions, p. 78.
3. 1981 Spiritual Axis (*Ling Shu Jing* 灵枢经), People's Health Publishing House, Beijing, first published *c*.100 BC, p. 111.
4. Classic of Difficulties, p. 80.
5. Simple Questions, p. 126.
6. 1981 Syndromes and Treatment of the Internal Organs (*Zang Fu Zheng Zhi* 脏腑证治), Tianjin Scientific Publishing House, Tianjin, p. 176.
7. Ibid., p. 176.
8. Ibid., p. 176.
9. The coating with 'root' grows out of the surface of the tongue like grass grows out of the soil. The coating 'without root' looks like grass that has been *added* to a bare patch of soil. Lack of root in the coating always indicates a weakness of Stomach-Qi and it is usually the stage preceding the total loss of coating (which indicates Stomach-Yin deficiency). Therefore, it is better to have a thick, yellow coating with root (pathological in colour and thickness but with root) than a thin coating without root: the former indicates that Stomach-Qi is still intact and the disease will be relatively easy to treat, while the latter indicates that Stomach-Qi is weak and the disease will be slow to heal.
10. Simple Questions, p. 126.
11. Spiritual Axis, p. 85.

SECTION 2 PART 2

The Functions of the Small Intestine — 14

Key contents

The Small Intestine controls receiving and transforming

The Small Intestine separates fluids

Other aspects of the Small Intestine
Mental aspect
Dreams
Relationship with the Heart

The Small Intestine receives food and drink after digestion by the Stomach and Spleen. This it transforms further by separating a 'clean' from a 'dirty' part. The 'Simple Questions' says in chapter 8: *'The Small Intestine is the official in charge of receiving, being filled and transforming.'*[1]

The functions of the Small Intestine and other aspects will be discussed under the following headings:

- The Small Intestine controls receiving and transforming
- The Small Intestine separates fluids
- Other aspects of the Small Intestine
  - Mental aspect
  - Dreams
  - Relationship with the Heart

THE SMALL INTESTINE CONTROLS RECEIVING AND TRANSFORMING

As we have seen, the Small Intestine receives food and drink from the Stomach to carry out its job of separating a 'clean' (i.e. reusable) part from a 'dirty' part. The clean part is then transported by the Spleen to all parts of the body to nourish the tissues. The 'dirty' part is transmitted to the Large Intestine for excretion as stools, and to the Bladder for excretion as urine (Fig. 14.1).

Box 14.1 summarizes the functions of the Small Intestine.

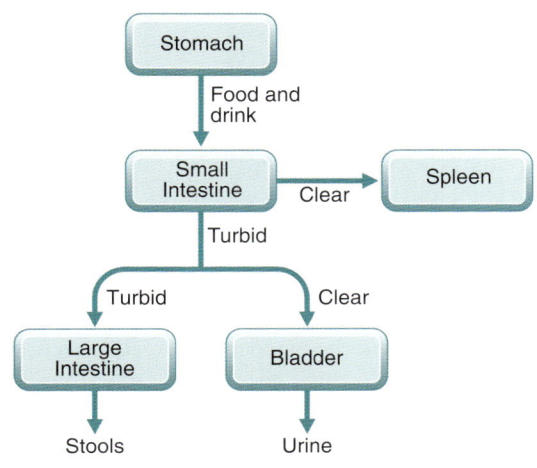

Figure 14.1 Small Intestine's separation of food and drink

Box 14.1 Functions of the Small Intestine

- The Small Intestine controls receiving and transforming
- The Small Intestine separates fluids
- Other aspects of the Small Intestine
  - Mental aspect
  - Dreams
  - Relationship with the Heart

Clinical note

The Small Intestine influences urination and its pathology may cause urinary problems, e.g. Damp-Heat in the Small Intestine or Small Intestine-Heat

From this it can be seen that the Small Intestine has a direct functional relation with the Bladder and it influences the urinary function. Indeed, in practice, the influence of the Small Intestine on urination is frequently seen and Small Intestine points can be used to treat urinary problems.

Box 14.2 summarizes this function of the Small Intestine.

> **Box 14.2 The Small Intestine controls receiving and transforming**
>
> - The Small Intestine receives food and drink from the Stomach
> - It separates these into a clear part, which goes to the Spleen, and a turbid part, which goes to the Large Intestine and Bladder

> **Box 14.3 The Small Intestine controls the separation of fluids**
>
> - The Small Intestine separates fluids received from the Stomach into a clear part, which goes to the Bladder for excretion as urine, and a turbid part, which goes to the Large Intestine, partly for reabsorption and partly for excretion in the stools
> - The Small Intestine's separation of fluids is aided by Kidney-Yang. which provides Qi and heat

THE SMALL INTESTINE SEPARATES FLUIDS

The Small Intestine plays an important role in the movement and transformation of fluids. This process is similar to the one outlined above in relation to food, although there is a slight difference. After the 'dirty' fluids are passed down from the Stomach, they are further separated by the Small Intestine into a 'clean' part, which goes to the Bladder for excretion as urine, and a 'dirty' part, which goes to the Large Intestine, partly for reabsorption and partly for excretion in the stools (Fig. 14.2).

The Small Intestine's function of separating fluids is controlled by the action of Kidney-Yang, which provides the Qi and the heat necessary for this separation to take place. If the Small Intestine's function is impaired, there may be excessive or scanty urination, depending on whether the organ is Cold or Hot.

The Small Intestine's role in separating fluids is a further reason why its physiology and pathology influence urination.

Box 14.3 summarizes this function of the Small Intestine.

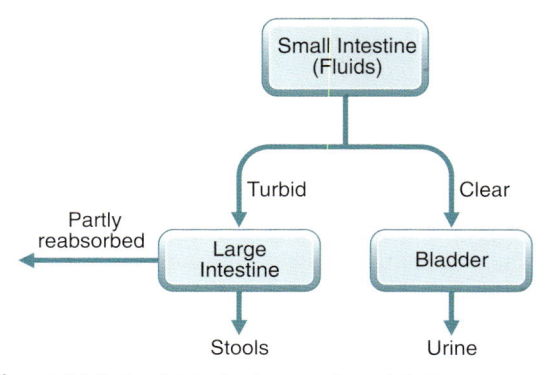

Figure 14.2 Small Intestine's separation of fluids

OTHER ASPECTS OF THE SMALL INTESTINE

The other aspects discussed are:

> - Mental aspect
> - Dreams
> - Relationship with the Heart

Mental aspect

From a psychological point of view, in my opinion, the Small Intestine has an influence on mental clarity and judgement. It is said that it helps us to distinguish our options in any situation clearly in order to come to a decision. Although it is the Gall Bladder that gives us the courage to make decisions, it is the Small Intestine that gives us the power of discernment: that is, the ability to distinguish relevant issues with clarity before we make a decision.

Dreams

The 'Simple Questions' in chapter 17 says: *'When one has small intestinal parasites, one will dream of crowds; when one has long intestinal parasites, one will dream of fights and mutual destruction.'*[2]

The 'Spiritual Axis' in chapter 43 says: *'When the Small Intestine is deficient, one dreams of large cities.'*[3]

Relationship with the Heart

The relationships between Yin and Yang organs within the Five Elements are not all equally close. For example, the relationship between Stomach and Spleen is very close indeed, as is that between the Liver and Gall Bladder. The relationship between Small Intestine and Heart, on the other hand, is rather tenuous. Chinese books normally say that Heart-Qi helps the

Small Intestine's function of separating, but it is not clear how this is achieved.

> The Small Intestine controls our capacity of discriminating between choices; the Gall Bladder gives us the decisiveness to act on a choice

In my opinion, the closest link between Heart and Small Intestine can probably be found on the psychological level. The Heart houses the Mind (*Shen*) and governs our mental and emotional life as a whole. Our mental activities all rely on our capacity for clear judgement and decisions, which are dependent on the Small Intestine. Conversely, the capacity of clear judgement must rely on our mental capacity and clarity as a whole, which is dependent on the Heart (Fig. 14.3).

There is a certain similarity between the Gall Bladder's role in helping us to make decisions and the Small Intestine's influence on judgement. However, there are some differences: the Gall Bladder gives us the courage to make decisions, while from the Small Intestine we derive the clarity of mind necessary to distinguish issues in order to make a choice in life.

When the Gall Bladder is deficient, the person will lack the courage and initiative to take decisions, whereas when the Small Intestine is deficient, the person cannot make a decision because he or she cannot distinguish the various options and make the right choices. The Gall Bladder and Small Intestine, in this respect, depend on each other since it is not enough to have the vision to see what is the right option if we then lack the courage to act on it (Fig. 14.4). The processes involved in decision making will be discussed further in chapter 16 with reference also to the role of the Liver and Kidneys (see Fig. 16.5).

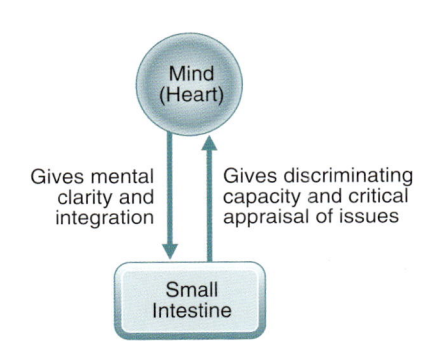

Figure 14.3 Relationship between the Heart and the Small Intestine on the mental level

> **Clinical note**
>
> In my experience, the best point to influence the Small Intestine's judgement and clarity is S.I.-5 Yanggu

The relationship between Heart and Small Intestine can sometimes be observed also in certain pathological situations when Heart-Fire can be transmitted to the Small Intestine, with such manifestations as thirst, bitter taste, tongue ulcers and blood in the urine.

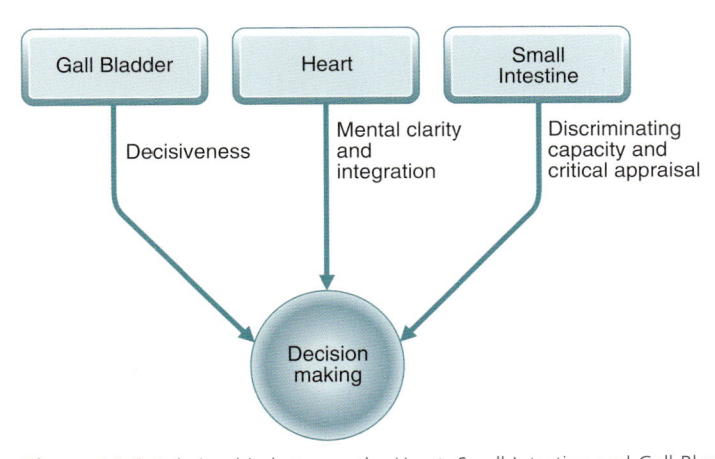

Figure 14.4 Relationship between the Heart, Small Intestine and Gall Bladder in decision making

Learning outcomes

In this chapter you will have learned:
- How the Small Intestine further transforms food received from the Stomach into 'clean' and 'dirty' parts
- The interaction between the Small Intestine and the Large Intestine, to which it transmits the 'dirty' for excretion
- The close relationship of the Small Intestine and the Bladder, to which it transmits fluids for excretion, and through which it influences urination
- The role of the Small Intestine in further separating 'dirty' fluids received from the Stomach, passing on the 'clean' part to the Bladder for excretion, and the 'dirty' to the Large Intestine for further processing
- The significance of Kidney-Yang in providing the Qi and heat for the separation of fluids in the Small Intestine
- The psychological influence of the Small Intestine, and its relationship with the Gall Bladder in decision making
- Dreams reflecting disharmonies of the Small Intestine
- The relationship between Small Intestine and the Heart

Self-assessment questions

1. Describe the path of the 'clean' and 'dirty' parts of food, once transformed by the Small Intestine.
2. What happens to turbid fluids which have been separated by the Small Intestine?
3. Give one symptom which might point to a pattern of Heat in the Small Intestine.
4. Describe the mental aspect of the Small Intestine and how this relates to the role of the Gall Bladder in the process of decision making.
5. Why might one might one see urinary symptoms such as blood in the urine in a patient presenting with a pattern of Heart-Fire?

See p. 1260 for answers

END NOTES

1. 1979 The Yellow Emperor's Classic of Internal Medicine – Simple Questions (*Huang Di Nei Jing Su Wen* 黄帝内经素问), People's Health Publishing House, Beijing, first published *c*.100 BC, p. 58.
2. Ibid., p. 103.
3. 1981 Spiritual Axis (*Ling Shu Jing* 灵枢经), People's Health Publishing House, Beijing, first published *c*.100 BC, p. 85.

The Functions of the Large Intestine

Key contents

The Large Intestine controls passage and conduction

The Large Intestine transforms stools and reabsorbs fluids

Other aspects of the Large Intestine
Mental aspect
Dreams
Relationship with the Lungs

The main function of the Large Intestine is to receive food and drink from the Small Intestine. Having reabsorbed some of the fluids, it excretes the stools.

Chinese medical theory is usually extremely brief with regard to the Large Intestine functions. This is not because its functions are unimportant, but because many of the functions attributed to the Large Intestine in Western medicine are attributed to the Spleen and Liver from a Chinese medical perspective.

The Spleen controls the transformation and transportation of food and fluids throughout the digestive system, including the Small and Large Intestine. For this reason, in disease, symptoms such as diarrhoea, loose stools, blood in the stools and mucus in the stools are usually attributed to a Spleen disharmony; symptoms such as abdominal distension and/or pain and constipation are often due to a Liver disharmony. In other words, in pathology, Large Intestine patterns are often sub-patterns of wider Spleen or Liver patterns.

The functions of the Large Intestine will be discussed under the following headings:

- The Large Intestine controls passage and conduction
- The Large Intestine transforms stools and reabsorbs fluids
- Other aspects of the Large Intestine
  - Mental aspect
  - Dreams
  - Relationship with the Lungs

Box 15.1 summarizes the functions of the Large Intestine.

> **Box 15.1 Functions of the Large Intestine**
> - Controls passage and conduction
> - Transforms stools and reabsorbs fluids
> - Other aspects
>   - Mental aspect
>   - Dreams
>   - Relationship with the Lungs

THE LARGE INTESTINE CONTROLS PASSAGE AND CONDUCTION

The Large Intestines receives digested food from the Small Intestine: it transforms it into stools and it ensures that the stools are moved along and conducted downwards: for this reason, it is said to control 'passage and conduction'. Chapter 8 of the 'Simple Questions' says: *'The Large Intestine is the official in charge of passage and conduction'*.[1]

Therefore, in the context of the 'Qi Mechanism' outlined in chapter 4, the Qi of the Large Intestine has a clear downward movement. Stagnation of Qi often affects the Large Intestine and this causes a disruption of the downward flow of Qi, resulting in abdominal distension and possibly constipation.

On the other hand, the Qi of the Large Intestine could 'sink', causing rectal prolapse or blood in the stools: this condition would always be associated with sinking of Spleen-Qi.

This function is summarized in Box 15.2.

> **Box 15.2 The Large Intestine controls passage and conduction**
>
> - The Large Intestine moves the digested food from the Small Intestine and conducts it downwards
> - It then conducts the stools downward for excretion

THE LARGE INTESTINE TRANSFORMS STOOLS AND REABSORBS FLUIDS

The Large Intestine performs the final transformation of the digested food to form stools, which are excreted. In forming stools, the Large Intestine reabsorbs some of the fluids; the reabsorption should be just right as, if it is too much, the stools will be dry, and if too little, the stools will be loose.

Chapter 10 of the 'Spiritual Axis' says: '*The Large Intestine ... causes Fluids diseases.*'[2] The book '10 Books by Dong Yuan' (*Dong Yuan Shi Shu*, published in 1529 but written three centuries earlier) says: '*The Large Intestine pertains to the Heavenly Stem Geng which is ruled by Dryness but it governs fluids ... it moves fuids.*'[3] This passage is interesting as it shows that the Large Intestine is 'ruled' by Dryness but it controls fluids: in other words, in Western medical terms, it reabsorbs fluids in the gut, thus achieving the right balance of fluids so that the bowels are neither too dry (resulting in constipation) nor too wet (resulting in loose stools).

This function is summarized in Box 15.3.

> **Box 15.3 The Large Intestine transforms stools and reabsorbs fluids**
>
> - The Large Intestine transforms digested food to form stools
> - It reabsorbs some of the fluids

OTHER ASPECTS OF THE LARGE INTESTINE

Other aspects discussed are:

- Mental aspect
- Dreams
- Relationship with the Lungs

Mental aspect

The main mental–emotional aspect of the Large Intestine is its influence on our capacity for 'letting go' and for not dwelling in the past. Several Large Intestine points affect our capacity for letting go and many also calm the Mind.

> **Clinical note**
>
> L.I.-4 Hegu is an excellent point to influence our capacity for 'letting go' and to calm the Mind

Dreams

The 'Spiritual Axis' in chapter 43 says: '*When the Large Intestine is deficient, one dreams of open fields.*'[4]

Relationship with the Lungs

The Lungs and Large Intestine channels are interiorly–exteriorly related. This relationship is important for the execution of common bodily functions as the descending Lung-Qi lends the Large Intestine the necessary Qi for the effort of defecation.

If Lung-Qi is deficient, it does not give enough Qi to the Large Intestine for the act of defecation, resulting in constipation. This is particularly common in old people with declining Lung-Qi.

Conversely, the Lung's ability to send Qi downwards depends on the Large Intestine's role in excreting waste food material. If this function is impaired, and there is constipation, the stagnation of food in the Large Intestine may impair the Lung descending function, giving rise to breathlessness (Fig. 15.1).

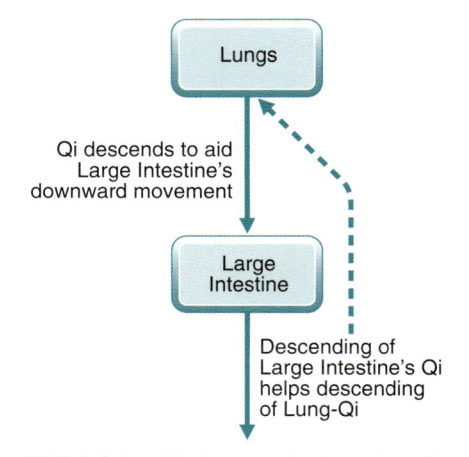

Figure 15.1 Relationship between the Large Intestine and the Lungs

The descending of Lung-Qi aids the downward movement of the Large Intestine and it therefore influences defecation

As the Lungs control the skin, the Large Intestine also has an influence on the skin. Chapter 47 of the 'Spiritual Axis' says: *'The Lungs are related to the Large Intestine which influences the skin. When the skin is thick [it indicates that] the Large Intestine is thick; when the skin is thin [it indicates that] the Large Intestine is thin; when the skin is loose [it indicates that] the Large Intestine is big and long; when the skin is tight [it indicates that] the Large Intestine is tight and short; when the skin is slippery [it indicates that] the Large Intestine is straight; when the skin and flesh cannot be separated [on palpation] [it indicates that] the Large Intestine is coiled.'*[5] This passage is interesting because it establishes a connection between the Large Intestine and skin (although the passage seems to refer specifically to the skin of the abdomen).

Learning outcomes

In this chapter you will have learned:
- Many symptoms attributed to Large Intestine pathology by Western medicine would be attributed to Spleen and/or Liver disharmony according to Chinese medical theory
- The role of the Large Intestine in the formation, 'passage' and 'conduction' of stools
- The significance of the downwards movement of the Qi of the Large Intestine
- The importance of balanced reabsorption of fluids in the Large Intestine
- The psychological influence of the Large Intestine on our capacity for 'letting go'
- Dreams reflecting disharmonies of the Large Intestine
- The relationship between Large Intestine and Lungs, particularly in terms of defecation, breathing and skin

Self-assessment questions

1. Give two symptoms which you might see if stagnation of Qi disrupts the downward flow of Qi of the Large Intestine.
2. The '10 Books by Dong Yuan' mentions that the Large Intestine 'governs fluids'. How does it do this?
3. Which acupuncture point might you use for someone who is unable to let go of issues from the past?
4. Describe how the Large Intestine and the Lung can affect each other in pathology.

See p. 1260 for answers

END NOTES

1. 1979 The Yellow Emperor's Classic of Internal Medicine – Simple Questions (*Huang Di Nei Jing Su Wen* 黄帝内经素问), People's Health Publishing House, Beijing, first published *c.*100 BC, p. 58.
2. 1981 Spiritual Axis (*Ling Shu Jing* 灵枢经), People's Health Publishing House, Beijing, first published *c.*100 BC, p. 31.
3. Cited in Wang Xue Tai 1988 Great Treatise of Chinese Acupuncture (*Zhong Guo Zhen Jiu Da Quan* 中国针灸大全), Henan Science Publishing House, p. 45.
4. Spiritual Axis, p. 85.
5. Ibid., p. 92.

SECTION 2 PART 2

Functions of the Gall Bladder   16

Key contents

The Gall Bladder stores and excretes bile

The Gall Bladder controls decisiveness

The Gall Bladder controls the sinews

Other aspects of the Gall Bladder
Mental aspect
Dreams
Relationship with the Liver

The Gall Bladder occupies a special place among the Yang organs because it is the only one that does not deal with food, drink and their waste products, but instead stores bile, which is a refined product. Furthermore, it neither communicates with the exterior directly, as all the other Yang organs do (via the mouth, rectum or urethra), nor does it receive food or transport nourishment, as do the other Yang organs. In fact, because it stores a refined substance, the Gall Bladder resembles a Yin organ. For this reason, the Gall Bladder is also one of the six Extraordinary Yang organs.

On a psychological level, the Gall Bladder is said to influence the capacity for making decisions and courage. The 'Simple Questions' in chapter 8 says: *'The Gall Bladder is the upright official that takes decisions.'*[1]

The functions of the Gall Bladder and other aspects will be discussed under the following headings:

- The Gall Bladder stores and excretes bile
- The Gall Bladder controls decisiveness
- The Gall Bladder controls the sinews
- Other aspects of the Gall Bladder
  - Mental aspect
  - Dreams
  - Relationship with the Liver

Box 16.1 lists the functions of the Gall Bladder.

THE GALL BLADDER STORES AND EXCRETES BILE

The Gall Bladder receives bile from the Liver, which it stores ready to excrete when needed during digestion. From this point of view, the function of the Gall Bladder is identical with that of Western medicine.

The Gall Bladder is the only Yang organ that stores a 'clean' fluid such as bile, instead of 'dirty' substances such as food, drink and their wastes. The 'purity' of the bile as a precious fluid has always been stressed by the ancient classics. Chapter 2 of the 'Spiritual Axis' calls the bile 'Central Essence' (*zhong jing*): *'The Gall Bladder is the organ of the Central Essence.'*[2] It should be noted here that 'essence' is used as a term to indicate a pure, refined fluid and it is not the Essence pertaining to the Kidneys.

The bile is produced by the Liver and stored by the Gall Bladder. The ancient Chinese were aware of this as the 'Pulse Classic' shows: *'The excess Qi of the Liver is discharged into the Gall Bladder and gathers to form bile.'*[3] Bile enters the Intestines to aid digestion (Fig. 16.1).

It is interesting that the ancient Chinese doctors referred to the Gall Bladder's function of aiding digestion as 'Gall Bladder-Qi' or also 'Gall Bladder-Fire'. 'Fire' should not be understood here as Fire in the context of the Five Elements, nor as pathological Fire.

Box 16.1 Functions of the Gall Bladder

- The Gall Bladder stores and excretes bile
- The Gall Bladder controls decisiveness
- The Gall Bladder controls the sinews
- Other aspects of the Gall Bladder
  - Mental aspect
  - Dreams
  - Relationship with the Liver

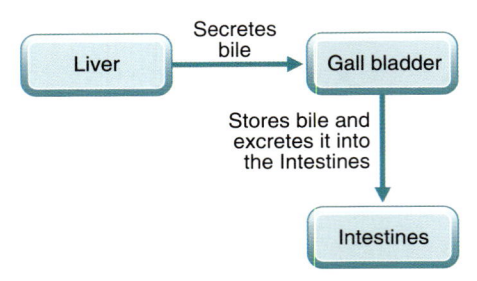

Figure 16.1 Storage and excretion of bile by the Gall Bladder

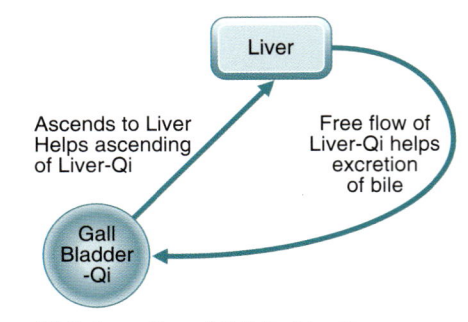

Figure 16.2 Ascending of Gall Bladder-Qi

'Fire' actually indicates the Minister Fire that arises from between the Kidneys and flows up to the Liver, Gall Bladder, Triple Burner and Pericardium. In this context, therefore, the Gall Bladder is like an emissary of the Minister Fire arising from the Kidneys: the Minister Fire of the Gall Bladder warms the Spleen and Intestines to aid digestion.

The Minister Fire communicates with the Gall Bladder, to which it provides heat to aid digestion

From a Five-Element perspective, Liver and Gall Bladder pertain to Wood and the Qi of the Gall Bladder is part of the free flow of Liver-Qi: the free flow of Liver-Qi promotes the secretion of bile into the Gall Bladder and also the discharge of bile into the Intestines. Gall Bladder-Qi helps the ascending of Liver-Qi, which has been mentioned in chapter 11 (relationship between Liver and Lungs).

On a physical level, Gall Bladder-Qi helps the ascending and free flow of Liver-Qi in relation to the Stomach and Spleen. As we have seen, under normal circumstances, the free flow of Liver-Qi helps Stomach-Qi to descend and Spleen-Qi to ascend (Fig. 16.2). In pathology, it can do the opposite. As we shall see below, the ascending of Gall Bladder-Qi has a psychological implication.

Under normal circumstances, the smooth flow of bile aids the Stomach and Spleen function of digestion. In disease, when Liver-Qi is stagnant and the bile does not flow smoothly, both Stomach and Spleen functions may be impaired. In particular, the Stomach ability to direct Qi downwards will be impaired, giving rise to nausea and belching.

> **Clinical note**
>
> The points to stimulate the free flow of Liver-Qi and the flow of bile are G.B.-34 Yanglingquan and G.B.-24 Riyue

This function of the Gall Bladder is summarized in Box 16.2.

Box 16.2 The Gall Bladder stores and excretes bile

- The Gall Bladder receives bile from the Liver and stores it to excrete it during digestion
- The Gall Bladder is the only Yang organ that stores a 'pure' substance, i.e. bile
- The Minister Fire reaches the Gall Bladder and warms it: the Gall Bladder transmits this heat to the digestive organs to aid digestion
- The flow of bile depends on the free flow of Liver-Qi
- Gall Bladder-Qi aids the ascending of Liver-Qi
- The smooth flow of bile helps the Stomach to digest and the Spleen to transform

THE GALL BLADDER CONTROLS DECISIVENESS

While the Liver is said to control the ability of planning one's life, the Gall Bladder controls the capacity to make decisions. The two functions have to be harmonized so that we can plan and act accordingly. Chapter 8 of the 'Simple Questions' says: *'The Gall Bladder is like an impartial judge from whom decisiveness emanates.'*[4] Chapter 9 of the 'Simple Questions' lists the functions of all the organs (omitting the Pericardium) and, at the end, it says: *'All the 11 organs depend on the decision-making of the Gall Bladder.'*[5]

This is an interesting statement because it implies not only that the Gall Bladder controls our capacity to take decisions but also that all the other internal organs depend on the Gall Bladder's 'decision making': in other words, the Gall Bladder is the organ that 'motivates' all others and Gall Bladder points can be used for this purpose.

> **Clinical note**
>
> Based on the idea that the Gall Bladder 'motivates' all other organs, some doctors in China use the point G.B.-40 to give impetus to other points combinations

This function of the Gall Bladder is summarized in Box 16.3.

> **Box 16.3 The Gall Bladder controls decisiveness**
>
> - The Gall Bladder controls the capacity to make decisions
> - The Gall Bladder's 'decision making' helps all other 11 Internal Organs

THE GALL BLADDER CONTROLS THE SINEWS

This function is almost identical to the Liver function of controlling sinews. The only slight difference is that, in so far as the Liver nourishes the sinews with its Blood, the Gall Bladder provides Qi to the sinews to ensure their proper movement and agility. This explains why the Gathering (*Hui*) point for sinews, G.B.-34 Yanglingquan, is on the Gall Bladder channel.

This function of the Gall Bladder is summarized in Box 16.4.

> **Box 16.4 The Gall Bladder controls the sinews**
>
> - The Gall Bladder provides Qi to the sinews to ensure their proper movement and agility
> - The Gathering (*Hui*) point for sinews is on the Gall Bladder channel, i.e. G.B.-34 Yanglingquan

OTHER ASPECTS OF THE GALL BLADDER

The other aspects discussed are:

- Mental aspect
- Dreams
- Relationship with the Liver

Mental aspect

As described above, the Gall Bladder is responsible for decisiveness, for the capacity of taking decisions.

Besides controlling decision making, the Gall Bladder is also said to give an individual courage and initiative. For this reason, in Chinese, there are several expressions such as 'big gall bladder', meaning 'courageous', and 'small gall bladder', meaning 'timid or fearful'.

This is an important function of the Gall Bladder on a psychological level. It controls the courage to take decisions and make changes. Although, as we have seen, the Kidneys also control the 'drive' and vitality, the Gall Bladder gives us the capacity to turn this drive and vitality into positive and decisive action. Thus a deficient Gall Bladder will cause indecision, timidity and the affected person will be easily discouraged at the slightest adversity.

The Gall Bladder provides the courage for the Mind (*Shen*), governed by the Heart, to carry out decisions (Fig. 16.3). This reflects the Mother–Child relationship existing between Gall Bladder and Heart, according to the Five Elements. In cases of weak Mind from Heart deficiency, it is often necessary to tonify the Gall Bladder to support the Heart. As a further confirmation of the relationship between the Gall Bladder and the Heart, the Gall Bladder Divergent channel flows through the heart. On the other hand, the Mind provides the clarity and, most of all, the integration and control necessary to somehow 'moderate' the decisiveness of the Gall Bladder: without the control and integration of the Mind, the decisiveness of the Gall Bladder may turn into recklessness.

Moreover, the Gall Bladder influences the mental–emotional life in yet another way. As described above,

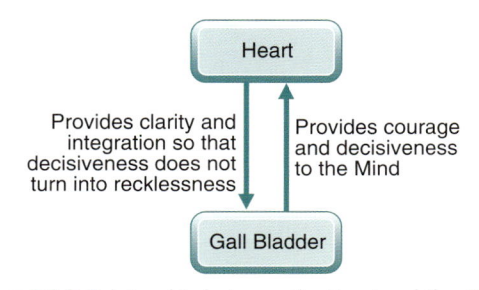

Figure 16.3 Relationship between the Heart and the Gall Bladder

Gall Bladder-Qi helps the ascending of Liver-Qi, which has been mentioned in chapter 11 (relationship between Liver and Lungs). On a physical level, Gall Bladder-Qi helps the ascending and free flow of Liver-Qi in relation to the Stomach and Spleen.

The ascending of Gall Bladder-Qi has a psychological implication in that it stimulates the ascending and free flow of Liver-Qi on a mental level. As we have seen, the Ethereal Soul, which is housed in the Liver, gives 'movement' to the Mind (*Shen*) of the Heart, providing it with inspiration, planning, ideas, initiative and creativity. This 'movement' of the Ethereal Soul depends on the physiological ascending of Liver-Qi, which, in turn, relies on Gall Bladder-Qi. If this 'movement' of the Ethereal Soul is lacking, the person will tend to be depressed: in this case, Liver-Qi is not ascending enough and Gall Bladder-Qi is weak (Fig. 16.4). If this movement is excessive, the person may be slightly manic.

Having now discussed the mental-emotional aspect of the Mind (Heart), Ethereal Soul (Liver), Will-power (Kidneys), Gall-Bladder and Small Intestine, we can build a picture of how these organs are involved and coordinated in decision making. Figure 14.4 in chapter 14 illustrates the role of the Heart, Small Intestine and Gall Bladder in decision making. Figure 16.5

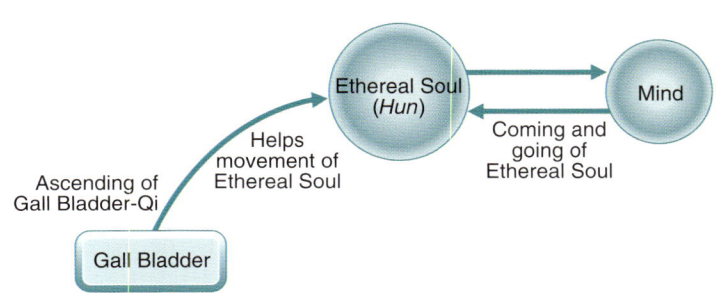

Figure 16.4 Relationship between the Gall Bladder and the Ethereal Soul

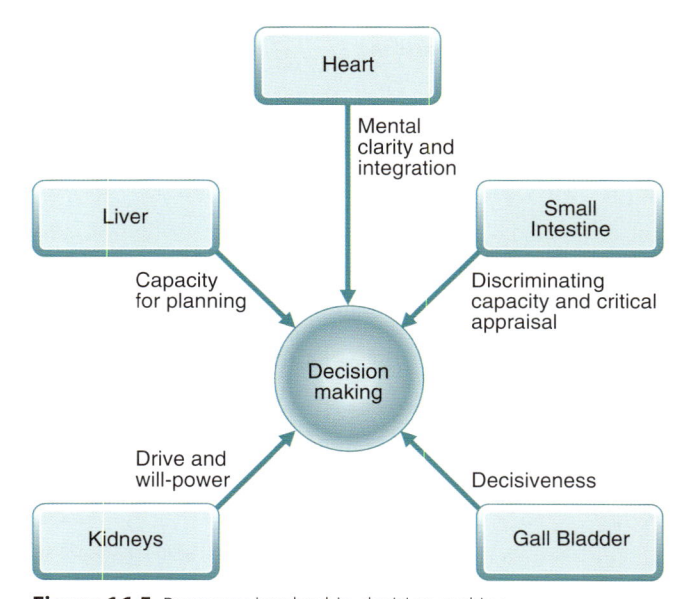

Figure 16.5 Processes involved in decision making

adds the role of the Kidneys and Liver in decision making. In order to make the 'right' decisions we need:

- The capacity of planning our life, to have 'dreams' and plans that is conferred by the Ethereal Soul (*Hun*) of the Liver
- The drive and will-power to want to make something of our lives that is conferred by the Will-power (*Zhi*) of the Kidneys
- The capacity to discriminate between issues, to analyse issues with clarity, to distinguish what is relevant and what is not that is conferred to us by the Small Intestine
- The capacity to take a decision with resoluteness once all issues have been analysed, and the courage to act that is conferred by the Gall Bladder
- The integration and direction provided by the Mind (*Shen*) of the Heart

Dreams

The Gall Bladder has an influence on the quality and length of sleep and, if it is deficient, a person will wake early in the morning and be unable to fall asleep again. The 'Spiritual Axis' in chapter 43 says: '*When the Gall Bladder is deficient one dreams of fights, trials and suicide.*'[6]

Relationship with the Liver

The relationship between the Liver and Gall Bladder is close both from the anatomical and the physiological point of view. The Liver and Gall Bladder depend on each other to perform their respective functions. The Gall Bladder function of storing and discharging bile depends on the Liver function of smooth flow of Qi. Conversely, the Liver relies on Gall Bladder-Qi to aid its function of smooth flow of Qi. Moreover, the ascending of Liver-Qi relies on Gall Bladder-Qi, which, as we have seen, has physical and mental–emotional implications.

On a psychological level, the Liver's influence on the planning of our life is dependent on the Gall Bladder's capacity to help us make decisions.

Learning outcomes

In this chapter you will have learned:
- The difference between the Gall Bladder and the other Yang organs
- The role of the Gall Bladder in storing and discharging bile to aid digestion
- The significance of the Gall Bladder in transmitting the warmth of the Minister Fire to the digestive organs
- The influence of the free flow of Liver-Qi on the appropriate discharge of bile by the Gall Bladder into the intestines
- How the healthy digestive functions of the Stomach and Spleen depend on a smooth flow of bile
- The importance of the Gall Bladder's function of controlling decisiveness, and how this affects the other organs
- The role of the Gall Bladder in providing Qi to the sinews for movement and agility
- The psychological manifestation of the Gall Bladder as courage, initiative and the ability to take decisive action
- The closeness of the relationship between the Liver and Gall Bladder

Self-assessment questions

1. Describe how the Gall Bladder differs from the other Yang organs.
2. Describe the role of the Gall Bladder in digestion.
3. How do the functions of the Gall Bladder and Liver differ in relation to the sinews?
4. How might a deficient Gall Bladder manifest psychologically?
5. Describe the relationship between Gall Bladder-Qi and the Ethereal Soul and Mind.
6. What is the capacity conferred by the Gall Bladder in the process of decision making?

See p. 1260 for answers

END NOTES

1. 1979 The Yellow Emperor's Classic of Internal Medicine – Simple Questions (*Huang Di Nei Jing Su Wen* 黄帝内经素问), People's Health Publishing House, Beijing, first published *c*.100 BC, p. 58.
2. 1981 Spiritual Axis (*Ling Shu Jing* 灵枢经), People's Health Publishing House, Beijing, first published *c*.100 BC, p. 8.
3. Cited in Wang Xue Tai 1988 Great Treatise of Chinese Acupuncture (*Zhong Guo Zhen Jiu Da Quan* 中国针灸大全), Henan Science Publishing House, p. 43.
4. Simple Questions, p. 58.
5. Ibid., p. 69.
6. Spiritual Axis, p. 85.

The Functions of the Bladder

SECTION 2 PART 2 — 17

> **Key contents**
>
> **The Bladder removes water by Qi transformation**
>
> **Other aspects of the Bladder**
> Mental aspect
> Dreams
> Relationship with the Kidneys

The Bladder has a wider sphere of activity in Chinese medicine than in Western medicine. It stores and excretes urine, but it also participates in the transformation of fluids necessary for the production of urine. The 'Simple Questions' in chapter 8 says: *'The Bladder is like a district capital, it stores fluids which are then excreted by the power of Qi transformation.'*[1]

The functions of the Bladder and other aspects will be discussed under the following headings:

- The Bladder removes water by Qi transformation
- Other aspects of the Bladder
  - Mental aspect
  - Dreams
  - Relationship with the Kidneys

THE BLADDER REMOVES WATER BY QI TRANSFORMATION

The clear part of fluids separated by the Small Intestine passes on to the Bladder, which further transforms them into urine. The Bladder subsequently stores and excretes urine. The Bladder's function of transforming fluids requires Qi and heat, which are provided by Kidney-Yang. In Chinese medicine this is usually called Bladder's function of 'Qi transformation': that is, the transformation of fluids by Qi (Fig. 17.1).

Box 17.1 lists this and other functions of the Bladder.

Although it is the Bladder that performs this function, the energy to do this is derived from the Kidney.

The Bladder can be seen as the Yang aspect of the Kidney and is therefore related to the Fire of the Gate of Life (*Ming Men*), from which it derives its energy. For this reason symptoms of Bladder deficiency are similar to those of deficiency of the Gate of Life: that is, abundant, clear urination.

It is worth noting that other organs besides the Kidneys work in conjunction with the Bladder to control urination: these are the Small Intestine, the Triple Burner, the Liver and the Lungs.

The Small Intestine and Bladder work together to move fluids in the Lower Burner as the Bladder receives the clean part of fluids separated by the Small Intestines. This explains the use of certain Small Intestine points, such as Qiangu S.I.-2, in urinary diseases.

> **Box 17.1 Functions of the Bladder**
>
> - The Bladder removes water by Qi transformation
> - Other aspects of the Bladder
>   - Mental aspect
>   - Dreams
>   - Relationship with the Kidneys

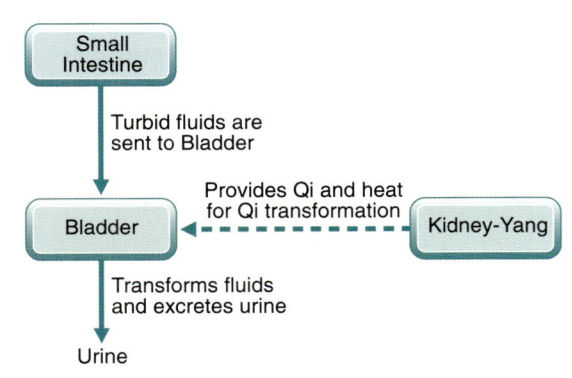

Figure 17.1 Relationship between the Small Intestine and Bladder

The Heart exerts an influence on urination as Heart-Qi needs to descend towards the Small Intestine and Bladder to help the excretion of urine. It is worth remembering that the Bladder Divergent channel flows through the Heart. The connection between the Small Intestine and the Bladder also explains how some Heart disharmonies can be transmitted to the Bladder via the Small Intestine (which is of course related to the Heart within the Five-Element model) and give rise to such urinary symptoms as blood in the urine (Fig. 17.2).

Other organs apart from the Kidneys assist the Bladder in urination, i.e. the Small Intestine, Triple Burner, and Lungs

The Bladder is assisted in its function of fluid transformation by the Triple Burner, or more precisely, the Lower Burner, which has the function of making sure the water passages in the lower part of the body are open and free. The Lower Burner is compared to a 'ditch' and its main function is to promote the transformation and excretion of fluids.

Clinical note

It is because of the relationship between the Bladder's fluid transformation and the Triple Burner's function of excretion that the point BL-39 Weiyang is the Lower He-Sea point of the Triple Burner

The Liver also exerts an influence on urination as its channel flows around the end of the urethra. The free flow of Liver-Qi in this area ensures smooth urination; Liver-Qi stagnation may lead to urinary dysfunction.

Finally, the Lungs are also related to the Bladder, via the Kidneys. Lung-Qi descends to the Kidneys to promote the transformation of fluids and excretion of urine. For this reason, a deficiency of Lung-Qi, particularly in the elderly, may cause urinary retention: this is due to the failure of Lung-Qi to descend to the Bladder to promote urination (Fig. 17.3).

Clinical note

The point LU-7 Lieque connects with the Bladder and stimulates the descending of fluids in urinary difficulty, especially in the elderly

Box 17.2 summarizes this function of the Bladder.

Box 17.2 The Bladder removes water by Qi transformation

- The Bladder receives clear fluids from the Small Intestine
- It transforms these fluids into urine, which is excreted
- The power for this transformation is called 'Qi transformation'
- The Qi and heat for this transformation are provided by Kidney-Yang

OTHER ASPECTS OF THE BLADDER

The other aspects of the Bladder functions are:

- Mental aspect
- Dreams
- Relationship with the Kidneys

Mental aspect

On a mental level, an imbalance in the Bladder can provoke negative emotions such as jealousy, suspicion and the holding of long-standing grudges.

Dreams

The 'Spiritual Axis' in chapter 43 says: '*When the Bladder is deficient one dreams of voyages.*'[2]

Relationship with the Kidneys

The relationship between the Bladder and the Kidneys is close. On the one hand, the Bladder derives the Qi

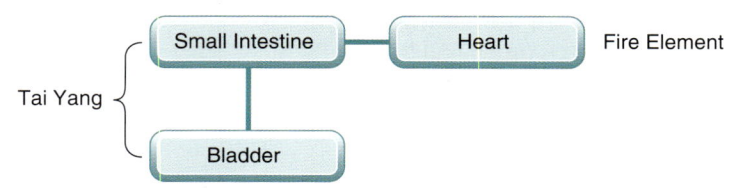

Figure 17.2 Relationship between the Bladder, Small Intestine and Heart

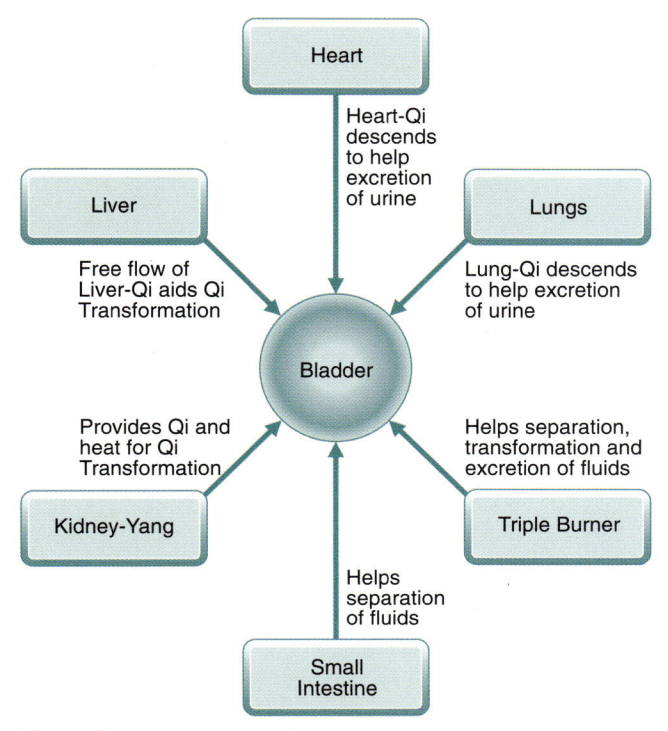

Figure 17.3 Organs involved in urination

- Heart → Heart-Qi descends to help excretion of urine
- Lungs → Lung-Qi descends to help excretion of urine
- Liver → Free flow of Liver-Qi aids Qi Transformation
- Kidney-Yang → Provides Qi and heat for Qi Transformation
- Triple Burner → Helps separation, transformation and excretion of fluids
- Small Intestine → Helps separation of fluids

and heat necessary for its function of fluids transformation from the Kidney and the Gate of Life. On the other hand, the Kidneys rely on the Bladder to move and excrete some of their 'dirty' fluids.

Learning outcomes

In this chapter you will have learned:
- The role of the Bladder in storing, transforming and excreting fluids
- The importance of Kidney-Yang in providing Qi and heat necessary for transformation of fluids in the Bladder
- The interaction of the Bladder with the Small Intestine, Triple Burner, Lungs and Liver in controlling urination
- The psychological influence of imbalance in the Bladder
- Dreams reflecting Bladder imbalance
- The closeness of the relationship between the Kidneys and the Bladder

Self-assessment questions

1. From where does the Bladder derive its energy for its function of 'Qi transformation'.
2. What symptom might suggest a deficiency of the Bladder?
3. Describe the relationship between the Heart and the Bladder.
4. Why might Lung-Qi deficiency cause urinary retention?
5. Describe the close relationship between the Kidney and Bladder.

See p. 1260 for answers

END NOTES

1. 1979 The Yellow Emperor's Classic of Internal Medicine – Simple Questions (*Huang Di Nei Jing Su Wen* 黄帝内经素问), People's Health Publishing House, Beijing, first published *c.*100 BC, p. 59.
2. 1981 Spiritual Axis (*Ling Shu Jing* 灵枢经), People's Health Publishing House, Beijing, first published *c.*100 BC, p. 85.

SECTION 2 PART 2

The Functions of the Triple Burner | 18

Key contents

Functions of the Triple Burner
Mobilizes the Original Qi (Yuan Qi)
Controls the transportation and penetration of Qi
Controls the Water passages and the excretion of fluids

Four views of the Triple Burner
The Triple Burner as one the six Yang organs
The Triple Burner as a 'mobilizer of the Original Qi'
The Triple Burner as the three divisions of the body
- The Upper Burner is like a mist
- The Middle Burner is like a maceration chamber
- The Lower Burner is like a ditch

The Triple Burner as body cavities

Other aspects of the Triple Burner
Mental aspect
Dreams
Relationship with the Pericardium

The Triple Burner is one of the most elusive topics of Chinese medicine and one which has been the subject of controversy for centuries. Although it is 'officially' one of the six Yang organs, Chinese doctors have always debated about the nature of the Triple Burner and in particular whether it has a 'form' or not: that is, whether it is an actual organ or a function.

After discussing the functions of the Triple Burner, it is appropriate to discuss four different views of the Triple Burner, which will throw light on its functions. Therefore, the discussion of the functions of the Triple Burner will be under the following topics:

- Functions of the Triple Burner
  - The Triple Burner mobilizes the Original Qi (*Yuan Qi*)
  - The Triple Burner controls the transportation and penetration of Qi
  - The Triple Burner controls the Water passages and the excretion of fluids
- Four views of the Triple Burner
  - The Triple Burner as one the six Yang organs
  - The Triple Burner as a 'mobilizer of the Original Qi'
  - The Triple Burner as the three divisions of the body
    - The Upper Burner is like a mist
    - The Middle Burner is like a maceration chamber
    - The Lower Burner is like a ditch
  - The Triple Burner as body cavities
- Other aspects of the Triple Burner
  - Mental aspect
  - Dreams
  - Relationship with the Pericardium

FUNCTIONS OF THE TRIPLE BURNER

The functions discussed are:

- The Triple Burner mobilizes the Original Qi
- The Triple Burner controls the transportation and penetration of Qi
- The Triple Burner controls the Water passages and the excretion of fluids

Box 18.1 lists the functions of the Triple Burner.

The Triple Burner mobilizes the Original Qi (*Yuan Qi*)

The Original Qi (*Yuan Qi*) is a transformation of the Pre-Heaven Essence with the input of the Post-Heaven Essence. The Original Qi represents the Essence 'in action' in the form of Qi. The Original Qi resides in between the Kidneys and is closely related to the Fire of the Gate of Life (*Ming Men*). Chapter 66 of the 'Classic of Difficulties' clarifies the relationship between

Box 18.1 Functions of the Triple Burner

1. Functions of the Triple Burner
   a) It mobilizes the Original Qi (*Yuan Qi*)
   b) It controls the transportation and penetration of Qi
   c) It controls the Water passages and the excretion of fluids
2. Four views of the Triple Burner
   a) The Triple Burner as one the six Yang organs
   b) The Triple Burner as a 'mobilizer of the Original Qi'
   c) The Triple Burner as the three divisions of the body
      i. The Upper Burner is like a mist
      ii. The Middle Burner is like a maceration chamber
      iii. The Lower Burner is like a ditch
   d) The Triple Burner as body cavities
3. Other aspects of the Triple Burner
   a) Mental aspect
   b) Dreams
   c) Relationship with the Pericardium

the Original Qi and the Triple Burner. It says: '*Below the umbilicus between the kidneys there is a Motive Force [Dong Qi] that is life-giving and is the root of the 12 channels: it is called Original Qi. The Triple Burner makes the Original Qi separate* [into its different functions] *and it controls the movement and passage of the 3 Qi* [of the Upper, Middle and Lower Burner] *through the 5 Yin and 6 Yang organs.*'[1]

Thus, the Triple Burner 'mobilizes' the Original Qi by making it differentiate into its different forms to perform different functions in different places and organs (Fig. 18.1). It is through the Triple Burner that the Original Qi can perform its functions. The Original Qi is closely related to the Gate of Life (*Ming Men*) and shares its role of providing the heat necessary to all the body's functional activities. The following are examples of functions carried out by the Original Qi which are aided by the Triple Burner:

- The Original Qi provides the heat necessary to the Spleen to transform and transport food essences and to the Kidneys to transform fluids. The Middle Burner makes sure that Original Qi reaches and assists the Spleen to transform and transport food essences and the Lower Burner ensures that Original Qi warms the Kidneys to transform fluids
- The Original Qi facilitates the transformation of Gathering Qi (*Zong Qi*) into True Qi (*Zhen Qi*). It can do this through the action of the Upper Burner in transporting Qi through the various passages in the chest.
- The Original Qi facilitates the transformation of Food-Qi (*Gu Qi*) into Blood in the Heart. The Upper Burner ensures the smooth passage and transportation of Qi in the chest for this transformation to take place

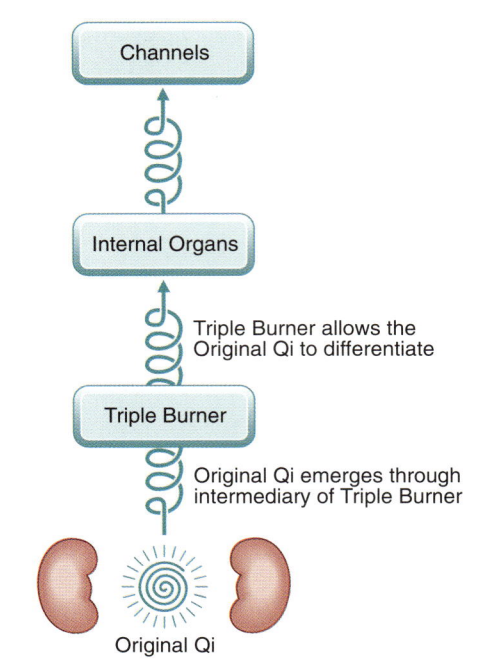

Figure 18.1 The Triple Burner as the mobilizer of the Original Qi

Thus, the Triple Burner helps the Original Qi to differentiate itself in different form to perform different functions in different places.

The Original Qi represents the transformation power of Qi in all Internal Organs: the Triple Burner allows the Original Qi to differentiate into its different forms to perform its functions in each organ

Thus the Original Qi represents the transformation power of Qi of all the Internal Organs. Chapter 38 of the 'Classic of Difficulties' says: '*The Triple Burner is the place where the Original Qi is separated: it supports all of the Qi.*'[2]

This function is summarized in Box 18.2.

Box 18.2 The Triple Burner mobilizes the Original Qi (*Yuan Qi*)

- The Triple Burner mobilizes the Original Qi by making it differentiate for different functions
- The Triple Burner allows the Original Qi to perform its various functions in relation to several organs

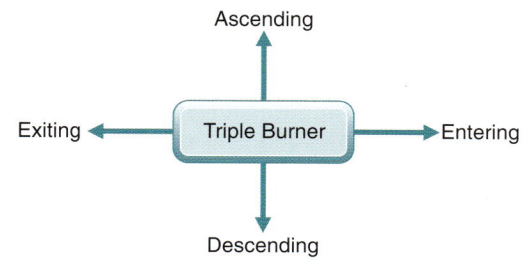

Figure 18.2 The Triple Burner and the Qi Mechanism

The Triple Burner controls the transportation and penetration of Qi

As we have seen in chapter 4, the movement of Qi to carry out its various functions is called the 'Qi Mechanism'. This Qi Mechanism relies on the ascending/descending and entering/exiting of Qi in different places and different organs. Each organ has a particular direction of flow of Qi (e.g. Spleen-Qi ascends while Stomach-Qi descends). In each channel, Qi flows in an upward or downward direction. Qi also enters and exits in and out of various structures and organs. For example, Qi enters and exits the space between skin and muscles, the Membranes, the joint capsules, and all other cavities (Fig. 18.2).

The Triple Burner controls the ascending/descending and entering/exiting of Qi in the Qi Mechanism. One of the words most frequently used in Chinese books to describe this function of the Triple Burner is *tong* 通, which means 'free passage', 'to pass through', 'penetrate': this describes the function of the Triple Burner in ensuring that Qi passes through in the Qi Mechanism, in all the cavities and in all organs. This whole process is called 'Qi Transformation by the Triple Burner': the result of the Qi transformation is the production of Nutritive Qi (*Ying Qi*), Defensive Qi (*Wei Qi*), Blood and Body Fluids. That is also why the Triple Burner is said to control 'all kinds of Qi'.

The 'Central Scripture Classic' (*Zhong Zang Jing*, Han dynasty) says: '*The Triple Burner is the three original Qi of the body, it is the Yang organ of clear [Qi], it controls the 5 Yin and 6 Yang organs, the Nutritive Qi and Defensive Qi, the channels and the Qi of the interior and exterior, left and right, above and below. When the Qi of the Triple Burner has free passage, Qi passes freely into interior, exterior, left, right, above and below. The Triple Burner irrigates the body, harmonizes interior and exterior, benefits the left and nourishes the right, it conducts upwards and descends downwards*'[3] (Fig. 18.3).

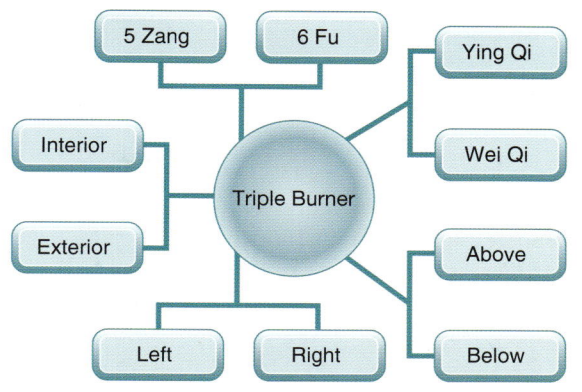

Figure 18.3 The Triple Burner according to *Zhong Zang Jing*

As mentioned above, chapter 66 of the 'Classic of Difficulties' confirms that the Triple Burner controls the movement of Qi in general: '*The Triple Burner makes the Original Qi separate [into its different functions] and it controls the movement and passage of the 3 Qi [of the Upper, Middle and Lower Burner] through the 5 Yin and 6 Yang organs.*'[4]

The 'three Qi' are the Qi of the Upper, Middle and Lower Burner: apart from referring generally to all the types of Qi in each Burner, this passage also refers specifically to the Gathering Qi (*Zong Qi*) in the Upper, Nutritive Qi (*Ying Qi*) in the Middle and Defensive Qi (*Wei Qi*) in the Lower Burner. Although the Defensive Qi exerts its influence primarily in the Upper Burner and the superficial layers of the body (the space between skin and muscles), it originates in the Lower Burner from the Gate of Life. Chapter 18 of the 'Spiritual Axis' says: '*The Nutritive Qi originates from the Middle Burner; the Defensive Qi originates from the Lower Burner.*'[5]

Chapter 38 of the 'Classic of Difficulties' confirms that the Triple Burner exerts its influence on all types of Qi: '*The Triple Burner is the place where the Original Qi is separated: it supports all of the Qi.*'[6] Chapter 31 confirms the influence of the Triple Burner on the movement of Qi in all parts of the body: '*The Qi of the Triple Burner gathers in the avenues of Qi [Qi Jie].*'[7] This means that the Triple Burner is responsible for the free passage of Qi in all channels but also all structures (such as cavities) of the body; *Qi Jie* is also an alternative name for the point ST-30.

> **Clinical note**
>
> T.B.-6 Zhigou stimulates the Triple Burner's function of transportation and penetration of Qi

With regard to the movement of Qi, it is useful to compare and contrast this function of the Triple Burner with those of Liver in ensuring the free flow of Qi and of the Lungs in governing Qi:

> **Triple Burner, Liver and Lungs: comparison and contrast**
>
> - The Liver ensures the free flow of Qi and this aids the ascending and descending of Qi, especially in the Stomach, Spleen and Intestines; the Triple Burner's influence on the ascending–descending and entering–exiting of Qi extends to all organs. The Triple Burner controls the entering and exiting of Qi in all parts of the body and especially the body cavities: the Liver has no such function in relation to the body cavities
> - The Lungs govern Qi in the sense of controlling the intake of air, breathing and the production of Gathering (*Zong*) Qi from Food-Qi (*Gu Qi*). The Triple Burner has no such function with regard to Qi. The Lungs also influence the ascending–descending and entering–exiting of Qi, but they do so mostly in the Upper Burner, while the Triple Burner's function of transporting Qi exerts its influence on all organs and all three Burners

This function of the Triple Burner is summarized in Box 18.3.

> **Box 18.3 The Triple Burner controls the transportation and penetration of Qi**
>
> - The Triple Burner controls the ascending–descending and entering–exiting of Qi in all organs and all parts of the body
> - The Triple Burner controls the movement and 'penetration' of Qi in general
> - The Triple Burner controls the three Qi: Gathering Qi (Upper Burner), Nutritive Qi (Middle Burner) and Defensive Qi (Lower Burner)
> - The Triple Burner controls all types of Qi and the avenues of Qi

The Triple Burner controls the Water passages and the excretion of fluids

Chapter 8 of the 'Simple Questions', which describes the functions of all the Internal Organs, comparing them to 'officials', says: '*The Triple Burner is the official in charge of ditches.*'[8] This means that just like the official who is in charge of irrigation, the Triple Burner is responsible for the transformation, transportation and excretion of fluids. This is one of the most important functions of the Triple Burner (Fig. 18.4).

The terms used in Chinese in connection with the Triple Burner's influence on the Body Fluids are often *shu* 疏, which means 'free flow', and *tong* 通, which means 'free passage'. Therefore the Triple Burner is like a system of canals and waterways to channel irrigation water through the proper fields and then out: this ensures that Body Fluids are transformed, transported and excreted properly.

The Triple Burner's function in relation to Body Fluids is closely dependent on its function of controlling the transportation and penetration of Qi. As described above, the Triple Burner influences the ascending–descending and entering–exiting of Qi in the Qi Mechanism: it is the coordinated and harmonized ascending–descending and entering–exiting of Qi in all organs and structures that ensures that the Body Fluids also ascend–descend and enter–exit in the proper way in all places. Essentially, the transformation and movement of fluids depends on Qi.

> **Clinical note**
>
> The best points to influence the Triple Burner's transformation and excretion of fluids are not on the Triple Burner channel itself but on the Directing Vessel (*Ren Mai*): i.e. Ren-17 Shanzhong for the Upper, Ren-9 Shuifen for the Middle and Ren-5 Shimen for the Lower Burner

The end result of the complex process of transformation, transportation and excretion of fluids leads to the formation of various Body Fluids in each of the three Burners. The fluids of the Upper Burner are primarily

Upper Burner	Diffusion of fluids
Middle Burner	Transformation and transportation of fluids
Lower Burner	Excretion of fluids

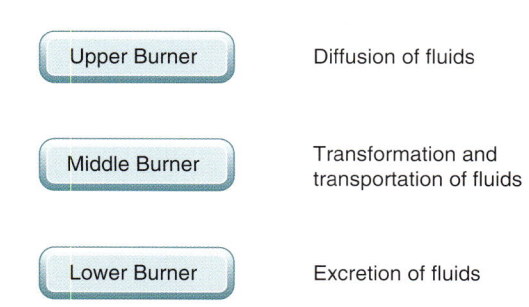

Figure 18.4 The Triple Burner and the metabolism of fluids

sweat, which flows in the space between skin and muscles; those of the Middle Burner are the fluids produced by the Stomach, which moisten the body and integrate Blood; those of the Lower Burner are primarily urine and the small amount of fluids in the stools.

This function is summarized in Box 18.4.

> **Box 18.4 The Triple Burner controls the Water passages and the excretion of fluids**
>
> - The Triple Burner is the official in charge of 'ditches'
> - It controls the transportation and excretion of fluids from the body
> - Its transportation and excretion of Body Fluids is closely dependent on its transportation and penetration of Qi
> - The transformation of fluids leads to sweat in the Upper Burner, Stomach fluids in the Middle Burner, and urine in the Lower Burner

FOUR VIEWS OF THE TRIPLE BURNER

Four views of the Triple Burner will be discussed:

- The Triple Burner as one of the six Yang Organs
- The Triple Burner as a mobilizer of the Original Qi (*Yuan Qi*)
- The Triple Burner as three divisions of the body
  - The Upper Burner is like a mist
  - The Middle Burner is like a maceration chamber
  - The Lower Burner is like a ditch
- The Triple Burner as body cavities

The Triple Burner as one of the six Yang organs

Historically, this view is derived from the 'Yellow Emperor's Classic'. The 'Simple Questions' in chapter 8 says: '*The Triple Burner is the official in charge of irrigation and it controls the water passages.*'[9] This comment about the Triple Burner is mentioned in the context of a list of functions of all the organs, from which it appears that the 'Simple Questions' considers the Triple Burner as one of the six Yang organs. If this is the case, the Triple Burner has a 'form', that is, it is substantial, like all the other organs. Its function is similar to that of the other Yang organs: that is, receiving food and drink, digesting and transforming it, transporting the nourishment and excreting the wastes.

The function of the Yang organs in general is often expressed in the Chinese word '*tong*' 通, which means 'making things go through' or 'ensuring a free passage', etc. The function of the Triple Burner, in addition, is often expressed in the Chinese word '*chu*' 出, meaning 'excreting' or rather 'letting out'. The Triple Burner performs this letting-out function in relation to the spreading of Defensive Qi (*Wei Qi*) in the Upper Burner, transportation of Nutritive Qi (*Ying Qi*) in the Middle Burner and excretion of Body Fluids in the Lower Burner. The 'Spiritual Axis' in chapter 18 says: '*The person receives Qi from food, food enters the stomach, then spreads to the Lungs and the 5 Yin organs and the 6 Yang organs, the clear part goes to the Nutritive Qi, the dirty part to the Defensive Qi.*'[10]

The capacity of the Nutritive and Defensive Qi to spread from the Stomach to the Lungs depends on the 'letting-out' function of the Triple Burner. In other words, the Triple Burner controls the movement of various types of Qi at the various stages of Qi and Blood production, in particular ensuring that the various types of Qi are 'let out' in a smooth way and that dirty fluids are excreted properly.

Thus, the Triple Burner is a three-stage passageway contributing to the production of Nutritive and Defensive Qi after the separation of food into a clear and dirty part and to the excretion of fluids. The Upper Burner lets out Defensive Qi (directing it to the Lungs), the Middle Burner lets out Nutritive Qi (directing it to all the organs) and the Lower Burner lets out waste fluids (directing them to the Bladder) (Fig. 18.5).

The 'Yellow Emperor's Classic' variously describes the function of the Triple Burner as 'opening up', 'discharging Qi' and 'letting Qi out'. Malfunctions of the Triple Burner are variously described as 'not flowing smoothly', 'overflowing' or 'being blocked'. In practice this means that an impairment of the Triple Burner function will manifest as a blockage of the various types of Qi or fluids in the three stages: a blockage of

Upper Burner 'Lets out' → Defensive Qi → Lungs

Middle Burner 'Lets out' → Nutritive Qi → All organs

Lower Burner 'Lets out' → Waste fluids → Bladder

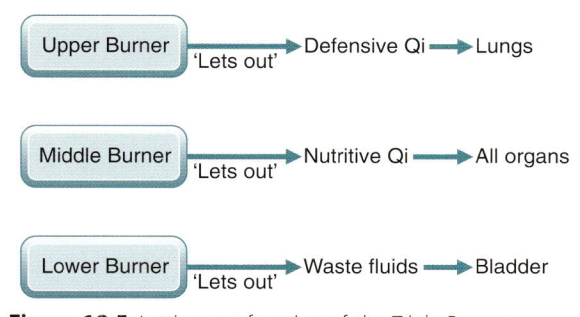

Figure 18.5 Letting-out function of the Triple Burner

Defensive Qi in the Upper Burner (impairment of the Lung diffusing function), a blockage of Nutritive Qi in the Middle Burner (impairment of the Spleen function of transportation) and a blockage of fluids in the Lower Burner (impairment of the Bladder function of Qi transformation). These situations would cause sneezing, abdominal distension and retention of urine, respectively.

This view of the Triple Burner is summarized in Box 18.5.

> **Box 18.5 The Triple Burner as one of the six Yang organs**
>
> - From this point of view, the Triple Burner is a Yang organ and 'has a form'
> - The Triple Burner has the function of maintaining free passage (*tong*) and of 'letting out', or excreting (*chu*)
> - The Triple Burner lets out Defensive Qi in the Upper, Nutritive Qi in the Middle, and fluids in the Lower Burner

The Triple Burner as a 'mobilizer of the Original Qi' (*Yuan Qi*)

This interpretation of the Triple Burner derives from the 'Classic of Difficulties', chapter 66.[11] According to this classic, the Triple Burner 'has a name but no form'; that is, it is not an organ but a collection of functions – it is insubstantial. As mentioned above, the 'Classic of Difficulties' states that the Original Qi resides in the lower abdomen between the two Kidneys, it spreads to the five Yin and six Yang organs via the Triple Burner; it then enters the 12 channels and emerges at the Source (*Yuan*) points (see Fig. 18.1). From this came the interpretation of the Triple Burner as a 'mobilizer of the Original Qi': that is, the channel for expression of the Original Qi. The Triple Burner mobilizes the Original Qi to perform its various functions in different organs and different parts of the body: it allows the Original Qi to separate and differentiate for its different functions around the body.[12]

Original Qi is also described in the same chapter as being the 'motive force (*Dong Qi*) between the Kidneys', activating all physiological functions of the body and providing heat for the digestion. This 'motive force between the Kidneys' can carry out its functions only through the intermediary and the mobilization of the Triple Burner. As mentioned before, Original Qi provides the heat necessary for the digestion and transformation of food. Because the Triple Burner is a 'mobilizer of the Original Qi', it obviously has an influence on the process of digestion.

This is clearly expressed in the 'Classic of Difficulties', in chapter 31, which states that the '*Triple Burner is the avenue of food and drink, the beginning and end of Qi.*'[13] It also states that the Upper Burner controls 'receiving but not excreting', the Middle Burner 'rotting and ripening of food and drink' and the Lower Burner 'excreting but not receiving'. All these expressions – 'receiving', 'rotting and ripening' and 'excreting' – describe a process of transportation, transformation and excretion of food and fluids by the Triple Burner.

From this point of view, there is therefore a convergence of views between the concept of Triple Burner in the 'Yellow Emperor's Classic' and the 'Classic of Difficulties', that is, between the Triple Burner as an organ or as a function, even though the starting point of these two classics is different. However, the 'Yellow Emperor's Classic' emphasizes the role of the Triple Burner in its 'letting-out' function, seeing the three Burners as three avenues of excretion or 'letting out'. The 'Classic of Difficulties', on the contrary, places emphasis on the work of 'receiving', 'rotting and ripening' and 'excretion' of food and fluids, seeing digestion as a process of 'Qi transformation' activated by the Original Qi through the intermediary action of the Triple Burner.

This view of the Triple Burner is summarized in Box 18.6.

> **Box 18.6 The Triple Burner as a mobilizer of the Original Qi**
>
> - According to this view, the Triple Burner 'has no form'
> - The Triple Burner mobilizes the Original Qi emerging from between the Kidneys to make it differentiate in its different forms in different parts of the body for different functions

The Triple Burner as the three divisions of the body

This view of the Triple Burner is derived from both the 'Classic of Difficulties' (ch. 31) and the 'Spiritual Axis' (ch. 18).[14] The three-fold division of the body is as follows: from the diaphragm upwards is the Upper Burner, between the diaphragm and the umbilicus is the Middle Burner, and below the umbilicus is the Lower Burner. As far as organs and anatomical parts are concerned, the Upper Burner includes Heart,

Lungs, Pericardium, throat and head; the Middle Burner includes Stomach, Spleen and Gall Bladder; and the Lower Burner includes Liver, Kidneys, Intestines and Bladder (Fig. 18.6).

The position of the Liver in the Lower Burner should be clarified. Anatomically, the Liver is in the Middle Burner and, indeed, some of its symptomatology occurs in the Middle Burner, such as hypochondrial pain, epigastric pain, belching, sour regurgitation, etc. However, as the Liver has many complex functions and a very long channel, energetically, it can also be placed in the Lower Burner. For example, from the point of view of gynaecology, the Liver's physiology and pathology are such that they place it definitely in the Lower Burner. Moreover, as one of the major functions of the Triple Burner is the transportation and transformation of food essences and fluids, this particular function in the Middle Burner is performed by the Stomach and Spleen, not the Liver, and that is why the Liver is usually placed in the Lower rather than Middle Burner.

The Upper Burner is like a mist

The main physiological process of the Upper Burner is that of distribution of fluids all over the body in the space between skin and muscles by the Lungs in the form of fine vapour. This is an aspect of the Lung diffusing function. For this reason the Upper Burner is compared to a *mist*[15] (Fig. 18.7).

The 'Spiritual Axis' in chapter 30 says: *'The Upper Burner opens outwards, spreads the 5 flavours of the food essences, pervades the skin, fills the body, moistens the skin and it is like mist.'*[16]

The Middle Burner is like a maceration chamber

The main physiological processes in the Middle Burner are those of digestion and transportation of food and drink (described as 'rotting and ripening') and the

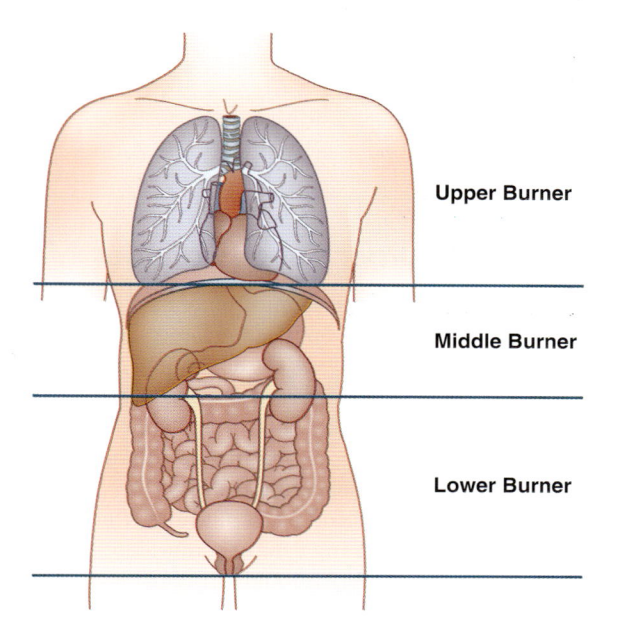

Figure 18.6 The three Burners as three divisions of the body (please note that the Liver is anatomically in the Middle Burner but that, energetically, it is usually placed in the Lower Burner)

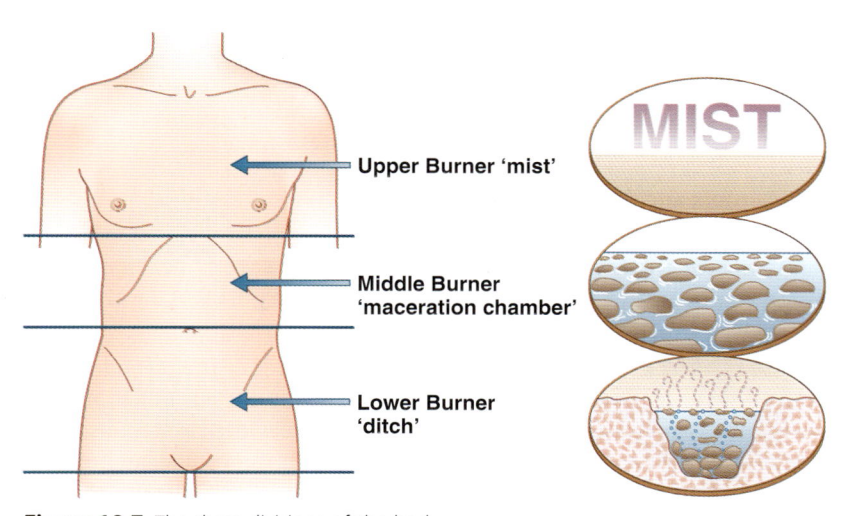

Figure 18.7 The three divisions of the body

transportation of the nourishment extracted from food to all parts of the body. For this reason the Middle Burner is compared to a 'maceration chamber' or a 'bubbling cauldron'[17] (see Fig. 18.7).

The 'Spiritual Axis' in chapter 18 says: *'The Middle Burner is situated in the Stomach ... it receives Qi, expels the wastes, steams the body fluids, transforms the refined essences of food and connects upwards with the Lungs.'*[18]

The Lower Burner is like a ditch

The main physiological process in the Lower Burner is that of separation of the essences of food into a clean and dirty part, with the excretion of the dirty part. In particular, the Lower Burner directs the separation of the clean from the dirty part of the fluids and facilitates the excretion of urine. For this reason the Lower Burner is compared to a 'drainage ditch'[19] (see Fig. 18.7).

The 'Spiritual Axis' in chapter 18 says: *'Food and drink first enter the stomach, the waste products go to the large intestine in the Lower Burner which oozes downwards, secretes the fluids and transmits them to the bladder.'*[20]

This aspect of the three Burners is summarized in Box 18.7.

In conclusion, the three-fold division of the Triple Burner is a summarization of the functions of all the Yang organs (but including also the Lungs and Spleen) in their work of receiving, digesting, transforming, absorbing, nourishing and excreting. The organs within each division are not separate from the three Burners themselves. From acupuncture's perspective, in particular, Lungs and Heart are the Upper Burner, Stomach and Spleen are the Middle Burner and Liver, Kidneys, Bladder and Intestines are the Lower Burner.

Box 18.8 summarizes Qi and the three Burners, while the three divisions of the body are summarized in Box 18.9. The three-fold division of the body can also be seen as a summarization of the mutual assistance and transformation into each other of the Gathering Qi (Upper Burner), Nutritive Qi (Middle Burner) and Original Qi (Lower Burner).

Box 18.7 The three Burners and fluids

- The Upper Burner is like a ***mist*** (sweat)
- The Middle Burner is like a ***maceration chamber*** (Stomach fluids)
- The Lower Burner is like a ***ditch*** (urine)

Box 18.8 The Qi of the three Burners

- The Upper Burner: Gathering Qi (*Zong Qi*)
- The Middle Burner: Nutritive Qi (*Ying Qi*)
- The Lower Burner: Original Qi (*Yuan Qi*)

Box 18.9 The Triple Burner as three divisions of the body

- Upper Burner: from the diaphragm upwards (Lungs, Heart and Pericardium)
- Middle Burner: between the diaphragm and the umbilicus (Stomach, Spleen and Gall Bladder)
- Lower Burner: below the umbilicus (Liver, Kidneys, Bladder, Small and Large Intestine)

The Triple Burner as body cavities

The Triple Burner is a system of body cavities. There are many cavities in the body, some large, some small: for example, the chest cavity, the abdominal cavity, the pelvic cavity, the joint cavities, the space between skin and muscles, the space above the diaphragm, the spaces in between the Membranes, and the spaces between these and the abdominal cavity.

Such cavities are called *Cou* 腠 in Chinese medicine, the term *Cou* usually being used in conjunction with *Li* 理, meaning 'texture'. Although the term *Cou Li* is often used to indicate the space between skin and muscles, this space is only one of the cavities of the body.

The body cavities are:
- The chest cavity
- The abdominal cavity
- The pelvic cavity
- The joint capsules
- The space between the skin and muscles
- The space above the diaphragm
- The spaces in between the Membranes
- The spaces between the Membranes and the abdominal cavity

The cavities of the body are generally irrigated and lubricated by various fluids and the Triple Burner controls these cavities also because it controls the transformation, transportation and excretion of fluids in all parts of the body. Moreover, the Triple Burner controls the movement of Qi in and out of such cavities. This movement is the 'entering and exiting' of Qi in the Qi Mechanism (see ch. 4). The entering and exiting of Qi in and out of the cavities is extremely important both for the proper circulation of Qi and for the transformation and transportation of Body Fluids in and out of such cavities (Fig. 18.8).

The abdominal cavity contains the Membranes (*Huang*); these include the superficial and deep fascia, the mesentery, the omentum and the stroma enveloping all internal organs. The superficial and deep fascia are connective tissues that envelop the muscles. The mesentery is the double layer of peritoneum attached to the abdominal wall and enclosing in its fold the abdominal viscera. The omentum is a fold of peritoneum passing from the stomach to another abdominal organ (Figs 18.9–18.12). The stroma is the framework, usually of connective tissue, of an organ. The Membranes have the function of wrapping, anchoring and connecting the organs. In other words, the organs in

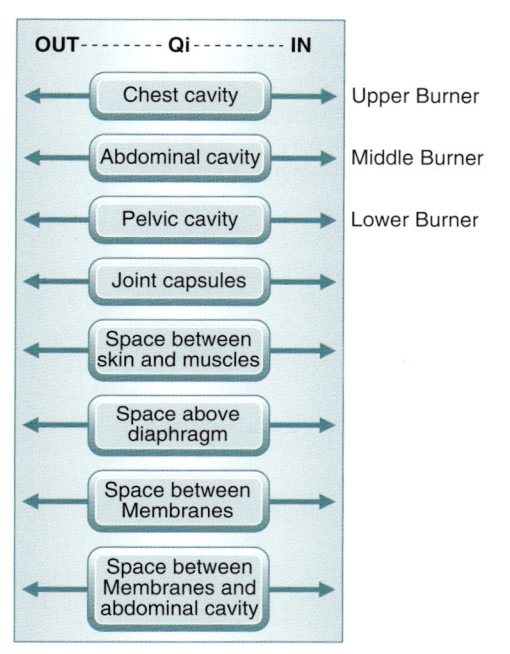

Figure 18.8 The entering and exiting of Qi in the body cavities

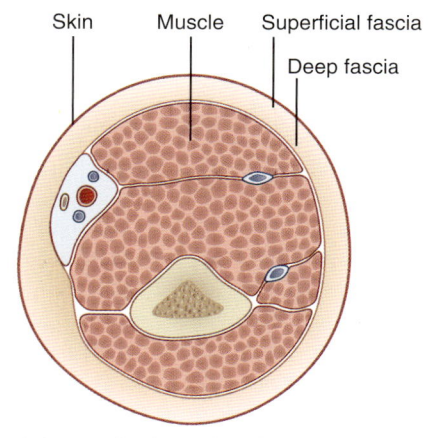

Figure 18.9 Superficial and deep fascia

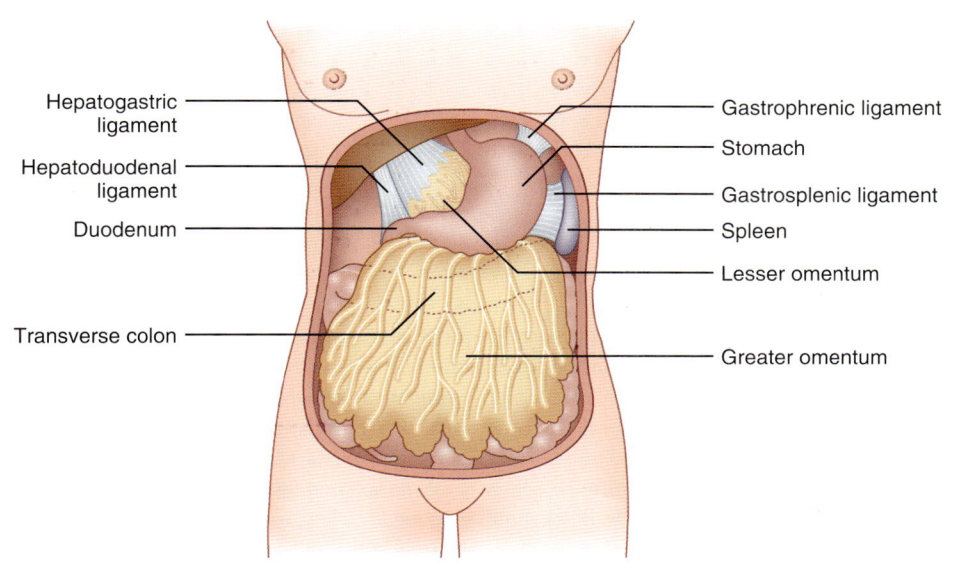

Figure 18.10 Omentum

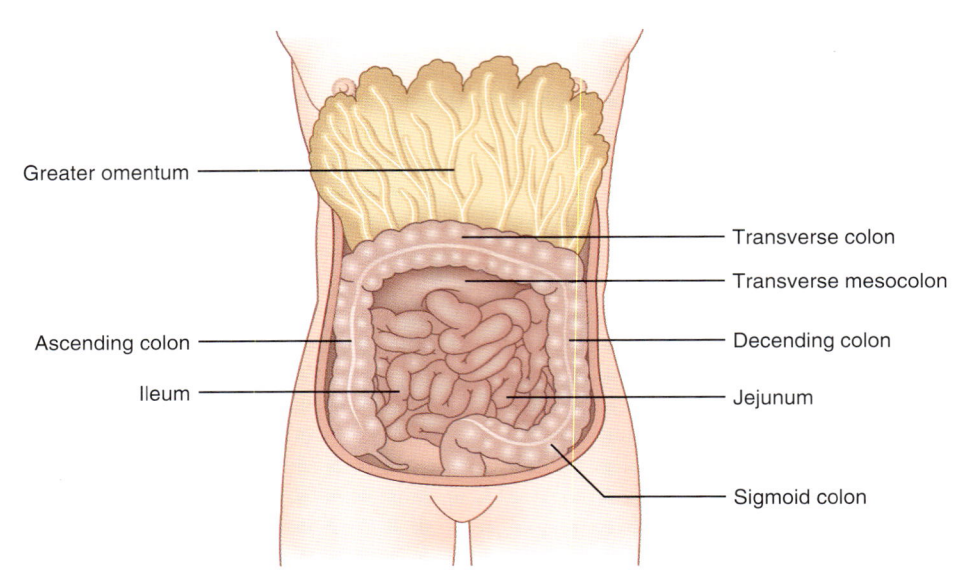

Figure 18.11 Greater Omentum

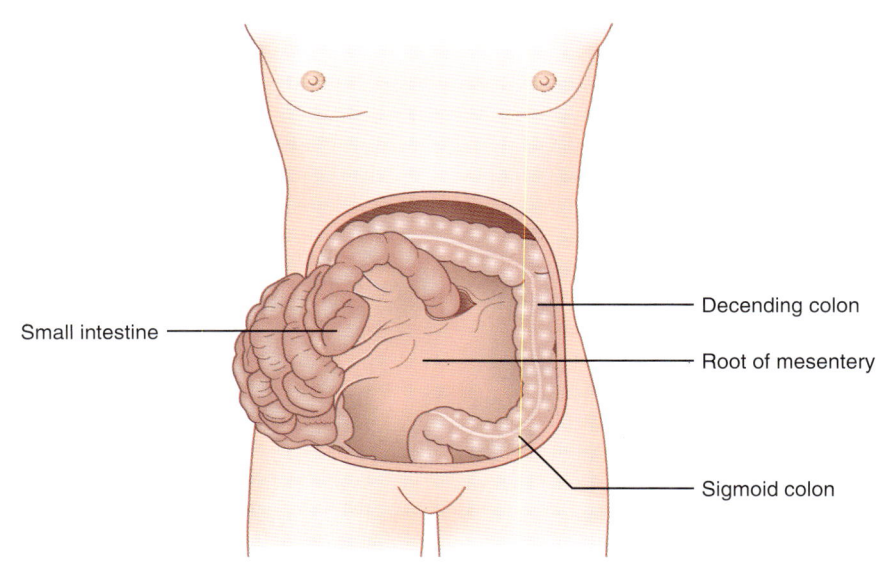

Figure 18.12 Mesentery

the abdominal cavity are not in a kind of vacuum connected by acupuncture channels. They occupy a solid space that is surrounded by Membranes. The Triple Burner is responsible for the movement of Qi in and out of the Membranes.

Therefore, when seen as a system of body cavities, the Triple Burner is not an organ but a complex of cavities outside or in between the Internal Organs. The 'Classic of Categories' (*Lei Jing*, 1624) by Zhang Jing Yue says: '*Outside the internal organs and inside the body [i.e. between the skin and the internal organs], wrapping the internal organs like a net, there is cavity that is a Fu. It has the name of a ditch but the shape of a Fu [Yang organ].*'[21] He also said: '*The Internal Organs have substance; the cavities are like a bag that contains that substance.*'[22]

The 'Selected Historical Theories of Chinese Medicine' (*Zhong Yi Li Dai Yi Lun Xuan*) says: '*There is a

Minister Fire in the body which moves within the cavities and up and down in between the Membranes: it is called the Triple Burner.'[23] The same book clarifies the relationship between the Triple Burner, Pericardium and cavities: '*The Heart is the Emperor who has a Minister. The Triple Burner cavities are like a capital which houses both the Emperor and the Minister. The Pericardium in the centre of the chest is like a palace that houses only the Emperor. The palace is inside and is Yin, the capital is outside and is Yang; hence the Triple Burner is a Yang organ and the Pericardium a Yin organ*'[24] (Fig. 18.13).

In the chest cavity, the Triple Burner controls the entering and exiting of Qi, which is governed by the Gathering Qi. In the abdominal and pelvic cavity, the Triple Burner controls the transportation and transformation of Qi in the Membranes. In the space between skin and muscles, the Triple Burner controls the diffusing of Defensive Qi and the entering and exiting of Qi in and out of that space. This function of the Triple Burner regulates the flow of Defensive Qi in this space, the opening and closing of pores and sweating. In the joint cavities, the Triple Burner controls the entering and exiting of Qi and fluids in the joint capsules: this contributes to irrigating and lubricating the synovial membranes.

This view of the Triple Burner is summarized in Box 18.10.

Box 18.10 The Triple Burner as body cavities

- The Triple Burner is a system of body cavities
- The Upper Burner is the chest cavity; the Middle Burner is the upper abdominal cavity; the Lower Burner is the lower abdominal and pelvic cavity
- The Triple Burner controls the 'penetration' of Qi in and out of the cavities and the entering–exiting of Qi
- In the abdominal cavity, the Triple Burner controls the entering–exiting of Qi in and out of the Membranes
- In the chest cavity, the Triple Burner controls the entering and exiting of the Gathering Qi (*Zong Qi*)
- In the space between skin and muscles, the Triple Burner controls the entering and exiting of Defensive Qi (*Wei Qi*)
- In the joint cavities, the Triple Burner controls the entering and exiting of Qi and fluids in the joint capsules

OTHER ASPECTS OF THE TRIPLE BURNER

Mental aspect

The mental–emotional aspect of the Triple Burner is determined by its dual nature as pertaining to the character of both Fire and Wood. The Triple Burner pertains to Fire as it is exteriorly–interiorly related to the Pericardium but also because it is the emissary of the Original Qi (*Yuan Qi*) and of the Fire of the Gate of Life (*Ming Men*). It partakes of the character of Wood as it is connected to the Gall Bladder within the Lesser Yang channels. These two aspects are not unrelated, since, as we have seen, the Minister Fire between the Kidneys ascends to connect with the Triple Burner, the Gall Bladder and the Pericardium (see Fig. 18.1).

In my experience, the Triple Burner's character of Fire means that this organ/channel is involved in assisting the Mind (*Shen*) and Ethereal Soul (*Hun*) especially in forming and maintaining relationships. As the Triple Burner is the 'hinge' between the Yang channels

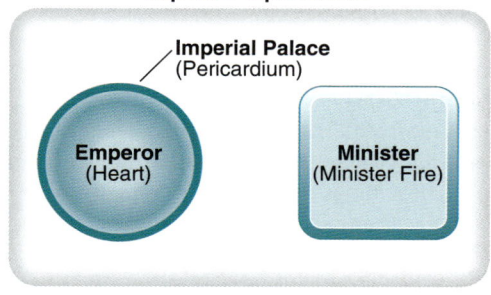

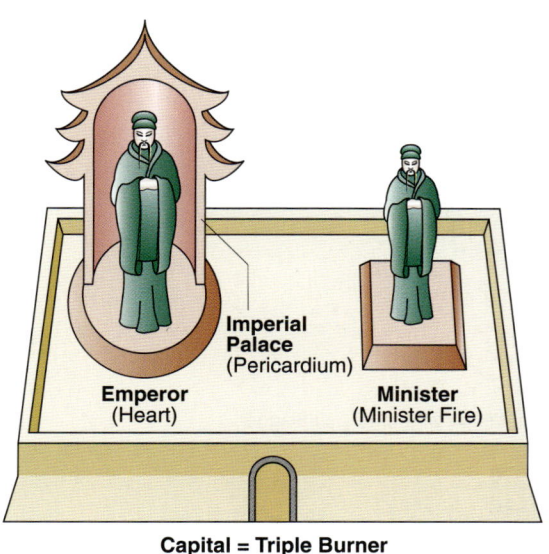

Figure 18.13 Relationship between Pericardium, Triple Burner and Heart

(with the Greater Yang opening onto the Exterior and the Bright Yang opening onto the Interior), it acts as the 'hinge' also on a psychic level, that is, in the emotional balance between the outgoing movement towards other people and relating and the inward movement towards oneself. The Pericardium also has this function within the Yin as it pertains to the Terminal Yin that is the 'hinge' between the Greater Yin and the Lesser Yin (Fig. 18.14).

In so far as it partakes the character of Wood, the Triple Burner has a similar mental–emotional influence as the Liver: that is, it also promotes the 'free flow' of emotions in a smooth way so that emotions are freely expressed and not repressed. Just as on a physical level, the Triple Burner controls the movement of Qi in all organs and structures, on a mental–emotional level, it controls the smooth flow of Qi between the Mind and the Ethereal Soul so that emotions do not turn into 'moods', which happens when Qi stagnates (Fig. 18.15).

Box 18.11 summarizes the mental aspect of the Triple Burner.

Box 18.11 Mental aspect of Triple Burner

Fire nature (with Pericardium)
As pertaining to Fire, the Triple Burner assists the Mind (*Shen*) and Ethereal Soul (*Hun*) in maintaining relationships

Wood nature (with Gall Bladder)
As pertaining to Wood, the Triple Burner assists the Liver in ensuring the smooth flow of emotions

---

Dreams

- Flying: Emptiness in the Lower Burner.[25]
- Falling: Fullness in the Lower Burner.[26]

Relationship with the Pericardium

Although they are interiorly–exteriorly related, the relationship between Pericardium and Triple Burner is somewhat tenuous. In the same way as for Heart and Small Intestine, the relationship between Triple Burner and Pericardium is more applicable to the channels, rather than to the interaction of the organs themselves.

The 'Yellow Emperor's Classic of Internal Medicine' and the 'Classic of Difficulties' always refer to the 'five Yin and six Yang organs' (omitting the Pericardium), but also to the '12 channels' (including the Pericardium). Originally the Pericardium was not thought to be separate from the Heart; the two were considered a single organ, which is perfectly logical considering their close anatomical relationship. In fact, when the 'Spiritual Axis' lists the Source points of the five Yin organs in chapter 1, it lists Daling (P-7) as the Source point of the Heart.[27]

A passage from Chapter 38 of the 'Classic of Difficulties' makes it clear that the Pericardium and Heart were, in those times, considered as one organ. It says: '*The Yin organs are 5; only the Yang organs are 6: why is that so? The Yang organs are 6 because of the Triple Burner ... it has a name but no form, and its channel pertains to the Hand Lesser Yang. [The Triple Burner] is a Yang organ and that is why these are 6.*'[28]

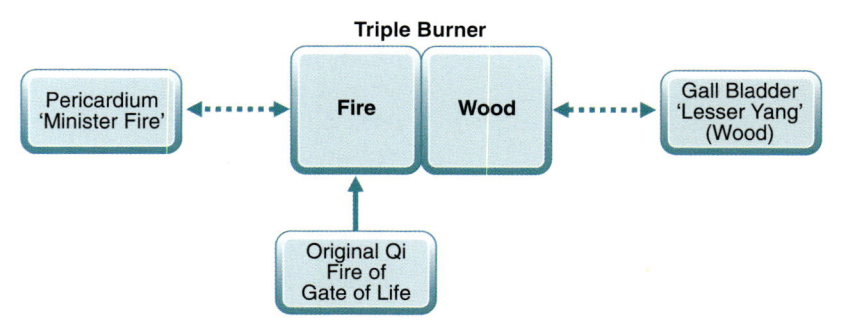

Figure 18.14 Relationship between Triple Burner, Pericardium and Gall Bladder

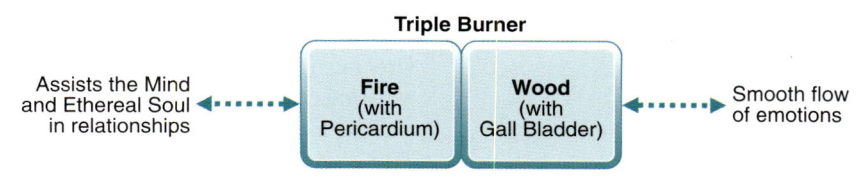

Figure 18.15 Emotional influence of Triple Burner

This passage is revealing because of its starting question: in fact, the very question '*the Yin organs are 5, why are there 6 Yang organs?*' implies that it is taken for granted that the Heart and Pericardium are part of the same organ and that therefore it is strange that the Yang organs are six. The answer explains that the Yang organs are six due to the existence of the Triple Burner. However, within the reply it says that the Triple Burner '*has a name but no form*', thus implying that the Triple Burner is different from the other regular Yang organs and their total only makes six only by adding the Triple Burner.[29]

Chapter 39 of the 'Classic of Difficulties' is even more specific about the fact that the Triple Burner is a Yang organ that is not actually associated with a Yin organ: '*Each of the Yin organs has a Yang one associated with it. The Triple Burner is also a Yang organ but it is not associated with any of the Yin organs. That is why some say that there are only 5 Yang organs.*'[30]

With the development of the channel theory, the Triple Burner was associated with the Pericardium (given their corresponding position on the arm) and their number totalled 12, including the Triple Burner and Pericardium channels.

Although the Pericardium and Triple Burner channels are exteriorly–interiorly related within the Five-Element scheme, there is hardly a close relationship between these two organs. In fact, some Chinese teachers and doctors go so far as saying that the Pericardium and Triple Burner organs are not interiorly–exteriorly related as the other organs are.

As channels, the Pericardium and Triple Burner channels have a close and symmetrical relationship. The Triple Burner belongs to the Lesser Yang channels, which are the 'hinge' between the Greater Yang and the Bright Yang channels; the Pericardium pertains to the Terminal Yin channels, which are the 'hinge' between the Greater Yin and Lesser Yin channels. Being the 'hinge' implies that these channels can connect the Yang and Yin channels: that is, the Triple Burner can connects the three Yang and the Pericardium the three Yin.

In my experience, being the 'hinge' on a psychological level means that these channels are 'mediators' in the sense that they can affect a person's capacity to relate to other people and the external world. The Triple Burner and Pericardium channels affect the mental–emotional state because the Minister Fire rises towards these two channels; therefore, when the Minister Fire is aroused by emotional problems, and it rises towards the Pericardium and Triple Burner channels, points of these channels can be used to clear Heat and calm the Mind.

Finally, the Pericardium and Triple Burner channels are symmetrical in so far as the former is the opening point of the Yin Linking Vessel (*Yin Wei Mai*) and the latter of the Yang Linking Vessel (*Yang Wei Mai*); this is another reason why these two channels connect the three Yin and three Yang, respectively.

The 'Medicine Treasure' even says that the Triple Burner is interiorly-exteriorly related to the Gate of Life (*Ming Men*).[31] Since the Gate of Life is also called the 'Minister Fire', this explains the attribution of Triple Burner to Fire and specifically Minister Fire in the Five-Element context. The Pericardium is obviously closely connected to the Heart and naturally belongs to the Fire Element; hence the connection between Pericardium and Triple Burner within the Fire Element and their name of 'Minister Fire'.

The 'Selected Historical Theories of Chinese Medicine' clarifies the relationship between the Triple Burner and Pericardium: '*The Heart is the Emperor who has a Minister. The Triple Burner cavities are like a capital which houses both the Emperor and the Minister. The Pericardium in the centre of the chest is like a palace that houses only the Emperor. The palace is inside and is Yin, the capital is outside and is Yang; hence the Triple Burner is a Yang organ and the Pericardium a Yin organ.*'[32]

Learning outcomes

In this chapter you will have learned:
- The role of the Triple Burner in 'mobilizing' Original Qi, enabling it to differentiate in order to perform its various functions in the different organs
- The influence of the Triple Burner on the Qi Mechanism, controlling the movement of all types of Qi and ensuring Qi passes freely through all cavities and organs
- The similarities and differences between the influence of the Triple Burner, the Liver and the Lungs on the movement of Qi
- The importance of the Triple Burner's function of controlling the transformation, transportation and excretion of fluids
- The four different views of the Triple Burner: as a Yang organ with form; as a mobilizer of the Original Qi without form; as a three-fold division of the body; as a system of cavities
- The mental–emotional influence of the Triple Burner, characterized by the qualities of both Fire and Wood
- Dreams reflecting disharmonies of the Triple Burner
- The relationship between the Triple Burner and the Pericardium, and questions which have historically surrounded this link

Self-assessment questions

1. Give three functions of the Original Qi which depend on the Triple Burner 'mobilizing' the Original Qi.
2. Complete the following from Chapter 18 of the 'Spiritual Axis': *The Nutritive Qi originates from the _____ Burner; the Defensive Qi originates from the _____ Burner.*
3. What is the metaphor used in Chapter 8 of the 'Simple Questions' to describe the Triple Burner's function of controlling fluids?
4. Which fluids result from the transformation process of the Triple Burner in the Upper, Middle and Lower Burners?
5. Give an example of the Triple Burner function of '*chu*' or 'letting out' for each of the three Burners.
6. How does the Triple Burner's 'mobilization' of the Original Qi influence digestion?
7. Complete the following sayings:
   a) 'The Upper Burner is like a _____'
   b) 'The Middle Burner is like a _____ _____'
   c) 'The Lower Burner is like a _____ _____.'
8. List the different Qi of the Three Burners, according to the three-fold division of the body.
9. What function does the Triple Burner have in relation to the joints of the body?
10. On a mental – emotional level, what is the significance of the Triple Burner's position as 'hinge' between the Greater Yang and Bright Yang channels?

See p. 1260 for answers

END NOTES

1. Nanjing College of Traditional Chinese Medicine 1979 A Revised Explanation of the Classic of Difficulties (*Nan Jing Jiao Shi* 难经校释), People's Health Publishing House, Beijing, first published *c*.AD 100, p. 144.
2. Ibid., p. 94.
3. Hua Tuo 1985 Classic of the Central Scripture (*Zhong Zang Jing*) (中藏经), Jiangsu Science Publishing House, Nanjing, p. 39. Written in Han dynasty.
4. Classic of Difficulties, p. 144.
5. 1981 Spiritual Axis (*Ling Shu Jing* 灵枢经), People's Health Publishing House, Beijing, first published *c*.100 BC, p. 52.
6. Classic of Difficulties, p. 94.
7. Ibid., p. 80.
8. 1979 The Yellow Emperor's Classic of Internal Medicine – Simple Questions (*Huang Di Nei Jing Su Wen* 黄帝内经素问), People's Health Publishing House, Beijing, first published *c*.100 BC, p. 59.
9. Ibid., p 59.
10. Spiritual Axis, p. 51.
11. Classic of Difficulties, p. 144.
12. Steve Clavey has proposed this interpretation of the passage of chapter 66 of the 'Classic of Difficulties'. The crucial sentence is: '*San Jiao zhe, Yuan Qi zhi bie shi*' 三焦者，原气之别使. The words '*bie shi*' are translated as 'emissary' or 'envoy' (for example, by Unschuld). Clavey proposes that '*bie shi*' has the meaning of 'to separate', i.e. the Triple Burner has the function of making the Original Qi separate and differentiate to assume different roles in different parts of the body. See Clavey S 2003 Fluid Physiology and Pathology in Traditional Chinese Medicine, Churchill Livingstone, Edinburgh, p. 35.
13. Classic of Difficulties, p. 79.
14. Spiritual Axis, p. 52 and Classic of Difficulties, p. 79.
15. Medicine Treasure, cited in Wang Xin Hua 1983 Selected Historical Theories of Chinese Medicine (*Zhong Yi Li Dai Yi Lun Xuan* 中医历代医论选), Jiangsu Scientific Publishing House, p. 2.
16. Spiritual Axis, p. 71.
17. Selected Historical Theories of Chinese Medicine, p. 2.
18. Spiritual Axis, p. 52.
19. Selected Historical Theories of Chinese Medicine, p. 2.
20. Spiritual Axis, p. 52.
21. Cited in Wang Xue Tai 1988 Great Treatise of Chinese Acupuncture, p. 46.
22. Selected Historical Theories in Chinese Medicine, p. 161.
23. Ibid., p. 159.
24. Ibid., p. 161.
25. Simple Questions, p. 102.
26. Ibid., p. 102.
27. Spiritual Axis, p 3.
28. Classic of Difficulties, p. 94.
29. Ibid., p. 94. To add to the confusion, chapter 39 even says that there are five Yang organs (excluding the Triple Burner) and six Yin organs (not, as one would expect, counting the Pericardium, but counting the Kidneys as two organs).
30. Ibid., p. 95.
31. Selected Historical Theories of Chinese Medicine, p. 2.
32. Ibid., p. 161.

SECTION 3

The Functions of the Six Extraordinary Yang Organs

INTRODUCTION

The Six Extraordinary Yang Organs complete and integrate the picture of the Internal Organs in Chinese medicine as they include structures and functions not falling under the umbrella of the Internal Organs, notably the Uterus and the Brain. They are called 'Extraordinary Yang Organs' because they function like a Yin organ (i.e. storing Yin essences and not excreting), but have the shape of a Yang organ (i.e. hollow).

All the Six Extraordinary Yang Organs store some form of refined essence, such as marrow, bile or blood; functionally, they are all directly or indirectly related to the Kidneys. Another characteristic they share is that most of them are cavities, for example the skull (containing the brain), the blood vessels, the bones, the gall bladder, and the spine.

The Six Extraordinary Yang Organs are:

1. The Uterus
2. The Brain
3. Marrow
4. The Bones
5. The Blood Vessels
6. The Gall Bladder

Each Extraordinary Yang Organ is related to a particular Internal Organ as follows:

Uterus = Kidneys and Liver
Brain = Kidneys
Marrow = Kidneys
Bones = Kidneys
Blood Vessels = Heart
Gall Bladder = Gall Bladder

SECTION 3 PART 2

19
The Functions of the Six Extraordinary Yang Organs (the Four Seas)

Key contents
The Uterus
The Brain
Marrow
The Bones
The Blood Vessels
The Gall Bladder
(The Four Seas)

- The Uterus
- The Brain
- Marrow
- The Bones
- The Blood Vessels
- The Gall Bladder

In addition, the Four Seas will be discussed.

Box 19.1 lists the Six Extraordinary Yang Organs.

Box 19.1 The Six Extraordinary Yang Organs
• Uterus
• Brain
• Marrow
• Bones
• Blood Vessels
• Gall Bladder

Besides the regular Yin and Yang organs, there are also Six Extraordinary Yang Organs which complete the picture of Chinese physiology. They are called 'Extraordinary Yang Organs' because they function like a Yin organ (i.e. storing Yin essence and not excreting), but have the shape of a Yang organ (i.e. hollow).

The Six Extraordinary Yang Organs are the Uterus, Brain, Bones, Marrow, Gall Bladder and Blood Vessels. The 'Simple Questions' in chapter 11 says: *'Brain, Marrow, Bones, Blood Vessels, Gall-Bladder and Uterus are generated by the Qi of Earth; they all store Yin essences but have the shape of Earth [i.e. a Yang, hollow organ]; they store and do not excrete, therefore they are called Extraordinary Yang organs'*.[1]

All the Six Extraordinary Yang Organs store some form of refined essence, such as marrow, bile or blood; functionally, they are all directly or indirectly related to the Kidneys. Another characteristic they share is that most of them are cavities: for example, the skull (containing the brain), the blood vessels, the bones, the gall bladder, and the spine (although the spine itself is not one of the Six Extraordinary Yang Organs, it pertains to Marrow).

The functions of the Six Extraordinary Yang Organs will be discussed under the following headings:

THE UTERUS

The Uterus was called *Zi Bao* in Chinese medicine. *Bao* is actually a structure that is common to both men and women and which is in the Lower Field of Elixir (*Dan Tian*): in men, *Bao* is the 'Room of Essence', in women, the Uterus (Fig. 19.1). Chapter 36 of the 'Classic of

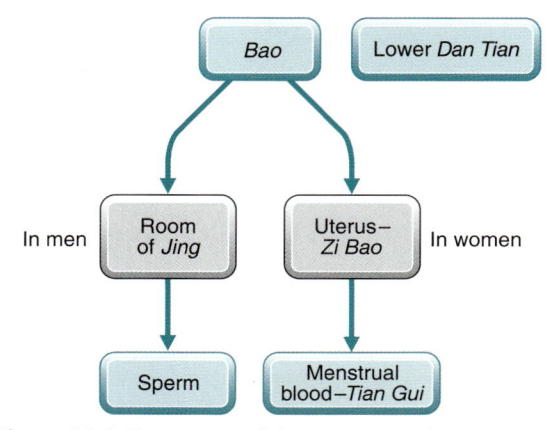

Figure 19.1 The Uterus and the Lower *Dan Tian*

Difficulties' says: *'The Gate of Life [Ming Men] is the residence of the Mind [Shen] and Essence [Jing] and it is connected to the Original Qi [Yuan Qi]: in men it houses the Sperm; in women the Uterus.'*[2]

The Uterus is the most important of the Six Extraordinary Yang Organs. It has the function of regulating menstruation, conception and pregnancy. Yin organs store essence and do not discharge; the Yang organs do not store but are constantly filled and constantly discharge. The Uterus functions as a Yin organ in that it stores Blood and the fetus during pregnancy; it functions as a Yang organ in that it discharges blood at menstruation and the baby in childbirth (Fig. 19.2).

The functions of the Uterus are:

- It regulates menstruation
- It houses the fetus during pregnancy

Before discussing these functions, we will discuss the relationship between the Uterus and Extraordinary Vessels and that between the Uterus and the Internal Organs.

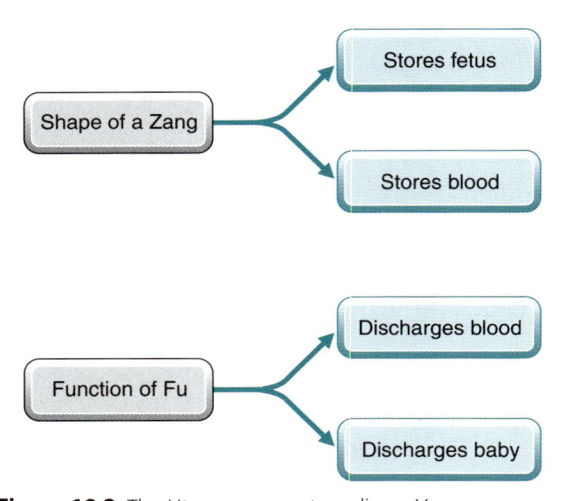

Figure 19.2 The Uterus as an extraordinary Yang organ

Relationship with the Directing and Penetrating Vessels

The Uterus is closely related to the Kidneys, the Directing Vessel (*Ren Mai*) and the Penetrating Vessel (*Chong Mai*). Both the Directing and Penetrating Vessels originate from the Kidneys and both flow through the Uterus, regulating menstruation, conception and pregnancy. In particular, the Directing Vessel provides Qi and Essence and the Penetrating Vessel Blood provides to the Uterus (Fig. 19.3).

Normal menstruation and pregnancy depend on the state of the Directing and Penetrating Vessels, which, in turn, depend on the state of the Kidneys. If Kidney-Essence is abundant, the Directing and Penetrating Vessels are strong and the Uterus is therefore adequately supplied with Blood and Essence, so that there will be normal menstruation and pregnancy. If Kidney-Essence is weak, the Directing and Penetrating Vessels will be empty, and the Uterus will be inadequately supplied with Blood and Essence, so that there may be irregular menstruation, amenorrhoea or infertility.

Remember: the Governing Vessel also has an important influence on the Uterus and menstruation as it brings Yang Qi to the Uterus (necessary for ovulation)

Although the Directing and Penetrating Vessels are the ones that influence the Uterus most directly, the influence of the Governing Vessel should not be underestimated. The menstrual cycle is like an ebb and flow of a tide of Kidney-Yin and Kidney-Yang with Yin increasing (and therefore Yang decreasing) in the first half of the cycle (follicular phase) and Yang increasing (and therefore Yin decreasing) in the second half of the cycle (luteal phase). In terms of channels, this tide of Yin and Yang occurs in channels that flow through the

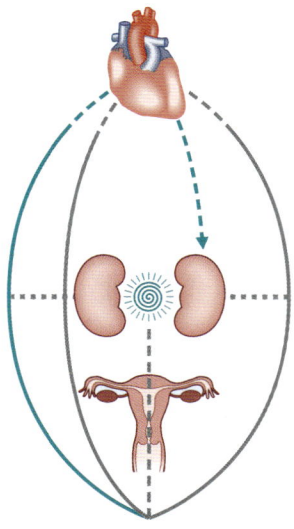

Figure 19.3 Relationship between Uterus and Directing and Penetrating Vessels

Uterus, that is, the Directing Vessel bringing Yin, the Penetrating Vessel also bringing Yin but more specifically Blood, and the Governing Vessel bringing Yang. From this point of view, the Governing Vessel is as important in menstruation as the Directing and Penetrating Vessels as it brings Yang Qi from Kidney-Yang to the Uterus in order to promote ovulation (ovulation needs heat).

Box 19.2 summarizes this relationship between the Uterus and the Directing and Penetrating Vessels.

Relationship with Internal Organs

Kidneys

The Uterus is connected to the Kidneys via a channel called the Uterus Channel (*Bao Luo*) and to the Heart via a channel called the Uterus Vessel (*Bao Mai*) (Fig. 19.4). The connection with the Kidneys is very important and well-known, that is, the Kidneys are the origin of menstrual blood (*Tian Gui*), they are the Mother of the Liver, which provides Blood to the Uterus, and closely connected to the Directing and Penetrating Vessels, which regulate Qi and Blood in the Uterus. Chapter 1 of the 'Simple Questions' explains the origin of menstrual blood: '*When a girl is 14, Tian Gui arrives, the Directing Vessel is open, the Penetrating Vessel is flourishing and she can conceive.*'[3] Thus, menstrual blood is not Blood in the same way as the Blood that nourishes the sinews for example, but it is a precious fluid deriving directly from the Kidney-Essence, and is equivalent to sperm in men.

Heart

The Heart is connected to the Uterus via the Uterus Vessel and this explains the strong influence of emotional problems on menstruation. More specifically, Heart-Qi and Heart-Blood descend towards the Uterus, promoting the discharge of menstrual blood during the bleeding phase and the discharge of the eggs during ovulation. The Heart also controls the two moments of transformation, that is, transformation of Yang to Yin with the beginning of bleeding and that of Yin to Yang with ovulation; in other words, the beginning of bleeding and ovulation are two moments of transformation during the tide of Yin and Yang, two moments of change from Yang to Yin and from Yin to Yang. The descending of Heart-Qi and Heart-Blood towards the Uterus ensures that these two moments of transformation occur smoothly and at the right time.

The Heart influences the Uterus also because it governs Blood and this indirectly nourishes the Uterus in a similar way as Liver-Blood does. For example, Heart-Blood deficiency may cause amenorrhoea, Heart-Blood Heat may cause menorrhagia and Heart-Blood stasis may cause painful periods.

Finally, the Heart influences menstruation as Heart-Yang descends to meet the Kidneys to contribute to forming *Tian Gui* (i.e. menstrual blood).

> **Box 19.2 Relationship between the Uterus and the Directing and Penetrating Vessels**
> - Both Directing and Penetrating Vessels flow through the Uterus
> - The Directing Vessel brings Qi, Yin and Essence to the Uterus
> - The Penetrating Vessel brings Blood to the Uterus

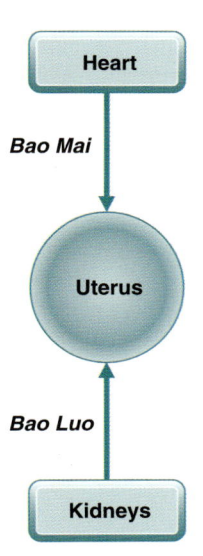

Figure 19.4 Relationship between Uterus, Kidneys and Heart

> **Clinical note**
>
> The Heart influences the Uterus and menstruation in four ways:
> 1. Heart-Qi and Heart-Blood descend to the Uterus to promote the discharge of menstrual blood during the period and of the eggs during ovulation
> 2. The descending of Heart-Qi and Heart-Blood bring about the transformation of Yang to Yin with the onset of the period and of Yin to Yang with ovulation
> 3. The Heart governs Blood and Heart-Blood nourishes the Uterus
> 4. Heart-Yang descends to meet the Kidney-Essence to form *Tian Gui*, i.e. menstrual blood

Spleen

The Spleen is the Root of Post-Heaven Qi and it is the source of Qi and Blood. As it is the source of Blood, it plays a role in relation to the Uterus and menstruation. However, this role is secondary to that of the Kidneys because the latter are the origin of menstrual blood (*Tian Gui*) and the Spleen plays only a secondary role in supplementing that Blood. In other words, menstrual blood is not quite 'Blood' but a precious fluids (equivalent to sperm in men) that derives directly from the Kidney-Essence.

Liver

Menstruation, conception and pregnancy depend on the state of the Blood, upon which the Uterus depends. The functional relationship between Uterus and Blood is very close: the Uterus relies on an abundant supply of Blood at all times. Since the Heart governs the Blood, while the Liver stores the Blood and the Spleen controls the Blood, these three Yin organs are physiologically related to the Uterus, but the Liver is clinically the most important one. For example, if the Liver does not store enough Blood, the Uterus is starved of Blood and this may cause amenorrhoea; if Liver-Blood is stagnant, this will affect the Uterus, causing painful periods with dark clotted blood. On the other hand, if the Spleen cannot produce enough Blood and Heart-Blood becomes deficient, the Uterus may lack Blood, resulting in amenorrhoea.

If the Blood stored by the Liver is hot, this may cause the Blood in the Uterus to flow out recklessly, causing menorrhagia or metrorrhagia. If Liver-Qi is stagnant, this may cause Liver-Blood stasis, which in turn, will affect the Blood of the Uterus, resulting in painful periods with dark clotted blood. In practice, the relationship between Uterus and Liver-Blood is extremely important and one which is very apparent in many pathological conditions. Because the Liver stores Blood and regulates the volume of Blood, menstrual irregularities are often due to a dysfunction of the Liver. For example, Liver-Qi stagnation often causes irregular periods; Liver-Blood stagnation often causes painful and/or irregular periods; Liver-Blood deficiency may cause scanty periods or absence of periods (Fig. 19.5).

Stomach

Among the Yang organs, the Uterus is closely related to the Stomach. This connection is via the Penetrating Vessel (*Chong Mai*). This vessel is closely related to the Stomach, and also flows through the Uterus, thus providing a link between Uterus and Stomach. Morning sickness during pregnancy and the nausea or vomiting which some women experience during menstruation are often caused by disruption of the Stomach (with

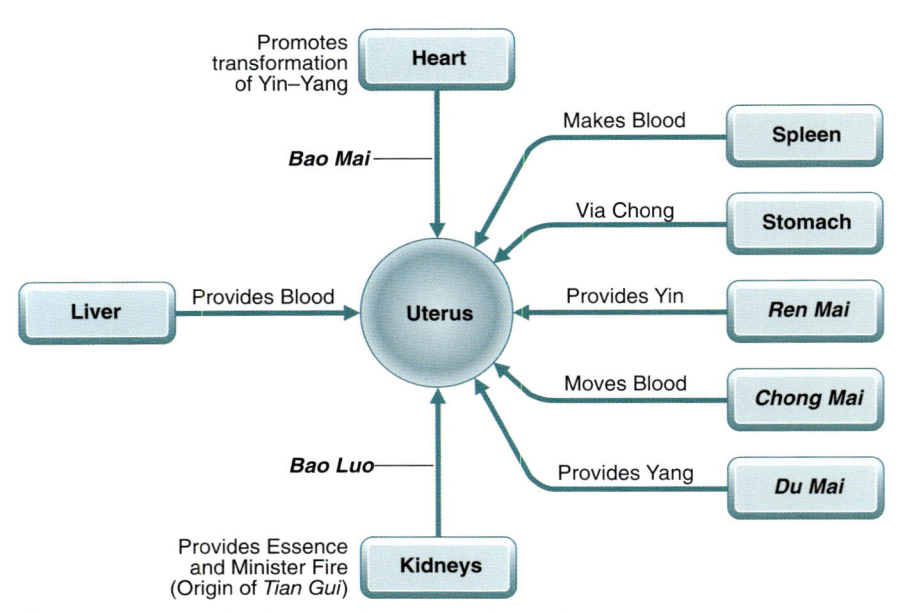

Figure 19.5 Relationship between the Uterus and Internal Organs

rebellious Qi) because of changes in the Penetrating Vessel in the Uterus.

The relationship between the Uterus and the Internal Organs is represented visually in Figure 19.5 and summarized in Box 19.3.

> **Box 19.3 The relationship between the Uterus and the Internal Organs**
>
> - **The Kidneys** are the origin of menstrual blood (*Tian Gui*)
> - **The Heart** governs Blood; Heart-Yang meets Kidney-Essence to form *Tian Gui*; Heart-Qi descends to promote discharge of menstrual blood and eggs; Heart-Qi descends to trigger transformation of Yang to Yin and vice versa in menstrual cycle
> - **The Liver** stores Blood, which fills the Uterus
> - **The Spleen** makes Blood, which supplements *Tian Gui*
> - **The Stomach** is related to the Uterus via the Penetrating Vessel

The Uterus regulates menstruation

The Uterus regulates menstruation. The two most important organs for this function are the Kidneys, because they are the origin of *Tian Gui* which forms menstrual blood, and the Liver, because it regulates Blood in the Uterus. The Liver influences the Uterus and menstruation in other ways too. Liver-Qi moves during the premenstrual phase, which brings about the movement of Blood and therefore the menstrual bleed.

One can distinguish four phases in the menstrual cycle (Fig. 19.6):

> Phase 1: bleeding phase. During this phase, Blood is moving. For bleeding to start at the right time and with the right amount, it is essential for Liver-Qi and Liver-Blood to move smoothly and for Heart-Qi and Heart-Blood to descend towards the Uterus
>
> Phase 2: postmenstrual phase. During this phase, Blood and Yin are *relatively* empty (i.e. not empty in absolute terms but only in relation to other phases), and Yin is beginning to grow. This represents the beginning of the follicular phase leading to ovulation
>
> Phase 3: intermenstrual phase. During this phase, Yin reaches its maximum with ovulation and therefore starts to decrease after that; on the other hand, Yang starts to grow and this produces the heat necessary for ovulation
>
> Phase 4: premenstrual phase. During this phase, Yang grows and reaches its maximum and Qi moves

The Uterus houses the fetus during pregnancy

The Uterus houses and nourishes the fetus during pregnancy. To do this, the Uterus needs the nourishment of Kidney-Essence (through the Directing and Penetrating Vessels) and that of Blood (through the Penetrating Vessel).

During pregnancy, the Uterus functions as a Yin organ (in that it 'stores' the fetus) and during childbirth it functions as a Yang organ (in that it 'discharges' the baby).

Box 19.4 summarizes the functions of the Uterus.

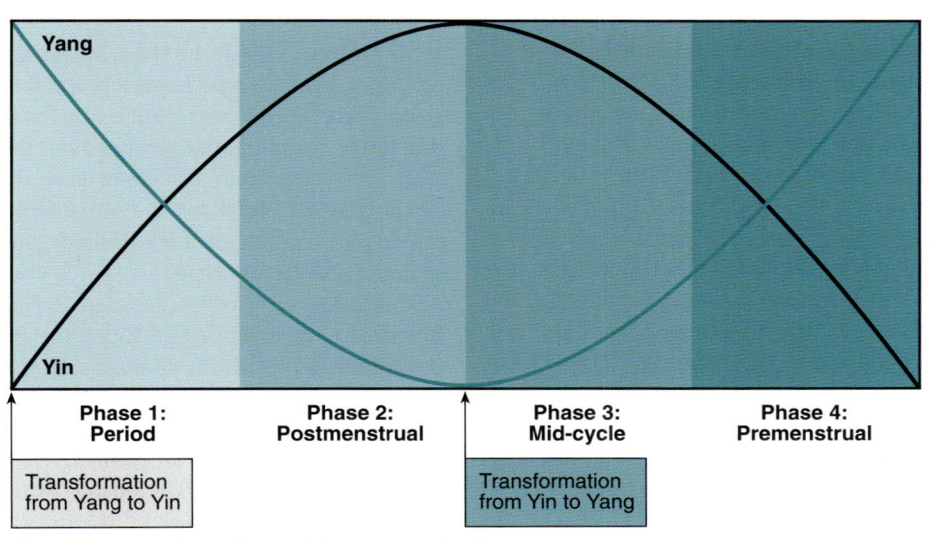

Figure 19.6 The four phases of the menstrual cycle

Box 19.4 Functions of the Uterus

- Regulates menstruation
- Houses the fetus in pregnancy

Men

Although the Uterus is one of the Six Extraordinary Yang Organs, there is a corresponding structure in men (see Fig. 19.1). It is said in Chinese medicine that *'The Uterus is related to the Kidneys, in males it is called Red Field (Dan Tian) or also Room of Essence, in females it is called Uterus.'*[4]

As mentioned above, the Uterus was called *Zi Bao* in Chinese medicine; *Bao* is actually a structure that is common to both men and women and which is in the Lower Field of Elixir (*Dan Tian*): in men, *Bao* is the 'Room of Essence'.

Bao is a structure in the Lower *Dan Tian* common to both men and women: in men, it is the Room of Essence, in women, the Uterus (called *Zi Bao*)

The 'Room of Essence' in men stores and produces sperm, and is closely related to the Kidneys and the Governing Vessel. If the Kidneys and the Governing Vessel (*Du Mai*) are empty, the production and storage of sperm by the Room of Essence will be affected, and this may cause impotence, premature ejaculation, clear and watery sperm, nocturnal emissions, spermatorrhoea, etc.

Obviously, while the Uterus is an actual organ occupying the space of the Lower Field of Elixir (*Dan Tian*), the Room of Essence is not an actual organ or structure as we know that sperm is made partly in the prostate and partly in the testicles. Although the prostate is not mentioned in ancient Chinese books, it could be postulated that the prostate is the male organ equivalent to the Uterus in women. Thus, we can postulate that the three extraordinary vessels Directing, Penetrating and Governing Vessels, which, in women, originate from the space between the Kidneys and flow downwards through the Uterus, in men, flow through the prostate.

In men, the prostate is the organ equivalent to the Uterus in women

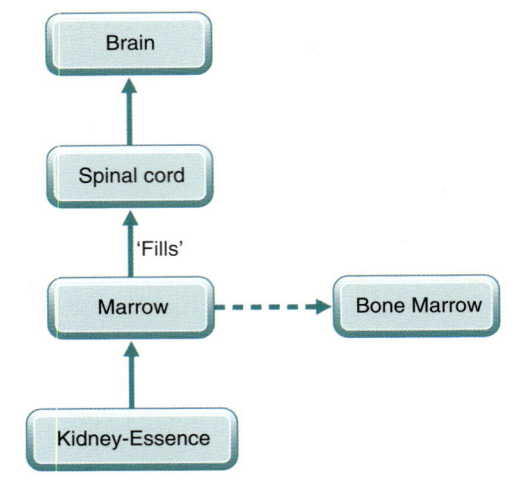

Figure 19.7 Relationship between Kidney-Essence, Marrow, spinal cord and Brain

THE BRAIN

The Brain is also called the 'Sea of Marrow'. The 'Spiritual Axis' in chapter 33 says: *'The Brain is the Sea of Marrow, extending from the top of the head to the point Fengfu (Du-16).'*[5] The 'Simple Questions' in chapter 10 says: *'The Marrow pertains to the Brain.'*[6]

In Chinese medicine, the Brain controls memory, concentration, sight, hearing, touch and smell. The 'Discussion on Stomach and Spleen' says: *'Sight, hearing, smelling, touch, intelligence all depend on the Brain.'*[7]

As we have seen in chapter 3, the Kidney-Essence produces Marrow, which gathers to fill the Brain and spinal cord. Since Marrow originates from the Kidneys, the Brain is functionally related to this Yin organ (Fig. 19.7). The brain also depends on the Heart, particularly Heart-Blood, for its nourishment, so that the physiological activities of the Brain depend on the state of both Kidneys and Heart.

The Kidneys store Essence and the Heart governs Blood. If both Essence and Blood are abundant, the Brain is in good health, vitality is good, the ears can hear properly and the eyes can see clearly. If Kidney-Essence and Heart-Blood are empty, the Brain is sluggish, memory is poor, vitality is low, hearing and sight may be decreased. The relationship of the Brain with Kidneys and Heart explains how in practice certain symptoms such as poor memory and concentration, dizziness and blurred vision can be due to deficiency of the Sea of Marrow (i.e. the Kidneys) or deficiency of Heart-Blood.

The 'Spiritual Axis' in chapter 33 says: *'If the Sea of Marrow is abundant, the vitality is good, the body feels light and agile and the body has endurance; if it is deficient, there will be dizziness, tinnitus, blurred vision, fatigue and great desire to lie down.'*[8]

The functions of the Brain are:

- It controls intelligence
- It is the Sea of Marrow and controls sight, hearing, smell and taste

The Brain controls intelligence

Chapter 17 of the 'Simple Questions' says: *'The Head is the Palace of Intelligence'*[9] ('palace' here, *Fu*, could also be translated as 'Yang organ'). Thus, in a similar way as in Western medicine, the Brain controls intelligence and mental clarity.

Many of the functions that Western medicine attributes to the brain are attributed to the Heart in Chinese medicine: the Heart houses the Mind (*Shen*), which is responsible for thinking, memory, perceptions, etc. However, during the course of development of Chinese medicine, too, there have been doctors who attributed mental functions to the brain rather than the Heart: in particular, Sun Si Miao of the Tang dynasty, Zhao You Qin of the Yuan dynasty, Li Shi Zhen of the Ming dynasty and especially Wang Qing Ren of the Qing dynasty.

For example, Li Shi Zhen said: *'The Brain is the Palace of the Original Shen.'*[10] Wang Qing Ren said specifically: *'Intelligence and memory reside not in the Heart but in the Brain.'*[11] Thus, the Brain controls intelligence, memory, thinking and consciousness. This is not in contradiction with the Heart being responsible for those functions: it simply means that there is an overlap between the Heart and Brain with regard to those functions.

However, in clinical practice, the relationship between the Heart and functions such as intelligence, memory, thinking and consciousness is more important than that of the Brain. Indeed, what it actually means in practice is that in order to stimulate those functions one can use points from the Heart channel or from the Governing Vessel on the head that act on the Brain.

> **Clinical note**
>
> To stimulate the Brain it is necessary to tonify the Kidneys with KI-3 Taixi and BL-23 Shenshu and the Governing Vessel with Du-20 Baihui and Du-16 Fengfu

The Brain is the Sea of Marrow and controls sight, hearing, smell and taste

Ancient Chinese medicine books related the functions of sight, hearing, smell and taste to the 'Sea of Marrow' (i.e. the Brain). Chapter 28 of the 'Spiritual Axis' says: *'When the Qi of the upper part of the body is insufficient, the Brain is not full and there may be hardness of hearing, tinnitus, drooping of the head and blurred vision.'*[12]

Wang Qing Ren was even more explicit: *'The two ears communicate with the Brain and therefore hearing depends on the Brain; the two eyes form a system like a thread that connects them to the Brain and therefore sight depends on the Brain; the nose communicates with the Brain and therefore smell depends on the Brain ... in small children the Brain grows gradually and that is why they can say a few words.'*[13]

Therefore the senses of sight, hearing, smell, taste and the function of speech all depend on the Brain.

Box 19.5 summarizes the functions of the Brain.

MARROW

'Marrow', the common matrix of bone marrow and Brain, is produced by the Kidney-Essence, and it fills the Brain, spinal cord and bones, forming bone marrow (see Fig. 19.7). The Kidney-Essence is the origin of Marrow but the Post-Heaven Qi also plays a role in the formation of Marrow. In fact, the 'Spiritual Axis' in chapter 36 says: *'The refined essence of food and drink is changed into fat, it enters the bone cavities and fills the Brain with Marrow.'*[14]

The Chinese concept of 'Marrow' should not be confused with bone marrow as defined by Western medicine. In Chinese medicine, the function of Marrow is to

> **Box 19.5 Functions of the Brain**
>
> - The Brain controls intelligence
> - The Brain is the Sea of Marrow and it controls the senses of sight, hearing, smell and taste

nourish the Brain and spinal cord and to form bone marrow: thus, it is the common matrix to brain, spinal cord and bone marrow (see Fig. 19.7).

> 'Marrow' in Chinese medicine is not the same as bone marrow in Western medicine. It is the common matrix to bone marrow, spinal cord and brain

Marrow is closely related to the Kidneys as the Kidney-Essence is the origin of Marrow. The 'Simple Questions' in chapter 34 says: *'If the Kidneys are deficient, Marrow cannot be abundant.'*[15]

The functions of Marrow are:

- It fills the bones
- It contributes to making Blood
- It nourishes the Brain

Marrow fills the bones

The 'Simple Questions' in chapter 17 says: *'The bones are the residence of Marrow.'*[16] Chapter 10 of the 'Spiritual Axis' says: *'In the beginning of life, Essence is formed: this, in turn, forms the Brain and Marrow.'*[17] Zhang Jie Bin (1563–1640) said: *'The Essence is stored in the Kidneys, the Kidneys communicate with the Brain, the Brain is Yin; Marrow fills the bones, and it also pertains to the Brain, therefore the Essence is the origin of both the Brain and the Marrow.'*[18]

The Marrow nourishes the Bones.

Marrow contributes to making Blood

Although modern Chinese books often say that bone marrow contributes to making Blood (in their desire to find parallels between Chinese and Western medicine), there are few references to the role of bone marrow in making Blood. Nevertheless, there are some. For example, the book 'Medical Transmission of Master Zhang' (*Zhang Shi Yi Tong*, 1695) says: *'The Qi that is not spent returns to the Kidneys to make Essence; the Essence that is not discharged returns to the Liver to make Blood.'*[19]

Chapter 5 of the 'Simple Questions' says: *'The Kidneys generate bone-marrow and this generates the Liver.'*[20] As the Liver stores Blood, it seems legitimate to assume that the ancient Chinese had some understanding of the role of bone marrow in making Blood. In any case, in clinical practice, the Kidney channel is indeed used to tonify Blood.

> **Clinical note**
>
> As the Kidney-Essence is the origin of Marrow and bone marrow, the Kidney channel can be used to nourish Blood

Marrow nourishes the Brain

Marrow fills the spinal cord and the Brain; the relationship between Marrow and Brain has already been described above under the Brain. Marrow's functions are summarized in Box 19.6.

Box 19.6 The functions of Marrow

- It contributes to making Blood
- It nourishes the Brain

THE BONES

The Bones were compared to a 'trunk' in the 'Yellow Emperor's Classic of Internal Medicine'; Chapter 10 of the 'Spiritual Axis' says: *'The Bones are like a trunk.'*[21] Thus, from this point of view, the Bones obviously have the same function as in Western anatomy. However, in Chinese medicine the Bones are more than a structural framework of the body. The Bones are the cavity that houses Marrow and, as such, they are also functionally related to the Kidneys. Moreover, the Bones are considered to be like an organ and Chinese books mention 'exhaustion' of the Bones.

For example, Chapter 17 of the 'Simple Questions' says: *'The Bones are the Palace of Marrow; if a person cannot stand for too long or walks in a wobbly way, it means that the Bones are exhausted.'*[22] In clinical practice, tonification of the 'Bones' can be achieved through the Kidneys.

The Bones, like all the other Extraordinary Yang Organs, are also related to the Kidneys and the Kidney-Essence. They are considered one of the Extraordinary Yang Organs because they store bone marrow. If Kidney-Essence and Marrow are deficient, the bones lose nourishment, they cannot sustain the body and there will be inability to walk or stand.

In clinical practice, the relationship between Kidneys and Bones is very important as a decline of

Kidney-Essence may cause osteoporosis in the elderly. During the menopause, tonification of the Kidneys may slow down the onset of osteoporosis in women. The relationship between the Kidneys and Bones can be exploited in practice also by treating the Kidneys to speed up the healing of bone fractures.

> **Clinical note**
>
> As the Kidneys control the bones, the Kidneys may be treated to strengthen the bones and prevent osteoporosis.

THE BLOOD VESSELS

Blood vessels are considered one of the Extraordinary Yang Organs because they are like a 'container' for Blood. They are also indirectly related to the Kidneys because Kidney-Essence (*Jing*) produces Marrow, which contributes to producing Blood, and also because the Original Qi (*Yuan Qi*) of the Kidneys contributes to the transformation of the Food-Qi into Blood.

Apart from this, the Blood Vessels are primarily influenced by the Heart as this governs Blood and controls blood vessels, but also by the Lungs as they control all channels and vessels.

The functions of the Blood Vessels are:

- They house Blood and are the vehicle for the circulation of Qi and Blood
- They transport the refined food essences, Qi and Blood all over the body

The Blood Vessels house Blood and are the vehicle for the circulation of Qi and Blood

The Blood Vessels are the organ that houses Blood. Chapter 17 of the 'Simple Questions' says: '*The Blood Vessels are the Palace of Blood.*'[23] Chapter 30 of the 'Spiritual Axis' says: '*The Blood Vessels contain Nutritive Qi so that it does not spill out.*'[24]

The Blood Vessels transport the refined food essences, Qi and Blood all over the body

Chapter 63 of the 'Spiritual Axis' says: '*The Blood Vessels are the passageways of the Middle Burner.*'[25] Thus, Blood Vessels transport the refined food essence, Qi and Blood produced in the Middle Burner all over the body to nourish all tissues. Although it is Blood that moves in the blood vessels, it relies on the power of Qi to circulate. Stagnation of Qi or Blood affects the Blood Vessels and causes stasis. Cold also easily affects the Blood Vessels, causing stasis. Chapter 39 of the 'Simple Questions' says: '*Cold can invade the Blood Vessels, Cold makes them contract and ... causes pain.*'[26]

The functions of the Blood Vessels are summarized in Box 19.7.

> **Box 19.7 The functions of the Blood Vessels**
>
> - They house Blood and are the vehicle for the circulation of Qi and Blood
> - They transport refined food essences, Qi and Blood all over the body

THE GALL BLADDER

The Gall Bladder is considered one of the Extraordinary Yang Organs because, unlike other Yang organs, it stores bile, which is a 'pure' fluid. The main significance of the Gall Bladder being one of the Extraordinary Yang Organs is on a psychological level.

Firstly, the Gall Bladder differs from the other Yang organs in that it is the only one that stores a 'pure' substance (bile) and does not deal with food, drink or waste products. For this reason, on a psychological level, the Gall Bladder affects our capacity of making decisions and our courage to act on decisions.

Secondly, the Gall Bladder's position as the Yang aspect of the Liver has psychological implications as the Qi of the Gall Bladder (this being a Yang organ) gives the Ethereal Soul (*Hun*) the capacity for 'movement': as we have seen, the Ethereal Soul provides 'movement' to the Mind (*Shen*) and is the source of inspiration, creativity, project, plans, aims, life dreams, sense of direction and purpose.

THE FOUR SEAS

The Four Seas are discussed in chapter 33 of the 'Spiritual Axis'. As often happens in acupuncture, the channel system is compared to an irrigation system. The channels are likened to rivers, which flow into the Four Seas: '*The body has 4 Seas and 12 River-channels;*

these flow into the Seas of which there is an East, West, North and South one.'²⁷

Box 19.8 lists the Four Seas.

The Four Seas are the Sea of Marrow, the Sea of Blood, the Sea of Qi and the Sea of Food. Each of these Seas is activated by specific 'upper' and 'lower' points. Chapter 33 of the 'Spiritual Axis' says: 'The Stomach is the Sea of Food: its upper point is ST-30 Qichong and its lower point is ST-36 Zusanli. The Penetrating Vessel [Chong Mai] is the Sea of the 12 Channels: its upper point is BL-11 Dashu and its lower points are ST-37 Shangjuxu and ST-39 Xiajuxu. The centre of the chest is the Sea of Qi: its upper points are Du-15 Yamen and Du-14 Dazhui and it also has a point in the front, ST-9 Renying. The Brain is the Sea of Marrow: its upper point is Du-20 Baihui and its lower point is Du-16 Fengfu.'²⁸ Although the text does not specifically say so, it is logical that Ren-17 Shanzhong is also a point of the Sea of Qi as the text refers to the Sea of Qi being in the 'centre of the chest'. The points are summarized in Box 19.9.

Each Sea can be adversely affected by Deficiency or Excess conditions as well as by conditions of rebellious Qi. Chapter 33 of the 'Spiritual Axis' says: 'When the Seas function harmoniously there is life; when they function against the normal flow there is disease. When the Sea of Qi is in excess, there is a feeling of fullness in the chest, breathlessness and red face; when the Sea of Qi is deficient, there is shortness of breath and dislike to speak. When the Sea of Blood is in excess, the person has the feeling of the body getting bigger and the person is unable to pin-point the trouble; when the Sea of Blood is deficient, the person has the feeling of the body getting smaller and is unable to pin-point the trouble. When the Sea of Food is in excess there is abdominal fullness; when the Sea of Food is deficient, the person is hungry but has no desire to eat. When the Sea of Marrow is full, the person feels agile with light limbs and great physical strength; when the Sea of Marrow is deficient, there is dizziness, tinnitus, blurred vision, weak legs and desire to lie down.'²⁹

The symptoms of the Four Seas are summarized in Box 19.10.

Although the main text mentions 'Excess' and 'Deficiency' of the Four Seas with the above symptoms, it also mentions the pathological condition of rebellious Qi (i.e. Qi flowing upwards instead of downwards). This is particularly evident in the case of the Sea of Qi as the symptoms of breathlessness, fullness of the chest and red face are symptoms of Lung-Qi rebelling upwards.

The Sea of Blood is synonymous with the Penetrating Vessel (*Chong Mai*), as the text makes clear. This is of great relevance in clinical practice and especially in gynaecology as we treat the Penetrating Vessel for disharmonies of Blood and especially Blood stasis.

The Sea of Marrow is synonymous with the Brain as it is Marrow that fills up the Brain. Its symptoms of deficiency are clearly related to obfuscation of the sense orifices due to not being nourished by Marrow. As the Kidney-Essence is the origin of Marrow, those symptoms are also symptoms of Kidney deficiency (dizziness, tinnitus, blurred vision, weak legs). The Sea of Marrow is related to the Governing Vessel (*Du Mai*), which flows in the spine and into the Brain: for this reason, the points of the Sea of Marrow (Du-20 Baihui and Du-16 Fengfu) are on the Governing Vessel.

Box 19.8 The Four Seas

- Sea of Qi
- Sea of Food
- Sea of Blood
- Sea of Marrow

Box 19.9 Points of the Four Seas

- **Sea of Food**: ST-30 Qichong (upper) and ST-36 Zusanli (lower)
- **Sea of Blood**: BL-11 Dashu (upper) and ST-37 Shangjuxu and ST-39 Xiajuxu (lower)
- **Sea of Qi**: Du-15 Yamen and Du-14 Dazhui (upper) and ST-9 Renying (front). Also Ren-17 Shanzhong
- **Sea of Marrow**: Du-20 Baihui (upper) and Du-16 Fengfu (lower)

Box 19.10 Symptoms of the Four Seas

Sea of Qi
 Excess: fullness of the chest, red face, breathlessness
 Deficiency: shortness of breath, dislike of speaking

Sea of Blood
 Excess: feeling of body getting bigger
 Deficiency: feeling of body getting smaller

Sea of Food
 Excess: abdominal fullness
 Deficiency: hungry but no desire to eat

Sea of Marrow
 Excess: light limbs and feeling of strength
 Deficiency: dizziness, tinnitus, blurred vision, weak legs, desire to lie down

The Sea of Food is synonymous with the Stomach and both of its points are on the Stomach channel. This is also of relevance in clinical practice as we always need to treat the Stomach in any disturbance of food absorption or digestion.

The Sea of Qi is clearly related to the Lungs and the Gathering Qi (*Zong Qi*) and its deficiency symptom (dislike of speaking) is a Lung-deficiency symptom.

Learning outcomes

In this chapter you will have learned:
- The main characteristics of the Six Extraordinary Yang Organs
- The importance of the Uterus in regulating menstruation, conception and pregnancy
- The close relationship between the Uterus and the Extraordinary Vessels
- The importance of the relationship between the Uterus and other Internal Organs: the Kidneys, Heart, Spleen, Liver and Stomach
- The 'Room of Essence' as the equivalent to the Uterus in men
- The role of the Brain in controlling intelligence, sight, hearing, smell and taste, and its relationship with the Heart and the Kidneys
- The significance of Marrow as the common matrix to bone marrow, spinal cord and brain, and its contribution to nourishing the Blood and the Brain
- The importance of the Bones in housing Marrow, and their relationship with the Kidneys
- The function of the Blood Vessels in storing Blood, and transporting food essences, Qi and Blood all over the body
- The inclusion of the Gall Bladder as an Extraordinary Yang organ as it stores a 'pure' fluid
- The role of the Four Seas, symptoms of their excess or deficiency, and their activating points

Self-assessment questions

1. Why are these Yang organs known as 'Extraordinary'?
2. Describe the pathology of amenorrhoea resulting from weak Kidney-Essence.
3. What is the origin of menstrual blood (*Tian Gui*)?
4. How does the Heart influence the Uterus?
5. How and why might the Liver be implicated if a patient suffers from painful periods with dark, clotted blood?
6. Which two Yin organs are most closely related to the Brain, and why?
7. Describe the pathology of osteoporosis in the elderly referring to Kidney-Essence, Marrow and bones.
8. Why are the Blood Vessels classed as an Extraordinary Yang organ?
9. What are the symptoms of a deficiency of the Sea of Qi?
10. Which points might you use to tonify the Sea of Marrow?

See p. 1260 for answers

END NOTES

1. 1979 The Yellow Emperor's Classic of Internal Medicine – Simple Questions (*Huang Di Nei Jing Su Wen* 黄帝内经素问), People's Health Publishing House, Beijing, first published c.100 BC, p. 77.
2. Nanjing College of Traditional Chinese Medicine 1979 A Revised Explanation of the Classic of Difficulties (*Nan Jing Jiao Shi* 难经校释), People's Health Publishing House, Beijing, first published c.AD 100, p. 90.
3. Simple Questions, p. 4.
4. 1978 Fundamentals of Chinese Medicine (*Zhong Yi Ji Chu Xue* 中医基础学), Shandong Scientific Publishing House, Jinan, p. 47.
5. 1981 Spiritual Axis (*Ling Shu Jing* 灵枢经), People's Health Publishing House, Beijing, first published c.100 BC, p. 73.
6. Simple Questions, p. 72.
7. Li Dong Yuan 1249 Discussion on Stomach and Spleen (*Pi Wei Lun* 脾胃论), cited in 1980 Concise Dictionary of Chinese Medicine (*Jian Ming Zhong Yi Ci Dian* 简明中医辞典), People's Health Publishing House, Beijing, p. 712.
8. Spiritual Axis, p. 73.
9. Simple Questions, p. 100.
10. Cited in Wang Xue Tai 1988 Great Treatise of Chinese Acupuncture (*Zhong Guo Zhen Jiu Da Quan* 中国针灸大全), Henan Science Publishing House, p. 49.
11. Ibid., p. 49.
12. Spiritual Axis, p. 68.
13. Ibid., p. 49.
14. Ibid. p. 77.
15. Ibid., p. 198.
16. Simple Questions, p. 100.
17. Spiritual Axis, p. 30.
18. Great Treatise of Chinese Acupuncture, p. 50.
19. Cited in Great Treatise of Acupuncture, p. 50.
20. Simple Questions, p. 41.
21. Spiritual Axis, p. 30.
22. Simple Questions, p. 100.
23. Ibid., p. 98.
24. Spiritual Axis, p. 71.
25. Ibid., p. 113.
26. Simple Questions, p. 218.
27. Spiritual Axis, p. 73.
28. Ibid., p. 73.
29. Ibid., p. 73.

PART 3

The Causes of Disease

INTRODUCTION

Identifying the cause of the patient's disharmony is an important part of Chinese medical practice. It is important not to consider the presenting disharmony as the cause of disease. For instance, if a person has loose stools, tiredness and no appetite, Spleen-Qi deficiency is not the cause of the disease, but simply an expression of the presenting disharmony. The cause of the disharmony itself is to be found in the person's dietary habits, lifestyle, exercise habits, etc.

Identifying the cause of the disharmony is important because only by doing that can we advise the patient on how to avoid it, minimize it or prevent its reoccurrence. If we give a treatment without addressing the cause of disease, it would be like pouring water into a container with a leak at the bottom (Fig. P3.1).

Chinese medicine stresses balance as a key to health: balance between rest and exercise, balance in diet, balance in sexual activity, balance in climate. Any long-term imbalance can become a cause of disease. For example, too much rest (not enough exercise) or too much physical exercise, too much work, too much sex or not enough sex, an unbalanced diet, an unbalanced emotional life, extreme climatic conditions, can all become causes of disease. This balance is relative to each person. What is too much exercise for one person may not be enough for another; what may constitute overeating for someone engaged in mental work in a sedentary job could be too little food to sustain someone engaged in heavy physical work.

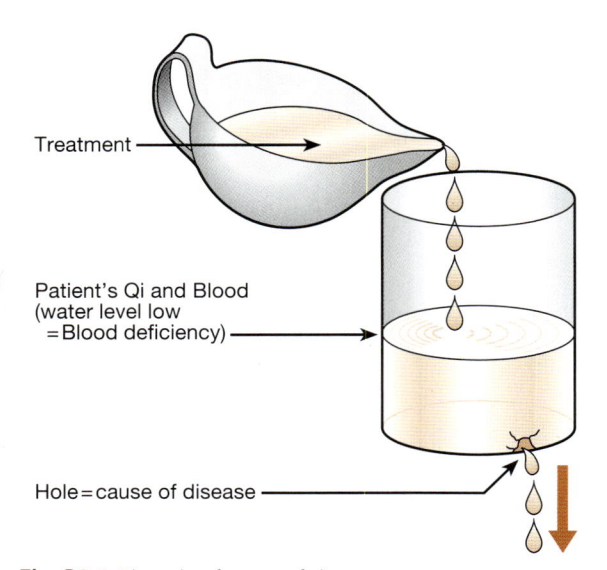

Fig. P3.1 The role of cause of disease

We should not, therefore, have in mind an ideal and rigid state of balance to which each patient should conform. It is important (and sometimes difficult) to make an assessment of the person's constitution and body–mind condition and relate these to their diet, lifestyle and climatic conditions.

Identifying the cause of the disharmony is necessary; otherwise, it will not be possible to advise the patient on specific changes which will restore harmony. If a person suffers from abdominal pain and distension from stagnation of Liver-Qi that is very evidently caused by emotional problems, there is no point in subjecting him or her to very strict diets in order to avoid the abdominal pain. This would only add to the person's misery. On the other hand, if a person suffers from pain in the hands and wrists from exterior Damp-Cold caused by a lifetime of hard work cleaning and washing things in cold water, there is no point in delving deeply into his or her emotional life.

Generally, the cause of disease is found by interrogation of the patient. I personally recommend first focusing the observation, interrogation and palpation on the pattern, not the cause, of disease. It is only after establishing the pattern of disease that I turn my attention to identifying the cause of the disease.

If a patient presents with a specific problem, for example abdominal pain, I focus first on identifying the pattern of disease: i.e. is the pain caused by Qi stagnation, Cold in the Intestines, Damp-Heat in the Intestines, etc. After identifying the pattern, I would then ask the patient about lifestyle issues to identify the cause of the disease (i.e. emotional stress, dietary irregularity, etc.).

The approach is somewhat different in the case of diseases caused by external pathogenic factors. In such cases, generally speaking, the cause of the disease is found by examination of the pattern rather than by interrogation. This is because the nature of the pattern is often related to its specific external cause of disease. In other words, if a person displays all the symptoms of an exterior attack of Wind-Heat, then we can say that Wind-Heat is the cause of the disease, no matter what climate the person was exposed to. We do not need to ask 'Were you exposed to wind?' In other words, identification of the cause (Wind-Heat) is achieved on the basis of the pattern, not the history.

In other cases, however, interrogation is necessary to identify the cause of disease. For example, if a person suffers from stagnation of Liver-Qi, we cannot know whether this is from emotional causes or from diet.

In trying to find a cause of the disease, it is convenient and useful to think of a person's life in three periods:

- The prenatal period
- From birth to about 18 years
- Adult life[1]

Differing causes of disease tend to characterize each of these three periods, whilst within each of these three time spans, a person is likely to be affected by similar aetiological factors. For example, if a disease started during early childhood, it is very frequently due to dietary factors as the digestive system of newborn babies is very vulnerable.

Thus, if we can pinpoint the beginning of the disharmony, we can have a first hint of what the likely cause might be.

The prenatal period

Chinese medicine stresses the importance of the parents' health in general, and at the time of conception specifically, for the health of the child. If the parents conceive when too old, or in poor health, the constitution of their child will be weak. This may also be the case if the mother suffered ill health or took excessive drugs during pregnancy.

If a mother suffers a shock during pregnancy, the health of the baby may be affected. This may manifest with a bluish tinge on the forehead and chin of the child and a Moving pulse (this is a pulse that is rapid, 'trembles' and feels as if it is shaped like a bean).

Childhood

This is the period from birth to the teenage years. A frequent cause of disease in early childhood is diet. Weaning a baby too early (as the tendency is more and more today) may cause Spleen deficiency. Feeding a child too much cow's milk may cause Dampness or Phlegm.

Emotions can be a cause of disease in childhood, although in a slightly different way than for adults. Young children (under 6 years) tend not to restrain their emotions, as they freely express them.

Children do suffer from emotional problems, but these are often caused by family situations, such as strain between the parents, a too strict upbringing, too demanding parents, or too much pressure at school.

All these situations can leave their mark on a child's psyche and be the cause for negative emotional patterns later in life. For example, headaches starting during childhood are often seen in bright children who are pushed too much by the parents to do well at school.

Accidents, traumas and falls are common causes of disease in childhood that can cause problems later in life. For example, a fall on the head in early childhood may cause headaches later, when another cause of disease is superimposed on the early one.

Excessive physical exercise at the time of puberty can cause menstrual problems in girls later in life, whilst too early sexual activity can cause urinary problems or painful periods in girls.

There are certain periods of life that are important watersheds as far as health is concerned: these are puberty for both sexes and, for women, childbirth and menopause. Particular care needs to be taken at those times, as they are important and delicate gateways when the body and mind are changing rapidly. The example of excessive physical exercise and sexual activity during puberty has already been mentioned.

Childbirth, is a very important time for a woman: it is a time when she can be considerably weakened, but also strengthened if she takes care. For example, if a woman resumes work too soon after childbirth, this may seriously weaken the Spleen and Kidneys. On the other hand, if she takes care to rest after childbirth, eat nourishing food and perhaps take herbal tonics, she can actually strengthen a previously weak constitution.

Adult life

Any of the usual causes of disease apply in this long period, paramount among them being emotional ones.

The causes of disease are usually divided into internal, external and others:

Internal: emotions
External: weather
Others: constitution, fatigue/overexertion, excessive sexual activity, diet, trauma, epidemics, parasites and poisons, wrong treatment

These are the causes of disease traditionally considered in Chinese medicine. In our times we obviously have many new causes of disease which did not exist in the times when Chinese medicine developed: for example radiation, pollution or chemicals in food. In practice it is important to keep these new causes in mind as possible causes of disease, and it might therefore be necessary in certain cases to integrate Chinese diagnosis with other Western diagnostic tests to find the cause of the disease.

The causes of disease will be discussed under the following headings:

1. Internal causes
    a) Anger
    b) Joy
    c) Sadness
    d) Worry and pensiveness
    e) Fear
    f) Shock
2. External causes
3. Other causes of disease
    a) Weak constitution
    b) Over-exertion
        i. Mental overwork
        ii. Physical overwork
        iii. Excessive physical exercise
        iv. Excessive sexual activity
    c) Diet
    d) Trauma
    e) Parasites and poisons
    f) Wrong treatment

END NOTES

1. This method of investigation for the cause of disease was suggested by Dr JHF Shen during one of his London lectures, and I am indebted to him for the subsequent personal communications on this subject of which he was a true master.

PART 3

Internal Causes of Disease   20

Key contents

Anger

Joy

Sadness

Worry

Pensiveness

Fear

Shock

- All emotions affect the Heart
- Effects of emotions on the body

The view of the Internal Organs as physical–mental–emotional spheres of influence is one of the most important aspects of Chinese medicine. Central to this is the concept of Qi as matter–energy that gives rise to physical, mental and emotional phenomena at the same time. Thus, in Chinese medicine, body, mind and emotions are an integrated whole with no beginning or end, in which the Internal Organs are the major sphere of influence.

For example, the 'Kidneys' of Chinese medicine correspond to the actual kidney organ on an anatomical level, to the Qi and Essence (*Jing*) associated with the Kidneys, to the Brain, will-power and drive on a mental level, and to fear on an emotional level. All these levels interact with each other simultaneously.

Please note that Chinese books (both ancient and modern) usually list these seven emotions as the main internal causes of disease. This should not be taken literally as there are many more emotions than these seven and these seven often encompass others. For example, under 'anger' I would include resentment, indignation and frustration.

Some of the emotions that I would consider to be missing from the above list of seven are envy, pride, shame, guilt, contempt, hopelessness, indignation, humiliation, regret, remorse, self-contempt, spite and vanity.

Any of these emotions can also be a cause of disease and most of them would cause Qi stagnation initially. Box 20.1 lists the internal–emotional causes of disease.

The 'internal' causes of disease are those due to emotional strain. Traditionally, internal, emotional causes of disease, injuring the internal organs directly, were contrasted to the external, climatic causes of disease, which affect the Exterior of the body first.

The internal causes of disease discussed are:

- Anger
- Joy
- Sadness
- Worry
- Pensiveness
- Fear
- Shock

The discussion of each emotion will be preceded by a general discussion of the role of the emotions as causes of disease in Chinese medicine as follows:

- Different view of emotions in Chinese and Western medicine
- When does an emotion become a cause of disease?
- Emotions as causes of disease
- Interaction of body and mind
- Positive counterpart of emotions
- The emotions and the Internal Organs

Different view of emotions in Chinese and Western medicine

There is a difference in the view of emotions between Chinese and Western medicine. While Western medicine also recognizes the interaction between body and

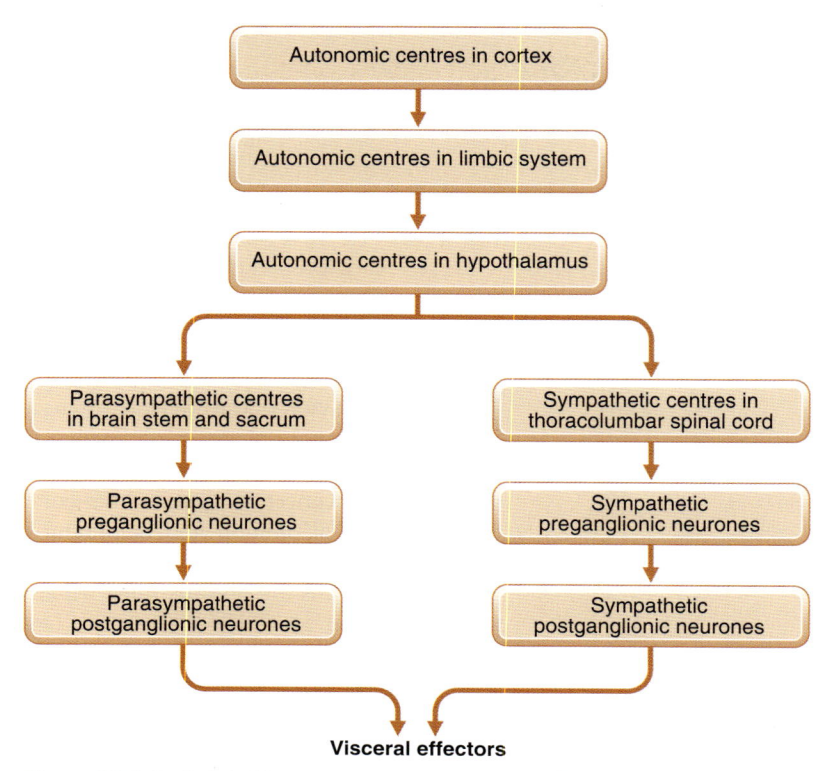

Figure 20.1 Body–Mind in Western medicine

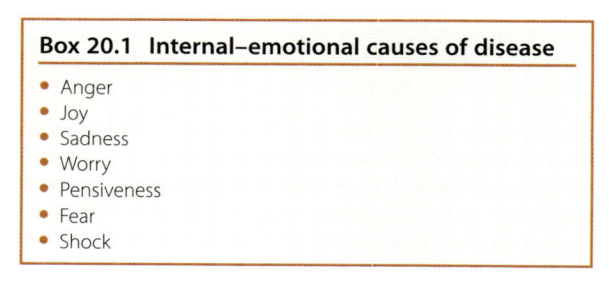

Box 20.1 Internal–emotional causes of disease
- Anger
- Joy
- Sadness
- Worry
- Pensiveness
- Fear
- Shock

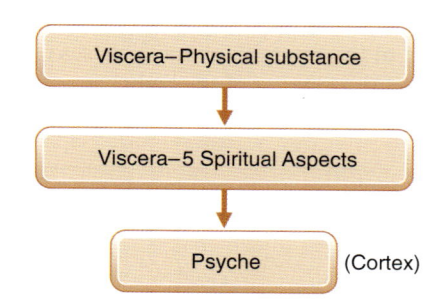

Figure 20.2 Body–Mind in Chinese medicine

emotions, it does so in a completely different way to Chinese medicine. In Western medicine, the brain is at the top of the body–mind pyramid. The emotions affect the limbic system within the brain, nerve impulses travel down the hypothalamus, through to the sympathetic and parasympathetic nerve centres, finally reaching the internal organs. Thus a nerve impulse, triggered off by an emotional upset, is transmitted to the relevant organ (Fig. 20.1).

The view of Chinese medicine is entirely different. The body–mind is not a pyramid, but a circle of interaction between the Internal Organs and their emotional aspects (Figs 20.2 and 20.3).

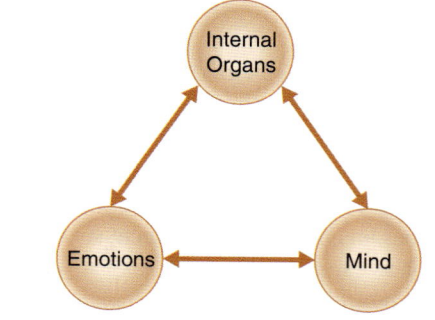

Figure 20.3 Interaction of body and mind in Chinese medicine

Whereas Western medicine tends to consider the influence of emotions on the organs as having a secondary or excitatory role rather than being a primary causative factor of disease, Chinese medicine sees the emotions as an integral and inseparable part of the sphere of action of the Internal Organs and also as direct causes of disease.

The interaction of body and mind in Chinese medicine is also expressed in the Three 'Treasures', i.e. Essence (*Jing*)–Qi–Mind (*Shen*), which were explained in chapter 3. Essence is the material basis of Qi and Mind, forming the foundation for a happy and balanced mental and emotional life (Fig. 20.4).

When does an emotion become a cause of disease?

The Chinese term for what we translate as 'emotion' is '*qing*' 情, which is based on the radical for 'heart'.

The word 'emotion' itself is not a good term to indicate the Chinese view of the 'emotional' causes of disease. The word 'emotion' derives from Latin and it refers to '*e-movere*' (i.e. to 'move out'); it is used to indicate any feeling of the mind as distinct from the cognitive or volitional states of consciousness. In this sense, the term 'emotion' may refer to any feeling such as fear, joy, hope, surprise, desire, aversion, pleasure, pain, etc.: it is therefore not entirely suitable as a term denoting the emotions as understood in Chinese medicine.

It is interesting to note that the word used to indicate a suffering of the mind was originally 'passion' rather than 'emotion'. The word 'passion' derives from the Latin verb '*patire*', which means 'to suffer'. The word 'emotion' replaced 'passion' only in the time between Descartes and Rousseau, i.e. between 1650 and 1750 (the former writer used the word 'passion' and the latter the word 'emotion').

> The emotions become causes of disease when we do not 'possess them' but they 'possess' us

The word 'passion' would also convey the idea of mental suffering better than 'emotion' because it implies the idea of something that is 'suffered', something that we are subject to. Indeed, feelings such as sadness, fear and anger become causes of disease when they take over our mind, when we no longer possess them but they 'possess' us. The Chinese expression most Chinese books use to describe the 'stimulation' or 'excitation' produced by the emotions is *ci ji* 刺激, where '*ji*' contains the radical for 'water' and means to 'swash, surge', as a wave does: that is, it denotes the surge of emotions like a wave that carries us away.

Emotions are mental stimuli that influence our affective life. Under normal circumstances, they are not a cause of disease. Hardly any human being can avoid being angry, sad, aggrieved, worried, or afraid at some time in his or her life but those states will not lead to any disharmony. For example, the death of a relative provokes a very natural feeling of grief.

Emotions become causes of disease only when they are either long-lasting, or very intense, or both. It is only when we are in a particular emotional state for a long time (months or years) that they become a cause of disease: for example, if a particular family or work situation makes us angry and frustrated in an ongoing way, this will affect the Liver and cause an internal disharmony. In a few cases, emotions can become a cause of disease in a very short time if they are intense enough: shock is the best example of such a situation.

Emotions as causes of disease

Chinese medicine is concerned with the emotions only when these are either the cause of disease, or when they themselves are the presenting symptoms. Chinese medicine neither ignores the emotions as causes of disease, nor places too much emphasis on them to the exclusion of other causes.

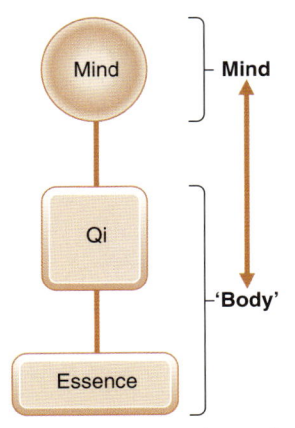

Figure 20.4 The Three Treasures as interaction of Body–Mind

In Chinese medicine, emotions (intended as causes of disease) are mental stimuli that disturb the Mind (*Shen*), the Ethereal Soul (*Hun*) and the Corporeal Soul (*Po*) and, through these, alter the balance of the Internal Organs and the harmony of Qi and Blood. For this reason, emotional stress is an internal cause of disease that injures the Internal Organs directly. Chapter 66 of the 'Spiritual Axis' says: '*Excessive joy and anger injure the Yin Organs ... when these are injured the disease is in the Yin.*'[1]

Emotions are internal causes of disease that cause an internal disharmony directly: this is contrasted with external, climatic factors, which can cause an internal disharmony only after passing through the stage of an Exterior disharmony. For example, sadness and grief deplete Lung-Qi directly and cause Lung-Qi deficiency. External Wind may invade the space between the skin and muscles (called the 'Exterior'), block the circulation of Defensive Qi and cause the typical exterior symptoms of aversion to cold and fever. It is only after passing through this Exterior stage, that the external Wind may become Interior (usually turning into Heat) and deplete Lung-Qi internally (Fig. 20.5).

Clinical note

Emotions injure the Internal Organs directly. External pathogenic factors (e.g. Wind) affect the Exterior (space between skin and muscles) first and then the Internal Organs (if the pathogenic factor is not expelled)

Box 20.2 summarizes emotions as causes of disease.

Box 20.2 Emotions as causes of disease

- Emotions are mental stimuli that influence our affective life but under normal circumstances are not a cause of disease
- Emotions become causes of disease when we do not 'possess them' but they 'possess us'
- Emotions become causes of disease when they are either long-lasting or very intense (or both)
- Emotional strain is an internal cause of disease that injures the Internal Organs directly

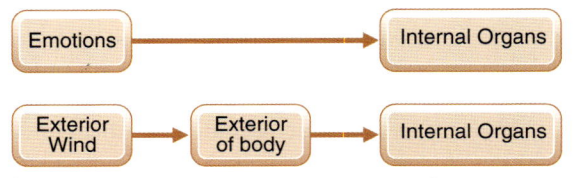

Figure 20.5 Internal versus external causes of disease

Interaction of body and mind

A very important feature of Chinese medicine is that the state of the Internal Organs affects our emotional state. For example, if Liver-Yin is deficient (perhaps from dietary factors) and causes Liver-Yang to rise, this may cause a person to become irritable all the time. Conversely, if a person is constantly angry about a certain situation or with a particular person, this may cause Liver-Yang to rise.

The 'Spiritual Axis' in chapter 8 clearly illustrates the reciprocal relationship between the emotions and the Internal Organs. It says: '*The Heart's fear, anxiety and pensiveness injure the Mind ... the Spleen's worry injures the Intellect ... the Liver's sadness and shock injure the Ethereal Soul ... the Lung's excessive joy injures the Corporeal Soul ... the Kidney's anger injures the Will-Power.*'[2] On the other hand, further on it says: '*If Liver-Blood is deficient there is fear, if it is in excess there is anger ... if Heart-Qi is deficient there is sadness, if it is in excess there is manic behaviour.*'[3] These two passages clearly show that on the one hand, emotional stress injures the Internal Organs and, on the other hand, disharmony of the Internal Organs causes emotional imbalance.

Since the body and mind form an integrated and inseparable unit, the emotions can not only cause a disharmony but can also be caused by it (Fig. 20.6). For example, a state of fear and anxiety over a long period of time may cause the Kidneys to become deficient; on the other hand, if the Kidneys become deficient through, say, overwork, this may cause a state of fear and anxiety. It is important in practice to be able to distinguish these two cases, as we should be able to advise and guide the patient. Patients are often reassured to know that their emotional state has a physical basis, or vice versa, to know that their disturbing physical symptoms are caused by their emotions. If we can make this distinction, then we can treat the disharmony properly and advise the patient accordingly.

Box 20.3 summarizes interactions of body and mind.

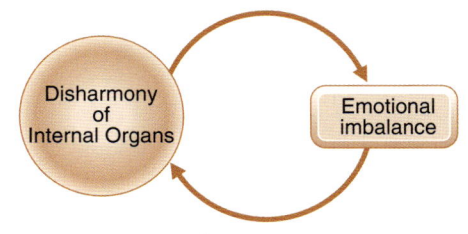

Figure 20.6 Interaction of Body–Mind

Positive counterpart of emotions

Each emotion reflects a particular mental energy that pertains to the relevant Yin organ. This, in fact, explains why a certain emotion affects a specific organ: that particular organ already produces a certain mental energy with specific characteristics, which, when subject to emotional stimuli, responds to or 'resonates' with a particular emotion. Thus emotions are not something that comes from outside the Internal Organs to attack them; the Internal Organs already have a positive mental energy which turns into negative emotions only when triggered by certain external circumstances.

> The nature of an Internal Organ 'resonates' with an emotion. Each Internal Organ has a positive mental nature that turns into negative emotions under the influence of emotional strain from life circumstances

For example, why does anger affect the Liver? If one considers the Liver's characteristics of free-going, easy and quick movement, its tendency for its Qi to rise, its correspondence to Spring when the powerful Yang energy bursts upwards and its correspondence to Wood with its expansive movement, it is easy to understand that the Liver would be affected by anger. This emotion, with its quick outbursts, the rising of blood to the head that one feels when very angry, the destructive, expansive quality of rage, mimics, on an affective level, the characteristics of the Liver and Wood outlined above. The same mental and affective qualities of the Liver that may give rise to anger and resentment over many years could be harnessed and used for creative mental development.

The emotions and the Internal Organs

The emotions taken into consideration in Chinese medicine have varied over the years. From a Five-Element perspective, the Yellow Emperor's Classic considered five emotions, each one affecting a specific Yin organ:

- Anger affecting the Liver
- Joy affecting the Heart
- Pensiveness affecting the Spleen
- Worry affecting the Lungs
- Fear affecting the Kidneys

Chapter 5 of the 'Simple Questions' says: '*Anger injures the Liver, sadness counteracts anger ... joy injures the Heart, fear counteracts joy ... pensiveness injures the Spleen, anger counteracts pensiveness ... worry injures the Lungs, joy counteracts worry ... fear injures the Kidneys, pensiveness counteracts fear.*'[4] An interesting feature of this passage is that each emotion is said to counteract another along the Controlling Sequence of the Five Elements. For example, fear pertains to the Kidneys and Water, Water controls Fire (Heart), the emotion related to the Heart is joy; hence fear counteracts joy. This thinking presents some interesting ideas, which are certainly true in practice, for example, that 'anger counteracts pensiveness' or that 'fear counteracts joy' (Fig. 20.7).

> **Box 20.3 Interaction of body and mind**
> - Emotional strain causes a disharmony of the Internal Organs
> - A disharmony of the Internal Organs may cause an emotional imbalance

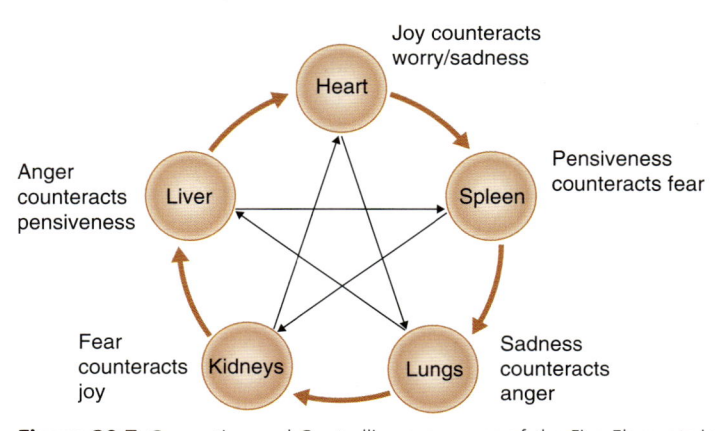

Figure 20.7 Generating and Controlling sequences of the Five Elements in emotions

However, these are not by any means the only emotions discussed in the Yellow Emperor's Classic. In other passages sadness and shock are added, giving seven emotions:

- Anger affecting the Liver
- Joy affecting the Heart
- Sadness affecting the Lungs and Heart
- Worry affecting the Lungs and Spleen
- Pensiveness affecting the Spleen
- Fear affecting the Kidneys
- Shock affecting the Heart

Effects of emotions on Qi

Each of the emotions has a particular effect on Qi and affects a certain organ:

- Anger makes Qi rise
- Joy slows Qi down
- Sadness dissolves Qi
- Worry knots Qi
- Pensiveness knots Qi
- Fear makes Qi descend
- Shock scatters Qi (Fig. 20.8)

Box 20.4 summarizes the effects of the seven emotions on the Internal Organs.

Each emotion is said to have a particular effect on the circulation of Qi. The 'Simple Questions' in chapter 39 says: '*Anger makes Qi rise, joy slows down Qi, sadness dissolves Qi, fear makes Qi descend ... shock scatters Qi ... pensiveness knots Qi.*'[5] Dr Chen Yan in 'A Treatise on the Three Categories of Causes of Diseases' (1174) says: '*Joy scatters, anger arouses, worry makes Qi unsmooth, pensiveness knots, sadness makes Qi tight, fear sinks, shock moves.*'[6]

The effect of each emotion on a relevant organ should not be interpreted too restrictively. There are passages from the Yellow Emperor's Classic which attribute the effect of emotions to organs other than the ones just mentioned. For example, the 'Spiritual Axis' in chapter 28 says: '*Worry and pensiveness agitate the Heart.*'[7] The 'Simple Questions' in chapter 39 says: '*Sadness agitates the Heart.*'[8]

The effect of an emotion also depends on other circumstances and on whether the emotion is manifested or repressed. For example, anger which is expressed affects the Liver (causing Liver-Yang rising), but anger which is repressed also affects the Heart. If one gets

Emotion	Effect on Qi
Anger	Makes Qi rise
Joy	Slows Qi
Sadness	Dissolves Qi
Worry	Knots Qi
Pensiveness	Knots Qi
Fear	Makes Qi descend
Shock	Scatters Qi

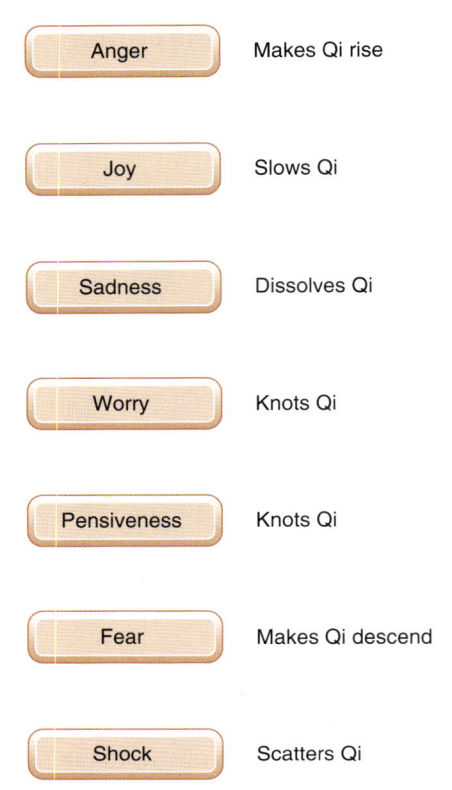

Figure 20.8 Effects of emotions on Qi

Box 20.4 The seven emotions and the Internal Organs

- Anger affects the Liver
- Joy affects the Heart
- Sadness affects the Lungs and Heart
- Worry affects the Lungs and Spleen
- Pensiveness affects the Spleen
- Fear affects the Kidneys
- Shock affects the Heart

angry at meal times (as sadly often happens in certain families), the anger will affect the Stomach and this will be manifested with a Wiry quality on the right Middle position of the pulse. The effect of an emotion will also depend on the constitutional trait of a person. For example, if a person has a tendency to a constitutional weakness of the Heart (manifested with a midline crack on the tongue extending all the way to the tip), fear will affect the Heart rather than the Kidneys.

Box 20.5 summarizes the effects of the emotions on Qi.

> **Box 20.5 Effect of emotions on Qi**
> - Anger makes Qi rise
> - Joy slows Qi down
> - Sadness dissolves Qi
> - Worry knots Qi
> - Pensiveness knots Qi
> - Fear makes Qi descend
> - Shock scatters Qi

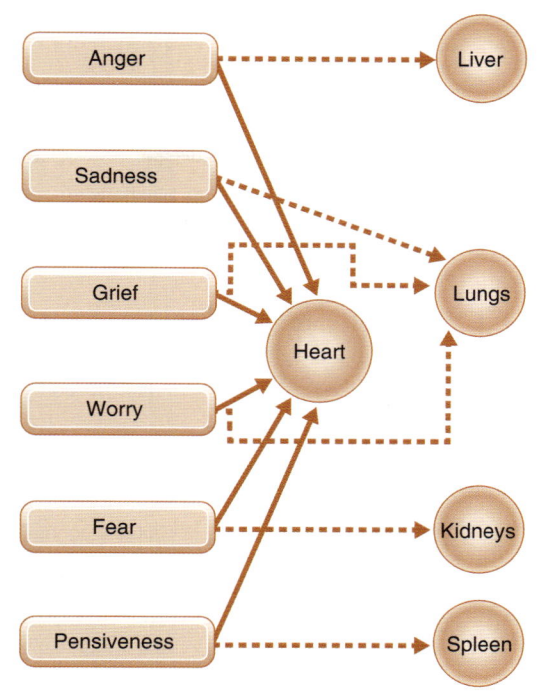

All emotions affect the Heart

All emotions, besides affecting the relevant organ directly, affect the Heart indirectly because the Heart houses the Mind. It alone, being responsible for consciousness and cognition, can recognize and feel the effect of emotional tension. Fei Bo Xiong (1800–1879) put it very clearly when he said: '*The seven emotions injure the 5 Yin organs selectively, but they all affect the Heart. Joy injures the Heart ... Anger injures the Liver, the Liver cannot recognize anger but the Heart can, hence it affects both Liver and Heart. Worry injures the Lungs, the Lungs cannot recognize it but the Heart can, hence it affects both Lungs and Heart. Pensiveness injures the Spleen, the Spleen cannot recognise it but the Heart can, hence it affects both Spleen and Heart.*'[9]

Yu Chang in 'Principles of Medical Practice' (1658) says: '*Worry agitates the Heart and has repercussions on the Lungs; pensiveness agitates the Heart and has repercussions on the Spleen; anger agitates the Heart and has repercussions on the Liver; fear agitates the Heart and has repercussions on the Kidneys. Therefore all the five emotions [including joy] affect the Heart.*'[10]

Chapter 28 of the 'Spiritual Axis' also says that all emotions affect the Heart: '*The Heart is the Master of the 5 Yin and 6 Yang Organs ... sadness, shock and worry agitate the Heart, when the Heart is agitated the 5 Yin and 6 Yang Organs are shaken.*'[11] Chinese writing clearly bears out the idea that all emotions affect the Heart since the characters for six of the seven emotions are based on the 'heart' radical. This is probably the most important aspect of the Heart functions and the main reason for it being compared to the 'monarch'.

The way that all emotions afflict the Heart also explains why a red tip of the tongue, indicating Heart-Fire, is so commonly seen, even in emotional problems related to other organs. Figure 20.9 illustrates the idea that all emotions affect the Heart (solid lines) as well as their relevant organ (dotted lines).

Figure 20.9 All emotions affect the Heart

> **Clinical note**
>
> As all emotions affect the Heart, I practically always use HE-7 Shenmen in emotional problems (in addition to other points)

> All emotions affect the Heart

Effects of emotions on the body

The first effect of emotional stress on the body is to affect the proper circulation and direction of Qi. Qi is non-substantial and the Mind, with its mental and emotional energies, is the most non-material type of Qi. It is therefore natural that emotional stress affecting the Mind impairs the circulation of Qi and disrupts the Qi Mechanism first of all (Fig. 20.10).

Although each emotion has a particular effect on Qi (e.g. anger makes it rise, sadness depletes it, etc.), all emotions have a tendency to cause some stagnation of Qi after some time. Even the emotions that deplete Qi, such as sadness, may have this effect because if Qi is

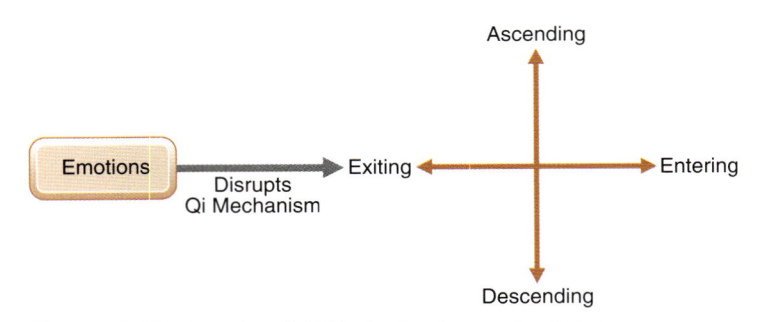

Figure 20.10 Disruption of Qi Mechanism by emotional strain

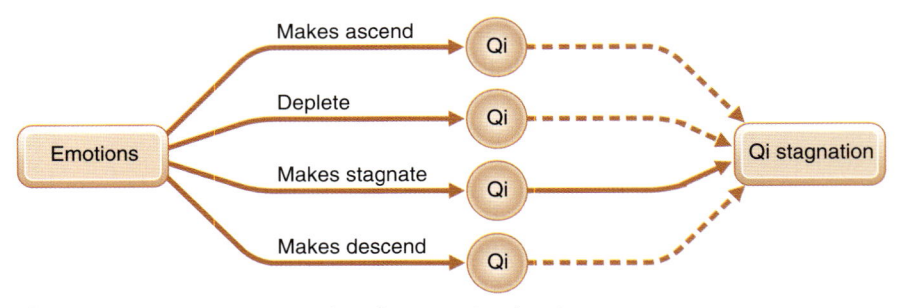

Figure 20.11 Qi stagnation resulting from emotional strain

deficient it cannot circulate properly and it therefore may tend to stagnate. For example, sadness depletes Lung-Qi in the chest: the deficient Qi in the chest fails to circulate properly and it causes some stagnation of Qi in the chest (Fig. 20.11).

> All emotions tend to cause Qi stagnation, even those that, like sadness, deplete Qi

When Qi stagnates, it may, in time, lead to Blood stasis, especially in women. Blood stasis affects particularly the Heart, Liver and Uterus.

Qi stagnation may also lead to Heat, and most of the emotions can, over a long period of time, give rise to Heat or Fire. There is a saying in Chinese medicine: 'The five emotions can turn into Fire'. This is because most of the emotions can cause stagnation of Qi and when Qi is compressed in this way over a period of time it creates Heat, just as the temperature of a gas increases when its pressure is increased.

For this reason, when someone has suffered from emotional problems for a long time, there are often signs of Heat, which may be in the Liver, Heart, Lungs or Kidneys (in the case of this last organ, Empty-Heat). This often shows on the tongue which becomes red or dark red and dry, and possibly has a red tip. A red tip of the tongue is a very common sign in practice which is always a reliable indicator that that patient is subject to some emotional stress.

With time, Heat may turn into Fire, which is more intense, more drying and affects the Mind more. Therefore emotional stress may in time cause Fire and this, in turn, harasses the Mind, causing agitation and anxiety.

The disruption of Qi caused by the emotions may in time also lead to the formation of Phlegm. As the proper movement of Qi in the right direction in the Qi Mechanism is essential to transform, transport and excrete fluids, the disruption in the movement of Qi may result in the formation of Phlegm. Phlegm, in turn, obstructs the Mind's orifices and becomes a further cause of emotional and mental disturbance.

Box 20.6 lists the effects of emotional strain on the body.

> Remember! Emotions do not cause Qi stagnation in the Liver only. They can cause Qi stagnation in most organs and especially Heart and Lungs

> **Box 20.6 Effects of emotional strain**
> - Qi stagnation
> - Blood stasis
> - Heat
> - Fire
> - Phlegm

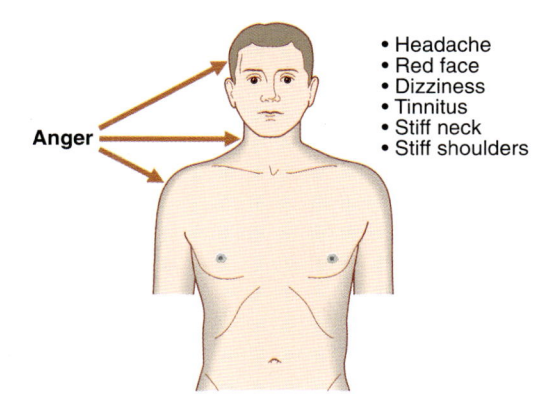

Anger →
- Headache
- Red face
- Dizziness
- Tinnitus
- Stiff neck
- Stiff shoulders

Figure 20.12 Effect of anger

ANGER

The term 'anger', perhaps more than any of the other emotions, should be interpreted very broadly to include several other allied emotional states, such as resentment, repressed anger, irritability, frustration, rage, hatred, indignation, animosity or bitterness.

If they persist for a long time, any of these emotional states can affect the Liver, causing stagnation of Liver-Qi or Liver-Blood, rising of Liver-Yang or blazing of Liver-Fire. These are the three most common Liver disharmonies arising out of the above emotional problems.

Anger (intended in the broad sense outlined above) makes Qi rise and many of the symptoms and signs will manifest in the head and neck, such as headaches, dizziness, tinnitus, neck stiffness, red blotches on the front part of the neck or a red face. One of the most common symptoms caused by anger is headache (Fig. 20.12).

Chapter 8 of the 'Spiritual Axis' says: '*Anger causes mental confusion.*'[12] The 'Simple Questions' in chapter 39 says: '*Anger makes Qi rise and causes vomiting of Blood and diarrhoea.*'[13] It causes vomiting of Blood because it makes Liver-Qi and Liver-Yang rise and it causes diarrhoea because it causes Liver-Qi to invade the Spleen. Chapter 3 of the 'Simple Questions' says: '*Severe anger severs body and Qi, Blood stagnates in the upper part and the person may suffer a syncope.*'[14]

The effect of anger on the Liver depends, on the one hand, on the person's reaction to the emotional stimulus and on the other hand, on other concurrent factors. If the anger is bottled up it will cause stagnation of Liver-Qi, whereas if it is expressed it will cause Liver-Yang rising or Liver-Fire blazing. In a woman stagnation of Liver-Qi may easily lead to stasis of Liver-Blood. If the person also suffers from some Kidney-Yin deficiency (perhaps from overwork), then he or she will develop Liver-Yang rising. If, on the other hand, the person has a tendency to Heat (perhaps from excessive consumption of hot foods), then he or she will tend to develop Liver-Fire blazing.

Anger does not always manifest outwardly with outbursts of anger, irritability, shouting, red face, etc. Some individuals may carry anger inside them for years without ever manifesting it. In particular, long-standing depression may be due to repressed anger or resentment. Because the person is very depressed, he or she may look very subdued and pale, walk slowly and speak with a low voice, all signs which one would associate with a depletion of Qi and Blood deriving from sadness or grief. However, when anger rather than sadness is the cause of disease, the pulse and tongue will clearly show it: the pulse will be Full and Wiry and the tongue will be Red with redder sides and with a dry yellow coating. This type of depression is most probably due to long-standing resentment, often harboured towards a member of that person's family.

In some cases anger can affect other organs, especially the Stomach. This can be due to stagnant Liver-Qi invading the Stomach. Such a condition is more likely to occur if one gets angry at meal times, which may happen if family meals become occasions for regular rows. It also happens when there is a pre-existing weakness of the Stomach, in which case the anger may affect the Stomach without affecting the Liver.

If one regularly gets angry an hour or two after meals, then the anger will affect the Intestines rather than the Stomach. This happens, for example, when one goes straight back to a stressful and frustrating job after lunch. In this case, stagnant Liver-Qi invades the Intestines and causes abdominal pain, distension and alternation of constipation with diarrhoea.

Finally, anger, like all other emotions, also affects the Heart. This is particularly prone to be affected by anger also because, from a Five-Element perspective, the Liver is the mother of the Heart and often Liver-Fire is transmitted to the Heart, giving rise to Heart-Fire. Anger makes the Heart full with blood rushing to it. With time, this leads to Blood-Heat affecting the Heart and therefore the Mind. Anger tends to affect the Heart, particularly when the person does a lot of jogging, hurrying or exercising.

Thus, in general, anger affects primarily the Liver and it may cause either stagnation of Liver-Qi or Liver-Yang rising. When advising patients on how to deal with their anger, we should note that if anger has caused stagnation of Liver-Qi, expressing the anger may be helpful. However, if anger has given rise to Liver-Yang rising, expressing it will not usually help: it is too late and expressing the anger forcefully may only make Liver-Yang rise even more.

The tongue gives a good indication of the pattern involved when anger is the causative factor. In Liver-Qi stagnation, the tongue may not change unless the stagnation is intense and long-lasting, in which case the sides may be slightly red. In Liver-Blood stasis, the tongue sides may be purple (Fig. 20.13). In Liver-Fire, the tongue is red, the sides redder and there is a yellow coating (Fig 20.14).

Finally, the pulse is an important indication when anger is the cause of the disease. In my opinion, when anger is the cause of the disease, the pulse is Wiry: if the pulse is not Wiry, then anger is not the cause of the disease.

When anger is the cause of disease, the pulse is Wiry; if the pulse is not Wiry, then it is not anger!

Clinical note

LIV-3 Taichong is a good point to deal with anger

Box 20.7 summarizes the effects of anger.

Box 20.7 Anger
- It affects the Liver
- It makes Qi rise
- Symptoms: headache, dizziness, tinnitus, red face, stiff neck
- It may cause Liver-Qi stagnation (if anger is repressed), Liver-Yang rising and Liver-Fire
- Anger may affect the Stomach and Intestines
- Wiry pulse

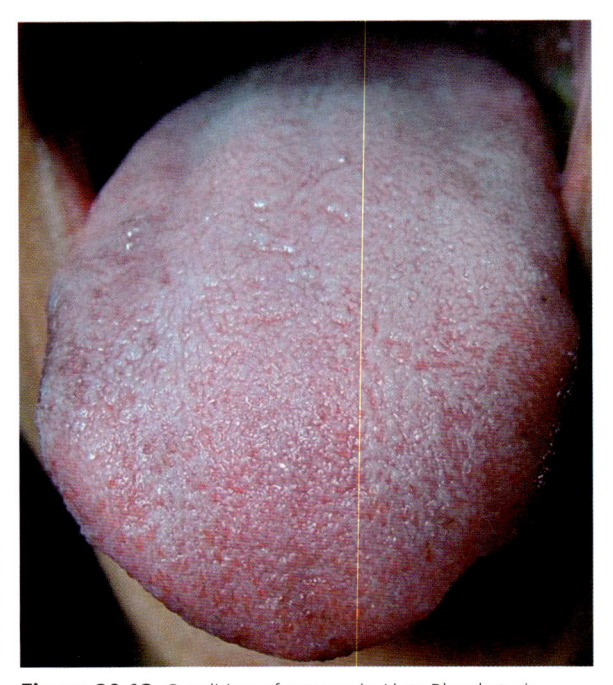

Figure 20.13 Condition of tongue in Liver-Blood stasis

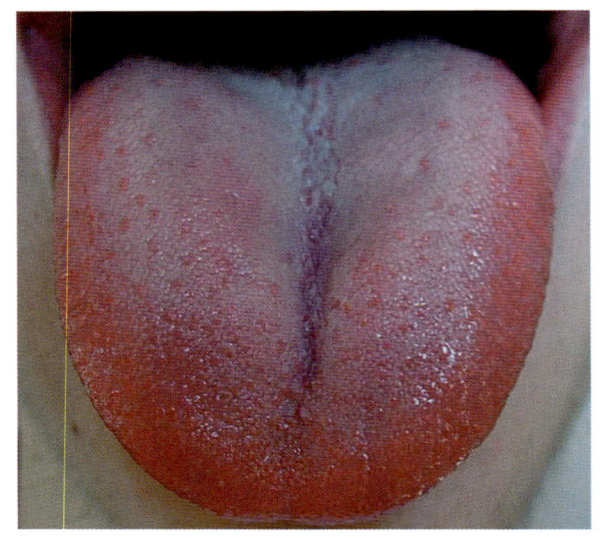

Figure 20.14 Condition of tongue in Liver-Fire

JOY

As with 'anger', the term 'joy' should also be interpreted broadly. Obviously joy is not in itself a cause of disease. In fact, the 'Simple Questions' in chapter 39 says: '*Joy makes the Mind peaceful and relaxed, it benefits the Nutritive and Defensive Qi and it makes Qi relax and slow down.*'[15]

The 'Simple Questions' in chapter 2 says: '*The Heart ... controls Joy, Joy injures the Heart, Fear counteracts Joy.*'[16] The 'Spiritual Axis' says in chapter 8: '*Excessive joy disperses the Mind out of its residence.*'[17]

What is meant by 'joy' as a cause of disease is obviously not a state of healthy contentment but one of excessive excitement and craving, which can injure the Heart. In particular, I think that, when considering Western patients, 'overstimulation' is probably the best interpretation of 'joy' as an emotional cause of disease. This is also akin to 'desire' as a cause of disease, which is stressed by the three main philosophies of China, namely Confucianism, Daoism and Buddhism.

Excessive stimulation disturbs the Mind (*Shen*) and it may even displace it from Heart-Blood. When considering our modern lifestyle, we do have plenty of factors leading to excessive stimulation, such as alcohol, recreational drugs, advertising, ambition, even sex. Excessive stimulation of the Heart can lead to Heart-Fire or Heart Empty-Heat, depending on the underlying condition.

Overstimulation is an aspect of the emotion 'joy' that stirs up the Minister Fire, which goes to harass the Mind.

Joy in the broad sense indicated above makes the Heart larger. This leads to excessive stimulation of the Heart, which, in time, may lead to Heart-related symptoms and signs. These may deviate somewhat from the classical Heart patterns. The main manifestations would be palpitations, overexcitability, insomnia, restlessness, talking a lot and a red tip of the tongue (Fig. 20.15). The pulse would typically be slow, slightly Overflowing but Empty on the left Front position.

Joy may also be marked out as a cause of disease when it is sudden; this happens, for example, on hearing good news unexpectedly. In this situation, 'joy' is akin to shock. Fei Bo Xiong (1800–1879) in 'Medical Collection from Four Families from Meng He' says: '*Joy injures the Heart ... [it causes] Yang Qi to float and the blood vessels to become too open and dilated.*'[18]

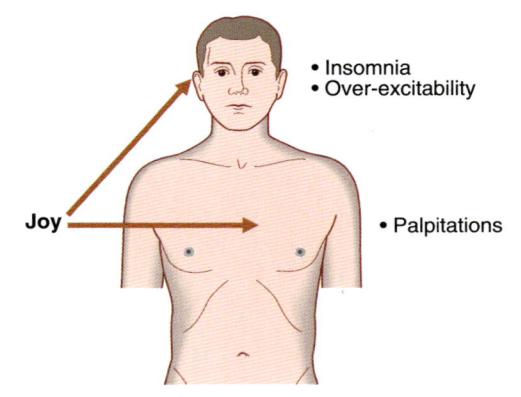

Figure 20.15 Effect of joy

Box 20.8 Joy

- It affects the Heart
- It slows down Qi
- 'Joy' should be interpreted as overstimulation
- Symptoms: palpitations, overexcitability, insomnia, restlessness, red tip of the tongue
- Sudden joy is akin to shock

In these cases of sudden joy and excitement the Heart dilates and slows down and the pulse becomes Slow and slightly Overflowing but Empty. In order to understand this, one can think of the fairly frequent situation when a migraine attack can be precipitated by a sudden excitement at hearing good news.[19] Another example of joy as a cause of disease is that of sudden laughter triggering a heart attack; this example also confirms the relationship existing between the Heart and laughter.

Finally, one can also get an idea of joy as an emotion of overexcitement in children, in whom overexcitement usually ends in tears.

Box 20.8 summarizes the effects of joy.

SADNESS

Sadness weakens the Lungs, but it also affects the Heart. In fact, according to the 'Simple Questions', sadness affects the Lungs via the Heart. It says in chapter 39: '*Sadness makes the Heart cramped and agitated, this pushes towards the lungs' lobes, the Upper Burner becomes obstructed, Nutritive and Defensive Qi cannot circulate freely, Heat accumulates and dissolves Qi.*'[20] According to this passage then, sadness primarily

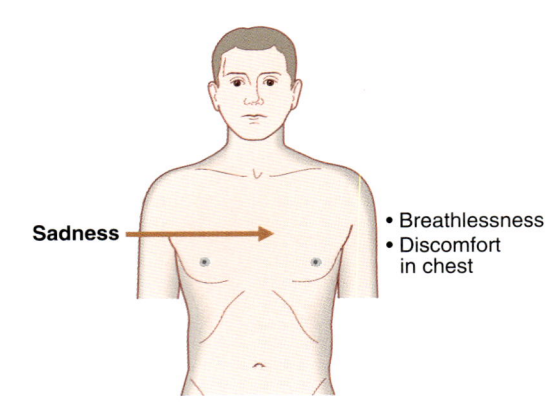

Figure 20.16 Effect of sadness

affects the Heart and the Lungs suffer in consequence, since heart and lungs are both in the Upper Burner.

Sadness includes the emotions of grief and regret, as when someone regrets a certain action or decision in the past and the Mind is constantly turned towards that time.

The Lungs govern Qi and sadness depletes Qi. This is often manifested on the pulse with a weakness of both Front positions (Heart and Lungs). In particular, the pulse has no 'wave' and does not flow smoothly towards the thumb.

Sadness leads to deficiency of Lung-Qi and may manifest in a variety of symptoms, such as breathlessness, tiredness, a feeling of discomfort in the chest, depression or crying (Fig. 20.16). In women, deficiency of Lung-Qi may lead to Blood deficiency and amenorrhoea.

Case history 20.1

A woman of 63 complained of anxiety, depression, sweating at night, feeling of heat in palms and chest and insomnia (waking up several times during the night). The tongue was dry and without coating. The pulse was Floating-Empty, especially in the Front position, and without wave.

On interrogation, it transpired that all the symptoms appeared after three deaths in the family in a short space of time (of mother, father and husband). In this case the profound sadness had 'dissolved' Lung-Qi and, after some time, this developed into Lung-Yin deficiency. This was apparent from the night sweating, the Floating-Empty pulse, the feeling of heat of palms and chest and the tongue without coating.

Although sadness and grief deplete Qi and therefore lead to deficiency of Qi, they may also, after a long time, lead to stagnation of Qi, because the deficient Lung- and Heart-Qi fail to circulate properly in the chest.

As mentioned before, each emotion can affect other organs apart from its 'specific' one. For example, the 'Spiritual Axis' in chapter 8 mentions injury of the Liver from sadness rather than anger: '*When sadness affects the Liver it injures the Ethereal Soul; this causes mental confusion ... the Yin is damaged, the tendons contract and there is hypochondrial discomfort.*'[21] In this case, sadness can naturally affect the Ethereal Soul (*Hun*) and therefore Liver-Blood and Liver-Yin. Sadness has a depleting effect on Qi and it therefore, in some cases, depletes Liver-Yin, leading to mental confusion, depression, lack of a sense of direction in life and inability to plan one's life.

Case history 20.2

A 40-year-old woman was under a great deal of stress due to her divorce, which caused her great sadness. She often felt weepy. She felt aimless and questioned her role in her relationships with men; she was at a turning point in her life and did not know what direction to take. She slept badly and her pulse was Choppy.

This is a clear example of sadness affecting the Liver and therefore the Ethereal Soul (*Hun*). She was treated, improving tremendously, with the Yin Linking Vessel (*Yin Wei Mai*) points (P-6 Neiguan on the right and SP-4 Gongsun on the left) and BL-23 Shenshu, BL-52 Zhishi and BL-47 Hunmen.

Finally, Dr Shen considers that grief that is unexpressed and borne without tears affects the Kidneys. According to him, when grief is held in without weeping, the fluids cannot come out (in the form of tears) and they upset the fluid metabolism within the Kidneys. This would happen only in situations when grief had been felt for many years.

Clinical note

LU-7 Lieque is a good point to deal with sadness

Box 20.9 summarizes the effects of sadness.

> **Box 20.9 Sadness**
>
> - It affects the Lungs and Heart
> - It dissolves Qi
> - Symptoms: breathlessness, tiredness, a feeling of discomfort in the chest, depression or crying
> - In some cases it may deplete Liver-Blood (only in women)

WORRY

Worry is one of the most common emotional causes of disease in our society. The extremely rapid and radical social changes that have occurred in Western societies in the past decades have created a climate of such insecurity in all spheres of life that only a Daoist sage could be immune to worry! Of course, there are also people who, because of a pre-existing disharmony of the Internal Organs, are very prone to worry, even about very minor incidents in life. For example, many people appear to be very tense and worry a lot. On close interrogation about their work and family life, often nothing of note emerges. They simply worry excessively about trivial everyday activities and they tend to do everything in a hurry and be pressed for time. This may be due to a constitutional weakness of the Spleen, Heart, or Lungs, or a combination of these.

Worry knots Qi, which means that it causes stagnation of Qi, and it affects both Lungs and Spleen: the Lungs because when one is worried breathing is shallow, and the Spleen because this organ is responsible for thinking and ideas. Chapter 8 of the 'Spiritual Axis' confirms that worry knots Qi: '*Worry causes obstruction of Qi so that Qi stagnates.*'[22]

Worry may affect the Spleen as well and Chapter 8 of the 'Spiritual Axis' confirms that: '*In the case of the Spleen, excessive worry injures the Intellect [Yi].*'[23] Worry is the pathological counterpart of the Spleen's mental activity in generating ideas. In a few cases, worry may also affect the Liver as a result of the stagnation of the Lungs; in a Five-Element sense that corresponds to Metal insulting Wood. When this happens, the neck and shoulders will tense up and become stiff and painful.

The symptoms and signs caused by worry will vary according to whether they affect the Lungs or the Spleen. If worry affects the Lungs it will cause an uncomfortable feeling of the chest, slight breathlessness, tensing of the shoulders, sometimes a dry cough, weak voice, sighing and a pale complexion (Fig. 20.17). The right Front pulse position (of the Lungs) may feel

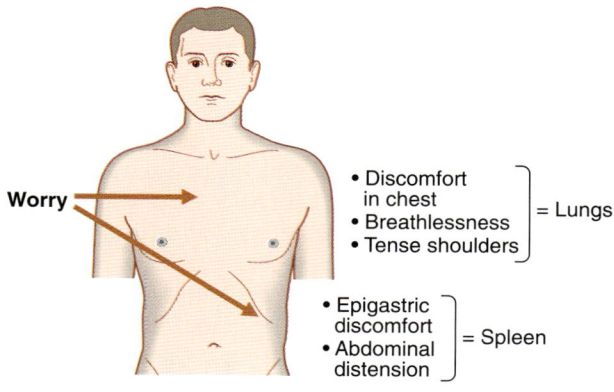

Figure 20.17 Effect of worry

> **Box 20.10 Worry**
>
> - It affects the Lungs and Spleen
> - It knots Qi
> - Symptoms (Lungs): uncomfortable feeling of the chest, slight breathlessness, tensing of the shoulders, a dry cough, weak voice, sighing, pale complexion
> - Symptoms (Spleen): poor appetite, slight epigastric discomfort, abdominal distension, tiredness, pale complexion

slightly Tight or Wiry, indicating the knotting action of worry on Qi.[24]

If worry affects the Spleen it may cause poor appetite, a slight epigastric discomfort, some abdominal pain and distension, tiredness and a pale complexion. The right Middle pulse position (Spleen) will feel slightly Tight but Weak. If worry affects the Stomach as well (which happens if one worries at meal times), the right Middle pulse may be Weak-Floating.

Finally, like all emotions, worry affects the Heart, causing stagnation of Heart-Qi. This will cause palpitations, a slight feeling of tightness of the chest and insomnia.

Worry is the emotional counterpart of the Spleen's mental energy, which is responsible for concentration and memorization. When the Spleen is healthy we can concentrate and focus on the object of our study or work; the same type of mental energy, when disturbed by worry, leads to constantly thinking, brooding and worrying about certain events of life.

Box 20.10 summarizes the effects of worry.

> **Clinical note**
>
> LU-7 Lieque is a good point to deal with worry

PENSIVENESS

Pensiveness is very similar to worry in its character and effect. It consists in brooding, constantly thinking about certain events or people (even though not worrying), nostalgic hankering after the past and generally thinking intensely about life rather than living it. In extreme cases, pensiveness leads to obsessive thoughts. In a different sense, pensiveness also includes excessive mental work in the process of one's work or study.

Pensiveness affects the Spleen and, like worry, it knots Qi. Chapter 39 of the 'Simple Questions' says: *'Pensiveness makes the Heart [Qi] accumulate, and causes the Mind to converge: the Upright Qi settles and does not move and therefore Qi stagnates.'*[25] Pensiveness will therefore cause similar symptoms to those outlined above for worry. In addition, it will cause a slight epigastric discomfort and the other difference will be that the pulse of the right side will not only feel slightly Tight, but will have no 'wave' (see ch. 25 on pulse diagnosis).[26] In the case of pensiveness, the pulse will lack a wave only on the right Middle position. A pulse without wave in the Front and Middle position indicates Sadness.

Pensiveness affects the Heart, causing stagnation of Qi of the Heart with symptoms such as palpitations, a slight feeling of tightness of the chest and insomnia (Fig. 20.18).

The positive mental energy corresponding to pensiveness is quiet contemplation and meditation. The same mental energy which makes us capable of meditation and contemplation will, if excessive and misguided, lead to pensiveness, brooding, or even obsessive thinking.

Box 20.11 summarizes the effects of pensiveness.

> **Clinical note**
>
> SP-3 Taibai is a good point to deal with pensiveness

FEAR

Fear includes both a chronic state of fear and anxiety and a sudden fright. Fear depletes Kidney-Qi and it makes Qi descend. The 'Simple Questions' in chapter 39 says: *'Fear depletes the Essence, it blocks the Upper Burner, which makes Qi descend to the Lower Burner.'*[27] Examples of Qi descending are nocturnal enuresis in children and incontinence of urine or diarrhoea in adults following a sudden fright (Fig. 20.19). Nocturnal enuresis is a common problem in children; it is often caused by fear or a feeling of insecurity in the child due to some family situation. Situations of chronic anxiety and fear will have different effects on Qi, depending on the state of the Heart.

In adults, however, fear and chronic anxiety more often cause deficiency of Kidney-Yin and rising of Empty-Heat within the Heart, with a feeling of heat in the face, night sweating, palpitations and a dry mouth and throat.

> **Box 20.11 Pensiveness**
>
> - It affects the Spleen
> - It knots Qi
> - Symptoms: poor appetite, slight epigastric discomfort, abdominal distension, tiredness, pale complexion

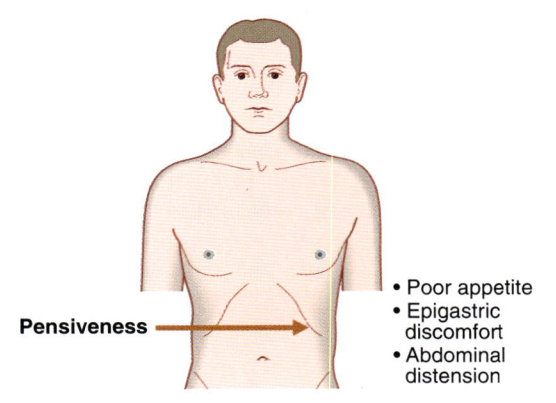

Figure 20.18 Effect of pensiveness

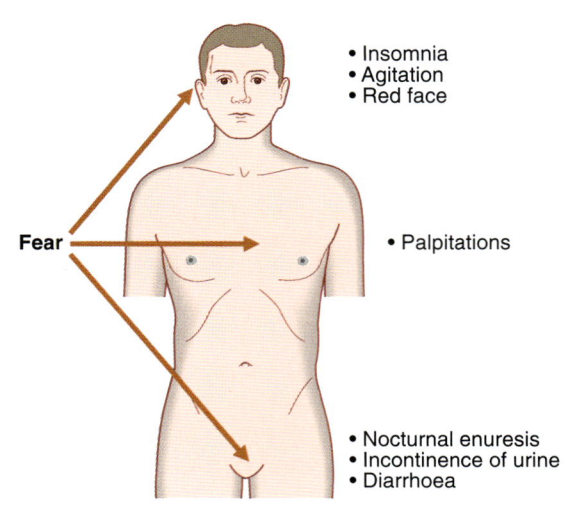

Figure 20.19 Effect of fear

> **Box 20.12 Fear**
> - It affects the Kidneys
> - It makes Qi descend
> - Symptoms: nocturnal enuresis, incontinence of urine, diarrhoea
> - In some cases, it may make Qi rise: palpitations, insomnia, night sweating, dry mouth, malar flush

If the Heart is strong, it will cause Qi to descend, but if the Heart is weak, it will cause Qi to rise in the form of Empty-Heat. This is more common in old people and in women as fear and anxiety weaken Kidney-Yin and give rise to Empty-Heat of the Heart with such symptoms as palpitations, insomnia, night sweating, a dry mouth, a malar flush and a Rapid pulse.

There are other causes of fear, not related to the Kidneys. Liver-Blood deficiency and a Gall Bladder deficiency can also make the person fearful.

Box 20.12 summarizes the effects of fear.

> **Clinical note**
>
> KI-9 Zhubin is a good point to deal with fear

SHOCK

Mental shock 'suspends' Qi and affects Heart and Kidneys. It causes a sudden depletion of Heart-Qi, makes the Heart smaller and may lead to palpitations, breathlessness and insomnia (Fig. 20.20). It is often reflected in the pulse with a so-called 'Moving' quality: that is, a pulse that is short, slippery, shaped like a bean, rapid and gives the impression of vibrating as it pulsates.

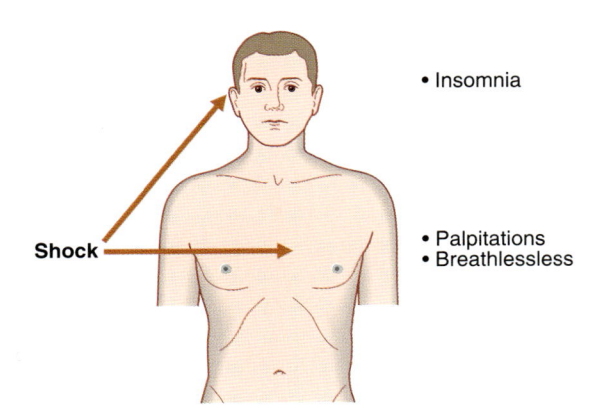

Figure 20.20 Effect of shock

> **Box 20.13 Shock**
> - It affects the Heart
> - It scatters Qi
> - Symptoms: palpitations, breathlessness, insomnia, Moving pulse

The 'Simple Questions' in chapter 39 says: '*Shock affects the Heart depriving it of residence, the Mind has no shelter and cannot rest, so that Qi becomes chaotic.*'[28]

Shock also 'closes' the Heart or makes the Heart smaller. This can be observed in a bluish tinge on the forehead and a Heart pulse which is Tight and Fine.

Box 20.13 summarizes the effects of shock.

> **Clinical note**
>
> HE-7 Shenmen is a good point to deal with shock

> **Learning outcomes**
>
> In this chapter you will have learned:
> - The importance of the concept in Chinese medicine of body, mind and emotions as an integrated whole, in which emotions are an integral of the sphere of action of the Internal Organs
> - The difference between the view of the emotions taken by Chinese and Western medicine
> - The problems in using the word 'emotion' to indicate the Chinese view of the 'emotional' causes of disease
> - That emotions become a cause of disease when they are either long-term or very intense
> - How emotions, unlike external causes, cause internal disharmonies directly
> - The importance of the reciprocal relationship between the emotions and the Internal Organs: emotional stress injures the Internal Organs; disharmony of the Internal Organs causes emotional imbalance
> - The role of the positive mental energies produced by the Internal Organs, which 'resonate' with emotions as a reaction to life events
> - The different effects produced by the various emotions on the circulation of Qi
> - That all emotions affect the Heart, as well as their relevant organ
> - The tendency of all emotions to cause stagnation of Qi, and thereafter Blood stasis, Heat, Fire or Phlegm
> - The effects of anger on Qi and the other organs
> - The effects of 'joy' on the Heart
> - The depleting and stagnating effects of sadness on Lung- and Heart-Qi
> - The effect of worry on the Lungs and Spleen
> - The effect of pensiveness, which knots Qi and affects the Spleen
> - The effect of fear, which makes Qi descend and affects the Kidneys
> - The effect of shock, which scatters Qi and affects the Heart

Self-assessment questions

1. What effect does anger have on Qi?
2. Which emotion makes Qi descend?
3. Why is a red tongue tip often present in patients with emotional problems related to other organs?
4. Explain the saying 'The five emotions can turn into Fire'.
5. Give three symptoms which might result from anger causing Qi to rise.
6. Give three symptoms which might manifest from overexcitement adversely affecting the Heart.
7. Complete the following: 'Sadness _____ Qi, and affects the _____ and the _____.'
8. A patient who worries excessively also complains of poor appetite, abdominal distension and tiredness. What effect has their worrying had on their Qi and internal organs?
9. How might fear and chronic anxiety lead to symptoms such as palpitations, insomnia, night sweats and a dry mouth in an elderly patient?
10. How might shock manifest on the pulse?

See p. 1261 for answers

END NOTES

1. 1981 Spiritual Axis (*Ling Shu Jing* 灵枢经), People's Health Publishing House, Beijing, first published *c*.100 BC, p. 121. It is interesting that the emotional causes of disease in this chapter are mentioned in the same breath as Wind and Dampness and the passage quoted says that the emotions injure the Yin, Wind injures the upper part and Dampness the lower part of the body.
2. Spiritual Axis, p. 24.
3. Ibid., p. 24.
4. 1979 The Yellow Emperor's Classic of Internal Medicine – Simple Questions (*Huang Di Nei Jing Su Wen* 黄帝内经素问), People's Health Publishing House, Beijing, first published *c*.100 BC, p. 37–41.
5. Simple Questions, p. 221.
6. Chen Yan 1174 A Treatise on the Three Categories of Causes of Diseases (*San Yin Ji Yi Bing Zheng Fang Lun*), cited in Theory of the Mind in Chinese Medicine, p. 55.
7. Ibid., p. 67.
8. Simple Questions, p. 221.
9. Fei Bo Xiong et al. 1985 Medical Collection from Four Families from Meng He (*Meng He Si Jia Yi Ji*), Jiangsu Science Publishing House, p. 40.
10. Principles of Medical Practice, cited in Theory of the Mind in Chinese Medicine, p. 34.
11. Spiritual Axis, p. 67.
12. Ibid., p. 24.
13. Simple Questions, p. 221.
14. Ibid., p. 17.
15. Simple Questions, p. 221.
16. Ibid., p. 38.
17. Spiritual Axis, p. 24.
18. Medical Collection from Four Families from Meng He, p. 40.
19. There is a common story in Chinese medicine which was related to me by two different teachers to illustrate this situation. According to this story, a certain promising young man had passed the examination to access the highest rank of the Imperial bureaucracy in the capital. As this man was walking in the Imperial palace, overjoyed about having passed the examination, a doctor friend of his saw him and, glancing at him, told him that he should immediately return to his native village because there was very bad news from his family there. The poor man became white in the face, and made preparations to leave straight away. Once he got to his village, his family told him that there was nothing wrong there and that they never sent for him. The young man returned to the capital and when he met his doctor friend again, he asked him in consternation, why on earth he had lied to him. The doctor told him that he saw on his face that he had had a sudden excitement and was overjoyed beyond measure: this could have seriously injured his heart. The only way to counteract this sudden excitement, was to instil fear in his heart, as fear counteracts joy.
20. Simple Questions, p. 221.
21. Spiritual Axis, p. 24.
22. Ibid., p. 24.
23. Ibid., p. 24.
24. When judging the quality of the Lung pulse, one should bear in mind that, in normal circumstances, this should naturally feel relatively soft (in relation to the other pulse positions). Thus a Lung pulse that feels as hard as a (normal) Liver pulse may well be Tight or Wiry.
25. Simple Questions, p. 222.
26. One can feel the normal pulse as a wave under the fingers moving from the Rear towards the Front position. The pulse without wave lacks this flowing movement from Rear to Front position and it is instead felt as if each individual position were separate from the others.
27. Simple Questions, p. 222.
28. Ibid., p. 222.

PART 3

External Causes of Disease   21

Key contents

Climate as a cause of disease

Bacteria and viruses in relation to 'Wind'

Historical background

Climatic factors as patterns of disharmony

Artificial 'climates' as causes of disease

Pathology and clinical manifestations

Aversion to cold and fever

Symptoms and signs of exterior pathogenic factors patterns
Wind
Cold
Summer-Heat
Dampness
Dryness
Fire

Consequences of invasion of exterior pathogenic factors
Invasions of exterior pathogenic factors resulting in an exterior pattern
Invasions of exterior pathogenic factors without an exterior pattern
Invasions of exterior pathogenic factors resulting in obstruction of muscles and channels

The six normal climates are called the 'Six Qi' (*Liu Qi*); when they become a cause of disease they were formerly called 'The Six Climates excessively victorious', but are now usually called the 'Six Excesses' (*Liu Yin*). As causes of disease, the exterior pathogenic factors are also called the 'Six Evils' (*Liu Xie*). I shall call these 'exterior pathogenic factors'.

Chapter 74 of the 'Simple Questions' states that the exterior pathogenic factors are the origin of many different diseases: '*100 diseases originate from Wind, Cold, Summer-Heat, Dampness, Dryness and Fire.*'[1] The pathogenic climates are closely related to the weather and the seasons. Chapter 25 of the 'Simple Questions' clearly states the close connection of a human being to the energies of the four seasons: '*A human being comes into being through the Qi of Heaven and Earth and its growth is governed by the 4 seasons.*'[2]

Box 21.1 lists the six climatic factors.

The external pathogenic factors will be discussed under the following headings:

- Climate as a cause of disease
- Bacteria and viruses in relation to 'Wind'
- Historical background
- Climatic factors as patterns of disharmony
- Artificial 'climates' as causes of disease
- Pathology and clinical manifestations of exterior pathogenic factors
- Aversion to cold and 'fever'
  - Aversion to cold
  - Fever

The external causes of disease are due to climatic factors, which are:

- Wind
- Cold
- Summer-Heat
- Dampness
- Dryness
- Fire

Box 21.1 The six climatic factors

- Wind
- Cold
- Summer-Heat
- Dampness
- Dryness
- Fire

- Symptoms and signs of exterior pathogenic factors patterns
  - Wind
  - Cold
  - Summer-Heat
  - Dampness
  - Dryness
  - Fire
- Consequences of invasion of exterior pathogenic factors
  - Invasions of exterior pathogenic factors resulting in an Exterior pattern
  - Invasions of exterior pathogenic factors without an exterior pattern
  - Invasions of exterior pathogenic factors resulting in obstruction of muscles and channels

CLIMATE AS A CAUSE OF DISEASE

Under normal circumstances, the weather will have no pathological effect on the body as it can adequately protect itself against exterior pathogenic factors. The weather becomes a cause of disease only when the equilibrium between the body and the environment breaks down, either because the weather is excessive or unseasonal (for instance too cold in summertime or too hot in wintertime), or because the body is weak relative to the climatic factor (Figs 21.1–21.3).

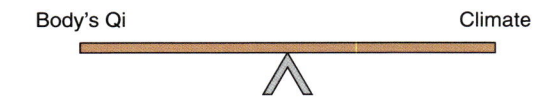

Figure 21.1 State of balance between the body's Qi and climate

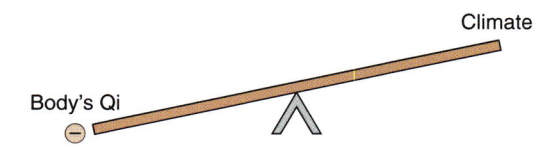

Figure 21.2 State of imbalance between body's Qi and climate due to relative weakness of the body's Qi

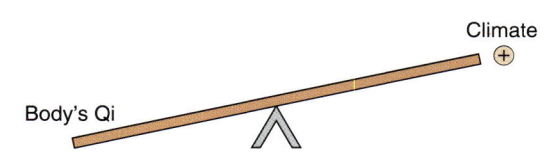

Figure 21.3 State of imbalance between body's Qi and climate due to relative excess of the climate

Another circumstance in which the climate may cause disease is when the weather changes very rapidly, giving the body no time to adapt properly. Indeed, Dr Shen used to say that the Chinese concept of 'Wind' actually refers to rapid changes in weather.

Either way, one can say that climatic factors become a cause of disease only when the body is weak in relation to them. It is important to stress here that the body is only *relatively* weak (i.e. in relation to the climatic factor), not necessarily fundamentally weak. In other words, one does not need to be very weak to be invaded by exterior pathogenic factors. A relatively healthy person can also be attacked by exterior pathogenic factors if these are stronger in relation to the body's energies *at that particular time*. So, the relative strength of climatic factors and Defensive Qi is all important.

Climatic factors become causes of disease only when there is a *relative* imbalance between the body's Qi and the exterior pathogenic factor

Climatic factors also include what the Chinese call exterior 'Warm epidemic pathogenic factors' (*Wen Yi*). These are not qualitatively different from other climatic factors, but they are infectious and are often more virulent. Always associated with Heat, they are a form of Warm Disease (*Wen Bing*) and they are highly infectious. In these cases, the exterior pathogenic factor is so strong that the majority of members of a community fall ill. Even in these cases, however, the strength of the body's Qi in relation to the pathogenic factor plays a role in the resistance to disease, as not every member of the community will fall ill.

Each of the six climatic factors is associated with a certain season during which it is more prevalent, as listed in Box 21.2.

Box 21.2 Climatic factors and seasons

- Wind – spring
- Cold – winter
- Summer-Heat – summer
- Dampness – late summer
- Dryness – autumn
- Fire – summer

In fact, with the exception of Summer-Heat, any of the climatic factors can arise in any season: it is not at all uncommon to have attacks of Wind-Heat in winter or Wind-Cold in summer. Summer-Heat, however, can arise only in the Summer. Living conditions also determine which climatic factor invades the body. For example, living in a damp house will cause invasion of exterior Damp irrespective of the season.

Remember: one can suffer an invasion of Wind-Heat in the middle of a very cold winter or an invasion of Wind-Cold in the summer

Fire is also a special case because, although it can be associated with the season of summer, it is actually primarily an internal pathogenic factor and therefore independent of seasons.

Each climate is also related to an internal organ. Chapter 38 of the 'Simple Questions' says: *Each of the 5 Yin Organs falls ill at a determinate time ... [if there is an external invasion] in the Autumn, it invades the Lungs; in the Spring, the Liver; in the Summer, the Heart; in Late Summer, the Spleen; and in Winter, the Kidneys.*[3] Chapter 74 of the 'Simple Questions' says: *Wind causing twitching and dizziness pertains to the Liver; Cold causing contraction and pulling pertains to the Kidneys; Qi stagnation pertains to the Lungs; Dampness causing a feeling of fullness and heaviness pertains to the Spleen; Heat causing mental confusion and tics pertains to Fire.*[4]

Box 21.3 summarizes climate as a cause of disease.

Box 21.3 Climate as a cause of disease

- Climate becomes a cause of disease only when it is either excessive or unseasonal
- Climate becomes a cause of disease when there is a temporary and relative imbalance between the body's Qi and the climatic factor
- Each climatic factor of disease is related to a particular season
- Each climatic factor is related to a Yin organ
  - Wind: Liver
  - Cold: Kidneys
  - Summer-Heat: Heart
  - Dampness: Spleen
  - Dryness: Lungs
  - Fire: Heart

BACTERIA AND VIRUSES IN RELATION TO 'WIND'

In Western medicine acute respiratory diseases are due to invasion of the body by bacteria or viruses. Ancient Chinese medicine did not have a knowledge of the existence of bacteria and viruses and acute respiratory infections were considered to be due to invasion of 'Wind' or other climatic pathogenic factors. The idea that climatic factors can be a *direct* cause of disease is of course a typical Chinese idea and one that is totally alien to modern Western medicine.[5] As we have indicated above, Chinese medicine holds that an exterior pathogenic factor invades the body when there is a temporary imbalance between a climatic factor and the body's Qi *at that particular time*.

Thus, while Western medicine places the emphasis on the external aspect of the disease (i.e. the invasion of bacteria and viruses), Chinese medicine places the emphasis on the temporary imbalance between the external causes of disease and the body's Qi. As a result, ancient Chinese medicine did not have a conception of infection until the early Qing dynasty (1644–1911). As it takes into account the strength of the body's Qi, this view of the pathology of exterior, acute diseases is more comprehensive than that of Western medicine and, most of all, it allows for *preventive* interventions by strengthening the body's Qi.

The ancient Chinese character for 'Wind' includes an 'insect' (i.e. a small organism carried by the wind and causing disease, equivalent to modern bacteria and viruses)

However, in later times, as described below, the 'Warm Disease' (*Wen Bing*) school of disease did understand the phenomenon of infection. Indeed, the character for 'Wind' contains within itself the one for 'insect': it could be construed that this is very early, primitive view of infection according to which disease is caused by small organisms ('insects', i.e. bacteria and viruses) carried by wind (Fig. 21.4).

Box 21.4 summarizes the difference between Western and Chinese approaches to bacteria and viruses as causes of disease.

風 *Feng* = Wind

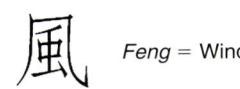

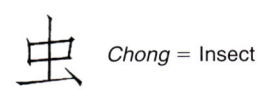

虫 *Chong* = Insect

Figure 21.4 Chinese character for 'Wind'

Box 21.4 'Wind' versus bacteria and viruses

- Western medicine sees infectious diseases as being caused by bacteria and viruses
- Chinese medicine sees them as being caused by exterior climatic factors
- Chinese medicine takes into consideration the state of the body's Qi in infectious diseases

---

Box 21.5 The Six Stages (*Shang Han*)

- Greater Yang (*Tai Yang*)
- Bright Yang (*Yang Ming*)
- Lesser Yang (*Shao Yang*)
- Greater Yin (*Tai Yin*)
- Lesser Yin (*Shao Yin*)
- Terminal Yin (*Jue Yin*)

HISTORICAL BACKGROUND

The study of the pathology and treatment of diseases caused by exterior pathogenic factors is dominated by two major schools of Chinese medicine. The earliest doctor who described the pathology of diseases from exterior pathogenic factors systematically was Zhang Zhong Jing (AD 150–219), the celebrated author of the 'Discussion of Cold-induced Diseases' (*Shang Han Lun*, c.AD 220). The pathology described in this book is mainly one of invasions of Wind-Cold and their consequences (some of which involve Heat).

Zhang Zhong Jing formulated the theory of the Six Stages, by which he classified the clinical manifestations of invasions of Wind-Cold according to the six channels: Greater Yang, Bright Yang, Lesser Yang, Greater Yin, Lesser Yin and Terminal Yin (Box 21.5). Zhang Zhong Jing's book 'Discussion of Cold-induced Diseases' dominated Chinese medicine, and in particular the treatment of diseases caused by exterior pathogenic factors, for 15 centuries; the school came to be known as the *Shang Han* school.

Towards the end of the Ming (1368–1644) and the beginning of the Qing (1644–1911) dynasty, a new school of thought regarding exterior diseases emerged. The three major representatives of this school were Wu You Ke (1592–1672), Ye Tian Shi (1667–1746) and Wu Ju Tong (1758–1836). This school concentrated on the study of the pathology and treatment of febrile diseases caused by exterior Wind-Heat and the school came to be known as the *Wen Bing* school: that is, the School of Warm Diseases. Warm Diseases are all caused by exterior Wind-Heat in the beginning stages but they present with special characteristics, the recognition of which was very innovative in Chinese medicine.

The characteristics of Warm Diseases are:

- They are all caused by Wind-Heat in the beginning stage
- They are characterized by fever
- The pathogenic factor penetrates through nose and mouth (as opposed to skin in the *Shang Han* school of Wind-Cold)
- The Wind-Heat has a strong tendency to turn into interior Heat rapidly
- They are characterized by rapid changes
- Once in the Interior, the Heat tends to injure Yin rather quickly

Ye Tian Shi formulated the brilliant theory of the Four Levels to describe the pathological changes resulting from invasion of Wind-Heat in a Warm Disease. The Four Levels are the Defensive Qi (*Wei*), Qi, Nutritive Qi (*Ying*) and Blood (*Xue*) levels (Fig. 21.5 and Box 21.6). The first level describes the pathological changes when the pathogenic factor (Wind-Heat) is on the Exterior. The other three levels all correspond to interior Heat: that is, the external Wind-Heat has become interior and transformed into Heat. However, the three levels Qi, Nutritive Qi and Blood reflect three different depths of penetration by the Heat (with Blood being the deepest). The clinical manifestations of the Four Levels are described in chapter 45.

Box 21.6 The Four Levels (*Wen Bing*)

- Defensive Qi (*Wei*)
- Qi (*Qi*)
- Nutritive Qi (*Ying*)
- Blood (*Xue*)

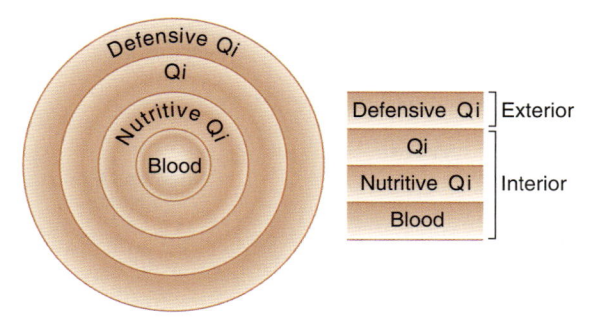

Figure 21.5 The Four Levels

Wu Ju Tong formulated the theory of the Three Burners to describe the pathological changes resulting from invasion of Wind-Heat in a Warm Disease. The clinical manifestations of the Three Burners are described in chapter 46.

Although a 'Warm Disease' presents with the pattern of Wind-Heat by definition, not every condition of invasion of Wind-Heat is a Warm Disease. Examples of Warm Diseases are influenza, mononucleosis, *rubeola* (measles), *rubella* (German measles), *varicella* (chicken pox), meningitis, polio, encephalitis and severe acute respiratory syndrome (SARS).

Box 21.7 summarizes the historical background.

> **Box 21.7 Historical background**
> - Originally diseases from exterior pathogenic factors were considered to be caused only by Cold
> - Zhang Zhong Jing, author of *Shang Han Lun*, was the first doctor to study systematically the pathology and treatment of diseases from exterior pathogenic factors
> - Zhang Zhong Jing formulated theory of Six Stages
> - Wen Bing school considered exterior diseases caused by invasion of Wind-Heat and understood the infectious nature of such diseases
> - Wen Bing school largely based on the theory of the Four Levels (Defensive Qi, Qi, Nutritive Qi and Blood)

CLIMATIC FACTORS AS PATTERNS OF DISHARMONY

Climatic factors differ somewhat from other causes of disease, in so far as they denote both causes and patterns of disease. When we say that a certain condition is due to exterior attack of Wind-Heat, we are saying two things: firstly, that exterior Wind-Heat has caused it and, secondly, that it manifests as Wind-Heat.

In clinical practice, these descriptions are more important as expressions of pathological conditions rather than as expressions of aetiological factors. For example, if a person has symptoms of a sore throat, sneezing, aversion to cold, fever, slight sweating, tonsillitis, thirst, and a Floating-Rapid pulse, we can certainly diagnose an exterior invasion of Wind-Heat. This diagnosis is not made on the basis of interrogation ('Have you been exposed to a hot wind?'), but through analysis of the symptoms and signs. In other words, if a person has the above symptoms and signs, these *are* Wind-Heat. We do not need to ask the patient whether he or she has been exposed to a hot wind in the hours previous to the arising of those symptoms. Hence, from this point of view, 'Wind-Heat' indicates a pathological pattern, rather than an aetiological factor.

The diagnosis of an invasion of an exterior pathogenic factor is made from the analysis of clinical manifestations, not from the interrogation of the patient

In the case of interior causes of disease, the situation is different as the causes are quite distinct from the disharmony pattern resulting from them. For example, if we diagnose the pattern of disharmony of Kidney-Yin deficiency in a patient, we cannot infer from this the cause of disease automatically but we can infer it only through interrogation of the patient. In this example, the two most likely causes of Kidney-Yin deficiency are overwork and excessive sexual activity and we cannot know which one it is except by enquiring about the patient's lifestyle. In contrast, if a patient presents with the pattern of disharmony bearing all the symptoms of invasion of Wind-Cold, then the aetiological factor *is* Wind-Cold and we do not need to ask whether the patient has been exposed to wind and cold (Fig. 21.6).

However, actual climatic elements do have a direct influence on the human body, giving rise to the clinical manifestations observed by Chinese doctors over many centuries: for example, if we are exposed to wind, cold and rain we will most probably suffer an invasion of 'Wind'; if we are exposed to damp weather we will suffer an invasion of 'Dampness'; and if we are exposed

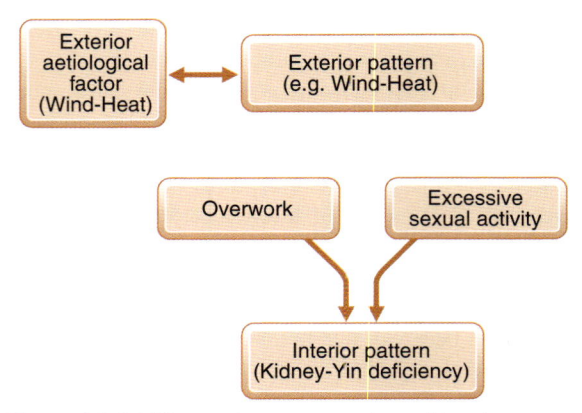

Figure 21.6 Difference between exterior and interior aetiological factors

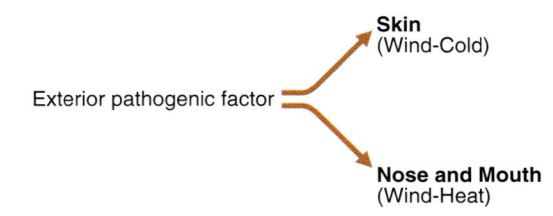

Figure 21.7 Penetration of exterior pathogenic factors

to intense heat in the summer, we will suffer an invasion of 'Summer-Heat'.

The underlying condition of the person partly determines the type of exterior pattern that will arise. A person with tendency to Heat will most likely display symptoms of Wind-Heat if he or she is invaded by exterior Wind. On the other hand, a person with a tendency to deficiency of Yang will display symptoms of Wind-Cold if he or she is attacked by exterior Wind. This explains how one can have symptoms of Wind-Heat in the middle of the coldest winter, or symptoms of Wind-Cold in the middle of the most torrid summer.

Box 21.8 summarizes climatic factors as patterns of disharmony.

> **Box 21.8 Climatic factors as patterns of disharmony**
>
> - Climatic factors denote both patterns of disharmony and aetiological factors (e.g. 'Wind-Heat' refers to a pattern and to an aetiological factor)
> - Diagnosis is made on the basis of clinical manifestations, not by interrogation of the patient
> - In interior causes of disease, the aetiological factor is quite distinct from the pattern of disharmony it causes

ARTIFICIAL 'CLIMATES' AS CAUSES OF DISEASE

Man-made climates can also cause disease. Air conditioning can cause symptoms of attack of exterior Wind.

For example, if someone enters an air-conditioned place coming from very hot outdoors, the person's skin pores will be open (from sweating) and the skin therefore more vulnerable to attack of 'Wind' (in this example, air conditioning).

The excessive heat and dryness of some centrally heated places can cause symptoms of attack of 'Wind-Heat'. Certain occupations are also prone to cause illness from exposure to artificial climates: for example those in the catering business who have to enter large refrigerated storerooms many times a day, steel workers who are exposed to very high temperatures at work or cooks who spend the whole day in very hot kitchens.

Box 21.9 summarizes artificial 'climates' as causes of disease.

> **Box 21.9 Artificial 'climates' as causes of disease**
>
> - Air conditioning
> - Refrigerated storerooms
> - Hot kitchens
> - Steel plants

PATHOLOGY AND CLINICAL MANIFESTATIONS OF EXTERIOR PATHOGENIC FACTORS

Exterior pathogenic factors enter the body either via the skin or via the nose and mouth (Fig. 21.7). Usually, Wind-Cold penetrates via the skin and Wind-Heat via nose and mouth.

Chapter 63 of the 'Simple Questions' describes clearly the penetration route of exterior pathogenic factors: '*When external evils invade the body, they invade the skin and hair first; if not expelled, they then invade the Minute Connecting channels [Sun Luo]; if not expelled, they then invade the Connecting channels [Luo, which are in the space between skin and muscles]; if not expelled, they* then invade the Main channels and then the 5 Yin Organs ... therefore external evils penetrate from the skin and hair to the 5 Yin Organs.'[6] This passage also clearly explains how exterior pathogenic factors can penetrate the five Yin organs (Fig. 21.8).

In the beginning stages of an invasion of external pathogenic factor, the pathogenic factor is in the space between the skin and muscles (*Cou Li* space) and in the channels as opposed to the Internal Organs: this is also called the 'Exterior' of the body and an 'exterior' pattern results from such invasion. The definition of 'exterior' is arrived at on the basis of the location of the pathogenic factor, not the aetiology (Fig. 21.9).

In other words a pattern is not called 'exterior' because it is caused by an exterior pathogenic factor, but because the pathogenic factor is located in the space between skin and muscles and channels: that is, the 'Exterior' of the body (Fig. 21.10). If an exterior pathogenic factor penetrates deeper to affect the internal organs (i.e. the 'Interior'), the resulting pattern of clinical manifestations is defined as an 'interior pattern', even though in this case it was caused originally by an exterior pathogenic factor.

> A pattern is not defined as 'exterior' when it is caused by an exterior pathogenic factor but when the pathogenic factor is *located* in the 'Exterior' of the body (space between skin and muscles). An exterior pathogenic factor can penetrate in the Interior and cause an interior pattern

Once inside the body, exterior pathogenic factors become interior if they are not expelled and they can completely change their nature. For example, Wind-Cold can turn into Heat, Dampness can easily generate Heat, Fire and Heat can cause Dryness while extreme Heat can give rise to Wind.

Each of the climatic factors causes certain clinical manifestations which are typical of that particular climate. An experienced practitioner of Chinese medicine will be able to infer the cause of the disease from the manifestations.

For example, exterior Wind causes symptoms and signs to arise suddenly and change rapidly. Cold contracts and causes pain and watery discharges. Dampness invades the body gradually and causes turbid, sticky discharges. Dryness obviously dries the Body Fluids. Heat and Fire give rise to sensations of heat, thirst and mental restlessness.

Figure 21.8 Penetration of exterior pathogenic factors according to the 'Yellow Emperor's Classic of Internal Medicine'

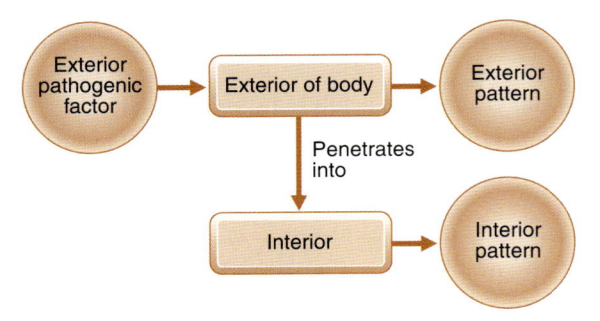

Figure 21.9 Exterior pathogenic factor giving rise to exterior or interior pattern

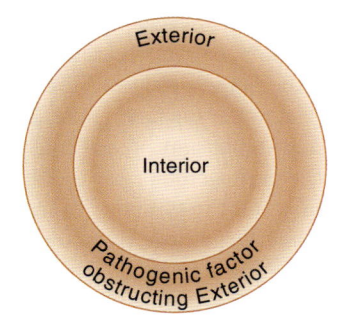

Figure 21.10 Location of pathogenic factor in Exterior determines exterior pattern

Although the climatic causes of disease are important, in practice, exterior pathogenic factors such as Wind-Heat or Wind-Cold are clinically more relevant as patterns of disharmony rather than as causes of disease. In other words, although the cause of a Wind-Heat pattern may be said to be in some cases climatic wind and heat, it is the pattern of Wind-Heat that is clinically significant and requiring treatment. For this reason, the clinical manifestations of these exterior pathogenic factors are discussed in the chapter on the Identification of Patterns according to Pathogenic Factors (ch. 43).

The two major symptoms of invasions of exterior pathogenic factors are 'aversion to cold' and 'fever' occurring *simultaneously* and it is therefore worth discussing these two symptoms in detail.

Box 21.10 summarizes pathology and clinical manifestations.

> **Box 21.10 Pathology and clinical manifestations**
> - Exterior pathogenic factors enter the body via the skin or via the nose and mouth
> - Exterior pathogenic factors invade the space between skin and muscles first (the 'Exterior' of the body)
> - If not expelled, an exterior pathogenic factor may penetrate into the Interior and cause an interior pattern

AVERSION TO COLD AND FEVER

'Aversion to cold' and 'fever' are the two major symptoms of invasion of most exterior pathogenic factors and it is worth discussing these two in detail. It is important to note that it is the *simultaneous* occurrence of aversion to cold and fever that denotes the invasion of an exterior pathogenic factor: that is, the patient feels cold *subjectively* but his or her body is *objectively* hot to the touch.

When the symptom of aversion to cold occurs simultaneously with the objective sign of the patient's body feeling hot to the touch (or having an actual fever), it indicates an acute invasion of external Wind and it denotes that the pathogenic factor is still on the Exterior. In particular, it is the symptom of aversion to cold that indicates that the pathogenic factor is on the Exterior: the moment the patient does not feel cold any longer but feels hot and, if in bed, he or she throws off the blankets, this means that the pathogenic factor is in the Interior and it has turned into Heat.

> A subjective aversion to cold by the patient and an objective 'fever' (or hot feeling of the patient's body on palpation) occurring *simultaneously* are the essential manifestations of an invasion of an exterior pathogenic factor

Aversion to cold

In the context of invasions of exterior pathogenic factors, 'aversion to cold' (*wu han*) refers to the typical cold feeling arising from an invasion of exterior Wind with a sudden onset. It is the cold, shivery feeling that we get when we catch a cold or a flu: it starts suddenly and we want to cover ourselves. If we go to bed, we like to be covered with blankets: however, it is a characteristic of 'aversion to cold' from exterior Wind that it is *not* relieved by covering oneself. Aversion to cold is a subjective feeling of the patient.

The acute 'aversion to cold' from an invasion of exterior Wind is obviously different from the general cold feeling experienced by someone suffering from Yang deficiency. The 'aversion to cold' from an exterior invasion has two characteristics: it arises suddenly and it is not relieved by covering oneself (the general cold feeling from Yang deficiency is chronic and is relieved by covering oneself).

The symptom of aversion to cold is due to the obstruction of the space between skin and muscles by exterior Wind. Defensive Qi circulates in the space between skin and muscles and it warms the muscles; if it is obstructed by exterior Wind, it cannot circulate well and it fails to warm the muscles: hence the 'aversion to cold'. The intensity of the aversion to cold is directly proportional to the strength of the pathogenic factor: the stronger the pathogenic factor, the more intense the aversion to cold (Fig. 21.11). Please note that aversion to cold occurs with both Wind-Cold and Wind-Heat.

Chinese medicine actually distinguishes four degrees of 'aversion to cold'. These are, in ascending order of severity:

- 'Aversion to wind' (*wu feng*, literally 'disliking wind')
- 'Fear of cold' (*wei han*)
- 'Aversion to cold' (*wu han*, literally 'disliking cold')
- 'Shivers' (*han zhan*)

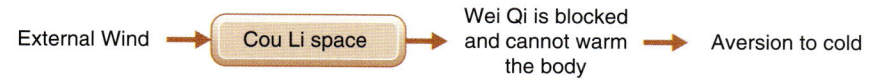

External Wind → Cou Li space → Wei Qi is blocked and cannot warm the body → Aversion to cold

Figure 21.11 Pathology of 'aversion to cold'

External Wind → Struggle ← Body's Qi → Fever

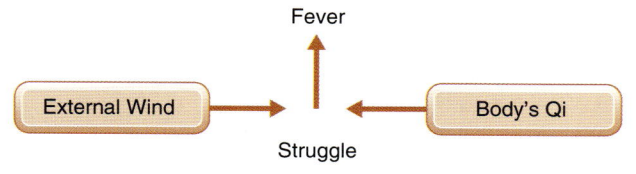

Figure 21.12 Pathology of 'fever'

Aversion to wind means that the patient has goose pimples, dislikes going out in the wind and wants to stay indoors.

Fear of cold means that the patient feels quite cold, wants to be indoors and near sources of heat and wants to cover up.

Aversion to cold means that the patient feels very cold, wants to say indoors and cover up in bed: this, however, does not relieve the cold feeling (Box 21.11).

Shivers means that the patient feels extremely cold, shivers and wants to cover up under several blankets in bed: this, however, does not relieve the cold feeling.

Box 21.11 Aversion to cold

- 'Aversion to cold' means that the patient feels subjectively cold quite suddenly, likes to stay indoors and likes to cover himself or herself with blankets
- Aversion to cold is due to the obstruction of the space between skin and muscles by the exterior pathogenic factor so that Defensive Qi cannot warm the muscles
- The intensity of the aversion to cold is directly proportional to the intensity of the pathogenic factor
- Aversion to cold is always a symptom of an invasion of an exterior pathogenic factor and it is a sign that the pathogenic factor is still on the Exterior
- When the aversion to cold goes and the patient feels hot, the pathogenic factor has penetrated into the Interior

---

Fever

'Fever' does not necessarily indicate an actual fever as measured by a thermometer. The term that we translate as 'fever' is actually *fa re*, which means 'emission of heat'. Thus, 'emission of heat' refers to the objective sensation of warmth emanating from the patient's body and felt by the physician on palpation. The patient's body feels hot, in severe cases almost burning to the touch: the areas touched are usually the forehead and especially the dorsum of the hands (as opposed to the palms which tend to reflect more Empty-Heat).

In fact, it is a characteristic of *fa re* (so-called 'fever') in the exterior stage of invasions of Wind that the dorsum of the hands feels hot compared with the palms and the upper back feels hot compared with the chest.[7] This objective hot feeling of the patient's body may or may not be accompanied by an actual fever. Thus, the 'aversion to cold' is subjective while the 'fever' is objective: that is, the patient's body feels hot on palpation.

> 'Fever' does not necessarily indicate a raised temperature: it indicates that the patient's forehead and dorsum of hands feel hot to the touch. The patient may or may not have an actual fever

Fever is produced by the struggle between the exterior pathogenic factor and the body's Qi (Fig. 21.12). Thus, the strength of the fever (or hot feeling of the body) reflects the intensity of this struggle: this depends on the relative strength of the external pathogenic factor and the strength of the Upright Qi. The stronger the external pathogenic factor, the higher the fever (or hot feeling of the body); likewise, the stronger the Upright Qi, the higher the fever (or hot feeling of the body). Thus the fever will be highest when both the external pathogenic factor and the Upright Qi are strong.

The relative strength of the pathogenic factor and the Upright Qi is only one factor which determines the intensity of the fever (or hot feeling of the body).

Another factor is simply the constitution of a person: a person with a Yang constitution (i.e. with predominance of Yang) will be more prone to a higher fever (or hot feeling of the body).

> The intensity of fever in exterior conditions is related to the struggle between the Upright Qi and the external pathogenic factor and has nothing to do with whether the pathogenic factor is Wind-Cold or Wind-Heat

Thus, there are three possible degrees of fever (or hot feeling of the body):

- Strong pathogenic factor and strong Upright Qi: high fever (or hot feeling of the body)
- Strong pathogenic factor with weak Upright Qi or vice versa: medium fever (or hot feeling of the body)
- Weak pathogenic factor and weak Upright Qi: low fever (or hot feeling of the body) or no fever at all

It is important to note that 'fever' or 'emission of heat' do not mean that the pathogenic factor is Wind-Heat (as opposed to Wind-Cold). The fever or emission of heat is due to the body's Qi fighting the pathogenic factor and can therefore occur also with invasions of Wind-Cold. If that was not the case, nobody would get invasions of Wind-Heat in winter, which is definitely not the case.

Box 21.12 summarizes fever.

> The fever or emission of heat (objective hot feeling of the patient's body) may occur both with Wind-Heat and Wind-Cold

Box 21.12 Fever

- 'Fever' indicates the objective hot feeling emanating from the patient's forehead and dorsum of hands and felt on palpation by the physician
- Fever is due to the struggle between the body's Qi and the exterior pathogenic factor
- The intensity of the fever is directly proportional both to the intensity of the pathogenic factor and to the strength of the body's Qi

SYMPTOMS AND SIGNS OF EXTERIOR PATHOGENIC FACTORS PATTERNS

The clinical manifestations arising from invasion of exterior pathogenic factors is discussed in detail in the chapter on the Identification of Patterns according to Pathogenic Factors (ch. 43). This is done for two reasons: firstly, because, as explained above, the exterior pathogenic factors are more relevant as patterns of disharmony than as causes of disease; secondly, because it is more logical to discuss the clinical manifestations of each pathogenic factor in both its exterior and interior form. For example, there are some similarities in the clinical manifestations of exterior and interior Wind, even though the two are completely different pathological conditions.

The following is therefore only a brief and necessarily broad description of the clinical manifestations arising from the invasion of each of the exterior pathogenic factors.

Wind

- Invading the space between the skin and muscles and the Lungs' Defensive Qi portion: aversion to cold, fever, sore throat, sneezing, runny nose, occipital stiffness, Floating pulse
- Invading the muscles and channels: stiffness, rigidity, contraction of the muscles with sudden onset
- Invading the joints: pain that moves from joint to joint, especially in the upper part of the body (Wind Painful Obstruction Syndrome)

Cold

- Invading the muscles and sinews: stiffness, contraction of muscles, pain, chilliness
- Invading the joints: severe pain in a joint (Cold Painful Obstruction Syndrome)
- Invading the Stomach, Intestines or Uterus: sudden epigastric pain with vomiting, sudden abdominal pain with diarrhoea, acute dysmenorrhoea

Summer-Heat

- Aversion to cold, fever, sweating, headache, dark urine, thirst, Floating-Rapid pulse

Dampness

- Invading muscles and sinews: a feeling heaviness of the limbs, dull ache of the muscles

- Invading the joints: pain, heaviness and swelling of the joints, especially of the lower part of the body (Damp Painful Obstruction Syndrome)
- Acute urinary discomfort, acute vaginal discharge, acute skin diseases with vesicles or papules, acute digestive upsets

Dryness

- Acute dry cough, aversion to cold, fever, dry mouth and nose

Fire

- Aversion to heat, high fever, sweating, mental confusion, thirst, Overflowing-Rapid pulse, Red tongue with yellow coating

CONSEQUENCES OF INVASION OF EXTERIOR PATHOGENIC FACTORS

A large variety of problems derive from invasion of exterior pathogenic factors. We can distinguish broadly three types of consequences of invasions of exterior pathogenic factors. These are as follows:

Invasions of exterior pathogenic factors resulting in an exterior pattern

Generally speaking, an invasion of an exterior pathogenic factor leads to an exterior pattern: that is, one characterized by the location of the pathogenic factor in the Exterior of the body (the space between skin and muscles and the channels) and by the simultaneous occurrence of aversion to cold and fever.

Examples of such invasions are upper respiratory infections, common cold, influenza, pharyngitis, laryngitis, ear infections, tonsillitis, etc. More serious diseases such as measles, mononucleosis, meningitis, etc., also start with symptoms of aversion to cold and fever and with an exterior pattern.

Invasions of exterior pathogenic factors without an exterior pattern

In a few cases, exterior Cold can penetrate some organs directly without the development of an exterior pattern with aversion to cold and fever. This happens when exterior Cold invades the Stomach, causing acute epigastric pain and vomiting; the Intestines, causing acute diarrhoea and abdominal pain; and the Uterus, causing acute dysmenorrhoea. In such cases, the patient will not go through a beginning stage characterized by aversion to cold and fever.

Invasions of exterior pathogenic factors resulting in obstruction of muscles and channels

In very many cases, exterior pathogenic factors invade the muscles, sinews and channels causing obstruction of Defensive Qi in the Connecting channels (*Luo*) and Muscle channels and therefore joint pain. This condition is called Painful Obstruction Syndrome (*Bi* Syndrome). It is extremely common and it is something that we see in our clinic every day.

For example, exterior Cold may invade the knees and cause knee pain; exterior Wind may invade the muscles of the neck and cause a stiff and painful neck; exterior Dampness may invade the wrist joints causing pain and swelling of the ankles, etc. Painful Obstruction Syndrome is generally caused primarily by Wind, Cold and Dampness in its initial stages.

The manifestations are the following:

- Wind: pain from joint to joint, affects more upper part of body
- Cold: intense pain in one joint
- Dampness: pain, swelling and feeling of heaviness of the joints, affects more the lower part of body

However, Painful Obstruction Syndrome may also start with an exterior pattern (with aversion to cold and fever) in its initial stages, but this is something we do not see frequently in the clinic.

Box 21.13 summarizes the consequences of invasion of exterior pathogenic factors.

Box 21.13 Consequences of invasion of exterior pathogenic factors

- Invasions of exterior pathogenic factors resulting in an exterior pattern: simultaneous aversion to cold and fever
- Invasions of exterior pathogenic factors without an exterior pattern: direct invasion of Cold in the Stomach, Intestine and Uterus
- Invasions of exterior pathogenic factors resulting in obstruction of muscles and channels: Painful Obstruction Syndrome (*Bi* Syndrome)

3

Learning outcomes

In this chapter you will have learned:

- How climatic factors become a cause of disease only when there is a *relative* imbalance between the body's Qi and the exterior pathogenic factor
- The seasons and organs associated with each of the six climatic factors
- The emphasis placed by Chinese medicine on considering the strength of the body's Qi in the prevention of infectious diseases
- The significance of Zhang Zhong Jing's 'Discussion of Cold-induced Diseases' and theory of Six Stages in the treatment of disease caused by exterior pathogenic factors
- The influence of the *Wen Bing* school on the treatment of febrile disease
- The importance of recognizing that climatic factors denote both patterns of disharmony as well as aetiological factors, with diagnosis made on signs and symptoms rather than enquiry about exposure to climatic factors
- The role of man-made climates as a modern cause of disease
- The definition of an 'exterior' pattern and the characteristic clinical manifestations caused by each of the exterior pathogenic factors
- The significance of symptoms of simultaneous aversion to cold and fever in exterior patterns
- The varying consequences of invasion of exterior pathogenic factors

Self-assessment questions

1. If a person's Defensive Qi is strong, how might they become ill through climatic causes?
2. Which organ and season are associated with the climatic factor of Dryness?
3. List the Four Levels as formulated by Ye Tian Shi. Which of these levels are classed as being on the Exterior and which are on the Interior?
4. A person with a tendency to Heat gets caught in the wind and rain in the middle of winter. What pattern are they likely to manifest?
5. How are Wind-Cold and Wind-Heat said to enter the body?
6. What is the definition of an exterior pattern?
7. How would you distinguish whether a patient who was averse to cold was presenting with an exterior pattern of Wind-Cold or Yang deficiency?
8. How would you tell if a patient was manifesting 'fever', or '*fa re*'?
9. Give three symptoms of Wind invading the space between the skin and muscles and the Lung's Defensive Qi portion.
10. Give three examples of exterior cold directly penetrating the body without causing an exterior pattern.

See p. 1261 for answers

END NOTES

1. 1979 The Yellow Emperor's Classic of Internal Medicine – Simple Questions (*Huang Ti Nei Jing Su Wen* 黄帝内经素问), People's Health Publishing House, Beijing, first published *c*.100 BC, p. 537.
2. Ibid., p. 158.
3. Ibid., p. 215.
4. Ibid., p. 538.
5. This has not always been so, as, before the onset of modern, biochemical medicine, Western medicine did recognize the influence of climatic factors as direct causes of disease. For example, Hippocrates studied the relationship between climate and organism in health and disease in great detail in his book 'Airs, Waters and Places'. Galen saw the relationship between air and disease. He considered harmful airs as causes of disease and examples of such harmful airs were those arising from swamps, marshes, sewers, putrefying animals and manure. He also considered weather changes as a cause of disharmony in the organism. The famous English doctor T Sydenham continued in the great Hippocratic tradition, seeing the relationship between weather and disease. He also considered weather as a direct of cause of disharmony.
6. Ibid., p. 344.
7. Deng Tie Tao 1988 Practical Chinese Diagnosis (*Shi Yong Zhong Yi Zhen Duan Xue* 实用中医诊断学), Shanghai Science Publishing House, Shanghai, p. 90.

PART 3

Miscellaneous Causes of Disease   22

Key contents

Weak constitution

Overwork

Excessive physical work (and lack of exercise)

Excessive sexual activity

Diet

Trauma

Parasites and poisons

Wrong treatment

Medicinal drugs

Drugs

Miscellaneous causes of disease are:

- Weak constitution
- Overwork
- Excessive physical work (and lack of exercise)
- Excessive sexual activity
- Diet
- Trauma
- Parasites and poisons
- Wrong treatment
- Medicinal drugs
- Drugs

WEAK CONSTITUTION

Every person is born with a certain constitution, which is dependent on the parents' health in general and their health at the time of conception specifically. It is also dependent on the mother's health during pregnancy.

The fusion of the parents' sexual essences at conception gives rise to a human being whose constitution is, to a large extent, determined at that time. The fetus is nourished by its Pre-Heaven Essence, which is the determinant of that individual's constitution. By and large, the constitution of a human being cannot be changed: for example, the immense power and stamina of certain of today's athletes is not only a matter of training but also of constitution, and those who are born with a relatively weak constitution can never hope to attain those outstanding athletic abilities.

The discussion on constitution will be conducted as follows:

- The importance of constitution in health and disease
- The hereditary constitution is not entirely fixed and unchangeable
- Causes of weak constitution
- Strong prenatal constitution
- Weak prenatal constitution
- Assessment of constitution

The importance of constitution in health and disease

We can verify the importance of constitution in our practices every day. The amount of morbidity people suffer in the course of their lifetime is largely dependent on their constitution and is affected only partly by causes of disease arising in the course of their life. It would impossible to quantify how much the constitution accounts for our quality of life but I personally would put it as high as 50%. We can verify this in our practice very frequently: there are many patients who may be struck by serious diseases (often caused by their lifestyle) and yet live to a ripe old age, enjoying good energy and good spirits. Conversely, there are patients who are very careful to lead a healthy life in terms of work, exercise and diet and yet are constantly plagued by distressing (albeit not serious) symptoms.

The hereditary constitution is a major factor determining the health and morbidity of a person throughout their lifetime

The hereditary constitution is not entirely fixed and unchangeable

A person's constitution is not entirely fixed and immutable. It can be changed and improved within certain limits. A healthy and balanced lifestyle, together with breathing exercises to develop one's Qi, can lead to an improvement in one's constitution.

As we know, the Pre-Heaven Essence (*Jing*), which is the basis of our inner strength and health, is not immutable, but is constantly replenished by Post-Heaven Qi. Whilst it is quite easy to weaken one's constitution through inadequate rest, overwork or excessive sexual activity, by taking care to achieve a balance in one's life it is possible to some extent to build up a weak constitution.

The broad field of Chinese medicine (including *Qi Gong* breathing exercises and certain forms of martial arts of the 'inner school' such as *Tai Ji Quan*), attaches great importance to the preservation of one's Essence and Qi and therefore the cultivation of one's constitution. This aim is implicit in the philosophy of and treatment by acupuncture and Chinese herbal medicine as well as the practice of traditional breathing exercises.

These practices and ideas have their origin in the ancient Daoist preoccupation with longevity and immortality. Due to the Daoist masters' research into herbal remedies, acupuncture and breathing exercises to attain 'immortality' or longevity, we now have a rich inheritance of herbal and acupuncture treatments as well as breathing exercises and life's 'hygiene' rules aimed at strengthening a weak constitution. The complex of such Daoist teachings is called *Yang Sheng* in Chinese: that is, 'nourishing life'. Indeed, some think that Chinese medicine developed as part of *Yang Shen* techniques.

Causes of weak constitution

The causes of weak constitution are to be found in the parents' health in general, in the parents' health at the time of conception or in events surrounding pregnancy. According to Chinese medicine, if the parents are too old, the child is more likely to have a poor constitution. The Chinese also believe this to be the case if the parents conceive in a state of drunkenness or if they are in poor health at the time of conception. Also, if the mother is under severe emotional stress and consumes alcohol or drugs or smokes during the pregnancy, this will adversely affect the child's constitution. There are also of course many medicinal drugs that affect the fetus adversely. A severe shock to the mother during pregnancy will affect the constitution of the baby, particularly its Heart. This is often manifested with a bluish tinge on the forehead and on the chin. Figure 22.1 shows the factors that affect hereditary constitution and Box 22.1 lists the causes of a weak constitution.

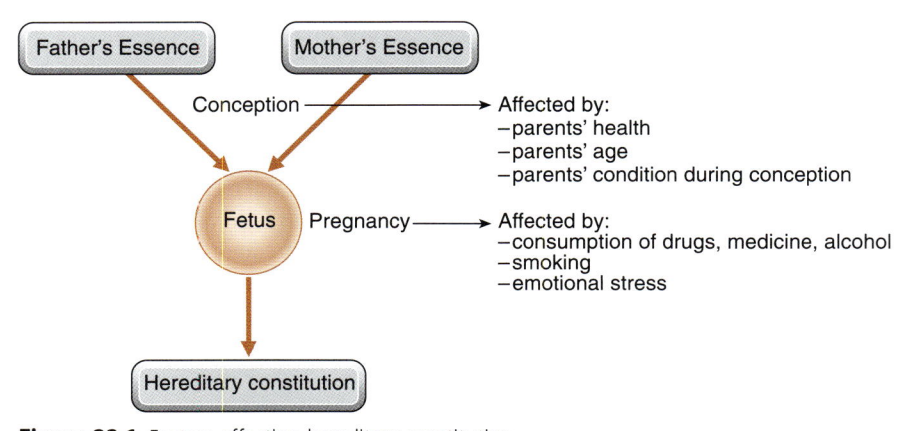

Figure 22.1 Factors affecting hereditary constitution

> **Box 22.1 Causes of weak constitution**
>
> - Parents' health in general
> - Parents' health at the time of conception
> - Parents too old
> - Events surrounding pregnancy (emotional stress, drugs, medicines, alcohol, smoking)

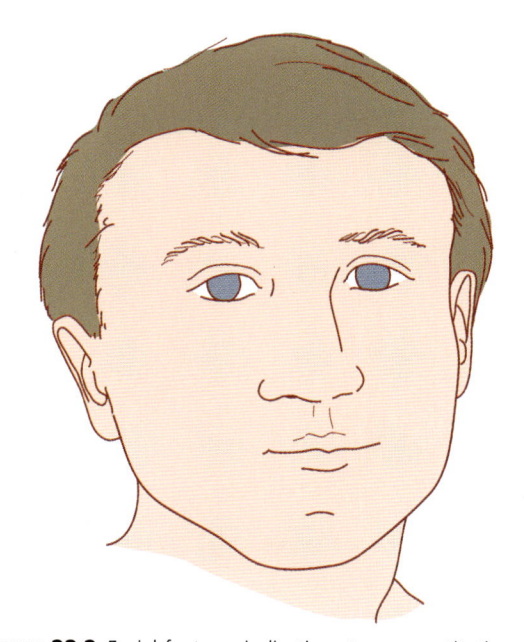

Figure 22.2 Facial features indicating strong constitution

Strong prenatal constitution

The main features indicating a good prenatal constitution are as follows (Fig. 22.2):

> - Broad forehead and glabella
> - Long and wide nose
> - Full cheeks
> - Strong lower jaw
> - Long ears with long ear lobes
> - Well-proportioned eyes, nose, ears and mouth
> - Long philtrum
> - Normal complexion with lustre
> - Firm muscles and skin

The above features indicate a good prenatal constitution: when this person is ill, the disease is easy to treat. Of course, it does not mean that people with a strong prenatal constitution will never be ill but, rather that, even if they do fall ill with a serious disease, they generally have a long life and they are able to survive even serious illnesses.

Chapter 37 of the 'Spiritual Axis' says: 'A life as long as 100 years can be expected if the forehead and glabella are full and broad; the cheek and the area from the cheek to the front of the ear have well-developed muscles and protrude from the face, connecting a strong lower jaw and long ear lobes together; the eyes, nose, ears and mouth are well spaced and well proportioned; the face colour is normal. These people have abundant Qi and Blood. Their skin and muscles are strong. They respond well to acupuncture treatment.'[1]

Chapter 54 of the 'Spiritual Axis' says: 'People with long life expectancy have long and deep nostrils. The muscles of the cheek and of the area from the cheek to the front of the ear are thick and high and well formed. The circulation of Nutritive and Defensive Qi is smooth. The upper, middle and lower parts of the face are in the right proportion, with well-developed and distinct muscles and prominent bones. People of this type can live out their normal life expectancy, or even up to the age of 100.'[2]

The chapter 'Keys to the Four Diagnostic Methods' in the 'Golden Mirror of Medicine' says: 'If the forehead is high, the glabella is full, the nose is high and straight, the cheeks are full and the skeleton is well built, the person will have a long life expectancy.'[3]

Weak prenatal constitution

The physical features of people with a weak prenatal constitution are as follows (Fig. 22.3):

> - Eyes, nose, ears and mouth close together
> - Narrow forehead
> - Small space between the eyebrows
> - Narrow nose with nostrils turned up and exposed
> - Short philtrum
> - Thin cheeks
> - Area between the cheek and the front of the ears narrow
> - Short and small ears that turn outwards
> - Flat, sunken, low and narrow lower jaw
> - Flabby muscles and loose skin

People with a poor prenatal constitution will have a tendency to suffer from a deficiency of Qi, Blood, Yin or Yang. Compared to people with a strong prenatal constitution, these people are more easily invaded by external pathogenic factors and, when this occurs, the treatment will be relatively more difficult. Having a weak prenatal constitution often also means that these

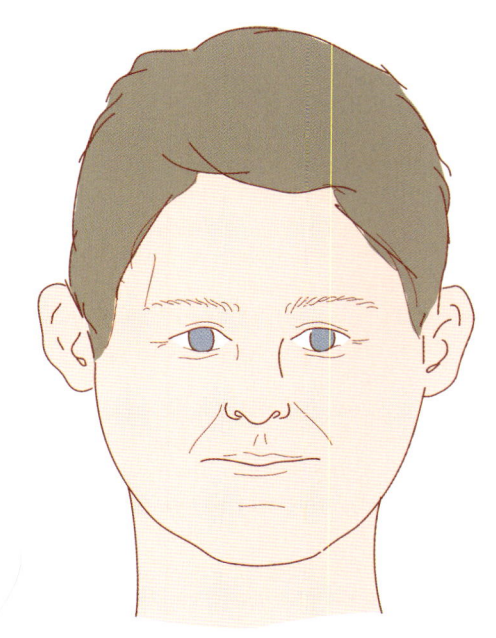

Figure 22.3 Facial features indicating weak constitution

people may suffer constantly from distressing (albeit not serious) symptoms throughout their life.

Chapter 37 of the 'Spiritual Axis' says: '*When the five senses are not sharp, the forehead and glabella are narrow, the nose is small, the area between the cheek and the front of the ears is narrow, the lower jaw is flat and the ears turn outwards, the prenatal constitution is poor even though the complexion and colour may be normal. These people are intrinsically unhealthy, even more so when they are ill.*'[4]

> **Clinical note**
>
> Although the prenatal constitution is predetermined, it is not entirely unchangeable. It can be assisted by treating primarily the Kidneys with Ren-4 Guanyuan and KI-3 Taixi

Assessment of constitution

The constitution of a person can be assessed also by examining the history, pulse, ears and tongue. A history of many childhood diseases, and in particularly whooping cough, indicates a weak constitution. Whooping cough, in particular, is often indicative of an inherited weakness of the Lungs. An inherited weakness of the Lungs, or tendency to Lung diseases (especially Lung tuberculosis) in the family, is often manifested by two signs: a pulse in the Front position (either side or both), which can be felt going medially up towards the thenar eminence, and one or two cracks on the tongue in the Lung area (Figs 22.4 and 22.5).

The face can show constitutional weaknesses, especially in the ears. Very small ears with short ear lobes show a poor constitution.

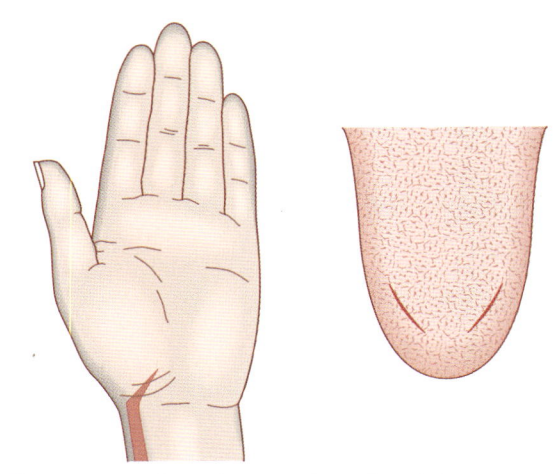

Figure 22.4 Pulse and tongue signs of weak Lung constitution

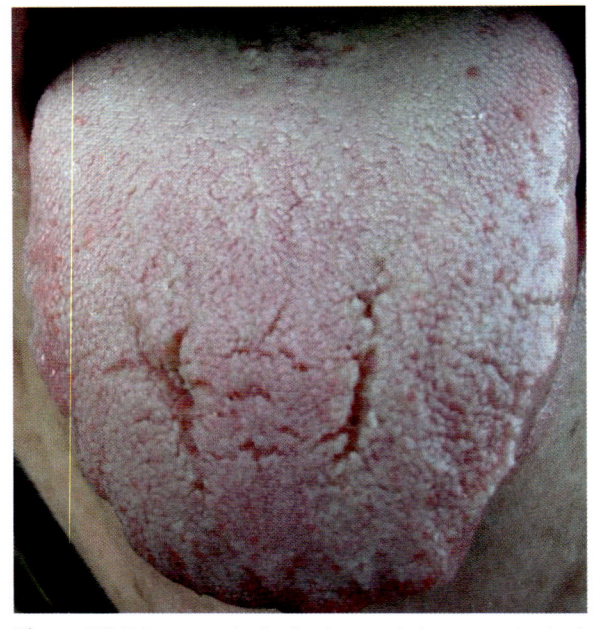

Figure 22.5 Lung cracks (indicating weak Lung constitution)

Box 22.2 Constitution

- Constitution depends on the parents' Kidney-Essence (*Jing*)
- Hereditary constitution is a very important factor in health and disease
- The hereditary constitution may be improved within certain limits
- The causes of a weak constitution lie in the parents' health in general and specifically at the time of conception
- The constitution of a person may be assessed by observation of facial features, ears, history, pulse and tongue

A Scattered, Minute or Leather pulse (see ch. 25) and a tongue without 'spirit' on the root (see ch. 23) are also indicative of a poor constitution.

An assessment of the constitution of a person is useful in clinical practice to make a realistic prognosis. It is always important to have a clear idea of what one can realistically expect to achieve with the treatment and, more importantly, to advise patients with poor constitution about diet, proper rest, sexual activity and breathing exercises.

Box 22.2 summarizes the essential points concerning the constitution.

OVERWORK

The discussion of overwork will proceed as follows:

- Definition
- Effects of overwork in relation to Qi and Yin

Definition

By 'overwork' I do not mean physical work, but working excessively long hours for many years. 'Overwork' becomes a cause of disease because the lifestyle associated with it usually also involves an irregular diet and some emotional stress (particularly worry). Very many people in modern Western countries lead a hectic life that severely depletes their Qi.

Chinese medicine and Chinese culture in general place great stress on the importance of a proper balance between work and rest, work and relaxation and a proper rhythm of work and rest. Very many people in the West have lost all sense of balance between work and rest. For example, among my patients, it is not at all uncommon to hear that someone gets up at 6 in the morning to catch a train at 6.30, travel to London to work in a hectic office for the whole day under conditions of stress, to then return home at 8 in the evening. Frequently, this also involves irregular eating, as very many people report that lunch consists of a quick sandwich consumed at one's desk while working. Moreover, frequently, such a person considers a frenetic, weekly game of squash as 'relaxation'. Such a working routine carried out over many years constitutes 'overwork'; it seriously depletes Qi and it is a major cause of disease in the West.

Many Western patients have lost all sense of balance between work and rest and, in my experience, overwork is a major cause of disease

Effects of overwork in relation to Qi and Yin

The question of balance between activity and rest affects Qi directly. Whenever we work or exercise, we are using up Qi; whenever we rest, Qi is restored. There are actually two levels of Qi to be considered here. On the one hand, there is Qi (the Post-Heaven Qi) that is formed by the Stomach and Spleen from food on a daily basis, is constantly replenished, and provides the energy for our daily activities; on the other hand, there are the Yin substances, which, being the foundation and nourishment of the body, determine our basic body nourishment and long-term resistance to disease.

In our daily activities of work and exercise, we normally use Qi, in particular Yang Qi. Yin substances provide the physiological basis for more long-term reservoirs of energy. Under normal circumstances, the Qi used up in normal work and exercise is quickly restored by proper diet and rest. If we take the pulse of a person who has been working very hard for a week, perhaps working towards exams, and who has been staying up until the early hours of the morning and eating poorly, the pulse will probably be weak and deep. If this person has adequate rest and a good diet, the pulse will return to normal in about 2 or 3 days. This shows that while Qi (Post-Heaven Qi) can be quickly used up, it can equally rapidly be restored by rest. In such a situation, the patient does not need any treatment but just rest.

If, however, one works extremely hard and for very long hours over many years without adequate rest, then the body has no chance of restoring the Post-Heaven Qi fast enough: before it has made up the lost Qi, the person is working again, using up more Qi. When one overworks beyond the point that Qi can keep up with the demands, then one is forced to draw on the Yin substances to face the demands of this lifestyle. At this point, the Yin will begin to be depleted and symptoms of Yin deficiency may appear.[5] When this point is reached, even adequate rest will not help the situation very quickly, and the situation will be rectified only by a radical change in routine and taking more rest on a *regular* basis. Most of these patients think that a short holiday in the sun will replenish their Qi after years of overwork: this is most definitely not so as their Yin will be replenished only gradually over a long period of time by modifying their lifestyle to work much shorter hours and taking more rest on a regular basis (Fig. 22.6).

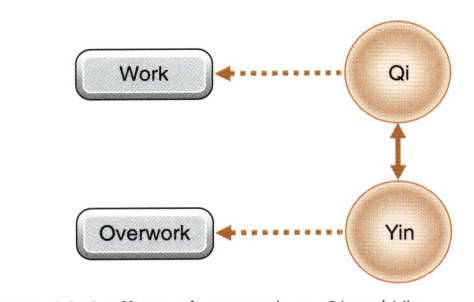

Figure 22.6 Effects of overwork on Qi and Yin

Qi and Yin represent two levels of energy. Qi is used up by working and replenished by rest. When a person overworks, Qi cannot be replenished fast enough and Yin is used instead

Overwork as described above, over many years, is a major cause of Yin deficiency and particularly Kidney-Yin deficiency. In some cases, it may also cause a Kidney-Essence (*Jing*) deficiency.

Mental overwork is a particular kind of overwork. In this case, the person does not necessarily lead a hectic life as described above but works long hours in a sedentary occupation involving mental work. Excessive mental work and concentration weakens the Spleen.

Box 22.3 summarizes overwork as a cause of disease.

Box 22.3 Overwork
- 'Overwork' consists in working long hours without adequate rest for years
- Overwork leads to Yin deficiency, especially Kidney-Yin deficiency

EXCESSIVE PHYSICAL WORK (AND LACK OF EXERCISE)

The discussion of excessive physical work will proceed as follows:

- Definition
- Effects of excessive physical work
- Lack of exercise

Definition

Excessive physical work includes physical work in the course of one's occupation (e.g. removal men), excessive physical exercise (e.g. gym work-out), excessive sport (e.g. football), excessive lifting, excessive ballet, etc.

A reasonable amount of exercise is of course beneficial and essential to good health. But exercise carried out to the point of exhaustion will deplete Qi. Excessive exercise is particularly harmful if carried out during puberty, especially for girls, who may later develop menstrual problems.

Certain types of exercise may also cause stagnation of Qi in a particular area. Weight-lifting affects the lower back, jogging the knees and tennis the elbows.

Excessive lifting, as happens frequently in the building or house removal trades, weakens the Kidneys and the lower back.

Excessive standing also weakens the Kidneys. The 'Simple Questions' in chapter 23 talks about the 'five exhaustions': '*Excessive use of the eyes injures the Blood [i.e. the Heart]; excessive lying down injures Qi [i.e. the Lungs]; excessive sitting injures the muscles [i.e. the Spleen]; excessive standing injures the bones [i.e. the Kidneys]; excessive exercise injures the sinews [i.e. the Liver]*.'[6]

Clinical note

'Simple Questions': '*Excessive use of the eyes injures the Blood [i.e. the Heart]; excessive lying down injures Qi [i.e. the Lungs]; excessive sitting injures the muscles [i.e. the Spleen]; excessive standing injures the bones [i.e. the Kidneys]; excessive exercise injures the sinews [i.e. the Liver].*'

Effects of excessive physical work

Excessive physical work in general depletes mostly the Spleen and the Liver, as the former controls the muscles and the latter the sinews. Excessive use of one part of the body will also cause stagnation of Qi in that particular part. For example, constant repetitive movement which may be associated with a certain job will tend to cause stagnation of Qi in that part: the aching arm of a hairdresser, the aching elbow of a bricklayer or the aching wrist of a word-processing operator.

Excessive jogging weakens the muscles and the bones and therefore the Spleen and Kidneys. Dr Shen thought that excessive jogging also weakens the Heart as it leads to a permanent dilation of the heart and a slowing down of circulation (as indicated by a slow pulse).

Lack of exercise

Lack of exercise is also a cause of disease. Regular exercise is essential for a proper circulation of Qi. Lack of exercise will lead to stagnation of Qi and, in some cases, Dampness. As mentioned above, chapter 23 of the 'Simple Questions' mentions lack of exercise as a cause of disease: '*Excessive sitting injures the muscles [i.e. the Spleen]*.'[7]

Oriental types of exercise such as Yoga or *Tai Ji Quan*, aimed at developing Qi rather than just the muscles, are very beneficial and should be recommended to patients suffering from deficiency of Qi who do not have enough energy to undertake vigorous exercises.

It is important (but difficult) to make patients understand that health and fitness are two different things and they do not necessarily coincide. A person may be very 'fit', i.e. able to sustain heavy exercise for long periods of time (e.g. run a marathon), but that does not necessarily mean that that person is healthy. This is because physical exercise generally develops muscles and sinews but does not necessarily 'nourish' the Internal Organs. By contrast, exercises such as Yoga, *Tai Ji Chuan*, *Ba Gua* and *Xing Yi* are aimed at developing muscles and sinews but also at nourishing the Internal Organs, promoting health.

Box 22.4 summarizes excessive (or insufficient) exercise as a cause of disease.

EXCESSIVE SEXUAL ACTIVITY

Since ancient times in China excessive sexual activity has been considered a cause of disease because it tends to deplete the Kidney-Essence. In the West, excessive sexual activity is hardly ever thought to be detrimental to health.

Excessive sexual activity is more often a cause of disease in men than in women: this is discussed in more detail below.

The discussion of excessive sexual activity will proceed as follows:

Box 22.4 Excessive (or insufficient) physical work

- Excessive physical work includes lifting, excessive gym work, excessive jogging, ballet, excessive sport activity, etc.
- Excessive physical work injures the muscles and sinews and therefore Spleen and Liver
- Repetitive physical work in one joint also causes Qi stagnation
- Excessive lifting injures the Kidneys
- Lack of exercise is also a cause of disease, which causes Qi stagnation and Dampness of Phlegm

---

- Sexual life and the Kidney-Essence
- Definition of 'excessive' sexual activity
- Differences between men's and women's sexuality
- Sexual causes of disease in women
- Insufficient sex as a cause of disease
- Sexual desire
- Beneficial effects of sexual activity

Sexual life and the Kidney-Essence

The sexual essences of both men and women are the outwards manifestation of the Kidney-Essence. For this reason, the loss of these sexual essences leads to a temporary loss of Kidney-Essence. Under normal circumstances, however, this loss is quickly made up, and normal sexual activity does not lead to disease. It is only when it is excessive that the loss of Essence (*Jing*) caused by sex is such that the body does not have time to recuperate and restore the Essence.

The *Tian Gui* that matures at puberty from the Kidney-Essence forms sperm in men and menstrual blood and ova in women.

Definition of 'excessive' sexual activity

Of course, it is difficult to define what a 'normal' or an 'excessive' sexual activity is as this is entirely relative and dependent on the person's constitution and strength of Essence. What may constitute 'excess sex' for a person with weak Kidneys may be normal for another. One can, quite simply, define sexual activity as 'excessive' if it results in marked fatigue afterwards, and even more so if it causes certain other specific symptoms, such as dizziness, blurred vision, a lower backache, weak knees and frequent urination.

> **Clinical note**
>
> Quite simply, 'excessive' sexual activity is one that results in marked fatigue, dizziness, blurred vision, a lower backache, weak knees and frequent urination afterwards. We should advise patients about sexual activity *before* it reaches this stage

The important thing to realize is that sexual activity should be adjusted according to age, physical condition and even the seasons.

That sexual activity ought to be adjusted according to one's age is an idea that is often totally alien to many people in our society. The book 'Classic of the Simple Girl' (Sui dynasty 581–618) gives an indication of the recommended frequency of ejaculation for men according to age and health condition (Table 22.1).[8]

Of course, this should not be taken literally, but only as a broad guideline. Another broad 'rule' regarding the frequency of sexual activity (somewhat less 'generous' than the one above) is that arrived at by dividing one's age in years by 5 to work out the interval in days between orgasms. For example, at 50, one should have sex no more than once every 10 days. We can therefore build a table as shown in Table 22.2.

Sexual activity should obviously be reduced if there is a deficiency of Qi or Blood, and particularly a deficiency of the Kidneys (Fig. 22.7).

Table 22.1 Recommended frequency of ejaculation for men in the 'Classic of the Simple Girl'

Age	In good health	Average health
15	2×/day	Once/day
20	2×/day	Once/day
30	Once/day	Every other day
40	Every 3 days	Every 4 days
50	Every 5 days	Every 10 days
60	Every 10 days	Every 20 days
70	Every 30 days	None

Table 22.2 Alternative recommendation for frequency of ejaculation for men*

Age	Interval in days
15	Once every 3 days
20	Once every 4 days
25	Once every 5 days
30	Once every 6 days
35	Once every 7 days
40	Once every 8 days
45	Once every 9 days
50	Once every 10 days
60	Once every 12 days
70	Once every 14 days

*A rough general guide, arrived at by dividing the age in years by 5.

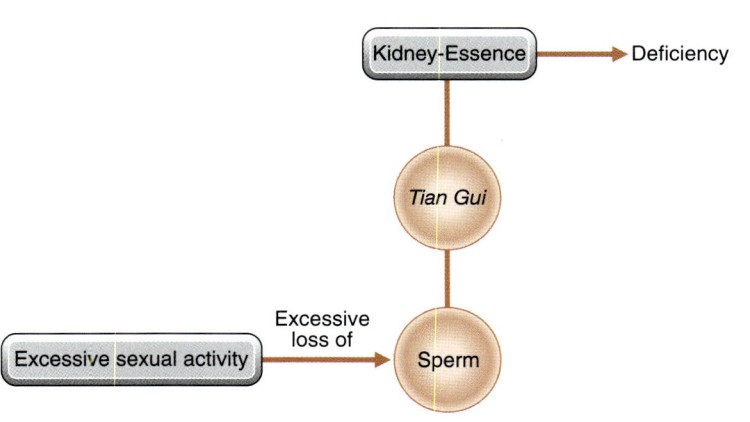

Figure 22.7 Effect of sexual activity on Kidney-Essence

Finally, sexual activity should also be adjusted according to seasons, increasing in spring and summer and declining in autumn and winter.

Although these 'rules' should be interpreted loosely, as practitioners of Chinese medicine, we should be able to advise our patients on this question.

In my practice I have seen patients who were engaging in levels of sexual activity which could not be described as 'normal' by any standard and yet were totally astounded when the idea was suggested that their sexual activity might have something to do with their problems.

In fact, many men's sexual problems, such as impotence or premature ejaculation, often require first of all a decrease in sexual activity if there is to be any chance of successful treatment.

Chinese medicine also considers the circumstances in which sexual activity takes place. For example, catching cold after sexual intercourse can weaken Kidney-Yang. As the energy of the Kidneys is temporarily and naturally weakened after intercourse, it is important not to be exposed to cold at this time in order not to aggravate such weakness.

Differences between men's and women's sexuality

Although excessive sexual activity affects both men and women, to a certain extent it affects men more.

There are also some important differences between men's and women's genital physiology from a Chinese medical perspective. In fact, sperm, called *Tian Gui*, is a direct manifestation of *Jing*. According to Chinese medicine, *Tian Gui* resides in the Room of Sperm (or Room of Jing) in men, which is in the Lower Dan Tian. In women, the Lower Dan Tian houses the Uterus. *Tian Gui* in women is menstrual blood and the ova (Fig. 22.8).

As described in chapter 3, the *Tian Gui* maturing at puberty (14 in girls and 16 in boys) is sperm in men and menstrual blood and ova in women. It follows that ejaculation is a more direct loss of Kidney-Essence than orgasm is for women as obviously there is no loss of menstrual blood or ova during orgasm in women. The equivalent to excessive loss of sperm in men, in women would be a massive loss of blood during childbirth or a chronic, heavy loss of blood from menorrhagia.[9]

Tian Gui (derived from the Kidney-Essence) is sperm in men and menstrual blood in women. As women do not lose menstrual blood during intercourse, they are not so affected by excessive sexual activity as men

In women, the Uterus is directly related to the Kidneys and any factor that weakens the Uterus eventually weakens the Kidneys, particularly Kidney-Yin.

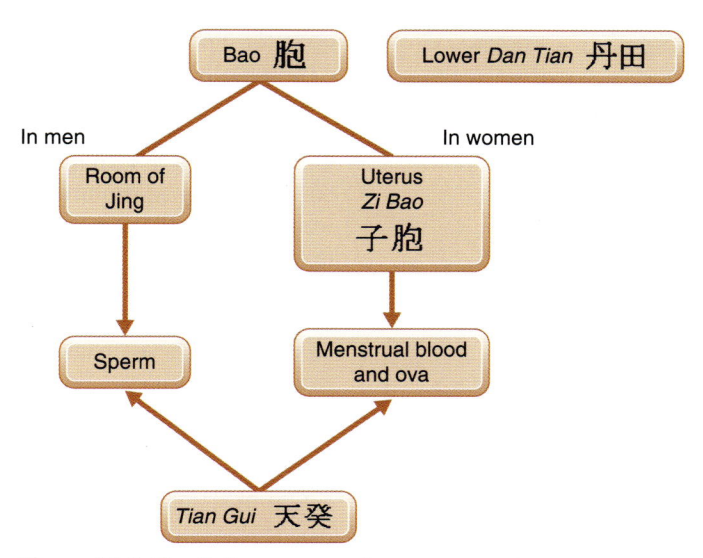

Figure 22.8 *Tian Gui* in women and men

In particular, too many childbirths in too short a time weakens the Uterus and the Kidneys in women: this is an important cause of depletion of Kidney-Essence in women, somewhat equivalent to excessive sexual activity in men. However, this is hardly a common cause of disease in modern Western countries, with their low birth rates.

Sexual causes of disease in women

There are some sexual activities, however, that are an important cause of disease in women. One is the practice of having sexual intercourse during the period. During the period, there is a downward movement of Qi and Blood; with sexual arousal, there is flaring up of the (physiological) Minister Fire, with, therefore, an upward movement of Qi. As the Qi flows downwards during the period but upwards with sexual arousal, these two opposing movements clash and cause stagnation of Qi and Blood in the Uterus (Fig. 22.9).

Fu Qing Zhu often mentions sexual intercourse during or soon after the end of the period as a cause of heavy menstrual bleeding. He says: '*Some women engage in sexual intercourse that leads to unstoppable bleeding ... If a woman has sexual intercourse during the period, sperm travels upwards along the [woman's] blood vessels ... One should know that the blood vessels are tender and should be protected from injury by sperm ... If sperm is ejaculated into the uterus when the menstrual flow is surging and gushing out, the blood will retreat and contract ... and the sperm will gather and transform Blood.*'[10] This passage clearly implies that sexual intercourse during the period causes stasis of Blood in the woman.

In another chapter, commenting on the fact that some women develop profuse menstrual bleeding after the period, Fu Qing Zhu says: '*When a woman is aroused the uterus is wide open and the Imperial and Minister Fire are stirred ... the Essence chamber is agitated and the Sea of Blood overflows and cannot be contained. The Liver, which likes storage, cannot store Blood; the Spleen, which likes containment, cannot contain Blood. Thus, menstrual flow follows sexual intercourse like an echo follows a sound.*'[11]

Another sexual cause of disease in women is beginning sexual activity too early, during puberty. During puberty, the Uterus is in a vulnerable state and it is easily affected by pathogenic factors. Sexual activity at too early an age damages the Penetrating (*Chong*) and Directing (*Ren*) Vessels and also leads not only to Blood stasis but also to Kidney deficiency.[12]

Insufficient sex as a cause of disease

Chinese medicine also considers lack of sex as a cause of disease, even though this will never be mentioned in modern China. The 'Classic of the Simple Girl' gives certain guidelines as to what the minimum recommended frequency of orgasm should be according to age, such as every 4 days for a 20-year-old, every 8 days for a 30-year-old, every 16 days for a 40-year-old, every 21 days for a 50-year-old and every 30 days for a 60-year-old.[13] Of course, these guidelines too should not be adhered to rigidly either.

Chinese medicine has always stressed the importance of excessive sexual activity as a cause of disease but not *insufficient* sexual activity. Especially in Western women, this is often a cause of disease somewhat akin to emotional stress. Sexual desire depends on the Minister Fire and a healthy sexual appetite indicates that this Fire is abundant. When sexual desire builds up, the Minister Fire blazes up and Yang increases: the orgasm is a release of such accumulated Yang energy and, under normal circumstances, it is a beneficial discharge of Yang-Qi and it promotes the free flow of Qi. When sexual desire builds up, the Minister Fire is stirred: this affects the Mind and, in terms of organs, specifically the Heart and Pericardium. The Heart is connected to the Uterus via the Uterus Vessel and the

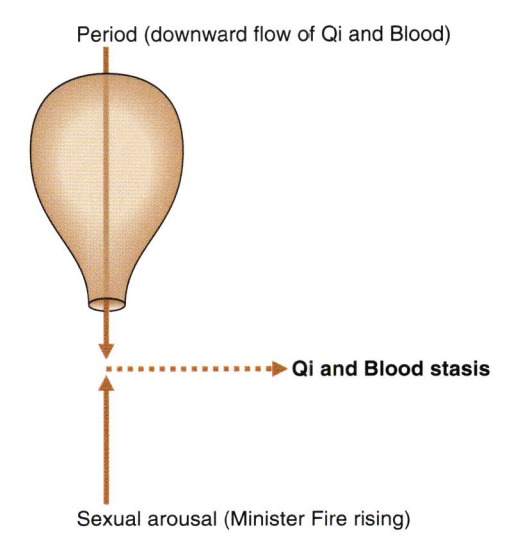

Figure 22.9 Effect of sexual activity during period

orgasmic contractions of the uterus discharge the accumulated Yang energy of the Minister Fire.

> **Clinical note**
>
> Although never mentioned in modern Chinese books, *lack* of sexual activity is also a cause of disease

When sexual desire is present but does not have an outlet in sexual activity and orgasm, the Minister Fire can accumulate and give rise both to Blood-Heat and to stagnation of Qi or Blood in the Lower Burner. This accumulated Heat will stir the Minister Fire further and harass the Mind, while the stagnation of Qi in the Lower Burner can give rise to gynaecological problems such as dysmenorrhoea.

Of course, if sexual desire is absent, then lack of sexual activity will not be a cause of disease. Conversely, if one abstains from sexual activity but the sexual desire is strong, this will also stir up the Minister Fire. Thus, the crucial factor is the mental attitude.

With regard to sexual frustration, the Qing dynasty's Chen Jia Yuan wrote very perceptively about some women's emotional longing and loneliness. Among the emotional causes of disease he distinguishes 'worry and pensiveness' from 'depression'. He basically considers depression, with its ensuing stagnation, due to emotional and sexual frustration and loneliness. He says: '*In women ... such as widows, Buddhist nuns, servant girls and concubines, sexual desire agitates [the mind] inside but cannot satisfy the Heart. The body is restricted on the outside and cannot expand with the mind [i.e. the mind longs for sexual satisfaction but the body is denied it]. This causes stagnation of Qi in the Triple Burner and the chest; after a long time there are strange symptoms such as a feeling of heat and cold as if it were malaria but it is not. This is depression.*'[14]

Although the above thoughts derive from Dr Chen's clinical experience with servant girls, Buddhist nuns and concubines and should therefore be seen in the social context of the Qing dynasty, they also have relevance to our times as he is essentially talking about sexual frustration and loneliness and his reference to widows confirms this (in old China widows were shunned and seldom remarried). He perceptively refers to sexual craving agitating the body but not finding a satisfaction in the Heart and Mind; besides sexual frustration, he is also referring to emotional frustration and craving for love. As sexual frustration in women is fairly common in our society (often deriving from men's sexual inadequacy or inexperience), Dr Chen's observations on the influence of sexual frustration on stagnation of Qi and depression (which apply to men too) acquire particular relevance.

It should be stressed that what has been said so far only concerns the relation between excessive sexual activity (with ejaculation and/or orgasm) and the Kidney energy, and that many other factors are involved in determining a happy sexual life. Although Chinese medicine is mostly concerned with excessive sexual activity as a cause of disease, an unhappy sexual life with inability to reach an orgasm, or lacking in warmth and affection, is also an important and frequent cause of disease. This often causes deep unhappiness or anxiety, which become causes of disease in themselves.

Sexual desire

Sexual desire itself is also related to the Kidney energy. A healthy sexual desire reflects a good and strong Kidney energy. If the Kidneys are weak and if, in particular, Kidney-Yang is deficient, there may be a lack of sexual desire or inability to enjoy sex and reach an orgasm. On the other hand, if Kidney-Yin is severely deficient, leading to the rising of Empty-Heat, there may be an excessive sexual desire with inability to be ever satisfied. Full-Heat of the Liver and/or Heart may also cause excessive sexual desire. The person may also have vivid sexual dreams resulting in nocturnal emissions in men and orgasms in women. For this reason, lack of sexual desire can be stimulated by strengthening Kidney-Yang and the Fire of the Gate of Life (*Ming Men*), and excessive sexual desire can be dampened by nourishing Kidney-Yin.

> **Clinical note**
>
> - Sexual desire (and performance) can be stimulated by the use of BL-23 Shenshu and Du-4 Mingmen to tonify the Fire of the Gate of Life
> - Sexual desire can be dampened by using KI-3 Taixi, KI-6 Zhaohai and SP-6 Sanyinjiao to nourish Kidney-Yin

Beneficial effects of sexual activity

Finally, although Chinese medicine traditionally stresses the importance of excessive sexual activity as a cause of disease, the broader Daoist tradition also considers the beneficial effects of sexual activity. Briefly, these emanate from the meeting of Water (women) and Fire (men), i.e. the quintessential Yin and Yang. Water and Fire are opposites but complementary and the exchange of energy occurring during the sexual act can be such that women absorb Yang energy and men Yin energy. Specifically, through kissing and genital contact during sex, there is a beneficial exchange of energy and fluids between the Governing and Directing Vessels (*Du* and *Ren Mai*) of the two partners. This also leads to the spanning of the 'bridge' in the Governing–Directing Vessel circuit in the mouth of both partners, with a beneficial mobilization of energy in these two vessels (Fig. 22.10).

Box 22.5 summarizes excessive sexual activity as a cause of disease.

Box 22.5 Excessive sexual activity

- Excessive sexual activity depletes the Kidney-Essence
- Sexual activity should be regulated according to age, health and seasons
- Men are far more affected by excessive sexual activity than women
- In women, having sexual intercourse during the period may cause Blood stasis
- In women, too early a start to sexual activity may damage the Penetrating and Directing Vessels
- Insufficient sexual activity is also a cause of disease
- Sexual desire depends on Kidney-Yang and the Fire of the Gate of Life
- According to Daoist practices, sexual activity has beneficial effects

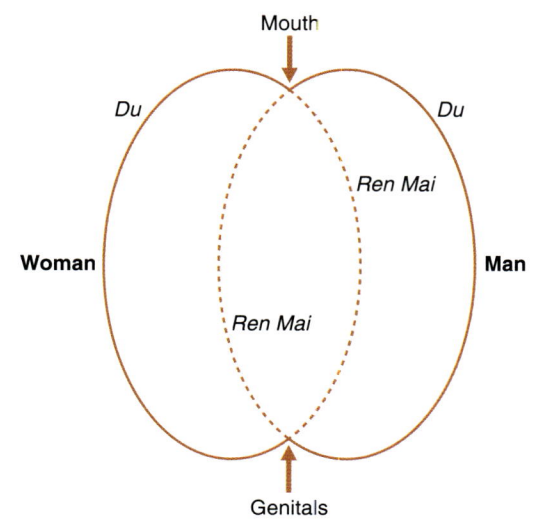

Figure 22.10 Effect of sexual intercourse on Directing and Governing Vessels

DIET

Diet is an important cause of disease, especially nowadays, and, probably more than for any other cause of disease, there are very important differences between the dietary causes of disease in ancient China and those in modern, Western countries.

Diet will be discussed under the following headings:

- Modern changes in food
- Insufficient eating
- Overeating
- Types of food and their energetic effect
  - Cold foods
  - Sweet foods and sugar
  - Hot foods
  - Greasy foods
- Conditions of eating

Modern changes in food

A great many discoveries have been made in recent years to completely revolutionize our ideas on diet. For example, the role of vitamins and minerals in health and disease have been discovered only relatively recently. On the other hand, food has never been subjected to so much chemical manipulation as in the past 30 years or so. Our food contains an incredible variety of chemicals, in the form of preservatives, flavourings, colourings, emulsifiers, nitrates, etc. Even worse, some drugs, such as hormones and antibiotics, are present in certain foods. To complete the picture, agricultural growing methods have also undergone a complete revolution with the abandonment of traditional ways of preserving the soil's fertility and controlling pests in favour of chemical pesticides and fertilizers. Residual amounts of pesticides and herbicides are inevitably present in food and water.

Because these changes in the production of food have been introduced relatively recently, Chinese ideas on diet do not take them into account. To give a very simple example, Chinese diet considers chicken meat to be beneficial to Blood. However, this does not take into account that battery chickens contain hormones and are raised in unhealthy conditions, so that the nutritional value of their meat is certainly not the same as it would have been in China 1000 years ago or even in our countries not so long ago.

All these modern changes in the production of food and modern research on food are important and need to be taken into account when considering diet as a cause of disease. However, a discussion of these aspects of foods would be entirely beyond the scope of this book, and I will therefore limit myself to a discussion of diet as a cause of disease from the traditional Chinese point of view.

Dietary habits can become a cause of disease if diet is unbalanced from either a quantitative or a qualitative point of view.

Insufficient eating

First of all, malnutrition is an obvious cause of disease. In its broad sense, malnutrition exists not only in poor Third World countries but also in rich industrialized countries where it is present in certain less obvious forms. For example, poor elderly people living alone often have a diet quite lacking in nutritive and caloric value. Other people may suffer from a mild form of malnutrition by adhering rigidly to very strict 'diets', the number and variety of which is becoming mind-boggling. Some of those who adhere to such strict diets may unwittingly lack essential nutrients in their diet. Another example of malnutrition in our society is in those who suffer from anorexia and/or bulimia, and yet another in those who regularly starve themselves in order to slim.[15]

Vegetarianism may also become a cause of disease, especially for women. Of course, a vegetarian diet by itself is not a cause of disease. However, being a vegetarian does necessitate being more aware of food combining to ensure an adequate intake of protein. From a Chinese perspective, this is important to ensure adequate production of Blood as meat is a potent Blood tonic. Moreover, from a Chinese perspective the effect of food on our body transcends the mere analysis of food in terms of protein, vitamins, minerals, etc. Chinese medicine holds that animal food has a certain 'quality' that makes it different from vegetable food and particularly nourishing to Blood. Li Shi Zhen said that animal products have 'qing' (i.e. 'feeling') and, for this reason, they nourish Blood. Therefore, a lack of animal food may induce a Blood deficiency, especially in women. This is all the more likely to occur if the woman has no clear understanding of food combining, as is often the case in young girls who become vegetarian. In fact, they tend to eat a lot of salads and cheese, both of which are cold in energy and, in addition, cheese also tends to lead to the formation of Dampness or Phlegm.

Insufficient eating causes deficiency of Qi and Blood and weakens the Spleen function of transformation and transportation, setting up a vicious circle because the lack of proper food weakens the Spleen while a weak Spleen fails to absorb the nutrients from what food is taken.

Of course, it should be stressed that a vegetarian diet with proper attention to food combining and a balance of hot and cold foods can be extremely healthy.

Overeating

Overeating is an even more common cause of disease in our society. Increasing affluence after the strictures of the Second World War has produced a great abundance and variety of food in rich industrialized countries and a dramatic increase in the average weight of the population. From the point of view of Chinese medicine, overeating also weakens the Spleen and Stomach, leading to accumulation of Dampness and Phlegm. Excessive consumption of sugar is also an important cause of Phlegm in Western countries.

Types of food and their energetic effect

All foods (and herbs) are classified according to their 'energy' into cold and hot foods. Foods are classified as 'cold' from two points of view: firstly, they have a 'cold' energy (e.g. lettuce); secondly, they are actually cold in temperature (e.g. iced water).

Cold foods

Excessive consumption of what Chinese medicine considers to be cold-energy foods and raw foods (such as salads, ice-creams, iced drinks or fruit) may weaken the Spleen, in particular Spleen-Yang. The idea that an excessive consumption of salads and fruit can be detrimental to health runs counter to all modern ideas about diet, according to which, by eating raw vegetables and fruit, we can absorb all the vitamins and minerals contained in them. This is true to a certain extent and a moderate consumption of these foods can be beneficial. However, from the Chinese point of view, the Spleen likes dryness and warmth in food and dislikes excess of fluids and cold: an excessive consumption of the above foods will be very difficult to digest and may weaken Spleen-Yang, causing diarrhoea, chilliness, cold mucus, abdominal pain and distension. Thus, particularly, those who have a tendency to Spleen deficiency should not consume raw and cold foods in excess.

Sweet foods and sugar

Excessive consumption of sweet foods and sugar, also extremely common in our society, blocks the Spleen function of transformation and transportation and gives rise to Dampness, with such symptoms as upper respiratory catarrh, abdominal distension and fullness, mucus in the stools and vaginal discharges.

Hot foods

Excessive consumption of hot-energy and spicy foods (such as curry, alcohol, lamb, beef or spices) gives rise to Heat symptoms, especially of the Stomach or Liver, such as a bitter taste, a burning sensation in the epigastrium and thirst.

Greasy foods

Excessive consumption of greasy and fried foods (such as any deep-fried foods, milk, cheese, butter, cream, ice-cream, banana, peanuts or fatty meats) gives rise to the formation of Phlegm or Dampness, which in turn obstructs the Spleen function of transformation and transportation. This may cause various Phlegm symptoms, such as sinusitis, a nasal discharge, a 'muzzy' feeling of the head, dull headaches, bronchitis and so on.

Conditions of eating

Chinese medicine considers not only what one eats but also how one eats it. One can eat the best-quality, perfectly balanced food available, but if it is eaten in the wrong circumstances it will also lead to disease. For example, eating in a hurry, discussing work while eating, going straight back to work after eating, eating late in the evening and eating in a state of emotional tension are all habits that interfere with a proper digestion of food and, in particular, lead to deficiency of Stomach-Yin. This manifests with a tongue with rootless coating, or no coating in the centre, thirst, epigastric pain and dry stools.

Box 22.6 summarizes diet as a cause of disease.

Box 22.6 Diet

- Modern food in industrialized countries is very different than it was in ancient China
- Insufficient eating leads to Qi and Blood deficiency
- Overeating weakens the Spleen and leads to Dampness and Phlegm
- Over-consumption of cold foods weakens Spleen-Yang
- Over-consumption of sweets and sugar leads to Dampness and Phlegm
- Over-consumption of hot foods leads to Heat
- Over-consumption of greasy foods leads to Dampness and Phlegm
- Irregular eating weakens Stomach-Yin

TRAUMA

This refers to physical traumas, as mental shock is included among the emotional causes of disease.

Physical traumas cause local stagnation of Qi or Blood in the area. A slight trauma causes stagnation of Qi and a severe one causes stasis of Blood. In either case, it gives rise to pain, bruising and swelling. Although trauma may seem only a transient cause of disease, in practice the effect of trauma can linger for a long time, manifesting with local stagnation of Qi and/or Blood in the area affected.

Old accidents and falls that the person may have completely forgotten can often be the cause of disease, or a contributory cause. This is especially true of headaches: as a rule of thumb, headaches that always occur in the same part of the head are often caused by a previous injury to that part of the head. This means that local treatment aimed at removing stasis of Blood in that area is particularly applicable.

Old traumas can also become a concurrent cause of disease when they overlap with a later trauma. For example, a trauma to a knee may seem to have cleared up completely, but when the person later in life contracts Painful Obstruction Syndrome caused by exposure to cold and damp conditions, the exterior pathogenic factor often will settle in that knee.

Box 22.7 summarizes trauma as a cause of disease.

Box 22.7 Trauma

- Light trauma causes Qi stagnation
- Severe trauma causes Blood stasis
- Trauma is often a concurrent cause of disease, overlapping with other causes

---

PARASITES AND POISONS

Very little needs to be said about these as they are self-evident as causes of disease.

Infestation of intestinal worms is more common in children and although worms are an external cause of disease, Chinese medicine regards poor diet as a contributory factor. An excessive consumption of greasy and sweet foods leads to Dampness, which makes for a favourable breeding ground for worms.

The symptoms of worms depend on the type of worm, but in general they are: white vesicles on the face, sallow complexion, emaciation, small white spots inside the lips, purple spots inside the eyelids, loss of appetite or desire to eat strange objects (such as wax, leaves, raw rice), abdominal pain, and itchy nose and anus.

WRONG TREATMENT

By 'wrong treatment' in Chinese books was obviously meant wrong herbal treatment.

As for Chinese medicine, wrong treatment can obviously be a cause of disease. Examples of 'wrong' treatments with herbal medicine are tonifying Yang when nourishing Yin is called for, or vice versa.

As for acupuncture, one of its great advantages as a form of treatment is that, in the right hands, it is a very safe therapy. Even if a wrong treatment is applied, in most cases, the energy rebalances itself out in a few days. This is not to say, however, that ill effects cannot arise from a wrong treatment. One of the situations in which acupuncture can be used wrongly is when one fails to distinguish an exterior from an interior condition. For example, if one gives a tonifying treatment during an acute exterior condition, this may actually push the exterior pathogenic factor inwards and lead to an aggravation. This is all the more likely to happen if moxa is used.

Acupuncture has less potential to cause side-effects and adverse reactions than herbal medicine

As far as Chinese herbal treatment is concerned, the possibility of ill effects arising from a wrong treatment is greater. This is because Chinese herbs have a more definite and somewhat less 'neutral' effect than acupuncture. For example, when tonifying the Kidneys with herbal treatment, it is essential to distinguish between Kidney-Yin and Kidney-Yang deficiency, as the herbs used in each case would be entirely different and the incorrect use of hot herbs for Kidney-Yin deficiency or cold herbs for Kidney-Yang deficiency would lead to a definite aggravation. In contrast, with acupuncture, one can use such a point as KI-3 Taixi in both Kidney-Yin or Kidney-Yang deficiency without any ill effects.

MEDICINAL DRUGS

A complete discussion of iatrogenic diseases caused by the side-effects of medicinal (Western) drugs is well beyond the scope of this book. Obviously, medicinal drugs are an important and frequent cause of disease as most of them lead to some side-effects and often to adverse reactions.

As practitioners of Chinese medicine, we should be aware of the side-effects and adverse reactions of medicines in order to diagnose the condition properly as we should be able to separate the symptoms that are caused by the drugs from those that are not.

Some drugs influence the pulse more and some the tongue. For example, beta-blockers affect the pulse deeply by making it slow and rather deep: in such a case, the pulse cannot be used for diagnosis at all. Tranquillizers also affect the pulse, making it somewhat 'sluggish' and 'reluctant', qualities that cannot be described in terms of the traditional 29 pulse qualities.

On the other hand, antibiotics clearly affect the tongue, making it peeled in patches: that is, with patches without coating (Figs 22.11 and 22.12). Whenever I see such a tongue (which indicates Stomach-Yin deficiency), I always ask the patient whether he or she is on antibiotics or has been on antibiotics up to 3 weeks before the consultation.

Oral steroids also change the tongue, tending to make it swollen and red.

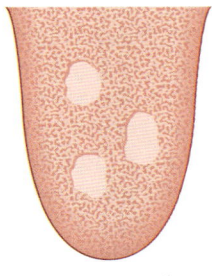

Figure 22.11 Tongue appearance after antibiotics

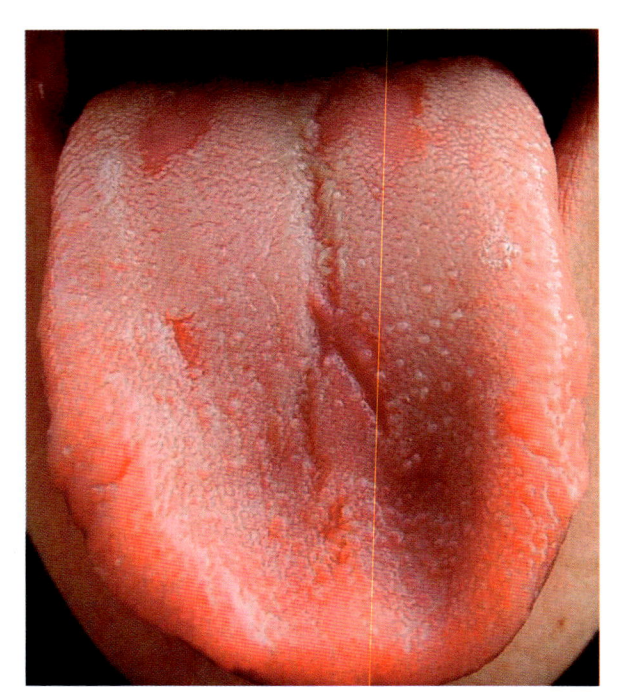

Figure 22.12 Tongue partially without coating (possibly from antibiotics)

DRUGS

By 'drugs' here I mean the so-called recreational drugs such as cannabis, cocaine, LSD and ecstasy.

Cannabis may cause anxiety, reduced motivation and occasionally psychosis.[16] Cannabis also impairs the conversion of short-term to long-term memory and concentration.[17] It also produces impairment of memory and judgement.[18] From a Chinese perspective, my opinion is that long-term use of cannabis seems to induce a Kidney deficiency and a weakness of *Zhi*, the Will-power of the Kidneys. It also affects Heart-Blood and the Spleen's Intellect (*Yi*), as evidenced by the poor memory and concentration.

Cocaine may lead to psychosis when taken consistently for some years.[19] In chronic abusers, psychological deterioration may eventually occur, resulting in loss of mental function, compulsive disorders, suicidal ideation, psychopathic disorders, and ultimately a psychosis resembling paranoid schizophrenia.[20] From the Chinese perspective, I think that long-term use of cocaine leads to the formation of Phlegm-Fire in the Heart.

LSD may cause the flashback phenomenon (recurrence of a previous effect of the drug) and rarely, psychosis.[21] From the Chinese perspective, my opinion is that LSD affects the Heart, possibly causing Heart-Fire.

Ecstasy may cause brain damage and immunosuppression after long-term use.[22] From the Chinese perspective, in my opinion Ecstasy weakens the Kidneys and obstructs the Heart's orifices.

Learning outcomes

In this chapter you will have learned:
- The influence of the constitution on predisposition to health or disease
- The causes of a weak constitution
- Lifestyles and practices that either further weaken or strengthen the constitution
- The diagnostic signs of a strong or weak constitution
- The role of overwork as a common cause of disease in modern Western society
- How excessive physical work and exercise can cause disease
- The importance of a balanced sex life in maintaining health
- The significance of poor diet and eating habits as a cause of disease
- The role of physical trauma, parasites and poisons in causing disease
- How wrong treatment with acupuncture or herbal medicine can cause disease
- The importance of being aware of the harmful effects of drugs, whether medicinal or recreational

Self-assessment questions

1. What are the causes of a poor constitution?
2. What signs of the ears indicate a poor constitution?
3. What effect will overwork over a period of years have on the body?
4. How does lack of exercise affect the Qi and cause disease?
5. Which patterns might present in patients experiencing either excessive sexual desire or else a lack of desire for sex?
6. Why do people following slimming diets based on eating a lot of salads and fruit frequently gain weight?
7. What effect do beta-blockers tend to have on the pulse?
8. What are the common effects of long-term cannabis use from the Chinese perspective?

See p. 1261 for answers

END NOTES

1. 1981 Spiritual Axis (*Ling Shu Jing* 灵枢经), People's Health Publishing House, Beijing, first published *c.*100 BC, p. 78.
2. Ibid., p. 102.
3. Wu Qian 1977 Golden Mirror of Medicine (*Yi Zong Jin Jian* 医宗金鉴), People's Health Publishing House, Beijing, first published 1742, vol. 2, p. 871.
4. Spiritual Axis, p. 78.

5. I compare Qi and Yang to a current bank account and Blood and Yin to a deposit account. We should meet our regular expenses with the income derived from our work, which goes into a current account. Any savings go into a deposit account, from which we derive interest. If we are able to meet all our expenses with the funds in the current account (Qi and Yang), our finances are in order. If, on the other hand, we find that our income is not enough to meet our expenses because we are spending too much (i.e. overwork), we then have to meet regular expenses with the funds in the deposit account (Yin). In the long run, this spells disaster as we will reach our old age without any savings (Yin).
6. 1979 The Yellow Emperor's Classic of Internal Medicine – Simple Questions (*Huang Di Nei Jing Su Wen* 黄 帝 内 经 素 问), People's Health Publishing House, Beijing, first published *c*.100 BC, p. 154.
7. Ibid., p. 154.
8. 1978 Classic of the Simple Girl (*Su Nu Jing* 素 女 经), French translation by Leung Kwok Po, Seghers, Paris, p. 106. This book is a translation of a Chinese text of the same title published in 1908 (first published in 1903). This text itself is a compilation from older texts on sexuality, the oldest dating back to the Tang dynasty.
9. Although some practitioners consider the lubricating fluids secreted by the Bartholin's glands during sexual arousal in women to be also a manifestation of Essence comparable to sperm, I tend to disagree because such fluids are secreted by glands in the vagina and not by sex glands (such as the ovaries in women or testicles/prostate in men): I would therefore consider these fluids precisely as a form of Body Fluids (*jin ye*) rather than a direct manifestation of Essence. In fact, the Bartholin's glands in the vagina are homologous to the Cowper's glands in men and their function is purely lubricative.
10. Fu Qing Zhu 1973 Fu Qing Zhu's Gynaecology (*Fu Qing Zhu Nu Ke* 傅 青 主 女 科), Shanghai People's Publishing House, Shanghai, p. 10. First published in 1827. Fu Qing Zhu was born in 1607 and died in 1684.
11. Ibid., p. 13.
12. Interestingly, this coincides with the Western medical view according to which excessive sexual activity at an early age predisposes girls to cervical cancer. In fact, during the teenage years, with the onset of ovulation and the change in vaginal pH, active squamous metaplasia is taking place in the cervix; during this time of cellular immaturity and vulnerability, a carcinogen is most likely to have an influence on the squamous epithelium and this predisposes the girl to cervical cancer later in life. This is in perfect agreement with the Chinese view of puberty as a very vulnerable and delicate stage in a woman's life.
13. Classic of the Simple Girl, p. 107.
14. Chen Jia Yuan 1988 Eight Secret Books on Gynaecology (*Fu Ke Mi Shu Ba Zhong* 妇 科 秘 书 八 种), Ancient Chinese Medicine Texts Publishing House, Beijing. Chen's book, written during the Qing dynasty (1644–1911) was entitled Secret Gynaecological Prescriptions (*Fu Ke Mi Fang* 妇 科 秘 方) and published in 1729, p. 152.
15. In passing, it is worth mentioning that some people who starve themselves to lose weight actually experience an increase in weight, whilst when they resume a balanced diet excess fat drops away. This apparent paradox is explained by the fact that starving weakens the Spleen, which fails to transform and transport food and fluids properly and this leads to weight gain. If proper food is eaten, the Spleen is strengthened, it transforms and transports food and fluids properly and this leads to loss of weight.
16. Grahame-Smith D G and Aronson J K 1995 Oxford Textbook of Clinical Pharmacology and Drug Therapy, Oxford University Press, Oxford, p. 480.
17. Laurence DR 1973 Clinical Pharmacology, Churchill Livingstone, Edinburgh, p. 14.29.
18. Reynolds JEF (Chief Editor) 1996 Martindale – The Extra Pharmacopoeia, Royal Pharmaceutical Society, London, p. 1685.
19. Clinical Pharmacology, p. 11.27.
20. Martindale – The Extra Pharmacopoeia, p. 1329.
21. Oxford Textbook of Clinical Pharmacology and Drug Therapy, p. 483.
22. Ibid., p. 481.

PART 4

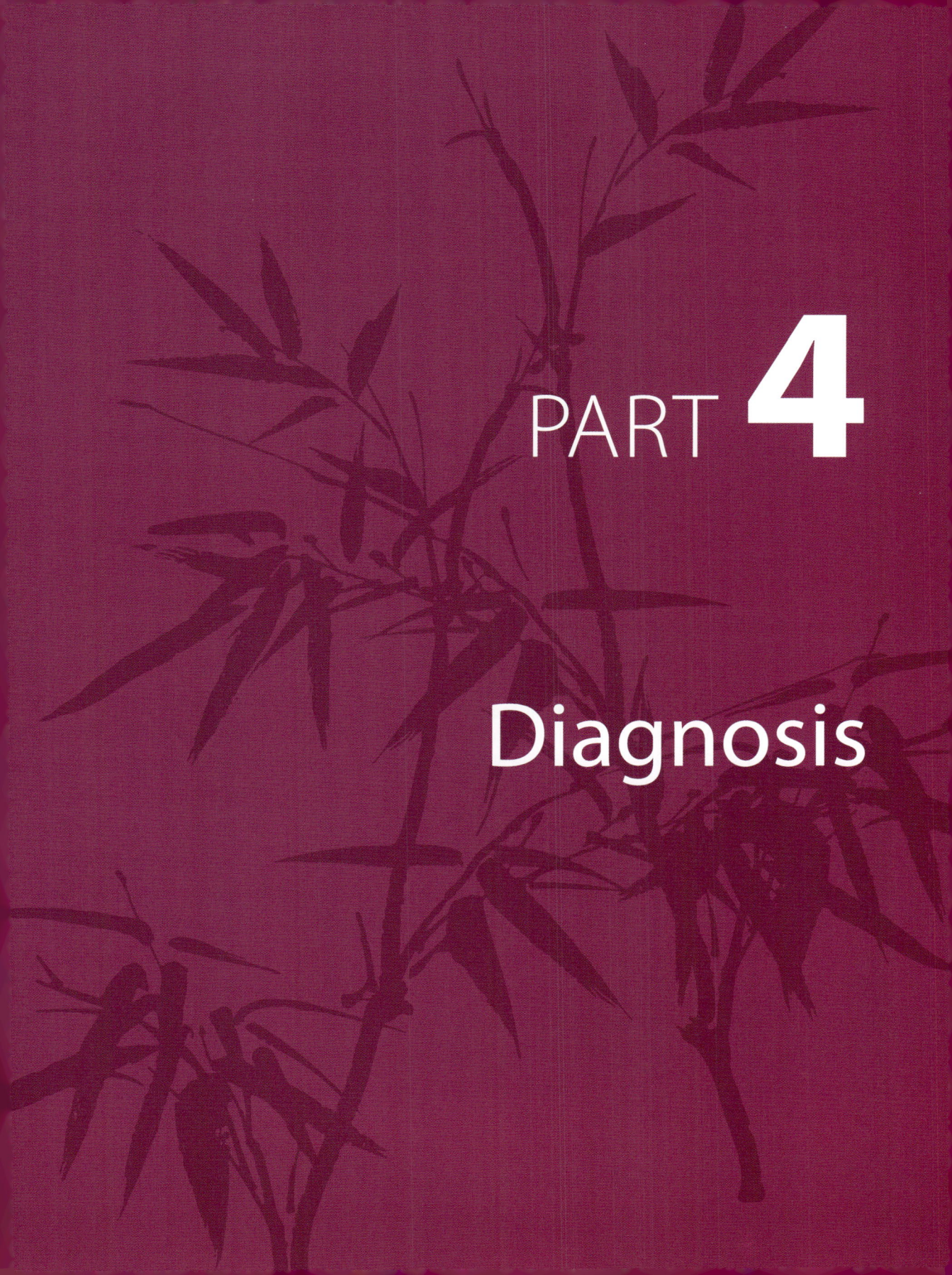

Diagnosis

INTRODUCTION

Chinese diagnostic methods have evolved continuously over more than 2000 years and reached a remarkable level of sophistication. Pulse diagnosis alone is a good example of the level of sophistication and subtlety of Chinese diagnostic methods.

One of the fundamental tenets of Chinese diagnosis is that the 'outer reflects the inner': that is, that the outer appearance of the patient, the pulse and his or her symptoms reflect the internal disharmony. Western medical diagnosis is very much based on 'looking inside' with X-rays, scans, blood tests, endoscopies, laparoscopies, etc. Chinese medical diagnosis is based on 'looking at the outer': that is, observing the complexion, the tongue, palpating the pulse and asking questions.[1]

Another fundamental principle of Chinese diagnosis is the correspondence between a part and the whole. Pulse and tongue diagnosis are a good example of this. The pulse is felt at the radial artery in three separate small sections and each section corresponds to a part of the body and its respective Internal Organs. The same goes for the tongue and many other aspects of Chinese diagnosis. Chinese diagnosis is based on an uncanny correspondence and 'resonance' between a part of the body and the whole body and also a resonance between the microcosm and macrocosm: the Five Elements are a good example of the latter.

Chinese diagnosis has traditionally four major parts: diagnosis by observation ('to look'), by interrogation ('to ask'), by palpation ('to touch') and by auscultation ('to hear and to smell').

The separation between observation and interrogation is made purely for didactic purposes and does not correspond to clinical reality where what is seen on observation and what is elicited on interrogation occurs simultaneously and may be integrated automatically. For example, the separation between dry skin (a sign in observation) and itchy skin (a symptom in interrogation) is artificial and unrealistic. Another good example is that of oedema of the ankles: the observation of this sign is immediately integrated with palpation of the area and interrogation of the patient about it.

The discussion of diagnosis will be conducted in the following chapters:

Chapter 23: Diagnosis by observation
  Spirit
  Body
  Demeanour and body movement
  Head and face
  Eyes
  Nose
  Ears
  Mouth and lips
  Teeth and gums
  Throat
  Limbs
  Skin
  Tongue
  Channels

Chapter 24: Diagnosis by interrogation
  Pain
  Food and taste
  Stools and urine
  Thirst and drink
  Energy levels
  Head, face and body
  Chest and abdomen
  Limbs
  Sleep
  Sweating
  Ears and eyes
  Feeling of cold, feeling of heat and fever
  Emotional symptoms
  Sexual symptoms
  Women's symptoms
  Children's symptoms

Chapter 25: Diagnosis by palpation
  Pulse
  Skin
  Limbs
  Chest
  Abdomen
  Points

Chapter 26: Diagnosis by hearing and smelling
  Hearing
    Voice
    Breathing
    Cough
    Vomiting
    Hiccup
    Borborygmi
    Sighing
    Belching
  Smelling
    Body odour

Odour of bodily secretions
    Breath
    Sweat
    Sputum
    Urine and stools
    Vaginal discharge and lochia
    Intestinal gas

END NOTES

1. In his typical pragmatic and effective way, Dr JHF Shen used to say that when one drives through a neighbourhood one can get a rather accurate idea of the socio-economic status of its inhabitants without the need to look inside the houses. He compared this to the way Chinese diagnosis works, i.e. it looks at the outer to get an idea of the inner. In contrast, Western medicine needs to look 'inside the houses' to form an appraisal of their inhabitants.

PART 4

Diagnosis by Observation 23

Key contents

Correspondence between an individual part and the whole

Observation of constitutional traits
Spirit
Body
Demeanour and body movement
Head and face
Eyes
Nose
Ears
Mouth and lips
Teeth and gums
Throat
Limbs
Skin
Tongue
Channels

INTRODUCTION

Before describing and discussing the various aspects of observation and their clinical significance, we should first highlight two important principles of diagnosis by observation: i.e. the principle of correspondence between individual parts of the body and the whole, and the importance of observing and assessing constitutional traits. The latter is important because there are various body types that do not reflect a patient's actual, present disharmonies but rather his or her constitutional traits.

This introduction will be set out under the following headings:

- Correspondence between an individual part and the whole
  - The face as a microsystem
  - The ear as a microsystem
  - The tongue as a microsystem
  - Microsystems over the whole body
- Observation of constitutional traits

After this introduction, the items of observation discussed are:

- Spirit
- Body
  - Five-Element body types
  - Five-Element correspondences
  - Body signs
- Demeanour and body movement
- Head and face
  - Hair
  - Face colour
    - Lustre and moisture of complexion
    - The four attributes of normal complexion
    - Pathological colours
      White
      Yellow
      Red
      Green
      Blue
      Black
    - Deep/floating, distinct/obscure, thin/thick, scattered/concentrated and moist/dry colour
  - Face areas
- Eyes
- Nose
- Ears
- Mouth and lips
- Teeth and gums
- Throat
  - Pharynx
  - Tonsils
- Limbs
  - Swelling of the joints of the four limbs
  - Oedema of the four limbs
  - Flaccidity of the four limbs

- Rigidity of the four limbs
- Paralysis of the four limbs
- Contraction of the four limbs
- Tremor or spasticity of the four limbs
- Nails
- Thenar eminence
- Index finger in babies
• Skin
• Tongue
  • Tongue-body colour
    - Pale
    - Red
    - Deep-Red
    - Purple
    - Blue
  • Tongue-body shape
    - Thin
    - Swollen
    - Stiff
    - Flaccid
    - Long
    - Short
    - Cracked
    - Quivering
    - Deviated
    - Toothmarked
  • Tongue coating
  • Moisture
• Channels

Correspondence between an individual part and the whole

One of the principles on which diagnosis by observation in Chinese medicine is based is that each single, small part of the body reflects the whole. Important examples of the application of this principle to diagnosis are diagnosis from the face, the tongue, the pulse and the ear.

The face as a microsystem

The face is a very important example of the principle or correspondence between a part of the body and the whole body, as it is a reflection both of the Internal Organs and of various parts of the body. Chapter 32 of the Simple Questions lists the correspondence of various parts of the face with Internal Organs, as follows: 'In Heat disease of the Liver, the left cheek becomes red; in Heat disease of the Heart, the forehead becomes red; in Heat disease of the Spleen, the nose becomes red; in Heat disease of the Lungs, the right cheek becomes red; in Heat disease of the Kidneys, the chin becomes red'[1] (Fig. 23.1).

Chapter 49 of the Spiritual Axis gives a more detailed map of the correspondence between Internal Organs and parts of the body and various areas of the face[2] (Fig. 23.2).

The ear as a microsystem

Ear acupuncture is a well-known application of the principle that a single, small part of the body reflects the whole: according to this theory, the ear resembles an upside-down fetus and there is a point in the ear pavilion that reflects a part or an organ of the body (Fig. 23.3).

The tongue as a microsystem

The tongue is a simple microsystem of the Internal Organs, with the Heart at the top (tip of the tongue), the Stomach and Spleen in the middle (centre of the tongue) and the Kidneys at the bottom (root of the tongue) (see Fig. 23.18 below).

Microsystems over the whole body

According to recent theories, each part of the body is a miniature replica of the whole and can therefore reflect pathological changes of the whole body.[3] This

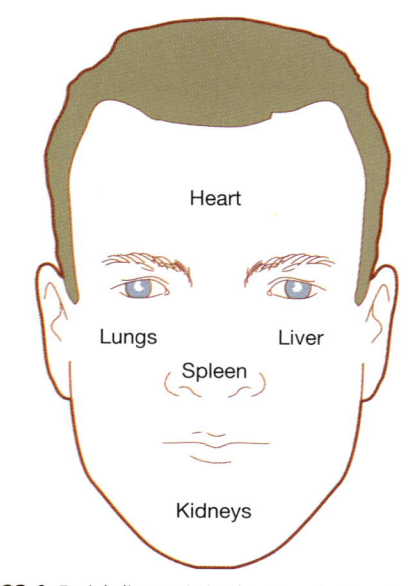

Figure 23.1 Facial diagnosis in the 'Simple Questions'

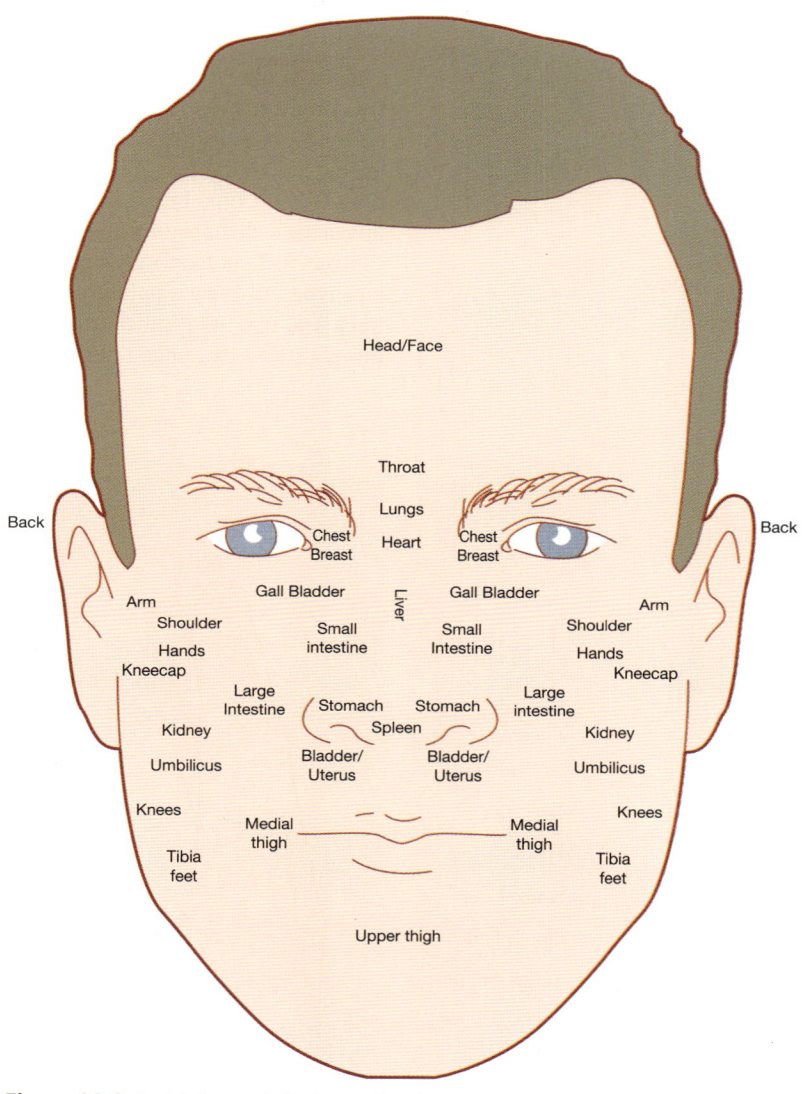

Figure 23.2 Facial diagnosis in the 'Spiritual Axis'

theory was first proposed by Zhang Ying Qing in 1973. In diagnosing and needling the side of the second metacarpal bone, he discovered that the points on this bone formed a pattern and constituted a miniature image of the whole body (Fig. 23.4).

Box 23.1 summarizes the correspondence between an individual part and the whole body.

After repeated research, Zhang Ying Qing discovered other microsystems all over the body (Fig. 23.5).

Box 23.1 Correspondence between a part and the whole

- Face
- Ear
- Tongue
- Body bones

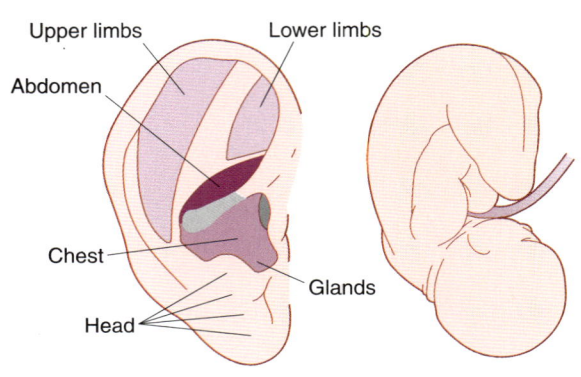

Figure 23.3 Correspondence between parts of the ear and the body

Observation of constitutional traits

The art of observation in Chinese medicine is based on two broad areas: observation of constitutional traits and observation of actual disharmony signs. For example, a tall, thin, sinewy body indicates a constitutional Wood type but it does not necessarily indicate any actual disharmony in the Liver or Gall Bladder. Conversely, a person may belong constitutionally to a Fire type but have a pale-greenish complexion, brittle nails and dry hair, indicating an actual Wood disharmony (in this example, Liver-Blood deficiency).

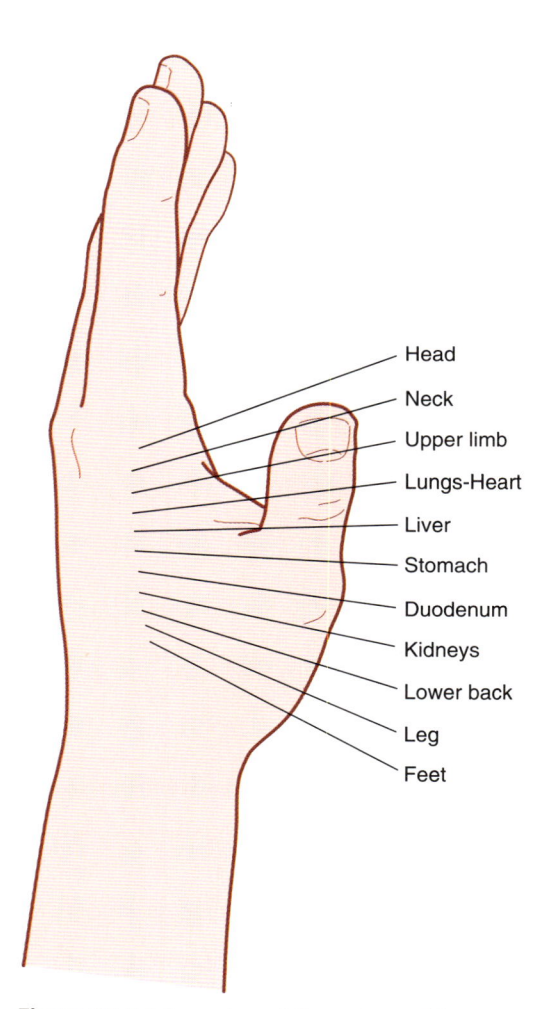

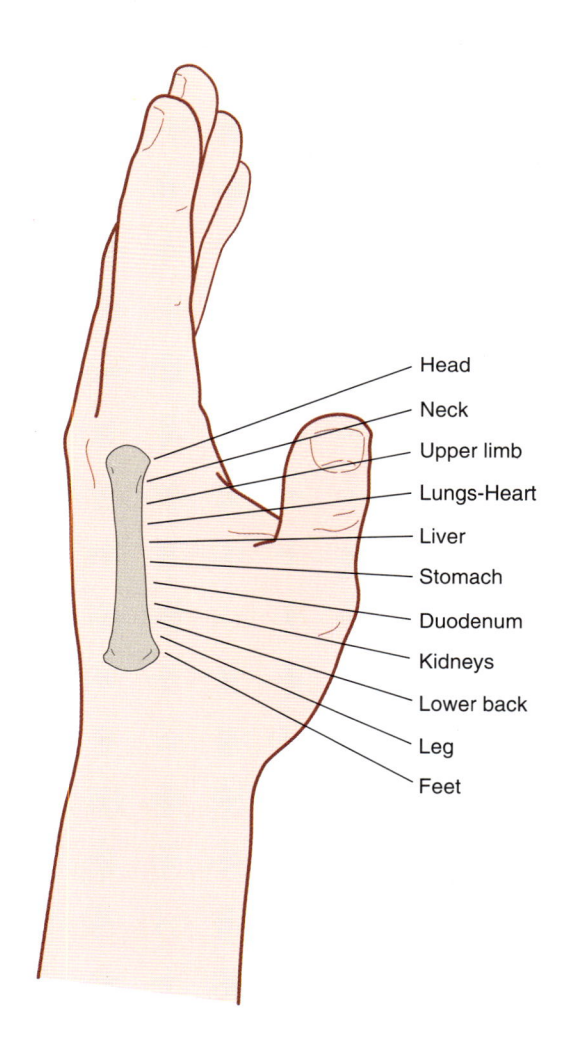

Figure 23.4 Microsystem of the metacarpal bone

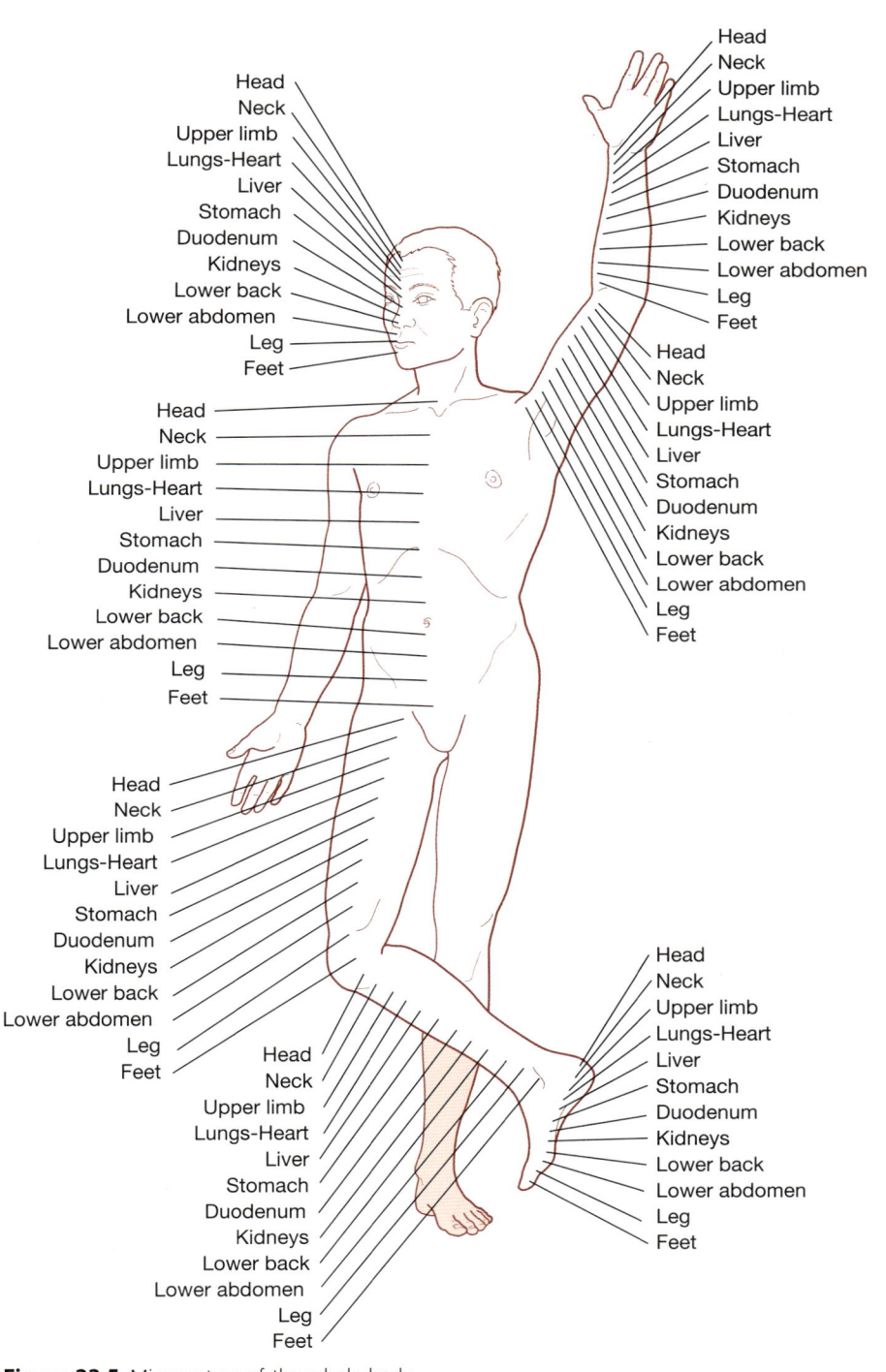

Figure 23.5 Microsystem of the whole body

Why is it necessary to observe constitutional traits if we need to treat the presenting disharmony? In the above example of a patient with a pale-greenish complexion, brittle nails and dry hair, we obviously need to nourish Liver-Blood, whatever the observation of constitutional characteristics might indicate.

However, observation of constitutional traits is important for various reasons, described below:

1. A constitutional type indicates the *tendency* to certain disharmonies and it therefore allows us to forecast, and accordingly to prevent, a possible pathological development. For example, if a person with constitutional Yang excess suffers an invasion of Wind-Heat and a febrile illness, we can expect that person to have a strong tendency to develop an intense Heat pattern. In terms of the Four Levels, we can foretell that that person might enter the Qi level more quickly and with more Heat than another person: this means that we should be prepared for this and administer strong cooling herbs.
2. Observation of a constitutional type and tendency allows us to put the presenting disharmony into perspective, helping us to gauge its severity. For example, if a person with constitutional Yang excess develops a Heat pattern, that is a less severe situation than a Heat pattern in a person with constitutional Yin excess or constitutional Yang deficiency.
3. Observation of constitutional traits and the deviation or conformity of a person to his or her constitutional type gives us an idea of the severity of a problem and therefore prognosis. For example, it is better for a Wood type to have a Wood rather than a Fire disharmony. So, if a Wood type suffers from a Fire disharmony, this indicates a worse prognosis than that of a Fire type suffering from a Fire disharmony or a Wood type suffering from a Wood disharmony.
4. Observation of constitutional types is important to give patients an underlying treatment, irrespective of the presenting disharmony. It is always important to bear in mind the constitutional type and treat it accordingly. In the above example, if a person of a Wood type suffers from a Fire disharmony, it is obviously necessary to treat the presenting disharmony, but, perhaps afterwards, it would be good to treat also the Element type (i.e. Wood). The treatment of the underlying Element type is an important aspect of the preventive potential of Chinese medicine and it should always be applied.
5. Treatment of the constitutional Element type is particularly useful in the case of mental–emotional problems. For example, a Wood type might display some typical emotional traits such as indecision and inability to plan one's life: treatment of the Wood Element would help the person on a mental–emotional level, whatever other disharmony that person might suffer from.
6. Observation of the constitutional type and tendency of a patient allows us to forecast the type of disharmony that such a patient might be subject to in the future: this means that the preventive potential of Chinese medicine can be exploited to the full. For example, if someone in their 40s displays signs of constitutional Yang excess and also pertains to the Wood type, we know that that person may have a strong tendency to develop Liver-Yang rising or Liver-Fire with signs such as hypertension. This allows us to actively subdue Yang and pacify Wood even in the absence of any clinical manifestations.
7. Observation of the Element type is useful when a person displays all the traits of a certain Element type except for one detail: this is a bad sign even if that person may not suffer any disharmony yet. For example, if a person displays all the characteristics of the Fire type but he or she walks slowly, this small detail tells us that something is amiss and that that person may develop a serious disharmony. This discrepancy might be particularly relevant in the case of the Fire type, as we know that a Fire type may have a tendency to develop a serious pathology very suddenly.

Box 23.2 summarizes the importance of observation of constitutional traits.

SPIRIT

'Spirit' (*shen*) is intended here in two different ways. Firstly, in a general sense, it indicates the vitality of a person: if this is thriving, the person 'has spirit'. The opposite, 'not having spirit', indicates a state of lack of vitality. The 'Simple Questions' says: '*If there is spirit the person thrives, if there is no spirit the person dies.*'[4] In this sense, such vitality or 'spirit' here indicates the attribute of '*shen*' that is often mentioned in the context

> **Box 23.2 The importance of observing constitutional traits**
>
> - A constitutional type indicates a *tendency* to certain disharmonies and therefore allows us to forecast and prevent a possible pathological development during the course of an illness
> - It allows us to put the presenting disharmony into perspective and helps us to gauge its severity
> - Deviation or conformity of a person to his or her constitutional type is a good measure of prognosis
> - It helps us to give patients a treatment appropriate to the underlying constitution, irrespective of the presenting disharmony
> - It is particularly useful in the treatment of mental–emotional problems
> - It allows us to forecast the type of disharmony that a patient might be subject to in the future and therefore to treat the patient preventatively
> - Deviation from an Element type in one detail may be a warning sign

of diagnosis. Having '*shen*' indicates a state of vitality and vibrancy as reflected outwardly in the lustre of the eyes, sheen of hair, lustre of complexion and 'spirit' of the tongue and pulse. Lacking '*shen*' indicates the opposite, a state of lack of vitality, and is reflected outwardly in a lack of lustre of eyes, hair and complexion.

In this sense, the presence or absence of spirit can be observed in the complexion, the eyes, the state of mind and the breathing.

If the person has spirit, the complexion is healthy and with lustre, the face colour is clear, the eyes have lustre and reveal inner vitality, the mind is clear and the breathing even.

Box 23.3 summarizes the observable signs of the 'spirit'.

If the person has no spirit, the complexion is dull and lacking in lustre, the eyes lack lustre, show no inner vitality and are not clear, the mind is unclear and the breathing is laboured or shallow.

> **Box 23.3 The observation of 'spirit' (*shen*)**
>
> - *Complexion* with spirit has lustre; without spirit, no lustre, dull
> - *Eyes* with spirit have lustre and brightness; without spirit, dull, clouded
> - *State of mind* with spirit is alert and clear; without spirit, dull and depressed
> - *Breathing* with spirit is even; without spirit is laboured

In a second sense, the 'spirit' of a person refers to the mental–emotional–spiritual state of that person. If the spirit is strong, the person has a clear voice that projects outwards well, the eyes and complexion have lustre (even if the complexion colour may be pathological), the expression is lively, the mind is clear and alert, the person walks with an erect posture and they have a naturally optimistic, enthusiastic and mentally strong attitude (even if he or she may have suffered emotional problems in the course of their life).

BODY

Observation of the body consists of observation of the Five-Element types and of various body signs.

Five-Element body types

Let us first consider the constitutional body shapes related to the Five Elements. Every individual is born with a certain constitution and, consequently, a certain body shape. There are a tremendous variety of body shapes even within the same race, not to mention between races. It is therefore important not to consider as a diagnostic sign a certain physical trait that is normal for that person.

Traditionally, five different constitutional body shapes are described, one for each Element. People of the Wood type have a subtle shade of green in their complexion, a relatively small head and long-shaped face, broad shoulders, straight back, tall, sinewy body and elegant hands and feet. In terms of personality, they have developed intelligence but their physical strength is poor. Hard workers, they think things over and tend to worry (Fig. 23.6 and Box 23.4).

People of the Fire type have a red, florid complexion, wide teeth, a pointed, small head, possibly with a pointed chin, hair that is either curly or scanty, well-developed muscles of the shoulders, back, hips and head and relatively small hands and feet. In terms of personality, they are keen thinkers. The Fire type is quick, energetic and active. They are short-tempered. They walk firmly and shake their body while walking. They tend to think too much and often worry. They have a good spirit of observation and they analyse things deeply (Fig. 23.7 and Box 23.5).

People of the Earth type have a yellowish complexion, round-shaped face, relatively big head, wide jaws, well-developed and nice-looking shoulders and back,

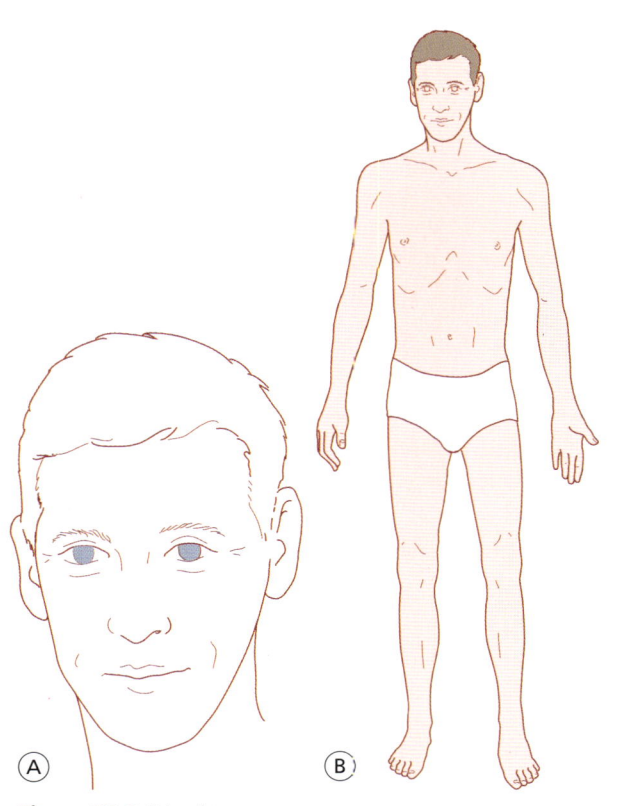

Figure 23.6 Wood type

> **Box 23.4 Wood type**
> - Greenish complexion
> - Small head
> - Long face
> - Broad shoulders
> - Straight back
> - Sinewy body
> - Tall
> - Small hands and feet

large abdomen, strong thigh and calf muscles, relatively small hands and feet, and well-built muscles of the whole body. They walk with firm steps without lifting their feet very high. The Earth type is calm and generous, has a steady character, likes to help people and is not over-ambitious. They are easy to get on with (Fig. 23.8 and Box 23.6).

People of the Metal type have a relatively pale complexion, a square-shaped face, a relatively small head, small shoulders and upper back, a relatively flat abdomen, and small hands and feet. They have a strong voice, move swiftly and have keen powers of thought.

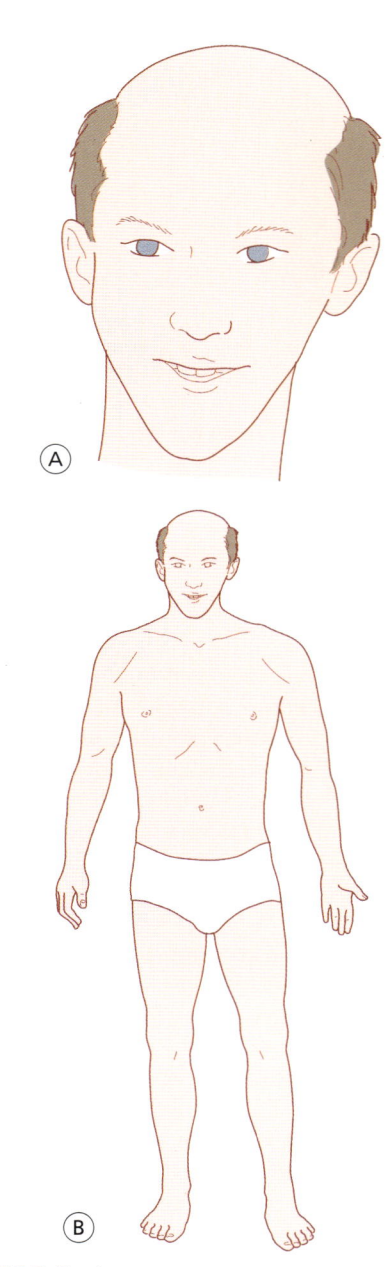

Figure 23.7 Fire type

> **Box 23.5 Fire type**
> - Red complexion
> - Wide teeth
> - Pointed, small head
> - Well-developed shoulder muscles
> - Curly hair or not much hair
> - Small hands and feet
> - Walking briskly

> **Box 23.6 Earth type**
>
> - Yellowish complexion
> - Round face
> - Wide jaws
> - Large head
> - Well-developed shoulders and back
> - Large abdomen
> - Large thighs and calf muscles
> - Well-built muscles

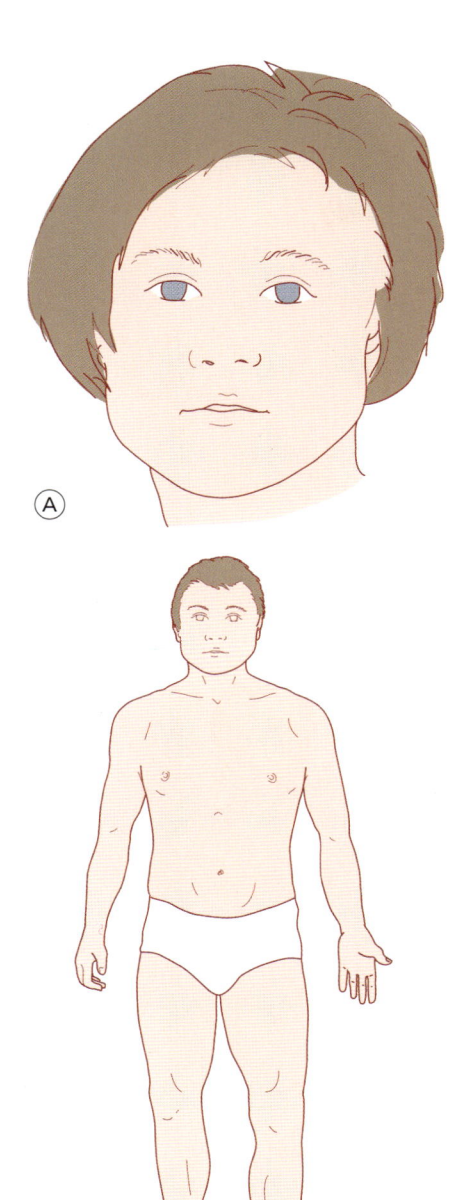

Figure 23.8 Earth type

They are honest and upright. They are generally quiet and calm in a solid way, but also capable of decisive action when necessary. They have a natural aptitude for leadership and management (Fig. 23.9 and Box 23.7).

People of the Water type have a relatively dark complexion, wrinkles, a relatively big head, a round face and body, broad cheeks, narrow and small shoulders and a large abdomen. They keep their body in motion while walking and find it difficult to keep still. They have a long spine. The Water type is sympathetic and slightly laid-back. They are good negotiators and loyal to their work colleagues. They are aware and sensitive (Fig. 23.10 and Box 23.8).

This typology can be used in diagnosis and prognosis. These portraits describe an archetype, but, in reality, due to the way people live their lives and other factors, there can be considerable variations from the types. For example, although a Wood type typically has a tall and slender body, if there is a tendency to overeat, he or she may obviously become fat and deviate from their type.

The Five-Element constitutional body types are useful in practice because they explain inherent differences between people which might otherwise be taken as pathological. For example, the Fire type is active and energetic and he or she walks fast: if we did not know about the Fire type, we might interpret these characteristics as pathological (i.e. Excess of Yang). Deviations from the Element type are also significant. For example, to stay with the Fire type, if all the characteristics of the body shape point to someone being a Fire type but he or she walks slowly, it indicates a problem. This is useful as this discrepancy may herald a future problem.

It should be borne in mind that a person may be a mixture of two or more types; one can have a mixed Earth–Wood type for example. As far as diagnosis and prognosis are concerned, it is the deviations from the ideal types that are important.

If a Wood type does not have a tall and slender body, it may indicate health problems. If they lose too much hair, it may indicate that there is too much Fire within Wood, 'burning' the hair on top of the head.

The Fire type should walk fast: if they do not, it indicates disease. Their strong point should be the Blood and blood vessels, but if it is not, they are then prone

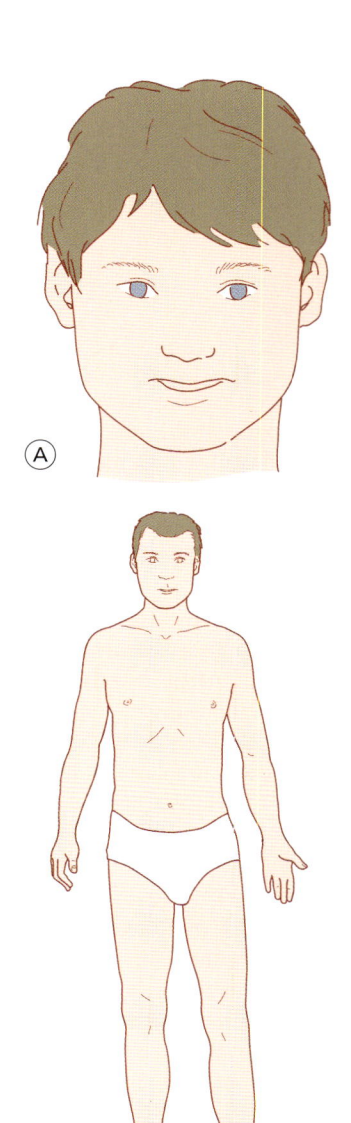

Figure 23.9 Metal type

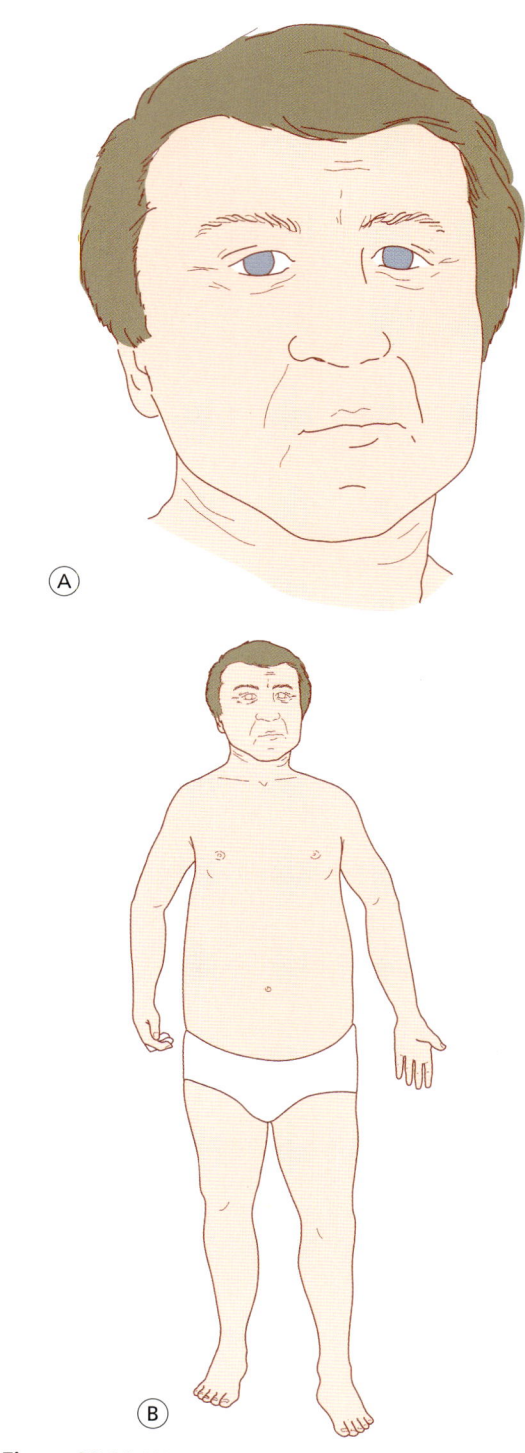

Figure 23.10 Water type

Box 23.7 Metal type

- Pale complexion
- Square face
- Small head
- Small shoulders and upper back
- Flat abdomen
- Strong voice

> **Box 23.8 Water type**
>
> - Dark complexion
> - Wrinkly skin
> - Large head
> - Broad cheeks
> - Narrow shoulders
> - Large abdomen
> - Long spine

to high blood pressure and heart disease. A poor Fire constitution may be indicated by a very weak and deep heart pulse and a central midline crack on the tongue running to the tip.

Metal types should walk slowly and deliberately: if they habitually walk fast, it may indicate a health problem. Their voice should be strong: if it is weak, it indicates a problem with their Lungs. A poor Metal constitution may be indicated by two small transverse cracks on the tongue in the Lung area and by a pulse that runs from the Front position up towards the base of the thumb medially (see ch. 25).

Earth types should have strong muscles. If they do not, it indicates problems, and they become prone to arthritis and rheumatism.

Water types tend to overindulge in sexual activity, and this may cause Kidney-Essence problems, which would be reflected in the eyes with a lack of lustre.

To sum up, each person must be observed carefully and the type assessed so that deviations from the type can be noted. If a person has a certain trait that is unrelated to that particular type, the prognosis is better than if that trait represents a deviation from the type. For example, the Fire type should walk fast. If they walk too fast, it is not so bad as a Metal type walking fast (as the Metal type should walk slowly). Or if a Metal type has a weak voice, it is worse than if another type has a weak voice.

Lastly, the Element types are important in prognosis. It is better for a person to suffer from a pattern of disharmony pertaining to his or her Element type than to a different one. This principle is more easily explained with an example: it is better for a Wood type to suffer from a Liver disharmony than from a Heart disharmony.

Five-Element correspondences

Other Five-Element correspondences are also useful in practice. The relationship between tissues and organs is of significance in practice: for example, any change in the sinews (such as weakness or stiffness) would reflect a disharmony of the Liver; a change in the blood vessels (such as hardening of the vessels, which can be felt as a very hard and Wiry pulse) indicates a problem of the Heart; a change in the muscles (such as weak and flaccid muscles) would reflect a deficiency of the Spleen; a change in the skin (such as flaccid skin) would indicate a deficiency of Lung-Qi; and a change in the bones (such as brittle bones) would indicate a Kidney deficiency.

> **Clinical note**
>
> The point G.B.-34 Yanglingquan can be used to nourish all the sinews

Box 23.9 summarizes observation of the body tissues.

> **Box 23.9 Observation of the body tissues**
>
> - *Sinews* (such as weakness or stiffness) = disharmony of the Liver
> - *Blood vessels* (such as hardening of the vessels) = disharmony of the Heart
> - *Muscles* (such as weak and flaccid muscles) = deficiency of the Spleen
> - *Skin* (such as flaccid skin) = deficiency of Lung-Qi
> - *Bones* (such as brittle bones) = Kidney deficiency

Body signs

Besides these constitutional body shapes, there can be long-term changes in the body shape that are not linked to the constitutional body shapes and which have a diagnostic significance. For example, a very large, barrel-like chest and epigastrium indicate an Excess condition of the Stomach (Fig. 23.11). Very large upper thighs, out of proportion with the rest of the body, indicate Spleen deficiency (Fig. 23.12). A thin and emaciated body usually indicates a long-standing deficiency of Blood or Yin (Fig. 23.13). An overweight body usually indicates deficiency of Spleen-Yang with retention of Dampness or Phlegm (Fig. 23.14). All these body changes would only take place over a long period of time.

Box 23.10 summarizes body signs.

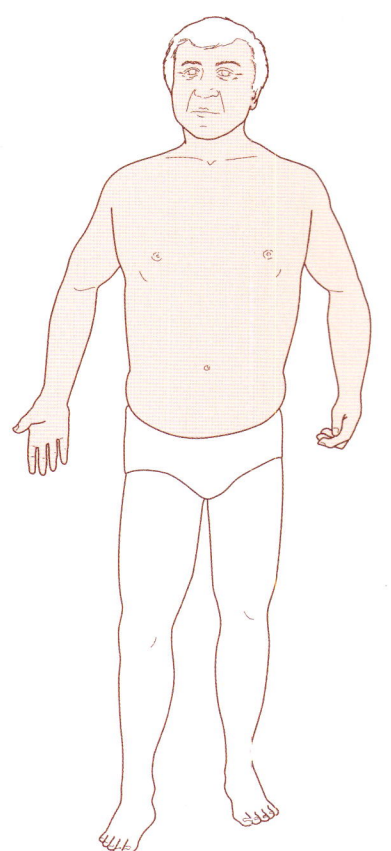

Figure 23.11 Body shape indicating Excess condition of Stomach

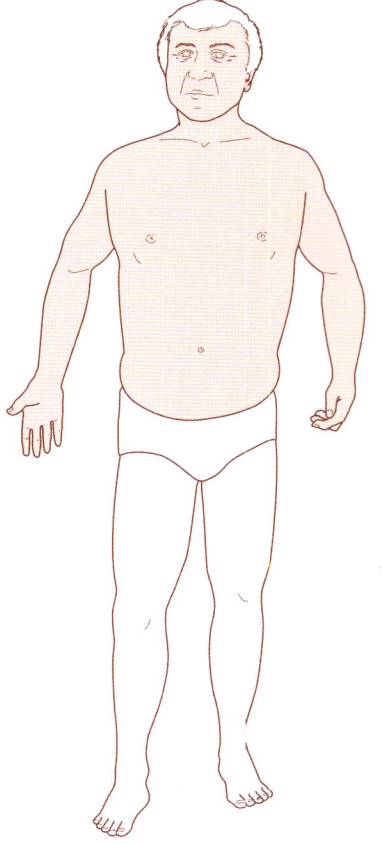

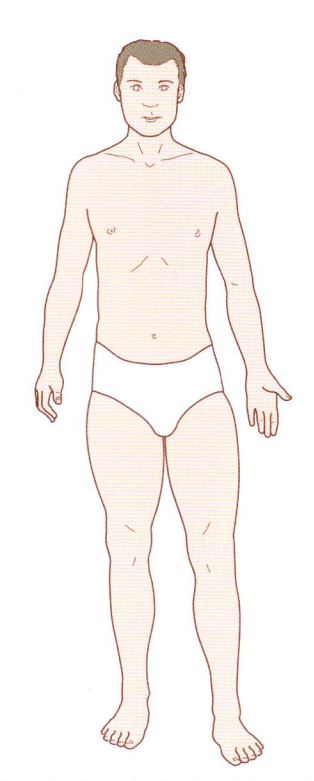

Figure 23.12 Body shape indicating Spleen deficiency

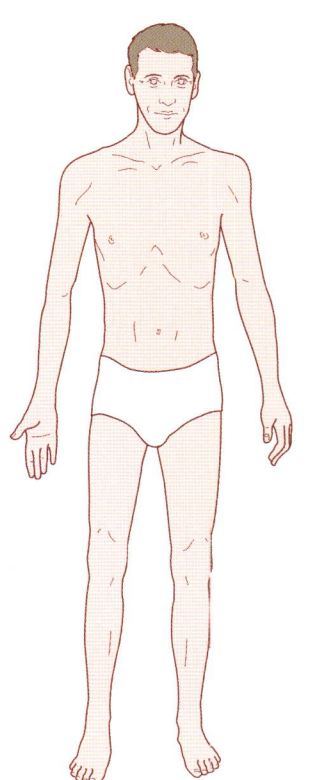

Figure 23.13 Body shape indicating Blood or Yin deficiency

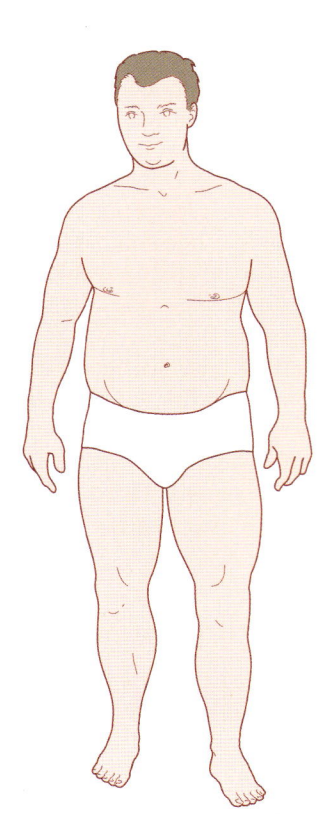

Figure 23.14 Body shape indicating Dampness or Phlegm

> **Box 23.10 Body signs**
> - Large, barrel-like chest and epigastrium: Full condition of Lungs and/or Stomach
> - Large, overweight thighs: Spleen deficiency
> - Thin body: Yin deficiency
> - Overweight body: Yang deficiency (and Phlegm)

> **Box 23.11 Demeanour and body movements**
> - Excess of movement: Yang/Full/Heat
> - Lack of movement: Yin/Empty/Cold
> - Quick movements, feeling of Heat: Excess of Yang
> - Slow movements, feeling cold: Deficiency of Yang
> - Small movements and continuous fidgeting, especially of the legs: Empty-Heat pattern of the Kidneys
> - Tremors, convulsions: Liver-Wind (Full-Wind)
> - Fine tremors, tics: Liver-Wind (Empty-Wind)
> - Paralysis: internal Wind
> - Stiffness and rigidity: Qi stagnation, Blood stasis, internal Wind

DEMEANOUR AND BODY MOVEMENTS

This includes the way the person moves, and also movement of individual parts of the body, such as eyes, face, mouth, limbs and fingers. Lack of movement, such as stiffness, rigidity or paralysis, is also considered here.

The general principle is that an excess of movement or rapid and jerky movements indicate Yang, Full or Hot patterns, while lack of movement or slow movements indicate Yin, Empty or Cold patterns.

The way a person moves has to be considered also in relation to the Five-Element body type. For example, the Fire type should move quickly; if he or she moves slowly, then it indicates some problem. The Metal type should move slowly and deliberately; if she or he moves quickly, then it indicates some problem.

If a person moves very quickly and when in bed throws off the bedclothes, it indicates an Excess pattern of Heat, often of the Liver or Heart. If a person moves very slowly, likes to lie down and feels generally cold, it indicates a Deficient pattern of Cold (Yang deficiency), usually of the Spleen and/or Kidneys.

Small movements and continuous fidgeting, especially of the legs, indicate an Empty-Heat pattern of the Kidneys.

Movements such as tremors or convulsions always indicate the presence of interior Wind of the Liver. These could be convulsions of the whole body, or just tremors of an eyelid or cheek. Generally, pronounced tremors or convulsions reflect Full-Wind (which often derives from Heat); small tremors or tics may indicate Empty-Wind (which usually arises from Blood and/or Yin deficiency).

Paralysis of a limb is also indicative of internal Wind, which is always related to the Liver. Stiffness and rigidity usually indicate a Full pattern, which may be Qi stagnation, Blood stasis or, in acute cases, external Wind.

Box 23.11 summarizes demeanour and body movements.

HEAD AND FACE

Hair

The state of the hair is related to the condition of Blood or Kidney-Essence. Falling hair may indicate a condition of Blood deficiency, while prematurely greying hair indicates a decline of Kidney-Essence.

The thickness and lustre of the hair depend on the Liver, and dull and brittle hair indicates deficiency of Liver-Blood.

Face colour

Observation of the face colour is an extremely important part of visual diagnosis. The face colour reflects the state of Qi and Blood and is closely related to the condition of the Mind.

The chapter 'On Observation of the Colour' in 'Principle and Prohibition for the Medical Profession' (Yi Men Fa Lu) says: *'When the five Yin organs are exhausted, the complexion colour becomes dark and lustreless ... So the complexion colour is like a flag of the Spirit, and the Yin organs are the residences of the Spirit. When the Spirit is gone, the Yin organs are worn out, and the complexion colour becomes dark and lustreless.'*[5]

As the above passage indicates clearly, observation of complexion colour is a very important diagnostic tool to assess the condition not only of Qi, Blood, Yin and Yang and of the Internal Organs but also of the Mind and Spirit. Indeed, from a Five-Element perspective, the facial complexion as a whole is a manifestation of the Heart and therefore the Mind and Spirit; this should never be forgotten in practice. Thus if, for example, a woman has a very dull, sallow complexion, it indicates Spleen-Qi deficiency and Dampness and possibly also Blood deficiency, but, at the same time, it also indicates that the Mind and Spirit are affected and suffering.

Yu Chang in 'Principles of Medical Practice' (1658) calls the complexion the 'banner of the Mind and Spirit' and he says: 'When the Mind and Spirit are flourishing, the complexion is glowing; when the Mind and Spirit are declining, the complexion withers. When the Mind is stable the complexion is florid.'[6]

Lustre and moisture of complexion

The normal complexion should have 'lustre' and 'moisture'. 'Lustre' means that the complexion colour should be bright, glowing and with a shine to it; 'moisture' means that the complexion should look moist and the skin firm, indicating that there is moisture underneath it. Therefore, 'moisture' also indicates that the complexion should have 'body'.

A complexion with lustre is said to have 'spirit' (*shen*); a complexion with moisture is said to have 'Stomach-Qi'. Thus, we can say that if the complexion has lustre there is spirit, if it has moisture there is Stomach-Qi.

Please note that having a 'spirit' and 'Stomach-Qi' or not is independent from the colour of the complexion, even if pathological. In other words, a complexion may have a pathological colour but this may be with or without 'spirit' and with or without 'Stomach-Qi'. Obviously, if a (pathological) complexion has 'spirit' and 'Stomach-Qi', this is a positive sign and indication of a good prognosis and the opposite (a poor prognosis) if it does not.

Box 23.12 summarizes the lustre and moisture of the complexion.

> **Box 23.12 Lustre and moisture of complexion**
>
> - Lustre: complexion is glowing, bright, lively, with sheen (indicates complexion has 'spirit')
> - Moisture: complexion is moist, has 'body', is firm (indicates complexion has 'Stomach-Qi')

The four attributes of normal complexion

Before describing the pathological colours of the complexion we should define the normal complexion. As 'normality' obviously varies from race to race, it is impossible to define a universal normal colour. We can, however, identify and define four essential characteristics of a normal complexion:

> - Lustre
> - A subtle, slightly reddish hue
> - 'Contained', 'veiled' colour
> - Moisture

The presence of *lustre* is an essential part of a normal complexion. Such a complexion is slightly shiny, vibrant in colour, lively, relatively bright and glowing. The presence of lustre in the complexion indicates that the Upright Qi is intact (even though there may be a pathology) and that the Mind and Spirit are healthy.

The normal complexion should have a subtle, slightly *reddish hue* because the facial colour as a whole reflects the state of the Heart and a reddish hue indicates a good supply of Heart-Blood (and by implication, a good state of the Mind).

The colour of the facial complexion should be '*contained*', as if there were a very thin, white silk veil over it. The book *Wang Zhen Zun Jing* describes the normal complexion colour as being bright and lustrous and says: '*The complexion is bright because of the embodiment of the Spirit. It is lustrous because of the nourishment of the Essence and Blood.*'[7]

The normal complexion should be *moist* and look firm (because of the fluids underneath): the moisture of the complexion indicates that the complexion has Stomach-Qi.

Apart from these four basic aspects of a normal complexion, the actual colour naturally varies enormously according to race and even within the same racial group. The normal complexion colour for Caucasian people is a mixed white and slightly reddish colour which is lustrous, bright and contained. Within the Caucasian race, however, there can be considerable variations in normal complexion: for example, the normal complexion of a Norwegian person will be quite different from that of a Spaniard as the Mediterranean complexion is naturally slightly darker and of a more earthy colour than that of the Northern European. The complexion of Chinese people is described in Chinese books as a mixed red and yellow colour, shown slightly, which is bright, lustrous and reserved. The normal complexion of African-American people varies from a light brown to dark brown and it should have the same four attributes of lustre, subtle, slightly reddish hue, a 'contained' colour, and moisture.

Box 23.13 summarizes the four attributes of a normal complexion.

> **Box 23.13 The four attributes of the normal complexion**
>
> - Lustre
> - A subtle, slightly reddish hue
> - 'Contained', 'veiled' colour
> - Moisture

Pathological colours

Various pathological colours are usually described, and these are:

- White
- Yellow
- Red
- Green
- Blue
- Black

White

White indicates Blood deficiency or Yang deficiency. A dull-pale-white complexion indicates Blood deficiency, while a bright-white complexion indicates Yang deficiency. A bluish-white complexion indicates Yang deficiency with pronounced Cold. Box 23.14 summarizes these variations.

Yellow

Yellow indicates Spleen deficiency, or Dampness, or both. A sallow yellow colour indicates Stomach and Spleen deficiency or Blood deficiency. A bright orange-yellow colour indicates Damp-Heat, with the prevalence of Heat rather than Dampness. A hazy, smoky yellow indicates Damp-Heat, with the prevalence of Dampness. A withered, dried-up yellow indicates Heat in Stomach and Spleen. A dull-pale yellow colour indicates Cold-Damp in Stomach and Spleen. An ash-like yellow colour indicates long-standing Dampness. A pale-yellow colour surrounded by red spots indicates Spleen deficiency and stasis of Liver-Blood. A clear and moist yellow colour in between the eyebrows indicates that Stomach-Qi is recovering after an illness affecting Stomach and Spleen. A dried-up and withered-looking yellow colour in the same area is a poor prognostic sign. Box 23.15 summarizes these points.

> **Box 23.14 White complexion**
>
> - Blood deficiency (dull-white)
> - Yang deficiency (bright-white)
> - Yang deficiency with Cold (bluish-white)

> **Box 23.15 Yellow complexion**
>
> - Spleen deficiency (sallow yellow)
> - Blood deficiency (sallow yellow)
> - Damp-Heat with prevalence of Heat (bright orange-yellow)
> - Damp-Heat with prevalence of Dampness (smoky, dull-yellow)
> - Heat in Stomach and Spleen (withered, dried-up yellow)
> - Cold-Dampness in Stomach and Spleen (dull-pale yellow)
> - Long-standing Dampness (ash-like yellow)
> - Spleen deficiency and stasis of Liver-Blood (pale yellow surrounded by red spots)
> - Stomach-Qi recovering after an illness affecting Stomach and Spleen (clear and moist yellow colour in between the eyebrows)
> - Poor prognostic sign: a dried-up and withered-looking yellow colour in between the eyebrows

Red

Red indicates Heat. This can be Full- or Empty-Heat. In Full-Heat, the whole face is red; in Empty-Heat only the cheekbones are red. Box 23.16 summarizes these points.

> **Box 23.16 Red complexion**
>
> - Full-Heat: whole face red
> - Empty-Heat: red cheek bones

Green

A green colour of the face indicates any of the following conditions: a Liver pattern, interior Cold, pain or interior Wind. A pale-greenish colour under the eyes indicates Liver-Qi stagnation. A greenish complexion on the cheeks denotes Liver-Qi stagnation, Liver-Blood stasis, Cold in the Liver channel or Liver-Wind. A green complexion with a red tinge is seen in the Lesser-Yang pattern. A green colour with red eyes indicates Liver-Fire. Yellowish-green cheeks denote Phlegm with Liver-Yang rising. A green colour on the nose indicates stagnation of Qi with abdominal pain. A dark-reddish green complexion indicates stagnant Liver-Qi turning into Heat. A pale-green colour under the eyes denotes Liver-Blood deficiency. Finally, a grass-like green colour indicates collapse of Liver-Qi. Box 23.17 summarizes a green complexion.

Box 23.17 Green complexion

- Liver patterns
- Interior Cold
- Pain
- Interior Wind
- Liver-Qi stagnation (pale-greenish colour under the eyes)
- Liver-Qi stagnation, Liver-Blood stasis, Cold in the Liver channel or Liver-Wind (greenish colour on the cheeks)
- Lesser-Yang pattern (green complexion with a red tinge)
- Liver-Fire (green complexion with red eyes)
- Phlegm with Liver-Yang rising (yellowish-green cheeks)
- Qi stagnation with abdominal pain (green colour on the nose)
- Stagnant Liver-Qi turning into Heat (dark-reddish green complexion)
- Liver-Blood deficiency (pale-green colour under the eyes)
- Collapse of Liver-Qi (grass-like green complexion)

Blue

A dark-bluish colour under the eyes indicates Cold in the Liver channel. A white-bluish complexion indicates Cold or chronic pain. A dull-bluish complexion indicates severe Heart-Yang deficiency with Blood stasis or chronic pain. A bluish complexion (in children) indicates Liver-Wind. Box 23.18 summarizes a blue complexion.

Box 23.18 Blue complexion

- Cold in Liver channel (dark-bluish under the eyes)
- Cold or chronic pain (white-bluish)
- Severe Heart-Yang deficiency with Blood stasis (dull-bluish)
- Liver Wind (bluish complexion, in children)

Black

'Black' complexion indicates a complexion that is greyish and very dark. A black complexion indicates Cold, pain, or Kidney disease, usually Kidney-Yin deficiency. A black and moist-looking colour indicates Cold, while a dried-up and burned-looking colour indicates Heat, usually Empty-Heat from Kidney-Yin deficiency. Box 23.19 summarizes a black complexion.

Box 23.19 Black complexion

- Cold (black and moist)
- Heat (black and dried-up, burned-looking)

Deep/floating, distinct/obscure, thin/thick, scattered/concentrated and moist/dry colour

Finally, irrespective of the actual shade, the colour can be described as being deep or floating, distinct or obscure, thin or thick, scattered or concentrated and moist or dry. Box 23.20 summarizes these attributes of the complexion.

A *floating* colour indicates an exterior, mild, Yang condition, while a *deep* colour indicates an interior, severe, Yin condition.

A *distinct* colour indicates a Yang condition and that the Upright Qi is still intact, while an *obscure* colour indicates a Yin condition and that the Upright Qi is exhausted.

A *thin* colour indicates a Deficiency, while a *thick* colour indicates a Full condition.

A *scattered* colour indicates a new disease, while a *concentrated* colour indicates an old disease.

A *moist* colour is a sign of good prognosis, while a *dry* colour is a sign of poor prognosis.

Box 23.20 Complexion colour types

- *Floating*: exterior, mild, Yang condition
- *Deep*: interior, severe, Yin condition
- *Distinct*: Yang condition, Upright Qi still intact
- *Obscure*: Yin condition, Upright Qi exhausted
- *Thin*: Deficiency
- *Thick*: Fullness
- *Scattered*: new disease
- *Concentrated*: old disease
- *Moist*: good prognosis
- *Dry*: poor prognosis

Face areas

Besides the colour, various areas of the face indicate the state of certain organs. There are two different arrangements of areas, one according to the 'Simple Questions' chapter 32 and the other according to the 'Spiritual Axis' chapter 49 (see Figs 23.1 and 23.2).

A careful observation of these face areas and their colours is an extremely important part of diagnosis by observation which should be always carried out. The correspondence between face areas and Internal Organs reveals three possible conditions:

- An actual disharmony, e.g. red cheeks may indicate Heat in the Lungs
- A constitutional trait, e.g. short earlobes may indicate weak Kidneys and short life
- An aetiological factor, e.g. a bluish colour on the forehead (related to the Heart according to the 'Simple Questions' correspondences) in a child may indicate prenatal shock

Observation of the face colour should be integrated with the face areas. For example, a bluish colour in the centre of the forehead (which corresponds to the Heart according to the 'Simple Questions') indicates that the Heart has suffered from a shock. A greenish colour on the nose may indicate Liver-Qi stagnation or Liver-Blood stasis. A red tip of the nose denotes Spleen deficiency. A very short chin indicates the possibility of Kidney deficiency.

The colour of the complexion in a particular area can also be interpreted in the light of the Five Elements. For example, a greenish colour on the tip of the nose (the face area corresponding to the Spleen) indicates that the Liver is invading the Spleen and that that particular Spleen disharmony is secondary to a Liver disharmony.

EYES

Observation of the eyes is an extremely important part of diagnosis. The eyes reflect the state of the Mind (Shen) and the Essence (Jing). The 'Spiritual Axis' says: *'The Essence of the five Yin and the six Yang organs ascends to the eyes.'*[3]

If the eyes are clear and have lustre, they indicate that the Mind and the Essences of the five Yin organs are in a good state of vitality. If the eyes are rather dull or clouded, it shows that the Mind is disturbed and the Essences of the five Yin organs have been weakened. It is very common to see very dull and clouded eyes in people who have been suffering from deep emotional problems for a long time.

Different parts of the eye are related to different organs. The corners of the eye are related to the Heart, the upper eyelid to the Spleen (or to the Greater Yang channels), the lower eyelid to the Stomach, the sclera to the Lungs, the iris to the Liver and the pupil to the Kidney (Fig. 23.15).

A red colour in the corners of the eye indicates Heart-Fire; a red colour in the sclera indicates Lung-Heat. A yellow colour of the sclera indicates Damp-Heat.

If the whole eye is red, painful and swollen, it indicates either an exterior invasion of Wind-Heat or rising of Liver-Fire.

A dull-white colour of the corners indicates Heat and a pale-white colour indicates Blood deficiency.

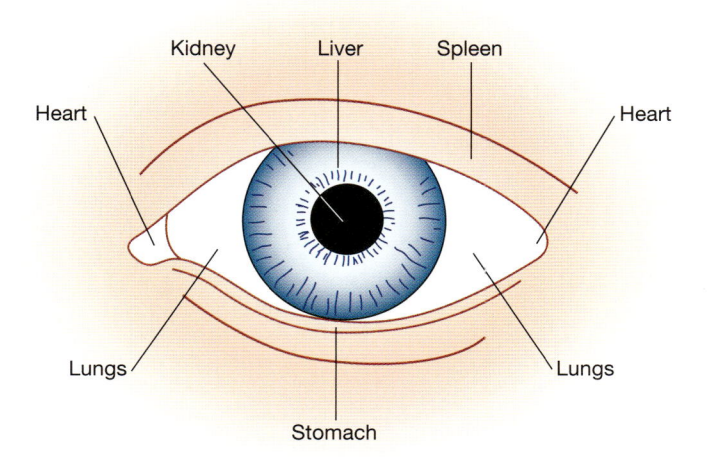

Figure 23.15 Correspondence between parts of the eye and the Internal Organs

A swelling under the eyes indicates Kidney deficiency.

Finally, according to modern research carried out at the Fujian College of Traditional Chinese Medicine, the sclera of the eye can reflect lesions of the back or chest.[9] Injuries of back and chest, such as internal haematomas, can be reflected on the sclera. If one draws a horizontal line across the centre of the eye, the upper part reflects the back and the lower part reflects the chest; also the right eye will reflect lesions on the right side and the left eye those on the left side (Fig. 23.16).

Box 23.21 summarizes these eye signs.

Green, blue, purple or red spots appearing at the end of red veins with purple blood spots on them indicate lesions within the back or chest. Such spots that are not directly connected to the veins have no diagnostic significance. Grey and scattered spots like clouds indicate injuries of Qi: that is, injuries causing only stagnation of Qi, without organic lesions. Deep-black spots like black sesame seeds indicate injury of Blood: that is, injuries causing stasis of Blood, a stage further than stagnation of Qi. Black spots surrounded by a grey, cloud-like halo indicate injuries of both Qi and Blood. If red veins are clearly visible and are spiral shaped, they indicate pain.

NOSE

The bridge of the nose reflects the state of the Liver, while the tip of the nose reflects the state of the Spleen. If the tip of the nose is green or blue it indicates abdominal pain from Cold in the Spleen. If it is yellow, it indicates Damp-Heat in the Spleen. A white colour of the tip indicates Blood deficiency. If it is red, it indicates Heat in Lungs and Spleen. If it is grey, it indicates an impairment of Water movement.

If the bridge of the nose is greenish, it indicates Liver-Qi stagnation; if it greyish or dark, it denotes Liver-Blood stasis; if it is red, it indicates Liver-Fire.

If the nose is slightly moist and shiny, it indicates that any disease there might be is not serious. If it is dry, it indicates Heat in the Stomach or Large Intestine. If it is dry and black, it indicates the presence of Toxic Heat.

A clear watery discharge from the nose indicates a Cold pattern; a thick-yellow discharge indicates a Heat pattern.

Flaring of the nostrils in a person with high fever indicates extreme Heat in the Lungs.

Box 23.22 summarizes these nose signs.

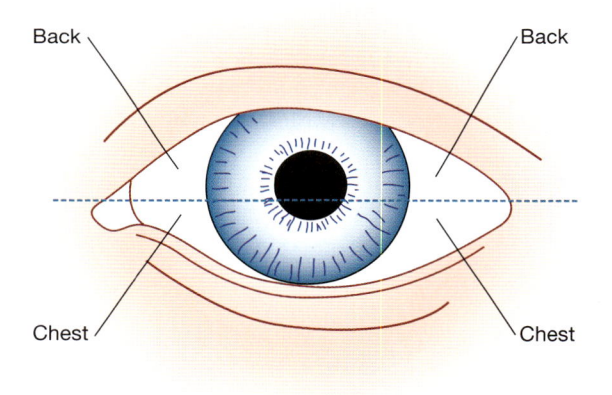

Figure 23.16 Correspondence between areas of the sclera and back and chest

Box 23.21 Eye signs

- Red corner of the eye: Heart-Fire
- Dull-white corners: Heat
- Pale-white corners: Blood deficiency
- Red sclera: Lung-Heat
- Yellow sclera: Damp-Heat
- Whole eye, red, painful, swollen: invasion of Wind-Heat or Liver-Fire
- Swelling under the eyes: Kidney deficiency

Box 23.22 Nose signs

- Green or blue tip of the nose: abdominal pain from Cold in the Spleen
- Yellow tip: Damp-Heat in the Spleen
- White tip: Blood deficiency
- Red tip: Heat in Lungs and Spleen
- Grey tip: impairment of Water movement
- Greenish bridge of the nose: Liver-Qi stagnation
- Greyish or dark bridge: Liver-Blood stasis
- Red bridge: Liver-Fire
- Nose slightly moist and shiny: good prognosis
- Dry nose: Heat in the Stomach or Large Intestine
- Dry and black nose: Toxic Heat
- Clear watery discharge: Cold pattern
- Thick yellow discharge: Heat pattern
- Flaring of the nostrils with high fever: extreme Heat in the Lungs

EARS

A white colour of the ears indicates a Cold pattern, while a bluish or black colour indicates pain. If the ear lobes are dry, withered and black, they indicate extreme exhaustion of Kidney-Qi.

The ear lobes are an indicator in assessing prognosis: if they are shiny and slightly moist, the prognosis is good; if they are dry and withered, the prognosis is bad.

Swelling and pain in the ear (or middle ear) are usually due to Heat in the Lesser Yang channels.

The shape of the ear also helps to distinguish Full from Empty patterns: a swollen ear indicates the presence of a pathogenic factor, hence a Full pattern. A thin ear indicates deficiency of Qi or Blood.

Apart from the above signs, the shape and size of the ear lobe is related to one's constitution and Kidney energy in Chinese facial diagnosis. A long and full lobe is indicative of strong Kidneys and good constitution; a thin and small lobe is indicative of a rather poor constitution.

Box 23.23 summarizes the ear signs.

Box 23.23 Ear signs

- White ears: Cold pattern
- Bluish or dark ears: pain
- Dry, withered, dark ear lobes: exhaustion of Kidney-Qi (usually Kidney-Yin)
- Shiny and moist ear lobes: good prognosis
- Dry and withered ear lobes: poor prognosis
- Swelling and pain of middle ear: Heat in Lesser Yang channels
- Swollen ear: pathogenic factor
- Thin ear: deficiency of Qi or Blood
- Long and full lobe: strong constitution
- Small lobe: poor constitution

MOUTH AND LIPS

The lips reflect the state of the Spleen, the mouth that of the Spleen and Stomach. The normal colour of the lips should be pale red and rather moist and shiny. If the lips are very pale, this indicates Deficiency of Blood or Yang. If they are too red and dry, this indicates Heat in the Spleen and Stomach. If the lips are purple or bluish, this indicates stasis of Blood.

If the mouth is always slightly open, it is a sign of an Empty pattern. If the person only breathes through the mouth, it indicates a deficiency of Lung-Qi (unless of course, it is due to a blocked nose).

A greenish colour around the mouth indicates Liver-Qi stagnation or stasis of Liver-Blood.

Box 23.24 summarizes the mouth and lip signs.

Box 23.24 Mouth and lips signs

- Pale-red, moist and shiny lips: normal, good state of Spleen
- Pale lips: Yang or Blood deficiency
- Red and dry lips: Heat in Stomach and Spleen
- Purple or bluish lips: Blood stasis
- Mouth slightly open: Empty pattern
- Breathing through mouth: Lung-Qi deficiency
- Greenish around the mouth: Liver-Blood stasis or Liver-Qi stagnation

TEETH AND GUMS

The teeth are considered an 'extension of the bones' and are under the influence of the Kidneys. The gums are under the influence of the Stomach.

If the gums are swollen and painful and perhaps bleeding, it indicates Heat in the Stomach. If there is no pain, it indicates Empty-Heat. If the gums are very pale, it indicates deficiency of Blood.

Moist teeth indicate a good state of the Body Fluids and Kidneys, whereas dry teeth indicate exhaustion of fluids and deficiency of Kidney-Yin.

If the teeth are bright and dry like a stone, it indicates Heat in the Bright Yang (in the context of exterior diseases). If they are dry and greyish like bones, it indicates Empty-Heat from Kidney-Yin deficiency.

If the teeth are bleeding, it indicates extreme Heat in the Stomach.[10]

Box 23.25 summarizes the teeth and gum signs.

Box 23.25 Teeth and gums signs

- Swollen and painful gums: Stomach-Heat
- Swollen but not painful gums: Empty-Heat of the Stomach
- Pale gums: Blood deficiency
- Moist teeth: good state of Kidneys
- Dry teeth: Kidney-Yin deficiency
- Bright and very dry teeth: Heat in Bright-Yang (febrile diseases)
- Dry and greyish teeth: Kidney-Yin deficiency

THROAT

Observation of the throat includes observation of the pharynx and tonsils.

Pharynx

Pain, redness and swelling of the throat indicate invasion of exterior Wind-Heat in acute cases or Stomach-Heat in chronic cases.

If the throat is only sore and dry but not swollen and red, it indicates deficiency of Lung- and/or Kidney-Yin with Empty-Heat. If the inside of the throat is pale red, it indicates Empty Heat affecting the Lung and/or Kidney channels.

Erosion, redness and swelling of the pharynx indicates Toxic Heat and this is seen more frequently in children suffering from acute upper respiratory infections.

Erosion, swelling and a yellowish-red colour of the pharynx, together with foul breath and a thick yellow tongue coating, indicates Full Heat in the Stomach and Intestines, which, again, is more common in children.

A chronic erosion of the pharynx that comes and goes is usually due to Empty-Heat, which may affect Stomach, Lungs or Kidneys.

Chronic erosion and dryness of the pharynx that comes and goes, with greyish ulcers, no swelling and a dry but not painful throat, indicate chronic, severe Yin deficiency.

Chronic erosion of the pharynx with ulcers that have raised, hard edges indicates Blood stasis mixed with Phlegm-Heat.

Box 23.26 summarizes the pharynx signs.

Tonsils

Swollen tonsils of a normal colour indicate retention of Dampness or Phlegm occurring against a background of Qi deficiency. This is seen frequently in children with retention of a residual pathogenic factor (e.g. Dampness or Phlegm) after repeated acute upper respiratory infections. If both tonsils are affected, it generally indicates a greater severity than if only one is affected.

Red and swollen tonsils indicate Heat or Toxic Heat, often in the Stomach and/or Large Intestine channel: in acute cases, this is usually due to invasion of Wind-Heat with accompanying Toxic Heat.

Chronic redness and swelling of the tonsils that comes and goes indicates either chronic Heat in the Stomach and/or Large Intestine channel (more common in children and often due to a residual pathogenic factor), or Empty-Heat in the Lung channel.

If both tonsils are affected, it generally indicates a greater severity than if only one is affected.

Red and swollen tonsils with exudate, usually seen during acute upper respiratory infections and more common in children, definitely indicate an invasion of Wind-Heat (as opposed to Wind-Cold), and this may be complicated by Toxic Heat in the Stomach and/or Large Intestine channel.

Greyish tonsils are often seen at the acute stage of glandular fever (mononucleosis).

Box 23.27 summarizes tonsil signs.

Box 23.26 Pharynx signs

- Deep red: Heat (interior or exterior)
- Pale red: Empty-Heat
- Acute pain, redness and swelling of throat: invasion of Wind-Heat
- Chronic pain, redness and swelling of the throat: Stomach-Heat
- Chronically sore and dry throat that is not swollen or red: Lung- and/or Kidney-Yin deficiency with Empty-Heat
- Pale-red throat: Empty-Heat affecting the Lung and/or Kidney channels
- Erosion, redness and swelling: Toxic Heat
- Erosion, swelling, yellowish-red: Heat in Stomach and Intestines
- Chronic erosion that comes and goes: Empty-Heat
- Chronic dryness and erosion with greyish ulcers: severe Yin deficiency
- Chronic erosion with ulcers that have raised, hard edges: Blood stasis with Phlegm-Heat

---

Box 23.27 Tonsil signs

- Swollen tonsils of a normal colour: retention of Dampness or Phlegm occurring against a background of Qi deficiency
- Chronically red and swollen tonsils: Heat or Toxic Heat often in the Stomach and/or Large Intestine channel
- Acutely red and swollen tonsils: invasion of Wind-Heat with accompanying Toxic Heat
- Chronic redness and swelling of the tonsils that come and go: either chronic Heat in the Stomach and/or Large Intestine channel or Empty-Heat in the Lung channel
- Acutely red and swollen tonsils with exudate: invasion of Wind-Heat (as opposed to Wind-Cold), complicated by Toxic Heat in the Stomach and/or Large Intestine channel
- Greyish tonsils: acute stage of glandular fever (mononucleosis)

LIMBS

In general, the limbs indicate the state of the Spleen and Stomach: the Spleen because it influences the muscles and the Stomach because it transports Food Essences to the limbs. Therefore, firm muscles indicate a good state of Stomach and Spleen, while flabby muscles indicate deficiency of the Stomach and Spleen.

A healthy colour and a firmness of the flesh around ankles and wrists indicates a good state of the Body Fluids. If the skin on these joints lacks lustre and is dry and the flesh shrivelled, it indicates exhaustion of Body Fluids.

The following limb signs will be discussed:

- Swelling of the joints of the four limbs
- Oedema of the four limbs
- Flaccidity of the four limbs
- Rigidity of the four limbs
- Paralysis of the four limbs
- Contraction of the four limbs
- Tremor or spasticity of the four limbs
- Nails
- Thenar eminence
- Index finger in babies

Swelling of the joints of the four limbs

A swelling of the joints of the four limbs is always due to Painful Obstruction (*Bi*) Syndrome, especially that deriving from Dampness; in chronic conditions, Dampness develops into Phlegm, which obstructs the joints and causes further swelling and bone deformities. In adult patients, and especially women, it is very common for Painful Obstruction Syndrome and swelling of the joints of the four limbs to occur against a background of Blood deficiency. If, in addition to being swollen, the joints are also red and hot to the touch, it indicates retention of Damp-Heat.

Box 23.28 summarizes swelling of the joints of the four limbs.

Box 23.28 Swelling of the joints of the four limbs

- Dampness Painful Obstruction Syndrome (*Bi*)
- Damp-Heat (joints red and hot)
- Dampness Painful Obstruction Syndrome (*Bi*) against a background of Liver-Blood deficiency

Oedema of the four limbs

There are two types of oedema, one called 'water oedema' (*shui zhong*) and the other 'Qi oedema' (*Qi zhong*). Water oedema is due to Yang deficiency and is always pitting oedema (i.e. the skin pits and it changes colour on pressure). Qi oedema is due to either Qi stagnation or Dampness and the skin neither nor changes colour on pressure.

Water oedema is generally due to deficient Yang; the fluids that it is unable to transform, transport and excrete properly accumulate in the space between the skin and muscles (*cou li*).

Yang deficiency is the most common cause of oedema of the limbs: Lung-Yang deficiency affects primarily the hands, Kidney-Yang deficiency primarily the feet and Spleen-Yang deficiency both. Oedema of the four limbs may also derive from retention of Dampness in the muscles, which may be associated with Cold or with Heat.

Qi stagnation affecting the muscles may also cause oedema of the limbs, in which case it will be of the non-pitting type. Finally, acute oedema of the hands and face only may be due to invasion of the Lungs by Wind-Water, which is a type of Wind-Cold.

Box 23.29 summarizes oedema of the four limbs.

Box 23.29 Oedema of the limbs

- Lung-Yang deficiency: oedema of the hands
- Kidney-Yang deficiency: oedema of the feet
- Spleen-Yang deficiency: oedema of the four limbs
- Dampness: oedema of the four limbs (non-pitting)
- Qi stagnation: oedema of the four limbs (non-pitting)
- Invasion of the Lungs by Wind-Water: acute oedema of the hands

Flaccidity of the four limbs

The term 'flaccidity' indicates that the muscles are flaccid, soft and limp but not atrophied (as in atrophy of the muscles).

In acute cases, flaccidity of the four limbs may be due to invasion of Wind-Heat in the Lungs, later becoming interior Heat and injuring the Body Fluids of the Stomach and Spleen. In chronic cases, the flaccidity may result from Damp-Heat affecting the Stomach and Spleen in Full cases or from a deficiency of the Stomach and Spleen in Empty conditions. In severe, chronic cases, flaccidity of the four limbs is often due to a deficiency of Kidney-Yin.

In severe cases, flaccidity may turn into atrophy of the muscles.

Box 23.30 summarizes flaccidity of the four limbs.

Box 23.30 Flaccidity of the limbs

- Lung-Heat injuring Body Fluids (acute)
- Damp-Heat in the Stomach and Spleen
- Stomach and Spleen deficiency
- Kidney-Yin deficiency

Rigidity of the four limbs

Rigidity of the four limbs means that the patient is unable to flex or extend the wrist, elbow, knee or ankle joints. It has many causes. In acute cases with sudden onset, it is due to invasion of Wind; such a rigidity is obviously of short duration and resolves itself once the Wind has been expelled.

In interior conditions, one common cause of rigidity of the four limbs is Liver-Yang rising or Liver-Wind in the elderly; another is of course seen in Painful Obstruction (Bi) Syndrome, especially when caused by Dampness complicated by Phlegm in chronic cases, in which case the limb rigidity is accompanied by swelling and pain of the joints.

In the elderly, an inability to flex the joints is often due to retention of Phlegm in the channels together with internal Wind. A rigidity of the limbs accompanied by pain in the joints and/or muscles, worsening at night, is due to Blood stasis.

In Empty conditions, rigidity of the limbs may be due to a deficiency of Liver- and Kidney-Yin or of Spleen- and Kidney-Yang and this is more common in the elderly.

Box 23.31 summarizes rigidity of the four limbs.

Box 23.31 Rigidity of the limbs

- Invasion of external Wind (acute)
- Liver-Yang rising
- Liver-Wind (elderly)
- Painful Obstruction Syndrome with Dampness and Phlegm
- Phlegm with internal Wind in the channels (elderly)
- Blood stasis
- Liver- and Kidney-Yin deficiency
- Spleen- and Kidney-Yang deficiency

Paralysis of the four limbs

Paralysis of the four limbs may range from a very slight limitation of movement, such as a tendency to drag a foot, to complete paralysis, as is seen in hemiplegia following a fracture of the spine.

The main causes of paralysis of the four limbs are a Stomach and Spleen deficiency, a general deficiency of Qi and Blood and a deficiency of Yin of the Liver and Kidneys. There are also Full causes of paralysis such as retention of Dampness in the muscles and Blood stasis.

The hemiplegia that occurs after a stroke is due to retention of Wind and Phlegm in the channels of the limbs on one side. The underlying pathology leading to a stroke is usually quite complex and includes Phlegm, internal Wind and Heat usually occurring against a background of deficiency of Qi and Blood or of Yin.

Box 23.32 summarizes paralysis of the four limbs.

Box 23.32 Paralysis of the limbs

- Stomach and Spleen deficiency
- Qi and Blood deficiency
- Liver- and Kidney-Yin deficiency
- Dampness in the muscles
- Blood stasis
- Phlegm and internal Wind in the channels

Contraction of the four limbs

In acute cases with sudden onset, contraction of the four limbs may be caused by invasion of Wind and this is always of short duration and self-resolving. In Full conditions, the contractions may be caused by Dampness obstructing the muscles or by Heat injuring the Body Fluids of the limb channels.

In Empty conditions, the most common cause of contraction of the four limbs is Liver-Blood or Liver-Yin deficiency. In the elderly, a common example usually deriving from Liver-Blood or Liver-Yin deficiency is the Dupuytren contracture, which usually involves either the ring finger or the little finger.

Box 23.33 summarizes contraction of the four limbs.

Box 23.33 Contraction of the four limbs

- Acute: invasion of Wind
- Dampness in the muscles
- Heat injuring fluids in muscles
- Liver-Blood or Liver-Yin deficiency

Tremor or spasticity of the four limbs

Tremor consists in a shaking, trembling or quivering of either the arms or the legs, or both. It ranges from a very pronounced shaking with wide amplitude to a quiver that is so fine and in amplitude so small that it is almost imperceptible. Tremor of the hands is more common than tremor of the legs. The cause is always Liver-Wind; as with convulsions, it may be either the Full or Empty type, the former being characterized by a pronounced shaking of the limbs and the latter by a fine tremor.

The most common cause of tremor of the four limbs, especially in the elderly, is a combination of Liver-Wind and Phlegm affecting the channels and sinews. Liver-Yang rising by itself may also give rise to internal Wind and tremors. Another common cause of tremors is Liver-Wind deriving from Liver-Blood deficiency; this is more common in women and will cause a fine tremor. Liver- and Kidney-Yin deficiency are also a common cause of tremors in the elderly.

A general deficiency of Qi and Blood failing to nourish the sinews and muscles may cause a mild, fine tremor of the limbs.

Spasticity and tremor of the limbs may also appear at the Blood Level (of the Four Levels) when the Heat generated by the febrile disease either leads to Liver-Wind or depletes the Yin so that Empty-Wind is generated.

Box 23.34 summarizes tremor or spasticity of the four limbs.

Box 23.34 Tremor or spasticity of the four limbs

- Tremor of the hands: Liver-Wind
- Tremor of the four limbs in the elderly: Liver-Wind and Phlegm affecting channels and sinews
- Fine tremor in women: Liver-Wind deriving from Liver-Blood deficiency
- Mild, fine tremor of the limbs: general deficiency of Qi and Blood
- Spasticity and tremor in febrile disease: Liver-Wind or Empty-Wind from Yin deficiency

---

Nails

Pale nails indicate deficiency of Blood; bluish nails indicate stasis of Blood (of the Liver). Ridged nails indicate deficiency of Liver-Blood.

Thenar eminence

The thenar eminence shows the state of the Stomach. A bluish colour of the venules on the thenar eminence of the thumb indicates Cold in the Stomach. Bluish and short venules indicate an Empty pattern. Red venules indicate Heat in the Stomach. Purple venules indicate Blood stasis in the Stomach. Box 23.35 summarizes the thenar eminence signs.

Box 23.35 Thenar eminence

Shows the state of the Stomach
- Bluish venules: Cold in the Stomach
- Bluish and short venules: Empty pattern
- Red venules: Heat in the Stomach
- Purple venules: Blood stasis in the Stomach

Index finger in babies

Examination of the venules on the index fingers of children under 2 is used for diagnosing infants. Usually the left index finger is examined in boys and the right one in girls. The creases at the metacarpophalangeal articulation and interphalangeal articulation are called 'gates', the first one at the base being the 'Gate of Wind', the second one the 'Gate of Qi', and the third one the 'Gate of Life' (Fig 23.17).

If after rubbing the finger towards the body, venules appear only beyond the 'Gate of Wind', this indicates an invasion by an exterior pathogenic factor and a mild disease. Venules extending beyond the 'Gate of Qi' indicates an interior and rather more severe disease. If they extend beyond the 'Gate of Life', this indicates

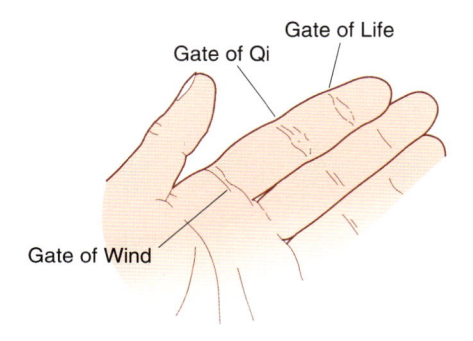

Figure 23.17 Index diagnosis in children

a serious and life-threatening disease. Furthermore, if the venules are bluish, they indicate a Cold pattern; if they are red, they indicate a Heat pattern.

SKIN

The skin is physiologically related to the Lungs within the Five-Element model. However, it is also related to the condition of Blood and, through this, to the Liver. Hence, not all skin diseases are related to the Lungs. Many skin conditions are due to Heat or stasis of Blood and are related to the condition of the Liver. Furthermore, Heat in the Blood can also derive from Stomach-Heat so that some skin diseases may also be related to the Stomach.

Dry skin usually indicates deficiency of Liver-Blood, whereas itchy skin is due to Wind, which, particularly in skin diseases, itself often derives from Liver-Blood.

A swelling of the skin which leaves a mark on pressure with a finger indicates oedema. This is called true oedema in Chinese medicine, or 'Water oedema', and is due to deficiency of Spleen- and/or Kidney-Yang as mentioned above.

A yellow colour of the skin may indicate jaundice and two different shades are distinguished. A bright and clear yellow colour indicates 'Yang jaundice', which is due to Damp-Heat. A dull-yellow colour indicates 'Yin jaundice', which is due to Damp-Cold.

The venules which frequently appear on the skin are considered to be an exterior manifestation of the Blood-Connecting channels. They indicate a state of Fullness of the secondary Connecting channels. If they are red they indicate Heat, if bluish they indicate Cold, if greenish they indicate pain and if purple they indicate stasis of Blood. They can be frequently seen on the posterior aspect of the legs in older people.

Papules usually indicate Heat in the Stomach and/or Lungs. Vesicles indicate Dampness; macules indicate a disharmony at the Blood level, denoting Heat in the Blood if they are red, Blood stasis if they are purple and Cold in the Blood if they are bluish.

Box 23.36 summarizes skin signs.

TONGUE[11]

Observation of the tongue is a pillar of diagnosis because it provides clearly visible clues to the patient's disharmony. Tongue diagnosis is remarkably reliable: whenever there are conflicting manifestations in a complicated condition, the tongue nearly always reflects the basic and underlying pattern.

Observation of the tongue is based on four main items: the tongue-body colour, the tongue-body shape, the tongue coating and the moisture:

Box 23.36 Skin signs

- Dry skin: Liver-Blood deficiency
- Itchy skin: Wind
- Pitting oedema: Kidney-Yang deficiency
- Non-pitting oedema: Qi stagnation
- Bright-yellow skin: Yang jaundice from Damp-Heat
- Dull-yellow skin: Yin jaundice from Damp-Cold
- Red venules: Heat in Blood
- Purple venules: Blood stasis
- Green venules: pain
- Blue venules: Cold in Blood
- Papules: Heat in Lungs and/or Stomach
- Vesicles: Dampness
- Macules: Blood level disharmony (red, Blood Heat; purple, Blood stasis; bluish, Cold in Blood)

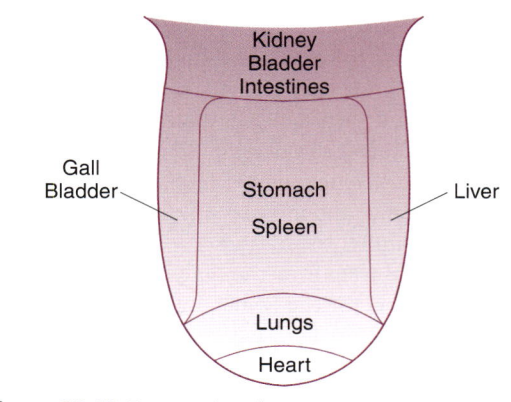

Figure 23.18 Topography of tongue

- The body colour indicates the conditions of Blood, Nutritive Qi and Yin organs: it reflects conditions of Heat or Cold, and Yin or Yang
- The body shape indicates the state of Blood and Nutritive Qi: it reflects conditions of Fullness or Deficiency
- The coating indicates the state of the Yang organs: it reflects conditions of Heat or Cold and of Fullness or Deficiency
- The moisture indicates the state of the Body Fluids

Various areas of the tongue reflect the state of the Internal Organs. A topography of the tongue in common use is as shown in Figure 23.18. As the figure

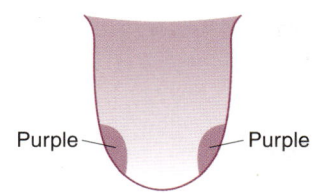

Figure 23.19 Chest areas on the tongue

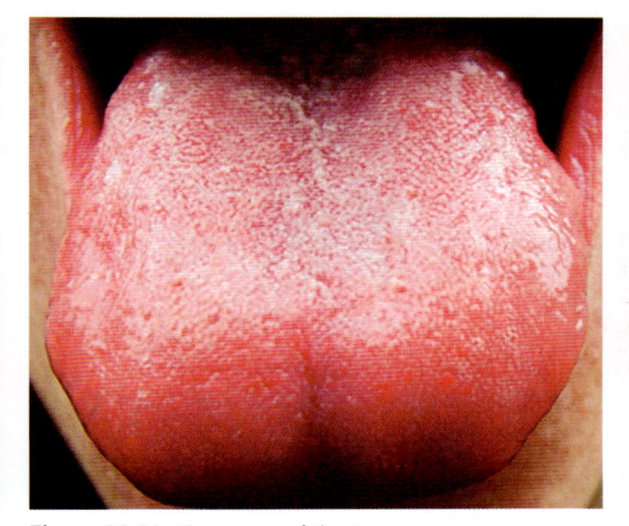

Figure 23.20 Chest areas of the tongue

shows, the sides of the tongue reflect the state of the Liver and Gall Bladder. However, the sides of the tongue towards the front reflect the chest area, which means the Heart, Lungs and breasts in women (Fig. 23.19 and Fig 23.20).

Box 23.37 summarizes items of observation in tongue diagnosis.

Box 23.37 Items of observation in tongue diagnosis

- Body colour: Blood, Nutritive Qi and Yin organs (Heat/Cold and Yin/Yang)
- Body shape: Blood and Nutritive Qi (Fullness/Deficiency)
- Coating: Yang organs (Heat/Cold and Fullness/Deficiency)
- Moisture: Body Fluids

Tongue-body colour

The normal body colour should be pale red. The body colour reflects the state of Blood and Nutritive Qi and the Yin organs; it reflects conditions of Heat or Cold and of Yin or Yang deficiency.

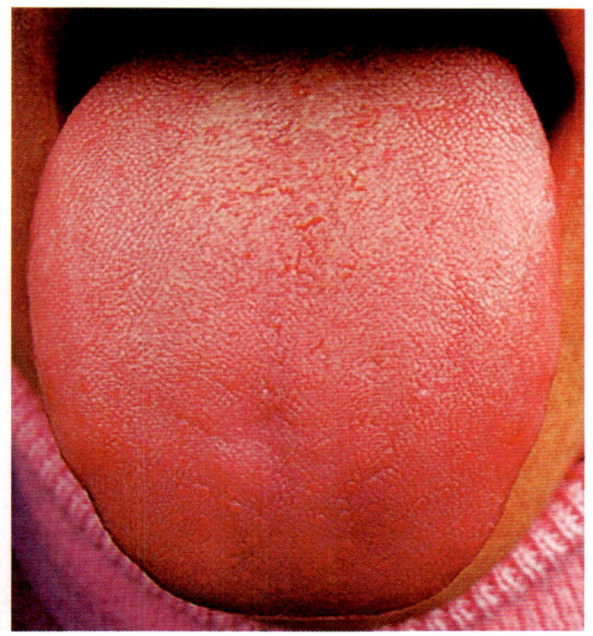

Figure 23.21 Pale tongue-body colour

There are five pathological colours: Pale, Red, Deep-Red, Purple, and Blue.

Pale

A pale body colour indicates either deficiency of Yang or deficiency of Blood. In deficiency of Yang the tongue is also usually slightly too wet, since deficient Yang Qi fails to transform and transport fluids. In deficiency of Blood the tongue tends to be somewhat dry (Fig. 23.21).

If the sides of the tongue are especially Pale, or in severe cases slightly orangey, it indicates deficiency of Liver-Blood.

Box 23.38 summarizes the Pale tongue colour.

Box 23.38 Pale tongue

- Yang deficiency (slightly wet)
- Blood deficiency (slightly dry)
- Pale sides: Liver-Blood deficiency
- Orangey sides: severe Liver-Blood deficiency

Red

By 'Red' is meant too red. A Red tongue body always indicates Heat. If the tongue has a coating, it indicates Full-Heat; if there is no coating, it indicates Empty-Heat (Fig. 23.22).

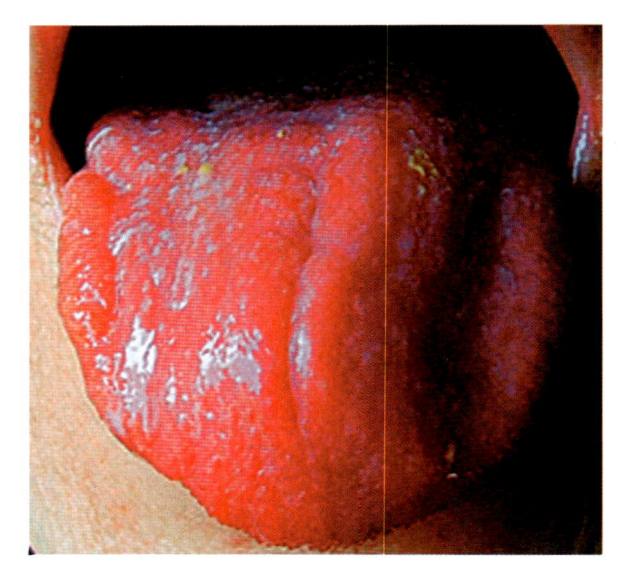

Figure 23.22 Red tongue-body colour

A Red tip, usually on a Red tongue, indicates Heart-Fire or Heart Empty-Heat, according to whether the tongue has a coating or not. In severe cases, the tip can also be swollen and have red points on it.

Red sides indicate Liver-Fire or Gall Bladder Heat if there is a coating, or Empty-Heat in the Liver if there is no coating. In severe cases they may also be swollen and display red points. A Red centre indicates Heat or Empty-Heat of the Stomach (depending on whether there is a coating or not).

Red tongues are likely to have red points or spots. These are raised papillae and always indicate Heat; if they are rather large (called 'spots' rather than 'points'), in addition to Heat, they also indicate stasis of Blood.

Red points or spots are frequently seen on the tip (Heart-Fire), on the sides (Liver-Fire), on the root (Heat in the Lower Burner) and around the centre (Stomach-Heat) (Fig. 23.23).

Box 23.39 summarizes Red tongue colour.

Deep-Red

This is simply a shade darker than Red and its clinical significance is the same as for the Red tongue, except that the condition is more severe.

Purple

A Purple tongue always indicates stasis of Blood. There are two types of Purple colour: Reddish-Purple and Bluish-Purple.

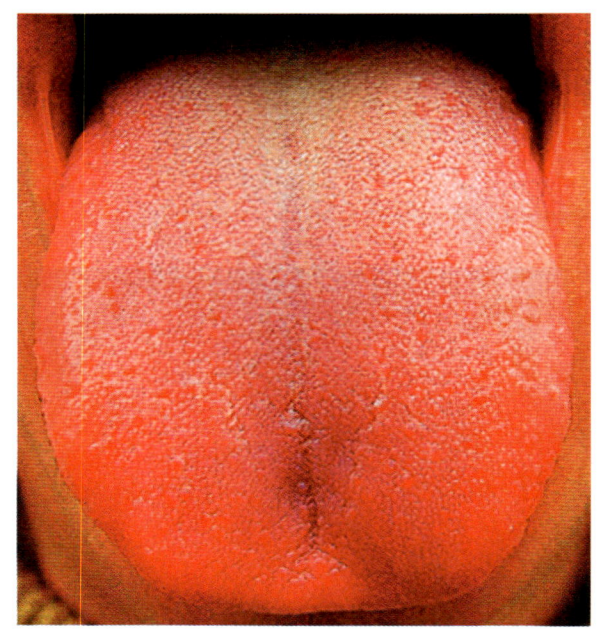

Figure 23.23 Red points on the tongue sides

Box 23.39 Red tongue

- Red: Heat
- Red with coating: Full-Heat
- Red without coating: Empty-Heat
- Red tip: Heart-Fire or Heart Empty-Heat (former with coating, latter without)
- Red sides with coating: Liver-Fire or Gall-Bladder Heat
- Red sides without coating: Liver-Yin deficiency with Empty-Heat
- Red centre: Heat or Empty-Heat of the Stomach (depending on whether there is a coating or not)
- Red points on the tip: Heart-Fire
- Red points on the sides: Liver-Fire
- Red spots on the root: Heat in the Lower Burner
- Red points in or around the centre: Stomach-Heat

A Reddish-Purple tongue indicates Heat and stasis of Blood, and it develops from a Red tongue (Fig 23.24).

A Bluish-Purple tongue indicates Cold and stasis of Blood, and it develops from a Pale tongue (Fig. 23.25).

A Purple colour is frequently seen on the sides, indicating Liver-Blood stasis, or in the centre, indicating stasis of Blood in the Stomach. A Purple colour on the sides may also reflect Blood stasis in women and, in such cases, it is usually Bluish-Purple.

Please note that most Chinese books say that a Purple tongue may indicates Qi stagnation: I do not

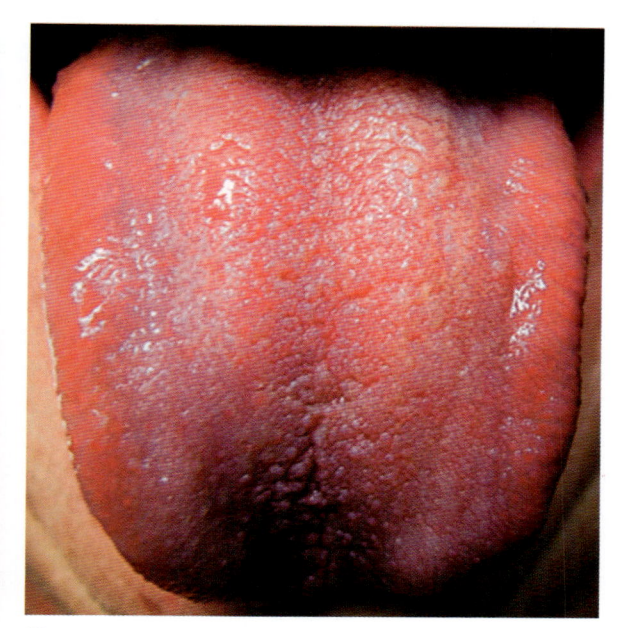

Figure 23.24 Reddish-Purple tongue

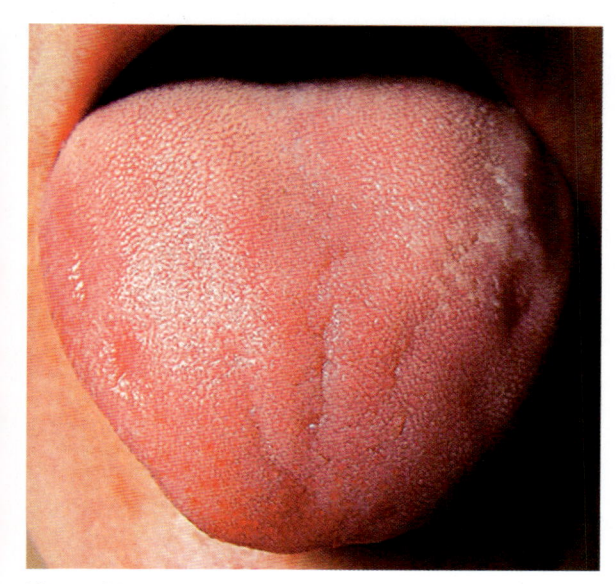

Figure 23.25 Bluish-Purple tongue

Box 23.40 Purple tongue

- Always indicates Blood stasis
- Reddish-Purple: Blood stasis from Heat
- Bluish-Purple: Blood stasis from Cold
- Reddish-Purple sides: Liver-Blood stasis
- Bluish-Purple sides in a woman: Blood stasis in the Uterus
- Purple in the centre: Blood stasis in the Stomach

Box 23.41 Tongue-body shape

- Thin: Blood or Yin deficiency (Pale or Red without coating, respectively)
- Swollen: Dampness or Phlegm
- Partially swollen: Heat
- Stiff: interior Wind or Blood stasis
- Flaccid: deficiency of Body Fluids
- Long: Heat
- Short: severe Yang or Yin deficiency (Pale or Red without coating, respectively)
- Cracked: Heat or Yin deficiency
- Quivering: Spleen-Qi deficiency
- Deviated: interior Wind
- Tooth-marked: Spleen-Qi deficiency

A Purple tongue reflects Blood stasis, not Qi stagnation

Blue

The significance of a Blue tongue is the same as a Bluish-Purple tongue: that is, Interior Cold giving rise to stasis of Blood.

Tongue-body shape

The body shape of the tongue gives an indication of Blood and Nutritive Qi and it reflects the Full or Empty character of a condition. Box 23.41 summarizes tongue-body shape.

Thin

A Thin body indicates either Blood deficiency if it is Pale, or Yin deficiency if it is Red and without coating. In both cases, it indicates that the condition is chronic.

Swollen

A Swollen tongue generally indicates retention of Dampness or Phlegm, especially the latter (Fig. 23.26).

agree. The tongue-body colour reflects Blood more than Qi and Qi stagnation often may not manifest on the tongue at all. In my experience, if the tongue is Purple, it always reflects Blood stasis.

Box 23.40 summarizes Purple tongue colour.

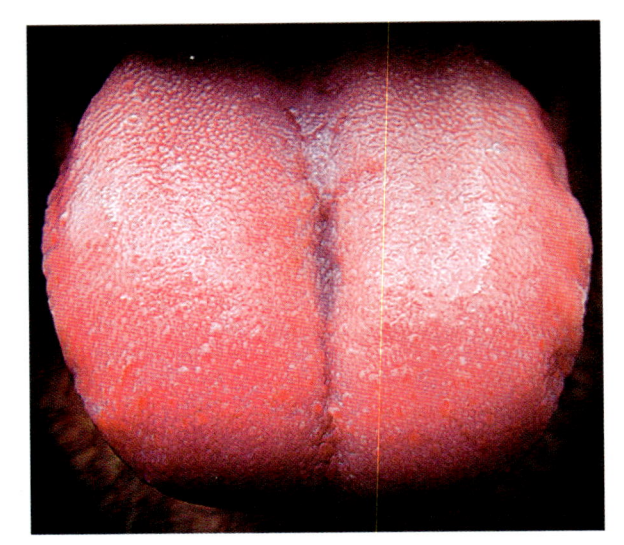

Figure 23.26 Swollen tongue

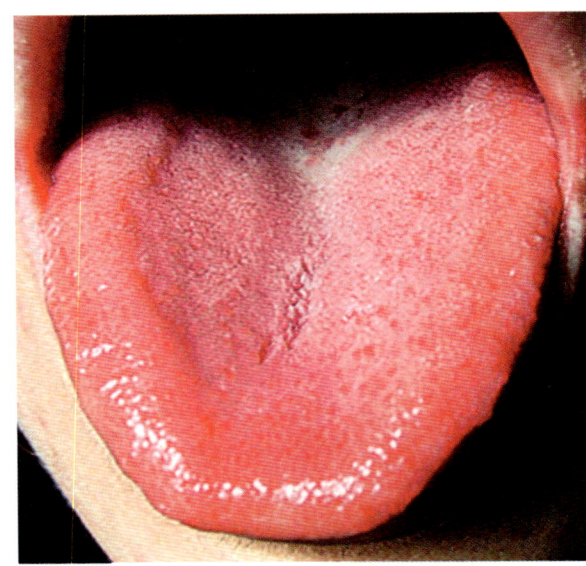

Figure 23.28 Swollen tongue sides (Spleen area)

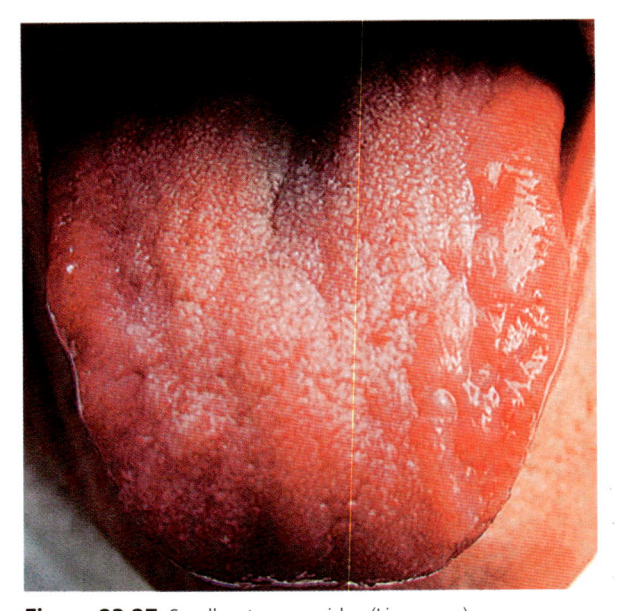

Figure 23.27 Swollen tongue sides (Liver area)

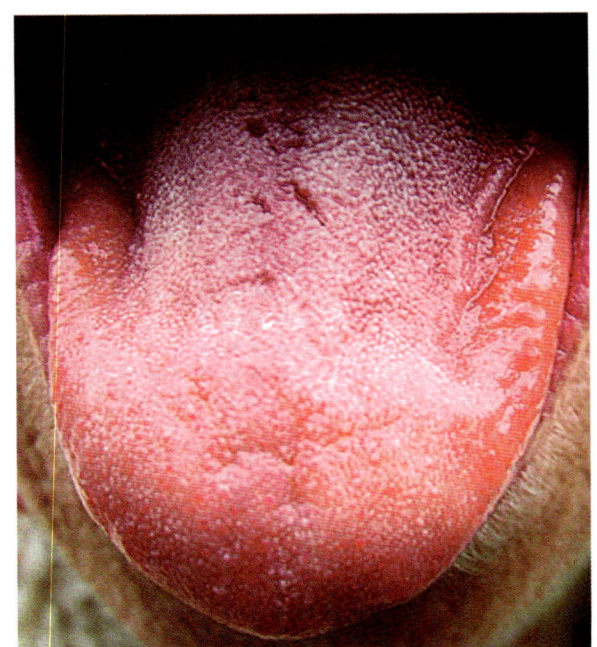

Figure 23.29 Swollen Lung area of tongue

A partial swelling usually indicates Heat. A swollen red tip indicates severe Heart-Fire while swollen and red sides indicate Liver-Fire (Fig. 23.27).

Swollen sides that are wider, usually on a Pale tongue, reflect Spleen deficiency (Fig. 23.28). A swelling in the front third of the tongue indicates Phlegm in the Lungs (Fig. 23.29).

Stiff

A Stiff tongue usually indicates interior Wind or Blood stasis (Fig. 23.30).

Flaccid

A Flaccid tongue indicates deficiency of Body Fluids.

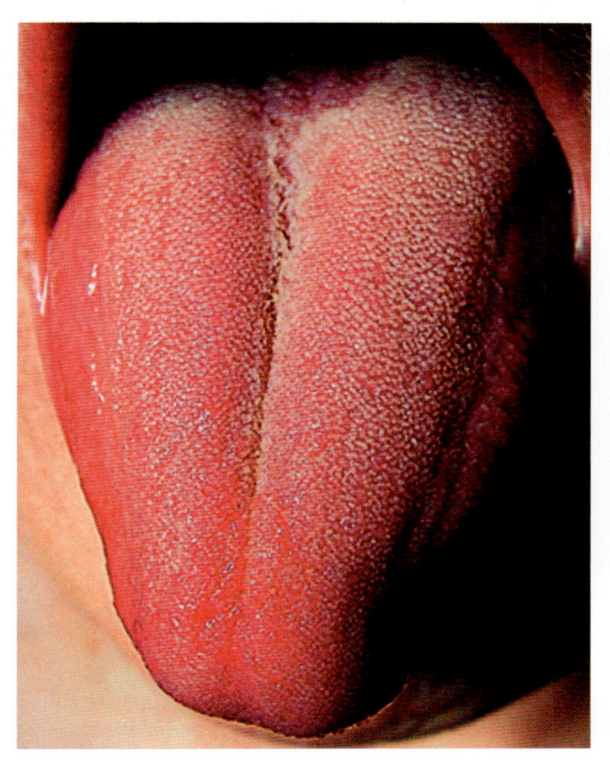

Figure 23.30 Stiff tongue

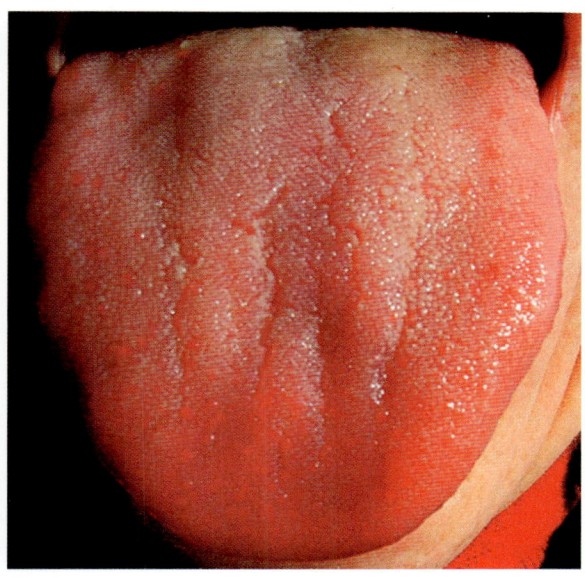

Figure 23.31 Stomach cracks

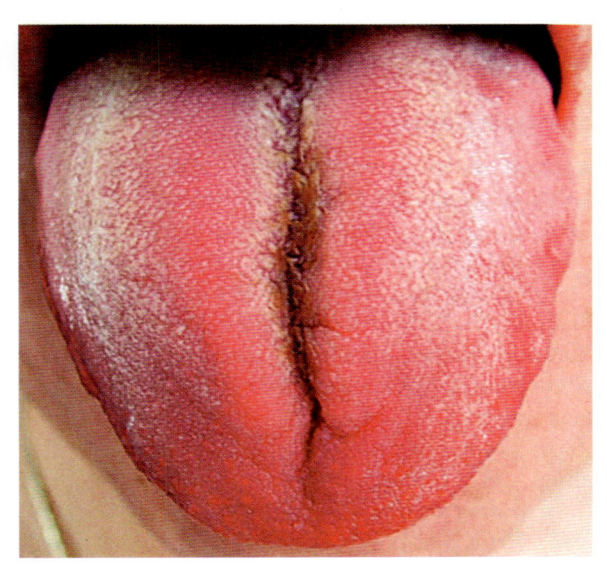

Figure 23.32 Heart crack

Long

A Long tongue indicates tendency to Heat, and in particular Heart-Heat.

Short

A Short tongue indicates interior Cold if it is Pale and wet, or extreme deficiency of Yin if it is Red and Peeled.

Cracked

Cracks indicate either Full-Heat or deficiency of Yin. Short horizontal or vertical cracks indicate Stomach-Yin deficiency (Fig. 23.31). A long-deep midline crack reaching the tip indicates a tendency to a Heart pattern: I call this a 'Heart crack' (Fig. 23.32).

A shallow, wide crack in the midline not reaching the tip indicates Stomach-Yin deficiency: I call this a 'Stomach crack' (Fig. 23.33).

Short, transverse cracks on the sides, in the middle section of the tongue, indicate chronic Spleen-Qi or Spleen-Yin deficiency.

Quivering

A Quivering tongue usually indicates Spleen-Qi deficiency.

Deviated

A Deviated tongue indicates interior Wind.

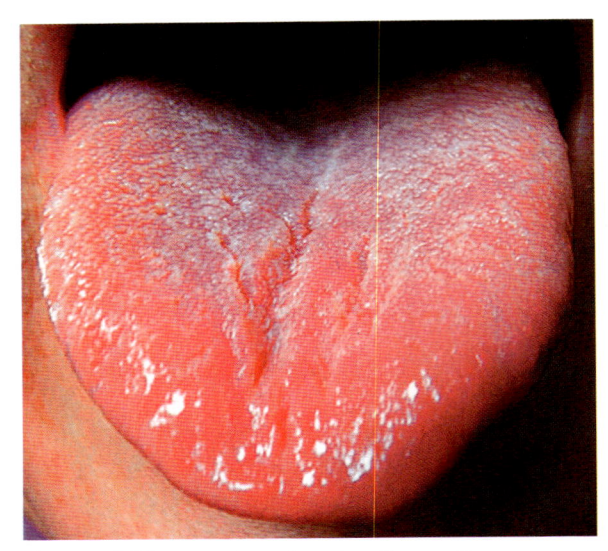

Figure 23.33 Stomach crack and rootless coating

Toothmarked

A tongue with teeth marks indicates Spleen-Qi deficiency.

Tongue coating

The tongue coating reflects the state of the Yang organs and in particular the Stomach. It reflects conditions of Heat or Cold and of Fullness or Deficiency.

A normal tongue should have a thin white coating. The tongue coating is formed from some residual 'dirty dampness', which is left over from the Stomach's digestion and reaches the tongue upwards. Thus, a thin white coating indicates that the Stomach is digesting food properly.

The coating gives an indication of the presence or absence of a pathogenic factor and of its strength. A thick coating always indicates the presence of a pathogenic factor and the thicker the coating the stronger the pathogenic factor. Such a pathogenic factor may be exterior or interior, such as exterior Wind, Dampness (interior or exterior), Cold, retention of Food, Phlegm, Heat, Fire.

A coating 'without root' looks as if the coating had been added to the tongue rather than growing out of it (see Fig. 23.33): this indicates deficiency of Stomach-Qi. The partial absence of coating indicates deficiency of Stomach-Yin (Fig. 23.34); the total absence of coating indicates deficiency of Stomach-Yin

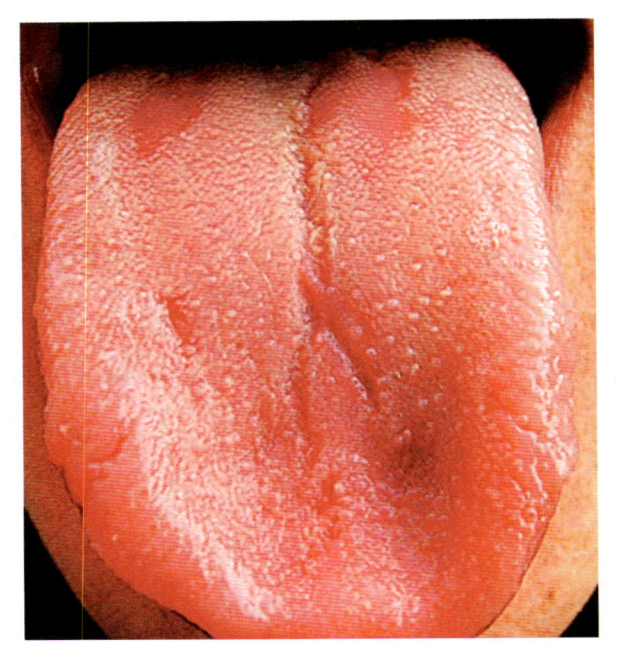

Figure 23.34 Partially peeled tongue

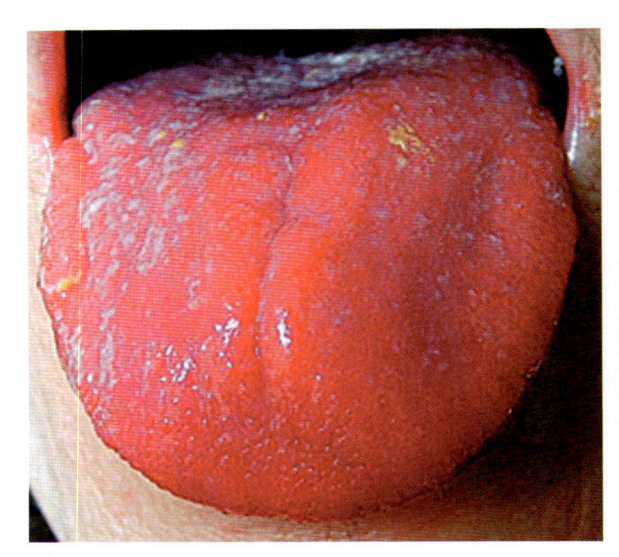

Figure 23.35 Completely peeled tongue

and/or Kidney-Yin (Fig. 23.35). If the tongue is also Red all over, it is a definite indication of deficient Kidney-Yin with Empty-Heat.

The pathological coating colours can be white, yellow, grey or black.

A white coating indicates a Cold pattern (unless of course, it is thin and white, in which case it is normal).

A yellow coating indicates a Full-Heat pattern.

A grey and black coating can indicate either extreme Cold or extreme Heat, according to whether the tongue is wet or dry.

Box 23.42 summarizes tongue coating signs.

Box 23.42 Tongue coating

- Reflects the state of the Yang organs and in particular the Stomach
- Reflects conditions of Heat/Cold and Fullness/Deficiency
- Normal coating is thin white
- Thick coating: pathogenic factor (the thicker the coating, the stronger the pathogenic factor)
- Absence of coating: Stomach-Yin deficiency
- Total absence of coating, Red tongue body: Stomach- and Kidney-Yin deficiency with Empty-Heat
- White coating: Cold pattern
- Yellow coating: Full-Heat pattern
- Grey and black coating: extreme Cold or extreme Heat (tongue wet or dry, respectively)

Moisture

The amount of moisture on a tongue gives an indication of the state of Body Fluids. Whenever the tongue is Red or Deep-Red, one should check the moisture: if the tongue is also dry, it means that the Heat has begun to injure the Body Fluids.

A normal tongue should be very slightly moist, indicating that the Body Fluids are intact and are being properly transformed and transported.

If the tongue is too wet, it indicates that Yang Qi is not transforming and transporting fluids and these accumulate to form Dampness.

If it is dry, it may indicate either Full-Heat or Empty-Heat, according to whether the tongue has a coating or not.

If the coating is sticky or slippery, it indicates retention of Dampness or Phlegm.

Box 23.43 summarizes tongue moisture signs.

Box 23.43 Moisture of tongue

- Indicates state of Body Fluids
- Normal tongue is slightly moist
- Too wet: Yang deficiency
- Too dry: Heat or Yin deficiency
- Sticky/slippery: Dampness and/or Phlegm

CHANNELS

Manifestations occurring along the channels can be an important aid to diagnosis. Any findings arising from channel diagnosis, however, should always be integrated with all the others, and treatment should never be solely based on subjective or objective manifestations appearing along a channel.

Apart from the 14 main channels, there are a great number of other secondary channels which form an intricate web distributing Qi and Blood all over the body. Channels should not be seen as 'lines' running in the body, but rather like areas of influence over a certain tridimensional section of the body.

The secondary channels are:

- The Connecting channels (*Luo Mai*)
- The Muscle channels (*Jing Jin*)
- The Divergent channels (*Jing Bie*)
- The Cutaneous regions

In addition, the Connecting channels branch out into two types of very minute channels, which are the Minute Connecting channels and the Superficial Connecting channels.[12] Moreover, the Connecting channels also have a deep level (beyond that of the Main channel) that is related to Blood: these are called the Deep, or Blood Connecting channels.

It is the superficial, capillary-like channels that are particularly important in producing the diagnostic signs that may appear along the course of a channel. Often their manifestations are a result of 'percolation' from the deep, Blood Connecting channels. For example, the small, purple distended venules appearing under the skin are, from the Chinese point of view, due to stasis of Blood in the Blood Connecting channels.

Channel diagnosis is based on both objective signs and subjective feelings experienced along the course of a channel. Objective signs include redness, white streaks, purple venules, purple spots, skin rashes following a definite channel pathway, flaccidity, hardness and a feeling of cold or heat. Anything that can be seen along a channel is due to the small Connecting channels, such as the Minute, Blood or Superficial Connecting channels. Generally speaking, the appearance of the above signs along the course of a channel by itself indicates an Excess condition of the channel. For example, a greenish colour indicates Qi stagnation in the channel or severe pain, a reddish colour indicates

Box 23.44 Connecting channel manifestations

- Greenish: Qi stagnation or pain
- Reddish: Heat in the channel
- Bluish: Cold in the channel

retention of Heat in the channels and a white colour indicates retention of Cold.

Box 23.44 summarizes Connecting Channel manifestations.

The objective feeling of heat or cold along a channel indicates retention of Heat or Cold, respectively. Flaccidity of the muscle along the course of a channel indicates a Deficient condition and that the channel is starved of Qi and Blood. This sign is often seen in Atrophy Syndrome. Rigidity or hardness of a muscle along the course of a channel indicates an Excess condition: this could be due to retention of Cold in the channel or to stagnation of Liver-Qi.

Learning outcomes

In this chapter you will have learned:

- The fundamental diagnostic principle that parts of the body reflect pathological changes of the whole
- The importance of paying attention to a patient's constitutional type
- How to observe the presence or absence of spirit in the patient's complexion, eyes, state of mind and breathing
- The signs and significance of the various constitutional body types
- The clinical meaning of changes in the tissues and other parts of the body
- How demeanour and body movement provide important diagnostic information
- Signs of health or disharmony in the hair, face colour and complexion
- The diagnostic significance of different areas of the face
- How observation of the patient's eyes provides valuable diagnostic information
- Signs of health and disharmony as manifested by the nose and ears
- Indications of disharmony manifested in the mouth, lips, teeth and gums
- The diagnostic significance of changes in the pharynx and tonsils
- How the limbs reflect pathological changes
- Diagnostic signs in the nails, thenar eminence and index finger of babies
- How the skin shows up various internal pathologies
- The importance of the tongue as a pillar of diagnosis, with information principally obtained by observing the body colour, body shape, coating and moisture
- Diagnostic signs as manifested along the channels

Self-assessment questions

1. Name four microsystems often used in diagnosis, where the whole is represented in microcosm in the part.
2. In which four main areas would one look to observe the presence of '*Shen*'?
3. Give three attributes which suggest a Fire constitutional body type.
4. Which two signs indicate a poor Metal constitution?
5. Which patterns might a thin and emaciated body point to?
6. Which pattern is suggested by continuous fidgeting of the legs?
7. A patient regularly experiences a twitching in her eyelid and cheek. Her tongue is rather Thin and Pale. Which pattern do you suspect?
8. Which two attributes of the complexion indicate 'Spirit' and 'Stomach-Qi', and thus a good prognosis?
9. You suspect the presence of Damp-Heat. Which colours might you look for on the face to confirm whether there is a prevalence of Dampness or Heat?
10. The tip of the nose reflects the state of which organ?
11. A patient's lips are red and chapped and he suffers from painful, bleeding gums. Which pattern do you suspect?
12. Describe the two different kinds of oedema and their significance.
13. Which internal pathogenic factors are the most common causes of tremor in the elderly?
14. The thenar eminence shows the state of which organ?
15. Purple venules on the skin suggest which pattern?
16. Which pattern is suggested by a tongue with a red central area and without coating?
17. Cracks on the tongue tend to indicate which patterns?
18. What does a thick tongue coating always indicate?
19. What pathological process is indicated by a very wet tongue?
20. What is the significance of flaccidity of muscles along the course of a channel?

See p. 1261 for answers

END NOTES

1. 1979 The Yellow Emperor's Classic of Internal Medicine – Simple Questions (*Huang Di Nei Jing Su Wen* 黄帝内经素问), People's Health Publishing House, Beijing, first published *c.*100 BC, p. 189.
2. 1981 Spiritual Axis (*Ling Shu Jing* 灵枢经), People's Health Publishing House, Beijing, first published *c.*100 BC, p. 97.
3. Zhang Shu Sheng 1995 Great Treatise of Diagnosis by Observation in Chinese Medicine (*Zhong Hua Yi Xue Wang Zhen Da Quan* 中华医学望诊大全), Shanxi Science Publishing House, Taiyuan, p. 38.
4. Simple Questions, p. 86.
5. Cited in Zhang Shu Sheng 1995 Great Treatise of Diagnosis by Observation in Chinese Medicine, p. 82.
6. Principles of Medical Practice, cited in Wang Ke Qin 1988 Theory of the Mind in Chinese Medicine (*Zhong Yi Shen Zhu Xue Shuo* 中医神主学说), Ancient Chinese Medical Texts Publishing House, Beijing, p. 56.
7. Cited in Great Treatise of Diagnosis by Observation in Chinese Medicine, p. 89.
8. Spiritual Axis, ch. 80, p. 151–152.

9. Guangdong College of Traditional Chinese Medicine 1964 A Study of Diagnosis in Chinese Medicine (*Zhong Yi Zhen Duan Xue* 中医诊断学), Shanghai Scientific Publishing House, p. 34–35.
10. Nanjing College of Traditional Chinese Medicine 1978 A Study of Warm Diseases (*Wen Bing Xue* 温病学), Shanghai Scientific Publishing House, p. 53.
11. This is only a brief account of tongue diagnosis. For a detailed discussion of tongue diagnosis in clinical practice see Maciocia G 1995 Tongue Diagnosis in Chinese Medicine, Eastland Press, Seattle.
12. Comprehensive Text, p. 90.

PART 4

Diagnosis by Interrogation   24

Key contents

Nature of diagnosis by interrogation

Nature of 'symptoms' in Chinese medicine

The art of interrogation: asking the right questions

Terminology problems in interrogation

Procedure for interrogation

Identification of patterns and interrogation

Tongue and pulse diagnosis: integration with interrogation

The 10 traditional questions

Three new questions for Western patients
Questions on emotional state
Questions about sexual life
Questions on energy levels

The 16 questions
 1. *Pain*
 2. *Food and taste*
 3. *Stools and urine*
 4. *Thirst and drink*
 5. *Energy levels*
 6. *Head, face and body*
 7. *Chest and abdomen*
 8. *Limbs*
 9. *Sleep*
 10. *Sweating*
 11. *Ears and eyes*
 12. *Feeling of cold, feeling of heat and fever*
 13. *Emotional symptoms*
 14. *Sexual symptoms*
 15. *Women's symptoms*
 16. *Children's symptoms*

Diagnosis by interrogation is one of the four pillars of the Chinese diagnostic methods and one that should always be carried out. If the patient is unconscious, or is a baby or a small child, the questions should be put to a close relative.

Before discussing each of the questions, I shall make some general remarks on the nature of diagnosis by interrogation and this discussion will include the following points:

- Nature of diagnosis by interrogation
- Nature of 'symptoms' in Chinese medicine
- The art of interrogation: asking the right questions
- Terminology problems in interrogation
- Procedure for interrogation
- Identification of patterns and interrogation
- Tongue and pulse diagnosis: integration with interrogation
- The 10 traditional questions
- Three new questions for Western patients
   - Questions on emotional state
   - Questions about sexual life
   - Questions on energy levels
- The 16 questions

After this initial discussion, the individual questions discussed are:

 1. Pain
    Aetiology and pathology of pain
 2. Food and taste
    Food
    Taste
    Vomit
 3. Stools and urine
    Stools
       Constipation
       Diarrhoea

Urine
  Function
  Pain
  Colour
  Amount
4. Thirst and drink
5. Energy levels
6. Head, face and body
  Head
    Headache
      Onset
      Time of day
      Location
      Character of pain
      Condition
    Dizziness
  Face
    Feeling of heat of the face
    Facial pain
    Runny nose
    Bleeding gums
    Mouth ulcers
    Cold sores
  Body
    Pain in the whole body
    Backache
    Numbness
7. Chest and abdomen
  Chest
  Hypochondrium
  Epigastrium
  Abdomen
  Hypogastrium
8. Limbs
  Weakness of the limbs
  Numbness/tingling of the limbs
  Generalized joint pain
  Muscle ache in the limbs
  Difficulty in walking
  Tremor of limbs
  Cold hands
  Weak knees
  Cold feet
  Feeling of heaviness of the limbs
9. Sleep
  Insomnia
  Lethargy
10. Sweating
  Area of body
  Time of day
  Condition of illness
  Quality of sweat
11. Ears and eyes
  Ears
    Tinnitus
      Onset
      Pressure
      Character of noise
    Deafness
  Eyes
    Eye pain
    Blurred vision
    Dry eyes
12. Feeling of cold, feeling of heat and fever
  Interior conditions
    Feeling of cold
    Feeling of heat
  Exterior conditions
    Aversion to cold
    'Fever'
    Simultaneous aversion to cold and fever
    Feeling of heat in diseases of exterior origin
    Alternating feeling of cold and feeling of heat
13. Emotional symptoms
  Depression
  Fear/anxiety
  Irritability/anger
  Worry/overthinking
  Sadness and grief
14. Sexual symptoms
  Men
    Impotence
    Lack of libido
    Premature ejaculation
    Tiredness and dizziness after ejaculation
  Women
    Lack of libido
    Headache soon after orgasm
15. Women's symptoms
  Menstruation
    Cycle
    Amount
    Colour
    Quality
    Pain
  Leucorrhoea
    Colour
    Consistency
    Smell

Pregnancy
Childbirth
16. Children's symptoms
Digestive symptoms
Respiratory symptoms and earache
Sleep
Immunizations

NATURE OF DIAGNOSIS BY INTERROGATION

We can distinguish two aspects to the interrogation: a general one and a specific one (Box 24.1).

In a **general** sense, the interrogation is the talk between doctor and patient to find out how the presenting problem arose, the living and working conditions of the patient and his or her emotional and family environment. The aim of an investigation of these aspects of the patient's life is ultimately to find the cause or causes of the disease rather than to identify the pattern; finding the causes of the disease is important in order for the patient and doctor to work together to try to eliminate or minimize such causes.

In a **specific** sense, the interrogation aims at identifying the prevailing pattern (or patterns) of disharmony in the light of whatever pattern identification is applicable (e.g. according to the Internal Organs, according to the channels, according to the Four Levels, etc.).

It is important not to blur the distinction between these two aspects of interrogation: enquiring about the patient's family situation, environment, work and relationships gives us an idea of the *cause*, not the *pattern* of the disharmony.

I personally concentrate first on the clinical manifestations to identify the patterns involved. It is only after I have come to a conclusion about the patterns involved that I ask general questions about lifestyle, work, emotions, sexual life, family life, diet, etc., in order to try and find the cause of the disease.

During the course of the interrogation, we ask about many symptoms which may be apparently unrelated to the presenting problem: we do this in order to find the pattern (or patterns) of disharmony which underlie the presenting problem.

Not all symptoms and signs add up to one pattern of disharmony: indeed, most patients will suffer from at least two *related* patterns of disharmony.

NATURE OF 'SYMPTOMS' IN CHINESE MEDICINE

Diagnosis by interrogation is based on the fundamental principle that symptoms and signs reflect the condition of the Internal Organs and channels. The concept of symptoms and signs in Chinese medicine is broader than in Western medicine. Whilst Western medicine mostly takes into account symptoms and signs as subjective and objective manifestations of a disease, Chinese medicine takes into account many different manifestations as parts of a whole picture, many of them not related to an actual disease process. Chinese medicine uses not only 'symptoms and signs' as such but also many other manifestations to form a picture of the disharmony present in a particular person.

Thus, the interrogation extends well beyond the 'symptoms and signs' pertaining to the presenting complaint. For example, if a patient presents with epigastric pain as the chief complaint, a Western doctor would enquire about the symptoms strictly relevant to that complaint: 'Is the pain better or worse after eating?', 'Does the pain come immediately after eating or 2 hours later?', 'Is there regurgitation of food?', etc.

A Chinese doctor would ask similar questions but many others too, such as 'Are you thirsty?', 'Do you have a bitter taste in your mouth?', 'Do you feel tired?', etc. Many of the so-called symptoms and signs of Chinese medicine would not be considered as such in Western medicine. For example, *absence* of thirst (which confirms a Cold condition), incapacity to make decisions (which points to a deficiency of the Gall Bladder), a dislike of speaking (which indicates a deficiency of the Lungs), a propensity to outbursts of anger (which confirms the rising of Liver-Yang or Liver-Fire), a desire to lie down (which indicates a weakness of the Spleen), a dull appearance of the eyes (which points to a disturbance of the mind and emotional problems), a deep midline crack on the tongue (which is a sign of propensity to deep emotional problems), and so on.

Whenever I refer to 'symptoms and signs' (which I shall also call 'clinical manifestations'), it will be in the above context.

Box 24.1 The two aspects of interrogation

- **General**: asking about lifestyle, work, emotions, diet, etc., to determine the cause of disease
- **Specific**: asking about clinical manifestations to determine the patterns of disharmony

4

THE ART OF INTERROGATION: ASKING THE RIGHT QUESTIONS

Diagnosis by interrogation is of course extremely important as, in the process of identifying a pattern, not all the information is given by the patient. Indeed, even if it were, it would still need to be organized in order to identify the pattern or patterns. Sometimes the absence of a certain symptom or sign is diagnostically determinant and patients, of course, would not report symptoms they do not experience. For example, in distinguishing between a Heat and a Cold pattern, it is necessary to establish whether a person is thirsty or not, and the absence of thirst would point to a Cold pattern. The patient would obviously not volunteer the information of '*not* being thirsty'.

The art of diagnosis by interrogation consists in asking relevant questions in relation to a specific patient and a specific condition. A certain pattern may be diagnosed only when the 'right' questions are asked: if we are not aware of a specific pattern and do not ask relevant questions, we will never arrive at a correct diagnosis. For example, if we do not know the existence of the pattern of Rebellious Qi of the Penetrating Vessel, we will obviously not ask the questions which might lead us to diagnose such a pattern (Fig. 24.1).

The interrogation should not consist of blindly following the traditional list of questions; it should be conducted in a flexible way following a 'lead', with our asking a series of questions to confirm or exclude a pattern (or patterns) of disharmony that comes to our mind during the exchange of question and response. Therefore, when we ask the patient a question, we should always ask ourselves *why* we are asking that question. During an interrogation, we should be constantly shifting or reviewing our hypotheses about the possible patterns of disharmony, trying to confirm or exclude certain patterns by asking the right questions.

Remember: the questions asked during the interrogation must always be guided by our attempt to confirm or exclude a pattern of disharmony

TERMINOLOGY PROBLEMS IN INTERROGATION

A potential problem for practitioners in the West is that the interrogation and the various expressions used to express symptoms are derived from Chinese experiences and culture; a Western patient would not necessarily use the same expressions. This is a problem, however, that can be overcome with experience. After some years of practice, we can learn to translate the Chinese way of expressing symptoms and find correlations more common to Western patients. For example, whereas a Chinese patient might spontaneously say that he has a 'distending pain', an English-speaking Western patient might say that he feels 'bloated' or 'bursting'. The words are different, but the symptom they describe is the same. With practice and acute observation we gradually build up a 'vocabulary' of symptoms as described by Western patients.

The translation from Chinese of the terms related to certain symptoms may also present some problems. The traditional terms are rich with meaning and sometimes very poetic and are more or less impossible to translate properly because Western language cannot convey all the nuances intrinsic in a Chinese character.

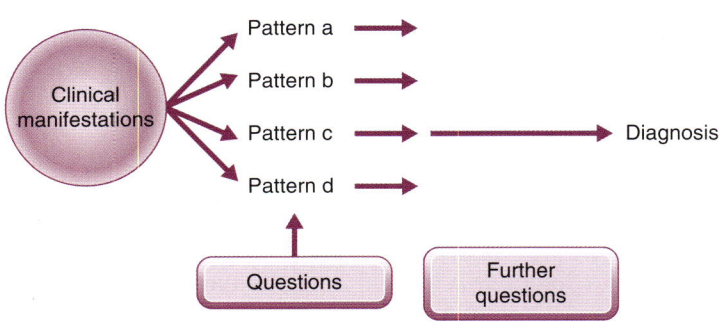

Figure 24.1 Asking the right questions

For example, I translate the word *men* as a 'feeling of oppression': an analysis of the Chinese character, however, which portrays a heart squashed by a door, conveys the feeling of oppression in a rich, metaphorical way. What cannot be adequately translated is the cultural use of this term in China often to imply that the person is rather 'depressed' (as we intend this term in the West) from emotional problems. As Chinese patients seldom admit openly to being 'depressed', they will often say they experience a feeling of *men* in the chest.

We should not, however, overemphasize the terminology problems caused by cultural differences between China and the West. Quite frequently, Western patients report symptoms exactly as they are in Chinese books. For example, a patient recently told me quite spontaneously '*I am often thirsty but I do not feel like drinking*'. This is of course a symptom of Damp-Heat as the Heat makes one thirsty and the Dampness makes one dislike drinking.

PROCEDURE FOR INTERROGATION

The interrogation generally follows on from the observation of the patient's facial colour, body shape and body movement and hearing the patient's voice and other sounds: thus observation precedes interrogation. As soon as the patient comes in, the diagnostic process has already started: we observe the movement of the patient (whether slow or quick, for example), the complexion, the body shape, to assess it in terms of Five Elements, the sound of the voice, and any smell emanating from the patient.

I usually start the interrogation by asking the patient about the main problems that brings him or her to me: I let the patient speak freely first without interrupting. I always make a note of any peculiar expressions the patient might use. As the patient is describing the main problem or problems, I am already thinking of various patterns of disharmony that might be causing it or them, and I therefore start asking questions to confirm or exclude the particular pattern of disharmony I had in mind.

After the patient has finished reporting the main problems for which he or she is seeking help, and after I have broadly decided on the patterns of disharmony involved, I then proceed to ask more questions, generally following either the traditional 10 questions or the 16 questions that are indicated below, but not in a rigid way. This is done for two reasons: first, because the answers to these further questions may confirm the patterns of disharmony diagnosed and, secondly, because they may bring up other problems that the patient has overlooked.

I generally look at the tongue and feel the pulse again towards the end of the interrogation to further confirm the patterns of disharmony. However, it is important to note that the tongue and pulse are not simply used to confirm the diagnosis of a pattern of disharmony: very often they clearly show the existence of other patterns which were not evident from the symptoms and signs. In this case, we should never discount the findings of the tongue and pulse but we should always ask further questions to confirm the patterns of disharmony shown by them.

Box 24.2 summarizes the procedure for interrogation.

IDENTIFICATION OF PATTERNS AND INTERROGATION

After the patient has finished describing the main problem or problems, we start asking questions to organize the presenting symptoms and signs into patterns. While we ask questions, we still observe the complexion, eyes, shape of facial features, sound of voice, smells, etc., to be integrated with the findings from the interrogation.

Once we are reasonably confident that we have identified the pattern or patterns involved, we must

---

Box 24.2 Procedure for interrogation

1. Observe first as the patient comes in (movement, complexion, eyes)
2. Listen to tone of voice
3. Ask about main problem
4. While asking, think about possible patterns
5. Ask specific questions to determine the pattern or patterns of disharmony causing the presenting problem or problems, trying to establish the time of onset accurately
6. Ask questions to confirm or exclude other patterns
7. Ask more questions broadly (not rigidly) following the 16 questions
8. Ask about past diseases and operations
9. Look at the tongue and feel the pulse
10. Ask about any family illness
11. Enquire about the patient's emotional life, family life and work conditions to try and establish the cause of the disease

continue the interrogation often to *exclude* or confirm the presence of other patterns that may stem from the existing ones. For example, if there is Liver-Blood deficiency, I would always check whether there is Heart-Blood deficiency (especially if the observation leads me to believe this); if there is a Liver deficiency, in women especially, I would always check whether there is a Kidney deficiency; if there is Liver-Qi stagnation, I would check whether this has given rise to some Heat; if there is a Spleen deficiency, I would check whether there is also a Stomach deficiency, etc.

TONGUE AND PULSE DIAGNOSIS: INTEGRATION WITH INTERROGATION

Finally, I look at the tongue and feel the pulse: this is done not only to *confirm* the pattern or patterns identified from the interrogation but also to see whether the tongue and pulse indicate the presence of patterns not evident from the clinical manifestations. This occurs frequently in practice and is the real value of tongue and pulse diagnosis: if tongue and pulse diagnosis were used simply to *confirm* a diagnosis, there would be no point in carrying out this step.

Very often the tongue and pulse add valuable information to the findings from interrogation and should never be discounted. For example, a patient may complain of various symptoms and we diagnose Liver-Qi stagnation: if the tongue has a deep Heart crack, this tells us that the patient has a constitutional tendency to Heart patterns and a constitutional tendency to be more affected by emotional problems.

Another very good example is when the pulse is very weak on both Kidney positions (this is especially common in women) and yet the patient (especially if still young) has no symptoms of Kidney deficiency whatsoever. I would always consider such a pulse picture indicative of a Kidney deficiency. I *never* discount what I find from the pulse.

Remember: the tongue and pulse may indicate the presence of patterns not evident from the clinical manifestations

In conclusion, this is the order I usually follow in my interrogation:

- Ask about the presenting problem, letting the patient speak freely
- Ask specific questions to determine the pattern or patterns causing the presenting problem or problems, trying to establish the time of onset accurately
- Ask questions to exclude or confirm other patterns
- Ask more questions, broadly following the 10 (or 16) questions
- Ask about past diseases and operations
- Look at the tongue and feel the pulse
- Ask about any family illnesses such as asthma, eczema, heart disease
- Inquire about the patient's emotional life, family life and working conditions to try to establish the *cause* of the disease

THE 10 TRADITIONAL QUESTIONS

The interrogation is traditionally carried out on the basis of 10 questions. This practice was started by Zhang Jing Yue (1563–1640), but the 10 questions used by subsequent doctors differed slightly from those found in Dr Zhang's book. The 10 questions proposed by Zhang Jing Yue were as follows:

1. Aversion to cold and fever
2. Sweating
3. Head and body
4. The two excretions (stools and urine)
5. Food and drink
6. Chest and abdomen
7. Deafness
8. Thirst
9. Previous illnesses
10. Causes of disease

Besides these questions, Zhang Jing Yue added two more: one regarding women's gynaecological history and the other regarding children, which makes a total of 12 questions.

The most commonly used areas of questioning mentioned in modern Chinese books are 10 + 2:

1. Aversion to cold and fever
2. Sweating
3. Head and body
4. Chest and abdomen
5. Food and taste
6. Stools and urine
7. Sleep
8. Hearing and tinnitus
9. Thirst and drink
10. Pain

The two additional areas of questioning are added for women and children, making a total of 12. It must be stressed that not all these questions need be asked in every situation; nor are these the only possible questions, since each situation requires an individual approach and other questions may be relevant.

It should be stressed also that the very order of the 10 questions reflects the huge influence of the Chinese medical text *Shang Han Lun* (Discussion on Cold-Induced Diseases, by Zhang Zhong Jing, c.AD 200). That is why the first question is about 'chills and fever' or 'aversion to cold and fever'. This is a crucial question that is asked in acute cases to establish whether there is an acute invasion of external Wind. There is no reason why this should be the first question and, indeed, unless we see a patient with an acute invasion of Wind, we do not need to ask this question at all.

Although these are usually referred to in Chinese books as 'questions', they rather represent areas of questioning. These have varied a lot over the centuries, as different doctors placed the emphasis on different questions.

One need not necessarily follow the above order of questioning. In fact, I personally never do because the order is strongly biased towards an interrogation of a patient suffering from an acute, Exterior condition, hence the prominent place afforded to the question about 'aversion to cold and fever', which in Chinese books always comes first. In Interior conditions, I do ask about sensation of heat or cold to establish or confirm whether there is internal Cold or internal Heat, but usually towards the end of the interrogation.

There is no reason why we should limit our interrogation rigidly to the traditional 10 questions. Each patient is different, with different causes of disease and different patterns of disharmony, and we need to adapt our questions to each patient's unique situation. Moreover, we need to respond to a patient's mental state during an interrogation with sensitivity and flexibility to put a patient at ease, especially during the first consultation. It would be wrong, therefore, to ask the 10 questions routinely without adapting one's approach to the concrete situation. For example, it might well be that a patient bursts into tears as soon as he or she describes his or her main problem and we should react to this situation in a sensitive and sympathetic manner.

Remember: do not follow the traditional 'questions' rigidly

THREE NEW QUESTIONS FOR WESTERN PATIENTS

The 10 questions (or rather 12 including questions on women and children), as the basis of the interrogation in Chinese diagnosis, were formulated during the early Qing dynasty in China, thus at a time and in a culture very different than ours. We should therefore not hesitate in changing the structure and contents of our interrogation to make it more suitable to our own time and culture.

I would therefore add the following to the traditional 10 (or 12) questions:

- Emotions
- Sexual symptoms
- Energy levels

In addition, I introduce a separate area of questioning concerning the limbs, which traditionally are included under 'Body'.

Questions on emotional state

An enquiry on the emotional life of the patient plays a role both in the general enquiry to find the *cause* of the disharmony and in the specific enquiry to find the *pattern* of disharmony. A prevailing emotional state is a clinical manifestation just like any other and it is therefore an important part of the pattern of disharmony. For example, a propensity to anger is a strong indication of Liver-Yang or Liver-Fire rising, sadness often indicates a Lung deficiency, obsessive thinking points to a Spleen pattern, etc.

It may be that, for cultural reasons, there is no specific question regarding the emotional state of the patient among the traditional 10 questions: Chinese patients tend not to talk about their emotions and often express them as physical symptoms, as a kind of agreed 'code' between patient and doctor.

For example, when I was in China, I noticed that when a patient said that they felt *men* (feeling of oppression in the chest), did not sleep well and felt thirsty, it basically meant that they were depressed.

Questions about sexual life

Modern Chinese doctors never ask about sexual symptoms due to the modern Chinese prudery in sexual matters. However, this should always form part of the interrogation as it provides further information on the symptomatology of the patient to arrive at a pattern of disharmony.

Questions on energy levels

An enquiry about energy levels is extremely important as it gives a very simple clue to the presence of a possible Deficiency pattern (excluding the few cases when a person may feel tired from Excess conditions). This question is all the more important since lack of energy is probably one of the main reasons for Western people to consult a practitioner of Chinese medicine.

Three new questions added to the traditional '10 questions':
1. Emotional state
2. Sexual life
3. Energy levels

THE 16 QUESTIONS

Thus, bearing in mind the three new questions on the emotional state, sexual symptoms and energy levels and a different order of questioning, I would therefore propose to revise the traditional 10 questions, making up a total of 16 questions as follows:

1. Pain
2. Food and taste
3. Stools and urine
4. Thirst and drink
5. Energy levels
6. Head, face and body
7. Chest and abdomen
8. Limbs
9. Sleep
10. Sweating
11. Ears and eyes
12. Feeling of cold, feeling of heat and fever
13. Emotional symptoms
14. Sexual symptoms
15. Women's symptoms
16. Children's symptoms

Box 24.3 The 16 questions

1. Pain
2. Food and taste
3. Stools and urine
4. Thirst and drink
5. Energy levels
6. Head, face and body
7. Chest and abdomen
8. Limbs
9. Sleep
10. Sweating
11. Ears and eyes
12. Feeling of cold, feeling of heat and fever
13. Emotional symptoms
14. Sexual symptoms
15. Women's symptoms
16. Children's symptoms

The 16 questions suggested are not different than the traditional 10 questions (plus two for women and children): they differ only in the addition of three new questions (on the emotional state, sexual symptoms and energy levels) and in the order in which they are discussed. I have changed the order of the questions to make it more relevant to a Western clinical setting. Finally, I have split some questions into two (for example, 'Food and Drink' into 'Food and Taste' and 'Thirst and Drink') (Box 24.3).

I have relegated the questions about aversion to cold and fever to 12th place in the list because they are usually asked towards the end of the interrogation to confirm the Hot or Cold nature of a particular pattern. The prominent place afforded to aversion to cold or fever in the traditional 10 questions is due to historical reasons, for in the times when the traditional 10 questions were formulated, febrile diseases were extremely common in China and would have formed the major part of a doctor's practice.

I have placed the questions on pain in first place in the revised 16 questions because that is by far the most common problem that Western patients present in a modern practice. The question on pain is followed by questions about food, bowels, urination and thirst, again because these questions cover a very large area of digestive and urinary problems in the patients we see. The order in which the questions are listed is not necessarily that in which they are asked: for example, in women, the questions about their gynaecological system would be asked fairly early in the interrogation.

The discussion that follows will often list the clinical significance of a given symptom (e.g. 'night-sweating indicates Yin deficiency' or 'thirst indicates Heat'). It should be pointed out that this approach actually contradicts the very essence of Chinese diagnosis and patterns according to which it is the *picture* formed by a number of symptoms and signs, rather than individual symptoms, that matters. No symptom or sign can be seen in isolation from the pattern of which it forms part: it is the landscape that counts, not individual features. Thus it is wrong to say 'night-sweating indicates Yin deficiency': we should say 'in the presence of malar flush, a Red tongue without coating and a dry throat at night, night sweating indicates Yin deficiency, while in the presence of a feeling of heaviness, a sticky taste, a bitter taste, epigastric fullness, night sweating indicates Damp-Heat'. It is only for didactic purposes that we need to list symptoms and signs in isolation with their possible diagnostic significance.

Strictly speaking, assigning a clinical significance to each individual symptom contradicts the spirit of Chinese diagnosis in which, what matters is the general 'picture' formed by the symptoms

1. Pain

Pain can be caused by Full or Empty conditions. The Full or Empty character of pain should always be ascertained, especially with relation to pain experienced in the head, chest or abdomen. As a general, reliable rule, pain from a Full condition is more intense and sharper than that from an Empty condition, which tends to be dull and much less intense.

Aetiology and pathology of pain

Pain can be due to the following *Full* conditions:

- Invasion of exterior pathogenic factors
- Interior Cold or Heat
- Stagnation of Qi or Blood
- Retention of food
- Obstruction by Phlegm

In all these conditions the pathology of pain is the same: that is, the above conditions cause an obstruction to the circulation of Qi in the channels and, therefore, pain. These are all Full types of pain. There is a saying in Chinese Medicine that goes: 'If the channels are free there is no pain; if the channels are obstructed there is pain.'

Pain can also be due to the following *Empty* conditions:

- Deficiency of Qi and Blood
- Consumption of Body Fluids from Yin deficiency

These conditions cause malnourishment of the channels and hence pain. This is an Empty type of pain and would tend to be duller than the previous type (Table 24.1).

Table 24.1 Factors affecting pain

	Empty	Full	Cold	Heat
Pressure	Alleviated	Aggravated	–	–
Food	Alleviated	Aggravated	–	–
Type	Dull, lingering	Sharp	Cramping	Burning
Temperature	–	–	Alleviated by heat	Alleviated by cold
Bowel movement	Aggravated	Alleviated	Aggravated	Alleviated
Posture	Better lying down	Better sitting up	–	–
Onset	Slow, gradual	Sudden	–	–
Vomiting	Aggravated	Alleviated	Aggravated	Alleviated
Rest/movement	Better with rest	Better with movement	Better with movement	Worse with movement

The most common causes of chronic pain in internal conditions are Qi stagnation, Blood stasis and Cold.

Stagnation of Qi causes distension more than pain, or a distending pain, having no fixed location. The pain from Qi stagnation often comes and goes according to the emotional state. Very common locations for pain from Qi stagnation are the epigastrium and abdomen. 'Distension' is a translation of the Chinese term *zhang* and Western, English-speaking patients would usually describe a 'bloating' sensation.

Liver-Yang rising may be seen as a type of Qi stagnation or rather Qi rebellious, i.e. Qi going in the wrong direction: Liver-Yang rising is a very frequent cause of chronic headaches and is characterized by a distending, throbbing pain.

Stasis of Blood causes a severe, boring or stabbing pain, with a fixed location in a small area. Common locations for pain from Blood stasis are the head, chest, epigastrium, abdomen and Uterus.

Cold (whether Full or Empty) causes a cramping, spastic pain that is typically aggravated by cold weather and cold foods/liquids and alleviated by the application of heat. Common locations of pain from Cold are the epigastrium, abdomen, Uterus and joints. Cold in the Uterus is a frequent cause of painful periods in young women.

Heat does not usually cause pain unless it is accompanied by Dampness. Damp-Heat causes a burning pain accompanied by a feeling of fullness and heaviness. Common locations of pain from Damp-Heat are the forehead, epigastrium, abdomen, Uterus, Bladder and joints.

Any *exterior pathogenic factor* may cause pain, but the two most likely to do so are Wind and Dampness. For example, Wind causes occipital headache and stiffness while Dampness causes pain in the joints or epigastrium.

Retention of food is usually a cause of pain that occurs mostly in children, causing epigastric and/or abdominal pain; the pain is intense and with a feeling of fullness.

Finally, *Phlegm* does not usually cause pain, but it may do so especially in the joints (as in rheumatoid arthritis).

The location of the various types of pain is highlighted in Table 24.2. Box 24.4 summarizes causes of pain.

Box 24.4 Causes of pain

- Qi stagnation: distension more than pain, or a distending pain, no fixed location, coming and going
- Liver-Yang rising: chronic headaches with a distending, throbbing pain
- Blood stasis: severe, boring or stabbing pain, with a fixed location
- Cold (Full or Empty): cramping, spastic pain aggravated by cold weather and cold foods/liquids and alleviated by the application of heat
- Damp-Heat: burning pain with a feeling of fullness and heaviness
- External Wind: occipital headache and stiffness
- External Dampness: pain in the joints or epigastrium
- Retention of food: intense pain with feeling of fullness (more in children)
- Phlegm: does not usually cause pain, but it may do so especially in the joints (as in rheumatoid arthritis)

Table 24.2 Location of pain

	Organs	Location
Qi stagnation	Liver, Stomach, Intestines	Epigastrium, abdomen
Blood stasis	Liver, Uterus, Heart, Stomach, Intestines	Head, chest, epigastrium, abdomen, Uterus
Liver-Yang rising	Liver	Head
Cold	Stomach, Uterus, Intestines	Epigastrium, Uterus, abdomen, joints
Damp-Heat	Stomach, Uterus, Intestines, Bladder, Gall Bladder	Hypochondrium, epigastrium, abdomen, hypogastrium, Uterus, forehead, joints
External Wind	None	Occiput
External Dampness	Stomach, Intestines, Uterus	Head, epigastrium, abdomen, Uterus, Bladder, joints
Retention of food	Stomach, Intestines	Epigastrium, abdomen
Phlegm	Stomach, Intestines, Uterus	Head, epigastrium, abdomen, joints

2. Food and taste

These are very important questions aimed at establishing the state of the Stomach and Spleen. The symptoms discussed are:

- Food
- Taste
- Vomit

Food

In general, a condition that is relieved by eating is of an Empty nature; if it is aggravated by eating, it is of a Full nature.

Lack of appetite indicates Spleen-Qi deficiency. Being always hungry indicates Heat in the Stomach.

A feeling of fullness after eating indicates retention of food or Dampness. A feeling of distension indicates Qi stagnation. A sharp pain indicates Blood stasis. A feeling of heaviness indicates Dampness. A preference for hot food (in terms of temperature) indicates a Cold pattern; preference for cold food indicates a Heat pattern.

Box 24.5 summarizes patterns connected to food.

Taste

A bitter taste indicates a Full-Heat pattern, either of Liver or Heart. If it is due to Liver-Fire, the bitter taste is more or less constant. If it is due to Heart-Fire, it is associated with insomnia and is only present in the morning after a sleepless night, and not after a good night's sleep.

A sweet taste indicates either Spleen deficiency or Damp-Heat.

A sour taste indicates retention of food in the Stomach or disharmony of Liver and Stomach.

Box 24.5 Food

- Condition relieved by eating: Empty
- Condition aggravated by eating: Full
- Lack of appetite: Spleen-Qi deficiency
- Excessive hunger: Stomach-Heat
- Feeling of fullness: Dampness or retention of food
- Feeling of distension: Qi stagnation
- Feeling of heaviness: Dampness
- Sharp pain: Blood stasis
- Preference for hot foods/drinks: Cold pattern
- Preference for cold foods/liquids: Heat pattern

A salty taste indicates Kidney-Yin deficiency. Lack of taste sensation indicates Spleen deficiency.

A pungent taste indicates Lung-Heat.

Box 24.6 summarizes questions about tastes.

Box 24.6 Taste

- Lack of taste sensation: Spleen and Stomach deficiency
- Bitter taste: Heat in Liver or Heart
- Sweet taste: Spleen deficiency or Damp-Heat
- Sour taste: retention of food or Liver invading Stomach
- Salty taste: Kidney-Yin deficiency
- Pungent taste: Lung-Heat

Vomit

Box 24.7 (unnumbered above)

- Sour vomiting: invasion of Stomach by Liver
- Bitter vomiting: Liver and Gall Bladder-Heat
- Clear watery vomiting: Cold in the Stomach with retention of fluids
- Vomiting soon after eating: Heat pattern

Any vomiting which is sudden and with a loud noise indicates a Full pattern. Any vomiting which is slow in coming and with a weak noise indicates an Empty pattern.

Box 24.7 summarizes questions about vomiting.

Box 24.7 Vomit

- Sour: invasion of Stomach by Liver
- Bitter: Liver and/or Gall Bladder-Heat
- Clear, watery: Cold in Stomach
- Soon after eating: Heat in Stomach
- Sudden with loud noise: Full
- Slow in coming with weak noise: Empty

3. Stools and urine

These are two important questions to establish the Full or Empty and Hot or Cold character of a condition. The symptoms discussed are:

- Stools
  - Constipation
  - Loose stools/diarrhoea
- Urine
  - Function
  - Pain
  - Colour
  - Amount

Stools

Constipation

Aggravation of a condition after a bowel movement suggests an Empty pattern; amelioration of a condition after a bowel movement suggests a Full condition.

Acute constipation with thirst and dry yellow coating indicates Heat in the Stomach and Intestines. Constipation in old people or women after childbirth is due to deficiency of Blood. Constipation with small, dry, bitty stools like goat's stools indicates stagnation of Liver-Qi and Heat in the Intestines.

If the stools are not dry, difficulty in performing a bowel movement indicates stagnation of Liver-Qi.

Constipation with abdominal pain indicates internal Cold, which may be Full or Empty.

Constipation with dry stools, with a dry mouth and a desire to drink in small sips indicates Yin deficiency, usually of Kidneys and/or Stomach.

Box 24.8 summarizes questions about constipation.

Alternation of constipation and diarrhoea indicates that stagnant Liver-Qi is invading the Spleen.

> **Box 24.8 Constipation**
>
> - Aggravation of a condition after a bowel movement: Empty pattern
> - Amelioration of a condition after a bowel movement: Full condition
> - Acute constipation with thirst and dry yellow coating: Heat in the Stomach and Intestines
> - Constipation in old people or women after childbirth: deficiency of Blood
> - Constipation with small, dry, bitty stools like goat's stools indicates stagnation of Liver-Qi and Heat in the Intestines
> - Difficulty in performing a bowel movement (stools not dry): stagnation of Liver-Qi
> - Constipation with abdominal pain: internal Cold, which may be Full or Empty
> - Constipation with dry stools, dry mouth, desire to drink in small sips: Yin deficiency, usually of Kidneys and/or Stomach
> - Alternation of constipation and diarrhoea: stagnant Liver-Qi invading the Spleen

Diarrhoea

The most common cause of chronic diarrhoea is either Spleen-Yang deficiency, or Kidney-Yang deficiency, or both. Chronic diarrhoea occurring every day in the very early morning is due to Kidney-Yang deficiency and is called 'cock-crow diarrhoea' or also '5th-hour diarrhoea'.

If the diarrhoea is accompanied by abdominal pain, it indicates the presence of interior Cold in the Intestines.

Diarrhoea with mucus in the stools indicates Dampness in the Intestines. If there is blood too, this usually indicates Damp-Heat in the Intestines, particularly if the blood is turbid and the anus feels heavy and painful. If the blood comes out first, is bright-red and splashes in all directions, it indicates Blood-Heat.

Loose stools with undigested food indicate Spleen-Qi deficiency. If the stools are not loose or only slightly loose but are very frequent and the person cannot hold them easily, it indicates deficiency of Middle Qi (i.e. the Qi of Stomach and Spleen); it also indicates sinking of Spleen-Qi.

Box 24.9 summarizes questions about loose stools and diarrhoea.

> **Box 24.9 Loose stools/diarrhoea**
>
> - Chronic loose stools/diarrhoea: Spleen- and/or Kidney-Yang deficiency
> - Chronic diarrhoea every day in the very early morning: Kidney-Yang deficiency
> - Diarrhoea with abdominal pain: interior Cold in the Intestines
> - Diarrhoea with mucus in the stools: Dampness in the Intestines
> - Diarrhoea with mucus and blood in the stools: Damp-Heat in the Intestines
> - Loose stools with undigested food: Spleen-Qi deficiency
> - Stools not loose or only slightly loose but very frequent, patient cannot hold them easily: deficiency of Central Qi, i.e. the Qi of Stomach and Spleen with sinking of Spleen-Qi
> - Black or very dark stools: stasis of Blood
> - Blood comes first, bright-red, splashing in all directions: Damp-Heat in the Intestines
> - Blood comes first and is turbid and the anus feels heavy and painful: Heat in the Blood
> - Stools come first and then the blood, which is watery: Spleen-Qi is deficient and unable to hold Blood
> - Pain accompanying diarrhoea: Liver involvement or Heat
> - Foul-smelling stools: Heat
> - Absence of smell: Cold
> - Borborygmi with loose stools: Spleen deficiency
> - Borborygmi with abdominal distension and without loose stools: stagnation of Liver-Qi
> - Flatulence: stagnation of Liver-Qi
> - Flatulence with foul smell: Damp-Heat in the Spleen or Heat in Intestines
> - Flatulence without smell: interior Cold from Spleen-Yang deficiency
> - Burning sensation in the anus while passing stools: Heat

Black or very dark stools indicate stasis of Blood. If the blood comes first, and is bright-red splashing in all directions, it indicates Damp-Heat in the Intestines.

If the blood comes first and is turbid and the anus feels heavy and painful, it indicates Heat in the Blood.

If the stools come first and then the blood, and this is watery, it indicates that Spleen-Qi is deficient and is unable to control Blood.

Pain accompanying diarrhoea always suggests involvement of the Liver or the presence of Heat.

The presence of a foul smell indicates Heat, while the absence of smell indicates Cold.

Borborygmi (gurgling sounds in the abdomen) with loose stools indicate Spleen deficiency.

Borborygmi with a feeling of abdominal distension and without loose stools, indicate stagnation of Liver-Qi.

Flatulence is generally due to stagnation of Liver-Qi. If there is a foul smell, it indicates Damp-Heat in the Spleen or Heat in the Intestines. If there is no smell, it indicates interior Cold from Spleen-Yang deficiency.

A burning sensation in the anus while passing stools indicates Heat.

Urine

The salient diagnostic features to be considered here are the function, pain, colour and amount of urine.

Function

Enuresis or incontinence of urine indicates Kidney deficiency. Retention of urine indicates Dampness in the Bladder or occasionally Lung-Qi deficiency.

Difficulty in urination indicates either Dampness in the Bladder or deficiency of Kidney (the latter is more common in old people).

Pain

Pain before urination indicates stagnation of Qi in the Lower Burner, pain during urination indicates Damp-Heat in the Bladder and pain after urination indicates deficiency of Qi.

Colour

Pale urine indicates a Cold pattern, usually of the Bladder and Kidneys. Dark urine indicates a Heat pattern.

Turbid or cloudy urine indicates Dampness in the Bladder. Copious, clear and pale urination during an exterior invasion of Wind-Cold or Wind-Heat indicates that the pathogenic factor has not penetrated into the Interior (if it had, the urine would be dark).

Box 24.10 Urine

1. Function

- Enuresis or incontinence of urine: Kidney deficiency
- Retention of urine: Dampness in the Bladder or occasionally Lung-Qi deficiency
- Difficulty in urination: either Dampness in the Bladder or deficiency of Kidney (the latter is more common in old people)

2. Pain

- Pain before urination: stagnation of Qi in the Lower Burner
- Pain during urination: Damp-Heat in the Bladder
- Pain after urination: deficiency of Qi

3. Colour

- Pale urine: Cold pattern, usually of the Bladder and Kidneys
- Dark urine: Heat pattern
- Turbid or cloudy urine: Dampness in the Bladder
- Copious, clear and pale urination during an exterior invasion of Wind-Cold or Wind-Heat: pathogenic factor has not penetrated into the Interior (if it had, the urine would be dark)

4. Amount

- Very frequent and copious urination: Kidney-Yang deficiency
- Frequent and scanty urination: Qi deficiency
- Scanty and dark urine: Kidney-Yin deficiency

Amount

Very frequent and copious urination indicates Kidney-Yang deficiency, frequent and scanty urination is usually caused by Qi deficiency. Scanty and dark urine is due to Kidney-Yin deficiency.

Box 24.10 summarizes questions about urine.

4. Thirst and drink

Thirst with desire to drink large amounts of cold water indicates a Full-Heat pattern, which can be of any organ. Thirst with desire to drink in small sips indicates Yin deficiency (usually of Stomach or Kidneys).

Absence of thirst indicates a Cold pattern, usually of the Stomach or Spleen. Thirst but with no desire to drink indicates Damp-Heat (the Heat gives rise to the thirst, but the Dampness makes one reluctant to drink).

The desire to drink cold liquids suggests a Heat pattern; the desire to drink warm liquids suggests a Cold pattern.

Box 24.11 summarizes questions about thirst and drink.

> **Box 24.11 Thirst and drink**
>
> - Thirst with desire to drink large amounts of cold water: Full-Heat pattern
> - Thirst with desire to drink in small sips: Yin deficiency (usually of Stomach or Kidneys)
> - Absence of thirst: Cold pattern, usually of the Stomach or Spleen
> - Thirst but with no desire to drink: Damp-Heat
> - Desire to drink cold liquids: Heat pattern
> - Desire to drink warm liquids: Cold pattern

5. Energy levels

This is not one of the traditional 10 questions of Chinese diagnosis. I have added it to the list of questions because tiredness is one of the most common symptoms reported by Western patients. In my practice, about 12% of patients seek treatment specifically and only for tiredness: to these should be added all the other patients who come for other symptoms or diseases but who also suffer from chronic tiredness.

I generally ask about tiredness quite early during the interrogation and as soon as I suspect a Deficiency pattern.

When enquiring about tiredness, it is very important to enquire about the patient's lifestyle. Many people have unrealistic expectations about their level of energy. If people in industrialized societies work too much and for far too long, a feeling of tiredness is entirely normal.

Our level of energy depends also on age: again very many people have unrealistic expectations about their desired level of energy and are surprised that they cannot do at 55 what they did when they were 25.

A chronic feeling of tiredness is usually due to a deficiency. This may be a deficiency of Qi, Yang, Blood or Yin. In some cases, tiredness may also be due to a Full condition, and especially Dampness, Phlegm or Qi stagnation.

The pulse is an important sign to differentiate Full from Empty types of tiredness: Full pulse, in general (often Slippery or Wiry), indicates that the tiredness is caused by a Full condition (usually Dampness, Phlegm or Qi stagnation).

Remember: tiredness is not always due to a condition of *Deficiency*. It can be, and it often is, due to a *Full* condition

Dampness and Phlegm are 'heavy' and weigh down the body so that the person feels heavy and tired. Qi stagnation may also make a person feel tired: this is not because there is not enough Qi but because, being stagnant, Qi does not circulate properly. This situation is more common in men and it often reflects a state of mental depression.

Chronic tiredness associated with a desire to lie down, poor appetite and loose stools indicates Spleen-Qi deficiency, which is probably the most common cause of it; if there are Cold symptoms, it is due to Spleen-Yang deficiency.

Chronic tiredness associated with a weak voice and a propensity to catching colds indicates Lung-Qi deficiency; if there are Cold symptoms, it is due to Lung-Yang deficiency.

Chronic tiredness associated with backache, lassitude, a feeling of cold, depression and frequent urination indicates Kidney-Yang deficiency.

Chronic tiredness associated with slight depression, dizziness and scanty periods indicates Liver-Blood deficiency.

Chronic tiredness associated with anxiety, insomnia, a dry mouth at night and a tongue without coating is due to Kidney-Yin deficiency.

Chronic tiredness associated with a feeling of heaviness of the body and muzziness of the head indicates retention of Dampness.

Chronic tiredness associated with a feeling of oppression of the chest, dizziness and muzziness of the head indicates retention of Phlegm.

Chronic tiredness in an anxious and tense person with a Wiry pulse indicates stagnation of Liver-Qi.

Box 24.12 summarizes questions concerning tiredness.

> **Box 24.12 Tiredness**
>
> - Chronic tiredness, desire to lie down, poor appetite, loose stools: Spleen-Qi or Spleen-Yang deficiency
> - Chronic tiredness, weak voice, propensity to catching colds: Lung-Qi or Lung-Yang deficiency
> - Chronic tiredness, backache, feeling cold, frequent urination: Kidney-Yang deficiency
> - Chronic tiredness, dizziness, blurred vision, scanty periods: Liver-Blood deficiency
> - Chronic tiredness, anxiety, dry mouth at night, tongue without coating: Kidney-Yin deficiency
> - Chronic tiredness, feeling of heaviness: Dampness
> - Chronic tiredness, feeling of heaviness, muzziness, dizziness: Phlegm
> - Chronic tiredness, abdominal distension, irritability, Wiry pulse: Liver-Qi stagnation
> - Short-term tiredness, alternating hot and cold feeling, irritability, unilateral tongue coating, Wiry pulse: Lesser Yang pattern

Short-term tiredness with alternating cold and hot feeling, irritability, unilateral tongue coating and a Wiry pulse indicates the Lesser Yang pattern (either of the Six Stages or of the Four Levels).

6. Head, face and body

The symptoms discussed are:

- Head
  - Headache
    - Onset
    - Time of day
    - Location
    - Character of pain
    - Condition
  - Dizziness
- Face
  - Feeling of heat in the face
  - Facial pain
  - Runny nose
  - Bleeding gums
  - Mouth ulcers
  - Cold sores
- Body
  - Pain in the whole body
  - Backache
  - Numbness

Head

The head is the area where all the Yang channels meet, bringing clear Yang to the head and to the orifices, thus enabling the person to have clear sight, hearing, taste and smell.

Headache

This can be distinguished according to onset, time, location, character of pain and condition.

Onset

- Recent onset, short duration: headache from exterior attack of Wind-Cold
- Gradual onset, in attacks: interior type

Box 24.13 summarizes questions concerning headaches.

Time of day

- Daytime: Qi or Yang deficiency
- Evening: Blood or Yin deficiency
- Night-time: Blood stasis

Location

- Nape of neck: Greater Yang channels (can be from exterior invasion of Wind-Cold, or from interior Kidney deficiency)
- Forehead: Bright Yang channels (can be from Stomach-Heat or Blood deficiency)
- Temples and sides of head: Lesser Yang channels (can be from exterior Wind in the Lesser Yang, or from interior Liver and Gall Bladder Fire rising)
- Vertex: Terminal Yin channels (usually from deficiency of Liver-Blood)
- Whole head: exterior invasion of Wind-Cold

Box 24.13   Headache

Onset

- Recent onset, short duration: headache from exterior attack of Wind-Cold
- Gradual onset, in attacks: interior type

Time of day

- Daytime: Qi or Yang deficiency
- Evening: Blood or Yin deficiency
- Night-time: Blood stasis

Location

- Nape of neck: Greater Yang channels (can be from exterior invasion of Wind-Cold, or from interior Kidney deficiency)
- Forehead: Bright Yang channels (can be from Stomach-Heat or Blood deficiency)
- Temples and sides of head: Lesser Yang channels (can be from exterior Wind in the Lesser Yang, or from interior Liver and Gall Bladder Fire rising)
- Vertex: Terminal Yin channels (usually from deficiency of Liver-Blood)
- Whole head: exterior invasion of Wind-Cold

Character of pain

- Heavy feeling: Dampness or Phlegm
- Pain which is 'inside' the head, 'hurting the brain': Kidney deficiency
- Distending, throbbing: rising of Liver-Yang
- Boring, like a nail in a small point: stasis of Blood
- With a feeling of muzziness and heaviness: Dampness
- With a feeling of muzziness, heaviness and dizziness: Phlegm

Condition

- With aversion to wind or cold: exterior invasion
- Aggravated by cold: Cold pattern
- Aggravated by heat: Heat pattern
- Aggravated by fatigue, improved by rest: Qi deficiency
- Aggravated by emotional tension: Liver-Yang rising
- Aggravated by sexual activity: Kidney deficiency

Character of pain
- Heavy feeling: Dampness or Phlegm
- Pain which is 'inside' the head, 'hurting the brain': Kidney deficiency
- Distending, throbbing: rising of Liver-Yang
- Boring, like a nail in a small point: stasis of Blood
- With a feeling of muzziness and heaviness: Dampness
- With a feeling of muzziness, heaviness and dizziness: Phlegm

Condition
- With aversion to wind or cold: exterior invasion
- Aggravated by cold: Cold pattern
- Aggravated by heat: Heat pattern
- Aggravated by fatigue, improved by rest: Qi deficiency
- Aggravated by emotional tension: Liver-Yang rising
- Aggravated by sexual activity: Kidney deficiency

Dizziness

Dizziness can be due to four factors, which can be summarized as Wind, Yang, Phlegm and Deficiency. Box 24.14 summarizes questions concerning dizziness.

The main way to distinguish the various types of dizziness is by integration with the accompanying symptoms and signs.

Severe giddiness when everything seems to sway and the person loses the balance is usually due to internal Wind.

Dizziness with throbbing headaches is due to Liver-Yang rising.

Dizziness accompanied by a feeling of heaviness and muzziness of the head indicates Phlegm obstructing the head and preventing the clear Yang from ascending to the head.

Slight dizziness aggravated when tired indicates Blood deficiency.

A sudden onset of dizziness points to a Full pattern. A gradual onset points to an Empty pattern.

Face

Feeling of heat in the face

It is important to ask if a patient suffers from a feeling of heat in the face, even if he or she feels cold in general. Especially in women, the two symptoms often coexist.

A feeling of heat in the face with contradictory Cold symptoms in women may be caused by:
- Simultaneous deficiency of Kidney-Yin and Kidney-Yang
- Blood deficiency with Empty-Heat
- Disharmony of the Penetrating Vessel (*Chong Mai*)
- Yin-Fire

Facial pain

The five main causes of facial pain are invasion of Wind-Heat, invasion of Wind-Cold, Damp-Heat, Liver-Fire and Qi deficiency with Blood stasis.

Box 24.15 summarizes questions concerning facial pain.

Box 24.14 Dizziness

- Severe giddiness when everything seems to sway and the person loses the balance: internal Wind
- Dizziness with throbbing headaches: Liver-Yang rising
- Dizziness accompanied by a feeling of heaviness and muzziness of the head: Phlegm obstructing the head
- Slight dizziness aggravated when tired: indicates Blood deficiency
- Sudden onset: Full pattern
- Gradual onset: Empty pattern

Box 24.15 Facial pain

- **Invasion of Wind-Heat**: acute onset, severe pain of the cheeks or jaws, feeling of heat in the face, face feels hot on palpation, headache, sore throat, aversion to cold, fever
- **Invasion of Wind-Cold**: acute onset, spastic pain of cheeks and jaws, sneezing, aversion to cold, dorsum of hands hot, runny nose
- **Damp-Heat**: severe pain in the cheeks and forehead, red cheeks, greasy skin, sticky-yellow or sticky-greenish nasal discharge, sticky-yellow tongue coating
- **Liver-Fire**: pain in the cheeks and forehead, red cheeks, thirst, bitter taste, Red tongue with redder sides, Wiry-Rapid pulse
- **Qi deficiency and Blood stasis**: intense, often unilateral pain of the cheeks, boring in nature and long in duration, dark complexion, Purple tongue

Trigeminal neuralgia is, of course, a type of facial pain: it is usually due to Liver-Fire combined with Liver- and Kidney-Yin deficiency.

Runny nose

A runny nose with an acute onset is due to an invasion of Wind, which may be Wind-Cold or Wind-Heat, but it is especially likely to occur with Wind-Cold. The severity of this symptom reflects directly the severity of the Cold (as opposed to Wind).

A chronic, runny nose with a thick sticky discharge, which is usually yellow, is generally due to Damp-Heat in the Stomach channel (often corresponding to sinusitis in Western medicine).

A chronic, profusely runny nose with a clear, watery discharge indicates a deficiency of Lung-Qi with Empty-Cold (often corresponding to allergic rhinitis in Western medicine). Such a profuse, watery discharge may also be due to a deficiency of Yang of both the Lungs and Kidneys and of the Governing Vessel.

Bleeding gums

The gums may bleed either from deficient Spleen-Qi not holding Blood or from Heat. This may be Stomach Full- or Empty-Heat or Empty-Heat from Kidney-Yin deficiency.

Box 24.16 summarizes patterns in bleeding gums.

Box 24.16 Bleeding gums

- **Deficient Spleen-Qi not holding Blood**: bleeding gums, tiredness, poor appetite, loose stools
- **Stomach Full-Heat**: inflamed, bleeding gums, feeling of heat, thirst
- **Stomach Empty-Heat**: bleeding gums, dry mouth, desire to drink in small sips
- **Kidney-Yin deficiency with Empty-Heat**: bleeding gums, dizziness, tinnitus, night sweating, malar flush

---

Mouth ulcers

As a general rule, mouth ulcers that recur very frequently or are even almost permanent indicate a Full condition, whereas ulcers that come and go usually indicate an Empty condition (Box 24.17).

The most common cause of ulcers is Heat. Full-Heat should be differentiated from Empty-Heat: in general, mouth ulcers from Full-Heat are very painful and have a red rim around them, while those from Empty-Heat are less painful and have a pale rim around them.

Box 24.17 Mouth ulcers

- Stomach Full-Heat: very painful, red-rimmed ulcers on the gums
- Stomach Empty-Heat: pale-rimmed ulcers on the gums
- Heart-Fire or Heart Empty-Heat: ulcers on the tip of the tongue
- Stomach-Heat: ulcers on the inside of the cheeks
- Disharmony of Directing Vessel: ulcers in pregnancy
- Kidney-Yin deficiency or Original-Qi deficiency: pale-rimmed ulcers aggravated by overwork

---

Mouth ulcers should be further differentiated according to their location: ulcers on the gums are due to Heat or Empty-Heat of the Stomach or Large Intestine (Stomach on the lower gum and Large Intestine on the upper gum); ulcers on the tongue are usually related to the Heart channel, especially if they occur on the tip; ulcers on the inside of the cheeks are usually related to the Stomach channel.

In women, and especially in pregnancy or after childbirth, a disharmony of the Directing Vessel may cause mouth ulcers; typically these occur on the floor of the mouth under the tongue.

Cold sores

Cold sores are generally related to the Stomach channel and reflect Full-Heat, Empty-Heat or Qi deficiency. When due to Stomach-Heat, the cold sores appear suddenly and cause a burning pain; when due to Stomach Empty-Heat they come in bouts, recurring over many years; when due to Qi deficiency, they occur in bouts over a long period of time, are usually pale in colour and are aggravated by overwork.

Body

Pain in the whole body

- Sudden onset, with aversion to cold and fever: exterior Wind invasion
- Ache all over, with feeling of tiredness: Qi-Blood deficiency
- In women after childbirth: if the pain is dull, Blood deficiency; if the pain is severe, Blood stasis
- Pain in arms and shoulders experienced only when walking: Liver-Qi stagnation
- Pain in all muscles, with hot sensation of the flesh: Stomach-Heat
- Dull ache in the muscles, especially of limbs, with feeling of heaviness: Dampness obstructing muscles

Backache

- Continuous, dull, better with rest: Kidney deficiency
- Recent onset, severe, with stiffness: sprain of back causing stasis of Blood
- Severe pain, aggravated during cold and damp weather, alleviated by application of heat: invasion of exterior Cold and Damp to the back channels
- Boring pain with inability to turn the waist: stasis of Blood
- Pain in the back extending up to the shoulders: exterior invasion of Wind

Numbness

- Numbness of arms and legs or only hands and feet on both sides: Blood deficiency
- Numbness of fingers, elbow and arm on one side only (especially of the first three fingers): internal Wind and Phlegm (this may indicate the possibility of impending Wind-stroke)

Box 24.18 summarizes body pain and numbness.

7. Chest and abdomen

The areas discussed are:

- Chest
- Hypochondrium
- Epigastrium
- Abdomen
- Hypogastrium

Chest

The chest is under the influence of Heart and Lungs, while the flanks are under the control of the Liver and Gall Bladder. The abdomen is influenced by the Liver, Intestines, Spleen, Kidneys and Bladder (Figs 24.2 and 24.3).

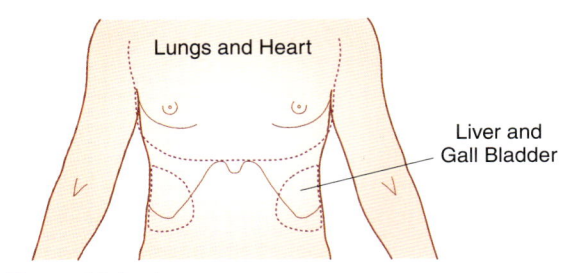

Figure 24.2 Chest

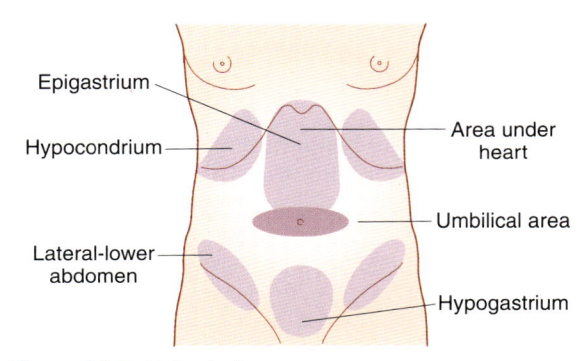

Figure 24.3 Abdominal areas

Box 24.18 Body

1. Pain in the whole body

- Sudden onset, with aversion to cold and fever: exterior Wind invasion
- Ache all over, with feeling of tiredness: Qi-Blood deficiency
- In women after childbirth: if the pain is dull, Blood deficiency; if the pain is severe, Blood stasis
- Pain in arms and shoulders experienced only when walking: Liver-Qi stagnation
- Pain in all muscles, with hot sensation of the flesh: Stomach-Heat
- Dull ache in the muscles, especially of limbs, with feeling of heaviness: Dampness obstructing muscles

2. Pain in joints

- Wandering from joint to joint: from Wind
- Fixed and very painful: from Cold
- Fixed, with swelling and numbness: from Dampness
- With swelling and redness of the joints: Damp-Heat
- Severe stabbing pain with rigidity: Blood stasis

3. Backache

- Continuous, dull, better with rest: Kidney deficiency
- Recent onset, severe, with stiffness: sprain of back causing stasis of Blood
- Severe pain, aggravated during cold and damp weather, alleviated by application of heat: invasion of exterior Cold and Damp to the back channels
- Boring pain with inability to turn the waist: stasis of Blood
- Pain in the back extending up to the shoulders: exterior invasion of Wind

4. Numbness

- Numbness of arms and legs or only hands and feet on both sides: Blood deficiency
- Numbness of fingers, elbow and arm on one side only (especially of the first three fingers): internal Wind and Phlegm

Pain in the chest is often due to stasis of Blood in the Heart, which, in turn is usually due to deficiency of Yang.

Chest pain accompanied by cough with profuse yellow sputum is due to Lung-Heat. A feeling of oppression of the chest is due either to Phlegm in the Lungs or to severe Liver-Qi stagnation.

Hypochondrium

A feeling of distension of the hypochondrium is due to stagnation of Liver-Qi. If the pain is stabbing, there is stasis of Liver-Blood.

Epigastrium

If epigastric pain is dull and alleviated by eating, it is of the Empty type; if it is severe and aggravated by eating, it is of the Full type. Severe epigastric pain can be due to many full patterns of the Stomach such as retention of food in the Stomach, Stomach-Heat, Damp-Heat in the Stomach, Fire or Phlegm-Fire in the Stomach, Blood stasis in the Stomach, or Liver-Qi invading the Stomach.

Dull epigastric pain is due to an Empty condition and often Stomach-Qi deficiency or Empty-Cold in the Stomach.

A feeling of fullness in the epigastrium is due to Dampness or to Spleen-Qi deficiency (in which case it is very slight). A feeling of distension of the epigastrium is due to Liver-Qi stagnation.

Abdomen

Lower abdominal pain can be due to many different causes, the most common of which are internal Cold, stagnation of Liver-Qi or Liver-Blood, Damp-Heat, stasis of Blood in the Intestines or Uterus. These various conditions can only be differentiated on the basis of the accompanying symptoms and signs.

An abdominal pain which is relieved by bowel movements is of a Full nature; if it is aggravated by bowel movements, it is of an Empty nature.

Box 24.19 summarizes questions about the chest and abdomen.

Hypogastrium

Hypogastric pain is usually due to Damp-Heat in the Bladder or sometimes Liver-Fire infusing downwards to the Bladder.

Box 24.19 Chest and abdomen

1. Chest
- Stabbing chest pain: stasis of Blood in the Heart
- Chest pain accompanied by cough with profuse yellow sputum : Lung-Heat
- A feeling of oppression of the chest: Phlegm in the Lungs or severe Liver-Qi stagnation

2. Hypochondrium
- A feeling of distension of the hypochondrium: stagnation of Liver-Qi
- Stabbing pain in hypochondrium: stasis of Liver-Blood

3. Epigastrium
- Dull epigastric pain alleviated by eating: Empty type
- Severe epigastric pain aggravated by eating: Full type
- Severe epigastric pain: Full patterns such as retention of food in the Stomach, Stomach-Heat, Damp-Heat in the Stomach, Fire or Phlegm-Fire in the Stomach, Blood stasis in the Stomach, Liver-Qi invading the Stomach
- Dull epigastric pain: Stomach-Qi deficiency or Empty-Cold in the Stomach
- Feeling of fullness in the epigastrium: Dampness
- Feeling of distension of the epigastrium: to Liver-Qi stagnation

4. Abdomen
- Lower abdominal pain can be due to many different causes, e.g. internal Cold, stagnation of Liver-Qi or Liver-Blood, Damp-Heat, stasis of Blood in the Intestines or Uterus
- Abdominal pain relieved by bowel movements: Full nature
- Abdominal pain aggravated by bowel movements: Empty nature

5. Hypogastrium
- Hypogastric pain: Damp-Heat in the Bladder or Liver-Fire infusing downwards to the Bladder

8. Limbs

Generally speaking, questions about the four limbs are asked only when the patient presents with a problem specific to them. The main exceptions to this are when a patient presents with symptoms of Blood deficiency, in which case I always ask about numbness of the limbs, or when a patient has symptoms of Dampness, in which case I ask about any feeling of heaviness in the limbs.

The symptoms discussed are:

- Weakness of the limbs
- Numbness/tingling of the limbs
- Generalized joint pain
- Muscle ache in the limbs
- Difficulty in walking
- Tremor of limbs
- Cold hands
- Weak knees
- Cold feet
- Feeling of heaviness of the limbs

Weakness of the limbs

Weakness of the limbs may be caused by Stomach-Qi deficiency, a general Qi and Blood deficiency and a deficiency of Kidney-Yang.

Numbness/tingling of the limbs

Numbness/tingling of the limbs may be due to:

- Blood deficiency
- Wind
- Phlegm
- Dampness or Damp-Heat
- Stagnation of Qi and Blood

Blood deficiency usually causes tingling, while Phlegm and Wind tend to cause more numbness: with Wind, the numbness is often unilateral. However, these are only general rules.

Box 24.20 summarizes numbness and tingling of the limbs.

Blood deficiency is a common cause of numbness/tingling of the limbs in younger people, especially women. In the elderly, a numbness of the limbs is very often caused by Wind or Wind-Phlegm obstructing the channels and, in the case of Wind, the numbness is often unilateral. Dampness or Damp-Heat may also cause numbness of the limbs and especially of the legs. In a few cases, numbness may be caused by stagnation of Qi and Blood in the limbs, in which case it is relieved by exercise.

Box 24.20 Numbness/tingling of the limbs

- Blood deficiency: common in women, more tingling
- Wind: more numbness, often unilateral, common in the elderly
- Phlegm: with feeling of heaviness
- Dampness: with swelling
- Stagnation of Qi and Blood: with pain

Generalized joint pain

Generalized joint pain is generally due to Wind (Wind Painful Obstruction Syndrome) combined with Dampness and/or Cold. If the site of the pain moves, affecting different joints every day, it strongly indicates Wind. A severe pain indicates Cold, while swelling of the joints indicates Dampness. In chronic conditions, Dampness frequently combines with Heat and causes a swelling, redness and heat of the joints.

Box 24.21 summarizes generalized joint pain.

Box 24.21 Generalized joint pain

- Pain wandering from joint to joint: Wind
- Severe pain in one joint: Cold
- Dull ache with swelling and heaviness: Dampness
- Pain with redness, swelling and heaviness: Damp-Heat

Muscle ache in the limbs

Muscle ache in the limbs is nearly always due to retention of Dampness in the space between skin and muscles. Muscle ache in the limbs is a common symptom in postviral fatigue syndrome.

Difficulty in walking (atrophy/flaccidity of limbs)

Difficulty in walking (atrophy/flaccidity of limbs) in the beginning stages is often due to a Stomach- and Spleen-Qi deficiency. In later stages, atrophy and/or flaccidity of the limbs is often due to a deficiency of Yin of the Liver and Kidneys or a deficiency of Yang of the Spleen and Kidneys.

Tremor of limbs

Tremor of limbs always indicates Liver-Wind: we should then establish the source of Liver-Wind and whether it is Full- or Empty-Wind. The root cause of Liver-Wind may be Heat during an acute febrile disease, Liver-Fire, Liver-Yang rising, a deficiency of Yin of the Liver and/or Kidneys and Liver-Blood deficiency. The last two types of Wind are of the Empty type, while all the others are of the Full type.

Full-Wind is characterized by pronounced tremors or convulsions (during an acute febrile disease), while Empty-Wind is characterized by fine tremors or tics.

Cold hands

Cold hands are due to three possible causes: Yang deficiency (the most common one); Blood deficiency; and Qi stagnation. Box 24.22 summarizes patterns in cold hands.

> **Box 24.22 Cold hands**
> - Cold hands ameliorated by heat: Yang deficiency
> - Cold hands with palpitations and dizziness: Heart-Blood deficiency
> - Cold fingers and toes: Liver-Qi stagnation

Weak knees

Weak knees are generally due to a deficiency of the Kidneys, especially Kidney-Yang.

Cold feet

Cold feet are generally due to Kidney-Yang deficiency. Another possible cause of cold feet, especially in women, is Liver-Blood deficiency.

Feeling of heaviness of the limbs

Feelings of heaviness of the limbs are more frequently experienced in the legs. A feeling of heaviness of the legs is always due to Dampness in the Lower Burner: Dampness may be combined with Heat or Cold and it may be Full or Empty. The feeling of heaviness from Full-Dampness is more pronounced than that from Dampness associated with Spleen-Qi deficiency.

When the Spleen-Qi deficiency is associated with Stomach-Qi deficiency, the feeling of heaviness is frequently experienced in all four limbs rather than just the legs. Similarly, when Phlegm causes a feeling of heaviness, it is experienced in all four limbs.

9. Sleep

The symptoms discussed are:

- Insomnia
- Lethargy

Insomnia

It is essential to ask every patient about their sleep because this gives an indication of the state of the Mind (*Shen*) and Ethereal Soul (*Hun*). A disturbance of the Mind and/or Ethereal Soul is of course extremely common in Western patients whose life is generally subject to a considerable amount of stress.

In general, sleep depends on the state of Blood and Yin, especially of the Heart and Liver, although the Blood and Yin of other organs also influence sleep. During the night Yin energy predominates and the Mind and the Ethereal Soul should be anchored in Heart-Blood and Liver-Blood, respectively (Fig. 24.4).

A sleep disturbance may be due to the Mind and/or the Ethereal Soul not being anchored in Heart-Blood (or Heart-Yin) and Liver-Blood (or Liver-Yin), respectively: this can happen either because there is not enough Blood or Yin to anchor the Mind and/or the Ethereal Soul or because a pathogenic factor (such as Heat) agitates them. The former is an Empty type of sleep disturbance, the latter a Full type. In both cases, the Mind and/or the Ethereal Soul is said to 'float' at night causing insomnia (Fig. 24.5).

The length of sleep needed varies according to age and, in general, it gradually decreases in one's lifetime, being highest in babies and lowest in the elderly. We

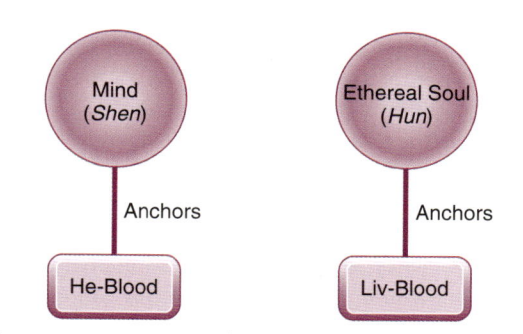

Figure 24.4 Mind and Ethereal Soul anchored in Heart and Liver

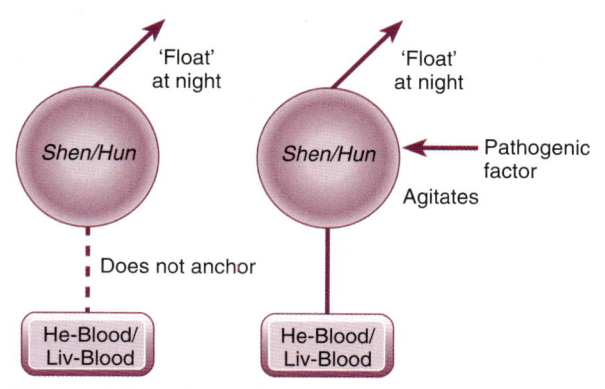

Figure 24.5 Mind and Ethereal Soul deprived of 'residence'

should therefore take age into account when judging whether the patient's sleep is adequate or not.

In general, in Deficiency conditions, a difficulty in falling asleep indicates a Blood deficiency of the Heart, Spleen or Liver, while difficulty in staying asleep and a tendency to wake up during the night indicate a Yin deficiency. Of course, waking up during the night may also be due to Full conditions, such as Heat, Fire, Phlegm-Fire or retention of food.

A difficulty in falling asleep generally indicates a deficiency of Blood or Yin, while waking during the night generally indicates Yin deficiency with Empty-Heat

When diagnosing sleep disturbances it is important to distinguish, first, a Full from an Empty condition and, secondly, a Heart from a Liver pattern. Full conditions are characterized by very restless sleep with a feeling of heat, agitation and excessive dreaming; Empty conditions are characterized by not being able to fall or stay asleep without any of the above symptoms. A Liver pattern causing insomnia is characterized by excessive dreaming and, when compared with a Heart pattern, a more severe restlessness.

However, the Heart and Liver are not the only organs that may cause insomnia: the Stomach, Spleen, Kidneys and Gall Bladder may all play a role in insomnia. For example, a deficiency of Spleen-Blood often accompanies a deficiency of Heart-Blood and contributes to causing insomnia (the famous formula Gui Pi Tang *Tonifying the Spleen Decoction* treats insomnia from these patterns). Kidney-Yin, like Liver-Yin, also needs to anchor the Mind and the Ethereal Soul at night and therefore a deficiency of Kidney-Yin, with or without Empty-Heat, is also a frequent cause of insomnia.

A deficiency of the Gall Bladder may cause someone to wake up early in the morning without being able to fall asleep again.

Insomnia in the sense of not being able to fall asleep, but sleeping well after falling asleep, indicates deficiency of Heart-Blood.

Insomnia in the sense of waking up many times during the night indicates deficiency of Yin, which may be of the Heart, Liver or Kidneys.

Insomnia with anxiety, dream-disturbed sleep and other symptoms of Qi and Blood deficiency may be due to deficiency of Blood of the Heart and Spleen.

Insomnia with difficulty in falling asleep, dizziness and blurred vision is due to Liver-Blood deficiency.

Insomnia, waking up frequently during the night with excessive dreams, together with night sweating and palpitations may be due to Heart- and Kidney-Yin deficiency with Empty-Heat.

Dream-disturbed sleep indicates Liver-Fire or Heart-Fire. Restless sleep with dreams indicates retention of food.

Waking up early in the morning and failing to fall asleep again indicates deficiency of Gall Bladder.

Box 24.23 summarizes patterns of insomnia.

Box 24.23 Insomnia

- For good sleep it is necessary for Mind and Ethereal Soul to be anchored in Heart- and Liver-Blood
- Deficient Blood not anchoring Mind and/or Ethereal Soul: Empty type
- Pathogenic factors agitating Mind and/or Ethereal Soul out of Blood: Full type
- Difficulty in falling asleep: deficiency of Heart-Blood
- Waking up many times during the night: deficiency of Yin, which may be of the Heart, Liver or Kidneys
- Insomnia with anxiety, dream-disturbed sleep and other symptoms of Qi and Blood deficiency: deficiency of Blood of the Heart and Spleen
- Insomnia with difficulty in falling asleep, dizziness, blurred vision: Liver-Blood deficiency
- Insomnia, waking up frequently during the night with excessive dreams together with night sweating and palpitations: Heart- and Kidney-Yin deficiency with Empty-Heat
- Dream-disturbed sleep: Liver-Fire or Heart-Fire
- Restless sleep with excessive dreams: retention of food
- Waking up early in the morning and failing to fall asleep again: deficiency of Gall Bladder

Lethargy

Feeling sleepy after eating indicates Spleen-Qi deficiency. A general feeling of lethargy and heaviness of the body indicates retention of Dampness. If there is also dizziness, it indicates Phlegm.

Extreme lethargy and lassitude with a feeling of cold indicates deficiency of Kidney-Yang.

Lethargic stupor with exterior Heat symptoms indicates invasion of Pericardium by Heat.

Lethargic stupor with rattling in the throat, a Slippery pulse and a sticky tongue coating indicates blurring of the mind by Phlegm.

Box 24.24 summarizes lethargy.

> **Box 24.24 Lethargy**
> - Feeling sleepy after eating: Spleen-Qi deficiency
> - General feeling of lethargy and heaviness of the body: retention of Dampness
> - General feeling of lethargy and heaviness of the body and dizziness: Phlegm
> - Extreme lethargy and lassitude with a feeling of cold: deficiency of Kidney-Yang
> - Lethargic stupor with exterior Heat symptoms: invasion of Pericardium by Heat
> - Lethargic stupor with rattling in the throat, a Slippery pulse and a sticky tongue coating: blurring of the mind by Phlegm

10. Sweating

Evaluation of symptoms of sweating must be made by considering if it is part of an exterior or interior pattern.

In the context of *exterior* conditions, sweating indicates a relatively deficient condition. I say 'relatively' because an invasion of an external pathogenic factor is a Full condition by definition. However, in some cases, if the Upright Qi is particularly deficient, there may be sweating: indeed, sweating is a sign that the Upright Qi is deficient.

Box 24.25 summarizes causes of sweating.

In invasions of Wind-Cold, there are two types of pattern, one characterized by predominance of Cold, the other by predominance of Wind: in the latter, there is some sweating, which indicates that the Upright Qi is somewhat deficient.

In the context of *interior* conditions, sweating may be caused either by a Full condition of Heat (or Damp-Heat) or by a Deficient condition, which may be of Yang or Yin.

The pathology of sweating in Full and Empty conditions is different. In Full conditions of Heat, sweating is caused by evaporation of Body Fluids by Heat. In Empty conditions, sweating is caused by the deficient Yang or Yin Qi not holding fluids, in the space between the skin and muscles in the former case and in the 'bones' in the latter.

One must distinguish sweating by the area of body, time of day, conditions and quality of sweat.

The areas and factors discussed are:

> - Area of body
> - Time of day
> - Condition of illness
> - Quality of sweat

Area of body

- Only on head: Heat in the Stomach or Damp-Heat
- Oily sweat on forehead: collapse of Yang
- Only on arms and legs: Stomach and Spleen deficiency
- Only on hands: Lung-Qi or Heart-Qi deficiency
- Whole body: Lung-Qi deficiency
- On palms, soles and chest: Yin deficiency (called 'five-palm sweat')

Box 24.26 summarizes patterns in sweating.

Time of day

- In daytime: Yang deficiency
- At night-time: Yin deficiency (in some cases it can also be from Damp-Heat)

> **Box 24.25 Causes of sweating**
>
> **Full**
> - Heat
> - Damp-Heat
>
> **Empty**
> - Deficiency of Yang
> - Deficiency of Yin

> **Box 24.26 Sweating**
>
> **Area of body**
> - Only on head: Heat in the Stomach or Damp-Heat
> - Oily sweat on forehead: collapse of Yang
> - Only on arms and legs: Stomach and Spleen deficiency
> - Only on hands: Lung-Qi or Heart-Qi deficiency
> - Whole body: Lung-Qi deficiency
> - On palms, soles and chest: Yin deficiency (called 'five-palm sweat').
>
> **Time of day**
> - In daytime: Yang deficiency
> - At night-time: Yin deficiency (in some cases it can also be from Damp-Heat)
>
> **Condition of illness**
> - Profuse cold sweat during a severe illness: collapse of Yang
> - Oily sweat on forehead, like pearls, not flowing: collapse of Yang, danger of imminent death
>
> **Quality of sweat**
> - Oily: severe Yang deficiency
> - Yellow: Damp-Heat

Condition of illness

- Profuse cold sweat during a severe illness: collapse of Yang
- Oily sweat on forehead, like pearls, not flowing: collapse of Yang, danger of imminent death

Quality of sweat

- Oily: severe Yang deficiency
- Yellow: Damp-Heat

11. Ears and eyes

The symptoms discussed are:

- Ears
  - Tinnitus
    - Onset
    - Pressure
    - Character of noise
  - Deafness
- Eyes
  - Eye pain
  - Blurred vision
  - Dry eyes

Ears

The Kidneys open into the ears, but not every ear problem is related to the Kidneys. The Lesser Yang channels flow to the ear and some exterior Heat conditions can cause ear problems. In addition, Dampness and Phlegm obstruct the rising of clear Yang to the upper orifices and this can affect the ears.

Box 24.27 summarizes patterns in the ears.

Tinnitus
Onset

A sudden onset suggests a Full condition (usually Liver-Fire, Liver-Yang rising or Liver-Wind). A gradual onset suggests an Empty condition (usually deficiency of the Kidneys).

Pressure

If the noise is aggravated by pressing with one's hands on the ears, it suggests a Full condition; if it is alleviated, it suggests an Empty condition.

Character of noise

A loud, high-pitched noise like a whistle indicates Liver-Yang, Liver-Fire or Liver-Wind rising. A low-pitched noise like rushing water indicates Kidney deficiency.

Box 24.27 Ears

Tinnitus

Onset

- Sudden onset: Full condition, Liver-Fire, Liver-Yang rising, Liver-Wind
- Gradual onset: Empty condition, Kidney deficiency

Pressure

- Noise aggravated by pressing with one's hands on the ears: Full condition
- Noise alleviated by pressing with one's hands on the ears: Empty condition

Character

- Loud, high-pitched noise, like whistle: Liver-Yang, Liver-Fire, Liver-Wind
- Low-pitched noise like rushing water: Kidney deficiency

Deafness

- Sudden onset: Full condition, Liver-Fire, Liver-Yang rising, Liver-Wind
- Gradual onset: Empty condition, deficiency of Kidneys, Heart-Blood or Qi of the Upper Burner

---

Deafness

A sudden onset suggests a Full condition (of the same type as for tinnitus) and a gradual onset suggests an Empty condition.

In chronic cases, apart from Kidney deficiency, deafness can also be due to:

- Heart-Blood deficiency
- Deficiency of Qi of the Upper Burner
- Yang Qi deficiency

Eyes

The eyes are the orifice of the Liver, but not every eye problem is related to the Liver as many other organs influence the eyes. For example, the Kidneys also nourish and moisten the eyes and the Heart nourishes them with Blood.

Box 24.28 summarizes patterns related to the eyes.

Eye pain

Pain like a needle and with redness of the eye associated with headache indicates Toxic Heat in the Heart channel.

Pain, swelling and redness of the eye indicate either invasion of the eye channels by exterior Wind-Heat, or interior Liver-Fire.

> **Box 24.28 Eyes**
>
> **Eye pain**
> - Pain like a needle, eye redness, headache: Toxic Heat in Heart channel
> - Pain, swelling and redness: invasion of the eye channels by Wind-Heat or Liver-Fire
> - Feeling of pressure: Kidney-Yin deficiency
>
> **Blurred vision**
> - With floaters: deficiency of Liver-Blood, Liver-Yin or Kidney-Yin
> - With photophobia: Liver-Blood deficiency or Liver-Yang rising
>
> **Dry eyes**
> - Liver- and/or Kidney-Yin deficiency

A feeling of pressure in the eyes indicates Kidney-Yin deficiency.

Blurred vision

Blurred vision and 'floaters' in the eyes indicate Liver-Blood or Liver-Yin deficiency. They may also be due to Kidney-Yin deficiency.

Photophobia indicates Liver-Blood deficiency or Liver-Yang rising.

Dry eyes

Dryness of the eyes indicates Liver- and/or Kidney Yin deficiency.

12. Feeling of cold, feeling of heat and fever

The symptoms discussed are:

> - Interior conditions
>   - Feeling of cold
>   - Feeling of heat
> - Exterior conditions
>   - Aversion to cold
>   - 'Fever'
>   - Simultaneous aversion to cold and 'fever'
>   - Feeling of heat in diseases of exterior origin
>   - Alternating feeling of cold and feeling of heat

In order to discuss the diagnostic significance of feelings of cold or of heat, it is essential to distinguish exterior from interior conditions.

> **Box 24.29 Clinical manifestations of Full-Cold**
> - Intense feeling of cold and shivers
> - Body feels noticeably cold and relatively hard to touch
> - Pain
> - Full pulse
> - Sudden onset

Interior conditions

Feeling of cold

In the context of interior diseases, if a person feels easily cold and experiences cold limbs, this clearly indicates either Full-Cold or Empty-Cold deriving from Yang deficiency. In patients with chronic diseases, Empty-Cold is more common than Full-Cold.

Full-Cold is characterized by an intense feeling of cold and shivers: the body also feels cold to the touch. Various parts of the body may feel particularly cold depending on the location of the Cold: if it is in the Stomach, the limbs and epigastrium will feel cold; if in the Intestines, the legs and lower abdomen are cold; if in the Uterus, the lower abdomen feels cold. Full-Cold has usually a sudden onset and may last only a few months at the most because Cold will inevitably injure Yang and lead to Yang deficiency and therefore Empty-Cold.

Box 24.29 summarizes the clinical manifestations of Full-Cold.

Empty-Cold derives from Yang deficiency of any organ and it may cause a cold feeling and/or cold limbs: it could be due especially to a deficiency of Yang of the Heart, Lungs, Spleen, Kidneys and Stomach. The cold feeling is both subjective and objective (i.e. the patient feels easily and frequently cold and his or her limbs or other parts of the body will feel cold to the touch).

A deficiency of Yang of the Lungs and/or Heart will manifest especially with cold hands, a deficiency of Spleen-Yang with cold limbs and abdomen and that of Kidney-Yang especially with cold legs, knees, feet and back. A deficiency of Stomach-Yang will manifest with cold epigastrium and cold limbs in a similar way to Spleen-Yang deficiency.

Box 24.30 summarizes the clinical manifestations of Empty-Cold.

There are, however, other causes of cold limbs (as opposed to a general cold feeling). One is Qi stagnation: when Qi stagnates it may fail to reach the hands and feet and these become cold. This is called the 'four

> **Box 24.30 Clinical manifestations of Empty-Cold**
>
> - Mild, persistent cold feeling or tendency to feeling cold
> - Body feels mildly cold to touch
> - No pain
> - Weak pulse
> - Slow, gradual onset

> **Box 24.31 Cold feeling/cold limbs**
>
> - Yang Deficiency of Heart and/or Lungs: cold hands, sweaty hands
> - Spleen-Yang/Stomach-Yang deficiency: cold limbs and abdomen
> - Kidney-Yang deficiency: cold legs, knees, feet, back
> - Qi stagnation: cold hands and feet, and especially the fingers
> - Heart-Blood deficiency: cold hands and chest
> - Liver-Blood deficiency: cold feet

rebellious syndrome' in which the 'four rebellious' indicate cold hands and feet: the famous formula Si Ni San *Four Rebellious Powder* is used for this pattern. An important difference if the cold limbs are due to Yang deficiency or Qi stagnation is that in the former case the whole limb will be cold, whereas in the latter case only the hands and feet, and especially the fingers, are cold.

Besides this, cold limbs in women may also derive from Blood deficiency and this is due to the deficient Blood not reaching the extremities. In cases of Heart-Blood deficiency, only the hands and chest will be cold, while in cases of Liver-Blood deficiency, the feet will be cold.

Box 24.31 summarizes feelings of cold and cold limbs.

In short, a cold feeling and cold limbs may be due to:

- Yang Deficiency of Heart and/or Lungs: cold hands, sweaty hands
- Spleen-Yang/Stomach-Yang deficiency: cold limbs and abdomen
- Kidney-Yang deficiency: cold legs, knees, feet, back
- Qi stagnation: cold hands and feet, and especially the fingers
- Heart-Blood deficiency: cold hands and chest
- Liver-Blood deficiency: cold feet

Feeling of heat

In interior conditions, a feeling of heat simply indicates a pattern of Heat, which may be Full- or Empty-Heat. Heat of any organ may cause a feeling of heat. Generally speaking, a feeling of heat that is experienced only in the afternoon/evening indicates Empty-Heat.

A low-grade fever getting worse in the afternoon, or only occurring in the afternoon in interior conditions, indicates Yin deficiency.

Box 24.32 summarizes the feeling of heat.

A constant low-grade temperature indicates a Damp-Heat pattern. A fever in the middle of the night in an adult indicates Yin deficiency, and in a child it indicates retention of food.

> **Box 24.32 Feeling of heat**
>
> - Feeling of heat in the afternoon or evening: Empty-Heat
> - Low-grade fever worse in the afternoon or only in the afternoon: Yin deficiency
> - Constant low-grade temperature: Damp-Heat
> - Fever in the middle of the night: in an adult Yin deficiency; in a child retention of food

Exterior conditions

Aversion to cold

In the context of exterior diseases, the subjective feeling of cold of the patient is associated with an objective hot feeling of the patient's body on palpation. The cold feeling experienced in invasions of exterior pathogenic factors is usually called 'aversion to cold': this means that the patient feels subjectively cold (with a sudden onset) and he or she is reluctant to go out. The aversion to cold can range from a very mild feeling to a very strong cold feeling with shivering.

In invasions of exterior pathogenic factors (especially Wind), Wind obstructs the space between the skin and muscles where the Defensive Qi circulates; as the Defensive Qi warms the muscles, when it is obstructed it cannot do so and the patient feels cold. Please note that the aversion to cold is due to invasion of Wind, whether this is Wind-Cold or Wind-Heat. Wind-Heat will also cause aversion to cold because it obstructs the space between the skin and muscles. The intensity of the aversion to cold is directly proportional to the intensity of the exterior pathogenic factor, i.e. the stronger the pathogenic factor, the more pronounced the aversion to cold.

'Fever'

At the same time as the patient invaded by Wind feels subjectively cold, his or her body (especially forehead and dorsum of hands) feels hot on palpation. This was called *fa re* in Chinese (literally 'emission of heat'). This is often translated as 'fever' but we should bear in mind that it does not necessarily indicate an actual fever as measured by a thermometer: it simply means that the patient's body feels hot on palpation. Of course, if a patient does have an actual fever in the course of an invasion of an exterior pathogenic factor, that is definitely *fa re*. I shall continue to use the term 'fever' on the above understanding to distinguish it from a subjective 'feeling of heat'.

'Fever' does not necessarily indicate a raised temperature: it indicates that the patient's forehead and dorsum of the hands feel hot to the touch. The patient may or may not have an actual fever

The 'fever' (or emission of heat) during the course of an exterior invasion is due to the struggle between the exterior pathogenic factor and the Upright Qi and the intensity of the 'fever' is directly proportional to the intensity of such a fight. Please bear in mind that the presence of 'fever' has nothing to do with the Wind-Cold or Wind-Heat character of the pathogenic factor: Wind-Cold may also cause an intense 'fever'. Thus, as far as the intensity of the 'fever' is concerned, three possible cases can be distinguished:

1. Pathogenic factor and Upright Qi both strong: high 'fever'
2. Pathogenic factor and Upright Qi both weak: low 'fever'
3. Pathogenic factor strong and Upright Qi weak or vice versa: medium 'fever'

The intensity of fever in exterior conditions is related to the struggle between the Upright Qi and the external pathogenic factor and has nothing to do with whether the pathogenic factor is Wind-Cold or Wind-Heat

Simultaneous aversion to cold and 'fever'

The *simultaneous* occurrence of aversion to cold and 'fever' is the cardinal symptom of an invasion of an exterior pathogenic factor. This corresponds to the pattern of Wind-Cold at the Greater Yang Stage of the identification of patterns according to the Six Stages or to the Defensive Qi Level of the identification of patterns according to the Four Levels.

Feeling of heat in diseases of exterior origin

In the context of acute exterior diseases, a (subjective) feeling of heat indicates that the pathogenic factor has entered into the Interior: indeed, a change from aversion to cold to a feeling of heat in the context of acute exterior diseases is the certain sign that the pathogenic factor has penetrated into the Interior. When this happens, the patient has both a subjective feeling of heat and his or her body is also objectively emanating heat (which may or may not be an actual fever).

Alternating feeling of cold and feeling of heat

Finally, if the patient suffers from alternating chills and (subjective) feeling of heat, this indicates an exterior invasion of Wind-Cold or Wind-Heat, and that the pathogenic factor is in the Lesser Yang Stage (within the Six-Stage pattern identification) or the Gall Bladder-Heat Level (within the Four-Level pattern identification). Please note that in this case, contrary to what happens in invasions of Wind in the Greater Yang, the feeling of heat is subjective.

Box 24.33 summarizes these feelings of cold and heat.

- 'Feeling of heat' in alternating cold and hot feeling is subjective
- 'Feeling of heat' (or fever) in simultaneous aversion to cold and fever is objective, i.e. the patient's body feels hot to the touch

Box 24.33 Feeling of cold and heat in exterior conditions

- Aversion to cold, fever: invasion of external Wind
- Feeling of heat, body emitting heat: pathogenic factor in the Interior
- Alternating feeling of heat and cold: Lesser-Yang pattern

13. Emotional symptoms

The area of questioning surrounding the emotions experienced by the patient is one of the most important, if not *the* most important. Emotional causes of disease play a very prominent role in the aetiology and clinical manifestations of most of our patients and therefore we should always ask patients about their emotional life. However, some patients may regard an enquiry about their emotional life as an intrusion and we should be sensitive about this.

The emotional state of the patient reflects of course the state of their Mind and Spirit and the findings from interrogation need to be carefully integrated with those gleaned from observation, particularly observation of the lustre (*shen*) of the eyes. In addition, the state of the patient's Mind and Spirit is an important prognostic factor.

If the emotional condition is not the presenting problem, I generally ask about a patient's emotional life towards the end of the consultation to try to find the cause of the disease. In many cases, however, the emotional state of the patient is the main presenting problem: for example, patients may come to us because they are depressed or anxious. In other cases, the emotional state of the patient is the underlying cause of physical symptoms: for example, a patient may complain of tiredness and digestive symptoms when frustration and resentment may be the cause of the condition.

It is important to be sensitive when asking about the emotional state of the patient (if this is not the presenting problem) and often it is observation that gives us a clue about this, in which case I would ask the patient about it. For example, a patient may come in complaining of tiredness and premenstrual breast distension: if the eyes of the patient lack lustre, I would suspect that emotional stress could be the cause of the problem and I would circumspectly ask the patient about it.

As mentioned above, we must use great sensitivity when asking patients about their emotions. First of all, we should ask questions only if they appear willing to talk about their emotions and respect their wishes if they do not want to do so. If I suspect that emotional stress is the cause of a problem, I ask questions such as 'Have you suffered any shock in the past?', 'Do you tend to feel irritable about some situation?' or 'Do you sometimes feel sad?', etc.

Of course, if the patient comes to us specifically for an emotional condition, the questioning is conducted differently as the patient will openly volunteer the information.

The symptoms discussed are:

- Depression
- Fear/anxiety
- Irritability/anger
- Worry/overthinking
- Sadness and grief

Depression

'Depression' is a modern Western term that indicates a change in mood that can range from a very mild feeling of despondency to the most abject depression and despair. Depression is twice as common in women as in men and its onset increases towards middle age. The main symptoms of depression are depressed mood, loss of interest, self-esteem or motivation, fatigue, anxiety, insomnia, loss of appetite.

Asking patients about feelings of depression should always be part of our questions about the patient's emotional state and it should be carried out with sensitivity and tact. In fact, some patients will not want to admit to being depressed; some will admit to being depressed but do not necessarily want to talk about it; and others may not even realize that they are in a state of depression. These patients will often complain only of physical symptoms such as extreme tiredness, lack of motivation and feeling cold, preferring not to face up to the fact that they may be depressed. In China this is more the norm than the exception as Chinese patients will seldom complain of feeling 'depressed' and somatization of their feelings of depression into bodily symptoms is often seen.

In Chinese medicine, mental depression was called *yu*, which means 'gloominess' or 'depression', or *yu zheng*, which means 'depression pattern'. *Yu* has the double meaning of 'depression' and 'stagnation', which implies that according to this theory, mental depression is always caused by a stagnation (which is *not* the case). Chinese books normally ascribe mental depression to Liver-Qi stagnation in its various manifestations, including Liver-Qi stagnation turning into Heat and Liver-Qi stagnation with Phlegm. In the later stages of mental depression, Empty patterns appear. Thus, although in Chinese medicine stagnation and depression are almost synonymous, Empty patterns may also cause depression.

In severe depression, the Liver is always involved due to its housing the Ethereal Soul (*Hun*). The Ethereal

Box 24.34 'Movement' of the Ethereal Soul

Lack of movement of the Ethereal Soul
- Liver-Qi stagnation
- Liver-Blood and Liver-Qi deficiency
- Spleen and Kidney deficiency

Excessive movement of the Ethereal Soul
- Fire
- Phlegm-Fire
- Liver-Blood and/or Liver-Yin deficiency

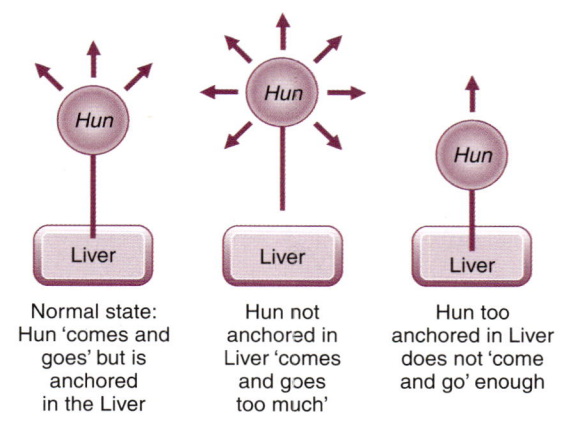

Figure 24.6 Patterns leading to deficient and excessive 'movement' of the Ethereal Soul

Normal state: Hun 'comes and goes' but is anchored in the Liver

Hun not anchored in Liver 'comes and goes too much'

Hun too anchored in Liver does not 'come and go' enough

Soul is responsible for our life's dreams, plans, ideas, projects, sense of purpose, relationship with other people, etc. The Ethereal Soul was often described as 'the coming and going of the Mind (*Shen*)': this means that the Ethereal Soul assists the Mind in giving it the capacity to have dreams, plans, ideas, projects, etc. In this sense, the Ethereal Soul gives the Mind 'movement', projection towards the outside and ability to form relationships with other people: hence its 'coming and going' described above. On the other hand, the Mind guides and controls the Ethereal Soul and, most of all, integrates the activity of the Ethereal Soul within the overall psychic life of the person.

Box 24.34 summarizes patterns relating to the 'movement' of the Ethereal Soul.

Thus, if the 'movement' of the Ethereal Soul is lacking (either through its lack of activity or the overcontrol of the Mind), the person is depressed; if the 'movement' of the Ethereal Soul is excessive (either through its overactivity or lack of control by the Mind), the person may display manic behaviour (bearing in mind that the latter may vary in intensity and seriousness from full-blown bipolar disease to much less severe manifestations that are relatively common also in mentally healthy individuals).

Figure 7.6 in chapter 7 illustrates the two states of the Ethereal Soul: when it 'comes and goes' too much; and when it does not 'come and go' enough.

The lack of 'movement' of the Ethereal Soul, and hence depression, may be due to pathogenic factors inhibiting the Ethereal Soul, such as Liver-Qi stagnation, or to a deficiency of the Liver, Spleen or Kidneys not stimulating the Ethereal Soul.

Figure 24.6 illustrates the patterns leading to excessive and deficient 'movement' of the Ethereal Soul.

The main Full patterns accompanying depression are:

- Liver-Qi stagnation
- Stagnant Liver-Qi turning into Heat
- Liver-Qi stagnation with Qi-Phlegm
- Phlegm-Fire harassing the Mind
- Blood stasis
- Gall Bladder-Heat

The main Empty patterns accompanying depression are:

- Spleen- and Heart-Blood deficiency
- Heart-Yang deficiency
- Liver-Blood deficiency
- Kidney- and Heart-Yin deficiency with Empty-Heat
- Kidney-Yang deficiency

Box 24.35 summarizes Full and Empty patterns in depression.

Fear/anxiety

A chronic feeling of anxiety (occurring on its own without depression) is very common in Western patients. A feeling of anxiety includes emotional states akin to the emotions of fear and worry (two of the seven emotions) in Chinese medicine. It may be accompanied or caused by a Deficiency (usually of Blood or Yin), by an Excess (usually Heat) or by a combination of Deficiency and Excess (usually Yin deficiency with Empty-Heat).

Box 24.36 summarizes patterns in anxiety.

When there is a deficiency of Blood or Yin, the Mind and Ethereal Soul lose their 'residence' in Heart-Blood

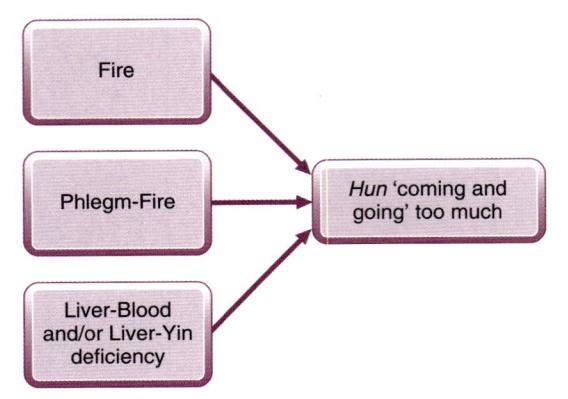

Figure 24.7 Full and Empty causes of anxiety

Box 24.35 Depression

Full

- Liver-Qi stagnation: depression, moodiness, irritability
- Stagnant Liver-Qi turning into Heat: depression, irritability, Red tongue
- Liver-Qi stagnation with Qi-Phlegm: depression, moodiness, feeling of a lump in the throat
- Phlegm-Fire harassing the Mind: depression, anxiety, agitation, expectoration of phlegm, Swollen tongue
- Heart-Blood stasis: depression, agitation, Purple tongue
- Gall Bladder-Heat: depression, irritability, bitter taste, hypochondrial fullness
- Diaphragm-Heat: depression, anxiety, feeling of stuffiness in the chest following an invasion of Wind-Heat

Empty

- Spleen- and Heart-Blood deficiency: depression, insomnia, palpitations, tiredness
- Heart-Yang deficiency: depression, palpitations, cold hands
- Liver-Blood deficiency: depression, lack of sense of direction, sadness
- Kidney- and Heart-Yin deficiency with Heart Empty-Heat: depression, anxiety, night sweating, palpitations, Red tongue without coating
- Kidney-Yang deficiency: depression, lack of motivation, lack of will-power, feeling cold, frequent urination

---

and Liver-Blood, respectively, and the person becomes anxious and sleeps badly. Conversely, pathogenic factors such as Qi stagnation, Blood stasis, Heat or Phlegm-Heat may 'agitate' the Mind and Ethereal Soul and lead to anxiety and insomnia. In some cases, of course, the Mind and Ethereal Soul are restless both from a deficiency (e.g. Yin deficiency) and a pathogenic factor (e.g. Empty-Heat). Figure 24.7 illustrates graphically the two causes of anxiety: a Deficiency leading to the Mind's not being 'anchored' or a pathogenic factor 'agitating' the Mind.

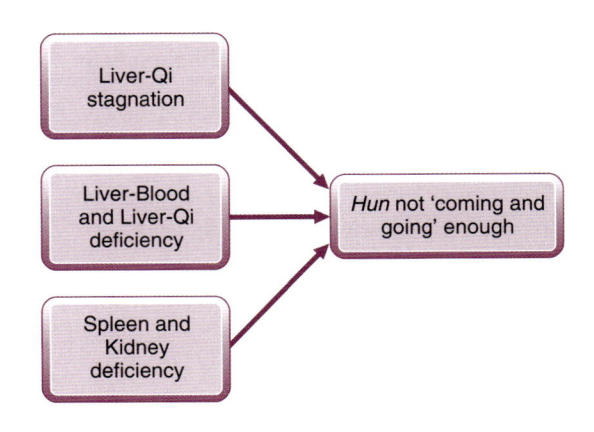

Box 24.36 Patterns in anxiety

Empty

- Deficiency of Blood
- Deficiency of Yin

Full

- Heat

Full/Empty

- Yin deficiency with Empty-Heat

As a general rule, the degree of anxiety or fear depends on whether it is caused by an Empty or a Full condition: in Empty conditions it is mild, while in Full conditions it is severe.

The main patterns accompanying anxiety and fear are (Box 24.37):

- Empty
  - Heart-Blood deficiency
  - Heart-Yin deficiency
  - Liver-Blood deficiency
  - Liver-Yin deficiency
  - Kidney-Yin deficiency
  - Deficiency of Qi of the Heart and Gall Bladder
- Full
  - Heart-Fire
  - Heart-Blood stasis
  - Phlegm-Fire harassing the Mind
  - Liver-Qi stagnation
  - Liver-Fire
  - Liver-Yang rising
  - Rebellious Qi of the Penetrating Vessel
  - Diaphragm-Heat
- Full/Empty
  - Kidney- and Heart-Yin deficiency with Heart Empty-Heat
  - Heart-Yin deficiency with Empty-Heat

> **Box 24.37 Fear/anxiety**
>
> **Empty**
> - Heart-Blood deficiency: mild anxiety, insomnia, palpitations
> - Heart-Yin deficiency: anxiety that is worse in the evening, palpitations, night sweating
> - Liver-Blood deficiency: mild anxiety, depression, insomnia
> - Liver-Yin deficiency: mild anxiety, depression, insomnia, tongue without coating
> - Kidney-Yin deficiency: anxiety that is worse in the evening, lack of will-power, dizziness, tinnitus
> - Deficiency of Qi of the Heart and Gall Bladder: mild anxiety, insomnia, timidity
>
> **Full**
> - Heart-Fire: severe anxiety, palpitations, Red tongue with coating
> - Heart-Blood stasis: severe anxiety, palpitations, Purple tongue
> - Phlegm-Fire harassing the Mind: severe anxiety, manic behaviour, Swollen tongue
> - Liver-Qi stagnation: anxiety, depression, irritability, hypochondrial distension
> - Liver-Fire: severe anxiety, headache, thirst, Red tongue, Wiry pulse
> - Liver-Yang rising: anxiety, headache, dizziness
> - Rebellious Qi of the Penetrating Vessel: anxiety, panicky feeling, feeling of constriction of the throat, palpitation, tightness of the chest, abdominal fullness, Firm pulse
> - Diaphragm-Heat: anxiety and feeling of stuffiness in the region under the heart following an invasion of Wind-Heat
>
> **Full/Empty**
> - Kidney- and Heart-Yin deficiency with Heart Empty-Heat: anxiety that is worse in the evening, dizziness, tinnitus, palpitations
> - Heart-Yin deficiency with Empty-Heat: anxiety that is worse in the evening, palpitations, Red tongue without coating

Irritability/anger

Irritability is a common emotional complaint. It includes feeling irritable frequently, flying off the handle easily, feeling frustrated, and similar emotional states. Of the traditional seven emotions, irritability is akin to 'anger' but it encompasses a broader range of emotional states and is generally not so intense. A propensity to anger is generally due to Liver patterns, while irritability may be caused by many different patterns affecting most organs.

In particular, the patterns that may cause irritability include:

> - Qi stagnation
> - Blood stasis
> - Liver-Yang rising
> - Blood deficiency
> - Yin deficiency (with or without Empty-Heat)
> - Heat (including Damp-Heat)
> - Empty-Heat

Therefore, irritability may be due to Full or Empty causes: in general the irritability from Empty causes is mild and somewhat vague, while that due to Full causes is more intense.

Box 24.38 summarizes irritability/anger patterns.

> **Box 24.38 Irritability/anger**
>
> - Qi stagnation
> - Blood stasis
> - Liver-Yang rising
> - Blood deficiency
> - Yin deficiency (with or without Empty-Heat)
> - Heat (including Damp-Heat)
> - Empty-Heat

Worry/overthinking

Many patients complain of a propensity to worry and overthinking and, even if it is not the presenting condition, many people profess to it when asked. The emotion of worry is related to the Lungs, and overthinking is more akin to the Spleen.

A propensity to worry and overthinking is most commonly caused by – and may in turn cause – an Empty condition. A deficiency of Spleen-Qi and/or -Blood is the most commonly seen pattern leading to worry and overthinking. However, Heart- and/or Liver-Blood deficiency may also lead to excessive worrying.

There are also cases where overthinking is caused by a mixed or Full condition, namely stagnation of Lung-Qi or Yin deficiency and Empty-Heat. Worry from a Full condition is usually more intense and consuming than that from an Empty condition, which a patient may describe as being more 'lurking in the background'.

Box 24.39 summarizes patterns underlying worry/overthinking.

> **Box 24.39 Worry/overthinking**
>
> - Heart- and Spleen-Qi deficiency: worry, slightly obsessive thinking, slight depression, overthinking, Pale tongue, Empty pulse
> - Lung-Qi deficiency: worry, depression, Pale tongue, Empty pulse
> - Lung-Qi stagnation: worry, mild irritability, depression, a feeling of lump in the throat, tongue slightly Red on the sides in the chest areas, pulse very slightly Tight on the Right-Front position
> - Heart-Blood deficiency: worry, depression, Pale and Thin tongue, Choppy or Fine pulse
> - Liver-Blood deficiency: worry which increases after the period in women, Pale tongue, Choppy or Fine pulse
> - Heart-Yin deficiency: worry, insomnia, dream-disturbed sleep, poor memory, anxiety, propensity to be startled, mental restlessness, uneasiness, 'feeling hot and bothered', Floating-Empty pulse, especially on the left-Front position
> - Heart-Yin deficiency with Empty-Heat: worry, especially in the evening, anxiety, propensity to be startled, mental restlessness, uneasiness, 'feeling hot and bothered', Red tongue, redder on the tip, no coating, Floating-Empty and Rapid pulse

Sadness and grief

'Sadness', which pertains to the Lungs, must be distinguished from a 'lack of joy', which pertains to the Heart. Sadness is an emotional state that weakens the Lungs and usually manifests with Lung-related symptoms such as a pale complexion and a weepy and weak voice. Lack of joy, on the other hand, is not an actual emotional state but a certain lack of vitality deriving from Heart deficiency: this manifests not with a sad demeanour, but with a flatness and lack of 'fire'.

Sadness depletes Lung- and Heart-Qi: however, with time, the deficiency of Qi in the chest may also give rise to some stagnation of Qi in the chest. This stagnation is associated with the Lungs and Heart and not the Liver. It manifests with a slight feeling of tightness of the chest, experiencing the sadness in the chest, sighing and slight palpitations.

The most likely Empty patterns giving rise to sadness are a deficiency of Lung-Qi or Liver- and/or Heart-Blood; when sadness is due to an Empty condition it is often accompanied by frequent crying. Sadness from Liver-Blood deficiency is more common in women and becomes worse after the period or after childbirth. Sadness with a feeling of lump in the throat may be due to Lung-Qi stagnation.

Grief is akin to sadness and usually derives from loss, separation or bereavement. Like sadness, it depletes Lung- and Heart-Qi but, with time, it may also give rise to some stagnation of Qi in the chest, causing similar symptoms to the ones mentioned above for sadness.

Box 24.40 summarizes patterns underlying sadness.

> **Box 24.40 Sadness**
>
> - Lung- and Heart-Qi deficiency: sadness, crying, depression, Pale tongue, Empty pulse
> - Liver-Blood deficiency: sadness, crying, mental confusion, aimlessness, Pale tongue, Choppy or Fine pulse
> - Heart-Blood deficiency: sadness, crying, depression, Pale and Thin tongue, Choppy or Fine pulse
> - Lung-Qi stagnation: sadness, mild irritability, depression, tongue slightly Red on the sides in the chest areas, pulse very slightly Tight on the Right-Front position

14. Sexual symptoms

An enquiry about the sexual life of the patient should always form part of the interrogation. This is not one of the traditional 10 questions from Chinese books, partly for cultural reasons. In fact, starting from the Ming period and especially during the Qing dynasty, Chinese medicine was heavily influenced by the prevalent Confucian morality, which condemned any talk or display of sexuality. Strangely, such *pruderie* continued in Communist China.

Questions about sexual symptoms are asked primarily to ascertain the state of the Kidneys and the Heart. In fact a Kidney deficiency is at the basis of many sexual symptoms, such as impotence, premature ejaculation and frigidity. A Heart deficiency also plays a prominent role in some sexual symptoms, such as impotence in men or inability to achieve an orgasm in women.

In men, apart from asking about any sexual problems such as impotence, it is important to establish whether any of their symptoms is aggravated by sexual activity or if they feel excessively tired after sexual activity. An aggravation of a symptom after sexual activity always indicates a Qi deficiency, often of the Kidneys. A Kidney deficiency is indicated also if a man feels especially tired after sexual activity and particularly if the tiredness is accompanied by dizziness, backache, weak knees, etc.

For obvious reasons, the practitioner needs to be particularly tactful when asking about sexual symptoms, especially when the practitioner and patient are of the opposite sex. In some cases, when I feel instinctively that the patient would not appreciate such questions, I do not ask them.

The sexual problems, and their clinical significance, of men and women will be discussed separately. These are:

- Men
  - Impotence
  - Lack of libido
  - Premature ejaculation
  - Tiredness and dizziness after ejaculation
- Women
  - Lack of libido
  - Headache soon after orgasm

Men

The sexual symptoms discussed are:

- Impotence
- Lack of libido
- Premature ejaculation
- Tiredness and dizziness after ejaculation

Impotence

Impotence is by far the most common sexual complaint in men and the first cause that would come to mind would be a Kidney deficiency and especially a Kidney-Yang deficiency. This is a common cause of impotence, especially in older men, in which case it is accompanied by backache, weak knees, dizziness, tinnitus and poor memory. In young men, however, it is my experience that impotence is more often related to a Heart pattern and anxiety. In a few cases, impotence may also be caused by Damp-Heat in the Liver channel. Box 24.41 summarizes impotence in men.

Box 24.41 Impotence

- Kidney-Yang deficiency: impotence, feeling cold, backache, abundant clear urine
- Heart-Blood deficiency: impotence, dizziness, palpitations, Choppy pulse
- Heart-Fire: impotence, palpitations, insomnia, dream-disturbed sleep, Rapid-Overflowing pulse
- Damp-Heat in the Liver channel: impotence, heaviness of the scrotum, urethral discharge, sticky yellow coating

Impotence in young men is caused more frequently by a Heart pattern rather than a Kidney deficiency

Lack of libido

Lack of libido in men is usually related to a deficiency of Qi or Yang, most frequently of the Kidneys: however, other organs may be relevant and a severe Qi deficiency of such organs as Spleen, Heart or Lungs may also cause lack of libido. In my experience, a deficiency of the Heart is a more common cause of lack of libido than deficiency of the Kidneys. Among Full conditions, Liver-Qi stagnation may also cause lack of libido. Box 24.42 summarizes lack of libido in men.

Box 24.42 Lack of libido

- Deficiency of Qi or Yang of the Kidneys
- Spleen deficiency
- Heart deficiency
- Lung deficiency
- Liver-Qi stagnation

Premature ejaculation

Premature ejaculation is usually related to a Kidney pattern and especially Kidney-Qi not Firm. It may also be due to a Heart pattern such as Heart-Qi or Heart-Blood deficiency. Box 24.43 summarizes premature ejaculation in men.

Tiredness and dizziness after ejaculation

A pronounced feeling of tiredness and dizziness after ejaculation is nearly always due to a deficiency of the Kidneys.

Box 24.43 Premature ejaculation

- Kidney-Qi not Firm
- Heart-Qi deficiency
- Heart-Blood deficiency

Women

The sexual symptoms discussed are as follows:

- Lack of libido
- Headache soon after orgasm

Lack of libido

Lack of libido

Lack of libido or an inability to reach an orgasm in women is usually related to a Kidney or Heart deficiency.

Generally, sexual desire depends on the state of Kidney-Yang and the Minister Fire: a deficient Minister Fire may cause a lack of sexual desire (and conversely, Fire of the Liver and/or Heart and Empty-Heat deriving from Kidney-Yin deficiency may cause an excessive sexual desire).

The Heart plays an important role in sexual arousal and orgasm in women. During sexual arousal, there is an arousal of the (physiological) Minister Fire of the Kidneys, which goes up towards the Heart and Pericardium: it is this upward flow of the Minister Fire towards the Heart that causes a flushed face and an increased heart rate. Thus, a lack of sexual desire is often due to a deficient Minister Fire and therefore Kidney-Yang.

During orgasm, the Minister Fire that was rising during sexual arousal is suddenly discharged downwards: this downward movement of the Minister Fire is controlled by the Heart (whose Qi naturally descends). Hence an inability to reach an orgasm may be due to a Heart deficiency (Fig. 24.8).

Of course, a woman's inability to reach an orgasm depends also on the man's performance during the sexual act. Therefore, when considering a woman's inability to reach an orgasm we should keep in mind the possibility that this is due to her partner's lack of skill rather than her own deficiency pattern.

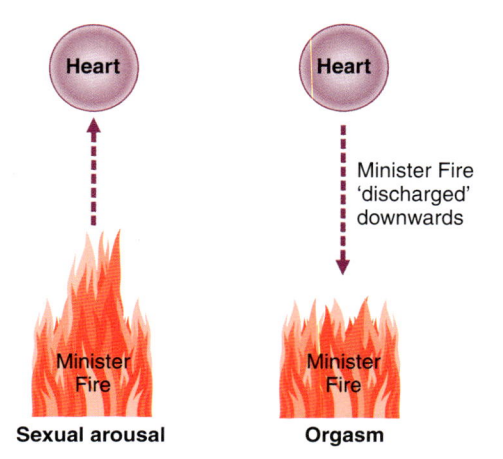

Figure 24.8 Role of Heart in sexual arousal and orgasm

Headache soon after orgasm

Headache soon after orgasm usually indicates rebellious Qi of the Penetrating Vessel. It may also indicate Heart-Fire.

15. Women's symptoms

Special questions need to be asked of women regarding menstruation, discharges, pregnancy and childbirth (Boxes 24.44 and 24.45).

The questions discussed are:

- Menstruation
  - Cycle
  - Amount
  - Colour
  - Quality
  - Pain
- Leucorrhoea
  - Colour
  - Consistency
  - Smell
- Pregnancy
- Childbirth

Menstruation

The condition of menstruation gives a very vivid idea of a woman's state of Qi and Blood. One must ask about the cycle, the amount of bleeding, colour of blood, quality and pain.

Cycle

If the periods are always early, it indicates either Heat in the Blood or Qi deficiency.

Box 24.44 Women's sexual symptoms

Lack of libido

- Lack of libido or inability to reach an orgasm: Kidney or Heart deficiency, Kidney-Yang deficiency
- Excessive sexual desire: Liver- or Heart-Fire, Empty-Heat from Kidney-Yin deficiency
- Inability to reach an orgasm: Heart deficiency

Headache soon after orgasm

- Rebellious Qi of the Penetrating Vessel (*Chong Mai*) or Heart-Fire

> **Box 24.45 Women's symptoms**
>
> **Menstruation**
>
> *Cycle*
> - Periods always early: Blood-Heat or Qi deficiency
> - Periods always late: Blood deficiency or stagnation of Blood or Cold
> - Periods irregular, sometimes early and sometimes late: stagnation of Liver-Qi or Liver-Blood, or Spleen deficiency
>
> *Amount*
> - Heavy loss of blood: Blood-Heat or Qi deficiency
> - Scanty periods: Blood deficiency or stagnation of Blood or Cold
>
> *Colour*
> - Dark-red or bright-red: Blood-Heat
> - Pale: Blood deficiency
> - Purple or blackish blood: stasis of Blood or Cold
> - Fresh-red: Empty-Heat from Yin deficiency
>
> *Quality*
> - Congealed blood with clots: stasis of Blood or Cold
> - Watery blood: Blood or Yin deficiency
> - Turbid blood: Blood-Heat or stagnation of Cold
>
> *Pain*
> - Before the periods: stagnation of Qi or Blood
> - During the periods: Blood-Heat or stagnation of Cold
> - After the periods: Blood deficiency
>
> **Leucorrhoea**
>
> *Colour*
> - White: Cold, Spleen- or Kidney-Yang deficiency, or exterior Cold-Damp
> - Yellow: Damp-Heat in the Lower Burner
> - Greenish: Damp-Heat in the Liver channel
> - Red and white: indicates Damp-Heat
> - Yellow with pus and blood after menopause: toxic Damp-Heat in the uterus
>
> *Consistency*
> - Watery: Cold-Damp
> - Thick: Damp-Heat
>
> *Smell*
> - Fishy: Damp-Cold
> - Leathery: Damp-Heat
>
> **Pregnancy**
> - Infertility: Blood or Kidney-Essence deficiency, Damp-Phlegm in the Lower Burner or stasis of Blood in the Uterus
> - Vomiting during pregnancy: Stomach and Penetrating Vessel deficiency
> - Miscarriage before 3 months: Blood or Essence deficiency
> - Miscarriage after 3 months: Liver-Blood stasis or sinking of Spleen-Qi
>
> **Childbirth**
> - Nausea and heavy bleeding after delivery: exhaustion of the Penetrating Vessel
> - Sweating and fever after delivery: exhaustion of Qi and Blood
> - Postnatal depression: Heart-Blood deficiency

If the periods always come late, it indicates either Blood deficiency of stagnation of Blood or Cold.

If the periods are irregular, coming sometimes early and sometimes late, it indicates stagnation of Liver-Qi or Liver-Blood, or Spleen deficiency.

Amount

A heavy loss of blood indicates either Heat in the Blood or Qi deficiency (see under colour of blood below).

Scanty periods indicate either Blood deficiency or stagnation of Blood or Cold.

Colour

A dark-red or bright-red colour indicates Heat in the Blood. Pale blood indicates Blood deficiency.

Purple or blackish blood indicates stasis of Blood or Cold. Fresh-red blood indicates Empty-Heat from Yin deficiency.

Quality

Congealed blood with clots indicates stasis of Blood or Cold. Watery blood indicates Blood or Yin deficiency.

Turbid blood indicates Blood-Heat or stagnation of Cold.

Pain

Pain before the periods indicates stagnation of Qi or Blood.

Pain during the periods indicates Blood-Heat or stagnation of Cold. Pain after the periods indicates Blood deficiency.

These questions and their answers have limited value with regard to women who take the contraceptive pill, or have had an intrauterine device fitted, or in multiparous women.

Leucorrhoea

This must be distinguished according to colour, consistency and smell.

Colour

A white discharge indicates a Cold pattern. This could be from Spleen- or Kidney-Yang deficiency, or exterior Cold-Damp, or sometimes from stagnation of Liver-Qi.

A yellow discharge indicates a Heat pattern, usually Damp-Heat in the Lower Burner.

A greenish discharge indicates Damp-Heat in the Liver channel. A red and white discharge also indicates Damp-Heat.

A yellow discharge with pus and blood in a woman after menopause indicates toxic Damp-Heat in the uterus.

Consistency

A watery consistency suggests a Cold-Damp pattern, whilst a thick consistency suggests a Damp-Heat pattern.

Smell

A fishy smell indicates Damp-Cold; a leathery smell indicates Damp-Heat.

Pregnancy

Infertility can be due to Empty conditions such as Blood or Kidney-Essence deficiency, or to Full conditions such as Damp-Phlegm in the Lower Burner or stasis of Blood in the uterus.

Vomiting during pregnancy indicates Stomach and Penetrating Vessel deficiency.

Miscarriage before 3 months indicates Blood or Essence deficiency and is associated with a Kidney deficiency; after 3 months it indicates Liver-Blood stasis or sinking of Spleen-Qi.

Childbirth

Nausea and heavy bleeding after delivery indicate exhaustion of the Penetrating Vessel. Sweating and fever after delivery indicate exhaustion of Qi and Blood.

Postnatal depression is usually due to Blood deficiency leading to Heart-Blood deficiency.

16. Children's symptoms

Interrogation of children does not differ substantially from that of adults, except that it needs to be carried out mostly with the child's parents.

There are several questions, however, which are peculiar to children's problems.

First of all, one needs to ask about the pregnancy, as emotional shocks or physical traumas can affect the constitution of the baby. Also the consumption of alcohol, smoking and use of drugs (both the medicinal and the 'recreational' kind) all affect the health of the baby adversely.

Traumas at birth, such as Caesarean delivery or very long birth, will affect the baby, particularly the baby's Lungs.

One also needs to ask about breast feeding and weaning. Weaning too early can lead to the retention of food and some skin diseases. Persistent sore throats and/or a runny nose in children often indicates too early weaning or too rich food consumed too early.

In older children, one must ask about childhood diseases such as whooping cough or measles. Whooping cough usually leaves the Lungs quite weakened, especially if it occurs in a severe form.

The symptoms discussed are:

- Digestive symptoms
- Respiratory symptoms and earache
- Sleep
- Immunizations

Digestive symptoms

Digestive symptoms are very common in children due to an inherently weak Spleen and Stomach at birth: the younger the child, the more common are digestive symptoms. The two most common causes of abdominal pain in children are retention of Cold in the Stomach and Intestines and stagnation of Qi in the Intestines. In babies, retention of food (called Accumulation Disorder in babies) is very common and it manifests with vomiting of milk and with colic.

Respiratory symptoms and earache

Questions concerning cough, wheezing, breathlessness and earache are always important in the child's interrogation because children are very prone to invasions of Wind, which may cause the above symptoms.

A history of repeated bouts of cough and wheezing nearly always indicates a residual pathogenic factor (usually Lung Phlegm-Heat) following invasions of external Wind. These give rise to a residual pathogenic factor when the Wind is not cleared properly, when antibiotics are used too frequently, or when the child has a weak constitution. In such cases the child will suffer from a chronic cough and/or wheezing and will be prone to frequent respiratory infections.

A history of chronic earache also indicates the presence of a residual pathogenic factor, which, in this case, is usually Damp-Heat in the Gall Bladder channel. This is also the result of frequent, acute ear infections, usually treated by the repeated administration of antibiotics, which only makes matters worse by promoting the development of a residual pathogenic factor.

The condition of chronic catarrh is very common in children and this is the consequence of a residual pathogenic factor after repeated invasions of Wind combined with a Spleen deficiency leading to the formation of Phlegm. A child with this condition will have a constantly runny nose or a blocked nose, cough and glue ear.

> **Box 24.46 Children's symptoms**
>
> **Digestive symptoms**
>
> - Abdominal pain: Cold in the Stomach and Intestines, Qi stagnation
> - Vomiting of milk and colic in babies: retention of food
>
> **Respiratory symptoms and earache**
>
> - Cough, wheezing, earache: invasion of Wind
> - Chronic cough, wheezing: residual Phlegm in Lungs
> - Chronic earache: residual Damp-Heat in Gall Bladder channel
> - Chronic mucus, blocked nose, cough, 'glue ear': residual Dampness
>
> **Sleep**
>
> - Disturbed sleep with crying in babies: retention of food or Stomach-Heat
> - Subdued crying at night: prenatal shock
> - Disturbed sleep in older children: Liver-Fire, Stomach-Heat
>
> **Immunizations**
>
> - Skin rash, insomnia, change in character: Latent Heat

Sleep

Disturbed sleep with crying in babies is often due to retention of food and Stomach-Heat, in which case the baby will cry out loudly. If the baby cries relatively quietly during the night, it may be due to a prenatal shock.

In older children disturbed sleep may be due to the same factors as in adults but the most common ones are Liver-Fire, Stomach-Heat and retention of food.

Immunizations

It is important to ask about immunizations as, in some cases, these may cause problems.

A full discussion on immunizations is beyond the scope of this book. To understand the effect of immunizations from a Chinese perspective, however, it is necessary to refer to the theory of the Four Levels (see ch. 45). When a pathogenic factor invades the body, it enters the Defensive Qi level first and, if not expelled, it progresses through the Qi, Nutritive Qi and Blood levels; the Four Levels represent four different energetic layers of penetration of Heat, with the Defensive Qi level being the most superficial and the Blood level the deepest.

From a Chinese perspective, therefore, immunizations basically consist in injecting a 'pathogenic factor' (i.e. the live or attenuated germ) directly at the Blood level. This may cause Latent Heat to develop at the Blood level, which may cause problems for the child both in the short term and in the long term.

In the short term, Latent Heat may cause a skin rash, insomnia and a temporary change in the child's character. The long-term effects of immunizations are more difficult to establish and the subject of great controversy. However, if immunizations lead to Latent Heat at the Blood level, it is quite possible that they may have serious long-term effects. These include brain damage, possibly autism, asthma, chronic cough, allergies and skin diseases later in life.

Box 24.46 summarizes children's symptoms.

Immunizations are a common cause of Latent Heat in children, which may persist into adulthood

4

Learning outcomes

In this chapter you will have learned:

- The different aspects of interrogation, in which the practitioner aims to uncover both the cause of the disease as well as pattern of disharmony itself
- The concept that signs and symptoms reflect the state of Internal Organs and channels
- That diagnosis takes into account many different manifestations as parts of a whole picture, many of them not related to an actual disease process
- The importance of asking the right questions in relation to a specific patient and specific condition, whilst constantly trying to confirm or exclude certain patterns
- The significance of terminology used by patients to describe their symptoms, which can differ between cultures
- How tongue and pulse diagnosis are used, not only to confirm suspected patterns but also to indicate the presence of patterns not evident from other signs and symptoms
- The importance of flexibility in following the traditional structure of questioning
- The reasons for making changes and additions to the traditional list of questions, in order to make the interrogation appropriate to a Western clinical setting
- How to question to differentiate the various patterns which cause pain
- How questions relating to food and taste provide important information, particularly about the state of Stomach and Spleen
- The importance of asking about stools and urine, especially to establish whether a condition is Full or Empty
- The role of asking about thirst and drink in the interrogation, particularly in indicating the presence of Heat and Cold
- The frequency of tiredness as a complaint in Western patients, and methods of questioning to ascertain the appropriate pattern
- How to question the patient to elicit information pertaining to headaches, dizziness, face (temperature, pain, nose, gums, mouth) and body (pain, backache, numbness)
- Questioning about the various areas of the chest and abdomen, and limbs
- The importance of asking patients about their sleep, which especially indicates the state of the Mind and the Ethereal Soul
- The clinical significance of sweating, which requires consideration of Interior and Exterior, Fullness and Emptiness, as well as the area of body, time of day, quality of sweat and condition of the illness
- How to ask about symptoms of the ears and eyes
- Clinical significance of feelings of cold, heat and fever and their different clinical significance in exterior and interior conditions
- The importance of questioning and observing the patient's emotional state
- The clinical significance of sexual symptoms in both women and men
- The significance of women's symptoms, including asking about menstruation, leucorrhoea, pregnancy and childbirth
- How to ask about children's symptoms, particularly in the areas of digestion, respiration, sleep and immunization

Self-assessment questions

1. List as many of the 16 diagnostic areas of questioning as you can.
2. Why was questioning about aversion to cold and fever traditionally placed at the beginning of the interrogation in the traditional '10 Questions'?
3. What is the basic pathology of pain due to a Full condition?
4. What are the characteristics of pain caused by Blood stasis?
5. In general, if a condition is aggravated by eating, what does this indicate?
6. What pattern is indicated by a constant bitter taste in the mouth?
7. If a condition gets worse after a bowel movement, what general pattern do you suspect?
8. Loose stools with undigested food indicate which pattern?
9. What is the likely pattern causing difficulty in urination in an elderly person?
10. The absence of thirst indicates which general pattern?
11. A patient reports long-term tiredness, and is also tense and anxious. Their pulse is Wiry. What pattern do you suspect?
12. A dull headache at the vertex of the head commonly comes from which pattern?
13. A patient complains of sinusitis, with a chronic, runny nose with a sticky yellow discharge. Which pattern is most likely?
14. What might mouth ulcers on the lower gum indicate?
15. Numbness of the fingers, elbow and arm on one side of the body indicates the presence of which pathogens?
16. Which patterns most commonly cause a feeling of fullness and distension of the epigastrium?
17. What are the three possible patterns causing cold hands?
18. What pattern is likely to be present if a patient wakes up frequently during the night?
19. Which organs do you suspect may be involved if a patient sweats only on their hands?
20. Tinnitus with a low-pitch noise like rushing water indicates what pattern?
21. Give three clinical manifestations of Full Cold.
22. What is meant by the term 'fever' in Chinese diagnosis in the context of exterior diseases?
23. A patient suffers from anxiety, which gets worse in the afternoon, and also suffers with insomnia, palpitations and night sweats. What is the likely presenting pattern?
24. Which two organs would you consider first in the diagnosis of a young man suffering with impotence?
25. Pain after a period indicates which pattern?

See p. 1261 for answers

PART 4

Diagnosis by Palpation   25

Key contents

Pulse diagnosis

Introduction
- Historical background
- Assignment of organs to pulse positions
- Reconciliation of contradictions
- The clinical significance of the pulse as a whole
- Organ vs channel in pulse diagnosis
- The three levels

Method for taking the pulse
- Time
- Levelling the arm
- Placing the fingers
- Arranging the fingers
- Regulating the fingers
- Using the fingers
- Moving the fingers
    - Lifting
    - Pressing
    - Searching
    - Pushing
    - Rolling
- Equalizing the breathing

Factors to take into account
- Season
- Gender
- Occupation

The normal pulse
- Stomach Qi
- Spirit
- Root

The pulse qualities
- Floating
- Deep
- Slow
- Rapid
- Empty
- Full
- Slippery
- Choppy
- Long
- Short
- Overflowing
- Fine
- Minute
- Tight
- Wiry
- Slowed-down
- Hollow
- Leather
- Firm
- Soggy (or Weak-floating)
- Weak
- Scattered
- Hidden
- Moving
- Hasty
- Knotted
- Intermittent
- Hurried

Palpating the skin

Temperature
Moisture and texture

Palpating the limbs

Palpation of hands and feet
Palpation and comparison of dorsum and palm
Palpating the hand

Palpating the chest

Palpating the apical beat
Palpating the area below the xiphoid process
Palpating the chest
Palpating the breast

Palpating the abdomen

Palpating points

Diagnosis by palpation includes palpation of the:

- Pulse
- Skin
- Limbs
- Chest
- Abdomen
- Points

PULSE DIAGNOSIS

The discussion of pulse diagnosis will include the following topics:

- Introduction
  - Historical background
  - Assignment of organs to pulse positions
  - Reconciliation of contradictions
  - The clinical significance of the pulse as a whole
  - Organ versus channel in pulse diagnosis
  - The three levels
- Method for taking the pulse
  - Time
  - Levelling the arm
  - Placing the fingers
  - Arranging the fingers
  - Regulating the fingers
  - Using the fingers
  - Moving the fingers
  - Equalizing the breathing
- Factors to take into account
  - Seasons
  - Gender
  - Occupation
- The normal pulse
  - Stomach-Qi
  - Spirit
  - Root
- The pulse qualities
  - Floating
  - Deep
  - Slow
  - Rapid
  - Empty
  - Full
  - Slippery
  - Choppy
  - Long
  - Short
  - Overflowing
  - Fine
  - Minute
  - Tight
  - Wiry
  - Slowed-down
  - Hollow
  - Leather
  - Firm
  - Soggy (or Weak-Floating)
  - Weak
  - Scattered
  - Hidden
  - Moving
  - Hasty
  - Knotted
  - Intermittent
  - Hurried

Introduction

Pulse diagnosis is an extremely complex subject with many ramifications, and the following will only be a simple discussion of it in the context of Chinese diagnosis.[1]

Pulse diagnosis is important for two reasons: firstly, because it can give very detailed information on the state of the internal organs, and secondly, because it reflects the whole complex of Qi and Blood. The pulse can be seen as a clinical manifestation, a sign like any other such as thirst, insomnia or a red face. The important difference is that, besides giving certain specific indications, the pulse also reflects the organism as a whole, the state of Qi, Blood and Yin, the Yin and Yang organs, all parts of the body, and even the constitution of a person.

Besides being a clinical manifestation like any other, the pulse reflects the state of Qi and Blood as a whole as well as the constitution of a person

The main drawback of pulse diagnosis is that it is an extremely subjective form of diagnosis, probably more than any other element of Chinese diagnosis. If a face is red, or if a tongue is red, these are quite objective signs and anyone can see them. Feeling the pulse is an extremely subtle skill and is very difficult to learn. Most students will be familiar with the frustrating experience of not being able to feel that a certain pulse is 'choppy' or 'slippery'.

The pulse can give very detailed information on the state of the internal organs, but it is also subject to external, short-term influences, which make its interpretation very difficult indeed and fraught with pitfalls. For example, if a person has been running upstairs the pulse becomes rapid very quickly, and it would be wrong to interpret that as a sign of a 'Heat pattern'. If a person has had an emotional upset or shock, the pulse will also change quickly. If a person works very hard and has very little sleep for a week or so, the pulse can become very weak and deep, but it is quickly restored with just a few days' rest. From this point of view, the tongue is less subject to such short-term influences.

Historical background

The practice of taking the pulse on the radial artery was started by the 'Classic of Difficulties'. Before that, the pulse was felt at nine different arteries, three on the head, three on the hands and three on the legs, reflecting the state of the energy of the Upper, Middle and Lower Burner, respectively. This location for pulse taking was described in the 'Simple Questions' in chapter 20.[2] These positions for pulse taking are all on acupuncture points that are situated near arteries. They are shown in Table 25.1.

As can be seen from the table, LIV-10 Wuli and SP-11 Jimen have an alternative position for pulse taking at LIV-3 Taichong and ST-42 Chongyang, respectively. This was done in ancient times in female patients to avoid the doctor (always a man) touching the thigh of his female patients.

Assignment of organs to pulse positions

The 'Classic of Difficulties' (AD 100) established for the first time the practice of taking the pulse at the radial artery: this pulse was variously called *Qi Kou* ('Portal of Qi'), *Cun Kou* ('Portal of Inch [Front pulse position]') and *Mai Kou* ('Portal of Pulse'). The 'Classic of Difficulties' says: '*The 12 main channels have their own arteries but the pulse can be taken only at the Portal of Inch [LU-9 position] reflecting the life and death of the 5 Yin and 6 Yang organs ... The Portal of Inch is the beginning and end point of the energy of the 5 Yin and 6 Yang organs and that is why we can take the pulse at this position only.*'[3]

The 'Classic of Difficulties' established the practice of feeling the pulse at the radial artery, dividing it into three areas and feeling it at three different levels: that is, superficial, middle and deep. The three sections of the pulse at the radial artery were called 'inch' (*cun*), 'gate' (*guan*) and 'foot' (*chi*). In this book they will be called 'Front', 'Middle' and 'Rear', respectively. Three levels at each of the three sections made the so-called 'nine regions'.[4]

The 'Classic of Difficulties' clearly relates the three sections of the pulse to the three Burners. It says: '*There are three positions, inch, bar and cubit and nine regions [each position being] superficial, middle and deep. The upper [distal] position corresponds to Heaven and reflects diseases from the chest to the head; the middle position corresponds to Person and reflects diseases between the diaphragm and umbilicus; the lower [proximal] position corresponds to Earth and reflects diseases from below the umbilicus to the feet*'[5] (Fig. 25.1).

Over the centuries, there have been several different attributions of organs to individual pulse positions.

Table 25.1 The nine regions of the pulse from the 'Simple Questions'

Area	Location	Region	Point	Organ or body part	Alternative
Upper	Head	Upper Middle Lower	Tai Yang ST-3 Juliao T.B.-21 Ermen	Qi of head Qi of mouth Qi of ears and eyes	
Middle	Hand	Upper Middle Lower	LU-8 Jingqu L.I.-4 Hegu HE-7 Shenmen	Lungs Centre of thorax Heart	
Lower	Leg	Upper Middle Lower	LIV-10 Wuli KI-3 Taixi SP-11 Jimen	Liver Kidneys Spleen and Stomach	LIV-3 Taichong ST-42 Chongyang

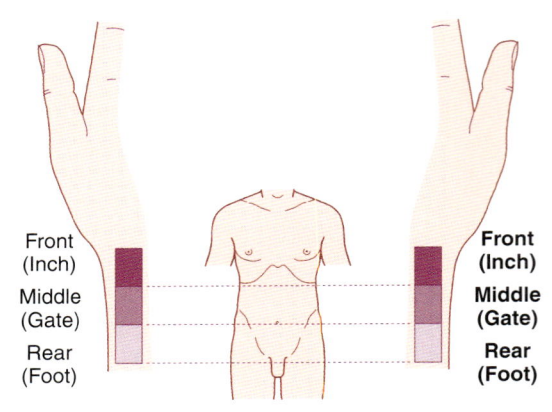

Figure 25.1 Correspondence of pulse positions to Three Burners

The most commonly used today are derived from the 'Pulse Classic' (*Mai Jing*, AD 280) of Wang Shu He, the 'Pulse Study of Bin-Hu Lake' (*Bin Hu Mai Xue*, 1564) by Li Shi Zhen and the 'Golden Mirror of Medical Tradition' (*Yi Zong Jin Jian*, 1742) by Wu Qian.

The pulse positions adopted in the 'Classic of Difficulties' are (Fig. 25.2):

	Left	Right
Front	Small Intestine/Heart	Lungs/Large Intestine
Middle	Gall Bladder/Liver	Spleen/Stomach
Rear	Bladder/Kidneys	Pericardium/Triple Burner

The 'Pulse Classic' discusses the correspondence of pulse positions to organs (or channels) in chapter 7 and these are:

	Left	Right
Front	Small Intestine/Heart	Lungs/Large Intestine
Middle	Gall Bladder/Liver	Spleen/Stomach
Rear	Bladder/Kidneys	Kidneys/Uterus/Triple Burner/Bladder

The pulse positions adopted in the 'Pulse Study of Bin-Hu Lake' (which omits the Yang organs) are:

	Left	Right
Front	Heart	Lungs
Middle	Liver	Spleen
Rear	Kidneys	Kidneys

Another widely used arrangement comes from the 'Golden Mirror of Medical Tradition' (*Yi Zong Jin Jian*, 1742) by Wu Qian. This includes positions for the Yang organs:

	Left	Right
Front	*Shanzhong*/Heart	Lungs/Chest
Middle	Gall Bladder/Liver	Spleen/Stomach
Rear	Bladder, Small Intestine/Kidneys	Large Intestine/Kidneys

The left Rear position is usually thought to reflect the Qi of Kidney-Yin and the right Rear position that of Kidney-Yang. *Shanzhong* here indicates the centre of the chest.

Reconciliation of contradictions

Contradictory though these different arrangements might seem, there is actually a common strand running through them. First of all, there is general agreement that the Front positions reflect the state of Qi in the Upper Burner, the Middle positions the Middle Burner and the Rear positions the Lower Burner (apart from the positioning of Large Intestine and Small Intestine in the Front positions, by the 'Classic of Difficulties' and by the 'Pulse Classic' of Wang Shu He, which will be explained shortly).

However, with regard to the Yang organs, there seem to be the most discrepancies. In fact, some doctors did not even consider that the state of the Yang organs could be reflected on the pulse.

In my opinion the differences are reconcilable because different pulse arrangements reflect the different therapeutic approaches of the herbalist and acupuncturist: this is especially clear with regard to the position of the Large Intestine and Small Intestine on the pulse. In fact, the assignment of these two organs to pulse positions is the one with the most striking contradictions: some assign them to the Upper Burner and some to the Lower Burner. Given that the pulse reflects the Qi of both organ and channel, the acupuncturist working on the channels would naturally assign the Small Intestine and Large Intestine to the same position as the Heart and Lungs (in the Upper Burner) to which their channels are connected.

The herbalist, on the other hand, would give more importance to the internal organs rather than channels, and assign the Small Intestine and Large Intestine

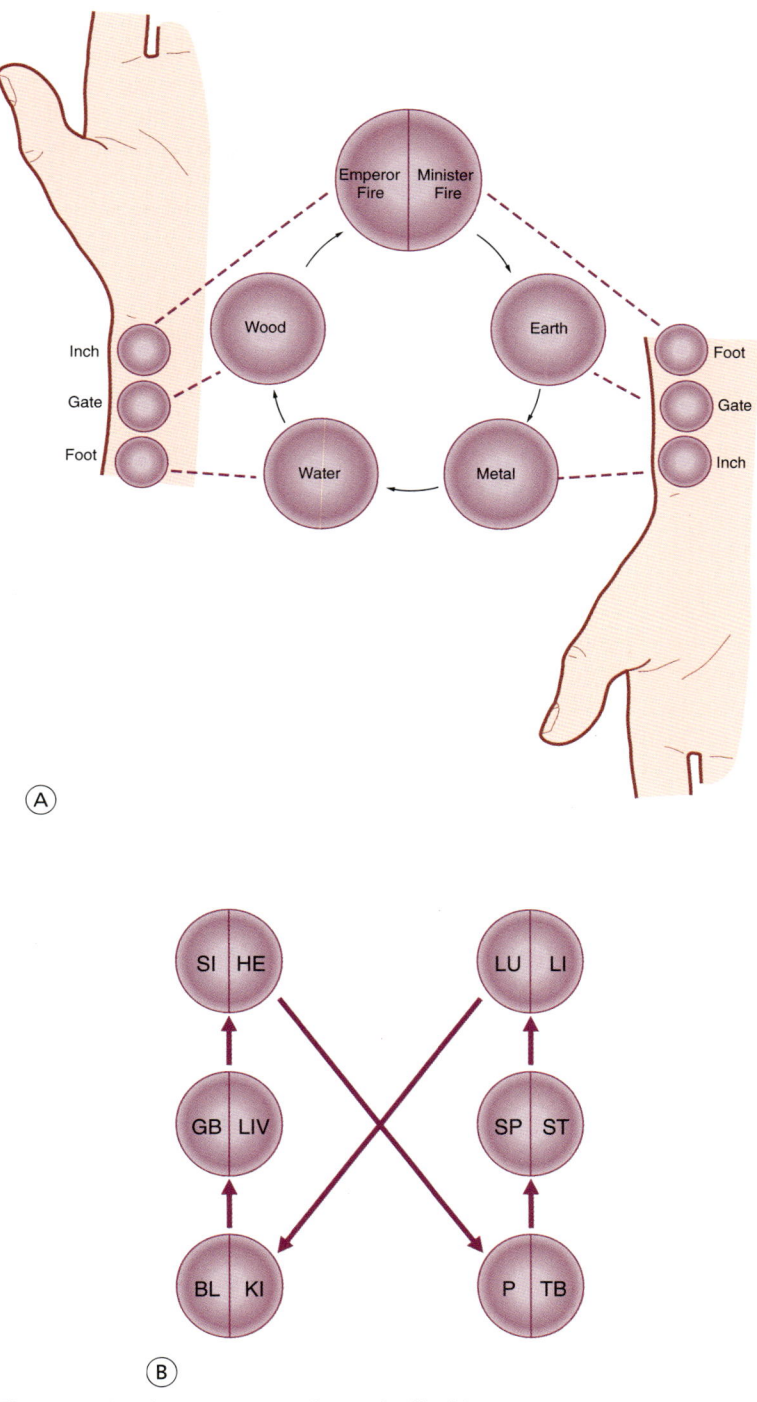

Figure 25.2 Pulse positions in 'Classic of Difficulties'

to the Rear position, i.e. the Lower Burner, which is where these organs are situated.

> The contradictory assignment of Large and Small Intestine to the Front (Upper Burner) or Rear (Lower Burner) position reflects the different perspective of the acupuncturist and herbalist, respectively

Another reason for the discrepancies is that the Small Intestine and Large Intestine organs are much less closely related to their respective channels than the other organs. These two organs are situated in the Lower Burner, while their channels are in the arms (all other organs in the Upper Burner have their respective channels on the arms, and those of the Middle or Lower Burner have their respective channels on the legs).

Moreover, the functions of the actual intestinal organs and their respective channels do not closely correspond for, although the Small Intestine and Large Intestine channel points can be used for their corresponding organ problems, they are frequently used to treat diseases of the Upper Burner areas (shoulders, neck, head) and invasions of exterior pathogenic factors affecting the shoulders, neck and head (Fig. 25.3).

Figure 25.3 illustrates two pathological conditions of the Large Intestine, one of the channel (tooth abscess), one of the organ (ulcerative colitis). Thus, a tooth abscess caused by Toxic Heat in the Large Intestine channel will be reflected on the right Front position, while ulcerative colitis, obviously affecting the Large Intestine organ, is reflected on the right Rear position (usually making the pulse here Wiry).

There is yet another discrepancy between the 'Classic of Difficulties' and all subsequent classics, in that the former attributes the right Rear position to the Triple Burner and Pericardium, while all other classics assign this position variously to the Kidneys, Uterus, Bladder, Large Intestine, all organs in the Lower Burner.

Again, I think this discrepancy reflects the different viewpoints of the acupuncturist and herbalist. From an acupuncture (and therefore channel) perspective, assigning the right Rear position to the Triple Burner and Pericardium maintains the symmetry between pulse positions and the 12 channels. From the organ point of view, the Rear position cannot possibly reflect channels that are in the Upper Burner and also an organ that is in the Upper Burner (Pericardium).

Indeed, chapter 18 of the 'Classic of Difficulties' assigns the right Rear position to the Pericardium and Triple Burner', but the *very same* chapter also says in a following paragraph that *'The pulse has three positions and 9 regions: to what do they correspond? The 3 positions are the cun, guan and chi. The 9 regions refer to Superficial, Middle and Deep [of each position]. The Upper position is ruled by Heaven and reflects diseases from the chest to the head; the Middle position is ruled by Person and reflects diseases between the diaphragm and umbilicus; the Lower position is ruled by Earth and reflects diseases from the*

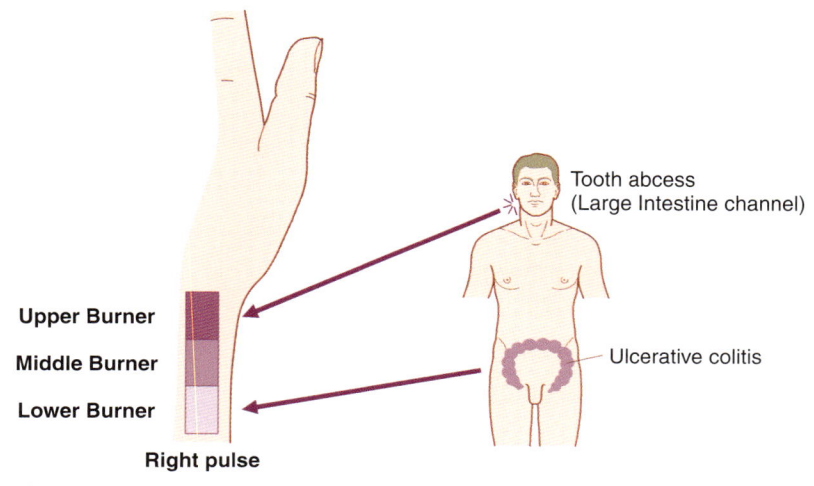

Figure 25.3 Organ versus channel in pulse diagnosis

umbilicus to the feet.'[6] Thus this passage clearly says that the Rear positions reflect diseases of the Lower Burner.

Please note that 'Earth' in this context is not the 'Earth' of the Five Elements, but the 'Earth' of the three-fold structure 'Heaven–Person–Earth'.

The clinical significance of the pulse as a whole

This aside, another aspect of pulse diagnosis also explains why we should not make too much of the different pulse positions assumed by different doctors. The pulse essentially reflects the state of Qi in the different Burners and at different energetic levels, which are dependent on the pathological condition. The pulse needs to be interpreted dynamically rather than mechanically. For this reason, we should not attach undue importance to the organ (or channel) positions on the pulse. The most important thing is to appraise how Qi is flowing; what is the relationship of Yin and Yang on the pulse; at what level Qi is flowing (i.e. is the pulse superficial or deep); whether the body's Qi is deficient; and whether there is an attack by an exterior pathogenic factor.

Organ versus channel in pulse diagnosis

Each pulse position can reflect different phenomena in different situations. For example, let us consider the left Middle pulse (Liver position): in a state of health, the Liver- and Gall Bladder-Qi will be balanced or, to put it differently, Yin and Yang within the Liver/Gall Bladder sphere are balanced. In this case, the pulse will be relatively soft and smooth and not particularly superficial or deep and the Gall Bladder influence on the pulse will not be felt. But if Liver-Yang is in excess and rises upwards affecting the Gall Bladder channel (causing severe temporal headaches), the rising Qi will be reflected on the pulse, which will be Wiry (harder than normal) and more superficial (it will be felt pounding under the finger). In interpreting this pulse we can say that Liver-Yang is rising, or, to put it differently, that the Gall Bladder-Qi is in Excess.

To give another example, if the right Front pulse (Lung pulse) is quite full, bigger than normal and rapid, it could indicate an emotional problem affecting the Lungs. Here, the pulse would reflect the state of the Lungs. But on another occasion exactly the same type of pulse may indicate something quite different when for example the patient has an acute, large, purulent tooth abscess. In such a case, the pulse reflects the state of the Large Intestine channel (where the abscess is) rather than a problem with the Lung organ.

The three levels

When feeling the pulse, one should assess it at three different depths: a superficial, middle and deep level. The superficial level is felt by just resting the fingers on the artery very gently; the deep level is felt by pressing quite hard to the point of nearly obliterating the pulse and then releasing very slightly; the middle level is felt in between these two pressures.

The three levels of the pulse give an immediate idea of the level of Qi in the pulse and therefore the kind of pathological condition that might be present. In particular:

- The Superficial level reflects the state of Qi (and the Yang organs)
- The Middle level reflects the state of Blood
- The Deep level reflects the state of Yin (and the Yin organs)

Thus, by examining the strength and quality of the pulse at the three levels, one can have an idea of the pathology of Qi, Blood or Yin, and also of the relative state of Yin and Yang.

The clinical significance of the three levels was interpreted differently by different doctors, but all these approaches are equally valid and should be borne in mind.

For example, besides reflecting Qi, Blood and Yin, the three levels also reflect the following:

- Superficial level: Exterior diseases
- Middle level: Stomach and Spleen diseases
- Deep level: Interior diseases

Li Shi Zhen gives yet another interpretation of the three levels, as follows:

- The Superficial level reflects the state of Heart and Lungs
- The Middle level reflects the state of Stomach and Spleen
- The Deep level reflects the state of Liver and Kidneys

With this slant, the Qi of the internal organs is not only reflected at the various positions, but also depths. The idea is that the Heart and Lungs (particularly the Lungs) can be said to control the Exterior of the body and their Qi is therefore felt at the superficial level. The

Table 25.2 Clinical significance of the three levels of the pulse

Level	Energy type	Energy level	Organ
Superficial	Qi (Yang organs)	Exterior	Heart and Lungs
Middle	Blood	Stomach and Spleen	Stomach and Spleen
Deep	Yin (Yin organs)	Interior	Kidneys

Stomach and Spleen make Blood and their Qi can therefore be felt at the Blood (middle) level. The Liver and Kidneys (particularly the Kidneys) control the Yin energies and their Qi is therefore felt at the Yin (deep) level.

Thus, the clinical significance of the three levels of depth on the pulse can be interpreted in three different ways, each of them meaningful (Table 25.2).

Conversely one can interpret the three positions Front, Middle and Rear as reflecting the energies Qi, Blood and Yin, respectively, as well as the three body areas of Upper, Middle and Lower and their respective organs (Table 25.3). Therefore, the three positions, Front, Middle and Rear of the pulse, may also reflect the three levels, with the Front representing the superficial level, the Middle the middle level and the Rear the deep level.

Table 25.3 Clinical significance of pulse positions

Position	Energy type	Burner	Organ
Superficial	Qi	Upper	Heart-Lungs
Middle	Blood	Middle	Stomach-Spleen
Deep	Yin	Lower	Kidney

Method for taking the pulse

Time

Traditionally, the best time for taking the pulse is in the early morning when the Yin is calm and the Yang has not yet come forth.

This is of course not always possible to achieve when patients are seen throughout the day.

Levelling the arm

The patient's arm should be horizontal and should not be held higher than the level of the heart. This means that if the patient is sitting up, the arm should rest horizontally on the table; if the patient is lying down, the arm should rest horizontally on the couch and not be held by the practitioner across the patient's body (Fig. 25.4).

Placing the fingers

Placing the fingers means that the practitioner's three fingers (index, middle and ring fingers) are placed simultaneously on the radial artery to make an initial assessment of the strength, level and quality of the pulse. To assess individual positions, it may be necessary to lift two of the fingers slightly, while interpreting the pulse with the third finger. Usually, one feels the pulse of the patient's right arm with one's left hand and vice versa and the index, middle and ring fingers are placed on the Front, Middle and Rear positions, respectively.

Arranging the fingers

Arranging the fingers means that the practitioner should either spread the fingers slightly or press them close together according to the size of the patient's arm. For example, when feeling the pulse of a 10-year-old child, we should press our fingers closer together to feel the three positions; the younger the child, the closer together our fingers should be and, in a baby under 1 year old, we feel the three positions with a single finger (by rolling it proximally and distally to feel the Rear and Front positions, respectively). When taking the pulse of a very tall man, we should spread the fingers out slightly to feel the three positions.

Regulating the fingers

Regulating the fingers means that the practitioner should place the finger tips on the three positions,

Ⓐ

Ⓑ

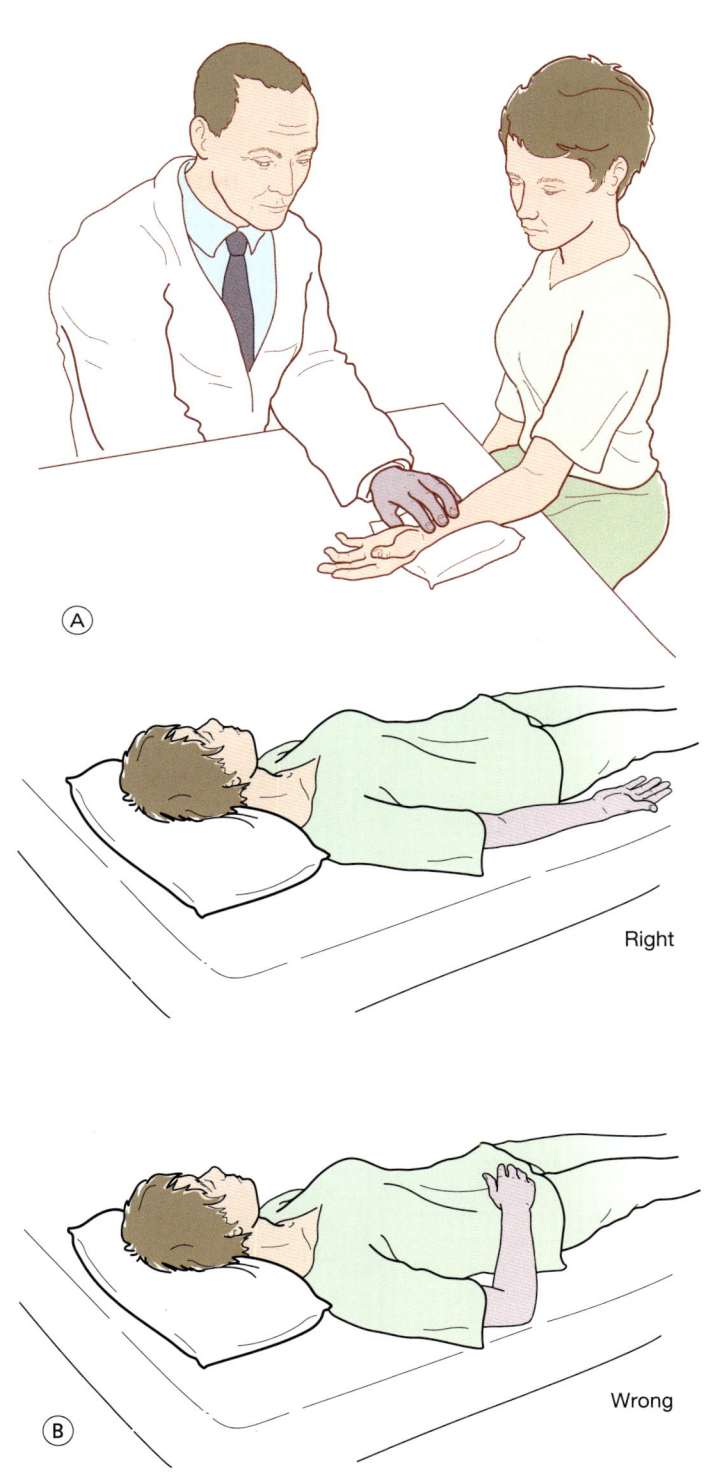

Figure 25.4 Levelling the arm

Right

Wrong

allowing for the different length of the fingers. In other words, the middle finger, being the longest, is slightly contracted. To feel the pulse, the pads rather than the tips of the fingers are used.

Using the fingers

Using the fingers means that the practitioner should bear in mind the subtle difference in sensitivity between the three fingers. Generally, the ring finger is slightly more sensitive than the others and we should take this into account when comparing the different strengths of the three positions: however, the difference in sensitivity is very small and not too important in clinical practice.

Moving the fingers

Moving the fingers means that the fingers should be moved in various directions when feeling the pulse. It is a common misconception that the pulse is felt by keeping the fingers absolutely still for a long time: in fact, the fingers are kept still only when counting the rate of the pulse to decide whether it is Slow, Rapid or normal. The movements are five:

1. **Lifting** consists of gently lifting the fingers to check the strength of the pulse at the superficial level and therefore whether the pulse is Floating, normal or deficient at that level
2. **Pressing** consists of gently pressing the fingers downwards to check the strength of the pulse at the middle and deep levels and therefore whether the pulse is Deep, normal or deficient at these levels: this is necessary to determine whether the pulse is Deep, Hollow, Hidden or empty at the deep level
3. **Searching** consists of not moving the fingers but keeping them still to count the rate of the pulse, to decide whether it is Slow, Rapid or normal
4. **Pushing** consists of gently moving the fingers from side to side (lateral–medial) in each position. This movement is necessary to interpret many pulse qualities, such as Slippery, Wiry, Leather, Tight, Choppy, Fine, Minute, etc. One can only identify these pulse qualities by moving the fingers in this way in order to feel *round* the pulse: it is only by feeling round the pulse that we can determine its shape
5. **Rolling** consists of moving the fingers back and forth (proximal–distal) in each position: this movement is necessary to determine whether the pulse is Short, Long or Moving or to read the pulse of a child under 1 year

Equalizing the breathing

Remember: the pulse is not felt with the fingers totally still but moving the fingers in four ways:
1. Lifting (upwards)
2. Pressing (downwards)
3. Pushing (from side to side)
4. Rolling (proximal–distal)

It is traditionally important for the practitioner to regulate and balance his or her own breathing pattern in order to be better attuned to the patient's Qi and to become more receptive.

Another reason for doing this was that the patient's pulse was correlated with the practitioner's breathing cycles in order to determine whether it was slow or rapid (Box 25.1).

Box 25.1 Method for taking the pulse

- Time (best in morning)
- Levelling the arm (patient's arm not higher than heart)
- Placing the fingers (placing fingers on artery in right place)
- Arranging the fingers (adjust fingers' spread to patient's size)
- Regulating the fingers (allow for different length of fingers)
- Using the fingers (allow for different sensitivity of fingers)
- Moving the fingers
  - *Lifting* (lift up to feel superficial level)
  - *Pressing* (press down to feel deep level)
  - *Searching* (finger still to count rate)
  - *Pushing* (move fingers laterally–medially)
  - *Rolling* (move fingers proximally–distally)
- Equalizing the breathing (calm and concentrate on one's own breathing)

Factors to take into account

Several factors should be taken into account in order to evaluate each pulse in its context and in relation to an individual patient.

Seasons

These influence the pulse, it being deeper in wintertime and more superficial in summertime.

Gender

Men's pulses are naturally slightly stronger than women's. Also, in men the left pulse should be very slightly stronger, and in women the right pulse should be slightly stronger. This is in accordance with the symbolism of Yin and Yang, following which the left side is Yang (hence male) and the right side is Yin (hence female).

In men, the Front position should be very slightly stronger, while in women the Rear position should be so. This also follows the Yin–Yang symbolism according to which upper is Yang (hence male) and lower is Yin (hence female). However, in practice this is hardly ever so.

Occupation

The pulse of those who are engaged in heavy physical work should be stronger than those who are engaged in mental work.

Box 25.2 summarizes factors to take into account.

The normal pulse

The pulse should have three qualities, which are described as having Stomach-Qi, having spirit and having a root.

Stomach-Qi

A pulse is said to have Stomach-Qi when it feels 'gentle', 'calm' and is relatively slow (four beats per respiratory cycle).

A pulse with Stomach-Qi is not rough. The Stomach is the Sea of Food, the Root of the Post-Heaven Qi and the origin of Qi and Blood. For this reason, it gives 'body' to the pulse. If the pulse feels too rough or hard, it indicates that the Stomach function is impaired. The 'Simple Questions' in chapter 19 says: *'The Stomach is the Root of the 5 Yin organs; the Qi of the Yin organs cannot reach the Lung channel [i.e. the radial artery on the Lung channel] by itself but it needs Stomach-Qi ... if the pulse is soft it indicates that it has Stomach-Qi and the prognosis is good.'*[7]

This particular quality of being 'soft' (but not too soft), 'gentle', 'calm' and 'not rough' is important: beginners often take a rough and hard quality of the pulse as being 'healthy'.

Box 25.2 Factors to take into account in pulse taking

- Season
- Gender
- Occupation

Box 25.3 The normal pulse

- Stomach-Qi (relatively soft, calm, gentle)
- Spirit (regular, soft)
- Root (clearly felt on deep level and third position)

Spirit

The pulse is said to have spirit when it is soft but with strength, neither big nor small, and regular. It should also be regular in its quality: that is, it should not change quality very easily and frequently. A pulse that has these qualities reflects a good state of Heart-Qi and Blood.

Root

A pulse is said to have root in two different senses. It has a root when the deep level can be felt clearly, and also when the Rear position can be felt clearly. Having a root indicates that the Kidneys are healthy and strong.

Thus a pulse that has spirit, Stomach-Qi and root indicates a good state of the Mind, Qi and Essence, respectively.

When interpreting the pulse one should therefore pay attention to the following elements and in this order (Boxes 25.3 and 25.4):

1. Feel the pulse as a whole
2. Feel whether the pulse has spirit, Stomach Qi and root
3. Feel the three levels and the three positions
4. Feel the strength of the pulse
5. Feel the overall quality of the pulse (if there is one)
6. Feel the quality of individual pulse positions

The pulse qualities

There are 28 pulse qualities, as follows.

1. Floating (*Fu*)

Feeling

This pulse can be felt with a light pressure of the fingers, just resting the fingers on the artery.

Box 25.4 Procedure for pulse taking

- Feel the pulse as a whole
- Feel whether the pulse has spirit, Stomach-Qi and root
- Feel the three levels and the three positions
- Feel the strength of the pulse
- Feel the overall quality of the pulse (if there is one)
- Feel the quality of individual pulse positions

Clinical significance
(Box 25.5)

In exterior conditions, this quality indicates the presence of an exterior pattern from invasion by an exterior pathogenic factor, such as Wind-Cold or Wind-Heat. If it is Floating and Tight, it indicates Wind-Cold; if it is Floating and Rapid, it indicates Wind-Heat.

In interior conditions, if the pulse is Floating at the superficial level but Empty at the deep level, it indicates deficiency of Yin.

In rare cases, the pulse can be Floating in other interior conditions, such as anaemia or cancer. In these cases, the pulse is Floating because Qi is very deficient and 'floats' to the surface of the body.

Box 25.5 Floating pulse

- Invasion of external Wind
- Yin deficiency (interior conditions)
---

2. Deep (*Chen*)

Feeling
This pulse is the opposite to the preceding one: it can only be felt with a heavy pressure of the fingers and is felt near the bone.

Clinical significance
(Box 25.6)

This quality indicates an interior condition, which could assume many different forms. It also indicates that the problem is in the Yin organs.

If it is Deep and Weak, it indicates deficiency of Qi and Yang. If it is Deep and Full, it indicates stasis of Qi or Blood in the Interior, or interior Cold or Heat.

Box 25.6 Deep pulse

- Pathogenic factor in the Interior (Deep-Full)
- Yang deficiency (Deep-Weak)
---

3. Slow (*Chi*)

Feeling
This pulse has three beats per respiration cycle (of the practitioner). In the old times the rate was referred to the practitioner's respiration cycle, but nowadays the pulse rate can also be counted conventionally using a watch.

Normal rates vary but they are roughly:

Age (year)	Rate (beat/min)
1–4	90 or more
4–10	84
10–16	78/80
16–35	76
35–50	72/70
50+	68

Clinical significance
(Box 25.7)

A Slow pulse indicates a Cold pattern. If it is Slow and Weak, it indicates Empty-Cold from deficiency of Yang. If it is Slow and Full, it indicates Full-Cold.

Box 25.7 Slow pulse

- Cold pattern
- Empty-Cold (Slow and Weak)
- Full-Cold (Slow and Full)
---

4. Rapid (*Shu*)

Feeling
This pulse has more than five beats per each respiration cycle, or has a higher rate than the ones indicated above.

Clinical significance
(Box 25.8)

A Rapid pulse indicates a Heat pattern. If it is Floating-Empty and Rapid, it indicates Empty-Heat from Yin deficiency. If it is Full and Rapid, it indicates Full-Heat.

Box 25.8 Rapid pulse

- Heat pattern
- Full-Heat (Rapid and Full)
- Empty-Heat (Rapid and Floating-Empty)
---

5. Empty (*Xu*)

Feeling
The Empty pulse feels rather big but soft. 'Empty' may suggest that nothing can be felt, but this is not so: this pulse is actually rather big but it feels empty on a slightly stronger pressure and is soft.

Clinical significance
(Box 25.9)

The Empty pulse indicates Qi deficiency.

> **Box 25.9 Empty pulse**
> - Qi deficiency

6. Full (*Shi*)

Feeling

This pulse feels full, rather hard and rather long. 'Full' is often used in two slightly different ways. On the one hand, it indicates a specific type of pulse, as described above; on the other hand, this term is often used to indicate any pulse of the Full type.

Clinical significance
(Box 25.10)

The Full pulse indicates a Full pattern. A Full and Rapid pulse indicates Full-Heat, and a Full and Slow pulse indicates Full-Cold.

> **Box 25.10 Full pulse**
> - Full pattern
> - Full-Heat (Full-Rapid)
> - Full-Cold (Full-Slow)

7. Slippery (*Hua*)

Feeling

A Slippery pulse feels smooth, rounded, slippery to the touch, as if it were oily. It slides under the fingers.

Clinical significance
(Box 25.11)

The Slippery pulse indicates Phlegm, Dampness, retention of food or pregnancy.

Generally speaking, the slippery pulse is Full by definition, but in some cases it can also be Weak, indicating Phlegm or Dampness with a background of Qi deficiency.

> **Box 25.11 Slippery pulse**
> - Phlegm
> - Dampness
> - Retention of food
> - Pregnancy

8. Choppy (*Se*)

Feeling

This pulse feels rough under the finger: instead of a smooth pulse wave, it feels as if it has a jagged edge to it. Choppy also indicates a pulse that changes rapidly both in rate and quality.

Clinical significance
(Box 25.12)

A Choppy pulse indicates deficiency of Blood. It may also indicate exhaustion of fluids and it may occur after profuse and prolonged sweating or vomiting.

> **Box 25.12 Choppy pulse**
> - Blood deficiency
> - Exhaustion of Body Fluids

9. Long (*Chang*)

Feeling

This pulse is basically longer than normal: it extends slightly beyond the normal pulse position.

Clinical significance
(Box 25.13)

It indicates a Heat pattern.

> **Box 25.13 Long pulse**
> - Heat pattern

10. Short (*Duan*)

Feeling

This pulse is the opposite of the previous one: it occupies a shorter space than the normal position.

Clinical significance
(Box 25.14)

The Short pulse indicates severe deficiency of Qi. It frequently appears on the Front positions of left or right.

It also specifically denotes deficiency of Stomach-Qi.

> **Box 25.14 Short pulse**
> - Severe Qi deficiency
> - Stomach-Qi deficiency

11. Overflowing (*Hong*)

Feeling

This pulse feels big. It extends beyond the pulse position. It is superficial and generally feels as if it overflows the normal pulse channel, like a river overflows during a flood.

Clinical significance
(Box 25.15)

The Overflowing pulse indicates extreme Heat. It frequently appears during a fever, but it is also felt in chronic diseases characterized by interior Heat.

If it is Overflowing but Empty on pressure, it indicates Empty-Heat from Yin deficiency.

Box 25.15 Overflowing pulse

- Full-Heat
- Empty-Heat (Overflowing-Empty)

---

12. Fine (*Xi*)
Feeling
This pulse is thinner than normal.

Clinical significance
(Box 25.16)

A Fine pulse indicates deficiency of Blood. It may also indicate internal Dampness with severe deficiency of Qi.

Box 25.16 Fine pulse

- Blood deficiency
- Dampness with severe Qi deficiency

---

13. Minute (*Wei*)
Feeling
This pulse is basically the same as the Fine one, just more so. It is extremely thin, small and difficult to feel.

Clinical significance
(Box 25.17)

The Minute pulse indicates severe deficiency of Qi and Blood.

Box 25.17 Minute pulse

- Severe deficiency of Qi and Blood

---

14. Tight (*Jin*)
Feeling
This pulse feels twisted like a thick rope.

Clinical significance
(Box 25.18)

A Tight pulse indicates Cold, which may be interior or exterior, such as invasion of exterior Wind-Cold. If it

---
Box 25.18 Tight pulse

- Cold
- Exterior Cold (Tight-Floating)
- Interior Full-Cold (Tight-Full-Deep)
- Interior Empty-Cold (Tight-Weak-Deep)
- Pain

---

is Tight and Floating, it indicates exterior Cold; if it is Tight, Full and Deep, it indicates interior Full-Cold; if it Tight, Weak and Deep, it denotes interior Empty-Cold.

This pulse is frequently felt in asthma from Cold in the Lungs, and in Stomach conditions from Cold.

The Tight pulse may also indicate pain from an interior condition.

15. Wiry (*Xian*)
Feeling
This pulse feels taut like a guitar string. It is thinner, more taut and harder than the Tight pulse. The Wiry pulse really hits the fingers.

Clinical significance
(Box 25.19)

The Wiry pulse can indicate three different conditions:

- Liver disharmony
- Pain
- Phlegm

Box 25.19 Wiry pulse

- Liver disharmony
- Pain
- Phlegm

---

16. Slowed-down (*Huan*)
Feeling
This pulse has four beats for each respiration cycle.

Clinical significance
(Box 25.20)

This is generally a healthy pulse and has no pathological significance.

Box 25.20 Slowed-down pulse

- Generally a healthy pulse

---

17. Hollow (Kou)

Feeling

This pulse can be felt at the superficial level, but if one presses slightly harder to find the middle level it is not there; it is then felt again at the deep level with a stronger pressure. In other words, it is Empty in the middle.

Clinical significance

(Box 25.21)

This pulse appears after a haemorrhage. If the pulse is rapid and slightly Hollow, it may indicate a forthcoming loss of blood.

> **Box 25.21 Hollow pulse**
> - Haemorrhage
> - Forthcoming haemorrhage (Hollow and Rapid)

18. Leather (Ge)

Feeling

This pulse feels hard and tight at the superficial level and stretched like a drum, but it feels completely Empty at the deep level. It is a large pulse, not thin.

Clinical significance

(Box 25.22)

The Leather pulse indicates severe deficiency of the Kidney-Essence or Yin.

> **Box 25.22 Leather pulse**
> - Severe deficiency of Kidney-Essence
> - Severe deficiency of Kidney-Yin

19. Firm (Lao)

Feeling

The Firm pulse is felt only at the deep level and it feels hard and rather wiry. It could be described as a Wiry pulse at the deep level.

Clinical significance

(Box 25.23)

The Firm pulse indicates Blood stasis, interior Cold (if it is also Slow) or pain.

> **Box 25.23 Firm pulse**
> - Blood stasis
> - Interior Cold (Firm and Slow)
> - Pain

20. Soggy (or Weak-Floating) (Ru)

Feeling

The Soggy pulse can be felt only on the superficial level. It feels very soft and is only slightly floating: that is, not as much as the Floating pulse. It disappears when a stronger pressure is applied to feel the deep level. It is similar to the Floating-Empty pulse, but it is softer and not so Floating.

Clinical significance

(Box 25.24)

The Soggy pulse indicates the presence of Dampness when this pathogenic factor occurs against a background of Qi deficiency.

It may also indicate deficiency of Yin or Essence.

> **Box 25.24 Soggy pulse**
> - Dampness with Qi deficiency
> - Deficiency of Yin
> - Deficiency of Essence

21. Weak (Ruo)

Feeling

A Weak pulse cannot be felt on the superficial level, but only at the deep level. It is also soft.

Clinical significance

(Box 25.25)

The Weak pulse indicates deficiency of Yang or sometimes deficiency of Blood.

> **Box 25.25 Weak pulse**
> - Yang deficiency
> - Blood deficiency

22. Scattered (San)

Feeling

This pulse feels very small and is relatively superficial. Instead of feeling like a wave, the pulse feels as if it were 'broken' in small dots.

Clinical significance

(Box 25.26)

This pulse indicates very severe deficiency of Qi and Blood, and in particular of Kidney-Qi. It always indicates a serious condition.

> **Box 25.26 Scattered pulse**
> - Severe deficiency of Qi and Blood
> - Severe deficiency of Kidney-Qi
> - Serious condition

23. Hidden (*Fu*)

Feeling

This pulse feels as if it were hidden beneath the bone. It is very deep and difficult to feel. It is basically an extreme case of a Deep pulse.

Clinical significance

(Box 25.27)

The Hidden pulse indicates extreme deficiency of Yang.

> **Box 25.27 Hidden pulse**
> - Severe Yang deficiency

24. Moving (*Dong*)

Feeling

The Moving pulse has a round shape like a bean; it is short and it 'trembles' under the finger. It has no definite shape, having no head or tail, just rising up in the centre. It feels as if it is shaking and is also somewhat slippery.

Clinical significance

(Box 25.28)

This pulse indicates shock, anxiety, fright or extreme pain. It is frequently found in persons with deep emotional problems, particularly from fear, or in those who have suffered an intense emotional shock, even if many years previously.

> **Box 25.28 Moving pulse**
> - Shock, anxiety, fright
> - Pain

25. Hasty (*Cu*)

Feeling

This pulse is Rapid and it stops at irregular intervals.

Clinical significance

(Box 25.29)

The Hasty pulse indicates extreme Heat and a deficiency of Heart-Qi. It is also felt with conditions of Heart-Fire.

> **Box 25.29 Hasty pulse**
> - Severe Heat
> - Deficiency of Heart-Qi
> - Heart-Fire

26. Knotted (*Jie*)

Feeling

This pulse is Slow and it stops at irregular intervals.

Clinical significance

(Box 25.30)

The Knotted pulse indicates Cold and deficiency of Heart-Yang.

> **Box 25.30 Knotted pulse**
> - Cold with deficiency of Heart-Yang

27. Intermittent (*Dai*)

Feeling

This pulse stops at regular intervals.

Clinical significance

(Box 25.31)

This pulse always indicates a serious internal problem of one or more Yin organs. If it stops every four beats or less, the condition is serious.

It can also indicate a serious heart problem (in a Western medical sense).

> **Box 25.31 Intermittent pulse**
> - Serious problem in Internal Organ
> - Heart problem (in Western medical sense)

28. Hurried (*Ji*)

Feeling

This pulse is very rapid, but it also feels very agitated and urgent.

Clinical significance

(Box 25.32)

This pulse indicates an Excess of Yang, with Fire in the body exhausting the Yin.

> **Box 25.32 Hurried pulse**
> - Fire exhausting Yin

The 28 pulse qualities can be grouped into six groups of pulses with similar qualities:

- *The Floating kind*: Floating – Hollow – Leather
- *The Deep kind*: Deep – Firm – Hidden
- *The Slow kind*: Slow – Knotted
- *The Rapid kind*: Rapid – Hasty – Hurried – Moving
- *The Empty kind*: Empty – Weak – Fine – Minute – Soggy – Short – Scattered
- *The Full kind*: Full – Overflowing – Wiry – Tight – Long

It may help us to understand the nature of pulse qualities if we realize that they reflect different aspects of the pulse: for example, Slow and Rapid clearly refer to an irregularity of the rate of the pulse, while Knotted, Hasty and Intermittent refer to an irregularity of the rhythm.

These different aspects are:

- *According to depth*: Floating – Deep – Hidden – Firm – Leather
- *According to rate*: Slow – Rapid – Slowed-down – Hurried – Moving
- *According to strength*: Empty – Full – Weak – Scattered
- *According to size*: Overflowing – Fine – Minute
- *According to length*: Long – Short – Moving
- *According to shape*: Slippery – Choppy – Wiry – Tight – Moving – Hollow – Firm
- *According to rhythm*: Knotted – Hasty – Intermittent

Of course, some pulse qualities escape such classification because they are defined according to more than one aspect. For example, the Soggy pulse is defined according to depth (it is floating), size (it is thin) and strength (it is soft).

Table 25.4 summarizes the 28 pulse qualities.

PALPATING THE SKIN

Palpating the skin includes feeling the temperature, moisture and texture of the skin.

Temperature

A cold feeling of the skin indicates a Cold pattern. If the four limbs feel cold, this usually indicates a deficiency of Yang of both Spleen and Stomach. If the loins, lower back or feet feel cold, it indicates a deficiency of Kidney-Yang. If the lower abdomen feels cold, it indicates a deficiency of Spleen-Yang.

Table 25.4 The 28 pulse qualities

No.	English	Pinyin	Literal translation	Chinese
1	Floating	Fu	Floating	浮
2	Deep	Chen	Deep (sinking)	沉
3	Slow	Chi	Slow, tardy	迟
4	Rapid	Shu	Several (in succession)	数
5	Empty	Xu	Empty	虚
6	Full	Shi	Solid	实
7	Slippery	Hua	Slippery	滑
8	Choppy	Se	Rough	涩
9	Long	Chang	Long	长
10	Short	Duan	Short	短
11	Overflowing	Hong	Big, vast, flood	洪
12	Fine	Xi	Thin, slender	细
13	Minute	Wei	Minute	微
14	Tight	Jin	Tight, taut	紧
15	Wiry	Xian	Bowstring	弦
16	Slowed-down	Huan	Slow, delay, postpone	缓
17	Hollow	Kou	Hollow	芤
18	Leather	Ge	Leather	革
19	Firm	Lao	Prison, firm, fastened	牢
20	Soggy	Ru	Immerse, moist	濡
21	Weak	Ruo	Weak, feeble	弱
22	Scattered	San	Break-up, disperse	散
23	Hidden	Fu	Hide	伏
24	Moving	Dong	To move	动
25	Hasty	Cu	Hurried, urgent	促
26	Knotted	Jie	Tie, knot, knit	结
27	Intermittent	Dai	Take the place of	代
28	Hurried	Ji	fast, rapid, urgent	疾

A subjective feeling of heat of a person does not always correspond to an objective heat feeling of the skin on palpation. If the skin actually feels hot to the touch, it often indicates the presence of Damp-Heat.

If the skin feels hot on first touch but, if the pressure of the fingers is maintained it ceases to feel hot, it indicates invasion of exterior Wind-Heat with the pathogenic factor still only on the Exterior.

If the skin over a blood vessel feels hot on medium pressure but not on heavy pressure, it indicates interior Heat in the Middle Burner or Heart.

If the skin feels hot on heavy pressure which nearly reaches the bone, it indicates Empty-Heat from Yin deficiency.

Box 25.33 summarizes skin temperature.

Moisture and texture

A moist feeling of the skin may indicate invasion of the Exterior by Wind-Cold or, more usually, by Wind-Heat.

If the skin feels moist in the absence of exterior symptoms, it indicates spontaneous sweating from deficiency of Lung-Qi.

If the skin feels dry, it indicates Blood deficiency or Lung-Yin deficiency. Skin which feels rough may indicate Painful Obstruction Syndrome from Wind. If the skin is scaly and dry, it indicates exhaustion of Body Fluids or severe deficiency and dryness of Liver-Blood.

If the skin is swollen and a pit is left visible after pressing with one's finger, it indicates oedema. If no pit

---

Box 25.33 Temperature of skin

Cold
- Cold feeling: Cold pattern
- Four limbs cold: deficiency of Yang of both Spleen and Stomach
- Loins, lower back or feet cold: deficiency of Kidney-Yang
- Lower abdomen cold: deficiency of Spleen-Yang

Heat
- Skin hot: Damp-Heat
- Skin hot on first touch but, if the pressure of the fingers is maintained it ceases to feel hot: invasion of exterior Wind-Heat with the pathogenic factor still only on the Exterior
- Skin over a blood vessel hot on medium pressure but not on heavy pressure: interior Heat in the Middle Burner or Heart
- Skin feels hot on heavy pressure, which nearly reaches the bone: Empty-Heat from Yin deficiency

---

Box 25.34 Moisture and texture

- Moist skin: invasion of exterior Wind
- Moist without exterior symptoms: deficiency of Lung-Qi
- Dry skin: Blood deficiency or Lung-Yin deficiency
- Rough skin: Painful Obstruction Syndrome from Wind
- Scaly and dry skin: exhaustion of Body Fluids or severe deficiency and dryness of Liver-Blood
- Swollen skin, pitting: 'Water swelling' from Spleen- and/or Kidney-Yang deficiency
- Swollen skin, not pitting: 'Qi swelling' from Dampness or Qi stagnation

---

is formed on pressing a swollen area, it indicates retention of Dampness or Qi stagnation and the swelling is called 'Qi swelling' as opposed to the former, called 'Water swelling'.

Box 25.34 summarizes moisture and texture.

PALPATING THE LIMBS

Palpation of hands and feet

Palpation of the hands and feet, particularly in regard to their temperature, is important to diagnose conditions of Heat and Cold. The most common cause of cold hands and cold feet is Yang deficiency; Lung- and Heart-Yang deficiency will cause coldness of the hands only; Spleen- and Kidney-Yang deficiency will cause coldness, particularly of the feet but often of both hands as well; Stomach-Yang deficiency may cause coldness both of hands and feet. With Spleen- and Kidney-Yang deficiency a particular feature is that not only the hands and feet but also the whole limbs are cold.

In women, cold hands and feet may also be caused by Blood deficiency; Heart-Blood deficiency may cause cold hands, while Liver-Blood deficiency may cause cold feet.

Stagnation of Liver-Qi may cause coldness of the hands and feet but particularly of the fingers and toes: in this case, the cold feeling is not due to a Yang deficiency but to Qi that is stagnant, being unable to reach the extremities.

There are other less common causes of cold hands and feet. One is Phlegm in the Interior, which may obstruct the circulation of Qi to the limbs and cause cold hands; this may happen also in the case of Phlegm-Heat, giving rise to contradictory hot and cold symptoms. Another less common situation of cold hands and feet is when there is a very pronounced and intense

> **Box 25.35 Cold hands and feet**
>
> **Common causes**
>
> - Cold hands and feet: Spleen- or Stomach-Yang deficiency
> - Cold hands: Lung- and/or Heart-Yang deficiency
> - Cold feet: Kidney-Yang deficiency
> - Cold hands and feet in women: Blood deficiency
> - Cold hands in women: Heart-Blood deficiency
> - Cold feet in women: Liver-Blood deficiency
> - Cold fingers and toes: Liver-Qi stagnation
>
> **Less common cause**
>
> - Cold hands and feet: Phlegm or interior Heat obstructing circulation of Qi

Heat in the Interior, obstructing the circulation of Qi so that it cannot warm the hands and feet; this condition will also give rise to contradictory hot and cold symptoms. An example of this situation is the condition of Heat in the Pericardium at the Nutritive Qi level within the Four Levels, which is characterized by symptoms and signs of intense Heat (Dark-Red tongue without coating, fever at night, mental restlessness, etc.) but cold hands.

Box 25.35 summarizes causes of cold hands and feet.

In cold hands and feet from Liver-Qi stagnation, it is particularly the fingers and toes that are cold

Palpation and comparison of dorsum and palm

When palpating the hands to feel their temperature, we should distinguish between the dorsum and the palm of the hand: a hot dorsum reflects more conditions of Full-Heat, while a hot palm reflects more conditions of Empty-Heat, though not exclusively so.

Hot dorsum of the hand indicates Full-Heat, while a hot palm usually indicates Empty-Heat

In the context of exterior invasions of Wind, palpation of the dorsum of the hands is important because it confirms the exterior nature of the condition. In fact, in exterior invasions of Wind (whether it is Wind-Cold or Wind-Heat) there is the characteristic contradiction between the patient's subjective sensation of cold ('aversion to cold') or even shivering and the objective hot feeling of the dorsum of the hands on palpation. The Chinese term *fa re*, which is often translated as 'fever' in the context of exterior invasions of Wind, actually refers precisely to this: that is, the *objective* hot feeling of the dorsum of the hands and forehead on palpation. The patient may or may not have an actual fever.

Therefore, the comparison between the temperature of the dorsum and the palms of the hands has two interpretations: on the one hand, it helps to distinguish Full- from Empty-Heat and, on the other hand, in the context of acute diseases, it confirms the exterior nature of it.

Chapter 74 of the 'Spiritual Axis' relates the temperature of the palm of the hand to the condition of the Intestines: if the palm is hot, it indicates Heat in the Intestines, while if it is cold, it indicates Cold in the Intestines.[8]

Palpating the hand

The palm of the hand reflects the state of most internal organs in a pattern similar to that found in the ear. The correspondence of various areas to internal organs can be visualized by superimposing the figure of a small baby on the palm of the hand (Fig. 25.5).[9]

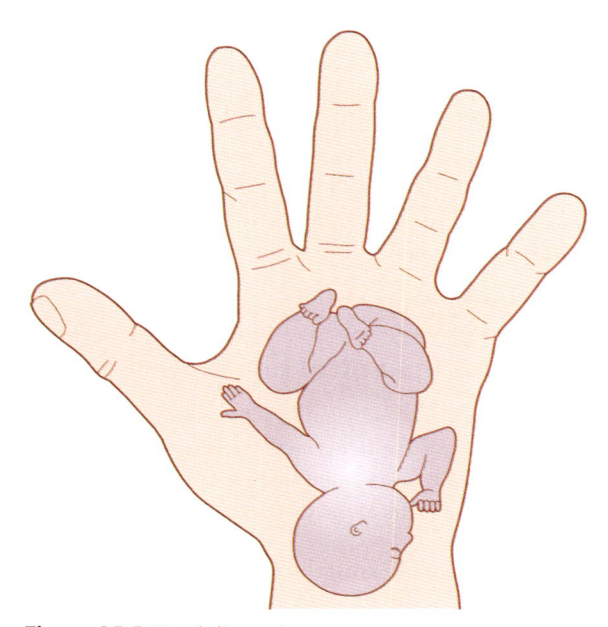

Figure 25.5 Hand diagnosis areas

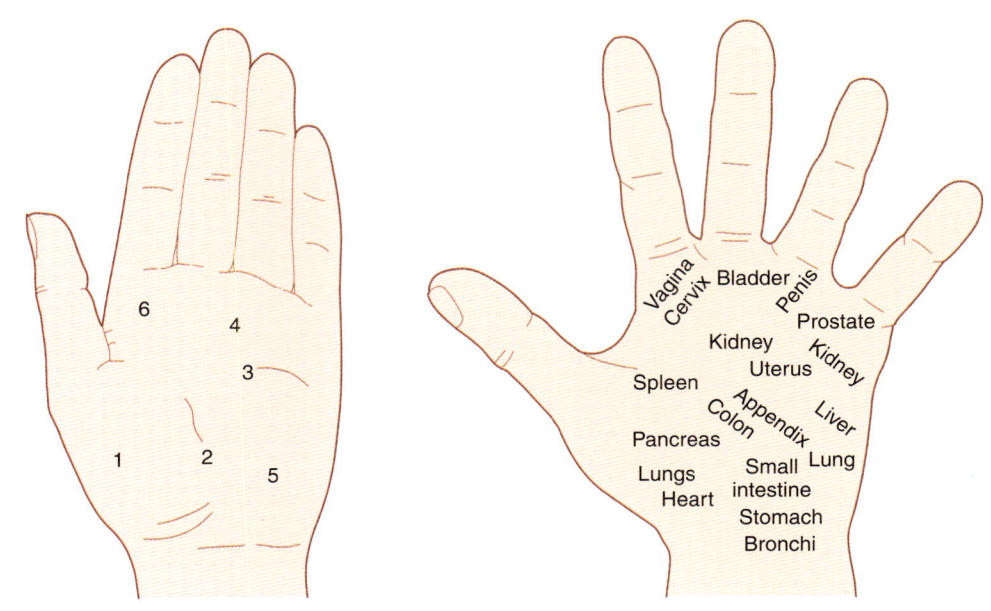

Figure 25.6 Organ positions in hand diagnosis

The major areas of correspondence are (Fig. 25.6):

1. Chest cavity organs
2. and 3. Abdominal cavity organs
4. Reproductive and urinary organs
5. Respiratory organs
6. Intestines, rectum

A more detailed representation of the correspondence with internal organs is shown in Figure 25.6.

Diagnosis is made by gently pressing the relevant areas: a sharp pain indicates a Full condition; a dull soreness indicates an Empty condition of the relevant organ.

PALPATING THE CHEST

Palpating the apical beat

First of all, one should palpate the area over the left ventricle apex of the heart, where the pulsation of the heart can be felt and sometimes even seen. This area is called 'Interior Emptiness' (*Xu Li*) in Chinese medicine (Fig. 25.7).

Box 25.36 summarizes the apical pulse.

Traditionally, this area is considered to be the end of the Stomach Great Connective Channel, starting in the

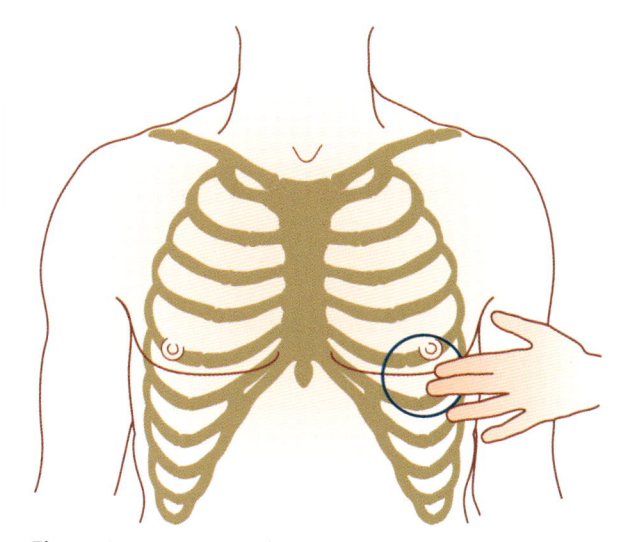

Figure 25.7 Palpation of apical beat

Box 25.36 Apical pulse

- Clearly felt, not hard, relatively slow: normal
- Feeble and without strength: deficiency of the Gathering Qi (*Zong Qi*)
- Strong and hard: excess condition of the Lungs and/or Heart
- Large but empty: Heart-Qi deficiency deficiency cond
- Stopping and starting: severe shock or alcoholism
- Discrepancy between apical and radial pulse: poor prognosis
- Rapid: shock, fright or outburst of anger

stomach itself. It is also considered to reflect the state of the Gathering Qi of the chest (Zong Qi). If the pulsation under this area is regular, and not tight nor rapid, it indicates a good state of the Gathering Qi. If the pulsation is faint but clear, it indicates deficiency of Gathering Qi. If the pulsation is too strong it indicates 'outpouring of Gathering Qi', i.e. a state of hyperactivity due to pushing oneself too much. If the pulsation cannot be felt, it indicates Phlegm or hiatus hernia.

Palpating the area below the xiphoid process

The feeling of this area on palpation should be compared to the rest of the abdomen: compared to the abdomen, the area below the xiphoid process should feel relatively soft (Fig. 25.8). The area just below the xiphoid process reflects the state of the Upper Burner Qi, i.e. Lung- and Heart-Qi and Gathering Qi. This area should be relatively softer than the rest, indicating a smooth flow of Lung- and Heart-Qi. If it feels hard and knotted, it indicates a stagnation of Lung- and Heart-Qi and a constriction of the Corporeal Soul due to bottled-up emotional tension.

If the same area feels too soft, it indicates a deficiency of the Heart.

Box 25.37 summarizes palpation of the area below the xiphoid process.

Box 25.37 Area below xiphoid process

- Should feel soft relative to the rest of the abdomen
- Hard on palpation: Full condition, Qi stagnation (from emotional problems)
- Too soft on palpation: Heart deficiency

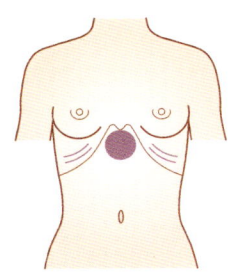

Figure 25.8 Area below the xiphoid process

Palpating the chest

The centre of the chest corresponds to the Heart and the rest of it to the Lungs. Palpation of the chest reveals the state of the Heart, Lungs and Pericardium and, generally speaking, tenderness on palpation indicates a Full condition of one of these organs. For example, if the chest feels very tender even on light palpation in the centre, in the area of Ren-17 Shanzhong, it may indicate Heart-Blood stasis (Box 25.38).

If the chest is tender on palpation in the areas around the centre, it usually indicates an Excess condition of the Lungs and often retention of Phlegm in the Lungs. By contrast, if palpation of the chest relieves discomfort, it indicates a Deficiency condition of the Heart or Lungs. If superficial palpation of the chest relieves a pain but the patient feels discomfort with a deeper pressure, it indicates a combined condition of Deficiency and Excess.

Box 25.38 Chest

- Tender with light palpation of Ren-17: Heart-Blood stasis
- Tender around the centre: excess condition of the Lungs
- Tenderness relieved by palpation: deficiency condition of Heart or Lungs
- Tenderness relieved by light palpation but elicited by deeper palpation: combined Deficiency and Excess

---

Palpating the breast

Palpation of the breasts in women is carried out when there are breast lumps. Breast lumps may be malignant or benign. It is important to stress that the purpose of breast palpation in Chinese medicine is never to replace the Western diagnosis but to identify the patterns causing the lump. We should *never* rely on palpation to distinguish benign from malignant lumps. The palpation of lumps should take into consideration their hardness, their edges and their mobility (Box 25.39).

Box 25.39 Breast lumps

- Relatively soft: Phlegm
- Relatively hard: Blood stasis
- Distinct edges: Phlegm
- Indistinct edges: Toxic Heat
- Mobile on palpation: Phlegm
- Immovable on palpation: Blood stasis or Toxic Heat

The key factors in palpation of breast lumps are listed in Box 25.39.

Small, movable lumps with distinct edges and which change size according to the menstrual cycle normally indicate fibrocystic disease of the breast, which is usually due to a combination of Phlegm and Qi stagnation. A single, relatively hard, movable lump with distinct edges which may be also slightly painful usually indicates a fibroadenoma, which, from the Chinese point of view, is due to a combination of Phlegm and Blood stasis. A single, hard, immovable lump with indistinct margins, without pain, may indicate carcinoma of the breast, which, in Chinese medicine, is usually due to a combination of Phlegm, Qi stagnation and Blood stasis occurring against a background of disharmony of the Penetrating and Directing Vessels.

Box 25.40 summarizes features of the most common breast lumps.

Box 25.40 Most common breast lumps

- Fibrocystic disease (Qi stagnation and Phlegm): small, multiple, movable lumps with distinct edges, changing size according to the menstrual cycle
- Fibroadenoma (Phlegm and Blood stasis): single, relatively hard, movable lump with distinct edges, possibly painful
- Carcinoma of the breast (Blood stasis and Phlegm): single, hard, immovable, painless lump with indistinct margins

---

PALPATING THE ABDOMEN

The elasticity and strength of the abdomen is important: it should feel solid but not hard, resilient but not tight, and elastic but not soft. If it feels like this, it indicates the good state of the Original Qi. If it feels too soft and flabby, it indicates deficiency of Original Qi.

In general, if the abdomen feels hard or if it is painful on palpation, it indicates a Full condition; if it feels too soft or if any ache is relieved by palpation, it indicates an Empty pattern.

The lower part of the abdomen below the umbilicus should feel relatively tenser (but nevertheless elastic) than the rest, indicating a good state of the Original Qi of the Kidneys. If it feels soft and flabby, it indicates a weakness of the Original Qi.

Abdominal masses that move under the fingers indicate stagnation of Qi: if they do not move and feel very hard, they indicates stasis of Blood.

Box 25.41 summarizes abdominal palpation.

Box 25.41 Abdominal palpation

- Hard: Full condition
- Too soft: Empty condition
- Ache relieved by palpation: Empty pattern
- Pain aggravated by palpation: Full pattern
- Lower abdomen soft and flabby: deficiency of Original Qi (*Yuan Qi*)
- Abdominal masses that come and go and move on palpation: Qi stagnation
- Fixed abdominal masses: Blood stasis

PALPATING POINTS

Channel and points diagnosis is based on objective or subjective reactions appearing at certain points. Generally speaking, any point can be used in diagnosis, following the general principles outlined above for the channels. However, certain points are particularly useful in diagnosis: these are the Back Transporting points (see ch. 51), the Front Collecting points (see ch. 51), the Lower Sea points (see ch. 50) and Ah Shi points.

The *Back Transporting points* are the places where the Qi and Blood of a particular organ 'infuses': they are directly related to their respective organ and very often manifest certain reactions when the organ is diseased.

As a general principle, any sharp pain (either spontaneous or on pressure) on these points indicates a Full condition of the relevant organ, and a dull soreness (either spontaneous or on pressure) indicates an Empty condition. Each Back Transporting point can reflect the condition of its relevant organ, for example BL-21 Weishu for the Stomach, BL-13 Feishu for the Lungs, etc.

In addition to the normal Back Transporting points, other points on the back are significant in palpatory diagnosis. BL-43 Gaohuangshu reflects the state of the Lungs, BL-53 Zhishi is often sore in Kidney diseases and BL-31 Shangliao, BL-32 Ciliao, BL-33 Zhongliao and BL-34 Xialiao reflect the state of the reproductive system, particularly in women.

The *Front Collecting points* are particularly reactive to pathological changes of the internal organs and are useful for diagnostic purposes. Each Front Collecting point reflects the state of an internal organ and a list is given in chapter 51. The general principle is the same: that is, if these points are tender on palpation they usually indicate a Full pattern, whereas if palpation relieves a tenderness it indicates an Empty pattern.

The *Lower Sea points* are also useful in diagnosing stomach or intestinal diseases: ST-36 Zusanli for the stomach, ST-37 Shangjuxu for the Large Intestine and ST-39 Xiajuxu for the Small Intestine. In addition, there is a special point between ST-36 Zusanli and ST-37 Shangjuxu that reflects the state of the appendix. Its location is variable and is situated wherever there is a soreness in between those two points. If this special point (called *'Lanweixue'*, meaning 'appendix point') is painful on pressure, it indicates inflammation of the appendix. If the appendix is healthy, there will be no reaction at this point.

Finally, *Ah Shi points* can be used for diagnosis. The theory of Ah Shi points was developed by Sun Si Miao (581–682) during the Tang dynasty. He said very simply that wherever there is soreness on pressure (whether on a channel or not), there is a point. This is obviously because the channel network is so dense that every area of the body is irrigated by a channel. As we have already seen, dull soreness on pressure indicates an Empty condition of the channel influencing that area, while a sharp pain on pressure indicates a Full condition of the channel.

Learning outcomes

In this chapter you will have learned:
- The role of the pulse in diagnosis: reflecting the organism as a whole, the state of Qi, Blood and Yin, the Yin and Yang organs, all parts of the body, and the constitution
- The problems inherent in pulse diagnosis: its subjective nature, subtlety and its short-term changeability
- The historical assignment of the different organs to pulse positions, and the reasons for discrepancies in these arrangements
- The importance of interpreting the pulse dynamically rather than mechanically
- How the pulse can reflect both the organ or the channel in different clinical situations
- The various theories of the clinical significance of the three levels of the pulse
- The importance of observing basic methodological guidelines on the method of pulse taking (positioning of patients arm, arranging fingers, moving fingers, etc.)
- Factors to take into account when evaluating the pulse (season, gender, occupation)
- The characteristics of a normal pulse: Stomach-Qi, spirit and root
- The different stages of a complete procedure for pulse taking

- The characteristics of the 28 pulse qualities
- How to recognize signs from palpating the temperature, moisture and texture of the skin
- The clinical significance of findings from palpating the limbs, the hands and the feet
- Palpation of the chest, including the apical beat, beneath the xiphoid process, and the breast
- How palpation of the abdomen provides valuable diagnostic information
- How to palpate points for both objective and subjective feedback, including the Back Transporting points, the Front Collecting points, Lower-Sea points and Ah Shi points

Self-assessment questions

1. List the three different ways of interpreting the three levels of the pulse (use the headings superficial, middle and deep).
2. List the four different ways the fingers are moved whilst taking the pulse, and the reasons for each movement.
3. How would you expect the pulse of a labourer to differ from that of an academic?
4. What is meant when it is said that a pulse has 'root'?
5. List the six basic stages of the procedure for pulse taking.
6. If the pulse is Floating and Tight, and the patient reports catching a cold, what is the likely diagnosis?
7. What does a Deep and Weak pulse indicate?
8. What are the indications of a pulse that is Slow and Weak? And a pulse that is Slow and Full?
9. What is the normal number of pulse beats per minute for a 55-year-old patient?
10. Which qualities would one expect to feel in a patient with symptoms of apparent Yin deficiency with Empty-Heat?
11. What are the four main indications of a Slippery pulse?
12. Give the two possible indications of a Fine pulse.
13. What are the three different conditions indicated by a Wiry pulse?
14. What does a Knotted pulse feel like, and what does it indicate?
15. Write down as many of the different pulse qualities as you can remember. Use the following groupings to guide you (the number of possible qualities in each group are given in parentheses): depth (5); rate (5); strength (4); size (4); length (3); shape (7); rhythm (3).
16. If a patient's four limbs feel cold to the touch, what might be indicated?
17. What is the particular feature of coldness in the limbs caused by Liver-Qi stagnation?
18. What does palpation of the area below the xiphoid process indicate?
19. If tenderness is felt upon light palpation of Ren-17 Shanzhong, what would you suspect?
20. What is indicated by a soft and flabby lower abdomen?

See p. 1262 for answers

END NOTES

1. For a more complete discussion of pulse diagnosis, see Maciocia G 2004 Diagnosis in Chinese Medicine, Elsevier, London.
2. 1979 The Yellow Emperor's Classic of Internal Medicine – Simple Questions (*Huang Di Nei Jing Su Wen* 黄帝内经素问), People's Health Publishing House, Beijing, first published *c*.100 BC, p. 129–135.
3. Nanjing College of Traditional Chinese Medicine 1979 A Revised Explanation of the Classic of Difficulties (*Nan Jing Jiao Shi* 难经校释), People's Health Publishing House, Beijing, first published *c*.AD 100, p. 1–2.
4. Classic of Difficulties, ch. 18, p. 46.
5. Ibid., p. 46
6. Ibid., p. 46.
7. Simple Questions, p. 127–128.
8. 1981 Spiritual Axis (*Ling Shu Jing* 灵枢经), People's Health Publishing House, Beijing, first published *c*.100 BC, p. 133.
9. Li Wen Chuan-He Bao Yi 1987 Practical Acupuncture (*Shi Yong Zhen Jin Xue* 实用针灸学), People's Health Publishing House, Beijing, p. 37.

PART 4

Diagnosis by Hearing and Smelling   26

> **Key contents**
>
> **Diagnosis by hearing**
> *Voice*
> *Breathing*
> *Cough*
> *Vomiting*
> *Hiccup*
> *Borborygmi*
> *Sighing*
> *Belching*
>
> **Diagnosis by smelling**
> *Body odour*
> *Odour of bodily secretions*
> - Breath
> - Sweat
> - Sputum
> - Urine and stools
> - Vaginal discharge and lochia
> - Intestinal gas

- Smelling
  - Body odour
  - Odour of bodily secretions
    - Breath
    - Sweat
    - Sputum
    - Urine and stools
    - Vaginal discharge and lochia
    - Intestinal gas

DIAGNOSIS BY HEARING

Diagnosis by hearing includes listening to the sound and pitch of the voice, cough, breathing, vomiting, hiccup, borborygmi, groaning, and indeed any other sound emitted by a person.

As a general principle, a loud sound is indicative of a Full pattern, while a weak sound is indicative of an Empty pattern.

Diagnosis by hearing will be discussed under the following headings:

> - Voice
> - Breathing
> - Cough
> - Vomiting
> - Hiccup
> - Borborygmi
> - Sighing
> - Belching

The same Chinese character '*wen*' means both 'to hear' and 'to smell'. Both hearing and smelling are used in Chinese diagnosis.

Diagnosis by hearing and smelling will be discussed under the following headings:

- Hearing
  - Voice
  - Breathing
  - Cough
  - Vomiting
  - Hiccup
  - Borborygmi
  - Sighing
  - Belching

Voice

A loud, coarse voice is indicative of an Excess pattern, while a weak and thin voice is indicative of a Deficiency pattern.

Reluctance to talk usually indicates either a Cold pattern or Lung-Qi deficiency, while incessant talking indicates a Heat pattern.

The type of voice can also be diagnosed according to the Five-Element scheme of correspondences, so that a shouting voice is indicative of a Liver disharmony, a laughing voice of a Heart disharmony, a singing voice of a Spleen disharmony, a whimpering voice of a Lung disharmony and a groaning voice of a Kidney disharmony (Fig. 26.1).

Sudden loss of voice is usually due to invasion of exterior Wind-Heat. A gradual loss of voice is due to deficiency of Lung-Qi or Lung-Yin.

Box 26.1 summarizes voice patterns.

Box 26.1 Voice

- Loud voice: Full pattern
- Weak voice: Empty pattern
- Reluctance to talk: Cold pattern or Lung-Qi deficiency
- Excessive talking: Heat
- Shouting voice: Wood
- Laughing voice: Fire
- Singing voice: Earth
- Weepy voice: Metal
- Groaning voice: Water
- Sudden loss of voice: invasion of Wind-Heat
- Gradual loss of voice: Lung-Qi or Lung-Yin deficiency

Breathing

A coarse, loud breathing sound indicates a Full pattern, while a weak, thin breathing sound indicates an Empty pattern.

Cough

A loud and explosive cough is indicative of a Full pattern, while a weak cough is indicative of an Empty pattern.

A dry cough indicates Lung-Yin deficiency.

Vomiting

Vomiting with a loud noise indicates a Full pattern, often with Heat (frequently Stomach-Heat), while vomiting with a low sound indicates an Empty pattern (frequently Stomach deficiency and Cold).

Hiccup

Hiccup with a loud sound indicates a Full pattern (frequently Liver-Qi invading the Stomach), while hiccup with a quiet, low sound denotes an Empty pattern (frequently Stomach-Qi or Stomach-Yin deficiency).

Borborygmi

Borborygmi (gurgling sound in the intestines) with a loud sound indicates a Full pattern, while borborygmi with a low sound indicates an Empty pattern.

Sighing

Sighing generally indicates Qi stagnation of the Liver or Lungs, usually deriving from emotional problems such as repressed anger or frustration if the Liver is involved or worry and sadness if the Lungs are involved. Sighing with a weak sound may also be due to deficiency of the Spleen and Heart deriving from sadness, grief or pensiveness.

Belching

Belching with a loud and long sound indicates a Full condition which, may be retention of food, Stomach-Heat or Liver-Qi invading the Stomach. Belching with a short and low sound indicates a deficient condition

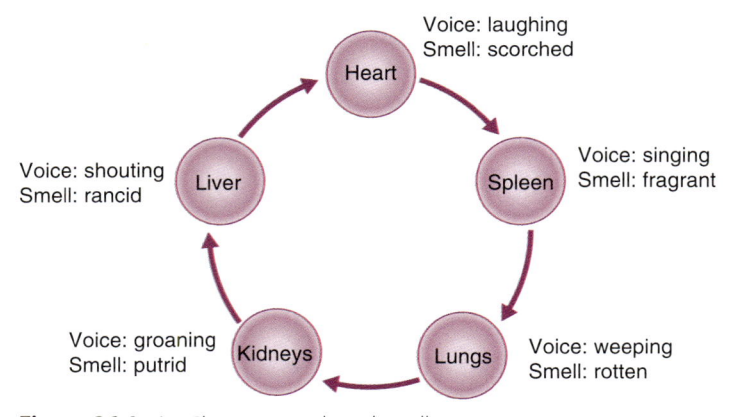

Figure 26.1 Five-Element sounds and smells

which may be Stomach-Qi deficiency or Stomach-Qi deficiency and Cold.

DIAGNOSIS BY SMELLING

Diagnosis by smelling is not a major part of the diagnostic process. It is used mostly to confirm our diagnosis and is seldom a clinching factor. The Five-Element smells mentioned below are useful mostly to correlate to the patient's Element type and to indicate accordance with or discordance from it. For example, a rancid smell in a Wood Element is a pathological exaggeration of a constitutional Wood smell and therefore is less serious than another smell would be. In other words, for a Wood type to have a putrid smell is more serious than for the same type to have a rancid smell.

Box 26.2 lists the Five-Element odours.

There are two quite distinct aspects to diagnosis by smelling: the first is the odour of the patient's body itself, which can give us an idea not only of the prevailing pattern of disharmony but also of the patient's constitutional type; the second is the odour of certain bodily secretions, which is used only to identify the prevailing pattern of disharmony.

Apart from the type of smell, as a general rule any strong, foul smell is indicative of Heat, while absence of smell is indicative of Cold.

Two main aspects of diagnosis by smelling are considered:

- Body odour
- Odour of bodily secretions
  - Breath
  - Sweat
  - Sputum
  - Urine and stools
  - Vaginal discharge and lochia
  - Intestinal gas

Body odour

From a Five-Element perspective, the five body odours are as follows: rancid for Wood, scorched for Fire,

Box 26.2 Five-Element odours

- Rancid: Wood
- Scorched: Fire
- Fragrant/ sweetish: Earth
- Rotten: Metal
- Putrid: Water

fragrant or sweetish for Earth, rotten for Metal and putrid for Water (Fig. 26.1). From this point of view, these body odours reflect a disharmony in the relevant Element which may be a Deficiency or an Excess. In most cases these odours are detected only when the patient undresses and especially on the back.

The body odour can be used diagnostically in two ways. In the absence of patterns of disharmony, accounting for a particular odour, the body odour reflects the patient's constitutional Element type in the same way as the body shape and facial structures do. Thus, a slightly rancid odour will emanate from a Wood type, a slightly scorched one from a Fire type, etc.

In addition to the constitutional body odour, a person's body odour reflects the patterns he or she is suffering from and these may not necessarily accord with the patient's Element type. For example, a Wood type may emanate a slightly scorched smell, indicating the presence of a Heart pattern. Indeed, if the body odour contradicts the constitutional Element type, this is a bad sign. In other words, it is worse for a Wood type to have a scorched odour (for example) than a rancid one.

Apart from the body odours related to the Five Elements, the body may emanate certain odours that reflect various patterns. For example, a strong, offensive body odour often indicates Damp-Heat.

Odour of bodily secretions

Diagnosis by smelling is based also on detecting the smell of bodily secretions. Obviously it is impractical for a practitioner to be able to smell a patient's urine or vaginal discharge. However, I usually ask patients if they have noticed a strong smell and most people are very aware if any of their bodily secretions are particularly smelly.

The following bodily secretions will be discussed:

- Breath
- Sweat
- Sputum
- Urine and stools
- Vaginal discharge and lochia
- Intestinal gas

Breath

The odour emanating from the mouth is closely related to the digestive system. Generally speaking, a strong, unpleasant breath indicates Stomach-Heat or retention of food. A sour-smelling breath indicates retention of food or, in children, Accumulation Disorder. A foul and somewhat pungent breath indicates Damp-Heat in the Stomach and Spleen. A rotten-smelling breath may indicate Damp-Heat in the Large Intestine which may be due to ulcerative colitis.

Box 26.3 summarizes the breath smells.

Sweat

The smell of sweat is often related to Dampness because the fluids forming sweat come from the space between the skin and muscles where Dampness often accumulates. Any strong-smelling sweat often indicates Damp-Heat. Putrid-smelling sweat may indicate a disease of the lungs, liver or kidneys.

Sputum

A strong-smelling sputum, often smelling rotten, indicates Heat in the Lungs and usually Phlegm-Heat or Toxic Heat. A fishy-smelling sputum may also indicate Lung-Heat. Sputum without smell indicates Cold.

Urine and stools

Foul-smelling stools always indicate Heat or Damp-Heat in the Intestines, while an irregularity of the bowel movement and an absence of smell indicates usually a Cold condition.

As for urine, strong-smelling urine indicates Damp-Heat in the Bladder, while absence of smell indicates Cold.

Vaginal discharge and lochia

A strong-smelling, leathery smell of vaginal discharge indicates Damp-Heat, while a fishy smell indicates Damp-Cold.

Strong-smelling lochia after childbirth may indicate Damp-Heat or Toxic Heat in the Uterus.

Box 26.3 Breath smells

- Strong, foul: Stomach-Heat or retention of food
- Sour: retention of food, Accumulation Disorder (in children)
- Foul, pungent: Damp-Heat in Stomach and Spleen
- Rotten: Damp-Heat in Large Intestine

Intestinal gas

A strong, foul-smelling intestinal gas indicates Damp-Heat in the Large Intestine. If the gas smells rancid and rotten like rotten eggs, it indicates Toxic Heat in the Large Intestines.

The release of gas without smell usually indicates Spleen-Qi deficiency.

Learning outcomes

In this chapter you will have learned:
- The general principle of diagnosis by hearing, where a loud sound indicates a Full pattern and a weak sound indicates an Empty pattern
- The significance of the voice in diagnosis, which can indicate Fullness and Emptiness as well as an Internal Organ disharmony (using the Five-Element scheme of correspondences)
- The diagnostic significance of the sounds of breathing, cough, vomiting, hiccup, borborygmi, sighing and belching
- The use of smell to confirm the main pattern of disharmony and the patient's constitutional type (using Five-Element theory)
- The general principle of diagnosis by smelling, where a strong, foul smell is indicative of Heat, while absence of smell is indicative of Cold
- The significance of the smell of bodily secretions: breath, sweat, sputum, urine and stools, vaginal discharge and lochia, and intestinal gas

Self-assessment questions

1. A patient feels tired and is reluctant to talk, as if it is a huge effort. What might this indicate?
2. What does a weak cough usually indicate?
3. An irritable patient suffers from frequent bouts of very loud hiccups. What pattern do you suspect?
4. What is the pattern most commonly associated with sighing?
5. If a patient presents with a strong and offensive body odour, what general pattern would you investigate?
6. A patient complains of foul-smelling breath. Which organs do you suspect may be involved?
7. Which pattern is commonly associated with foul-smelling flatulence?

See p. 1262 for answers

PART 5

Pathology

INTRODUCTION

Pathology explains how a disease process arises, how its manifestations change and how they are resolved. 'Pathology' in Chinese medicine has a very different meaning than in Western medicine. Chinese medicine does not analyse pathological changes at a microscopic level, nor does it take into account the changes taking place in the tissues and chemistry of the body. Chinese medicine pathology is concerned only with the broad disease processes and changes in the light of general, broad factors, such as pathogenic factors versus the body's Qi and the balance of Yin and Yang.

For example, if a patient falls ill with an upper respiratory infection which later causes a chest infection with symptoms of fever, chest ache, profuse cough with purulent sputum, Western medicine would want to analyse the pathology of this disease process by determining which particular bacterium is causing it: this might be pneumonia, bronchitis or even SARS (Severe Acute Respiratory Syndrome).

Chinese medicine does not analyse the pathogenic factor in such detailed, microscopic fashion but is concerned only with the broad picture: in the case example outlined above, according to Chinese medicine pathology, the exterior pathogenic factor has penetrated the Interior and has become stronger. Chinese medicine would also want to look at the general picture of clinical manifestations to assess the relative strength of pathogenic factor and body's Qi: this is crucial to determine the treatment principle and method and prognosis.

One can see how the two approaches, although quite different, can be complementary because Western medicine could benefit from the assessment of the broad picture provided by Chinese medicine. For example, examination of the tongue of the above patient may show the presence of several, dense, bright-red points on the tongue: this indicates that the pathogenic factor is very strong and might alert the Western doctor to the seriousness of the situation and therefore the necessity of using antibiotics early in the disease process.

The discussion of pathology will be centred around three broad subjects:

Chapter 27   The relative strength of pathogenic factor and body's Qi (Upright Qi)
Chapter 28   The imbalance of Yin and Yang
Chapter 29   The derangement of the ascending – descending movement of Qi

PART 5

The Pathology of Full and Empty Conditions

27

Key contents

Introduction

Nature of 'pathogenic factor' in Chinese medicine
External pathogenic factors
Internal pathogenic factors

Full conditions

Empty conditions

Full/Empty conditions
No pathogenic factor–normal Upright Qi
No pathogenic factor–deficient Upright Qi
Strong pathogenic factor–strong Upright Qi
Strong pathogenic factor–deficient Upright Qi
Weak pathogenic factor–strong Upright Qi
Weak pathogenic factor–deficient Upright Qi

Interaction between pathogenic factors and Upright Qi

The pathology of Full and Empty conditions depends on the relative strength of pathogenic factors and Upright Qi. The discussion of the relative strength of pathogenic factors and Upright Qi will be under the following headings:

- Introduction
- Nature of 'pathogenic factor' in Chinese medicine
- Full conditions
- Empty conditions
- Full/Empty conditions
- Interaction between pathogenic factors and Upright Qi

INTRODUCTION

The relative strength of pathogenic factors and Upright Qi is probably the most important factor in treatment with Chinese medicine. In treatment, it is absolutely essential to determine whether a condition is Full, Empty or Full/Empty. The importance of diagnosing correctly the Full or Empty (or Full/Empty) character of a condition cannot be overestimated: such diagnosis influences the principle of treatment and the therapeutic results (see also ch. 69).

It would be completely wrong to tonify the Upright Qi (*Zheng Qi*) in a Full condition or to expel pathogenic factors in an Empty condition. In Full/Empty conditions, diagnosing the relative importance and balance of pathogenic factors and Upright Qi is still very important.

In Full/Empty conditions it is not simply a matter of simultaneously expelling pathogenic factors and tonifying the Upright Qi: in such conditions, the treatment principle must be based on a careful assessment of the relative strength of pathogenic factors and Upright Qi and of the pathology of each individual case. Although balanced between expelling pathogenic factors and tonifying the Upright Qi, the treatment will nevertheless always place the emphasis on one or the other.

NATURE OF 'PATHOGENIC FACTOR' IN CHINESE MEDICINE

'Pathogenic factor' (called *xie qi* in Chinese) has a broad meaning in Chinese medicine. This may be an external pathogenic factor such as external Wind or external Dampness or an internal pathogenic factor such as Phlegm or Blood stasis.

External pathogenic factors

External climatic factors derive from the environment and, when they invade the body's Exterior, they become 'external pathogenic factors'; external pathogenic factors can become internal (usually changing their

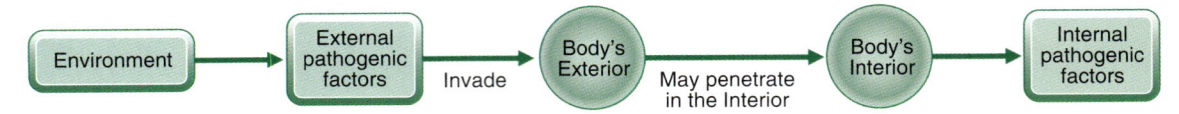

Figure 27.1 External pathogenic factors

nature in the process): for example, external Wind may turn into Heat and become internal (Fig. 27.1).

> Diagnosing the Full or Empty (or Full/Empty) character of the condition is the most important factor in deciding the treatment principle

Examples of external pathogenic factors are:

- Wind
- Dampness
- Summer-Heat
- Cold

External pathogenic factors were discussed as causes of disease in chapter 20. They are further discussed as pathogenic factors in chapter 43. Please note that the names are the same ('Wind', 'Cold', etc.) when these are discussed as aetiological factors or as pathogenic factors.

As aetiological factors, they are important for any practitioner to know about in order to counsel patients about their lifestyle: for example, about the importance of avoiding exposure to artificial types of 'wind' such as strong fans or air conditioning, or advising young women about not going out in cold weather with their abdomen exposed (Cold).

Pathogenic factors represent the pathology rather than the aetiology. If a woman has very painful periods with small, dark clots, a pronounced cold feeling during the period, and the period pain is relieved by the application of heat, then the pathology is that of Cold in the Uterus. The diagnosis is done on the basis of clinical manifestations and we do not need to ask whether she was exposed to cold.

Box 27.1 summarizes external pathologenic factors.

> **Box 27.1 External pathogenic factors**
>
> - External pathogenic factors derive from the environment
> - External pathogenic factors can become internal
> - External pathogenic factors include Wind, Dampness, Summer-Heat and Cold

Internal pathogenic factors

Internal pathogenic factors are either internally generated (e.g. Phlegm deriving from a Spleen and Kidney deficiency) or a transformation of an external pathogenic factor. In only three cases can an external pathogenic factor penetrate the Interior from the beginning without going through an exterior stage, thus becoming internal pathogenic factors as soon as they invade the body: this happens in invasions of Cold in the Stomach (acute epigastric pain and vomiting), Intestines (acute abdominal pain and diarrhoea) and Uterus (acute dysmenorrhoea).

> In only three cases does an external pathogenic factor penetrate the body's Interior from the beginning without causing exterior symptoms:
> - Invasion of Cold in the Stomach
> - Invasion of Cold in the Intestines
> - Invasion of Cold in the Uterus

Internal pathogenic factors are internally generated, i.e. they form because of an internal disharmony (Fig. 27.2). For example, a deficiency of the Lungs, Spleen and Kidneys may give rise to Phlegm, a deficiency of Yang may lead to (Empty) Cold, a deficiency of the Spleen may lead to Dampness, etc.

Examples of internal pathogenic factors are:

- Qi stagnation
- Blood stasis
- Internal Wind
- Internal Dampness
- Internal Cold
- Phlegm
- Heat
- Fire

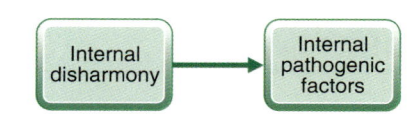

Figure 27.2 Internal pathogenic factors

Qi stagnation

Qi stagnation is an extremely common pathogenic factor. Qi stagnation may be caused by emotional strain, irregular eating, excessive physical work and lack of exercise. Emotional strain is the most common cause of Qi stagnation in Western patients. Some emotions, such as anger, frustration, resentment, worry and pensiveness, may cause Qi stagnation directly. However, all emotions, even those that deplete Qi, may eventually lead to Qi stagnation. For example, sadness and grief deplete Qi, especially of the Lungs; this will impair the circulation of Qi in the chest and some Qi stagnation in this area will ensue.

The chief symptom of stagnation is 'distension' (*zhang*). English-speaking patients seldom use this term and will often describe this feeling as 'bloating'. Distension may be experienced in the abdomen, hypochondrium, chest, women's breasts, throat and head. Distension is a subjective and objective sensation. Subjectively, the patient feels bloated, distended, 'like a balloon'; objectively, the abdomen is distended, i.e. protruding, rather hard but also elastic, like a balloon.

Qi stagnation may also cause pain, in which case the pain is accompanied by a pronounced feeling of distension. Other symptoms of Qi stagnation include irritability, symptoms that come and go according to the emotional state, a gloomy feeling, frequent mood swings, frequent sighing, Wiry pulse, tongue body either normal-coloured or slightly Red on the sides.

Distension is the cardinal symptom of Qi stagnation

Other symptoms and signs depend on the organ involved. The Liver is the main organ affected by Qi stagnation and, indeed, Liver-Qi stagnation is very commonly seen in practice. However, it should be stressed that other organs suffer from Qi stagnation, for example Heart, Lungs, Stomach and Intestines.

The clinical manifestations of Liver-Qi stagnation are described in chapter 34. It is important to note that Qi stagnation is a 'non-substantial' pathogenic factor: in this, it differs for example, from Dampness or Phlegm. For this reason, abdominal distension affecting the Liver and the Intestines is not relieved by the bowel movement. In contrast, abdominal fullness and pain caused by Dampness or retention of food is relieved by the bowel movement.

> **Box 27.2 Qi stagnation**
> - Feeling of distension
> - Distending pain that moves from place to place
> - Mental depression
> - Irritability
> - Gloomy feeling
> - Frequent mood swings
> - Frequent sighing
> - Wiry pulse
> - Tongue body either normal-coloured or slightly Red on the sides

Remember: Qi stagnation does not affect only the Liver! It may also affect Lungs, Heart, Stomach, Spleen and Intestines.

Another important characteristic of Qi stagnation, when compared to Blood stasis, is that it cannot cause any serious diseases from the point of view of Western medicine. For example, Qi stagnation cannot cause cancer, heart disease or stroke; in contrast, Blood stasis is involved in all the above diseases.

Box 27.2 summarizes the manifestations of Qi stagnation.

Blood stasis

While Qi stagnation causes distension, Blood stasis causes pain (although it also occurs without causing pain). The pain from Blood stasis is typically stabbing, fixed and boring. Blood stasis is associated with a purple or dark colour: for example, a dark complexion, purple lips, purple nails, bleeding with dark blood and dark clots, dark menstrual blood with dark clots, Purple tongue. The pulse qualities associated with Blood stasis are Wiry, Choppy or Firm. Blood stasis is also described in chapter 31.

The organ that is most frequently affected by stasis of Blood is the Liver. Other affected organs are the Heart, Lungs, Stomach, Intestines and Uterus. The symptoms of Blood stasis in each of these organs are described in chapter 31.

In contrast to Qi stagnation, which may not cause serious biomedical diseases, Blood stasis is potentially the cause of serious diseases: for example, cancer, abdominal masses, myoma, endometriosis, heart disease and stroke. Of course, that is not to say that such diseases inevitably appear whenever there is Blood stasis.

While Qi stagnation may arise directly as a consequence of emotional strain, Blood stasis does not arise directly as a result of an aetiological factor. For example, there is no emotional state that leads to Blood stasis directly: some will do so after first causing Qi stagnation. Blood stasis usually derives from other pathological conditions and the main ones are:

- Qi stagnation
- Cold
- Heat
- Qi deficiency
- Blood deficiency
- Phlegm

Blood stasis is also an important pathogenic factor because it becomes itself the cause of further disharmonies. In fact, Blood stasis may cause the following pathological conditions (Fig. 27.3):

- Heat
- Dryness
- Blood deficiency
- Qi deficiency
- Bleeding (haemorrhage)

> **Clinical note**
>
> General points for Blood stasis are BL-17 Geshu and SP-10 Xuehai

Box 27.3 Blood stasis

- Stabbing, fixed or boring pain
- Dark complexion
- Purple lips
- Purple nails
- Bleeding with dark blood and dark clots
- Dark menstrual blood with dark clots
- Purple tongue
- Wiry, Choppy or Firm pulse

Box 27.3 summarizes the manifestations of Blood stasis.

Internal Wind

Internal Wind is characterized by involuntary movements. The main clinical manifestations of interior Wind are tremors, tics, severe dizziness, vertigo and numbness. In severe cases, they are convulsions, unconsciousness, opisthotonos, hemiplegia and deviation of mouth.

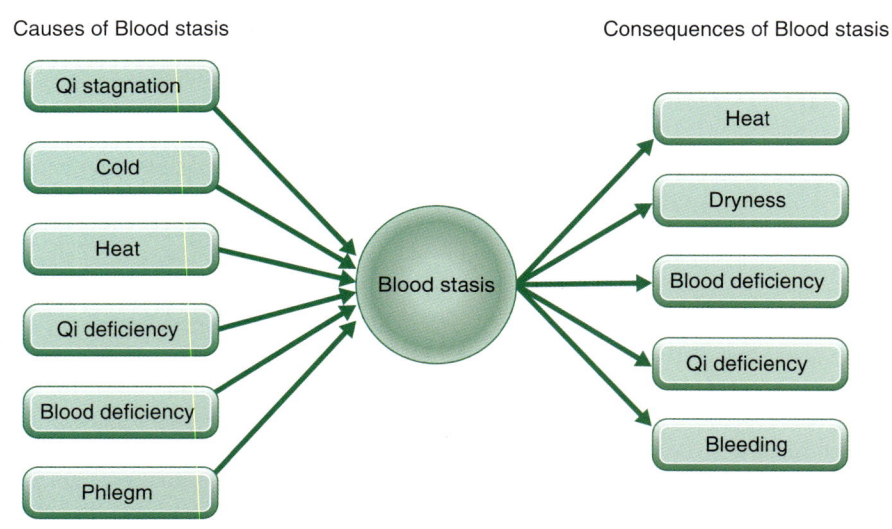

Figure 27.3 Causes and consequences of Blood stasis

Interior Wind is always related to a Liver disharmony. It can arise from several different conditions:

- *Extreme Heat can give rise to Liver-Wind*. This happens in the late stages of febrile diseases when the Heat enters the Blood portion and generates Wind. The clinical manifestations are a high fever, delirium, convulsion, coma and opisthotonos.
- *Liver-Yang rising can give rise to Liver-Wind in prolonged cases*. The clinical manifestations are severe dizziness, vertigo, headache, tremors, tics and irritability.
- *Liver-Fire can give rise to Liver-Wind*.
- *Deficiency of Liver-Blood and/or Liver-Yin can give rise to Liver-Wind*. This is due to the deficiency of Blood creating an empty space within the blood vessels which is taken up by interior Wind. The clinical manifestations are numbness, dizziness, blurred vision, tics and slight tremors.

With the exception of internal Wind occurring in the late stages of febrile diseases in children (in the form of convulsions), internal Wind is much more common in the elderly. For example, internal Wind is the cause of Wind-stroke and Parkinson's disease.

Internal Wind is discussed in more detail in chapter 43. Box 27.4 summarizes the manifestations of internal Wind.

Clinical note

General points for internal Wind are LIV-3 Taichong and Du-16 Fengfu

Internal Dampness

Internal Dampness is an extremely common pathogenic factor. It derives either from an internal disharmony (Spleen-Qi deficiency) or from the transformation of external Dampness. Dampness is responsible for a wide range of diseases affecting many different systems. For example, it is the cause of many skin diseases, digestive diseases, urinary diseases, sinus problems, menstrual problems, postviral fatigue syndrome and others.

The main clinical manifestations of internal Dampness are a feeling of fullness in the abdomen, a feeling of heaviness, lethargy, turbid urine, excessive vaginal discharge, muscle ache, sinus problems, a sticky taste, a sticky tongue coating and a Slippery or Soggy pulse.

These are only the general manifestations of Dampness and other symptoms and signs depend on the organ involved. Many organs may suffer from internal Dampness, for example Stomach, Spleen, Bladder, Intestines, Gall Bladder, Liver, Kidneys and Uterus. Apart from the Internal Organs, Dampness is frequently located in various structures such as the joints, the channels, the muscles, the space between the skin and muscles, the skin, the head.

The various clinical manifestations can be correlated to the main characteristics of Dampness as follows:

- *Heaviness*: this causes a feeling of tiredness, heaviness of limbs or head, or a 'muzzy' (fuzzy) feeling of the head
- *Dirtiness*: Dampness is dirty and is reflected in dirty discharges, such as cloudy urine, vaginal discharges or skin diseases characterized by thick and dirty fluids oozing out, such as in certain types of eczema
- *Stickiness*: Dampness is sticky and this is reflected in a sticky tongue coating, sticky taste and Slippery pulse

Dampness is discussed in detail in chapter 43. Box 27.5 summarizes the manifestations of internal Dampness.

Clinical note

General points for Dampness are Ren-12 Zhongwan, Ren-9 Shuifen, SP-9 Yinlingquan, Ren-5 Shimen and BL-22 Sanjiaoshu

Box 27.4 Internal wind

- Tremors
- Tics
- Severe dizziness
- Vertigo and numbness
- Convulsions
- Unconsciousness
- Opisthotonos
- Hemiplegia and deviation of mouth

Box 27.5 Dampness

- Feeling of fullness in the abdomen
- Feeling of heaviness
- Lethargy
- Turbid urine
- Excessive vaginal discharge
- Muscle ache
- Sinus problems
- Sticky taste
- Sticky tongue coating
- Slippery or Soggy pulse

> **Box 27.6 Cold**
>
> - Pain of a crampy nature that is alleviated by the consumption of hot drinks or the application of heat
> - A feeling of cold
> - The absence of thirst
> - Thin clear discharges
> - Cold limbs
> - Bright-white complexion
> - White tongue coating
> - Slow pulse

Internal Cold

Internal Cold derives either from Yang deficiency (in which case it is Empty-Cold) or from a transformation of external Cold (in which case it is Full-Cold). Internal Cold causes pain of a crampy nature that is alleviated by the consumption of hot drinks or the application of heat, a feeling of cold, the absence of thirst, thin clear discharges, cold limbs, bright-white complexion, white tongue coating and Slow pulse.

The clinical manifestations of Full- and Empty-Cold are very similar as they are the same in nature. The main difference is that Full-Cold is characterized by an acute onset, severe pain and a tongue and pulse of the Excess type: for example, the tongue has a thick white coating and the pulse is Full and Tight. In Empty-Cold, the pain is less intense, the tongue is Pale with a thin white coating and the pulse is Slow-Deep-Weak.

Cold is described in more detail in chapter 43. Box 27.6 summarizes the manifestations of internal Cold.

> **Clinical note**
>
> The best treatment for Cold is moxa either in the form of moxa stick or direct moxa cones or moxa box

Phlegm

Phlegm is a very important and common internal pathogenic factor. Like Blood stasis, it is also potentially the cause of serious diseases such as cancer, heart disease and stroke. Phlegm is at the same time a pathological condition and an aetiological factor. In fact, Phlegm that is retained over a long period of time becomes itself a cause of disease.

The main cause for the formation of Phlegm is Spleen deficiency. If the Spleen fails to transform and transport Body Fluids, these will accumulate and change into Phlegm. The Lungs and Kidneys are also involved in the formation of Phlegm. If the Lungs fail to diffuse and make fluids descend and if the Kidneys fail to transform and excrete fluids, these may accumulate into Phlegm.

The essential signs of Phlegm are a Swollen tongue body, a sticky tongue coating and a Slippery or Wiry pulse. Other symptoms may include a feeling of oppression of the chest, nausea, a feeling of heaviness, a feeling of muzziness (fuzziness) of the head and dizziness.

Other signs of chronic Phlegm are:

- Lack of lustre (*shen*) of the eyes
- Dark eye sockets
- Corners of the eyes have very slight cracks with exudate
- Sallow complexion
- Swollen body, puffy face, obesity
- Greasy skin
- Sweaty external genitalia, axillae or palms and soles
- Enlarged fingers and toes
- Thick thumbs

> **Clinical note**
>
> General points for Phlegm are Ren-12 Zhongwan, Ren-9 Shuifen, SP-9 Yinlingquan, ST-40 Fenglong, Ren-5 Shimen and BL-22 Sanjiaoshu

Box 27.7 summarizes essential manifestations of Phlegm.

Phlegm is a Yin pathogenic factor and it injures Yang

Phlegm is a pathological accumulation of fluids which occurs when there is a disruption to:

- Lung-Qi diffusing and descending
- Heart-Qi moving and transporting
- Spleen-Yang transforming and transporting
- Kidney-Yang warming, transforming and excreting
- Liver-Qi free flow

> **Box 27.7 Essential manifestations of Phlegm**
>
> - **Tongue and pulse:** Swollen tongue body with sticky tongue coating; Slippery or Wiry pulse
> - **Other symptoms:** a feeling of oppression of the chest, expectoration of phlegm, nausea, a feeling of heaviness, a feeling of muzziness (fuzziness) of the head and dizziness

The warming, movement, transportation, transformation and excretion of fluids depends of Yang Qi. Thus, when Yang is deficient, Yin prevails, fluids accumulate and form Phlegm. Conversely, as Phlegm is an accumulation of Yin, it injures Yang.

Phlegm is sticky and obstructs the Qi mechanism

Because Phlegm is sticky, it causes symptoms such as:

- Sticky phlegm
- Sticky mouth
- Sticky saliva at the corners of the mouth
- Nausea, vomiting
- Phlegm in throat
- Swallowing and spitting
- Mucus in stools

Because it is sticky and obstructs the Qi Mechanism, Phlegm is difficult to remove, becomes chronic and gives rise to slow pathological changes. Because it obstructs the Qi Mechanism, very often Qi-moving herbs are added to prescriptions that resolve Phlegm.

Phlegm causes lumps

As Phlegm is an accumulation of fluids and it is Yin in nature, it may give rise to lumps, swellings, nodules, lumps under skin, lumps in the abdominal cavity or in organs. Lumps deriving from Phlegm are generally relatively soft on palpation and usually painless. By contrast, lumps deriving from Blood stasis are usually hard on palpation and painful.

Many diseases characterized by lumps are due to Phlegm:

Luo Li = scrofula
Ying Liu = goitre
Pi Kuai = *Pi* masses
Zheng Jia = abdominal masses
Tan He = nodules
Ru Pi = breast lumps

Phlegm flows and moves, always changing

Phlegm always flows and moves, follows Qi in its ascending/descending and entering/exiting, and goes round the body on the Exterior and to the Internal Organs. It is stored in the Lungs, it is amassed in the Stomach, it obstructs the Heart orifices, it harasses the Liver and Gall Bladder, and it settles in the channels.

Phlegm often harbours stasis

After it has been formed, Phlegm follows Qi and Blood, it is in the Interior in the Internal Organs and in the Exterior in the channels; because it obstructs, it may give rise to or aggravate Blood stasis, also because of the interaction between fluids and Blood. In fact, on the one hand, there is a relationship of mutual exchange between Body Fluids and Blood (ch. 3) and therefore Bloods stasis affects the Fluids; on the other hand, Phlegm is an accumulation of pathological fluids and it therefore aggravates Blood stasis. However, just as Phlegm may aggravate Blood stasis, the latter may also contribute to the former due to the interaction between fluids and Blood: thus the two reinforce each other and establish a vicious circle (Fig. 27.4).

Zhu Dan Xi says: '*When the Lungs are distended and there is a cough and the patient cannot lie down, it is due to Phlegm harbouring Blood stasis.*' Zhang Lu says: '*Phlegm harbours dead Blood, it follows Qi to attack, it flows and causes pain.*' Li Yong Cui says: '*The Blood in the Stomach may stagnate with accumulation of Phlegm day and night; this leads to the diseases of Yi Ge and Fan Wei.*'

Many of the diseases of Western medicine are considered to be due to Phlegm and Blood stasis, such and lymphoma, cancer, brain haemorrhage, coronary heart disease and some mental illness.

The interaction between Phlegm and Blood stasis may cause the following manifestations:

- Dark nails
- Dark complexion
- Purple lips
- Purple and swollen tongue
- Dark rings under the eyes

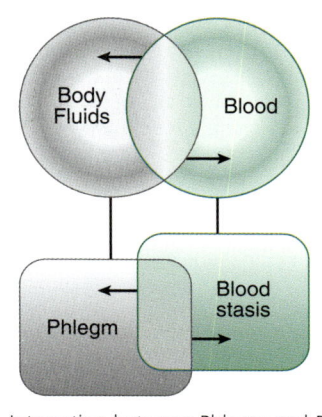

Figure 27.4 Interaction between Phlegm and Blood stasis

Phlegm is the origin of many diseases, many diseases have Phlegm

Phlegm is the origin of many diseases, its clinical scope is very wide and it usually gives rise to complicated diseases. 'Phlegm syndrome' indicates a condition where Phlegm is the cause of most pathological changes; thus, just because there is Phlegm, it does not mean that there is a 'Phlegm syndrome'.

Phlegm assumes many different forms, which contributes to its causing very many different problems: for example, Wind-Phlegm, Cold-Phlegm, Phlegm-Heat, etc. These are described in chapter 31.

Phlegm easily damages Stomach and Spleen

Phlegm obstructs the Middle Burner and very easily leads to deficiency of the Stomach and Spleen. In particular, the Stomach is affected by Phlegm and prescriptions that resolve Phlegm often have herbs that 'harmonize the Stomach'. On the tongue, chronic Phlegm often manifests with a Stomach crack with a sticky dry coating inside it.

Phlegm easily mixes with other pathogenic factors

Phlegm often mixes with Wind, Cold, Heat and Dampness. These combinations are described in chapter 31.

Chinese doctors give various guidelines to follow in complicated clinical situations that often harbour Phlegm. The following are some of them:

- *In strange diseases treat Phlegm.* This refers to complicated clinical patterns with symptoms and signs that do not seem to fit into any pattern. For example: a strongly built man wakes up frequently during the night, dreams a lot, has a voracious appetite, and the tongue is Swollen: this condition is most probably due to Phlegm. Another example could be that of an elderly woman with palpitations, constipation, thirst, insomnia and bitter taste: these manifestations could be due to Phlegm-Heat.
- *In complicated syndromes treat Phlegm.*
- *In acute, serious diseases treat Phlegm.* Example: Wind-stroke, heart infarction, cancer.
- *If you can see phlegm, treat Phlegm.*

Heat

The term 'Heat' is generally used with at least two different meanings. On the one hand, 'Heat' is a general term that includes any manifestations characterized by Heat, which may be interior Heat, exterior Wind-Heat, or Fire. In this sense, 'Fire' comes under the general umbrella of 'Heat'.

In a more narrow definition, 'Heat' denotes a pathogenic factor that is differentiated from Fire. Although Heat and Fire share many common characteristics and the same nature, these two pathogenic factors differ in the degree of intensity (i.e. Fire is more intense than Heat) and their clinical manifestations (and treatment) are somewhat different. From this point of view, therefore, Heat is different and separate from Fire.

There is another important terminology difference between Heat and Fire. While Heat always denotes pathological Heat, the term 'Fire' can denote the physiological Fire of the body (the Minister Fire or the Fire of the Gate of Life) or pathological Fire (as in 'Liver-Fire'). In the 'Yellow Emperor's Classic of Internal Medicine', the physiological Fire of the body is sometimes called 'Lesser Fire' (*Shao Huo*) and the pathological Fire 'Exuberant Fire' (*Zhuang Huo*) (see Fig. 43.10).

Heat, therefore, denotes a state of Excess Yang: it may affect practically every organ and it is either internally generated or the transformation of external Heat. The main internal causes of Heat are emotional strain and diet. As described above, all emotions can give rise to Qi stagnation, and this in turn often leads to Heat as stagnant Qi 'implodes', generating Heat.

The general clinical manifestations of Heat are a feeling of heat, red face, thirst, mental restlessness, Red tongue and an Overflowing-Rapid pulse. Other clinical manifestations depend on the organ involved and whether it is Full- or Empty-Heat.

Heat is an extremely common pathogenic factor and one that can also coexist with Cold. For example, it is not unusual to have Kidney-Yang deficiency (and therefore Empty-Cold) and Damp-Heat in the Bladder.

Heat frequently combines with Dampness, giving rise to Damp-Heat, which is the source of many clinical manifestations in many different organs and places of the body. Damp-Heat is discussed in chapter 43.

Box 27.8 summarizes the manifestations of Heat.

Box 27.8 Heat

- A feeling of heat, red face, thirst, mental restlessness, Red tongue, Overflowing-Rapid pulse. Other clinical manifestations depend on the organ involved and whether it is Full- or Empty-Heat

Fire

Fire is primarily an internal pathogenic factor. The only type of 'external Fire' could be considered to be that seen in Warm Diseases. Fire can derive from the transformation of other exterior pathogenic factors (e.g. Wind, Cold, Summer-Heat, Dampness), but once it affects the Internal Organs, it is an interior pathogenic factor.

Internal causes of Fire are the excessive consumption of hot foods and alcohol, emotional stress (stagnant Qi turns into Fire) and smoking (see Fig. 43.11).

The general clinical manifestations of Fire are red face, red eyes, swelling and pain of the eyes, tongue ulcers, mouth ulcers, scanty dark urine, dry stools, bleeding, insomnia, mental restlessness, pronounced irritability, propensity to outbursts of anger (in Liver-Fire), agitation, Red tongue with a dry, dark-yellow coating and a Deep-Full-Rapid pulse.

As mentioned above, when used in a narrow sense the term 'Heat' denotes a milder form of Fire. Heat and Fire have obviously the same nature and share similar characteristics; they will both cause thirst, a feeling of heat, some mental restlessness, a Red tongue and a Rapid pulse. However, there are some important differences in the clinical manifestations, possible complications and treatment.

Fire is more 'solid' than Heat, it tends to move and dry out more than Heat, and this nature of Fire causes dark scanty urine and dry stools. Fire moves upwards (causing mouth ulcers for example) or damages the blood vessels (causing bleeding). Also, Fire tends to affect the Mind more than Heat, causing anxiety, mental agitation, insomnia or mental illness.

Box 27.9 summarizes the main characteristics of Fire.

The nature of Fire therefore is to:

- Rise to the head
- Dry fluids
- Injure Blood and Yin
- Cause bleeding
- Affect the Mind

Clinical note

In general, the Ying points (second points) of every channel clear Heat or drain Fire. For example, LIV-2 Xingjian, HE-8 Shaofu, BL-66 Tonggu, etc.

> **Box 27.9 Main characteristics of Fire (as opposed to Heat)**
>
> - It blazes upwards
> - It is very drying
> - It damages Blood and Yin
> - It may cause bleeding
> - It has the potential to general Wind
> - It affects the Mind
> - It causes ulcers with swelling

FULL CONDITIONS

It is the presence of a pathogenic factor that determines a 'Full' or 'Excess' condition; the term 'Excess' here refers to the pathogenic factor, not the Upright Qi; that is, in an 'Excess' condition there is not an excess of Upright Qi, but the presence of a pathogenic factor. A 'Full' or 'Excess' condition is called *shi* in Chinese, which means 'solid': this term describes the situation well as the condition is characterized by the presence of a pathogenic factor and it is therefore 'solid' with it.

It should be noted that the conditions necessary to define a pattern as purely 'Full' are not only that there is a pathogenic factor but also that the Upright Qi is relatively intact and is fighting the pathogenic factor. In fact, if the Upright Qi were deficient in the presence of a pathogenic factor, the condition would be defined as a mixed 'Full/Empty' condition (Fig. 27.5).

A Full condition will manifest by definition with symptoms that are relatively severe and intense. For example, if a patient is suffering from a severe, intense pain which stops him or her from conducting normal activities, such a pain must definitely be caused by a Full condition. Please note that a Full condition may be acute or chronic and that 'acute' is not synonymous with an external condition (Fig. 27.6). An example of an acute, Full, external condition is that of invasion of external Wind; an example of an acute, Full, internal condition is an acute episode of Liver-Yang rising causing a severe migraine attack.

Box 27.10 summarizes the characteristics of a Full condition.

EMPTY CONDITIONS

An Empty condition is characterized by 'emptiness': that is, a deficiency of the Upright Qi. It should be remembered that 'Upright Qi' is a general term that

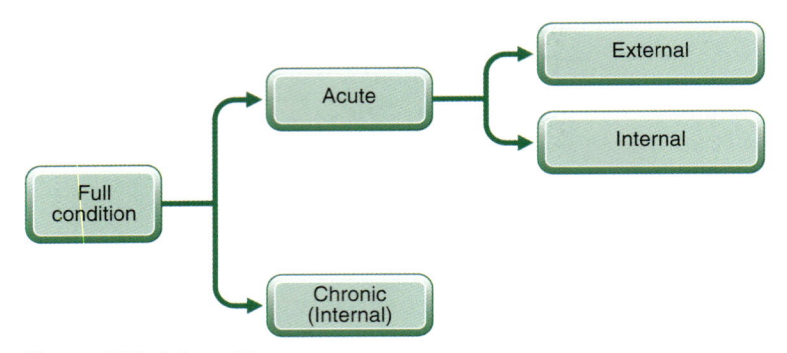

Figure 27.5 Full conditions

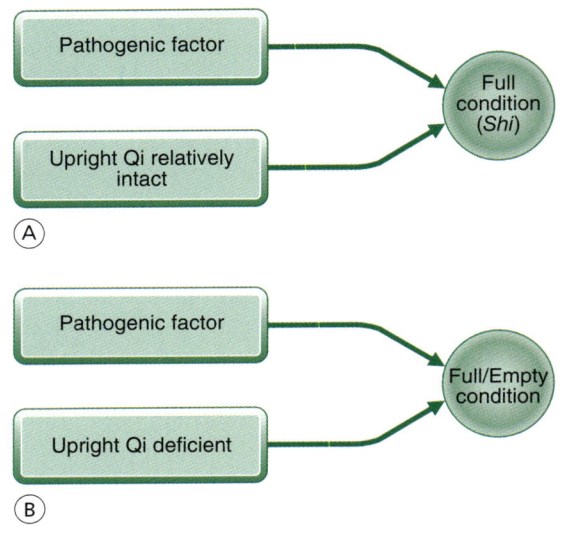

Figure 27.6 Full/Empty conditions

Box 27.10 Full condition

- A 'Full' or 'Excess' (*shi*) condition is characterized by the presence of a pathogenic factor (while the Upright Qi is relatively intact)

includes all types of Qi as well as Blood and that it essentially denotes the body's resistance to pathogenic factors; the term 'Upright Qi' (*Zheng Qi*) is, in fact, used in conjunction with and in opposition to the term 'pathogenic factor' (*Xie Qi*).

The clinical manifestations of an Empty condition are much milder than those of a Full condition. Pain is a good symptom to use to compare and contrast a Full versus an Empty condition: in a Full condition the pain is severe and intense, while in an Empty condition it is mild and more an ache than a pain.

Box 27.11 Empty condition

- An 'Empty' or 'Deficient' condition is characterized by a deficiency of the Upright Qi

Like a Full condition, an Empty condition may be chronic or acute but it is much more frequently the former. For example, a Spleen deficiency will develop gradually and slowly over years (generally due to irregular eating); the same for a Kidney deficiency (generally due to overwork). Examples of acute Empty conditions are the Yin deficiency induced by an acute febrile disease, the Blood deficiency following a heavy blood loss or the Qi deficiency that follows heavy sweating. The overwhelming majority of patients with Empty conditions that we see suffer from an internal, chronic, gradually developing deficiency.

Box 27.11 summarizes the characteristics of an Empty condition.

FULL/EMPTY CONDITIONS

A condition is defined as a mixed 'Full/Empty' condition when there is a pathogenic factor and the Upright Qi is deficient and it is therefore not fighting the pathogenic factor adequately or, in serious cases, not at all. In most chronic, internal conditions, it is actually the deficiency of the Upright Qi that leads to the formation of the pathogenic factor (e.g. Spleen and Kidney deficiency leading to the formation of Phlegm).

Pathogenic factors and Upright Qi constantly interact with each other. Generally speaking, when one has the supremacy, the other goes down (Fig. 27.7). For example, if Phlegm (a pathogenic factor) grows in intensity, it will inevitably weaken the Spleen and possibly also the Kidneys; vice versa, if the Spleen and

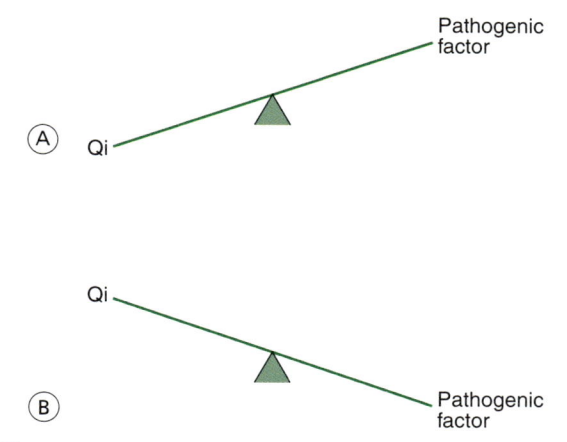

Figure 27.7 Balance between pathogenic factor and Upright Qi

Table 27.1 Six situations of relative strength of pathogenic factors and upright Qi

Pathogenic factor	Upright Qi	Result
None	Normal	Health
None	Deficient	Empty condition
Strong	Strong	Full condition
Strong	Deficient	Full/Empty condition
Weak	Strong	Full/Empty condition
Weak	Deficient	Full/Empty condition

Box 27.12 Full/Empty condition

- A 'Full/Empty' condition is characterized by the presence of a pathogenic factor while the Upright Qi is deficient

Kidneys become stronger, the Phlegm will be reduced. Chapter 28 of the 'Simple Questions' says: '*When pathogenic factors are strong, the condition is Full; the Upright Qi is deprived and becomes deficient*'.[1]

Box 27.12 summarizes the characteristics of a Full/Empty condition.

We can hypothesize six different situations with differing relative strength of pathogenic factors and Upright Qi. These are (Table 27.1):

1. No pathogenic factor–normal Upright Qi = health
2. No pathogenic factor–deficient Upright Qi = Empty condition
3. Strong pathogenic factor–strong Upright Qi = Full condition
4. Strong pathogenic factor–deficient Upright Qi = Full/Empty condition
5. Weak pathogenic factor–strong Upright Qi = Full/Empty condition
6. Weak pathogenic factor–deficient Upright Qi = Full/Empty condition

Let us discuss these six situations in detail.

No pathogenic factor–normal Upright Qi

This is of course a (rare) state of perfect health (Box 27.13).

Box 27.13 No pathogenic factor–normal Upright Qi

- Health

No pathogenic factor–deficient Upright Qi

This is a purely Deficient condition, usually seen in chronic, internal conditions. For example, a chronic Spleen-Qi deficiency developing gradually and slowly from irregular diet, a chronic Kidney-Yang deficiency developing gradually and slowly from overwork, etc.

Although this may seem to be a very common situation, it is, in fact, not that common because, in the majority of cases, there will be some kind of pathogenic factor in addition to (or as a result of) the deficiency (e.g. Dampness deriving from Spleen deficiency).

Box 27.14 summarizes the characteristics of this condition.

Strong pathogenic factor–strong Upright Qi

This is a classic, purely Full condition: the patient suffers from a pathogenic factor (which may be internal or external, acute or chronic) and his or her

Box 27.14 No pathogenic factor–deficient Upright Qi

- Purely Empty condition
- Mild symptoms
- Long, protracted, chronic disease developing gradually
- Can only be internal

> **Box 27.15 Strong pathogenic factor–strong Upright Qi**
>
> - Purely Full condition
> - Can be external or internal
> - Very intense, heightened symptoms
> - If external, high fever

> **Box 27.16 Strong pathogenic factor–deficient Upright Qi**
>
> - Mixed Full/Empty condition
> - May be external or internal
> - If external, moderate fever
> - Frequently seen in postviral fatigue syndrome

Upright Qi is strong and fighting the pathogenic factor strongly. This is the situation that produces strong, intense clinical manifestations, especially in acute, external conditions. For example, if a person with a strong Upright Qi is invaded by a strong external Wind, the clinical manifestations will be very intense and heightened, such as in a high fever, very pronounced body aches, etc.

Whilst it is easy to postulate an exterior, acute condition when both the pathogenic factor and the Upright Qi are strong, this situation also occurs in chronic, internal conditions. For example, a person may develop a strong Qi stagnation (a Full condition) from emotional problems and his or her Upright Qi is strong: this will induce a purely Full condition that is internal and chronic. Indeed such a situation is often seen in patients who, although encumbered by a strong pathogenic factor, have a good constitution that makes the Upright Qi strong and who therefore often live to a ripe old age, despite such strong pathogenic factors.

Box 27.15 summarizes the condition of strong pathogenic factor–strong Upright Qi.

Strong pathogenic factor–deficient Upright Qi

Although the three situations of strong pathogenic factor–deficient Upright Qi, weak pathogenic factor–strong Upright Qi and weak pathogenic factor–deficient Upright Qi all lead to a Full/Empty condition, they are in fact quite different, and I will explain the differences with examples.

When the pathogenic factor is strong and the Upright Qi is deficient, the condition is a mixed Full/Empty condition that may be external or internal and is extremely common. An example of such an external Full/Empty condition is that of a person with a deficient Upright Qi (extremely common) who is invaded by a strong external Wind. As the Upright Qi is deficient, the clinical manifestations will be less intense than the previous case (i.e. when the pathogenic factor and the Upright Qi are both strong). Contrary to the previous case, if the patient has a fever, in this case it will be quite low.

An example of an interior condition with a strong pathogenic factor and a deficient Upright Qi is that of a person suffering from postviral fatigue syndrome characterized by a pronounced, intense Dampness but a deficient Upright Qi: this situation is very common. In such cases, the Upright Qi is still trying to fight off the pathogenic factor but it does so ineffectually. This is exactly what happens in postviral fatigue syndrome when the patient's Upright Qi is ineffective in fighting off the pathogenic factor: this results in a very protracted, chronic condition that for long periods gets neither better nor worse.

Another example of an interior condition with strong pathogenic factor and deficient Upright Qi is that of patient suffering from a serious condition of Phlegm and a simultaneous deficiency of the Spleen and Kidneys: this situation is rather common and it is one that, in the elderly, may potentially lead to serious diseases.

Box 27.16 summarizes the condition of strong pathogenic factor–deficient Upright Qi.

Weak pathogenic factor–strong Upright Qi

This situation also leads to a mixed Full/Empty condition which may be external or internal. Although this is a Full/Empty condition in a similar way to the previous situation (with strong pathogenic factor and deficient Upright Qi), its manifestations will be quite different and generally milder (because the pathogenic factor is weak).

An example of an exterior condition with these characteristics is that of a patient with a strong Upright Qi who is invaded by a mild external Wind: in such a case, the clinical manifestations will be very mild, there will be no fever and the patient will generally be able to work through such a condition.

> **Box 27.17 Weak pathogenic factor–strong Upright Qi**
>
> - Mixed Full/Empty condition
> - Symptoms mild
> - If external, moderate fever

An example of an interior condition with weak pathogenic factor and strong Upright Qi is that of a patient suffering from a mild condition of Dampness but with a strong Upright Qi: in this case, too, the clinical manifestations will be mild.

Box 27.17 summarizes the condition of weak pathogenic factor–strong Upright Qi.

Weak pathogenic factor–deficient Upright Qi

It may seem strange that such a condition (when both pathogenic factor and Upright Qi are 'weak') is also defined as Full/Empty. It is described as such because, although weak, there is a pathogenic factor. This condition, too, may be external or internal and the clinical manifestations will be the mildest of the last three cases.

An example of such a situation in exterior conditions is that of patient with a deficient Upright Qi who suffers an invasion of a mild exterior Wind: the clinical manifestations will be very mild and there will be no fever.

An example of such a situation in interior conditions is that of patient suffering from a chronic deficiency of the Upright Qi and the simultaneous presence of mild Dampness or Phlegm. The situation with a weak pathogenic factor and a deficient Upright Qi is one that causes the symptoms to linger for many years without getting better or worse.

Box 27.18 summarizes the condition of weak pathogenic factor–deficient Upright Qi.

> **Box 27.18 Weak pathogenic factor–deficient Upright Qi**
>
> - Mixed Full/Empty condition
> - Very mild symptoms
> - Long, protracted, chronic disease
> - If external, no fever

INTERACTION BETWEEN PATHOGENIC FACTORS AND UPRIGHT QI

Pathogenic factors and Upright Qi are not fixed entities but are constantly interacting with each other. This is because every pathogenic factor evolves and frequently changes nature and also because each pathogenic factor tends to injure the Upright Qi in one way or another. For example, external Wind frequently changes into Heat and becomes interior (this happens when an upper respiratory infection progresses to a chest infection). Qi stagnation frequently leads to Blood stasis. Dampness may lead to Phlegm.

Box 27.19 summarizes Upright Qi versus pathogenic factors.

Besides changing their nature, pathogenic factors also have a strong tendency to injure the Upright Qi in various ways. For example, Heat dries up Body Fluids and may injure Yin; Dampness or Phlegm encumbers Qi and causes Qi deficiency; severe Blood stasis may cause dryness of Body Fluids; Qi stagnation interferes with the proper ascending/descending of Qi; Cold congeals Blood and causes Blood stasis; Cold also tends to weaken Yang Qi.

On the other hand, the Upright Qi interacts with pathogenic factors because, if they are external, it will attempt to fight them off, and, if they are internal, it will influence them and attempt to eliminate them. For example, in invasions of external Wind, the Upright Qi fights the pathogenic factor and fever is a result of such a fight.

In internal conditions, too, the Upright Qi is fighting the pathogenic factor: for example, if a patient is encumbered by Dampness, by its very nature Qi will attempt to transform, resolve and excrete Dampness. Whether such an attempt succeeds or not depends on the relative strength of Dampness and the Upright Qi: generally, the longer a condition is rooted in the body, the more difficult it will be for the body's Qi to resolve it. Given a chance, the Upright Qi can and does expel pathogenic factors. For example, if a patient is encumbered by Dampness, a simple change in dietary habits

> **Box 27.19 Pathogenic factors evolution**
>
> - Pathogenic factors evolve and change
> - Pathogenic factors tend to injure the Upright Qi

may be all that is needed to give the Upright Qi a chance to resolve Dampness even without treatment with acupuncture or herbs (Fig. 27.8 and Box 27.20).

The interaction between pathogenic factors and Upright Qi may become very intricate as they affect each other so that, for example, a pathogenic factor may injure Qi, which, in turn, may either strengthen the original pathogenic factor itself or lead to another, new pathogenic factor (Figs 27.9 and 27.10).

For example, an invasion of external Wind may obstruct Qi and this, in turn, may lead to Dampness (this happens frequently in children). Qi deficiency may lead to Dampness and this, turn, weakens Qi even more. Figures 27.11–27.14 illustrate examples of complex interactions between pathogenic factors and Upright Qi.

> **Box 27.20 Upright Qi versus pathogenic factors**
> - In invasions of external pathogenic factors, Upright Qi fights them off
> - In internal pathogenic factors, the Upright Qi influences them and attempts to eliminate them

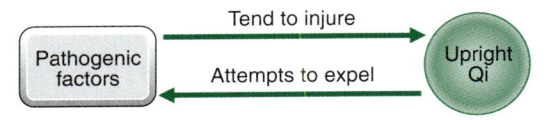

Figure 27.8 Interaction between pathogenic factors and Upright Qi

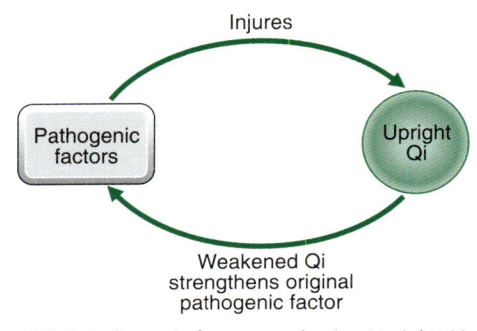

Figure 27.9 Pathogenic factors weakening Upright Qi

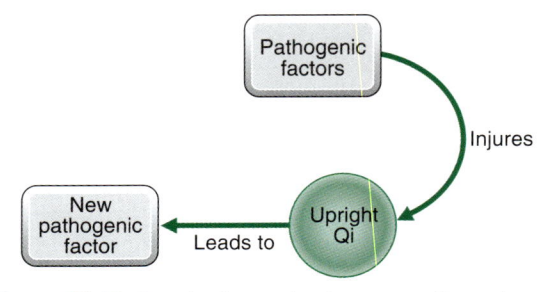

Figure 27.10 Complex interaction between pathogenic factors and Upright Qi

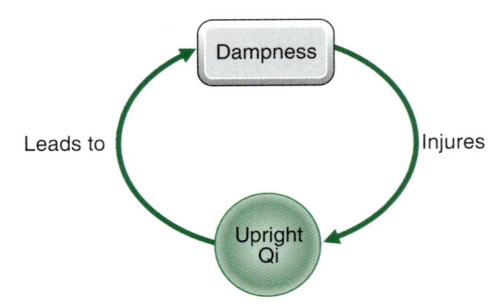

Figure 27.11 Interaction between Dampness and Qi

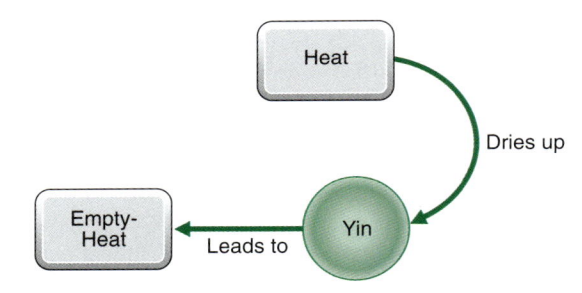

Figure 27.12 Interaction between Heat, Yin and Empty-Heat

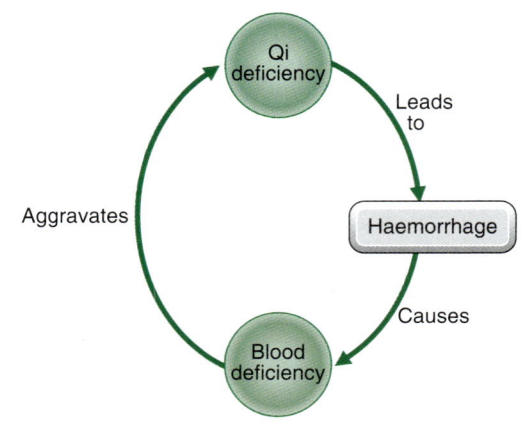

Figure 27.13 Interaction between Qi deficiency, haemorrhage and Blood deficiency

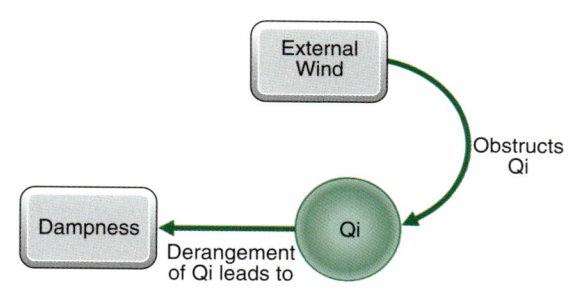

Figure 27.14 Interaction between external Wind, Qi and Dampness

Learning outcomes

In this chapter you will have learned:

- The importance of diagnosing correctly the Full/Empty character of a condition
- The nature of 'pathogenic factor' in Chinese medicine, both external and internal
- The nature of the 'Full' or 'Excess' condition
- The nature of the 'Empty' or 'Deficient' condition
- The nature of the mixed 'Full/Empty' condition
- The six different hypothetical situations which, depending on the relative strength of the pathogenic factor and the Upright Qi, lead to either Full, Empty or mixed Full/Empty conditions
- The dynamics of the interaction between pathogenic factors and Upright Qi

Self-assessment questions

1. What are the three ways an external pathogenic factor can directly penetrate the Interior of the body?
2. Give three examples of internal pathogenic factors.
3. What conditions are required to define a pattern as Full?
4. How would the manifestations of pain differ between a Full and an Empty condition?
5. What conditions are required to define a pattern as mixed Full/Empty?
6. Describe the type of condition and the general severity of symptoms of someone with deficient Upright Qi who is invaded by a strong External Wind.
7. Why might a person with deficient Upright Qi, and the presence of mild Dampness, suffer from lingering symptoms over many years?
8. How does Heat in the body injure the Upright Qi?

See p. 1262 for answers

END NOTE

1. 1979 The Yellow Emperor's Classic of Internal Medicine – Simple Questions (*Huang Di Nei Jing Su Wen* 黄帝内经素问), People's Health Publishing House, Beijing, first published c.100 BC, p. 173–174.

PART 5

The Pathology of Yin–Yang Imbalance

28

Key contents

- Imbalance of Yin and Yang
- Yin–Yang imbalance and Heat–Cold patterns
- Transformation and interaction between Yin and Yang
- Excess of Yang
- Deficiency of Yang
- Excess of Yin
- Deficiency of Yin
- Principles of treatment

- An Excess of Yang
- A Deficiency of Yang
- An Excess of Yin
- A Deficiency of Yin

This chapter will discuss the pathology of an imbalance between Yin and Yang and the discussion will focus on the following points:

- Imbalance of Yin and Yang
- Yin–Yang imbalance and Heat-Cold patterns
- Transformation and interaction between Yin and Yang
- Excess of Yang
- Deficiency of Yang
- Excess of Yin
- Deficiency of Yin
- Principles of treatment

IMBALANCE OF YIN AND YANG

An imbalance between Yin and Yang is a fundamental aspect of Chinese pathology. Indeed, it could be said that all clinical manifestations and all types of pathology ultimately boil down to an imbalance between Yin and Yang: that is, every pathological situation could be described as one of four situations (see Figs 1.7, 1.11–1.15 in ch. 1):

For example, Heat or Fire are an Excess of Yang; deficiency of Yang of the Spleen and/or Kidneys is of course a type of Yang deficiency; Full-Cold is an Excess of Yin; deficiency of Kidney-Yin is a type of Yin deficiency.

Please note that the parameters used when describing 'Excess of Yang' and 'Deficiency of Yang' (similarly for 'Excess of Yin' and 'Deficiency of Yin') are *not* the same. In fact, 'Excess of Yang' indicates *not* an 'excess' of normal Yang Qi, but the presence of a Yang pathogenic factor (i.e. Heat). In contrast, 'Deficiency of Yang' denotes a deficiency, a lack of normal Yang Qi. In other words, 'Yang' in 'Excess of Yang' indicates a pathological Heat; 'Yang' in 'Deficiency of Yang' indicates a physiological Heat.

Similarly, 'Excess of Yin' indicates *not* an 'excess' of normal Yin substances, but the presence of a Yin pathogenic factor, i.e. Cold, Dampness, Blood stasis or Phlegm. In contrast, 'Deficiency of Yin' denotes a deficiency of Yin substances, fluids and Essence. Blood is also a type of Yin substance and Blood deficiency is a type of 'Deficiency of Yin'. In other words, 'Yin' in 'Excess of Yin' indicates pathological Cold, Dampness, Blood stasis or Phlegm; 'Yin' in 'Deficiency of Yin' indicates the physiological Yin substances, the fluids, the Essence and Blood.

Please note that these four pathological situations are not necessarily mutually exclusive. For example, a deficiency of Yang of the Spleen and Kidneys often leads to the formation of Phlegm, which, in itself, is a form of 'Excess of Yin' as it is a pathological accumulation of fluids (although it should be stressed that

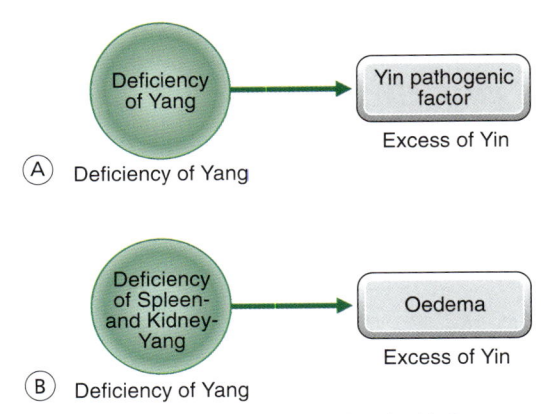

Figure 28.1 Deficiency of Yang associated with Excess of Yin

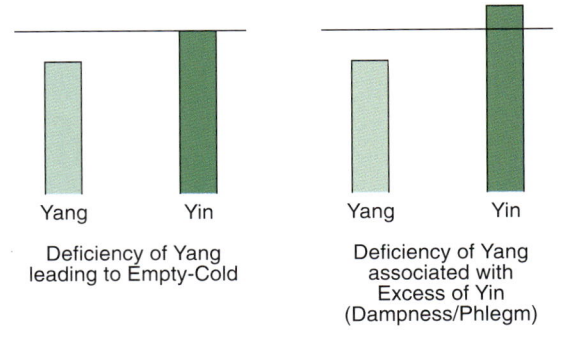

Figure 28.2 Deficiency of Yang resulting in Empty-Cold and deficiency of Yang associated with Full-Cold

Box 28.1 The four imbalances of Yin–Yang

- Excess of Yang
- Deficiency of Yang
- Excess of Yin
- Deficiency of Yin

Phlegm can be associated with Heat, but this usually happens as a long-term development of Phlegm). Similarly, a deficiency of Yang of the Spleen and Kidneys often leads to the formation of oedema, which, in itself, is a form of 'Excess of Yin' as it is a pathological accumulation of fluids (Fig. 28.1).

Box 28.1 summarizes the four imbalances of Yin–Yang.

YIN–YANG IMBALANCE AND HEAT–COLD PATTERNS

Thus, a deficiency of Yang usually generates Empty-Cold but it also be associated with Excess of Yin as, for example, when it generates Dampness or Phlegm. These two situations can be represented as shown in Figure 28.2.

The relative balance of Yin and Yang is reflected in conditions of Heat or Cold: Heat is an Excess of Yang and Cold is an Excess of Yin. We can therefore postulate the correspondence between Yin/Yang, Cold/Heat and Full/Empty as follows:

- Excess of Yang = Full-Heat
- Deficiency of Yang = Empty-Cold
- Excess of Yin = Full-Cold
- Deficiency of Yin = Empty-Heat

Box 28.2 Yin–Yang imbalance and Heat–Cold patterns

- Excess of Yang = Full-Heat
- Deficiency of Yang = Empty-Cold
- Excess of Yin = Full-Cold
- Deficiency of Yin = Empty-Heat

Box 28.2 summarizes Yin–Yang imbalance and Heat–Cold patterns.

TRANSFORMATION AND INTERACTION BETWEEN YIN AND YANG

There is a tendency for both Full-Cold and Full-Heat to eventually lead to Empty-Cold and Empty-Heat, respectively. In fact, Full-Cold tends to weaken Yang Qi; this leads to Yang deficiency, which, in turn, will lead to Empty-Cold. Full-Heat tends to injure Yin Qi; this leads to Yin deficiency, which, in turn, will lead to Empty-Heat (Fig. 28.3).

Deficiency of Yang and Deficiency of Yin are not mutually exclusive and may occur simultaneously. Generally, this happens only in Kidney deficiency. As the Kidneys are the root, the origin of all the Yin and Yang energies of the body and the source of the physiological Fire and Water, a Kidney deficiency often (but not always) involves a deficiency of both Yin and Yang. This is especially common in women over 45.

Yin and Yang mutually consume each other and this is very apparent especially in pathology. Excess of Yin (i.e. Cold, Dampness or Phlegm) tends to injure Yang (because it obstructs the movement and transformation of Yang) and Excess of Yang (i.e. Heat) tends to injure Yin (because it tends to dry up Yin).

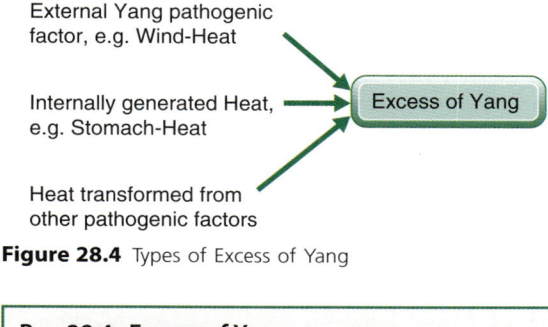

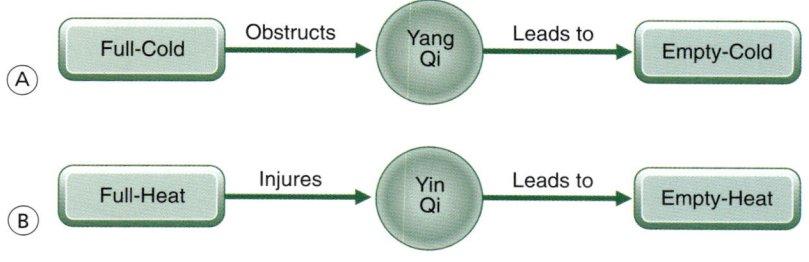

Figure 28.3 Interactions between (A) Full-Cold and Empty-Cold and between (B) Full-Heat and Empty-Heat

---

Box 28.3 Transformation and interaction of Yin–Yang

- Both Full-Cold and Full-Heat eventually lead to Empty-Cold and Empty-Heat
- Deficiency of Yang and Deficiency of Yin are not mutually exclusive and may occur simultaneously (especially in the Kidneys)
- Yin and Yang mutually consume each other
- Excess of Yin (i.e. Cold, Dampness or Phlegm) tends to injure Yang
- Excess of Yang (i.e. Heat) tends to injure Yin

Box 28.3 summarizes transformation and interaction of Yin and Yang.

EXCESS OF YANG

'Excess of Yang' is a general, abstract term. In practice, what forms can 'Excess of Yang' take and how does it originate? There are basically three types of 'Excess of Yang':

- It can be an external Yang pathogenic factor such as Wind-Heat or Summer-Heat
- It can be Heat that is internally generated (usually from emotional stress or diet), e.g. Heart-Fire, Liver-Fire
- It can be Heat that derives from the transformation of other pathogenic factors (even Cold), e.g. external Wind (even Wind-Cold) turning into interior Heat (Fig. 28.4).

Excess of Yang causes symptoms of Heat such as feeling of heat, thirst and dark urine. The main organs that suffer from Excess of Yang are the Heart, Liver, Lungs and Stomach.

Box 28.4 summarizes Excess of Yang.

DEFICIENCY OF YANG

As mentioned above, while 'Excess of Yang' denotes the excess of pathological Heat, 'Deficiency of Yang'

Figure 28.4 Types of Excess of Yang

Box 28.4 Excess of Yang

- It can be an external Yang pathogenic factor such as Wind-Heat or Summer-Heat
- It can be Heat that is internally generated, e.g. Heart-Fire, Liver-Fire
- It can be Heat that derives from the transformation of other pathogenic factors
- Excess of Yang causes symptoms of Heat such as feeling of heat, thirst and dark urine
- Excess of Yang of internal origin may be caused by emotional stress or dietary irregularity
- The main organs that suffer from Excess of Yang are the Heart, Liver, Lungs and Stomach

---

denotes the deficiency of physiological heat (i.e. Yang Qi). It is one of the functions of Qi to warm the body as this relies on physiological heat to perform its functions. Deficiency of Yang leads to Empty-Cold and there will therefore be some Cold symptoms such as feeling cold, desiring warmth, cold limbs, pale urine, etc.

Deficiency of Yang may be caused by dietary factors (excessive consumption of cold foods), excessive physical work or overwork. Deficiency of Yang may also be caused by Full-Cold; in fact, when Full-Cold stays in the body, after some time (generally in terms of months) this injures Yang Qi and leads to Yang deficiency.

The main organs that suffer from Yang deficiency are the Heart, Spleen, Lungs, Kidneys and Stomach.

Box 28.5 summarizes Deficiency of Yang.

> **Box 28.5 Deficiency of Yang**
>
> - 'Deficiency of Yang' denotes the deficiency of physiological heat, i.e. Yang Qi
> - Deficiency of Yang leads to Empty-Cold
> - There are Cold symptoms such as feeling cold, desiring warmth, cold limbs, pale urine, etc.
> - Deficiency of Yang may be caused by dietary factors (excessive consumption of cold foods), excessive physical work or overwork
> - Deficiency of Yang may also be caused by Full-Cold
> - The main organs that suffer from Yang deficiency are the Heart, Spleen, Lungs, Kidneys and Stomach

EXCESS OF YIN

'Excess of Yin' denotes the excess of Yin pathogenic factors such as Cold. In a broad sense it may include also Dampness and Phlegm as these pathogenic factors often originate from a deficiency of Yang (although it should be stressed that both Dampness and Phlegm often associate with Heat).

There are basically four types of 'Excess of Yin':

- It can be an external Yin pathogenic factor such as Wind-Cold or Cold-Dampness
- It can be external Cold that invades the Interior of the body directly without going through an Exterior stage (this happens in the Stomach, Intestines and Uterus)
- It can be external Cold that invades the channels and joints (causing Painful Obstruction Syndrome)
- It can be internally generated Dampness or Phlegm. Although these two pathogenic factors generally derive from a Yang deficiency, Dampness and Phlegm in themselves are Yin pathogenic factors and a type of 'Excess Yin' (in this case, therefore, there is a simultaneous 'Excess of Yin' and 'Deficiency of Yang')

Please note that, even when they are combined with Heat, Dampness and Phlegm are still 'Yin' pathogenic factors because they are an accumulation of pathological fluids.

The clinical manifestations of Excess of Yin will involve Cold symptoms such as feeling cold, cold limbs, pain, pale urine, etc. (Fig. 28.5).

The organs that are most affected by Excess of Yin are the Stomach, Lungs, Intestines and Uterus.

Box 28.6 summarizes Excess of Yin.

DEFICIENCY OF YIN

Deficiency of Yin involves the excessive consumption of body fluids, the Yin substances of each organ, the

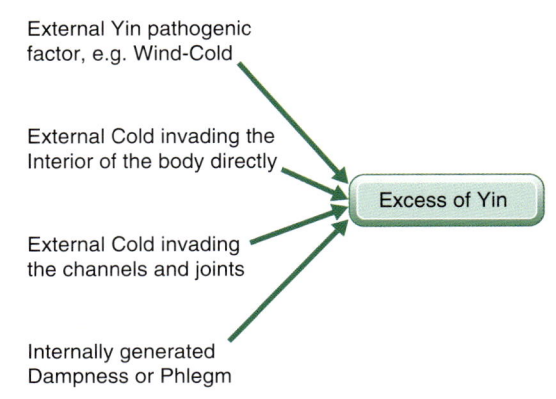

Figure 28.5 Types of Excess of Yin

> **Box 28.6 Excess of Yin**
>
> - 'Excess of Yin' denotes the excess of Yin pathogenic factors such as Cold (also Dampness and Phlegm)
> - There are four types of 'Excess of Yin':
>   - It can be an external Yin pathogenic factor such as Wind-Cold or Cold-Dampness
>   - It can be external Cold that invades the Interior of the body directly without going through an Exterior stage (this happens in the Stomach, Intestines and Uterus)
>   - It can be external Cold that invades the channels and joints (causing Painful Obstruction Syndrome)
>   - It can be internally generated Dampness of Phlegm
> - The clinical manifestations of Excess of Yin will involve Cold symptoms such as feeling cold, cold limbs, pain, pale urine, etc.
> - The organs that are most affected by Excess of Yin are the Stomach, Lungs, Intestines and Uterus

Essence and Blood. The main cause of Yin deficiency in Western patients is overwork, as defined in chapter 22. Yin deficiency usually develops very gradually and slowly over several years. The only exception to this is the Yin deficiency that can develop rapidly in febrile diseases when pathological Heat consumes body fluids and Yin.

The clinical manifestations of Yin deficiency involve dryness, such as a dry mouth in the afternoon, dry skin, dry eyes, etc.

If Yin deficiency persists for a long time, it eventually leads to the development of Empty-Heat. The clinical manifestations will therefore involve Heat, such as a feeling of heat in the afternoon, a dry mouth with desire to drink in small sips, etc. It is important to note that, although Yin deficiency *eventually* causes Empty-Heat, it may exist for years without generating Empty-Heat. The tongue reflects these situations very accurately. Deficiency of Yin manifests on the tongue with a lack of coating: that is, a tongue without coating but of a normal colour indicates Yin deficiency (without Empty-Heat). A Red tongue without coating indicates Yin deficiency with Empty-Heat.

The organs that are most subject to Yin deficiency are the Heart, Lungs, Kidneys, Liver and Stomach.

Box 28.7 summarizes Deficiency of Yin.

Box 28.7 Deficiency of Yin

- Deficiency of Yin involves the excessive consumption of body fluids, the Yin substances of each organ, the Essence and Blood
- The main cause of Yin deficiency is overwork
- Deficiency of Yin may be caused by Full-Heat
- The clinical manifestations of Yin deficiency involve dryness, such as a dry mouth in the afternoon, dry skin, dry eyes, etc.
- If Yin deficiency persists for a long time, it eventually leads to the development of Empty-Heat
- The clinical manifestations will involve Heat, such as a feeling of heat in the afternoon, a dry mouth with desire to drink in small sips, etc.
- The organs that are most subject to Yin deficiency are the Heart, Lungs, Kidneys, Liver and Stomach

---

PRINCIPLES OF TREATMENT

An understanding of the pathology of imbalances between Yin and Yang is crucial to determine the correct treatment principle and method.

The treatment principle is intimately related not only to the imbalance of Yin–Yang but also to the Hot–Cold and Full–Empty nature of the pathology. Put simply, there are only four basic treatment principles:

- In Excess of Yang, clear Heat
- In Deficiency of Yang, tonify Yang
- In Excess of Yin, expel Cold
- In Deficiency of Yin, nourish Yin

In Excess of Yang and Excess of Yin, the emphasis is on 'clearing' and 'expelling' pathogenic factors, while in Deficiency of Yang and Deficiency of Yin, the emphasis is on 'tonifying' and 'nourishing' the body's Qi. It should be noted here that 'expel Cold' in Excess of Yin should be interpreted in a broad sense, including resolving Dampness and Phlegm (which are also an Excess of Yin).

Box 28.8 summarizes principles of treatment.

Box 28.8 Treatment principles

- Excess of Yang: clear Heat
- Deficiency of Yang: tonify Yang
- Excess of Yin: expel Cold
- Deficiency of Yin: nourish Yin
- Empty-Cold: expel Cold, tonify and warm Yang
- Empty-Heat: clear Heat, nourish Yin

Moreover, the Yin–Yang imbalance determines also the method of treatment in acupuncture as follows:

- In Excess of Yang, clear Heat and do not use moxa
- In Deficiency of Yang, tonify Yang and use moxa
- In Excess of Yin, expel Cold and use moxa
- In Deficiency of Yin, nourish Yin and do not use moxa

Box 28.9 summarizes Yin–Yang imbalance and acupuncture treatment method.

Box 28.9 Yin–Yang imbalance and acupuncture treatment method

- Excess of Yang: clear Heat and do not use moxa
- Deficiency of Yang: tonify Yang and use moxa
- Excess of Yin: expel Cold and use moxa
- Deficiency of Yin: nourish Yin and do not use moxa

So far we have discussed the treatment principle in Full-Heat (Excess of Yang) and Full-Cold (Excess of Yin), but what of Empty-Heat and Empty-Cold? In Empty-Heat, one must simultaneously nourish Yin and clear Heat (and use no moxa); in Empty-Cold, one must simultaneously tonify and warm Yang and expel Cold (with moxa).

Learning outcomes

In this chapter you will have learned:
- The importance of understanding how all clinical manifestations and pathology can be described in terms of Yin–Yang imbalance
- The four basic pathological situations of Yin–Yang imbalance
- The difference between the pathological Yin in 'Excess of Yin' and the physiological Yin of 'Deficiency of Yin' (and the same for Yang)
- The correspondences of Yin–Yang imbalance in terms of Cold/Heat and Full/Empty
- The transformation and interaction of Yin–Yang
- The various forms taken by 'Excess of Yang' and 'Deficiency of Yang' and their causes
- The forms taken by 'Excess of Yin' and 'Deficiency of Yin' and their causes
- The relationship between the nature of the Yin–Yang imbalance and the required treatment principle and method

Self-assessment questions

1. What are the four basic pathological situations in terms of Yin–Yang, Cold/Heat and Full/Empty?
2. Complete the following sentence: 'Full-Cold tends to _____ Yang Qi; this leads to ____ _____ which, in turn, will lead to _____ ____.'
3. What are the three basic types of 'Excess of Yang'.
4. Give three possible causes of Deficiency of Yang.
5. What is the main cause of Yin deficiency in Western patients?
6. What is the characteristic clinical manifestation associated with Yin deficiency?
7. Complete the following: 'In Excess of Yang, _____ ____. In Deficiency of Yang, _____ _____. In Excess of Yin, _____ ____. In Deficiency of Yin, _____ ___.'

See p. 1262 for answers

PART 5

Pathology of the Qi Mechanism | 29

> **Key contents**
>
> **Pathology of the ascending/descending of Qi**
>
> Pathology of ascending/descending of Qi in the Internal Organs
> - Spleen
> - Stomach
> - Lungs
> - Heart
> - Liver
> - Kidneys
> - Bladder
> - Small Intestine
> - Large Intestine
>
> Pathology of ascending/descending of Qi in the channels
> Pathology of ascending/descending of Qi in orifices and sense organs
>
> **Pathology of the entering/exiting of Qi**
>
> Pathology of the entering/exiting of Qi in the channels
> Pathology of the entering/exiting of Qi in the space between the skin and muscles
> Pathology of the entering/exiting of Qi in the Triple Burner cavities
> Pathology of the entering/exiting of Qi in the organs
> Pathology of the entering/exiting of Qi in the joints
> Pathology of the entering/exiting of Qi in the orifices
> Pathology of the entering/exiting of Qi in the Essence
> Pathology of the entering/exiting of Qi in the Mind
> Pathology of the entering/exiting of Qi in the Membranes
> Pathology of the entering/exiting of Qi in the Fat Tissue

The 'Qi Mechanism' (*Qi Ji*) is the complex of all movements of Qi, in every organ and in every part of the body. In particular, the Qi Mechanism consists of the ascending/descending and entering/exiting of Qi (see ch. 4). As was discussed in chapter 4, the harmonious ascending/descending and entering/exiting of Qi is essential for the movement and transformation of Qi in every part of the body and at every stage of the process leading to the making of Qi and Blood; such movements are essential also for the metabolism of body fluids.

The Qi Mechanism relies on four fundamental movements of Qi (see Fig. 4.7 in ch. 4):

> 1. Ascending (a Yang movement)
> 2. Descending (a Yin movement)
> 3. Exiting (a Yang movement)
> 4. Entering (a Yin movement)

In pathology, excessive ascending or exiting represents a pathology of Yang (not an 'Excess' of Yang but an excessive Yang *movement*), while excessive descending or entering represents a pathology of Yin (not an 'Excess' of Yin but an excessive Yin *movement*). A derangement of the ascending/descending and entering/exiting of Qi has important repercussions in every organ and every pathological process.

- Excessive ascending or exiting: Yang pathology
- Excessive descending or entering: Yin pathology

Chapter 68 of the 'Simple Questions' says: '*If there is no ascending/descending, there is no birth, growth, maturation and decline. If there is no entering/exiting, there is no birth, growth, transformation, receiving and storage. If the Qi Mechanism functions well there is room for birth and transformation; if the Qi Mechanism is disrupted, there is fragmentation and no birth or transformation.*'[1]

The 'Notes on Reading Medical Books' (Du Yi Sui Bi, 1891) by Zhou Xue Hai says: '*The faculties of seeing, hearing, smelling, tasting and thinking all depend on the smooth ascending/descending and entering/exiting of Qi; if

Qi is obstructed [in its ascending/descending and entering/exiting] those faculties are not normal.'[2]

'If there is no ascending/descending, there is no birth, growth, maturation and decline. If there is no entering/exiting, there is no birth, growth, transformation, receiving and storage.' ('Simple Questions', ch. 68)

In pathology, a derangement of the Qi Mechanism causes pathological changes in every organ and every part of the body and in particular in the following structures or processes:

- Internal Organs
- Channels
- Yin and Yang
- Qi and Blood
- Body Fluids
- Nutritive Qi (*Ying Qi*) and Defensive Qi (*Wei Qi*)
- Orifices and sense organs

It is important to study and understand the pathology of the ascending/descending and entering/exiting of Qi because it adds another dimension beyond that of Full–Empty and Yin–Yang. In fact, some of the pathologies of the ascending/descending and entering/exiting of Qi escape a definition in terms of Fullness–Emptiness, Heat–Cold or Yin–Yang. The pathology of Liver-Yang rising is a good example of this. In Liver-Yang rising, the Qi of the Liver is rising excessively, causing headaches and dizziness. How should we classify this pathology in terms of Full–Empty, Heat–Cold and Yin–Yang? It is neither Full nor Empty as it is simply a derangement of the movement of Qi; it is neither Hot nor Cold (there are a few, mild symptoms of heat with Liver-Yang but it is *not* Full-Heat in the same way as Liver-Fire); for the same reason, it is not a pathology of Excess of Yang; neither is it a pathology of Empty-Heat. How to classify and, more importantly, how to understand then the pathology of Liver-Yang rising? It is simply a pathology of the Qi Mechanism and, more specifically, of the ascending/descending of QI: that is, Liver-Qi is rising too much (also called 'rebelling upwards'). The key words in the pathology of the Qi Mechanism are not 'Deficiency' or 'Excess' but rather 'derangement', 'disruption', 'counterflow' and 'obstruction' of Qi.

Let us now discuss the pathology of the ascending/descending and entering/exiting of Qi. Although the pathology of ascending/descending and entering/exiting of Qi are discussed separately, it is important to understand that the two processes are interrelated and influence each other.

The 'Notes on Reading Medical Books' (*Du Yi Sui Bi*, 1891) by Zhou Xue Hai says: '*Without ascending/descending there is no entering/exiting; without entering/exiting there is no ascending/descending. The ascending/descending and entering/exiting of Qi mutually influence each other.*'[3]

Generally speaking, in internal diseases, there is more of a disruption of the ascending/descending of Qi, while in external diseases there is more of a disruption of the entering/exiting of Qi. For example, Liver-Yang rising, an internal disease, is characterized by a derangement of the ascending/descending of Qi; in contrast, an invasion of external Wind in the Exterior (an exterior disease) is characterized by a disruption of the entering/exiting of Qi.

Box 29.1 summarizes the general pathology of the Qi Mechanism.

Box 29.1 Pathology of Qi Mechanism

- The Qi Mechanism relies on the four movements of ascending, descending, entering and exiting
- The Qi Mechanism influences the fluid metabolism
- Ascending and exiting are Yang movements; descending and entering are Yin movements
- A derangement of the Qi Mechanism affects every organ, every process and every part of the body
- A pathology of the ascending/descending and entering/exiting movements escapes definition in terms of Full–Empty or Heat–Cold
- Key words in Qi Mechanism pathology are 'obstruction', 'disruption', 'counterflow' and 'derangement'

PATHOLOGY OF THE ASCENDING/DESCENDING OF QI

In certain physiological processes Qi needs to ascend, in others to descend: this applies to every organ and every part of the body. For example, Spleen-Qi ascends while Stomach-Qi descends (the movement of Qi for each organ is discussed in ch. 3). Ascending is a Yang movement, while descending is a Yin one. For example, the ascending of Spleen-Qi is Yang and, in fact, the Qi of the Spleen fails to ascend when Spleen-Yang of Spleen-Qi is deficient.

What causes the disruption of the ascending/descending of Qi? The two most common causes are emotional and dietary. Indeed, the very first effect of all emotions is to disrupt the movement of Qi; for example, worry knots Qi, fear makes Qi descend, while anger makes it rise. We could therefore say that the very first effect of each emotion is to disrupt the ascending/descending of Qi. For example, anger makes Liver-Qi rise, while fear makes Kidney-Qi descend.

The main dietary causes of a disruption of the ascending/descending of Qi lie in eating habits rather than in what one eats. For example, eating too fast or working immediately after eating make Qi ascend.

I shall discuss the pathology of the ascending/descending of Qi in three main areas:

- Organs
- Channels
- Orifices and sense organs

Pathology of ascending/descending of Qi in the Internal Organs

The proper ascending/descending of Qi in the Internal Organs is essential for their proper functioning and for the transformation of Qi that leads to the production of Qi and Blood. Each Internal Organ's Qi flows in a certain proper direction ('proper' being the translation of the Chinese term *shun*, which means 'in the same direction as' but which also conveys Confucian ideas of 'conforming' and 'obeying'). The proper directions of flow of Qi in each organ are as follows:

- Spleen-Qi ascends
- Stomach-Qi descends
- Lung-Qi descends (but in one respect it ascends)
- Heart-Qi descends
- Liver-Qi ascends and extends in all directions
- Kidney-Qi descends (but in certain respects it also ascends)
- Bladder, Small and Large Intestine Qi all descend

As already discussed in chapter 4, the Stomach and Spleen are at the centre of the crossroads of Qi and their descending and ascending, respectively, is crucial to regulate the whole Qi Mechanism.

The 'improper' direction of Qi is called '*ni*' in Chinese, which means 'rebellious' or 'counterflow' (again, 'rebellious' conjures up Confucian ideas of lack of conformity and lack of obeying). I shall call the counterflow direction of Qi 'rebellious Qi'.

Let us now describe the pathology of rebellious Qi in each organ.

Spleen

The Spleen sends Qi upwards (to Lungs and Heart) and its Food-Qi (*Gu Qi*) to the Lungs to combine with air to generate Gathering Qi (*Zong Qi*) (Fig. 29.1; see also Fig. 3.18 in ch. 3).

When Spleen-Qi descends instead of ascending, it cannot ascend to the chest and the Lungs to carry Food-Qi and therefore the whole production of Qi is disrupted and this may result in Qi deficiency. Moreover, when Spleen-Qi descends, it may cause loose stools or prolapse of the organs.

> **Clinical note**
>
> Ren-12 Zhongwan and Du-20 Baihui stimulate the ascending of Spleen-Qi

Stomach

The Stomach sends impure Qi downwards towards the Intestines (Fig. 29.2; see also Fig. 3.18 in ch. 3). When Stomach-Qi ascends instead of descending, it causes hiccups, nausea, vomiting and belching. As the Stomach carries Food essences to the whole body and the limbs especially, the ascending of Stomach-Qi also

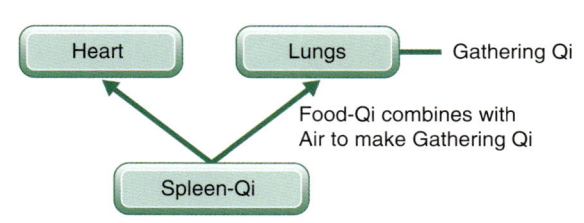

Figure 29.1 Ascending of Spleen-Qi

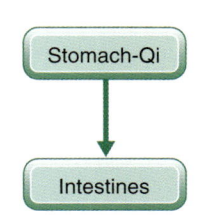

Figure 29.2 Descending of Stomach-Qi

disrupts the production of Qi and Blood and may result in Qi deficiency.

> **Clinical note**
>
> Ren-10 Xiawan stimulates the descending of Stomach-Qi

Lungs

The Lungs are the uppermost organ and their Qi therefore naturally descends. Lung-Qi descends towards the Kidneys: when Lung-Qi descends, breathing is normal. Lung-Qi also descends to communicate with the Bladder (Fig. 29.3; see also Fig. 3.13 in ch. 3).

In pathology, if Lung-Qi ascends instead of descending, it may cause cough, breathlessness and occasionally, especially in the elderly, urinary retention (see Fig. 3.13).

In one respect, Lung-Qi ascends to carry Defensive Qi (*Wei Qi*) to the space between skin and muscles: this is called the diffusing of Lung-Qi. In pathology, if Lung-Qi fails to ascend towards the space between skin and muscles, Defensive Qi becomes deficient and the space between the skin and muscles becomes too 'open': this will make the person prone to invasion of external pathogenic factors.

> **Clinical note**
>
> LU-7 Lieque stimulates the descending of Lung-Qi

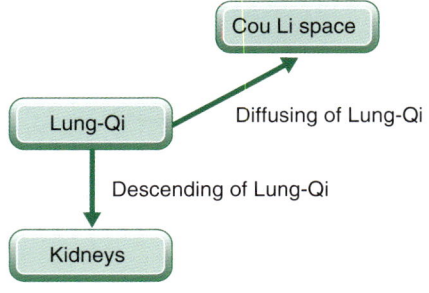

Figure 29.3 Descending and diffusing of Lung-Qi

Heart

In health, Heart-Qi descends towards the Kidneys (Fig. 29.4; see also Fig. 3.19 in ch. 3). If Heart-Qi ascends instead of descending, it affects the Mind, causing anxiety, mental restlessness and insomnia. The ascending of Heart-Qi may also cause nausea.

The descending of Heart-Qi and Heart-Blood is also important to promote the transformation of Yang to Yin and the discharge of blood at the beginning of the period, and that of Yin to Yang and the discharge of eggs at ovulation. A failure of Heart-Qi and Heart-Blood to descend may cause menstrual irregularities.

> **Clinical note**
>
> HE-5 Tongli stimulates the descending of Heart-Qi

Liver

In health, Liver-Qi ascends towards the Heart and Lungs and the eyes. This ascending movement of Liver-Qi is coordinated with the descending of Lung-Qi. Besides this, Liver-Qi extends in all directions, assisting Internal Organs in channelling their Qi in the proper direction. For example, Liver-Qi facilitates the ascending of Spleen-Qi and descending of Stomach-Qi (Fig. 29.5; see also Fig. 3.14 in ch. 3).

In pathology, Liver-Qi can fail to ascend towards the Heart and this would have primarily mental–emotional repercussions, making the person depressed and aimless. It will be remembered that the Ethereal Soul (*Hun*, housed in the Liver) 'comes and goes', giving the

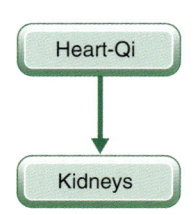

Figure 29.4 Descending of Heart-Qi

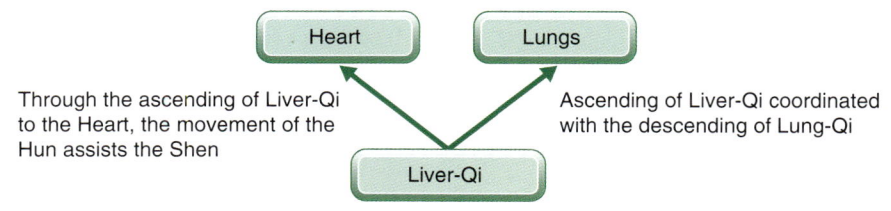

Figure 29.5 Ascending of Liver-Qi

Mind (*Shen*, housed in the Heart) the capacity for relationships, and for projecting outwards: this influences a person's capacity for planning and for having ideas, plans, inspiration, etc. Therefore when Liver-Qi fails to ascend, the Ethereal Soul does not 'come and go' enough and the person is depressed. On a physical level, when Liver-Qi fails to ascend to the eyes, clear Qi does not reach this sense orifice and the person has blurred vision.

Conversely, in pathology, Liver-Qi could ascend too much, causing what is called 'Liver-Yang rising': this causes irritability, propensity to outbursts of anger, headache and dizziness. On a mental–emotional level, when Liver-Qi ascends too much (and especially with Liver-Fire), the Ethereal Soul will 'come and go' too much, giving the Mind excessive 'movement': this will result in slightly manic behaviour.

The physiological ascending of Liver-Qi is coordinated with the descending of Lung-Qi. Energetically (though obviously not anatomically) the Liver is on the left side and its Qi ascends, and the Lungs are on the right side and their Qi descends. The ascending of Liver-Qi and descending of Lung-Qi mutually influence each other and depend on each other.

Clinical note

- G.B.-40 Qiuxu stimulates the physiological ascending of Liver-Qi
- LIV-3 Taichong subdues rebellious Liver-Qi

Kidneys

Kidney-Qi descends to the Bladder to promote urination (Fig. 29.6; see also Fig. 3.16 in ch. 3). In pathology, if Kidney-Qi fails to descend towards the Bladder, there may be urinary retention. When Kidney-Qi fails to descend, it cannot 'grasp' Lung-Qi and this may cause breathlessness.

In other respects, the Kidneys have an ascending movement in so far as Kidney-Yang vaporizes the fluids and sends them up to the Lungs. If Kidney-Qi fails to ascend in this respect, the Lungs will suffer from dryness and the person will experience a dry cough.

Clinical note

Ren-4 Guanyuan stimulates the descending of Kidney-Qi

Bladder

The Qi of the Bladder descends to promote the excretion of urine. If the Qi of the Bladder fails to descend, there will be urinary retention.

Small Intestine

The Qi of the Small Intestine descends to promote the movement of the products of digestion towards the Large Intestine and the fluids towards the Bladder. If the Qi of the Small Intestine fails to descend, there will be abdominal distension and pain.

Large Intestine

The Qi of the Large Intestine descends to promote the excretion of stools. If the Qi of the Large Intestine fails to descend, there will be constipation and abdominal distension.

Pathology of ascending/descending of Qi in the channels

The proper ascending/descending of Qi in the channels is extremely important to regulate the movement of Qi in the whole body, outside the Internal Organs.

As we have seen, the ascending/descending of Qi in the Internal Organs is disrupted primarily from emotional stress and irregular eating. How is the ascending/descending of Qi in the channels disrupted? This occurs mostly as a result either of invasion of external pathogenic factors in the channels or of local stagnation in the channels from a trauma or repetitive strain.

For example, if a channel is invaded by external Cold or Dampness, this will create a local stagnation in a joint and it will prevent the normal ascending/descending of Qi in that channel. When the normal upwards and downwards circulation of Qi in a channel is obstructed, pain results. Thus the pain is due to the disruption of the ascending/descending of Qi in that channel (Fig. 29.7).

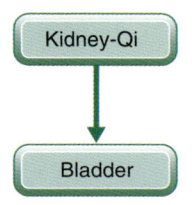

Figure 29.6 Descending of Kidney-Qi

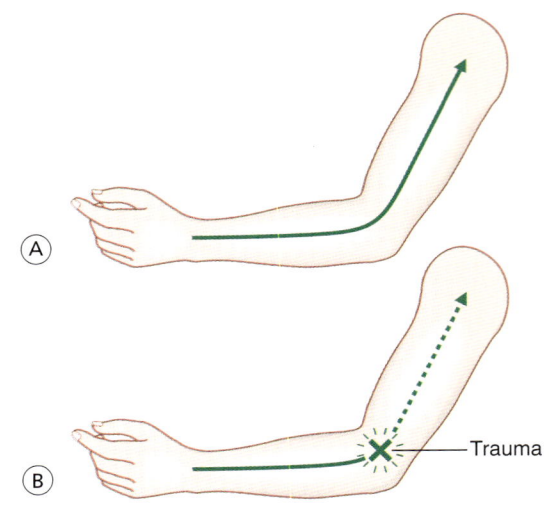

Figure 29.7 Disruption of ascending/descending of Qi in a channel

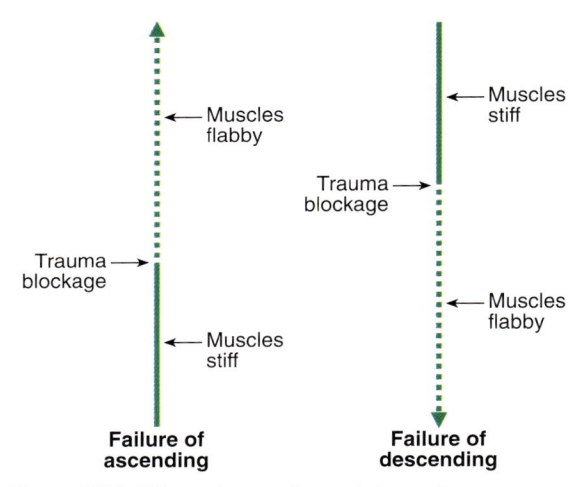

Figure 29.8 Failure of ascending and descending

Generally speaking, if Qi fails to ascend in a channel from a particular area that has been subjected to trauma or repetitive strain, the muscles below that area will feel stiff while those above the area will feel flabby. Similarly, if Qi fails to descend in a channel from a particular area that has been subjected to trauma or repetitive strain, the muscles above that area will feel stiff while those below the area will feel flabby (Fig. 29.8).

Every channel has a proper ascending or descending movement of Qi: for example, in the arm, the Qi of the Yang channels ascends towards the head, while that of the Yin channels descends from the chest towards the hands in the following scheme:

- Arm Yang channels ascend from the fingertips to the head
- Arm Yin channels descend from the chest to the fingertips
- Leg Yang channels descend from the head to the toes
- Leg Yin channels ascend from the toes to the chest

Therefore it follows that the ascending/descending of Qi in the channels can be disrupted in the following ways:

- Yang channels of arm: failing to ascend properly
- Yin channels of arm: failing to descend properly
- Yang channels of leg: failing to descend properly
- Yin channels of leg: failing to ascend properly

I will give an example from each of the above groups. If a person suffers a repetitive strain of the elbow (perhaps from playing tennis) in the Large Intestine channel, this will prevent the Qi of the Large Intestine from ascending properly and pain in the elbow will result. On careful palpation, and if the condition is long-lasting, one will probably find that the muscles below the elbow will feel stiff while those above will feel flabby.

If a person suffers from a repetitive strain or trauma in the pectoral muscle on the Lung channel, this will prevent the Qi of the Lung channel from descending towards the hand. This will create a local stagnation in the pectoral muscle and therefore pain.

If a person suffers from a trauma or repetitive strain in the thigh muscle along the Stomach channel, the Qi of the Stomach channel will fail to descend properly: this will create a local stagnation and therefore pain. On careful palpation, and if the condition is long-lasting, one will probably find that the muscles above the stagnation area on the thigh will feel stiff while those below will feel flabby.

If a person suffers from a trauma or repetitive strain in the calf muscle along the Spleen channel, the Qi of the Spleen channel will fail to ascend properly: this will create a local stagnation and therefore pain. On careful palpation, and if the condition is long-lasting, one will probably find that the muscles below the stagnation area on the calf will feel stiff while those above will feel flabby.

Therefore, we can say that in every channel problem (i.e. a local problem not involving the Internal Organs) caused by trauma or invasion of external pathogenic factors, there is a disruption of the ascending/descending of Qi which causes local stagnation and therefore pain.

Pathology of ascending/descending of Qi in orifices and sense organs

The ascending/descending of Qi is crucial to bring Qi to the orifices: this 'brightens' them and enables our sense organs of sight, hearing, smell and taste. Please bear in mind that the Mind is, in this respect, also considered an 'orifice' of the Heart and therefore the ascending/descending of Qi is crucial also for normal brain functioning.

It is worth repeating here the passage from the 'Notes on Reading Medical Books' mentioned above: *'The faculties of seeing, hearing, smelling, tasting and thinking all depend on the smooth ascending/descending and entering/exiting of Qi; if Qi is obstructed [in its ascending/descending and entering/exiting] those faculties are not normal.'*[4] This clearly states that the ascending/descending of Qi is crucial to the normal functioning of the sense organs and of the brain. Chapter 5 of the 'Simple Questions' says: *'The clear Yang ascends to the upper orifices; turbid Yin descends from the lower orifices.'*[5]

The upper orifices (eyes, nose, ears, mouth and Mind) rely on the ascending of Qi to bring clear Yang upwards: this 'brightens' the orifices and enables the relevant sense organs (Fig. 29.9). Just as the ascending of clear Qi is important, the descending of turbid Qi is equally important. Indeed, sometimes the problem in the pathology of these sense organs is not so much that the clear Qi is not ascending as that the turbid Qi is not descending.

In fact, the pathology and clinical manifestations due to the failure of Qi to ascend to the upper orifices are not the same as those due to the failure of Qi to descend: in the former case, clear Qi fails to ascend to brighten the orifices, in the latter turbid Qi fails to descend from the orifices.

Table 29.1 presents the clinical manifestations due to the failure of ascending or descending of Qi in each upper orifice.

The lower orifices (urethra and anus) rely on the descending of (turbid) Qi for a normal excretion of urine and stools. In pathology, the failure of the descending of Qi will cause urinary retention or constipation (Fig. 29.10).

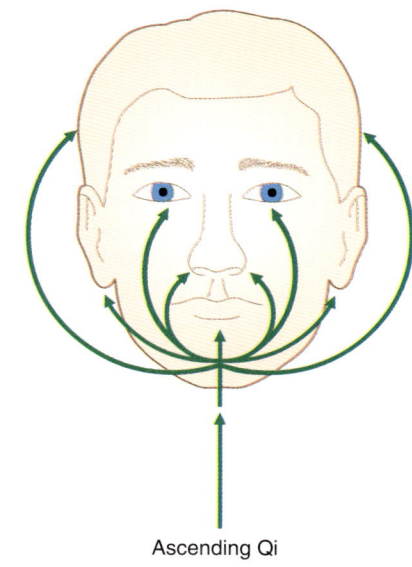

Figure 29.9 Qi ascending to the upper orifices

Table 29.1 Clinical manifestations of failure of ascending or descending of Qi in the upper orifices

	Qi not ascending	Qi not descending
Eyes	Blurred vision	Sticky eyes, pain in eyes
Ears	Hardness or hearing	Excessive wax production
Nose	Diminished or absent sense of smell	Blocked nose, runny nose
Mouth	Lack of taste sensation	Sticky taste
Mind	Thinking not clear, muzziness, poor memory	A feeling of heaviness, muzziness and dizziness of the head

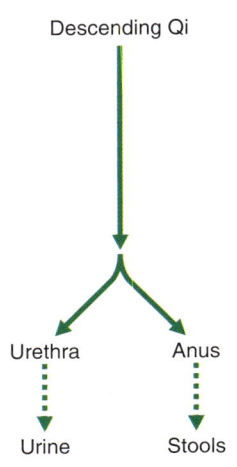

Figure 29.10 Qi descending to the lower orifices

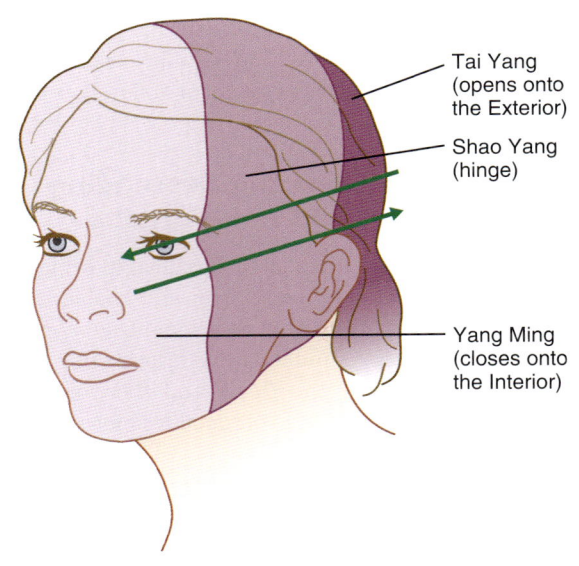

Figure 29.11 Yang channels of the face

PATHOLOGY OF THE ENTERING/EXITING OF QI

The entering/exiting of Qi is the second aspect of the Qi Mechanism. The ascending/descending of Qi provides a vertical dimension to the Qi Mechanism while the entering/exiting of Qi provides a horizontal dimension (see Fig. 3.12 in ch. 3). The entering/exiting of Qi is an essential process of the Qi Mechanism that takes place in every organ, every tissue and every part of the body. As we shall see, the entering/exiting of Qi is particularly important for the movement, transformation and excretion of fluids and, therefore, in pathology, its disruption leads to Dampness, Phlegm or oedema.

The physiology of the entering/exiting of Qi was described in chapter 4. The discussion of the pathology of the entering/exiting of Qi will be under the following headings:

- Channels
- Space between skin and muscles
- Triple Burner cavities
- Organs
- Joints
- Orifices
- Essence (*Jing*)
- Mind (*Shen*)
- Membranes (*Huang*)
- Fat Tissue (*Gao*)

Pathology of the entering/exiting of Qi in the channels

As discussed in chapter 4, the entering–exiting of Qi is an important aspect of the movement among the three Yang energetic layers of Greater Yang (*Tai Yang*), Lesser Yang (*Shao Yang*) and Bright Yang (*Yang Ming*) and among the three Yin energetic layers of Greater Yin (*Tai Yin*), Terminal Yin (*Jue Yin*) and Lesser Yin (*Shao Yin*). Grouped as above, the channels are at different depths, as follows (see Fig. 4.9 in ch. 4):

	Yang	Yin
Superficial	Greater Yang	Greater Yin
'Hinge'	Lesser Yang	Terminal Yin
Deep	Bright Yang	Lesser Yin

There is a 'horizontal' movement between the three levels of channels within the Yang and within the Yin channels: for example<in the case of the Yang channels, a movement between Greater Yang, Bright Yang and Lesser Yang channels. As the Greater Yang channels are superficial and the Bright Yang ones deep (within the Yang channels), this movement of Qi is part of the entering/exiting of Qi.

A good example of such movement is on the face. The face is richly supplied by all the Yang channels, illustrated broadly in Figure 29.11 (bearing in mind that the figure illustrates only the superficial pathway of the channels and not the deep one, which is more complex). (Another example based on the channels of the shoulder is illustrated in Fig. 4.10 in ch. 4.)

On the face, as an example, there is a 'horizontal' movement of Qi (see Fig. 29.11) between the Greater Yang, Bright Yang and Lesser Yang channels that is part of the entering/exiting of Qi.

A disruption of the entering/exiting of Qi in the channels causes local stagnation and pain. Therefore, it is worth noting that local stagnation and pain may be caused by a disruption of either the ascending/descending of Qi or of the entering/exiting of Qi.

Box 29.2 summarizes the pathology of entering/exiting of Qi in the channels.

> **Box 29.2 Pathology of entering/exiting of Qi in the channels**
>
> - Three different depths within the Yang and Yin channels (Greater Yang and Greater Yin more external, Bright Yang and Lesser Yin more internal in the Yang and Yin, respectively)
> - The horizontal movement of Qi between the three energetic layers is an expression of the entering/exiting of Qi
> - A disruption of this horizontal movement creates local stagnation

Pathology of the entering/exiting of Qi in the space between the skin and muscles

The space between the skin and muscles is one of the Triple Burner cavities called *Cou Li*. I translate the term *Cou Li* as 'Spaces and Texture' (see Fig. 4.11 in ch. 4). Thus, although we usually translate the term *Cou Li* as the 'space between skin and muscles', strictly speaking such a space is only one of the *Cou Li* spaces.

The space between the skin and muscles is an energetic layer corresponding to the surface of the body, also called the 'Exterior' of the body. The physiology of this space has been discussed in chapter 4.

In pathology, excessive 'exiting' of Qi in the space between the skin and muscles implies excess Yang movement: this will make the space between the skin and muscles too 'tight', sweating is reduced and, if the patient is invaded by an external pathogenic factor, he or she will develop a high fever. Excessive 'entering' of Qi in the space between the skin and muscles implies excess of Yin movement: this will make the space between the skin and muscles too 'relaxed', Defensive Qi does not circulate well, the pores are too open and the patient will be prone to invasions of pathogenic factors (even weak ones) (Fig. 29.12).

Box 29.3 summarizes pathology of entering and exiting of Qi in the space between the skin and the muscles.

Pathology of the entering/exiting of Qi in the Triple Burner cavities

The Triple Burner has been discussed in greater detail in chapter 18 and its relation to the entering/exiting of Qi in chapter 4. The Triple Burner is a system of body cavities and 'spaces' ranging from very large ones to very small ones. All these cavities are called *Cou* (as in *Cou Li*, 'Spaces and Texture'). In particular, the Three Burners are the three large cavities of the chest (Upper Burner), the upper abdominal cavity (Middle Burner) and the lower abdominal and pelvic cavities (Lower Burner). The space between the skin and muscles is one of the Triple Burner cavities and so are the joint cavities (see Fig. 4.13 in ch. 4).

In relation to the entering/exiting of Qi in and out of the body cavities, the Triple Burner makes sure that all passages and cavities are open, and that Qi enters and exits in and out of these cavities in a balanced way. As one of the main functions of the Triple Burner is to ensure and regulate the transformation, transportation and excretion of fluids, the entering/exiting of Qi in and out of the Triple Burner cavities is essential for a proper fluid metabolism. A disruption of the entering/exiting of Qi in the Triple Burner cavities will therefore result in the formation of Dampness, Phlegm or oedema.

Box 29.4 summarizes the pathology of the entering and exiting of Qi in the Triple Burner cavities.

Pathology of the entering/exiting of Qi in the organs

The entering/exiting of Qi in the organs is the way in which the Internal Organs influence their respective tissues, That is:

> - Lungs – skin
> - Spleen – muscles
> - Liver – sinews
> - Heart – blood vessels
> - Kidneys – bones

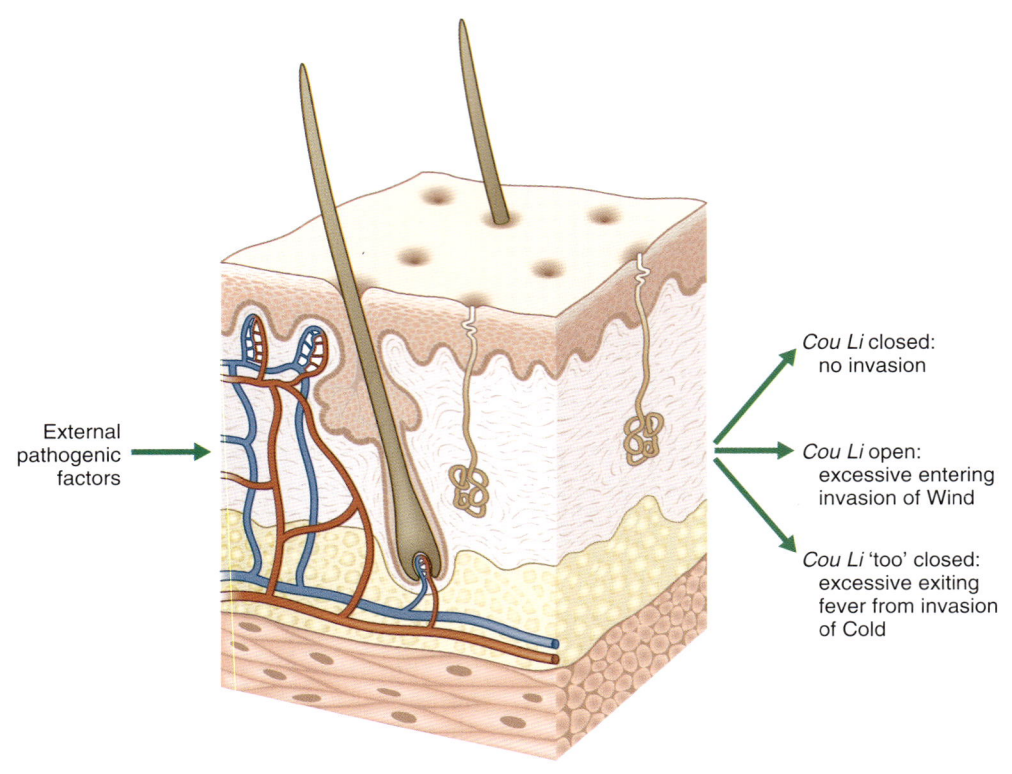

Figure 29.12 Pathology of the entering/exiting of Qi in the space between skin and muscles

Box 29.3 Pathology of entering/exiting of Qi in the space between the skin and muscles

- The space between the skin and muscles is part of the Triple Burner cavities called *Cou Li*
- The space between the skin and muscles is the 'Exterior' of the body
- Defensive Qi and sweat are in the space between the skin and muscles
- Excessive exiting of Qi makes the space between skin and muscles too 'tight'
- Excessive entering of Qi makes the space between the skin and muscles too 'open'

Box 29.4 Pathology of the entering/exiting of Qi in the Triple Burner cavities

- The Triple Burner is a system of 'cavities' (such as chest, abdominal and pelvic cavity)
- A disruption of the entering/exiting of Qi in the Triple Burner cavities causes a dysfunction of the fluids metabolism

Therefore the entering/exiting of Qi in each organ ensures the communication between each organ and its relevant tissue. In pathology, a disruption of the entering/exiting of Qi between an organ and its respective tissue leads to a pathology of the relevant tissue as illustrated in Table 29.2.

Pathology of the entering/exiting of Qi in the joints

The joint capsules are also spaces or cavities where Qi enters and from which it exits. The movement of Qi in and out of the joints is controlled primarily by whatever channels course through that joint. However, it is also influenced in general by the Liver (because it controls all sinews) and the Triple Burner (because it controls all cavities). The entering/exiting of Qi in a joint is illustrated in Figure 4.13 in chapter 4.

Table 29.2 Pathology of the entering/exiting of Qi between each organ and its relevant tissue

Organ	Tissue	Excessive exiting	Excessive exiting
Lungs	Skin	Space between skin and muscles too tight	Space between skin and muscles too lax
Spleen	Muscles	Muscles stiff	Muscles flaccid
Liver	Sinews	Contraction of sinews, cramps	Sinews too soft, prone to injury
Heart	Blood vessels	Hardening of vessels	Slackness of vessels (e.g. varicose veins)
Kidneys	Bones	Night sweating	Blood stasis

If Qi enters and exits from the joints in a balanced way, the joint will be free of pain and its movement unrestricted. In pathology, if there is excessive exiting of Qi, the joint will be rigid, painful and extension will be difficult; if there is excessive entering of Qi, the joint will be weak, achy and adduction will be difficult.

Box 29.5 summarizes the pathology of the entering and exiting of Qi in the joints.

> **Box 29.5 Pathology of the entering/exiting of Qi in the joints**
>
> - The joints are cavities pertaining to the Triple Burner
> - Qi enters and exits from joint cavities ensuring health of joints
> - Excessive exiting of Qi in joints will cause rigidity; excessive entering will cause weakness

Pathology of the entering/exiting of Qi in the orifices

The entering/exiting of Qi is very important for the health of the orifices and relevant sense organs. As we have seen above, the ascending/descending of Qi is important for the health of the orifices as the ascending of Qi ensures that clear Yang reaches the upper orifices. The entering/exiting of Qi affects the orifices and in particular the sense organs as it ensures that Qi flows in and out of the sense organs, thus allowing proper sensations of sight, hearing, smell and taste. In other words, the ascending of clear Qi to the upper orifices is the necessary precondition for a proper functioning of the senses, but the proper entering/exiting of Qi in and out of the orifices is the way in which the sense organs communicate with the external world in seeing, hearing, smelling and tasting.

In pathology, a disruption of the entering/exiting of Qi in the orifices will affect the relevant sense organs.

Table 29.3 Pathology of entering/exiting of Qi in the orifices

Orifice	Excessive exiting	Excessive entering
Eyes	Red, painful	Blurred vision
Ears	Ear discharge, pain	Tinnitus
Nose	Nasal discharge, blocked nose	Runny nose with profuse, watery discharge
Mouth	Sticky taste	Lack of taste sensation

> **Box 29.6 Pathology of entering/exiting of Qi in the orifices**
>
> - The entering/exiting of Qi in the orifices ensures health of sense organs
> - Disruption of the entering/exiting of Qi in the orifices will diminish acuity of sense organs

The clinical manifestations of such a disruption are listed in Table 29.3. Box 29.6 summarizes the pathology of entering/exiting of Qi in the orifices.

Pathology of the entering/exiting of Qi in the Essence

The Corporeal Soul (*Po*) is often described as the 'the entering and exiting of the Essence' (*Jing*). This 'entering and exiting' of the Corporeal Soul is another aspect of the general entering/exiting of Qi.

The Corporeal Soul (*Po*) is the 'entering and exiting of the Essence'.

In pathology, a disruption of the entering/exiting of Qi in relation to the Essence affects the way in which the Essence promotes and participates in various physiological activities. This will manifest primarily in the area of resistance to pathogenic factors and in the sexual area.

In the area of resistance to pathogenic factors, excessive exiting of the Corporeal Soul in relation to the Essence causes an over-reaction of the Upright Qi to external pathogenic factors: this is often seen in allergic diseases such as allergic asthma and allergic rhinitis. Excessive entering of the Corporeal Soul in the relation to the Essence will cause a lack of reaction of the Upright Qi to external pathogenic factors: this will make the person prone to invasion of external pathogenic factors.

In the sexual area, excessive exiting of the Corporeal Soul in relation to the Essence causes excessive sexual desire, while excessive entering will cause lack of sexual desire or, in men, impotence.

Box 29.7 summarizes pathology of the entering and exiting of Qi in the Essence.

> **Box 29.7 Pathology of the entering/exiting of Qi in the Essence**
> - The Corporeal Soul is the 'entering and exiting' of the Essence
> - A disruption of the entering and exiting of the Corporeal Soul affects the Essence
> - Excessive exiting of the Corporeal Soul may cause allergic reactions or excessive sexual desire
> - Excessive entering of the Corporeal Soul may cause propensity to colds or impotence

Pathology of the entering/exiting of Qi in the Mind (*Shen*)

As discussed in chapter 4, the entering and exiting of Qi in and out of the Mind must be seen in the context of the coordination between the Mind of the Heart and the Ethereal Soul (*Hun*) of the Liver. The Ethereal Soul is sometimes defined as the 'coming and going of the Mind': that is, it is always searching, dreaming (in terms of life dreams), exploring, making plans and being inspired. Hence, on a psychic level, this constitutes the 'entering and exiting of Qi' (i.e. the 'coming and going') in and out of the Mind.

The Ethereal Soul (*Hun*) is the 'coming and going' (i.e. exiting/entering) of the Mind (*Shen*)

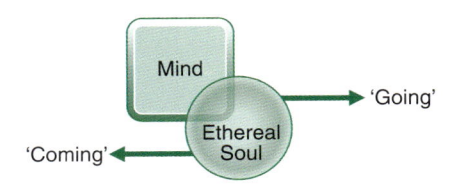

Figure 29.13 Pathology of the entering/exiting of Qi between the Mind and the Ethereal Soul

In pathology, if there is excessive 'exiting of Qi' (i.e. 'going'), the Ethereal Soul's natural movement is out of control (which could occur because the control and integration of the Mind is insufficient), the person has too many life dreams, too many projects that often do not come to fruition and too many ideas that often result in chaos; in serious cases, it may turn into manic behaviour. If there is excessive 'entering of Qi' ('coming'), the Ethereal Soul's natural movement is defective (which could occur because the control of the Mind is too rigid), the person will tend to be depressed, to be confused about life's direction, and to lack vision, aims, life dreams and inspiration (Fig. 29.13).

> **Clinical note**
>
> G.B.-40 Qiuxu can stimulate the 'going' of the Ethereal Soul and LIV-3 Taichong the 'coming' of it (i.e. restrain its movement)

Box 29.8 summarizes the pathology of the entering and exiting of Qi in the Mind.

> **Box 29.8 Pathology of the entering/exiting of Qi in the Mind**
> - The Ethereal Soul is the 'coming and going' of the Mind
> - 'Coming and going' is a form of entering/exiting
> - Excessive exiting of the Ethereal Soul may cause a rather chaotic state of the Mind
> - Excessive entering of the Ethereal Soul may cause depression

Pathology of the entering/exiting of Qi in the Membranes (*Huang*)

As discussed in chapter 4, '*Huang*' literally means 'membranes' and it refers to membranes which cover the whole body with a superficial layer below the skin and an inner layer. Membranes have the function of *wrapping* and *anchoring* the organs, muscles and bones and of *connecting* the organs among themselves.

Membranes are found only in the abdomen and they broadly correspond to the fascia (superficial and deep), the peritoneum, mesenterium and omentum. The stroma (i.e. the framework of connective tissue or organs) is also an example of Membranes.

Proper entering and exiting of Qi in and out of the Membranes ensures a smooth circulation of Qi in the abdomen and also a smooth metabolism of fluids.

In pathology, if there is excessive exiting of Qi, there will be stagnation of Qi in the Membranes, resulting in abdominal distension and pain; if there is excessive entering of Qi, there will be a deficiency and possibly sinking of Qi with a slackening of the Membranes and possibly oedema.

The pathology of rebellious Qi in the Penetrating Vessel (*Chong Mai*) is a disruption of the entering and exiting of Qi in and out of the Membranes of the abdomen (see ch. 53).

Box 29.9 summarizes the pathology of the entering and exiting of Qi in the Membranes.

Box 29.9 Pathology of the entering/exiting of Qi in the Membranes

- The Membranes (*Huang*) are the fascia, peritoneum, mesenterium, omentum and stroma
- The entering/exiting of Qi in the Membranes ensures smooth movement of Qi in the abdomen and contributes to a healthy fluid metabolism
- Excessive exiting of Qi in the Membranes will cause Qi stagnation in the abdomen
- Excessive entering of Qi in the Membranes will cause slackening of abdominal muscles and oedema

Pathology of the entering/exiting of Qi in the Fat Tissue (*Gao*)

Fat Tissue is called *Gao* in Chinese. It broadly corresponds to adipose tissue in Western medicine, but it has a slightly different meaning. While from a Western perspective adipose tissue is distributed all over the body, Fat Tissue (*Gao*) in Chinese medicine refers primarily to the adipose tissue in the abdomen (in both men and women) and breasts in women and it also includes the peritoneal membranes that encapsulate the organs (the peritoneal membranes are connective, not adipose, tissue).

The entering and exiting of Qi in and out of the Fat Tissue relies primarily on the Spleen; a balanced entering and exiting of Qi in and out of the Fat Tissue will result in normal tissues.

In pathology, excessive entering of Qi may result in the accumulation of fat and obesity, while excessive exiting of Qi may result in loss of weight.

Box 29.10 summarizes the pathology of the entering and exiting of Qi in the Fat Tissue.

Box 29.10 Pathology of the entering/exiting of Qi in the Fat Tissue

- Fat Tissue (*Gao*) broadly corresponds to adipose tissue in the abdomen and breasts
- Excessive exiting of Qi in the Fat Tissue may cause obesity, while excessive entering may cause loss of weight

Learning outcomes

In this chapter you will have learned:
- The importance of understanding the pathology of ascending/descending and entering/exiting of Qi, in addition to Full/Empty, Heat/Cold and Yin–Yang
- Why excessive ascending or exiting of Qi is a Yang pathology, while excessive descending or entering is a Yin pathology
- How some pathologies of ascending/descending or entering/exiting escape definition in terms of Full–Empty or Heat–Cold
- The main causes of disruption of the ascending/descending of Qi
- The various pathologies of ascending/descending of Qi in the Internal Organs, channels, orifices and sense organs
- The pathology of the entering/exiting of Qi in the channels, particularly the 'horizontal' movement between the three energetic layers of the Yang and Yin channels
- How excessive entering or exiting of Qi in the space between the skin and muscles can cause this cavity to become to 'tight' or too 'open'
- How a disruption of entering/exiting of Qi in the Triple Burner cavities results in improper fluid metabolism and the formation of Dampness, Phlegm or oedema
- The pathology of entering/exiting of Qi in the organs, and how this affects their respective tissues
- How excessive entering or exiting of Qi in the joints affects the health of the joint
- The importance of correct entering/exiting of Qi in the orifices to ensure proper functioning of the sense organs
- The results of a disruption of the entering/exiting of the Corporeal Soul in relation to the Essence, particularly in the resistance to pathogenic factors and sexual function
- The role of the Ethereal Soul in the 'coming and going' (entering/exiting) of the Mind, and problems which result from a derangement of this process
- The pathology of excessive entering/exiting of Qi in and out of the Membranes and the Fat Tissue

Self-assessment questions

1. Complete the following sentence: 'The key words in the pathology of the Qi Mechanism are not 'Deficiency' or 'Excess' but rather '_____,' '_____' and '_____' of Qi.
2. What are the two most common causes of disruption of ascending/descending of Qi?
3. In which direction does the Stomach send its Qi? Give three symptoms which might arise if Stomach-Qi should counterflow.
4. What might be the psychological symptoms of Liver-Qi failing to ascend?
5. What might you expect to feel on palpation of the arm of a person who has strained their elbow, preventing the Qi of the Large Intestine channel from ascending properly?
6. How does the ascending of Qi affect the upper orifices?
7. What would be the result of excessive 'entering' of Qi in the space between the skin and muscles?
8. Why does a dysfunction of the entering/exiting of Qi of the Triple Burner cavities result in the formation of Dampness, Phlegm or oedema?
9. How does excessive entering/exiting of the Corporeal Soul affect sexual function?
10. How would excessive exiting of Qi affect the Membranes in the abdomen?

See p. 1262 for answers

END NOTES

1. 1979 The Yellow Emperor's Classic of Internal Medicine – Simple Questions (*Huang Di Nei Jing Su Wen* 黄帝内经素问), People's Health Publishing House, Beijing, first published *c.*100 BC, p. 173–174.
2. Cited in Wang Xue Tai 1988 Great Treatise of Chinese Acupuncture (*Zhong Guo Zhen Jiu Da Quan* 中国针灸大全), Henan Science Publishing House, p. 162.
3. Ibid., p. 163.
4. Ibid., p. 162.
5. Simple Questions, p. 32.

PART 6

Identification of patterns

The discussion of identification of patterns will be based on the following topics:

- Introduction
- Concept of 'pattern'
- Concept of 'disease' in Chinese medicine
- The relationship between diseases and patterns
- The concept of 'disease' in Chinese medicine compared to diseases in Western medicine
- Characteristics of 'symptoms' in Chinese medicine
- Identifying patterns
- Methods of identification of patterns

INTRODUCTION

'Identification of patterns' (*bian zheng* in Chinese) indicates the process of identifying the basic disharmony that underlies all clinical manifestations. This is the essence of Chinese medical diagnosis and pathology. Identifying a pattern involves discerning the underlying pattern of disharmony by considering the picture formed by all symptoms and signs.

Rather than analyzing symptoms and signs one by one in trying to find a cause for them, as Western medicine does, Chinese medicine forms an overall picture taking all symptoms and signs into consideration to identify the underlying disharmony (Box P6.1). In this respect, Chinese medicine does not look primarily for causes but patterns. Thus, when we say that a certain patient presents the pattern of deficient Kidney-Yin, this is not the cause of the disease (which has to be looked for in the person's life), but the disharmony underlying the disease or the way the condition presents itself. Of course, in other respects, after identifying the pattern, Chinese medicine does go a step further in trying to identify a cause for the disharmony.

CONCEPT OF 'PATTERN'

Therefore the '*pattern*' (also called 'syndrome') is a picture formed by the clinical manifestations of the patient which point to the character, the site and the pathology of the condition. The art of the identification of pattern lies in seeing the picture formed by the clinical manifestations of the patient: this is done using the tools described in Part 4 on Diagnosis (Fig. P6.1).

For example, if a patient complains of poor appetite, loose stools, tiredness, weak voice, propensity to catching colds and dislike to speak, we can identify here two patterns. The first (manifesting the first three symptoms) is Spleen-Qi deficiency and the other Lung-Qi deficiency. By defining the patterns as such we are identifying the pathology (Qi deficiency) and the site of the disease (the Spleen and Lungs).

CONCEPT OF 'DISEASE' IN CHINESE MEDICINE

The concept of '*disease*' is different in Chinese medicine than in Western medicine. In Chinese medicine, a 'disease' is actually a 'symptom' in Western medicine. For example, in gynaecology, 'Painful Periods' is a disease category, whereas in Western medicine, it is a symptom (and Western medicine would attempt to find a 'disease', such as endometriosis, causing the symptom of 'painful periods') (Fig. P6.2). Other examples of 'diseases' in Chinese medicine are Diarrhoea, Constipation, Cough, Breathlessness, Dizziness, Headaches, Epigastric Pain, Abdominal Pain, etc. As can be seen these are all symptoms rather than 'diseases' in Western medicine.

> **Box P6.1 Identification of patterns**
>
> - Indicates the process of identifying the basic disharmony underlying the patient's clinical manifestations
> - Chinese medicine does not look for causes but patterns

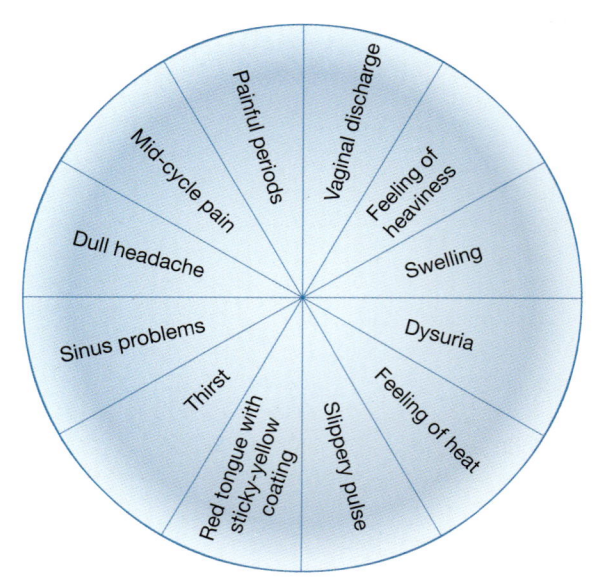

Figure P6.1 Pattern of Chinese medicine (Damp-Heat)

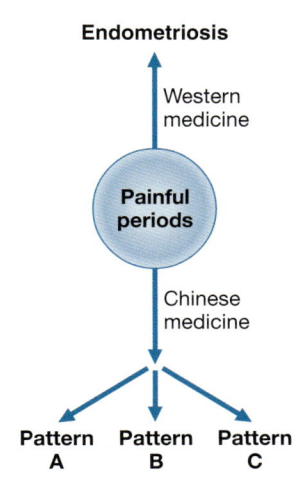

Figure P6.2 Relationship between Chinese disease and patterns

Box P6.2 Concept of 'disease' in Chinese medicine

- A 'disease' in Chinese medicine (e.g. Painful Periods) is actually a symptom in Western medicine
- The discussion of 'diseases' may be found already in the 'Yellow Emperor's Classic of Internal Medicine'

However, there is no reason why it should not be possible to apply Chinese-style pattern differentiation to Western medical diseases and indeed many modern Chinese medicine books do just that.[1] For example, the Western medical disease of 'coronary heart disease' broadly corresponds to 'Chest Painful Obstruction Syndrome' (*Chest Bi*) in Chinese medicine. If we were to examine and perform a Chinese medical diagnosis on a large enough number of patients suffering from coronary heart disease we would be able to identify the most common patterns displayed by those patients. Given the hospital structures existing for Chinese medicine in China and the large number of patients using them, modern Chinese doctors are in a position to apply Chinese pattern differentiation to Western medical diseases.

Another example that springs to mind is that of endometriosis. As the chief symptom of endometriosis is painful periods, we can treat this disease by referring to the Chinese disease 'Painful Periods'. However, if we analyze the patterns displayed by a large number of women with endometriosis, it is equally possible to make a Chinese pattern differentiation of endometriosis. Indeed, in some cases, a pattern differentiation according to a Western, rather than Chinese, medical disease can enhance our treatment. Endometriosis is a good case in point. There is a general consensus in modern China that the migration of the endometrial tissue outside the Uterus must be seen as a case of Blood stasis. If we rely purely on Chinese diagnosis and pattern identification, in many women with endometriosis we may not see signs of Blood stasis (the tongue is not Purple, the periods are not very painful, there are no abdominal masses, etc.) and therefore not apply the important treatment method of invigorating Blood.

The concept of 'disease' is very ancient in Chinese medicine and can be seen already in the 'Yellow Emperor's Classic of Internal Medicine'. For example, the 'Spiritual Axis' discusses Manic Depression (*Dian Kuang*) in chapter 22 and Painful Obstruction Syndrome (*Bi*) in chapter 27. The 'Simple Questions' discusses Cough in chapter 38 and Painful Obstruction Syndrome (*Bi*) in chapter 43.

Of course, there is some correspondence between Chinese and Western diseases. For example, the Chinese disease 'Epigastric Pain' obviously may correspond to Western digestive diseases such as gastric ulcer which presents with epigastric pain. However, there is never a direct, one-to-one correspondence between a Chinese and a Western disease. In the above example, very many people will suffer from epigastric pain without having a gastric ulcer.

Finally, in a few cases there is a direct correspondence between Chinese and Western diseases with the two entities coinciding entirely. Example of such identification between Chinese and Western diseases are epilepsy (*dian xian*), malaria (*nue ji*), dysentery (*li ji*) and measles (*ma zhen*).

Box P6.2 summarizes the concept of 'disease' in Chinese medicine.

THE RELATIONSHIP BETWEEN CHINESE MEDICINE DISEASES AND PATTERNS

It is an important and fundamental principle of Chinese medicine that the same disease may manifest with different patterns and the same pattern may give rise to many different diseases. This is summed up in the saying 'one disease, many patterns; one pattern, many

Figure P6.3 'One disease, many patterns; one pattern, many diseases'

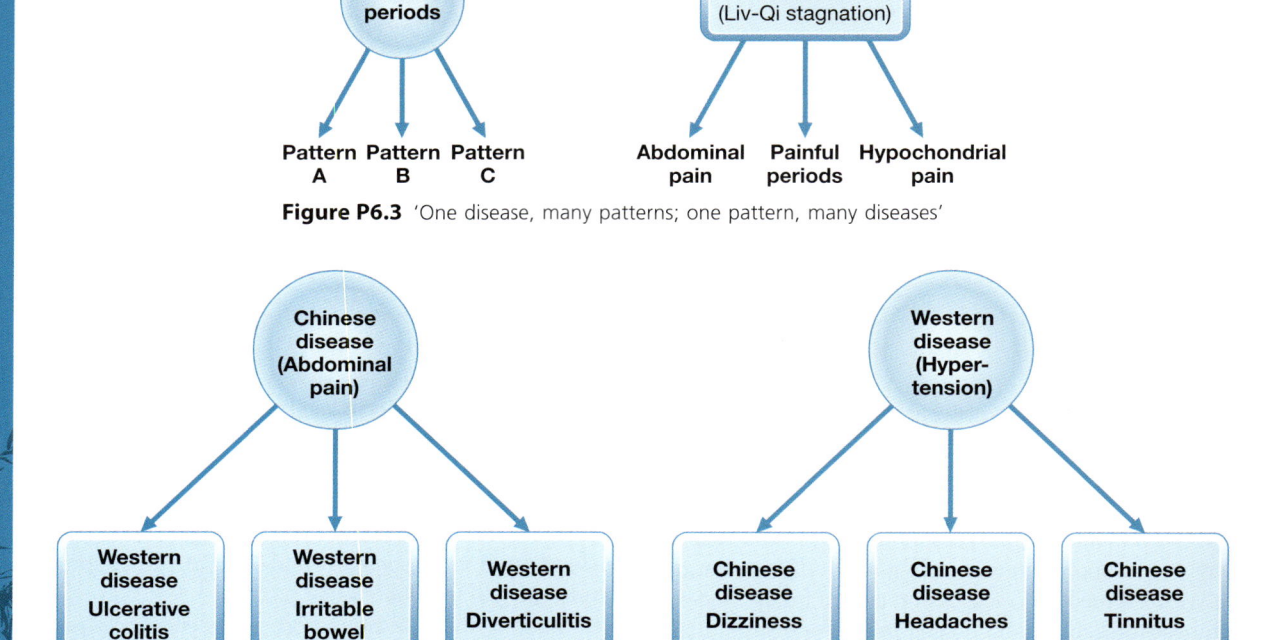

Figure P6.4 'One Chinese disease, many Western diseases; one Western disease, many Chinese diseases'

diseases' (Fig. P6.3). Please bear in mind that this saying applies to Chinese, not Western 'diseases'. For example, the 'disease' of Painful Periods may manifest with several different patterns, such as Qi stagnation, Blood stasis, Cold in the Uterus, Damp-Heat in the Uterus, etc. This is a very important principle of Chinese medicine which ensures that each patient is treated individually and there is no standard treatment for 'Painful Periods'.

On the other hand, one pattern may be seen in many different diseases. For example, the pattern of Liver-Qi stagnation may be a factor in Painful Periods, Premenstrual Syndrome, Epigastric Pain, Abdominal Pain, Hypochondrial Pain, etc.

Box P6.3 summarizes the relationship between diseases and patterns.

THE CONCEPT OF 'DISEASE' IN CHINESE MEDICINE COMPARED TO DISEASES IN WESTERN MEDICINE

The same principle of 'one disease, many patterns; one pattern, many diseases' applies to the relationship between Chinese and Western diseases and we could

Box P6.3 Relationship between diseases and patterns

- One disease manifests with different patterns; one pattern may be seen in many different diseases

coin a modern saying 'one Chinese disease, many Western diseases; one Western disease, many Chinese diseases' (Fig. P6.4).

For example, the Chinese 'disease' of Abdominal Pain may correspond to several Western diseases such as ulcerative colitis, irritable bowel, diverticulitis, etc. Conversely, one Western disease may correspond to several Chinese diseases. For example, the disease of hypertension may correspond to Dizziness, Headaches and Tinnitus in Chinese medicine; ulcerative colitis may correspond to Abdominal Pain or Diarrhoea (Box P6.4).

CHARACTERISTICS OF 'SYMPTOMS' AND 'SIGNS' IN CHINESE MEDICINE

'Symptoms and signs' in Chinese Medicine have a rather different meaning than in Western medicine.

> **Box P6.4 Relationship between Chinese and Western diseases**
>
> - One Chinese disease (e.g. Abdominal Pain) corresponds to different Western diseases (ulcerative colitis, irritable bowel, diverticulitis)
> - One Western disease (e.g. hypertension) corresponds to different Chinese diseases (e.g. Dizziness, Headaches, Tinnitus)

> **Box P6.5 'Symptoms and signs' in Chinese medicine**
>
> - Chinese medicine takes into account many symptoms and signs that would not be such in Western medicine (e.g. inability to take decisions, small ears, dull eyes, etc.)

They are different from the relatively narrow area explored by Western medicine despite its battery of laboratory tests and scans. Instead, the doctor of Chinese medicine widens his or her view to assess changes in a broad range of common bodily functions (in addition to the presenting symptoms) such as urination, defecation, sweating, thirst and so on.

Furthermore, the doctor of Chinese medicine takes into account many clinical manifestations ranging from certain facial and bodily signs to psychological and emotional traits which are not really 'symptoms' or 'signs' as such, but rather expressions of a certain disharmony. Many of the clinical manifestations contributing to form a picture of an underlying disharmony would not be considered as 'symptoms' or 'signs' in Western medicine.

For example, absence of thirst, inability to make decisions, a dull appearance of the eyes, thirst with desire to drink in small sips or small ears, all of which are meaningful manifestations in Chinese medicine, would not be considered as such in Western medicine. Thus, whenever the words 'symptoms' and 'signs' occur, they should be interpreted in this broad way. Over many centuries of accumulated clinical experience by countless doctors, Chinese medicine has developed a comprehensive and extremely effective diagnostic system and symptomatology to identify disease patterns and the underlying disharmonies.

Box P6.5 summarizes 'symptoms' and 'signs' in Chinese medicine.

IDENTIFYING PATTERNS

Identifying patterns also follows the typical way of Chinese natural philosophy, which looks for relationships rather than causes. Each symptom and sign has a meaning only in relation to all the others: one symptom can mean different things in different situations. For example, a dry tongue accompanied by a feeling of heat in the evening, dry mouth with desire to drink in small sips, night sweating and a Floating-Empty pulse indicates Yin deficiency (the more common cause of a dry tongue), while a dry tongue accompanied by a feeling of cold, absence of thirst, cold hands and profuse pale urination indicates Yang deficiency (a rarer cause of a dry tongue).

Identifying the pattern of disharmony blends diagnosis, pathology and treatment principle all in one. When we say that a certain pattern is characterized by deficiency of Spleen-Yang with retention of Dampness, we are defining the nature of the condition (Yang deficiency and Dampness), the site (the Spleen) and, by implication, the treatment principle (tonify Yang and resolve Dampness).

In the particular case of exterior patterns, by identifying the pattern we also identify the 'cause'. For example, if we say that a certain complex of clinical manifestations forms the pattern of exterior invasion of Wind-Cold, we are simultaneously identifying the cause (Wind-Cold), the type of pattern and by implication the treatment principle, which in this case would be to release the Exterior and expel Cold.

Identifying the pattern allows us to find the nature and character of the condition, the site of the disease, the treatment principle and the prognosis.

As the 'Essentials of Chinese Acupuncture' points out, *'identification [of the pattern] is made not from a simple list of symptoms and signs, but from a reflection on the pathogenesis of the disease'*.[2]

In other words, we should not only identify the pattern but also understand how it arose and how different aspects of it interact with each other. For example, if we identify the pattern of Liver-Qi stagnation and also one of Spleen-Qi deficiency, we should go a step further and find out how these two patterns interact and whether one can be considered the cause of the other.

Box P6.6 summarizes pattern identification in Chinese medicine.

METHODS OF IDENTIFICATION OF PATTERNS

There are several methods used to identify patterns. These are applicable in different situations and were

> **Box P6.6 Identifying patterns**
> - Identification of patterns looks for relationships rather than causes
> - Identification of patterns blends diagnosis, pathology and treatment principle all in one
> - In exterior diseases, the identification of patterns identifies the cause as well (e.g. external Wind)
> - Apart from identifying the pattern, we should understand its origin, development and relationship with other patterns

formulated at different times in the development of Chinese medicine. The various modes of identifying patterns are:

- Identification of patterns according to the Eight Principles
- Identification of patterns according to Qi, Blood and Body Fluids
- Identification of patterns according to the Internal Organs
- Identification of patterns according to pathogenic factors
- Identification of patterns according to the 12 Channels
- Identification of patterns according to the Eight Extraordinary Vessels
- Identification of patterns according to the Five Elements
- Identification of patterns according to the Six Stages
- Identification of patterns according to the Four Levels
- Identification of patterns according to the Three Burners

The discussion of the identification of patterns will be divided into the following headings:

Section 1: Identification of patterns according to the Eight Principles and Qi–Blood–Body Fluids
    Chapter 30   Identification of patterns according to the Eight Principles
    Chapter 31   Identification of patterns according to Qi–Blood–Body Fluids

Section 2: Identification of patterns according to the Internal Organs
    Chapter 32   Heart patterns
    Chapter 33   Pericardium patterns
    Chapter 34   Liver patterns
    Chapter 35   Lung patterns
    Chapter 36   Spleen patterns
    Chapter 37   Kidney patterns
    Chapter 38   Stomach patterns
    Chapter 39   Small Intestine patterns
    Chapter 40   Large Intestine patterns
    Chapter 41   Gall Bladder patterns
    Chapter 42   Bladder patterns

Section 3: Identification of patterns according to pathogenic factors
    Chapter 43   Identification of patterns according to pathogenic factors
    Chapter 44   Identification of patterns according to the Six Stages
    Chapter 45   Identification of patterns according to the Four Levels
    Chapter 46   Identification of patterns according to Three Burners

Section 4: Identification of patterns according to the 12 channels and the Five Elements
    Chapter 47   Identification of patterns according to the 12 channels
    Chapter 48   Identification of patterns according to the Eight Extraordinary Vessels
    Chapter 49   Identification of patterns according to the Five Elements

Each of these is applicable in different cases and the following is a brief discussion of the applicability of each of the methods for pattern identification. A more detailed discussion of each method will be found in the relevant chapters.

Identification of patterns according to the Eight Principles

Elements of this identification are found throughout Chinese medical texts starting from the 'Yellow Emperor's Classic of Internal Medicine' and the 'Discussion on Cold-induced Diseases'. In its present form, this method of identifying patterns was formulated by Cheng Zhong Ling in the early Qing dynasty.

The identification of patterns according to the Eight Principles is based on the categories of Interior/Exterior, Hot/Cold, Full/Empty and Yin/Yang. It is the summarization of all other modes of identification and is applicable in all cases, for both interior and exterior diseases. This method of identification of patterns is discussed in chapter 30.

Identification of patterns according to Qi, Blood and Body Fluids

This method of identification of patterns describes the basic disharmonies of Qi, Blood and Body Fluids, such as deficiency, stagnation and rebellion of Qi, deficiency, stasis, Heat and loss of Blood and deficiency of fluids, oedema and Phlegm.

This particular method is very important and constantly used in clinical practice, especially for internal diseases. It is integrated with the method of identification according to the Internal Organs and that according to the Eight Principles. This method of identification is discussed in chapter 31.

Identification of patterns according to the Internal Organs

Again, elements of this process of identification of patterns are found throughout Chinese medical texts from the earliest times, but, in its present form, it was formulated during the early Qing dynasty.

This method of identification is based on the pathological changes occurring in the Internal Organs, and is the most important of all the various systems for the diagnosis and treatment of internal diseases.

The method of identification of patterns according to the Internal Organs basically consists in the application of the Eight Principles to specific Internal Organs. For example, according to the Eight Principles, a condition may be due to Full-Heat, but, applying the process of identification according to the Internal Organs, we can identify the organ affected by the Full-Heat, for example Liver-Fire. This identification is discussed in chapters 32 to 42.

Identification of patterns according to pathogenic factors

This method of pattern identification is based on the pathological changes occurring when the body is invaded by pathogenic factors such as Wind, Dampness, Cold, Heat, Dryness and Fire. Each of these pathogenic factors may be exterior or interior. This method of identification is discussed in chapter 43.

Identification of patterns according to the Six Stages

This was formulated by Zhang Zhong Jing (born c.AD 158) in his 'Discussion on Cold-induced Diseases'. This method of identification is used primarily for the diagnosis and treatment of diseases from exterior Cold, but many of its recommended herbal prescriptions are still used nowadays to treat internal, Hot conditions.

This method of identification has been the bible of Chinese doctors, especially in North China, for about 16 centuries, to be supplanted, especially in South China, by the method of identification according to the Four Levels and Three Burners. This method of identification is discussed in chapter 44.

Identification of patterns according to the Four Levels

This was devised by Ye Tian Shi (1667–1746) in his book 'Discussion of Warm Diseases' and it describes the pathological changes caused by exterior Wind-Heat. It is the most important and most widely used method of identification of patterns for the treatment of febrile infectious diseases that start with invasion of exterior Wind-Heat. I personally find this method of identification of patterns extremely important and useful for the treatment of exterior diseases and their consequences. This method of identification is discussed in chapter 45.

Identification of patterns according to the Three Burners

This was formulated by Wu Ju Tong (1758–1836) in his book 'A Systematic Identification of Febrile Diseases'. This method of identification of patterns is usually combined with the previous one for the diagnosis and treatment of febrile infectious diseases starting with invasion of Wind-Heat. This method of identification is discussed in chapter 46.

These last three methods of identifications of patterns are deeply rooted in the tradition of herbal medicine, rather than acupuncture: they can only really be understood and put into perspective within the context of herbal medicine.

Identification of patterns according to the 12 channels

This is the oldest of all modes of identification of patterns. Reference to it occurs in the 'Spiritual Axis'.[3] This method of identification of patterns, discussed in chapter 47, describes the symptoms and signs related to each channel, rather than the organ.

This way of identifying patterns comes into its own when an acupuncturist treats a condition which is caused by damage to a channel rather than an internal organ or even by damage to an internal organ manifesting along its corresponding channel. For this reason, it is not used much for the treatment of internal conditions, as it does not give the doctor enough information to make a diagnosis or formulate a method of treatment. When treating an internal condition, that is, a disease of an internal organ, the identification of patterns according to the Internal Organs is the preferred method.

IDENTIFICATION OF PATTERNS ACCORDING TO THE EIGHT EXTRAORDINARY VESSELS

This method of identification of patterns is based on the interpretation of clinical manifestations arising from a disharmonies of the Eight Extraordinary Vessels. These are discussed in chapter 48 and the pathology of the Eight Extraordinary Vessels is also discussed in chapters 52 and 53.

IDENTIFICATION OF PATTERNS ACCORDING TO THE FIVE ELEMENTS

This method of identification of patterns is based on the interpretation of clinical manifestations according to the Generating, Overacting and Insulting sequences of the Five Elements. These will be described in chapter 49.

END NOTES

1. Hu Xi Ming 1989 Great Treatise of Secret Formulae in Chinese Medicine (*Zhong Guo Zhong Yi Mi Fang Da Quan* 中国中医秘方大全), Literary Publishing House, Shanghai. This book is only an example of many modern Chinese books presenting a pattern identification applied to Western medical diseases.
2. Beijing, Shanghai and Nanjing College of Traditional Chinese Medicine 1980 Essentials of Chinese Acupuncture, Foreign Languages Press, Beijing, p. 60.
3. 1981 Spiritual Axis (*Ling Shu Jing* 灵枢经), People's Health Publishing House, Beijing, first published c.100 BC, p. 30–39.

SECTION 1

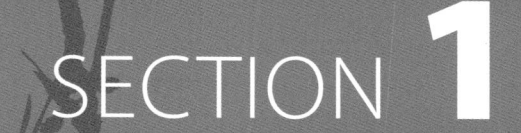

Identification of Patterns according to the Eight Principles and Qi–Blood–Body Fluids

INTRODUCTION

Section 1 includes two methods of identification of patterns:

> Chapter 30 Identification of patterns according to the Eight Principles
> Chapter 31 Identification of patterns according to Qi–Blood–Body Fluids

IDENTIFICATION OF PATTERNS ACCORDING TO THE EIGHT PRINCIPLES

The identification of patterns according to the Eight Principles is based on the categories of Interior/Exterior, Hot/Cold, Full/Empty and Yin/Yang. It is the summarization of all other modes of identification and is applicable in all cases, for both interior and exterior diseases. This method of identification of patterns is discussed in chapter 30.

The discussion of the Eight-Principle patterns is divided as follows:

1. Interior–Exterior
    a) Exterior
    b) Interior
2. Hot–Cold
    a) Hot
        i. Full-Heat
        ii. Empty-Heat
    b) Cold
        i. Full-Cold
        ii. Empty-Cold
3. Combined Hot and Cold
    a) Cold on the Exterior, Heat on the Interior
    b) Heat on the Exterior, Cold in the Interior
    c) Heat Above, Cold Below
    d) Combination of Hot and Cold patterns
    e) True Cold, False Heat and True Heat, False Cold
4. Full–Empty
    a) Empty Qi
    b) Empty Yang
    c) Empty Blood
    d) Empty Yin
5. Yin–Yang
    a) Collapse of Yin
    b) Collapse of Yang

IDENTIFICATION OF PATTERNS ACCORDING TO QI, BLOOD AND BODY FLUIDS

This method of identification of patterns describes the basic disharmonies of Qi, Blood and Body Fluids, such as deficiency, stagnation and rebellion of Qi, deficiency, stasis, Heat and loss of Blood and deficiency of fluids, oedema and Phlegm.

This particular method is very important and constantly used in clinical practice especially for internal diseases. It is integrated with the method of identification according to the Internal Organs and that according to the Eight Principles. This method of identification is discussed in chapter 31.

The discussion of the patterns of the pathology of Qi, Blood and Body Fluids is divided into the following parts:

1. Qi pattern identification
    a) Qi deficiency
    b) Qi sinking
    c) Qi stagnation
    d) Rebellious Qi
2. Blood pattern identification
    a) Deficiency of Blood
    b) Stasis of Blood
        i. Liver
        ii. Heart
        iii. Lungs
        iv. Stomach
        v. Intestines
        vi. Uterus
    c) Heat in the Blood
    d) Loss of blood
3. Body Fluid pattern identification
    a) Deficiency of Body Fluids
        i. Lungs
        ii. Stomach
        iii. Kidneys
        iv. Large Intestine
    b) Oedema
    c) Phlegm
        i. Substantial versus non-substantial Phlegm
            Substantial Phlegm
            Non-substantial Phlegm
                Under the skin
                In the channels

      Misting the Heart
      In Gall Bladder or Kidneys
      In the joints
  ii. Types of Phlegm according to nature
      Damp-Phlegm
      Phlegm-Heat
      Cold-Phlegm
      Wind-Phlegm
      Qi-Phlegm
      Phlegm-Fluids
         In the Stomach and Intestines
         In the hypochondrium
         In the limbs
         Above the diaphragm

SECTION 1   PART 6

Identification of Patterns according to the Eight Principles

30

Key contents

Interior–Exterior
Exterior
Interior

Hot–Cold
Hot
- Full-Heat
- Empty-Heat

Cold
- Full-Cold
- Empty-Cold

Combined Hot and Cold
Cold on the Exterior–Heat on the Interior
Heat on the Exterior–Cold in the Interior
Heat above–Cold below
Combination of Hot and Cold patterns
True Cold–False Heat and True Heat–False Cold

Full–Empty
Empty Qi
Empty Yang
Empty Blood
Empty Yin

Yin–Yang
Collapse of Yin
Collapse of Yang

The Identification of Patterns according to the Eight Principles is the foundation for all the other methods of pattern formulation. It is the basic groundwork of pattern identification in Chinese medicine, allowing the practitioner to identify the location and nature of the disharmony, as well as establish the principle of treatment.

Although the term 'Eight Principles' is relatively recent in Chinese medicine (early Qing dynasty), their main aspects were discussed both in the 'Yellow Emperor's Classic of Internal Medicine' and in the 'Discussion on Cold-induced Diseases'. Both these classics contain many references to the Interior/Exterior, Hot/Cold, Full/Empty and Yin/Yang character of diseases.

For example, chapter 62 of the 'Simple Questions' says: '*When Yang is deficient there is external Cold, when Yin is deficient there is internal Heat, when Yang is in Excess there is external Heat, when Yin is in Excess there is internal Cold.*'[1] This succinct and terse statement embodies all the Eight Principles: that is, Heat and Cold, Interior and Exterior, Full and Empty and Yin and Yang.

The same chapter of the 'Simple Questions' says: '*In the human body there is Essence, Qi, Body Fluids, the 4 limbs, the 9 orifices, the 5 Yin Organs, the 16 areas, 365 points, all of which are subject to the 100 diseases and these arise from either Emptiness or Fullness [Xu-Shi].*'[2] Again, this brief statement highlights very effectively how all conditions are characterized by either Fullness or Emptiness.

Doctor Zhang Jing Yue (1563–1640) (also called Zhang Jie Bin) discussed the identification of patterns according to the above principles and called it the 'Six Changes' (*Liu Bian* 六 变), these being Interior/Exterior, Full/Empty and Hot/Cold.

During the early Qing dynasty, at the time of Emperor Kang Xi (1661–1690), Doctor Cheng Zhong Ling wrote the 'Essential Comprehension of Medical Studies' (*Yi Xue Xin Wu* 医 学 心 悟), in which he, for the first time, used the term 'Eight Principles' (*Ba Gang* 八 纲).

The method of identification of patterns according to the Eight Principles differs from all the others in so far as it is the theoretical basis for all of them and is applicable in every case. For example, the method of identification of patterns according to the Channels is applicable only in channel problems, and that according to the Internal Organs in organ problems, but the identification of patterns according to the Eight Principles is applicable in every case because it allows us to distinguish Exterior from Interior, Hot from Cold and Full from Empty. It therefore allows us to decide which method of identification of patterns applies to a particular case. No condition is too complex to fall outside the scope of identification according to the Eight Principles.

It is important to realize that identifying a pattern according to the Eight Principles does not mean rigidly 'categorizing' the disharmony in order to 'fit' the clinical manifestations into pigeonholes. An understanding of the Eight Principles, on the contrary, allows us to unravel complicated patterns and identify the basic contradictions within them, reducing the various disease manifestations to the bare relevant essentials.

> Identifying patterns does not mean categorizing them into pigeonholes. It involves understanding the pathogenesis, development and relationship of patterns

Although this process might seem rigid and somewhat forced in the beginning, after a few years of practice, it will become completely natural and spontaneous.

The Eight Principles should not be seen in terms of 'either–or'. It is not at all unusual to see conditions that are Exterior and Interior simultaneously, or Hot and Cold, or Full and Empty or Yin and Yang. It is even possible for a condition to be all of these at the same time. The purpose of applying the Eight Principles is not to categorize the disharmony, but to understand its genesis and nature. It is only by understanding this that we can decide on treatment for a particular disharmony.

> The Eight Principles are not 'either–or' but all interrelated. A condition could be characterized by both Hot and Cold patterns, or by both Full and Empty patterns.

Moreover, not every condition need have all four characteristics (Interior or Exterior, Hot or Cold, Full or Empty and Yin or Yang). For example, a condition need not necessarily be either hot or cold. Deficiency of Blood is a case in point as it does not involve any Hot or Cold symptoms.

Finally, although the Identification of Patterns according to the Eight Principles is the foundation of all other methods, it is not one that is applied rigidly and mechanically in practice. In most cases, the Identification of Patterns according to the Eight Principles is implicit to the Identification of Patterns according to the Internal Organs or that according to Qi, Blood and Body Fluids.

For example, if we are presented with a patients suffering from tiredness, loose stools, poor appetite, feeling cold, cold limbs, abdominal fullness, a feeling of heaviness, a Soggy pulse and a sticky tongue coating, according to the Internal Organs pathology, this is a fairly obvious case of Spleen-Yang deficiency and retention of Dampness. We would identify the patterns in this way without actually thinking about 'classifying' them according to the Eight Principles as such classification is implicit. In this case, Spleen-Yang deficiency represents an Empty condition and Dampness a Full condition; as the condition affects the Spleen it is Interior; as there are Cold symptoms, it is a Cold condition (Empty-Cold); finally, from the Yin–Yang point of view, there is Yang deficiency. As mentioned above, such classification is implicit in that of Spleen-Yang deficiency and Dampness.

However, it is still important to evaluate the disharmony from the point of view of the Eight Principles to get a sense of priority between Full and Empty (i.e. which is the predominant aspect of the disharmony). The Identification of Patterns according to the Eight Principles provides the tools for that evaluation.

The Eight Principles are:

- Interior–Exterior
- Hot–Cold
- Full–Empty (or Excess–Deficiency)
- Yin–Yang

The discussion of the Identification of Patterns according to the Eight Principles will be divided into the following headings:

- Exterior–Interior
  - Exterior
  - Interior
- Hot–Cold
  - Hot
    - Full-Heat
    - Empty-Heat

- Cold
  - Full-Cold
  - Empty-Cold
- Combined Hot and Cold
  - Cold on the Exterior–Heat in the Interior
  - Heat on the Exterior–Cold in the Interior
  - Heat above–Cold below
  - Combination of Heat and Cold patterns
  - True Cold–False Heat and True Heat–False Cold
- Full–Empty
  - Full conditions
  - Mixed Full–Empty conditions
  - Empty conditions
    - Empty Qi
    - Empty Yang
    - Empty Blood
    - Empty Yin
- Yin–Yang
  - Collapse of Yin
  - Collapse of Yang

EXTERIOR–INTERIOR

The differentiation of Exterior and Interior is not made on the basis of what caused the disharmony (aetiology), but on the basis of the location of the disease. For example, a disease may be caused by an exterior pathogenic factor, but if this is affecting the Internal Organs, the condition will be classified as interior. Therefore, a disease is classified as 'exterior' not because it derived from an exterior pathogenic factor but because its manifestations are such that they are located in the 'Exterior' of the body.

The Eight Principles are listed in Box 30.1.

> **Box 30.1 The Eight Principles**
> 1. Interior–Exterior
> 2. Hot–Cold
> 3. Full–Empty (or Excess–Deficiency)
> 4. Yin–Yang

Exterior

Definition

We should first define the 'Exterior' of the body. 'Exterior' of the body comprises the skin, muscles and channels. More specifically, the 'Exterior' refers to the space between skin and muscles: this is the space where Defensive Qi (*Wei Qi*) and sweat are located and it is also the space that is first invaded by external pathogenic factors. This space is also sometimes called the 'Lung's Defensive Qi portion'.

A condition is defined as 'exterior' when the pathogenic factors are located in the 'Exterior' as defined above. At the risk of being repetitive: a condition is therefore defined as 'exterior' according to its location (i.e. the 'Exterior') and not according to the aetiology (e.g. external Wind). The diagnosis of 'exterior' condition is therefore made on the basis of its clinical manifestations.

Skin, muscles and channels are the 'Exterior' of the body, and the Internal Organs the 'Interior'.

Exterior patterns

The clinical manifestations arising from invasion of the Exterior by a pathogenic factor are called an 'exterior pattern', while the manifestations arising from a disharmony of the Internal Organs is called an 'interior pattern'.

When we say that an exterior condition affects the skin, muscles and channels, we mean that these areas have been invaded by an exterior pathogenic factor, giving rise to typical 'exterior' clinical manifestations. However, it would be wrong to assume that any problem manifesting on the skin is an 'exterior pattern'. In fact, most chronic skin problems are due to an interior pattern manifesting on the skin.

There are two types of exterior conditions: those that affect skin and muscles and are caused by an exterior pathogenic factor having an acute onset (such as in invasion of Wind-Cold or Wind-Heat), and those that affect the channels and have a slower onset (such as in Painful Obstruction Syndrome).

Clinical manifestations of exterior patterns

When an exterior pathogenic factor invades skin and muscles it gives rise to a typical set of symptoms and signs which are described as an 'exterior pattern'. It is difficult to generalize as to what these symptoms and signs are, as it depends on the other characters: that is, whether they are of the Cold or Hot type, and the Empty or Full type. However, fever and aversion to cold occurring simultaneously always indicate an invasion from an exterior pathogenic factor. These have been discussed in chapter 21. To remind the reader briefly, 'aversion to cold' indicates the sudden chilliness that occurs when we fall ill with a cold or other acute exterior diseases: this is a subjective feeling of cold. 'Fever' (*fa re* in Chinese) does not necessarily indicate an actual fever, but rather the objective feeling of the heat of the patient's body on palpation.

Generally speaking, we can say that the main symptoms of an exterior pattern are 'fever', aversion to cold, aching body, a stiff neck and a Floating pulse. The onset is acute and the correct treatment will usually induce a swift and marked improvement of the condition.

Box 30.2 summarizes the clinical manifestations of exterior patterns.

If the condition is one of Cold (such as Wind-Cold), the symptoms are a slight 'fever', pronounced aversion to cold, severe aches in the body, severe stiff neck, no sweating, no thirst, a Floating-Tight pulse and a thin white tongue coating.

Box 30.3 summarizes the clinical manifestations of exterior Cold patterns.

If the condition is one of Heat (such as Wind-Heat), the symptoms are fever, aversion to cold, slight sweating, thirst, a Floating-Rapid pulse, a thin white tongue coating and, sometimes, redness of the tongue on the sides and/or front. In this case the body aches are not so pronounced.

Box 30.4 summarizes the clinical manifestations of exterior Heat patterns.

The main factors in differentiating the Hot or Cold character of an exterior pattern are:

- Thirst (Hot) or its absence (Cold)
- Tight (Cold) or Rapid (Hot) pulse

The character of an exterior pattern will further depend on its Full or Empty character. If a person has a tendency to deficiency of Qi or Blood, the exterior pattern will have an Empty character. This is also described as an exterior pattern from Wind-Cold with prevalence of Wind. It should be noted that 'Empty' here should be intended in a relative sense: that is, the pattern is still Full (because there is a pathogenic factor) but it is *relatively* Empty (compared to other patterns). In fact, an exterior pattern is characterized by Fullness by definition, as it consists of an invasion by an exterior pathogenic factor. The person's Qi is still relatively intact and the pathogenic factor fights against the body's Qi. It is precisely this that defines a Full condition: that is, one characterized by the presence of a pathogenic factor and the resulting struggle with the body's Qi. Thus an exterior condition must, by definition, be Full. However, according to a person's pre-existing condition, one can further differentiate an exterior condition between Full and Empty, but only in relative terms.

The clinical manifestations of an exterior Empty pattern are slight or no fever, sweating, aversion to wind, slight body aches, a Floating-Slow pulse and a thin white tongue coating (Box 30.5).

If a person has a tendency to Fullness, the exterior pattern will have a Full character. The clinical manifestations of such an exterior Full pattern are fever, no sweating, severe body aches, aversion to cold, a Floating-Tight pulse and a thin white tongue coating (Box 30.6)

Box 30.2 Clinical manifestations of exterior patterns

Aversion to cold, 'fever', aching body, a stiff neck and a Floating pulse

---

Box 30.3 Clinical manifestations of exterior Cold pattern

Slight 'fever', pronounced aversion to cold, severe aches in the body, severe stiff neck, no sweating, no thirst, a Floating-Tight pulse and a thin white tongue coating

---

Box 30.4 Clinical manifestations of exterior Heat pattern

Aversion to cold, 'fever', slight sweating, thirst, a Floating-Rapid pulse, a thin white tongue coating and sometimes redness of the tongue on the sides and/or front

---

Box 30.5 Clinical manifestations of exterior Empty pattern

Slight or no fever, sweating, aversion to wind, slight body aches, a Floating-Slow pulse and a thin white tongue coating

---

Box 30.6 Clinical manifestations of exterior Full pattern

Fever, no sweating, severe body aches, aversion to cold, a Floating-Tight pulse and a thin white tongue coating

The main factors in differentiating an Empty from Full Exterior condition are:

- Sweating (Empty) or its absence (Full)
- Pulse (Slow in Empty and Tight in Full)
- Severity of body aches (severe in Fullness, less severe in Emptiness)

Case history 30.1

A young girl of 13 fell ill with what was described as 'influenza'. She had a temperature of 102°F (38.8°C), a sore throat, cough, headache, aches in all joints, slight thirst and slight sweating. Her tongue was slightly red on the sides and the Pulse was Floating in both Front positions.

This is a clear example of invasion of exterior Wind-Heat.

The second kind of exterior pattern is that occurring when an exterior pathogenic factor invades the channels in a gradual way causing Painful Obstruction Syndrome. This is characterized by obstruction to the circulation of Qi in channels and joints by a pathogenic factor, which can be Cold, Dampness, Wind or Heat.

In obstruction from Cold, usually only one joint is affected, the pain is severe and is relieved by application of heat. In obstruction from Wind, the pain moves from joint to joint. In obstruction from Dampness, there will be swelling of the joints, while in obstruction from Heat, the pain is severe and the joints are swollen and hot.

Interior

A disharmony is defined as interior when the Internal Organs are affected. This may have arisen from an exterior pathogenic factor, but once the disease is located in the Interior, it is defined as an interior pattern, and treated as such (Fig. 30.1).

It is impossible to generalize to give the clinical manifestations of interior conditions as these will depend on the organ affected, and whether the condition is Hot or Cold and Full or Empty.

When an interior condition starts with the invasion of an exterior pathogenic factor, the most important symptoms that mark the change from the exterior to the interior stage are the disappearance of aversion to cold and the onset of aversion to heat. For example, if a patient suffers an invasion of Wind (whether it is Wind-Cold or Wind-Heat), in the beginning stage the pathogenic factor is on the Exterior and the condition is defined as exterior: the two chief symptoms that denote this are aversion to cold and 'fever' (as defined in ch. 21). At this stage, the pathogenic factor is either expelled completely and the patient recovers or it penetrates into the Interior: when this happens, the condition is interior. The main change that denotes this progression of the pathogenic factor to the interior is the disappearance of aversion to cold and the onset of aversion to heat.

Most of the Internal Organ patterns described in chapters 32–42 are internal ones. These are caused mostly by internal causes of disease such as emotional stress, diet and overwork.

Interior patterns of the Hot or Cold and Full or Empty type will be described shortly.

HOT–COLD

Hot and Cold describe the nature of a pattern, and their clinical manifestations depend on whether they are combined with a Full or Empty condition.

Hot

Full-Heat

Full-Heat can be external (as in Wind-Heat) or internal. The manifestations of invasion of Wind-Heat have already been described above. Full-Heat (whether external or internal) is a manifestation of Excess Yang (Fig. 30.2).

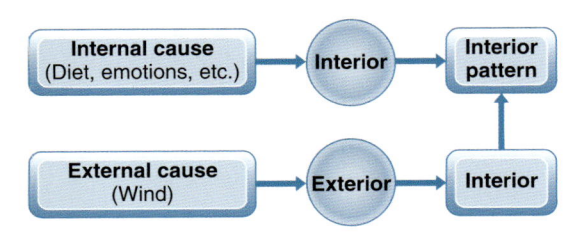

Figure 30.1 Origin of interior pattern

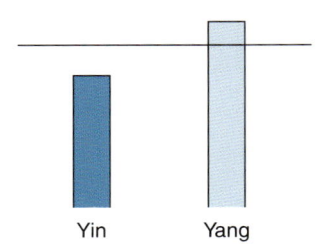

Figure 30.2 Full-Heat from Excess of Yang

The main manifestations of Full-Heat in an internal condition are thirst, a feeling of heat, some mental restlessness, red face, dry stools, scanty dark urine, a Rapid-Full pulse, and a Red tongue with yellow coating. Beyond these, it is difficult to generalize as other manifestations will depend on the organ affected.

Aside from the above clinical manifestations, there are other diagnostic guides which indicate Heat.

Any raised, red skin eruption which feels hot indicates Heat. For example, acute urticaria normally takes this form. As for pain, any burning sensation indicates Heat: for example, the burning sensation of cystitis, or a burning feeling in the stomach. Any loss of blood, with large quantities of dark-red blood, indicates Heat in the Blood. As far as the mind is concerned, any condition of extreme restlessness or manic behaviour indicates Heat in the Heart. Of course, a subjective feeling of heat also indicates Heat.

Aetiology

Internal Full-Heat may derive directly from the excessive consumption of hot-energy foods (e.g. red meats, spices and alcohol) or, indirectly, from emotional stress. In fact, emotional stress tends to cause Qi stagnation in its early stages; if Qi stagnates for some time, it usually gives rise to some Heat. With further passage of time, Heat may turn into Fire. Finally, Internal Full-Heat may also derive from the transformation of a pathogenic factor which penetrates the Interior and turns into Heat as it does so (Fig. 30.3 and Box 30.7).

Case history 30.2

A woman of 50 suffered from burning pain in the epigastrium. She also complained of nausea with occasional vomiting, bleeding of the gums, bad breath, thirst and insomnia. Her tongue was Red, had a crack in the centre with a sticky, dry, yellow coating and was dry. Her pulse was Full and slightly Rapid.

These manifestations indicate Full-Heat in the Stomach.

Empty-Heat

From the Yin–Yang point of view, Empty-Heat arises from Deficiency of Yin (Fig. 30.4). If the Yin energy is deficient for a long period of time, the Yin is consumed and the Yang is relatively in Excess. Please note that Yin may be deficient for years before giving rise to Empty-Heat. Therefore, Empty-Heat always derives

---

Box 30.7   Full-Heat

Manifestations

- Thirst, a feeling of heat, mental restlessness, red face, dry stools, scanty dark urine, Rapid-Full pulse, Red tongue with yellow coating (Internal Full-Heat)

Aetiology

- Emotional problems
- Diet (too much red meat, spices, alcohol)
- An external pathogenic factor that has penetrated into the Interior and transformed into Heat

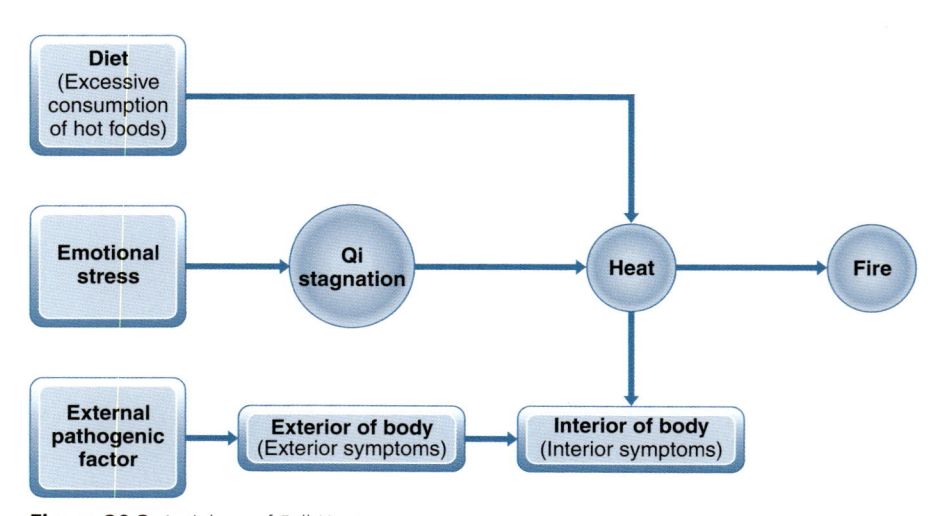

Figure 30.3 Aetiology of Full-Heat

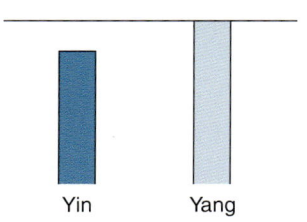

Figure 30.4 Empty-Heat from Deficiency of Yin

from Yin deficiency but this may occur without Empty-Heat. The tongue will show the difference clearly: in Yin deficiency, the tongue lacks a coating but it has a normal colour; in Yin deficiency with Empty-Heat, the tongue lacks a coating and is red.

The main general manifestations of Empty-Heat are a feeling of heat in the afternoon/evening, a dry mouth with desire to drink in small sips, a dry throat at night, night sweating, a feeling of heat in the chest and palms and soles (also called 'five-palm heat'), dry stools, scanty dark urine, a Floating-Empty and Rapid pulse and a Red tongue without coating.

Again, these are only the general symptoms and signs; others depend on which organ is mostly affected. Empty-Heat frequently arises from deficiency of Kidney-Yin. Because Kidney-Yin is the foundation for all the Yin energies of the body, when this is deficient it can affect the Yin of the Liver, Heart and Lungs. A long-standing deficiency of Yin in any of these organs can give rise to Empty-Heat manifesting with various symptoms, such as mental restlessness and insomnia when Heart-Yin is deficient, irritability and headaches when Liver-Yin is deficient and malar flush and dry cough when Lung-Yin is deficient.

Aside from these manifestations, from a mental–emotional point of view Empty-Heat can often be recognized from a typical feeling of mental restlessness, fidgeting and vague anxiety. The person feels that something is wrong but is unable to describe what or how. Empty-Heat restlessness is quite different from that of Full-Heat and one can almost visually perceive the Emptiness underlying the Heat.

> **Clinical note**
>
> - *Full-Heat* causes severe mental restlessness, agitation, anxiety, insomnia with agitated sleep
> - *Empty-Heat* causes a vague mental restlessness that is worse in the evening, an anxiety with fidgeting, and waking up frequently during the night

In practice, it is important to differentiate Full-Heat from Empty-Heat as the treatment method in the former case is to clear the Heat, while in the latter case it is to nourish Yin (Table 30.1).

It is worth noting also that Empty-Heat is no less 'real' than Full-Heat. The term 'Empty' in 'Empty-Heat' may give the false impression that this is not 'real' Heat: in fact, Empty-Heat produces as much heat as Full-Heat, albeit in different forms.

Aetiology

Empty-Heat derives from Yin deficiency: therefore the causes of Empty-Heat are the same as those that cause Yin deficiency. These causes are:

- Overwork (in the sense of working long hours)
- Irregular eating
- Excessive sexual activity
- Persistent, heavy blood loss (such as in menorrhagia)

Box 30.8 summarizes the manifestations and aetiology of Empty-Heat.

Case history 30.3

A woman of 54 suffered from severe anxiety, insomnia, dizziness, tinnitus, soreness of the lower back, a feeling of heat in the evening, a dry mouth and night sweating. Her face was flushed on the cheekbones. Her pulse was Floating-Empty and slightly Rapid and her tongue was Red and Peeled.

This is an example of Empty-Heat (dry mouth, feeling of heat, flushed cheekbones, night sweating, Rapid pulse and Red-Peeled tongue) arising from Kidney-Yin deficiency (soreness of the back, dizziness and tinnitus). The Empty-Heat was affecting the Heart as indicated by the anxiety and insomnia.

Cold

Full-Cold

The main manifestations are feeling cold, cold limbs, no thirst, pale face, abdominal pain aggravated on pressure, desire to drink warm liquids, loose stools, clear abundant urination, Deep-Full-Tight pulse and a Pale tongue with thick white coating.

These are the clinical manifestation of interior Full-Cold as exterior Cold (in the form of Wind-Cold) has already been described above.

Table 30.1 Comparison between Full-Heat and Empty-Heat

	Full-Heat	**Empty-Heat**
Face	Whole face red	Malar flush
Thirst	Desire to drink cold water	Desire to drink in small sips
Eyelid	Red all over inside eyelid	Thin red line inside eyelid
Taste	Bitter taste	No bitter taste
Feeling of heat	All day	In the afternoon or evening
Fever	High fever	Low-grade fever in the afternoon
Mind	Very restless and agitated	Vague anxiety, fidgeting
Bowels	Constipation, abdominal pain	Dry stools, no abdominal pain
Bleeding	Profuse	Slight
Sleep	Dream-disturbed, very restless	Waking up frequently during the night or early morning
Skin	Red, hot painful skin eruptions	Scarlet-red, not raised painless skin eruptions
Pulse	Full-Rapid-Overflowing	Floating-Empty, Rapid
Tongue	Red with yellow coating	Red and Peeled
Treatment method	Clear Heat	Nourish Yin, clear Empty-Heat

Box 30.8 Empty-Heat

Manifestations

- A feeling of heat in the afternoon or evening, a dry mouth with desire to drink in small sips, a dry throat at night, night sweating, a feeling of heat in the chest, palms and soles (five-palm heat), dry stools, scanty dark urine, Floating-Empty and Rapid pulse, Red tongue without coating

Aetiology

- Overwork (in the sense of working long hours)
- Irregular eating
- Excessive sexual activity
- Persistent, heavy blood loss (such as in menorrhagia)

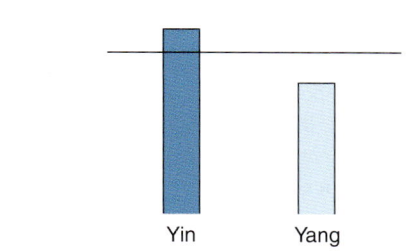

Figure 30.5 Full-Cold from Excess of Yin

Cold contracts and obstructs and this often causes pain. Hence pain, especially abdominal pain, is a frequent manifestation of Full-Cold. Also, anything that is white or bluish-purple may indicate Cold. For example, a pale face or pale tongue, a white tongue coating, a bluish-purple tongue and bluish lips or fingers and toes.

From the Yin–Yang point of view, Full-Cold arises from Excess of Yin (Fig. 30.5).

Exterior Cold can sometimes penetrate into the Interior directly. In particular, exterior Cold can invade the Stomach (causing vomiting and epigastric pain), the Intestines (causing diarrhoea and abdominal pain) and the Uterus (causing acute dysmenorrhoea). All these conditions would have an acute onset. Cold can also invade the Liver channel, causing swelling and pain of the scrotum.

Aetiology

Interior Full-Cold may be caused by the excessive consumption of cold-energy foods (such as salads, fruit

Box 30.9 Full-Cold

Manifestations

- Feeling cold, cold limbs, no thirst, pale face, abdominal pain aggravated on pressure, desire to drink warm liquids, loose stools, clear abundant urination, Deep-Full-Tight pulse and a Pale tongue with thick white coating (Internal Full-Cold)

Aetiology

- Cold foods (salads, fruit, iced drinks)
- External Cold that penetrates into the Interior

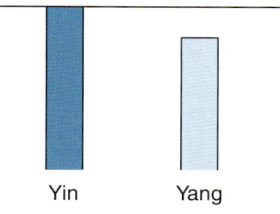

Figure 30.6 Empty-Cold from Deficiency of Yang

Table 30.2 Comparison between Full-Cold and Empty-Cold

	Full-Cold	Empty-Cold
Face	Bright-white	Dull-white
Pain	Sharp, worse on pressure	Dull, better on pressure
Bowels	Better after bowel movement	Worse after bowel movement
Pulse	Full-Tight-Deep	Weak-Slow-Deep
Tongue	Thick white coating	Thin white coating

and iced drinks) or by external Cold. When external Cold invades the body, it will invade the channels first and then the organs. For example, invasion of external Cold in the Spleen is common: when in the channel, it is still exterior Cold, when in the Spleen it is internal Cold.

Box 30.9 summarizes the manifestations and aetiology of Full-Cold.

Case history 30.4

A woman of 24 had a sudden attack of severe, spastic abdominal pain. Her stools became loose, her tongue had a thick, white, sticky coating, and her pulse was Deep and Tight.

These manifestations clearly indicated an attack of exterior Cold and Dampness. They are a case of Full-Cold. The severity and sudden onset of the pains indicates a Full condition, as does the thick tongue coating (in case of Empty-Cold it would have been thin). The Cold and Dampness come from the exterior but have attacked the Interior directly, in this case the Intestines. The Cold character of the pattern is apparent from the white coating and the Tight pulse. The presence of Dampness with the Cold is indicated by the stickiness of the tongue coating and the loose stools (due to Dampness obstructing the Spleen function of transformation, although Cold by itself may also cause loose stools).

Empty-Cold

From the Yin–Yang point of view, Empty-Cold arises from deficiency of Yang (Fig. 30.6).

The main manifestations are feeling cold, cold limbs, a dull pale face, no thirst, listlessness, sweating, loose stools, clear abundant urination, a Deep-Slow or Weak pulse and a Pale tongue with thin white coating.

Empty-Cold develops when Yang Qi is weak and fails to warm the body. It is mostly related to Spleen-Yang and/or Kidney-Yang deficiency. The most common cause is Spleen-Yang deficiency. When this is deficient, the Spleen fails to warm the muscles, hence the feeling of cold. The Spleen needs heat for its function of transformation of food, and when Yang is deficient, food is not transformed properly and loose stools result.

Table 30.2 illustrates the difference between Full-Cold and Empty-Cold.

Aetiology

The cause of Empty-Cold is Yang deficiency. The main causes of Yang deficiency are:

- Excessive physical work
- Diet, i.e. inadequate consumption of hot foods
- Excessive sexual activity (Kidney-Yang)
- Internal Cold injuring Yang

Box 30.10 summarizes manifestations and aetiology of Empty-Cold.

> **Box 30.10 Empty-Cold**
>
> **Manifestations**
>
> - Feeling cold, cold limbs, a dull pale face, no thirst, listlessness, sweating, loose stools, clear abundant urination, a Deep-Slow or Weak pulse and a Pale tongue with thin white coating
>
> **Aetiology**
>
> - Excessive physical work
> - Diet, i.e. inadequate consumption of hot foods
> - Excessive sexual activity (Kidney-Yang)
> - Internal Cold injuring Yang

Case history 30.5

A woman of 31 suffered from tiredness, weight gain, constipation and chilliness. In the past, she had also developed a swelling of the thyroid gland. Her tongue was very Pale and Swollen, and the pulse was very Fine, Deep and Slow.

This is a clear case of Yang deficiency with internal Empty-Cold. The tiredness, chilliness, Pale and Swollen tongue and Deep-Slow pulse all indicate deficiency of Spleen-Yang. The deficiency of Spleen-Yang has given rise to internal Dampness, manifested by weight gain, the Swollen tongue and the swelling of the thyroid gland. The constipation is, in this case, due to deficiency of Yang, since deficient Yang Qi is unable to promote the descending function of the Intestines. This is a less common type of constipation, as normally deficiency of Yang will cause loose stools.

COMBINED HOT AND COLD

A condition can often be characterized by the presence of both Heat and Cold. These can be:

- Cold on the Exterior and Heat in the Interior
- Heat on the Exterior and Cold in the Interior
- Heat above and Cold below
- Combination of Heat and Cold patterns
- False Heat–True Cold and False Cold–True Heat

Cold on the Exterior–Heat in the Interior

This condition is found when a person has a pre-existing condition of interior Heat and is subsequently invaded by exterior Wind-Cold.

The symptoms and signs would include a fever with aversion to cold, no sweating, a headache and stiff neck, aches throughout the body (manifestations of exterior Cold), irritability and thirst (manifestations of interior Heat).

This situation also occurs in attacks of Latent Heat combined with a new invasion of Wind-Cold. According to the theory of Warm diseases (from exterior Wind-Heat), a person can be attacked by Cold in wintertime without developing any manifestations of it. The Cold can lie dormant in the Interior and change into Heat. In the Spring, with the rising of Yang energy, the interior Heat may be pulled towards the Exterior, especially in combination with a new attack of Wind-Cold. Because of this, the person would have symptoms and signs of an attack of Wind-Cold, but also signs of interior Heat such as a thirst, irritability and a Fine-Rapid pulse, as described above.

Heat on the Exterior–Cold in the Interior

This situation simply occurs when a person with a Cold condition is attacked by exterior Wind-Heat. There will therefore be some symptoms of exterior invasion of Wind-Heat (such as a fever with aversion to cold, a sore throat, thirst, a headache and a Floating-Rapid pulse) and some symptoms of interior Cold (such as loose stools, chilliness and profuse pale urine).

Heat above–Cold below

In some cases there is Heat above (as Heat tends to rise) and Cold below. The manifestations of this situation might be thirst, irritability, sour regurgitation, bitter taste, mouth ulcers (manifestations of Heat above), loose stools, borborygmi and profuse pale urine (manifestations of Cold below).

Combination of Heat and Cold patterns

The most common situation in which there are manifestations of both Heat and Cold is when these patterns simply coexist. This is an extremely common situation in practice. For example, it is common for a person to suffer from Kidney-Yang deficiency and Damp-Heat in the Bladder, or Spleen-Yang deficiency and Liver-Fire.

We should therefore not be surprised when we observe contradictory Hot and Cold symptoms in practice: in most cases, they are due to the coexistence of Hot and Cold patterns. To return to the above example, if a patient suffers from Spleen-Yang deficiency, he or she may feel generally cold but have a red face and thirst.

True Cold–False Heat and True Heat–False Cold

In some cases there may be contradictory Hot and Cold signs and symptoms, one of them being due to a 'false' appearance. This usually only happens in extreme conditions and is quite rare. It is important not to confuse this phenomenon with common situations when Heat and Cold are simply combined, as described in the point above. For example, it is perfectly possible for someone to have a condition of Damp-Heat in the Bladder and Cold in the Spleen. This is simply a combination of Hot and Cold signs in two different organs, and does not fall under the category of False Heat and True Cold or vice versa.

In cases of False Heat and False Cold, tongue diagnosis shows its most useful aspect as the tongue-body colour nearly always reflects the true condition. If the tongue-body colour is Red it indicates Heat, if it is Pale it indicates Cold.

It is worth mentioning here that False Heat and False Cold are not the same as Empty-Heat and Empty-Cold. Empty-Heat and Empty-Cold arise from deficiency of Yin or Yang, respectively, but there is nevertheless Heat or Cold. In False Heat and False Cold, the appearance is false: that is, there is no Heat or Cold, respectively.

The clinical manifestations of False Heat and False Cold are best illustrated by Table 30.3.

FULL–EMPTY

The differentiation between Fullness and Emptiness is an extremely important one. The distinction is made according to the presence or absence of a pathogenic factor and to the strength of the body's energies. It is important to define Full and Empty conditions clearly. The clinical manifestations of Full and Empty conditions are also described in chapter 27 on Pathology.

A *Full* condition is characterized by the presence of a pathogenic factor (which may be interior or exterior) of any kind and by the fact that the body's Qi is relatively intact. It therefore battles against the pathogenic factor and this results in the rather plethoric character of the symptoms and signs. Therefore 'Fullness' denotes fullness of a pathogenic factor not fullness of Qi.

An *Empty* condition is characterized by weakness of the body's Qi and the absence of a pathogenic factor.

If the body's Qi is weak but a pathogenic factor lingers on, the condition is of Empty character complicated with Fullness.

Box 30.11 summarizes the characteristics of Full, Empty and Full-Empty conditions.

Box 30.11 Full–Empty

1. **Full** condition is characterized by the presence of a pathogenic factor while the Upright Qi is relatively intact and actively fighting against the pathogenic factor
2. **Empty** condition is characterized by an Emptiness (Deficiency) of the Upright Qi and the absence of a pathogenic factor
3. **Full–Empty** condition is characterized by an Emptiness of the Upright Qi with the presence of a lingering pathogenic factor that the Upright Qi is not fighting effectively

Table 30.3 Clinical manifestations of false Heat and false Cold

Diagnostic signs	True Cold–false Heat	True Heat–false Cold
By observation	Red cheeks, but red colour is like powder, rest of face white; irritability but also listlessness, desire to lie with body curled-up; Pale and wet tongue	Dark face, bright eyes with 'spirit', red-dry lips, irritability, strong body tongue-body colour Red-dry
By hearing	Breathing quiet; low voice	Breathing noisy; loud voice
By interrogation	Thirst but no desire to drink, or desire to drink warm fluids, body feels hot but he or she likes to be covered; sore throat but without redness or swelling; pale urine	Thirst with desire to drink cold fluids: scanty dark urine, constipation, burning sensation in anus
By palpation	Pulse Rapid, Floating and Big but Empty	Pulse Deep, Full; cold limbs but chest is hot

The findings from observation are often important to distinguish between Full and Empty conditions. A strong, loud voice, an excruciating pain, a very red face, profuse sweating, restlessness, throwing off the bedclothes and outbursts of temper are all signs of a Full condition. A weak voice, a dull lingering pain, a very pale face, slight sweating, listlessness, curling up in bed and quiet disposition are all signs of an Empty condition.

Full conditions

Although it is difficult to generalize, the main clinical manifestations of a Full condition are acute disease, restlessness, irritability, a strong voice, coarse breathing, pain aggravated by pressure, high-pitch tinnitus, scanty urination, constipation and a pulse of the Full type.

As usual, it is difficult to generalize and some of the above symptoms cannot, strictly speaking, be categorized as Full symptoms. Just to give one example, constipation is included among the Full symptoms because it is often caused by stagnation or by Heat, but there are also Deficient causes of constipation, such as Blood or Yin deficiency.

Moreover, the above symptoms are broad generalizations, indeed too general to be of use in clinical practice.

Many examples could be given of Full conditions. First of all, any exterior condition due to invasion of exterior Cold, Wind, Damp or Heat is Full by definition, as it is characterized by the presence of those exterior pathogenic factors.

Any interior pathogenic factor also gives rise to a Full condition, provided the body's Qi is strong enough to engage in a struggle against such pathogenic factors. Examples of these are interior Cold, Heat, Dampness, Wind, Fire and Phlegm. Stagnation of Qi and Stasis of Blood are also Full conditions.

Box 30.12 summarizes the clinical manifestations of a Full condition.

> **Box 30.12 Full conditions**
>
> Acute onset, restlessness, irritability, a strong voice, coarse breathing, pain aggravated by pressure, high-pitched tinnitus, scanty urination, constipation, Full pulse

Mixed Full–Empty conditions

Conditions characterized by a combination of Emptiness and Fullness arise when there is a pathogenic factor but its influence is not very strong, while the body's Qi is weak and not reacting properly against it. Examples of conditions of Emptiness complicated with Fullness are Kidney-Yin deficiency with rising of Liver-Yang, Kidney-Yin deficiency with flaring up of Heart Empty-Heat, Spleen-Qi deficiency with retention of Dampness or Phlegm, deficiency of Blood with stasis of Blood and deficiency of Qi with stasis of Blood.

Box 30.13 gives examples of mixed Full–Empty conditions.

Empty conditions

It is impossible to generalize the clinical manifestations of Empty conditions as these depend on the organ and the Vital Substance involved. Generally, the most common manifestations are tiredness, loose stools, weak voice, desire to lie down, slightly Pale tongue and Weak pulse.

The clinical manifestations of Empty conditions, and specifically Qi and Blood deficiency, are also discussed in chapter 31.

We can distinguish four types of Emptiness:

> 1. Empty Qi
> 2. Empty Yang
> 3. Empty Blood
> 4. Empty Yin

Empty Qi

The clinical manifestations are a pale face, a weak voice, slight sweating (in daytime), slight shortness of breath, tiredness, lack of appetite and an Empty pulse.

These are only the symptoms of Lung- and Spleen-Qi Emptiness, which are those customarily given in

> **Box 30.13 Mixed Full–Empty conditions**
>
> **Examples**
> - Kidney-Yin deficiency with Liver-Yang rising
> - Liver-Blood deficiency with Liver-Yang rising
> - Spleen-Qi deficiency with Phlegm
> - Deficiency of Blood with Blood stasis
> - Kidney-Yang deficiency with Dampness

Chinese books, as it is the Spleen that produces Qi and the Lungs that govern Qi. However, there can be many other symptoms of Emptiness of Qi, according to which organ is involved, in particular Heart or Kidneys. These will be described in the chapter on the Identification of Patterns according to the Internal Organs (see chs 32–42).

Emptiness of Qi is the first and least severe deficiency from which one can suffer. Most of the above symptoms arise from weakness of Lung-Qi failing to control breathing, and weakness of Spleen-Qi failing to transform and transport.

Box 30.14 summarizes manifestations of Empty Qi.

Box 30.14 Empty Qi

- Pale face, weak voice, slight sweating, slight shortness of breath, tiredness, loose stools, poor appetite, Empty pulse

Case history 30.6

A man of 30 suffered from tiredness, lack of appetite and persistent catarrh in the nose and throat. His pulse was Empty and the tongue was slightly Pale and slightly Swollen.

These manifestations indicate Spleen-Qi deficiency, complicated by the presence of Dampness (causing the mucus).

Empty Yang

The main clinical manifestations are, in addition to those of Emptiness of Qi: chilliness, a bright pale face, cold limbs, no thirst, a desire for hot drinks, loose stools, frequent pale urination, a Weak pulse and a Pale and wet tongue.

Qi is part of Yang, and Emptiness of Qi is similar in nature to Emptiness of Yang. In fact, the two are practically the same, just emphasizing different aspects of the functions of Qi. In Emptiness of Qi, it is the Qi function of transformation that is mostly at fault, while in Emptiness of Yang, it is the Qi function of warming and protecting that is impaired.

The organs which most commonly suffer from Yang deficiency are the Spleen, Kidneys, Lung, Heart and Stomach. The patterns for each of these are discussed in the chapter on the Internal Organs patterns (see chs 32–42).

Case history 30.7

A woman of 30 suffered from tiredness, chilliness, chronic soreness of the lower back, frequent and pale urination and loose stools. Her pulse was Weak, especially on the right side, and her tongue was Pale and wet.

These manifestations clearly indicate Deficiency of Spleen and Kidney-Yang.

Box 30.15 summarizes the clinical manifestations of Empty Yang.

Box 30.15 Empty Yang

- Chilliness, a bright pale face, cold limbs, no thirst, a desire for hot drinks, loose stools, frequent pale urination, a Weak pulse and a Pale and wet tongue (in addition to the manifestations of Empty Qi)

Empty Blood

The main manifestations of Emptiness of Blood are a dull pale face, pale lips, blurred vision, dry hair, tiredness, poor memory, numbness or tingling, insomnia, scanty periods or amenorrhoea, a Fine or Choppy Pulse and a Pale-Thin tongue.

The above symptoms are due to dysfunction of various organs. Emptiness of Liver-Blood causes blurred vision, tiredness, numbness or tingling and scanty periods. Emptiness of Heart-Blood causes pale face, pale lips, Pale tongue and insomnia.

Blood is part of Yin and a long-standing Emptiness of Blood gives rise to dryness, causing dry hair and nails.

The organs which are most likely to suffer from Blood Emptiness are the Heart, Liver and Spleen. These patterns are described in chapters 32, 34 and 36.

Case history 30.8

A woman of 27 suffered from tiredness, poor memory, scanty menstruation, constipation and insomnia. Her pulse was Choppy and her tongue was Pale and Thin.

These manifestations indicate deficiency of Blood of the Liver (scanty menstruation, tiredness, constipation) and the Heart (poor memory, insomnia).

Box 30.16 summarizes the clinical manifestations of Empty Blood.

> **Box 30.16 Empty Blood**
>
> - Dull pale face, pale lips, blurred vision, dry hair, tiredness, poor memory, numbness or tingling, insomnia, scanty periods, Fine or Choppy pulse, Pale-Thin tongue

Empty Yin

The main manifestations of Emptiness of Yin are a feeling of heat in the afternoon or evening, a dry throat at night, night sweating, thin body, a Floating-Empty pulse and a tongue without coating.

Again, the above are only the general symptoms of Emptiness of Yin, other symptoms depending on which organ is mostly involved. The organs most likely to suffer from Yin Emptiness are the Kidneys, Lung, Heart, Liver and Stomach.

Other symptoms also depend on whether there is Empty-Heat or not. If the Yin deficiency is severe, after some time, Empty-Heat will develop, causing (in addition to the above symptoms of Yin deficiency) the following symptoms: a low-grade fever, a feeling of heat in the evening, five-palm heat and a Red tongue.

Yin also moistens, hence the symptoms of dryness such as dry throat and tongue.

Box 30.17 summarizes the clinical manifestations of Empty Yin.

> **Box 30.17 Empty Yin**
>
> - Feeling of heat in the afternoon or evening, a dry throat at night, night sweating, thin body, a Floating-Empty pulse and a Red-Peeled and dry tongue

Case history 30.9

A woman of 45 suffered from dizziness, night sweating, soreness of the lower back and a slight tinnitus. Her pulse was Fine and her tongue was of a normal colour with a rootless coating.

These manifestations point to deficiency of Kidney-Yin and Stomach-Yin (the 'rootless' coating indicates deficiency of Stomach-Yin).

Case history 30.10

A young woman of 31 had had a severe abdominal and hypogastric pain 6 months prior to examination. During that attack she doubled up in spasms and had a slight temperature. Afterwards her stools became loose and she felt very weak. The abdominal pain would occasionally return after exertion, in the right iliac fossa, and was worse with pressure. She also developed a vaginal discharge. Her appetite was poor and her legs felt weak and she was exhausted in general. During the last 2 months she had experienced some bleeding in between periods and a slight swelling of the ankles. The tongue was peeled except for some thin yellow coating in the centre. There were ice-floe cracks on the root while the tongue body was thin. Her pulse was Rapid, Slippery, slightly Floating-Empty and both Rear positions were Fine but also slightly Wiry. Her voice was very weak and she generally appeared weak and withdrawn.

This rather complicated case is introduced here to illustrate the intricate web of Emptiness and Fullness appearing simultaneously. First of all, the sudden onset of abdominal pain with slight temperature probably indicated an invasion of exterior Damp-Heat. However, she must have obviously suffered from previous Spleen-Qi deficiency: this is apparent by the Empty and Fine pulse, the general exhaustion and the weak voice. The Spleen-Qi deficiency had led to the formation of Dampness, hence the vaginal discharge.

Besides the Spleen deficiency, she must have also suffered from Kidney-Yin deficiency: this is apparent from the peeled tongue, the cracks on the root of the tongue, the Floating-Empty and Rapid pulse and the swollen ankles. This last sign is usually a sign of Kidney-Yang deficiency, but as explained before, it is not at all unusual to have a mixture of symptoms and signs from Kidney-Yin and -Yang deficiency: this happens because Kidney-Yin and Kidney-Yang share the same root and a deficiency of one often causes a secondary deficiency of the other. In this case there is a primary deficiency of Kidney-Yin and a secondary deficiency of Kidney-Yang (swollen ankles). How can a young person of 31 suffer from such severe Kidney-Yin deficiency? On interrogation, it became apparent that, for many years, she had worked very hard and long hours. Her work also involved a lot of lifting, which, over a long period of time, injured the Kidneys while overworking injured Kidney-Yin. However, lifting can also cause stagnation of Qi in the Lower Burner. This concurrent factor (together with the exterior Damp-Heat) accounts for her severe abdominal pain. Had the pain been caused only by Damp-Heat, it would have been less severe.

The bleeding in between periods more recently was due to deficiency of Qi and Yin failing to hold Blood.

To summarize, this case shows a mixture of Emptiness of Qi (Spleen) and Yin (Kidneys) with Fullness in the form of Damp-Heat. It also shows a mixture of exterior and interior conditions, as the Damp-Heat originally arose from an exterior invasion, but, due to the previously present Spleen-Qi deficiency, was transformed into interior Dampness.

YIN–YANG

The categories of Yin and Yang within the Eight Principles have two meanings: in a general sense, they are a summarization of the other six, whilst in a specific sense they are used mostly in Emptiness of Yin and Yang and Collapse of Yin and Yang.

Yin and Yang are a generalization of the other six Principles since Interior, Emptiness and Cold are Yin and Exterior, Fullness and Heat are Yang in nature.

In a specific sense, the categories of Yin and Yang can define two kinds of Emptiness and also two kinds of Collapse. Emptiness of Yin and Yang have already been described above.

Collapse of Yin or Yang simply indicates an extremely severe and sudden state of Emptiness. It also implies a complete separation of Yin and Yang from each other. Collapse of Yin or Yang is often, but not necessarily, followed by death.

Collapse of Yin

The main manifestations are abundant perspiration, skin hot to the touch, hot limbs, a dry mouth with desire to drink cold liquids in small sips, retention of urine, constipation, a Floating-Empty and Rapid pulse and a Red-Peeled, Short and Dry tongue.

Collapse of Yang

The main manifestations are chilliness, cold limbs, weak breathing, profuse sweating with an oily sweat, no thirst, frequent profuse urination or incontinence, loose stools or incontinence, a Minute-Deep pulse and a Pale-Wet-Swollen-Short tongue.

The following are two rather complicated case histories to illustrate the interaction of the Eight Principles in the same condition.

Case history 30.11

A woman of 45 suffered from persistent and profuse uterine bleeding. The bleeding started with each period and then continued for 3 weeks. The blood was dark at first and then clear-coloured and there was pain. She also experienced premenstrual tension, irritability (she said 'she could kill someone') and swelling of the breasts. She felt very tired most of the time, did not sleep well and sweated at night. She also complained of frequent urination, having to pass water twice at night. Her bowels had been loose for 3 years and she felt thirsty. Asked whether she felt either hot or cold she answered 'both'. She was overweight. Her pulse was Deep, Weak and both Rear positions were very Weak. Her tongue was slightly Red tending to Purple, but also slightly Pale on the sides. It was peeled in the centre and there was a rootless coating on the root, and the root itself had no 'spirit'. There were cracks in the centre and root.

These clinical manifestations paint a very complicated picture. What is apparent from the pulse and tongue first is deficiency of Stomach- and Kidney-Yin: the absence of 'spirit' on the root, the rootless coating on the root, the cracks on the root, the night sweating and the thirst all point to Kidney-Yin deficiency. The peeled and cracked centre indicates Stomach-Yin deficiency. The Kidney deficiency is also confirmed by the very Deep and Weak pulse on the Rear positions. Contradicting the Yin deficiency are frequent urination, pale sides of the tongue, sometimes feeling cold, and the diarrhoea. The frequent urination, nocturia, feeling cold and diarrhoea are due to Kidney-Yang deficiency. It is not at all uncommon to have both Kidney-Yin and -Yang deficiency as they share the same root and a deficiency of one often causes a lesser deficiency of the other. In this case, the deficiency of Kidney-Yin is predominant at the moment (judging from tongue and pulse). The deficiency of both Kidney-Yin and -Yang explains why she feels hot sometimes and cold other times.

The reddish-purple colour of the tongue, the painful periods with dark blood initially and premenstrual tension indicate stagnation of Liver-Qi and -Blood. The stasis of Liver-Blood was probably a consequence of a long-standing deficiency of Liver-Blood, which is apparent from the pale colour of the sides of the tongue and her tiredness.

The profuse and persistent bleeding is caused by deficiency of Qi and Yin unable to hold blood. This is a Deficient type of bleeding, hence the clear colour of the blood after the initial darkness.

In conclusion, this case shows Deficiency (of Kidneys, Stomach and Liver-Blood), Excess (stasis of Blood), Yin deficiency (of Kidneys and Stomach), Yang deficiency (of Kidneys too), Cold symptoms (diarrhoea, frequent urination, feeling cold) and Hot symptoms (feeling hot). Thus it shows Fullness and Emptiness, Heat and Cold, Yin and Yang simultaneously.

Case history 30.12

A young man of 18 had suffered from epilepsy since the age of 11. The attacks were characterized by severe convulsions and passing out with foaming at the mouth. He also suffered from migraine headaches, tinnitus and irritability. His pulse was Fine, Rapid and slightly Wiry. His tongue was Red, redder at the sides, Stiff and with a thick, sticky, yellow coating.

There was some contradiction between the pulse, the tongue and the symptoms. The tongue indicates a Full-Heat condition (Red with coating) and the presence of Phlegm (sticky coating). It also indicates Liver-Fire (redder on the sides). Both of these are Full patterns (Liver-Fire and Phlegm). The pulse is Fine, which indicates deficiency of Blood.

The Phlegm originates from a long-standing deficiency of Spleen-Qi' which means that he fails to produce Blood and this causes Liver-Blood deficiency (hence the Fine pulse). The deficiency of Liver-Blood leads to the rising of Liver-Yang and the stirring of Liver-Wind, hence the epileptic convulsions. His epilepsy is therefore traceable to two concurrent causes: the stirring up of Liver-Wind and Phlegm misting the brain. The stirring of Liver-Wind causes the convulsions, while the Phlegm misting the brain causes unconsciousness during the attacks.

In conclusion, this condition is characterized by Emptiness (of Spleen-Qi and Liver-Blood) and Fullness (Liver-Wind and Phlegm).

Learning outcomes

In this chapter you will have learned:
- The historical background of identifying patterns according to the Eight Principles
- How identification of patterns according to the Eight Principles can always be applied in all cases
- The importance of not being too rigid in the application of the Eight Principles, and to avoid an 'either/or' approach
- How to identify a disharmony in terms of Exterior–Interior, according to the location of the disease
- The definition of the 'Exterior' of the body and 'exterior' patterns with their typical clinical manifestations
- The definition of 'interior' patterns, and changes which happen when a pathogenic factor moves from the Exterior to the Interior of the body
- How to recognize the causes and manifestations of Hot and Cold patterns, according to whether they are combined with a Full or Empty pattern
- The identification of patterns characterized by the simultaneous presence of Heat and Cold
- How to identify the Full/Empty nature of a condition, according to the presence or absence of a pathogenic factor and the strength of the body's Qi
- The clinical manifestations of different Empty patterns: Empty Qi, Empty Yang, Empty Blood and Empty Yin
- Identification of patterns according to Yin and Yang, both in summary of the other six principles, and specifically to identify Collapse of Yin and Yang

Self-assessment questions

1. Define the 'Exterior' of the body and explain what is meant by an 'exterior' pattern.
2. What are the two most characteristic clinical manifestations arising from invasion of the Exterior by a pathogenic factor?
3. What are the main signs that differentiate the Hot or Cold character of an exterior pattern?
4. How might you tell whether an exterior pattern is Full or Empty?
5. What symptom would tell you that a pathogenic factor had progressed into the Interior?
6. Give three clinical manifestations of an internal condition of Full-Heat.
7. How do the mental–emotional symptoms characterizing Full-Heat differ from those of Empty-Heat?
8. Give as many clinical manifestations of internal Full-Cold as you can.

9. A patient presents feeling cold, with loose stools, a pale and swollen tongue and a Deep and Slow pulse. What pattern do you suspect and what is its nature in terms of Hot/Cold and Full/Empty?
10. How would you describe the following clinical manifestations in terms of the Eight Principles: thirst, irritability, sour regurgitation, bitter taste, mouth ulcers, loose stools, borborygmi and profuse pale urine.
11. Define the Full and the Empty condition.
12. Give three general signs of an Empty condition.
13. Give three manifestations of Empty Blood.

See p. 1263 for answers

END NOTES

1. 1979 The Yellow Emperor's Classic of Internal Medicine – Simple Questions (*Huang Di Nei Jing Su Wen* 黄帝内经素问), People's Health Publishing House, Beijing, first published *c.*100 BC, p. 341.
2. Ibid., p. 334.

Identification of Patterns according to Qi–Blood–Body Fluids

SECTION 1 PART 6

31

Key contents

Qi pattern identification
Qi deficiency
Qi sinking
Qi stagnation
Rebellious Qi

Blood pattern identification
Deficiency of Blood
Stasis of Blood
- Liver
- Heart
- Lungs
- Stomach
- Intestines
- Uterus

Heat in the Blood
Loss of Blood

Body Fluid pattern identification
Deficiency of Body Fluids
- Lungs
- Stomach
- Kidneys
- Large Intestine

Oedema
Phlegm
- Substantial versus non-substantial Phlegm
  - Substantial Phlegm
  - Non-substantial Phlegm
    - Under the skin
    - In the channels
    - Misting the Heart
    - In Gall Bladder or Kidneys
    - In the joints

- Types of Phlegm according to nature
  - Damp-Phlegm
  - Phlegm-Heat
  - Cold-Phlegm
  - Wind-Phlegm
  - Qi-Phlegm
  - Phlegm-Fluids
    - In the Stomach and Intestines
    - In the hypochondrium
    - In the limbs
    - Above the diaphragm

Pattern identification according to Qi, Blood and Body Fluids is based on the pathological changes of these Vital Substances. These patterns describe the clinical manifestations arising when Qi, Blood or Body Fluids are in a pathological state.

There is some overlap between these patterns and those according to the Eight Principles and Internal Organs. For example, the pattern of Qi deficiency is essentially the same as Qi deficiency according to the Eight Principles. The patterns according to Qi, Blood and Body Fluids are important as they complete the clinical picture emerging from the Eight-Principle and Internal Organ patterns.

Identification of patterns according to Qi–Blood–Body Fluids will be discussed under the following headings:

- Qi pattern identification
  - Qi deficiency
  - Qi sinking
  - Qi stagnation
  - Rebellious Qi

- Blood pattern identification
  - Deficiency of Blood
  - Stasis of Blood
    - Liver
    - Heart
    - Lungs
    - Stomach
    - Intestines
    - Uterus
  - Heat in the Blood
  - Loss of Blood
- Body Fluid pattern identification
  - Deficiency of Body Fluids
    - Lungs
    - Stomach
    - Kidneys
    - Large Intestine
  - Oedema
  - Phlegm
    - Substantial versus non-substantial Phlegm
      - Substantial Phlegm
      - Non-substantial Phlegm
        - Under the skin
        - In the channels
        - Misting the Heart
        - In Gall Bladder or Kidneys
        - In the joints
    - Types of Phlegm according to nature
      - Damp-Phlegm
      - Phlegm-Heat
      - Cold-Phlegm
      - Wind-Phlegm
      - Qi-Phlegm
      - Phlegm-Fluids
        - Phlegm-Fluids in the Stomach and Intestines
        - Phlegm-Fluids in the hypochondrium
        - Phlegm-Fluids in the limbs
        - Phlegm-Fluids above the diaphragm

QI PATTERN IDENTIFICATION

The pathological patterns of Qi disharmonies can be:

- Deficiency of Qi
- Sinking of Qi
- Stagnation of Qi
- Rebellious Qi

Qi deficiency

Clinical manifestations: these include slight shortness of breath, weak voice, spontaneous sweating, poor appetite, loose stools, tiredness, Empty pulse.

These are the symptoms and signs of Lung- and Spleen-Qi deficiency. Obviously, there can be Qi deficiency of other organs too. Heart-Qi deficiency is marked by palpitations, whilst Kidney-Qi deficiency leads to frequent urination. As mentioned in the chapter on the Eight Principles (ch. 30), it is customary to list only the symptoms of Lung- and Spleen-Qi deficiency: first, because they are more common and, secondly, because the Lungs govern Qi and the Spleen is the source of Qi through its activity of transformation and transportation. The patterns of Qi deficiency of the Heart and Kidneys are discussed in chapters 32 and 37.

Clinical note

Ren-6 Qihai and ST-36 Zusanli can tonify Qi in general

Box 31.1 summarizes Qi deficiency.

Box 31.1 Qi deficiency

- Slight shortness of breath, weak voice, spontaneous sweating, poor appetite, loose stools, tiredness, Empty pulse

Qi sinking

Clinical manifestations: these include feeling of bearing down, tiredness, listlessness, mental depression, prolapse of organs (stomach, uterus, intestines, anus, vagina or bladder), Empty pulse.

In addition to the above symptoms, there can be any of the other symptoms of Qi deficiency. 'Qi sinking' is, in fact, only a particular aspect of Qi deficiency and not essentially separate from it. In 'Qi sinking' therefore, Qi deficiency is implicit.

This distinction needs to be made, however, as when it comes to treatment, it is necessary not only to tonify but also to raise Qi. There are particular herbs and acupuncture points (such as Du-20 Baihui with moxa) that have this effect.

Box 31.2 summarizes Qi sinking.

Clinical note

The point Du-20 Baihui may be used with moxa to raise Qi in cases of Qi sinking

---

Box 31.2 Qi sinking

- Slight shortness of breath, weak voice, spontaneous sweating, poor appetite, loose stools, tiredness, a feeling of bearing down, mental depression, listlessness, prolapse of an organ, Empty pulse

---

Qi stagnation

Clinical manifestations: these include feeling of distension, distending pain that moves from place to place, mental depression, irritability, gloomy feeling, frequent mood swings, frequent sighing, Wiry pulse, tongue body either normal-coloured or slightly Red on the sides.

These are only the general but essential and distinctive symptoms of Qi stagnation. The feeling of distension (called *zhang* in Chinese), which can affect the throat, hypochondrium, chest, epigastrium, abdomen and hypogastrium, is the most characteristic and important of the symptoms of Qi stagnation. (English-speaking patients would generally use the word 'bloating' rather than 'distension'.) Emotional symptoms are very characteristic and frequent in stagnation of Qi, particularly of Liver-Qi.

Distension is the cardinal symptom of Qi stagnation

Other symptoms and signs depend on the organ involved. The Liver is the main organ affected by Qi stagnation and, indeed, Liver-Qi stagnation is very commonly seen in practice. However, it should be stressed that other organs suffer from Qi stagnation, for example the Heart, Lungs, Stomach and Intestines.

Box 31.3 summarizes Qi stagnation. Qi stagnation is also discussed in chapter 27.

Rebellious Qi

Rebellious Qi occurs when Qi flows in the wrong direction (i.e. a direction different from its normal physiological one). Although Qi sinking may be seen as a type

---

Box 31.3 Qi stagnation

- Feeling of distension, distending pain that moves from place to place, mental depression, irritability, gloomy feeling, frequent mood swings, frequent sighing, Wiry pulse, tongue body either normal-coloured or slightly Red on the sides

---

of rebellious Qi in so far as it is wrong flow of Spleen-Qi (downwards instead of upwards), the term 'rebellious' Qi is usually used to refer to the wrong upwards flow of Qi.

The normal direction of Qi varies from organ to organ, as each has its own normal direction of flow of Qi, but the majority of them flow downwards. This has been described in chapters 3 and 4. To summarize briefly, the normal direction of flow of each organ is as follows:

- Spleen-Qi: upwards
- Stomach-Qi: downwards
- Lung-Qi: downwards
- Heart-Qi: downwards
- Liver-Qi: in all directions and upwards
- Intestines Qi: downwards
- Kidney-Qi: downwards (but from some aspects also upwards)
- Bladder-Qi: downwards

The different kinds of rebellious Qi and their clinical manifestations are summarized in Table 31.1 and directions and manifestation of these are illustrated in Figures 31.1–31.6.

As in the case of sinking Qi, the identification of rebellious Qi is important from the point of view of treatment as there are herbs and specific acupuncture points to subdue rebellious Qi. A well-known acupuncture point that subdues Qi is at the opposite end of Du-20 Baihui (which lifts Qi): that is, KI-1 Yongquan.

The pathology of rebellious Qi is discussed also in chapter 29.

BLOOD PATTERN IDENTIFICATION

The Blood pathology patterns are:

- Deficiency of Blood
- Stasis of Blood
- Heat in the Blood
- Loss of Blood

Table 31.1 Rebellious Qi types

Organ	Normal Qi direction	Pathological Qi direction	Symptoms and signs
Stomach	Downwards	Upwards	Belching, hiccup, nausea, vomiting
Spleen	Upwards	Downwards	Diarrhoea, prolapse
Liver	Upwards	i) Excessive upwards ii) Horizontally – to Stomach – to Spleen – to Intestines iii) Downwards	Headache, dizziness, irritability Nausea, belching, vomiting Diarrhoea Dry stools Burning urination
Lungs	Downwards	Upwards	Cough, asthma
Kidneys	Downwards	Upwards	Asthma
Heart	Downwards	Upwards	Mental restlessness, insomnia

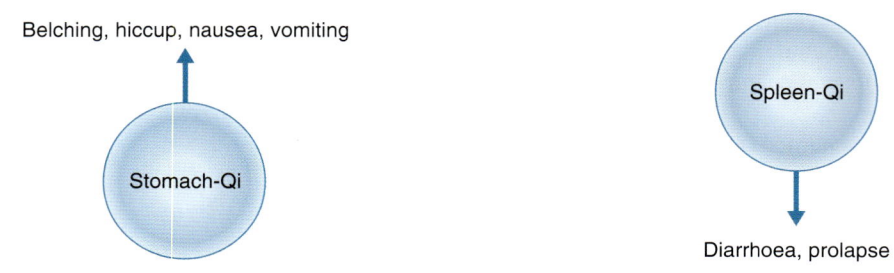

Figure 31.1 Rebellious Qi of Stomach

Figure 31.2 Rebellious Qi of Spleen

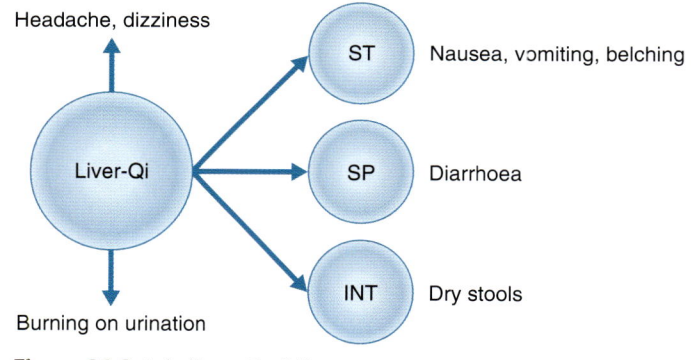

Figure 31.3 Rebellious Qi of Liver

Figure 31.4 Rebellious Qi of Lungs

Figure 31.5 Rebellious Qi of Kidneys

Anxiety, mental restlessness, insomnia

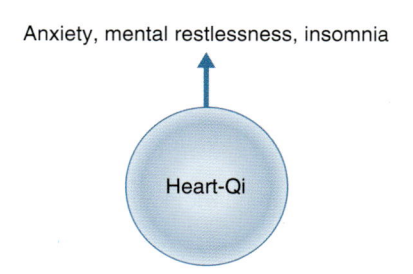

Heart-Qi

Figure 31.6 Rebellious Qi of Heart

Deficiency of Blood

Clinical manifestations: these include dull-white-sallow complexion, dizziness, poor memory, numbness or tingling, blurred vision, insomnia, pale lips, scanty periods or amenorrhoea, depression, slight anxiety, Pale and slightly dry tongue, Choppy or Fine pulse.

Several organs are involved in the making of Blood and chiefly the Spleen, Kidneys and Liver: therefore Blood deficiency is usually combined with a deficiency of one or more of these organs. Liver-Blood deficiency is the most common one and it is especially common in women.

Once Liver-Blood becomes deficient, it may affect particularly the Heart. The above symptoms are mixed symptoms of deficiencies of Liver-Blood (numbness, blurred vision, dizziness, scanty periods) and Heart-Blood (sallow complexion, poor memory, insomnia, depression, slight anxiety).

In severe and long-standing cases, deficiency of Blood can further lead to some dryness as Blood is part of Yin. This manifests with a particularly dry tongue, dry skin, dry hair and withered nails. In other cases, the long-standing dryness of the Blood can give rise to Wind in the skin, which, combined with dryness, can cause some skin diseases characterized by dry and itchy skin.

Liver-Blood deficiency is a frequent cause of Liver-Yang rising (especially in women); finally, Liver-Blood deficiency may also give rise to internal Wind, which manifests with vertigo, tics and fine tremors (Fig. 31.7).

Clinical note

Ren-4 Guanyuan, ST-36 Zusanli, LIV-8 Ququan and SP-6 Sanyinjiao can nourish Blood in general

Box 31.4 summarizes Blood deficiency.

> **Box 31.4 Blood deficiency**
> - Dull-white sallow complexion, dizziness, poor memory, numbness or tingling, blurred vision, insomnia, pale lips, scanty periods or amenorrhoea, depression, slight anxiety, Pale and slightly dry tongue, Choppy or Fine pulse

Stasis of Blood

Clinical manifestations: these include dark complexion, purple lips, pain which is boring, fixed and stabbing in character, abdominal masses that do not move, purple nails, bleeding with dark blood and dark clots, painful periods with dark clots, Purple tongue, Wiry, Firm or Choppy pulse.

These are only the general symptoms of stasis of Blood, without specific reference to particular organs. One of the main distinguishing symptoms of stasis of Blood is pain that is fixed in one place, and is of

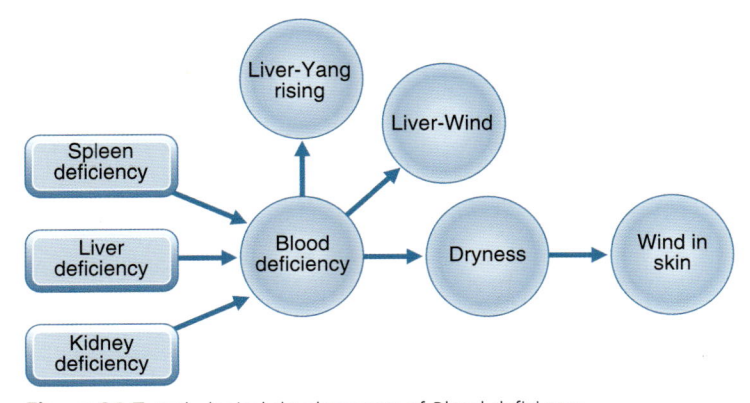

Figure 31.7 Pathological developments of Blood deficiency

a boring or stabbing character. It is useful here to compare and contrast stagnation of Qi with stasis of Blood (Table 31.2).

The organ that is most frequently affected by stasis of Blood is the Liver. Other affected organs are the Heart, Lungs, Stomach, Intestines and Uterus. The symptoms and signs for each of these organs are as follows:

Liver

Purple nails, dark face, painful periods with dark menstrual blood with dark clots, abdominal pain, premenstrual pain, Purple tongue especially on the sides, Wiry or Firm pulse.

Heart

Purple lips, stabbing or pricking pain in the chest, mental restlessness, Purple tongue on the sides towards the front, purple and distended veins under the tongue, Choppy or Knotted pulse.

Lungs

Feeling of oppression of the chest, coughing of dark blood, tongue purple on the sides towards the front part, purple and distended veins under the tongue.

Stomach

Epigastric pain, vomiting of dark blood, dark blood in stools, tongue Purple in the centre.

Intestines

Severe abdominal pain, dark blood in stools.

Uterus

Painful periods, premenstrual pain, dark menstrual blood with dark clots, amenorrhoea, fixed abdominal masses, Purple tongue, Wiry or Firm pulse.

Box 31.5 summarizes Blood stasis.

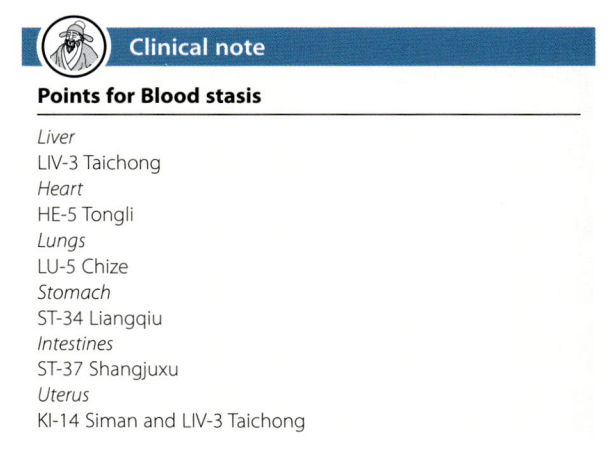

> **Clinical note**
>
> **Points for Blood stasis**
>
> *Liver*
> LIV-3 Taichong
> *Heart*
> HE-5 Tongli
> *Lungs*
> LU-5 Chize
> *Stomach*
> ST-34 Liangqiu
> *Intestines*
> ST-37 Shangjuxu
> *Uterus*
> KI-14 Siman and LIV-3 Taichong

Stasis of Blood can derive from (Fig. 31.8):

1. *Stagnation of Qi*: this is the most common cause of stasis of Blood. Qi moves Blood, if Qi stagnates Blood stagnates

Table 31.2 Comparison between Stagnation of Qi and Stasis of Blood

	Stagnation of Qi	Stasis of blood
Pain/distension	More distension than pain	More pain than distension
Location	Moving pain	Fixed pain
Character	Distending pain	Boring or stabbing pain
Abdominal masses	Appearing and disappearing	Fixed
Skin	Not appearing on skin	May manifest with purple blotches or bruises
Face	May be unchanged	Dark colour or bluish-green
Tongue	Normal colour or slightly red	Purple on the sides
Pulse	Wiry	Wiry, Firm or Choppy

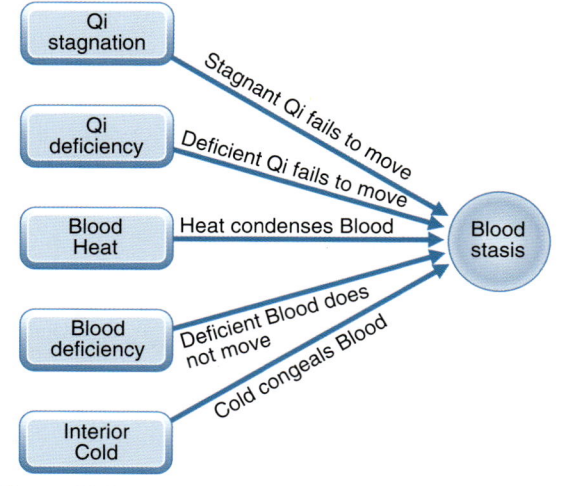

Figure 31.8 Causes of Blood stasis

Box 31.5 Stasis of Blood

Dark complexion, purple lips, pain which is boring, fixed and stabbing in character, abdominal masses that do not move, purple nails, bleeding with dark blood and dark clots, painful periods with dark clots, Purple tongue, Wiry, Firm or Choppy pulse.

Liver

Purple nails, dark face, painful periods with dark menstrual blood with dark clots, abdominal pain, premenstrual pain, Purple tongue especially on the sides, Wiry or Firm pulse

Heart

Purple lips, stabbing or pricking pain in the chest, mental restlessness, Purple tongue on the sides towards the front, purple and distended veins under the tongue, Choppy or Knotted pulse

Lungs

Feeling of oppression of the chest, coughing of dark blood, tongue Purple on the sides towards the front part, purple and distended veins under the tongue

Stomach

Epigastric pain, vomiting of dark blood, dark blood in stools, tongue Purple in the centre

Intestines

Severe abdominal pain, dark blood in stools

Uterus

Painful periods, premenstrual pain, dark menstrual blood with dark clots, amenorrhoea, fixed abdominal masses, Purple tongue, Wiry or Firm pulse

---

2. *Deficiency of Qi:* deficiency of Qi over a long period of time may cause stasis of Blood as Qi becomes too weak to move Blood
3. *Heat in the Blood:* Heat in the Blood may cause the Blood to condense and stagnate
4. *Blood deficiency:* if Blood is deficient over a long period of time, it will induce Qi deficiency and subsequently stasis of Blood, from impairment of the Qi moving function
5. *Interior Cold:* this slows down the circulation of Blood and congeals Blood (see Fig. 31.8)
6. *Phlegm:* although Phlegm does not directly cause Blood stasis, it aggravates it

Heat in the Blood

Clinical manifestations: these include feeling of heat, skin diseases with red eruptions, thirst, bleeding, Red tongue, Rapid pulse.

These are only the general symptoms of Blood Heat. Others may be present according to the organ involved.

If Heart-Blood has Heat, there will be anxiety, mental restlessness and mouth ulcers. If Liver-Blood has Heat, there will be skin diseases characterized by itching, heat and redness. This is one of the most common types of skin diseases.

If the Blood Heat affects the Uterus and the Penetrating Vessel, there will be excessive blood loss during the periods. If there is Blood Heat in the Intestines, there will be blood in the stools.

Blood stasis is discussed also in chapter 27. Figure 31.9 illustrates the manifestations of Blood Heat and Box 31.6 summarizes Blood Heat.

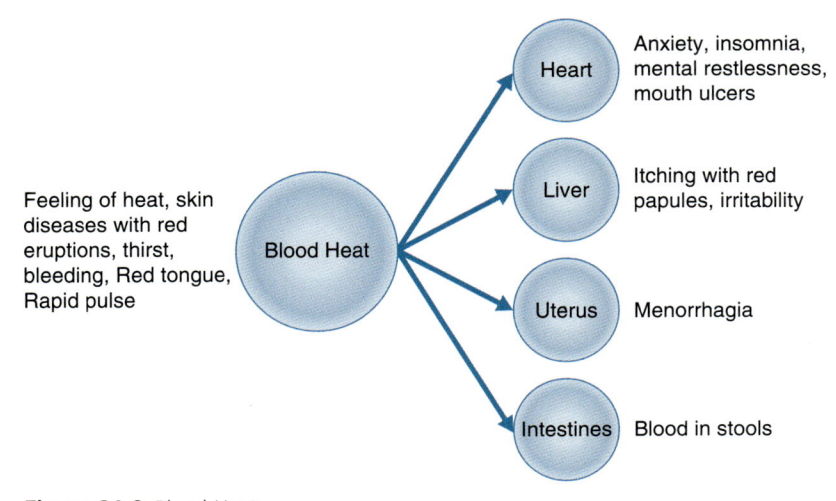

Figure 31.9 Blood Heat

Box 31.6 Blood Heat

Feeling of heat, skin diseases with red eruptions, thirst, bleeding, Red tongue, Rapid pulse

Heart-Blood Heat

Anxiety, mental restlessness and mouth ulcers

Liver-Blood Heat

Skin diseases characterized by itching, heat and redness

Blood Heat in Uterus

Excessive blood loss during the periods

Blood Heat in the Intestines

Blood in the stools

> **Clinical note**
>
> The points LIV-2 Xingjian and SP-10 Xuehai can cool Blood. Another combination is LIV-3 Taichong with KI-2 Rangu.

Loss of Blood

Clinical manifestations: these include epistaxis, haematemesis, haemoptysis, melaena, menorrhagia, metrorrhagia, haematuria.

Loss of Blood can occur from two main causes: either because deficient Qi is unable to hold Blood, or because Blood Heat pushes blood out of the vessels. The former is a Deficiency type, the latter an Excess type of loss of Blood. Two other less common causes of bleeding are stasis of Blood and Yin deficiency. These can be differentiated (Table 31.3).

Box 31.7 summarizes loss of Blood.

Table 31.3 Differentiation of causes of haemorrhage

Cause	Colour of blood	Quantity
Heat in blood	Fresh red or dark	Heavy loss
Stasis of blood	Very dark with clots	Scanty loss
Qi deficiency	Pale	Heavy loss, prolonged
Yin deficiency	Bright-red	Scanty

Box 31.7 Loss of Blood

- Epistaxis, haematemesis, haemoptysis, melaena, menorrhagia, metrorrhagia, haematuria

BODY FLUID PATTERN IDENTIFICATION

The Body Fluids pathological patterns are:

- Deficiency of Body Fluids
- Oedema
- Phlegm

Dampness is also a pathology of Body Fluids but, as it can also be of external origin, this will be discussed in chapter 43 (Identification of patterns according to pathogenic factors).

Deficiency of Body Fluids

Clinical manifestations: these include dry skin, mouth, nose, cough, lips, dry tongue.

Body Fluids are part of Yin and their deficiency always causes a condition of dryness. This is not quite the same as Yin deficiency and it can be the condition preceding Yin deficiency. Deficiency of Body Fluids may be considered as a mild form of Yin deficiency.

Deficiency of Body Fluids can also, on the other hand, derive from Yin deficiency: if Yin is deficient over a long period of time, Body Fluids will become deficient too.

Deficiency of Body Fluids may be caused by dietary factors (excessive consumption of drying foods such as baked foods, or irregular eating). Deficiency of Body Fluids may also arise from a heavy and prolonged loss of fluids such as in sweating (as during a febrile disease), vomiting and diarrhoea.

As there is a constant interchange between fluids and Blood, deficiency of fluids can also derive from a heavy, acute loss of Blood, such as during childbirth, or from a heavy, chronic loss of Blood such as in menorrhagia.

Finally, severe and chronic deficiency of Blood can cause dryness and deficiency of fluids (Fig. 31.10).

Deficiency of fluids affects mostly the Lungs, Stomach, Kidneys and Large Intestine.

> **Clinical note**
>
> In deficiency of Body Fluids, I nourish first of all Stomach-Yin with Ren-12 Zhongwan, ST-36 Zusanli and SP-6 Sanyinjiao.

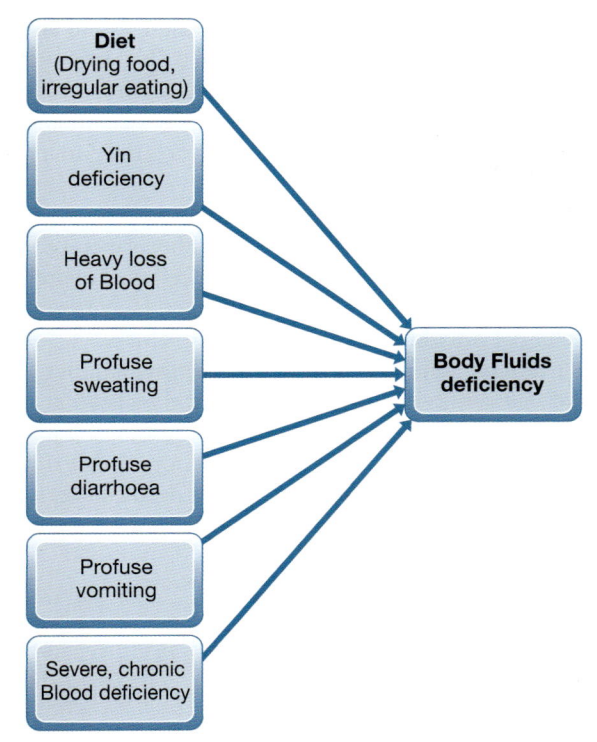

Figure 31.10 Causes of Body Fluids deficiency

Box 31.8 Deficiency of Body Fluids

Dry skin, mouth, nose, cough, lips, dry tongue

Lungs

Dry skin and dry cough

Stomach

Dry tongue with horizontal cracks and a dry mouth but without desire to drink, or with a desire to drink in small sips

Kidneys

Scanty urination, a dry mouth at night and a dry throat

Large Intestine

Dry stools

Lungs

The main symptoms are dry skin and dry cough.

Stomach

The Stomach is the origin of fluids and a deficiency of Stomach-Qi and particularly Stomach-Yin will induce a deficiency of Body Fluids. The main symptoms are a dry tongue with horizontal cracks and a dry mouth but without desire to drink, or with a desire to drink in small sips.

Kidneys

The Kidneys govern Water and deficiency of Kidney-Yin causes dryness and deficiency of Body Fluids. The main symptoms are scanty urination, a dry mouth at night and a dry throat.

Large Intestine

The Large Intestine is related to the Stomach within the Bright Yang and a deficiency of fluids of the Stomach is easily transmitted to the Large Intestine. The main symptoms are dry stools.

Box 31.8 summarizes deficiency of Body Fluids.

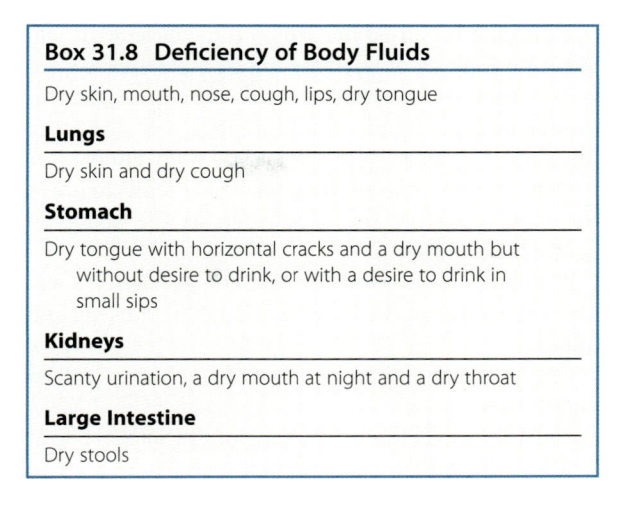

Oedema

Oedema consists of swelling due to the retention of fluids outside the cells. From the Chinese perspective, it is due to the leaking of fluids from their normal pathways into the space between skin and muscles. The swelling from oedema is usually pitting: that is, if we press with a finger, it leaves a dip that takes a long time to disappear.

Oedema arises from a Yang deficiency of either Spleen, Lungs or Kidneys or all three of them. Lungs, Spleen and Kidneys are the three organs that are mostly involved in the transformation and transportation of fluids. If one or more of these organs is deficient, the Body Fluids are not transformed properly; they overflow out of the channels and settle in the space under the skin. This is the origin of oedema (Fig. 31.11).

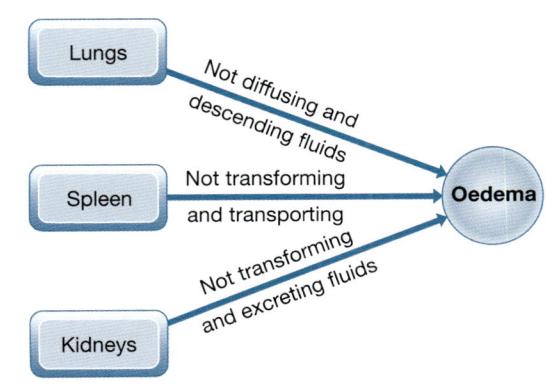

Figure 31.11 Causes of oedema

If oedema is caused by Lung-Yang deficiency it will affect the top part of the body, for example the face and hands. This type of oedema can also be caused by invasion of exterior Wind-Cold interfering with the Lung function of diffusing and descending Body Fluids.

Oedema from Spleen-Yang deficiency tends to affect the middle part of the body, such as the abdomen (ascites) and limbs.

If oedema is caused by Kidney-Yang deficiency, it will affect the lower part of the body, such as the legs and ankles.

Box 31.9 summarizes oedema of the Lungs, Spleen and Kidneys.

Oedema from deficiency of Yang of the Spleen, Lungs and Kidneys is the most common type. There are two other, less common causes of oedema, namely Qi stagnation and Dampness: in these two cases, the oedema is non-pitting.

> **Clinical note**
>
> The main points for oedema are Ren-9 Shuifen, Ren-5 Shimen, SP-9 Yinlingquan and BL-22 Sanjiaoshu.

Box 31.10 summarizes oedema.

Phlegm

The concept of Phlegm is very wide-ranging and important in Chinese medicine. It is extremely frequent in clinical practice. Phlegm is at the same time a pathological condition and an aetiological factor. In fact, Phlegm which is retained over a long period of time becomes itself a cause of disease.

The main cause for the formation of Phlegm is Spleen deficiency. If the Spleen fails to transform and transport Body Fluids, these will accumulate and change into Phlegm. The Lungs and Kidneys are also involved in the formation of Phlegm. If the Lungs fail to diffuse and lower fluids, and if the Kidneys fail to transform and excrete fluids, these may accumulate into Phlegm. However, the Spleen is always the primary factor in the formation of Phlegm.

The essential signs of Phlegm are a Swollen tongue body, a sticky tongue coating and a Slippery or Wiry pulse. Other symptoms may include a feeling of oppression of the chest, nausea, a feeling of heaviness, a feeling of muzziness of the head and dizziness.

There are many ways of classifying Phlegm; here I will describe two of them. The first classification is according to the distinction between substantial and non-substantial Phlegm; the second is according to the association of Phlegm with other pathogenic factors.

Substantial versus non-substantial Phlegm

There are two types of Phlegm, one 'substantial', one 'non-substantial'. In the old classics, these were described as Phlegm 'having a form' and Phlegm 'without a form'.

Substantial Phlegm can be seen, such as the sputum that collects in the Lungs and is spat out during bronchitis or other lung diseases.

Non-substantial Phlegm can be retained subcutaneously or in the channels. It can obstruct the Heart orifices or the Gall Bladder or Kidneys in the form of stones. It can settle in the joints in the form of arthritic bone deformities.

The two types of Phlegm can be summarized as follows.

Substantial Phlegm

Substantial Phlegm is Phlegm in the Lungs.

Non-substantial Phlegm
Under the skin

This takes the form of lumps under the skin (although not all lumps are due to Phlegm), nerve ganglia swellings, swelling of lymph nodes, swelling of the thyroid and lipomas.

In the channels

Phlegm in the channels is not visible as a swelling, but it causes numbness. This is more common in old people and is frequently seen in Wind-stroke.

Box 31.9 Lung, Spleen and Kidney oedema

- *Lung-Yang deficiency:* oedema of face and hands
- *Spleen-Yang deficiency:* abdomen and limbs
- *Kidney-Yang deficiency:* lower part of the body, the legs and ankles

---

Box 31.10 Oedema

- *Pitting:* deficiency of Yang of Spleen, Lungs and/or Kidneys
- *Non-pitting:* Qi stagnation or Dampness

> **Box 31.11 Essential manifestations of Phlegm**
>
> - *Tongue and pulse*: Swollen tongue body with sticky tongue coating; Slippery or Wiry pulse
> - *Other symptoms*: a feeling of oppression of the chest, nausea, a feeling of heaviness, a feeling of muzziness of the head and dizziness

Box 31.11 summarizes the essential manifestations of Phlegm.

Misting the Heart

Non-substantial Phlegm can obstruct the Heart orifices and mist the Mind (*Shen*). In severe cases, this gives rise to some types of mental illness such as schizophrenia and manic depression and also to epilepsy. However, Phlegm misting the Mind may also occur in milder forms and cause mental confusion, depression or anxiety.

In Gall Bladder or Kidneys

Gall bladder or kidney stones are considered as a form of Phlegm, arising from the 'steaming and brewing' of Phlegm by Heat over a long period of time.

In the joints

The bone deformities that occur in chronic rheumatoid arthritis are seen as a form of Phlegm. When the fluids are not transformed and accumulate in the joints over a long period of time, they can give rise to Phlegm, and this can further condense to form bone growths.

Box 31.12 summarizes non-substantial Phlegm.

> **Box 31.12 Non-substantial Phlegm**
>
> **Under the skin**
>
> Lumps under the skin, nerve ganglia swellings, swelling of lymph nodes, swelling of the thyroid, lipoma
>
> **In the channels**
>
> Numbness
>
> **Misting the Heart**
>
> Mental illness
>
> **In Gall Bladder or Kidneys**
>
> Gall bladder or kidney stones
>
> **In the joints**
>
> Bone deformities in chronic rheumatoid arthritis

Phlegm (both substantial and non-substantial) can assume different forms, according to its associations with other pathogenic factors.

Types of Phlegm according to nature

The types of Phlegm discussed are (Table 31.4):

- Damp-Phlegm
- Phlegm-Heat
- Cold-Phlegm
- Wind-Phlegm
- Qi-Phlegm
- Phlegm-Fluids

Damp-Phlegm

This is manifested with expectoration of very profuse phlegm that is white and sticky and relatively easy to expectorate, a feeling of oppression of the chest and epigastrium, nausea, a sticky taste, no thirst, Swollen tongue with a sticky tongue coating and a Slippery pulse.

This form of Phlegm is seen in Lung patterns.

Phlegm-Heat

This is manifested with expectoration of sticky yellow phlegm, a feeling of oppression of the chest, nausea, a red face, dry mouth, restlessness, a Red and Swollen tongue with sticky yellow coating and a Rapid-Slippery pulse.

This form of Phlegm affects the Lungs, the Stomach or the Heart.

Table 31.4 Types of Phlegm

	Area affected
Damp-Phlegm in the Lungs	Internal Organs
Phlegm-Fire in the Stomach	Internal Organs
Phlegm misting the Heart	Internal Organs
Phlegm blocking the channels	Limbs
Phlegm under the skin	Skin
Phlegm in the joints	Joints

Cold-Phlegm

This is manifested with expectoration of white watery phlegm, a feeling of oppression of the chest, cold limbs, nausea, a Pale and Swollen tongue with white wet coating and a Deep-Slippery-Slow pulse.

This form of Phlegm is often seen in Stomach or Lung patterns.

Wind-Phlegm

This causes dizziness, nausea, vomiting, numbness of the limbs (especially unilateral), coughing of phlegm, a feeling of oppression of the chest, a rattling sound in the throat and aphasia, Swollen and Deviated tongue with sticky coating and a Wiry pulse.

This form of Phlegm is seen in Wind-stroke.

Qi-Phlegm

This type of Phlegm is non-substantial and is manifested with a feeling of swelling in the throat (but no actual swelling), a difficulty in swallowing, a feeling of oppression of chest and diaphragm, irritability, moodiness, depression and a Wiry pulse.

This form of Phlegm is usually associated with stagnation of Qi in the throat. It is caused by emotional problems giving rise to (or deriving from) stagnation of Liver-Qi. The typical feeling of constriction of the throat is called 'plum-stone syndrome' in Chinese medicine and this feeling appears and disappears according to mood swings.

Phlegm-Fluids

Finally, another form of Phlegm is called 'Yin' in Chinese medicine, which simply means 'fluids' or 'watery'. The term for 'Phlegm' (*tan yin*) is in fact composed of the two terms, *tan* being sticky, and *yin* being watery: the two terms *tan yin* together indicate either what I call 'Phlegm-Fluids' in general or the specific Phlegm-Fluids in the Stomach and Intestines. Clavey calls these 'thin mucus'.[1]

This is a type of substantial Phlegm characterized by white, very watery and thin sputum. It can sometimes actually be heard splashing in the body.

There are four kinds of Phlegm-Fluids:

1. Phlegm-Fluids in Stomach and Intestines

This is called *tan yin* in Chinese, meaning 'phlegm and fluids'. This is manifested with abdominal fullness and distension, vomiting of watery fluids, a dry tongue and mouth without desire to drink, a splashing sound in the stomach, a feeling of fullness of the chest, loose stools, loss of weight, a Deep-Slippery or Wiry pulse and a Swollen tongue with sticky coating.

2. Phlegm-Fluids in the hypochondrium

This is called *xuan yin* in Chinese, meaning 'suspended fluids'. This is manifested with hypochondrial pain that is worse on coughing and breathing, a feeling of distension of the hypochondrium, shortness of breath, a Swollen tongue with a sticky coating and a Deep-Wiry pulse.

3. Phlegm-Fluids in the limbs

This is called *yi yin* in Chinese, meaning 'flooding fluids'. This is manifested with a feeling of heaviness of the body, a pain in the muscles, no sweating, no desire to drink, a cough with abundant white sputum, a Swollen tongue with a sticky white coating and a Wiry pulse.

4. Phlegm-Fluids above the diaphragm

This is called *zhi yin* in Chinese, meaning 'prodding fluids'. This is manifested with a cough, asthma, oedema, a feeling of oppression of the chest, dizziness, abundant white sputum, a Swollen tongue with a sticky, thick white coating and a Wiry pulse. All the symptoms are aggravated by exposure to cold.

Phlegm is also discussed in chapter 27. Box 31.13 summarizes Phlegm.

> **Clinical note**
>
> The main points for Phlegm are Ren-9 Shuifen, Ren-5 Shimen, SP-9 Yinlingquan, ST-40 Fenglong and BL-22 Sanjiaoshu

Case history 31.1

A man of 32 suffered from tiredness, poor appetite, a feeling of muzziness (fuzziness) and heaviness of the head. He also experienced a feeling of oppression of the chest, lack of concentration and dizziness. His pulse was Empty but also slightly Slippery and his tongue was Pale and Swollen with a sticky coating.

These manifestations are due to deficiency of Spleen-Qi, leading to the formation of Phlegm (the non-substantial kind). The Phlegm causes the muzziness, heaviness, dizziness and inability to think clearly, as it obstructs the rising of clear Yang Qi to the head.

Box 31.13 Phlegm

Damp-Phlegm

Expectoration of very profuse, sticky white phlegm, a feeling of oppression of the chest and epigastrium, nausea, a sticky taste, no thirst, Swollen tongue with a sticky tongue coating and a Slippery pulse

Phlegm-Heat

Expectoration of sticky yellow phlegm, a feeling of oppression of the chest, nausea, a red face, dry mouth, restlessness, a Red and Swollen tongue with sticky yellow coating and a Rapid-Slippery pulse

Cold-Phlegm

Expectoration of white-watery phlegm, a feeling of oppression of the chest, cold limbs, nausea, a Pale and Swollen tongue with white wet coating and a Deep-Slippery-Slow pulse

Wind-Phlegm

Dizziness, nausea, vomiting, numbness of the limbs (especially unilateral), coughing of phlegm, a feeling of oppression of the chest, a rattling sound in the throat, aphasia, Swollen and Deviated tongue with sticky coating and a Wiry pulse

Qi-Phlegm

Feeling of swelling in the throat (but no actual swelling), a difficulty in swallowing, a feeling of oppression of chest and diaphragm, irritability, moodiness, depression, Wiry pulse

Phlegm-Fluids

Expectoration of very thin, watery sputum, dizziness, Swollen tongue with sticky coating, Wiry pulse

Learning outcomes

In this chapter you will have learned:
- How to identify the four pathological patterns of Qi disharmony: Qi deficiency, Qi sinking, Qi stagnantion and rebellious Qi
- Why Qi deficiency is characterized by symptoms of Lung- and Spleen-Qi deficiency
- The relationship between Qi sinking and Qi deficiency
- The importance of distension as a characteristic of Qi stagnation
- The various types of rebellious Qi
- How to identify the four Blood pathology patterns: Deficiency of Blood, Stasis of Blood, Heat in the Blood, loss of Blood
- The characteristics of various types of Blood stasis: of the Liver, Heart, Lungs, Stomach, Intestines and Uterus
- The causes of Blood stasis: Qi stagnation, Qi deficiency, Heat in the Blood, Blood deficiency or Internal Cold
- The various types of Heat in the Blood: Heart-Blood Heat, Liver-Blood Heat, Blood Heat in the Uterus and Blood Heat in the Intestines
- The causes and symptoms of loss of Blood
- How to identify the three types of pathological Body Fluid patterns: Deficiency of Body Fluids, Oedema and Phlegm
- The causes of deficiency of Body Fluids, and the importance of dryness as an identifying symptom
- The importance of Yang deficiency of the Lungs, Spleen and Kidneys in causing Oedema
- The significance of the concept of Phlegm in Chinese medicine, and its frequency in clinical practice
- The role of the Spleen, Lungs and Kidneys in the production of Phlegm
- The difference between substantial and non-substantial Phlegm
- How to identify the different types of Phlegm

Self-assessment questions

1. List the four pathological patterns of Qi disharmony.
2. Give three symptoms of Qi stagnation.
3. A patient presents with a sallow complexion, poor memory, insomnia, depression and slight anxiety. What pattern do you suspect?
4. Which organ is most frequently affected by stasis of Blood?
5. What are the characteristic manifestations of Liver-Blood Heat?
6. What dietary factors might lead to deficiency of Body Fluids?
7. What are the essential *signs* of Phlegm?
8. What is the main symptom of non-substantial Phlegm in the channels?
9. Which organs are commonly affected by Phlegm-Heat?
10. What are the main signs and symptoms of Qi-Phlegm?

See p. 1263 for answers

END NOTE

1. Clavey S 2003 Fluid Physiology and Pathology in Traditional Chinese Medicine. Churchill Livingstone, Edinburgh. This book is highly recommended as the most thorough discussion of Dampness, Phlegm and oedema.

SECTION 2

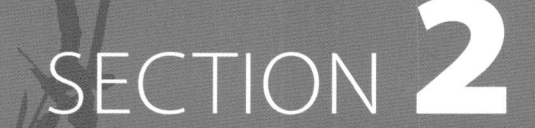

Identification of patterns according to the Internal Organs

INTRODUCTION

The identification of patterns according to the Internal Organs is based on the symptoms and signs arising when the Qi and Blood of the Internal Organs are out of balance.

This method of identification of patterns is used mostly for interior and chronic conditions, but it also includes a few exterior and acute patterns.

The Internal Organs patterns are an application of the Eight-Principle method of pattern identification to the particular disharmony of a specific Internal Organ. For example, according to the Eight-Principle identification the symptoms and signs of Qi deficiency are slight shortness of breath, a weak voice, a pale face, tiredness and lack of appetite. Although useful to diagnose a condition of Qi deficiency, this is not detailed enough and does not identify which organ is involved. It is therefore too general to give an indication of the treatment needed.

According to the Internal-Organ pattern identification, the above symptoms can be further classified as Lung-Qi deficiency (shortness of breath and weak voice) and Spleen-Qi deficiency (tiredness and lack of appetite). This is more useful in clinical practice because it gives concrete indications as to which organ needs to be treated (Fig. P6-S2.1).

The identification of patterns according to the Internal Organs is the most important one in clinical practice, particularly for interior chronic diseases.

Although the identification of patterns according to the Internal Organs is the result of a relatively recent systematization (early Qing dynasty), elements of it have existed in Chinese medicine since early times. For example, the 'Discussion of Prescriptions of the Golden Chest' (*Jin Gui Yao Lue Fang Lun*, AD 220) says: '*When Wind invades the Lungs the patient will suffer cough, dry mouth, breathlessness, dry throat without thirst, spitting of saliva and shivering.*'[1] Although the symptoms described are somewhat different to those we would normally ascribe to an external invasion of Wind, the above passage is nevertheless an example of pattern identification according to the Internal Organs (in this case the Lungs).

To give another example, the 'Dictionary of Origin of Diseases' (*Bing Yuan Ci Dian*) gives the symptoms and signs of various patterns such as 'Cold in the Heart', 'Deficiency of the Pericardium' and 'Empty Heat in the Heart'.[2]

The 'Discussion of the Origin of Symptoms in Diseases' (*Zhu Bing Yuan Hou Lun*, AD 610) by Chao Yuan Fang describes patterns throughout the text. For example, the chapter on Exhaustion (*Xu Lao*) gives the symptoms for the patterns of Lung deficiency, Liver deficiency, etc.[3] Generally speaking, Internal Organs patterns are mentioned in the ancient books primarily in relation to the relevant herbal formulae and such patterns therefore pertain more to the herbal than to the acupuncture tradition.

Let us now look at some of the characteristics of this method of identification of patterns.

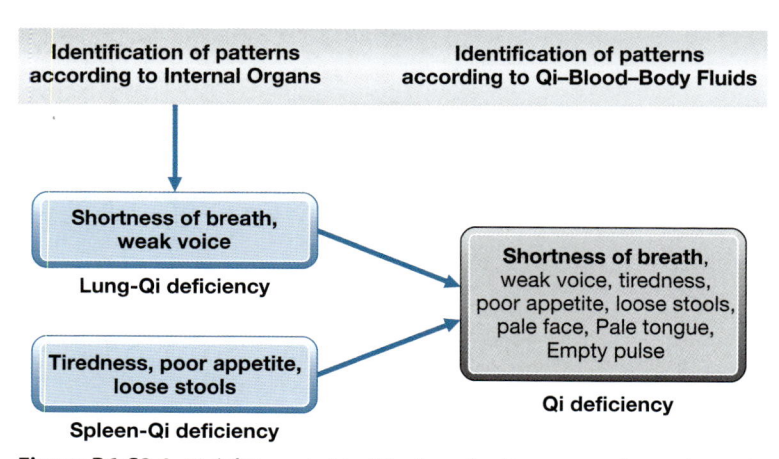

Figure P6-S2.1 Qi deficiency in identification of patterns according to Internal Organs and to Qi, Blood and Body Fluids

A pattern may consist of only a few symptoms

In the following pages the patterns of each organ will be described in detail. It is important to realize that, in practice, not all the symptoms and signs described need necessarily appear simultaneously. What these patterns describe are actually advanced cases of a particular organ disharmony. In some cases, even only two symptoms will be sufficient to identify a specific Internal Organ pattern. In fact, the real art of Chinese diagnosis consists in being able to detect a certain disharmony from a minimum of symptoms and signs.

Not all clinical manifestation listed under each pattern need to appear to diagnose that pattern

The patterns are not pigeon holes

The organ patterns are not 'pigeon holes' into which we fit certain symptoms and signs. In practice, it is essential to have an understanding of the aetiology and pathology of a given disharmony. The aim of this method, therefore, is not to 'classify' symptoms and signs according to organ patterns, but to understand how the symptoms and signs arise and how they interact with each other, in order to identify the prevailing organ disharmony.

Patterns are not just a collection of symptoms and signs, but an expression of the disharmony prevailing in a person. Symptoms and signs are used to identify the character and nature of the disharmony which, in itself, gives an indication as to the strategy and method of treatment needed. Essential in organ patterns is the relationship between the symptoms and signs forming the picture of a disharmony.

There is no correspondence between the organ patterns of Chinese medicine and organ diseases of Western medicine

The organ patterns are not 'pigeon holes' into which we fit certain symptoms and signs. It is essential to have an understanding of the aetiology and pathology of a given disharmony

The Organ patterns are not 'diseases' of the organs in a Western medical sense

The organ patterns are not diseases in a Western medical sense. There is no correspondence between the organ patterns of Chinese medicine and organ diseases of Western medicine. For example, a patient can suffer from Kidney-Yin deficiency without any recognizable kidney disease from the Western medical point of view. Vice versa, a patient may suffer from a kidney inflammation from a Western point of view not corresponding to a Kidney pattern from the Chinese medical point of view.

Organ patterns as they are listed describe advanced cases of such disharmonies

Organ patterns appear in different degrees of severity, and the symptoms and signs listed under each pattern usually only describe the advanced cases of a given organ disharmony. In practice, if a pattern is only just developing, its symptoms and signs will be few and mild. Identifying an organ pattern as it is arising with only a few symptoms and signs releases the full potential of Chinese medicine in the prevention of disease.

For example, the symptoms and signs of Kidney-Yin deficiency are tinnitus, dizziness, night sweating, a dry mouth at night, backache, a Red tongue without coating and a Floating-Empty and Rapid Pulse. In fact, what this picture of symptoms and signs describes is quite an advanced case of Kidney-Yin deficiency. In practice, if a Kidney-Yin deficiency is just developing, a patient might only suffer from backache, slight night sweating and have a tongue with a slightly rootless coating: these manifestations would be enough to warrant a diagnosis of Kidney-Yin deficiency.

Organ patterns appear in different degrees of severity, and the symptoms and signs listed under each pattern usually only describe the advanced cases of a given organ disharmony. In practice, if a pattern is only just developing, its symptoms and signs will be few and mild

Combination of patterns

In practice several patterns may occur simultaneously. The combinations can be:

- Two or more patterns from the same Yin organ (e.g. Liver-Qi stagnation and Liver-Fire)
- Two or more patterns from different Yin organs (e.g. Liver-Fire and Heart-Fire)
- One or more patterns of a Yin organ with one or more patterns of a Yang organ (e.g. Spleen-Qi deficiency and Bladder Damp-Heat)
- An interior and an exterior pattern (e.g. retention of Damp-Phlegm in the Lungs and exterior attack of Wind-Cold in the Lungs)
- An interior organ pattern and a Channel pattern (e.g. Lung-Qi deficiency and Painful Obstruction Syndrome of the Large Intestine channel)

Tongue and pulse abnormalities may be the only clinical manifestations of a pattern

It is important to remember that the tongue and pulse signs are an important part of the picture of a disharmony and they should never be used in diagnosis simply to 'confirm' the existence of a particular pattern.

This raises two separate issues: the first is that, as mentioned above, we should not use the tongue and pulse signs simply to confirm a diagnosis, that is, we should be open-minded and be prepared to explore and explain why the tongue and pulse may be contradicting the prevailing pattern (e.g. the patient has Liver-Fire but the pulse is Slow).

The second issue is that occasionally even the tongue or pulse by themselves may be enough to diagnose an organ pattern. For example, if a patient's Kidney pulse is consistently quite Weak on both Rear positions, this definitely indicates a Kidney deficiency even in the absence of any Kidney symptoms. This is, in fact, quite frequent in practice and it allows us to treat the patient for the *prevention* of illness.

The tongue and pulse signs are an important part of the picture of a disharmony: they should never be used simply to 'confirm' the existence of a particular pattern and, sometimes, may be the only manifestations of a particular pattern

Patterns of Yin deficiency: differentiation from Empty-Heat

For the patterns of Yin deficiency, I have separated the clinical manifestations of Yin deficiency itself from those due to Empty-Heat (which arises from Yin deficiency). I have done this to highlight the fact that, although Empty-Heat derives from Yin deficiency, it does so only in long-standing and severe cases. In other words, a patient may suffer from Yin deficiency for many years without developing symptoms of Empty-Heat. I see this in particular in patients who may present, over several years, with the pattern of Stomach-Yin deficiency manifested by a tongue with deep Stomach cracks (see Figures 23.31 and 23.33) and yet no symptoms of Empty-Heat.

Patterns are not cast in stone

Finally, it should be noted that patterns are not cast in stone, that is, different authors may report slightly different clinical manifestations for the same pattern. For example, 'insomnia' is sometimes listed as a clinical manifestation of Liver-Blood deficiency and sometimes it is not. So we should not be surprised if textbooks differ in their listing of the patterns.

In the discussion of each organ pattern the following points will be discussed:

A brief summary of the functions of the organ

This is only a brief summary of the functions of the organ to remind the reader of them without the need to refer back to the chapters on the functions of the organs.

It is important to be reminded of the functions of the organs as the patterns of the organs reflect what happens when their functions are impaired so that the clinical manifestations do not become mere 'lists' to be memorized but a logical development from the impairment of physiological functions.

The clinical manifestations

This section will include the clinical manifestations in as comprehensive fashion as possible. I have separated the clinical manifestations of Yin deficiency from those of Empty-Heat to emphasize that Yin deficiency can occur without Empty-Heat.

The main sources for the clinical manifestations are:

> 1981 Syndromes and Treatment of the Internal Organs (*Zang Fu Zheng Zhi* 脏腑证治), Tianjin Scientific Publishing House, Tianjin.
> 1979 Patterns and Treatment of Kidney Diseases (*Shen Yu Shen Bing de Zheng Zhi* 肾与肾病的证治), Hebei People's Publishing House, Hebei.
> Beijing College of Traditional Chinese Medicine 1980 Practical Chinese Medicine (*Shi Yong Zhong Yi Xue* 实用中医学), Beijing Publishing House, Beijing.
> Anwei College of Traditional Chinese Medicine 1979 Clinical Manual of Chinese Medicine (*Zhong Yi Lin Chuang Shou Li* 中医临床手册), Anwei Scientific Publishing House, Anwei.
> Lu Fang 1981 Identification of Diseases and Patterns in Internal Medicine (*Nei Ke Bian Bing Yu Bian Zheng* 内科辨病与辨证), Heilongjiang People's Publishing House, Harbin.
> Cheng Shao An 1994 Diagnosis, Patterns and Treatment in Chinese Medicine (*Zhong Yi Zheng Hou Zhen Duan Zhi Liao Xue* 中醫证候诊断治疗学), Beijing Science Publishing House, Beijing.
> Zhao Jin Ze 1991 Differential Diagnosis and Patterns in Chinese Medicine (*Zhong Yi Zheng Hou Jian Bie Zhen Duan Xue* 中醫证候鉴别诊断学), People's Health Publishing House, Beijing.
> Zhao Jin Duo 1985 Identification of Patterns and Diagnosis in Chinese Medicine (*Zhong Yi Zheng Zhuang Jian Bie Zhen Duan Xue* 中醫证状鉴别诊断学), People's Health Publishing House, Beijing.

The aetiology

This section will include the most usual causes of each pattern according to my experience.

The pathology

This section explains how the clinical manifestations arise and the pathological process behind it. For example, cough is due to the failure of Lung-Qi to descend, sneezing is due to the failure of Lung-Qi to diffuse, withered nails are due to deficient Liver-Blood not nourishing nails, etc.

Pathological precursors of the pattern

This section explores the patterns or other pathological processes that might lead to the pattern in question. For example, Heart-Blood deficiency frequently derives from Liver-Blood deficiency.

Pathological developments from the pattern

This section will indicate the pattern or patterns that may develop as a result of the pattern in question. For example, Liver-Blood deficiency often leads to Heart-Blood deficiency or to Liver-Yang rising, etc.

The treatment with acupuncture

With regard to treatment with acupuncture, the most useful acupuncture points will be mentioned for each pattern. However, it should be understood that these are not point prescriptions, but simply the best points to use according to their functions. Not all the points mentioned, therefore, would necessarily be used in each case.

Furthermore, when the functions of each point are explained, only those functions which are relevant to the pattern in question will be mentioned. For example, in the pattern of Heart-Yang collapse Du-20 Baihui is recommended for its function of restoring consciousness, even though it has many other functions which are not listed under that pattern. The functions of the points are described in detail in chapters 54 to 68.

Finally, with regard to needling method, whenever the reducing method is indicated, it is understood that this is to be replaced by the even method in all the usual cases, i.e.:

- When the illness is chronic
- When the patient is in a very weak condition or is very old
- When there is a mixed pattern of Deficiency and Excess

Herbal formula

This section will give the suggested herbal formula for each pattern.

END NOTES

1. 1981 Discussion of Prescriptions of the Golden Chest (*Jin Gui Yao Lue Fang Lun* 金匮要略方论), Zhejiang Scientific Publishing House, Zhejiang, first published c.AD 220, p. 51.
2. Wu Ke Qian Origin of Diseases Dictionary (*Bing Yuan Ci Dian* 病源辞典), Tianjin Ancient Texts Publishing House, Tianjin, 1988, p. 87 and p. 92.
3. Chao Yuan Fang 1991 Discussion of the Origin of Symptoms in Diseases (*Zhu Bing Yuan Hou Lun* 诸病源候论), People's Health Publishing House, Beijing, first published AD 610, p. 87.

Heart Patterns 32

Key contents

General aetiology
Exterior pathogenic factors
Emotions
- Joy
- Sadness and grief
- Anger
- Worry

Deficiency patterns
Heart-Qi deficiency
Heart-Yang deficiency
Heart-Yang Collapse
Heart-Blood deficiency
Heart-Yin deficiency

Excess patterns
Heart-Fire blazing
Phlegm-Fire harassing the Heart
Phlegm misting the Mind
Heart-Qi stagnation
Heart vessel obstructed

Deficiency–Excess patterns
Heart-Blood stasis

Combined patterns
Heart- and Liver-Blood deficiency (discussed under Liver patterns, ch. 34)
Heart- and Spleen-Blood deficiency (discussed under Spleen patterns, ch. 36)
Heart- and Lung-Qi deficiency (discussed under Lung patterns, ch. 35)
Kidneys and Heart not harmonized (discussed under the Kidney patterns, ch. 37).

The functions of the Heart (ch. 6) are:

- It governs Blood
- It controls the blood vessels
- It manifests in the complexion
- It houses the Mind
- It opens into the tongue
- It controls sweat

The most important of these functions are those of governing Blood and housing the Mind (*Shen*). Most of the pathological changes of the Heart reflect this and involve the Blood and the Mind.

Governing Blood and housing the Mind are complementary functions, mutually influencing each other. Blood and Yin are the 'residence' for the Mind: if Blood and Yin are flourishing, the Mind will be in a good state and the person will feel mentally happy and vital. If Blood and Yin are deficient, the Mind will suffer, the person will feel unhappy, depressed and lack vitality. Conversely, if the Mind is disturbed from emotional upsets, this can induce a weakness of Blood or Yin and therefore lead to symptoms of Heart-Blood or Heart-Yin deficiency.

The discussion of Heart patterns will be preceded by a discussion of the general aetiology under the following headings:

GENERAL AETIOLOGY
- Exterior pathogenic factors
- Emotions
  - Joy
  - Sadness and grief
  - Anger
  - Worry

The patterns discussed are:
DEFICIENCY PATTERNS
- Heart-Qi deficiency
- Heart-Yang deficiency
- Heart-Yang Collapse
- Heart-Blood deficiency
- Heart-Yin deficiency

EXCESS PATTERNS
- Heart-Fire blazing
- Phlegm-Fire harassing the Heart
- Phlegm misting the Mind
- Heart-Qi stagnation
- Heart vessel obstructed

DEFICIENCY–EXCESS PATTERNS
- Heart-Blood stasis

COMBINED PATTERNS
Heart- and Liver-Blood deficiency (discussed under Liver patterns, ch. 34)
Heart- and Spleen-Blood deficiency (discussed under Spleen patterns, ch. 36)
Heart- and Lung-Qi deficiency (discussed under Lung patterns, ch. 35)
Kidneys and Heart not harmonized (discussed under the Kidney patterns, ch. 37)

GENERAL AETIOLOGY

The aetiological factors discussed are:

- Exterior pathogenic factors
- Emotions
  - Joy
  - Sadness and grief
  - Anger
  - Worry
- Diet
- Overwork

Box 32.1 summarizes the general aetiology of Heart patterns.

Exterior pathogenic factors

Generally speaking, exterior climatic factors do not affect the Heart directly. Of all the climatic factors, Fire and Heat are the ones that most affect the Heart, but even those do not affect it directly. Chinese medicine maintains that exterior pathogenic factors do not affect the Heart directly, but instead affect the Pericardium. The 'Spiritual Axis' in chapter 71 says: '*If*

Box 32.1 General aetiology of Heart patterns

- Exterior pathogenic factors
- Emotions
  - Joy
  - Sadness and grief
  - Anger
  - Worry
- Diet
- Overwork

---

exterior pathogenic factors attack the Heart, they penetrate the Pericardium instead.'[1] Thus, if exterior Heat invades the body, it will affect the Pericardium rather than the Heart. This pattern will be discussed in chapter 33.

Exterior pathogenic factors as causes of disease are discussed in chapter 21.

Exterior pathogenic factors do not usually affect the Heart directly, but the Pericardium instead

Emotions

Joy

The Heart is related to 'joy' within the Five-Element correspondence scheme. Under normal circumstances, a happy state of mind is obviously beneficial to the Mind and the body. It is only when joy is excessive that it becomes a cause of disease and it can injure the Heart. (The significance of 'joy' as a cause of disease was discussed in ch. 20.)

Excess joy and overstimulation can injure the Heart and, more specifically, make Heart Qi slow down and become deficient, and they dilate the Heart.

Sadness and grief

Although related to the Lungs within the Five-Element scheme, sadness and grief deeply affect Heart-Qi. The Lungs and Heart are very closely related as one governs Qi and the other Blood; they mutually assist each other and they are both situated in the chest.

Sadness and grief induce Qi deficiency of the Lungs, which, in time, affects the Heart and makes Heart-Qi deficient. The 'Simple Questions' in chapter 39 says: '*Sadness dissolves Qi*'.[2]

Sadness and grief are very common causes of Heart-Qi deficiency and when they affect both Lungs and Heart, they can often be manifested on the pulse, with a very weak pulse on both Front positions (i.e. Heart and Lung positions).

Prolonged sadness and grief causing deficiency of Qi over a long period of time may lead to stagnation of Qi, which, in turn, can turn into Heat. When this happens, they will cause Heart-Heat.

> **Clinical note**
>
> Qi deficiency of the Heart and Lungs can give rise to Qi stagnation in these organs so that Qi deficiency and stagnation coexist

Anger

What is termed 'anger' in Chinese medicine includes feelings of frustration and resentment (see ch. 20 on the causes of disease).

Although anger affects the Liver directly, it may also affect the Heart indirectly. Anger causes the rising of Liver-Yang or Liver-Fire, and this can easily be transmitted to the Heart, causing Heart-Fire. This is manifested on the tongue with a Red body colour on the sides and tip and possibly with red points on the tip.

Worry

Worry is one of the most common emotional causes of disease in our society. Worry knots Qi, which means that it causes stagnation of Qi, and it affects both Lungs and Spleen: the Lungs because when one is worried breathing is shallow and the Spleen because this organ is responsible for thinking and ideas. Chapter 8 of the 'Spiritual Axis' confirms that worry knots Qi: '*Worry causes obstruction of Qi so that Qi stagnates.*'[3]

However, worry also affects the Heart deeply, causing Qi stagnation in the Heart and the chest, causing palpitations, a slight feeling of tightness of the chest and insomnia.

Please note that worry also affects the Liver and may cause Liver-Yang to rise. Zhang Jing Yue said: '*Worry makes Qi rise and can affect the Liver; the Liver becomes overactive and it invades the Spleen.*'[4]

Emotions as causes of disease are discussed in chapter 20. Effects of emotions on the Heart are illustrated in Figure 32.1 and summarized in Box 32.2. Box 32.3 summarizes symptoms and signs giving a 'feel' for Heart pathology.

Joy → Slows down the Heart, makes Heart larger

Sadness and Grief → Depletes Heart-Qi

Anger → May cause Heart-Fire

Worry → Causes Heart-Qi stagnation

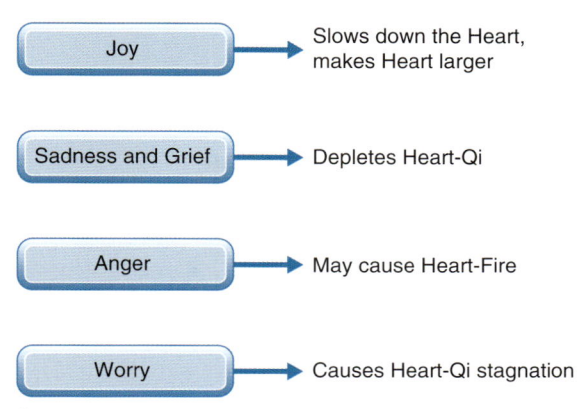

Figure 32.1 Emotions affecting the Heart

> **Box 32.2 Emotions affecting the Heart**
>
> - Joy (slows down Heart-Qi)
> - Sadness (depletes Heart-Qi)
> - Grief (depletes Heart-Qi)
> - Anger (makes Heart-Qi rise)
> - Worry (knots Heart-Qi)

> **Box 32.3 A 'feel' for Heart pathology**
>
> - Mental–emotional symptoms
> - Pathology of Mind reflected in the '*shen*' of the eyes
> - Depression, anxiety, insomnia
> - Palpitations

DEFICIENCY PATTERNS

Heart-Qi deficiency

Clinical manifestations

Palpitations, shortness of breath on exertion, pale face, spontaneous sweating, tiredness, slight depression (Fig. 32.2).

Tongue: Pale or normal colour.
Pulse: Empty. In severe cases, the Heart pulse could feel slightly Overflowing and Empty (i.e. it feels very superficial and somewhat pounding with a light pressure of the finger but empty with a heavier pressure).
Key symptoms: palpitations, tiredness, Empty pulse.

Aetiology

Emotional problems

Emotional problems, particularly from sadness or grief, can lead to deficiency of Heart-Qi.

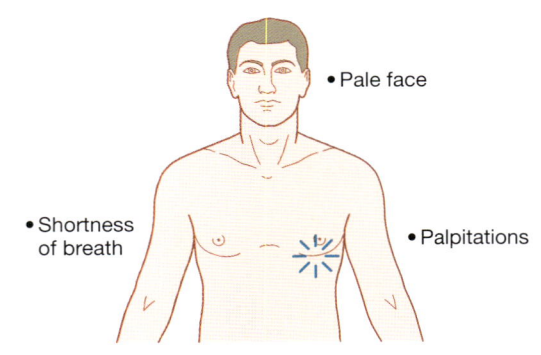

Figure 32.2 Heart-Qi deficiency

- Pale face
- Shortness of breath
- Palpitations

Blood loss

This pattern may be caused by a chronic illness, particularly after a serious haemorrhage or after a prolonged chronic haemorrhage (such as from menorrhagia). The Heart governs Blood and, as Blood is the Mother of Qi, any severe or prolonged blood loss will cause a deficiency of Heart-Blood, which, in turn, will lead to deficiency of Heart-Qi.

Pathology

This pattern includes general signs of Qi deficiency (such as shortness of breath, sweating, pallor, tiredness and Empty pulse) and palpitations, which is the cardinal sign of Heart-Qi deficiency. In this case the palpitations will be only light and occasional.

It is important to define 'palpitations' here. 'Palpitations' indicates a *subjective* feeling of the patient in being aware of the heart beating in an uncomfortable way. We are not usually aware of our heart's beating, but if we become aware of it and it is a vaguely unpleasant sensation, this is called 'palpitations'.

It should be noted that 'palpitations' has nothing to do with the rate or rhythm of the heart. The patient may often experience 'palpitations' as if the heart were beating more rapidly but this is not necessarily so. Vice versa, someone's pulse may be rapid but, if they are not aware of it, this symptom would not be defined as 'palpitations'. It is therefore important, when we ask about 'palpitations', to explain to the patient what we mean. If we ask a patient 'do you experience palpitations?', most patients would assume we are asking whether the heart beats faster. For this reason, I usually ask 'are you ever aware of your heart beat in an uncomfortable way?'

'Palpitations' is a subjective feeling of the patient who is uncomfortably aware of the heart beating; it has nothing to do with the objective rate or rhythm of the heart.

Pathological precursors of pattern

Heart-Qi deficiency may derive from a deficiency of Kidney-Qi. In some cases, Heart-Qi deficiency may also be the result of Gall Bladder-Qi deficiency (Fig. 32.3).

Pathological developments from pattern

Heart-Qi deficiency frequently leads to Heart-Yang deficiency. It may also affect the Lungs and become associated with Lung-Qi deficiency: this happens especially when there is emotional stress (see Fig. 32.3).

Treatment

Principle of treatment: tonify Heart-Qi.

Acupuncture

Points: HE-5 Tongli, P-6 Neiguan, BL-15 Xinshu, Ren-17 Shanzhong, Ren-6 Qihai, Du-14 Dazhui.
Method: all with reinforcing method.
Explanation
- HE-5 tonifies Heart-Qi.
- P-6 also tonifies Heart-Qi and it would be particularly useful if sadness is the cause of pattern.
- BL-15 is the Back Transporting point and it tonifies Heart-Qi. Direct moxa should be used on this point.

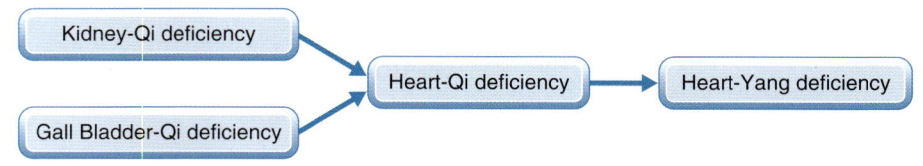

Figure 32.3 Heart-Qi deficiency pattern: precursors and developments

- Ren-17 is the Gathering point for Qi and it tonifies the Qi of the Upper Burner and therefore Heart-Qi. This point would also be particularly useful if sadness is the cause of disease as it will tonify both Lung- and Heart-Qi.
- Ren-6 tonifies the whole body's Qi and will therefore strengthen Heart-Qi. This point would be particularly useful in case the Heart deficiency derives from a chronic illness with general deficiency of Qi.
- Du-14, with direct moxa cones, tonifies Heart-Qi.

Herbal formula

Bao Yuan Tang *Preserving the Source Decoction*.

Three Treasures

Calm the Shen (variation of Gui Pi Tang).

Heart-Yang deficiency

Clinical manifestations

Palpitations, shortness of breath on exertion, tiredness, spontaneous sweating, a slight feeling of stuffiness or discomfort in the heart region, feeling of cold, cold hands, bright-pale face, slightly dark lips.
Tongue: Pale, slightly wet.
Pulse: Deep-Weak, in severe cases Knotted (Fig. 32.4 and Box 32.4).
Key symptoms: palpitations, cold hands, Deep-Weak pulse.

Aetiology

This is basically the same as for Heart-Qi deficiency. Heart-Yang deficiency may therefore be indirectly caused by any of the causes of Kidney-Yang deficiency (see ch. 37).

Pathology

Some of the symptoms are the same as for Heart-Qi deficiency (palpitations, shortness of breath, tiredness, sweating and pale face): this is because Heart-Qi deficiency could be considered as included within Heart-Yang deficiency. In other words, it is not possible to have a deficiency of Yang without a deficiency of Qi.

Feelings of cold and cold hands are due to Heart-Yang not transporting Blood to the extremities to warm them. The slight feeling of stuffiness in the chest region

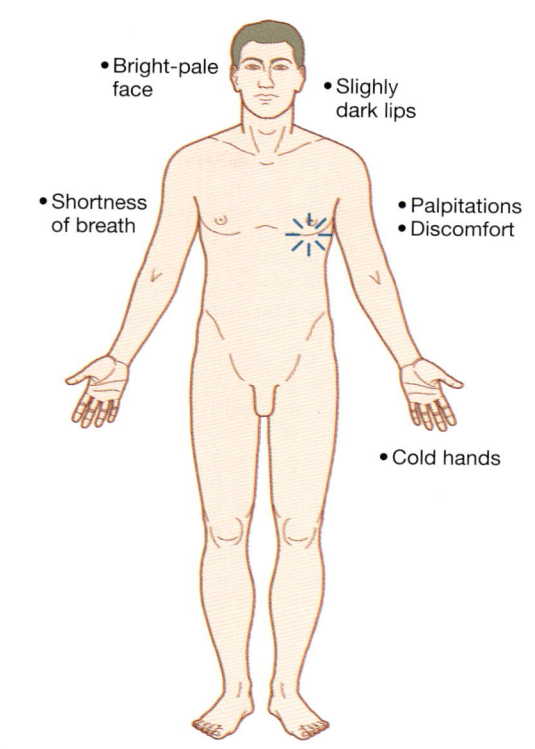

Figure 32.4 Heart-Yang deficiency

Box 32.4 Heart-Qi deficiency

Clinical manifestations

Palpitations, shortness of breath on exertion, pale face, spontaneous sweating, tiredness, slight depression, Pale tongue, Empty pulse

Treatment

HE-5 Tongli, P-6 Neiguan, BL-15 Xinshu, Ren-17 Shanzhong, Ren-6 Qihai, Du-14 Dazhui

---

is due to Heart-Yang not moving Qi in the chest and hence leading to a slight stagnation of Qi in the chest.

The bright-pale face is typical of Yang deficiency (in Blood deficiency the face would be dull-pale).

The lips are slightly dark because deficient Heart-Yang fails to move Qi and Blood and this may cause a slight Blood stasis. Please note that this sign would appear only in severe and advanced cases of Heart-Yang deficiency.

The tongue is Pale because Heart-Yang cannot transport enough Blood to the tongue, and it is slightly wet because Heart-Yang cannot transform the fluids, which therefore accumulate on the tongue.

The Deep and Weak pulse reflects the deficiency of Yang. A Knotted pulse (a Slow pulse that stops at irregular intervals) might be found in severe cases.

Pathological precursors of pattern

Heart-Yang deficiency may derive indirectly from a chronic deficiency of Kidney-Yang as Kidney-Yang is the source of all Yang energies of the body.

The Stomach and Spleen also influence the Heart directly (see ch. 2) and a deficiency of Yang of the Stomach and/or Spleen is a frequent cause of Heart-Yang deficiency.

Heart-Yang deficiency may develop also from Heart-Qi deficiency (Fig. 32.5).

Pathological developments from pattern

The most clinically important potential consequence of Heart-Yang deficiency is Heart-Blood stasis. Deficient Heart-Yang fails to move Qi in the chest; this may lead first to Heart-Qi stagnation and then to Heart-Blood stasis. This pattern is clinically important because it is involved in Western medical diseases such as angina pectoris and coronary heart disease (see Fig. 32.5).

Treatment

Principle of treatment: tonify and warm Heart-Yang.

Acupuncture

Points: HE-5 Tongli, P-6 Neiguan, BL-15 Xinshu, Ren-17 Shanzhong, Ren-6 Qihai, Du-14 Dazhui.
Method: all with reinforcing method, moxa is applicable.
Explanation
- HE-5 and P-6 tonify Heart-Qi (see above).
- BL-15 tonifies Heart-Yang if moxa is used.
- Ren-17 also tonifies Heart-Yang if moxa is used. This point would be particularly useful if there is stuffiness of the chest.
- Ren-6 with moxa also tonifies all Yang energies of the body and is particularly useful if the Heart-Yang deficiency results from Kidney-Yang deficiency.
- Du-14 with direct moxa tonifies Heart-Yang.

Herbal formula

Rou Fu Bao Yuan Tang *Cinnamomum–Aconitum Preserving the Source Decoction*.

Box 32.5 summarizes Heart-Yang deficiency.

Box 32.5 Heart-Yang deficiency

Clinical manifestations

Palpitations, shortness of breath on exertion, tiredness, spontaneous sweating, a slight feeling of stuffiness or discomfort in the heart region, feeling of cold, cold hands, bright-pale face, slightly dark lips, Pale tongue, Deep-Weak pulse

Treatment

HE-5 Tongli, P-6 Neiguan, BL-15 Xinshu, Ren-17 Shanzhong, Ren-6 Qihai, Du-14 Dazhui

---

Heart-Yang Collapse

Clinical manifestations

Palpitations, shortness of breath, weak and shallow breathing, profuse sweating, cold limbs, cyanosis of lips, greyish-white complexion, in severe cases coma (Fig. 32.6).
Tongue: Very Pale or Bluish-Purple, Short.
Pulse: Hidden-Minute-Knotted.
Key symptoms: cyanosis of lips, Hidden-Minute pulse, cold limbs.

Aetiology

This is the same as for Heart-Yang deficiency. Heart-Yang Collapse, however, always derives from a chronic and severe deficiency of Kidney-Yang. Thus, any of the

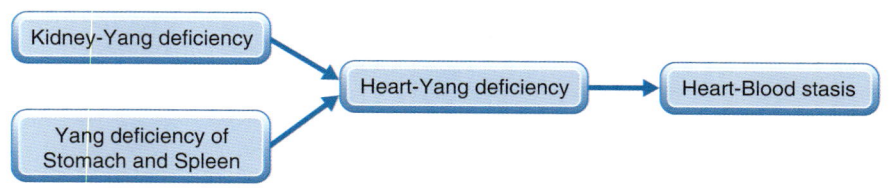

Figure 32.5 Heart-Yang deficiency pattern: precursors and developments

causes of Kidney-Yang deficiency, are indirectly causes of Heart-Yang Collapse: these can be excessive sexual activity, overwork over a long period of time, or a chronic illness.

Pathology

This pattern is an extreme case of Heart-Yang deficiency and is not substantially different from it. The clinical manifestations are basically the same as for Heart-Yang deficiency, only more severe. In addition to these, there is cyanosis of lips, which is due to deficient Yang Qi not moving the Blood, hence resulting in severe stasis of Blood.

The coma is caused by the complete collapse of Heart-Qi, hence the Mind has no 'residence'. This coma is of the Deficiency type.

The tongue may be Short (i.e. cannot be extended much out of the mouth) because the deficiency of Yang is so severe that Yang Qi cannot move the tongue muscle at all. Also, the deficiency of Yang generates internal Cold, which contracts the muscles; hence the tongue cannot be stuck out.

The Hidden pulse is an extreme case of the Deep pulse and reflects the severe deficiency of Yang. The Knotted pulse reflects the severe deficiency of Yang not giving the Heart enough energy to beat regularly.

Pathological precursors of pattern

Heart-Yang Collapse always derives from a chronic and severe deficiency of Kidney-Yang. The total collapse of Qi (whether it is Yin or Yang Qi) always derives from the collapse of Kidney energy (whether Kidney-Yin or Kidney-Yang), which is the foundation of all energies of the body (Fig. 32.7).

A general deficiency of Yang, especially of the Spleen and Stomach, is also a frequent precursor to this pattern. Stomach-Yang is particularly important because the Stomach channel controls the Great Connecting Channel of the Stomach (also called *Xu Li*), which beats in the fifth intercostal space. The pulsation of the left ventricle that can be felt in the fifth intercostal space was called the 'beat of *Xu Li*' (see ch. 51).

Pathological developments from the pattern

Heart-Yang Collapse is a very severe, serious, acute condition corresponding broadly to cardiac infarction in Western medicine. When it does not cause death, the main consequence is severe Blood stasis (see Fig. 32.7).

Treatment

Principle of treatment: rescue Yang, restore consciousness, stop sweating.

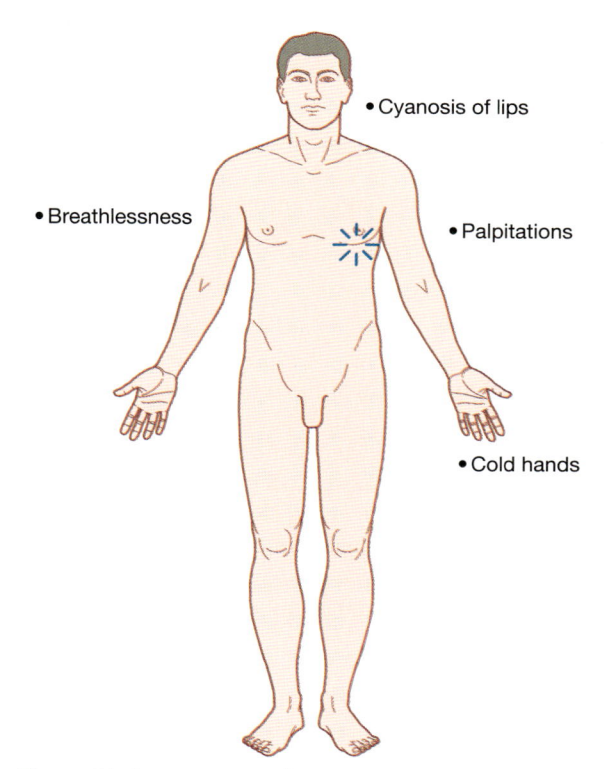

Figure 32.6 Heart-Yang Collapse

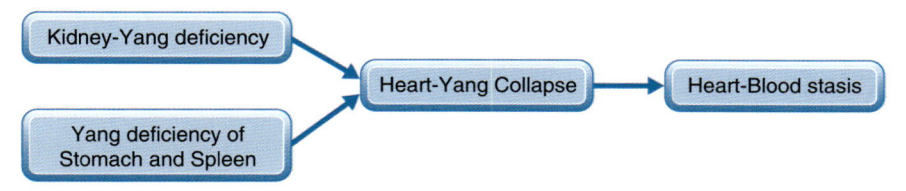

Figure 32.7 Heart-Yang Collapse pattern: precursors and developments

Acupuncture

Points: Ren-6 Qihai, Ren-4 Guanyuan, Ren-8 Shenque, Du-4 Mingmen, ST-36 Zusanli, P-6 Neiguan, BL-23 Shenshu, Du-20 Baihui, Du-14 Dazhui, BL-15 Xinshu.

Method: all with reinforcing method, no retention of needle, moxa must be used.

Explanation
- Ren-4, Ren-6 and Ren-8 rescue Yang Qi and stop sweating if indirect moxibustion on ginger or aconite is applied.
- Du-4 with moxa tonifies Kidney-Yang.
- ST-36 and P-6 strengthen Heart-Yang.
- BL-23 with moxa strengthens Kidney-Yang.
- Du-20 is the meeting point of all the Yang channels: it rescues Yang and promotes resuscitation if used with direct moxibustion.
- Du-14 and BL-15 combined together can tonify Heart-Yang if direct moxibustion is applied.

It is important to stop sweating because profuse sweating will further weaken the Heart in two ways. Firstly, a loss of sweat implies loss of Defensive Qi, which represents a further loss of Yang. Secondly, a loss of fluids from sweating leads to a deficiency of Blood because of the interchange relation between Body Fluids and Blood. The resulting deficiency of Blood will further weaken the Heart.

Herbal formula

Shen Fu Tang *Ginseng–Aconitum Decoction*.

Box 32.6 summarizes Heart-Yang Collapse.

Box 32.6 Heart-Yang Collapse

Clinical manifestations

Palpitations, shortness of breath, weak and shallow breathing, profuse sweating, cold limbs, cyanosis of lips, greyish-white complexion, in severe cases coma, very Pale or Bluish tongue, Hidden-Minute-Knotted pulse

Treatment

Ren-6 Qihai, Ren-4 Guanyuan, Ren-8 Shenque, Du-4 Mingmen, ST-36 Zusanli, P-6 Neiguan, BL-23 Shenshu, Du-20 Baihui, Du-14 Dazhui, BL-15 Xinshu

---

Heart-Blood deficiency

Clinical manifestations

Palpitations, dizziness, insomnia, dream-disturbed sleep, poor memory, anxiety, propensity to be startled, dull-pale complexion, pale lips (Fig. 32.8).

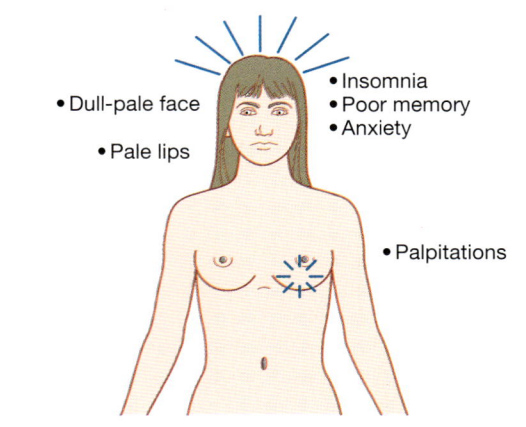

Figure 32.8 Heart-Blood deficiency

Tongue: Pale, Thin, slightly dry.
Pulse: Choppy or Fine.
Key symptoms: palpitations, insomnia, poor memory, Pale tongue.

Aetiology

Diet

A diet lacking in nourishment or in Blood-producing foods (such as meat) can lead to Spleen-Qi deficiency. Food-Qi (*Gu Qi*) produced by the Spleen is the basis for the production of Blood; hence Spleen-Qi deficiency over a long period of time may lead to Blood deficiency. Blood deficiency, in turn, can weaken the Heart and cause Heart-Blood deficiency. For this reason, Heart-Blood deficiency is often associated with Spleen-Qi deficiency.

Emotional stress

Sadness, grief, anxiety and worry over a long period of time can disturb the Mind, which, in turn, can depress the Heart function. Since the Heart governs Blood, this eventually leads to Heart-Blood deficiency.

Severe blood loss

A severe haemorrhage (such as during childbirth) can lead to Blood deficiency, since the Heart governs Blood. This, in time, can lead to Heart-Blood deficiency. In fact, Chinese medicine holds this to be the main cause of postnatal depression.

Pathology

The Heart governs Blood: if Blood is deficient the Heart suffers and the Mind is deprived of its 'residence', hence the insomnia, dream-disturbed sleep, anxiety and propensity to be startled. The Heart also controls the mental faculties and if Heart-Blood is deficient thinking will be dull and the memory poor.

Blood is the mother of Qi: if Heart-Blood is deficient, Heart-Qi also becomes deficient, causing palpitations. There is a subtle difference between the palpitations from Heart-Qi or from Heart-Blood deficiency. In the former case, it is the Qi of the Heart that is deficient and fails to control the Blood. In the latter case, it is the Blood of the Heart that is deficient and fails to nourish Qi. Although they are both described as palpitations, the clinical appearance of the symptoms will be different in each case. In the case of Heart-Qi deficiency, the palpitations will occur more in the daytime and may occur on exertion without any other particular feeling. In the case of Heart-Blood deficiency, the palpitations will occur more in the evening, even at rest, and with a slight feeling of uneasiness in the chest or anxiety.

> **Clinical note**
>
> Palpitations from Heart-Qi deficiency occur more in daytime, those from Heart-Blood deficiency occur more commonly in the afternoon/evening

Dizziness is a general symptom of Blood deficiency and is caused by Blood not nourishing the brain.

Dull-pale complexion reflects the deficiency of Blood (in deficiency of Yang, it is bright-pale).

The tongue is the offshoot of the Heart; when Heart-Blood is deficient, not enough Blood reaches the tongue, which becomes Pale. The slight dryness (related to the deficiency of Blood) distinguishes this tongue from that of Heart-Yang deficiency, which is wet. When not enough Blood reaches the tongue over a long period of time, this becomes also Thin.

The Choppy or Fine pulse reflects deficiency of Blood.

Pathological precursors of pattern

Liver-Blood deficiency is the most common precursor of Heart-Blood deficiency for two reasons. Firstly, when Blood is deficient, this usually starts with Liver-Blood deficiency: as the Heart governs Blood, Heart-Blood becomes deficient too. Secondly, as the Liver is the Mother of the Heart in the Five-Element scheme, a Liver pathology is easily transferred to the Heart; for example, just as Liver-Blood deficiency can affect the Heart, Liver-Fire may also affect the Heart, causing Heart-Fire (Fig. 32.9).

Pathological development from pattern

Heart-Blood deficiency may eventually lead to Heart-Yin deficiency as Blood is part of Yin.

Although on a physical level it is the Spleen that affects the Heart (Food-Qi produced by the Spleen is the origin of Blood), on a mental–emotional level, Heart-Blood deficiency may affect the Spleen (as the Heart is the Mother of the Spleen in the Five-Element scheme) causing pensiveness and brooding (see Fig. 32.9).

Treatment

Principle of treatment: nourish Blood, tonify the Heart, calm the Mind.

Acupuncture

Points: HE-7 Shenmen, Ren-14 Juque, Ren-15 Jiuwei, Ren-4 Guanyuan, BL-17 Geshu (with moxa), BL-20 Pishu.

Method: all with reinforcing method. Moxa can be used.

Explanation
- HE-7 nourishes Heart-Blood and calms the Mind.

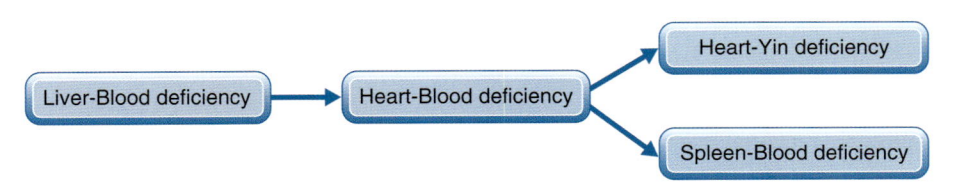

Figure 32.9 Heart-Blood deficiency pattern: precursors and developments

- Ren-14 and Ren-15 tonify Heart-Blood and calm the Mind. They are particularly useful if there is pronounced anxiety.
- Ren-4, BL-17 and BL-20 tonify Blood. BL-17 is the Gathering (*Hui*) point for Blood and BL-20 is the Back Transporting point for the Spleen and it tonifies Spleen-Qi to produce more Blood.

Herbal formula

Shen Qi Si Wu Tang *Ginseng–Astragalus–Four Substances Decoction*.

Three Treasures

Calm the Shen (variation of Gui Pi Tang).

Case history 32.1

A 51-year-old lady suffered from poor circulation in hands and feet, poor memory, dizziness, numbness of fingers, dull headaches on the vertex, palpitations and insomnia. Her tongue was Pale, slightly orangey on the sides and her pulse was Choppy.

This is a clear example of deficiency of Blood of both Heart and Liver (the orangey colour of the tongue on the sides indicates long-standing deficiency of Liver-Blood).

Box 32.7 summarizes Heart-Blood deficiency.

Box 32.7 Heart-Blood deficiency

Clinical manifestations

Palpitations, dizziness, insomnia, dream-disturbed sleep, poor memory, anxiety, propensity to be startled, dull-pale complexion, pale lips, Pale and Thin tongue, Choppy or Fine pulse

Treatment

HE-7 Shenmen, Ren-14 Juque, Ren-15 Jiuwei, Ren-4 Guanyuan, BL-17 Geshu (with moxa), BL-20 Pishu

---

Heart-Yin deficiency

Clinical manifestations

Palpitations, insomnia, dream-disturbed sleep, propensity to be startled, poor memory, anxiety, mental restlessness, 'uneasiness', 'fidgetiness', dry mouth and throat, night sweating (Fig. 32.10).
Tongue: no coating, deep midline crack reaching the tip.
Pulse: Floating-Empty.
Key symptoms: palpitations, mental restlessness, night sweating, tongue without coating.

Empty-Heat

Malar flush, feeling of heat especially in the evening, 'feeling hot and bothered', five-palm heat.
Tongue: Red without coating, redder tip with red points.
Pulse: Floating-Empty and Rapid or Fire-Rapid.

Aetiology

Emotional stress

Long-standing anxiety, worry and fear may injure Heart-Yin, usually injuring Heart-Blood first.

Overwork

Overwork (in the sense of working long hours and under stress as described in ch. 22) injures Yin. When overwork is accompanied by emotional stress and anxiety, the Mind becomes disturbed and Heart-Yin deficiency develops. This is a very common situation in the type of patients we see in the West where our hectic lifestyle is particularly conducive to Yin deficiency.

External Heat injuring Yin

Heart-Yin deficiency can also arise after an attack of exterior Heat consuming the Body Fluids and exhausting the Yin of the Heart. However, this usually only happens in very hot countries.

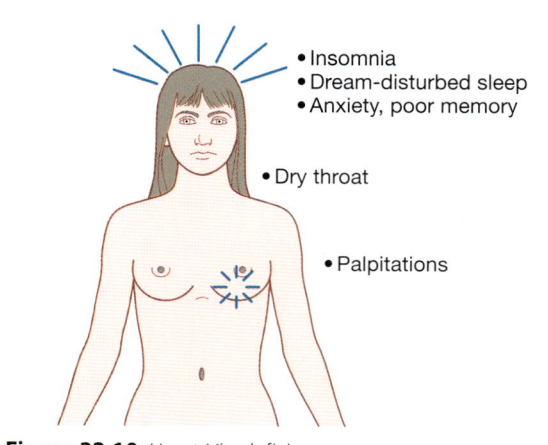

Figure 32.10 Heart-Yin deficiency

Pathology

As can be noticed, the pattern of Heart-Yin deficiency includes that of Heart-Blood deficiency. In other words, it is not possible to have Heart-Yin deficiency without Heart-Blood deficiency because Yin embodies Blood. The symptoms common to Heart-Blood deficiency are insomnia, dream-disturbed sleep, propensity to be startled, poor memory and anxiety. There is a slight difference in the insomnia, however. In Heart-Blood deficiency the patient will find it difficult to fall asleep, but once asleep, will sleep well. In Heart-Yin deficiency the patient will find it difficult to fall asleep *and* will wake up many times during the night.

'Mental restlessness' is a translation of the Chinese expression *xin fan*, which literally means 'heart feels vexed'. It indicates the feeling of mental irritability or uneasiness typical of Yin deficiency. The patient feels uneasy, fidgety or fretful without any apparent reason. This is accompanied by a feeling of heat in the face, typically in the late evening.

The malar flush, five-palm heat (a feeling of heat in palms, soles and chest), feeling of heat, are all due to Empty-Heat deriving from Yin deficiency.

This pattern is more common in middle-aged or old people as Yin deficiency usually arises then. The pattern of Heart-Blood deficiency is more common in young people, especially young women.

A tongue without coating but with normal colour indicates Yin deficiency. It is only when Empty-Heat is pronounced that the tongue becomes Red and completely without coating. The red tip with red points reflects the flaring of Empty-Heat within the Heart (the tip reflects the condition of the Heart).

The Floating-Empty or Fine pulse reflects Yin deficiency. The pulse is often Weak on both Rear positions, reflecting the deficiency of Kidney-Yin, and Overflowing on both Front positions, reflecting the flaring up of Heart Empty-Heat. When Empty-Heat is pronounced, the pulse becomes Rapid.

Remember: although Yin deficiency eventually leads to Empty-Heat, it can occur for a long time without Empty-Heat

Pathological precursors of pattern

Heart-Yin deficiency is often accompanied or caused by Kidney-Yin deficiency. This causes the Water to be deficient so that Kidney-Yin cannot rise to nourish and cool the Heart. Since Heart-Yin loses the nourishment of Kidney-Yin, this eventually leads to the flaring up of Empty-Heat of the Heart (Fig. 32.11).

Liver-Yin deficiency may also lead to the pattern of Heart-Yin deficiency.

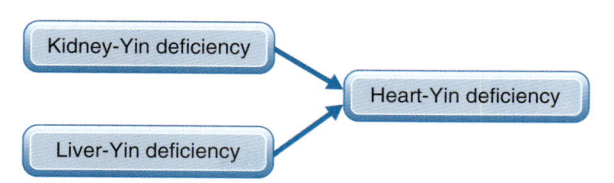

Figure 32.11 Heart-Yin deficiency pattern: precursors and developments

Pathological developments from pattern

Heart-Yin deficiency does not normally lead specifically to other patterns, other than (when the Yin deficiency is pronounced) Empty-Heat (see Fig. 32.11).

Treatment

Principle of treatment: nourish Heart-Yin, calm the Mind. If Empty-Heat is pronounced, clear Empty-Heat.

Acupuncture

Points: HE-7 Shenmen, Ren-14 Juque, Ren-15 Jiuwei, Ren-4 Guanyuan, HE-6 Yinxi, SP-6 Sanyinjiao, KI-7 Fuliu.
Method: all with reinforcing method, no moxa.
Explanation
- HE-7 nourishes Heart-Blood and Heart-Yin and calms the Mind.
- Ren-14 and Ren-15 calm the Mind. In particular, Ren-15 is an excellent point to calm the Mind if there is marked anxiety and mental restlessness.
- Ren-4 nourishes Yin and 'grounds' the Mind.
- HE-6 nourishes Heart-Yin and, in combination with KI-7, stops night sweating.
- SP-6 nourishes Yin and calms the Mind.
- KI-7 tonifies Kidneys and, in combination with HE-6, stops night sweating.

Herbal formula

Tian Wang Bu Xin Dan *Heavenly Emperor Tonifying the Heart Pill*.

Box 32.8 Heart-Yin deficiency

Clinical manifestations

Palpitations, insomnia, dream-disturbed sleep, propensity to be startled, poor memory, anxiety, mental restlessness, 'uneasiness', 'fidgetiness', dry mouth and throat, night sweating, tongue without coating, Floating-Empty pulse

Treatment

HE-7 Shenmen, Ren-14 Juque, Ren-15 Jiuwei, Ren-4 Guanyuan, HE-6 Yinxi, SP-6 Sanyinjiao, KI-7 Fuliu

Women's Treasure

Heavenly Empress (variation of Tian Wang Bu Xin Dan).

Box 32.8 summarizes Heart-Yin deficiency.

Case history 32.2

A 50-year-old lady suffered from night sweating, lower backache, a feeling of heat in the face in the evenings and dry mouth at night. Her tongue was Red, redder on the tip and Peeled and her pulse was Weak and very Deep and Weak in both Rear positions.

This is a case of Yin deficiency of Heart and Kidneys with Empty-Heat in the Heart.

EXCESS PATTERNS

Heart-Fire blazing

Clinical manifestations

Palpitations, thirst, mouth and tongue ulcers, mental restlessness, feeling agitated, feeling of heat, insomnia, dream-disturbed sleep, red face, dark urine or blood in urine, bitter taste (after a bad night's sleep) (Fig. 32.12).
Tongue: Red, tip redder and swollen with red points, yellow coating. There may be a midline crack reaching to the tip.
Pulse: Full-Rapid-Overflowing especially on the left Front position. It could also be Hasty (Rapid and stopping at irregular intervals).
Key symptoms: tongue ulcers, thirst, palpitations, Red tongue.

Aetiology

Emotional stress

Emotional problems such as chronic anxiety, constant worrying and depression can lead to Heart-Fire. These

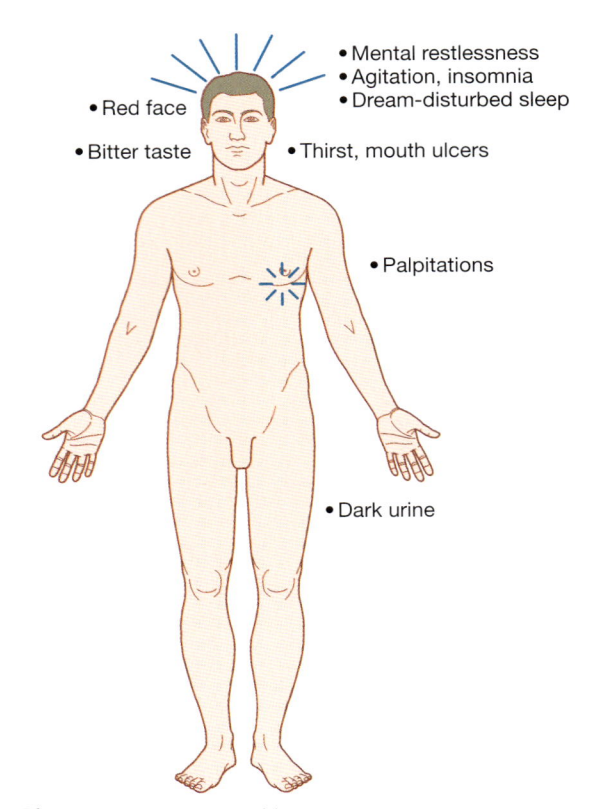

Figure 32.12 Heart-Fire blazing

emotions, over a long period of time, can lead to stagnation of Qi, and when Qi stagnates over many years, it may give rise to Fire. In particular, long-term stagnation of Qi associated with mental depression can turn into Fire, causing the appearance of the pattern of Heart-Fire blazing.

Diet

Excessive consumption of hot-energy foods (spices and red meat), but especially alcohol, may contribute to causing this pattern.

Pathology

This is an Excess pattern of Full-Heat in the Heart, and it contrasts with the previous one of Heart-Yin deficiency where there is Empty-Heat in the Heart. There are several symptoms of Heat, such as thirst, red face, feeling of heat, Red tongue and Rapid-Overflowing or Hasty Pulse.

The tongue is the offshoot of the Heart and, when this has Fire, the excess Heat may flare upward to the tongue, causing ulcers. These ulcers will have a red and raised rim around them and will be very painful (ulcers with a white rim around them can be due to Empty-Heat from Yin deficiency).

The mental restlessness is very pronounced and is due to the excess Heat in the Heart disturbing the Mind. This 'mental restlessness' differs from that of Heart-Yin deficiency in that it is more severe and the patient appears more restless, more agitated, hotter and generally more plethoric.

The insomnia is due to Heat in the Heart disturbing the Mind at night. The patient will wake up frequently and have disturbing dreams, typically of fires and flying.

The red face is due to the flaring of Heat upwards and manifesting on the complexion, which is the outward manifestation of the Heart. This can be differentiated from the redness of Empty-Heat of the Heart deriving from Yin deficiency when only the cheekbones are flushed (malar flush), whereas in the case of Heart-Fire blazing, the whole face is red.

The bitter taste is a symptom of Full-Heat in the Heart since the Heart opens into the tongue and controls taste. The bitter taste of Heart-Fire can be differentiated from that of Liver-Fire by the fact that the former appears only in the morning and is related to the quality of sleep: if the patient has a sleepless night there will be bitter taste in the morning, if he or she has a better night there will be no bitter taste.

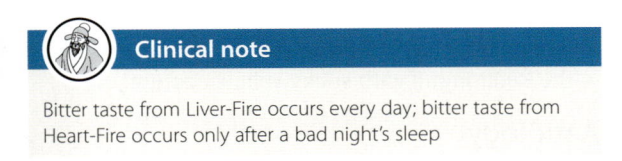

> **Clinical note**
>
> Bitter taste from Liver-Fire occurs every day; bitter taste from Heart-Fire occurs only after a bad night's sleep

The dark urine or blood in the urine are due to the transmission of Heart-Fire to the Small Intestine (to which the Heart is interiorly–exteriorly related), and from this to the Bladder (to which the Small Intestine is related within the Greater Yang).

The tongue is Red with a coating, reflecting Full-Heat. The red and swollen tip shows the localization of the Heat in the Heart.

The Rapid pulse shows Heat and its Overflowing quality, especially in the Front position, shows the presence of Heart-Fire.

Pathological precursors of pattern

Heart-Fire is often transmitted from Liver-Fire as the Liver is the Mother of the Heart within the Five-Element scheme. The transmission from the Liver is also due to the emotional origin of both these patterns. In fact, anger, frustration and resentment may lead to Liver-Fire and, as the Heart houses the Mind which recognizes and feels such emotions, Liver-Fire is transmitted to the Heart, leading to Heart-Fire (Fig. 32.13).

Pathological developments from pattern

Heart-Fire may affect the Spleen and lead to Spleen-Heat. It may also affect the Stomach and lead to Stomach-Fire.

If Heart-Fire persists for many years, the Fire may injure Yin and lead to Heart-Yin deficiency with complex symptoms and signs due to the coexistence of Fire and Yin deficiency (see Fig. 32.13).

Treatment

Principle of treatment: clear the Heart, drain Fire, calm the Mind.

Acupuncture

Points: HE-9 Shaochong, HE-8 Shaofu, HE-7 Shenmen, Ren-15 Jiuwei, SP-6 Sanyinjiao, KI-6 Zhaohai, L.I.-11 Quchi, Du-24 Shenting, Du-19 Houding.

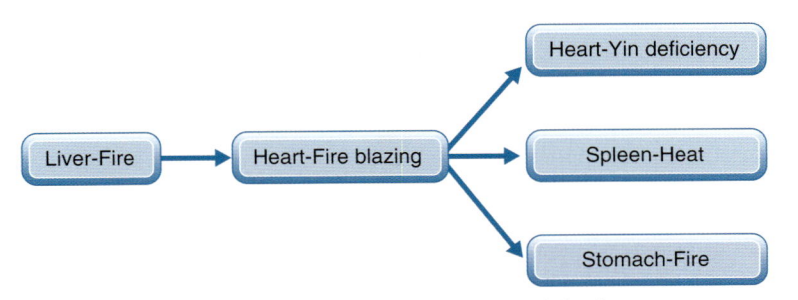

Figure 32.13 Heart-Fire blazing pattern: precursors and developments

Method: All with reducing method, except SP-6 and KI-6 to be reinforced. No moxa.

Explanation
- HE-9 and HE-8 clear Heart-Fire.
- HE-7 calms the Mind.
- Ren-15 calms the Mind and clears Heat.
- SP-6 and KI-6 are used to promote Yin and cool Fire, even though there may be no Yin deficiency.
- L.I.-11 clears Heat.
- Du-24 and Du-19 calm the Mind.

Herbal formula

Xie Xin Tang *Draining the Heart Decoction*.

Three Treasures

Drain Fire (variation of Long Dan Xie Gan Tang). Box 32.9 summarizes Heart-Fire blazing.

Case history 32.3

A woman of 34 suffered from severe anxiety, insomnia, worrying and brooding, palpitations and mental restlessness. She also had headaches affecting the right eye and side of the head along the Gall Bladder channel. The headaches were severe and throbbing in character. Her periods came irregularly, sometimes late and sometimes early, were heavy, and the blood was dark with clots. She also experienced premenstrual irritability. Her pulse was Wiry but Fine and her tongue was Deep-Red with red points along the sides and the tip, the tip was redder and swollen and there was a thick yellow coating.

These manifestations are rather complicated. The pattern on the whole is one of Full-Heat as the tongue is Red and has a coating. There is Liver-Fire, which is causing the headaches. This is evident also from the Wiry quality of the pulse and the Red colour of the tongue with red points on the sides. Liver-Fire over a long period of time can easily be transmitted to the Heart and cause Heart-Fire: this was the cause of the anxiety, insomnia, palpitations, worrying, mental restlessness and a red and swollen tip of the tongue with red points. In addition, there was also stasis of Liver-Blood as evidenced by the premenstrual irritability and the irregularity of her periods with dark-clotted blood.

Box 32.9 Heart-Fire blazing

Clinical manifestations

Palpitations, thirst, mouth and tongue ulcers, mental restlessness, feeling agitated, feeling of heat, insomnia, dream-disturbed sleep, red face, dark urine or blood in urine, bitter taste, Red tongue, tip redder and swollen with red points, yellow coating, Full-Rapid-Overflowing pulse

Treatment

HE-9 Shaochong, HE-8 Shaofu, HE-7 Shenmen, Ren-15 Jiuwei, SP-6 Sanyinjiao, KI-6 Zhaohai, L.I.-11 Quchi, Du-24 Shenting, Du-19 Houding

---

Phlegm-Fire harassing the Heart

Clinical manifestations

Palpitations, thirst, red face, bitter taste, a feeling of oppression of the chest, expectoration of phlegm, rattling sound in the throat, mental restlessness, insomnia, dream-disturbed sleep, agitation, incoherent speech, mental confusion, rash behaviour, tendency to hit or scold people, uncontrolled laughter and crying, shouting, muttering to oneself, mental depression and dullness, manic behaviour (Fig. 32.14).

Tongue: Red, Swollen, yellow dry sticky coating, deep Heart crack. The tip may be redder and swollen with red points.

Pulse: Full-Rapid-Slippery or Rapid-Overflowing-Slippery or Rapid-Full-Wiry.

Key symptoms: all the various mental symptoms and the Red tongue with sticky yellow coating.

Aetiology

Emotional stress

Severe emotional problems and depression leading to stagnation of Qi, which, over a long period of time, turns into Fire.

Diet

Excessive consumption of hot greasy foods creates Heat and Phlegm.

Pathology

This is an Excess pattern characterized by the presence of Fire harassing the Heart and Phlegm obstructing it. All the mental symptoms are due to Phlegm obstructing the Heart orifices and disturbing the Mind.

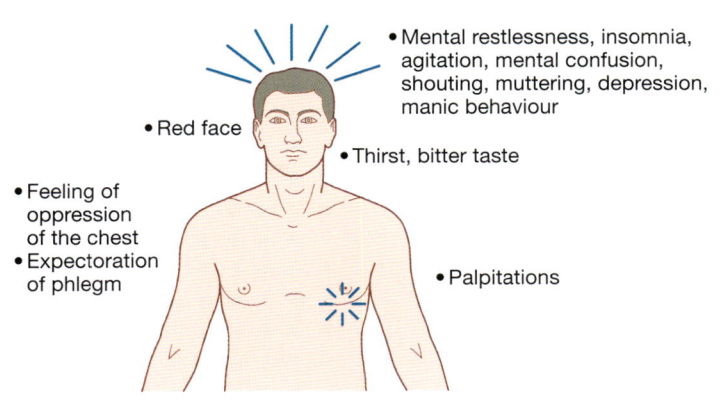

Figure 32.14 Phlegm-Fire harassing the Heart

- Mental restlessness, insomnia, agitation, mental confusion, shouting, muttering, depression, manic behaviour
- Red face
- Thirst, bitter taste
- Feeling of oppression of the chest
- Expectoration of phlegm
- Palpitations

Although the main manifestations derive from dysfunction of the Heart, this pattern is also characterized by deficient Spleen-Qi being unable to transform and transport fluids, which accumulate into Phlegm. The interior Heat facilitates this process by condensing the fluids into Phlegm.

It is interesting to compare this pattern with the previous one from the mental point of view. Heart-Fire agitates the Mind and the person suffers from insomnia, dream-disturbed sleep, anxiety, agitation, etc., but the Mind is not clouded: that is, there is no loss of insight. With Phlegm and Fire in the Heart, the Fire agitates the Mind as in the previous case but Phlegm obstructs the Mind: it is this obstruction that leads to a loss of insight and mental disturbances such as manic depression.

There are actually two separate aspects to this pattern, which may appear separately or alternately (as in manic depression):

1. Mental depression and dullness, muttering to oneself: this is called *Dian* in Chinese, meaning 'insanity'
2. Uncontrolled laughter or crying, shouting, violent behaviour, hitting or scolding people, incoherent speech: this is called *Kuang* in Chinese, meaning 'violent behaviour'

Both these patterns are of the Excess type and are caused by Phlegm and Fire obstructing the Heart and Mind. It is important not to be misled by the Yin nature of the symptoms in the *Dian* type and think that it is a Deficiency pattern requiring tonification.

The yellow sticky coating on the tongue reflects the presence of Phlegm and the Red body colour reflects the presence of Heat.

The Slippery quality of the Pulse indicates Phlegm.

Please note that the clinical manifestations outlined above are from Chinese books and they basically describe a patient with bipolar disease (incoherent speech, mental confusion, rash behaviour, tendency to hit or scold people, uncontrolled laughter or crying, shouting, muttering to oneself, mental depression and dullness, manic behaviour). It is important to note, however, that this pattern can and does occur without bipolar disease. Very many patients may suffer from Phlegm-Fire harassing the Heart without suffering from bipolar disease.

Clinical note

Phlegm obstructs the Mind, causing either mental dullness or mental illness (the latter if the Phlegm is combined with Fire). P-5 and ST-40 resolve Phlegm from the Mind

Pathological precursors of pattern

As this pattern is characterized by the presence of Phlegm, there must be an underlying deficiency of the Spleen and possibly Lungs and Kidneys too. It is the Spleen deficiency that leads to the formation of Phlegm. However, Fire, by condensing body fluids, contributes to the formation of Phlegm (Fig. 32.15).

Pathological developments from pattern

This pattern may have several pathological developments. Heart-Fire may injure Yin and lead to Yin deficiency: this will lead to a very complex clinical picture with Fire, Phlegm and Yin deficiency.

Phlegm obstructs Qi and therefore may lead to Spleen-Qi deficiency or aggravate it. As Phlegm is a

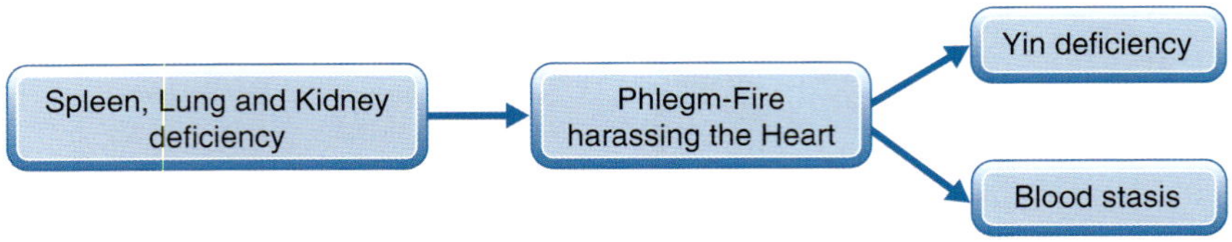

Figure 32.15 Phlegm-Fire harassing the Heart pattern: precursors and developments

pathological accumulation of Body Fluids, it may actually lead to dryness.

Finally, as Fire condenses Blood and Phlegm is connected to Blood through Body Fluids, both Fire and Phlegm may lead to Blood stasis, which will further obstruct the Mind (see Fig. 32.15).

Treatment

Principle of treatment: clear the Heart, drain Fire, resolve Phlegm, calm the Mind, open the Mind's orifices.

Acupuncture

Points: P-5 Jianshi, HE-7 Shenmen, HE-8 Shaofu, HE-9 Shaochong, P-7 Daling, Ren-15 Jiuwei, BL-15 Xinshu, Ren-12 Zhongwan, ST-40 Fenglong, SP-6 Sanyinjiao, BL-20 Pishu, LIV-2 Xingjian, GB-13 Benshen, Du-24 Shenting, GB-17 Zhengying.

Method: all with reducing method, except Ren-12 and BL-20, which should be reinforced. No moxa.

Explanation
- P-5 resolves Phlegm from the Heart and clears orifices.
- HE-7 calms the Mind.
- HE-8 and HE-9 clear Heart-Fire.
- P-7 calms the Mind and clears Heart-Fire.
- Ren-15 pacifies the Mind.
- BL-15 clears Heart-Fire.
- Ren-12 tonifies the Spleen to resolve Phlegm.
- ST-40 resolves Phlegm.
- SP-6 resolves Phlegm and calms the Mind.
- BL-20 tonifies the Spleen to resolve Phlegm.
- LIV-2 subdues Fire to conduct it downwards.
- GB-13 and Du-24 calm the Mind.
- GB-17 opens the Mind's orifices.

Ancient prescription

There is an ancient prescription for manic behaviour from Sun Si Miao (581–682), the eminent doctor of the Tang dynasty, author of the 'Thousand Golden Ducat Prescriptions'. This is: Du-26 Renzhong, LU-11 Shaoshang, SP-1 Yinbai, P-7 Daling, BL-62 Shenmai, Du-16 Fengfu, ST-6 Jiache, Ren-24 Chengjiang, P-8 Laogong, Du-23 Shangxing, Ren-1 Huiyin, LI-11 Quchi, extra point Haiquan (on the sublingual veins). These points should be needled one by one in this order, without retention of needle with reducing method: use the left side in men and the right side in women.

These points are called the '13 Ghost points' and are discussed in chapter 51.

Herbal formula

Wen Dan Tang *Warming the Gall Bladder Decoction*.

Three Treasures

Clear the Soul (variation of Wen Dan Tang).

Box 32.10 summarizes Phlegm-Fire harassing the Heart.

Case history 32.4

A 37-year-old woman suffered from what had been diagnosed as manic depression since her teenage years. The symptoms differed according to whether she was at the manic or depressive phase.

In the manic phase symptoms were palpitations, uncontrolled activity, 'cannot stop', talking very fast, overexcited, uncontrolled laughter, obsessional thoughts. In the depressive phase symptoms were frightened of failure, frustration, depressed mood, does not want to see people, tiredness, inability to work, mentally unclear. The tongue was Red, with a tip redder and swollen with red points, and a thick sticky yellow coating. The Pulse was Full and Overflowing.

All these manifestations point to obstruction of the Heart orifices and misting of the Mind by Fire and Phlegm. The Red tongue, Overflowing pulse and the mental symptoms all indicate Fire, while the sticky tongue coating denotes the presence of Phlegm.

> **Box 32.10 Phlegm-Fire harassing the Heart**
>
> **Clinical manifestations**
>
> Palpitations, thirst, red face, bitter taste, a feeling of oppression of the chest, expectoration of phlegm, rattling sound in the throat, mental restlessness, insomnia, dream-disturbed sleep, agitation, incoherent speech, mental confusion, rash behaviour, tendency to hit or scold people, uncontrolled laughter or crying, shouting, muttering to oneself, mental depression and dullness, manic behaviour, Red tongue, redder and swollen tip with red points, yellow dry sticky coating, deep Heart crack, Full-Rapid-Slippery or Rapid-Overflowing-Slippery or Rapid-Full-Wiry pulse
>
> **Treatment**
>
> P-5 Jianshi, HE-7 Shenmen, HE-8 Shaofu, HE-9 Shaochong, P-7 Daling, Ren-15 Jiuwei, BL-15 Xinshu, Ren-12 Zhongwan, ST-40 Fenglong, SP-6 Sanyinjiao, BL-20 Pishu, Du-20 Baihui, LIV-2 Xingjian, GB-13 Benshen, GB-17 Zhengying, Du-24 Shenting

Case history 32.5

A woman of 67 had been suffering from manic depression for a long time. She had bouts of depression alternating with bouts of manic behaviour. These symptoms appeared after the death of her husband. During the depressive phase she felt extremely gloomy, had no interest in life, did not wash or speak to anyone. During the manic phase she would have lots of energy, go for several days without sleep and spend money uncontrollably. Her pulse was Wiry and Overflowing on the Front positions. Her tongue was Red with a sticky yellow coating all over, and the tip was redder and swollen.

All the manifestations point to Phlegm and Fire stirring the Heart and obstructing the Heart orifices, causing her mental symptoms.

Phlegm misting the Mind

Clinical manifestations

Mental confusion, unconsciousness, lethargic stupor, incoherent speech, slurred speech, aphasia, vomiting of phlegm, rattling sound in the throat, mental depression, very dull eyes (Fig. 32.16).
Tongue: Swollen with thick sticky coating, midline crack reaching the tip (Heart crack).
Pulse: Slippery.
Key symptoms: mental confusion, rattling sound in throat, Swollen tongue with sticky coating.

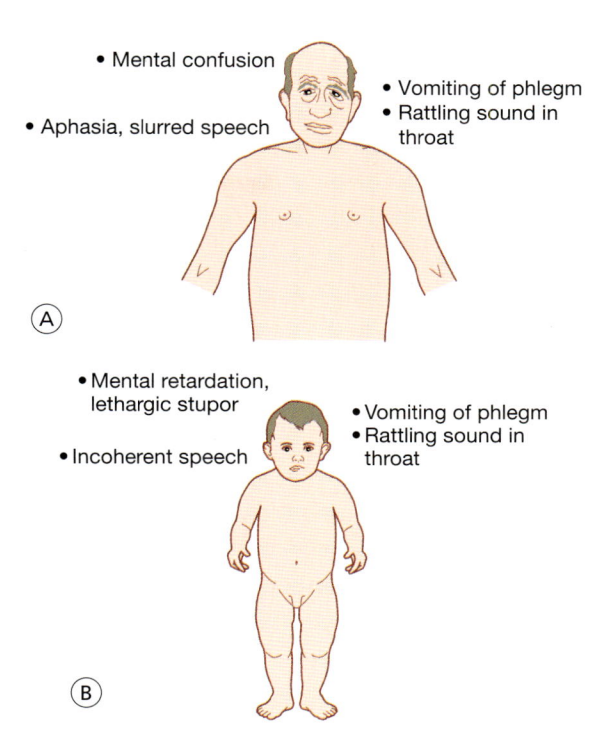

Figure 32.16 Phlegm misting the Mind

Aetiology

Constitution

In children, this pattern is constitutional.

Diet

In adults this pattern can be caused by excessive consumption of greasy cold raw foods leading to the formation of Phlegm. However, for the Phlegm to obstruct the Heart, the dietary origin of this pattern is usually combined with severe emotional problems such as long-standing anxiety.

Pathology

This pattern is also called 'Phlegm obstructing the Heart orifices'. This pattern is of the Excess type and is very similar to the previous one, except for the absence of Fire. Although similar, the two patterns occur in different types of patients and situations. The pattern of Phlegm misting the Mind is seen in children, when it can be a cause of mental retardation or speech difficulties, and in adults after an attack of Wind-stroke, when Wind associates with Phlegm, causing coma, paralysis and aphasia. In both these cases all the severe mental symptoms of the previous pattern are absent.

The mental confusion, lethargic stupor and unconsciousness are all due to Phlegm obstructing the Heart and therefore the Mind.

The Heart opens into the tongue and the Phlegm prevents the tongue from moving, hence the aphasia. The obstructive effect of the Phlegm on the Heart prevents Heart-Qi from opening into the tongue and Heart-Blood from housing the Mind: hence the Heart 'orifices' (Mind and tongue) are obstructed.

Vomiting and the rattling sound in the throat are due to Phlegm obstructing the chest.

The Swollen tongue body with sticky coating and Slippery pulse reflect the presence of Phlegm.

Pathological precursors of pattern

A deficiency of the Spleen, Lungs and Kidneys leading to Phlegm is often at the root of this pattern in adults (Fig. 32.17).

Pathological developments from pattern

Obstruction of Qi by Phlegm may tend to cause Qi deficiency and long-standing retention of Phlegm may lead to dryness and Blood stasis, especially in the elderly (see Fig. 32.17).

Treatment

Principle of treatment: open the Heart, resolve Phlegm, open the Mind's orifices.

Acupuncture

Points: P-5 Jianshi, HE-9 Shaochong, BL-15 Xinshu, ST-40 Fenglong, Du-26 Renzhong, Ren-12 Zhongwan, BL-20 Pishu, Du-14 Dazhui.
Method: all with reducing method except for Ren-12 Zhongwan and BL-20 Pishu, which should be reinforced.
Explanation
- P-5 resolves Phlegm from the Heart. This is the main point for this pattern.
- HE-9 clears the Heart and opens its orifices. In case of unconsciousness it could be bled.
- BL-15 clears the Heart and is particularly useful in children to clear Phlegm from the Heart: it will stimulate the child's intellectual capacities and speech.
- ST-40 resolves Phlegm.
- Du-26 is used to restore consciousness if necessary.
- Ren-12 and BL-20 tonify the Spleen to resolve Phlegm.
- Du-14 clears the Heart and tonifies Heart-Yang. Heart-Yang is stimulated to mobilize the Phlegm.

Herbal formula

Di Tan Tang *Scouring Phlegm Decoction*.
Gun Tan Wan *Vapourizing Phlegm Pill*.

Box 32.11 summarizes Phlegm misting the Mind.

Box 32.11 Phlegm misting the Mind

Clinical manifestations

Mental confusion, unconsciousness, lethargic stupor, incoherent speech, vomiting of phlegm, rattling sound in the throat, mental depression, emotional lability, aphasia, very dull eyes, Swollen tongue with thick-sticky coating, Heart crack, Slippery pulse

Treatment

P-5 Jianshi, HE-9 Shaochong, BL-15 Xinshu, ST-40 Fenglong, Du-26 Renzhong, Ren-12 Zhongwan, BL-20 Pishu, Du-14 Dazhui

---

Heart-Qi stagnation

Clinical manifestations

Palpitations, a feeling of distension or oppression of the chest, depression, a slight feeling of lump in the throat, slight shortness of breath, sighing, poor appetite, slight nausea, cold limbs, slightly purple lips, pale complexion (Fig. 32.18).

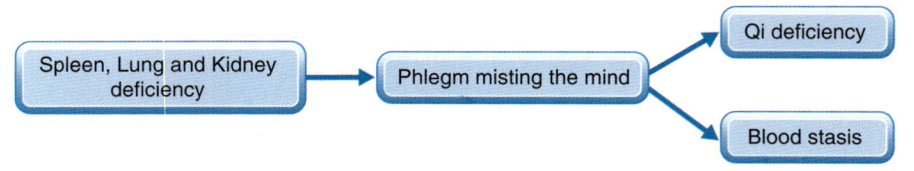

Figure 32.17 Phlegm misting the Mind pattern: precursors and developments

- Slightly purple lips
- Depression
- Sighing
- Feeling of lump in the throat
- Feeling of distension or oppression of the chest
- Shortness of breath
- Palpitations
- Cold hands

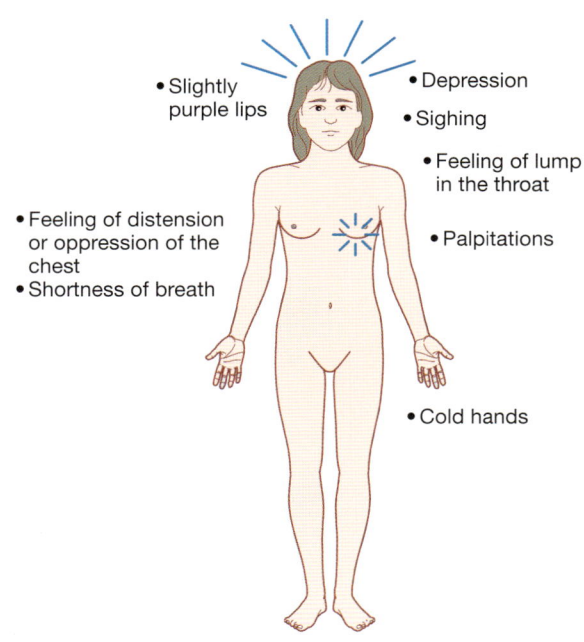

Figure 32.18 Heart-Qi stagnation

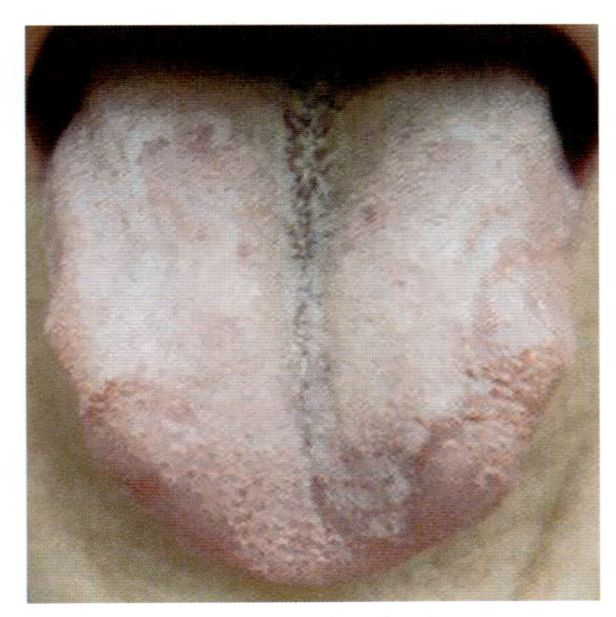

Figure 32.19 Slightly Pale-Purple in chest/breast area on the left

Tongue: slightly Pale-Purple on the sides in the chest area (see Fig. 23.19 in chapter 23 and Fig. 32.19).
Pulse: Empty but very slightly Overflowing on the left Front position.

Aetiology

Emotional stress

Emotional stress is the only cause of this pattern. Sadness, grief and worry affect the Heart and may make Heart-Qi stagnate in the chest. This is, in fact, the very first effect of those emotions. After some time, the Qi stagnation will lead to Heat and give rise to Heart-Heat.

Why would these emotions cause Qi stagnation in some patients and, more commonly, Qi deficiency in others? Generally speaking, it depends on three factors. Firstly, if a patient has a robust constitution and a tendency to Full patterns, he or she will develop Heart-Qi stagnation rather than deficiency when subject to that emotional stress. Secondly, Qi stagnation is more likely to happen when the person tends to suppress and hide his or her emotions. Thirdly, Heart-Qi stagnation is more likely to develop when there is a pre-existing Liver-Qi stagnation, but it should be stressed that Heart-Qi stagnation can and does occur without Liver-Qi stagnation.

Pathology

The feeling of distension of the chest, slight feeling of lump in the throat and sighing all indicate Qi stagnation. As Heart-Qi stagnates, there will be some slight shortness of breath caused by stagnation rather than deficiency of Qi. The Qi stagnation also causes the lips to become slightly purple. The complexion is pale not so much because of Qi deficiency but because the stagnant Heart-Qi in the chest fails to ascend to the face.

The symptom of poor appetite (normally due to a Spleen deficiency) is due to Heart-Qi not descending towards the Stomach. The slight nausea is due to Heart-Qi not descending because it is stagnating.

The slightly Overflowing quality of the Heart pulse is an important indication of this pattern.

Pathological precursors of pattern

Liver-Qi stagnation is a possible precursor of this pattern. When Liver-Qi stagnates, if may affect the free flow of Qi in any organ and, when subject to emotional stress, the Heart-Qi is easily affected.

This pattern may also derive from Heart-Qi deficiency when this is caused by sadness or grief. In fact, when Qi is deficient it does not circulate properly and it may lead to a secondary Qi stagnation: thus, Qi can be both deficient and stagnant (Fig. 32.20).

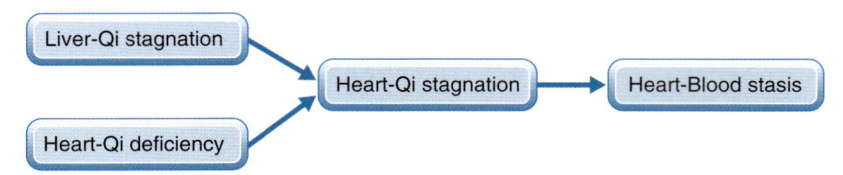

Figure 32.20 Heart-Qi stagnation pattern: precursors and developments

Pathological developments from pattern

Heart-Qi stagnation may easily lead to Heart-Blood stasis, which is potentially a more serious pattern. Stagnation of Heart-Qi in the chest may also affect the Liver and cause Liver-Qi stagnation (see Fig. 32.20).

Treatment

Principle of treatment: move Heart-Qi, open the chest, calm the Mind.

Acupuncture

Points: P-6 Neiguan, HE-5 Tongli, HE-7 Shenmen, Ren-15 Jiuwei, Ren-17 Shanzhong, LU-7 Lieque, ST-40 Fenglong.
Method: all with reducing method.
Explanation
- P-6 opens the chest, moves Qi and calms the Mind.
- HE-5 moves Heart-Qi and calms the Mind.
- HE-7 calms the Mind.
- Ren-15 opens the chest and calms the Mind.
- Ren-17 moves Qi in the chest.
- LU-7 moves Qi in the chest.
- ST-40 is used here not to resolve Phlegm but to open the chest and move Qi in the chest.

Herbal formula

Mu Xiang Liu Qi Yin *Aucklandia Flowing Qi Decoction*.
Ban Xia Hou Po Tang *Pinellia–Magnolia Decoction*.

Three Treasures

Open the Heart (Variation of Ban Xia Hou Po Tang). Box 32.12 summarizes Heart-Qi stagnation.

Heart vessel obstructed

Clinical manifestations

Palpitations, shortness of breath with inability to lie down, depression, mental restlessness, a feeling of oppression of the chest, stabbing or pricking pain in the heart region which comes and goes and which may radiate to the upper back or shoulder, pain aggravated by exposure to cold and alleviated by heat, expectoration of phlegm, a feeling of heaviness, dislike to speak, cold hands, sighing, purple lips, face and nails (Fig. 32.21).
Tongue: Purple on the sides in the chest area, Swollen with a sticky coating.
Pulse: Wiry, Choppy or Knotted; Slippery if Phlegm is predominant.

Aetiology

Emotional stress

Emotional stress such as worry, anxiety and anger may lead to Heart-Qi stagnation, which, in time, leads to Heart-Blood stasis.

Diet

Excessive consumption of dairy foods and greasy foods leads to the formation of Phlegm, which is one of the pathogenic factors in this pattern.

Excessive physical work

Excessive physical work injures Kidney- and Heart-Yang; deficient Heart-Yang fails to move Qi and Blood in the chest and leads to Blood stasis from Cold.

Box 32.12 Heart-Qi stagnation

Clinical manifestations

Palpitations, a feeling of distension or oppression of the chest, depression, a slight feeling of lump in the throat, slight shortness of breath, sighing, poor appetite, slight nausea, cold limbs, slightly purple lips, pale complexion, tongue slightly Pale-Purple on the sides in the chest area, pulse Empty but very slightly Overflowing on the left Front position

Treatment

P-6 Neiguan, HE-5 Tongli, HE-7 Shenmen, Ren-15 Jiuwei, Ren-17 Shanzhong, LU-7 Lieque, ST-40 Fenglong

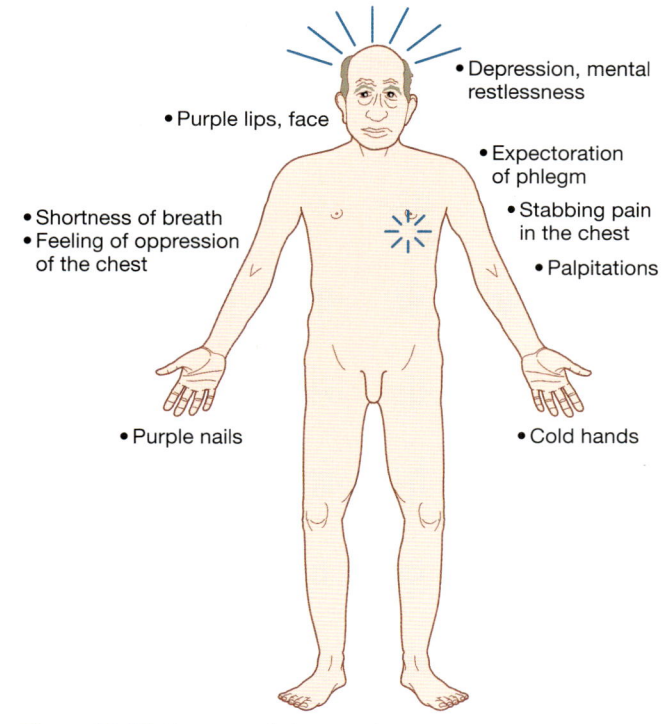

Figure 32.21 Heart vessel obstructed

- Depression, mental restlessness
- Purple lips, face
- Expectoration of phlegm
- Stabbing pain in the chest
- Palpitations
- Shortness of breath
- Feeling of oppression of the chest
- Purple nails
- Cold hands

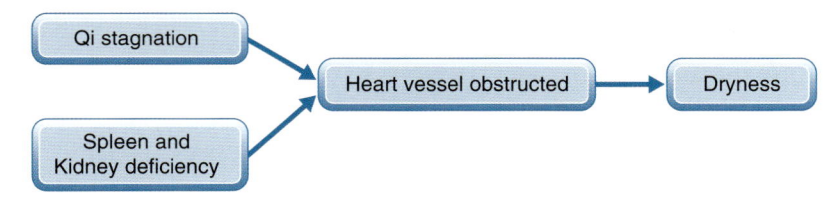

Figure 32.22 Heart vessel obstructed pattern: precursors and developments

Qi stagnation → Heart vessel obstructed → Dryness
Spleen and Kidney deficiency →

Pathology

This is a complex condition characterized by Blood stasis, Phlegm, Qi stagnation and Cold.

Phlegm obstructs the chest and causes a feeling of oppression of the chest, expectoration of phlegm, feeling of heaviness, shortness of breath with inability to lie down, and a Swollen tongue.

Blood stasis obstructs the chest and causes the stabbing of pricking pain as well as the purple lips, face and nails and Purple tongue.

Cold contracts and congeals and this causes the feeling of cold and cold hands. The mental–emotional symptoms (depression, mental restlessness) are caused by both Qi stagnation and Blood stasis.

Clinical note

This pattern and the next one, Heart-Blood stasis, are the only two Heart patterns that involve chest pain

Pathological precursors of pattern

Qi stagnation generally precedes this pattern as Blood stasis often derives from Qi stagnation.

A deficiency of the Spleen and/or Kidneys is usually also at the root of this pattern as this leads to the formation of Phlegm.

Yang deficiency is also a precursor of this patterns as it leads to Cold (Fig. 32.22).

Pathological developments from pattern

There may be pathological developments from both Blood stasis and Phlegm. In fact, both Blood stasis and Phlegm may lead to dryness. Phlegm also obstructs Qi and may therefore make the Qi and Yang deficiency worse (see Fig. 32.22).

Treatment

Principle of treatment: move Heart-Qi and Heart-Blood, eliminate stasis, open the chest, resolve Phlegm, expel Cold, calm the Mind.

Acupuncture

Points: P-6 Neiguan, HE-5 Tongli, HE-7 Shenmen, Ren-15 Jiuwei, Ren-17 Shanzhong, LU-7 Lieque, ST-40 Fenglong, L.I.-4 Hegu, BL-15 Xinshu, BL-17 Geshu, Ren-12 Zhongwan.
Method: all with reducing method except for Ren-12, which should be reinforced.
Explanation
– P-6 opens the chest, moves Qi and Blood and calms the Mind.
– HE-5 moves Heart-Qi and Heart-Blood and calms the Mind.
– HE-7 calms the Mind.
– Ren-15 opens the chest and calms the Mind.
– Ren-17 moves Qi in the chest.
– LU-7 and L.I.-4 regulate the ascending and descending of Qi in the chest and therefore move Qi.
– ST-40 resolves Phlegm.
– BL-15 moves Heart-Qi.
– BL-17 moves Blood.
– Ren-12 tonifies the Spleen to resolve Phlegm.

Herbal formula

Zhi Shi Gua Lou Gui Zhi Tang *Citrus–Trichosanthes–Ramulus Cinnamomi Decoction* plus Dan Shen *Radix Salviae miltiorrhizae*.
Box 32.13 summarizes Heart vessel obstructed.

DEFICIENCY–EXCESS PATTERNS

Heart-Blood stasis

Clinical manifestations

Palpitations, stabbing or pricking pain in the chest which may radiate to the inner aspect of the left arm or to the shoulder, a feeling of oppression or constriction of the chest, cyanosis of lips and nails, cold hands (Fig. 32.23).
Tongue: Purple in its entirety or only on the sides in the chest area.
Pulse: Choppy, Wiry or Knotted.
Key symptoms: stabbing pain in the chest, cyanosis of lips, purple tongue.

Aetiology

Emotional stress

Emotional problems, particularly anxiety, grief or worry over a long period of time, can lead to stasis of Blood in the chest. The chest is a part of the body where pent-up emotions are frequently kept and they therefore easily lead to impairment in the circulation of Qi or Blood in this area. Furthermore, all these emotions disturb the Mind. Heart-Blood is the physiological basis for the Mind and any emotional problem that constrains the Mind may lead to stagnation of Qi and/or Blood of the Heart.

Pathology

This pattern does not occur on its own, but is derived from other Heart patterns, mostly Heart-Yang deficiency, Heart-Blood deficiency or Heart-Qi stagnation. The symptoms and signs will therefore vary according to the origin of the pattern. The symptoms and signs described above are only those related to the stasis of

---

Box 32.13 Heart vessel obstructed

Clinical manifestations

Palpitations, shortness of breath with inability to lie down, depression, mental restlessness, a feeling of oppression of the chest, stabbing or pricking pain in the heart region which comes and goes and which may radiate to the upper back or shoulder, pain aggravated by exposure to cold and alleviated by heat, expectoration of phlegm, a feeling of heaviness, dislike to speak, cold hands, sighing, purple lips, face and nails
Tongue: Purple on the sides in the chest area, Swollen with a sticky coating
Pulse: Wiry, Choppy or Knotted; Slippery if Phlegm is predominant

Treatment

P-6 Neiguan, HE-5 Tongli, HE-7 Shenmen, Ren-15 Jiuwei, Ren-17 Shanzhong, LU-7 Lieque, ST-40 Fenglong, L.I.-4 Hegu, BL-15 Xinshu, BL-17 Geshu, Ren-12 Zhongwan

- Cyanosis of lips
- Stabbing chest pain
- Feeling of constriction of the chest
- Palpitations
- Pain inner aspect of left arm
- Cyanosis of nails
- Cold hands

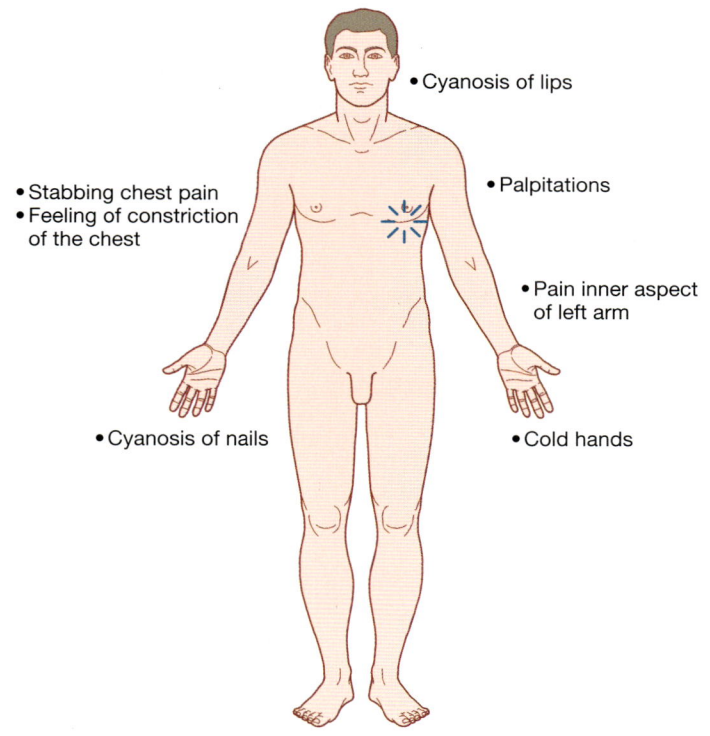

Figure 32.23 Heart-Blood stasis

Heart-Blood and, in practice, there would be in addition some symptoms of Heart-Yang deficiency, Heart-Blood deficiency or Heart-Qi stagnation.

If it is due to Heart-Yang or Heart-Blood deficiency, this pattern is a combined Deficiency/Excess pattern. In most cases, it is derived from Heart-Yang deficiency.

Yang Qi moves and transports. If Heart-Yang is deficient, it cannot move Blood in the chest: hence Blood stagnates in this area and causes the pain and feeling of constriction. The intensity of the pain can vary from a mild pricking sensation to an intense stabbing pain. Chest pain is the key symptom of this pattern, which only one other Heart pattern has (Heart vessel obstructed). The pain typically comes in repeated bouts and is elicited by exertion or cold weather.

The cyanosis of lips and nails and the cold hands are due to stagnant Heart-Blood not reaching the face and hands. The stasis of Blood in the chest also obstructs the circulation of Gathering Qi, which normally has the function of helping the movement of Lung- and Heart-Qi to the hands, resulting in cold hands.

The Purple colour of the tongue body reflects the stasis of Blood. In most cases, this will be Bluish-Purple reflecting the internal Cold from Deficiency of Yang causing stasis of Blood.

The Choppy or Wiry pulse reflects Blood stasis. If there is Yang deficiency with Cold the pulse may be Knotted. The irregularity of it is due to the stagnation of Blood, which prevents it from circulating properly.

Pathological precursors of pattern

This pattern may be derived from other Heart patterns, particularly Heart-Yang deficiency. Therefore, any of the causes leading to Heart-Yang deficiency can, in the long run, lead to Heart-Blood stasis.

Heart-Qi stagnation is also a frequent precursor of this pattern as when Qi stagnates it fails to move Blood and Blood stasis frequently occurs.

For the same reasons, Liver-Qi stagnation may be a precursor to this pattern. The Liver channel affects the chest and the loss of the free flow of Liver-Qi may easily affect the Heart, leading to Heart-Qi stagnation first and then Heart-Blood stasis (Fig. 32.24).

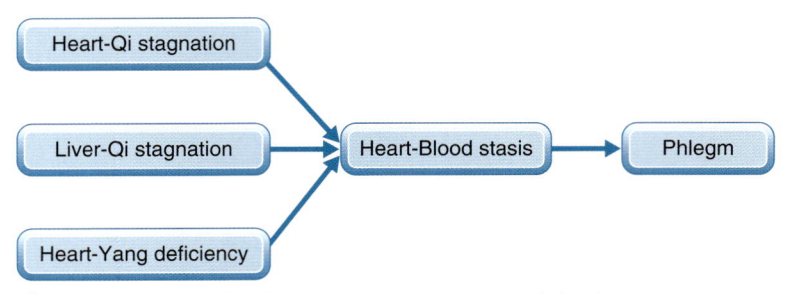

Figure 32.24 Heart-Blood stasis pattern: precursors and developments

Pathological developments from pattern

Heart-Blood stasis may lead to the formation of Phlegm because of the interaction between these two pathogenic factors. A long-term consequence of Blood stasis, especially in the elderly, can be dryness (see Fig. 32.24).

Treatment

Principle of treatment: move Blood, eliminate stasis, tonify and warm Heart-Yang, calm the Mind.

Acupuncture

Points: P-6 Neiguan, P-4 Ximen, HE-5 Tongli, Ren-17 Shanzhong, BL-14 Jueyinshu, BL-17 Geshu, SP-10 Xuehai, KI-25 Shencang.
Method: all with reducing method during an attack, or even method in between the attacks. Moxa is applicable if there is Heart-Yang deficiency.
Explanation
- P-6 moves Heart-Blood and opens the chest. This is the main point.
- P-4 is the Accumulation point and is particularly useful to stop chest pain.
- HE-5 moves Heart-Blood and calms the Mind.
- Ren-17 moves Qi and Blood in the chest and stimulates the circulation of Gathering Qi. Moxa after needling can be used if there is Heart-Yang deficiency.
- BL-14 moves Heart-Blood.
- BL-17 moves Blood and eliminates stasis.
- SP-10 moves Blood.
- KI-25 is a local chest point to move Qi and Blood in the chest. It is particularly useful if the Heart-Yang deficiency is associated with Kidney-Yang deficiency.

Herbal formula

Xue Fu Zhu Yu Tang *Blood-Mansion Eliminating Stasis Decoction*.

Box 32.14 Heart-Blood stasis

Clinical manifestations

Palpitations, stabbing or pricking pain in the chest which may radiate to the inner aspect of the left arm or to the shoulder, a feeling of oppression or constriction of the chest, cyanosis of lips and nails, cold hands, tongue Purple in its entirety or only on the sides in the chest area, Choppy, Wiry or Knotted pulse

Treatment

P-6 Neiguan, P-4 Ximen, HE-5 Tongli, Ren-17 Shanzhong, BL-14 Jueyinshu, BL-17 Geshu, SP-10 Xuehai, KI-25 Shencang

---

Three Treasures

Red Stirring (Variation of Xue Fu Zhu Yu Tang).
Box 32.14 summarizes Heart-Blood stasis.

Case history 32.6

A 52-year-old lady had been suffering from bouts of severe palpitations and stabbing pain in the chest radiating to the left arm for 30 years. During the attacks her lips became cyanotic and she felt cold. The tongue was Bluish-Purple and the pulse Knotted.

This is an example of stasis of Heart-Blood from deficiency of Heart-Yang.

Case history 32.7

A 77-year-old man suffered from a more or less permanent sensation of constriction of the chest elicited by exertion. The tongue was Reddish-Purple and the pulse was Wiry.

This is an example of stasis of Heart-Blood from Heart-Fire.

COMBINED PATTERNS

- Heart- and Liver-Blood deficiency (discussed under Liver patterns, ch. 34)
- Heart- and Spleen-Blood deficiency (discussed under Spleen patterns, ch. 36)
- Heart- and Lung-Qi deficiency (discussed under Lung patterns, ch. 35)
- Kidneys and Heart not harmonized (discussed under the Kidney patterns, ch. 37)

Learning outcomes

In this chapter you will have learned:
- The concept that the Heart is not affected directly by exterior climatic factors
- The way in which excessive excitement, sadness and grief, anger and worry affect the Heart
- How to identify the following Deficiency patterns:
  - *Heart-Qi deficiency:* light palpitations and other Qi deficiency symptoms
  - *Heart-Yang deficiency:* similar to Heart-Qi deficiency with cold hands and stuffy chest
  - *Heart-Yang Collapse:* extreme Heart-Yang deficiency with cyanosis of lips
  - *Heart-Blood deficiency:* insomnia, anxiety and poor memory due to the Mind being deprived of its residence, with palpitations from Heart-Qi deficiency
  - *Heart-Yin deficiency:* similar to Heart-Blood deficiency with mental restlessness, night sweating and other symptoms of Empty-Heat
- How to identify the following Excess patterns:
  - *Heart-Fire blazing:* tongue ulcers, palpitations and heat symptoms
  - *Phlegm-Fire harassing the Heart:* mental symptoms due to Phlegm (loss of insight) and Fire (agitation) obstructing the Heart orifices and disturbing the Mind
  - *Phlegm misting the Mind:* mental confusion and rattling in the throat due to obstruction from Phlegm
  - *Heart-Qi stagnation:* distension in chest, a lump in the throat, depression and sighing due to emotions causing stagnation in the chest
  - *Heart-Vessel obstructed:* oppression and pain in the chest from Blood stasis, Phlegm, Qi stagnation and Cold
  - *Heart-Blood stasis:* stabbing pain in chest and cyanosis of lips usually deriving from Heart-Yang deficiency

Learning tips

- Remember, all Heart patterns start with 'palpitations' (except for 'Phlegm misting the Mind'); therefore that is the first word you should write when asked to list a Heart pattern
- Next, think of the Heart functions and work out some symptoms accordingly. The most important Heart function is that of housing the Mind and therefore put some mental–emotional symptoms accordingly, bearing in mind the difference between Full and Empty conditions. For example, in Heart-Blood deficiency, write 'mild anxiety'; in Heart-Fire write 'agitation'
- Remember the orifices related to the Heart, i.e. tongue (e.g. tongue ulcers in Heart-Fire)
- Remember that Heart-Blood stasis is the only pattern that manifests with pain ('pain in the chest')
- As for all other patterns, remember the general symptoms that are 'safe' to add to any pattern, e.g. 'feeling of heat' in case of Fire patterns, 'feeling of cold' in Yang deficiency, 'pale face' in Qi and Yang deficiency, tiredness in Empty patterns
- Finally, remember the pulse qualities, e.g. Empty for Qi deficiency, Weak and Deep for Yang deficiency, Floating-Empty for Yin deficiency and Choppy or Fine for Blood deficiency

Self-assessment questions

1. What are the six functions of the Heart according to Chinese medical theory?
2. How might prolonged sadness and grief lead eventually to Heat in the Heart?
3. Describe the pulse you might find in a severe case of Heart-Qi deficiency.
4. Describe the pathology of the feeling of 'stuffiness in the chest' associated with Heart-Yang deficiency. What is the most clinically important potential consequence of this symptom?
5. In treating a collapse of Heart-Yang, why is it important to stop sweating?
6. How does long-term sadness lead to Blood deficiency?
7. How do palpitations from Heart-Qi deficiency differ from those from Heart-Blood deficiency?
8. Describe the possible pulse pictures associated with Heart-Yin deficiency.
9. What tongue usually accompanies the pattern Heart-Fire blazing?
10. Apart from the Heart, what is the other main organ implicated in the pattern Phlegm-Fire harassing the Heart?
11. When is the pattern Phlegm misting the Mind commonly seen in adults?
12. What tongue picture is associated with the pattern Heart-Qi stagnation?
13. What is the key symptom in diagnosing Heart-Blood stasis?

See p. 1263 for answers

END NOTES

1. 1981 Spiritual Axis (*Ling Shu Jing* 灵枢经), People's Health Publishing House, Beijing, first published *c.*100 BC, p. 128.
2. 1979 The Yellow Emperor's Classic of Internal Medicine – Simple Questions (*Huang Di Nei Jing Su Wen* 黄帝内经素问), People's Health Publishing House, Beijing, first published *c.*100 BC, p. 221.
3. Spiritual Axis, p. 24.
4. 1982 Zhang Jing Yue 'Classic of Categories' (*Lei Jing* 类经), People's Health Publishing House, Beijing, first published 1624, p. 464.

SECTION 2 PART 6

Pericardium Patterns 33

> **Key contents**
>
> **The Pericardium in invasions of exterior pathogenic factors**
> Heat in the Pericardium
>
> **The Pericardium as the 'house' of the Mind**
> Blood deficiency of the Pericardium
> Pericardium-Fire
> Phlegm-Fire harassing the Pericardium
>
> **The Pericardium as the 'centre of the thorax'**
> Qi stagnation in the Pericardium
> Blood stasis of the Pericardium

As mentioned in chapter 11, the Pericardium is not as well defined in its functions as the other Yin organs; as a consequence, its pathology is also less well defined.

In pathology, the Heart and Pericardium are very closely related but what differentiates Pericardium from Heart patterns is the involvement of the Pericardium as a *channel* in the chest. Therefore, in the Pericardium patterns generated by mental–emotional strain, the prevailing pathology is reflected in the involvement of Pericardium channel with symptoms at the chest level: for example, a feeling of oppression of the chest, a feeling of stuffiness of the chest, or a feeling of distension of the chest and chest pain.

Another characteristic that differentiates Pericardium from Heart patterns is the involvement of the Lung channel. As mentioned in chapter 11, the Pericardium is the centre of the thorax, where it influences both the Heart and Lungs and therefore the Gathering Qi (*Zong Qi*): the Pericardium channel, therefore, is like the propulsive agent for the Qi and Blood of both Heart and Lungs. For this reason, Pericardium patterns may present with symptoms such as shortness of breath and cold hands.

A third characteristics that differentiates Heart from Pericardium patterns is that the latter patterns often involve the Liver channel as well. This is due to two reasons: firstly because the Liver and Pericardium are related within the Terminal Yin channels (*Jue Yin*); secondly because, in its upward rising (from emotional problems), the Minister Fire affects the Liver, Gall Bladder and Pericardium.

A fourth characteristic that distinguishes Heart from Pericardium patterns is that the latter is involved in the pathology of acute fevers. For example, one of the two patterns of the Nutritive Qi (*Ying*) Level of the Four Levels in *Wen Bing* diseases is 'Heat in the Pericardium'. This is an aspect of the Chinese view that the Pericardium 'takes the knocks for the Heart': that is, it is invaded by exterior pathogenic factors aimed at the Heart (see below).

We can identify three main areas of Pericardium pathology:

> - The Pericardium as the 'protector' of the Heart: invasions of exterior pathogenic factors
>   - Heat in the Pericardium
> - The Pericardium as the house of the Mind: mental–emotional problems
>   - Blood deficiency of the Pericardium
>   - Pericardium Fire
>   - Phlegm-Fire harassing the Pericardium
> - The Pericardium as the 'centre of the thorax': channel pathology
>   - Qi stagnation in the Pericardium
>   - Blood stasis in the Pericardium

THE PERICARDIUM IN INVASIONS OF EXTERIOR PATHOGENIC FACTORS

Generally speaking, exterior climatic factors do not affect the Heart directly. Of all the climatic factors, Fire and Heat are the ones that most affect the Heart, but even those do not affect it directly. Chinese medicine maintains that exterior pathogenic factors do not affect the Heart directly, but instead affect the Pericardium. The 'Spiritual Axis' in chapter 71 says: '*If exterior pathogenic factors attack the Heart, they penetrate the Pericardium instead.*'[1] Thus, if exterior Heat invades the body, it will easily affect the Pericardium.

Box 33.1 summarizes factors that might give a 'feel' for Pericardium pathology.

Clinical note

Four main factors differentiating Pericardium from Heart patterns:
1. Involvement of Pericardium channel in the chest: feeling of stuffiness, oppression, distension or pain of the chest
2. Involvement of Lung channel: shortness of breath, cold hands
3. Often involvement of Liver channel: irritability, headache
4. Involvement of the Pericardium in acute fevers

The pattern of invasion of the Pericardium by Heat is especially significant in the context of the Chinese herbal treatment of infectious diseases caused by exterior Heat. It denotes a condition of rapid invasion of exterior Heat at the Nutritive Qi (*Ying*) Level (within the Four Levels), manifesting with very high temperature, delirium and, in severe cases, coma. Invasion of the Pericardium by Heat mists the Mind and causes coma. This pattern is called 'Heat in the Pericardium' and is one of the two patterns at the Ying Level. This pattern is the same as the pattern of Heat in the Pericardium at the Upper Burner Stage within the Three Burners Pattern Identification (Fig 33.1).

The clinical manifestations of these two patterns are almost identical and I will therefore list only one pattern.

Heat in the Pericardium

(Nutritive Qi Level within the Four Levels or Upper Burner Stage within the Three Burners.) (See ch. 45.)

Clinical manifestations

Fever at night, mental confusion, incoherent speech or aphasia, delirium, body hot, hands and feet cold, macules (Fig. 33.2).
Tongue: Red and dry without coating.
Pulse: Fine-Rapid.
Key symptoms: fever at night, delirium, Red tongue without coating.

Diagnostic tip

Fever at night, delirium and a Red tongue without coating are enough to diagnose Heat in the Pericardium

Aetiology

This is due to invasion of Wind-Heat that penetrates into the Interior and transforms into interior Heat,

Box 33.1 A 'feel' for pericardium pathology

- Mental-emotional problems, especially from relationships
- Chest symptoms: stuffiness, distension, oppression, tightness, pain

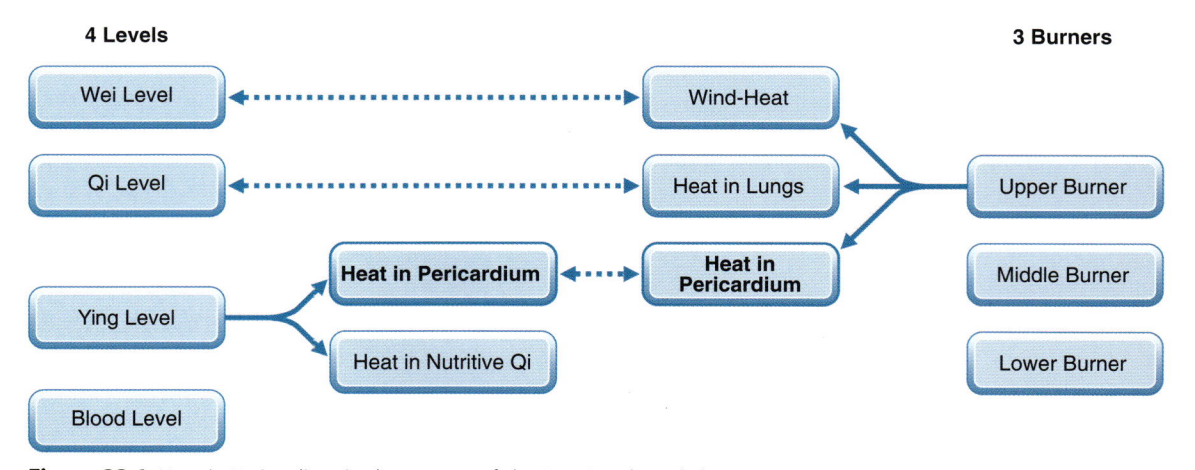

Figure 33.1 Heat in Pericardium in the context of the Four Levels and Three Burners

going through the Defensive Qi and Qi Levels before reaching the Nutritive Qi Level (see Fig. 33.1).

Pathology

This is Heat at the Nutritive Qi (*Ying*) Level. Within the Four Levels, interior Heat is further classified as being at the Qi, Nutritive Qi and Blood Level, this progression reflecting the depth of the Heat.

When Heat penetrates the Nutritive Qi Level, it has begun to injure Yin and dry up the Body Fluids, hence the tongue has no coating and is dry. Heat clouds the Mind and gives rise to delirium. Fever at night is characteristic of Heat at the Nutritive Qi Level.

The hands and feet are cold from False Cold: this phenomenon is due to the fact that the Heat is so intense that it impairs the circulation of Qi to the limbs, leading to cold hands and feet. This is an example of False Cold–True Heat.

Pathological precursors of pattern

The only precursor of this pattern is Heat at the Qi level (Fig. 33.3).

Pathological developments from pattern

Heat in the Pericardium can progress to the next level, leading to Heat at the Blood Level. At this level, internal Wind may develop, causing convulsions (see Fig. 33.3).

Treatment

Principle of treatment: clear Nutritive Qi Level Heat.

Acupuncture

Points: P-9 Zhongchong, P-8 Laogong, HE-9 Shaochong, KI-6 Zhaohai, SP-6 Sanyinjiao.
Method: reducing method except for KI-6, which should be reinforced.
Explanation
- P-9 and P-8 clear Heat in the Pericardium.
- HE-9 clears Heat in the Pericardium and clears the Mind.
- KI-6 and SP-6 nourish fluids to prevent further injury of Yin.

Herbal formula

Qing Ying Tang *Clearing the Nutritive Qi [Heat] Decoction*.

Box 33.2 summarizes Heat in the Pericardium.

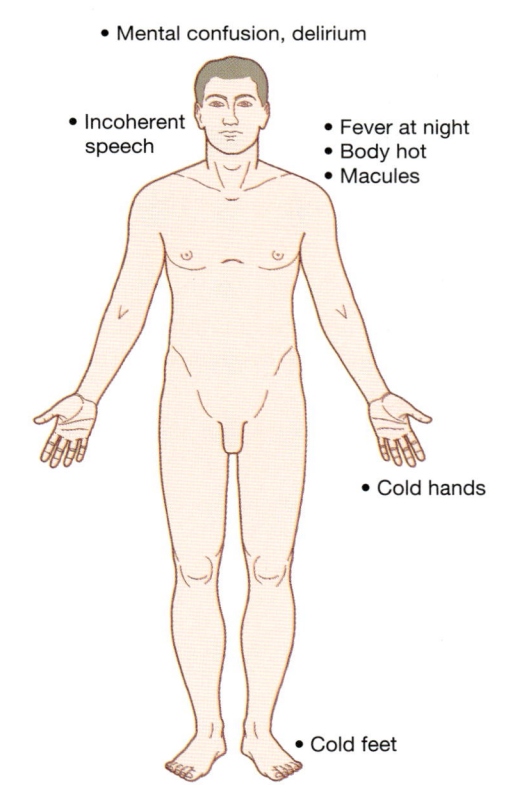

Figure 33.2 Heat in Pericardium
- Mental confusion, delirium
- Incoherent speech
- Fever at night
- Body hot
- Macules
- Cold hands
- Cold feet

Box 33.2 Heat in the Pericardium

(Nutritive Qi Level of the Four Levels or Upper Burner Stage within the Six Burners)

Clinical manifestations

Fever at night, mental confusion, incoherent speech or aphasia, delirium, body hot, hands and feet cold, macules, Red and dry tongue without coating, Fine-Rapid pulse.

Treatment

P-9 Zhongchong, P-8 Laogong, HE-9 Shaochong, KI-6 Zhaohai, SP-6 Sanyinjiao

---

Heat at the Qi level → Heat in the Pericardium → Heat at the Blood level

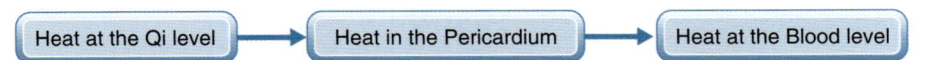

Figure 33.3 Heat in Pericardium pattern: precursors and developments

THE PERICARDIUM AS THE 'HOUSE' OF THE MIND

The 'Simple Questions' in chapter 8 says: '*The Pericardium is the ambassador and from it joy and happiness derive.*'[2] Incidentally, in this passage, the Pericardium is actually called the 'centre of the chest' (*Shan Zhong*).

Like the Heart, the Pericardium houses the Mind and it therefore influences our mental–emotional state deeply. It could be said that the protective function of the Pericardium in relation to the Heart, mentioned above, is reflected primarily in the mental–emotional sphere where the 'Minister Fire' of the Pericardium protects the 'Emperor Fire' of the Heart.

Two main areas differentiate Pericardium from Heart patterns in the mental–emotional sphere: the first is the involvement of the Pericardium channel in the chest, the second is the frequent manifestation of mental–emotional strain due to relationship problems.

The second factor is probably the psychic equivalent of the above-mentioned function of the Pericardium in the chest with regard to moving Qi and Blood of Heart and Lungs: just as it does that on a physical level, on a mental–emotional level, the Pericardium is responsible for 'movement' towards others (i.e. in relationships). Given that the Pericardium is related to the Liver within the Terminal-Yin channels, this 'movement' is also related to the 'movement' of the Ethereal Soul (*Hun*) from the self towards others in social, relationships and familial interactions (Fig. 33.4).

The patterns discussed are:

- Blood deficiency of the Pericardium
- Pericardium-Fire
- Phlegm-Fire harassing the Pericardium

Blood deficiency of the Pericardium

Clinical manifestations

A feeling of stuffiness and discomfort of the chest, dull ache in the chest, very slight shortness of breath, palpitations, anxiety, insomnia, dizziness, dream-disturbed sleep, poor memory, propensity to be startled, dull-pale complexion, pale lips, cold hands, scanty periods, amenorrhoea (Fig. 33.5).
Tongue: Pale, Thin, slightly dry.
Pulse: Choppy or Fine but very slightly hard on the left Front position.
Key symptoms: discomfort of the chest, palpitations, insomnia, Choppy pulse.

> **Diagnostic tip**
>
> Discomfort of the chest, palpitations and insomnia are enough to diagnose Blood deficiency of the Pericardium

Aetiology

The aetiology of this pattern is from emotional strain such as sadness and grief, frequently from the break-up of relationships.

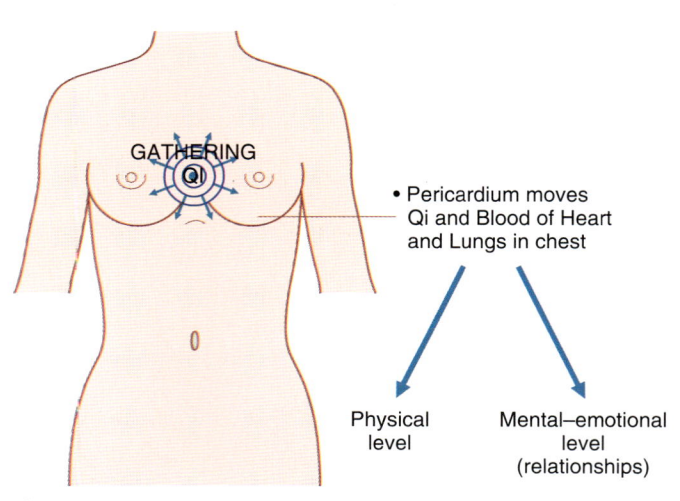

Figure 33.4 Pericardium and Gathering Qi (*Zong Qi*)

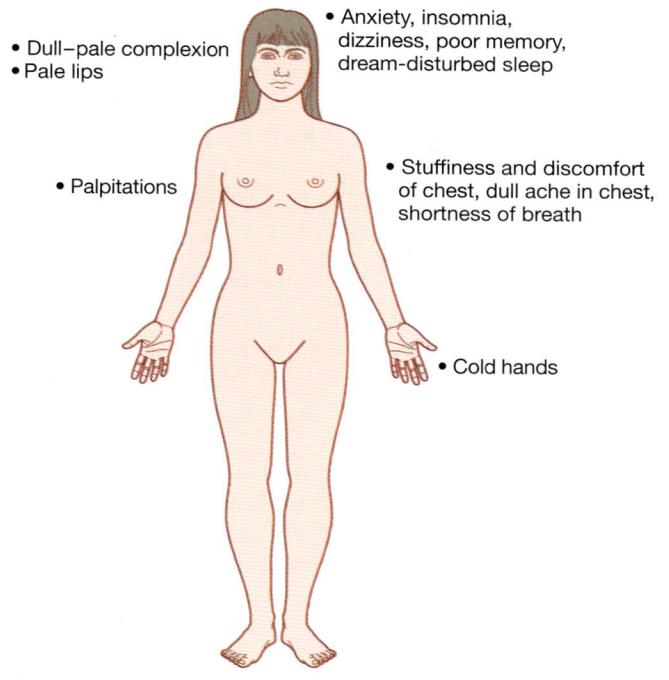

Figure 33.5 Blood deficiency of the Pericardium

- Dull–pale complexion
- Pale lips
- Anxiety, insomnia, dizziness, poor memory, dream-disturbed sleep
- Palpitations
- Stuffiness and discomfort of chest, dull ache in chest, shortness of breath
- Cold hands

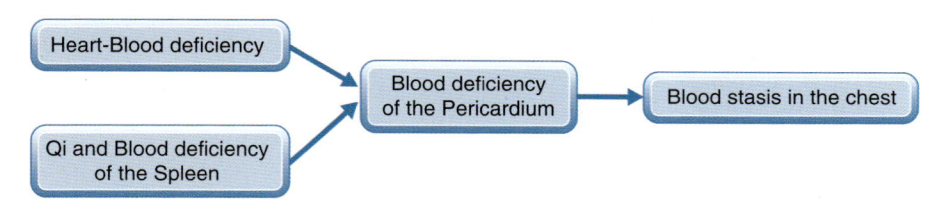

Figure 33.6 Blood deficiency of the Pericardium pattern: precursors and developments

Heart-Blood deficiency → Blood deficiency of the Pericardium → Blood stasis in the chest
Qi and Blood deficiency of the Spleen → Blood deficiency of the Pericardium

Pathology

Heart and Pericardium house the Mind: when Blood of the Heart and Pericardium is deficient, the Mind lacks its residence and therefore it is agitated, resulting in insomnia, dream-disturbed sleep, propensity to be startled and anxiety. Heart-Blood is one of the factors contributing to memory and a deficiency of Blood of the Pericardium will result in poor memory.

When Blood is deficient, both Qi and Blood fail to circulate properly in the Pericardium channel, resulting in a feeling of stuffiness and discomfort of the chest or a dull ache in the chest. As the Pericardium is the propulsive agent for both Heart- and Lung-Qi in the middle of the chest, deficiency of Blood of the Pericardium may result in shortness of breath. As Blood is deficient, it fails to circulate properly to the hands and this results in cold hands.

Given the relationship between the Pericardium and the Uterus (ch. 11), deficiency of Blood of the Pericardium in women may cause scanty periods or amenorrhoea.

The pulse on the Heart position will characteristically be very slightly hard (although the pulse as a whole may be Choppy or Fine), indicating the involvement of the Pericardium channel.

Pathological precursors of pattern

Obviously Heart-Blood deficiency itself may be the precursor of this pattern. A deficiency of Qi and Blood of the Spleen is also a common precursors of this pattern (Fig. 33.6).

Pathological developments from pattern

Deficiency of Blood of the Pericardium may lead to Blood stasis in the chest (see Fig. 33.6).

Treatment

Principle of treatment: nourish Blood, strengthen the Heart and Pericardium, move Qi and Blood in the chest.

Acupuncture

Points: P-6 Neiguan, HE-7 Shenmen, Ren-14 Juque, Ren-15 Jiuwei, Ren-4 Guanyuan, BL-17 Geshu (with moxa), BL-20 Pishu, BL-14 Jueyinshu, Ren-17 Shanzhong, P-6 Neiguan and SP-4 Gongsun in combination (*Yin Wei Mai*).

Method: reinforcing method.

Explanation
- P-6 tonifies the Pericardium and moves Qi.
- HE-7 nourishes Heart-Blood and calms the Mind.
- Ren-14 and Ren-15 nourish Heart-Blood and calm the Mind.
- Ren-4 nourishes Blood in general.
- BL-17 with direct moxa nourishes Blood.
- BL-20 is used if there is a Spleen deficiency to nourish Blood.
- BL-14 tonifies the Pericardium.
- Ren-17 tonifies the Heart, Lungs and Pericardium and moves Qi and Blood in the chest.
- P-6 and SP-4 in combination open the Yin Linking Vessel (*Yin Wei Mai*), nourish Blood and calm the Mind.

Herbal formula

Shen Qi Si Wu Tang *Ginseng–Astragalus–Four Substances Decoction*.

Box 33.3 summarizes Blood deficiency of the Pericardium.

Pericardium-Fire

Clinical manifestations

Palpitations, a feeling of tightness and heat of the chest, slight chest ache, rapid breathing, thirst, mouth and tongue ulcers, mental restlessness, feeling agitated, feeling of heat, insomnia, dream-disturbed sleep, red face, bitter taste (after a bad night's sleep), heavy periods (Fig. 33.7).

Box 33.3 Blood deficiency of the Pericardium

Clinical manifestations

A feeling of stuffiness and discomfort of the chest, dull ache in the chest, very slight shortness of breath, palpitations, anxiety, insomnia, dizziness, dream-disturbed sleep, poor memory, propensity to be startled, dull-pale complexion, pale lips, cold hands, tongue Pale, Thin, slightly dry, pulse Choppy or Fine but very slightly hard on the left Front position

Treatment

P-6 Neiguan, HE-7 Shenmen, Ren-14 Juque, Ren-15 Jiuwei, Ren-4 Guanyuan, BL-17 Geshu (with moxa), BL-20 Pishu, BL-14 Jueyinshu, Ren-17 Shanzhong, P-6 Neiguan and SP-4 Gongsun in combination (Yin Linking Vessel)

Tongue: Red, tip redder and swollen with red points, yellow coating. There may be a midline crack reaching to the tip.

Pulse: Full-Rapid-Overflowing especially on the left Front position. It could also be Hasty (Rapid and stopping at irregular intervals).

Key symptoms: palpitations, a feeling of tightness of the chest, thirst, bitter taste, insomnia.

Diagnostic tip

Palpitations, a feeling of tightness of the chest, bitter taste and insomnia are enough to diagnose Pericardium-Fire

Aetiology

Emotional strain

Any of the emotions that affect the Heart cause some Qi stagnation in the Heart: after some time, this may turn into Heat and then Fire. Emotions that cause this may be sadness, grief, worry, anger, frustration, resentment and guilt.

Diet

The excessive consumption of hot foods (red meat) and alcohol may contribute to the formation of Fire and therefore to this pattern.

Pathology

Fire in the Pericardium harasses the Mind and causes the insomnia, mental restlessness, feeling agitated, dream-disturbed sleep. The mental–emotional manifestations will be much more plethoric and agitated than those of Blood deficiency of the Pericardium.

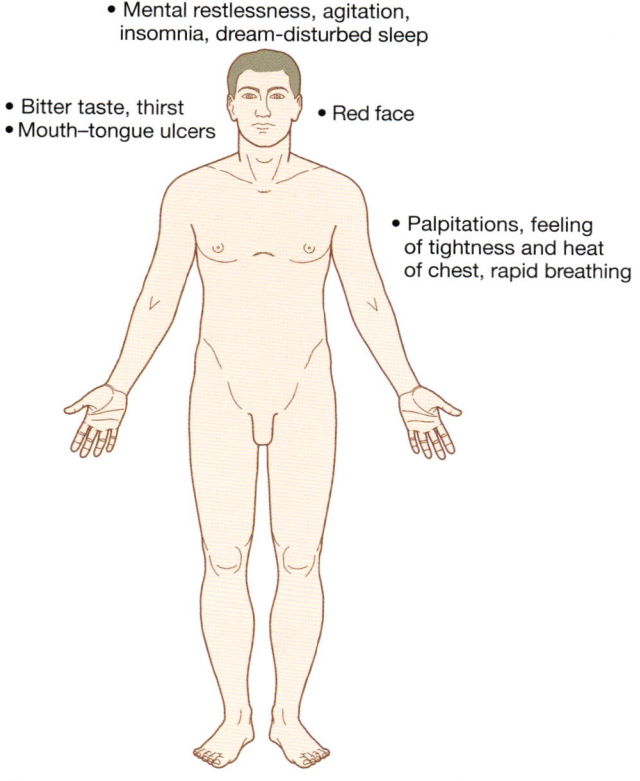

Figure 33.7 Pericardium-Fire

- Mental restlessness, agitation, insomnia, dream-disturbed sleep
- Bitter taste, thirst
- Mouth–tongue ulcers
- Red face
- Palpitations, feeling of tightness and heat of chest, rapid breathing

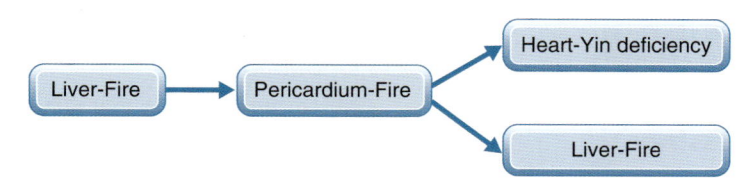

Figure 33.8 Pericardium-Fire pattern: precursors and developments

Liver-Fire → Pericardium-Fire → Heart-Yin deficiency / Liver-Fire

The Pericardium affects the mouth and tongue and Fire may therefore cause mouth ulcers, thirst and bitter taste.

The involvement of the Pericardium channel in the chest causes the feeling of tightness and heat of the chest and slight chest ache. The rapid breathing is due to the influence of the Pericardium on the Lungs.

Given the relationship between the Pericardium and the Uterus (ch. 11), Pericardium-Fire may heat the Blood and cause heavy periods from Blood-Heat.

Pathological precursors of pattern

Liver-Fire may be a precursor of this pattern, particularly so because the Liver and Pericardium channel are related within the Terminal Yin (*Jue Yin*) channels (Fig. 33.8).

Pathological developments from pattern

Pericardium-Fire may injure Yin and lead to Heart-Yin deficiency. Because of the above-mentioned relationship between the Liver and Pericardium, Pericardium-Fire may also lead to Liver-Fire (see Fig. 33.8).

Treatment

Principle of treatment: drain Fire of the Heart and Pericardium.

Acupuncture

Points: P-8 Laogong, HE-8 Shaofu, BL-14 Jueyinshu, Ren-15 Jiuwei, Ren-14 Juque, Ren-17 Shanzhong, L.I.-11 Quchi, Du-24 Shenting, Du-19 Houding, SP-6 Sanyinjiao, LIV-2 Xingjian.

Method: reducing except for SP-6, which should be reinforced.

Explanation
- P-8 and HE-8 drain Fire of the Pericardium and Heart.
- BL-14 clears Pericardium-Heat.
- Ren-14 and Ren-15 clear Heart-Heat and calm the Mind.
- Ren-17, Front-Collecting point of the Pericardium, clears Pericardium-Heat.
- L.I.-11 is used to clear Heat if the symptoms of Fire are very pronounced.
- Du-24 and Du-19 calm the Mind.
- SP-6 is used to nourish Yin to reduce Fire.
- LIV-2 drains Liver-Fire and is used to help to drain Pericardium-Fire in view of the above-mentioned relationship between the Liver and Pericardium channels. This point is particularly useful if the pattern is caused by anger, frustration or resentment.

Herbal formula

Xie Xin Tang *Draining the Heart Decoction*.
Box 33.4 summarizes Pericardium-Fire

Phlegm-Fire harassing the Pericardium

Clinical manifestations

Palpitations, feeling of oppression and heat of the chest, chest pain, rapid breathing, thirst, red face, bitter taste, expectoration of phlegm, rattling sound in the throat, mental restlessness, insomnia, dream-disturbed sleep, agitation, incoherent speech, mental confusion, rash behaviour, tendency to hit or scold people, uncontrolled laughter or crying, shouting, muttering to oneself, mental depression and dullness, manic behaviour (Fig. 33.9).

Tongue: Red, Swollen with yellow, dry sticky coating, deep Heart crack. The tip may be redder and swollen with red points.

Pulse: Full-Rapid-Slippery or Rapid-Overflowing-Slippery or Rapid-Full-Wiry.

Box 33.4 Pericardium-Fire

Clinical manifestations

Palpitations, a feeling of tightness and heat of the chest, slight chest ache, rapid breathing, thirst, mouth and tongue ulcers, mental restlessness, feeling agitated, feeling of heat, insomnia, dream-disturbed sleep, red face, bitter taste (after a bad night's sleep), tongue Red, tip redder and swollen with red points, yellow coating, pulse Full-Rapid-Overflowing especially on the left Front position

Treatment

P-8 Laogong, HE-8 Shaofu, BL-14 Jueyinshu, Ren-15 Jiuwei, Ren-14 Juque, Ren-17 Shanzhong, L.I.-11 Quchi, Du-24 Shenting, Du-19 Houding, SP-6 Sanyinjiao, LIV-2 Xingjian

---

Key symptoms: feeling of oppression and pain of the chest, all the mental symptoms, Red and Swollen tongue with sticky yellow coating.

> **Diagnostic tip**
>
> Feeling of oppression and pain of the chest, all the mental symptoms, and a Red and Swollen tongue with sticky yellow coating are enough to diagnose Phlegm-Fire harassing the Pericardium

Aetiology

Emotional strain

Any of the emotions that affect the Heart cause some Qi stagnation in the Heart: after some time, this may turn into Heat and then Fire. Emotions that cause this may be sadness, grief, worry, anger, frustration and resentment.

Diet

Excessive consumption of greasy hot foods leads to the formation of Phlegm.

Pathology

Fire harasses the Mind and causes mental restlessness, insomnia, dream-disturbed sleep, agitation. Phlegm obstructs the Mind and causes mental confusion, rash behaviour, tendency to hit or scold people, uncontrolled laughter or crying, shouting, muttering to oneself, mental depression and dullness, manic behaviour.

The feeling of oppression and heat of the chest and chest pain are due to involvement of the Pericardium

- Red face
- Thirst, bitter taste
- Mental restlessness, agitation, insomnia, dream-disturbed sleep, incoherent speech, mental confusion, rash behaviour, uncontrolled laughter or crying, muttering to oneself, depression, mania
- Rattling sound in throat
- Palpitations, feeling of oppression and heat of the chest, rapid breathing, expectoration of phlegm

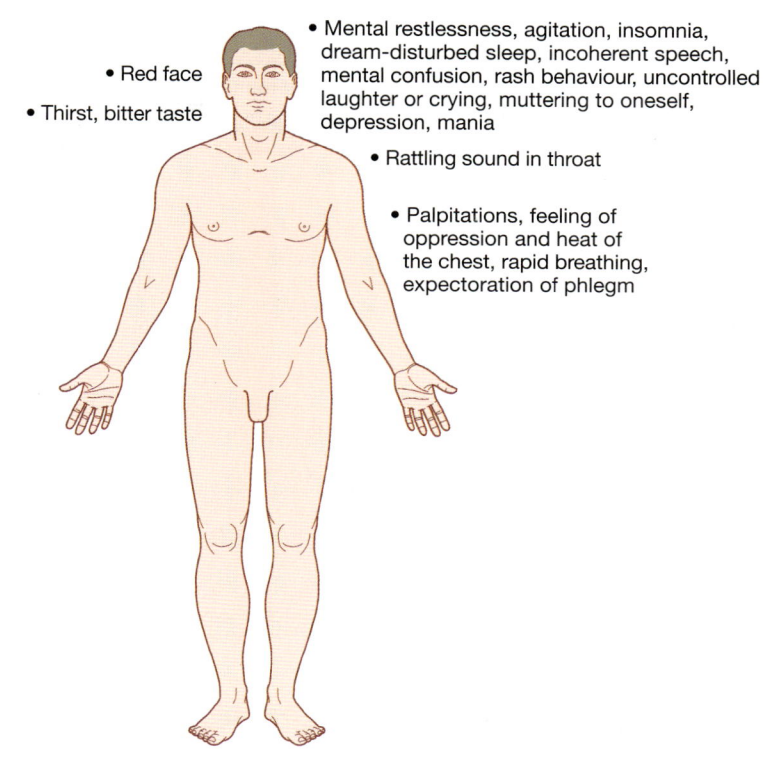

Figure 33.9 Phlegm-Fire harassing the Pericardium

Spleen deficiency → Phlegm-Fire harassing the Pericardium → Yin deficiency / Spleen-Qi deficiency / Dryness / Blood stasis

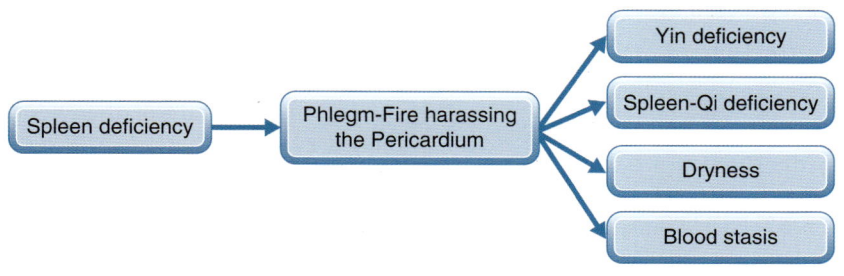

Figure 33.10 Phlegm-Fire harassing the Pericardium pattern: precursors and developments

channel. Rapid breathing is due to the influence of the Pericardium on the Lung channel.

As I mentioned for the pattern of Phlegm-Fire harassing the Heart, the clinical manifestations described here are those of full-blown bipolar disease. In practice, this pattern also occurs in patients not suffering from such a disease. Therefore, the symptoms may be milder than those described under the present pattern.

Pathological precursors of pattern

A Spleen deficiency leading to the formation of Phlegm is often the precursor of this pattern. Fire, by condensing Body Fluids, contributes to the formation of Phlegm (Fig. 33.10).

Pathological developments from pattern

This pattern may have several pathological developments. Pericardium-Fire may injure Yin and lead to Yin deficiency: this will lead to a very complex clinical picture with Fire, Phlegm and Yin deficiency.

Phlegm obstructs Qi and therefore may lead to (or aggravate) Spleen-Qi deficiency. As Phlegm is a pathological accumulation of Body Fluids, it may actually lead to dryness.

Finally, as Fire condenses Blood and because Phlegm is connected to Blood through Body Fluids, both Fire and Phlegm may lead to Blood stasis, which will further obstruct the Mind (see Fig. 33.10).

Treatment

Principle of treatment: drain Fire of the Pericardium and Heart, resolve Phlegm, open the Mind's orifices, calm the Mind.

Acupuncture

Points: P-5 Jianshi, HE-7 Shenmen, HE-8 Shaofu, HE-9 Shaochong, P-7 Daling, Ren-15 Jiuwei, BL-15 Xinshu, BL-14 Jueyinshu, Ren-17 Shanzhong, Ren-12 Zhongwan, ST-40 Fenglong, SP-6 Sanyinjiao, BL-20 Pishu, LIV-2 Xingjian, GB-13 Benshen, Du-24 Shenting, GB-17 Zhengying.

Method: all with reducing method, except Ren-12 and BL-20, which should be reinforced. No moxa.

Explanation
- P-5 resolves Phlegm from the Heart and clears orifices.
- HE-7 calms the Mind.
- HE-8 and HE-9 clear Heart-Fire.
- P-7 calms the Mind and clears Heart-Fire.
- Ren-15 calms the Mind.
- BL-15 clears Heart-Fire.
- BL-14 and Ren-17, Back-Transporting and Front-Collecting point of the Pericardium, respectively, drain Fire and calm the Mind.
- Ren-12 tonifies the Spleen to resolve Phlegm.
- ST-40 resolves Phlegm.
- SP-6 resolves Phlegm and calms the Mind.
- BL-20 tonifies the Spleen to resolve Phlegm.
- LIV-2 subdues Fire to conduct it downwards.
- GB-13 and Du-24 calm the Mind.
- GB-17 opens the Mind's orifices.

Herbal formula

Wen Dan Tang *Warming the Gall Bladder Decoction*.

Box 33.5 summarizes Phlegm-Fire harassing the Pericardium.

Box 33.5 Phlegm-Fire harassing the Pericardium

Clinical manifestations

Palpitations, feeling of oppression and heat of the chest, chest pain, rapid breathing, thirst, red face, bitter taste, expectoration of phlegm, rattling sound in the throat, mental restlessness, insomnia, dream-disturbed sleep, agitation, incoherent speech, mental confusion, rash behaviour, tendency to hit or scold people, uncontrolled laughter or crying, shouting, muttering to oneself, mental depression and dullness, manic behaviour.

Tongue: Red, Swollen with yellow, dry sticky coating, deep Heart crack. The tip may be redder and swollen with red points.

Pulse: Full-Rapid-Slippery or Rapid-Overflowing-Slippery or Rapid-Full-Wiry.

Treatment

P-5 Jianshi, HE-7 Shenmen, HE-8 Shaofu, HE-9 Shaochong, P-7 Daling, Ren-15 Jiuwei, BL-15 Xinshu, BL-14 Jueyinshu, Ren-17 Shanzhong, Ren-12 Zhongwan, ST-40 Fenglong, SP-6 Sanyinjiao, BL-20 Pishu, LIV-2 Xingjian, GB-13 Benshen, GB-17 Zhengying, Du-24 Shenting.

THE PERICARDIUM AS THE 'CENTRE OF THE THORAX'

The Pericardium channel goes to the centre of the thorax, and this area, called *Shan Zhong*, is under the influence of the Pericardium. Chapter 35 of the 'Spiritual Axis' says: '*The centre of the thorax [shan zhong] is the palace of the Pericardium [Xin Zhu].*'[3]

Being in the centre of the chest, the Pericardium influences the Gathering Qi (*Zong Qi*) and therefore both Heart and Lungs. The Pericardium in this area acts as the agent of propulsion for the Qi and Blood of both Heart and Lungs; for this reason, Pericardium patterns are characterized by clinical manifestations along the chest channels, causing tightness, distension, oppression or pain of the chest.

The patterns discussed are:

- Qi stagnation in the Pericardium
- Blood stasis in the Pericardium

Qi stagnation in the Pericardium

Clinical manifestations

A feeling of distension and slight pain of the chest, feeling of tightness of the chest, slight shortness of breath, sighing, a feeling of lump in the throat, palpitations, depression, irritability, poor appetite, weak and cold limbs, slightly purple lips, pale complexion (Fig. 33.11).

Tongue: slightly Pale-Purple on the sides in the chest area (see Fig. 23.19 in ch. 23).
Pulse: Empty but very slightly Overflowing on the left Front position.
Key symptoms: palpitations, a feeling of distension of the chest.

> **Diagnostic tip**
>
> Palpitations and a feeling of distension of the chest are enough to diagnose stagnation of Qi of the Pericardium

Aetiology

The aetiology of this pattern is always from emotional strain. Sadness, grief, worry and guilt knot Qi in the chest and lead to Qi stagnation in this area.

Pathology

The feeling of distension and slight pain of the chest and feeling of tightness of the chest are due to Qi stagnation along the Pericardium channel. Sighing and slight shortness of breath are due to Qi stagnation of the Lung channel (affected by the Pericardium channel).

Depression and irritability are due to Qi stagnation. All the other symptoms are due to Qi stagnation in the Heart and they have already been explained under the pattern of Heart-Qi stagnation in chapter 32.

Pathological precursors of pattern

Liver-Qi stagnation may be a precursor of this pattern (Fig. 33.12).

Pathological developments from pattern

If it is not a precursor of it, stagnation of Qi in the Pericardium may lead to Liver-Qi stagnation. Long-term Qi stagnation may also lead to Blood stasis and

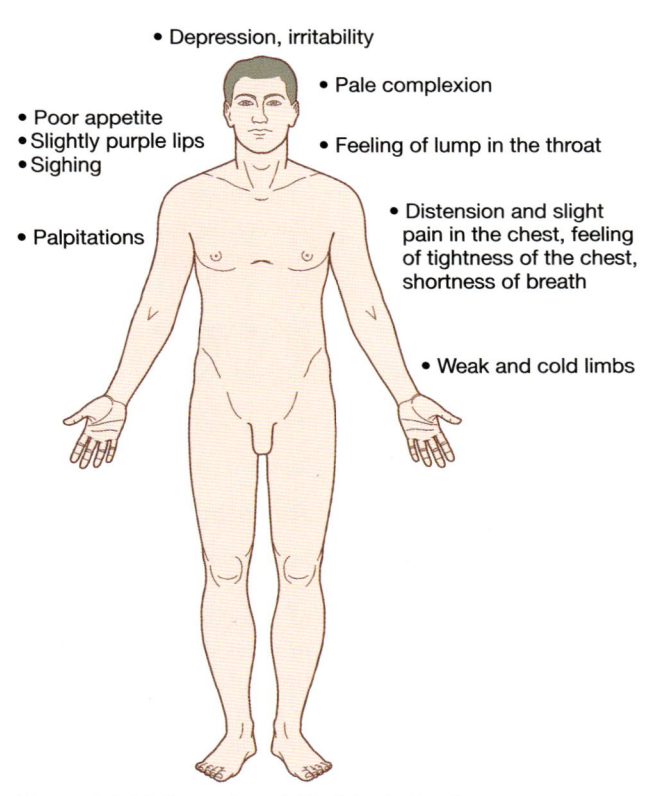

Figure 33.11 Stagnation of Qi of the Pericardium

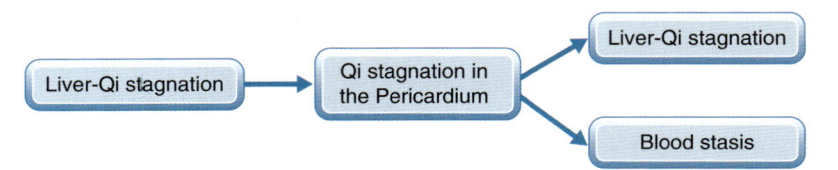

Figure 33.12 Stagnation of Qi of the Pericardium pattern: precursors and developments

this is even more likely to happen when Qi stagnation affects the Pericardium as well as the Heart (see Fig. 33.12).

Treatment

Principle of treatment: move Qi in the chest, regulate the Pericardium and Heart, calm the Mind.

Acupuncture

Points: P-6 Neiguan, HE-5 Tongli, HE-7 Shenmen, Ren-14 Juque, Ren-15 Jiuwei, Ren-17 Shanzhong, BL-14 Jueyinshu, LU-7 Lieque, ST-40 Fenglong, L.I.-4 Hegu.

Method: reducing.

Explanation

- P-6 opens the chest, moves Qi and calms the Mind.
- HE-5 moves Heart-Qi and calms the Mind.
- HE-7 calms the Mind.
- Ren-14 and Ren-15 open the chest and calm the Mind.
- Ren-17, Front-Collecting point of the Pericardium, moves Qi in the Pericardium channel in the chest.
- BL-14, Back-Transporting point of the Pericardium, moves Qi in the Pericardium.
- LU-7 moves Qi in the chest.
- ST-40 is used here not to resolve Phlegm but to open the chest and move Qi in the chest.
- L.I.-4 regulates the ascending and descending of Qi and therefore moves Qi.

Herbal formula

Mu Xiang Liu Qi Yin *Aucklandia Flowing Qi Decoction*.
Ban Xia Hou Po Tang *Pinellia–Magnolia Decoction*.

Box 33.6 summarizes Qi stagnation in the Pericardium.

Blood stasis of the Pericardium

Clinical manifestations

Palpitations, stabbing or pricking pain in the chest which may radiate to the inner aspect of the left arm or to the shoulder, a feeling of oppression or constriction of the chest, shortness of breath, cyanosis of lips and nails, cold hands, painful periods with dark clots (Fig. 33.13).

Tongue: Purple in its entirety or only on the sides in the chest area.
Pulse: Choppy, Wiry or Knotted.
Key symptoms: stabbing chest pain, purple lips.

> **Diagnostic tip**
>
> Stabbing chest pain and purple lips are enough to diagnose Blood stasis in the Pericardium

Aetiology

Emotional problems, particularly anxiety, grief, worry and guilt over a long period of time, can lead to stasis of Blood in the chest. The chest is the most likely part of the body where pent-up emotions are kept and they therefore easily lead to impairment in the circulation of Qi or Blood in this area. Furthermore, all these emotions disturb the Mind. Heart-Blood is the physiological basis for the Mind and any emotional problem that constrains the Mind may lead to stagnation of Qi and/or Blood of the Heart.

Box 33.6   Qi stagnation in the Pericardium

Clinical manifestations

A feeling of distension and slight pain of the chest, feeling of tightness of the chest, slight shortness of breath, sighing, a feeling of lump in the throat, palpitations, depression, poor appetite, weak and cold limbs, slightly purple lips, pale complexion, tongue slightly Pale-Purple on the sides in the chest area, pulse Empty but very slightly Overflowing on the left Front position

Treatment

P-6 Neiguan, HE-5 Tongli, HE-7 Shenmen, Ren-14 Juque, Ren-15 Jiuwei, Ren-17 Shanzhong, BL-14 Jueyinshu, LU-7 Lieque, ST-40 Fenglong, L.I.-4 Hegu

Pathology

The pathology of this pattern has already been explained under the pattern of Heart-Blood stasis in chapter 32. The pain in the chest and arm are due to Blood stasis in the Pericardium channel. The shortness of breath is due to Blood stasis in the Lung channel.

Given the relationship between the Pericardium and the Uterus (ch. 11), Blood stasis of the Pericardium may cause painful periods with dark, clotted menstrual blood.

Pathological precursors of pattern

Qi stagnation in the Pericardium channel is nearly always the precursor of this pattern; Liver-Qi stagnation may also be a precursor to this pattern. The Liver channel affects the chest and the loss of the free flow of Liver-Qi may easily affect the Pericardium (to which the Liver is related within the Terminal Yin channels) leading to Qi stagnation first and then Blood stasis (Fig. 33.14).

Pathological developments from pattern

Blood stasis in the Pericardium may lead to the formation of Phlegm because of the interaction between these two pathogenic factors. A long-term consequence of Blood stasis, especially in the elderly, can be dryness.

Blood stasis in the Pericardium may also lead to Blood stasis in the Liver due to the relationship between these two channels within the Terminal Yin (*Jue Yin*) channels (see Fig. 33.14).

Treatment

Principle of treatment: move Blood in the chest, regulate the Pericardium and Heart, calm the Mind.

Acupuncture

Points: P-6 Neiguan, P-4 Ximen, HE-7 Shenmen, Ren-14 Juque, Ren-17 Shanzhong, BL-14 Jueyinshu, BL-17 Geshu, SP-10 Xuehai.
Method: reducing.
Explanation
- P-6 moves Blood in the Pericardium channel and opens the chest. This is the main point.
- P-4 is the Accumulation point and is particularly useful to stop chest pain.
- HE-7 calms the Mind.
- Ren-14 moves Heart-Blood.
- Ren-17, Front-Collecting point of the Pericardium, moves Qi and Blood in the chest and stimulates the circulation of Gathering Qi.
- BL-14, Back-Transporting point of the Pericardium, moves Blood in the Pericardium.
- BL-17 moves Blood and eliminates stasis.
- SP-10 moves Blood.

- Cyanosis of lips
- Palpitations, stabbing chest pain, feeling of oppression or constriction of chest, shortness of breath
- Cold hands
- Cyanosis of nails

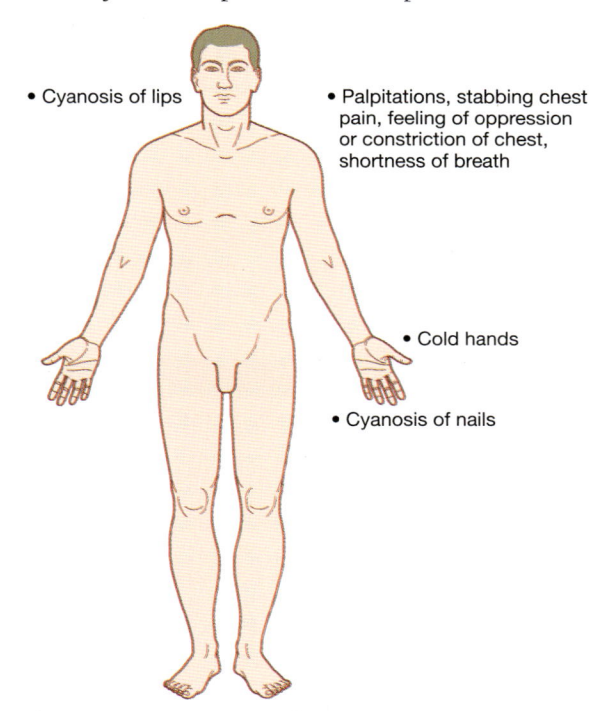

Figure 33.13 Blood stasis of the Pericardium

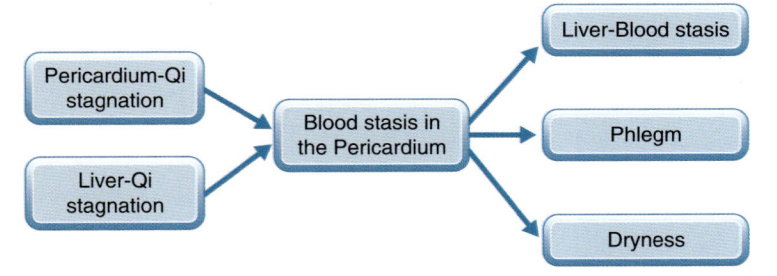

Figure 33.14 Blood stasis of the Pericardium pattern: precursors and developments

Box 33.7 Blood stasis in the Pericardium

Clinical manifestations

Palpitations, stabbing or pricking pain in the chest which may radiate to the inner aspect of the left arm or to the shoulder, a feeling of oppression or constriction of the chest, shortness of breath, cyanosis of lips and nails, cold hands, tongue Purple in its entirety or only on the sides in the chest area, pulse Choppy, Wiry or Knotted

Treatment

P-6 Neiguan, P-4 Ximen, HE-7 Shenmen, Ren-14 Juque, Ren-17 Shanzhong, BL-14 Jueyinshu, BL-17 Geshu, SP-10 Xuehai

Box 33.7 summarizes Blood stasis of the Pericardium

Herbal formula

Xue Fu Zhu Yu Tang *Blood-Mansion Eliminating Stasis Decoction.*

Three Treasures

Red Stirring (Variation of *Xue Fu Zhu Yu Tang*).

Learning outcomes

In this chapter you will have learned:
- The factors which differentiate Pericardium patterns from Heart patterns, particularly chest symptoms (Pericardium channel) and involvement of Lung and Liver channels
- The characteristic three main areas of Pericardium pathology: invasions of exterior pathogenic factors, mental–emotional problems and channel pathology in the thorax
- How to identify the following pattern arising from an invasion of exterior Heat:
  Heat in the Pericardium: fever at night, delirium and a red tongue without coating
- How to differentiate pathology of the Pericardium from that of the Heart in the mental–emotional sphere (involvement of the Pericardium channel and problems 'relating')
- How to identify the following patterns relating to the Pericardium function of housing the Mind:
  Blood deficiency of the Pericardium: discomfort of the chest, palpitations and insomnia
  Pericardium-Fire: palpitations, tightness of chest, thirst, bitter taste and insomnia
  Phlegm-Fire harassing the Pericardium: oppression and pain of chest, mental symptoms, and a Red and Swollen tongue with a sticky yellow coating
- The role of the Pericardium as 'centre of the thorax', and as the agent of propulsion for the Qi and Blood of the Heart and Lungs
- The significance of tightness, distension, oppression and pain of the chest in Pericardium pathology
- How to identify the following patterns relating to the Pericardium's role as 'centre of the thorax':
  Qi stagnation in the Pericardium: palpitations and a feeling of distension of the chest
  Blood stasis of the Pericardium: stabbing chest pain and purple lips

Learning tips

Pericardium patterns

- First of all, when thinking of the Pericardium, think of 'chest'. Therefore Pericardium patterns have more chest symptoms than Heart patterns, e.g. chest pain, feeling of oppression, distension or stuffiness of the chest, discomfort of the chest
- The Pericardium 'takes the blows' for the Heart and is affected by external Heat. Pericardium-Heat patterns appear in febrile diseases causing obstruction of the Mind, hence delirium, high fever, fever at night, aphasia, mental confusion, unconsciousness
- The Pericardium affects Blood and causes Blood-Heat, hence skin diseases with red macular rashes
- The Pericardium houses the Mind and it is especially affected by Heat and Phlegm-Heat, hence insomnia, mental restlessness, agitation, manic behaviour
- The Pericardium affects the Uterus especially in Blood-Heat, hence menorrhagia

Self-assessment questions

1. By what mechanism is the Lung channel often involved in Pericardium pathology?
2. Why is there no tongue coating associated with the pattern Heat in the Pericardium?
3. Describe the mental–emotional characteristics of Pericardium pathology.
4. A patient presents with insomnia, palpitations and a stuffy, uncomfortable chest. What is your diagnosis?
5. Explain the pathology of the symptom of rapid breathing in the pattern Pericardium-Fire.
6. What are the two probable pathological precursors to the pattern Phlegm-Fire harassing the Pericardium?
7. How would you expect the tongue to appear in a patient presenting with the pattern Blood stasis of the Pericardium?

See p. 1263 for answers

END NOTES

1. 1981 Spiritual Axis (*Ling Shu Jing* 灵枢经), People's Health Publishing House, Beijing, first published *c.*100 BC, p. 128.
2. 1979 The Yellow Emperor's Classic of Internal Medicine – Simple Questions (*Huang Di Nei Jing Su Wen* 黄帝内经素问), People's Health Publishing House, Beijing, first published *c.*100 BC, p. 58.
3. Spiritual Axis, p. 75.

SECTION 2 PART 6

Liver Patterns 34

Key contents

General aetiology
Exterior pathogenic factors
Emotions
- Anger
- Worry
- Sadness

Diet
Blood loss

Full patterns
Liver-Qi stagnation
Stagnant Liver-Qi turning into Heat
Rebellious Liver-Qi
Liver-Blood stasis
Liver-Fire blazing
Damp-Heat in the Liver
Stagnation of Cold in the Liver channel

Empty patterns
Liver-Blood deficiency
Liver-Yin deficiency

Full/Empty patterns
Liver-Yang rising
Liver-Wind
- Extreme Heat generating Wind
- Liver-Yang rising generating Wind
- Liver-Fire generating Wind
- Liver-Blood deficiency generating Wind

Combined patterns
Rebellious Liver-Qi invading the Spleen
Rebellious Liver-Qi invading the Stomach
Liver-Fire insulting the Lungs
Liver- and Heart-Blood deficiency
Liver- and Kidney-Yin deficiency (this is discussed under Kidneys, Combined patterns, in ch. 37)

The functions of the Liver (ch. 7) are:

- It stores Blood
- It ensures the smooth flow of Qi
- It controls the sinews
- It manifests in the nails
- It opens into the eyes
- It controls tears
- It houses the Ethereal Soul (*Hun*)
- It is affected by anger

The two most important functions of the Liver are those of ensuring the smooth flow of Qi and storing Blood. The smooth flow of Liver-Qi influences all organs and many different parts of the body. It helps the Spleen to transform and transport food essences and the Stomach to rot and ripen food. Liver-Qi also helps Spleen-Qi to ascend and Stomach-Qi to descend. It stimulates the Gall Bladder secretion of bile and it ensures the smooth flow of Qi in the Intestines and the Uterus, thus influencing menstruation.

Moreover, the smooth flow of Liver-Qi has a paramount influence on the emotional state: it ensures a 'smooth flow' of our emotional life. If Liver-Qi is constrained over a long period of time, our emotional life will be characterized by depression, frustration, irritability and emotional tension generally.

As the Liver ensures the smooth flow of Qi but has no part in the actual production and supply of Qi, it seldom suffers from deficiency of Qi (although it does have patterns of deficiency of Blood and Yin). In relation to Qi, the most important and common pattern is that of stagnation of Liver-Qi. However, Liver-Qi deficiency does occur and it manifests primarily on a psychological level with depression, timidity and lack of initiative.

Whilst Liver-Qi is seldom deficient, Liver-Blood and Liver-Yin are often deficient. The Liver stores Blood and this can easily be depleted, leading to symptoms of Blood deficiency and scanty periods. Liver-Blood can also become stagnant: this is usually a consequence of stagnation of Liver-Qi. Qi is the 'commander of Blood': when Qi stagnates, Blood congeals.

The functional relationship between the Liver and the sinews often manifests in pathological circumstances with physical tiredness and weakness or contraction of the tendons.

Liver pathology is also characterized by rapid changes such as skin rashes that appear quickly, sudden tinnitus, sudden outbursts of anger, or in severe cases, sudden collapse and coma.

Box 34.1 summarizes possible indications of Liver pathology.

The discussion of Liver patterns will be preceded by a discussion of the general aetiology of Liver disharmonies presented under the following headings:

GENERAL AETIOLOGY
- Exterior pathogenic factors
- Emotions
  - Anger
  - Worry
  - Sadness
- Diet
- Blood loss

The Liver patterns discussed are:

FULL PATTERNS
- Liver-Qi stagnation
- Stagnant Liver-Qi turning into Heat
- Rebellious Liver-Qi
- Liver-Blood stasis
- Liver-Fire blazing
- Damp-Heat in the Liver
- Stagnation of Cold in the Liver channel

EMPTY PATTERNS
- Liver-Blood deficiency
- Liver-Yin deficiency

FULL/EMPTY PATTERNS
- Liver-Yang rising
- Liver-Wind agitating within
  - Extreme Heat generating Wind
  - Liver-Yang rising generating Wind
  - Liver-Fire generating Wind
  - Liver-Blood deficiency generating Wind

COMBINED PATTERNS
- Rebellious Liver-Qi invading the Spleen
- Rebellious Liver-Qi invading the Stomach
- Liver-Fire insulting the Lungs
- Heart- and Liver-Blood deficiency
- Liver- and Kidney-Yin deficiency (this is discussed under Kidneys, Combined patterns, ch. 37)

Note

After discussing the Liver patterns, I will discuss the frequent combinations of Liver patterns seen in practice.

Each Liver pattern will be discussed with the following headings:

- Clinical manifestations
- Aetiology
- Pathology
- Pathological precursors of pattern
- Pathological developments from pattern
- Treatment
  - Acupuncture
  - Herbal formula

GENERAL AETIOLOGY

Exterior pathogenic factors

The two pathogenic factors which affect the Liver are Wind and Dampness.

Exterior Wind does not attack the Liver directly (it invades the Lung's Defensive Qi portion) but it can aggravate a situation of interior Wind of the Liver; it could, for instance, precipitate an attack of interior Liver-Wind, causing a Wind-stroke.

In some cases, exterior Wind can aggravate an internal Liver disharmony (such as Liver-Yang rising), causing stiff neck and headaches.

Clinical note

External Wind can aggravate an interior Liver disharmony (e.g. Liver-Yang rising, Liver-Wind)

Box 34.1 A 'Feel' for Liver pathology

- Rapid changes (e.g. in skin diseases)
- Up and down fluctuation (e.g. level of energy, mood)
- Emotionally up and down
- Moodiness, irritability
- Eye problems
- A feeling of 'distension'
- Gynaecological problems

Exterior Wind can also stir the Blood stored in the Liver and manifest with skin rashes that start suddenly and move quickly, such as in urticaria. In such cases, the Wind usually combines with Heat to cause Heat in Liver-Blood at the superficial levels of the Blood-Connecting channels. The sudden onset and quick changes are typical of Wind as a pathogenic factor.

Exterior pathogenic factors as causes of disease are discussed in chapter 21.

> **Clinical note**
>
> Exterior Wind may affect Liver-Blood and either cause or aggravate skin diseases

Emotions

Anger

This is the emotion which is most directly related to the Liver. As mentioned previously (ch. 20, Internal causes of disease), 'anger' is a broad term used in Chinese medicine which includes feelings of frustration, repressed anger, resentment and irritation. As always in Chinese medicine, the relationship between a certain emotion and organ is mutual: the Liver function of ensuring a smooth flow of Qi has a profound influence on the emotional state, and conversely, the emotional state will influence the Liver function.

Thus if the Liver is functioning well and its Qi flowing smoothly, the emotional state will be happy and free-going and the person will be in good spirits and freely express his or her emotions. If Liver-Qi stagnates and does not flow freely and unimpeded, it will stagnate and affect the emotional state, causing anger and irritability.

Over a long period of time, stagnation of Liver-Qi will severely impair the circulation of Qi giving rise to a gloomy emotional state of constant resentment, repressed anger or depression. On a physical level, these constrained emotions could be 'carried' in the chest, hypochondrium, epigastrium, abdomen or throat. The person will then experience a feeling of tightness of the chest, or distension of the hypogastrium, or tension in the stomach area, or abdominal distension or a feeling of lump in the throat with difficulty in swallowing. The person will tend to sigh frequently.

If Liver-Qi rebels upward causing the rising of Liver-Yang, the person will be very irritable, 'fly off the handle' easily and suffer from headaches.

Stagnation of Qi over a long period of time can lead to Heat as the implosion of Qi caused by emotional constraint generates Heat. This situation is often manifested on the tongue with red sides and tip, possibly with red points on the tip.

Box 34.2 summarizes the effects of anger.

Worry

Worry affects primarily the Lungs but it can affect the Liver as well, causing Liver-Qi stagnation. This happens particularly if the worry is work-related and it occurs in conjunction with frustration.

In my experience, worry may also cause Liver-Yang to rise.

Sadness

Although in Chinese books the Liver is always and only related to anger, sadness can affect the Liver too and this happens especially in women. The 'Spiritual Axis' in chapter 8 says: *'The Liver's sadness and shock injure the Ethereal Soul.'*[1] In the same chapter it also says: *'When sadness affects the Liver it injures the Ethereal Soul; this causes mental confusion ... the Yin is damaged, the tendons contract and there is hypochondrial discomfort.'*[2]

Diet

An excessive consumption of hot-energy foods (such as red meat, spices and alcohol) can lead to Liver-Fire. An excessive consumption of greasy foods (such as dairy foods and fried foods) can lead to Dampness in the Liver (and usually in the Gall Bladder as well).

An inadequate consumption of warming and Blood-nourishing foods, such as meat and grains, can lead to a state of Blood deficiency, which can lead to deficiency of Liver-Blood. This is more common in women who particularly need an adequate supply of Blood-forming foods at certain times of their life, such as at puberty and after childbirth, as well as, to a lesser degree, after each period.

Diet as a cause of disease is discussed in chapter 22.

> **Box 34.2 Anger**
>
> - 'Anger' includes frustration and resentment
> - Anger may cause Liver-Qi stagnation or Liver-Yang rising
> - Anger makes Qi rise and is a frequent cause of headaches from Liver-Yang rising

Blood loss

A severe blood loss, such as one occurring after childbirth, can lead to deficiency of Liver-Blood.

Box 34.3 summarizes the general aetiology of Liver patterns.

FULL PATTERNS

Liver-Qi stagnation

Clinical manifestations

- Feeling of distension of hypochondrium, chest, epigastrium or abdomen, sighing

> **Box 34.3 General aetiology of Liver patterns**
> - Exterior pathogenic factors
> - Emotions
>   - Anger
>   - Worry
>   - Sadness
> - Diet
> - Blood loss

- Melancholy, depression, moodiness, fluctuation of mental state, 'feeling wound-up', feeling of lump in the throat
- Irregular periods, distension of breasts before the periods, premenstrual tension and irritability (Fig. 34.1)

Tongue: the body colour may be normal. In severe cases, it may be slightly Red on the sides.
Pulse: Wiry, especially on the left side.
Key symptoms: feeling of distension, depression, moodiness, Wiry pulse.

> **Diagnostic tip**
>
> A feeling of distension and a Wiry pulse by themselves are enough to diagnose Liver-Qi stagnation

Aetiology

Emotional stress

Problems in the emotional life are by far the most important (if not the only) cause of Liver-Qi stagnation.

- Depression, moodiness melancholy
- Feeling of lump in the throat
- Premenstrual breast distension and irritability
- Distension of hypochondrium, chest, epigastrium, abdomen
- Irregular periods
- Cold hands

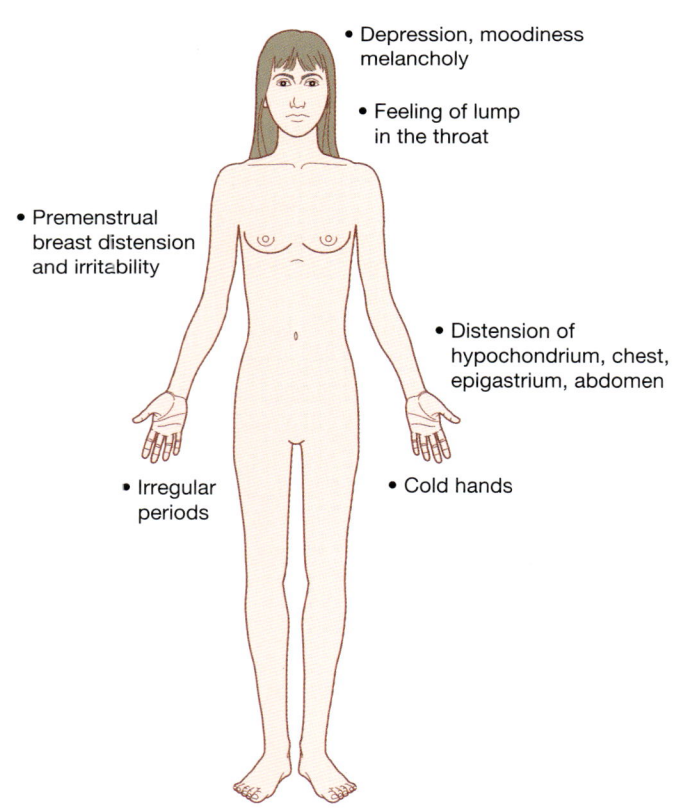

Figure 34.1 Liver-Qi stagnation

As mentioned before, a state of frustration, repressed anger or resentment over a long period of time can cause the flow of Qi to be impeded so that Qi does not flow smoothly and it becomes stuck, resulting in stagnation of Liver-Qi.

Pathology

This is by far the most common of the Liver patterns and also one of the most common patterns in general (although in my opinion it does tend to be over-diagnosed). Obviously not all the above manifestation need be present to warrant a diagnosis of Liver-Qi stagnation. I have arranged the manifestations in three different groups to highlight the different pathology of each group. Stagnation of Liver-Qi is very far-reaching and manifests its influence in a wide range of symptoms and signs.

On a physical level, stagnation of Liver-Qi can manifest in the hypochondrium, chest, epigastrium and abdomen. The stagnation manifests with a characteristic feeling of distension. 'Distension' is a translation of the Chinese word *zhang*. Distension refers to a subjective bloated feeling of the patient but, in the epigastrium and abdomen, it can also be seen and palpated objectively. On observation, the abdomen does look distended and on palpation, it feels somewhat hard but elastic (like a balloon). Sighing is a spontaneous way to release the stagnant Qi in the chest.

> **Clinical note**
>
> 'Distension' (*zhang*) is the chief symptom of Qi stagnation. Most English-speaking patients would use the term 'bloating'

The second group of symptoms includes several emotional manifestations, which are very common and typical of Liver-Qi stagnation. These are due to the lack of flow of Qi at a psychic level. Stagnation of Liver-Qi impedes the 'coming and going' of the Ethereal Soul (*Hun*) with a resulting depression, feeling of aimlessness, lack of projects, dreams, etc. The Qi stagnation also causes a feeling of irritability.

The stagnation of Liver-Qi in the throat (where the Liver channel also flows) gives rise to the feeling of a lump in the throat (this is described in Chinese medicine as like a feeling of 'plum stone in the throat'). The feeling comes and goes according to the emotional state. Typically, the emotional symptoms fluctuate: the person goes through periods of depression when all the physical symptoms also appear, and periods when the depression is lifted and the physical symptoms disappear. This fluctuation is typical of Liver-Qi stagnation.

Finally, stagnation of Liver-Qi can impair the movement of Qi and Blood in the Directing and Penetrating Vessels (*Ren Mai* and *Chong Mai*), thus affecting the Uterus, resulting in irregular periods and premenstrual tension with distension of the breasts (which are also under the influence of the Liver channel).

This pattern is of the Full type and one should not be misled by the emotional state of the person, which may appear to be 'deficient' (i.e. the person is depressed, moody and quiet). In spite of its appearance, it is caused by an 'implosion' of Qi due to the stagnation of Liver-Qi and, as such, it is to be treated as an Excess pattern. In such situations when the patient suffers from Liver-Qi stagnation but appears subdued, the Wiry pulse is an essential symptom that points to Liver-Qi stagnation.

It is important to discuss the tongue appearance in Liver-Qi stagnation. Most Chinese books say that the tongue in Liver-Qi stagnation is Purple or has purple sides. I disagree and I think that a change in the colour of the tongue body reflects a change in the state of Blood more than of Qi. Therefore, if the tongue is Purple, I always attribute that to Blood stasis. In Qi stagnation, the tongue body may actually not change colour at all so that this pathology does not show on the tongue; in severe cases of Qi stagnation, the tongue may be slightly Red on the sides.

> **Clinical note**
>
> The tongue in Qi stagnation may be normal-coloured; it is *not* purple. In severe cases it may be red on the sides

The pulse quality associated with Qi stagnation is Wiry and this is a very frequent finding in practice. Indeed, I would say that if the pulse is *not* Wiry (or at least partially Wiry), then it is not Liver-Qi stagnation.

Please note that in women, Liver-Qi stagnation may sometimes arise as a consequence of Liver-Blood deficiency, or it may be associated with it. When that happens, the pattern is a combination of Excess (Qi stagnation) and Deficiency (Liver-Blood). The symptoms and signs will be slightly different and generally of the Deficient type; most of all, the pulse may be generally Fine and only slightly Wiry on the left.

Indeed, the famous formula Xiao Yao San *Free and Easy Wanderer Powder* is for this pattern, whereas when Liver-Qi stagnation occurs independently, Yue Ju Wan *Gardenia-Ligusticum Pill* is indicated (see below).

> **Clinical note**
>
> In women, Liver-Qi stagnation is often deriving from or associated with Liver-Blood deficiency:
> - The symptoms and signs will be slightly different and generally of the Deficient type
> - There will be depression rather than irritability
> - The pulse may be generally Fine and only slightly Wiry on the left
> - Xiao Yao San is for Liver-Qi stagnation deriving from or associated with Liver-Blood deficiency
> - Yue Ju Wan is for 'pure' Liver-Qi stagnation

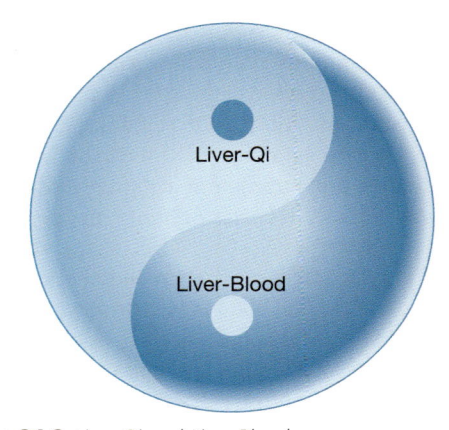

Figure 34.2 Liver-Qi and Liver-Blood

Pathological precursors of pattern

There are few pathological precursors of Liver-Qi stagnation as this pattern itself is usually the beginning stage of a pathological process deriving from emotional stress. However, this pattern may arise as a secondary consequence of Liver-Blood deficiency: this is because Liver-Qi and Liver-Blood are the Yang and Yin aspect of the Liver, respectively, and they mutually influence each other (Figs 34.2 and 34.3).

As the Kidneys are the Mother of the Liver in the Five-Element scheme, a deficiency of the Kidneys may induce a secondary Liver-Qi stagnation.

Pathological developments from pattern

As Qi is 'the commander of Blood' and 'when Qi stagnates Blood congeals', stagnation of Liver-Qi over a long period of time can easily induce stasis of Liver-Blood. This is the most important consequence of Liver-Qi stagnation, which will be discussed as a separate pattern.

With time, stagnation of Liver-Qi frequently leads to Liver-Heat (see Fig. 34.3).

Treatment

Principle of treatment: smooth the Liver and move Qi.

Acupuncture

Points: GB-34 Yanglingquan, LIV-3 Taichong, LIV-13 Zhangmen, LIV-14 Qimen, T.B.-6 Zhigou, P-6 Neiguan.

Method: reducing method, no moxa.

Explanation
- GB-34 moves Liver-Qi and it particularly influences the hypochondrial region.
- LIV-3 also moves Liver-Qi and it particularly affects the throat and head.
- LIV-13 regulates Liver-Qi in the Middle Burner, particularly when it invades the Spleen.
- LIV-14 regulates Liver-Qi in the Middle Burner, particularly when it affects the Stomach.
- T.B.-6 moves Liver-Qi and it particularly affects the sides of the body.
- P-6 moves Liver-Qi (by virtue of the relationship between Liver and Pericardium channels within the Terminal Yin). This point would be particularly well indicated when the stagnation of Liver-Qi is caused by emotional problems.

Herbal formula

Yue Ju Wan *Gardenia-Ligusticum Pill* (for Liver-Qi stagnation arising independently).

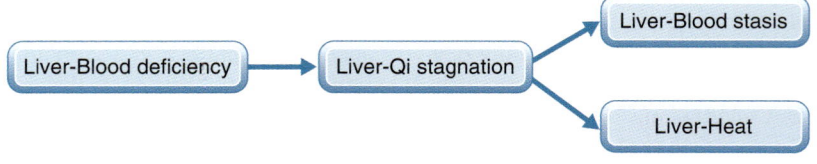

Figure 34.3 Liver-Qi stagnation pattern: precursors and developments

Xiao Yao San *Free and Easy Wanderer Powder* (for Liver-Qi stagnation secondary to Liver-Blood deficiency).

Three Treasures and Women's Treasure

Release Constraint (variation of Yue Ju Wan).
Freeing the Moon (variation of Xiao Yao San).

Box 34.4 summarizes Liver-Qi stagnation.

Case history 34.1

A woman of 50 suffered from tiredness, depression, pronounced mood swings, premenstrual depression and irritability, distension of the breasts before a period and a swelling of the thyroid gland with a feeling of constriction in the throat. The pulse was Wiry, the tongue-body colour was normal and only slightly Red on the sides.

The above manifestations indicate stagnation of Liver-Qi manifesting more in the throat, rather than the hypochondrium. The depression, mood swings and premenstrual irritability with distension of the breasts, the Wiry pulse, the slightly red colour on the sides of the tongue, all clearly point to stagnation of Liver-Qi. Had the periods been painful with dark clotted blood and the tongue been purple, one would have diagnosed stasis of Liver-Blood.

Case history 34.2

A woman of 34 suffered from epigastric and abdominal pain of a spastic character, indigestion, belching, a feeling of fullness and distension of the abdomen and nausea. Her bowel movements alternated between constipation with small, bitty stools and diarrhoea. The pulse was Wiry and the tongue was Red with redder sides and a yellow coating.

These symptoms and signs show stagnation of Liver-Qi, with Liver-Qi invading the Stomach (epigastric pain and distension, belching, nausea), the Spleen (diarrhoea, abdominal pain and distension) and the Intestines (constipation with small bitty stools). The Wiry pulse and red colour of the sides of the tongue confirms the involvement of the Liver. Thus, in this case, the symptoms and signs appear in three organs (Stomach, Spleen and Intestines) but all stem from the primary factor of Liver-Qi stagnation. The Red colour of the tongue shows that the stagnation of Liver-Qi is beginning to transform into Heat, as often happens after a prolonged period.

Box 34.4 Liver-Qi stagnation

Clinical manifestations

1. Feeling of distension of hypochondrium, chest, epigastrium or abdomen, sighing
2. Melancholy, depression, moodiness, fluctuation of mental state, 'feeling wound-up', feeling of lump in the throat
3. Irregular periods, distension of breasts before the periods, premenstrual tension and irritability

Tongue: the body colour may be normal. In severe cases, it may be slightly Red on the sides
Pulse: Wiry, especially on the left side

Treatment

GB-34 Yanglingquan, LIV-3 Taichong, LIV-13 Zhangmen, LIV-14 Qimen, T.B.-6 Zhigou, P-6 Neiguan

---

Stagnant Liver-Qi turning into Heat

Clinical manifestations

Hypochondrial or epigastric distension, a slight feeling of oppression of the chest, irritability, melancholy, depression, moodiness, a feeling of lump in the throat, a feeling of heat, red face, thirst, propensity to outbursts of anger, premenstrual tension, irregular periods, premenstrual breast distension, heavy periods (Fig. 34.4).

Tongue: Red on the sides.
Pulse: Wiry, especially on the left side, and slightly Rapid.
Key symptoms: feeling of distension, irritability, feeling of heat, Wiry pulse, Red sides of the tongue.

> **Diagnostic tip**
>
> A feeling of distension, a Wiry pulse and red sides of the tongue would be enough to diagnose stagnant Liver-Qi turning into Heat

Aetiology

Emotional stress

The aetiology of this pattern is exactly the same as that for Liver-Qi stagnation.

Diet

The excessive consumption of hot-energy foods (such as red meat, spices and alcohol) may facilitate the development of Heat from Qi stagnation.

- Red face, feeling of heat
- Thirst
- Premenstrual tension and breast distension
- Irregular periods, heavy periods
- Irritability, depression, moodiness, outbursts of anger
- Feeling of lump in the throat
- Hypochondrial/epigastric distension

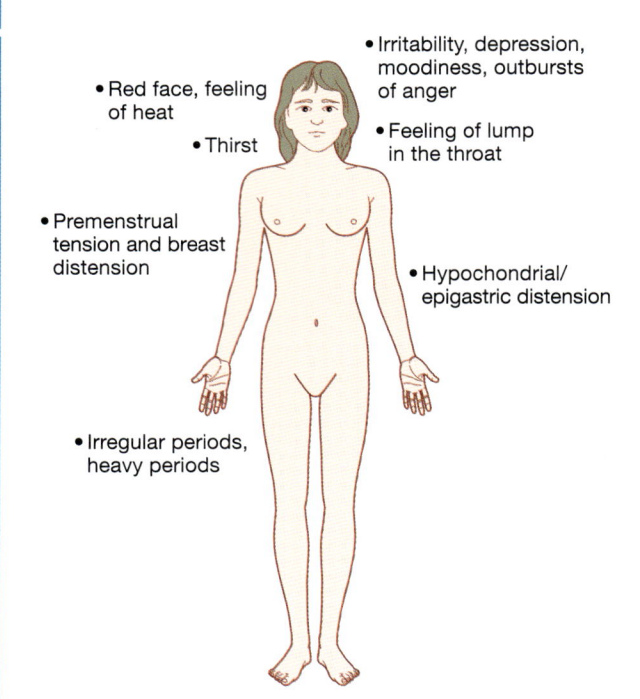

Figure 34.4 Liver-Qi stagnation turning into Heat

Pathology

The pathology of Qi stagnation is the same for this pattern as for the previous one. In this pattern, there is some Heat deriving from Qi stagnation manifesting with a feeling of heat, a red face, thirst, Red sides of the tongue and slightly Rapid pulse.

On an emotional level, the presence of Heat makes the person more prone to outbursts of anger and to anxiety, whereas Liver-Qi stagnation makes the person repress the anger more and become moody.

Pathological precursors of pattern

The pathological precursor of this pattern is Liver-Qi stagnation. This pattern is more likely to arise from Qi stagnation when it arises independently rather than as a consequence of Liver-Blood deficiency or Kidney deficiency (Fig. 34.5).

Pathological developments from pattern

The Heat generated by the Liver-Qi stagnation can, in time, turn into Liver-Fire. In this pattern, the Heat is more intense (see below) (see Fig. 34.5).

Treatment

Principle of treatment: smooth the Liver, move Qi, lightly clear Heat.

Acupuncture

Points: GB-34 Yanglingquan, LIV-3 Taichong, LIV-13 Zhangmen, LIV-14 Qimen, T.B.-6 Zhigou, P-6 Neiguan, LIV-2 Xingjian.
Method: reducing method, no moxa.
Explanation
- The actions of the first six points have already been explained under the previous patterns. Please note that when Heat derives from Qi stagnation, the main treatment principle is to smooth the Liver and clear Qi rather than directly clearing Heat.
- LIV-2 is used if the symptoms and signs of Liver-Heat are pronounced.

Herbal formula

Dan Zhi Xiao Yao San Moutan *Gardenia Free and Easy Wanderer Powder*.

Three Treasures

Freeing the Sun (variation of Dan Zhi Xiao Yao San).

Box 34.5 summarizes stagnant Liver-Qi turning into Heat.

Rebellious Liver-Qi

Clinical manifestations

Hypochondrial or epigastric distension, hiccup, sighing, nausea, vomiting, belching, 'churning feeling in the stomach', irritability; in women, breast distension (Fig. 34.6).

Liver-Qi stagnation → Stagnant Liver-Qi turning into Heat → Liver-Fire

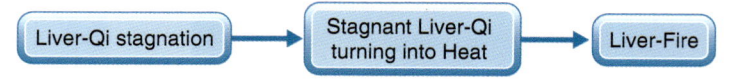

Figure 34.5 Liver-Qi stagnation turning into Heat pattern: precursors and developments

> **Box 34.5 Stagnant Liver-Qi turning into Heat**
>
> **Clinical manifestations**
>
> Hypochondrial or epigastric distension, a slight feeling of oppression of the chest, irritability, melancholy, depression, moodiness, a feeling of lump in the throat, a feeling of heat, red face, thirst, propensity to outbursts of anger, premenstrual tension, irregular periods, premenstrual breast distension, heavy periods, tongue Red on the sides, Wiry pulse
>
> **Treatment**
>
> GB-34 Yanglingquan, LIV-3 Taichong, LIV-13 Zhangmen, LIV-14 Qimen, T.B.-6 Zhigou, P-6 Neiguan, LIV-2 Xingjian

Tongue: in light cases the tongue-body colour may not change; in severe cases the sides will be Red.
Pulse: Wiry. It may be particularly Wiry on the Liver and Stomach positions.

> **Diagnostic tip**
>
> Belching, irritability and a Wiry pulse would be enough to diagnose rebellious Liver-Qi

Aetiology

Emotional stress

Anger, frustration, worry and resentment may all cause Liver-Qi to rebel.

Diet

Eating in a hurry or when under stress, eating while working, getting angry at meal times and eating standing up may all lead to Liver-Qi rebelling horizontally.

Pathology

In this pattern, Liver-Qi 'rebels' horizontally: that is, its horizontal movement in the epigastrium (which under physiological conditions assists the function of the Stomach and Spleen) becomes excessive and it impairs the descending of Stomach-Qi.

Please note that this is a different pathological mechanism than Qi stagnation. In Qi stagnation, the free flow of Liver-Qi is impaired and there are very pronounced emotional symptoms; in rebellious Liver-Qi, the horizontal movement of Liver-Qi is actually *accentuated* and the emotional symptoms are fewer. By

- Irritability
- Hiccup, sighing, nausea, vomiting, belching
- In women, breast distension
- Hypochondrial/epigastric distension

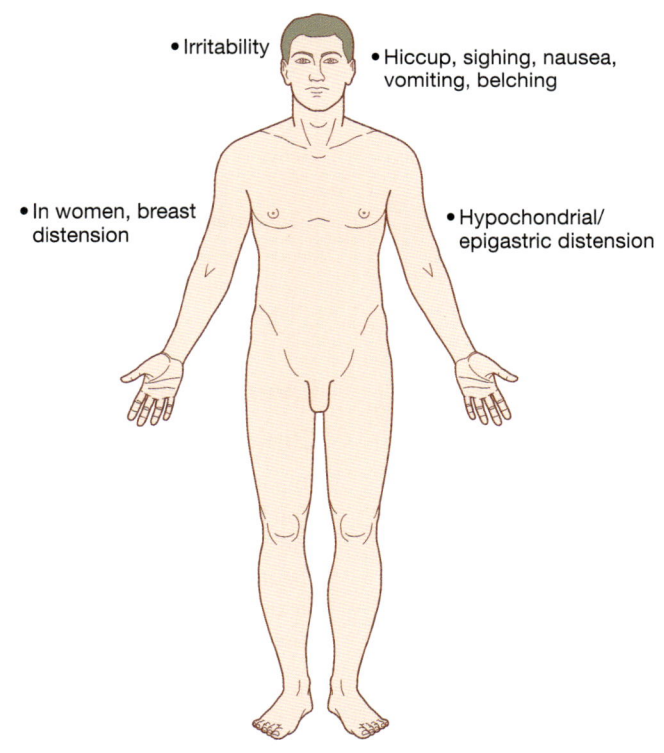

Figure 34.6 Rebellious Liver-Qi

contrast, there are many more digestive symptoms (Fig. 34.7).

Besides the feeling of distension, most of the symptoms in this pattern are due to the impairment of the descending of Stomach-Qi by the rebellious Liver-Qi. These are: hiccup, belching, nausea, vomiting.

In women, there can be breast distension due to Liver-Qi rebelling upwards in the chest and affecting the breasts.

A typical pulse presentation for this pattern is a pulse that is Wiry on both Middle positions (i.e. in the Liver and Stomach positions).

Pathological precursors of pattern

Stagnant Liver-Qi may become rebellious (but not vice versa): therefore the pattern of Liver-Qi stagnation may precede this (Fig. 34.8).

Pathological developments from pattern

Rebellious Liver-Qi may easily give rise to Liver-Yang rising, in which case, the symptoms manifest on the head (headaches, dizziness, tinnitus) (see Fig. 34.8).

Treatment

Principle of treatment: smooth the Liver, subdue Liver-Qi.

Acupuncture

Points: LIV-14 Qimen, P-6 Neiguan, G.B.-34 Yanglingquan, LIV-3 Taichong, T.B.-6 Zhigou, L.I.-4 Hegu, ST-21 Liangmen, ST-19 Burong.
Method: reducing method, no moxa.

Explanation
- LIV-14 is the main point to subdue Liver-Qi when it invades the Stomach, i.e. it harmonizes Liver and Stomach.
- P-6 subdues rebellious Liver-Qi, makes Stomach-Qi descend and calms the Mind.
- G.B.-34 smoothes the Liver and moves Qi. It acts on the hypochondrium.
- LIV-3 smooths the Liver, moves Qi, calms the Mind and settles the Ethereal Soul.
- T.B.-6 moves Liver-Qi.
- L.I.-4 regulates the ascending and descending of Qi and therefore helps to subdue Liver-Qi.
- ST-21 and ST-19 make Stomach-Qi descend.

Herbal formula

Chai Hu Shu Gan Tang *Bupleurum Soothing the Liver Decoction*.
Yi Gan San *Restrain the Liver Powder*.
Si Ni San *Four Rebellious Powder*.

Box 34.6 summarizes rebellious Liver-Qi. Table 34.1 compares and contrasts Liver-Qi stagnation with Rebellious Liver-Qi.

Box 34.6 Rebellious Liver-Qi

Clinical manifestations

Hypochondrial or epigastric distension, hiccups, sighing, nausea, vomiting, belching, 'churning feeling in the stomach', irritability, in women, breast distension, tongue normal or slightly Red on the sides, Wiry pulse

Treatment

LIV-14 Qimen, P-6 Neiguan, G.B.-34 Yanglingquan, LIV-3 Taichong, T.B.-6 Zhigou, L.I.-4 Hegu, ST-21 Liangmen, ST-19 Burong

---

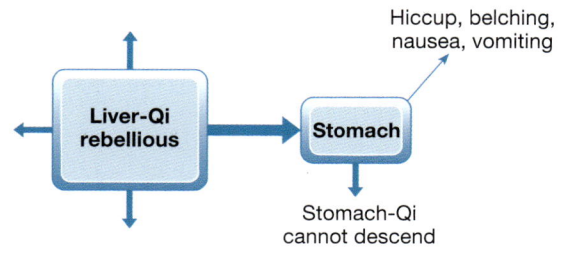

Figure 34.7 Rebellious Liver-Qi invading the Stomach

Liver-Blood stasis

Clinical manifestations

Hypochondrial pain, abdominal pain, vomiting of blood, epistaxis, painful periods, irregular periods, dark and clotted menstrual blood, infertility, masses in the abdomen, purple nails, purple lips, purple or dark complexion, dry skin (in severe cases), purple petechiae (Fig. 34.9).

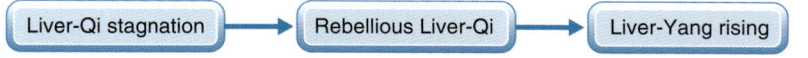

Figure 34.8 Rebellious Liver-Qi pattern: precursors and developments

Table 34.1 Comparison between Liver-Qi stagnation and rebellious Liver-Qi

	Liver-Qi stagnation	Liver-Qi rebellious
Five Elements	Wood underactive	Wood overactive
Pathology	Lack of free flow	Liver-Qi overactive, flow in wrong direction
Manifestations	Depression, moodiness, unhappiness, gloominess, distension of hypochondrium, chest, epigastrium, abdomen, feeling of fullness and *oppression*	Distension of hypochrondium, chest, epigastrium, abdomen, belching, nausea, vomiting, hiccups
Pulse	Wiry and 'reluctant'	Wiry, especially on both Middle positions
Development	Liver-Fire. Can turn into rebellious Liver-Qi	
Treatment principle	Move Qi, eliminate stagnation with pungent herbs	Subdue rebellious Liver-Qi with sweet herbs
Ethereal Soul	Stimulate its coming and going	Restrain its coming and going
Acupuncture	LIV-14, LIV-3, GB-34, TB-6, P-6, Du-24, GB-13	LIV-14, P-6, G.B.-34, LIV-3, T.B.-6, L.I.-4, ST-21, ST-19
Prescriptions	1. Yue Ju Wan 2. Xiao Yao San	1. Chai Hu Shu Gan Tang 2. Yi Gan San 3. Si Ni San

- Epistaxis
- Dark face
- Purple lips
- Vomiting of blood
- Hypochondrial pain
- Abdominal pain
- Masses in abdomen
- Painful periods with dark clots
- Purple nails

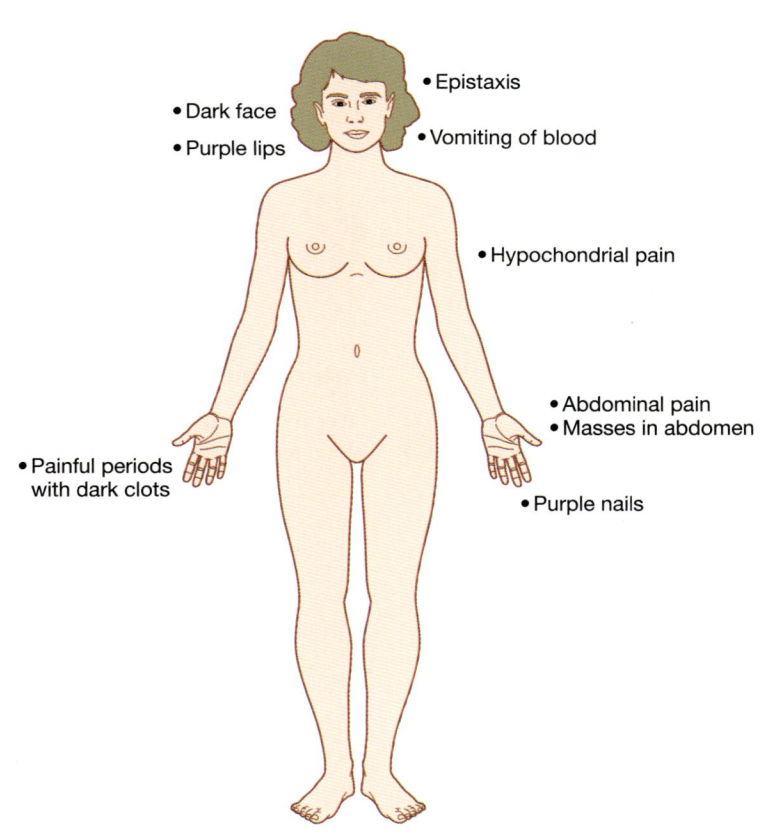

Figure 34.9 Liver-Blood stasis

Tongue: Purple especially, or only, on the sides. In severe cases, there will be purple spots on the sides.
Pulse: Wiry or Firm.
Key symptoms: dark and clotted menstrual blood, Purple tongue.

> **Diagnostic tip**
>
> Stabbing pain and a Purple tongue are enough to diagnose Blood stasis

Aetiology

Blood stasis does not have direct aetiological factors as it is a pathology that develops from other pathological conditions, chiefly Qi stagnation, Cold or Heat. The most common cause of Liver-Blood stasis is Liver-Qi stagnation and, therefore, the aetiological factors leading to Liver-Qi stagnation may, in the long run, lead to Liver-Blood stasis.

Pathology

This pattern often derives from that of stagnation of Liver-Qi. When Qi stagnates, in the long run it leads to stasis of Blood. The Liver stores Blood and is particularly affected by stasis of Blood.

When Liver-Blood stagnates, the Blood in the Directing and Penetrating Vessels (*Ren* and *Chong Mai*) will also stagnate and affect the menstrual function. The chief manifestation of stasis of Blood in the Uterus is dark and clotted menstrual blood and painful periods. Blood stasis leads to pain, and, just as distension is the chief symptom of Qi stagnation, pain is for Blood stasis.

> **Clinical note**
>
> Blood stasis frequently causes a severe pain. Blood stasis may occur without pain but a severe, stabbing pain always indicates Blood stasis

Stasis of Blood of the Liver may cause pain not only during (or before) the periods but also generally in the abdomen at other times and it affects men too. The pain from stasis of Blood is usually fixed in one place and is boring or stabbing in character. This may also be accompanied by a swelling or mass in the abdomen which is fixed (stagnation of Qi can also be manifested with abdominal masses that come and go).

Vomiting of blood and epistaxis are caused by stasis of Blood in the Liver channel.

The Liver manifests on the nails and their purple colour reflects the stasis of Blood in the Liver. General stasis of Blood also causes purple lips and complexion. In severe cases, stagnant Blood obstructs the circulation of fluids (due to the interchange between Body Fluids and Blood) and the skin becomes dry. Petechiae (of a purple colour) are due to bleeding under the skin caused by Blood stasis in the Blood Connecting channels.

The Purple colour of the tongue body reflects stasis of Blood. In severe cases there will also be purplish spots, usually on the sides. The Firm pulse is typical of Blood stasis.

> **Clinical note**
>
> Blood stasis *can* occur without a Purple tongue

Blood stasis is a very important pathology in practice because it potentially leads to serious diseases; by contrast, Qi stagnation by itself cannot lead to serious diseases. For example, coronary heart disease, stroke and cancer are all characterized by the presence of Blood stasis (in addition to other patterns).

> Blood stasis *potentially* leads to serious diseases (Qi stagnation cannot)

Pathological precursors of pattern

Liver-Blood stasis always derives from other patterns. Blood stasis may derive from the following patterns:

- Qi stagnation
- Cold
- Heat
- Qi deficiency
- Blood deficiency
- Phlegm

The first three patterns are the most common precursors of Liver-Blood stasis. Qi stagnation is probably the most common precursor of Blood stasis. Qi is the commander of Blood: when Qi moves, Blood moves. Conversely, when Qi stagnates, Blood stagnates.

Cold also frequently leads to Blood stasis as it congeals Blood. Cold is a frequent cause of Blood stasis in the Uterus.

Heart leads to Blood stasis by condensing Blood. Qi deficiency may cause Blood stasis as the deficient Qi fails to move Blood. Blood deficiency may also lead to Blood stasis as deficient Blood leads to deficient Qi, which fails to move Blood. In women, the combination of Blood deficiency and Blood stasis is relatively common: it would, for example, manifest with scanty but painful periods.

Finally, Phlegm interacts with Blood stasis and they mutually aggravate each other. This happens due to the interrelationship between Blood and Body Fluids. Phlegm is a pathological accumulation of Body Fluids: given the interchange between Body Fluids and Blood, this pathological accumulation may aggravate Blood stasis. The interaction between Phlegm and Blood stasis is more common in the elderly and it is particularly pernicious as it is present in serious modern diseases such as coronary heart disease, stroke and cancer.

> **Clinical note**
>
> Blood stasis and Phlegm occur frequently in the elderly and they are seen in serious diseases such as coronary heart disease, stroke and cancer

Pathological developments from pattern

Liver-Blood stasis in the long run can give rise to dryness. This happens because of the interchange between Blood and Body Fluids so that when Blood stagnates it impairs the production of Body Fluids and leads to dryness (see Fig. 34.10).

Treatment

Principle of treatment: smooth the Liver, move Qi, move Blood, eliminate stasis.

Acupuncture

Points: GB-34 Yanglingquan, LIV-3 Taichong, BL-18 Ganshu, BL-17 Geshu, SP-10 Xuehai, Ren-6 Qihai, SP-4 Gongsun and P-6 Neiguan (opening points of the Penetrating Vessel *Chong Mai*), ST-29 Guilai, KI-14 Siman, LIV-5 Ligou, LIV-6 Zhongdu.

Method: reducing method, no moxa.

Explanation
- GB-34 moves Liver-Qi; in order to move Blood, it is necessary to move Qi.
- LIV-3 moves Liver-Qi and Blood.
- BL-18 moves Liver-Blood.
- BL-17 is the Gathering (*Hui*) point for Blood and it can move Blood (when used with needle only, without moxa).
- SP-10 moves Blood. These two points, BL-17 and SP-10, are often used in combination to move Blood, in the Upper and Lower Burner, respectively.
- Ren-6 moves Qi (apart from tonifying Qi) and is used to move Qi and Blood in the abdomen, in cases of abdominal pain.
- SP-4 Gongsun and P-6 Neiguan open the Penetrating Vessel (*Chong Mai*). This extraordinary vessel is the Sea of Blood and its major use is to move Blood in Blood stasis.
- ST-29 Guilai moves Blood in the Lower Burner and Uterus.
- KI-14 Siman is a point of the Penetrating Vessel that moves Bloods.
- LIV-5 Ligou and LIV-6 Zhongdu move Liver-Qi and Liver-Blood.

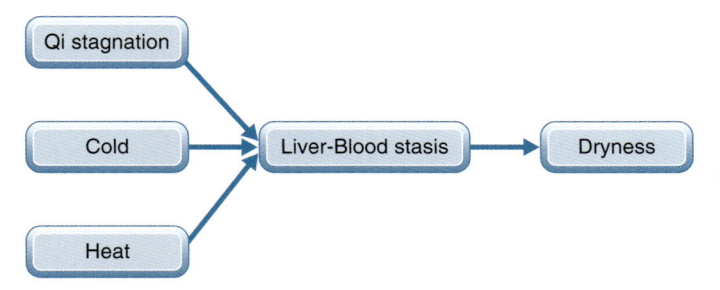

Figure 34.10 Liver-Blood stasis pattern: precursors and developments

> **Box 34.7 Liver-Blood stasis**
>
> **Clinical manifestations**
>
> Hypochondrial pain, abdominal pain, vomiting of blood, epistaxis, painful periods, irregular periods, dark and clotted menstrual blood, infertility, masses in abdomen, purple nails, purple lips, purple or dark complexion, dry skin (in severe cases), purple petechiae, Purple tongue, Wiry or Firm pulse
>
> **Treatment**
>
> GB-34 Yanglingquan, LIV-3 Taichong, BL-18 Ganshu, BL-17 Geshu, SP-10 Xuehai, Ren-6 Qihai, SP-4 Gongsun and P-6 Neiguan (opening points of the Penetrating Vessel), ST-29 Guilai, KI-14 Siman, LIV-5 Ligou, LIV-6 Zhongdu

Herbal formula

Ge Xia Zhu Yu Tang *Eliminating Stasis below the Diaphragm Decoction*.
Shi Xiao San *Breaking into a Smile Powder*.
Yan Hu Suo Tang *Corydalis Decoction*.

Womens's Treasure

Stir Field of Elixir (variation of Ge Xia Zhu Yu Tang).
Box 34.7 summarizes Liver-Blood stasis.

Case history 34.3

A 35-year-old woman suffered from very painful periods with dark clotted blood, premenstrual distension of breasts, a thin white vaginal discharge, a feeling of heaviness and bearing down sensation, chilliness, floaters in eyes and dizziness. She also experienced abdominal pain in mid-cycle. Her pulse was Deep and Choppy and her tongue was Bluish-Purple and Swollen and had a dirty sticky coating.

The pain during and before the periods with dark clotted blood and the purple colour of the tongue body indicated stasis of Blood. With stasis of Liver-Blood there was also some stagnation of Liver-Qi as indicated by the premenstrual distension of breasts. Pre-existing the stasis of Liver-Blood there was also deficiency of Liver-Blood, as indicated by the Choppy pulse, Pale tongue (a Bluish-Purple colour develops from a Pale colour), the floaters and the dizziness.

Besides this Liver disharmony, there was also Spleen-Yang deficiency leading to the retention of Dampness, as indicated by the chilliness, the white vaginal discharge, the Swollen tongue body, the feeling of heaviness and bearing down sensation and the dirty sticky tongue coating. Deficient Spleen-Yang generated internal Cold, which congealed Blood. Stasis of Blood is, in this case, caused by internal Cold, and the chilliness and Bluish-Purple tongue are important factors in determining this. Had the tongue been Reddish-Purple, the diagnosis would have been different.

Case history 34.4

A woman of 43 had a very large subserous fibroid in the uterus. She experienced pain before and sometimes during the periods, which were heavy and in which the blood was dark with clots. She also had headaches before her periods. For 6 weeks the previous year she had suffered from what was diagnosed as thyroiditis, manifesting with a rapid pulse, a swelling of the neck and an earache. Her pulse was Deep and Wiry and her tongue was Reddish-Purple and Stiff.

All these symptoms and signs are due to stasis of Liver-Blood, which is further confirmed by the pulse and tongue. The fibroid is also a manifestation of stasis of Liver-Blood: when Liver-Qi stagnates over a long period of time, Liver-Blood becomes stagnant, and this affects the Directing and Penetrating Vessels (*Ren Mai* and *Chong Mai*) which flow through the Uterus. The thyroiditis is also a manifestation of stasis of Liver-Qi and Liver-Blood affecting the neck.

Liver-Fire blazing

Clinical manifestations

Irritability, propensity to outbursts of anger, tinnitus, deafness, temporal headache, dizziness, red face and eyes, thirst, bitter taste, dream-disturbed sleep, constipation with dry stools, dark-yellow urine, epistaxis, haematemesis, haemoptysis (Fig. 34.11).

Tongue: Red body, redder on the sides, dry yellow coating.
Pulse: Full-Wiry-Rapid.
Key symptoms: headache, irritability, red face, red eyes, Red tongue with yellow coating.

> **Diagnostic tip**
>
> A Red tongue with redder sides and a dry yellow coating would be enough to diagnose Liver-Fire

- Headache
- Dizziness
- Epistaxis
- Red face, red eyes
- Thirst, bitter taste
- Irritability, outbursts of anger, dream-disturbed sleep
- Tinnitus, deafness
- Dry stools
- Dark urine

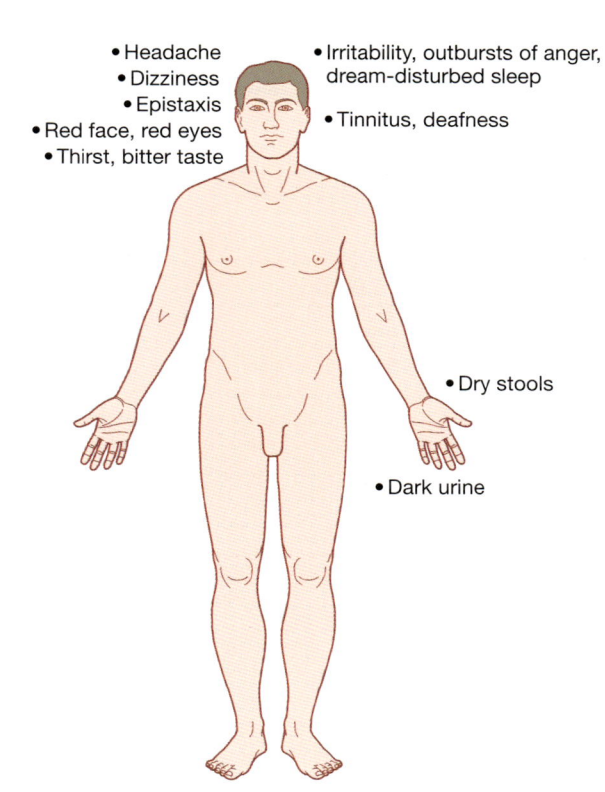

Figure 34.11 Liver-Fire blazing

> **Box 34.8 Fire**
>
> 1. Fire dries up fluids (thirst, dark urine, dry stools)
> 2. Fire agitates the Mind (agitation, insomnia, restlessness)
> 3. Fire may cause bleeding (menorrhagia, epistaxis)

Aetiology

Emotional stress

The most common cause of this pattern is a long-standing emotional state of anger, resentment, repressed anger or frustration. The emotional repression makes Qi stagnate and implode, giving rise to Heat.

Diet

Excessive consumption of alcohol, fried foods and red meat can contribute to the formation of Heat in the Liver.

Pathology

This pattern is characterized by Full-Heat in the Liver. Liver-Fire has a natural tendency to flare upwards; hence many of the symptoms and signs reflect the rising of Liver-Fire towards the head, such as red face and eyes, temporal headache, dizziness, dream-disturbed sleep and irritability. Fire agitates the Mind and the mental–emotional symptoms will be more pronounced than those of Liver-Yang rising or Liver-Qi stagnation. The patient will be more prone to outbursts of anger.

Liver-Fire ascends to the ears and clouds the ear orifices, causing tinnitus and deafness, which, in this case, will be characterized by a sudden onset. The tinnitus will be experienced as a high-pitched whistle.

The headache is caused by the rising upwards of Liver-Yang and Liver-Fire and will be very intense, throbbing in character, usually on the temple or in the eye.

The bitter taste is caused by the rising of Liver-Fire towards the throat and mouth. Bitter taste can also be caused by Heart-Fire, in which case it manifests only in the mornings after a bad night's sleep (it will not be present after a good night's sleep). If bitter taste is caused by Liver-Fire it will be present for the whole day and not just in the morning.

Liver-Fire dries up Body Fluids, resulting in constipation with dry stools and a concentrated, dark urine.

In a few cases, Liver-Fire heats the Blood and causes it to extravasate, resulting in epistaxis or vomiting or coughing of blood.

The Red tongue body reflects the Heat and the redder colour of the sides reflects the location of Heat in the Liver. The dry yellow coating confirms that it is Full-Heat.

The Full-Rapid quality of the Pulse reflects Full-Heat and its Wiry quality reflects the location of Heat in the Liver.

Box 34.8 summarizes the effects of Fire.

Pathological precursors of pattern

Liver-Fire often derives from long-standing Liver-Qi stagnation: when Qi stagnates for a long time, it 'implodes' and gives rise to Heat, which can then transform into Fire.

Liver-Yang rising could also transform itself into Liver-Fire, especially when there are dietary aetiological factors (Fig. 34.12).

Pathological developments from pattern

Liver-Fire can dry up Yin and may therefore induce a deficiency of Liver-Yin. Liver-Fire is also easily transmitted to the Heart, giving rise to Heart-Fire: this is

```
Liver-Qi stagnation → Liver-Fire blazing → Liver-Yin deficiency
                                        → Heart-Fire
```

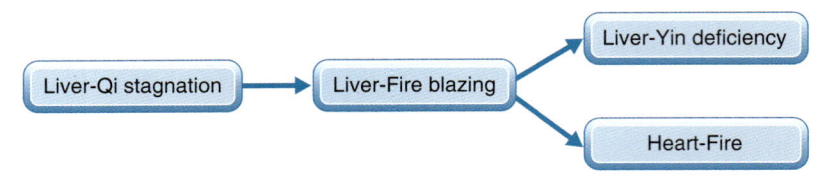

Figure 34.12 Liver-Fire blazing pattern: precursors and developments

more likely to happen when severe emotional stress is the cause of the problem (see Fig. 34.12).

Treatment

Principle of treatment: clear the Liver, drain Fire.

Acupuncture

Points: LIV-2 Xingjian, LIV-3 Taichong, GB-20 Fengchi, Taiyang, GB-13 Benshen, LI-11 Quchi, G.B.-1 Tongziliao, G.B.-9 Tianchong, G.B.-8 Shuaigu, G.B.-6 Xuanli, SP-6 Sanyinjiao, LIV-1 Dadun.

Method: reducing method, no moxa.

Explanation
- LIV-2 is the main point to use: it is specific to drain Liver-Fire.
- LIV-3 drains the Liver.
- GB-20 drains Liver-Fire and subdues ascending Liver-Qi. A very important point to use in case of eye problems or headaches caused by Liver-Fire.
- Taiyang (extra point) clears Liver-Fire and is used for temporal headache.
- GB-13 subdues ascending Liver-Yang and calms the Mind.
- L.I.-11 clears Heat.
- G.B.-1, G.B.-9, G.B.-8 and G.B.-6 are important local points for Liver-Fire ascending to the head to be used only if there are headaches.
- SP-6 is used to nourish Yin, which will help to drain Fire.
- LIV-1 clears the Liver and subdues rising Liver-Yang and Liver-Fire.

Herbal formula

Long Dan Xie Gan Tang *Gentiana Draining the Liver Decoction*.

Dang Gui Long Hui Tang *Angelica-Gentiana-Aloe Decoction*.

Three Treasures

Drain Fire (variation of Long Dan Xie Gan Tang). Box 34.9 summarizes Liver-Fire blazing.

Box 34.9 Liver-Fire blazing

Clinical manifestations

Irritability, propensity to outbursts of anger, tinnitus, deafness, temporal headache, dizziness, red face and eyes, thirst, bitter taste, dream-disturbed sleep, constipation with dry stools, dark-yellow urine, epistaxis, haematemesis, haemoptysis, Red tongue, redder on the sides, dry yellow coating, Full-Wiry-Rapid pulse

Treatment

LIV-2 Xingjian, LIV-3 Taichong, GB-20 Fengchi, Taiyang, GB-13 Benshen, LI-11 Quchi, G.B.-1 Tongziliao, G.B.-9 Tianchong, G.B.-8 Shuaigu, G.B.-6 Xuanli, SP-6 Sanyinjiao, LIV-1 Dadun

---

Damp-Heat in the Liver

Clinical manifestations

Fullness of the hypochondrium, abdomen or hypogastrium, bitter taste, sticky taste, poor appetite, nausea, feeling of heaviness of the body, yellow vaginal discharge, vaginal itching, vulvar eczema or sores, midcycle bleeding and/or pain, pain, redness and swelling of the scrotum, genital, papular or vesicular skin rashes and itching, urinary difficulty, burning on urination, dark urine (Fig. 34.13).

Tongue: Red body with redder sides, sticky yellow coating.

Pulse: Slippery-Wiry-Rapid.

Key symptoms: fullness of hypochondrium and abdomen, feeling of heaviness, nausea, bitter and sticky taste, sticky yellow coating, Slippery pulse.

Diagnostic tip

A feeling of fullness and heaviness and a sticky yellow tongue coating are enough to diagnose Damp-Heat. Together with red sides of the tongue they are enough to diagnose Liver Damp-Heat

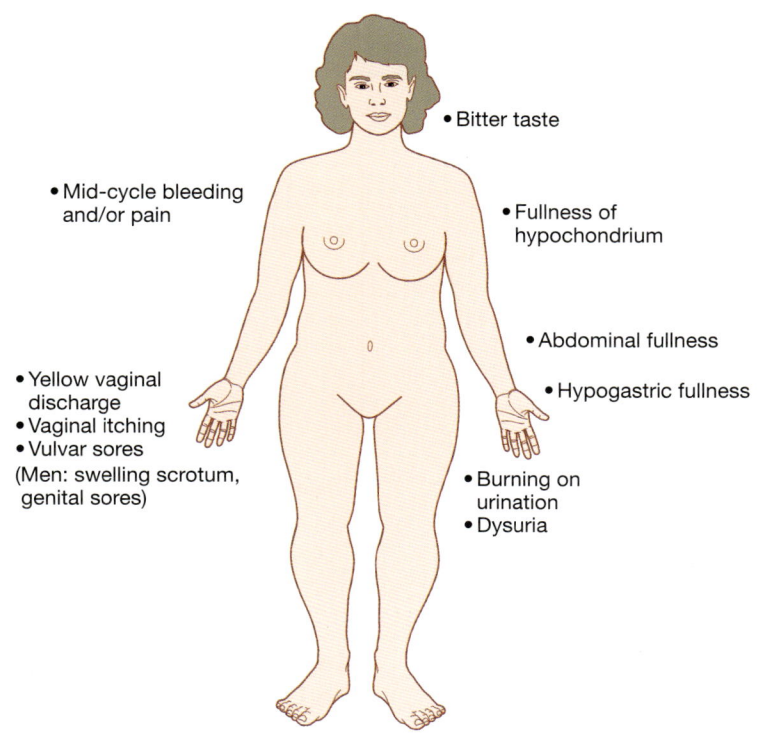

Figure 34.13 Damp-Heat in the Liver

- Bitter taste
- Mid-cycle bleeding and/or pain
- Fullness of hypochondrium
- Abdominal fullness
- Hypogastric fullness
- Yellow vaginal discharge
- Vaginal itching
- Vulvar sores
(Men: swelling scrotum, genital sores)
- Burning on urination
- Dysuria

Aetiology

Diet

Excessive consumption of dairy foods and greasy foods or an irregular diet leads to the formation of Dampness.

External pathogenic factors

External Dampness is a frequent cause for the formation of Damp-Heat. External Dampness invades the channels of the legs (in this case the Liver) and can then easily settle in the organs. With time, Dampness frequently combines with Heat to give rise to Damp-Heat. In hot tropical countries, external Dampness and Heat invade the body, causing Damp-Heat from the beginning.

Pathology

This pattern arises from a combination of Heat in the Liver and Dampness. A feeling of *fullness* is typical of Dampness.

Dampness is 'sticky' and this causes the sticky taste, the vaginal discharge and vaginal sores. Dampness infuses downwards and for this reason it often manifests in the genitals with sores or eczema in this area.

Dampness obstructs the Middle Burner, impairing the descending of Stomach Qi: this causes nausea and poor appetite. Dampness is 'heavy' and it causes a typical feeling of heaviness of the body.

Dampness infuses downwards and may obstruct the urinary passages, causing burning on urination and difficulty in urination.

The stickiness of the tongue coating is indicative of the presence of Dampness and the Slippery pulse also reflects Dampness. The pulse may also be Wiry, reflecting the Liver disharmony.

Box 34.10 summarizes the characteristics of Dampness.

> **Box 34.10 Dampness**
>
> Dampness is characterized by:
> - *Fullness* (feeling of fullness, epigastrium or abdomen)
> - *Heaviness* (feeling of heaviness)
> - *Stickiness* (sticky taste, oozing skin lesions, sticky stools)

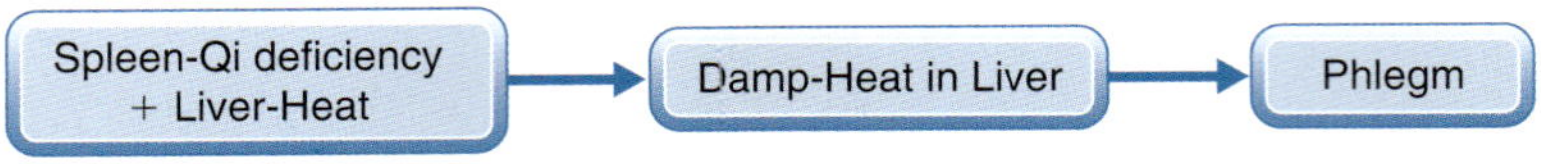

Figure 34.14 Damp-Heat in the Liver pattern: precursors and developments

Pathological precursors of pattern

Spleen-Qi deficiency may be the precursor to this pattern as Dampness may form when the Spleen fails in its function of transportation and transformation.

Long-term stagnation of Liver-Qi can lead to Liver Heat, which combines with the Dampness. Any of the causes of Liver-Qi stagnation (excessive anger, etc.), therefore, can contribute to this pattern (Fig. 34.14).

Pathological developments from pattern

Dampness may lead to the formation of Phlegm when it persists for some years (see Fig. 34.14).

Treatment

Principle of treatment: resolve Dampness, clear the Liver, clear Heat.
Points: LIV-14 Qimen, GB-34 Yanglingquan, BL-18 Ganshu, Ren-12 Zhongwan, SP-9 Yinlingquan, SP-6 Sanyinjiao, LI-11 Quchi, LIV-2 Xingjian.
Method: reducing method on all points except Ren-12, which should be tonified.
Explanation
- LIV-14 regulates Liver-Qi in the hypochondrium and epigastrium.
- GB-34 resolves Dampness in Liver and Gall Bladder.
- BL-18 resolves Dampness from the Liver.
- Ren-12 tonifies the Spleen to resolve Dampness.
- SP-9 and SP-6 resolve Dampness. In particular, SP-9 and SP-6 resolve Dampness from the Lower Burner.
- LI-11 resolves Dampness and clears Heat.
- LIV-2 clears Liver-Heat.

Herbal formula

Long Dan Xie Gan Tang *Gentiana Draining the Liver Decoction*.
Box 34.11 summarizes Damp-Heat in the Liver.

Box 34.11 Damp-Heat in the Liver

Clinical manifestations

Fullness of the hypochondrium, abdomen or hypogastrium, bitter taste, sticky taste, poor appetite, nausea, feeling of heaviness of the body, yellow vaginal discharge, vaginal itching, vulvar eczema or sores, mid-cycle bleeding and/or pain, pain, redness and swelling of the scrotum, genital, papular or vesicular skin rashes and itching, urinary difficulty, burning on urination, dark urine, Red tongue with redder sides, sticky yellow coating, Slippery-Wiry-Rapid pulse

Treatment

LIV-14 Qimen, G.B.-34 Yanglingquan, BL-18 Ganshu, Ren-12 Zhongwan, SP-9 Yinlingquan, SP-6 Sanyinjiao, LI-11 Quchi, LIV-2 Xingjian

Stagnation of Cold in the Liver channel

Clinical manifestations

Fullness and distension of the hypogastrium with pain which refers downwards to the scrotum and testis and upwards to the hypochondrium, the pain is alleviated by warmth, straining of the testis or contraction of the scrotum, vertical headache, feeling of cold, cold hands and feet, vomiting of clear watery fluid or dry vomiting (Fig. 34.15). In women there can be shrinking of the vagina.
Tongue: Pale and wet with a white coating.
Pulse: Deep-Wiry-Slow.
Key symptoms: hypogastric pain referring to scrotum, cold hands and feet, Wiry-Deep-Slow Pulse.

Aetiology

This pattern is due to invasion of exterior Cold.

Pathology

This is caused by invasion of the Liver channel by cold. The Liver channel flows around the external genitalia, Cold contracts, hence the pain and contraction of the scrotum.

The Pulse is Deep reflecting the presence of interior Cold, Wiry reflecting affection of the Liver and Slow reflecting the presence of Cold.

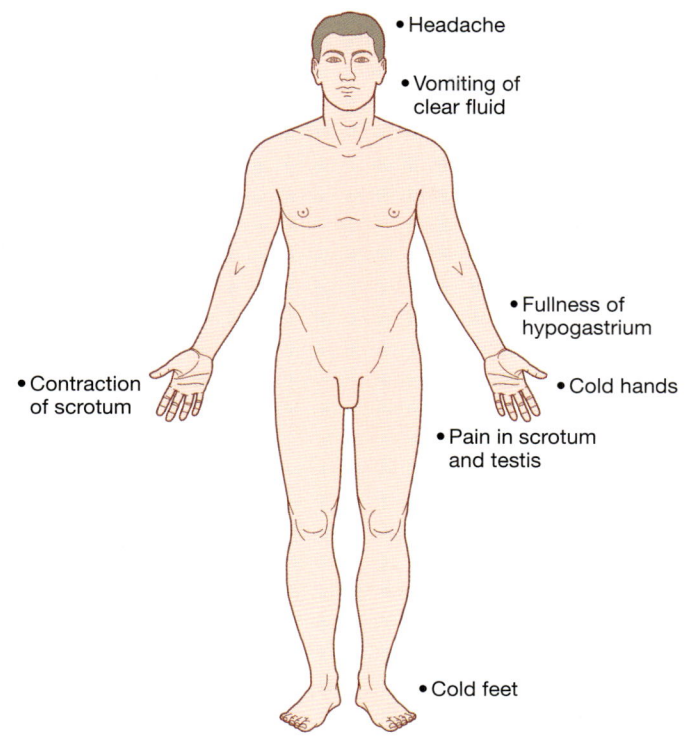

Figure 34.15 Stagnation of Cold in the Liver channel

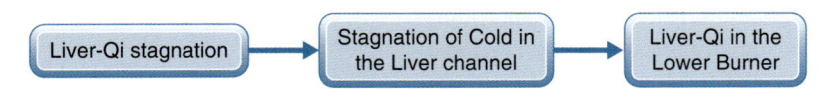

Figure 34.16 Stagnation of Cold in the Liver channel pattern: precursors and developments

Pathological precursors of pattern

A pre-existing internal state of Liver-Qi stagnation may predispose the patient to develop this pattern after invasion of Cold (Fig. 34.16).

Pathological developments from pattern

Stagnation of Cold in the Liver channel may lead to stagnation of Liver-Qi in the Lower Burner (see Fig. 34.16).

Treatment

Principle of treatment: clear the Liver, expel Cold.

Acupuncture

Points: Ren-3 Zhongji, LIV-5 Ligou, LIV-1 Dadun, LIV-3 Taichong. Moxa is applicable.

Method: reducing method, moxa is applicable.
Explanation
- Ren-3 with moxa disperses Cold from the Lower Burner.
- LIV-5, Connecting point of the Liver-Connecting channel which flows around the genitals, can disperse Cold from the Liver channel.
- LIV-1 clears Liver channel and removes obstruction of Cold from the Lower Burner.
- LIV-3 resolves spasms and helps to relieve contraction.

Herbal formula

Nuan Gan Jian *Warming the Liver Decoction*.

Box 34.12 summarizes stagnation of Cold in the Liver channel.

> **Box 34.12 Stagnation of Cold in the Liver channel**
>
> **Clinical manifestations**
>
> Fullness and distension of the hypogastrium with pain which refers downwards to the scrotum and testis and upwards to the hypochondrium, the pain is alleviated by warmth, straining of the testis or contraction of the scrotum, vertical headache, feeling of cold, cold hands and feet, vomiting of clear watery fluid or dry vomiting. In women there can be shrinking of the vagina, Pale and wet tongue with a white coating, Deep-Wiry-Slow pulse
>
> **Treatment**
>
> Ren-3 Zhongji, LIV-5 Ligou, LIV-1 Dadun, LIV-3 Taichong

EMPTY PATTERNS

Liver-Blood deficiency

Clinical manifestations

Dizziness, numbness or tingling of limbs, insomnia, blurred vision, 'floaters' in eyes, diminished night vision, scanty menstruation or amenorrhoea, dull-pale complexion without lustre, pale lips, muscular weakness, cramps, withered and brittle nails, dry hair and skin, depression, a feeling of aimlessness (Fig. 34.17).
Tongue: Pale body, especially on the sides, which, in extreme cases, can assume an orangey colour, Thin and slightly dry.
Pulse: Choppy or Fine.
Key symptoms: blurred vision, scanty periods, dull-pale complexion, Pale tongue.

> **Diagnostic tip**
>
> Blurred vision, a Pale tongue and a Choppy pulse are enough to diagnose Liver-Blood deficiency

Aetiology

Diet

A diet poor in nourishment or lacking in Blood-forming foods (such as meat and grains) can weaken the Spleen, which, in turn, cannot make enough Blood. When not enough Blood is produced by the Spleen, not enough Blood is stored by the Liver.

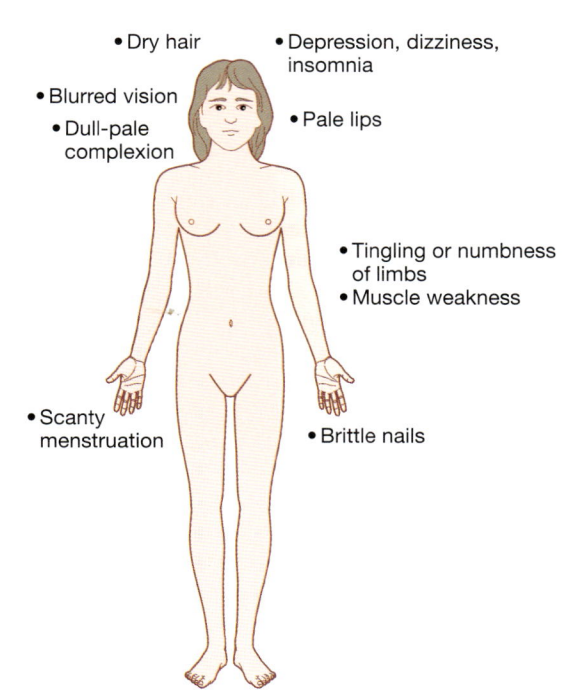

Figure 34.17 Liver-Blood deficiency

Emotional stress

Emotions such as sadness and grief can deplete Liver-Blood directly, as indicated above under 'General aetiology'. Emotional stress may also lead to Blood deficiency by initially depleting Qi, which then fails to make enough Blood.

Excessive physical exercise

Excessive physical exercise injures primarily the Yang of the Spleen and Kidneys. As the Spleen and Kidneys become weaker, they may induce a Blood deficiency as the Food-Qi of the Spleen is the precursor of Blood and the Kidneys are the origin of *Tian Gui*, which makes menstrual Blood. This is the reason why women athletes often develop amenorrhoea.

However, excessive exercise also injures the sinews and therefore the Liver: in the long run, this may lead to Liver-Blood deficiency.

Blood loss

A serious haemorrhage (such as during childbirth) can also lead to deficiency of Liver-Blood.

Pathology

Liver-Blood deficiency is much more common in women than men. The Liver stores Blood and any deficiency of Blood often manifests in the Liver sphere. As the Liver opens into the eyes, when Liver-Blood is deficient the eyes will lack nourishment and moisture so that they cannot see clearly.

The Liver controls the sinews and when Liver-Blood is deficient these will lack nourishment and moistening and the person will experience muscular weakness, cramps or tingling.

Dizziness, pale lips, dull-pale complexion are all signs of general Blood deficiency. As the Liver manifests in the nails, when Liver-Blood is deficient they will lose nourishment and become withered and brittle.

Liver-Blood is closely related to the Directing and Penetrating Vessels (*Ren Mai* and *Chong Mai*), which are dependent on the Liver for their Blood supply. Thus, when Liver-Blood is deficient, the Directing and Penetrating Vessels will also lack Blood, resulting in scanty periods or no periods at all.

The Liver houses the Ethereal Soul (*Hun*) and Liver-Blood in particular 'anchors' the Ethereal Soul at night. When Liver-Blood is deficient, this may fail to anchor the Ethereal Soul at night and the patient cannot sleep well or dreams a lot.

The Ethereal Soul is responsible for the 'coming and going' of the Mind and is responsible for the capacity of planning, having projects, projecting towards the others, life dreams, etc. When Liver-Blood is deficient, the Ethereal Soul is not rooted in Liver-Blood and this may result in its excessive 'coming and going': this causes insomnia, anxiety and a tendency to have too many projects, aims, dreams, plans in a rather 'scattered' way. By contrast, when both Liver-Blood and Liver-Qi are deficient, there is not enough 'coming and going' of the Ethereal Soul and the person may become depressed and have a feeling of aimlessness.

> When Liver-Blood is deficient, the Ethereal Soul (*Hun*) is not rooted in Liver-Blood and this may result in its excessive 'coming and going': this causes insomnia, anxiety and a tendency to have too many projects, aims, dreams, plans in a rather 'scattered' way. By contrast, when both Liver-Blood and Liver-Qi are deficient, there is not enough 'coming and going' of the Ethereal Soul and the person may become depressed and have a feeling of aimlessness

Clinical note

Liver-Blood nourishes:
- Eyes: blurred vision
- Sinews: tingling, cramps
- Nails: ridged nails
- Uterus: scanty periods
- Ethereal Soul: insomnia, dreaming

The tongue is Pale and its slight dryness indicates Blood deficiency. In severe cases, the tongue would also be Thin. It is worth noting here that, although Blood deficiency does tend to make the tongue Thin, in practice, a Thin tongue is not seen frequently and the Swollen tongue is much more common. This is because Dampness and Phlegm (which make the tongue Swollen) are such pervasive and common pathogenic factors: therefore, although the patient may have Blood deficiency, the swelling of the tongue 'masks' it.

The Choppy or Fine pulse are typical of Blood deficiency.

Clinical note

Liver-Blood deficiency is much more common in women than men

Pathological precursors of pattern

The Kidneys play a role in the formation of Blood and a deficiency of the Kidneys can lead to deficiency of Blood (Fig. 34.18).

Pathological developments from pattern

Liver-Blood deficiency often leads to Heart-Blood deficiency, especially when the patient is subject to emotional stress.

As Blood plays a role in the formation of Essence and the Liver and Kidneys share a very close physiological relationship, a deficiency of Liver-Blood may lead to a Kidney deficiency (or vice versa, as noted above).

In women, Liver-Blood deficiency often leads to a secondary stagnation of Liver-Qi, in which case the symptoms of Qi stagnation are milder, there is premenstrual depression rather than irritability and the pulse is only slightly Wiry and often Fine.

Finally, in women too, Liver-Blood deficiency is the most common cause of the rising of Liver-Yang,

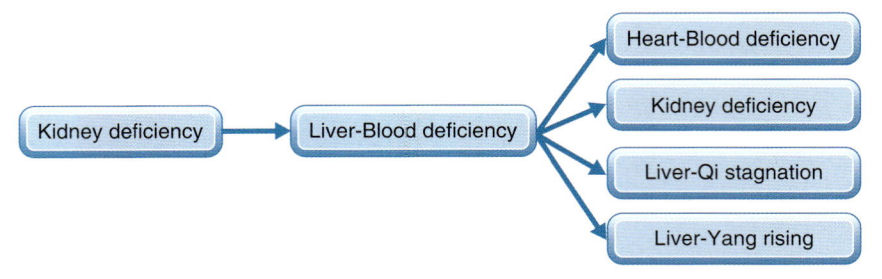

Figure 34.18 Liver-Blood deficiency pattern: precursors and developments

Box 34.13 Consequences of Liver-Blood deficiency

1. May lead to Heart-Blood deficiency
2. May lead to Kidney deficiency
3. May lead to secondary Liver-Qi stagnation
4. May lead to Liver-Yang rising

leading to headaches. Typically, the woman will have two kinds of headaches, a dull one from Liver-Blood deficiency and occasional attacks of a severe, throbbing headache from Liver-Yang rising (see Fig. 34.18).

Box 34.13 summarizes the consequences of Liver-Blood deficiency.

Treatment

Principle of treatment: tonify the Liver, nourish Blood.

Acupuncture

Points: LIV-8 Ququan, SP-6 Sanyinjiao, ST-36 Zusanli, Ren-4 Guanyuan, BL-18 Ganshu, BL-20 Pishu, BL-23 Shenshu, BL-17 Geshu, Yuyao extra point.
Method: reinforcing, moxa can be used.
Explanation
– LIV-8 nourishes Liver-Blood.
– ST-36 and SP-6 tonify the Post-Heaven Qi to produce Blood. The combination of these three points, LIV-8, ST-36 and SP-6, is excellent to nourish Blood.
– Ren-4 (with direct moxa) nourishes Blood and especially menstrual Blood.
– BL-18 tonifies the Liver.
– BL-20 tonifies the Spleen to produce Blood.
– BL-23 tonifies the Kidneys to produce Blood.
– BL-17 with direct moxa, nourishes Blood.
– Yuyao is a good local point for dull headaches or blurred vision from Liver-Blood deficiency.

Box 34.14 Liver-Blood deficiency

Clinical manifestations

Dizziness, numbness or tingling of limbs, insomnia, blurred vision, 'floaters' in eyes, diminished night vision, scanty menstruation or amenorrhoea, dull-pale complexion without lustre, pale lips, muscular weakness, cramps, withered and brittle nails, dry hair and skin, depression, a feeling of aimlessness, Pale tongue, Thin and slightly dry, Choppy or Fine pulse

Treatment

LIV-8 Ququan, SP-6 Sanyinjiao, ST-36 Zusanli, Ren-4 Guanyuan, BL-18 Ganshu, BL-20 Pishu, BL-23 Shenshu, BL-17 Geshu, Yuyao extra point

Herbal formula

Bu Gan Tang *Tonifying the Liver Decoction*.

Three Treasures

Brocade Sinews.
Brighten the Eyes.
Precious Sea (variation of Ba Zhen Tang).

Box 34.14 summarizes Liver-Blood deficiency.

Case history 34.5

A woman of 38 suffered from poor memory, tiredness, a tingling sensation in the limbs, dry hair and constipation with slightly dry stools. Her pulse was Choppy and her tongue was Pale, Thin and slightly dry.

All these symptoms and signs are due to deficiency of Liver-Blood.

Liver-Yin deficiency

Clinical manifestations

Dizziness, numbness or tingling of limbs, insomnia, blurred vision, 'floaters' in eyes, dry eyes, diminished

night vision, scanty menstruation or amenorrhoea, dull-pale complexion without lustre but with red cheekbones, muscular weakness, cramps, withered and brittle nails, very dry hair and skin, depression, a feeling of aimlessness (Fig. 34.19).
Tongue: normal-coloured without coating or with rootless coating.
Pulse: Floating-Empty.
Key symptoms: blurred vision, dry eyes, tongue without coating.

Empty-Heat

Malar flush, anxiety, a feeling of heat in the evening, night sweating, five-palm heat, thirst with desire to drink in small sips, heavy menstrual bleeding.
Tongue: Red without coating.
Pulse: Floating-Empty and slightly Rapid.

Diagnostic tip

Dry eyes and tongue without coating would be enough to diagnose Liver-Yin deficiency

Aetiology

The aetiology of Liver-Yin deficiency is exactly the same as that for Liver-Blood deficiency.

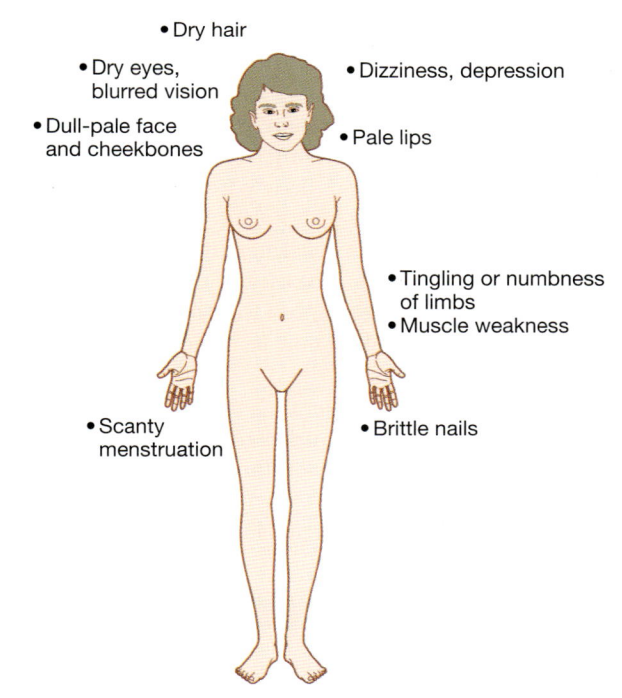

Figure 34.19 Liver-Yin deficiency

Pathology

Liver-Yin deficiency is very closely related to Liver-Blood deficiency. As can be seen from the list of clinical manifestations, Liver-Yin deficiency includes all the same symptoms and signs as Liver-Blood deficiency.

The main clinical manifestations distinguishing Liver-Yin from Liver-Blood deficiency are dry eyes, red cheekbones and tongue without coating.

Dry eyes are due to deficient Liver-Yin not nourishing and moistening the eyes. Red cheekbones are due to Empty-Heat arising from Yin deficiency, although the cheeks may be pale from a pre-existing Liver-Blood deficiency.

The lack of coating on the tongue is an important sign distinguishing this pattern. Please note that the tongue may not necessarily be Red as it becomes so only when Empty-Heat is pronounced.

When Yin deficiency is advanced, Empty-Heat develops and this causes the cheekbones to become redder, thirst with desire to drink in small sips, night sweating and five-palm heat. Empty-Heat also affects the patient from a mental–emotional point of view. When there is Liver-Yin deficiency and Empty-Heat, this agitates the Ethereal Soul (which lacks root as Liver-Yin is deficient) so that it 'comes and goes' too much, causing anxiety, insomnia, mental restlessness and an excessive mental activity in terms or plans, projects, dreams, aims which are pursued in a rather 'scattered' way.

Pathological precursors of pattern

Liver-Blood deficiency is nearly always the precursor of Liver-Yin deficiency. A deficiency of Kidney-Yin also facilitates the development of Liver-Yin deficiency from Liver-Blood deficiency (Fig. 34.20).

Pathological developments from pattern

Liver-Yin deficiency may affect the Kidneys and lead to Kidney-Yin deficiency. Liver-Yin deficiency may also easily give rise to Liver-Yang rising.

Finally, Liver-Yin affects Heart-Yin and therefore Liver-Yin deficiency may cause Heart-Yin deficiency (see Fig. 34.20).

Box 34.15 summarizes the consequences of Liver-Yin deficiency.

Treatment

Principle of treatment: tonify the Liver, nourish Yin, clear Empty-Heat if necessary.

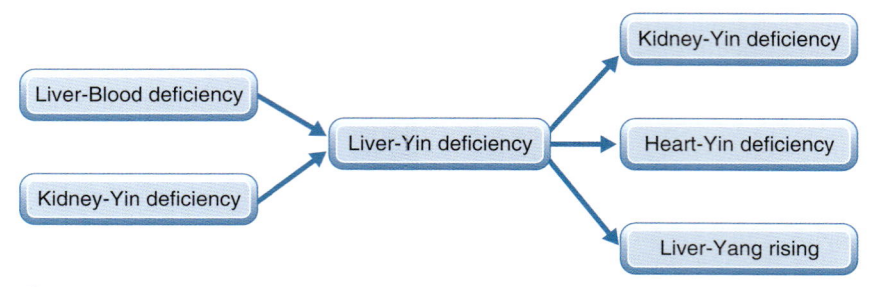

Figure 34.20 Liver-Yin deficiency pattern: precursors and developments

---

Box 34.15 Consequences of Liver-Yin deficiency

1. May lead to Kidney-Yin deficiency
2. May lead to Liver-Yang rising
3. May lead to Heart-Yin deficiency

Acupuncture

Points: LIV-8 Ququan, SP-6 Sanyinjiao, ST-36 Zusanli, Ren-4 Guanyuan, KI-3 Taixi, KI-6 Zhaohai, LIV-2 Xingjian.

Method: reinforcing (except for LIV-2), no moxa.

Explanation
- The first four points, LIV-8, ST-36, SP-6 and Ren-4 are the same as those used to nourish Liver-Blood.
- KI-3 and KI-6 are used to nourish Kidney- and Liver-Yin.
- LIV-2, with reducing method, is used if there is Empty-Heat.

Herbal formula

Yi Guan Jian *One Linking Decoction*.

Three Treasures

Root the Spirit (variation of Yin Mei Tang).
Nourish the Soul (variation of Suan Zao Ren Tang).

Box 34.16 summarizes manifestations and treatment of Liver-Yin deficiency.

FULL/EMPTY PATTERNS

Liver-Yang rising

Clinical manifestations

Headache, which may be on the temples, eyes or lateral side of the head, dizziness, tinnitus, deafness, blurred vision, dry mouth and throat, insomnia, irritability, feeling worked-up, propensity to outbursts of anger, stiff neck (Fig. 34.21).

Tongue: the tongue presentation may vary widely depending on the underlying condition causing Liver-Yang rising. If this derives from Liver-Blood deficiency the tongue-body colour will be Pale; if it derives from Liver-Yin deficiency the tongue will be without coating. In some cases, Liver-Yang rising may develop from rebellious Liver-Qi: in this case the tongue-body colour may be normal or slightly red on the sides.

Pulse: Wiry. However, if there is a background of Liver-Blood or Liver-Yin deficiency, the pulse may be Wiry only on one side or it may also be Wiry but Fine.

Key symptoms: headache, irritability, Wiry Pulse.

Box 34.16 Liver-Yin deficiency

Clinical manifestations

Dizziness, numbness or tingling of limbs, insomnia, blurred vision, 'floaters' in eyes, dry eyes, diminished night vision, scanty menstruation or amenorrhoea, dull-pale complexion without lustre but with red cheekbones, muscular weakness, cramps, withered and brittle nails, very dry hair and skin, depression, a feeling of aimlessness, normal-coloured tongue without coating or with rootless coating, Floating-Empty pulse

Treatment

LIV-8 Ququan, SP-6 Sanyinjiao, ST-36 Zusanli, Ren-4 Guanyuan, KI-3 Taixi, KI-6 Zhaohai, LIV-2 Xingjian

---

Diagnostic tip

Throbbing headaches and a Wiry pulse would be enough to diagnose Liver-Yang rising

- Blurred vision
- Insomnia, outbursts of anger
- Headache, dizziness, tinnitus, deafness

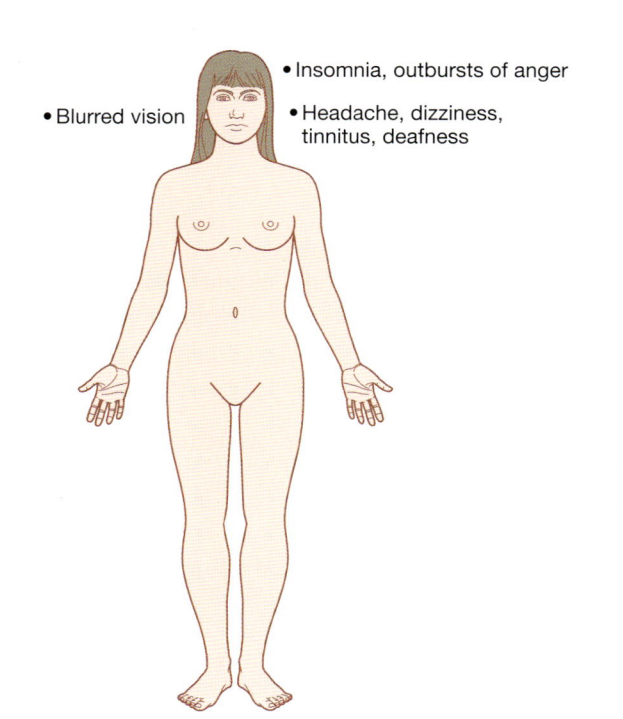

Figure 34.21 Liver-Yang rising

Aetiology

Emotional stress

The most common cause of rising of Liver-Yang is from emotional problems, in particular anger, frustration and resentment over a long period of time. Anger makes Qi rise and this causes Liver-Qi to have an excessive upward movement.

Diet

Eating in a hurry, getting angry at meal times and eating while working may all cause Liver-Qi to rise, causing the pattern of Liver-Yang rising.

Pathology

This is a mixed Deficiency/Excess pattern as it derives from deficiency of Liver-Yin and/or Kidney-Yin or Liver-Blood causing the rising of Liver-Yang. When Liver-Yang derives from a Kidney deficiency, in Five-Element terms, Water is deficient and fails to nourish and 'submerge' Wood, which becomes too dry and causes the upwards rising of Liver-Yang.

This pattern is therefore characterized by an imbalance between Liver-Yin (which is deficient) and Liver-Yang (which is in excess). This pattern is a type of rebellious Liver-Qi characterized by the excessive rise of Liver-Yang. Although there are a few symptoms of Heat (such as dry throat), this pattern is not a Full-Heat pattern, but simply an imbalance between Yin and Yang with excessive rising of Qi.

The manifestations described above are only those of the rising of Liver-Yang. In practice, they would normally appear together with some symptoms and signs of Liver- and/or Kidney-Yin deficiency or Liver-Blood deficiency.

The main difference between the pattern of Liver-Yang rising and that of Liver-Fire blazing is that in Liver-Fire blazing there is 'solid' Fire drying up the Body Fluids and causing symptoms and signs of dryness such as constipation, scanty-dark urine, red eyes and face and bitter taste which are absent in Liver-Yang rising. Liver-Fire blazing is a purely Excess pattern, while Liver-Yang rising is a combined Deficiency/Excess pattern characterized by an imbalance between Yin and Yang and by rising of Qi, without 'solid' Fire.

Most of the manifestations are due to the rising of Liver-Yang to the head: tinnitus, deafness (both of sudden onset), propensity to outbursts of anger and headache. The headache is one of the most common and distinctive signs of rising of Liver-Yang and, conversely, Liver-Yang rising is the most common cause of chronic headaches.

> **Clinical note**
>
> Liver-Yang rising is the most common cause of chronic headaches

The headache from Liver-Yang rising is typically on either temple, but it can also be on the lateral side of the head (Gall Bladder channel) or in or just above the eye. It is usually unilateral. With regard to headaches, Chinese medicine holds that an Excess condition more often manifests on the right side, whereas a Deficient condition more often manifests on the left side. In case of Liver-Yang rising, therefore, it would manifest more often on the right side, but this is by no means an absolute rule. The headache has a characteristic throbbing nature.

The tongue and pulse can have many different appearances depending on the condition underlying the rising of Liver-Yang.

Table 34.2 illustrates the differences between Liver-Yang rising and Liver-Fire.

> **Clinical note**
>
> The characteristics of the pathology of Liver-Yang rising are:
> - Imbalance between Yin and Yang
> - Excessive rising of Liver-Qi
> - Not a Heat pattern

Pathological precursors of pattern

Liver-Yang rising always derives from another condition, which may be Liver-Yin deficiency, Kidney-Yin deficiency, Liver- and Kidney-Yin deficiency or Liver-Blood deficiency. When arising from a Kidney deficiency, usually Liver-Yang rising is a result of Kidney/Liver-Yin deficiency, but in practice, it can also arise from Kidney-Yang deficiency. This is because Kidney-Yin and Kidney-Yang have the same root, and a deficiency of one always implies a deficiency of the other (albeit to a lesser degree). Therefore, when Kidney-Yang is deficient, Kidney-Yin will also be deficient to a certain extent and may give rise to symptoms of rising of Liver-Yang (Fig. 34.22).

Pathological developments from pattern

Liver-Yang rising may, in time, develop into Liver-Fire, especially if the patient has a diet consisting in excessive consumption of hot-energy foods.

Liver-Yang rising may also in time cause the development of Liver-Wind, especially in the elderly (see Fig. 34.22).

Treatment

Principle of treatment: subdue Liver-Yang, nourish Yin or Blood.

Acupuncture

Points: LIV-3 Taichong, T.B.-5 Waiguan, P-6 Neiguan, L.I.-4 Hegu, G.B.-43 Xiaxi, G.B.-38 Yangfu, G.B.-20 Fengchi, BL-2 Zanzhu, Taiyang extra point, G.B.-9 Tianchong, G.B.-8 Shuaigu, G.B.-6 Xuanli. In case of Liver-Blood or Liver-Yin deficiency: SP-6 Sanyinjiao, LIV-8 Ququan, ST-36 Zusanli, KI-3 Taixi, KI-6 Zhaohai.

Table 34.2 Comparison between Liver-Yang rising and Liver-Fire

	Liver-Yang rising	Liver-Fire	Common characteristic
Aetiology	Emotional stress	Emotional stress and diet	Excessive ascending of Liver-Qi
Pathology	Imbalance between Yin and Yang, excessive ascending of Liver-Qi, no real Heat	Full-Heat	
Eight Principles	–	Full-Heat	
Symptoms	Headaches	Headaches and eye problems	
Treatment principle	Subdue Liver-Yang	Drain Fire	
Herbal treatment method	Sweet herbs to correct flow of Liver-Qi, sinking herbs to subdue Yang	Bitter-cold herbs to drain Fire	

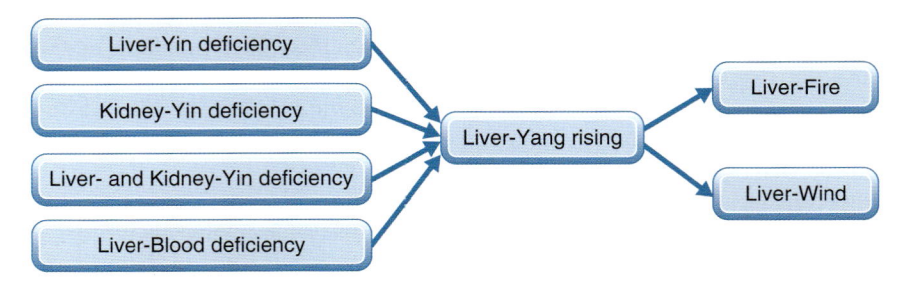

Figure 34.22 Liver-Yang rising pattern: precursors and developments

Method: reducing method on points to subdue Liver-Yang and tonifying method on points to nourish Yin or Blood.

Explanation
- LIV-3 subdues Liver-Yang. This is the main distal point to use.
- T.B.-5 subdues Liver-Yang and is particularly indicated for headaches along the Gall Bladder channel.
- P-6 helps to subdue Liver-Yang and calms the Mind.
- L.I.-4 regulates the ascending and descending of Qi and therefore helps to subdue Liver-Yang.
- G.B.-43 is the main distal point for headaches around the eye or temple.
- G.B.-38 is a distal point to subdue Liver-Yang and is often used for chronic and stubborn migraine headaches.
- G.B.-20 is an important adjacent point to subdue Liver-Yang.
- BL-2, Taiyang, G.B.-9, G.B.-8 and G.B.-6 are all important local points for headaches from Liver-Yang rising, chosen according to the location of the headache.
- SP-6, LIV-8 and ST-36 nourish Liver-Blood and Liver-Yin.
- KI-3 and KI-6 are used if there is a Kidney-Yin deficiency.

Herbal formula

Tian Ma Gou Teng Yin *Gastrodia–Uncaria Decoction*.
Ling Jiao Gou Teng Tang *Cornu Antelopis–Uncaria Decoction*.

Box 34.17 summarizes Liver-Yang rising.

Box 34.17 Liver-Yang rising

Clinical manifestations

Headache, which may be on the temples, eyes or lateral side of the head, dizziness, tinnitus, deafness, blurred vision, dry mouth and throat, insomnia, irritability, feeling worked-up, propensity to outbursts of anger, stiff neck, tongue Pale if there is Liver-Blood deficiency or without coating if there is Yin deficiency, pulse Wiry.

Treatment

LIV-3 Taichong, T.B.-5 Waiguan, P-6 Neiguan, L.I.-4 Hegu, G.B.-43 Xiaxi, G.B.-38 Yangfu, G.B.-20 Fengchi, BL-2 Zanzhu, Taiyang extra point, G.B.-9 Tianchong, G.B.-8 Shuaigu, G.B.-6 Xuanli. In case of Liver-Blood or Liver-Yin deficiency: SP-6 Sanyinjiao, LIV-8 Ququan, ST-36 Zusanli, KI-3 Taixi, KI-6 Zhaohai

---

Three Treasures

Bend Bamboo.

Case history 34.6

A woman of 35 had suffered from headaches since the age of 14. The headaches occurred on the right temple and in the eye socket, were of a throbbing character and were accompanied by nausea and blurred vision. Her periods were rather scanty and she felt often tired. She also had dry hair, poor memory and insomnia. Her pulse was Choppy but slightly Wiry on the left, and her tongue was Pale, but with red spots on the sides.

This case illustrates well the rising of Liver-Yang caused by deficiency of Liver-Blood. Her symptoms of Liver-Yang rising are headache, nausea, a Wiry pulse on the left and red spots on the sides of the tongue. Her symptoms of Liver-Blood deficiency are scanty periods, dry hair, poor memory, insomnia, a Choppy pulse and a Pale tongue. The poor memory and insomnia also show that the deficiency of Blood has affected the Heart.

Liver-Wind agitating within

There are four distinct types of Liver-Wind from four different causes. These are:

---

1. Extreme Heat generating Wind
2. Liver-Yang rising generating Wind
    a) Liver-Yang rising deriving from Liver-Yin deficiency
    b) Liver-Yang rising deriving from Liver- and Kidney-Yin deficiency
    c) Liver-Yang rising deriving from Liver-Blood deficiency
3. Liver-Fire generating Wind
4. Liver-Blood deficiency generating Wind

The general clinical manifestations of Liver-Wind are tremor, tic, numbness, dizziness and convulsions or paralysis (Fig. 34.23). Internal Wind signs are characterized by movement or the absence of it, hence the tremor and convulsions or paralysis (as in Wind-stroke). Internal Wind is always related to the Liver as the convulsions and tremors are explained in Chinese medicine as 'shaking' of the sinews, which are controlled by the Liver.

Each of the above four types of Liver-Wind will be discussed separately. I shall not give the pathological precursors or pathological developments of internal Wind as, generally speaking, these have been discussed

- Facial tic
- Dizziness, vertigo, tinnitus, headache
- Numbness of limbs
- Tremor

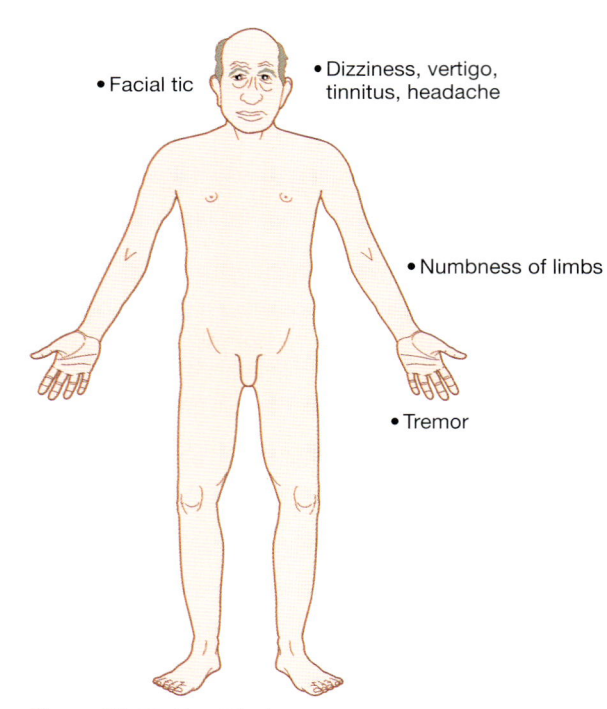

Figure 34.23 Liver-Wind

Box 34.18 Internal Wind

- Tremor
- Tic
- Numbness/tingling
- Dizziness
- Convulsions
- Paralysis

---

under the relevant patterns. Also, for the three subpatterns of Liver-Yang rising generating Wind, I shall not give the aetiology or pathology as this is the same as for the patterns discussed above.

Box 34.18 summarizes internal Wind.

> **Diagnostic tip**
>
> 'If it moves involuntarily, it is Wind'

Extreme Heat generating Wind

Clinical manifestations

High temperature, convulsions, rigidity of the neck, tremor of limbs, opisthotonos, in severe cases coma.
Tongue: Deep-Red, Stiff, dry yellow coating.
Pulse: Wiry-Rapid.

Aetiology

This pattern is due to an invasion of exterior Wind-Heat, then transforming into interior Heat. When Heat reaches the Blood level, it may lead to the development of internal Wind (see ch. 45). This type of Wind is seen in febrile diseases such as meningitis.

Pathology

When Heat reaches the Blood level in febrile diseases, it injures the Yin and the Yin deficiency gives rise to internal Wind.

Treatment

Treatment principle: cool Blood, nourish Yin, extinguish Wind.

Acupuncture

Points: LIV-3 Taichong, Shixuan extra points, Du-20 Baihui, Du-16 Fengfu, G.B.-20 Fengchi, Du-8 Jinsuo, Du-14 Dazhui.
Method: reducing method, bleed the Shixuan points.
Explanation
  – LIV-3 extinguishes Liver-Wind.
  – The Shixuan points (at the tips of each finger) extinguish Wind and cool Blood when they are pricked to cause bleeding.
  – Du-20, Du-16 and G.B.-20 extinguish Wind.
  – Du-8 relieves spasms to stop convulsions.
  – Du-14 is pricked to cool Blood.

Herbal formula

Ling Jiao Gou Teng Tang *Cornu Antelopis–Uncaria Decoction*.
Da Ding Feng Zhu Big *Stopping Wind Pearl* (for febrile disease Heat injuring Yin).

Box 34.19 summarizes extreme Heat generating Wind.

Box 34.19 Extreme Heat generating Wind

Clinical manifestations

High temperature, convulsions, rigidity of the neck, tremor of limbs, opisthotonos, in severe cases coma
Tongue: Deep-Red, Stiff, dry yellow coating
Pulse: Wiry-Rapid

Treatment

LIV-3 Taichong, Shixuan extra points, Du-20 Baihui, Du-16 Fengfu, G.B.-20 Fengchi, Du-8 Jinsuo, Du-14 Dazhui

Liver-Yang rising generating Wind

Liver-Yang rising may generate Wind if it persists for some years. This usually happens only in the elderly. We can distinguish the clinical manifestations according to the cause of Liver-Yang rising, that is:

- Liver-Yang rising deriving from Liver-Yin deficiency
- Liver-Yang rising deriving from Liver- and Kidney-Yin deficiency
- Liver-Yang rising deriving from Liver-Blood deficiency

Liver-Yang rising deriving from Liver-Yin deficiency

Clinical manifestations

Tremor, facial tic, severe dizziness, tinnitus, headache, hypertension, dry throat, dry eyes, blurred vision, numbness or tingling of limbs, poor memory.
Tongue: normal-coloured without coating.
Pulse: Wiry-Fine.

Treatment

Principle of treatment: subdue Liver-Yang, extinguish Wind, nourish Liver-Yin.

Acupuncture

Points: LIV-3 Taichong, G.B.-20 Fengchi, L.I.-4 Hegu, T.B.-5 Waiguan, Du-19 Houding, SP-6 Sanyinjiao, LIV-8 Ququan, KI-3 Taixi.
Method: reducing on the points that extinguish Wind and reinforcing on the points that nourish Liver-Yin.
Explanation
 – LIV-3 subdues Liver-Yang and extinguishes Wind.
 – G.B.-20 extinguishes Wind and subdues Yang.
 – L.I.-4 helps to subdue Yang.
 – T.B.-5 subdues Liver-Yang.
 – Du-19 extinguishes Wind.
 – SP-6, LIV-8 and KI-3 nourish Liver-Yin.

Box 34.20 summarizes Liver-Yang rising resulting from Liver-Ying deficiency.

Herbal formula

San Jia Fu Mai Tang *Three Carapaces Restoring the Pulse Decoction*.

Box 34.20 Liver-Yang rising deriving from Liver-Yin deficiency

Clinical manifestations

Tremor, facial tic, severe dizziness, tinnitus, headache, hypertension, dry throat, dry eyes, blurred vision, numbness or tingling of limbs, poor memory
Tongue: normal-coloured without coating
Pulse: Wiry-Fine

Treatment

LIV-3 Taichong, G.B.-20 Fengchi, L.I.-4 Hegu, T.B.-5 Waiguan, Du-19 Houding, SP-6 Sanyinjiao, LIV-8 Ququan, KI-3 Taixi

---

Liver-Yang rising deriving from Liver- and Kidney-Yin deficiency

Clinical manifestations

Tremor, facial tic, severe dizziness, tinnitus, headache, dry throat, dry eyes, blurred vision, numbness or tingling of limbs, poor memory, backache, scanty urination, night sweating, possibly hypertension.
Tongue: normal-coloured without coating.
Pulse: Wiry-Fine.

Treatment

Principle of treatment: subdue Liver-Yang, extinguish Wind, nourish Liver- and Kidney-Yin.

Acupuncture

Points: LIV-3 Taichong, G.B.-20 Fengchi, L.I.-4 Hegu, T.B.-5 Waiguan, Du-19 Houding, SP-6 Sanyinjiao, LIV-8 Ququan, KI-3 Taixi, KI-6 Zhaohai, Ren-4 Guanyuan.
Method: reducing on points that extinguish Wind and subdue Yang and reinforcing on points that nourish Liver- and Kidney-Yin.
Explanation
 – The first eight points have been explained under the previous pattern.
 – KI-6 and Ren-4 nourish Kidney-Yin.

Herbal formula

Zhen Gan Xi Feng Tang *Pacifying the Liver and Subduing Wind Decoction*.
Jian Ling Tang *Constructing Roof Tiles Decoction*.

Box 34.21 summarizes Liver-Yang rising deriving from Liver- and Kidney-Yin deficiency.

> **Box 34.21 Liver-Yang rising deriving from Liver- and Kidney-Yin deficiency**
>
> **Clinical manifestations**
>
> Tremor, facial tic, severe dizziness, tinnitus, headache, dry throat, dry eyes, blurred vision, numbness or tingling of limbs, poor memory, backache, scanty urination, night sweating, possibly hypertension
> *Tongue*: normal-coloured without coating
> *Pulse*: Wiry-Fine
>
> **Treatment**
>
> LIV-3 Taichong, G.B.-20 Fengchi, L.I.-4 Hegu, T.B.-5 Waiguan, Du-19 Houding, SP-6 Sanyinjiao, LIV-8 Ququan, KI-3 Taixi, KI-6 Zhaohai, Ren-4 Guanyuan

> **Box 34.22 Liver-Yang rising deriving from Liver-Blood deficiency**
>
> **Clinical manifestations**
>
> Tremor, dizziness, tinnitus, headache, hypertension, dry throat, blurred vision, numbness or tingling of limbs, poor memory, insomnia
> *Tongue*: Pale and Thin
> *Pulse*: Wiry-Fine
>
> **Treatment**
>
> LIV-3 Taichong, G.B.-20 Fengchi, L.I.-4 Hegu, T.B.-5 Waiguan, Du-19 Houding, SP-6 Sanyinjiao, LIV-8 Ququan, KI-3 Taixi, BL-17 Geshu, Ren-4 Guanyuan

Liver-Yang rising deriving from Liver-Blood deficiency

Clinical manifestations

Tremor, dizziness, tinnitus, headache, hypertension, dry throat, blurred vision, numbness or tingling of limbs, poor memory, insomnia.
Tongue: Pale and Thin.
Pulse: Wiry-Fine.

Treatment

Principle of treatment: subdue Liver-Yang, extinguish Wind, nourish Liver-Blood.

Acupuncture

Points: LIV-3 Taichong, G.B.-20 Fengchi, L.I.-4 Hegu, T.B.-5 Waiguan, Du-19 Houding, SP-6 Sanyinjiao, LIV-8 Ququan, KI-3 Taixi, BL-17 Geshu, Ren-4 Guanyuan.
Method: reducing on points that subdue Yang and extinguish Wind, reinforcing on points that nourish Liver-Blood.
Explanation
 – The first eight points have been explained under the previous pattern.
 – BL-17 nourishes Blood.
 – Ren-4 nourishes Blood.

Herbal formula

E Jiao Ji Zi Huang Tang *Gelatinum Corii Asini–Egg Yolk Decoction*.

Three Treasures

Bend Bamboo combined with **Nourish the Root**.

Box 34.22 summarizes Liver-Yang rising deriving from Liver-Blood deficiency.

Liver-Fire generating Wind

Clinical manifestations

Tremor, irritability, propensity to outbursts of anger, tinnitus and/or deafness (with sudden onset), temporal headache, dizziness, red face and eyes, thirst, bitter taste, dream-disturbed sleep, constipation with dry stools, dark-yellow urine, epistaxis, haematemesis, haemoptysis.
Tongue: Red with redder sides and dry yellow coating.
Pulse: Wiry-Rapid.

Aetiology

The aetiology of this pattern is the same as that for the pattern of Liver-Fire discussed above.

Pathology

Liver-Fire may generate Wind when it persists for some years: this is more likely to occur in the elderly. This phenomenon can be compared to a forest fire that fans winds. This is a Full-Heat pattern.

Treatment

Principle of treatment: clear the Liver, drain Fire, extinguish Wind.

Acupuncture

Points: LIV-2 Xingjian, LIV-3 Taichong, G.B.-20 Fengchi, L.I.-11 Quchi, G.B.-1 Tongziliao, SP-6 Sanyinjiao, LIV-1 Dadun, Du-8 Jinsuo.
Method: reducing method, no moxa.
Explanation
 – LIV-2 drains Liver-Fire.
 – LIV-3 extinguishes Liver-Wind.
 – G.B.-20 extinguishes Wind.

> **Box 34.23 Liver-Fire generating Wind**
>
> **Clinical manifestations**
>
> Tremor, irritability, propensity to outbursts of anger, tinnitus and/or deafness (with sudden onset), temporal headache, dizziness, red face and eyes, thirst, bitter taste, dream-disturbed sleep, constipation with dry stools, dark-yellow urine, epistaxis, haematemesis, haemoptysis
> *Tongue*: Red with redder sides and dry yellow coating
> *Pulse*: Wiry-Rapid
>
> **Treatment**
>
> LIV-2 Xingjian, LIV-3 Taichong, G.B.-20 Fengchi, L.I.-11 Quchi, G.B.-1 Tongziliao, SP-6 Sanyinjiao, LIV-1 Dadun, Du-8 Jinsuo

- L.I.-11 drains Fire.
- G.B.-1 extinguishes Liver-Wind.
- SP-6 is used to nourish Yin to help to drain Fire.
- LIV-1 extinguishes Liver-Wind.
- Du-8 relieves spasms and tremors.

Box 34.23 summarizes Liver-Fire generating Wind.

Herbal formula

Ling Jiao Gou Teng Tang *Cornu Antelopis–Uncaria Decoction* plus Long Dan Cao *Radix Gentianae scabrae*.

Liver-Blood deficiency generating Wind

Clinical manifestations

Fine tremor, facial tic, dizziness, blurred vision, numbness or tingling of limbs, poor memory, insomnia, scanty periods.
Tongue: Pale and Thin.
Pulse: Wiry-Fine.

Aetiology

The aetiology of this pattern is the same as that for Liver-Blood deficiency.

Pathology

Liver-Blood deficiency may lead to the development of internal Wind as the place normally occupied by Blood in the vessels is 'taken up' by Wind. Whereas the previous pattern of Wind (Liver-Fire generating Wind) can be compared to the wind generated by a forest fire, in this pattern, the Wind can be compared to the strong draughts generated by the empty spaces in underground (subway) stations.

With Wind deriving from Liver-Blood deficiency, the tremors are less marked than in Full Wind.

> **Box 34.24 Liver-Blood deficiency generating Wind**
>
> **Clinical manifestations**
>
> Fine tremor, facial tic, dizziness, blurred vision, numbness or tingling of limbs, poor memory, insomnia, scanty periods
> *Tongue*: Pale and Thin
> *Pulse*: Wiry-Fine
>
> **Treatment**
>
> LIV-3 Taichong, G.B.-20 Fengchi, L.I.-4 Hegu, T.B.-5 Waiguan, Du-19 Houding, SP-6 Sanyinjiao, LIV-8 Ququan, KI-3 Taixi, BL-17 Geshu, Ren-4 Guanyuan

Treatment

Principle of treatment: nourish Liver-Blood, extinguish Wind.

Acupuncture

Points: LIV-3 Taichong, G.B.-20 Fengchi, L.I.-4 Hegu, T.B.-5 Waiguan, Du-19 Houding, SP-6 Sanyinjiao, LIV-8 Ququan, KI-3 Taixi, BL-17 Geshu, Ren-4 Guanyuan.
Method: reducing on points that extinguish Wind, reinforcing on points that nourish Liver-Blood. Moxa on BL-17 is applicable.
Explanation
- LIV-3 and G.B.-20 extinguish Wind.
- L.I.-4 helps to subdue Yang and therefore extinguish Wind.
- T.B.-5 and Du-19 extinguish Liver-Wind.
- SP-6, LIV-8 and KI-3 nourish Liver-Blood.
- Ren-4 and BL-17 nourish Blood.

Herbal formula

E Jiao Ji Zi Huang Tang *Gelatinum Corii Asini–Egg Yolk Decoction*.

Box 34.24 summarizes Liver-Blood deficiency generating Wind.

COMBINED PATTERNS

The Liver combined patterns are:

- Rebellious Liver-Qi invading the Spleen
- Rebellious Liver-Qi invading the Stomach
- Liver-Fire insulting the Lungs
- Heart- and Liver-Blood deficiency

Rebellious Liver-Qi invading the Spleen

Clinical manifestations

Irritability, abdominal distension and pain, alternation of constipation and diarrhoea, stools sometimes dry and bitty (small pieces) and sometimes loose, flatulence, tiredness (Fig. 34.24).
Tongue: normal-coloured or slightly Red on the sides.
Pulse: Wiry on the left and Weak on the right.
Key symptoms: alternation of constipation and diarrhoea, abdominal distension and pain, Wiry pulse.

> **Diagnostic tip**
>
> Alternation of constipation and loose stools and a Wiry pulse would be enough to diagnose rebellious Liver-Qi invading the Spleen

Aetiology

Emotional stress

This pattern is usually caused by emotional problems which affect the Liver, such as anger, frustration and resentment. These emotions, over a long period of time, cause Liver-Qi to stagnate and this interferes with the Spleen functions, preventing Spleen-Qi from rising.

Diet

Irregular eating and especially eating in a hurry, when worried, when angry or while working can cause Liver-Qi to rebel towards the Spleen and the Spleen's function of transportation and transformation to be impaired.

Pathology

The Liver is responsible for the smooth flow of Qi throughout the body. When Liver-Qi becomes rebellious (i.e. its horizontal movement towards the Spleen is accentuated), it often disturbs the Spleen function of transformation and transportation and it prevents Spleen-Qi from rising: in Chinese medicine terms, it is said that the 'Liver invades the Spleen', or that 'Liver and Spleen are not harmonized'.

In Five-Element terms, it corresponds to Wood over-acting on Earth. In Eight-Principle terms, it is a pattern of mixed Deficiency and Excess: Excess of the Liver (rebellious Liver-Qi) and Deficiency of Spleen-Qi.

- Irritability
- Alternation of constipation and loose stools, flatulence
- Abdominal distension and pain

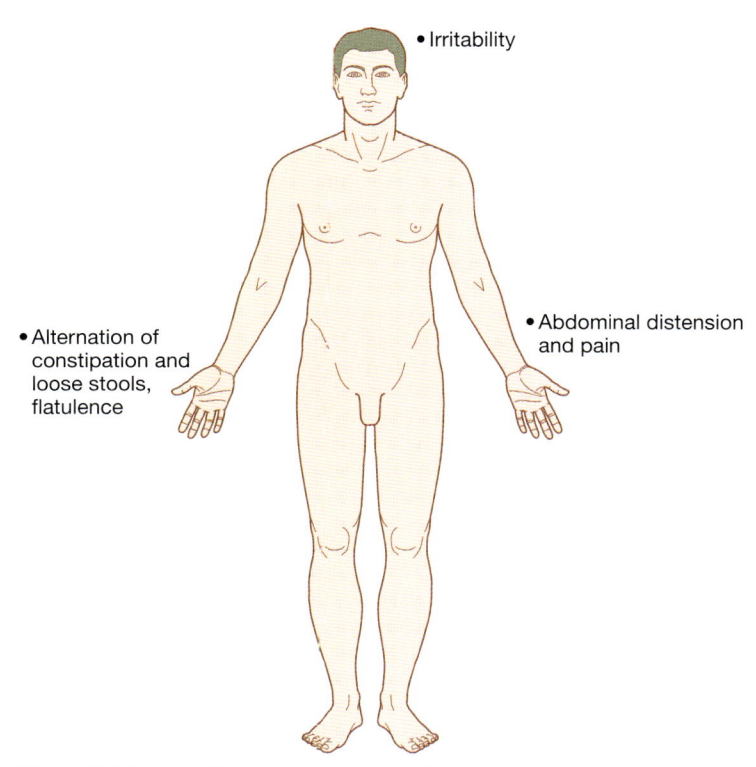

Figure 34.24 Rebellious Liver-Qi invading the Spleen

When the rebellious Liver-Qi predominates, there is constipation with dry, difficult and bitty stools. When the deficiency of the Spleen predominates, there are loose stools. The distension and pain of the abdomen are caused by the stagnation of Liver-Qi in the abdomen. Distension is the most characteristic symptom of rebellious Liver-Qi. There may be some pain too (typically 'distending pain'), but not severe.

This pattern can present itself with two different situations characterized by a different emphasis. In one situation the Liver is primarily in Excess and rebellious and it actively 'invades' the Spleen, interfering with its transformation and transportation function. This pattern is therefore primarily an Excess pattern: there is constipation more frequently than diarrhoea and the abdominal distension and pain are quite marked.

In another situation the Spleen is primarily deficient and 'allows' itself to be invaded by the Liver. This pattern is primarily a Deficiency pattern: there are loose stools more often than constipation and the abdominal pain is only slight.

> **Clinical note**
>
> When rebellious Liver-Qi invades the Spleen there are two distinct situations:
> 1. The Liver is overactive and it invades the Spleen
> 2. The Spleen is weak and 'allows' itself to be invaded by the Liver (even when the Liver is not overactive)

This explains why the tongue could either be Red on the sides or normal coloured. In the first case, when the Liver actively invades the Spleen, it would be Red on the sides. In the latter case, when the Spleen is weak and allows itself to be invaded by the Liver, the tongue would be normal-coloured.

> **Clinical note**
>
> Rebellious Liver-Qi invading the Spleen is frequently seen in irritable bowel syndrome

Pathological precursors of pattern

Rebellious Liver-Qi can develop from stagnation of Liver-Qi (Fig. 34.25).

Pathological developments from pattern

When it persists for a long time rebellious Liver-Qi can weaken the Spleen, causing Spleen-Qi deficiency and, in some cases, even Spleen-Yin deficiency.

The combination of rebellious Liver-Qi with subsequent loss of free flow of Qi and Spleen-Qi deficiency may lead to an impairment of the transportation and transformation of fluids and the formation of Dampness. The combination of these three factors, rebellious Liver-Qi, Spleen deficiency and Dampness are very common in irritable bowel syndrome (see Fig. 34.25).

Treatment

Principle of treatment: subdue rebellious Qi, tonify the Spleen.

Acupuncture

Points: LIV-13 Zhangmen, LIV-14 Qimen, LIV-3 Taichong, G.B.-34 Yanglingquan, Ren-6 Qihai, T.B.-6 Zhigou, P-6 Neiguan, ST-25 Tianshu, SP-15 Daheng, Ren-12 Zhongwan, ST-36 Zusanli, SP-6 Sanyinjiao, SP-4 Gongsun and P-6 Neiguan in combination (*Chong Mai*).

Method: reducing for points to harmonize the Liver, reinforcing for points to tonify the Spleen.

Explanation
- LIV-13 harmonizes Liver and Spleen.
- LIV-14 harmonizes the Liver and promotes the smooth flow of Liver-Qi.
- LIV-3 promotes the smooth flow of Liver-Qi and calms abdominal pain.
- G.B.-34 promotes the smooth flow of Liver-Qi and, in combination with Qihai Ren-6, calms abdominal pain.
- Ren-6 stops abdominal pain and, in combination with Yanglingquan G.B.-34, moves Qi in the abdomen.

Liver-Qi stagnation → Rebellious Liver-Qi invading the Spleen → Spleen-Qi deficiency

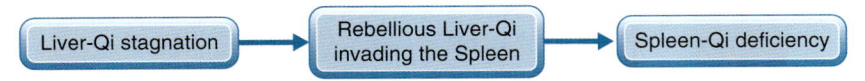

Figure 34.25 Rebellious Liver-Qi invading the Spleen pattern: precursors and developments

> **Box 34.25 Rebellious Liver-Qi invading the Spleen**
>
> **Clinical manifestations**
>
> Irritability, abdominal distension and pain, alternation of constipation and diarrhoea, stools sometimes dry and bitty (small pieces) and sometimes loose, flatulence, tiredness
> *Tongue*: normal coloured or slightly Red on the sides
> *Pulse*: Wiry on the left and Weak on the right
>
> **Treatment**
>
> LIV-13 Zhangmen, LIV-14 Qimen, LIV-3 Taichong, G.B.-34 Yanglingquan, Ren-6 Qihai, T.B.-6 Zhigou, P-6 Neiguan, ST-25 Tianshu, SP-15 Daheng, Ren-12 Zhongwan, ST-36 Zusanli, SP-6 Sanyinjiao, SP-4 Gongsun and P-6 Neiguan in combination

- T.B.-6 and P-6 move Liver-Qi and calm the Mind.
- ST-25 and SP-15 harmonize the Liver and Spleen and treat both constipation and loose stools.
- Ren-12, ST-36 and SP-6 tonify the Spleen. SP-6 also harmonizes Liver and Spleen and stops abdominal pain.
- SP-4 and P-6 in combination open the Penetrating Vessel (*Chong Mai*) and harmonize the Liver and Spleen, particularly in digestive diseases.

Box 34.25 summarizes rebellious Liver-Qi invading the Spleen.

Herbal formula

Xiao Yao San *Free and Easy Wanderer Powder*.

Women's Treasure

Freeing the Moon (Variation of Xiao Yao San).

Rebellious Liver-Qi invading the Stomach

Clinical manifestations

Irritability, epigastric and hypochondrial distension and pain, a feeling of oppression in the epigastrium, sour regurgitation, hiccups, belching, nausea, vomiting, sighing, weak limbs (Fig. 34.26).
Tongue: normal-coloured or slightly Red on the sides.
Pulse: Wiry on the left and Weak on the right or Wiry on both Middle positions.

- Irritability
- Sour regurgitation, hiccups, belching, nausea, vomiting, sighing
- Hypochondrial/epigastric distension and pain

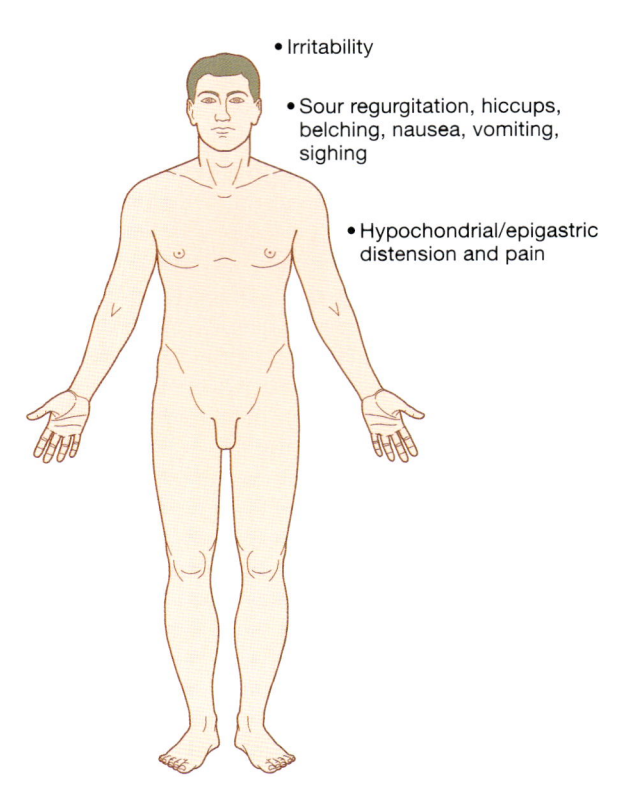

Figure 34.26 Rebellious Liver-Qi invading the Stomach

Aetiology

This is also caused by emotional problems combined with irregular diet and overwork in the same way as for the previous pattern.

Pathology

This pattern is characterized by rebellious Liver-Qi invading the Stomach and interfering with the descending of Stomach-Qi: this results in the ascending of Stomach-Qi, hence the belching, nausea and vomiting.

The rebellious Liver-Qi in the Middle Burner also interferes with the Stomach rotting and ripening of food, resulting in distension in the epigastrium and sour regurgitation.

The rebellious Liver-Qi causes distension, pain and irritability. The same things that were said about Liver invading the Spleen apply to this pattern with regard to the two possible situations in the tongue manifestation. For this reason, the tongue could be Red on the sides if it is Liver-Qi that primarily invades the Stomach,

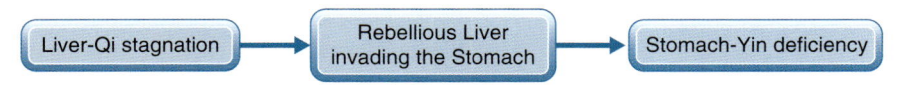

Figure 34.27 Rebellious Liver-Qi invading the Stomach pattern: precursors and developments

or normal-coloured if the Stomach is primarily weak and allows itself to be invaded by the Liver.

Pathological precursors of pattern

Rebellious Liver-Qi may develop from stagnation of Liver-Qi (Fig. 34.27).

Pathological developments from pattern

Rebellious Liver-Qi may weaken the Stomach if it persists for a long time to the point of injuring Stomach-Yin (see Fig. 34.27).

Treatment

Principle of treatment: subdue rebellious Liver-Qi and tonify the Stomach.

Acupuncture

Points: LIV-14 Qimen, G.B.-34 Yanglingquan, Ren-13 Shangwan, Ren-10 Xiawan, ST-21 Liangmen, ST-19 Burong, ST-36 Zusanli, ST-34 Liangqiu, BL-21 Weishu.
Method: reducing for points to harmonize the Liver and reinforcing for points to tonify the Stomach.
Explanation
 - LIV-14 harmonizes the Liver in the Middle Burner. In particular, LIV-14 harmonizes Liver and Stomach.
 - G.B.-34 harmonizes the Liver, stimulates the smooth flow of Liver-Qi, particularly in the hypochondrium.
 - Ren-13 subdues rebellious ascending Stomach-Qi.
 - Ren-10 stimulates the descending of Stomach-Qi.
 - ST-21 and ST-19 make Stomach-Qi descend.
 - ST-36 tonifies the Stomach.
 - ST-34 stops epigastric pain.
 - BL-21 tonifies the Stomach and is particularly important in chronic cases.

Herbal formula

Si Mo Tang *Four Milled-Herb Decoction*.
Xuan Fu Dai Zhe Tang *Inula–Haematite Decoction*.

> **Box 34.26 Rebellious Liver-Qi invading the Stomach**
>
> **Clinical manifestations**
>
> Irritability, epigastric and hypochondrial distension and pain, a feeling of oppression in the epigastrium, sour regurgitation, hiccups, belching, nausea, vomiting, sighing, weak limbs
> *Tongue*: normal-coloured or slightly Red on the sides
> *Pulse*: Wiry on the left and Weak on the right or Wiry on both Middle positions
>
> **Treatment**
>
> LIV-14 Qimen, G.B.-34 Yanglingquan, Ren-13 Shangwan, Ren-10 Xiawan, ST-21 Liangmen, ST-19 Burong, ST-36 Zusanli, ST-34 Liangqiu, BL-21 Weishu

Ju Pi Zhu Ru Tang *Citrus–Bambusa Decoction*.
Ding Xiang Shi Di Tang *Caryophyllum–Diospyros Decoction*.
Ban Xia Hou Po Tang *Pinellia–Magnolia Decoction* plus Zuo Jin Wan *Left Metal Pill*.

Box 34.26 summarizes rebellious Liver-Qi invading the Stomach.

Liver-Fire insulting the Lungs

Clinical manifestations

Breathlessness, asthma, a feeling of fullness and distension of the chest and hypochondrium, cough with a yellow or blood-tinged sputum, headache, dizziness, red face, thirst, bitter taste, bloodshot eyes, scanty dark urine, constipation (Fig. 34.28).
Tongue: Red with redder sides and dry yellow coating.
Pulse: Wiry.
Key symptoms: breathlessness, asthma, fullness of hypochondrium, headache, Wiry pulse.

Aetiology

This pattern is caused by anger, which causes the formation of Liver-Fire, usually after a prolonged time of Liver-Qi stagnation.

It is also compounded by the excessive consumption of hot and greasy foods, which tend to create Heat.

Pathology

The Liver controls the smooth flow of Qi: this has an influence on the descending of Lung-Qi. If Liver-Qi stagnates over a long period of time, it turns into Liver-Fire. Fire tends to rise and therefore Liver-Qi rebels upwards towards the chest. Here it prevents Lung-Qi from descending, resulting in breathlessness and asthma.

The stagnation of Liver-Qi causes a feeling of distension of the chest and hypochondrium.

The rising of Liver-Fire causes headache, dizziness, red face, bloodshot eyes, thirst and bitter taste. Fire in the body condenses the fluids and causes scanty dark urine and constipation; if Fire enters the Blood, it heats the Blood and this causes bleeding and therefore blood-tinged sputum.

From the Five-Element point of view, this pattern is described as Wood insulting Metal.

The red colour of the sides of the tongue reflects the presence of Liver-Fire.

Pathological precursors of pattern

Generally, Liver-Fire may develop (but not necessarily) from long-term Liver-Qi stagnation. Liver-Yang rising may also turn into Liver-Fire (Fig. 34.29).

Pathological developments from pattern

This pattern may give rise to various pathological consequences because of its relatively complex pathology. Firstly, Liver-Fire may dry up Body Fluids and lead to Yin deficiency. By condensing Body Fluids, Fire may also lead to the formation of Phlegm; this process would be facilitated by the disruption of the Qi Mechanism with the impairment of the descending of Lung-Qi and the excessive ascending of Liver-Qi.

Given the Five-Element Mother–Child relationship between Wood and Fire, the Liver affects the Heart and therefore Liver-Fire often gives rise to Heart-Fire (see Fig. 34.29).

Treatment

Principle of treatment: clear the Liver, drain Fire, subdue Liver-Qi, stimulate the descending of Lung-Qi.

Acupuncture

Points: LIV-2 Xingjian, LIV-3 Taichong, LIV-14 Qimen, Ren-17 Shanzhong, Ren-22 Tiantu, P-6 Neiguan, LU-7 Lieque, LI-11 Quchi.
Method: reducing.
Explanation
  – LIV-2 clears Liver-Fire.
  – LIV-3 subdues Liver-Qi.
  – LIV-14 harmonizes Liver-Qi in the chest.

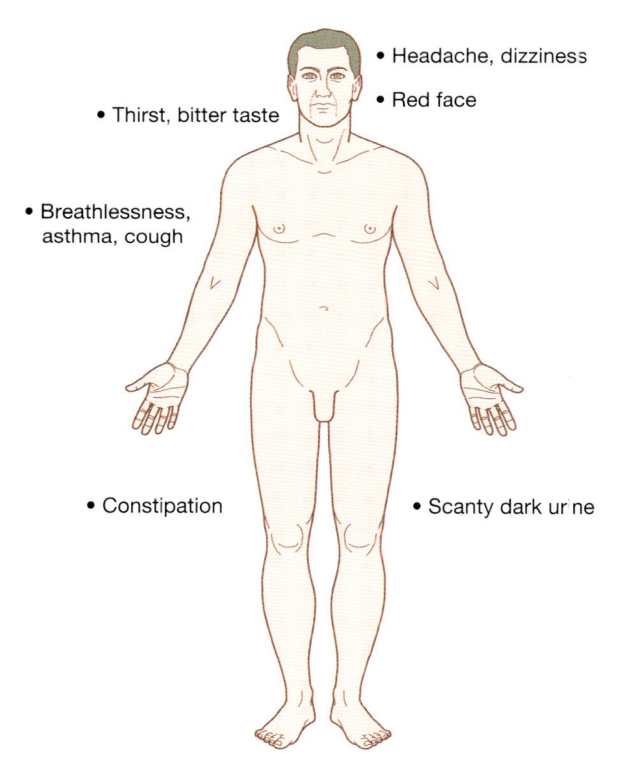

Figure 34.28 Liver-Fire insulting the Lungs

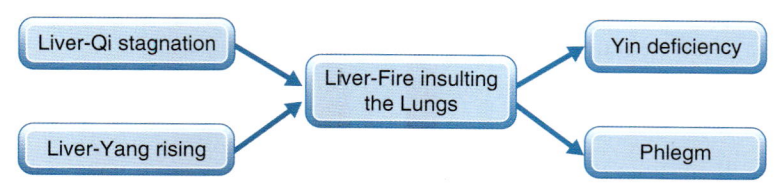

Figure 34.29 Liver-Fire insulting the Lungs pattern: precursors and developments

> **Box 34.27 Liver-Fire insulting the Lungs**
>
> **Clinical manifestations**
>
> Breathlessness, asthma, a feeling of fullness and distension of the chest and hypochondrium, cough with a yellow or blood-tinged sputum, headache, dizziness, red face, thirst, bitter taste, bloodshot eyes, scanty dark urine, constipation
> *Tongue*: Red with redder sides and dry yellow coating
> *Pulse*: Wiry
>
> **Treatment**
>
> LIV-2 Xingjian, LIV-3 Taichong, LIV-14 Qimen, Ren-17 Shanzhong, Ren-22 Tiantu, P-6 Neiguan, LU-7 Lieque, LI-11 Quchi

- Ren-17 and Ren-22 stimulate the descending of Lung-Qi.
- P-6 harmonizes Liver-Qi in the chest (by virtue of the relation between Liver and Pericardium within the Terminal Yin) and stimulates the descending of Lung-Qi.
- LU-7 stimulates the descending of Lung-Qi.
- LI-11 clears Heat.

Box 34.27 summarizes Liver-Fire insulting the Lungs.

Herbal formula

Long Dan Xie Gan Tang *Gentiana Draining the Liver Decoction*.

Liver- and Heart-Blood deficiency

Clinical manifestations

Palpitations, dizziness, insomnia, dream-disturbed sleep, poor memory, anxiety, propensity to be startled, dull-pale complexion, pale lips, blurred vision, floaters in eyes, diminished night vision, tingling or numbness of limbs, scanty periods or amenorrhoea, cramps, muscular weakness, dry hair and skin, depression, a feeling of aimlessness, withered and brittle nails (Fig. 34.30).
Tongue: Pale, Thin, slightly dry.
Pulse: Choppy or Fine.
Key symptoms: palpitations, dizziness, blurred vision, insomnia, poor memory, Pale tongue.

> **Diagnostic tip**
>
> Blurred vision, palpitations, a Pale tongue and a Choppy pulse are enough to diagnose Liver- and Heart-Blood deficiency

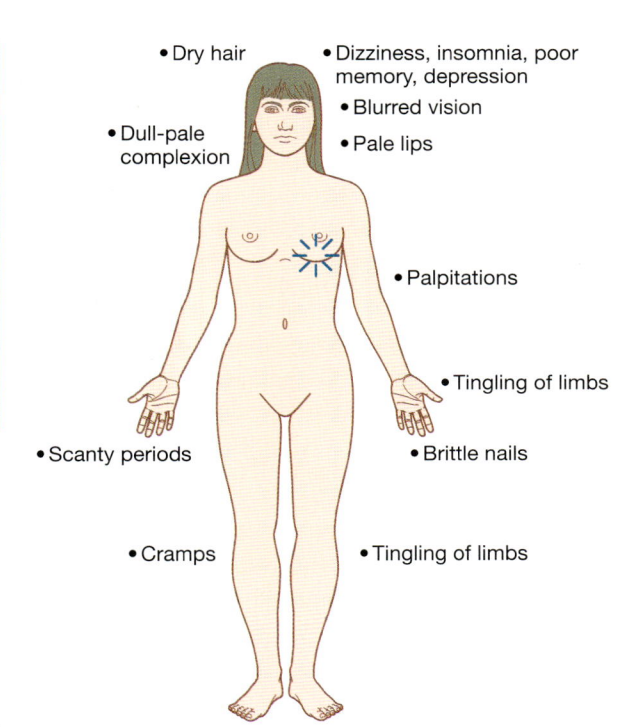

Figure 34.30 Liver- and Heart-Blood deficiency

Aetiology

Emotional stress

Anxiety, worry, sadness and grief affect the Heart and may cause Heart-Blood deficiency. Both worry and sadness can affect the Liver too, causing Liver-Blood deficiency.

Diet

A diet poor in nourishment and Blood-nourishing foods may lead to Liver-Blood deficiency.

Excessive physical work

Excessive physical work may injure the sinews and therefore Liver-Blood. Excessive jogging may injure Heart-Blood.

Blood loss

A severe blood loss such as that which may occur in childbirth may deplete Liver-Blood and this, in turn, may lead to Heart-Blood deficiency.

Pathology

The pathology of the individual patterns of Heart-Blood and Liver-Blood deficiency is discussed under the relevant patterns (ch. 32 for the Heart patterns).

The combination of Heart- and Liver-Blood deficiency is very common, especially in women. Indeed, the Heart and Liver are the two main organs to suffer from Blood deficiency as the Heart governs and the Liver stores Blood.

Heart-Blood and Liver-Blood interact with each other and, for some of the clinical manifestations, there is an overlap so that they may be attributed to either organ's pathology. For example, insomnia may be attributed to Heart-Blood or Liver-Blood deficiency as both the Mind (*Shen*) and the Ethereal Soul (*Hun*) play a role in sleep. The Mind is anchored in Heart-Blood and the Ethereal Soul in Liver-Blood: when either is deficient, the Mind or the Ethereal Soul 'wander' at night, causing insomnia. The insomnia due to Liver-Blood is characterized by more dreaming.

Dizziness is another symptom for which there is an overlap as it may be caused by either Heart-Blood or Liver-Blood deficiency (Fig. 34.31).

The two key symptoms of Heart-Blood and Liver-Blood deficiency, respectively, are palpitations and blurred vision.

Diagnostic tip

Even just blurred vision and palpitations might be enough to diagnose Liver- and Heart-Blood deficiency

Generally speaking, this combination of patterns is more likely to start with Liver-Blood rather than Heart-Blood deficiency. As women are more prone to Liver-Blood deficiency than men are, this combination of patterns is more common in women, where scanty menstruation is a symptom of Liver-Blood deficiency.

The combination of Heart-Blood and Liver-Blood deficiency is frequently seen in postnatal depression. If the woman suffers a severe blood loss at childbirth (or 'severe' relatively to her pre-existing levels of Liver-Blood), this may induce Liver-Blood deficiency; as the Liver is the Mother of the Heart, this may induce a deficiency of Heart-Blood. Deficient Heart-Blood may fail to house the Mind and the woman becomes depressed and suffers from insomnia.

Clinical note

Liver- and Heart-Blood deficiency is particularly common in women, causing scanty periods and postnatal depression

Pathological precursors of pattern

A Kidney deficiency may sometimes be the precursor of this combination of patterns, especially in women, and especially in gynaecological conditions. The Kidneys are the Mother of the Liver and the Kidney-Essence nourishes Liver-Blood. Moreover, although the Liver stores Blood (and therefore menstrual blood as well), it is the Kidneys that are the origin of menstrual blood (*Tian Gui*) as described in chapter 3.

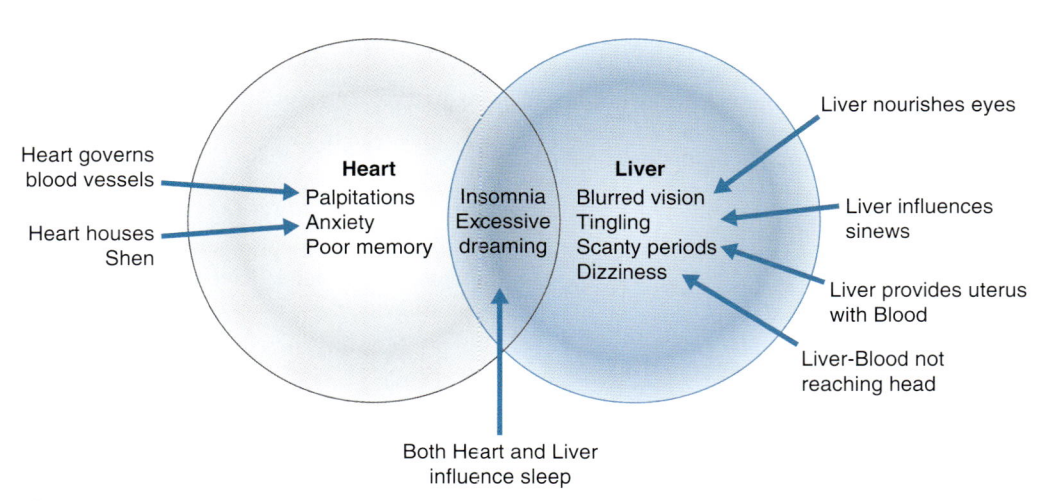

Figure 34.31 Pathology of Liver- and Heart-Blood deficiency

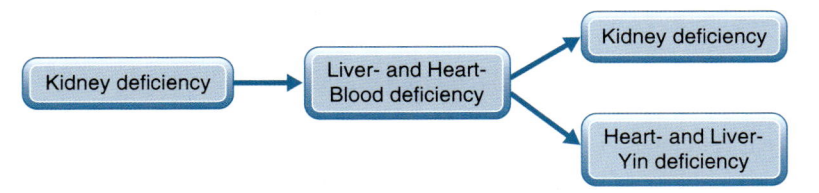

Figure 34.32 Liver- and Heart-Blood deficiency pattern: precursors and developments

---

Box 34.28 Consequences of Liver- and Heart-Blood deficiency

1. May lead to a Kidney deficiency
2. Leads to dryness
3. May lead to Yin deficiency of Liver and Heart

Box 34.29 Liver- and Heart-Blood deficiency

Clinical manifestations

Palpitations, dizziness, insomnia, dream-disturbed sleep, poor memory, anxiety, propensity to be startled, dull-pale complexion, pale lips, blurred vision, floaters in eyes, diminished night-vision, tingling or numbness of limbs, scanty periods or amenorrhoea, cramps, muscular weakness, dry hair and skin, depression, a feeling of aimlessness, withered and brittle nails.
Tongue: Pale, Thin, slightly dry.
Pulse: Choppy or Fine.

Treatment

HE-7 Shenmen, Ren-14 Juque, Ren-15 Jiuwei, Ren-4 Guanyuan, BL-17 Geshu (with moxa), BL-20 Pishu, LIV-8 Ququan, SP-6 Sanyinjiao, ST-36 Zusanli, BL-18 Ganshu, BL-23 Shenshu

---

Please remember that in many young women a Kidney deficiency may sometimes manifest simply with a Weak pulse on both Rear positions (Fig. 34.32).

Pathological developments from pattern

Although a Kidney deficiency may be the root of this combination of patterns, equally, Liver- and Heart-Blood deficiency may themselves lead to a Kidney deficiency, especially in women.

Long-term Blood deficiency of the Heart and Liver leads to dryness manifesting with dry hair, dry skin, dry and withered nails and dry lips.

Finally, long-term Blood deficiency of the Heart and Liver will lead to Yin deficiency of these two organs (see Fig. 34.32).

Box 34.28 describes the consequences of Liver- and Heart-Blood deficiency.

Treatment

Principle of treatment: nourish Blood, tonify Heart and Liver, calm the Mind and settle the Ethereal Soul.

Acupuncture

Points: HE-7 Shenmen, Ren-14 Juque, Ren-15 Jiuwei, Ren-4 Guanyuan, BL-17 Geshu (with moxa), BL-20 Pishu, LIV-8 Ququan, SP-6 Sanyinjiao, ST-36 Zusanli, BL-18 Ganshu, BL-23 Shenshu.
Method: all with reinforcing method. Moxa can be used.
Explanation
- HE-7 nourishes Heart-Blood and calms the Mind.
- Ren-14 and Ren-15 nourish Heart-Blood and calm the Mind. They are particularly useful if there is pronounced anxiety.
- Ren-4, BL-17 and BL-20 nourish Blood. BL-17 is the Gathering point for Blood and BL-20 is the Back Transporting point for the Spleen and it tonifies Spleen-Qi to produce more Blood.
- LIV-8, ST-36 and SP-6 nourish Liver-Blood.
- BL-18 and BL-23 nourish Liver-Blood, particularly in gynaecological conditions.

Herbal formula

Gui Pi Tang *Tonifying the Spleen Decoction.*
Sheng Yu Tang *Sage Healing Decoction.*
Bu Gan Tang *Tonifying the Liver Decoction.*
Dang Gui Ji Xue Teng Tang *Angelica–Ji Xue Teng Decoction.*

Box 34.29 summarizes Heart- and Liver-Blood deficiency.

Note on frequent combinations of Liver patterns

The Liver is rather different from other organs in that its patterns frequently occur in combination. In practice, it is not unusual to see two, often three, and sometimes even four Liver patterns occurring together. This combination of patterns is much more frequent for the Liver than for other organs. For example, it is not unusual to see a patient suffering from Liver-Qi stagnation, Liver-Blood stasis and Liver-Yang rising; in contrast, I have never seen a patient who suffers (for example) from Heart-Fire, Heart-Blood stasis and Heart-Yin deficiency.

In a way, the frequent combination of various Liver patterns is the pathological counterpart of the free flow of Liver-Qi. Just as in health Liver-Qi flows freely in all directions, in all organs and every part of the body, in pathology, this flow of Liver-Qi in all directions and parts of the body causes the appearance of several patterns simultaneously.

I shall discuss below some frequent combinations of Liver patterns.

Liver-Qi stagnation and Liver-Blood deficiency

The combination of Liver-Qi stagnation and Liver-Blood deficiency is very common in women (see Figs 34.2 and 34.33). They may simply either occur together or Liver-Blood deficiency may lead to Liver-Qi stagnation. Liver-Blood is the Yin and Liver-Qi the Yang of the Liver: the two need to mutually support each other and 'merge' harmoniously with each other.

When Liver-Qi stagnation occurs as a result of Liver-Blood deficiency, the pattern is one of mixed Fullness and Emptiness and the symptoms of Liver-Qi stagnation are milder than in what I call 'pure' Liver-Qi stagnation: that is, one that arises independently from emotional stress.

The combination of Liver-Qi stagnation and Liver-Blood deficiency is seen frequently in women suffering from premenstrual problems. When Liver-Qi stagnation derives from or is associated with Liver-Blood deficiency, the main premenstrual symptoms will be depression (more than irritability), crying, a feeling of aimlessness, slight or no breast distension, a Pale tongue and a pulse that either Choppy or Fine in general and slightly Wiry on the left.

Liver-Qi stagnation and Liver-Yang rising

The combination of Liver-Qi stagnation and Liver-Yang rising is common. The patient would suffer from a feeling of abdominal distension, depression, moodiness and from chronic throbbing headaches (Fig. 34.34).

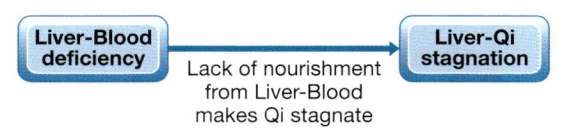

Liver-Blood deficiency, Liver-Qi stagnation, Liver-Blood stasis, Liver-Yang rising

In this case there are four patterns. For example, a woman may suffer from scanty periods, blurred vision and tingling (Liver-Blood deficiency); premenstrual tension and breast distension (Liver-Qi stagnation); painful periods with dark clots (Liver-Blood stasis); and premenstrual headaches of a throbbing nature with nausea, vomiting and visual disturbances (Liver-Yang rising) (Fig. 34.35).

Liver-Blood deficiency, Liver-Yang rising, rebellious Liver-Qi

In this case there are three patterns. For example, a woman might suffer from digestive problems with indigestion, belching, nausea and sour regurgitation (rebellious Liver-Qi); tiredness, blurred vision and dry hair and skin (Liver-Blood deficiency); and chronic, throbbing headaches (Liver-Yang rising) (Fig. 34.36).

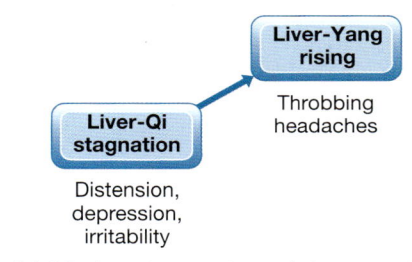

Figure 34.33 Liver-Blood deficiency and Liver-Qi stagnation

Figure 34.34 Liver-Qi stagnation and Liver-Yang rising

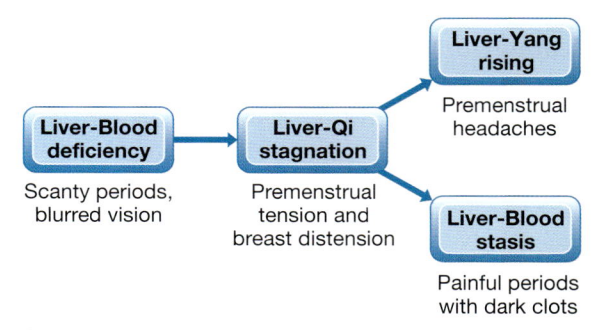

Figure 34.35 Liver-Blood deficiency, Liver-Qi stagnation, Liver-Yang rising and Liver-Blood stasis

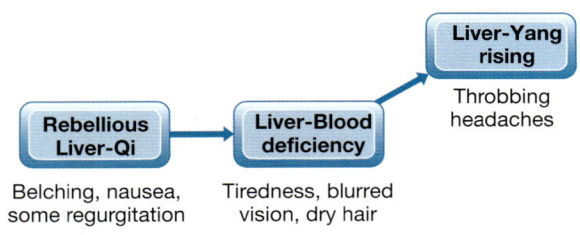

Figure 34.36 Rebellious Liver-Qi, Liver-Blood deficiency and Liver-Yang rising

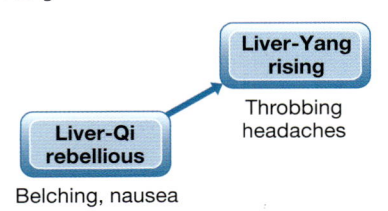

Figure 34.37 Rebellious Liver-Qi and Liver-Yang rising

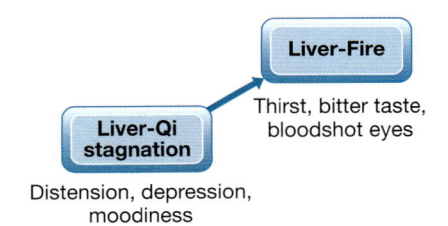

Figure 34.38 Liver-Qi stagnation and Liver-Fire

Rebellious Liver-Qi, Liver-Yang rising

The combination of rebellious Liver-Qi and Liver-Yang rising is common as when Liver-Qi rebels horizontally, it is likely to rebel upwards as well. The patient would suffer from indigestion, belching, sour regurgitation and throbbing headaches (Fig. 34.37).

Liver-Qi stagnation, Liver-Fire

The combination of Liver-Qi stagnation and Liver-Fire is common as long-term Qi stagnation may lead to Heat and then Fire. The symptoms would be a feeling of distension, irritability, moodiness, depression (Liver-Qi stagnation) and a feeling of heat, thirst, bitter taste, bloodshot eyes (Liver-Fire) (Fig. 34.38).

In women, the combination of these two patterns often causes chronic urinary problems from the infusing of Liver-Fire downwards with symptoms such as frequency and burning on urination. Although Liver-Fire naturally blazes upwards (hence the bitter taste, thirst, bloodshot eyes), it may also infuse to the Lower Burner downwards and this happens particularly when it is combined with Liver-Qi stagnation.

Learning outcomes

In this chapter you will have learned:
- The wide sphere of influence of the Liver on other Internal Organs: the Spleen, Stomach, Gall Bladder, Intestines and Uterus
- The general characteristics of Liver pathology
- The effect of exterior Wind and Dampness on the Liver
- How anger, worry and sadness can affect the Liver
- The role of diet as a cause of Liver imbalance
- How to identify the following Excess patterns:
  Liver-Qi stagnation: distension, depression/moodiness, menstrual problems and a Wiry pulse
  Stagnant Liver-Qi turning into Heat: distension, more pronounced irritability, a feeling of heat and Red sides to the tongue
  Rebellious Liver-Qi: Liver-Qi rebels horizontally causing distension, hiccup and belching
  Liver-Blood stasis: dark, clotted menstrual blood, stabbing menstrual pain and a Purple tongue
  Liver-Fire Blazing: headache, irritability, red face and eyes and other Heat signs
  Damp-Heat in Liver: a feeling of fullness and heaviness, nausea and a sticky yellow tongue coat
  Stagnation of Cold in Liver Channel: hypogastric pain referring to scrotum and a Wiry-Deep-Slow pulse
- How to identify the following Deficiency patterns:
  Liver-Blood deficiency: blurred vision, scanty periods, a dull-pale face and a Pale tongue, more common in women
  Liver-Yin deficiency: blurred vision, dry eyes and a tongue without coating
- How to identify the following Full/Empty patterns:
  Liver-Yang rising: headache, irritability and a Wiry pulse deriving from deficiency of Liver- or Kidney-Yin or Liver-Blood
  Extreme Heat generating Wind: convulsions and high temperature
  Liver-Yang rising generating Wind (Liver-Yin deficiency): tremor, dizziness, headache
  Liver-Yang rising generating Wind (Liver- and Kidney-Yin deficiency): tremor, backache and night sweats
  Liver-Yang rising generating Wind (Liver-Blood deficiency): tremor, blurred vision and numbness
  Liver-Fire generating Wind: tremor, irritability, red face and eyes, more common in elderly
  Liver-Blood deficiency generating Wind: fine tremor, tic, numbness and scanty periods
- How to identify the following combined patterns:
  Rebellious Liver-Qi invading the Spleen: abdominal distension, alternating constipation and diarrhoea due to Wood overacting on Earth
  Rebellious Liver invading the Stomach: epigastric pain and oppression, hiccups, and belching due to Liver-Qi interfering with descending of Stomach-Qi
  Liver-Fire insulting the Lungs: asthma, fullness of hypochondrium, headache and Wiry pulse

Continued

Heart- and Liver-Blood deficiency: palpitations, blurred vision, insomnia and a Pale tongue
- Awareness of the following combinations of Liver patterns:
  Liver-Qi stagnation and Liver-Blood deficiency
  Liver-Qi stagnation and Liver-Yang rising
  Liver-Blood deficiency, Liver-Qi stagnation, Liver-Blood stasis and Liver-Yang rising
  Liver-Blood deficiency, Liver-Yang rising and rebellious Liver-Qi
  Rebellious Liver-Qi and Liver-Yang rising
  Liver-Qi stagnation and Liver-Fire

Self-assessment questions

1. What are the functions of the Liver?
2. Give three general characteristics of Liver pathology.
3. What are the two most important signs/symptoms to diagnose Liver-Qi stagnation?
4. How might the tongue tell you that Liver-Qi stagnation had turned into Heat?
5. If Liver-Qi 'rebels' horizontally into the epigastrium, what pattern might you diagnose, and give two key symptoms of this pattern.
6. What is the main acupuncture point to use if Liver-Qi invades the Stomach?
7. What are the most important symptoms of stagnant Blood in the Uterus?
8. What is the pathology of the dry stools and constipation in the pattern Liver-Fire blazing?
9. Which signs/symptoms would enable you to diagnose Damp-Heat in the Liver?
10. What sign would you look for on the hands if you suspect Liver-Blood deficiency?
11. A patient presents with blurred vision, dry eyes and a tongue without coating. Which pattern do you suspect?
12. What are the treatment principles to treat Liver-Yang rising?
13. Give three symptoms of internal Wind.
14. Which points on the Directing Vessel (*Ren Mai*) might you use to help the descending of Stomach-Qi if Liver-Qi has invaded the Stomach?
15. A patient presents with blurred vision and palpitations. What is the likely pattern?

See p. 1263 for answers

END NOTES

1. 1981 Spiritual Axis (*Ling Shu Jing* 灵枢经), People's Health Publishing House, Beijing, first published *c.*100 BC, p. 24.
2. Ibid., p. 24.

SECTION 2 PART 6

Lung Patterns 35

Key contents

General aetiology
Exterior pathogenic factors
Diet
Emotions
- Sadness and grief
- Worry

Life habits

Empty patterns
Lung-Qi deficiency
Lung-Yin deficiency
Lung Dryness

Full patterns
Exterior
- Invasion of Lungs by Wind-Cold
- Invasion of Lungs by Wind-Heat
- Invasion of Lungs by Wind-Water

Interior
- Lung-Heat
- Damp-Phlegm in the Lungs
- Cold-Phlegm in the Lungs
- Phlegm-Heat in the Lungs
- Dry Phlegm in the Lungs
- Phlegm-Fluids Obstructing the Lungs

Combined patterns
Lung- and Heart-Qi deficiency
Lung-Qi and Kidney-Yang deficiency (see Kidney deficiency, Water overflowing to the Lungs, or Kidney failing to receive Qi in ch. 37)
Lung- and Kidney-Yin deficiency (see under Kidney combined patterns, ch. 37)
Liver-Fire insulting the Lungs (see under Liver combined patterns, ch. 34)
Lung- and Spleen-Qi deficiency (see under Spleen combined patterns, ch. 36)

The functions of the Lungs are (see ch. 8):

- They govern Qi and respiration
- They control channels and blood vessels
- They control diffusing and descending of Qi
- They regulate all physiological activities
- They regulate Water passages
- They control skin and hair
- They open into the nose
- They control nasal mucus
- They house the Corporeal Soul

The main Lung function is that of governing Qi and deficiency of Qi is the most common Deficiency pattern of the Lungs.

The Lungs have a diffusing and descending function in relation to Body Fluids and Defensive Qi (*Wei Qi*) and they are the most 'exterior' organ controlling the skin and Defensive Qi. This means that the Lungs are the first organ to be affected by exterior pathogenic factors such as Wind-Cold and Wind-Heat. For this reason, three of the patterns discussed are exterior patterns: that is, they do not involve injury of the Lung organ itself but only of its 'Exterior portion'.

Box 35.1 summarizes the factors that give a 'feel' for Lung pathology.

Box 35.1 A 'feel' for Lung pathology

- Qi deficiency (weak voice, shortness of breath)
- Pallor
- Thin chest
- Sadness
- Skin problems such as eczema
- Atopic constitution (allergic asthma and eczema)
- Phlegm
- Exterior invasions of Wind (aversion to cold, sneezing, runny nose)
- No gynaecological connection

The discussion of Lung patterns will be preceded by a discussion of the general aetiology of Lung disharmonies discussed under the following headings:
GENERAL AETIOLOGY
- Exterior pathogenic factors
- Diet
- Emotions
  - Sadness and grief
  - Worry
- Life habits

The Lung patterns discussed are:
EMPTY PATTERNS
- Lung-Qi deficiency
- Lung-Yin deficiency
- Lung Dryness

FULL PATTERNS: EXTERIOR
- Invasion of Lungs by Wind-Cold
- Invasion of Lungs by Wind-Heat
- Invasion of Lungs by Wind-Water

FULL PATTERNS: INTERIOR
- Lung-Heat
- Damp-Phlegm in the Lungs
- Cold-Phlegm in the Lungs
- Phlegm-Heat in the Lungs
- Dry Phlegm in the Lungs
- Phlegm-Fluids obstructing the Lungs

COMBINED PATTERNS
- Lung- and Heart-Qi deficiency
- Lung-Qi and Kidney-Yang deficiency (see 'Kidney deficiency, Water overflowing to the Lungs' or 'Kidney failing to receive Qi' patterns under the Kidney patterns, ch. 37)
- Lung- and Kidney-Yin deficiency (see under Kidney, Combined patterns, ch. 37)
- Liver-Fire insulting the Lungs (see under Liver, Combined patterns, ch. 34)
- Lung- and Spleen-Qi deficiency (see under Spleen, Combined patterns, ch. 36)

GENERAL AETIOLOGY

Exterior pathogenic factors

Wind

The Lungs control the skin, they are the most 'exterior' of the organs and influence Defensive Qi: for all these reasons, the Lungs are the organ that is most easily and directly affected by exterior pathogenic factors, particularly Wind, Heat, Fire, Cold, Dampness and Dryness.

The Lungs are sometimes called the 'delicate' organs because of their susceptibility to invasion by exterior pathogenic factors.

> **Clinical note**
>
> The Lungs are called the 'delicate' organs as they are the most likely to be invaded by exterior pathogenic factors

Exterior pathogenic factors engage in a fight with Defensive Qi and impair the diffusing and descending of Lung-Qi. All the symptoms and signs arising from these Full patterns are a reflection of the impairment of the diffusing and descending of Lung-Qi (headache, aches of the body, aversion to cold, sneezing, blocked nose, cough, etc.).

Wind usually combines with other pathogenic factors, notably Cold and Heat, to form Wind-Cold and Wind-Heat: these are the two most common exterior pathogenic factors to attack the Lungs. When the Lungs are attacked by these exterior pathogenic factors, it is the Lung Exterior portion (or Lung Defensive Qi portion) that is invaded, not the Lung organ itself. The pattern is therefore an exterior one, even though there may be such symptoms as cough.

> **Clinical note**
>
> When the Lungs are invaded by exterior pathogenic factors, it is only the 'Exterior portion' that is affected, not the Lung itself

Dryness

The Lungs are also easily injured by Dryness as they need a certain amount of moisture to function properly (one can think of the moistening fluid in the pleural cavity). Excessively dry weather can therefore cause the Lungs to become dry, resulting in such symptoms as a dry cough, a dry throat, dry skin.

Bear in mind that artificial dryness (e.g. very dry, centrally heated environments) also affects the Lungs in the same way as a dry climate.

Dampness

Dampness does not usually attack the Lungs directly, except when combined with Wind, in which case it will impair not only the Lungs' diffusing and descending functions, giving rise to the usual exterior symptoms mentioned above, but also their function of regulating the Water passages, giving rise to facial oedema.

Exterior pathogenic factors as causes of disease are discussed in chapter 21.

Diet

Diet has an important influence on the Lung function. The excessive consumption of cold and raw foods can generate internal Dampness and Phlegm, which derives from Spleen dysfunction and is often 'stored' in the Lungs. It is said in Chinese medicine that 'the Spleen creates Phlegm and the Lungs store it'. In this case there would be profuse sputum in the Lungs. For this reason, an excessive consumption of cold and raw foods is contraindicated in cases of asthma due to retention of Damp-Phlegm in the Lungs.

Apart from cold and raw foods, an excessive consumption of greasy foods and dairy foods have the same effect on the Lungs, giving rise to Phlegm.

Diet as a cause of disease is discussed in chapter 22.

Emotions

Sadness and grief

Sadness and grief deplete Lung-Qi. In particular, sadness and grief cause deficiency of Lung-Qi: this is often manifested with a pulse that is Weak on both Front positions. With time, deficient Qi in the chest fails to circulate properly and Qi stagnation in the chest may result. Thus, deficiency and stagnation of Qi can, and often do, occur simultaneously (Fig. 35.1).

Worry

Worry 'knots' Qi and causes stagnation of Qi in the chest, which affects the Lungs. This manifests with a slight feeling of tightness of the chest, a slight breathlessness, sighing and a Lung pulse that is very slightly Tight.

Emotions as causes of disease are discussed in chapter 20.

> **Clinical note**
>
> In my experience, sadness and grief (from loss and separation) are major and very common emotional causes of disease in Western patients

Life habits

Sitting for long periods of time bent over a desk to read or write can weaken Lung-Qi (because the chest is impeded and proper breathing impaired).

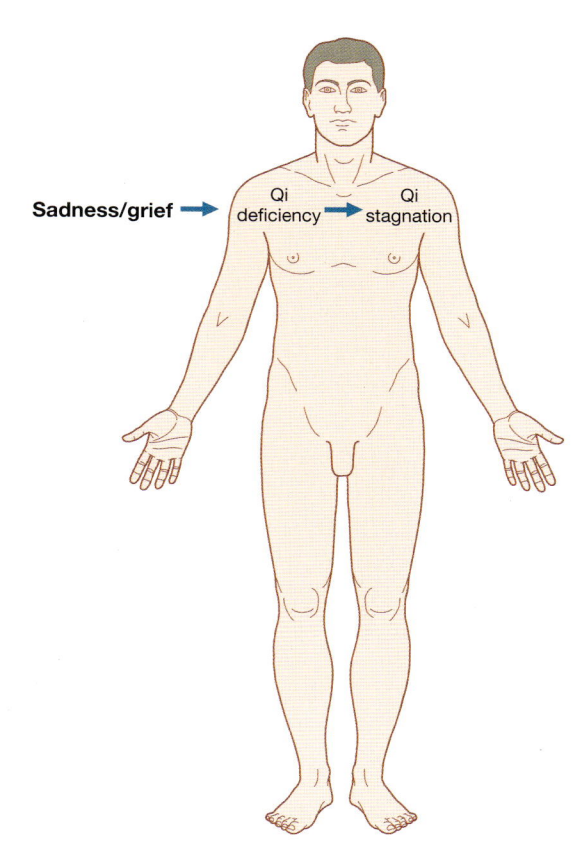

Figure 35.1 Influence of sadness and grief on Lung-Qi

Smoking (cigarettes or marijuana) dries up the Lungs and damages the Lung fluids.

Box 35.2 summarizes the general aetiology of Lung patterns.

> **Box 35.2 General aetiology of Lung patterns**
>
> - Exterior pathogenic factors
> - Diet
> - Emotions
>   - Sadness and grief
>   - Worry
> - Life habits

EMPTY PATTERNS

Lung-Qi deficiency

Clinical manifestations

Slight shortness of breath, slight cough, weak voice, spontaneous daytime sweating, dislike of speaking,

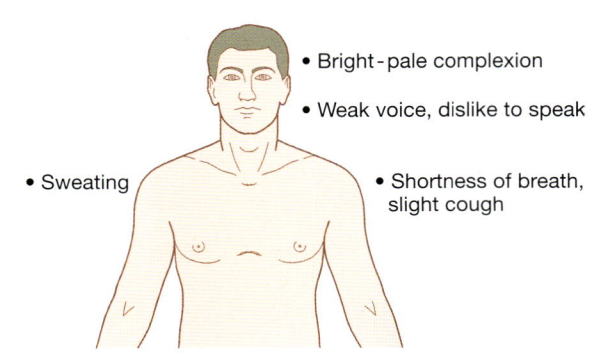

Figure 35.2 Lung-Qi deficiency

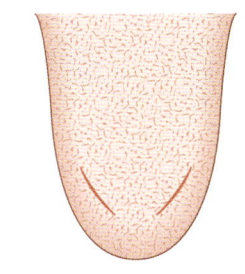

Figure 35.3 Lung cracks

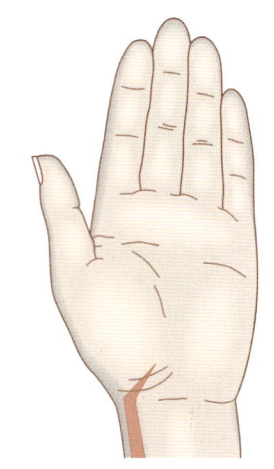

Figure 35.4 'Special' Lung position on pulse

bright-pale complexion, propensity to catch colds, tiredness, dislike of cold (Fig. 35.2).
Tongue: Pale.
Pulse: Empty, especially on the Right-Front position.
Key symptoms: shortness of breath, weak voice, Empty Pulse.

> **Diagnostic tip**
>
> A slight shortness of breath and an Empty Lung pulse are enough to diagnose Lung-Qi deficiency

Aetiology

Constitution

First of all, this pattern could be due to hereditary Lung weakness, particularly if one of the parents suffered from tuberculosis of the Lungs. In these cases the tongue often has one or two small transversal cracks in the Lung area (Fig. 35.3 and Plate 22.6), and the Pulse can be felt further up the wrist in a position medial to the normal Front position. When the pulse can be felt in this position, it often has a Slippery and slightly Wiry quality (Fig. 35.4).

Emotional stress

Sadness and grief deplete Lung-Qi and cause Lung-Qi deficiency. With time, deficient Qi fails to move in the chest and Qi stagnation results.

Life habits

Lung-Qi deficiency can also be induced by prolonged stooping over a desk for long hours. This constricts breathing and, in the long run, will cause Lung-Qi deficiency.

Lung-Qi deficiency may also be induced by excessive use of the voice over many years (e.g. teachers).

Exterior pathogenic factors

The pattern of Lung-Qi deficiency can also be the result of an exterior attack of Wind-Cold or Wind-Heat that is not treated properly, so that some pathogenic factor remains in the body and, in the long run, causes Lung-Qi deficiency.

Pathology

The Lungs govern Qi and respiration, and when Qi is deficient, breathing is short, especially on exertion. The shortness of breath in this case is only slight (not like the one seen in bronchitis or asthma) and mostly on exertion.

The Lungs send Qi downwards and if Lung-Qi is deficient, Qi cannot descend and will cause cough.

The tone and strength of voice is an expression of the strength of the Gathering Qi (*Zong Qi*), which, in turn, depends on Lung-Qi, hence the weak voice and dislike of speaking in this pattern.

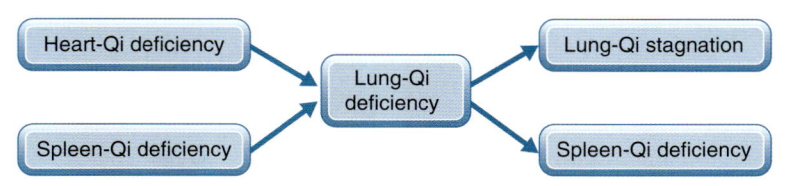

Figure 35.5 Lung-Qi deficiency pattern: precursors and developments

Lung-Qi influences the skin and controls Defensive Qi, which regulates the opening and closing of the pores. When Lung-Qi is weak, the Defensive Qi is weak in the space between skin and muscles; this space is too 'open', the pores become flaccid and let sweat out.

Defensive Qi warms the skin and muscles, hence the dislike of cold in the Lung-Qi deficiency pattern.

The bright-pale complexion reflects deficiency of Yang (which in the case of the Lungs is synonymous with deficiency of Qi).

Finally, Defensive Qi protects the body from exterior pathogenic factors; when Lung-Qi is deficient, Defensive Qi is not strong enough and is not diffused properly by the Lungs so that it cannot protect the body properly and it becomes prone to invasion of exterior Wind.

The Empty Pulse reflects the deficiency of Qi.

Pathological precursors of pattern

Earth is the Mother of Metal and Spleen-Qi deficiency often leads to Lung-Qi deficiency. Heart-Qi deficiency may also lead to Lung-Qi deficiency given the close relationships between these two organs in the chest: this is a common situation, especially when emotional stress is the cause of the disease (Fig. 35.5).

Pathological developments from pattern

First of all, Lung-Qi deficiency in time may lead to stagnation of Lung-Qi. Although Spleen-Qi may lead to Lung-Qi deficiency as discussed above, the reverse is also possible, so that Lung-Qi deficiency may lead to Spleen-Qi deficiency (see Fig. 35.5).

Treatment

Principle of treatment: tonify Lung-Qi, warm Yang.

Acupuncture

Points: LU-9 Taiyuan, LU-7 Lieque, Ren-6 Qihai, BL-13 Feishu, Du-12 Shenzhu, ST-36 Zusanli, Ren-12 Zhongwan.

Method: reinforcing method, moxa is applicable.

Explanation
- LU-9 is the Source point of the Lung and it tonifies Lung-Qi.
- LU-7 tonifies Lung-Qi and stimulates the descending of Lung-Qi. For this reason, it is particularly useful if there is a cough or a residual pathogenic factor from a previous attack of Wind-Cold or Wind-Heat.
- Ren-6 tonifies Qi. The deep pathway of the Lung channel reaches this point where it connects with the Large Intestine channel.
- BL-13 tonifies Lung-Qi.
- Du-12 tonifies Lung-Qi and is particularly important to use in chronic cases.
- ST-36 and Ren-12 tonify Stomach- and Spleen-Qi. It is often necessary to tonify the Stomach and Spleen in order to nourish the Lungs. In Five-Element terms this corresponds to 'Tonifying Earth to nourish Metal'. The deep pathway of the Lung channel starts in the region of Ren-12.

Herbal formula

Ren Shen Bu Fei Tang *Ginseng Tonifying the Lungs Decoction*.

Box 35.3 summarizes Lung-Qi deficiency.

Box 35.3 Lung-Qi deficiency

Clinical manifestations

Slight shortness of breath, slight cough, weak voice, spontaneous daytime sweating, dislike of speaking, bright-pale complexion, propensity to catch colds, tiredness, dislike of cold, Pale tongue, Empty pulse, especially on the Right-Front position

Treatment

LU-9 Taiyuan, LU-7 Lieque, Ren-6 Qihai, BL-13 Feishu, Du-12 Shenzhu, ST-36 Zusanli, Ren-12 Zhongwan

Lung-Yin deficiency

Clinical manifestations

Cough which is dry or with scanty sticky sputum, weak and/hoarse voice, dry mouth and throat, tickly throat, tiredness, dislike of speaking, thin body or thin chest, night sweating (Fig. 35.6).
Tongue: normal-coloured, dry without coating (or with rootless coating) in the front part.
Pulse: Floating-Empty.
Key symptoms: dry cough, weak hoarse voice, dry throat, night sweating.

Empty Heat

Feeling of heat in the evening, afternoon fever, five-palm heat, malar flush.
Tongue: Red without coating.
Pulse: Floating-Empty and Rapid.

> **Diagnostic tip**
>
> A dry cough and a rootless tongue coating in the front area (Lung area) are enough to diagnose Lung-Yin deficiency

Aetiology

Emotional stress

Sadness and grief normally deplete Qi: however, when a person has a pre-existing constitutional tendency to Yin deficiency, these emotions may deplete Lung-Yin.

Life habits

Excessive use of the voice over many years may lead to Lung-Yin deficiency. Smoking is an important contributory factor to Lung-Yin deficiency as tobacco or cannabis have a drying effect.

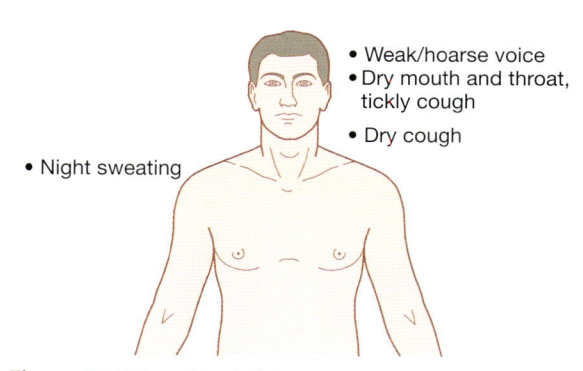

> **Clinical note**
>
> Tobacco is hot in energy and has a drying effect. It is a major cause of Lung-Yin deficiency

Pathology

This is characterized by deficiency of Body Fluids and ensuing dryness. Hence the dry cough, dry throat and mouth, tickly throat and hoarse voice.

When Yin deficiency is pronounced and long-lasting, Empty-Heat is produced, causing a low-grade fever, a feeling of heat in the evening, malar flush, five-palm heat (a feeling of heat of the chest, palms of hands and soles of feet), and a Rapid pulse.

The Red tongue without coating is indicative of Yin deficiency with Empty-Heat. It must be emphasized that a tongue that is Red and completely without coating appears only in the late stages of Yin deficiency with Empty Heat, whereas in the beginning stages and in a young person, the tongue may not be Red and may not be completely without coating. The transversal cracks in the Lung area are even more likely to appear in Lung-Yin deficiency than in Lung-Qi deficiency.

Lung-Yin deficiency generally occurs in middle-aged and elderly people as a result of overwork, irregular diet and smoking. However, it can also occur in a child after whooping cough.

Pathological precursors of pattern

This pattern can develop from Lung-Qi deficiency after a long period of time. Any of the causes of Lung-Qi deficiency, therefore, can lead to Lung-Yin deficiency.

Lung-Yin deficiency is often associated with Stomach- and/or Kidney-Yin deficiency. An irregular diet, such as eating late at night, or eating in a hurry, can cause Stomach-Yin deficiency, while overwork over a long period of time can cause Kidney-Yin deficiency.

Lung-Yin deficiency can also develop from a condition of Dryness of the Lungs, which, in turn, may originate internally or externally (Fig. 35.7).

Pathological developments from pattern

Firstly, Lung-Yin deficiency, in time, leads to Empty-Heat in the Lungs. Although Lung-Yin deficiency frequently derives from Kidney-Yin deficiency as mentioned above, the reverse is also true as Lung-Yin

- Night sweating
- Weak/hoarse voice
- Dry mouth and throat, tickly cough
- Dry cough

Figure 35.6 Lung-Yin deficiency

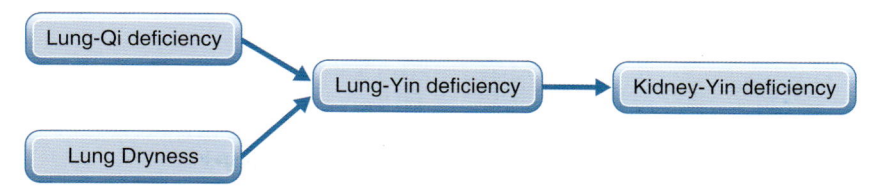

Figure 35.7 Lung-Yin deficiency pattern: precursors and developments

deficiency may lead to Kidney-Yin deficiency (see Fig. 35.7).

Treatment

Principle of treatment: tonify Lung-Yin, nourish Body Fluids, if necessary clear Empty-Heat.

Acupuncture

Points: LU-9 Taiyuan, Ren-17 Shanzhong, BL-43 Gaohuangshu, BL-13 Feishu, Du-12 Shenzhu, Ren-4 Guanyuan, KI-6 Zhaohai, Ren-12 Zhongwan, SP-6 Sanyinjiao, LU-10 Yuji, L.I.-11 Quchi.

Method: reinforcing on all points except LU-10 and L.I.-11, which should be reduced, no moxa.

Explanation
- LU-9 is the Source point and it can tonify Lung-Yin.
- Ren-17 tonifies Qi and Lung-Yin.
- BL-43 tonifies Lung-Yin and is particularly important in chronic cases.
- BL-13 and Du-12 tonify Lung Qi and Yin.
- Ren-4 tonifies Kidney-Yin and is particularly necessary when the Lung-Yin deficiency is associated with Kidney-Yin deficiency. Ren-4 also conducts Empty-Heat downwards.
- KI-6 tonifies Kidney-Yin and benefits the throat. It is particularly useful if there is a dry throat and cough. It can be combined with Lieque LU-7 to open the Directing Vessel (*Ren Mai*). The combination of these two points tonifies Lung-Qi and Lung-Yin, stimulates the descending of Lung-Qi, tonifies Kidney-Yin, benefits the throat and re-establishes the communication between Lungs and Kidneys.
- Ren-12 tonifies the Stomach and nourishes fluids (as the Stomach is the origin of fluids).
- SP-6 nourishes Yin.
- LU-10 is used with reducing method to clear Empty-Heat from the Lungs.
- L.I.-11 is used if there is Empty Heat.

Herbal formula

Yang Yin Qing Fei Tang *Nourishing Yin and Clearing the Lungs Decoction*.

Three Treasures

Jade Spring (variation of Sha Shen Mai Dong Tang). Box 35.4 summarizes Lung-Yin deficiency.

Box 35.4 Lung-Yin deficiency

Clinical manifestations

Cough which is dry or with scanty sticky sputum, weak and/or hoarse voice, dry mouth and throat, tickly throat, tiredness, dislike of speaking, thin body or thin chest, night sweating, normal-coloured tongue, dry without coating (or with rootless coating) in the front part, Floating-Empty pulse

Treatment

LU-9 Taiyuan, Ren-17 Shanzhong, BL-43 Gaohuangshu, BL-13 Feishu, Du-12 Shenzhu, Ren-4 Guanyuan, KI-6 Zhaohai, Ren-12 Zhongwan, SP-6 Sanyinjiao, LU-10 Yuji, L.I.-11 Quchi

---

Lung Dryness

Clinical manifestations

Dry cough, dry skin, dry throat, dry mouth, thirst, hoarse voice (Fig. 35.8).

Tongue: dry.
Pulse: Empty, especially on the Right-Front position.
Key symptoms: dry cough, dry throat, hoarse voice, dry tongue which is not Red.

> **Diagnostic tip**
>
> A dry cough, dry throat and hoarse voice are enough to diagnose Lung Dryness

Aetiology

Exterior dryness

Exterior dryness, during long spells of dry and hot weather or in particularly dry environments (such as the American South-West or the Australian interior), can cause Lung Dryness. Please note that Lung Dryness may also be caused by 'artificial' exterior factors such as very dry and hot workplaces.

> Dryness of the Lungs may also be caused by artificial 'dryness' such as that in very dry and hot working conditions

Irregular diet

Irregular eating with irregular meal times, eating late at night, worrying about work while eating, etc., can induce Lung Dryness.

Pathology

This is a state of dryness of the Lungs, with deficiency of Body Fluids. It is a stage preceding Yin deficiency. It is characterized by dryness but not yet Yin deficiency.

Pathological precursors of pattern

Stomach-Yin deficiency is the most common precursor of Lung Dryness (Fig. 35.9).

Pathological developments from pattern

Dryness will eventually lead to Lung-Yin deficiency (see Fig. 35.9).

Treatment

Principle of treatment: moisten the Lungs, nourish fluids.

Acupuncture

Points: LU-9 Taiyuan, Ren-4 Guanyuan, KI-6 Zhaohai, SP-6 Sanyinjiao, Ren-12 Zhongwan, ST-36 Zusanli.
Method: reinforcing method. No moxa.
Explanation
- LU-9 moistens the Lungs.
- Ren-4 tonifies Kidney-Yin and nourishes fluids.
- KI-6 nourishes fluids and benefits the throat.
- SP-6 nourishes fluids.
- Ren-12 and ST-36 tonify the Stomach and nourishes fluids.

Herbal formula

Bai He Gu Jin Tang *Lilium Consolidating Metal Decoction*.

Box 35.5 summarizes Lung Dryness.

Box 35.5 Lung Dryness

Clinical manifestations

Dry cough, dry skin, dry throat, dry mouth, thirst, hoarse voice, dry tongue, Empty pulse, especially on the Right-Front position

Treatment

LU-9 Taiyuan, Ren-4 Guanyuan, KI-6 Zhaohai, SP-6 Sanyinjiao, Ren-12 Zhongwan, ST-36 Zusanli

---

- Dry mouth, thirst
- Hoarse voice
- Dry cough
- Dry throat
- Dry skin

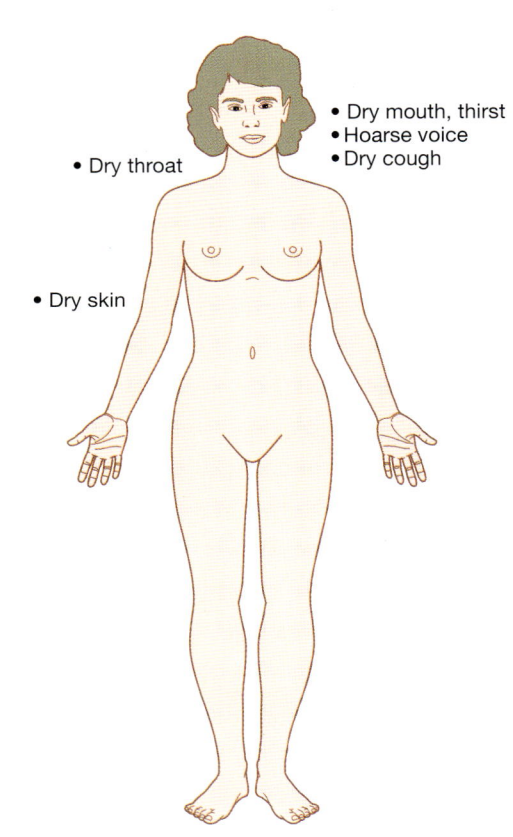

Figure 35.8 Lung Dryness

Stomach-Yin deficiency → Lung Dryness → Lung-Yin deficiency

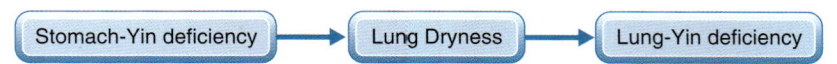

Figure 35.9 Lung Dryness pattern: precursors and developments

FULL PATTERNS: EXTERIOR

Invasion of Lungs by Wind-Cold

Clinical manifestations

Aversion to cold, fever, cough itchy throat, slight breathlessness, blocked or runny nose with clear, watery discharge, sneezing, occipital headache, body aches (Fig. 35.10).
Tongue: thin-white coating.
Pulse: Floating-Tight.
Key symptoms: aversion to cold, sneezing, Floating pulse.

> **Diagnostic tip**
>
> Aversion to cold and 'fever' are the cardinal manifestations of external invasion of Wind

Aetiology

This is caused by exposure to wind and cold: this is due to an invasion of an exterior pathogenic factor and this is therefore its only aetiological factor. As was discussed in chapter 21, diagnosis of this pattern is done not according to aetiology but to pathology. In other words, if a patient displays all or some of the above symptoms and signs, we can diagnose an invasion of the Lungs by Wind-Cold and we do not need to enquire about the person's probable exposure to wind and cold.

Furthermore, invasion of the Lungs by Wind-Cold is due to the relative weakness of the body's Qi in relation to the pathogenic factor at that particular time. Thus the person need not have been exposed to extremes of wind and cold to develop the above symptoms and signs. This explains why we can catch a cold in any season, even during a hot summer, and not just in wintertime.

Finally, as previously discussed (see ch. 21), there are artificial sources of 'Wind-Cold' such as air conditioning, draughts or refrigerated store-rooms which can cause this pattern.

As the body's Qi is only relatively weak in comparison to the pathogenic factor, this pattern is of Excess nature which calls for a reducing treatment method. To think that we need to tonify the body's Qi because it has succumbed to the exterior pathogenic factor due to its weakness would be wrong and would make the patient worse.

> Invasion of the Lungs by Wind-Cold may also be caused by artificial 'wind-cold', such as that in very draughty and cold working conditions

Pathology

This corresponds to the Greater Yang stage of the Identification of Patterns according to the Six Stages, from the 'Discussion on Cold-induced Diseases' by Zhang Zhong Jing (see ch. 44).[1]

Aversion to cold is due to the obstruction of the space between skin and muscles by exterior Wind so that the Defensive Qi does not circulate well and fails to warm the muscles. At this stage the exterior Wind-Cold attacks the Defensive Qi layer of the Lung system and the exterior Wind engages in a fight with the Defensive Qi. Fever results from this fight. However, if the pathogenic factor is not too strong, or if the Defensive Qi does not react to it, there may not be a fever. As discussed in chapter 21, please remember that 'fever' does not necessarily indicate an actual temperature as measured by

- Blocked or runny nose
- Occipital headache
- Itchy throat
- Aversion to cold fever
- Cough, slight breathlessness
- Body aches

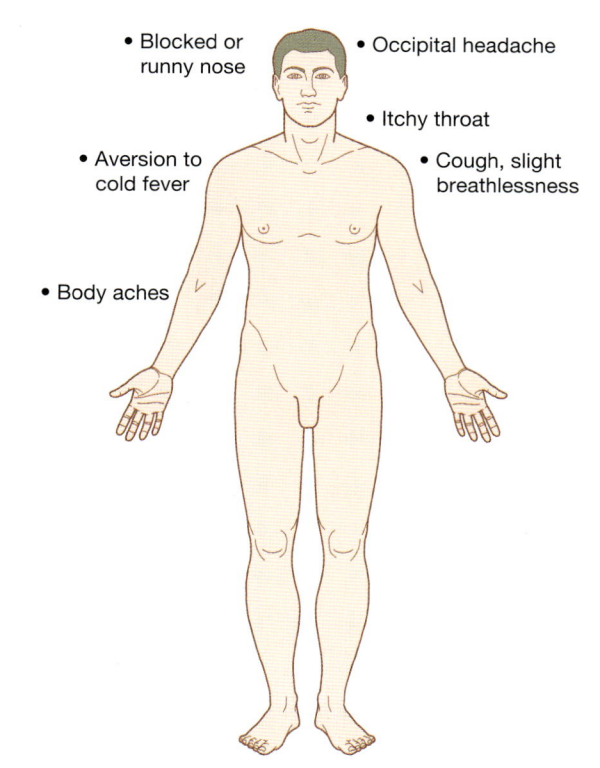

Figure 35.10 Invasion of Lungs by Wind-Cold

a thermometer but rather denotes an objective emission of heat (*fa re*) of the patient's body felt on palpation by the doctor.

> 'Fever' does not necessarily indicate a raised temperature but the objective 'emission of heat' of the patient's body that can be felt on palpation

The exterior Wind obstructs the Lung's Defensive Qi system and impairs the descending of Lung-Qi, causing a cough and a blocked or runny nose, and the dispersing of Lung-Qi, causing sneezing.

The exterior Wind also obstructs the circulation of Defensive Qi, resulting in occipital headache and body aches as Defensive Qi does not circulate properly in the space between skin and muscles.

The headache is typically on the occiput along the Greater Yang channels (Small Intestine and Bladder), or it could be in the whole head.

The tongue may not show much at all in the beginning stages. The body colour will be unchanged and there might only be a thin white coating, white indicating Cold and thin indicating that the pathogenic factor is at the beginning stage.

The Pulse will be Floating, reflecting the rush of the body's Qi to the exterior layers to fight the pathogenic factor. It might be Floating in all positions, or only in the Front ones, or even only in the right Front position (Lungs).

Pathological precursors of pattern

As this is an exterior pattern from invasion of exterior Wind, there are no pathological precursors. However, if the Defensive Qi is weak, the person will be particularly prone to invasions of exterior pathogenic factors (Fig. 35.11).

Pathological developments from pattern

When Wind invades the body, it causes an exterior pattern: that is, the pathogenic factor is located on the Exterior and it does not affect the Internal Organs (see Fig. 35.11). When this happens, there can be only three possible outcomes (Fig. 35.12):

1. The exterior pathogenic factor is expelled and the patient recovers completely
2. The exterior pathogenic factor penetrates into the Interior
3. The exterior pathogenic factor appears to recede but the patient is left with a residual pathogenic factor (often Damp-Phlegm or Phlegm-Heat in the Lungs in the case of invasion by Wind-Cold)

Treatment

Principle of treatment: release the Exterior, expel Cold, stimulate the descending and diffusing of Lung-Qi.

Acupuncture

Points: LU-7 Lieque, BL-12 Fengmen, Du-16 Fengfu.
Method: reducing method, moxa is applicable after needling.
Explanation
- LU-7 expels Wind, releases the Exterior and stimulates the descending and diffusing of Lung-Qi.

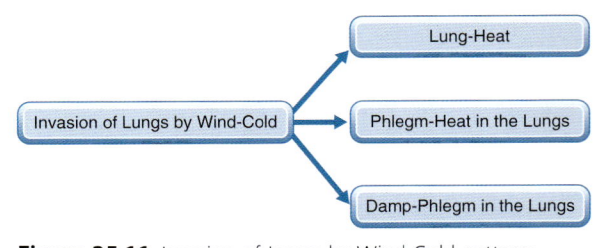

Figure 35.11 Invasion of Lungs by Wind-Cold pattern: precursors and developments

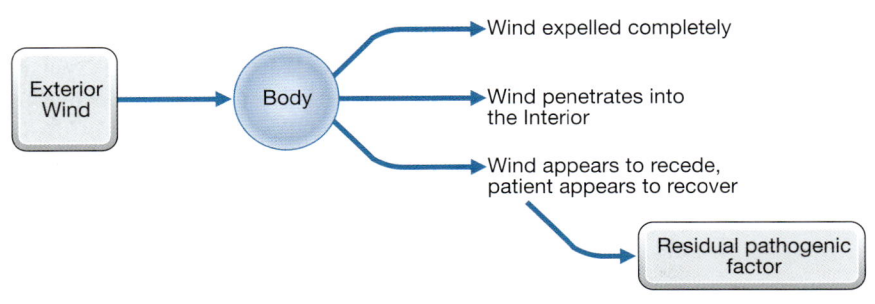

Figure 35.12 Development of residual pathogenic factor

- BL-12 releases the Exterior and expels Wind. Moxa can be used on this point after needling. Cupping this point is extremely effective to expel Wind.
- Du-16 expels Wind, and is particularly useful if there is a headache.

Herbal formula

Ma Huang Tang *Ephedra Decoction*.

Three Treasures

Expel Wind-Cold (variation of Jing Fang Jie Biao Tang).

Box 35.6 summarizes invasion of Lungs by Wind-Cold.

Box 35.6 Invasion of Lungs by Wind-Cold

Clinical manifestations

Aversion to cold, fever, cough, itchy throat, slight breathlessness, stuffed or runny nose with clear, watery discharge, sneezing, occipital headache, body aches, thin white tongue coating, Floating-Tight pulse

Treatment

LU-7 Lieque, BL-12 Fengmen, Du-16 Fengfu

Invasion of Lungs by Wind-Heat

Clinical manifestations

Aversion to cold, fever, cough, sore throat, blocked or runny nose with yellow discharge, sneezing, headache, body aches, slight sweating, slight thirst, swollen tonsils (Fig. 35.13).

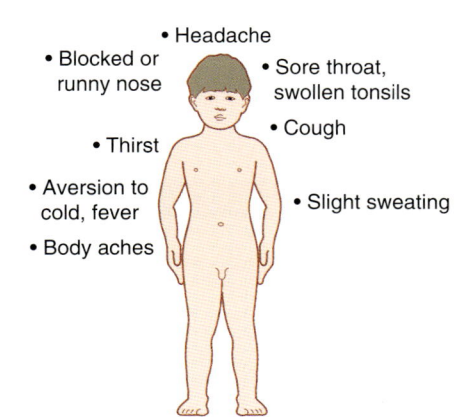

Figure 35.13 Invasion of Lungs by Wind-Heat

Tongue: slightly Red on the sides in the chest areas or on the front part.
Pulse: Floating-Rapid.
Key symptoms: fever, aversion to cold, sore throat, Floating-Rapid pulse.

> **Diagnostic tip**
>
> Aversion to cold and 'fever' are the cardinal manifestations of external invasion of Wind

Aetiology

This is due to exposure to climatic wind and heat. For a discussion of the aetiology of this pattern refer to the pattern of Wind-Cold discussed above.

Similarly, as for Wind-Cold, there are many artificial factors that may cause invasion of Wind-Heat, such as central heating and certain other artificial sources of heat at the place of work (e.g. for cooks or steelworkers).

Pathology

This is the same as for invasion of Wind-Cold, with the only difference that Wind in this case combines with Heat. In invasion of Wind-Heat there is more often a fever.

In invasion of Wind-Heat the person also experiences an aversion to cold, similar to invasion of Wind-Cold. This is because the pathogenic factor obstructs the circulation of the Defensive Qi, which therefore cannot warm the muscles.

Exterior Heat dries up Body Fluids, resulting in thirst and a sore throat.

The tongue coating can be white (even though white usually indicates Cold) because in the very beginning stage of invasion of Wind-Heat there is not enough time for the Heat to turn the coating yellow.

Pathological precursors of pattern

As this is an exterior pattern from invasion of exterior Wind, there are no pathological precursors. However, if the Defensive Qi is weak, the person will be particularly prone to invasions of exterior pathogenic factors (Fig. 35.14).

Pathological developments from pattern

When Wind invades the body, it causes an exterior pattern: that is, the pathogenic factor is located on the

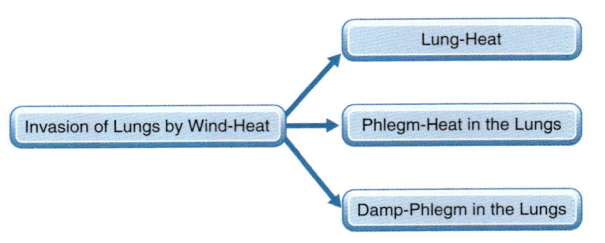

Figure 35.14 Invasion of Lungs by Wind-Heat pattern: precursors and developments

Exterior and it does not affect the Internal Organs (see Fig. 35.14). When this happens, there can be only three possible outcomes:

1. The exterior pathogenic factor is expelled and the patient recovers completely
2. The exterior pathogenic factor penetrates into the Interior
3. The exterior pathogenic factor appears to recede but the patient is left with a residual pathogenic factor (often Phlegm-Heat in the Lungs in the case of invasion by Wind-Heat)

Treatment

Principle of treatment: release the Exterior, clear Heat, stimulate the descending and diffusing of Lung-Qi.

Acupuncture

Points: LU-7 Lieque, L.I.-4 Hegu, L.I.-11 Quchi, LU-11 Shaoshang, Du-14 Dazhui, BL-12 Fengmen (with cupping), Du-16 Fengfu, G.B.-20 Fengchi, T.B.-5 Waiguan.
Method: reducing method, no moxa.
Explanation
 – LU-7 stimulates the diffusing of Lung-Qi to expel Wind.
 – L.I.-4 and L.I.-11 release the Exterior and clear Heat.
 – LU-11 (pricked for bleeding) is especially indicated for a sore throat and swollen tonsils.
 – Du-14 clears Heat.
 – BL-12, Du-16 and GB-20 expel exterior Wind.
 – T.B.-5 expels Wind-Heat and releases the Exterior.

Herbal formula

Sang Ju Yin *Morus–Chrysanthemum Decoction*.
Yin Qiao San *Forsythia–Lonicera Powder*.

Three Treasures

Expel Wind-Heat (variation of Yin Qiao San).

> **Clinical note**
>
> The formula Yin Qiao San (by Wu Ju Tong) is a very effective formula for invasions of Wind-Heat. No household with children should be without it!

Box 35.7 summarizes invasion of Lungs by Wind-Heat.

> **Box 35.7 Invasion of Lungs by Wind-Heat**
>
> **Clinical manifestations**
>
> Aversion to cold, fever, cough, sore throat, stuffed or runny nose with yellow discharge, headache, body aches, slight sweating, slight thirst, swollen tonsils, tongue slightly Red on the sides in the chest areas or on the front part, Floating-Rapid pulse
>
> **Treatment**
>
> LU-7 Lieque, L.I.-4 Hegu, L.I.-11 Quchi, LU-11 Shaoshang, Du-14 Dazhui, BL-12 Fengmen (with cupping), Du-16 Fengfu, G.B.-20 Fengchi, T.B.-5 Waiguan

Invasion of Lungs by Wind-Water

Clinical manifestations

Sudden swelling of eyes and face gradually spreading to the whole body, bright shiny complexion, scanty and pale urination, aversion to wind, fever, cough, slight breathlessness (Fig. 35.15).
Tongue: sticky white coating.
Pulse: Floating-Slippery.
Key symptoms: sudden swelling of face, aversion to Wind, Floating-Slippery pulse.

> **Diagnostic tip**
>
> Aversion to cold and 'fever' are the cardinal manifestations of external invasion of Wind

Aetiology

This is due to exposure to exterior Wind-Cold and Dampness.

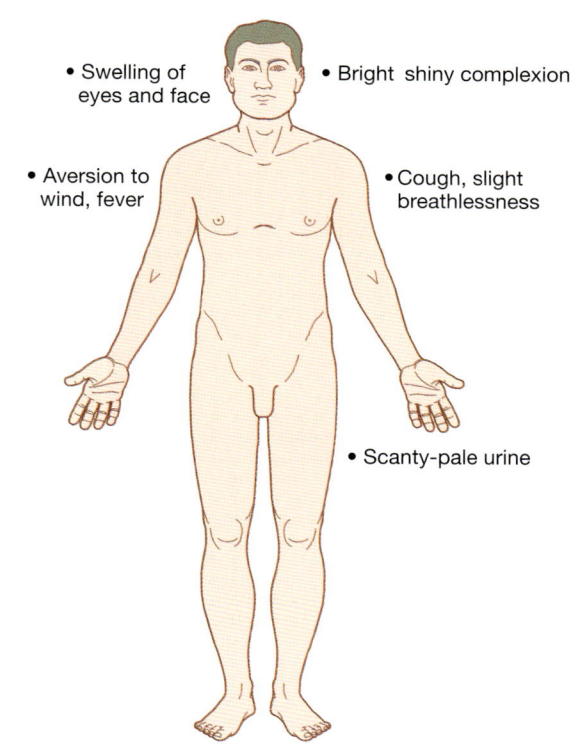

Figure 35.15 Invasion of Lungs by Wind-Water

- Swelling of eyes and face
- Bright shiny complexion
- Aversion to wind, fever
- Cough, slight breathlessness
- Scanty-pale urine

Pathology

This is an exterior pattern due to attack of Wind-Cold and Dampness. It differs from a normal attack of Wind-Cold in that it impairs the Lung function of controlling Water passages, resulting in facial oedema.

Since the Lung-Defensive Qi portion is obstructed by the exterior Wind-Cold-Damp, the Lungs cannot direct fluids downwards: this also causes facial oedema and scanty urination.

The bright shiny complexion and pale urine reflect deficiency of Yang, as Defensive Qi is obstructed by the exterior Wind-Cold-Damp.

Aversion to wind is due to failure of Defensive Qi to warm the muscles. 'Aversion to wind' is basically the same as 'aversion to cold' except for a difference of degree of intensity, aversion to cold being stronger. Some doctors say that aversion to cold is experienced even indoors, whereas aversion to wind is only experienced outdoors.

The fever reflects the struggle between the Defensive Qi and the exterior Wind-Cold-Damp.

Invasion of Lungs by Wind-Water → Dampness in Spleen and/or Kidneys

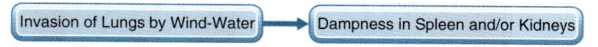

Figure 35.16 Invasion of Lungs by Wind-Water: precursors and developments

The cough and breathlessness are due to the impairment of the descending of Lung-Qi.

The sticky tongue coating reflects the presence of Dampness. The Slippery quality of the pulse also reflects Dampness. The Floating quality of the pulse reflects the presence of a pathogenic factor on the Exterior.

Pathological precursors of pattern

There are no pathological precursors to this pattern as it is due to an invasion of an exterior pathogenic factor (Fig. 35.16).

Pathological developments from pattern

As this pattern is characterized by Dampness, it may lead to the obstruction of the Spleen and/or Kidneys by Dampness (see Fig. 35.16).

Treatment

Principle of treatment: release the Exterior, expel Cold, resolve Dampness, restore the descending of Lung-Qi and open the Water passages.

Acupuncture

Points: LU-7 Lieque, L.I.-6 Pianli, L.I.-7 Wenli, L.I.-4 Hegu, BL-12 Fengmen, Ren-9 Shuifen, BL-13 Feishu, Du-26 Renzhong.

Method: reducing method.

Explanation

- LU-7 releases the Exterior, stimulates the descending of Lung-Qi and opens the Water passages.
- L.I.-6 opens the Lung Water passages.
- L.I.-7 is the Accumulation point of the Large Intestine channel and is used for acute conditions.
- L.I.-4 releases the Exterior and opens the Water passages.
- BL-12 and BL-13 release the Exterior and stimulate the descending of Lung-Qi.
- Ren-9 opens the Water passages and resolves oedema.
- Du-26 (also called Shuigou, which means 'water ditch') opens the Water passages of the Upper Burner.

Herbal formula

Xiao Qing Long Tang *Small Green Dragon Decoction*.

Box 35.8 summarizes invasion of Lungs by Wind-Water.

Box 35.8 Invasion of the Lungs by Wind-Water

Clinical manifestations

Sudden swelling of eyes and face gradually spreading to the whole body, bright shiny complexion, scanty and pale urination, aversion to wind, fever, cough, slight breathlessness, sticky white tongue coating, Floating-Slippery pulse

Treatment

LU-7 Lieque, L.I.-6 Pianli, L.I.-7 Wenli, L.I.-4 Hegu, BL-12 Fengmen, Ren-9 Shuifen, BL-13 Feishu, Du-26 Renzhong

---

FULL PATTERNS: INTERIOR

Lung-Heat

Clinical manifestations

Cough, slight breathlessness, feeling of heat, chest ache, flaring of nostrils, thirst, red face (Fig. 35.17).
Tongue: Red with yellow coating.
Pulse: Overflowing-Rapid.
Key symptoms: cough, feeling of heat, thirst, Red tongue with yellow coating.

> **Diagnostic tip**
>
> A cough with feeling of heat and red tongue are enough to diagnose Lung-Heat

Aetiology

Lung-Heat may be either acute or chronic. When it is acute, it usually derives from an invasion of external Wind that becomes internal and turns into Heat.

Chronic Lung-Heat may be either a residual Heat or it may derive from the combination of a diet rich in hot foods together with smoking (as tobacco has a hot and drying nature).

Pathology

Heat in the Lungs impairs the descending of Lung-Qi and it causes cough and breathlessness. There are general symptoms of Heat such as thirst, red face and a feeling of heat. Obstruction of the chest by Heat causes the ache in the chest.

- Flaring of nostrils
- Thirst
- Feeling of heat
- Red face
- Cough, slight breathlessness, chest ache

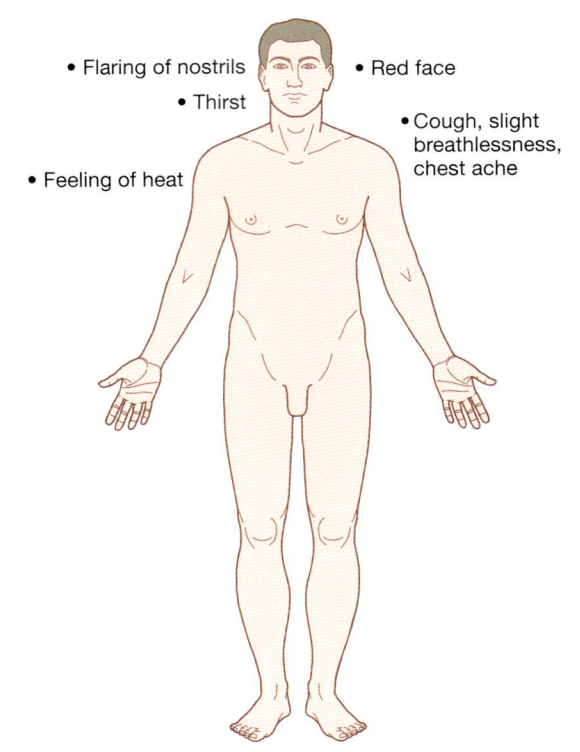

Figure 35.17 Lung-Heat

Flaring of the nostrils is caused by Lung-Heat as the Lungs opens into the nose: this symptom is seen only in acute cases.

In acute cases of Lung-Heat, there is usually also a fever and this pattern corresponds to the Heat in the Lungs pattern within the Qi Level of the Identification of Patterns according to the Four Levels (ch. 45).

In chronic cases, this pattern is usually due to retention of a residual pathogenic factor. This occurs when a person is subject to an invasion of external Wind, appears to recover (often after the use of antibiotics), but there is a leftover Heat in the Lungs (in the Interior). This often manifests with a red colour in the front part of the tongue (Lung area).

Pathological precursors of pattern

Lung-Heat may derive from an exterior pathogenic factor that penetrates the Interior and turns into Heat (Fig. 35.18).

Pathological developments from pattern

Lung-Heat dries up the fluids and it may lead to Lung-Yin deficiency (see Fig. 35.18).

External Wind → Lung-Heat → Lung-Yin deficiency

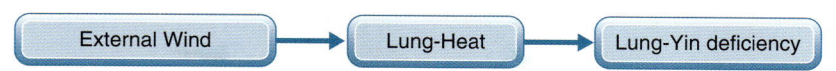

Figure 35.18 Lung-Heat pattern: precursors and developments

Treatment

Principle of treatment: clear Lung-Heat, restore the descending of Lung-Qi.

Acupuncture
Points: LU-5 Chize, LU-10 Yuji, LU-7 Lieque, L.I.-11 Quchi, LU-1 Zhongfu, BL-13 Feshu.
Method: reducing method, no moxa.
Explanation
- LU-5 and LU-10 clear Lung-Heat.
- LU-7 restores the descending of Lung-Qi.
- L.I.-11 clears Heat.
- LU-1 and BL-13 clear Lung-Heat and restore the descending of Lung-Qi.

Herbal formula
Ma Xing Shi Gan Tang *Ephedra–Prunus–Gypsum–Glycyrrhiza Decoction*.
Box 35.9 summarizes Lung-Heat.

Box 35.9 Lung-Heat

Clinical manifestations

Cough, slight breathlessness, feeling of heat, chest ache, flaring of nostrils, thirst, red face, Red tongue with yellow coating, Overflowing-Rapid pulse

Treatment

LU-5 Chize, LU-10 Yuji, LU-7 Lieque, L.I.-11 Quchi, LU-1 Zhongfu, BL-13 Feshu

---

Damp-Phlegm in the Lungs

Clinical manifestations

Chronic cough coming in bouts with profuse sticky white sputum which is easy to expectorate, white pasty complexion, phlegm in the throat, a feeling of oppression in the chest, shortness of breath, dislike of lying down, wheezing, nausea, a feeling of heaviness, muzziness (fuzziness) and dizziness of the head (Fig. 35.19).
Tongue: Swollen with a sticky white coating.
Pulse: Slippery or Soggy.

- Dizziness, muzziness, heaviness
- Pasty-white complexion
- Phlegm in throat
- Nausea
- Cough with profuse, sticky white sputum
- Feeling of oppression of the chest, shortness of breath, wheezing

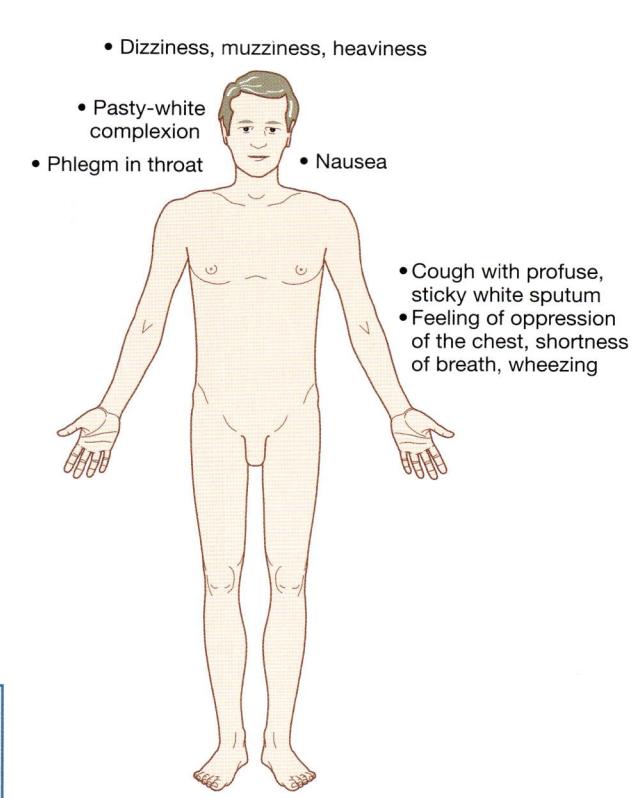

Figure 35.19 Damp-Phlegm in the Lungs

Key symptoms: chronic cough with profuse white sputum, thick sticky white tongue coating.

> **Diagnostic tip**
>
> A cough with profuse expectoration of sticky sputum is enough to diagnose Damp-Phlegm in the Lungs

> **Diagnostic tip**
>
> In all the Phlegm patterns of the Lungs, phlegm in the throat and a Swollen tongue would be enough to diagnose such patterns

Aetiology

Exterior pathogenic factors

Recurrent attacks of exterior pathogenic factors may weaken the Lungs and Spleen, leading to the formation of Phlegm, which settles in the Lungs.

Diet

Excessive consumption of dairy foods, greasy foods and/or cold and raw foods leads to the formation of Phlegm and can therefore contribute to the arousal of this pattern.

Pathology

This is a Full pattern of a chronic nature. From the Eight-Principle point of view, it is an Excess-Interior-Cold pattern. It is characterized by the presence of Phlegm retained in the Lungs. This Phlegm is associated with or deriving from Dampness. The Dampness 'quality' of this type of Phlegm is manifested by the stickiness of the coating and by the fact that the sputum is expectorated easily.

However, this is seldom a purely Excess pattern because the Phlegm usually arises from a chronic dysfunction of the Spleen in transforming and transporting fluids, which accumulate to form Phlegm. As mentioned before, the Spleen produces Phlegm and the Lungs store it.

The presence of Phlegm is clearly indicated by the profuse sputum and the feeling of oppression of the chest.

Phlegm obstructs the Lungs and impairs the descending of Lung-Qi, hence the cough and shortness of breath. Inability to lie down is due to the obstruction of the Upper Burner by Phlegm. The patient dislikes lying flat and prefers to sit up or lie propped up because the obstruction of Phlegm in the chest is made worse by the horizontal position. This is a typical sign of a Full pattern.

The white complexion reflects deficiency of Yang of the Spleen and Lung, whilst its pasty quality reflects the presence of Phlegm and Dampness.

The feeling of oppression of the chest is caused by the obstruction of Phlegm in the chest and it is a typical, distinctive symptom of Phlegm.

The feelings of muzziness and heaviness of the head and dizziness are caused by obstruction of the head's orifices by Phlegm.

The swelling of the tongue reflects the presence of Phlegm, while the stickiness of the tongue coating reflects the Dampness.

The Pulse would be Slippery in a purely Full pattern when the person's Qi is not weakened. However, in chronic cases, when the person's Qi has been weakened, the Pulse would be Soggy, reflecting the presence of Dampness and weakness of Qi.

This pattern can be acute or chronic. In acute cases, it usually follows an invasion of Wind in the Lungs that is not treated properly and the patient develops an acute cough with profuse sputum. In chronic cases, it derives from a deficiency of the Spleen, leading to Dampness and Phlegm that are stored in the Lungs.

Pathological precursors of pattern

A deficiency of Spleen-Qi or Spleen-Yang is usually a precondition for the arousal of this pattern because it predisposes the patient to the formation of Dampness and/or Phlegm.

In the elderly, a deficiency of Kidney-Yang is also a frequent precursor of this pattern (Fig. 35.20).

Pathological developments from pattern

Although a Spleen deficiency is often the precursor of this pattern, this pattern itself may also aggravate a

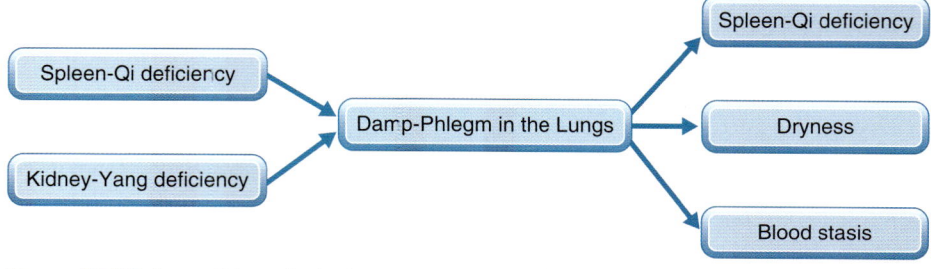

Figure 35.20 Damp-Phlegm in the Lungs: precursors and developments

Spleen deficiency because of the obstruction of the Spleen by Dampness and Phlegm.

Long-term retention of Phlegm, especially in the elderly, may lead to Dryness. Also in the elderly, Phlegm may either lead to or aggravate Blood stasis (see Fig. 35.20).

Treatment

Principle of treatment: resolve Dampness and Phlegm, restore the descending of Lung-Qi.

Acupuncture

Points: LU-5 Chize, LU-7 Lieque, LU-1 Zhongfu, Ren-17 Shanzhong, ST-40 Fenglong, P-6 Neiguan, Ren-22 Tiantu, Ren-12 Zhongwan, BL-20 Pishu, Ren-9 Shuifen, BL-13 Feishu.

Method: reducing method on all points except BL-20 Pishu and Ren-12 Zhongwan, which should be reinforced.

Explanation
– LU-5 expels Phlegm from the Lungs.
– LU-7 restores the descending of Lung-Qi and stops cough.
– LU-1 stops cough, restores the descending of Lung-Qi and resolves Phlegm.
– Ren-17 restores the descending of Lung-Qi.
– ST-40 resolves Phlegm.
– P-6 opens the chest and expels Phlegm from the chest.
– Ren-22 expels Phlegm from the throat and LU-7 restores the descending of Lung-Qi and stops cough.
– Ren-12 and BL-20 tonify the Spleen to resolve Phlegm.
– Ren-9 stimulates the Spleen's function of transformation and transportation and resolves Dampness and Phlegm.
– BL-13 restores the descending of Lung-Qi.

Herbal formula

Er Chen Tang *Two Old Decoction*.
Box 35.10 summarizes Damp-Phlegm in the Lungs.

Three Treasures

Limpid Sea (variation of Er Chen Tang).

Box 35.10 Damp-Phlegm in the Lungs

Clinical manifestations

Chronic cough coming in bouts with profuse sticky white sputum which is easy to expectorate, white pasty complexion, a feeling of oppression in the chest, phlegm in the throat, shortness of breath, dislike of lying down, wheezing, nausea, a feeling of heaviness, muzziness and dizziness of the head, Swollen tongue with a sticky white coating, Slippery or Soggy pulse

Treatment

LU-5 Chize, LU-7 Lieque, LU-1 Zhongfu, Ren-17 Shanzhong, ST-40 Fenglong, P-6 Neiguan, Ren-22 Tiantu, Ren-12 Zhongwan, Ren-9 Shuifen, BL-20 Pishu, BL-13 Feishu

---

Cold-Phlegm in the Lungs

Clinical manifestations

Cough with expectoration of white, watery sputum, aggravated by exposure to cold, feeling cold, cold hands, phlegm in the throat, dizziness, a feeling of oppression of the chest, a feeling of cold of the chest, a feeling of heaviness, muzziness and dizziness of the head (Fig. 35.21).

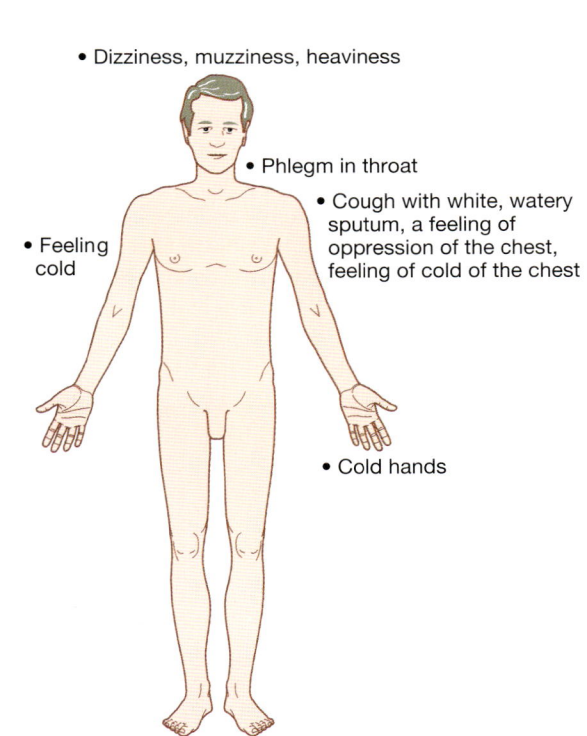

Figure 35.21 Cold-Phlegm in the Lungs

Tongue: Swollen and wet tongue with a sticky white coating.
Pulse: Slippery-Slow.
Key symptoms: cough with white, watery sputum, phlegm in throat, Swollen tongue with sticky white coating.

> **Diagnostic tip**
>
> A cough with expectoration of white, watery sputum is enough to diagnose Cold-Phlegm in the Lungs

Aetiology

External pathogenic factors
Repeated invasions of Wind-Cold may weaken the Lungs and Spleen and lead to the formation of Cold-Phlegm. This would happen particularly if the person has a pre-existing Yang-deficiency constitution.

Diet
Excessive consumption of dairy foods, cold and raw foods and iced drinks may lead to Cold-Phlegm.

Pathology
The pathology of this pattern is similar to the previous one of Damp-Phlegm in the Lungs. The main difference lies in the character of the Phlegm: in this case, Phlegm is associated with Cold. This makes the sputum white and watery and causes the cold symptoms of cold hands, cold feeling and feeling of cold of the chest.

The sputum in the throat and feeling of oppression of the chest are typical of Phlegm. Dizziness, a feeling of heaviness and muzziness of the head are caused by the obstruction of the head orifices by Phlegm.

Pathological precursors of pattern
A deficiency of Spleen-Yang is usually a precondition for the arousal of this pattern because it predisposes the patient to the formation of Dampness and/or Phlegm.

In the elderly, a deficiency of Kidney-Yang is also a frequent precursor of this pattern (Fig. 35.22).

Pathological developments from pattern
Although a Spleen deficiency is often the precursor of this pattern, this pattern itself may also aggravate a Spleen deficiency because of the obstruction of the Spleen by Dampness and Phlegm.

Long-term retention of Phlegm, especially in the elderly, may lead to Dryness. Also in the elderly, Phlegm may either lead to or aggravate Blood stasis (see Fig. 35.22).

Treatment
Principle of treatment: resolve Phlegm, expel Cold, warm Yang, restore the descending of Lung-Qi.

Acupuncture
Points: LU-5 Chize, LU-7 Lieque, LU-1 Zhongfu, Ren-17 Shanzhong, ST-40 Fenglong, P-6 Neiguan, Ren-22 Tiantu, Ren-12 Zhongwan, BL-20 Pishu, Ren-9 Shuifen, BL-13 Feishu, BL-23 Shenshu.
Method: reducing method on all points except BL-20 Pishu, Ren-12 Zhongwan and BL-23 Shenshu, which should be reinforced. Moxa should be used.
Explanation
– LU-5 expels Phlegm from the Lungs.
– LU-7 restores the descending of Lung-Qi and stops cough.
– LU-1 stops cough, restores the descending of Lung-Qi and resolves Phlegm.
– Ren-17 restores the descending of Lung-Qi.
– ST-40 resolves Phlegm.
– P-6 opens the chest and expels Phlegm from the chest.

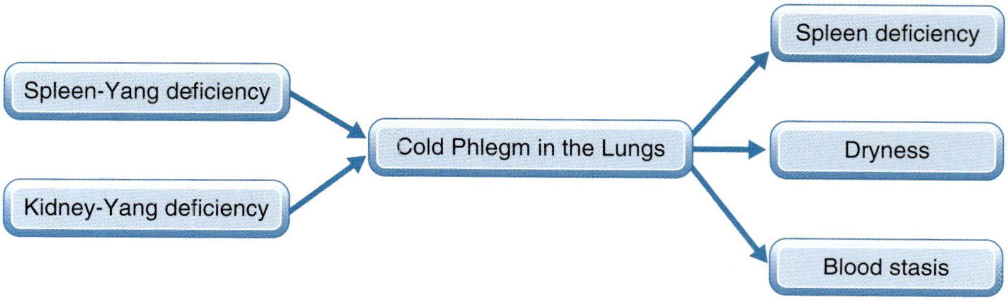

Figure 35.22 Cold-Phlegm in the Lungs: precursors and developments

- Ren-22 expels Phlegm from the throat and LU-7 restores the descending of Lung-Qi and stops cough.
- Ren-12 and BL-20 tonify the Spleen to resolve Phlegm.
- Ren-9 stimulates the Spleen's function of transformation and transportation and resolves Phlegm.
- BL-13 restores the descending of Lung-Qi.
- BL-23 is reinforced to tonify Kidney-Yang.

Herbal formula

She Gan Ma Huang Tang *Belamcanda–Ephedra Decoction.*

Ling Gui Zhu Gan Tang *Poria–Ramulus Cinnamomi–Atractylodis–Glycyrrhiza Decoction.*

Ling Gan Wu Wei Jiang Xin Tang *Poria–Glycyrrhiza–Schisandra–Zingiberis–Asarum Decoction.*

San Zi Yang Qin Tang *Three-Seed Nourishing the Ancestors Decoction.*

Box 35.11 summarizes Cold-Phlegm in the Lungs.

Box 35.11 Cold-Phlegm in the Lungs

Clinical manifestations

Cough with expectoration of white, watery sputum, aggravated by exposure to cold, feeling cold, cold hands, phlegm in the throat, dizziness, a feeling of oppression of the chest, a feeling of cold of the chest, a feeling of heaviness, muzziness and dizziness of the head, Swollen and wet tongue with a sticky white coating, Slippery-Slow pulse

Treatment

LU-5 Chize, LU-7 Lieque, LU-1 Zhongfu, Ren-17 Shanzhong, ST-40 Fenglong, P-6 Neiguan, Ren-22 Tiantu, Ren-12 Zhongwan, Ren-9 Shuifen, BL-20 Pishu, BL-13 Feishu, BL-23 Shenshu

---

Phlegm-Heat in the Lungs

Clinical manifestations

Barking cough with profuse sticky yellow or green sputum, shortness of breath, wheezing, a feeling of oppression of the chest, phlegm in the throat, a feeling of heat, thirst, insomnia, agitation, a feeling of heaviness and muzziness (fuzziness) of the head, dizziness (Fig. 35.23).

Tongue: Red, Swollen with a sticky yellow coating.
Pulse: Slippery-Rapid.
Key symptoms: cough, yellow or green sputum, thick sticky yellow coating, Rapid-Slippery pulse.

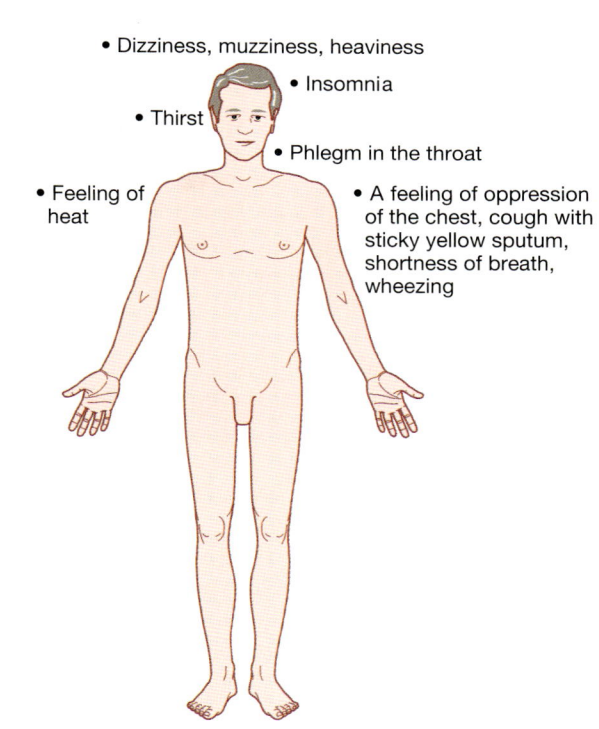

Figure 35.23 Phlegm-Heat in the Lungs

- Dizziness, muzziness, heaviness
- Insomnia
- Thirst
- Phlegm in the throat
- Feeling of heat
- A feeling of oppression of the chest, cough with sticky yellow sputum, shortness of breath, wheezing

Diagnostic tip

A barking cough with expectoration of sticky yellow sputum is enough to diagnose Phlegm-Heat in the Lungs

Aetiology

Diet

This pattern can be due to excessive consumption of greasy and hot foods (such as fried meats, alcohol, greasy and pungent foods), leading to the formation of Phlegm and Heat.

Irregular eating disrupts the ascending of Spleen-Qi and descending of Stomach-Qi, leading to the formation of Phlegm.

Life habits

Smoking can also be a factor leading to the pattern, since tobacco has a hot and dry energy from the point of view of Chinese medicine. On the one hand, the hot energy of tobacco leads to Heat and, on the other, the drying effect of tobacco condenses the Body Fluids into Phlegm.

Exterior pathogenic factors

This pattern can also be precipitated or aggravated by invasion of exterior Wind-Heat. Phlegm-Heat in the Lung is often the consequence of an invasion of Wind going from the Defensive Qi to the Qi Level.

In chronic conditions, Phlegm-Heat in the Lungs is a residual pathogenic factor remaining after an invasion of Wind. This is very common in children.

Emotional stress

Anger, frustration and resentment lead to Qi stagnation, which, in turn may lead to the formation of Heat.

Pathology

This is a chronic condition, similar to the previous one of Damp-Phlegm, but accompanied by Heat. In chronic conditions, Phlegm can easily combine with Heat. The underlying condition is also in this case a deficiency of Spleen-Qi leading to the formation of Phlegm.

From the Eight-Principle point of view, this is an Excess-Hot-Interior condition. In acute cases, this pattern is seen frequently when exterior Wind (usually Wind-Heat) is not expelled and it penetrates the Interior, transforming into Heat. The disruption from external Wind impairs the Qi Mechanism and leads to the production of Phlegm. Phlegm-Heat settles in the Lungs and causes an acute chest infection, often with a fever.

In chronic cases, Phlegm results from a dysfunction of the Lungs, Spleen and Kidneys and the pattern of Phlegm-Heat is seen more in middle-aged or elderly people. In chronic cases, Phlegm-Heat in the Lungs is frequently a residual pathogenic factor remaining after an invasion of Wind.

Pathological precursors of pattern

A deficiency of Spleen-Qi is usually a precondition for the arousal of this pattern because it predisposes the patient to the formation of Dampness and/or Phlegm.

In the elderly, a deficiency of the Kidneys is also a frequent precursor of this pattern. Long-term Qi stagnation may lead to Heat and contribute to the formation of this pattern (Fig. 35.24).

Pathological developments from pattern

Although a Spleen deficiency is often the precursor of this pattern, the pattern itself may also aggravate a Spleen deficiency because of the obstruction of the Spleen by Dampness and Phlegm.

Long-term retention of Phlegm, especially in the elderly, may lead to Dryness. Also in the elderly, Phlegm may either lead to or aggravate Blood stasis.

The Heat part of Phlegm-Heat may dry up the Body Fluids and lead to Yin deficiency (see Fig. 35.24).

Treatment

Principle of treatment: resolve Phlegm, clear Heat, stimulate the descending of Lung-Qi.

Acupuncture

Points: LU-5 Chize, LU-7 Lieque, LU-10 Yuji, L.I.-11 Quchi, LU-1 Zhongfu, BL-13 Feishu, Ren-12 Zhongwan, ST-40 Fenglong.

Method: reducing method, except for Ren-12, which should be needled with even method.

Explanation
 – LU-5 clears Heat and Phlegm from the Lungs.
 – LU-7 restores the descending of Lung-Qi and stops cough.
 – LU-10 clears Heat from the Lung.
 – L.I.-11 clears Heat.
 – LU-1 restores the descending of Lung-Qi and clears Lung-Heat.
 – BL-13 clears Lung-Heat.
 – Ren-12 resolves Phlegm (with even method).
 – ST-40 resolves Phlegm.

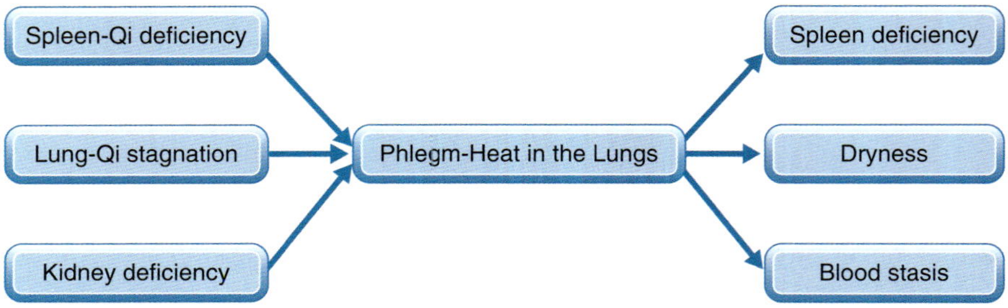

Figure 35.24 Phlegm-Heat in the Lungs pattern: precursors and developments

Herbal formula

Wen Dan Tang *Warming the Gall Bladder Decoction*.
Qing Qi Hua Tan Tang *Clearing Qi and Resolving Phlegm Decoction*.

Three Treasures

Clear the Soul (variation of Wen Dan Tang).
Ringing Metal (variation of Qing Qi Hua Tan Tang).
Box 35.12 summarizes Phlegm-Heat in the Lungs.

Box 35.12 Phlegm-Heat in the Lungs

Clinical manifestations

Barking cough with profuse sticky yellow or green sputum, shortness of breath, wheezing, a feeling of oppression of the chest, phlegm in the throat, a feeling of heat, thirst, insomnia, agitation, a feeling of heaviness and muzziness of the head, dizziness, Red, Swollen tongue with a sticky yellow coating, Slippery-Rapid pulse

Treatment

LU-5 Chize, LU-7 Lieque, LU-10 Yuji, L.I.-11 Quchi, LU-1 Zhongfu, BL-13 Feishu, Ren-12 Zhongwan, ST-40 Fenglong

---

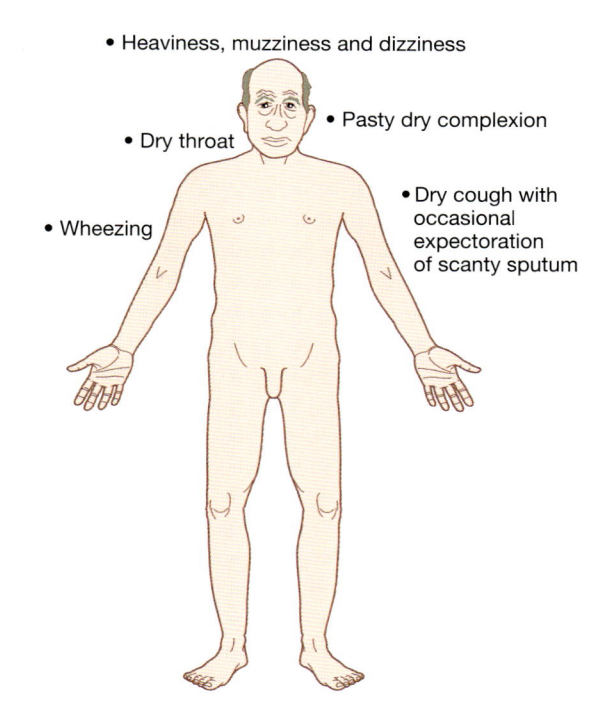

Figure 35.25 Dry-Phlegm in the Lungs
- Heaviness, muzziness and dizziness
- Pasty dry complexion
- Dry throat
- Dry cough with occasional expectoration of scanty sputum
- Wheezing

Dry-Phlegm in the Lungs

Clinical manifestations

Dry cough but with occasional, difficult expectoration of scanty sputum, shortness of breath, a feeling of oppression of the chest, scanty phlegm in the throat, a feeling of heaviness and muzziness of the head, dizziness, dry throat, wheezing, pasty dry complexion (Fig. 35.25).
Tongue: Swollen with a dry sticky coating or without coating.
Pulse: Fine-Slippery.
Key symptoms: Dry cough with occasional expectoration of scanty sputum, a feeling of oppression of the chest.

Diagnostic tip

A dry cough with difficult expectoration of scanty phlegm is enough to diagnose Dry-Phlegm in the Lungs.

Aetiology

Diet

The excessive consumption of greasy foods and dairy foods can lead to the formation of Phlegm. Irregular eating over many years can also lead to the formation of Phlegm, irrespective of what one eats.

Pathology

Dry-Phlegm usually occurs only in the elderly. It is always the result of a rather long pathological process. Dry-Phlegm is formed either because Phlegm leads to Dryness or because Phlegm occurs in a patient with a pre-existing Yin deficiency. Dryness and Phlegm may seem contradictory but they are not because Phlegm is an accumulation of *pathological* fluids while Dryness is a deficiency of *physiological* fluids.

A typical symptom of Dry-Phlegm is a dry cough with the occasional, difficult expectoration of scanty sputum. There are all the clinical manifestations of Phlegm such as feeling of oppression of the chest, scanty phlegm in the throat, a feeling of heaviness and muzziness of the head, dizziness.

Dryness causes a dry throat and dry tongue.

Pathological precursors of pattern

Phlegm itself (which may be Damp-Phlegm, Cold-Phlegm or Phlegm-Heat) may lead to Dryness when it persists for years (Fig. 35.26).

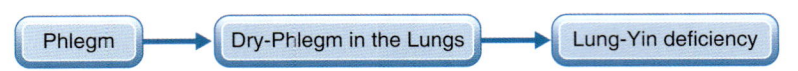

Figure 35.26 Dry-Phlegm in the Lungs pattern: precursors and developments

Phlegm → Dry-Phlegm in the Lungs → Lung-Yin deficiency

Pathological developments from pattern

The pattern of Dry-Phlegm may lead to full-blown Lung-Yin deficiency combined with Phlegm (see Fig. 35.26).

Treatment

Principle of treatment: resolve Phlegm, nourish fluids, nourish Lung-Yin, restore the descending of Lung-Qi.

Acupuncture

Points: LU-9 Taiyuan, LU-7 Lieque and KI-6 Zhaohai in combination, Ren-12 Zhongwan, ST-36 Zusanli, SP-6 Sanyinjiao, ST-40 Fenglong, BL-13 Feishu, Ren-17 Shanzhong.
Method: reinforcing on the points that nourish fluids and Lung-Yin, reducing on the others. No moxa.
Explanation
 – LU-9 nourishes Lung-Yin.
 – LU-7 restores the descending of Lung-Qi.
 – LU-7 and KI-6 in combination open the Directing Vessel (*Ren Mai*) and nourish Yin.
 – Ren-12, ST-36 and SP-6 nourish fluids.
 – ST-40 resolves Phlegm.
 – BL-13 and Ren-17 restore the descending of Lung-Qi.

Herbal formula

Bei Mu Gua Lou San *Fritillaria–Trichosanthes Powder*. Box 35.13 summarizes Dry-Phlegm in the Lungs.

Box 35.13 Dry-Phlegm in the Lungs

Clinical manifestations

Dry cough but with occasional, difficult expectoration of scanty sputum, shortness of breath, a feeling of oppression of the chest, scanty phlegm in the throat, a feeling of heaviness and muzziness of the head, dizziness, dry throat, wheezing, pasty dry complexion, Swollen tongue with a dry sticky coating, Fine-Slippery pulse

Treatment

LU-9 Taiyuan, LU-7 Lieque and KI-6 Zhaohai in combination, Ren-12 Zhongwan, ST-36 Zusanli, SP-6 Sanyinjiao, ST-40 Fenglong, BL-13 Feishu, Ren-17 Shanzhong

---

Phlegm-Fluids obstructing the Lungs

Clinical manifestations

Cough with expectoration of white, watery sputum, breathlessness, splashing sound in the chest, vomiting of white, watery, frothy sputum, a feeling of oppression of the chest, a feeling of heaviness and muzziness of the head, dizziness, feeling cold, coughing which may be elicited by a scare (Fig. 35.27).
Tongue: Pale with thick sticky white coating.
Pulse: Fine-Slippery or Soggy or Wiry.
Key symptoms: cough with white, watery, frothy sputum.

> **Diagnostic tip**
>
> A cough with the expectoration of white, watery, foamy sputum in an elderly person is enough to diagnose Phlegm-Fluids in the Lungs

- Heaviness, muzziness, dizziness
- Vomiting of white, watery fluids
- Cough with expectoration of white, watery, frothy sputum, splashing sound in chest, feeling of oppression of the chest
- Feeling cold

Figure 35.27 Phlegm-Fluids in the Lungs

```
Spleen-, Lung- and          Phlegm-Fluids           'Water overflowing
Kidney-Yang deficiency  →   obstructing the Lungs  →  to the Heart'
```

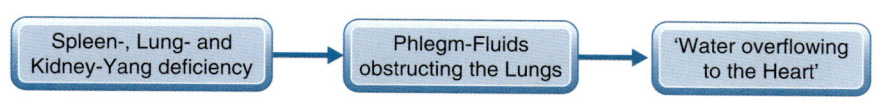

Figure 35.28 Phlegm-Fluids obstructing the Lungs pattern: precursors and developments

Aetiology

Diet

The excessive consumption of greasy foods and dairy foods can lead to the formation of Phlegm.

Excessive physical work

Excessive physical work weakens Spleen- and Kidney-Yang: this leads to the formation of Phlegm.

Pathology

This is a chronic condition of Phlegm in the Lungs. This pattern is characterized by a particular kind of Phlegm which is very watery, dilute and frothy. I call this 'Phlegm-Fluids' (*Tan Yin*): it always indicates that the condition is chronic and that the body is weak. It is also characterized by deficiency of Yang of the Spleen, Lungs and Kidneys (hence the cold feeling and Pale tongue-body).

This pattern is usually only seen in the elderly.

Pathological precursors of pattern

The underlying condition for this pattern is a chronic deficiency of Yang of the Spleen, Lungs and Kidneys (Fig. 35.28).

Pathological developments from pattern

Phlegm-Fluids are particularly obstructive and they aggravate the Yang deficiency of the Spleen, Lungs and Kidneys.

Phlegm-Fluids may, in particular, obstruct Heart-Yang and lead to the pattern of 'Water overflowing to the Heart' (see under Kidney patterns, ch. 37) (see Fig. 35.28).

Treatment

Principle of treatment: resolve Phlegm, tonify Spleen-, Lung- and Kidney-Yang.

Acupuncture

Points: LU-5 Chize, LU-9 Taiyuan, Ren-17 Shanzhong, BL-13 Feishu, ST-40 Fenglong, BL-43 Gaohuangshu, Ren-12 Zhongwan, ST-36 Zusanli, Ren-9 Shuifen, SP-9 Yinlingquan, BL-20 Pishu and BL-23 Shenshu.

Method: reducing on LU-5, ST-40, SP-9 and Ren-9; even on BL-13, Ren-17 and LU-5; tonifying on all the other points. Moxa is applicable.

Explanation
- LU-5 clears Phlegm from the Lungs.
- LU-9 tonifies Lung-Qi and resolves Phlegm. It is particularly indicated for chronic conditions.
- Ren-17 restores the descending of Lung-Qi.
- BL-13 restores the descending of Lung-Qi.
- ST-40 resolves Phlegm.
- BL-43 tonifies Lung-Qi and is indicated in chronic conditions.
- Ren-12 resolves Phlegm.
- ST-36 and BL-20 tonify Spleen-Qi.
- Ren-9 resolves Phlegm by promoting the transformation and transportation of fluids.
- BL-23 tonifies Kidney-Yang

Herbal formula

Ling Gan Wu Wei Jiang Xin Tang *Poria–Glycyrrhiza–Schisandra–Zingiberis–Asarum Decoction*.

Box 35.14 summarizes Phlegm-Fluids in the Lungs.

Box 35.14 Phlegm-Fluids in the Lungs

Clinical manifestations

Cough with expectoration of white, watery sputum, breathlessness, splashing sound in the chest, vomiting of white, watery, frothy sputum, a feeling of oppression of the chest, a feeling of heaviness and muzziness of the head, dizziness, feeling cold, coughing which may be elicited by a scare, Pale tongue with thick sticky white coating, Fine-Slippery or Soggy or Wiry pulse

Treatment

LU-5 Chize, LU-9 Taiyuan, Ren-17 Shanzhong, BL-13 Feishu, ST-40 Fenglong, BL-43 Gaohuangshu, Ren-12 Zhongwan, ST-36 Zusanli, Ren-9 Shuifen, SP-9 Yinlingquan, BL-20 Pishu and BL-23 Shenshu

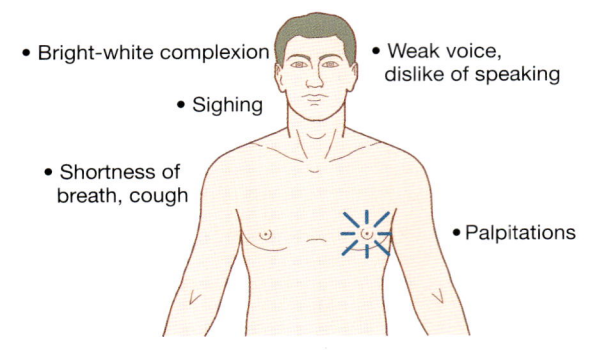

Figure 35.29 Heart- and Lung-Qi deficiency

COMBINED PATTERNS

Lung- and Heart-Qi deficiency

Clinical manifestations

Slight shortness of breath, slight cough, weak voice, dislike of speaking, bright-white complexion, propensity to catch colds, tiredness, palpitations, depression, spontaneous sweating, sighing (Fig. 35.29).
Tongue: Pale.
Pulse: Empty, especially on both Front positions.

Aetiology

Emotional problems

Emotional problems, particularly from sadness or grief, can lead to deficiency of Heart-Qi. The same emotions and worry can lead to Lung-Qi deficiency.

Overwork

Overwork may injure Qi of the Heart and Lungs: this is especially likely to happen if the person is in an occupation requiring constant use of the voice (e.g. teachers). A Qi deficiency is the first pathological consequence of overwork as, in the long run, this will end by causing Yin deficiency.

> **Clinical note**
>
> A simultaneous deficiency of Lung- and Heart-Qi is seen frequently when the patient is affected by emotional problems such as sadness and grief

Pathology

The pathology of Heart-Qi deficiency has already been described in chapter 32 and that of Lung-Qi deficiency has been discussed above.

A simultaneous deficiency of both Heart-Qi and Lung-Qi is very common and it occurs especially when the patient is subject to emotional stress.

The slight shortness of breath and cough are due to deficient Lung-Qi not descending: this is only a slight shortness of breath.

The Lungs control the voice (also through their influence on Gathering Qi) and when the Lungs are deficient the voice is weak and the patient dislikes talking.

The Lungs diffuse Defensive Qi in the space between skin and muscles, which determines a person's resistance to pathogenic factors: when Lung-Qi is deficient, it does not diffuse Defensive Qi adequately, Defensive Qi does not circulate properly in the space between skin and muscles and this space is easily invaded by external pathogenic factors.

There is an overlap in the clinical manifestation of spontaneous sweating as this can be due either to deficient Lung-Qi not consolidating Body Fluids in the space between skin and muscles or to deficient Heart-Qi not holding sweat.

Pathological precursors of pattern

Kidney-Qi deficiency may be a precursor of this pattern (Fig. 35.30).

Pathological developments from pattern

Heart-Qi and Lung-Qi deficiency may lead to Heart-Blood deficiency as the deficient Qi fails to make enough Blood.

Especially when emotional stress is the cause of the condition, Heart-Qi and Lung-Qi deficiency may lead to Qi stagnation in the chest as the deficient Qi fails to move in the chest. As mentioned above, Qi deficiency and Qi stagnation can occur simultaneously. In the long-term, stagnation of Qi in the chest may lead to Blood stasis in the chest (see Fig. 35.30).

Treatment

Principle of treatment: tonify Qi, strengthen the Heart and the Lungs, calm the Mind.

Acupuncture

Points: LU-9 Taiyuan, LU-7 Lieque, Ren-6 Qihai, BL-13 Feishu, Du-12 Shenzhu, ST-36 Zusanli, Ren-12 Zhongwan, HE-5 Tongli, P-6 Neiguan, BL-15 Xinshu, Ren-17 Shanzhong.
Method: all with reinforcing method. Moxa can be used.

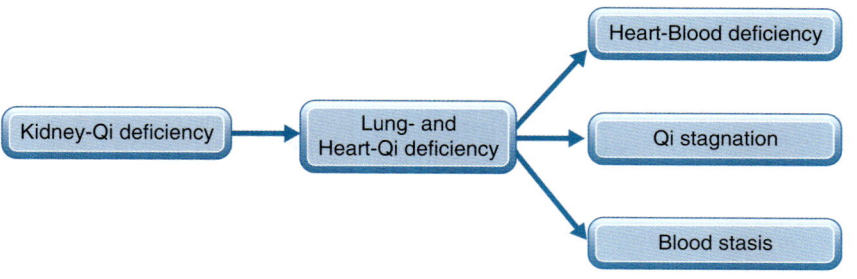

Figure 35.30 Heart- and Lung-Qi deficiency pattern: precursors and developments

---

Box 35.15 Heart- and Lung-Qi deficiency

Clinical manifestations

Slight shortness of breath, slight cough, weak voice, dislike of speaking, bright-white complexion, propensity to catch colds, tiredness, palpitations, shortness of breath on exertion, depression, spontaneous sweating, sighing, Pale tongue, Empty pulse

Treatment

LU-9 Taiyuan, LU-7 Lieque, Ren-6 Qihai, BL-13 Feishu, Du-12 Shenzhu, ST-36 Zusanli, Ren-12 Zhongwan, HE-5 Tongli, P-6 Neiguan, BL-15 Xinshu, Ren-17 Shanzhong

---

Explanation
- LU-9, LU-7, BL-13 and Du-12 tonify Lung-Qi.
- Ren-6 tonifies Qi in general but also specifically Lung-Qi (the Lung channel originates from that area).
- ST-36 and Ren-12 are used to tonify Qi in general. They also specifically help Lung-Qi because Earth is the Mother of Metal.
- HE-5, P-6 and BL-15 tonify Heart-Qi.
- Ren-17 tonifies the Gathering Qi (*Zong Qi*) and therefore both Lung- and Heart-Qi.

Herbal formula

Si Jun Zi Tang *Four Gentlemen Decoction plus Huang Qi Radix Astragali membranacei.*
Bao Yuan Tang *Preserving the Source Decoction.*
Bu Fei Tang *Tonifying the Lungs Decoction.*
Sheng Mai San *Generating the Pulse Powder.*

Box 35.15 summarizes Lung- and Heart-Qi deficiency.

Other combined patterns are:
- Lung-Qi and Kidney-Yang deficiency (see 'Kidney deficiency, Water overflowing to the Lungs' or 'Kidney failing to receive Qi' patterns in ch. 37)
- Lung- and Kidney-Yin deficiency (see under Kidney combined patterns, ch. 37)
- Liver-Fire insulting the Lungs (see under Liver combined patterns, ch. 34)
- Lung- and Spleen-Qi deficiency (see under Spleen combined patterns, ch. 36)

Learning outcomes

In this chapter you will have learned:
- How exterior Wind (combined with Heat or Cold) can invade the Lung Exterior portion to cause exterior patterns
- The effects of Dryness and Dampness on the Lungs
- The importance of diet in Lung disease, particularly Phlegm-forming foods
- How sadness, grief and worry can cause a Lung disharmony
- The significance of posture and smoking in the aetiology of Lung disharmonies
- How to identify the following Deficiency patterns:
  Lung-Qi deficiency: slight shortness of breath, a weak voice and an empty Lung pulse
  Lung-Yin deficiency: a dry cough, night sweating and a rootless tongue coating in the front area of the tongue
  Lung Dryness: dry cough, dry throat, a hoarse voice and a dry tongue
- How to identify the following Excess patterns:
  Exterior:
  Invasion of the Lungs by Wind-Cold: aversion to cold, sneezing, fever and a Floating pulse
  Invasion of the Lungs by Wind-Heat: aversion to cold, fever and a Floating-Rapid pulse
  Invasion of the Lungs by Wind-Water: aversion to Wind, sudden swelling of face and a Floating-Slippery pulse
  Interior:
  Lung-Heat: cough, feeling of heat and a Red tongue with a yellow coating
  Damp-Phlegm in the Lungs: chronic cough with profuse white sputum and a sticky white tongue coating

Continued

- *Cold-Phlegm in the Lungs*: cough with white, watery sputum, phlegm in the throat and a Swollen tongue with a sticky white coating
- *Phlegm-Heat in the Lungs*: barking cough with sticky yellow or green sputum
- *Dry-Phlegm in the Lungs*: dry cough with difficult expectoration of scanty phlegm
- *Phlegm-Fluids obstructing the Lungs*: cough with expectoration of white, watery, foamy sputum
- How to identify the following combined pattern:
  Lung- and Heart-Qi deficiency: shortness of breath, weak voice, palpitations and an Empty pulse
- Awareness of the following combinations of Lung patterns:
  Lung-Qi and Kidney-Yang deficiency
  Lung- and Kidney-Yin deficiency
  Liver-Fire insulting the Lungs
  Lung- and Spleen-Qi deficiency

Learning tips

Lung-Qi deficiency

- First, think of the general symptoms of Qi deficiency: tiredness, Empty pulse, Pale tongue
- Then add the Qi deficiency symptoms that are Lung-related, bearing in mind the influence of the Lungs on breathing and voice: slight shortness of breath, weak voice
- The Lungs influence the Defensive Qi: hence spontaneous sweating and propensity to catching cold

Lung-Yin deficiency

- First, think of the general symptoms of Yin deficiency: night sweating, dry mouth, tongue without coating, Floating-Empty pulse
- Remember that the Lungs influence breathing, voice and throat: dry cough, hoarse voice, dry throat

Lungs invaded by Wind

- First, remember the cardinal symptoms of invasion of exterior Wind: *simultaneous aversion to cold* and *fever*
- Lungs control breathing: cough
- The Lungs open into the nose: sneezing, nasal congestion
- When external Wind is involved, think always of invasion of the Greater-Yang channels, hence occipital stiffness and headache

Phlegm in the Lungs

- First, remember the general manifestations of Phlegm: a feeling of oppression of the chest, sputum in the throat, nausea, feeling of heaviness, dizziness, muzziness of the head, Swollen tongue with sticky coating and Slippery pulse
- In all Phlegm patterns of the Lungs there is cough with expectoration of sputum
- Differentiate the sputum, i.e. profuse and sticky in Damp-Phlegm, watery white in Cold-Phlegm and sticky yellow in Phlegm-Heat

Self-assessment questions

1. What is the main function of the Lungs?
2. Why are the Lungs sometimes called the 'delicate' organ?
3. How might patients be affected by Dryness in damp climates?
4. What kind of foods would encourage the formation of Phlegm in the Lungs?
5. What pulse picture might you expect in someone who has deficient Lung-Qi from long-term sadness and grief?
6. What life habits might contribute to Lung-Qi deficiency?
7. What are the key signs and symptoms for diagnosis of the pattern invasion of the Lungs by Wind-Cold?
8. What is the pathology of the symptom 'aversion to cold' in an exterior invasion?
9. Explain the swelling of the face in the pattern invasion of the Lungs by Wind-Water.
10. Which lifestyle factors would you wish to investigate in a patient presenting the pattern of Lung-Heat?
11. Which two clinical manifestations would show the presence of Phlegm in any Lung pattern?
12. Describe the various appearances of the sputum in the five Phlegm patterns of the Lungs.
13. What is the most common cause of Heart- and Lung-Qi deficiency?

See p. 1264 for answers

END NOTE

1. Nanjing College of Traditional Chinese Medicine, Shang Han Lun Research Group 1980 Discussion on Cold-induced Diseases (*Shang Han Lun* 伤寒论) by Zhang Zhong Jing, Shanghai Scientific Publishing House, Shanghai, first published c.AD 220.

Spleen Patterns

SECTION 2 PART 6

36

Key contents

General aetiology
Exterior pathogenic factors
Emotional strain
- Pensiveness
- Worry

Diet

Empty patterns
Spleen-Qi deficiency
Spleen-Yang deficiency
Spleen-Qi sinking
Spleen not controlling Blood
Spleen-Blood deficiency

Full patterns
Cold-Dampness invading the Spleen
Damp-Heat invading the Spleen

Combined patterns
Spleen- and Heart-Blood deficiency
Spleen- and Lung-Qi deficiency
Spleen- and Liver-Blood deficiency
Obstruction of Spleen by Dampness with stagnation of Liver-Qi
Spleen- and Stomach-Qi deficiency (discussed under Stomach patterns, ch. 38)

The Spleen's functions (ch. 9) are:

- Governs transformation and transportation
- Controls the ascending of Qi
- Controls Blood
- Controls the muscles and the four limbs
- Opens into the mouth
- Manifests in the lips
- Controls saliva
- Controls the raising of Qi
- Houses the Intellect (*Yi*)
- The Spleen is affected by pensiveness

The most important Spleen function is that of transporting and transforming food and fluids. Any Spleen disharmony will therefore always influence the digestive process, with such symptoms as abdominal distension, lack of appetite and loose stools.

The Spleen controls muscles and is responsible for transporting Food-Qi (*Gu Qi*) to the muscles throughout the body, and in particular to the four limbs. A disharmony in this sphere often causes tiredness, which is an extremely common symptom of Spleen deficiency.

Finally, the Spleen controls Blood and a weakness of Spleen-Qi often causes bleeding. This is a frequent Deficient-type cause of bleeding.

A 'feel' for spleen pathology

- Tiredness
- Digestive disorders
- Dull-yellow complexion
- Abdominal distension

The discussion of the Spleen patterns will be preceded by a discussion of the general aetiology of the Spleen's disharmonies as follows:
GENERAL AETIOLOGY
- Exterior pathogenic factors
- Emotional strain
  - Pensiveness
  - Worry
- Diet

The Spleen patterns discussed are:
EMPTY PATTERNS
- Spleen-Qi deficiency
- Spleen-Yang deficiency
- Spleen-Qi sinking
- Spleen not controlling Blood
- Spleen-Blood deficiency

FULL PATTERNS
- Cold-Dampness invading the Spleen
- Damp-Heat invading the Spleen

COMBINED PATTERNS
- Spleen- and Heart-Blood deficiency
- Spleen- and Lung-Qi deficiency
- Spleen- and Liver-Blood deficiency
- Obstruction of Spleen by Dampness with stagnation of Liver-Qi
- Spleen- and Stomach-Qi deficiency (discussed under Stomach patterns, ch. 38)

GENERAL AETIOLOGY

Exterior pathogenic factors

The Spleen is easily attacked by external Dampness. This can invade the body in different ways due to environmental circumstances or life habits, such as living in a damp area or a damp house, wearing wet clothes after swimming or exercising, sitting on damp surfaces, wading in water. Women are particularly prone to exterior Dampness especially at certain times of their life: namely, during puberty, during each period and after childbirth.[1]

An invasion of the Spleen by exterior Dampness will give rise to abdominal fullness, lack of appetite, nausea, a feeling of heaviness, a thick sticky tongue coating and a Slippery pulse.

Exterior Dampness can be combined with Heat or Cold, giving rise to symptoms of Damp-Heat or Cold-Dampness.

Exterior pathogenic factors as causes of disease are discussed in chapter 21.

> **Clinical note**
>
> Invasion of the Spleen by Dampness is an extremely common occurrence in practice. SP-9 Yinlingquan and SP-6 Sanyinjiao resolve Dampness

Emotional strain

Pensiveness

'Pensiveness' refers to thinking too much, brooding, thinking about the past and, in extreme cases, obsessive thinking. Pensiveness makes Qi stagnate and it affects primarily the Spleen but also the Lungs.[2] In certain circumstances when the patient's diet is irregular, pensiveness may lead to Spleen-Qi deficiency.

Included under the term of 'pensiveness' is also the excessive use of the mind in studying, concentrating and memorizing, which, over a long period of time, tends to weaken the Spleen.

Worry

Worry injures the Lungs primarily but also the Spleen. Worry 'knots' Qi, which means that it makes Qi stagnate, but, if the person's diet is irregular, it may also lead to Spleen-Qi deficiency. When it affects the Spleen, it will cause primarily stagnation in the digestive system with symptoms such as abdominal distension and pain.

Emotions as causes of disease are discussed in chapter 20.

Diet

Since the Spleen is in charge of transforming and transporting food, diet plays an extremely important role in Spleen disharmonies. The Spleen is said to prefer warm and dry foods. By 'warm' is meant warm in terms of both temperature and food energy. All foods can be classified as warm (or hot) or cool (or cold). Examples of warm foods are meat (and especially red meat) and most spices. Examples of cold foods are all raw foods (salads), fruit (with few exceptions), vegetables (with few exceptions) and icy-cold drinks.

An excessive consumption of cold foods will impair the Spleen transformation and transportation function, causing digestive problems and interior Dampness.

Diet as cause of disease is discussed in chapter 22.

Box 36.1 summarizes the general aetiology of Spleen patterns.

> **Box 36.1 General aetiology of Spleen patterns**
>
> - Exterior pathogenic factors
> - Emotional strain
>   - Pensiveness
>   - Worry
> - Diet

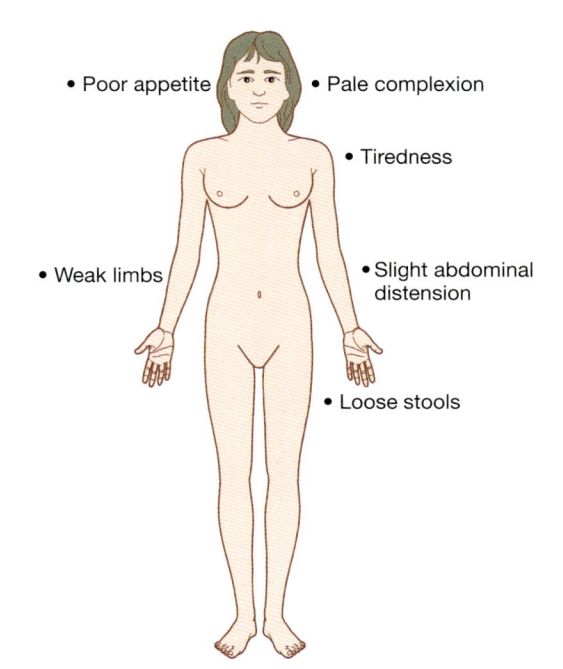

Figure 36.1 Spleen-Qi deficiency

Labels on figure:
- Poor appetite
- Pale complexion
- Tiredness
- Weak limbs
- Slight abdominal distension
- Loose stools

EMPTY PATTERNS

Spleen-Qi deficiency

Clinical manifestations

Poor appetite, slight abdominal distension after eating, tiredness, lassitude, desire to lie down, pale complexion, weakness of the limbs, loose stools (Fig. 36.1).
Tongue: Pale.
Pulse: Empty.
Key symptoms: poor appetite, tiredness, loose stools.

> **Diagnostic tip**
>
> Tiredness and loose stools would be enough to diagnose Spleen-Qi deficiency.

Aetiology

Diet

As mentioned before, excessive consumption of cold and raw foods can hinder the Spleen function of transformation and transportation and lead to Spleen-Qi deficiency. The Spleen prefers warm foods. Eating at irregular times or excessive eating can also strain the Spleen capacity and lead to Spleen-Qi deficiency. Eating too little or eating a protein-deficient diet can also cause Spleen deficiency.

> The Spleen likes warm (both in terms of energy and temperature) and dry foods and dislikes cold (both in terms of energy and temperature) and wet foods

Emotional strain

Pensiveness (as described above) and worry may weaken the Spleen and lead to Spleen-Qi deficiency.

Climate

Prolonged exposure to dampness (either from weather or from the place of living) can weaken the Spleen and lead to Spleen-Qi deficiency.

> Dampness is a climatic factor that affects the Spleen very frequently

Chronic disease

Any protracted disease will tend to weaken the Spleen and lead to Spleen-Qi deficiency. This is the reason why Dampness and Phlegm are a frequent consequence of protracted diseases, as Spleen-Qi is weakened and this leads to the formation of Dampness or Phlegm.

Pathology

This is by far the most common Spleen disharmony and probably the most common pattern in general, no doubt because of our irregular dietary habits and excessive use of the mind in studying, working, etc.

The pattern of Spleen-Qi deficiency is also central to all Spleen disharmonies as all its other Deficiency patterns are but a variation of it. For example, the pattern of Spleen-Yang deficiency is nothing but a further stage of Spleen-Qi deficiency; the pattern of Spleen-Qi sinking is a type of Spleen-Qi deficiency characterized by sinking of Qi; the pattern of Spleen not holding Blood is simply the same as Spleen-Qi deficiency when deficient Spleen-Qi fails to hold Blood in the vessels; the pattern of Spleen-Blood deficiency describes the clinical manifestations occurring when deficient Spleen-Qi

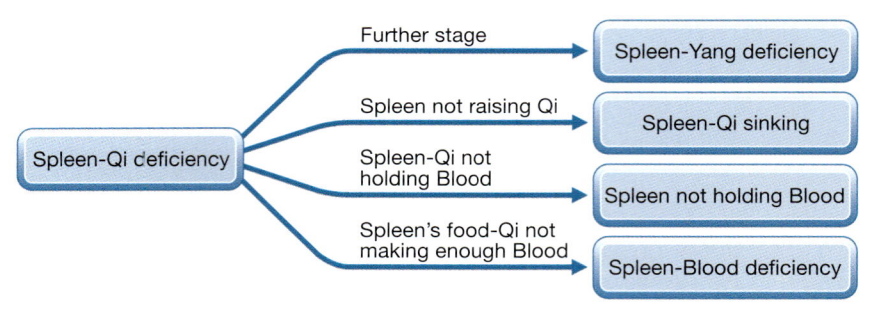

Figure 36.2 Variations of Spleen-Qi deficiency

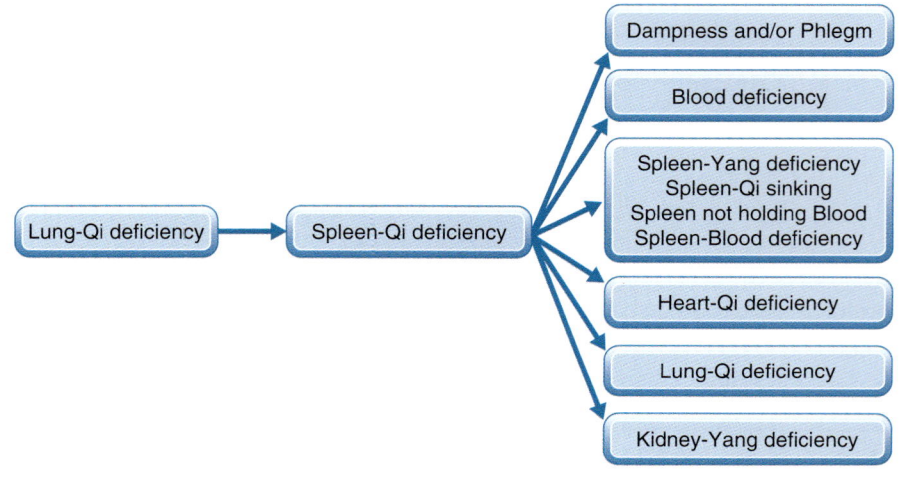

Figure 36.3 Spleen-Qi deficiency pattern: precursors and developments

and its Food-Qi (*Gu Qi*) are defective in making Blood (Fig. 36.2).

> **Clinical note**
>
> Spleen-Yang deficiency, Spleen-Qi sinking, Spleen not holding Blood and Spleen-Blood deficiency are all variations of Spleen-Qi deficiency

The impairment of the Spleen transformation and transportation function causes the various digestive symptoms, such as abdominal distension, loose stools and lack of appetite. As the Spleen is responsible for transporting Food-Qi to the four limbs, when Spleen-Qi is deficient, the limbs will be deprived of nourishment and feel weak. The Spleen also transports Food-Qi throughout the body, hence the tiredness and lassitude experienced when Spleen-Qi is deficient. When Spleen-Qi is deficient, typically the patient desires to lie down.

If Spleen-Qi is deficient over a long period of time, the inability of Spleen-Qi in transforming fluids can give rise to Dampness and Phlegm, which may cause obesity.

The Empty pulse reflects deficiency of Qi.

> **Clinical note**
>
> Spleen-Qi deficiency is one of the most common patterns in practice. It is the most common cause of chronic tiredness

Pathological precursors of pattern

There are not many patterns that are a precursor of this pattern, as Spleen-Qi deficiency itself is a 'first-line' pattern, i.e. one that arises first and that itself is the precursor to other patterns. However, Lung-Qi deficiency may be the precursor of Spleen-Qi deficiency (Fig. 36.3).

Pathological developments from pattern

As mentioned above, Spleen-Qi deficiency is a precursor to many other patterns. First of all, a chronic Spleen-Qi deficiency may lead to the formation of Dampness and/or Phlegm.

A Spleen-Qi deficiency may often lead to Blood deficiency as the deficient Food-Qi (*Gu Qi*) fails to produce enough Blood: this situation is much more common in women in whom a Spleen-Qi deficiency frequently leads to Blood deficiency. This leads to the pattern of 'Spleen-Blood deficiency' that is discussed below (see Fig. 36.3).

A Spleen-Qi deficiency is the precursor of Spleen-Yang deficiency, Spleen-Qi sinking, Spleen not holding Blood and Spleen-Blood deficiency.

A Spleen-Qi deficiency may also affect the Heart, leading to Heart-Qi (and often Heart-Blood) deficiency, and the Lungs, leading to Lung-Qi deficiency. A chronic Spleen-Qi deficiency may also lead to Kidney-Yang deficiency, especially if there is Dampness. Figure 36.4 illustrates the various potential consequences of Spleen-Qi deficiency.

Treatment

Principle of treatment: tonify Spleen-Qi.

Acupuncture

Points: Ren-12 Zhongwan, ST-36 Zusanli, SP-3 Taibai, SP-6 Sanyinjiao, BL-20 Pishu, BL-21 Weishu.

Method: reinforcing method. Moxa is applicable.
Explanation
- Ren-12 tonifies Spleen-Qi.
- ST-36 tonifies Spleen-Qi. The Stomach and Spleen are very closely related and points on the Stomach channel are often used to tonify the Spleen.
- SP-3 is the Source point of the Spleen and tonifies Spleen-Qi.
- SP-6 tonifies Spleen-Qi. The use of ST-36 and SP-6 bilaterally with moxa on the needles is an extremely effective tonification of the Spleen that gives the patient more energy almost immediately.
- BL-20 and BL-21 can tonify Spleen-Qi. The combination of these two points is particularly important to treat chronic conditions of both Spleen and Stomach deficiency.

Herbal formula

Si Jun Zi Tang *Four Gentlemen Decoction*.
Liu Jun Zi Tang *Six Gentlemen Decoction* (if there is some Dampness).

Three Treasures

Prosperous Earth (variation of Liu Jun Zi Tang).

Clinical note

The use of ST-36 and SP-6 bilaterally with moxa on the needles is an extremely effective tonification of the Spleen that gives the patient more energy almost immediately.

Box 36.2 summarizes Spleen-Qi deficiency.

Box 36.2 Spleen-Qi deficiency

Clinical manifestations

Poor appetite, slight abdominal distension after eating, tiredness, lassitude, desire to lie down, pale complexion, weakness of the limbs, loose stools, Pale tongue, Empty pulse

Treatment

Ren-12 Zhongwan, ST-36 Zusanli, SP-3 Taibai, SP-6 Sanyinjiao, BL-20 Pishu, BL-21 Weishu

---

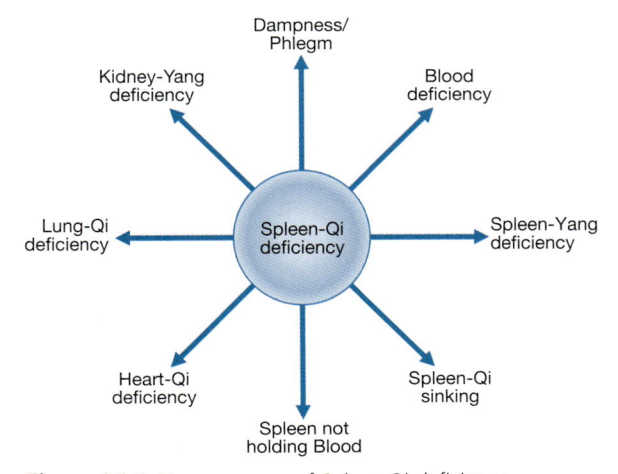

Figure 36.4 Consequences of Spleen-Qi deficiency

- Poor appetite
- Tiredness, desire to lie down
- Slight abdominal distension
- Weak and cold limbs
- Feeling cold
- Loose stools
- Oedema

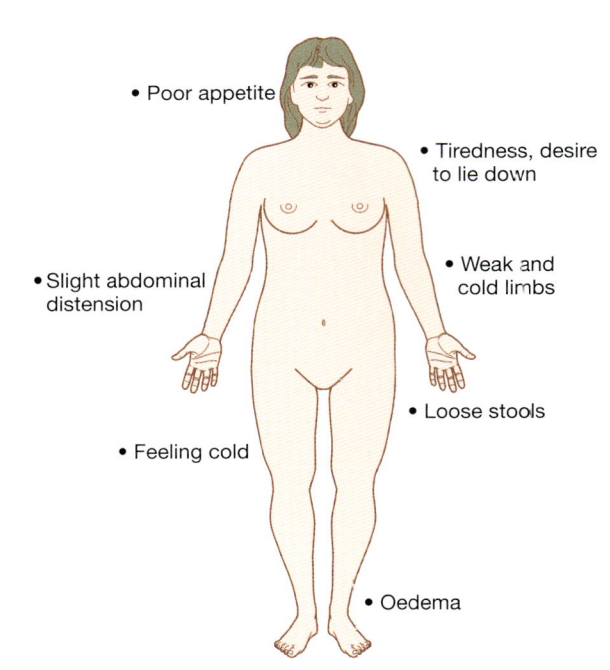

Figure 36.5 Spleen-Yang deficiency

Spleen-Yang deficiency

Clinical manifestations

Poor appetite, slight abdominal distension after eating, tiredness, lassitude, desire to lie down curled up, pale complexion, weakness of the limbs, loose stools, feeling cold, cold limbs, oedema (Fig. 36.5).
Tongue: Pale and wet.
Pulse: Deep-Weak.
Key symptoms: loose stools, feeling cold, cold limbs and tiredness.

> **Diagnostic tip**
>
> Loose stools, feeling cold and tiredness are enough to diagnose Spleen-Yang deficiency

Aetiology

The aetiology of this pattern is exactly the same as for Spleen-Qi deficiency, the only difference being that this pattern is more likely to be caused by exposure to a cold and damp environment.

Pathology

This pattern is substantially the same as Spleen-Qi deficiency with the addition of Cold symptoms, such as feeling cold and cold limbs. These are due to the failure of Spleen-Yang to warm the body.

The oedema is due to the impairment of the Spleen function in transforming and transporting fluids; when fluids cannot be transformed, they may accumulate under the skin, giving rise to oedema.

The tongue is Pale from the deficiency of Yang, and wet because the impairment in the Spleen function of fluid transportation leads to accumulation of fluids on the tongue.

The Pulse is Deep and Weak, reflecting the deficiency of Yang.

Pathological precursors of pattern

Spleen-Yang deficiency generally always derives from Spleen-Qi deficiency (Fig. 36.6).

Pathological developments from pattern

The pathological developments of this pattern are the same as those for Spleen-Qi deficiency. Spleen-Yang deficiency is even more likely than Spleen-Qi deficiency to lead to the formation of Dampness and/or Phlegm (see Fig. 36.6).

Treatment

Principle of treatment: tonify and warm Spleen-Yang.

Acupuncture

Points: the same as for Spleen-Qi deficiency, with the addition of SP-9 Yinlingquan, Ren-9 Shuifen, ST-28 Shuidao, BL-22 Sanjiaoshu, which should all be reduced if there is Dampness.
Method: reinforcing method. Moxa must be used.
Explanation
- SP-9 resolves Dampness in the Lower Burner.
- Ren-9, ST-28 and BL-22 can all stimulate the Spleen to transform and transport fluids and resolve oedema.

Herbal formula

Li Zhong Tang *Regulating the Centre Decoction*.
Box 36.3 summarizes Spleen-Yang deficiency.

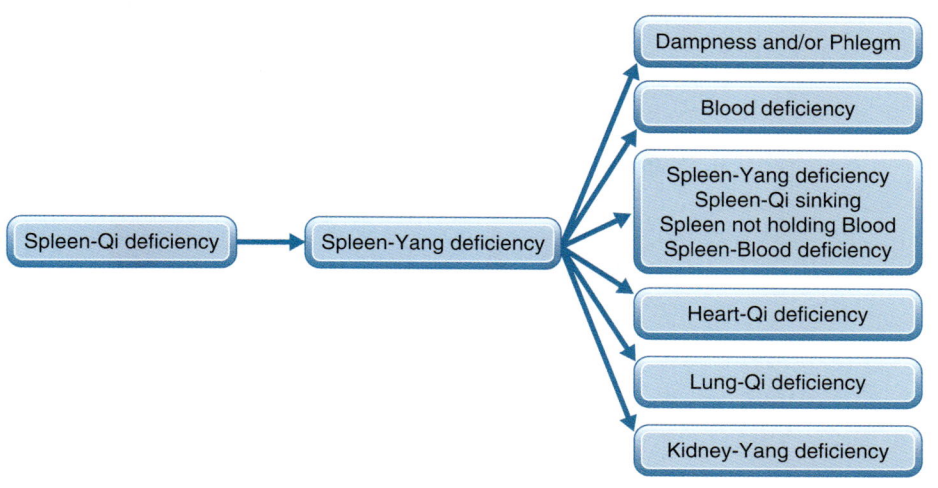

Figure 36.6 Spleen-Yang deficiency pattern: precursors and developments

Spleen-Qi deficiency → Spleen-Yang deficiency →
- Dampness and/or Phlegm
- Blood deficiency
- Spleen-Yang deficiency / Spleen-Qi sinking / Spleen not holding Blood / Spleen-Blood deficiency
- Heart-Qi deficiency
- Lung-Qi deficiency
- Kidney-Yang deficiency

Box 36.3 Spleen-Yang deficiency

Clinical manifestations

Poor appetite, slight abdominal distension after eating, tiredness, lassitude, desire to lie down curled up, pale complexion, weakness of the limbs, loose stools, feeling cold, cold limbs, oedema, Pale and wet tongue, Deep-Weak pulse

Treatment

Ren-12 Zhongwan, ST-36 Zusanli, SP-3 Taibai, SP-6 Sanyinjiao, BL-20 Pishu, BL-21 Weishu. SP-9 Yinlingquan, Ren-9 Shuifen, ST-28 Shuidao, BL-22 Sanjiaoshu

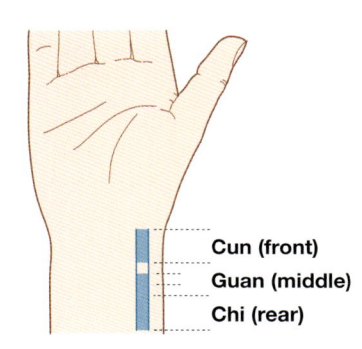

Figure 36.7 Spleen-Qi sinking

- Cun (front)
- Guan (middle)
- Chi (rear)

Spleen-Qi sinking

Clinical manifestations

Poor appetite, slight abdominal distension after eating, tiredness, lassitude, pale complexion, weakness of the limbs, loose stools, depression, tendency to obesity, a bearing-down sensation in the abdomen, prolapse of stomach, uterus, anus or bladder, frequency and urgency of urination, menorrhagia (Fig. 36.7).
Tongue: Pale.
Pulse: Weak. When the stomach is prolapsed, this can be felt on the middle right position on the pulse. If we divide the Stomach position on the pulse in three parts, the upper part will simply not be felt when the stomach is prolapsed.
Key symptoms: bearing down sensation, Weak Pulse.

> **Diagnostic tip**
>
> A bearing-down sensation and a Weak pulse are enough to diagnose sinking of Spleen-Qi

> Spleen-Qi sinking is the main cause of organ prolapse

Aetiology

This is the same as for Spleen-Qi deficiency. In addition, persons who, because of their work, have to stand for long hours every day, are more prone to this pattern if there are other factors in their life that cause Spleen-Qi deficiency.

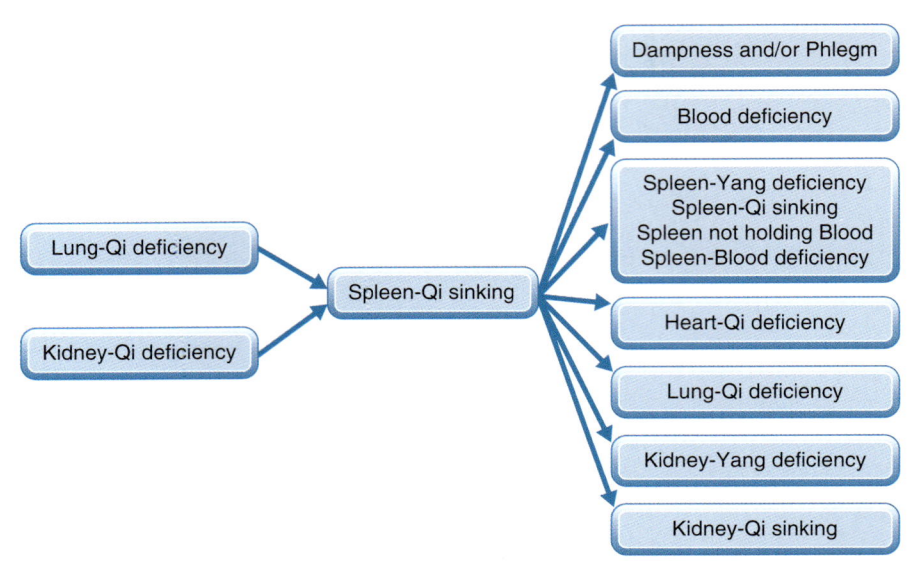

Figure 36.8 Spleen-Qi sinking pattern, precursors and developments

Pathology

This is exactly the same as for Spleen-Qi deficiency. The main difference is that this pattern reflects the impairment of the Spleen function of raising Qi.

The frequency and urgency of urination are due to the sinking of Qi unable to control urine. This happens particularly if there is also sinking of Kidney-Qi. Sinking of Spleen-Qi may also lead to excessive menstrual bleeding, although this is more likely to happen if there is also sinking of Kidney-Qi.

> **Clinical note**
>
> Especially in urinary and menstrual bleeding problems, sinking of Spleen-Qi is frequently accompanied by sinking of Kidney-Qi

Pathological precursors of pattern

These are the same as for Spleen-Qi deficiency. In addition, sinking of Kidney-Qi may lead to this pattern (Fig. 36.8).

Pathological developments from pattern

These are the same as for Spleen-Qi deficiency. In addition, sinking of Spleen-Qi may lead to sinking of Kidney-Qi (see Fig. 36.8).

Treatment

Principle of treatment: tonify Spleen-Qi, raise Qi.

Acupuncture

Points: all the same as for Spleen-Qi deficiency, plus Du-20 Baihui, Ren-6 Qihai, ST-21 Liangmen, Du-1 Chengqiang.
Method: reinforcing. Moxa is applicable.
Explanation
– Du-20 raises Qi. When used to raise Qi, moxa cones should be applied. It is particularly useful for prolapse of the uterus.
– Ren-6 tonifies and raises Qi. It is used for all prolapses.
– ST-21 tonifies Stomach and is used for prolapse of stomach.
– Du-1 is used for prolapse of anus.

Herbal formula

Bu Zhong Yi Qi Tang *Tonifying the Centre and Benefiting Qi Decoction*.

Three Treasures

Tonify Qi and Ease the Muscles (variation of Bu Zhong Yi Qi Tang).

> **Clinical note**
>
> The three main points to lift Spleen-Qi are Du-20 Baihui, Ren-12 Zhongwan and Ren-6 Qihai

Box 36.4 summarizes Spleen-Qi sinking.

> **Box 36.4 Spleen-Qi sinking**
>
> **Clinical manifestations**
>
> Poor appetite, slight abdominal distension after eating, tiredness, lassitude, pale complexion, weakness of the limbs, loose stools, depression, tendency to obesity, a bearing-down sensation in the abdomen, prolapse of stomach, uterus, anus or bladder, frequency and urgency of urination, menorrhagia, Pale tongue, Weak pulse
>
> **Treatment**
>
> Ren-12 Zhongwan, ST-36 Zusanli, SP-3 Taibai, SP-6 Sanyinjiao, BL-20 Pishu, BL-21 Weishu, Du-20 Baihui, Ren-6 Qihai, ST-21 Liangmen, Du-1 Chengqiang

Spleen not controlling Blood

Clinical manifestations

Poor appetite, slight abdominal distension after eating, tiredness, lassitude, pale sallow complexion, weakness of the limbs, loose stools, depression, blood spots under the skin, blood in the urine or stools, excessive uterine bleeding (Fig. 36.9).

Tongue: Pale.
Pulse: Weak or Fine.
Key symptoms: Fine Pulse, Pale tongue and bleeding.

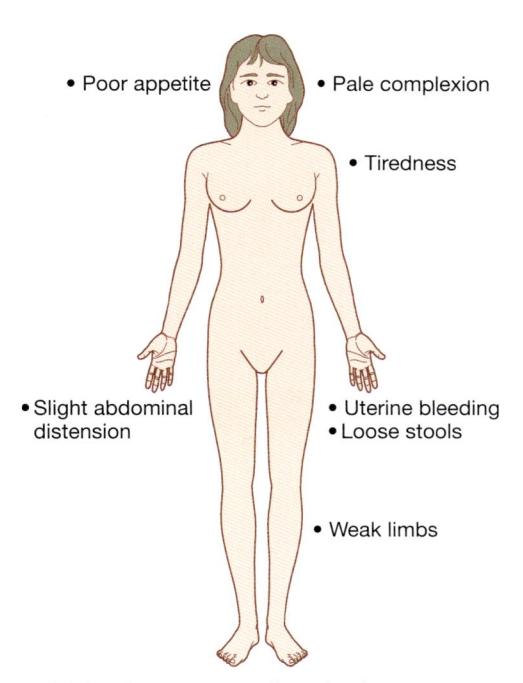

Figure 36.9 Spleen not controlling Blood

> **Diagnostic tip**
>
> A Fine pulse, Pale tongue and bleeding are enough to diagnose Spleen-Qi not controlling Blood

Aetiology

This is the same as for Spleen-Qi deficiency.

Pathology

All these symptoms are due to the impairment of the Spleen function of controlling Blood. When Spleen-Qi is deficient, it cannot hold the blood in the vessels and bleeding appears from various sources, such as under the skin, in the stools or urine or from the uterus. This is bleeding of a Deficient nature, as opposed to the bleeding from Heat in the Blood, which is of an Excess nature.

> **Clinical note**
>
> In bleeding, roughly half the cases are due to Spleen not holding Blood and half to Blood-Heat

Pathological precursors of pattern

The precursors of this pattern are the same as those for Spleen-Qi deficiency (Fig. 36.10).

Pathological developments from pattern

The pathological developments from this pattern are the same as for Spleen-Qi deficiency. In addition, if bleeding persists for some years, it may lead to Blood deficiency and/or Qi deficiency (as Blood is the mother of Qi) (see Fig. 36.10; Fig. 36.11).

Treatment

Principle of treatment: tonify Spleen-Qi, stop bleeding.

Acupuncture

Points: the same as for Spleen-Qi deficiency, plus: SP-10 Xuehai, BL-17 Geshu, SP-1 Yinbai, SP-4 Gongsun.
Method: reinforcing. Moxa is applicable.
Explanation
  – SP-10 strengthens the Spleen function of holding Blood and returns Blood to the blood vessels.
  – BL-17 tonifies Blood and stops bleeding, if needled.
  – SP-1 with moxa cones, strengthens the Spleen function of holding Blood and stops uterine

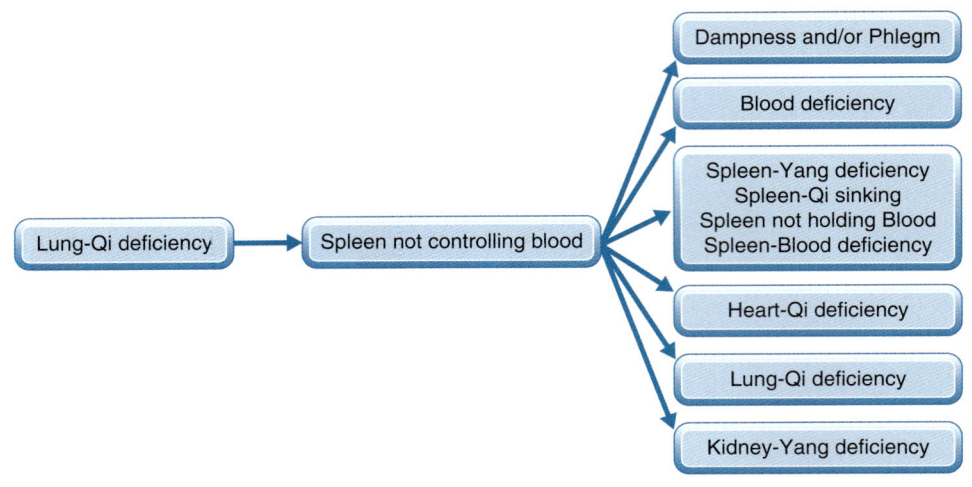

Figure 36.10 Spleen not controlling Blood pattern: precursors and developments

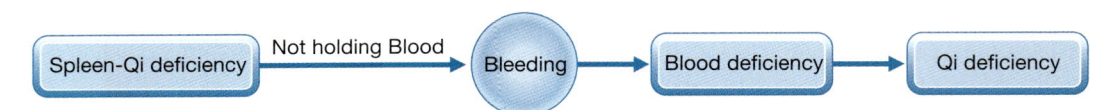

Figure 36.11 Consequences of bleeding from Spleen-Qi deficiency

bleeding. Moxa can only be applied to this point to stop bleeding when it derives from Spleen-Qi deficiency.
– SP-4 stops bleeding related to the Spleen.

Herbal formula
Gui Pi Tang *Tonifying the Spleen Decoction*.

> **Clinical note**
>
> The main points to use to stop bleeding from deficient Spleen-Qi not holding Blood are Du-20 Baihui, Ren-12 Zhongwan, Ren-6 Qihai and SP-10 Xuehai

Box 36.5 summarizes Spleen not controlling Blood.

Spleen-Blood deficiency
Clinical manifestations
Poor appetite, slight abdominal distension after eating, tiredness, lassitude, dull-pale complexion, weakness of the limbs, loose stools, depression, thin body, scanty periods or amenorrhoea, insomnia (Fig. 36.12).
Tongue: Pale, Thin and slightly dry.
Pulse: Choppy or Fine.

Box 36.5 Spleen not controlling Blood

Clinical manifestations

Poor appetite, slight abdominal distension after eating, tiredness, lassitude, pale-sallow complexion, weakness of the limbs, loose stools, depression, blood spots under the skin, blood in the urine or stools, excessive uterine bleeding, Pale tongue, Weak or Fine pulse

Treatment

Ren-12 Zhongwan, ST-36 Zusanli, SP-3 Taibai, SP-6 Sanyinjiao, BL-20 Pishu, BL-21 Weishu, SP-10 Xuehai, BL-17 Geshu, SP-1 Yinbai, SP-4 Gongsun

---

Key symptoms: tiredness, slight abdominal distension, scanty periods, Pale tongue.

> **Diagnostic tip**
>
> Tiredness, slight abdominal distension and scanty periods are enough to diagnose Spleen-Blood deficiency

Aetiology
The aetiology of this pattern is the same as that for Spleen-Qi deficiency. Diet plays a particularly important role in the aetiology of Spleen-Blood deficiency: the inadequate consumption of Blood-producing foods

- Depression, insomnia
- Poor appetite
- Dull-pale complexion
- Tiredness
- Slight abdominal distension
- Joint ache
- Scanty periods
- Weak limbs

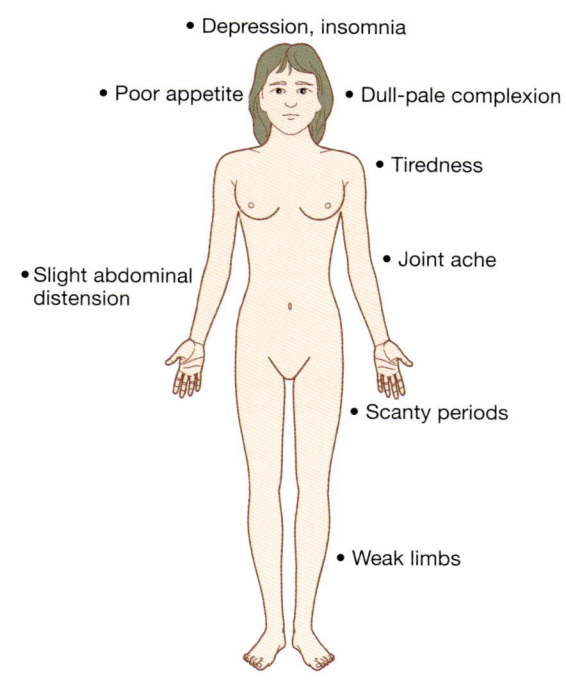

Figure 36.12 Spleen-Blood deficiency

(such as meat and grains) is a frequent aetiological factor in the development of this pattern.

Pathology

Strictly speaking, there is no such entity as 'Spleen-Blood' as the Spleen is not related to Blood in the same way as the Heart or Liver are. The Heart governs Blood and the Liver stores Blood, hence we can refer to 'Heart-Blood' and 'Liver-Blood'. In contrast, the Spleen is related to Qi and, indeed, Qi deficiency nearly always involves Spleen-Qi deficiency. However, the Food-Qi (*Gu Qi*) produced by the Spleen is the precursor of Blood as Food-Qi is transformed into Blood with the help of Lungs and Heart.

Therefore, 'Spleen-Blood deficiency' simply indicates a deficiency of Spleen-Qi that leads to deficient Blood: as mentioned above, a diet lacking in Blood-nourishing foods is often the cause of this condition.

This pattern therefore presents all the clinical manifestations of Spleen-Qi deficiency such as poor appetite, slight abdominal distension after eating, tiredness, lassitude, dull-pale complexion, weakness of the limbs and loose stools. In addition, there will be symptoms of Blood deficiency such as scanty or no periods, a thin tongue and a Choppy or Fine pulse.

Note that there is some depression and insomnia as the deficiency of Blood may affect the Heart and that the body is likely to be thin (from Blood deficiency) rather than tending to obesity as it is in Spleen-Qi deficiency.

The tongue and the pulse also reflect Blood deficiency as the tongue is thin and slightly dry (rather than slightly wet as in Spleen-Yang deficiency) and the pulse is Choppy or Fine (rather than Empty or Weak as in Spleen-Qi and Spleen-Yang deficiency, respectively).

Pathological precursors of pattern

The pathological precursors of this pattern are the same as those for Spleen-Qi deficiency. In addition, a deficiency of Liver-Blood often facilitates the development of Spleen-Blood deficiency (Fig. 36.13).

Pathological developments from pattern

The pathological developments from this pattern are the same as those for Spleen-Qi deficiency. In addition, Spleen-Blood deficiency can easily lead to Heart-Blood and Liver-Blood deficiency (see Fig. 36.13).

Treatment

Principle of treatment: tonify Spleen-Qi, nourish Blood.

Acupuncture

Points: Ren-12 Zhongwan, ST-36 Zusanli, SP-3 Taibai, SP-6 Sanyinjiao, BL-20 Pishu, BL-21 Weishu, Ren-4 Guanyuan, BL-17 Geshu (with direct moxa).

Method: reinforcing method. Moxa is applicable.

Explanation
- Ren-12, ST-36, SP-3, SP-6, BL-20 and BL-21 tonify the Spleen.
- Ren-4 nourishes Blood, especially in relation to the Uterus.
- BL-17 with direct moxa cones nourishes Blood.

Herbal formula

Gui Pi Tang *Tonifying the Spleen Decoction*.

Three Treasures

Calm the Shen (variation of Gui Pi Tang).
Precious Sea (variation of Ba Zhen Tang).

Box 36.6 summarizes Spleen-Blood deficiency.

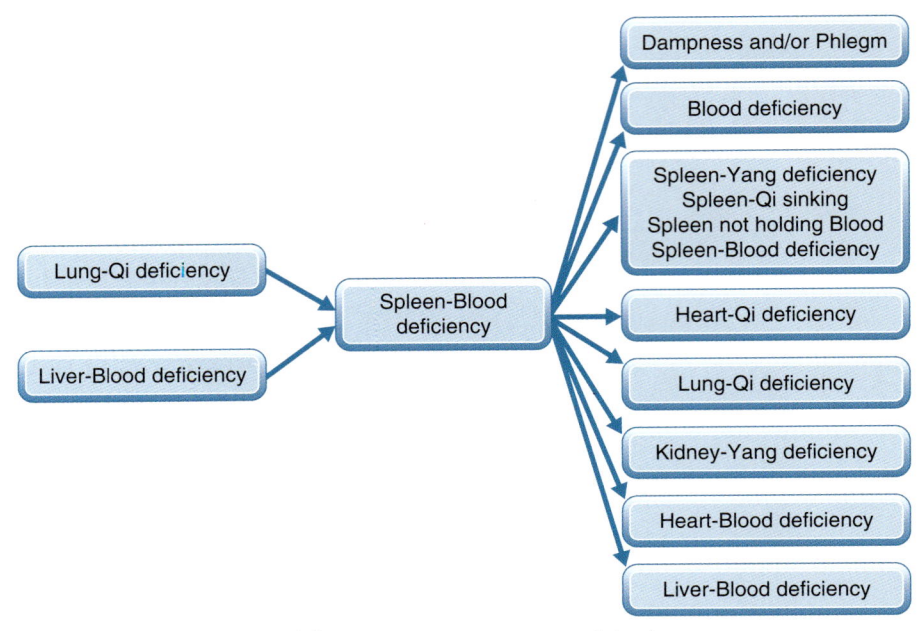

Figure 36.13 Spleen-Blood deficiency pattern: precursors and developments

---

Box 36.6 Spleen-Blood deficiency

Clinical manifestations

Poor appetite, slight abdominal distension after eating, tiredness, lassitude, dull-pale complexion, weakness of the limbs, loose stools, depression, thin body, scanty periods or amenorrhoea, insomnia, Pale, Thin and slightly dry tongue, Choppy or Fine pulse

Treatment

Ren-12 Zhongwan, ST-36 Zusanli, SP-3 Taibai, SP-6 Sanyinjiao, BL-20 Pishu, BL-21 Weishu, Ren-4 Guanyuan, BL-17 Geshu

---

FULL PATTERNS

Cold-Dampness invading the Spleen

Clinical manifestations

Poor appetite, a feeling of fullness of the epigastrium and/or abdomen, a feeling of cold in the epigastrium which improves with the application of heat, a feeling of heaviness of the head and body, a sweetish taste or absence of taste, no thirst, loose stools, lassitude, tiredness, nausea, oedema, dull-white complexion, excessive white vaginal discharge (Fig. 36.14).

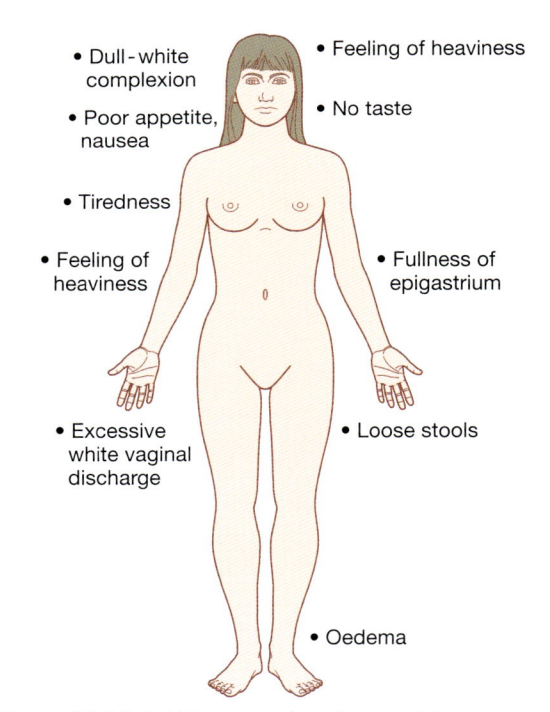

Figure 36.14 Cold-Dampness invading the Spleen

Tongue: Pale with a sticky white coating.
Pulse: Slippery-Slow.
Key symptoms: abdominal fullness, feeling of heaviness, sticky white tongue coating.

> **Diagnostic tip**
>
> Abdominal fullness and a sticky white tongue coating would be enough to diagnose Cold-Dampness invading the Spleen

Aetiology

This is from exposure to exterior Dampness, which would derive either from the weather or living conditions. Please note that, although this pattern is of exterior origin (i.e. it is caused by exterior Dampness), once in the Spleen, this is interior Dampness and an interior pattern.

Pathology

This is an Excess pattern occurring when the Spleen is invaded by exterior Dampness. The above manifestations correspond to the acute stage, but the pattern can also be chronic. The clinical manifestations would be different in chronic cases, particularly with regard to tongue and pulse. The tongue would be more Pale and the pulse partly Weak or Soggy.

Dampness obstructs the chest and epigastrium and prevents the normal movement of Qi, causing the typical feeling of fullness. Dampness is a 'heavy' pathogenic factor and it obstructs the muscles, hence the characteristic feeling of heaviness of the body.

Dampness prevents the clear Yang from ascending to the head, causing the feeling of heaviness of the head.

Nausea is caused by the obstruction of Dampness in the epigastrium preventing Stomach-Qi from descending.

The Spleen opens into the mouth and when Dampness obstructs the Spleen, it affects the taste.

Dampness is heavy and has a tendency to infuse downwards: when this happens, it will cause vaginal discharge.

The sticky or slippery tongue coating is highly indicative of Dampness, as is the Slippery Pulse. The pulse would be Slow only when Cold is pronounced.

The pattern presented here derives from invasion of the Spleen by exterior Dampness, but very similar manifestations can arise from a chronic deficiency of Spleen-Qi, which leads to the formation of Dampness. The main differentiating features will be the pulse and tongue. In case of Dampness from chronic Spleen-Qi deficiency, the pulse would be Weak and only slightly Slippery (rather than Full-Slippery), and the tongue would be Pale and have a thin coating (rather than a thick coating).

> **Clinical note**
>
> SP-9 Yinlingquan, SP-6 Sanyinjiao, Ren-9 Shuifen, Ren-5 Shimen and BL-22 Sanjiaoshu are five important points to resolve Dampness

Pathological precursors of pattern

In acute cases, there are no pathological precursors of this pattern as it is caused by an exterior invasion of Dampness. However, in reality, there is nearly always a pre-existing deficiency of Spleen-Qi, which predisposes the patient to an invasion of exterior Dampness (Fig. 36.15).

Pathological developments from pattern

When Dampness obstructs the Spleen for some time, it inevitably leads to (or aggravates) a deficiency of the Spleen. Cold-Dampness may also lead to deficiency of Kidney-Yang if it persists for a long time.

Finally, in some cases, Dampness in the Spleen may interfere with the free flow of Liver-Qi and lead to Liver-Qi stagnation (see Fig. 36.15).

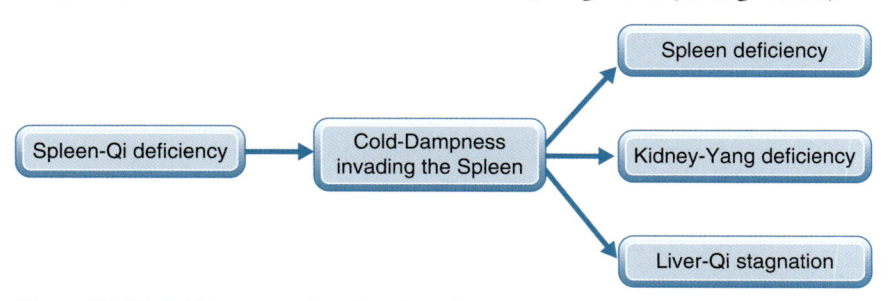

Figure 36.15 Cold-Dampness invading the Spleen pattern: precursors and developments

Treatment

Principle of treatment: resolve Dampness, expel Cold.

Acupuncture

Points: SP-9 Yinlingquan, SP-6 Sanyinjiao, SP-3 Taibai, Ren-12 Zhongwan, ST-8 Touwei, BL-22 Sanjiaoshu, BL-20 Pishu, Ren-9 Shuifen, Ren-11 Jianli, ST-22 Guanmen, ST-28 Shuidao.

Method: reducing or even except on the points that tonify the Spleen, which should be needled with reinforcing method.

Explanation
- SP-9 resolves Dampness from the Lower Burner.
- SP-6 and SP-3 resolve Dampness.
- Ren-12 tonifies the Spleen to resolve Dampness.
- ST-8 resolves Dampness from the head. It is particularly indicated for a feeling of heaviness of the head or headache from Dampness.
- BL-22 resolves Dampness, particularly from the Lower Burner.
- BL-20 tonifies the Spleen.
- Ren-9 resolves Dampness. In particular, in combination with Ren-11 and ST-22, it resolves Dampness from the Middle Burner.
- ST-28 resolves Dampness from the Lower Burner and the Uterus.

Herbal formula

Ping Wei San *Balancing the Stomach Powder*.

Three Treasures

Drain Fields (variation of Huo Po Xia Ling Tang).

Box 36.7 summarizes Cold-Dampness invading the Spleen.

Box 36.7 Cold-Dampness invading the Spleen

Clinical manifestations

Poor appetite, a feeling of fullness of the epigastrium and/or abdomen, a feeling of cold in the epigastrium which improves with the application of heat, a feeling of heaviness of the head and body, a sweetish taste or absence of taste, no thirst, loose stools, lassitude, tiredness, nausea, oedema, dull-white complexion, excessive white vaginal discharge, Pale tongue with a sticky white coating, Slippery-Slow pulse

Treatment

SP-9 Yinlingquan, SP-6 Sanyinjiao, Ren-12 Zhongwan, SP-3 Taibai, ST-8 Touwei, BL-22 Sanjiaoshu, BL-20 Pishu, Ren-9 Shuifen, Ren-11 Jianli, ST-22 Guanmen, ST-28 Shuidao

---

Damp-Heat invading the Spleen

Clinical manifestations

A feeling of fullness of the epigastrium and/or lower abdomen, epigastric and/or abdominal pain, poor appetite, a feeling of heaviness, thirst without desire to drink, nausea, vomiting, loose stools with offensive odour, burning sensation in the anus, a feeling of heat, scanty dark urine, low-grade fever, dull headache with feeling of heaviness of the head, dull-yellow complexion like tangerine peel, yellow sclera of the eyes, oily sweat, bitter taste, itchy skin or skin eruptions (papules or vesicles), sweating which does not relieve the fever and does not lead to the clearing of Heat (Fig. 36.16).

Tongue: Red with sticky yellow coating.
Pulse: Slippery-Rapid.
Key symptoms: abdominal fullness, feeling of heaviness, sticky yellow coating.

> **Diagnostic tip**
>
> Abdominal fullness and a sticky yellow tongue coating would be enough to diagnose Damp-Heat invading the Spleen

- Dull-yellow complexion
- Nausea, vomiting, bitter taste
- Feeling of heat
- Feeling of heaviness
- Scanty-dark urine
- Dull headache, feeling of heaviness
- Yellow sclera
- Thirst with no desire to drink
- Skin eruptions
- Fullness of epigastrium
- Loose stools
- Burning sensation of anus

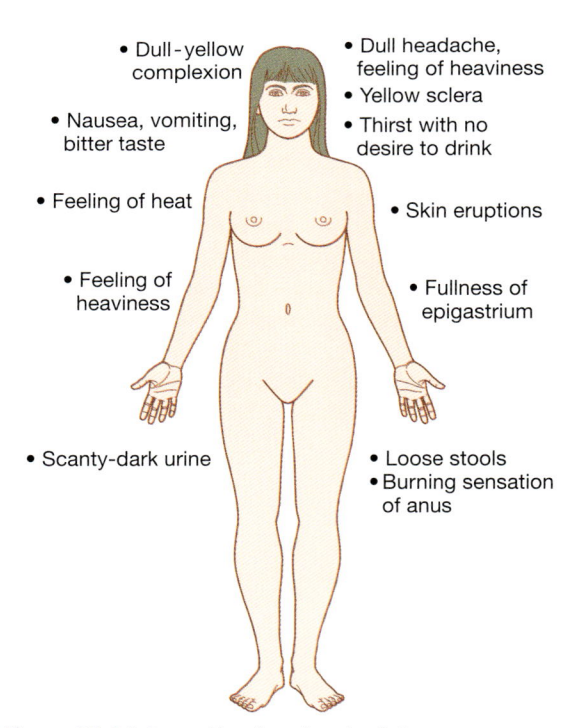

Figure 36.16 Damp-Heat invading the Spleen

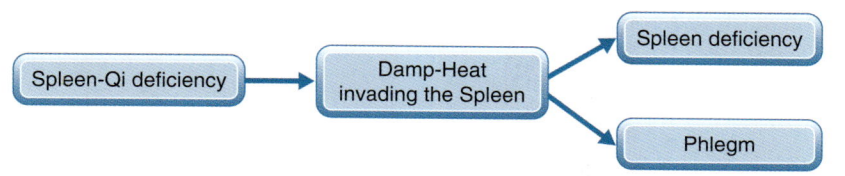

Figure 36.17 Damp-Heat invading the Spleen pattern: precursors and developments

Aetiology

This is usually due to exterior Damp-Heat (i.e. exposure to hot and humid weather). It can also be due to eating unclean or contaminated food.

Pathology

The pathology is essentially the same as for Cold-Dampness invading the Spleen, with the difference that in this case there is Heat. Most of the symptoms can be analysed in the same way as those of Cold-Dampness. For example, the feeling of fullness of the epigastrium and/or abdomen, the feeling of heaviness, the nausea, the sticky tongue coating and Slippery pulse are all due to Dampness.

The low-grade fever is caused by the steaming of Damp-Heat and is constant throughout the day (contrary to the low-grade fever from Yin deficiency which only appears in the afternoon or early evening).

The offensive odour of the stools, the bitter taste, the burning sensation of the anus and the scanty dark-yellow urination are indicative of Heat.

It should be stressed that the pattern as it is described above applies only to a relatively acute case of invasion of Damp-Heat. In most chronic cases we see in practice, many of the above symptoms will be missing: for example, the fever, the burning sensation of the anus and the tangerine-like skin. However, such symptoms may be seen in chronic cases: for example, in ulcerative colitis.

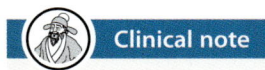

> **Clinical note**
>
> Damp-Heat is an extremely common cause of urinary problems and/or skin diseases

Pathological precursors of pattern

In acute cases, there are no pathological precursors of this pattern as it is caused by an exterior invasion of Dampness. However, in reality, there is nearly always a pre-existing deficiency of Spleen-Qi, which predisposes the patient to an invasion of exterior Dampness (Fig. 36.17).

In chronic cases, this pattern can develop from a combination of Spleen deficiency and Heat (often in the Stomach).

Pathological developments from pattern

The Dampness part of Damp-Heat may obstruct the Spleen and cause or aggravate a Spleen deficiency. The Heat part of Damp-Heat can further aggravate the Dampness by condensing fluids or it may also, in time, lead to the formation of Phlegm (see Fig. 36.17).

Treatment

Principle of treatment: resolve Dampness, clear Heat.

Acupuncture

Points: SP-9 Yinlingquan, SP-6 Sanyinjiao, Du-9 Zhiyang, L.I.-11 Quchi, BL-20 Pishu, G.B.-34 Yanglingquan, Ren-9 Shuifen, Ren-11 Jianli, ST-22 Guanmen, ST-28 Shuidao, BL-22 Sanjiaoshu.

Method: reducing method, except on the points that tonify the Spleen which should be reinforced. No moxa.

Explanation
- SP-9 and SP-6 resolve Dampness and Damp-Heat from the Lower Burner.
- Du-9 resolves Damp-Heat.
- L.I.-11 clears Heat and resolves Dampness.
- BL-20 tonifies the Spleen.
- G.B.-34 resolves Damp-Heat.
- Ren-9 resolves Dampness by stimulating the transformation and transportation of fluids.

- Ren-9, Ren-11 and ST-22 resolve Dampness from the Middle Burner.
- ST-28 and BL-22 resolve Dampness from the Lower Burner.

Herbal formula
Lian Po Yin *Coptis–Magnolia Decoction*.

Three Treasures
Ease the Muscles (variation of Lian Po Yin).

Box 36.8 summarizes Damp-Heat invading the Spleen.

Box 36.8 Damp-Heat invading the Spleen

Clinical manifestations

A feeling of fullness of the epigastrium and/or lower abdomen, epigastric and/or abdominal pain, poor appetite, a feeling of heaviness, thirst without desire to drink, nausea, vomiting, loose stools with offensive odour, burning sensation in the anus, a feeling of heat, scanty dark urine, low-grade fever, dull headache with feeling of heaviness of the head, dull-yellow complexion like tangerine peel, yellow sclera of the eyes, oily sweat, bitter taste, itchy skin or skin eruptions (papules or vesicles), sweating which does not relieve the fever and does not lead to the clearing of Heat, Red tongue with sticky yellow coating, Slippery-Rapid pulse

Treatment

SP-9 Yinlingquan, SP-6 Sanyinjiao, Du-9 Zhiyang, L.I.-11 Quchi, BL-20 Pishu, G.B.-34 Yanglingquan, Ren-9 Shuifen, Ren-11 Jianli, ST-22 Guanmen, ST-28 Shuidao, BL-22 Sanjiaoshu

---

COMBINED PATTERNS

Spleen- and Heart-Blood deficiency

Clinical manifestations

Palpitations, dizziness, insomnia, dream-disturbed sleep, poor memory, anxiety, propensity to be startled, dull-pale complexion, pale lips, tiredness, weak muscles, loose stools, poor appetite, scanty periods (Fig. 36.18).
Tongue: Pale and Thin.
Pulse: Choppy or Fine.
Key symptoms: palpitations, insomnia, tiredness, loose stools, scanty periods.

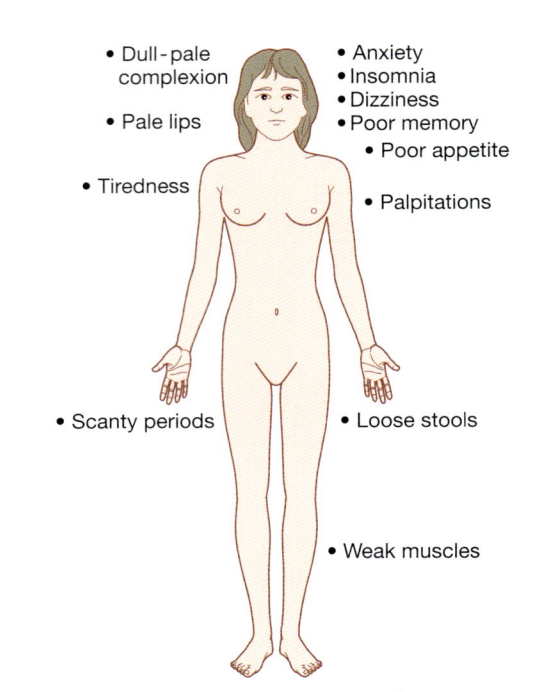

Figure 36.18 Spleen- and Heart-Blood deficiency

- Dull-pale complexion
- Pale lips
- Tiredness
- Scanty periods
- Anxiety
- Insomnia
- Dizziness
- Poor memory
- Poor appetite
- Palpitations
- Loose stools
- Weak muscles

> **Diagnostic tip**
>
> Palpitations, insomnia, loose stools and scanty periods would be enough to diagnose Spleen- and Heart-Blood deficiency

Aetiology

Diet

A diet lacking in nourishment and Blood-producing foods (such as meat) leads to Blood deficiency in general and Spleen-Blood deficiency specifically.

Emotional stress

Sadness, grief, anxiety and worry over a long period of time can disturb the Mind, which, in turn, can depress the Heart function. Since the Heart governs Blood, this eventually may lead to Heart-Blood deficiency.

Excessive physical work

Excessive physical work may injure the muscles and therefore the Spleen: when the Spleen is deficient for a long time, Spleen-Blood deficiency may develop as Food-Qi is the precursor of Blood.

The aetiology of Spleen- and Heart-Blood deficiency is usually a combination of the above three factors.

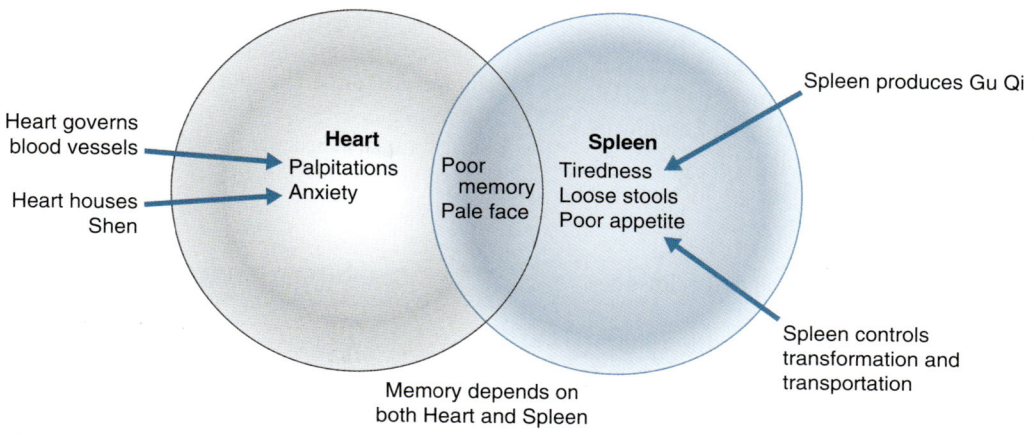

Figure 36.19 Pathology of Spleen- and Heart-Blood deficiency

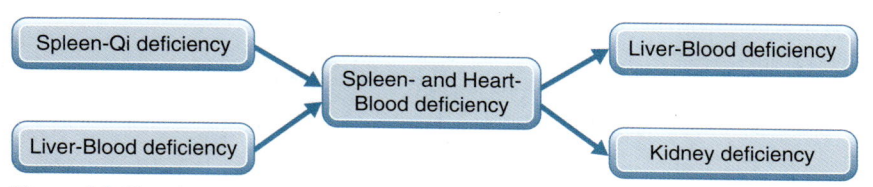

Figure 36.20 Spleen- and Heart-Blood deficiency pattern: precursors and developments

Severe blood loss

A severe haemorrhage (such as during childbirth) can lead to Blood deficiency, since the Heart governs Blood. This, in time, can lead to Heart-Blood deficiency. As Spleen-Qi holds Blood, blood loss also weakens Spleen-Qi and eventually Spleen-Blood.

Pathology

The pathology of Heart-Blood deficiency has already been discussed above. 'Spleen-Blood deficiency' arises from Spleen-Qi deficiency and it describes the pathological changes when Food-Qi (*Gu Qi*) produced by the Spleen does not produce enough Blood. The clinical manifestations related to 'Spleen-Blood' are basically the same as for Spleen-Qi deficiency when this leads to not enough Blood being made.

Tiredness and weak muscles are due to deficient Spleen-Qi not transporting food essences to the muscles. Loose stools occur when Spleen-Qi descends rather than ascends and the Spleen's transportation and transformation of food essences is impaired.

When Food-Qi produced by the Spleen does not produce enough Blood, Spleen-Blood becomes deficient and this may lead to scanty periods. Please note that this is only one factor involved in the pathology of scanty periods. From a different perspective, the Kidneys are the source of *Tian Gui*, menstrual Blood (Fig. 36.19).

Pathological precursors of pattern

Spleen-Blood deficiency is always preceded by Spleen-Qi deficiency: it is not possible to have the former without the latter.

Liver-Blood deficiency may lead to Heart- and/or Spleen-Blood deficiency, so that a deficiency of Blood of all three organs (Heart, Liver and Spleen) may occur (Fig. 36.20).

Pathological developments from pattern

Heart- and Spleen-Blood deficiency may lead to Liver-Blood deficiency and to a Kidney deficiency (see Fig. 36.20).

Treatment

Principle of treatment: nourish Blood, tonify the Heart and the Spleen, calm the Mind.

Acupuncture

Points: HE-7 Shenmen, P-6 Neiguan, Ren-14 Juque, Ren-15 Jiuwei, Ren-4 Guanyuan, BL-17 Geshu (with moxa), BL-20 Pishu, Ren-12 Zhongwan, ST-36 Zusanli, SP-6 Sanyinjiao.

Method: all with reinforcing method. Moxa can be used.

Explanation
- HE-7 nourishes Heart-Blood and calms the Mind.
- P-6 tonifies Heart-Qi and calms the Mind.
- Ren-14 and Ren-15 tonify Heart-Blood and calm the Mind. They are particularly useful if there is pronounced anxiety.
- Ren-4, BL-17 and BL-20 tonify Blood. BL-17 is the Gathering point for Blood and BL-20 is the Back Transporting point for the Spleen and it tonifies Spleen-Qi to produce more Blood.
- BL-20, Ren-12, ST-36 and SP-6 tonify Spleen-Qi and Spleen-Blood.

Herbal formula

Gui Pi Tang *Tonifying the Spleen Decoction*.

Three Treasures

Calm the Shen (variation of Gui Pi Tang).

Box 36.9 summarizes Spleen- and Heart-Blood deficiency.

Spleen- and Lung-Qi deficiency

Clinical manifestations

Poor appetite, slight abdominal distension after eating, tiredness, lassitude, pale complexion, weakness of the limbs, loose stools, tendency to obesity, slight shortness of breath, slight cough, weak voice, spontaneous daytime sweating, dislike of speaking, propensity to catch colds, dislike of cold (Fig. 36.21).

Tongue: Pale.
Pulse: Empty, especially on the right side.
Key symptoms: no appetite, tiredness and breathlessness.

> **Diagnostic tip**
>
> Poor appetite, tiredness and shortness of breath would be enough to diagnose Spleen- and Lung-Qi deficiency

Aetiology

Diet

Irregular eating or a diet lacking in nourishment may lead to Spleen-Qi deficiency.

Life habits

A sedentary lifestyle with stooping over a desk may lead to Lung-Qi deficiency. A profession that involves much talking (e.g. teaching) may weaken Lung-Qi.

In pathological situations, deficiency of one often affects the other: a diet poor in nourishment will

---

Box 36.9 Spleen- and Heart-Blood deficiency

Clinical manifestations

Palpitations, dizziness, insomnia, dream-disturbed sleep, poor memory, anxiety, propensity to be startled, dull-pale complexion, pale lips, tiredness, weak muscles, loose stools, poor appetite, scanty periods, Pale and Thin tongue, Choppy or Fine pulse

Treatment

HE-7 Shenmen, P-6 Neiguan, Ren-14 Juque, Ren-15 Jiuwei, Ren-4 Guanyuan, BL-17 Geshu (with moxa), BL-20 Pishu, Ren-12 Zhongwan, ST-36 Zusanli, SP-6 Sanyinjiao

---

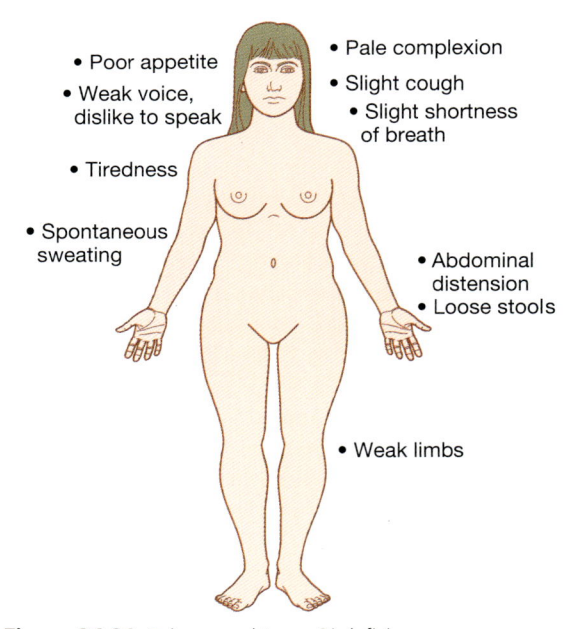

Figure 36.21 Spleen- and Lung-Qi deficiency

- Poor appetite
- Weak voice, dislike to speak
- Tiredness
- Spontaneous sweating
- Pale complexion
- Slight cough
- Slight shortness of breath
- Abdominal distension
- Loose stools
- Weak limbs

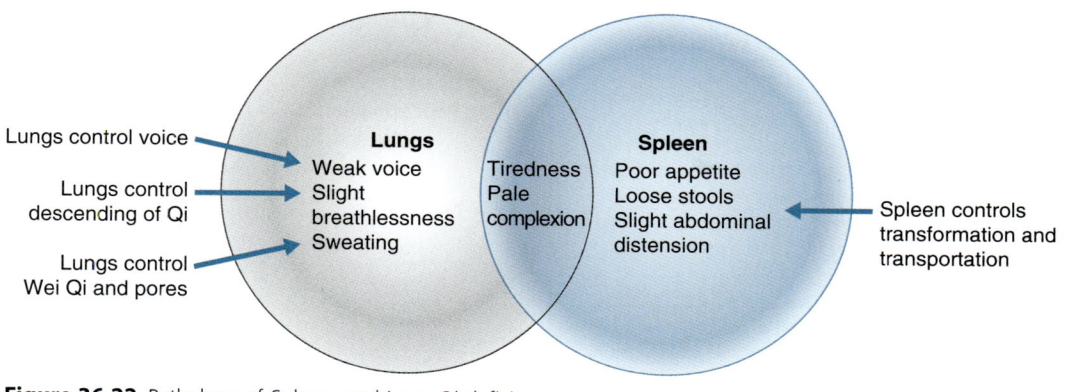

Figure 36.22 Pathology of Spleen- and Lung-Qi deficiency

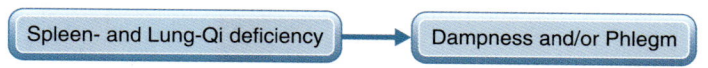

Figure 36.23 Spleen- and Lung-Qi deficiency pattern: precursors and developments

weaken the Spleen and eventually affect the Lungs, because they will not receive enough Food-Qi. On the other hand, poor breathing, lack of exercise, excessive stooping over a desk for many years, all weaken Lung-Qi: not enough air is taken in, Lung-Qi weakens and therefore not enough Qi from the Lungs is available to produce True Qi (*Zhen Qi*).

Pathology

Both Spleen and Lungs are involved in the production of Qi and they influence each other in health and disease (Fig. 36.22).

The Spleen is the source of Food-Qi from which all Qi is produced; the Lungs control breathing and the taking in of air, which combines with Food-Qi to produce True Qi. Thus they both determine the crucial stages of the production of Qi. There is a saying in Chinese medicine: '*The Spleen is the source of Qi and the Lungs are the pivot of Qi.*'[3]

Pathological precursors of pattern

Both Spleen- and Lung-Qi deficiency are usually 'first-line' patterns and therefore do not often have pathological precursors as they themselves are usually precursor patterns (Fig. 36.23).

Pathological developments from pattern

Long-term Spleen-Qi deficiency often leads to the formation of Dampness and/or Phlegm. Lung-Qi deficiency, especially when combined with Spleen-Qi deficiency may contribute to forming Phlegm (see Fig. 36.23).

Treatment

Principle of treatment: tonify Lung- and Spleen-Qi.

Acupuncture

Points: LU-9 Taiyuan, BL-13 Feishu, LU-7 Lieque, Du-12 Shenzhu, Ren-6 Qihai, ST-36 Zusanli, Ren-12 Zhongwan, SP-3 Taibai, SP-6 Sanyinjiao, BL-20 Pishu, BL-21 Weishu.

Method: reinforcing.

Explanation
- LU-9 and BL-13 tonify Lung-Qi.
- LU-7 tonifies Lung-Qi and restores the descending of Lung-Qi.
- Du-12 tonifies Lung-Qi, particularly for chronic conditions.
- Ren-6 tonifies Qi in general. The Lung channel flows down to the region of this point.
- ST-36, Ren-12, SP-3, SP-6, BL-20 and BL-21 tonify Spleen-Qi.

Herbal formula

Si Jun Zi Tang *Four Gentlemen Decoction* plus Huang Qi Radix *Astragali membranacei*.

Liu Jun Zi Tang *Six Gentlemen Decoction* plus Huang Qi *Radix Astragali membranacei*.

> **Box 36.10 Spleen- and Lung-Qi deficiency**
>
> **Clinical manifestations**
>
> Poor appetite, slight abdominal distension after eating, tiredness, lassitude, pale complexion, weakness of the limbs, loose stools, tendency to obesity, slight shortness of breath, slight cough, weak voice, spontaneous daytime sweating, dislike of speaking, propensity to catch colds, dislike of cold, Pale tongue, Empty pulse, especially on the right side
>
> **Treatment**
>
> LU-9 Taiyuan, LU-7 Lieque, Ren-6 Qihai, BL-13 Feishu, Du-12 Shenzhu, ST-36 Zusanli, Ren-12 Zhongwan, SP-3 Taibai, SP-6 Sanyinjiao, BL-20 Pishu, BL-21 Weishu

Box 36.10 summarizes Spleen- and Lung-Qi deficiency.

Spleen- and Liver-Blood deficiency

Clinical manifestations

Poor appetite, slight abdominal distension after eating, tiredness, lassitude, dull-pale complexion, weakness of the limbs, loose stools, thin body, scanty periods or amenorrhoea, insomnia, dizziness, numbness of limbs, blurred vision, 'floaters' in eyes, diminished night vision, pale lips, muscular weakness, cramps, withered and brittle nails, dry hair and skin, slight depression, a feeling of aimlessness (Fig. 36.24).

Tongue: Pale body especially on the sides, which, in extreme cases, can assume an orange colour, and dry.

Pulse: Choppy or Fine.

Key symptoms: loose stools, scanty periods, blurred vision and pale sides of the tongue.

> **Diagnostic tip**
>
> Loose stools, scanty periods and blurred vision would be enough to diagnose Spleen- and Liver-Blood deficiency

Aetiology

This pattern is usually due to dietary factors: either a diet lacking in nourishment or excessive in cold and raw foods.

Pathology

The Spleen is the origin of Blood because Food-Qi (*Gu Qi*) produced by the Spleen is the basis for the formation

- Depression, insomnia, dizziness
- Dry hair
- Blurred vision
- Poor appetite
- Dull-pale complexion
- Pale lips
- Tiredness
- Abdominal distension
- Loose stools
- Brittle nails
- Scanty periods
- Numbness of limbs
- Cramps
- Weak limbs

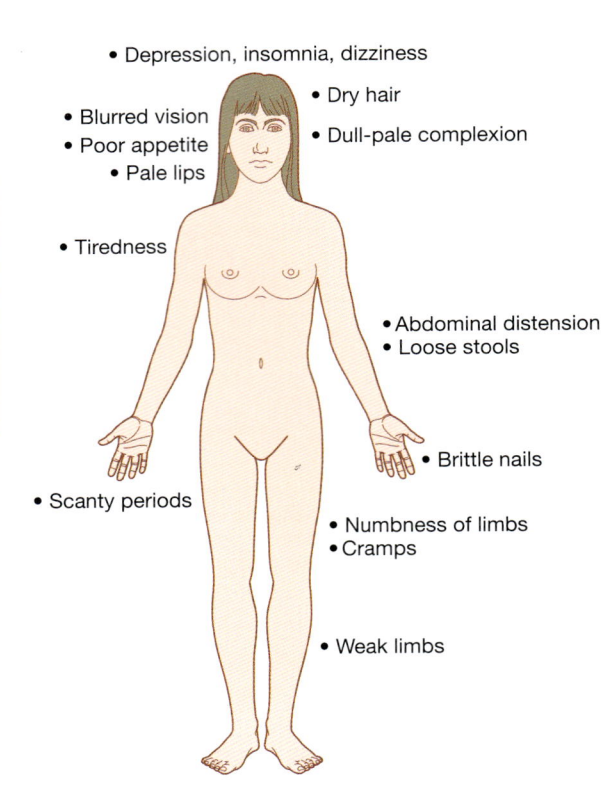

Figure 36.24 Spleen- and Liver-Blood deficiency

of Blood. If Spleen-Qi is deficient, not enough Blood is produced. Since the Liver stores Blood, when this is deficient, there will be lack of Blood in the Liver. This will cause dizziness, blurred vision, numbness, scanty periods and a pale or orangey colour of the sides of the tongue.

The slight depression and feeling of aimlessness are due to the lack of 'movement' of the Ethereal Soul (*Hun*) housed in the Liver.

The other symptoms, such as loose stools, poor appetite and weak limbs, are typical of Spleen-Qi deficiency (Fig. 36.25).

Pathological precursors of pattern

Spleen-Qi deficiency always precedes Spleen-Blood deficiency (Fig 36.26).

Pathological developments from pattern

Both Spleen-Blood and Liver-Blood deficiency may lead to Heart-Blood deficiency (see Fig 36.26).

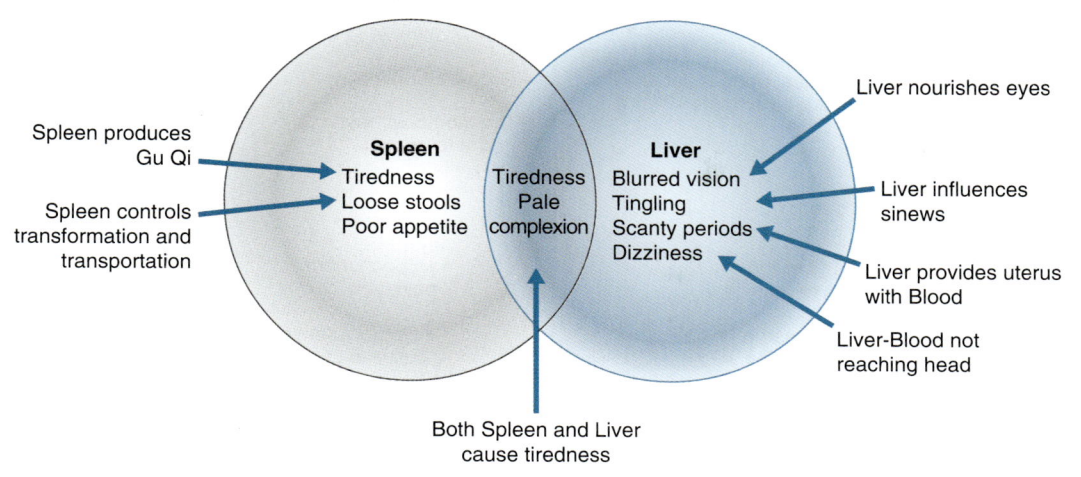

Figure 36.25 Pathology of Spleen- and Liver-Blood deficiency

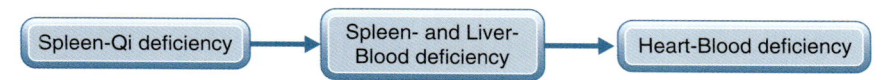

Figure 36.26 Spleen- and Liver-Blood deficiency pattern: precursors and developments

Treatment

Principle of treatment: tonify Spleen-Qi, nourish Liver-Blood.

Acupuncture

Points: LIV-8 Ququan, SP-6 Sanyinjiao, Ren-4 Guanyuan, BL-18 Ganshu, BL-23 Shenshu, Ren-12 Zhongwan, ST-36 Zusanli, SP-3 Taibai, BL-20 Pishu, BL-21 Weishu, BL-17 Geshu (with direct moxa).
Method: reinforcing, moxa is applicable
Explanation
– LIV-8 and SP-6 tonify Liver-Blood.
– Ren-4 nourishes Blood.
– BL-18 and BL-23 nourish Liver-Blood.
– Ren-12, ST-36, SP-3, BL-20 and BL-21 tonify Spleen-Qi.
– BL-17 nourishes Blood (with direct moxa).

Herbal formula

Gui Pi Tang *Tonifying the Spleen Decoction*.

Three Treasures

Calm the Shen (Variation of Gui Pi Tang).
Box 36.11 summarizes Spleen- and Liver-Blood deficiency.

Box 36.11 Spleen- and Liver-Blood deficiency

Clinical manifestations

Poor appetite, slight abdominal distension after eating, tiredness, lassitude, dull-pale complexion, weakness of the limbs, loose stools, thin body, scanty periods or amenorrhoea, insomnia, dizziness, numbness of limbs, blurred vision, 'floaters' in eyes, diminished night vision, pale lips, muscular weakness, cramps, withered and brittle nails, dry hair and skin, slight depression, a feeling of aimlessness, Pale tongue especially on the sides, dry, Choppy or Fine pulse

Treatment

LIV-8 Ququan, SP-6 Sanyinjiao, Ren-4 Guanyuan, BL-18 Ganshu, BL-23 Shenshu, Ren-12 Zhongwan, ST-36 Zusanli, SP-3 Taibai, BL-20 Pishu, BL-21 Weishu, BL-17 Geshu

---

Obstruction of Spleen by Dampness with stagnation of Liver-Qi

Clinical manifestations

A feeling of oppression and fullness of the epigastrium, nausea, no appetite, loose stools, a feeling of heaviness, dry mouth without desire to drink, sallow complexion, hypochondrial pain, a sticky taste, epigastric and hypochondrial distension, irritability (Fig. 36.27).

- Irritability
- Nausea, poor appetite, sticky-bitter taste
- Sallow complexion
- Dry mouth without desire to drink
- Feeling of heaviness
- Hypochondrial pain
- Epigastric distension
- Oppression and fullness of epigastrium
- Loose stools

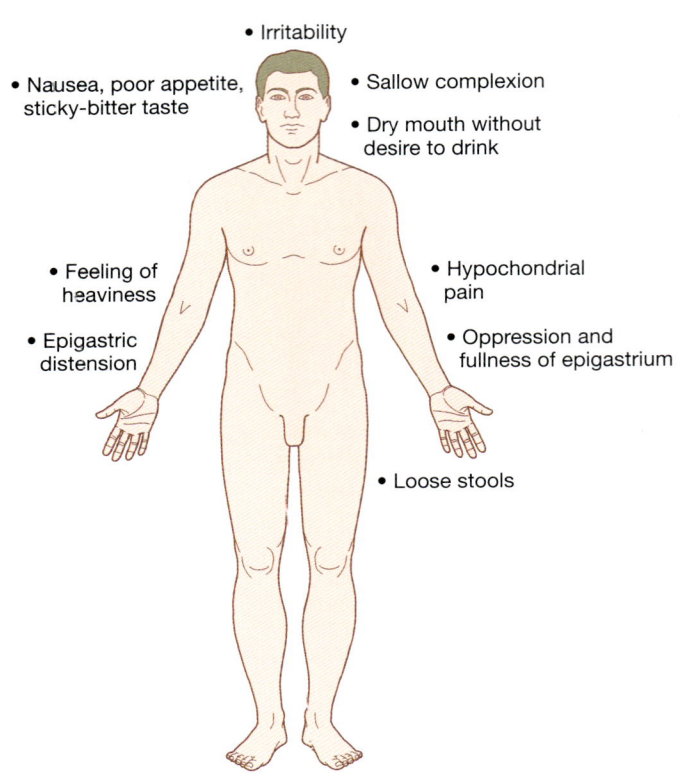

Figure 36.27 Obstruction of the Spleen by Dampness with stagnation of Liver-Qi

Tongue: thick sticky yellow coating.
Pulse: Slippery-Wiry.
Key symptoms: fullness of epigastrium, hypochondrial distension and a thick sticky yellow tongue coating.

Diagnostic tip

Fullness of epigastrium, hypochondrial distension and a thick sticky yellow tongue coating.

Aetiology

This pattern is caused by the excessive consumption of greasy foods and dairy foods, which tend to create Dampness in the Spleen.

Pathology

When the Spleen is deficient and fails in its function of transformation and transportation, fluids accumulate into Dampness. Dampness obstructs the flow of Qi in the Middle Burner, interfering with the proper direction of flow of Qi (ascending of Spleen-Qi, descending of Stomach-Qi and smooth flow of Liver-Qi). After a long period of time, the obstruction of Dampness gives rise to Heat. Dampness begins to interfere with the smooth flow of Liver-Qi and the flow of bile: Liver-Qi stagnates in the Middle Burner and the Gall Bladder cannot secrete bile.

From a Five-Element perspective, this corresponds to Earth insulting Wood.

Pathological precursors of pattern

Spleen-Qi deficiency may lead to the formation of Dampness: this obstructs the Middle Burner and may interfere with the free flow of Liver-Qi (Fig. 36.28).

Pathological developments from pattern

Dampness in the Middle Burner may, in time, give rise to Phlegm. Stagnation of Liver-Qi may lead to Liver-Blood stasis or to Heat (see Fig. 36.28).

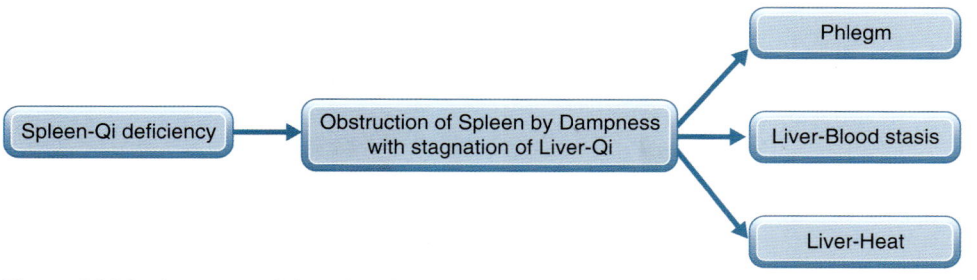

Figure 36.28 Obstruction of the Spleen by Dampness with stagnation of Liver-Qi pattern: precursors and developments

Treatment

Principle of treatment: resolve Dampness, promote the smooth flow of Liver-Qi, clear Heat.

Acupuncture

Points: Ren-12 Zhongwan, SP-6 Sanyinjiao, SP-3 Taibai, SP-9 Yinlingquan, BL-20 Pishu, LIV-13 Zhangmen, LIV-14 Qimen, G.B.-24 Riyue, G.B.-34 Yanglingquan, LIV-3 Taichong, ST-19 Burong,.

Method: reducing for points of Liver and Gall Bladder channels as well as for SP-6, LIV-13 and SP-3 (to resolve Dampness); reinforcing for the other points (to tonify the Spleen).

Explanation
- Ren-12 tonifies the Spleen to resolve Dampness.
- SP-6, SP-3 and SP-9 resolve Dampness.
- BL-20 tonifies the Spleen to resolve Dampness.
- LIV-13 promotes the smooth flow of Liver-Qi and resolves Dampness from the Middle Burner.
- LIV-14 promotes the smooth flow of Liver-Qi.
- G.B.-24 promotes the smooth flow of Liver-Qi and the secretion of bile.
- G.B.-34 promotes the smooth flow of Liver-Qi in the Middle Burner.
- LIV-3 promotes the smooth flow of Liver-Qi.
- ST-19 eliminates Dampness from the Middle Burner.

Herbal formula

Ping Wei San *Balancing the Stomach Powder* plus Mu Xiang *Radix Aucklandiae lappae* and Xiang Fu *Rhizoma Cyperi rotundi*.

Huo Xiang Zheng Qi San *Agastache Upright Qi Powder* plus Mu Xiang *Radix Aucklandiae lappae* and Xiang Fu *Rhizoma Cyperi rotundi*.

Yi Jia Jian Zheng Qi San *First Variation of Upright Qi Powder*.

Box 36.12 summarizes obstruction of the Spleen by Dampness with stagnation of Liver-Qi.

Box 36.12 Obstruction of the Spleen by Dampness with stagnation of Liver-Qi

Clinical manifestations

A feeling of oppression and fullness of the epigastrium, nausea, no appetite, loose stools, a feeling of heaviness, dry mouth without desire to drink, sallow complexion, hypochondrial pain, bitter taste, a sticky taste, epigastric and hypochondrial distension, irritability, thick sticky yellow tongue coating, Slippery-Wiry pulse

Treatment

Ren-12 Zhongwan, SP-6 Sanyinjiao, SP-3 Taibai, SP-9 Yinlingquan, BL-20 Pishu, LIV-13 Zhangmen, LIV-14 Qimen, G.B.-24 Riyue, G.B.-34 Yanglingquan, LIV-3 Taichong, ST-19 Burong

Learning outcomes

In this chapter you will have learned:
- The significance of Dampness (exterior or interior) in causing a Spleen imbalance, and its frequency in clinical practice
- The effects of worry and pensiveness on Spleen-Qi
- How diet can benefit or adversely affect the Spleen
- How to identify the following Deficiency patterns:
  Spleen-Qi deficiency: tiredness and loose stools, with a Pale tongue and an Empty pulse
  Spleen-Yang deficiency: loose stools, tiredness and feeling cold, with a Pale, Wet tongue
  Spleen-Qi sinking: bearing-down sensation, Weak pulse and other symptoms of Spleen-Qi deficiency
  Spleen not controlling the Blood: Fine pulse, Pale tongue and bleeding
  Spleen-Blood deficiency: tiredness, slight abdominal distension and scanty periods

- How to identify the following Excess patterns:
  Cold-Dampness invading the Spleen: abdominal fullness and a sticky white tongue coating
  Damp-Heat invading the Spleen: abdominal fullness and a sticky yellow tongue coating
- How to identify the following combined patterns:
  Spleen- and Heart-Blood deficiency: palpitations, insomnia, loose stools and scanty periods
  Spleen- and Lung-Qi deficiency: poor appetite, tiredness and shortness of breath
  Spleen- and Liver-Blood deficiency: loose stools, scanty periods and blurred vision
  Obstruction of Spleen by Dampness with stagnation of Liver-Qi: fullness of the epigastrium, hypochondrial distension and a thick sticky yellow tongue coating
- Awareness of the following combination Spleen patterns: Spleen- and Stomach-Qi deficiency (discussed under Stomach patterns, ch. 38)

Learning tips

Spleen-Qi deficiency

First, think of the general manifestations of Qi deficiency: tiredness, Pale tongue, Empty pulse

With the Spleen, digestive symptoms are paramount, hence poor appetite, loose stools

Spleen-Qi deficiency is the nucleus of all other Spleen Deficiency patterns, i.e.:
– Spleen-Yang deficiency: cold limbs
– Spleen-Qi sinking: prolapse
– Spleen not controlling Blood: bleeding
– Spleen-Blood deficiency: scanty periods

Dampness in the Spleen

First, think of the general manifestations of Dampness: feeling of heaviness, abdominal fullness, sticky tongue coating, Slippery pulse

Next, as in all Spleen patterns, digestive symptoms are paramount, hence nausea, poor appetite, epigastric fullness

In Cold Dampness add cold limbs and feeling cold; in Damp-Heat add feeling of heat and thirst without desire to drink

Remember that Dampness is a Full pattern and that is reflected on the tongue coating (thick sticky) and the pulse (Slippery-Full)

Self-assessment questions

1. When might a woman be particularly prone to an invasion of exterior Dampness?
2. What eating habits can cause Spleen-Qi deficiency?
3. What is the pathology of weak limbs and tiredness in the pattern of Spleen-Qi deficiency?
4. Why is a wet tongue associated with Spleen-Yang deficiency?
5. What is the most important aetiological factor leading to Spleen-Blood deficiency?
6. A female patient presents with poor appetite, abdominal fullness, a feeling of heavy head and body, vaginal discharge and has a pale tongue with a sticky white coating. Which pattern do you suspect?
7. What is a common clinical precursor to a chronic pattern of Damp-Heat invading the Spleen?
8. What key symptoms would you look for to diagnose the pattern Spleen- and Heart-Blood deficiency?
9. What is the pathology of Heat symptoms in the combined pattern Obstruction of Spleen by Dampness with stagnation of Liver-Qi?

See p. 1264 for answers

END NOTES

1. The idea that women should pay great attention to not catching Dampness during each period and particularly after childbirth is deeply rooted in Chinese culture. Even today, in rural areas some women follow the custom of not washing at all for a month after childbirth. In all parts of China, both rural areas and cities, women often do not wash their hair at the time of menstruation.
2. Some modern Chinese textbooks, such as the 'Essentials of Chinese Acupuncture', call the emotion related to the Spleen 'meditation'. This is obviously a mistranslation of the Chinese character which simply indicates 'thinking' or 'pensiveness'. Far from being a cause of disease, meditation is very beneficial to the Spleen and Heart.
3. 1981 Syndromes and Treatment of the Internal Organs (*Zang Fu Zheng Zhi* 脏 腑 证 治), Tianjin Scientific Publishing House, Tianjin, p. 291.

SECTION 2 PART 6

Kidney Patterns 37

Key contents

General aetiology
Hereditary weakness
Emotional strain
Excessive sexual activity
Chronic illness
Overwork
Old age

Empty patterns
Kidney-Yang deficiency
Kidney-Yin deficiency
Kidney-Qi not Firm
Kidney failing to receive Qi
Kidney-Essence deficiency

Empty/Full patterns
Kidney-Yang deficiency, Water overflowing
Kidney-Yin deficiency, Empty-Heat blazing

Combined patterns
Kidney- and Liver-Yin deficiency
Kidneys and Heart not harmonized
Kidney- and Lung-Yin deficiency
Kidney- and Spleen-Yang deficiency

The functions of the Kidneys (ch. 10) are:

- Store the Essence (*Jing*) and govern birth, growth, reproduction and development
- Produce Marrow, fill up the brain and control bones
- Govern Water
- Control the reception of Qi
- Open into the ears
- Manifest in the hair
- Control spittle
- Control the two lower orifices
- House the Will-power (*Zhi*)
- Control the Gate of Life (Minister Fire, *Ming Men*)

The main Kidney function is that of storing Essence and governing birth, growth and reproduction. Since the Essence of the Kidneys can never be in excess but can only be deficient, Chinese medical theory holds that the Kidneys do not have Excess patterns but only Deficiency ones. There is, however, an exception as acute Damp-Heat can affect Bladder and Kidneys. In chronic conditions, though, all Kidney patterns are either of the Deficiency type or the combined Deficiency/Excess type.

Central to any Kidney pathology is the duality of Kidney-Yin and Kidney-Yang. Although this duality can be observed in both physiology and pathology, it is in disease that it becomes very apparent.

Kidney-Yin represents the Essence (*Jing*) and the fluids within the Kidneys. Kidney-Yang is the motive force of all physiological processes and it is the root of transformation and movement: it is the physiological Fire. Kidney-Yin is the material foundation for Kidney-Yang, and Kidney-Yang is the exterior manifestation of Kidney-Yin.

Every pathological condition of the Kidneys will necessarily manifest itself as a deficiency of Kidney-Yin or Kidney-Yang. For example, the patterns of Kidney-Qi not Firm and Kidneys failing to receive Qi are variations of Kidney-Yang deficiency while the pattern of Kidney-Essence deficiency is a type of Kidney-Yin deficiency (although it may sometimes present with symptoms of Kidney-Yang deficiency). Hence:

Kidney-Yang deficiency	Kidney-Yin deficiency
Kidney-Qi not Firm	Kidney-Essence deficiency
Kidney failing to receive Qi	

However, as mentioned in the chapter on the Kidney functions (ch. 10), Kidney-Yin and Kidney-Yang have the same root and they are but two manifestations of the same entity. It follows that in pathological

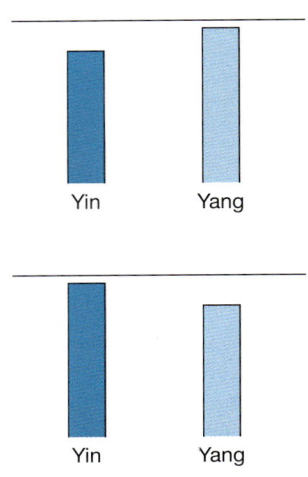

Figure 37.1 Deficiency of both Kidney-Yin and Kidney-Yang

conditions, a deficiency of Yin of the Kidneys will also necessarily imply, to a lesser degree, a deficiency of the Yang of the Kidneys and vice versa. In many cases, and especially in women over 45, a deficiency of the Kidneys nearly always involves both Kidney-Yin and Kidney-Yang. However, it must be stressed that the deficiency will always be primarily either of Yin or Yang: it can never be 50% Yin and 50% Yang deficient. This can be expressed in diagrammatic form (Fig. 37.1).

It will be noted that this diagram differs from those usually presented in so far as the column for Yin is below the normal mark in Yang deficiency, and the column for Yang is below the normal mark in Yin deficiency. This is a visual representation of the fact that Kidney-Yin and Kidney-Yang have the same origin and one cannot be deficient without the other also being slightly (but to a lesser degree) deficient.

This situation is very common in practice. How often do we see a patient who has a malar flush, dark urine, night sweating, tinnitus (Kidney-Yin deficiency) but also swollen ankles (Kidney-Yang deficiency)? Or how often do we see a patient whose urination is frequent and pale, who feels chilly, has a lower back ache (Kidney-Yang deficiency) but also suffers from night sweating (Kidney-Yin deficiency)?

The simultaneous deficiency of Kidney-Yin and Kidney-Yang is very common in practice and especially in women over 45 years of age

Clinical note

1. Kidney-Yang and Kidney-Yin deficiency with predominance of the former: lower backache, feeling cold, cold knees, abundant and frequent urination, night sweating
2. Kidney-Yang and Kidney-Yin deficiency with predominance of the latter: dizziness, tinnitus, night sweating, dry throat at night, cold feet, swollen ankles

The Kidneys are called the 'Root of Pre-Heaven Qi' because they store Essence. The Kidneys are nearly always affected in chronic diseases. There is a saying in Chinese medicine: 'A chronic disease will inevitably reach the Kidneys.'

The Kidneys are nearly always affected in chronic diseases

The Kidneys are also the root of all the other organs, as Kidney-Yin is the foundation for the Yin of Liver and Heart, whilst Kidney-Yang is the foundation for the Yang of Spleen and Lungs. Thus most chronic diseases will eventually manifest with a Kidney disharmony, either Kidney-Yin or Kidney-Yang deficiency. Since the Kidneys are the foundation for the Yin and Yang energies of all other organs, the combined patterns of the Kidneys with other organs will be discussed in this chapter.

Kidney-Yin is root of:	Kidney-Yang is root of:
Liver	Spleen
Heart	Lungs
Lungs	Heart

Box 37.1 summarizes factors that might indicate Kidney pathology.

The discussion of the Kidney patterns will be preceded by a discussion of the general aetiology of Kidney disharmony as follows:
GENERAL AETIOLOGY
- Hereditary weakness
- Emotional strain

> **Box 37.1 A 'feel' for Kidney pathology**
> - Backache
> - Tendency to obesity in Kidney-Yang deficiency
> - Thinness in Kidney-Yin deficiency
> - Emotionally, a tendency to depression
> - Sexual issues
> - Exhaustion
> - Long, protracted problems

- Excessive sexual activity
- Chronic illness
- Overwork
- Old age

The Kidney patterns discussed are:

EMPTY PATTERNS
- Kidney-Yang deficiency
- Kidney-Yin deficiency
- Kidney-Qi not Firm
- Kidney failing to receive Qi
- Kidney-Essence deficiency

EMPTY/FULL PATTERNS
- Kidney-Yang deficiency, Water overflowing
- Kidney-Yin deficiency, Empty-Heat blazing

COMBINED PATTERNS
- Kidney- and Liver-Yin deficiency
- Kidney and Heart not harmonized
- Kidney- and Lung-Yin deficiency
- Kidney- and Spleen-Yang deficiency

GENERAL AETIOLOGY

Hereditary weakness

The Pre-Heaven Qi of each person is formed at conception from the union of the parents' Kidney-Essences (sperm and ova are but an external manifestation of Kidney-Essence). It follows that the inherited constitution will depend on the strength and quality of the parents' Essences in general and at the time of conception in particular.

Chinese medicine has always placed great emphasis on the relation between the parents' Essences and the hereditary constitution of their offspring. Some ancient texts even stated the most auspicious or unfavourable times of conception in great detail.[1]

If the parents' Essences are weak, the child's Kidneys will also be weak. This may manifest with poor bone development, some mental retardation, a pigeon chest, a weak back, incontinence, enuresis, loose teeth and thin hair.

One of the most important factors in the parents' condition is their age. As Kidney-Essence declines with age, if the parents conceive when they are too old, their child's constitution might suffer. Similarly, if the parents are in a state of exhaustion at the time of conception, this may also induce a hereditary weakness of their child. This may explain the sometimes striking difference in physical appearance and personality amongst siblings.

Hereditary weakness as a cause of disease is discussed in chapter 22.

Emotional strain

The emotion pertaining to the Kidneys is fear. This includes fear, anxiety and shock. It is said in Chinese medicine that fear makes Qi descend. In children this will be manifested by enuresis: in fact, very often enuresis is caused by a situation of anxiety or insecurity in the family for the child.

In adults, however, very often fear and anxiety do not make Qi descend but rise. Very often a long-standing situation of anxiety may induce Empty-Heat within the Kidneys, which rises to the head, causing dry mouth, malar flush, mental restlessness and insomnia.

The Kidneys are also affected by worry and guilt.

Emotions as a cause of disease are discussed in chapter 20.

Excessive sexual activity

This is modestly referred to in Chinese books as 'unregulated affairs of the bedroom' or 'excessive labours of the bedroom'. Traditionally, the idea that excessive sexual activity can weaken the Kidneys is very old and can be found in the 'Yellow Emperor's Classic of Internal Medicine'.[2]

As mentioned in the chapter on Miscellaneous causes of disease (ch. 22), excessive sexual activity weakens the Kidney energy because sexual essences are a manifestation of the Kidney-Essence, and the orgasm quite simply tends to deplete the Kidney-Essence. It should be clarified here that by 'excessive sexual activity' is meant actual ejaculation for men and orgasm for women. Sexual activity without ejaculation or orgasm does not have a depleting effect on the Kidney-Essence. 'Excessive sexual activity' also includes masturbation, which affects the Kidney energy as much as sex with a partner.

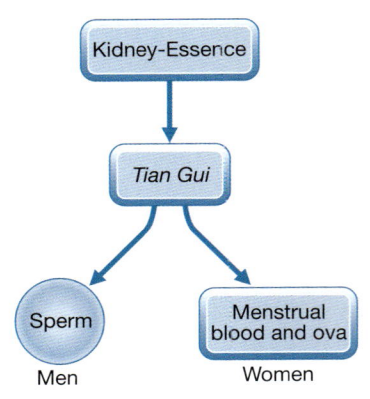

Figure 37.2 Sexual differences between men and women

However, there is an important difference in the effect of sexual activity on the Kidney-Essence between men and women. Sperm (called *Tian Gui* in the first chapter of the 'Simple Questions') is a direct manifestation of Kidney-Essence and, for this reason, too frequent ejaculation may weaken the Kidney-Essence. In women, *Tian Gui* is menstrual blood and ova: as there is no loss of these substances during sexual activity in women, there is no corresponding loss of Kidney-Essence. It follows that sexual activity is not depleting of Kidney-Essence in women as it is in men (Fig. 37.2).

However, there are two important sexual causes of disease in women: the first is having sexual intercourse during the period, which causes Blood stasis in the abdomen; the second is too early sexual activity (during puberty or around puberty), which seriously damages the Directing and Penetrating Vessels (*Ren Mai* and *Chong Mai*). These are discussed in chapter 22.

Chronic illness

As mentioned before, most chronic diseases eventually affect the Kidneys. In the late stages of a chronic disease a pattern of Kidney-Yin or Kidney-Yang deficiency can nearly always be seen. For example, if a person suffers from a Spleen-Yang deficiency for many years, this is very likely to lead to Kidney-Yang deficiency.

Overwork

This is intended both in a physical and mental sense. Excessive physical work or exercise over a long period of time will weaken Kidney-Yang. Overwork in the sense of working long hours without adequate rest for many years under conditions of stress will eventually weaken Kidney-Yin. This is, in fact, the most common cause of Kidney-Yin deficiency in Western industrialized societies.

A lifetime of work under conditions of stress, lack of relaxation, long hours of work, hurried meals, irregular eating schedule, eating late at night, discussing business while eating, excessive mental work not balanced with physical exercise, all these factors combine to erode the Yin energies because the body is never given a chance to recuperate. The result is that, instead of using Yang energies, which are quickly replenished by the Post-Heaven Qi, the body starts using the Yin essences, which are stored in the Kidneys. This eventually causes Kidney-Yin deficiency. If, in addition, there is great stress, worry and anxiety usually associated with overwork, this may also give rise to Empty-Heat (see Fig. 22.5 in ch. 22).

Overwork as a cause of disease is discussed in chapter 22.

A normal amount of work balanced with rest uses up Yang energies, which are constantly replenished (by rest). Overwork uses up Yin energies, which are not easily replenished

Old age

Kidney-Essence declines with age and, in fact, Chinese medicine sees the process of ageing as the result of the decrease of Kidney-Essence throughout our life. Old age is therefore not really a 'cause of disease' as the physiological decline of Kidney-Essence.

For this reason, many elderly people will suffer from a deficiency of Kidney-Essence and, indeed, the symptoms of old age are due to the decline of Kidney-Essence. Hearing decreases because Kidney-Essence cannot reach the ears, bones become brittle and weak because Kidney-Essence fails to nourish bones and bone marrow, and the sexual function decreases because the declining Kidney-Essence and the Fire of the Gate of Life cannot nourish the sexual organs.

Box 37.2 summarizes the general aetiology of Kidney patterns.

Box 37.2 General aetiology of Kidney patterns

- Hereditary weakness
- Emotional strain
- Excessive sexual activity
- Chronic illness
- Overwork
- Old age

EMPTY PATTERNS

Kidney-Yang deficiency

Clinical manifestations

Lower backache, dizziness, tinnitus, cold and weak knees, sensation of cold in the lower back, feeling cold, weak legs, bright-white complexion, tiredness, lassitude, abundant clear urination, urination at night, apathy, oedema of the legs, infertility in women, loose stools, depression, impotence, premature ejaculation, low sperm count, decreased libido (Fig. 37.3).
Tongue: Pale and wet.
Pulse: Deep-Weak.
Key symptoms: backache, feeling of cold, abundant clear urination, Pale tongue, Deep Pulse.

> **Diagnostic tip**
>
> Backache, a feeling of cold and a Weak Kidney pulse are enough to diagnose a Kidney-Yang deficiency

- Bright-white complexion
- Abundant clear urination
- Backache
- Weak legs
- Cold and weak knees
- Oedema of legs

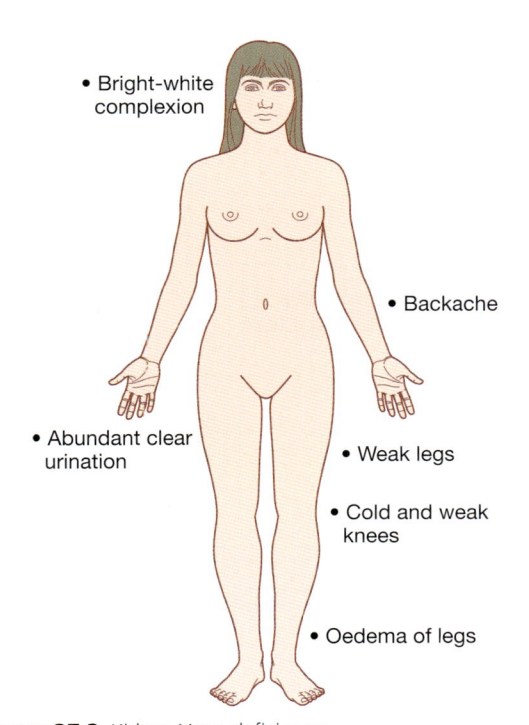

Figure 37.3 Kidney-Yang deficiency

Aetiology

Chronic illness

A chronic illness, and especially one manifesting with Spleen-Yang deficiency, can cause Kidney-Yang deficiency after a protracted period of time.

Excessive sexual activity

Excessive sexual activity can also cause Kidney-Yang deficiency. This happens in particular if one is exposed to cold immediately after intercourse.

In women, too early sexual activity during puberty may weaken Kidney-Yang.

Excessive physical work

Excessive physical work or exercise may weaken Kidney-Yang.

Diet

Excessive consumption of cold and raw foods may weaken Spleen- and Kidney-Yang.

Pathology

This is the classic pattern of Yang deficiency and it is therefore characterized by interior Cold symptoms.

When Kidney-Yang is deficient, the Fire of the Gate of Life (*Ming Men*) fails to warm the body, causing the feeling of cold in the back and knees and the general cold feeling.

When Kidney-Yang is deficient, the Kidneys do not have enough Qi to give strength to bones and the back, hence the soreness of the back and weakness of the legs and knees.

Deficient Kidney-Yang fails to warm the Essence, hence the sexual energy is deprived of the nourishment of the Essence and warmth of Kidney-Yang. This results in impotence, premature ejaculation, low sperm count, cold and thin sperm in men, infertility in women or lack of libido in both men and women.

> A deficiency of Kidney-Yang causes lack of libido. Conversely, Empty-Heat within the Kidneys causes an excessive sexual desire

When Kidney-Yang is deficient it fails to transform the fluids, which therefore accumulate, resulting in abundant and clear urination. In special cases when

Kidney-Yang is so deficient that it cannot move the fluids at all, there may be the opposite: that is, scanty (but clear) urination. If the fluids accumulate under the skin there will be oedema of the legs. The accumulation of fluids in the tongue makes it wet.

Deficient Kidney-Yang fails to nourish the Spleen, hence the muscles lack nourishment: this causes the tiredness, lassitude and Pale tongue. From a psychological point of view, it is manifested with apathy, lack of will-power and depression.

Deficient Kidney-Yang not brightening the brain causes dizziness and not brightening the ears causes tinnitus.

Pathological precursors of pattern

Spleen-Yang deficiency is the most common precursor of this pattern. Retention of Dampness (resulting from Spleen deficiency) over a long period of time will eventually affect the Kidneys by obstructing the movement of fluids and therefore leading to deficiency of Kidney-Yang.

A deficiency of Kidney-Yang may also evolve from Kidney-Yin deficiency, in which case both Yin and Yang will be deficient (although with a predominance of Yang deficiency) (Figs 37.4 and 37.5).

Pathological developments from pattern

Kidney-Yang deficiency may induce a Yang deficiency of various organs and especially the Spleen, Stomach, Lungs and Heart. Indeed, in chronic conditions, a long-standing deficiency of Kidney-Yang will always affect one or more of the above organs (see Fig. 37.5).

Treatment

Principle of treatment: tonify and warm the Kidneys, strengthen the Fire of the Gate of Life.

Acupuncture

Points: BL-23 Shenshu, Du-4 Mingmen, Ren-4 Guanyuan, Ren-6 Qihai, KI-3 Taixi, KI-7 Fuliu, BL-52 Zhishi, Jinggong extra point (0.5 cun lateral to BL-52 Zhishi).

Method: reinforcing, moxa should be used.

Explanation
- BL-23 tonifies Kidney-Yang.
- Du-4 strengthens the Fire of the Gate of Life. Moxa is applicable.
- Ren-4 (with moxa) tonifies Kidney-Yang and the Original Qi.
- Ren-6 (with moxa) tonifies Kidney-Yang.
- KI-3 tonifies the Kidneys.
- KI-7 is specific to tonify Kidney-Yang.
- BL-52 tonifies the Kidneys and in particular their mental aspect, i.e. the Will-power.
- Jinggong tonifies Kidney-Yang and warms the Essence.

Herbal formula

You Gui Wan *Restoring the Right [Kidney] Pill*.
Jin Gui Shen Qi Wan *Golden Chest Kidney-Qi Pill*.

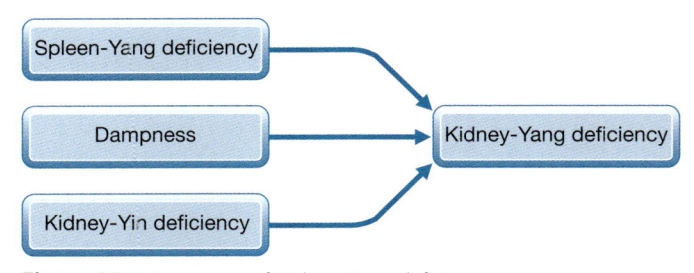

Figure 37.4 Precursors of Kidney-Yang deficiency

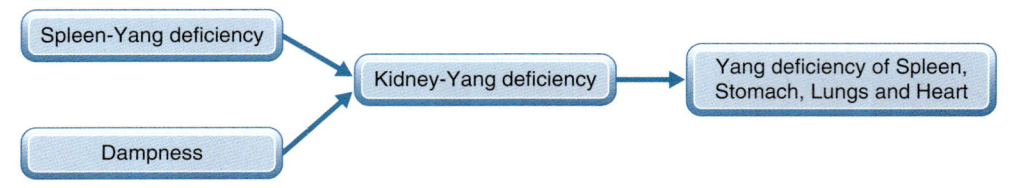

Figure 37.5 Kidney-Yang deficiency pattern: precursors and developments

Three Treasures

Strengthen the Root (variation of You Gui Wan).
  Box 37.3 summarizes Kidney-Yang deficiency.

> **Box 37.3 Kidney-Yang deficiency**
>
> **Clinical manifestations**
>
> Lower backache, cold and weak knees, sensation of cold in the lower back, feeling cold, weak legs, bright-white complexion, tiredness, lassitude, abundant clear urination, urination at night, apathy, oedema of the legs, infertility in women, loose stools, depression, impotence, premature ejaculation, low sperm count, decreased libido, Pale and wet tongue, Deep-Weak pulse
>
> **Treatment**
>
> BL-23 Shenshu, Du-4 Mingmen, Ren-4 Guanyuan, Ren-6 Qihai, KI-3 Taixi, KI-7 Fuliu, BL-52 Zhishi, Jinggong extra point

Kidney-Yin deficiency

Clinical manifestations

Dizziness, tinnitus, vertigo, poor memory, hardness of hearing, night-sweating, dry mouth and throat at night, lower backache, ache in bones, nocturnal emissions, constipation, dark scanty urine, infertility, premature ejaculation, tiredness, lassitude, depression, slight anxiety (Fig. 37.6).
Tongue: normal-coloured without coating.
Pulse: Floating-Empty.
Key symptoms: backache, night sweating.

Empty-Heat

Five-palm heat, a feeling of heat in the evening, malar flush, menopausal hot flushes, thirst with desire to drink in small sips, pronounced anxiety in the evening, nocturnal emissions with dreams.
Tongue: Red without coating; in severe cases also cracked.
Pulse: Floating-Empty and slightly Rapid.

> **Diagnostic tip**
>
> Even just backache and night sweating are enough to diagnose Kidney-Yin deficiency

Aetiology

Overwork

Overwork, in the sense described in chapter 22, over a period of several years weakens Kidney-Yin.

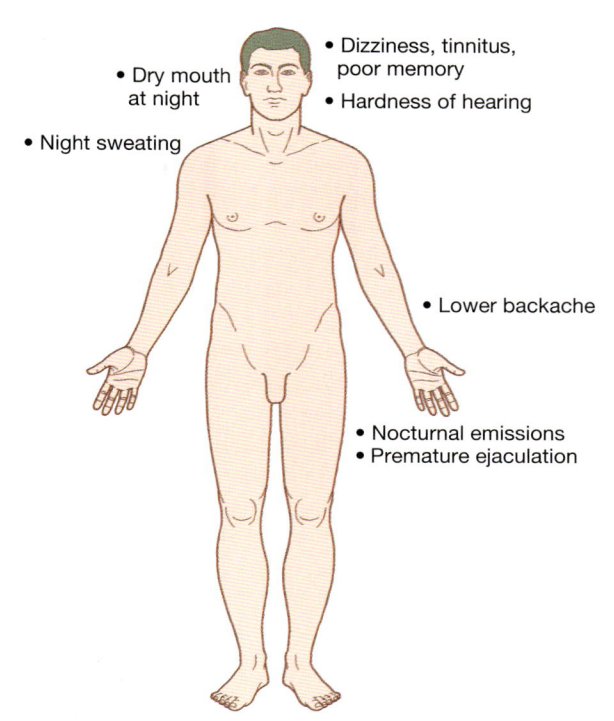

Figure 37.6 Kidney-Yin deficiency

Excessive sexual activity

Excessive sexual activity depletes Kidney-Essence and Kidney-Yin.

Loss of body fluids

Depletion of Body Fluids, which can be consumed by Heat after a febrile disease, may lead to Kidney-Yin deficiency.

Loss of blood

Loss of blood over a long period of time (such as from menorrhagia) can cause deficiency of Liver-Blood, which, in turn, can lead to deficiency of Kidney-Yin. It is said in Chinese medicine that Liver and Kidney share the same root.

Chronic illness

A long, chronic illness, usually transmitted from the Liver, Heart or Lungs, may lead to Kidney-Yin deficiency.

Overdosage of Chinese herbs

Overdosage of Chinese herbal medicines to strengthen Kidney-Yang or administration of wrong medicine (to strengthen Kidney-Yang when Kidney-Yin should be strengthened) leads to Kidney-Yin deficiency. The former situation is very common in China and Hong Kong as the habit of taking medicines to strengthen Kidney-Yang as middle-age approaches is ingrained in Chinese culture. If this is overdone and Kidney-Yang is overstimulated by the administration of too hot herbal medicines, Kidney-Yin will be injured.[3]

Pathology

This pattern is characterized by deficiency of Yin and also Essence of the Kidneys, as Essence is part of Kidney-Yin.

Deficient Kidney-Yin fails to produce enough Marrow to fill the brain, resulting in dizziness, tinnitus, vertigo and poor memory. The dizziness would be slight and the tinnitus would be of gradual and slow onset with a sound like rushing water.

The deficiency of Kidney-Yin leads to lack of Body Fluids and ensuing dryness, resulting in a dry mouth at night, constipation and scanty dark urine.

Night sweating is due to Yin being deficient and failing to hold Defensive Qi (*Wei Qi*) in the body at night (Defensive Qi retires into the Yin at night), so that the precious Yin nutritive essences come out with the sweat. Thus night sweating is very different from daytime sweating as, with the former, the Yin nutritive essences are lost, whilst with the latter, Yang fluids are lost. Night sweating is also called 'evaporation from the bones', whilst daytime sweating is called 'evaporation from the muscles'. The term for night sweating is also 'rob sweating', probably to indicate that with it the body is robbed of precious Yin essences.

> **Clinical note**
>
> Kidney-Yin deficiency often causes night sweating, which represents a loss of Yin fluids. Night sweating is 'evaporation from the bones', i.e. a loss of deep, precious fluids. It was called 'rob sweating' because it robs the body of precious Yin essences.

> Please note that, although Yin deficiency is the most common cause, night sweating is not always due to Yin deficiency (it may be sometimes due to Damp-Heat)

Kidney-Yin deficiency may cause deficiency of Essence, which results in nocturnal emissions.

The sore back and ache in the bones are due to the failure of Kidney-Essence in nourishing bones.

Deficient Kidney-Yin induces a deficiency of willpower and depression ensues. There is a slight anxiety as the Yin deficiency leads to some rising of Empty-Heat. The anxiety is more pronounced if there is fullblown Empty-Heat.

Pathological precursors of pattern

A deficiency of Liver-Yin may lead to Kidney-Yin deficiency as the Liver and Kidneys share a common root. However, deficiency of Yin of the Heart or Lungs may also lead to Kidney-Yin deficiency.

In women, a long-standing deficiency of Liver-Blood may also lead to Kidney-Yin deficiency.

A deficiency of Kidney-Yin may also evolve from Kidney-Yang deficiency, in which case both Yin and Yang will be deficient (although with a predominance of Yin deficiency) (Fig. 37.7).

Pathological developments from pattern

Kidney-Yin deficiency may lead to Yin deficiency of various organs and particularly Liver, Heart, Lungs and Stomach (see Fig. 37.7).

Treatment

Principle of treatment: nourish Kidney-Yin.

Acupuncture

Points: Ren-4 Guanyuan, KI-3 Taixi, KI-6 Zhaohai, KI-10 Yingu, KI-9 Zhubin, SP-6 Sanyinjiao, Ren-7

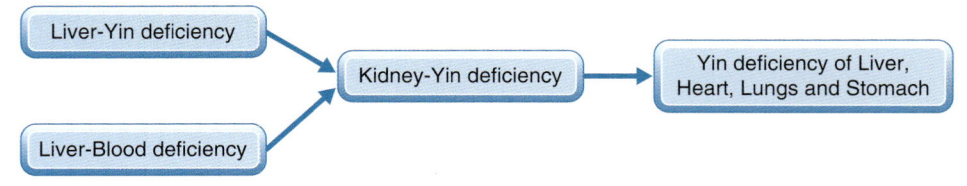

Figure 37.7 Kidney-Yin deficiency pattern: precursors and developments

Yinjiao, LU-7 Lieque and KI-6 Zhaohai in combination (opening points of the Directing Vessel).

Method: reinforcing method, no moxa.

Explanation
- Ren-4 without moxa tonifies Kidney-Yin and Kidney Essence (with moxa it can tonify Kidney-Yang).
- KI-3 tonifies the Kidneys.
- KI-6 is specific to tonify Kidney-Yin and it benefits the throat (particularly indicated for dry mouth at night).
- KI-10 is specific to tonify Kidney-Yin.
- KI-9 tonifies Kidney-Yin, particularly useful in case of anxiety and emotional tension of Kidney origin.
- SP-6 tonifies Liver- and Kidney-Yin and calms the mind.
- Ren-7 nourishes Yin.
- LU-7 and KI-6 in combination open the Directing Vessel (*Ren Mai*) and nourish Kidney-Yin.

Herbal fomula

Zuo Gui Wan *Restoring the Left [Kidney] Pill.*
Liu Wei Di Huang Wan *Six-Ingredient Rehmannia Pill.*

Three Treasures

Nourish the Root (variation of Zuo Gui Wan).

Box 37.4 summarizes Kidney-Yin deficiency.

Case history 37.1

A man of 50 suffered from a severe pain in the left loin, with very dark and scanty urine, dry mouth and night sweating. This pain came in bouts and was caused by a kidney stone lodged in the ureter. The tongue was Deep-Red and nearly completely without coating, the tip was redder, it had an extremely deep crack in the midline with smaller cracks arising out of it and it was dry. The pulse at the time of examination was Deep and Wiry (when a pulse has these two qualities it is also called Firm).

The night sweating, dry mouth and very dark and scanty urine point to Kidney-Yin deficiency. This is confirmed by the tongue, which is completely peeled: this always indicates Kidney-Yin deficiency. It is also indicated by its dryness. The deep crack in the midline with smaller cracks also indicates severe Kidney-Yin deficiency. The Deep-Red colour of the tongue indicates that Kidney-Yin deficiency has given rise to Empty-Heat. The pulse in this case is affected by the acute episode and it reflects the internal stagnation of Qi and Blood and intense pain caused by the stone in the ureter.

From interrogation, it transpired that this person had been very worried and anxious about job insecurity for the past years. The anxiety was reflected in the red tip of the tongue indicating Heart Empty-Heat. Presumably, the anxiety, fear and insecurity caused the Kidney deficiency.

> **Box 37.4 Kidney-Yin deficiency**
>
> **Clinical manifestations**
>
> Dizziness, tinnitus, vertigo, poor memory, hardness of hearing, night sweating, dry mouth and throat at night, lower backache, ache in bones, nocturnal emissions, constipation, dark scanty urine, infertility, premature ejaculation, tiredness, lassitude, depression, slight anxiety, normal-coloured tongue without coating, Floating-Empty pulse
>
> **Treatment**
>
> Ren-4 Guanyuan, KI-3 Taixi, KI-6 Zhaohai, KI-10 Yingu, KI-9 Zhubin, SP-6 Sanyinjiao, Ren-7 Yinjiao, LU-7 Lieque and KI-6 Zhaohai in combination (opening points of the Directing Vessel).

Kidney-Qi not Firm

Clinical manifestations

Soreness and weakness of the lower back, weak knees, clear frequent urination, weak-stream urination, abundant urination, dribbling after urination, incontinence of urine, enuresis, urination at night, nocturnal emissions without dreams, premature ejaculation, spermatorrhoea, tiredness, feeling cold, cold limbs, in women prolapse of uterus, chronic white vaginal discharge, a dragging-down feeling in the lower abdomen, recurrent miscarriage (Fig. 37.8).

Tongue: Pale.
Pulse: Deep-Weak, especially in the Rear positions.
Key symptoms: dribbling after urination, chronic vaginal discharge, backache.

> **Diagnostic tip**
>
> Dribbling after urination, chronic vaginal discharge and backache are enough to diagnose Kidney-Qi not Firm

- Lower backache
- Prolapse of uterus, chronic vaginal discharge, dragging-down feeling in abdomen
- Clear frequent urination, weak-stream urination, dribbling after urination, incontinence of urine
- Weak knees

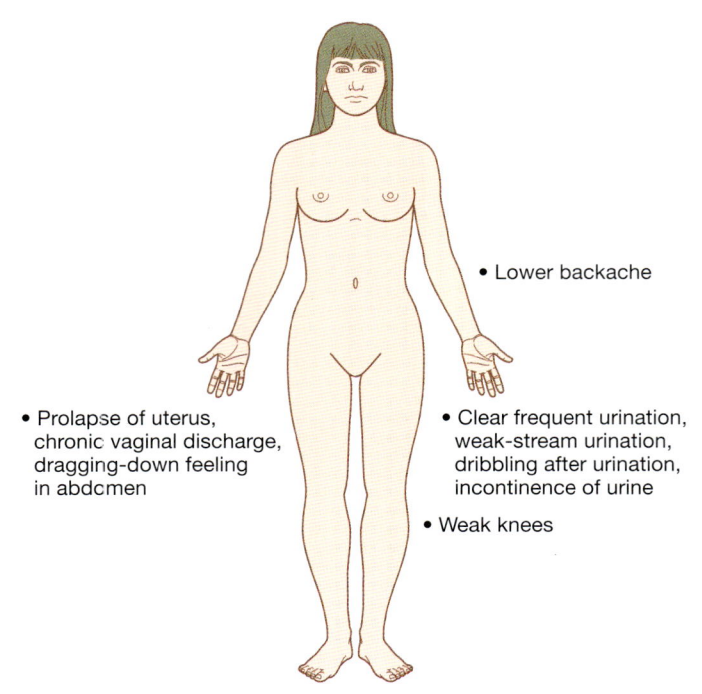

Figure 37.8 Kidney-Qi not Firm

Aetiology

Excessive sexual activity

In men, excessive sexual activity is the most important and frequent cause of this pattern.

Childbirth

In women, too many childbirths too close together can cause this pattern to arise. This may also happen if childbirth is prolonged and depletes Qi severely.

Excessive physical work

Excessive physical work or exercise depletes Spleen- and Kidney-Yang and may lead to Kidney-Qi not Firm.

Pathology

Two characteristics are evident in this pattern. First of all, it is a type of Kidney-Yang deficiency, hence the cold symptoms. Secondly, it is a type of sinking of Qi of the Kidneys, hence the many 'leaking' downwards symptoms.

This pattern is characterized by a weakness of one of the two 'lower Yin orifices' (i.e. the urethra and the 'Sperm Gate' in men), leading to manifestations of 'leaking'. The symptoms broadly fall into two categories of urinary and sexual manifestations. This pattern is also called 'Lower Original Qi [*Yuan Qi*] not Firm', to indicate that it is also caused by a weakness of the Original Qi and the Fire of the Gate of Life (*Ming Men*). Original Qi is weak in the Lower Burner, and Qi cannot hold fluids and sperm, hence the leaking character of most of the manifestations.

When Kidney-Qi and Original Qi are weak, the Kidneys cannot provide enough Qi to the Bladder for its function of Qi transformation, hence the urine cannot be held and this causes frequent urination, incontinence, enuresis, weak-stream urination and dribbling after urination.

When Kidney-Qi is deficient it cannot hold the sperm (or vaginal secretions in women), and this causes spermatorrhoea, premature ejaculation, nocturnal emissions without dreams and chronic vaginal discharge. The nocturnal emissions are without dreams because they are caused by a totally Deficient condition, so that the sperm leaks out because Kidney-Qi cannot hold it in. If nocturnal emissions are accompanied by vivid sexual dreams, this indicates that there is some Empty-Heat within the Kidneys arousing sexual desire.

Kidney-Yang deficiency → Kidney-Qi not Firm → Kidney-Yang deficiency

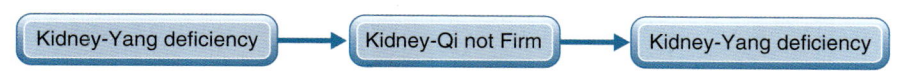

Figure 37.9 Kidney-Qi not Firm pattern: precursors and developments

There is urination at night because Yang Qi is not Firm, Yang cannot control the Yin at night, hence Yin predominates and the person needs to urinate during the night.

When Kidney-Yang is deficient, Qi may sink and this may cause prolapse of the uterus and a dragging-down feeling in the lower abdomen. The chronic vaginal discharge can also be seen to be a manifestation of the sinking of Qi from chronic Kidney and Spleen deficiency.

Pathological precursors of pattern

Kidney-Yang deficiency is a precursor of this pattern. A long-standing, chronic deficiency of Spleen-Yang may also lead to Kidney-Qi not Firm (Fig. 37.9).

Pathological developments from pattern

Kidney-Qi not Firm may easily lead to full-blown Kidney-Yang deficiency (see Fig. 37.9).

Treatment

Principle of treatment: reinforce and stabilize Kidney-Qi, raise Qi, and tonify Kidney-Yang.

Acupuncture

Points: BL-23 Shenshu, Du-4 Mingmen, KI-3 Taixi, BL-52 Zhishi, Ren-4 Guanyuan, Jinggong extra point, Ren-6 Qihai, Du-20 Baihui, KI-13 Qixue, BL-32 Ciliao.
Method: reinforcing, moxa is applicable.
Explanation
- BL-23 tonifies Kidney-Yang and firms Qi.
- Du-4 tonifies Kidney-Yang and the Fire of the Gate of Life. It is an important point to stop incontinence, enuresis, excessive urination, etc.
- KI-3 tonifies the Kidneys.
- BL-52 tonifies Kidney-Yang and strengthens Will-power.
- Ren-4 with moxa, tonifies Kidney-Yang and the Original Qi.
- Jinggong tonifies Kidney-Yang and firms the Sperm Gate.
- Ren-6 tonifies and firms Qi.
- Du-20 raises sinking Qi.
- KI-13 strengthens the Sperm Gate and tonifies the Kidneys.
- BL-32 firms Qi in the sexual organs.

Herbal formula

You Gui Wan *Restoring the Right [Kidney] Pill* plus Huang Qi *Radix Astragali membranacei* and Qian Shi *Semen Euryales ferocis*.
Jin Suo Gu Jing Wan *Metal Lock Consolidating the Essence Pill*.
Fu Tu Dan *Poria–Cuscuta Pill*.

Box 37.5 summarizes Kidney-Qi not Firm.

Box 37.5 Kidney-Qi not Firm

Clinical manifestations

Soreness and weakness of the lower back, weak knees, clear frequent urination, weak-stream urination, abundant urination, dribbling after urination, incontinence of urine, enuresis, urination at night, nocturnal emissions without dreams, premature ejaculation, spermatorrhoea, tiredness, feeling cold, cold limbs, in women prolapse of uterus, chronic white vaginal discharge, a dragging-down feeling in the lower abdomen, recurrent miscarriage, Pale tongue, Deep-Weak pulse especially in the Rear positions

Treatment

BL-23 Shenshu, Du-4 Mingmen, KI-3 Taixi, BL-52 Zhishi, Ren-4 Guanyuan, Jinggong extra point, Ren-6 Qihai, Du-20 Baihui, KI-13 Qixue, BL-32 Ciliao

---

Kidneys failing to receive Qi

Clinical manifestations

Shortness of breath on exertion, rapid and weak breathing, difficulty in inhaling, chronic cough and/or asthma, spontaneous sweating, cold limbs, cold limbs after sweating, swelling of the face, thin body, mental listlessness, clear urination during asthma attack, lower backache, dizziness, tinnitus (Fig. 37.10).
Tongue: Pale.
Pulse: Deep-Weak-Tight.
Key symptoms: shortness of breath on exertion, lower backache, clear urination.

- Dizziness, tinnitus
- Swelling of face
- Shortness of breath on exertion, cough, asthma
- Sweating
- Cold limbs
- Lower backache
- Clear urination during asthma attack

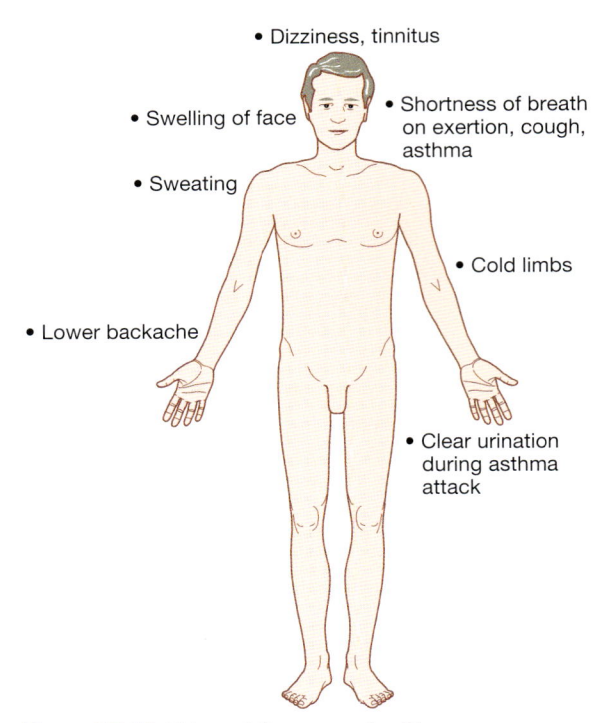

Figure 37.10 Kidneys failing to receive Qi

> **Diagnostic tip**
>
> Shortness of breath on exertion, lower backache and clear urination are enough to diagnose Kidneys failing to receive Qi

Aetiology

Hereditary weakness

Hereditary weakness of Lungs and Kidneys may be the predisposing factor to the development of this pattern.

Chronic illness

A long-standing, chronic disease, which inevitably reaches the Kidneys, particularly if transmitted from the Lungs, may cause this pattern.

Excessive physical work

Excessive physical work or exercise particularly during puberty and excessive lifting and standing may lead to this pattern.

Pathology

This is basically an impairment of the Kidney function of reception of Qi, and is also to be considered as a type of Kidney-Yang deficiency pattern.

When the Kidneys are weak and fail to receive and hold Qi down, Qi accumulates above, resulting in Excess above, in the chest, and Deficiency below, in the abdomen, hence the shortness of breath and asthma. Kidneys control inhalation, hence the asthma is characterized by difficulty in inhalation more than exhalation (the Lungs control exhalation).

When Kidney-Yang is deficient, all the Yang energies of the body are deficient, including Defensive Qi, hence the sweating and cold limbs.

Deficiency of Kidney-Yang also causes the abundant and clear urination, typically during an asthma attack.

This pattern can only appear in long-standing, chronic conditions, hence the general lassitude, thin body and mental exhaustion.

This pattern is also characterized by a failure of communication between Lung and Kidneys. As explained before, Lungs and Kidneys have to communicate with each other and assist each other particularly in the function of respiration (Lung controls exhalation and Kidneys control inhalation) and movement of fluids. When Kidney-Yang is deficient, the fluids cannot be transformed and this can give rise to oedema, which, in this case, is localized in the face because of the Lung involvement.

Pathological precursors of pattern

A deficiency of Kidney-Yang may lead to this pattern. A deficiency of Lung-Qi may also lead to this pattern if it is very prolonged (Fig. 37.11).

Pathological developments from pattern

The pattern of Kidneys failing to receive Qi may lead to the formation of Phlegm, which, itself, would aggravate the breathlessness (see Fig. 37.11).

Treatment

Principle of treatment: tonify and warm the Kidneys, stimulate the Kidney's receiving of Qi, stimulate the descending of Lung-Qi.

Acupuncture

Points: KI-7 Fuliu, KI-3 Taixi, LU-7 Lieque and KI-6 Zhaohai in combination (opening points of the Directing Vessel *Ren Mai*), ST-36 Zusanli, BL-23 Shenshu, Du-4 Mingmen, Ren-6 Qihai,

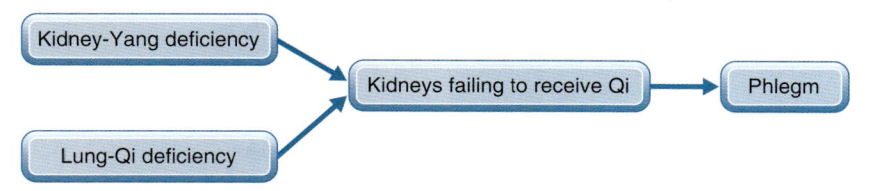

Figure 37.11 Kidney failing to receive Qi pattern: precursors and developments

Ren-17 Shanzhong, KI-25 Shencang, Du-12 Shenzhu, BL-13 Feishu, Ren-4 Guanyuan, KI-13 Qixue.

Method: reinforcing. Moxa is applicable.

Explanation
- KI-7 strengthens the Kidney's receiving of Qi.
- KI-3 tonifies the Kidneys.
- LU-7 and KI-6 in combination open the Directing Vessel, stimulate the descending of Lung-Qi and the Kidney's reception of Qi and benefit the throat.
- ST-36 tonifies Qi in general and is important to use in chronic conditions.
- BL-23 and Du-4 tonify Kidney-Yang.
- Ren-6 tonifies Kidney-Yang (used with moxa) and draws Qi down to the abdomen.
- Ren-17 tonifies Qi and stimulates the descending of Lung-Qi.
- KI-25 is an important local chest point of the Kidney channel to stimulate the Kidney reception of Qi and improve breathing.
- Du-12 and BL-13 tonify Lung Qi, important in chronic conditions.
- Ren-4 and KI-13 tonify the Kidneys and KI-13 specifically strengthens the Kidney's receiving of Qi.

Herbal formula

You Gui Wan *Restoring the Right [Kidney] Pill* plus Dong Chong Xia Cao *Sclerotium Cordicipitis chinensis* and Wu Wei Zi *Fructus Schisandrae chinensis*.

Shen Ge San *Ginseng–Gecko Powder*.

Su Zi Jiang Qi Tang *Perilla-Seed Subduing Qi Decoction*.

Three Treasures

Strengthen the Root (variation of You Gui Wan).
Box 37.6 summarizes Kidneys failing to receive Qi.

Box 37.6 Kidneys failing to receive Qi

Clinical manifestations

Shortness of breath on exertion, rapid and weak breathing, difficulty in inhaling, chronic cough and/or asthma, spontaneous sweating, cold limbs, cold limbs after sweating, swelling of the face, thin body, mental listlessness, clear urination during asthma attack, lower backache, dizziness, tinnitus, Pale tongue, Deep-Weak-Tight pulse

Treatment

KI-7 Fuliu, KI-3 Taixi, LU-7 Lieque and KI-6 Zhaohai in combination (opening points of the Directing Vessel), ST-36 Zusanli, BL-23 Shenshu, Du-4 Mingmen, Ren-6 Qihai, Ren-17 Shanzhong, KI-25 Shencang, Du-12 Shenzhu, BL-13 Feishu, Ren-4 Guanyuan, KI-13 Qixue

---

Kidney-Essence deficiency

Clinical manifestations

In children: poor bone development, late closure of fontanelle, deafness, mental dullness or retardation (Fig. 37.12).

In adults: softening of bones, weakness of knees and legs, poor memory, loose teeth, falling hair or premature greying of hair, weakness of sexual activity, lower backache, infertility, sterility, primary amenorrhoea, dizziness, tinnitus, deafness, blurred vision, absent-mindedness, decreased mental sharpness (Fig. 37.13).

- Mental retardation
- Late closure of fontenelle
- Deafness
- Poor bone development

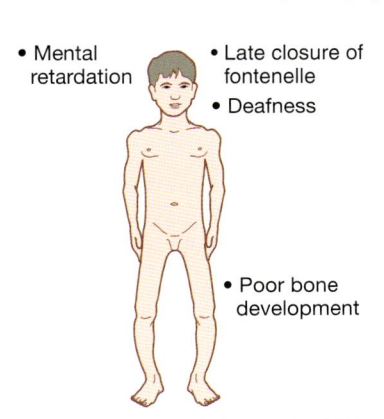

Figure 37.12 Kidney-Essence deficiency in children

- Dizziness
- Blurred vision
- Loose teeth
- Poor memory
- Falling hair
- Tinnitus, deafness
- Lower backache
- Weak sexual activity
- Weak legs
- Softening of bones

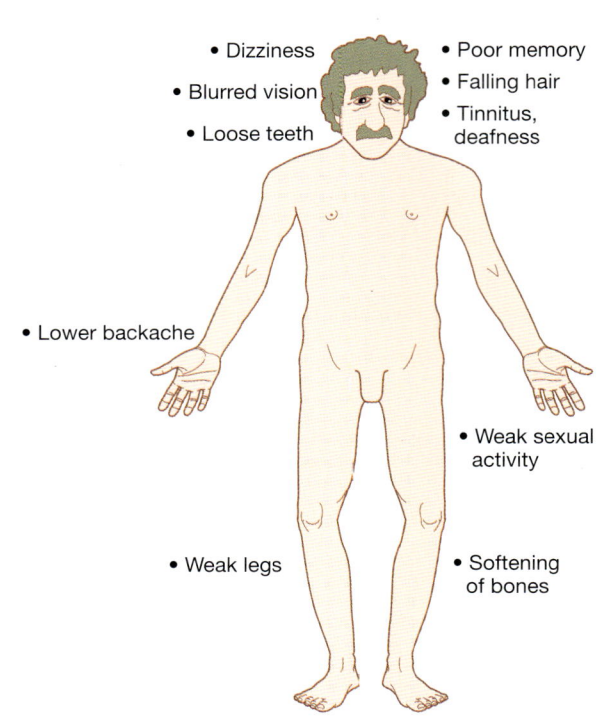

Figure 37.13 Kidney-Essence deficiency in adults

Tongue: without coating if this pattern occurs against a background of Kidney-Yin deficiency; Pale if against a background of Kidney-Yang deficiency.
Pulse: Floating-Empty or Leather.
Key symptoms: children: poor bone development; adults: weak knees, falling hair, weak sexual activity.

> **Diagnostic tip**
>
> Poor bone development in children; weak knees, falling hair and weak sexual activity in adults are enough to diagnose Kidney-Essence deficiency

Aetiology

Hereditary weakness

In children, this pattern is always caused by a hereditary weakness of the Kidney-Essence (which can be due to parents being too old or in poor health at the time of conception).

Excessive sexual activity

In adults, the pattern of Kidney-Essence deficiency may be caused by excessive sexual activity.

Loss of blood

In women, a Kidney-Essence deficiency may be caused by prolonged loss of blood occurring over many years, such as that occurring in a woman suffering from heavy periods.

Childbirth

Too many children too close together may cause a Kidney-Essence deficiency in a woman but in Western industrialised countries this is now a rare occurrence.

Pathology

This pattern can be considered as a type of Kidney-Yin deficiency pattern, as Kidney-Essence is part of Yin. However, there is also a Yang aspect to Kidney-Essence, so that a deficiency of Kidney-Essence can also occur against a background of Kidney-Yang deficiency. In this case the Tongue would be Pale.

> **Clinical note**
>
> Although the Essence is a Yin substance, a deficiency of Kidney-Essence may occur against a background of both Kidney-Yin and Kidney-Yang deficiency (more commonly the former)

When this pattern is present against a background of Kidney-Yin deficiency, there may be other symptoms of Yin deficiency such as tinnitus and dizziness.

This pattern is characterized by a deficiency of Essence: its manifestations therefore affect growth, reproduction and bones, all of which are under the control of Essence. When the Kidney-Essence is deficient, it will fail to generate Marrow and nourish the bones, hence the poor bone development, late closure of fontanelle, softening of bones and weakness of knees and legs. Teeth are seen as an extension of bone tissue, hence the looseness of teeth.

The Kidney-Essence generates Marrow, which fills the Brain; if the Essence is deficient, not enough Marrow is generated to fill the Brain, hence the poor memory in adults and mental dullness or retardation in children.

The Kidney-Essence also dominates the growth of head hair, hence the falling of hair or premature greying of hair.

The Kidney-Essence is the material basis for a healthy sexual function, hence the weakness of sexual activity.

Pathological precursors of pattern

Both Kidney-Yin and Kidney-Yang deficiency may lead to Kidney-Essence deficiency (Fig. 37.14).

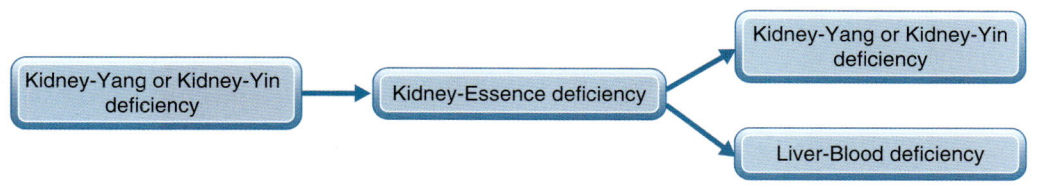

Figure 37.14 Kidney-Essence deficiency pattern: precursors and developments

Pathological developments from pattern

Kidney-Essence deficiency may lead to Kidney-Yin or Kidney-Yang deficiency. In women, it may also lead to Liver-Blood deficiency as the Essence plays a role in making Blood (see Fig. 37.14).

Treatment

Principle of treatment: nourish the Essence, tonify the Kidneys.

Acupuncture

Points: KI-3 Taixi, KI-6 Zhaohai, Ren-4 Guanyuan, KI-13 Qixue, BL-23 Shenshu, Du-4 Mingmen, GB-39 Xuanzhong, Du-20 Baihui, BL-15 Xinshu, BL-11 Dashu, Du-17 Naohu, Du-16 Fengfu.

Method: reinforcing. Moxa is applicable unless there is marked Yin deficiency with Empty-Heat.

Explanation
- KI-3 tonifies Kidney-Yin and Essence.
- KI-6 tonifies Kidney-Yin.
- Ren-4 and KI-13 tonify the Essence.
- BL-23 tonifies the Kidneys.
- Du-4 tonifies the Yang aspect of the Essence. This point would only be used if the Kidney-Essence deficiency occurs on a background of pronounced Yang deficiency.
- GB-39 tonifies the Bone Marrow.
- Du-20 stimulates the Marrow to fill the Brain.
- BL-15 tonifies the Heart to house the Mind, hence it tonifies the brain.
- BL-11 nourishes the Bones.
- Du-17 and Du-16 are points of the Sea of Marrow and therefore stimulate the nourishment of the Brain by Marrow.

Herbal formula

Zuo Gui Wan *Restoring the Left [Kidney] Pill*.

Three Treasures

Nourish the Root (Variation of Zuo Gui Wan).
Box 37.7 summarizes Kidney-Essence deficiency.

Box 37.7 Kidney-Essence deficiency

Clinical manifestations in children

Poor bone development, late closure of fontanelle, deafness, mental dullness or retardation

Clinical manifestations in adults

Softening of bones, weakness of knees and legs, poor memory, loose teeth, falling hair or premature greying of hair, weakness of sexual activity, lower backache, infertility, sterility, primary amenorrhoea, dizziness, tinnitus, deafness, blurred vision, absent-mindedness, decreased mental sharpness, tongue without coating if there is Kidney-Yin deficiency; Pale if there is Kidney-Yang deficiency, Floating-Empty or Leather pulse

Treatment

KI-3 Taixi, KI-6 Zhaohai, Ren-4 Guanyuan, KI-13 Qixue, BL-23 Shenshu, Du-4 Mingmen, GB-39 Xuanzhong, Du-20 Baihui, BL-15 Xinshu, BL-11 Dashu, Du-17 Naohu, Du-16 Fengfu.

EMPTY/FULL PATTERNS

Kidney-Yang deficiency, Water overflowing

Clinical manifestations

Oedema, especially of the legs and ankles, cold feeling in legs and back, fullness and distension of abdomen, soreness of lower back, feeling cold, scanty clear urination (Fig. 37.15).

Water overflowing to the Heart: the above symptoms plus palpitations, breathlessness, cold hands.

Water overflowing to the Lungs: the above symptoms plus thin watery frothy sputum, cough, asthma and breathlessness on exertion

Tongue: Pale, Swollen and wet with a white coating.
Pulse: Deep-Weak-Slow.
Key symptoms: oedema of ankles, Deep-Weak pulse, Pale-Swollen tongue.
  Water overflowing to the Heart: all the above plus palpitations.
  Water overflowing to the Lungs: all the above plus thin watery frothy sputum.

- Feeling cold
- Watery sputum, cough, asthma
- Palpitations, breathlessness
- Abdominal fullness and distension
- Cold feeling in back
- Lower backache
- Scanty clear urination
- Oedema

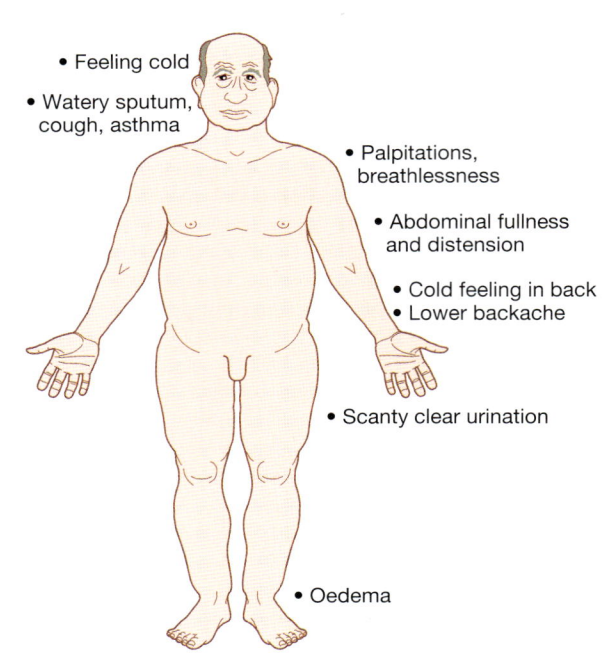

Figure 37.15 Kidney-Yang deficiency, Water overflowing

Diagnostic tip

Oedema of ankles, breathlessness, Deep-Weak-Slow pulse and Pale-Swollen tongue are enough to diagnose Kidney-Yang deficiency, Water overflowing.

Aetiology

Diet

Excessive consumption of cold and raw foods may weaken Spleen- and Kidney-Yang.

Excessive physical work

Excessive physical work or exercise, and especially lifting, weakens Spleen- and Kidney-Yang.

Excessive sexual activity

Excessive sexual activity in men weakens Kidney-Yang.

Hereditary weakness

Kidney-Yang deficiency may be due to poor hereditary constitution.

Chronic illness

A chronic illness, and especially one manifesting with Spleen-Yang deficiency, can cause Kidney-Yang deficiency after a protracted period of time.

Pathology

This is a severe case of Kidney-Yang deficiency, when Kidney-Yang fails to transform the fluids which accumulate under the skin and form oedema. From the Eight-Principle point of view, this is a Deficiency/Excess pattern since Kidney-Yang deficiency leads to the accumulation of fluids, which, in itself, is an Excess condition.

Besides affecting the Kidney itself, in certain cases the deficiency of Yang can affect the Heart or the Lungs as well. If it affects the Heart it will be manifested with palpitations and cold hands, which are due to deficiency of Heart-Yang.

If it affects the Lungs, it will be manifested with a thin watery frothy sputum, which is indicative of Phlegm-Fluids formation. This is due to deficiency of Lung-Qi over a long period of time. In addition, the deficiency of Kidney-Yang implies a failure of the Kidney's receiving of Qi, hence the cough and asthma. This is necessarily a very chronic condition.

Pathological precursors of pattern

Chronic, long-standing retention of Dampness which interferes with the Kidney function of transformation of fluids may lead to this pattern.

This pattern may be transmitted from long-term Spleen-Yang deficiency, especially when there is also Dampness.

In the case of Water overflowing to Heart this pattern may be transmitted from Heart-Yang deficiency.

In the case of Water overflowing to Lungs this pattern may be transmitted from Lung-Qi deficiency together with Phlegm-Fluids in the Interior.

Figures 37.16 and 37.17 summarize the precursors of Kidney-Yang deficiency, Water overflowing.

Pathological developments from pattern

This pattern is an extreme pattern, which, itself, usually derives from other patterns (see Fig. 37.17).

Treatment

Principle of treatment: tonify and warm the Kidneys, transform Water, and warm and tonify Spleen-Yang. In case of Water overflowing to Heart or Lungs, warm and tonify Heart-Yang or Lung-Qi, respectively.

Acupuncture

Points: Du-4 Mingmen, BL-23 Shenshu, BL-22 Sanjiaoshu, BL-20 Pishu, Ren-9 Shuifen, ST-28

Shuidao, SP-9 Yinlingquan, SP-6 Sanyinjiao, KI-7 Fuliu.
For Water overflowing to the Heart: Du-14 Dazhui (moxa), BL-15 Xinshu.
For Water overflowing to the Lungs: LU-7 Lieque, BL-13 Feishu, Du-12 Shenzhu.

Method: reinforcing on points to tonify Kidney-Yang and Spleen-Yang (BL-23, Du-4, BL-20, KI-7) or Heart-Yang (Du-14, BL-15) or Lung-Qi (BL-13, LU-7, Du-12). Reducing method on all the other points in order to resolve Dampness and transform Water. Moxa is applicable. Use thick needles and leave the points open after withdrawal so that a few drops of fluid come out.

Explanation
- Du-4 strengthens the Fire of the Gate of Life (*Ming Men*), which promotes the transformation of Water.
- BL-23 tonifies Kidney-Yang.
- BL-22 stimulates the transformation of fluids in the Lower Burner.
- BL-20 tonifies Spleen-Yang (with moxa).
- Ren-9 promotes the transformation of fluids.
- ST-28 promotes the transformation of fluids in the Lower Burner.
- SP-9 and SP-6 resolve Dampness from the Lower Burner.
- KI-7 tonifies Kidney-Yang and resolves oedema.
- Du-14 with direct moxa tonifies Heart-Yang.
- BL-15 with moxa tonifies Heart-Yang.
- LU-7 stimulates the Lung function of dominating Water passages and resolves oedema.
- BL-13 and Du-12 tonify Lung-Qi.

Herbal formula

Jin Gui Shen Qi Wan *Golden Chest Kidney-Qi Pill* plus Wu Ling San *Five 'Ling' Powder*.

Box 37.8 summarizes Kidney-Yang deficiency, Water overflowing.

Box 37.8 Kidney-Yang deficiency, Water overflowing

Clinical manifestations

Oedema especially of the legs and ankles, cold feeling in legs and back, fullness and distension of abdomen, soreness of lower back, feeling cold, scanty clear urination
Water overflowing to the Heart: the above symptoms plus palpitations, breathlessness, cold hands
Water overflowing to the Lungs: the above symptoms plus thin watery frothy sputum, cough, asthma and breathlessness on exertion
Tongue: Pale, Swollen and wet with a white coating
Pulse: Deep-Weak-Slow

Treatment

Du-4 Mingmen, BL-23 Shenshu, BL-22 Sanjiaoshu, BL-20 Pishu, Ren-9 Shuifen, ST-28 Shuidao, SP-9 Yinlingquan, SP-6 Sanyinjiao, KI-7 Fuliu
For Water overflowing to the Heart: Du-14 Dazhui (moxa), BL-15 Xinshu
For Water overflowing to the Lungs: LU-7 Lieque, BL-13 Feishu, Du-12 Shenzhu

---

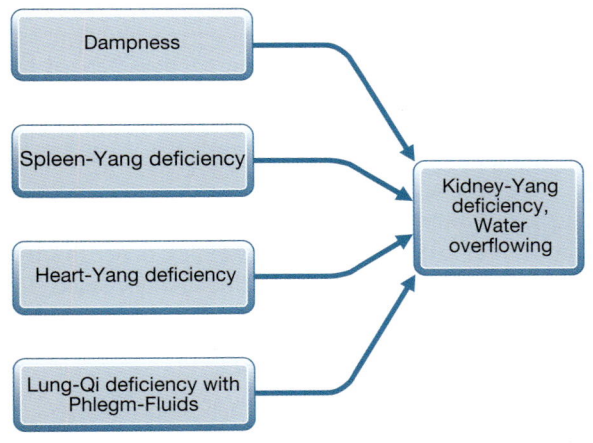

Figure 37.16 Precursors of Kidney-Yang deficiency, Water overflowing

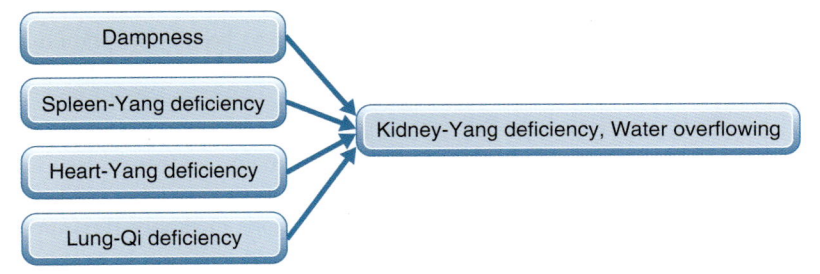

Figure 37.17 Kidney-Yang deficiency, Water overflowing pattern: precursors and developments

Kidney-Yin deficiency, Empty-Heat blazing

Clinical manifestations

Malar flush, mental restlessness, insomnia, night sweating, low-grade fever, afternoon fever, five-palm heat, feeling of heat in the afternoon and/or evening, scanty dark urine, blood in the urine, dry throat especially at night, thirst with desire to drink in small sips, dizziness, tinnitus, hardness of hearing, lower backache, nocturnal emissions with dreams, excessive sexual desire, dry stools (Fig. 37.18).

Tongue: Red, cracked with a red tip, without coating.
Pulse: Floating-Empty and Rapid.
Key symptoms: malar flush, dizziness, tinnitus, feeling of heat in the afternoon, Red tongue without coating.

> **Diagnostic tip**
>
> Even only tinnitus and a Red tongue without coating would be enough to diagnose Kidney-Yin deficiency with Empty-Heat

- Malar flush
- Dry throat at night
- Mental restlessness, insomnia, dizziness
- Tinnitus
- Night sweating
- Feeling of heat in the afternoon
- Lower backache
- Scanty dark urine, blood in urine
- Dry stools

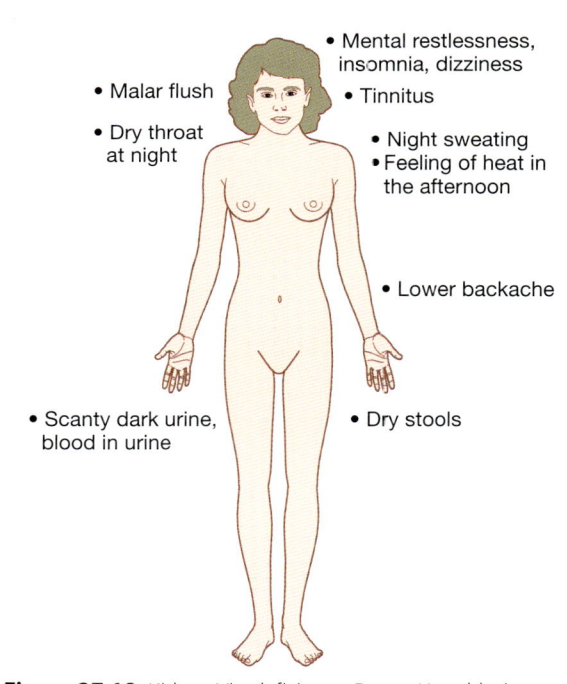

Figure 37.18 Kidney-Yin deficiency, Empty-Heat blazing

Aetiology

This is the same as for Kidney-Yin deficiency with the addition of emotional problems such as chronic anxiety and worry.

Pathology

This pattern corresponds to an advanced stage of Kidney-Yin deficiency that has given rise to pronounced Empty-Heat: it is therefore a combined Deficiency/Excess pattern, the Empty-Heat representing the Excess condition.

Most of the symptoms are caused by the flaring of Empty-Heat and dryness from Yin deficiency.

The malar flush is a redness of the face, but only on the small area of the cheekbones, not the whole cheek. The afternoon fever is typical of Empty-Heat; it can also simply be a feeling of heat in the afternoon, rather than an actual fever.

The Empty-Heat arising from Kidney-Yin deficiency can ascend to disturb the Heart and therefore the Mind, hence the insomnia and mental restlessness. This is described as 'heart feels vexed' in Chinese, and it describes a state of fidget, uneasiness and vague anxiety which is undefinable but very real and distressing to the patient. The insomnia is characterized by falling asleep easily but waking up in the middle of the night several times, or also in the early hours of the morning.

The deficiency of Yin leads to the exhaustion of Body Fluids and therefore Dryness; the Empty-Heat further contributes to drying up the Body Fluids, hence the dry throat at night, concentrated urine and dry stools. In severe cases, the Empty-Heat can also cause Blood to rush out of the blood vessels, resulting in blood in the urine.

The deficiency of Yin leads to deficiency of Essence, hence the nocturnal emissions. These are accompanied by vivid sexual dreams because the Empty-Heat agitates the mind and creates a strong sexual desire.

The tongue is Red because of the Empty-Heat and without coating because of the Yin deficiency. The cracks also reflect deficiency of Yin.

The Floating-Empty quality reflects Yin deficiency and the Rapid quality of the pulse reflects Empty-Heat.

The manifestations of Empty-Heat are summarized in Figure 37.19.

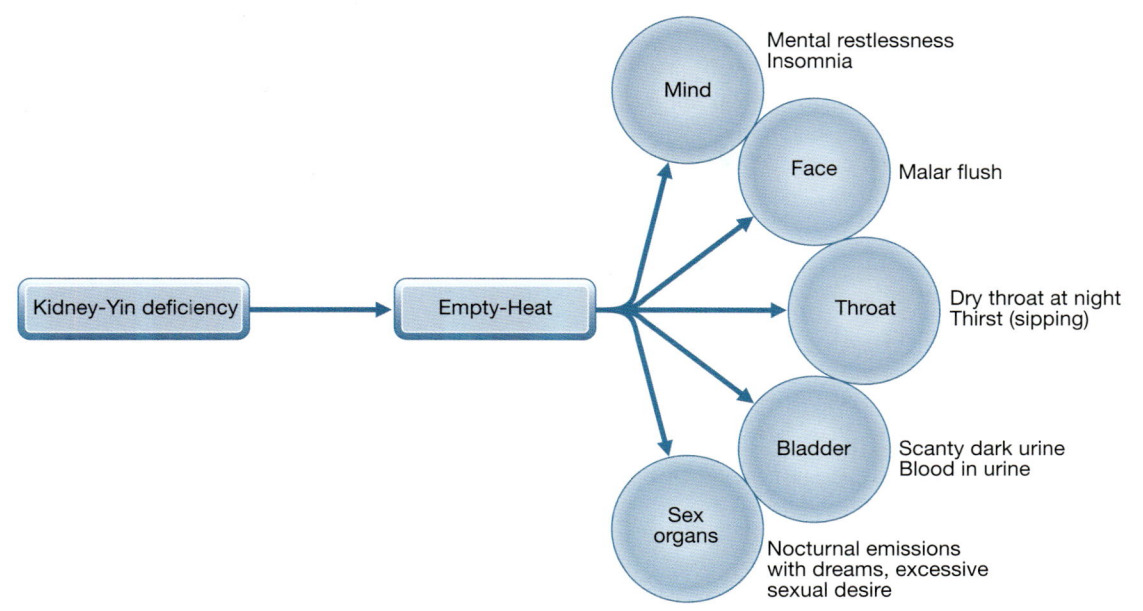

Figure 37.19 Manifestations of Empty-Heat

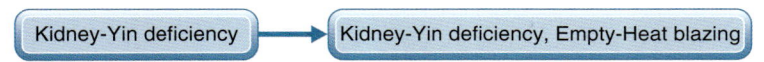

Figure 37.20 Kidney-Yin deficiency, Empty-Heat blazing pattern: precursors and developments

Pathological precursors of pattern

This pattern always derives from Kidney-Yin deficiency (Fig. 37.20).

Pathological developments from pattern

This pattern does not have many pathological developments as it is itself an end-result pattern. If Empty-Heat is pronounced, it leads to bleeding (see Fig. 37.20).

Treatment

Principle of treatment: nourish Kidney-Yin, clear Empty-Heat, calm the Mind.

Acupuncture

Points: KI-3 Taixi, KI-6 Zhaohai, KI-10 Yingu, KI-9 Zhubin, Ren-4 Guanyuan, KI-2 Rangu, SP-6 Sanyinjiao, HE-5 Tongli, LU-7 Lieque, LU-10 Yuji, HE-6 Yinxi, Du-24 Shenting, L.I.-11 Quchi.

Method: reinforcing on points to nourish Kidney-Yin (KI-3, -6, -9, -10, Ren-4, SP-6) and reducing method on the others. Positively no moxa.

Explanation
- KI-3 tonifies the Kidneys.
- KI-6 and KI-10 nourish Kidney-Yin.
- KI-9 tonifies Kidney-Yin and calms the Mind.
- Ren-4 nourishes Kidney-Yin and calms the Mind.
- KI-2 clears Empty-Heat from the Kidneys.
- SP-6 nourishes Kidney-Yin and calms the Mind.
- HE-5 and LU-7 are used to conduct Heat downwards away from the head (where it disturbs the Mind).
- LU-10 clears Lung-Heat and is used if there are symptoms of Heat in the Lungs (dry cough, bloody sputum). It also conducts Heat downwards away from the head.
- HE-6 clears Empty-Heat and calms the Mind.
- Du-24 calms the Mind.
- L.I.-11 clears Heat.

Herbal formula

Liu Wei Di Huang Wan *Six-Ingredient Rehmannia Pill* plus Di Gu Pi *Cortex Lycii radicis* and Zhi Mu *Radix Anemarrhenae asphodeloidis*.

Box 37.9 summarizes Kidney-Yin deficiency, Empty-Heat blazing.

Box 37.9 Kidney-Yin deficiency, Empty-Heat blazing

Clinical manifestations

Malar flush, mental restlessness, insomnia, night sweating, low-grade fever, afternoon fever, five-palm heat, feeling of heat in the afternoon and/or evening, scanty dark urine, blood in the urine, dry throat especially at night, thirst with desire to drink in small sips, dizziness, tinnitus, hardness of hearing, lower backache, nocturnal emissions with dreams, excessive sexual desire, dry stools
Tongue: Red, cracked with a red tip, without coating
Pulse: Floating-Empty and Rapid

Treatment

KI-3 Taixi, KI-6 Zhaohai, KI-10 Yingu, KI-9 Zhubin, Ren-4 Guanyuan, KI-2 Rangu, SP-6 Sanyinjiao, HE-5 Tongli, LU-7 Lieque, LU-10 Yuji, HE-6 Yinxi, Du-24 Shenting, L.I.-11 Quchi

---

COMBINED PATTERNS

Kidney- and Liver-Yin deficiency

Clinical manifestations

Dizziness, tinnitus, hardness of hearing, lower backache, dull occipital or vertical headache, insomnia, numbness or tingling of limbs, dry eyes, blurred vision, dry throat, dry hair and skin, brittle nails, dry vagina, night sweating, dry stools, nocturnal emissions, scanty menstruation or amenorrhoea, delayed cycle, infertility (Fig. 37.21).
Tongue: normal-coloured without coating or with rootless coating.
Pulse: Floating-Empty.
Key symptoms: dry eyes, dry throat, night sweating, scanty menstruation, tongue without coating.

Empty-Heat

Five-palm heat, a feeling of heat in the evening, menopausal hot flushes.
Tongue: Red without coating.
Pulse: Floating-Empty and slightly Rapid.

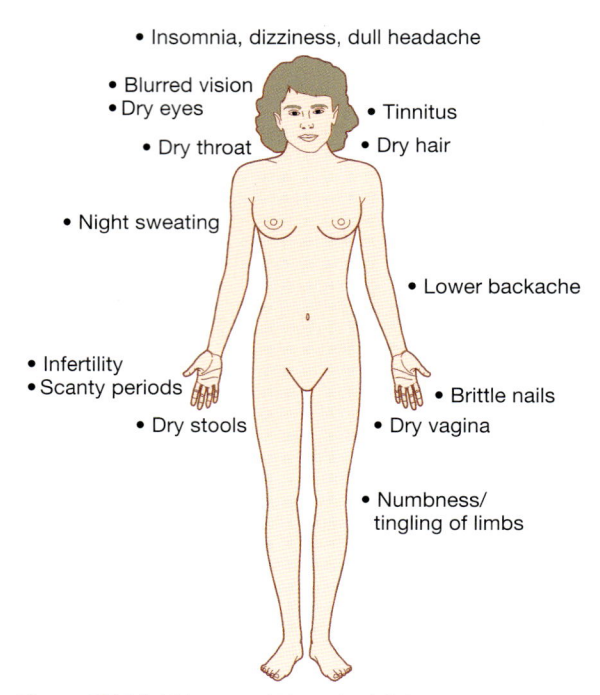

Figure 37.21 Kidney- and Liver-Yin deficiency

- Insomnia, dizziness, dull headache
- Blurred vision
- Dry eyes
- Dry throat
- Tinnitus
- Dry hair
- Night sweating
- Lower backache
- Infertility
- Scanty periods
- Brittle nails
- Dry stools
- Dry vagina
- Numbness/tingling of limbs

Diagnostic tip

Even just dry eyes, dry throat, backache and a tongue without coating are enough to diagnose Kidney- and Liver-Yin deficiency

Aetiology

This is the same as for Kidney-Yin deficiency and Liver-Blood deficiency, but with the additional component of emotional problems due to anger, frustration and depression.

Pathology

This pattern includes symptoms and signs of both Liver- and Kidney-Yin deficiency, bearing in mind that Liver-Yin deficiency embodies Liver-Blood deficiency. The Kidneys correspond to Water and should nourish the Liver, which corresponds to Wood. Thus the Yin and Blood of the Liver are dependent on the nourishment of Kidney-Yin and Kidney-Essence (Fig. 37.22).

Dry eyes are a symptom of Liver-Yin deficiency, due to the Yin of the Liver being unable to moisten the eyes. Indeed, dry eyes are one of the most distinctive

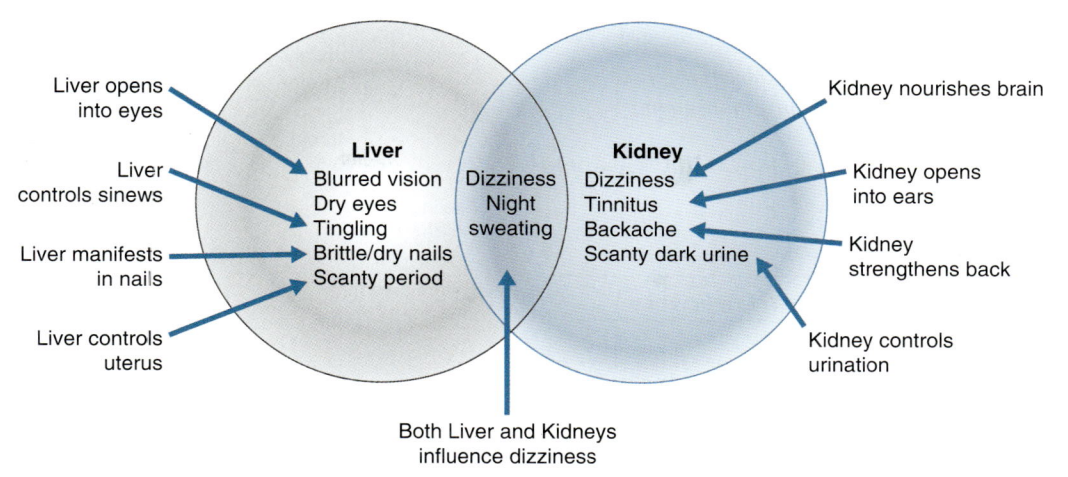

Figure 37.22 Pathology of Kidney- and Liver-Yin deficiency

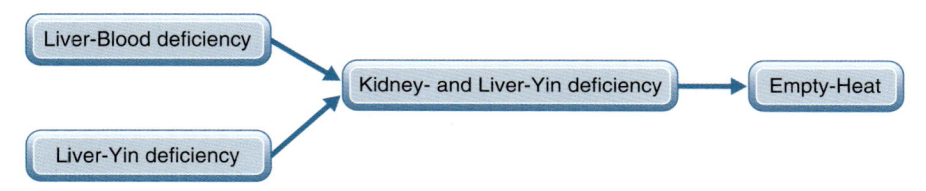

Figure 37.23 Kidney- and Liver-Yin deficiency pattern: precursors and developments

symptoms of Liver-Yin deficiency. Dream-disturbed sleep, insomnia, numbness, blurred vision and scanty menstruation or amenorrhoea are all symptoms of Liver-Blood deficiency, which is part of Liver-Yin deficiency.

The headache is also due to Liver-Blood deficiency and would be either on the occiput (related to the Kidney) or on the vertex of the head (related to the Liver channel). When Liver-Yin is deficient, Liver-Yang may ascend, in which case the headache would be on the temples and be of a throbbing rather than dull character.

All the other symptoms are due to deficiency of Yin of the Kidneys, all of which have already been explained.

The infertility in women would be due both to deficient Liver-Blood failing to nourish the Uterus, and to deficient Kidney-Essence unable to promote conception.

The pulse is Floating-Empty, reflecting the Yin deficiency. The absence of coating on the tongue reflects Yin deficiency.

Pathological precursors of pattern

This pattern may develop from Liver-Blood and Liver-Yin deficiency (Fig. 37.23).

Pathological developments from pattern

The most common consequence of this pattern is the development of Empty-Heat (see Fig. 37.23).

Treatment

Principle of treatment: nourish Liver- and Kidney-Yin.

Acupuncture

Points: KI-3 Taixi, KI-6 Zhaohai, LIV-8 Ququan, Ren-4 Guanyuan, BL-23 Shenshu, KI-13 Qixue, SP-6 Sanyinjiao, BL-10 Tianzhu.

Method: reinforcing.

Explanation
– KI-3 tonifies the Kidneys.
– KI-6 tonifies Kidney-Yin.
– LIV-8 tonifies Liver-Blood and Liver-Yin.
– Ren-4 tonifies Kidney-Yin, Liver-Yin and Kidney-Essence.
– BL-23 tonifies the Kidneys in chronic conditions.
– KI-13 nourishes Kidney-Yin.
– SP-6 nourishes Liver- and Kidney-Yin.
– BL-10 can be used for occipital headache.

Herbal formula

Zuo Gui Wan *Restoring the Left [Kidney] Pill.*
Qi Ju Di Huang Wan *Lycium–Chrysanthemum– Rehmannia Pill.*

Box 37.10 summarizes Kidney- and Liver-Yin deficiency.

Box 37.10 Kidney- and Liver-Yin deficiency

Clinical manifestations

Dizziness, tinnitus, hardness of hearing, lower backache, dull occipital or vertical headache, insomnia, numbness or tingling of limbs, dry eyes, blurred vision, dry throat, dry hair and skin, brittle nails, dry vagina, night sweating, dry stools, nocturnal emissions, scanty menstruation or amenorrhoea, delayed cycle, infertility, normal-coloured tongue without coating or with rootless coating, Floating-Empty pulse

Treatment

KI-3 Taixi, KI-6 Zhaohai, LIV-8 Ququan, Ren-4 Guanyuan, BL-23 Shenshu, KI-13 Qixue, SP-6 Sanyinjiao, BL-10 Tianzhu

---

Kidneys and Heart not harmonized

Clinical manifestations

Palpitations, mental restlessness, insomnia, dream-disturbed sleep, anxiety, poor memory, dizziness, tinnitus, hardness of hearing, lower backache, nocturnal emissions with dreams, a feeling of heat in the evening, dry throat at night, thirst with desire to drink in small sips, night sweating, five-palm heat, scanty dark urine, dry stools (Fig. 37.24).

Tongue: Red with redder tip without coating, midline Heart crack.
Pulse: Floating-Empty and Rapid or Deep-Weak on both Rear positions and relatively Overflowing on both Front positions.
Key symptoms: palpitations, dizziness, tinnitus, night sweating, Red tongue with redder tip and midline crack and without coating.

> **Diagnostic tip**
>
> Palpitations, tinnitus, night sweating and a Red tongue with redder tip and midline crack and without coating are enough to diagnose Heart and Kidneys not harmonized

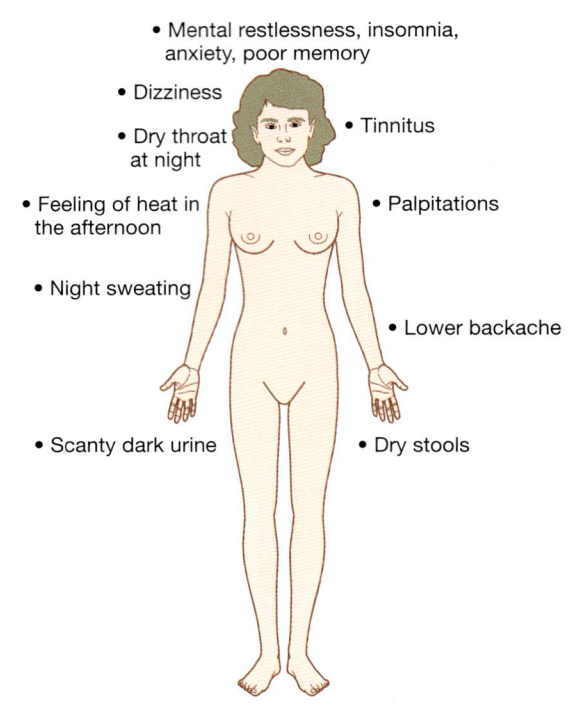

Figure 37.24 Kidneys and Heart not harmonized

- Mental restlessness, insomnia, anxiety, poor memory
- Dizziness
- Dry throat at night
- Tinnitus
- Feeling of heat in the afternoon
- Palpitations
- Night sweating
- Lower backache
- Scanty dark urine
- Dry stools

Aetiology

The same as for Kidney-Yin deficiency, with the additional component of emotional problems such as anxiety, sadness and depression. Emotional shocks and the ensuing sadness from break-up of relationships are a common cause of Heart-Yin deficiency in this pattern.

Pathology

This pattern is basically characterized by Kidney-Yin deficiency failing to nourish Heart-Yin, which also becomes deficient. This leads to the flaring up of Heart Empty-Heat: therefore this pattern of Yin deficiency includes manifestations of Empty-Heat of the Heart (Fig. 37.25).

From a mental point of view, Essence (*Jing*) is the foundation for the Mind. If Essence is deficient, the Mind suffers. Thus the relationship of mutual assistance between Kidneys and Heart finds expression also in the relationship between the Essence and the Mind.

When Kidney-Yin is weak and Heart-Yin is deficient, Empty-Heat flares within the Heart, resulting in mental restlessness, insomnia (waking up several times during the night), palpitations and a red tip of the tongue.

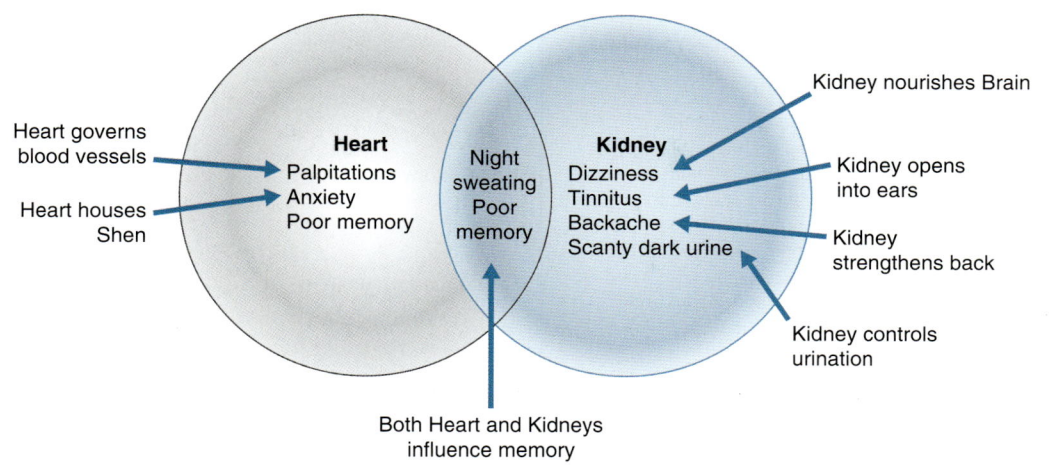

Figure 37.25 Pathology of Kidneys and Heart not harmonized

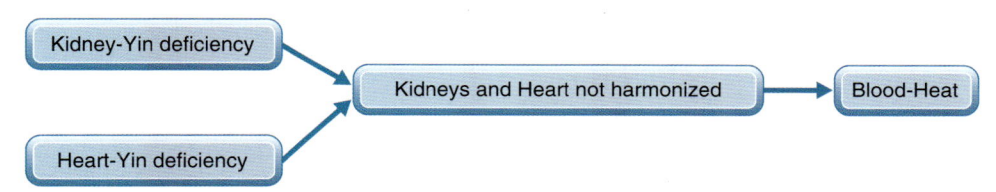

Figure 37.26 Kidneys and Heart not harmonized pattern: precursors and developments

Poor memory, dizziness, tinnitus and deafness are all due to deficiency of Kidney-Yin failing to nourish the brain and open into the ear.

The feeling of heat in the evening, dark urine, Red tongue and Rapid pulse are all due to the flaring of Empty-Heat.

Pathological precursors of pattern

This pattern usually develops from Kidney-Yin deficiency. It may also develop from chronic Heart-Yin deficiency (Fig. 37.26).

Pathological developments from pattern

The flaring of Empty-Heat may heat the Blood and cause bleeding (see Fig. 37.26).

Treatment

Principle of treatment: nourish Kidney- and Heart-Yin, clear Heart Empty-Heat, calm the Mind.

Acupuncture

Points: HE-7 Shenmen, HE-6 Yinxi, HE-5 Tongli, Yintang extra point, BL-15 Xinshu, Ren-15 Jiuwei, Du-24 Shenting, KI-3 Taixi, KI-10 Yingu, KI-9 Zhubin, KI-6 Zhaohai, Ren-4 Guanyuan, SP-6 Sanyinjiao.

Method: reinforcing on the points to nourish Kidney-Yin (KI-3, -6, -9, 10, Ren-4, SP-6), reducing method on the points to clear Heart Empty-Heat (HE-5, -6, -7, BL-15), even method on the others (Yintang, Ren-15, Du-24).

Explanation

- HE-7 calms the Mind.
- HE-6 clears Empty-Heat and nourishes Heart-Yin (it is specific for night sweating combined with KI-7 Fuliu).
- HE-5 clears Heart Empty-Heat and conducts Heat downwards away from the head.
- Yintang calms the Mind.
- BL-15 clears Heart-Heat.
- Ren-15 calms the Mind and nourishes Heart-Yin.
- Du-24 calms the Mind.
- KI-3, KI-9 and KI-10 tonify Kidney-Yin. KI-9, in particular, calms the Mind.
- KI-6 nourishes Kidney-Yin.

> **Box 37.11 Kidneys and Heart not harmonized**
>
> **Clinical manifestations**
>
> Palpitations, mental restlessness, insomnia, dream-disturbed sleep, anxiety, poor memory, dizziness, tinnitus, hardness of hearing, lower backache, nocturnal emissions with dreams, a feeling of heat in the evening, dry throat at night, thirst with desire to drink in small sips, night sweating, five-palm heat, scanty dark urine, dry stools, Red tongue with redder tip without coating, midline Heart crack, Floating-Empty and Rapid pulse or Deep-Weak on both Rear positions and relatively Overflowing on both Front positions
>
> **Treatment**
>
> HE-7 Shenmen, HE-6 Yinxi, HE-5 Tongli, Yintang extra point, BL-15 Xinshu, Ren-15 Jiuwei, Du-24 Shenting, KI-3 Taixi, KI-6 Zhaohai, KI-10 Yingu, KI-9 Zhubin, Ren-4 Guanyuan, SP-6 Sanyinjiao

- Ren-4 nourishes Kidney-Yin and Kidney-Essence and conducts Heat downwards.
- SP-6 nourishes Yin and calms the Mind.

Herbal formula

Tian Wang Bu Xin Dan *Heavenly Emperor Tonifying the Heart Pill*.

Women's Treasure

Heavenly Empress (variation of Tian Wang Bu Xin Dan).

Box 37.11 summarizes Kidneys and Heart not harmonized.

Kidney- and Lung-Yin deficiency

Clinical manifestations

Dry cough which is worse in the evening, dry throat and mouth, thin body, breathlessness on exertion, lower backache, night sweating, dizziness, tinnitus, hardness of hearing, scanty urination (Fig. 37.27).
Tongue: normal-coloured without coating or with rootless coating.
Pulse: Floating-Empty.
Key symptoms: dry cough, dizziness, tinnitus, night sweating, tongue without coating.

Empty-Heat

Feeling of heat in the evening, five-palm heat, afternoon fever, malar flush.
Tongue: Red without coating.
Pulse: Floating-Empty and slightly Rapid.

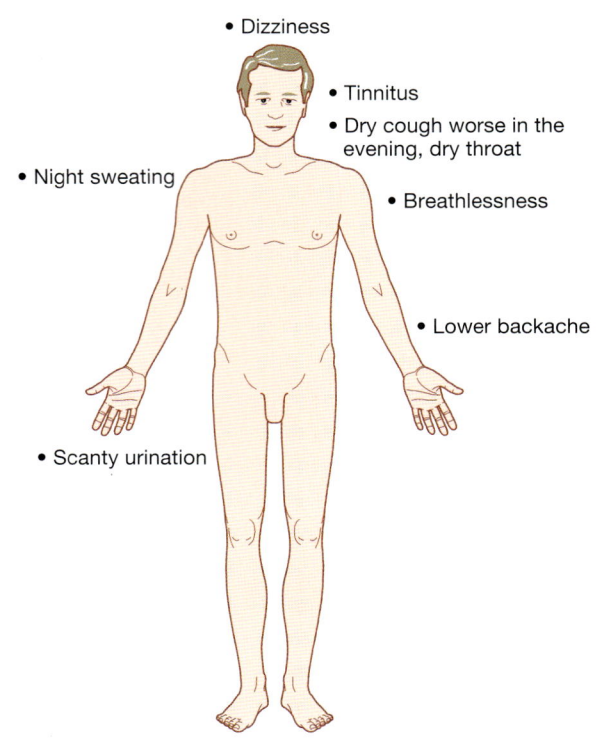

Figure 37.27 Kidney- and Lung-Yin deficiency

> **Diagnostic tip**
>
> A dry cough, tinnitus and a tongue without coating would be enough to diagnose Kidney- and Lung-Yin deficiency

Aetiology

The aetiology of this pattern is the same as for Kidney-Yin deficiency, with the additional component of worrying over a long period of time leading to injury of the Lung energy.

Pathology

This pattern is characterized by both Lung- and Kidney-Yin deficiency. It is not to be confused with the pattern of 'Kidneys failing to receive Qi', which is characterized by deficiency of Kidney-Yang and Lung-Qi (Fig. 37.28).

The Yin deficiency leads to exhaustion of Body Fluids and ensuing dryness, hence the dry cough and dry mouth.

The breathlessness on exertion is caused by the failure of the Kidney in receiving and holding Qi.

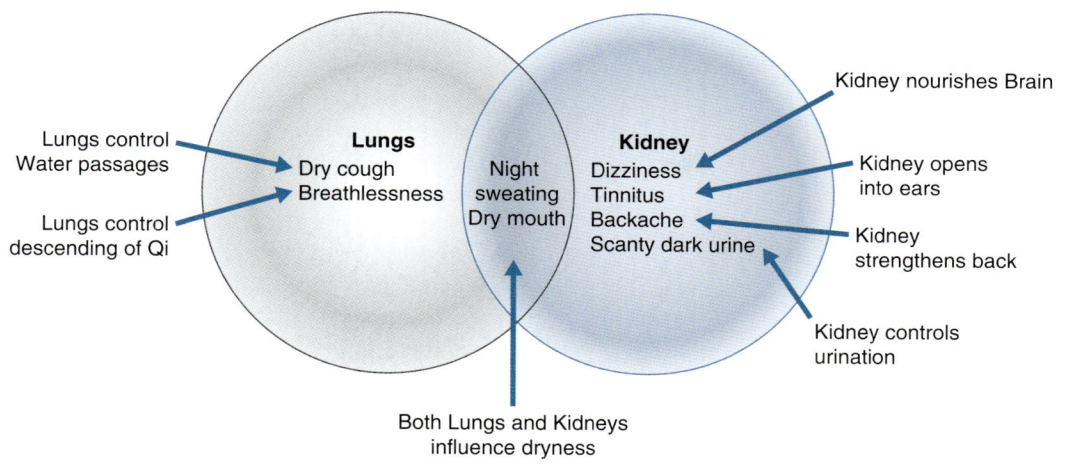

Figure 37.28 Pathology of Kidney- and Lung-Yin deficiency

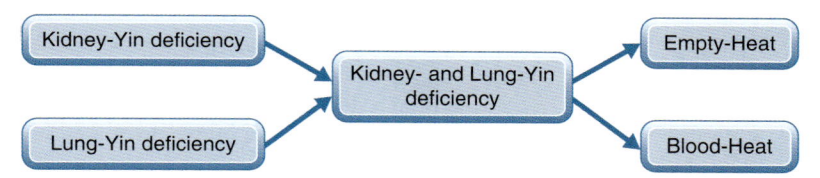

Figure 37.29 Kidney- and Lung-Yin deficiency pattern: precursors and developments

This pattern only occurs in very chronic conditions and is therefore characterized by exhaustion of the body's Qi, which causes weakness of the limbs and a thin body.

All the other symptoms are typical of Kidney-Yin deficiency (night sweating, dizziness, tinnitus, hardness of hearing, scanty urination).

Pathological precursors of pattern

Obviously this pattern usually derives from Kidney-Yin deficiency; however, it may also develop from a chronic condition of Lung-Yin deficiency (Fig. 37.29).

Pathological developments from pattern

This pattern will eventually lead to the development of Empty-Heat and therefore the possibility of bleeding from Blood-Heat (see Fig. 37.29).

Treatment

Principle of treatment: nourish Lung- and Kidney-Yin, nourish Body Fluids.

Acupuncture

Points: KI-3 Taixi, KI-6 Zhaohai, LU-7 Lieque and KI-6 Zhaohai in combination (opening points of the Directing Vessel *Ren Mai*), Ren-4 Guanyuan, KI-13 Qixue, LU-9 Taiyuan, LU-1 Zhongfu, SP-6 Sanyinjiao, BL-43 Gaohuangshu.

Method: reinforcing, no moxa.

Explanation

– KI-3 tonifies Kidney-Yin.
– LU-7 and KI-6 in combination open the Directing Vessel, benefit the throat, stimulate the Kidney reception of Qi and tonify Lung- and Kidney-Yin.
– Ren-4 and KI-13 nourish Kidney-Yin and -Essence.
– LU-9 nourishes Lung-Yin.
– LU-1 nourishes Lung-Yin, restores the descending of Lung-Qi and stops cough.
– SP-6 nourishes Kidney-Yin and promotes fluids.
– BL-43 tonifies Lung-Yin and is specific for chronic conditions.

Herbal formula

Ba Xian Chang Shou Wan *Eight Immortals Longevity Pill*.

Box 37.12 summarizes Kidney- and Lung-Yin deficiency.

Box 37.12 Kidney- and Lung-Yin deficiency

Clinical manifestations

Dry cough which is worse in the evening, dry throat and mouth, thin body, breathlessness on exertion, lower backache, night sweating, dizziness, tinnitus, hardness of hearing, scanty urination, normal-coloured tongue without coating or with rootless coating, Floating-Empty pulse

Treatment

KI-3 Taixi, KI-6 Zhaohai, LU-7 Lieque and KI-6 Zhaohai in combination (opening points of the Directing Vessel), Ren-4 Guanyuan, KI-13 Qixue, LU-9 Taiyuan, LU-1 Zhongfu, SP-6 Sanyinjiao, BL-43 Gaohuangshu

---

Kidney- and Spleen-Yang deficiency

Clinical manifestations

Lower backache, cold and weak knees, sensation of cold in the back, feeling cold, weak legs, bright-white complexion, impotence, premature ejaculation, low sperm count, cold and thin sperm, decreased libido, tiredness, lassitude, abundant clear urination, scanty clear urination, urination at night, apathy, oedema of the legs, infertility in women, loose stools, depression, poor appetite, slight abdominal distension, desire to lie down, early morning diarrhoea, chronic diarrhoea (Fig. 37.30).
Tongue: Pale and wet.
Pulse: Deep-Weak.
Key symptoms: lower backache, feeling of cold, loose stools, Deep-Weak pulse.

> **Diagnostic tip**
>
> Lower backache, feeling of cold, loose stools and Deep-Weak pulse are enough to diagnose Kidney- and Spleen-Yang deficiency

Aetiology

The aetiology of this pattern is the same as for Kidney-Yang deficiency, with the additional component of excessive consumption of cold and raw foods.

Pathology

This is always a chronic condition. It represents a stage further than Spleen-Yang deficiency, from which it usually develops (Fig. 37.31).

The Spleen is the Root of Post-Heaven Qi and, when it is deficient, it fails to nourish the muscles, resulting in lack of strength. The general deficiency of Qi causes the tiredness, lassitude and desire to lie down.

When Spleen-Yang is deficient it cannot transport nourishment to the limbs, which will feel cold. Furthermore, the deficiency of Kidney-Yang implies a weakness of the Fire of the Gate of Life (*Ming Men*), which further contributes to the various cold symptoms (feeling of cold in back and legs).

Deficient Kidney-Yang cannot transform Water and fluids accumulate, hence the oedema and the abundant urination. In severe cases, the opposite could manifest as well, i.e. scanty urination. This happens when the Yang is so deficient that it cannot move the fluids at all.

Deficient Kidney-Yang fails to transform the fluids in the abdomen and help the Spleen to transport and transform, resulting in chronic diarrhoea.

Deficient Spleen-Yang fails to transform and transport, hence the abdominal distension.

Pathological precursors of pattern

This pattern develops frequently from a chronic condition of Spleen-Yang deficiency (Fig. 37.32).

Pathological developments from pattern

When it persists for a long time, this pattern frequently leads to the formation of Dampness and/or Phlegm. Also, if this combined pattern is chronic, it may lead to the pattern of Kidney-Yang deficiency, Water overflowing (see Fig. 37.32).

Treatment

Principle of treatment: tonify and warm Spleen- and Kidney-Yang.

Acupuncture

Points: BL-23 Shenshu, Du-4 Mingmen, Ren-4 Guanyuan, Ren-6 Qihai, KI-3 Taixi, KI-7 Fuliu, BL-52 Zhishi, Ren-12 Zhongwan, ST-36 Zusanli, SP-3 Taibai, BL-20 Pishu, BL-21 Weishu, Ren-9 Shuifen, ST-37 Shangjuxu, ST-25 Tianshu, BL-25 Dachangshu.

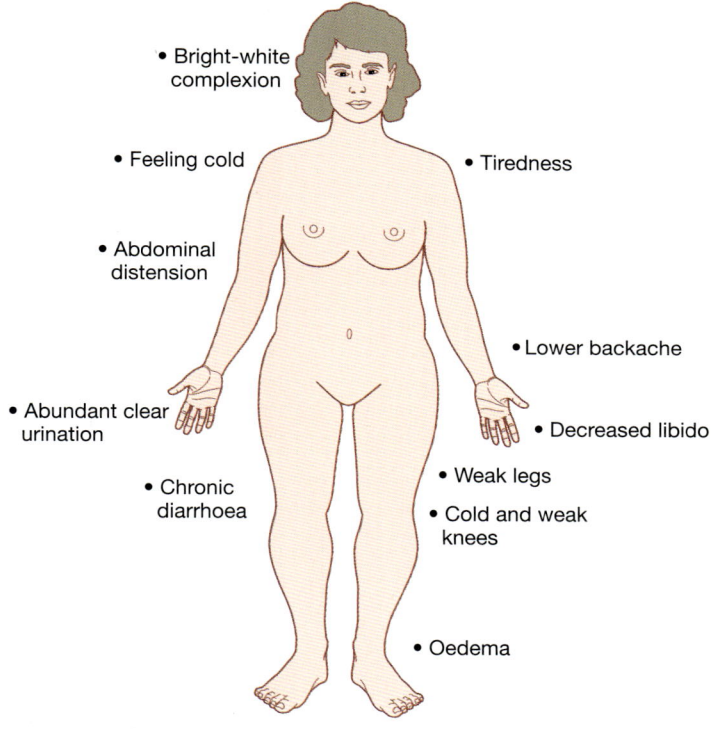

Figure 37.30 Kidney- and Spleen-Yang deficiency

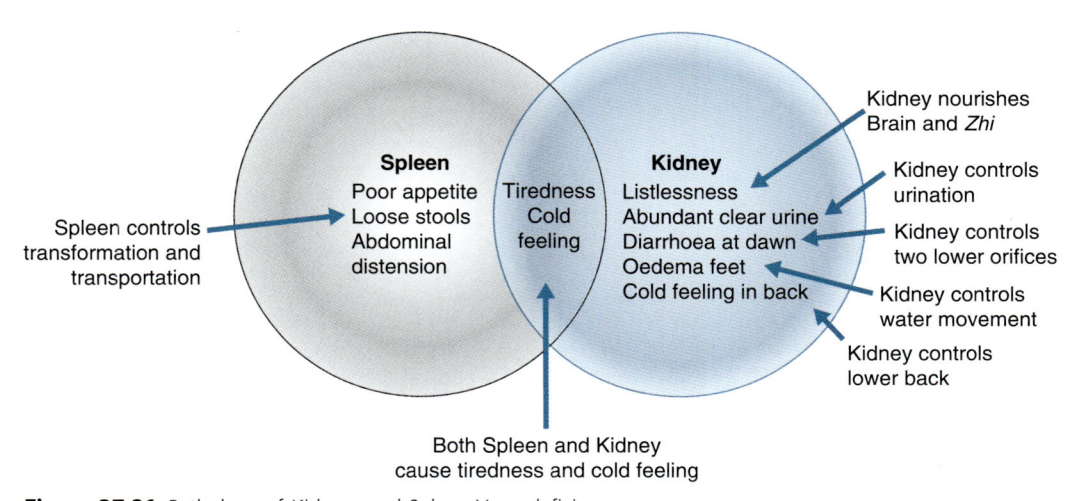

Figure 37.31 Pathology of Kidney- and Spleen-Yang deficiency

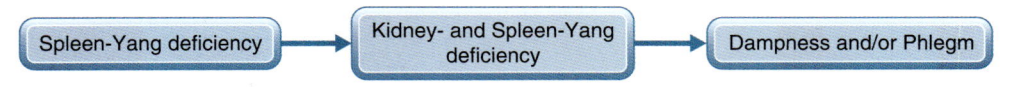

Figure 37.32 Kidney- and Spleen-Yang deficiency pattern: precursors and developments

Method: reinforcing, moxa must be used.
Explanation
- BL-23 tonifies Kidney-Yang.
- Du-4 strengthens the Fire of the Gate of Life.
- Ren-4 tonifies Kidney-Yang (with direct moxa cones).
- Ren-6 tonifies Qi in general and Yang if used with direct moxa. It is an important point for chronic diarrhoea.
- KI-3 tonifies the Kidneys.
- KI-7 tonifies Kidney-Yang and resolves oedema.
- BL-52 tonifies Kidney-Yang, strengthens the Will-power and nourishes the Essence: this point is good for depression from Kidney-Yang deficiency.
- Ren-12, ST-36 and SP-3 tonify Spleen-Yang.
- BL-20 and BL-21 tonify Spleen-Yang.
- Ren-9 promotes the transformation and transportation of fluids to resolve Dampness.
- ST-37 is the Lower Sea point for the Large Intestine and is specific to stop chronic diarrhoea.
- ST-25 stops diarrhoea.
- BL-25 is the Back Transporting point for the Large Intestine and it stops diarrhoea.

Herbal formula

Li Zhong Wan *Regulating the Centre Pill* plus Jin Gui Shen Qi Wan *Golden Chest Kidney-Qi Pill*.

Box 37.13 summarizes Kidney- and Spleen-Yang deficiency.

Box 37.13 Kidney- and Spleen-Yang deficiency

Clinical manifestations

Lower backache, cold and weak knees, sensation of cold in the back, feeling cold, weak legs, bright-white complexion, impotence, premature ejaculation, low sperm count, cold and thin sperm, decreased libido, tiredness, lassitude, abundant clear urination, scanty clear urination, urination at night, apathy, oedema of the legs, infertility in women, loose stools, depression, poor appetite, slight abdominal distension, desire to lie down, early morning diarrhoea, chronic diarrhoea, Pale and wet tongue, Deep-Weak pulse

Treatment

BL-23 Shenshu, Du-4 Mingmen, Ren-4 Guanyuan, Ren-6 Qihai, KI-3 Taixi, KI-7 Fuliu, BL-52 Zhishi, Ren-12 Zhongwan, ST-36 Zusanli, SP-3 Taibai, BL-20 Pishu, BL-21 Weishu, Ren-9 Shuifen, ST-37 Shangjuxu, ST-25 Tianshu, BL-25 Dachangshu

Learning outcomes

In this chapter you will have learned:
- The theory that the Kidneys can never be in Excess but only Deficient
- The significance of the duality of Kidney-Yin and Kidney-Yang in Kidney pathology
- The frequency in clinical practice of a simultaneous deficiency of Kidney-Yin and Kidney-Yang
- How the Kidneys are affected by any chronic disease, as they are the root of all the other organs
- The importance of heredity in determining the strength of a child's Kidneys
- The adverse effects of fear, anxiety and shock on Kidney-Qi
- How sexual activity, chronic illness and overwork can cause a Kidney deficiency
- The role of the Kidney-Essence in the ageing process
- How to identify the following Deficiency patterns:
  Kidney-Yang deficiency: backache, a feeling of cold and a Weak Kidney pulse
  Kidney-Yin deficiency: backache and night sweating
  Kidney-Qi not Firm: dribbling after urination, chronic vaginal discharge and backache
  Kidney failing to receive Qi: shortness of breath on exertion, lower backache, pale urine
  Kidney-Essence deficiency: poor bone development in children, weak knees, falling hair and weak sexual activity in adults
- How to identify the following Empty/Full patterns:
  Kidney-Yang deficiency, Water overflowing: oedema of the ankles, breathlessness, Deep-Weak-Slow pulse and Pale-Swollen tongue
  Kidney-Yin deficiency, Empty-Heat blazing: malar flush, dizziness, tinnitus, a feeling of heat in the afternoon and a Red-Peeled tongue
- How to identify the following combined patterns:
  Kidney- and Liver-Yin deficiency: dry eyes, dry throat, night sweating, backache and a tongue without coating
  Kidneys and Heart not harmonized: palpitations, tinnitus, night sweating and a Red tongue without coating and a redder tip and a midline crack
  Kidney- and Lung-Yin deficiency: dry cough, tinnitus and a tongue without coating
  Kidney- and Spleen-Yang deficiency: lower backache, feeling of cold, loose stools and a Deep-Weak pulse

Learning tips

Kidney deficiency

In all Kidney patterns, start off by listing the three general manifestations of lower backache, dizziness, tinnitus.

In Yang deficiency, add cold knees, feeling cold, Pale tongue, Deep-Weak pulse

In Yin deficiency, add feeling of heat in the evening and night sweating, tongue without coating and Floating-Empty pulse

In Essence, deficiency add symptoms from three main areas:
- Brain: poor memory, dizziness
- Bones: weak bones
- Hair: loss of hair, premature greying of hair

In Kidney-Qi not Firm, remember that everything is 'leaking out': frequent urination, incontinence of urine, premature ejaculation, seminal emissions, urethral discharge

In Kidney not receiving Qi, the focus is on breathing: chronic asthma, breathlessness, difficulty in breathing in

Self-assessment questions

1. Complete the following: 'Kidney-Yin is the root of the _____, _____ and Lungs. Kidney-Yang is the root of the _____, the _____ and the Heart.'
2. What main factors determine the hereditary strength of a child's Kidney-Qi?
3. What effect does long-standing fear and anxiety tend to have on the Qi of adults?
4. What is the most common cause of Kidney-Yin deficiency in Western industrialized societies?
5. Why does sexual function decrease with age?
6. What are the possible aetiological factors causing Kidney-Yang deficiency?
7. What is the pathology of dizziness and vertigo in Kidney-Yin deficiency?
8. Why does night sweating happen, and why is it potentially damaging to the body?
9. What key symptoms would you look for in a woman to diagnose Kidney-Qi not Firm?
10. What characterizes the breathing of asthma caused by deficient Kidney-Yang?
11. What symptoms would you expect in an adult presenting with Kidney-Essence deficiency?
12. If Kidney-Yang deficiency affects the Heart, what symptoms might you expect?
13. What are the characteristics of the insomnia in an advanced stage of Yin deficiency?
14. What is the pathology of infertility in women in the combined pattern Kidney- and Liver-Yin deficiency?
15. What pulse picture might you expect in the pattern Kidneys and Heart not harmonized?

See p. 1264 for answers

END NOTES

1. Sou Nu King (Classic of the Simple Girl), La sexualité taoiste de la Chine ancienne, translated by Leung Kwok Po, Seghers, Paris, 1978, p. 108.
2. 1979 The Yellow Emperor's Classic of Internal Medicine – Simple Questions (*Huang Di Nei Jing Su Wen* 黄帝内经素问), People's Health Publishing House, Beijing, first published c.100 BC, p. 2: '*Nowadays ... people have sex in a state of drunkenness ... hence they barely reach the age of 50*'.
3. Ancient Chinese alchemists of the Daoist school searched for the elixir of immortality or longevity. Most of these prescriptions contained very hot, sometimes toxic, herbs to tonify the Fire of the Gate of Life. These herbal pills became very popular during the Ming dynasty and some emperors actually died from an overdose of such preparations. The first emperor of a unified Chinese empire, Qin Shi Huang Di, also died taking 'elixirs of immortality'.

Stomach Patterns

Key contents

General aetiology

Diet
- The nature of food eaten
- The regularity of meal times
- The conditions of eating

Emotional strain

Exterior pathogenic factors

Empty patterns

Stomach-Qi deficiency
Stomach Deficient and Cold
Stomach-Yin deficiency

Full patterns

Stomach-Qi stagnation
Stomach-Heat (or Phlegm-Heat)
Cold invading the Stomach
Stomach-Qi rebelling upwards
Damp-Heat in the Stomach
Retention of Food in the Stomach
Stasis of Blood in the Stomach

Combined patterns

Stomach- and Spleen-Qi deficiency
Stomach- and Spleen-Yin deficiency
Liver-Qi invading the Stomach (discussed in ch. 34 under the Liver patterns)

The functions of the Stomach are (ch. 13):

- It controls 'receiving'
- It controls the 'rotting and ripening' of food
- It controls the transportation of food essences
- It controls the descending of Qi
- It is the origin of fluids

The main Stomach function is that of 'rotting and ripening' food: that is, transforming and digesting it so that the Spleen can separate the distilled food essences. It is therefore natural that all Stomach patterns involve some digestive symptoms.

The Stomach, together with the Spleen, occupies a central position in the Middle Burner and is at the centre of all Qi pathways of other organs, some of which are ascending and some descending. Stomach-Qi itself normally descends in order to send the digested food downwards, while Spleen-Qi ascends to direct Food-Qi upwards to the Lungs and Heart.

Because of the intricate crossing of Qi pathways in the Middle Burner, the Stomach occupies a strategic position and has a crucial role in ensuring the smooth flow of Qi in the Middle Burner. In disease, the Stomach is often affected by stagnation of Qi, rebellious Qi (i.e. ascending instead of descending) or retention of food.

The Stomach, with the Spleen, is the Root of the Post-Heaven Qi: this means that it is the source of all the Qi which is produced by the body after birth. If the Stomach is deficient, not enough Qi is produced by the body, and a person will experience tiredness and weakness, which are very common Stomach symptoms. Tiredness deriving from both Stomach- and Spleen-Qi deficiency is one of the most common clinical symptoms encountered in practice.

Clinical note

Tiredness deriving from both Stomach- and Spleen-Qi deficiency is one of the most common clinical symptoms encountered in practice

The Stomach and Spleen, Root of Post-Heaven Qi, are so fundamental to our health that Stomach-Qi came to be identified with 'life' and lack of Stomach-Qi with 'death'. Of course, this should not be taken literally. It simply means that, as long as there is Stomach-Qi, every disease can be conquered; if Stomach-Qi is weak, every disease will be more difficult

Coating with root: Stomach-Qi good

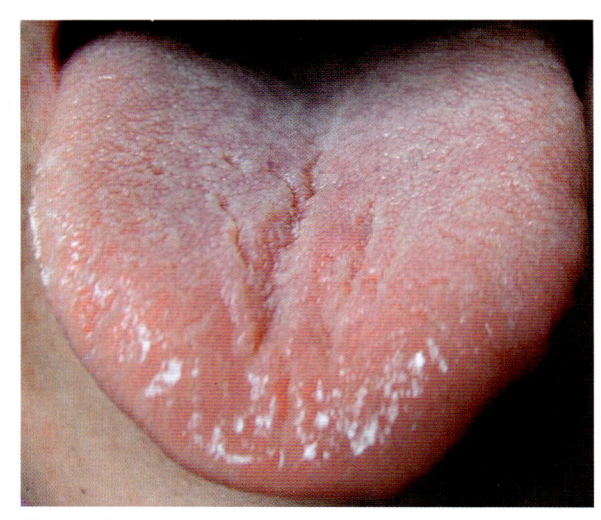

Coating without root: Stomach-Qi deficiency

No coating Stomach-Yin deficiency

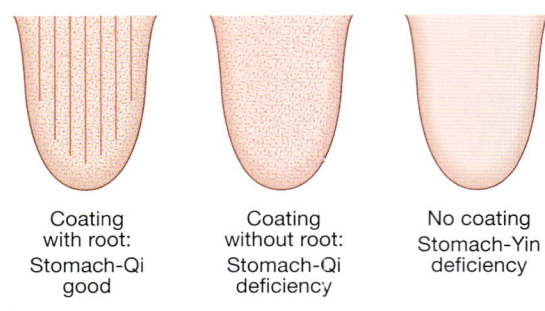

Figure 38.1 Tongue coating in Stomach-Qi and Stomach-Yin deficiency

to treat. Thus, the relative strength of Stomach-Qi is an essential factor in prognosis.

The state of Stomach-Qi may be observed in the tongue and in the pulse. On the tongue, Stomach-Qi manifests with a coating with root; a rootless coating is the beginning stage of Stomach-Qi deficiency and a total lack of coating is a clear indication of deficiency of Stomach-Yin (Fig. 38.1).

A coating without root is formed when the Stomach is weak and ceases to send its 'dirty dampness' (which is the normal by-product of its activity of rotting and ripening) up to the tongue: no new coating is being formed and the old coating therefore loses its root. A coating without root looks patchy, as if it had been sprinkled on top of the tongue, rather than arising out of the tongue surface, as the normal coating does (Fig. 38.2). A coating with root cannot be scraped away while a coating without root can.

On the pulse, a pulse with Stomach-Qi is gentle and relatively soft; a pulse that lack such qualities and deviates from them either way (i.e. too hard or too soft) is said not to have 'Stomach-Qi'.

Another sign of Stomach deficiency on the tongue is a Stomach crack. A Stomach crack is rather wide and it is mostly in the central section of the tongue (Middle Burner), in contrast to a Heart crack that is rather narrow and all along the tongue (from Lower to Upper Burner). Figure 23.33 shows a Stomach crack, while Figure 23.32 shows a Heart crack.

Clinical note

Whenever I see signs of Stomach deficiency (which could be a Stomach crack or a coating without root), I tonify the Stomach also in the absence of any digestive symptom. I use Ren-12 Zhongwan, ST-36 Zusanli and SP-6 Sanyinjiao

Figure 38.2 Coating without root: Stomach-Qi deficiency

Box 38.1 The Stomach

- The main Stomach function is that of rotting and ripening
- The Stomach occupies a central position in the Middle Burner and its Qi descends
- A failure of the smooth flow of Stomach-Qi in the Middle Burner results in Stomach-Qi stagnation or Stomach-Qi rebelling upwards
- The Stomach and Spleen are the Root of Post-Heaven Qi
- Stomach-Qi is identified with 'life' (i.e. good prognosis) and its absence with 'death' (i.e. poor prognosis)
- A coating without root indicates Stomach-Qi deficiency; absence of coating indicates Stomach-Yin deficiency
- A pulse with Stomach-Qi is gentle and appropriately soft
- The School of Stomach and Spleen (Li Dong Yuan) emphasized the central role of the Stomach and Spleen in health and disease

The importance of the Stomach and Spleen in health and disease is such that a whole school stressing the importance of the Stomach and Spleen in physiology, pathology and treatment arose during the Yuan dynasty. This was the 'School of Stomach and Spleen', of which the most famous representative was Li Dong Yuan (1180–1251), author of the important work 'Discussion on Stomach and Spleen' (*Pi Wei Lun*, 1246).

Finally, it should be remembered that the Stomach is the origin of fluids, as all the drink ingested has to be transformed and digested by it. It follows that the Stomach can be affected by Yin deficiency and, indeed, Stomach-Yin deficiency is usually the beginning of a Yin deficiency pathology that later affects other organs.

Box 38.1 summarizes the information detailed above.

The discussion of Stomach patterns will be preceded by a discussion of the aetiology of Stomach patterns as follows:

- General aetiology
  - Diet
    - The nature of food eaten
    - The regularity of meal times
    - The conditions of eating
  - Emotional strain
  - Exterior pathogenic factors

GENERAL AETIOLOGY

Diet

Diet is obviously the main cause of disease for the Stomach. This can be approached from many viewpoints concerning the nature of the food eaten, the regularity of eating times and the conditions of eating.

The nature of food eaten

This is a very complex subject which cannot be dealt with here in depth, as the nature of the food eaten should take into account many variables such as the character of the food, the season, the constitution, state of health and occupation of the person. Dietary irregularity as a cause of disease was discussed in chapter 22.

Generally speaking, the Stomach prefers foods which are moist and not too dry (the Spleen prefers the opposite, i.e. foods that are dry). Soups and porridge are examples of moist foods preferred by the Stomach; foods that are baked for a long time (including bread) are 'dry'.

If the person eats foods which are too dry (such as baked and broiled foods), the Stomach may become dry and eventually suffer from Yin deficiency.

Besides this, the Stomach may suffer from excessive consumption of foods that are either too hot or too cold in terms of energy. Excessive consumption of hot foods (which includes meat and especially red meat, spices and alcohol) may cause Heat in the Stomach.

Of course, one cannot define in absolute terms what is an 'excessive' consumption of these foods, as this is relative to the constitution of the person, the season and the occupation. If a person suffers from a deficiency of Yang, it is appropriate to eat more of the heated foods. These are also more appropriate in wintertime in cold countries. If the person is engaged in heavy physical work, it is also appropriate to eat more of the hot foods.

Excessive consumption of cold foods (such as vegetables, especially raw, fruit and cold drinks) may cause Cold in the Stomach. Similar to what was said for the hot foods, a heavier consumption of cold foods could be appropriate for someone suffering from excess of Heat, or living in a very hot country.

Box 38.2 summarizes the Stomach in relation to the nature of the food eaten.

Box 38.2 The nature of food and the Stomach

- The Stomach prefers moist foods (porridge, soups)
- The Stomach dislikes dry foods (baked or broiled foods, bread)
- Excessive consumption of meat, spices and alcohol (hot foods) causes Stomach-Heat
- Excessive consumption of raw vegetables, fruit and cold drinks (cold foods) causes Cold in the Stomach

The regularity of meal times

The Chinese traditionally stress the importance of eating at regular times. This is because the body has a natural rhythm of flow of Qi in different organs at different times, and it would be inappropriate to eat at a time when Stomach-Qi is quiescent. The Stomach would obviously not be able to digest food properly. Advice to eat at regular times may sound very old-fashioned to some patients, but experience shows that irregular eating does produce Stomach disorders. It is therefore important:

- To have meals at regular times
- To eat a proper breakfast (in some countries people have just a small cup of strong coffee)
- Not to over- or undereat
- Not to nibble between meals
- Not to eat late at night
- Not to eat too fast

Overeating prevents the Stomach from digesting food properly, so that it stagnates in the Middle Burner and Stomach-Qi cannot descend.

Undereating or a form of malnourishment due to too-strict unsuitable diets leads to Stomach and Spleen deficiency.

Constant nibbling or eating too fast does not give the Stomach time to digest food properly and leads to retention of food.

Eating late at night, a time of Yin, forces the Stomach to use its Yin energy and leads to deficiency of Stomach-Yin.

Box 38.3 summarizes information about the regularity of meal times.

> **Box 38.3 The regularity of meal times and the Stomach**
>
> - Overeating prevents the Stomach from digesting food properly and causes retention of food
> - Undereating or too strict or unsuitable diets lead to Stomach and Spleen deficiency
> - Constant nibbling or eating too fast lead to retention of food
> - Eating late at night leads to deficiency of Stomach-Yin

The conditions of eating

Apart from the nature and amount of food eaten and the time at which it is eaten, the accompanying circumstances are also extremely important. One might eat the purest and most balanced food at absolutely regular times, but if this is eaten in a negative frame of mind, such as when one is very sad, angry or worried, it will not do one any good.

The emotional frame of mind at meal times is important. If one eats while worrying about something (such as one's work), it will lead to stagnation of Qi in the Stomach or Stomach-Qi rebelling upwards. If one eats in a state of sadness, it may lead to Stomach-Qi deficiency.

If meal times are a regular opportunity for family rows (as sadly is sometimes the case), even the best of foods will not be digested and will cause retention of food in the Stomach and stagnation of Qi in the Middle Burner or Stomach-Qi rebelling upwards. Eating on the run, grabbing a quick bite during a short lunch hour and eating while working also cause stagnation of Qi in the Stomach or Stomach-Qi rebelling upwards. Reading while eating leads to deficiency of Stomach-Qi.

Diet as a cause of disease is discussed in chapter 22. Conditions of eating are summarized in Box 38.4.

Emotional strain

The Stomach is mostly affected by worry and excessive thinking in a similar way to the Spleen. Worry will cause stagnation of Qi in the Stomach and will manifest with a niggling, burning pain, belching and nausea.

> **Box 38.4 Conditions of eating and the Stomach**
>
> - Eating while worried causes Stomach-Qi stagnation or Stomach-Qi rebelling upwards
> - Eating while sad causes Stomach-Qi deficiency
> - Eating while angry causes Stomach-Qi rebelling upwards or Stomach-Qi stagnation
> - Eating on the run and in a hurry causes Stomach-Qi stagnation
> - Reading while eating leads to deficiency of Stomach-Qi

Excessive mental work or pensiveness over a period of many years leads to deficiency of Stomach-Qi.

Anger also affects the Stomach, either directly or indirectly via the Liver. Anger, frustration and resentment cause stagnation of Liver-Qi, which invades the Stomach, resulting in nausea, belching or distending pain.

Emotional strain as a cause of disease is discussed in chapter 20. Box 38.5 summarizes emotional strain in relation to the Stomach.

> **Box 38.5 Emotional strain and the Stomach**
>
> - Worry causes stagnation of Qi in the Stomach
> - Excessive mental work leads to deficiency of Stomach-Qi
> - Anger may affect the Stomach directly
> - Anger, frustration and resentment cause stagnation of Liver-Qi, which invades the Stomach

Exterior pathogenic factors

The Stomach can be affected by climatic factors directly, in particular by Cold. Cold can invade the Stomach directly (bypassing the Exterior layers of the body) and give rise to Interior Cold in the Stomach, with symptoms of sudden acute pain and vomiting.

Exterior pathogenic factors as causes of disease are discussed in chapter 21.

The Stomach patterns discussed are:
EMPTY PATTERNS
- Stomach-Qi deficiency
- Stomach Deficient and Cold
- Stomach-Yin deficiency

FULL PATTERNS
- Stomach-Qi stagnation
- Stomach Heat (or Phlegm-Heat)
- Cold invading the Stomach
- Stomach-Qi rebelling upwards
- Damp-Heat in the Stomach
- Retention of Food in the Stomach
- Stasis of Blood in the Stomach

> **Box 38.6 General aetiology of Stomach patterns**
>
> - Diet
>   - The nature of food eaten
>   - The regularity of meal times
>   - The conditions of eating
> - Emotional strain
> - Exterior pathogenic factors

COMBINED PATTERNS
- Stomach- and Spleen-Qi deficiency
- Stomach- and Spleen-Yin deficiency
- Liver-Qi invading the Stomach (discussed in ch. 34 under the Liver patterns)

Boxes 38.6 and 38.7 provide summaries of the general aetiology of Stomach patterns and factors which may give a 'feel' for Stomach pathology.

> **Box 38.7 A 'feel' for Stomach patterns**
>
> - Tiredness
> - Digestive complaints
> - Weak limbs
> - Stomach-Qi and Stomach-Yin reflected directly on tongue coating

EMPTY PATTERNS

Stomach-Qi deficiency

Clinical manifestations

Uncomfortable feeling in the epigastrium, no appetite, lack of taste sensation, loose stools, tiredness especially in the morning, weak limbs (Fig. 38.3).
Tongue: Pale.
Pulse: Empty, especially on the Right-Middle position.
Key symptoms: tiredness in the morning, uncomfortable feeling in the epigastrium, Empty pulse on the Stomach position.

> **Clinical note**
>
> Stomach-Qi deficiency is one of the most common patterns encountered in practice and a common cause of chronic tiredness

> **Diagnostic tip**
>
> Tiredness in the morning and a Weak Stomach pulse are enough to diagnose Stomach-Qi deficiency

- No appetite, lack of taste
- Tiredness in the morning
- Uncomfortable feeling in epigastrium
- Loose stools
- Weak limbs

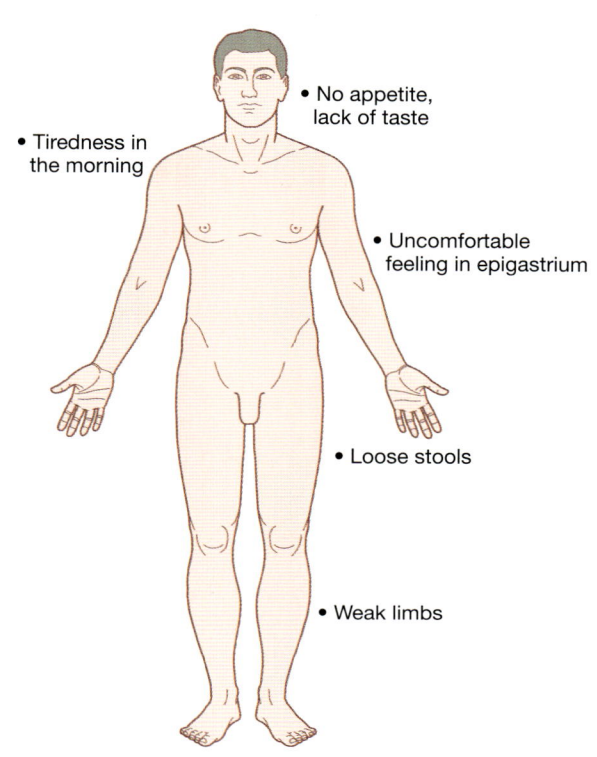

Figure 38.3 Stomach-Qi deficiency

Aetiology

Diet

The most common cause of Stomach disharmonies is dietary. A diet lacking in nourishment and protein, or plain undereating (due to 'dieting'), can cause deficiency of Stomach-Qi.

Irregular eating habits as described above can also cause a Stomach-Qi deficiency.

Chronic illness

Stomach-Qi deficiency can also arise as a consequence of a chronic disease, which weakens Qi in general. For example, it is very common to see Stomach-Qi deficiency after a prolonged illness such as mononucleosis (glandular fever).

Pathology

The Stomach is the Root of Post-Heaven Qi and the beginning stage in the production of Qi from food: if the Stomach is weak, therefore, Qi will be deficient and all other organs will suffer. Tiredness will be the main

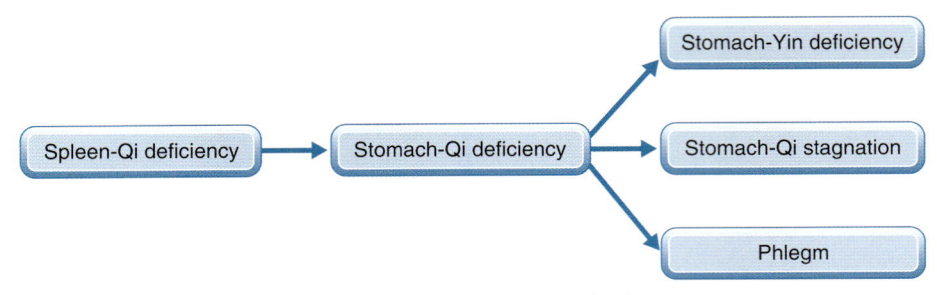

Figure 38.4 Stomach-Qi deficiency pattern: precursors and developments

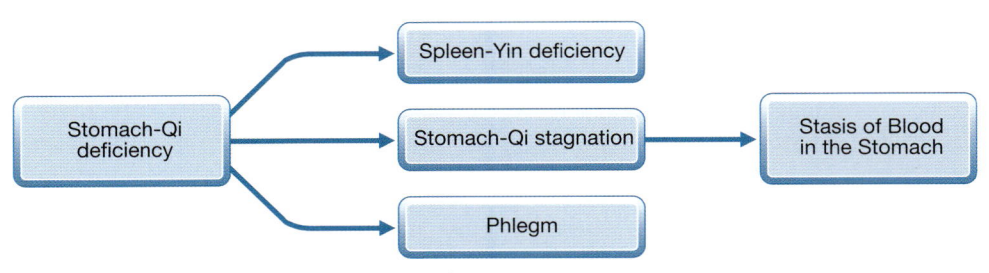

Figure 38.5 Consequences of Stomach-Qi deficiency

symptom of Stomach deficiency. It will be worse in the mornings in correspondence with the peak of activity of the Stomach between 7 and 9 a.m.

Deficient Stomach-Qi will fail to descend, causing a vaguely uncomfortable feeling in the epigastrium, indicative of a Deficiency condition (if it was from an Excess condition, it would be a strong feeling of discomfort or pain).

When Stomach-Qi is deficient, Spleen-Qi is also often deficient as Stomach and Spleen are so closely intertwined. This results in lack of appetite, loose stools, lack of taste and a Pale tongue.

When Stomach-Qi is weak, it cannot transport the food essences to the limbs, resulting in a feeling of weakness of the limbs.

Pathological precursors of pattern

Spleen-Qi deficiency frequently leads to the pattern of Stomach-Qi deficiency (Fig. 38.4).

Pathological developments from pattern

Stomach-Qi deficiency is usually the beginning stage of a pathological process with several possible outcomes. First of all, Stomach-Qi deficiency may lead to Stomach-Yin deficiency after some years.

Stomach-Qi deficiency sometimes leads to Qi stagnation and, later, to Blood stasis. The impairment of the descending of Stomach-Qi (which occurs often with Stomach-Qi deficiency) may lead to the formation of Phlegm (Figs 38.4 and 38.5).

Treatment

Principle of treatment: tonify Stomach Qi.

Acupuncture

Points: ST-36 Zusanli, Ren-12 Zhongwan, BL-21 Weishu, Ren-6 Qihai.
Method: reinforcing, moxa is applicable.
Explanation
– ST-36 is the main point to tonify Stomach-Qi. Using moxa on the needle is especially effective.
– Ren-12 tonifies Stomach- and Spleen-Qi.
– BL-21 tonifies Stomach-Qi. It is an important point in case of extreme tiredness. Moxa is also applicable.
– Ren-6 tonifies Qi in general, and is indicated for chronic cases of Stomach-Qi deficiency, especially with loose stools.

Herbal formula

Si Jun Zi Tang *Four Gentlemen Decoction*.

> **Box 38.8 Stomach-Qi deficiency**
>
> **Clinical manifestations**
>
> Uncomfortable feeling in the epigastrium, no appetite, lack of taste sensation, loose stools, tiredness especially in the morning, weak limbs, Pale tongue, Empty pulse, especially on the Right-Middle position
>
> **Treatment**
>
> ST-36 Zusanli, Ren-12 Zhongwan, BL-21 Weishu, Ren-6 Qihai

Three Treasures

Prosperous Earth (variation of Liu Jun Zi Tang).
  Box 38.8 summarizes Stomach-Qi deficiency.

> **Diagnostic tip**
>
> Both Spleen-Qi deficiency and Stomach-Qi deficiency are a common cause of chronic tiredness. They can be distinguished, as Spleen-Qi deficiency will cause a slight abdominal distension and often loose stools while Stomach-Qi deficiency will cause a slight discomfort in the epigastrium (and generally more upper digestive symptoms) and also weak limbs

Stomach Deficient and Cold

Clinical manifestations

Discomfort or dull pain in the epigastrium, better after eating and better with pressure or massage, no appetite, preference for warm drinks and foods, vomiting of clear fluid, no thirst, cold and weak limbs, tiredness, pale complexion (Fig. 38.6).
Tongue: Pale and wet.
Pulse: Deep-Weak-Slow, especially on the Right-Middle position.
Key symptoms: discomfort in the epigastrium which is better after eating, tiredness, cold limbs.

> **Diagnostic tip**
>
> Discomfort in the epigastrium, which is better after eating, tiredness and cold limbs are enough to diagnose Stomach Deficient and Cold

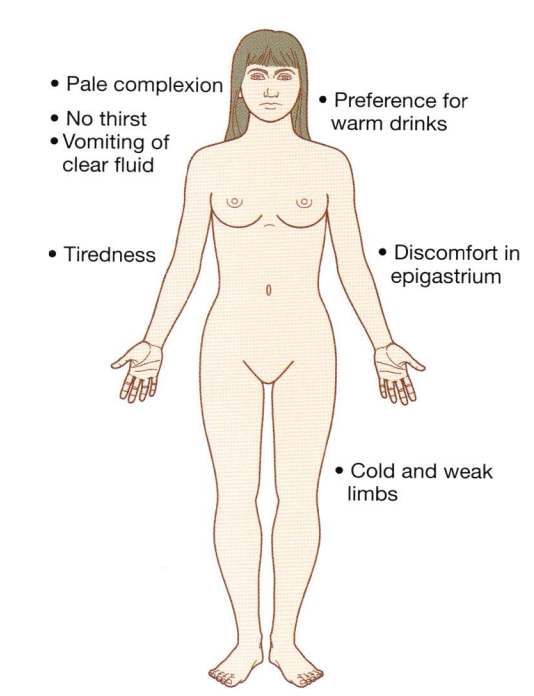

Figure 38.6 Stomach Deficient and Cold

- Pale complexion
- No thirst
- Vomiting of clear fluid
- Preference for warm drinks
- Tiredness
- Discomfort in epigastrium
- Cold and weak limbs

Aetiology

Diet

A diet lacking in nourishing foods such a protein may lead to the pattern Stomach Deficient and Cold. It may also be due to excessive consumption of cold foods and drinks, ice-creams, salads, fruit and iced drinks.

Exterior pathogenic factors

Exterior Cold can invade the Stomach, and if it is not expelled, after some time it will interfere with the Stomach function and cause Stomach-Qi deficiency.

Pathology

This is similar to the previous pattern, with the addition of Empty-Cold symptoms. Normally this pattern is associated with Spleen-Yang deficiency, which leads to internal Cold, resulting in cold limbs, loose stools, vomiting of clear fluids, no thirst, preference for warm drinks and foods and a Weak pulse.

When Stomach-Qi is deficient, it may be made worse by the bowel movement (because of the relationship between Stomach and Large Intestine with the Bright-Yang), hence the aggravation of the feeling of discomfort in the epigastrium after a bowel movement.

Because the discomfort is caused by a Deficiency condition, it is better with eating and better for pressure or massage.

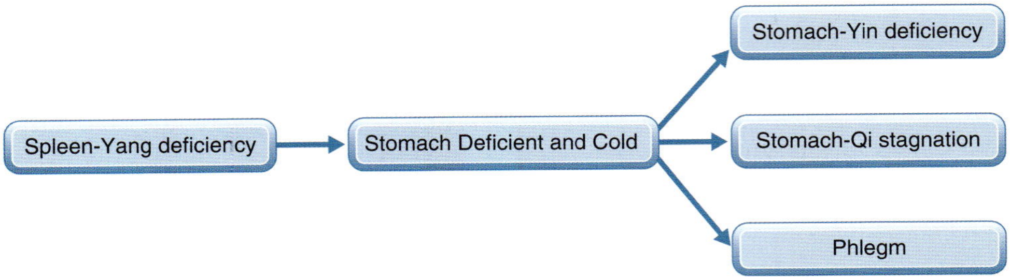

Figure 38.7 Stomach Deficient and Cold pattern: precursors and developments

Pathological precursors of pattern

This pattern can be the consequence of Spleen-Yang deficiency (Fig. 38.7).

Pathological developments from pattern

Stomach Deficient and Cold may lead to Qi stagnation and, later, Blood stasis. It may also lead to the formation of Phlegm (see Fig. 38.7).

Treatment

Principle of treatment: tonify and warm Stomach- and Spleen-Qi.

Acupuncture

Points: ST-36 Zusanli, Ren-12 Zhongwan, BL-20 Pishu, BL-21 Weishu, Ren-6 Qihai.
Method: reinforcing, moxa must be used.
Explanation
 – ST-36 tonifies Stomach-Qi.
 – Ren-12 tonifies Stomach- and Spleen-Qi.
 – BL-20 tonifies Spleen-Qi.
 – BL-21 tonifies Stomach-Qi.
 – Ren-6 tonifies Qi in general. Moxa on ginger can be used on this point: this is the best method for Empty-Cold in the Stomach.

Herbal formula

Huang Qi Jian Zhong Tang *Astragalus Strengthening the Centre Decoction*.
Xiao Jian Zhong Tang *Small Strengthening the Centre Decoction*.
Box 38.9 summarizes Stomach Deficient and Cold.

Stomach-Yin deficiency

Clinical manifestations

No appetite or slight hunger but no desire to eat, constipation (dry stools), dull or slightly burning epigastric pain, dry mouth and throat, especially in the afternoon, with desire to drink in small sips, slight feeling of fullness after eating (Fig. 38.8).
Tongue: without coating in the centre, or with rootless coating, normal body colour.
Pulse: Floating-Empty on the Right-Middle position.
Key symptoms: dull epigastric pain, dry mouth, tongue without coating or with rootless coating in the centre.

Empty-Heat

Thirst with desire to drink in small sips, feeling of hunger, night sweating, five-palm heat, bleeding gums, feeling of heat in the evening.
Tongue: Red and without coating in the centre.
Pulse: Floating-Empty on the Right-Middle position and slightly Rapid.

Box 38.9 Stomach Deficient and Cold

Clinical manifestations

Discomfort or dull pain in the epigastrium, better after eating and better with pressure or massage, no appetite, preference for warm drinks and foods, vomiting of clear fluid, no thirst, cold and weak limbs, tiredness, pale complexion, Pale and wet tongue, Deep-Weak-Slow pulse, especially on the Right-Middle position

Treatment

ST-36 Zusanli, Ren-12 Zhongwan, BL-20 Pishu, BL-21 Weishu, Ren-6 Qihai

---

Diagnostic tip

Even just the absence of coating in the centre of the tongue is enough to diagnose Stomach-Yin deficiency

- No appetite or slight hunger without desire to eat
- Dry mouth and throat
- Dull epigastric pain, fullness after eating
- Dry stools

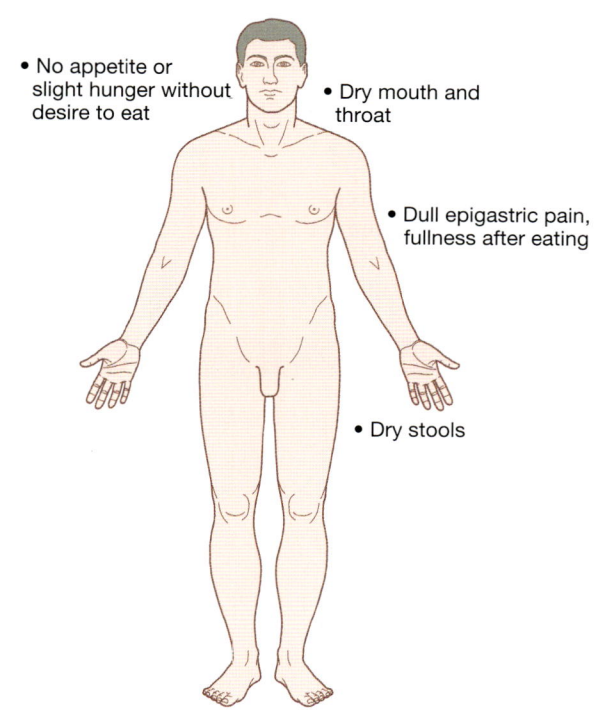

Figure 38.8 Stomach-Yin deficiency

Aetiology

Diet

The most common cause of Stomach-Yin deficiency is an irregular diet and eating habits, mostly due to eating late at night, skipping meals, 'grabbing a quick bite' during a short and hectic lunch hour, worrying about work while eating, going straight back to work immediately after a meal, eating while working at one's desk, as described at the beginning of this chapter. All these habits seriously deplete Stomach-Qi and, if they persist over a long period of time, they will begin to weaken Stomach-Yin. In particular, eating late at night depletes Stomach-Yin.

Constitution

In some cases, Stomach-Yin deficiency may be constitutional and, for this reason, it is occasionally seen in young people, teenagers and even children.

Fevers

A high fever during the course of an infectious disease may cause Stomach-Yin deficiency in an acute way. However, this is normally not long-lasting and Stomach-Yin reverts to normal a few days or weeks after the end of the disease. In a few cases, however, it may persist.

Drugs

Antibiotics may injure Stomach-Qi and Stomach-Yin, causing the coating of the tongue to fall off. If the course of antibiotics is not too long, normally Stomach-Yin reverts back to normal after the antibiotics are discontinued.

Pathology

The Stomach is the origin of fluids and when its Yin is deficient there will be dryness, causing dry stools, dry mouth and throat and thirst. The dry mouth in Stomach-Yin deficiency is peculiar in so far as it is with a desire to drink in small sips. Because the thirst is due to deficiency of Yin, the person likes to drink in small sips or sometimes even likes to drink warm liquids.

> **Diagnostic tip**
>
> A dry mouth with desire to drink in small sips is typical of Stomach-Yin deficiency

The feeling of heat in the afternoon is due to deficiency of Yin. The most significant sign of deficiency of Stomach-Yin is a tongue that is either without coating or has a rootless coating in the centre (Stomach area).

Pathological precursors of pattern

Stomach-Yin deficiency always derives from Stomach-Qi deficiency (unless it is caused by antibiotics) (Fig. 38.9).

Pathological developments from pattern

Stomach-Yin deficiency often leads to Kidney-Yin deficiency or Yin deficiency of other organs if it persists for some years (see Fig. 38.9).

> **Clinical note**
>
> Stomach-Yin deficiency is nearly always the precursor of Kidney-Yin deficiency

Treatment

Principle of treatment: nourish Stomach-Yin, nourish fluids.

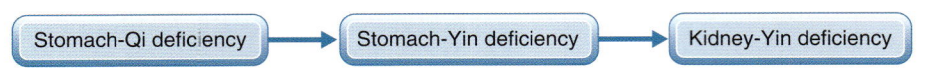

Figure 38.9 Stomach-Yin deficiency pattern: precursors and developments

Stomach-Qi deficiency → Stomach-Yin deficiency → Kidney-Yin deficiency

Acupuncture

Points: Ren-12 Zhongwan, ST-36 Zusanli, SP-6 Sanyinjiao, SP-3 Taibai.
Method: reinforcing, no moxa.
Explanation
- Ren-12 tonifies Stomach-Yin.
- ST-36 tonifies Stomach-Qi and Stomach-Yin.
- SP-6 tonifies Stomach-Yin and nourishes fluids.
- SP-3 nourishes fluids.

Herbal formula

Sha Shen Mai Dong Tang *Glehnia–Ophiopogan Decoction*.
Shen Ling Bai Zhu San *Ginseng–Poria–Atractylodes Powder*.
Yi Wei Tang *Benefitting the Stomach Decoction*.

Three Treasures

Central Mansion (variation of Shen Ling Bai Zhu San).
Jade Spring (variation of Sha Shen Mai Dong Tang).
Box 38.10 summarizes Stomach-Yin deficiency.

Box 38.10 Stomach-Yin deficiency

Clinical manifestations

No appetite or slight hunger but no desire to eat, constipation (dry stools), dull or slightly burning epigastric pain, dry mouth and throat especially in the afternoon, with desire to drink in small sips, slight feeling of fullness after eating
Tongue: without coating in the centre, or with rootless coating, normal body colour
Pulse: Floating-Empty on the Right-Middle position

Treatment

ST-36 Zusanli, Ren-12 Zhongwan, SP-6 Sanyinjiao, SP-3 Taibai

FULL PATTERNS

Stomach-Qi stagnation

Clinical manifestations

Epigastric pain and distension, belching, nausea, vomiting, hiccups, irritability (Fig. 38.10).

Tongue: no particular signs on the tongue except that in severe cases it may be Red on the sides in the central section.
Pulse: Wiry on the Right-Middle position.

> **Diagnostic tip**
>
> Epigastric distension, belching and irritability are enough to diagnose Stomach-Qi stagnation

Aetiology

Diet

Eating in a hurry, working while eating, eating in a state of tension or while upset, eating standing up: all these habits lead to this pattern.

Emotional strain

Anger, frustration and resentment (the same emotions that affect the Liver) may affect the Stomach and cause Stomach-Qi stagnation. They are more likely to affect the Stomach when the person also has irregular eating habits.

> **Clinical note**
>
> A combination of dietary irregularity and emotional strain causes Stomach-Qi stagnation; emotional strain by itself will tend to cause Liver-Qi stagnation

Pathology

Epigastric distension is the cardinal symptom of Stomach-Qi stagnation. The Qi stagnation in the Middle Burner also causes Stomach-Qi to ascend and this causes belching, nausea, vomiting and hiccups. Irritability is due to stagnation of Qi.

The tongue may not show much in this pattern except that, in severe cases, it may be slightly Red on the sides in the central section.

Pathological precursors of pattern

Liver-Qi stagnation may be transmitted to the Stomach causing Stomach-Qi stagnation (Fig. 38.11).

- Irritability
- Belching, nausea, vomiting, hiccup
- Epigastric distension and pain

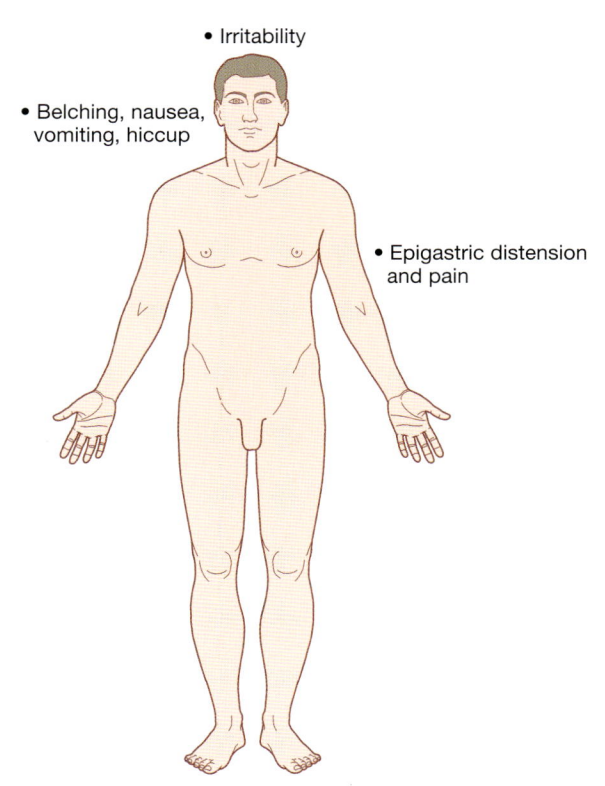

Figure 38.10 Stomach-Qi stagnation

Pathological developments from pattern

Stomach-Qi stagnation may give rise to Blood stasis in the Stomach if the condition persists for a long time.

Stomach-Qi stagnation may also generate Heat and lead to Stomach-Fire or Stomach-Heat. In long-standing conditions, the Qi stagnation may also contribute to the formation of Phlegm and lead to Phlegm-Fire in the Stomach (Figs 38.11 and 38.12).

Treatment

Principle of treatment: move Stomach-Qi, eliminate stagnation, restore the descending of Stomach-Qi.

Acupuncture

Points: ST-34 Liangqiu, ST-21 Liangmen, ST-19 Burong, KI-21 Youmen, T.B.-6 Zhigou, P-6 Neiguan, SP-4 Gongsun with P-6 Neiguan (opening points of the Penetrating Vessel *Chong Mai*), G.B.-34 Yanglingquan with Ren-12 Zhongwan, ST-40 Fenglong.

Explanation
- ST-34 is the Accumulation point of the Stomach channel; it moves Stomach-Qi and it is used for Full conditions.

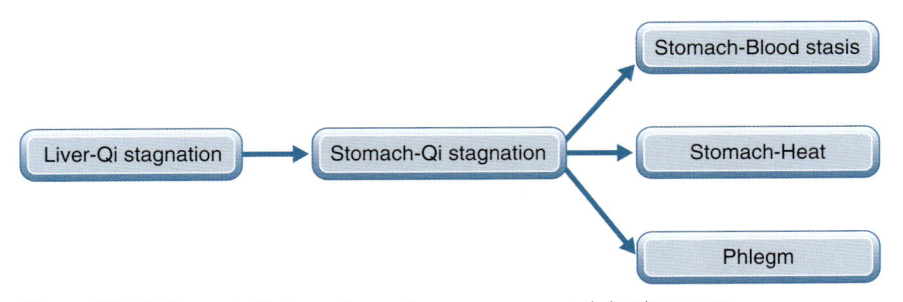

Figure 38.11 Stomach-Qi stagnation pattern: precursors and developments

Liver-Qi stagnation → Stomach-Qi stagnation → Stomach-Blood stasis / Stomach-Heat / Phlegm

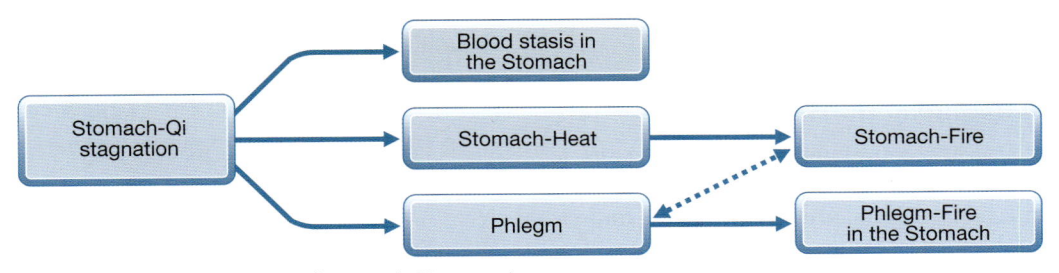

Figure 38.12 Consequences of Stomach-Qi stagnation

Stomach-Qi stagnation → Blood stasis in the Stomach / Stomach-Heat → Stomach-Fire / Phlegm → Phlegm-Fire in the Stomach

- ST-21 and ST-19 restore the descending of Stomach-Qi.
- KI-21, a point of the Penetrating Vessel (*Chong Mai*), restores the descending of Stomach-Qi and eliminates stagnation from the Middle Burner.
- T.B.-6 moves Qi and eliminates stagnation in the Middle Burner.
- P-6 restores the descending of Stomach-Qi and calms the Mind.
- SP-4 and P-6 in combination open the Penetrating Vessel (*Chong Mai*) and move Qi in the Middle Burner.
- G.B.-34 in combination with Ren-12 moves Qi and eliminates stagnation in the Middle Burner.
- ST-40 moves Stomach-Qi, restores the descending of Stomach-Qi and calms the Mind.

Herbal formula

Chen Xiang Jiang San *Aquilaria Subduing Qi Powder*.
Ban Xia Hou Po Tang *Pinellia–Magnolia Decoction*.
Zuo Jin Wan *Left Metal Pill*.

Box 38.11 summarizes Stomach-Qi stagnation.

Box 38.11 Stomach-Qi stagnation

Clinical manifestations

Epigastric pain and distension, belching, nausea, vomiting, hiccups, irritability, no particular signs on the tongue except that in severe cases it may be Red on the sides in the central section, pulse Wiry on the Right-Middle position

Treatment

ST-34 Liangqiu, ST-21 Liangmen, ST-19 Burong, KI-21 Youmen, T.B.-6 Zhigou, P-6 Neiguan, SP-4 Gongsun with P-6 Neiguan (opening points of the Penetrating Vessel), G.B.-34 Yanglingquan with Ren-12 Zhongwan, ST-40 Fenglong

---

Stomach-Heat (or Phlegm-Heat)

Clinical manifestations

Burning epigastric pain, intense thirst with desire to drink cold liquids, mental restlessness, dry stools, dry mouth, mouth ulcers, sour regurgitation, nausea, vomiting soon after eating, excessive hunger, foul breath, a feeling of heat (Fig. 38.13).

- Mental restlessness
- Bleeding gums, foul breath
- Intense thirst, mouth ulcers
- Sour regurgitation, nausea, vomiting, excessive hunger
- Burning epigastric pain
- Dry stools

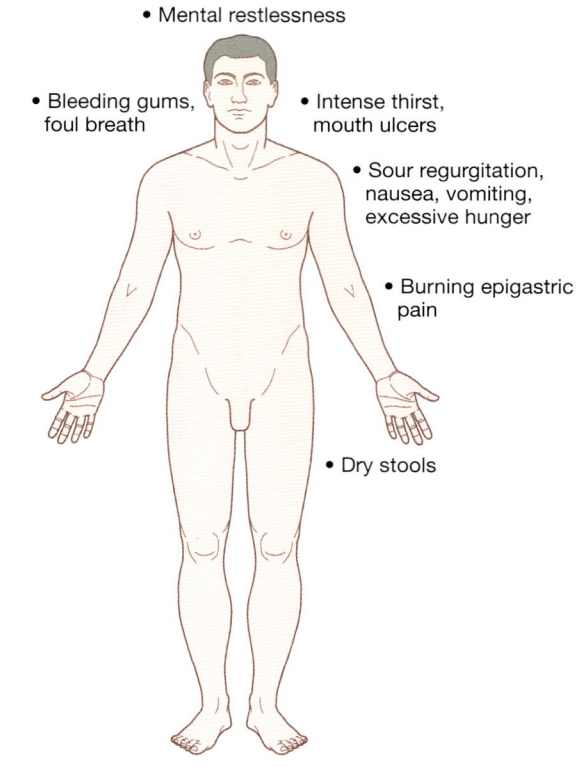

Figure 38.13 Stomach-Heat

Tongue: Red in the centre with a dry yellow or dark-yellow coating.
Pulse: Rapid and slightly Overflowing on the Right-Middle position.
Key symptoms: burning sensation in the epigastrium, thirst with desire to drink cold liquids, thick yellow coating, Red tongue.

Phlegm-Heat

In addition to the above symptoms: a feeling of oppression of the chest and epigastrium, mucus in stools, expectoration of phlegm, mental derangement.
Tongue: Red with a sticky yellow coating.
Pulse: Rapid-Slippery-Overflowing.

Diagnostic tip

A burning sensation in the epigastrium, thirst with a desire to drink cold liquids and a Red tongue with a thick yellow coating are enough to diagnose Stomach-Heat

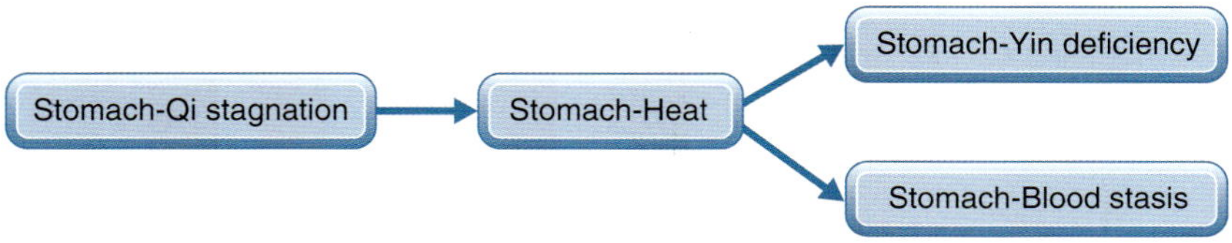

Figure 38.14 Stomach-Heat pattern: precursors and developments

Aetiology

Diet

This pattern can be due to excessive consumption of hot foods in the sense described above (i.e. meat, spices and alcohol) and to smoking (tobacco has a hot energy). In case of Phlegm-Heat, it is caused by excessive consumption of hot greasy foods, such as deep-fried foods.

Emotional strain

Anger, frustration and resentment lead to stagnation of Stomach-Qi, which, in turn may lead to Stomach-Heat.

Pathology

This is a pattern of interior Full-Heat in the Stomach. Heat in the Stomach burns the fluids, hence the intense thirst, constipation and dry tongue.

Heat makes the Blood extravasate in the Stomach channel, resulting in bleeding from the gums. The swelling and pain in the gums is due to Heat rising in the Stomach channel.

Full-Heat obstructs the Stomach and interferes with the descending of Stomach-Qi, hence the sour regurgitation, nausea and vomiting. The fluid regurgitated is 'sour' because the Heat ferments the Stomach fluids. Excessive hunger is caused by Stomach-Heat.

In case of Phlegm-Heat, Phlegm is more obstructive, causing the feeling of oppression of the epigastrium and chest.

Phlegm and Heat in the Stomach can affect the Mind and cause severe mental symptoms such as manic depression.

Please note that the above clinical manifestations are those of Stomach-Heat, which is a less severe form of Stomach-Fire. In case of Stomach-Fire, the symptoms are more severe. For example, there would be bleeding gums, the tongue would be redder and the coating darker and drier.

> **Clinical note**
>
> Compared to Heat, Fire has distinguishing characteristics:
> - It is more intense (intense thirst)
> - It dries up fluids more (dry stools, dark urine)
> - It may cause bleeding (bleeding gums)
> - It disturbs the Mind more (mental restlessness)
> - The tongue has a drier and darker coating

Pathological precursors of pattern

Stomach-Heat usually derives from other patterns such as Stomach-Qi stagnation (Fig. 38.14).

Pathological developments from pattern

Stomach-Heat dries up the Body Fluids and may lead to Stomach-Yin deficiency. In some cases, Stomach-Heat may also condense Blood and lead to Blood stasis in the Stomach (see Fig. 38.14).

Treatment

Principle of treatment: clear Stomach-Heat, stimulate the descending of Stomach-Qi.

Acupuncture

Points: ST-44 Neiting, ST-34 Liangqiu, ST-21 Liangmen, Ren-13 Shangwan, L.I.-11 Quchi, L.I.-4 Hegu, Ren-11 Jianli, SP-15 Daheng.

Method: reducing method, except on Ren-12 and Ren-13, on which even method should be used.

Explanation
- ST-44 clears Stomach-Heat.
- ST-34 is the Accumulation point of the Stomach and it is used in Full conditions. It also stops bleeding (in case of bleeding gums).
- ST-21 clears Stomach-Heat and stimulates the descending of Stomach-Qi.
- Ren-13 subdues rebellious Stomach-Qi.
- L.I.-11 clears Heat in general.
- L.I.-4 clears Stomach-Heat

> **Box 38.12 Stomach-Heat**
>
> **Clinical manifestations**
>
> Burning epigastric pain, intense thirst with desire to drink cold liquids, mental restlessness, bleeding gums, dry stools, dry mouth, mouth ulcers, sour regurgitation, nausea, vomiting soon after eating, excessive hunger, foul breath, a feeling of heat, tongue Red in the centre with a dry yellow or dark-yellow (or even black) coating, Rapid and slightly Overflowing pulse on the Right-Middle position
>
> **Treatment**
>
> ST-44 Neiting, ST-34 Liangqiu, ST-21 Liangmen, Ren-13 Shangwan, L.I.-11 Quchi, L.I.-4 Hegu, Ren-11 Jianli, SP-15 Daheng

- Ren-11 clears Stomach-Heat.
- SP-15 stimulates the bowel movement and is used if there is constipation.

Herbal formula

Tiao Wei Cheng Qi Tang *Regulating the Stomach Conducting Qi Decoction*.
Qing Wei San *Clearing the Stomach Powder*.
Liang Ge San *Cooling the Diaphragm Powder*.
  Box 38.12 summarizes Stomach-Heat.

Case history 38.1

A woman of 60 had lost her sense of smell and taste 2 years previously. For the past 10 years, she had also suffered from epigastric pain, a sensation of 'knot' in the stomach and nausea. She was often very thirsty and drank large amounts of water every day. Occasionally she experienced bleeding of the gums. She also complained of a lack of appetite and loose stools. Her pulse was Full and Wiry, especially on the Right-Middle position, and her tongue was red in the centre and had a dry yellow coating.

This patient suffered from Stomach-Heat ('knot' in the stomach, thirst and bleeding gums) and deficiency of Spleen-Qi (lack of appetite and loose stools). The loss of taste and smell is due to Spleen deficiency, but also to Stomach-Heat 'burning' upwards.

Cold invading the Stomach

Clinical manifestations

Sudden severe pain in the epigastrium, a feeling of cold, cold limbs, preference for warmth, vomiting of clear fluids (which may alleviate the pain), nausea, feeling worse after swallowing cold fluids, which are quickly vomited, preference for warm liquids (Fig. 38.15).
Tongue: thick white coating.
Pulse: Deep-Tight-Slow.
Key symptoms: sudden pain in epigastrium, vomiting, feeling cold, Deep-Tight Pulse.

- Vomiting of clear fluids
- Feeling cold
- Sudden, severe epigastric pain
- Cold limbs

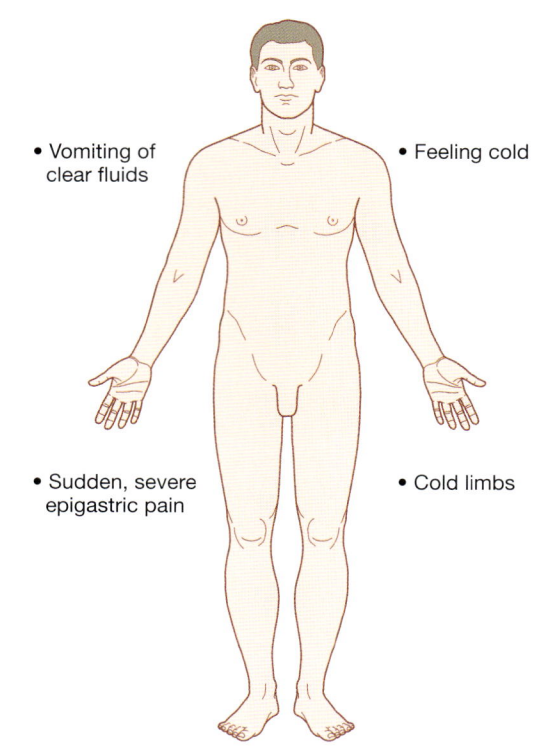

Figure 38.15 Cold invading the Stomach

> **Diagnostic tip**
>
> Sudden pain in epigastrium and a Tight pulse are enough to diagnose Cold invading the Stomach

Aetiology

This is caused by invasion of the Stomach by exterior Cold, due to exposure to cold and excessive consumption of cold foods and iced drinks.

Pathology

This is a pattern of interior Full-Cold. It is an acute pattern caused by the invasion of the Stomach by exterior Cold. The Stomach is one of three organs

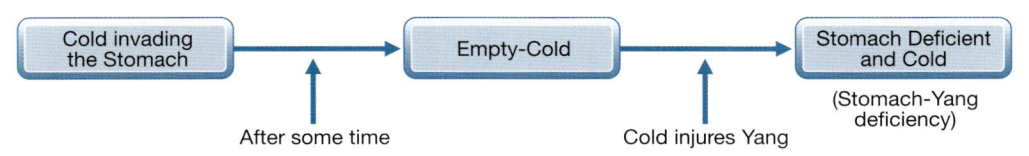

Figure 38.16 Consequences of Cold invading the Stomach

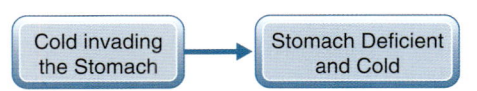

Figure 38.17 Cold invading the Stomach pattern: precursors and developments

> **Box 38.13 Cold invading the Stomach**
>
> **Clinical manifestations**
>
> Sudden severe pain in the epigastrium, a feeling of cold, cold limbs, preference for warmth, vomiting of clear fluids (which may alleviate the pain), nausea, feeling worse after swallowing cold fluids which are quickly vomited, preference for warm liquids, thick white tongue coating, Deep-Tight-Slow pulse
>
> **Treatment**
>
> ST-21 Liangmen, SP-4 Gongsun, Ren-13 Shangwan, ST-34 Liangqiu

(with Intestines and Uterus) that can be attacked by exterior Cold directly, bypassing the exterior layers of the body.

Exterior Cold blocks the Stomach and prevents Stomach-Qi from descending, hence the vomiting and the pain.

Cold impairs the Yang of the Stomach and Spleen and prevents the food essences from reaching the body, hence the feeling of cold, Slow pulse, preference for warm liquids and aggravation from cold liquids.

Please note that the above clinical manifestations describe the acute stage of an invasion of Cold in the Stomach. If the Cold is not expelled and we see the patient a few weeks or months after the initial invasion, the symptoms will be characterized by Empty-Cold: in this case, the epigastric pain is less intense, the tongue coating less thick and the pulse less Full. As Cold injures Yang, if this situation persists, the Stomach will suffer from Empty-Cold and Yang deficiency (i.e. the pattern of Stomach Deficient and Cold described above). Therefore the present pattern of Cold invading the Stomach may lead to Stomach Deficient and Cold (Fig. 38.16).

Pathological precursors of pattern

There are no pathological precursors of this pattern as this is an invasion of external Cold. However, a pre-existing Yang deficiency is often the predisposing factor (Fig. 38.17).

Pathological developments from pattern

As described above under Pathology, the pattern of Cold invading the Stomach may, after some months, lead to the pattern of Stomach Deficient and Cold because Cold injures Yang (see Fig. 38.17).

Treatment

Principle of treatment: expel Cold, warm the Stomach, stimulate the descending of Stomach-Qi.

Acupuncture

Points: ST-21 Liangmen, SP-4 Gongsun, Ren-13 Shangwan, ST-34 Liangqiu.

Method: reducing method, moxa can be used in conjunction with needling (not on its own). Even method if the condition is subacute.

Explanation
- ST-21 expels Stomach-Cold if used with moxa after needling.
- SP-4 expels Stomach-Cold, stimulates the descending of Stomach-Qi, clears obstruction from the Stomach.
- Ren-13 subdues rebellious Stomach-Qi.
- ST-34 is the Accumulation point and therefore suitable for acute and painful patterns. It will clear obstructions from the Stomach and stop pain.

Herbal formula

Liang Fu Wan *Alpinia–Cyperus Pill*.

Box 38.13 summarizes Cold invading the Stomach.

Stomach-Qi rebelling upwards

Clinical manifestations

Nausea, difficulty in swallowing, belching, vomiting, hiccups (Fig. 38.18).
Tongue: no changes.
Pulse: Tight or Wiry on the Right-Middle position.
Key symptoms: nausea, belching.

Aetiology

Diet

Eating in a hurry, working while eating, eating in a state of tension or while upset, eating standing up: all these habits lead to this pattern.

- Nausea, difficulty in swallowing, belching, vomiting, hiccup

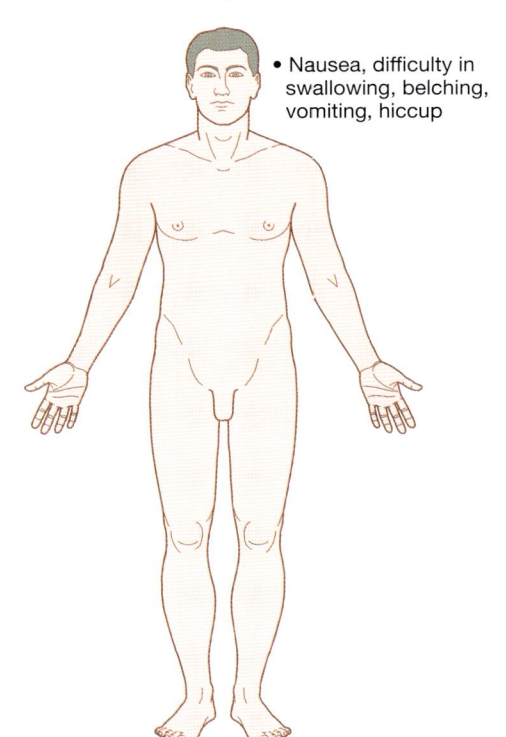

Figure 38.18 Stomach-Qi rebelling upwards

Emotional strain

Anger, frustration and resentment (the same emotions which affect the Liver) may affect the Stomach and cause Stomach-Qi to rebel upwards. They are more likely to affect the Stomach when the person also has irregular eating habits.

Pathology

This pattern is an expression of the impairment of the descending of Stomach-Qi. It is frequently not a pattern appearing on its own, but accompanying other patterns, such as Stomach-Fire, Stomach-Qi stagnation or Cold invading the Stomach.

All the symptoms are caused by the failure of Stomach-Qi to descend and rebelling upwards instead.

Pathological precursors of pattern

Practically every Stomach pattern could be a precursor of this pattern: for example, Stomach-Qi stagnation, Cold invading the Stomach, Stomach-Fire, Stomach Phlegm-Fire, etc.

Liver-Qi also has an important influence on this pattern and rebellious Liver-Qi may lead to Stomach-Qi rebelling upwards (Fig. 38.19).

Pathological developments from pattern

Stomach-Qi rebelling upwards may affect the Penetrating Vessel (*Chong Mai*) and cause rebellious Qi in the Penetrating Vessel (see Fig. 38.19).

Treatment

Principle of treatment: subdue rebellious Qi, stimulate the descending of Stomach-Qi.

Acupuncture

Points: Ren-13 Shangwan, Ren-10 Xiawan, P-6 Neiguan, SP-4 Gongsun, ST-21 Liangmen, ST-19 Burong.
Method: reducing.

Most Stomach patterns → Stomach-Qi rebelling upwards → Rebellious Qi of Chong Mai
Liver-Qi rebelling upwards →

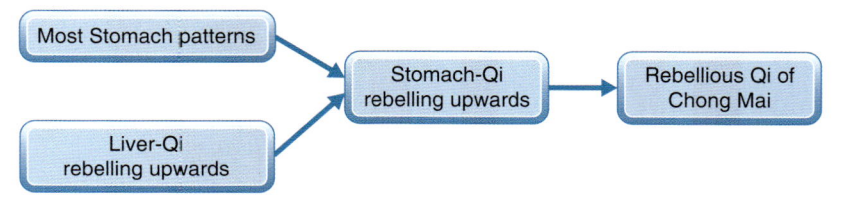

Figure 38.19 Stomach-Qi rebelling upwards pattern: precursors and developments

Explanation
- Ren-13 subdues rebellious Stomach-Qi.
- Ren-10 stimulates the descending of Stomach-Qi.
- P-6 and SP-4 stimulate the descending of Stomach-Qi.
- ST-21 and ST-19 stimulate the descending of Stomach-Qi.

Herbal formula

Ding Xiang Shi Di Tang *Caryophyllum–Diospyros Decoction*.
Huo Xiang Zheng Qi San *Agastaches Upright-Qi Powder*.
Ban Xia Hou Po Tang *Pinellia–Magnolia Decoction*.

Box 38.14 summarizes Stomach-Qi rebelling upwards.

Box 38.14 Stomach-Qi rebelling upwards

Clinical manifestations

Nausea, difficulty in swallowing, belching, vomiting, hiccups, no changes on tongue, pulse Tight or Wiry on the Right-Middle position

Treatment

Ren-13 Shangwan, Ren-10 Xiawan, P-6 Neiguan, SP-4 Gongsun, ST-21 Liangmen, ST-19 Burong

---

Damp-Heat in the Stomach

Clinical manifestations

A feeling of fullness and pain of the epigastrium, a feeling of heaviness, facial pain, blocked nose or thick sticky nasal discharge, thirst without desire to drink, nausea, a feeling of heat, dull-yellow complexion, a sticky taste (Fig. 38.20).
Tongue: Red with sticky yellow coating.
Pulse: Slippery-Rapid.
Key symptoms: epigastric fullness, a feeling of heaviness, nausea, sticky yellow coating.

Diagnostic tip

Epigastric fullness, nausea and sticky yellow coating are enough to diagnose Damp-Heat in the Stomach

Aetiology

Diet

The excessive consumption of dairy foods and greasy fried foods may lead to the formation of Damp-Heat.

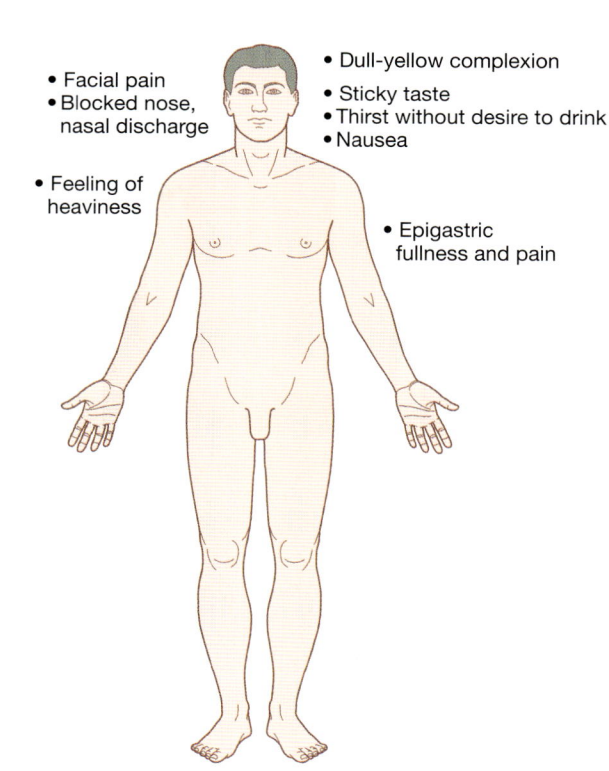

Figure 38.20 Damp-Heat in the Stomach

Greasy fried foods are especially likely to cause this pattern as greasy foods tend to create Dampness and frying makes food hotter so that it may lead to Heat.

Emotional strain

Emotional strain due to anger, frustration and resentment, which leads to Stomach-Qi stagnation, may, in time, lead to Heat as stagnant Qi often produces Heat.

Pathology

Dampness obstructs the Middle Burner and prevents the descending of Stomach-Qi: this causes nausea and a feeling of fullness of the epigastrium.

Dampness is 'sticky', hence the sticky taste and sticky tongue coating. A feeling of heaviness is caused by Dampness as this obstructs the muscles. The blocked nose and yellow nasal discharge are due to Dampness in the Stomach channel on the face. This is a common cause of chronic sinusitis.

The Heat part of Damp-Heat causes a thirst but the obstruction of the Middle Burner by Dampness makes the patient reluctant to drink: this may seem a strange symptom but patients do report it.

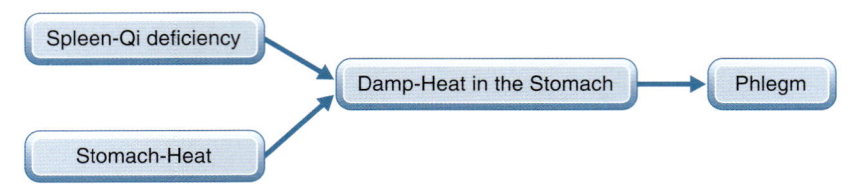

Figure 38.21 Damp-Heat in the Stomach pattern: precursors and developments

The dull-yellow complexion and Slippery pulse reflect Dampness.

> **Clinical note**
>
> Damp-Heat in the Stomach frequently causes symptoms on the face (due to Stomach channel) such as facial pain and nasal discharge (as in sinusitis)

Pathological precursors of pattern

Spleen-Qi deficiency nearly always precedes this pattern as the deficient Spleen-Qi fails to transform and transport and leads to Dampness. Stomach-Heat is also often a precursor of this pattern not only because Heat combines with Dampness but also because Heat itself may contribute to the formation of Dampness by condensing fluids (Fig. 38.21).

Pathological developments from pattern

Damp-Heat in the Stomach may give rise to Phlegm (often Phlegm-Heat) (see Fig. 38.21).

Treatment

Principle of treatment: resolve Dampness, clear Heat, restore the descending of Stomach-Qi.

Acupuncture

Points: ST-44 Neiting, ST-34 Liangqiu, ST-21 Liangmen, Ren-12 Zhongwan, Ren-13 Shangwan, L.I.-11 Quchi, L.I.-4 Hegu, Ren-11 Jianli, ST-25 Tianshu, ST-40 Fenglong, SP-9 Yinlingquan, Ren-9 Shuifen.
Method: reducing or even (if chronic), except for Ren-12, which should be reinforced. No moxa.
Explanation
- ST-44 clears Stomach-Heat.
- ST-34, Accumulation point, is used for Full conditions.
- ST-21 restores the descending of Stomach-Qi.
- Ren-12 tonifies the Spleen to resolve Dampness.
- Ren-13 subdues rebellious Stomach-Qi: this is used if the nausea is pronounced.
- L.I.-11 clears Heat.
- L.I.-4 clears Stomach-Heat and restores the descending of Stomach-Qi.
- Ren-11 clears Stomach-Heat.
- ST-25 clears Stomach-Heat.
- ST-40 restores the descending of Stomach-Qi.
- SP-9 resolves Dampness.
- Ren-9 promotes the transformation and transportation of fluids and so resolves Dampness.

Herbal formula

Lian Po Yin *Coptis–Magnolia Decoction*.

Three Treasures

Ease the Muscles (variation of Lian Po Yin).
Box 38.15 summarizes Damp-Heat in the Stomach.

Box 38.15 Damp-Heat in the Stomach

Clinical manifestations

A feeling of fullness and pain of the epigastrium, a feeling of heaviness, facial pain, blocked nose or thick sticky nasal discharge, thirst without desire to drink, nausea, a feeling of heat, dull-yellow complexion, a sticky taste, Red tongue with sticky yellow coating, Slippery-Rapid pulse

Treatment

ST-44 Neiting, ST-34 Liangqiu, ST-21 Liangmen, Ren-12 Zhongwan, Ren-13 Shangwan, L.I.-11 Quchi, L.I.-4 Hegu, Ren-11 Jianli, ST-25 Tianshu, ST-40 Fenglong, SP-9 Yinlingquan, Ren-9 Shuifen

---

Retention of Food in the Stomach

Clinical manifestations

Fullness, pain and distension of the epigastrium which are relieved by vomiting, nausea, vomiting of sour

fluids, foul breath, sour regurgitation, belching, insomnia, loose stools or constipation, poor appetite (Fig. 38.22).
Tongue: thick coating (which could be white or yellow).
Pulse: Full-Slippery.
Key symptoms: epigastric fullness, sour regurgitation, thick tongue coating.

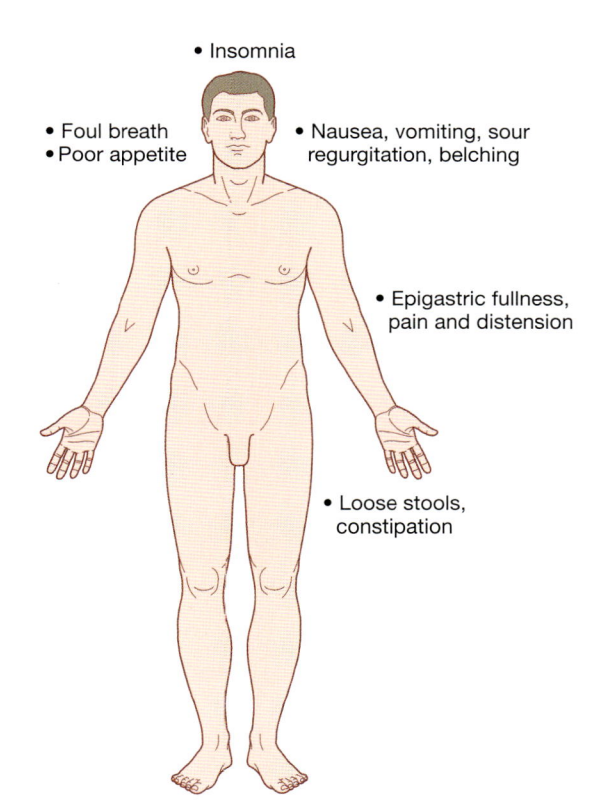

> **Diagnostic tip**
>
> Epigastric fullness, sour regurgitation and a thick tongue coating are enough to diagnose retention of Food in the Stomach

Aetiology

The main cause of this pattern is dietary. This pattern could be simply due to overeating. It can also be due to eating too quickly, or eating in a hurry or worrying while eating.

This pattern is common in babies and children as their Stomach and Spleen are inherently weak in the first years of life and food easily accumulates in the Stomach.

Pathology

This is an interior Full pattern. It could be associated either with Cold or Heat, in which case the tongue coating would be white or yellow, respectively.

Most of the symptoms are caused by the obstruction of food in the Stomach, preventing Stomach-Qi from descending, hence the nausea, vomiting, feeling of fullness, belching and sour regurgitation.

The foul breath is due to the fermentation of food in the Stomach for too long.

The prolonged retention of food in the Stomach creates an obstruction in the Middle Burner and prevents Heart-Qi from descending. This causes the Mind to be disturbed at night, resulting in insomnia.

The Slippery pulse indicates the presence of undigested food.

Pathological precursors of pattern

A deficiency of Spleen-Qi is a frequent precursor to this pattern (Fig. 38.23).

Figure 38.22 Retention of Food in the Stomach

- Insomnia
- Foul breath
- Poor appetite
- Nausea, vomiting, sour regurgitation, belching
- Epigastric fullness, pain and distension
- Loose stools, constipation

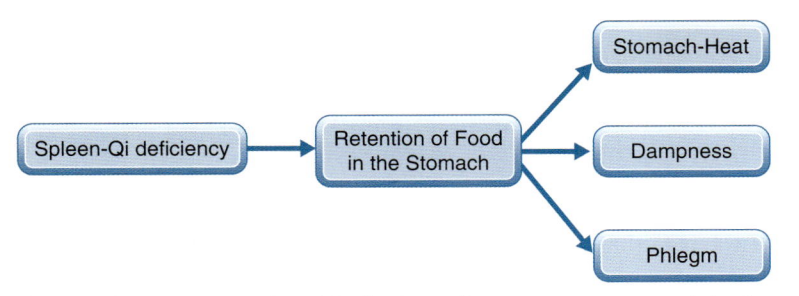

Figure 38.23 Retention of Food in the Stomach pattern: precursors and developments

Spleen-Qi deficiency → Retention of Food in the Stomach → Stomach-Heat / Dampness / Phlegm

Pathological developments from pattern

Retention of Food in the Stomach is likely to generate Heat and lead to Stomach-Heat. The undigested food, together with the impairment of the descending of Stomach-Qi may also lead to the formation of Dampness or Phlegm (see Fig. 38.23).

Treatment

Principle of treatment: resolve retention of Food, stimulate the descending of Stomach-Qi.

Acupuncture

Points: Ren-13 Shangwan, Ren-10 Xiawan, ST-21 Liangmen, ST-44 Neiting, ST-45 Lidui, SP-4 Gongsun, P-6 Neiguan, ST-40 Fenglong, ST-19 Burong, KI-21 Youmen, Ren-12 Zhongwan.
Method: reducing.
Explanation

- Ren-13 subdues rebellious Stomach-Qi.
- Ren-10 stimulates the descending of Stomach-Qi.
- ST-21 stimulates the descending of Stomach-Qi and resolves stagnant food.
- ST-44 resolves stagnant food and clears Heat.
- ST-45 resolves stagnant food and calms the Mind (if there is insomnia).
- SP-4 resolves stagnant food.
- P-6 stimulates the descending of Stomach-Qi.
- ST-40 restores the descending of Stomach-Qi.
- ST-19 and KI-21 Youmen restore the descending of Stomach-Qi. ST-19 is specific to resolve retention of Food.
- Ren-12 resolves retention of Food.

Herbal formula

Bao He Wan *Preserving and Harmonizing Pill*.
Zhi Shi Dao Zhi Wan *Citrus Eliminating Stagnation Pill*.

Box 38.16 summarizes retention of Food in the Stomach.

Stasis of Blood in the Stomach

Clinical manifestations

Severe, stabbing epigastric pain that may be worse at night, dislike of pressure, nausea, vomiting, possibly vomiting of blood, vomiting of food looking like coffee grounds (Fig. 38.24).

Tongue: Purple.
Pulse: Wiry.
Key symptoms: stabbing pain in the epigastrium, vomiting of dark blood.

Diagnostic tip

A stabbing pain in the epigastrium and a tongue that is purple in the centre are enough to diagnose stasis of Blood in the Stomach

Box 38.16 Retention of Food in the Stomach

Clinical manifestations

Fullness, pain and distension of the epigastrium which are relieved by vomiting, nausea, vomiting of sour fluids, foul breath, sour regurgitation, belching, insomnia, loose stools or constipation, poor appetite
Tongue: thick coating (which could be white or yellow)
Pulse: Full-Slippery

Treatment

Ren-13 Shangwan, Ren-10 Xiawan, ST-21 Liangmen, ST-44 Neiting, ST-45 Lidui, SP-4 Gongsun, P-6 Neiguan, ST-40 Fenglong, ST-19 Burong, KI-21 Youmen, Ren-12 Zhongwan

- Nausea, vomiting, vomiting of blood
- Stabbing epigastric pain

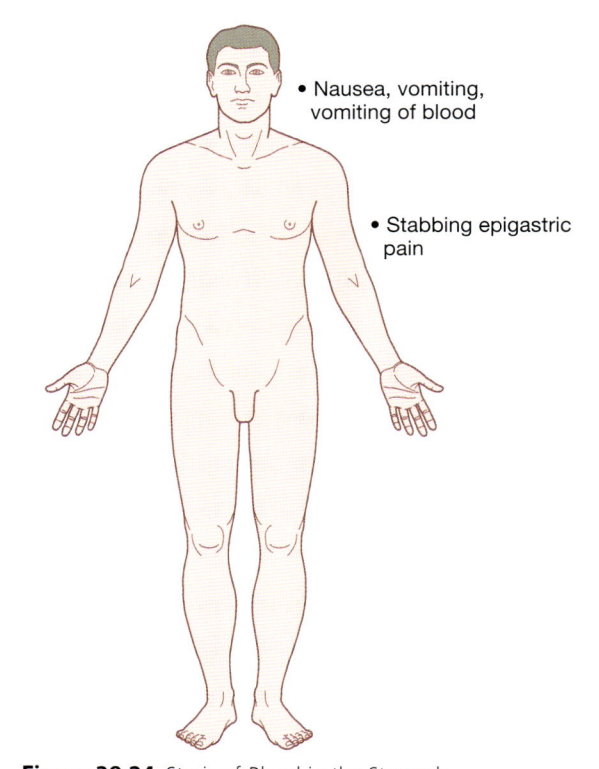

Figure 38.24 Stasis of Blood in the Stomach

Aetiology

As Blood stasis is a pathological condition that always derives from other pathological conditions, it has no specific aetiology. For example, we cannot say that such and such an emotion or diet leads to Blood stasis. Blood stasis normally derives from the three main conditions of Qi stagnation, Cold and Heat. Aetiological factors which cause these three pathological conditions are therefore *indirectly* causes of Blood stasis.

Pathology

Stasis of Blood often causes a pain of a stabbing or boring nature, hence the stabbing epigastric pain. This pain is much more intense than in any of the other Stomach patterns.

Stasis of Blood always manifests with dark-coloured blood, hence the vomiting of dark blood.

Since the Stomach is related to the Large Intestine, the stasis of Blood extends to it and is manifested with blood in the stools.

The Purple tongue reflects the stasis of Blood. Please note that the tongue may not necessarily be Purple: if a patient has clear manifestations of Blood stasis but the tongue is not Purple, it simply means that the Blood stasis is not severe.

Clinical note

Blood stasis is a very important pathology because it *potentially* gives rise to serious diseases, such as cancer, heart disease and stroke. For example, one cannot get carcinoma of the Stomach purely from Stomach-Qi stagnation, but one can from Blood stasis in the Stomach

Pathological precursors of pattern

This is always a chronic condition, resulting from various pathological conditions. In general, Blood stasis may derive from Qi stagnation, Cold or Heat. With specific reference to the Stomach, four Stomach patterns are therefore most likely to cause Blood stasis: namely, Stomach-Qi stagnation, Cold invading the Stomach, Stomach Deficient and Cold and Stomach-Heat. However, most Stomach Full patterns may lead to Blood stasis in the Stomach, for example retention of Food in the Stomach, Stomach-Qi rebelling upwards, Damp-Heat in the Stomach and Liver-Qi invading the Stomach (Fig. 38.25).

Pathological developments from pattern

Stasis of Blood in the Stomach is the consequence of other patterns and it is not therefore itself a cause of other patterns (see Fig. 38.25).

Treatment

Principle of treatment: invigorate Blood, eliminate stasis, stimulate the descending of Stomach-Qi.

Acupuncture

Points: ST-34 Liangqiu, ST-21 Liangmen, ST-19 Burong, KI-21 Youmen, T.B.-6 Zhigou, P-6 Neiguan, SP-4 Gongsun with P-6 Neiguan (opening points of the Penetrating Vessel *Chong Mai*), G.B.-34 Yanglingquan with Ren-12 Zhongwan, ST-40 Fenglong, BL-17 Geshu, SP-10 Xuehai, L.I.-4 Hegu, Ren-11 Jianli.

Method: reducing, no moxa.

Explanation
- ST-34, Accumulation point, moves Qi and Blood in the channel.
- ST-21 and ST-19 restore the descending of Stomach-Qi.
- KI-21 restores the descending of Stomach-Qi and invigorates Blood (as it is a point of the Penetrating Vessel (*Chong Mai*) which is the Sea of Blood).

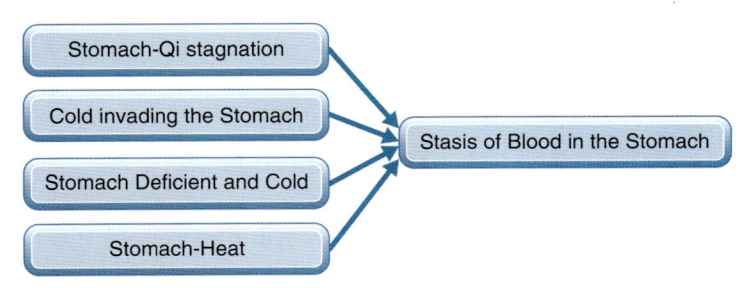

Figure 38.25 Stasis of Blood in the Stomach pattern: precursors and developments

- T.B.-6 moves Qi in the Middle Burner.
- P-6 invigorates Blood and restores the descending of Stomach-Qi.
- SP-4 and P-6 in combination open the Penetrating Vessel (*Chong Mai*), invigorate Blood and restore the descending of Stomach-Qi.
- G.B.-34 with Ren-12 moves Qi in the Middle Burner.
- ST-40 restores the descending of Stomach-Qi.
- BL-17 and SP-10 invigorate Blood.
- L.I.-4 restores the descending of Stomach-Qi.
- Ren-11 restores the descending of Stomach-Qi.

Herbal formula

Shi Xiao San *Breaking into a Smile Powder*.
Dan Shen Yin *Salvia Decoction*.
Ge Xia Zhu Yu Tang *Eliminating Stasis below the Diaphragm Decoction*.
Tong You Tang *Penetrating the Depth Decoction*.

Three Treasures

Red Stirring (variation of Xue Fu Zhu Yu Tang).

Box 38.17 summarizes stasis of Blood in the Stomach.

Box 38.17 Stasis of Blood in the Stomach

Clinical manifestations

Severe, stabbing epigastric pain that may be worse at night, dislike of pressure, nausea, vomiting, possibly vomiting of blood, vomiting of food looking like coffee grounds, Purple tongue, Wiry pulse

Treatment

ST-34 Liangqiu, ST-21 Liangmen, ST-19 Burong, KI-21 Youmen, T.B.-6 Zhigou, P-6 Neiguan, SP-4 Gongsun with P-6 Neiguan (opening points of the Penetrating Vessel), G.B.-34 Yanglingquan with Ren-12 Zhongwan, ST-40 Fenglong, BL-17 Geshu, SP-10 Xuehai, L.I.-4 Hegu, Ren-11 Jianli

---

COMBINED PATTERNS

Stomach- and Spleen-Qi deficiency

Clinical manifestations

Poor appetite, slight abdominal distension after eating, tiredness, lassitude, pale complexion, weakness of the limbs, loose stools, uncomfortable feeling in the epigastrium, lack of taste sensation (Fig. 38.26).

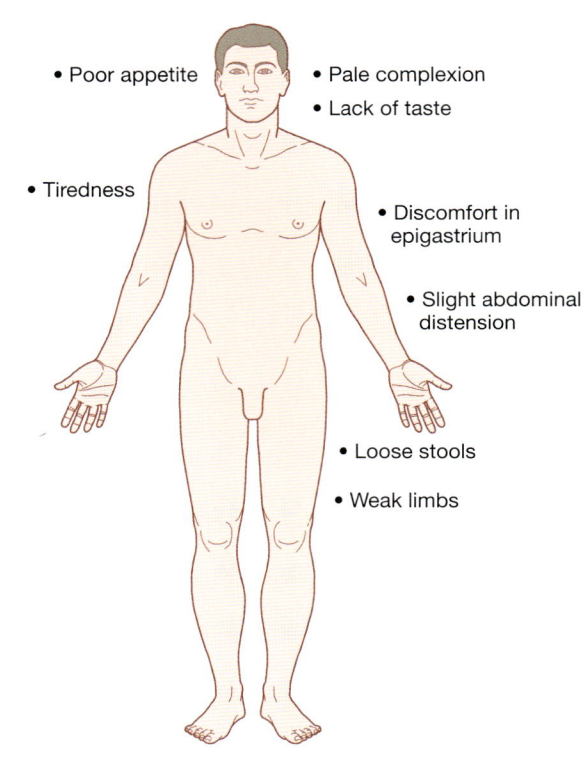

Figure 38.26 Stomach- and Spleen-Qi deficiency

Tongue: Pale.
Pulse: Empty, especially on the Right-Middle position.
Key symptoms: poor appetite, epigastric discomfort, tiredness.

Diagnostic tip

Poor appetite, epigastric discomfort and tiredness are enough to diagnose Stomach- and Spleen-Qi deficiency

Aetiology

The aetiology of this pattern is the same as that for Spleen-Qi deficiency and Stomach-Qi deficiency: that is, primarily dietary.

Pathology

The pathology of this pattern has already been explained in the relevant patterns of Spleen-Qi deficiency and Stomach-Qi deficiency.

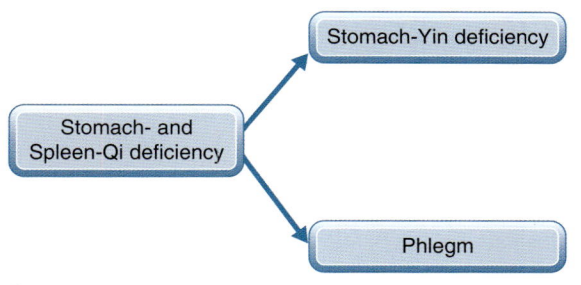

Figure 38.27 Stomach- and Spleen-Qi deficiency pattern: precursors and developments

Clinical note

The simultaneous deficiency of Stomach- and Spleen-Qi is extremely common in practice

Pathological precursors of pattern

There is no pathological precursor of this pattern as this pattern itself is often at the root of other patterns.

A simultaneous Qi deficiency of both Stomach and Spleen is very common (Fig. 38.27).

Pathological developments from pattern

A Qi deficiency of both Stomach and Spleen may give rise to a Yin deficiency of one or both these organs.

This pattern may also lead to the formation of Dampness or Phlegm (see Fig. 38.27).

Treatment

Principle of treatment: tonify Stomach- and Spleen-Qi.

Acupuncture

Points: Ren-12 Zhongwan, ST-36 Zusanli, SP-3 Taibai, SP-6 Sanyinjiao, BL-20 Pishu, BL-21 Weishu, Ren-6 Qihai.
Method: reinforcing. Moxa is applicable.
Explanation
- Ren-12, ST-36, SP-3 and SP-6 tonify the Stomach and Spleen.
- BL-20 tonifies the Spleen, especially indicated in chronic conditions.
- BL-21 tonifies the Stomach, especially indicated in chronic conditions.
- Ren-6 tonifies Qi in general.

Herbal formula

Si Jun Zi Tang *Four Gentlemen Decoction*.
Shen Ling Bai Zhu San *Ginseng–Poria–Atractylodes Powder*.

Three Treasures

Prosperous Earth (variation of Liu Jun Zi Tang).
Central Mansion (variation of Shen Ling Bai Zhu Tang).

Box 38.18 summarizes Stomach- and Spleen-Qi deficiency.

Box 38.18 Stomach- and Spleen-Qi deficiency

Clinical manifestations

Poor appetite, slight abdominal distension after eating, tiredness, lassitude, pale complexion, weakness of the limbs, loose stools, uncomfortable feeling in the epigastrium, lack of taste sensation, Pale tongue, Empty pulse, especially on the Right-Middle position

Treatment

Ren-12 Zhongwan, ST-36 Zusanli, SP-3 Taibai, SP-6 Sanyinjiao, BL-20 Pishu, BL-21 Weishu, Ren-6 Qihai

---

Stomach- and Spleen-Yin deficiency

Clinical manifestations

Poor appetite, dry mouth, thirst with desire to drink in small sips, dry stools, dry lips, slight nausea, tiredness, uncomfortable feeling in the epigastrium, lack of taste sensation (Fig. 38.28).
Tongue: without coating.
Pulse: Floating-Empty, especially on the Right-Middle position.
Key symptoms: dry mouth, dry lips, epigastric discomfort, tiredness.

Diagnostic tip

Dry mouth, dry lips, epigastric discomfort and a tongue without coating are enough to diagnose Stomach- and Spleen-Yin deficiency

Aetiology

The aetiology of this pattern is the same as that for Spleen-Qi deficiency and Stomach-Qi deficiency: that is, primarily dietary. It particularly derives from eating while working, eating late at night, eating in a hurry, etc.

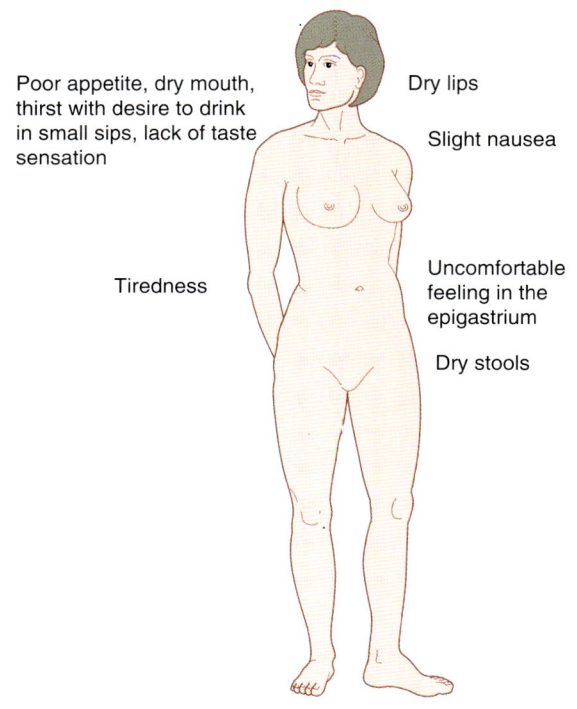

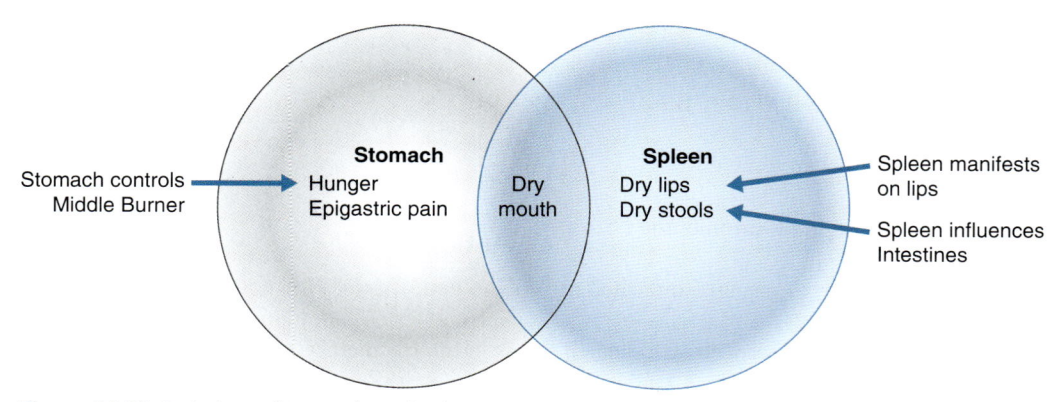

Pathology

Stomach- and Spleen-Yin deficiency usually derive from Stomach- and Spleen-Qi deficiency. As the Stomach is the source of Yin, it causes a dry mouth and a thirst: the desire to drink in small sips is typical of Yin deficiency. The dry lips are a very distinctive sign of Spleen-Yin deficiency. As the Spleen affects the Intestines, the stools are dry (Fig. 38.29).

Clinical note

The simultaneous deficiency of Stomach- and Spleen-Yin is extremely common in practice

Pathological precursors of pattern

This pattern practically always derives from Stomach- and Spleen-Qi deficiency (Fig. 38.30).

Pathological developments from pattern

Stomach-Yin deficiency often leads to Kidney-Yin deficiency (see Fig. 38.30).

Treatment

Principle of treatment: tonify Stomach- and Spleen-Yin.

Acupuncture

Points: Ren-12 Zhongwan, ST-36 Zusanli, SP-6 Sanyinjiao.
Method: reinforcing. Moxa.
Explanation
– Ren-12, ST-36 and SP-6 tonify the Yin of Stomach and Spleen.

Herbal formula

Shen Ling Bai Zhu San *Ginseng–Poria–Atractylodes Powder*.

Box 38.19 summarizes Stomach- and Spleen-Yin deficiency.

The combined pattern of Liver-Qi invading the Stomach is discussed in chapter 34 under the Liver patterns.

Figure 38.28 Stomach- and Spleen-Yin deficiency

Figure 38.29 Pathology of Stomach- and Spleen-Yin deficiency

```
Stomach- and Spleen-    →    Stomach- and Spleen-    →    Kidney-Yin
Qi deficiency                Yin deficiency               deficiency
```

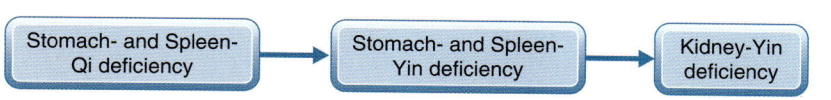

Figure 38.30 Stomach- and Spleen-Yin deficiency pattern: precursors and developments

Box 38.19 Stomach- and Spleen-Yin deficiency

Clinical manifestations

Poor appetite, dry mouth, thirst with desire to drink in small sips, dry stools, dry lips, slight nausea, tiredness, uncomfortable feeling in the epigastrium, lack of taste sensation
Tongue: without coating
Pulse: Floating-Empty, especially on the Right-Middle position

Treatment

Ren-12 Zhongwan, ST-36 Zusanli, SP-6 Sanyinjiao

Learning outcomes

In this chapter you will have learned:

- The importance of the Stomach, both in terms of its central position in the Middle Burner, and its role as the Root of Post-Heaven Qi
- The significance of Stomach-Qi in prognosis, and how it manifests on tongue and pulse
- The historical importance attributed to the Stomach by Li Dong Yuan and his 'School of Stomach and Spleen'
- The role of diet as the main cause of Stomach pathology, in particular the type of food eaten, regularity of eating, and the conditions of eating
- How emotional strain and exterior Cold can affect the Stomach and lead to disease
- How to identify the following Deficiency patterns:
  Stomach-Qi deficiency: tiredness in the morning, uncomfortable feeling in epigastrium and a Weak Stomach pulse
  Stomach Deficient and Cold: discomfort in the epigastrium which is better after eating, tiredness and cold limbs
  Stomach-Yin deficiency: dull epigastric pain, dry mouth, tongue without coat or with rootless coating in the centre
- How to identify the following Full patterns:
  Stomach-Qi stagnation: epigastric distention, belching and irritability
  Stomach-Heat (or Phlegm-Heat): burning sensation in the epigastrium, thirst with desire to drink cold liquids and a Red tongue with a thick yellow coating (Phlegm-Heat also has mental derangement, mucus in stools and expectoration of phlegm and a sticky yellow tongue coating)

  Cold Invading the Stomach: sudden pain in the epigastrium, vomiting, Deep-Tight pulse
  Stomach-Qi rebelling upwards: nausea, belching and hiccup
  Damp-Heat in the Stomach: epigastric fullness, nausea, and a sticky yellow tongue coating
  Retention of Food in the Stomach: epigastric fullness, sour regurgitation, thick tongue coating
  Stasis of Blood in the Stomach: stabbing pain in epigastrium and tongue with purple centre
- How to identify the following combined patterns:
  Stomach- and Spleen-Qi deficiency: poor appetite, epigastric discomfort and tiredness

Self-assessment questions

1. What is the main function of the Stomach?
2. Why is the position of the Stomach so important?
3. What is the pathology of tiredness, when Stomach-Qi is deficient?
4. How is the Stomach-Qi manifested in the tongue and the pulse?
5. What sort of foods is the Stomach said to prefer?
6. Why is it important to eat at regular times?
7. What is the main symptom of Stomach-Qi deficiency?
8. Why might a bowel movement aggravate epigastric discomfort in the pattern Stomach Deficient and Cold?
9. What would the tongue look like in the pattern Stomach-Yin deficiency?
10. Which two aetiological factors combine to cause the pattern Stomach-Qi stagnation?
11. What is the pathology of nausea and vomiting in Stomach-Heat?
12. What will happen to an invasion of Cold in the Stomach if it is not treated?
13. Why is there often facial pain and sinusitis presenting with the pattern Damp-Heat in the Stomach.
14. A patient presents with the pattern retention of Food in the Stomach, and is unable to sleep. Explain the pathology of the insomnia.
15. Why is it so important that Blood stasis in the Stomach is properly treated?

See p. 1264 for answers

Small Intestine Patterns

Key contents

General aetiology
Diet
Emotional strain

Full patterns
Full-Heat in the Small Intestine
Small Intestine-Qi pain
Small Intestine-Qi tied
Infestation of worms in the Small Intestine

Empty pattern
Small Intestine Deficient and Cold

- General aetiology
  - Diet
  - Emotional strain
    - Sadness
    - Worry
    - Anger

The functions of the Small Intestine are (ch. 14):

- It controls receiving and transforming
- It separates fluids

The main function of the Small Intestine is that of receiving and transforming food by separating the clean from the dirty part. It also has an important function in relation to movement of fluids as it separates clean from dirty fluids. To carry out this function in relation to fluids, the Small Intestine is in direct communication with the Bladder, helping the Bladder function of Qi transformation.

The Small Intestine transforms food in coordination with the Spleen, whilst it transforms fluids in coordination with the Bladder- and Kidney-Yang. In both cases, the Small Intestine's role is subordinate to that of the Spleen- and Kidney-Yang. For this reason, most of the Small Intestine patterns are different manifestations of Spleen- or Kidney-Yang patterns.

Before discussing the patterns, I shall discuss the general aetiology of Small Intestine patterns as follows:

GENERAL AETIOLOGY

Diet

The Small Intestine is easily and readily affected by the type and energy of food eaten. An excessive consumption of cold and raw foods can create Cold in the Small Intestine, whilst an excessive consumption of hot foods can create Heat.

Emotional strain

The Small Intestine is affected by the same emotional stress that affects the Spleen and Liver. The Small Intestine may be affected by sadness that grips a person and destroys the mental clarity and capacity of sound judgement for which this organ is responsible.

Worry also affects the Small Intestine, leading to Qi stagnation in this organ. Anger, frustration and resentment also cause Qi stagnation in the Small Intestine.

Box 39.1 summarizes the general aetiology of Small Intestine patterns.

The patterns discussed are:

FULL PATTERNS
- Full-Heat in the Small Intestine
- Small Intestine-Qi pain
- Small Intestine-Qi tied
- Infestation of worms in the Small Intestine

EMPTY PATTERN
- Small Intestine Deficient and Cold

In order to understand the pathology of the Small Intestine, it is important to distinguish its channel from

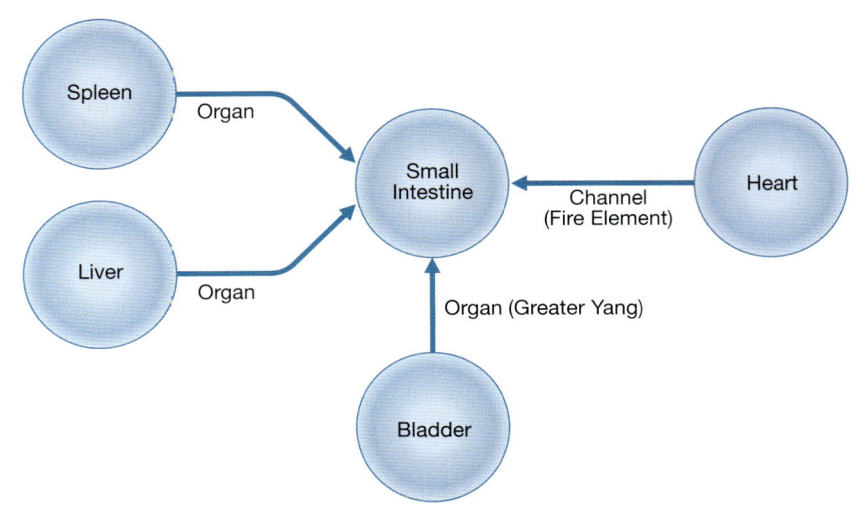

Figure 39.1 Small Intestine's connections with other organs

Box 39.1 General aetiology of Small Intestine patterns

- Diet
- Emotional strain
  - Sadness
  - Worry
  - Anger

Box 39.2 A 'feel' for Small Intestine pathology

- Bowel problems
- Borborygmi
- Issues with mental clarity and discrimination

---

its organ associations with other organs. In other words, some of its patterns can be explained in the light of a channel connection and others in the light of an organ connection with a particular organ. For example, its relationship with the Heart is based on a channel relationship: the pattern of Full-Heat in the Small Intestine presents some symptoms of Heart-Fire such as tongue ulcers and insomnia (due to the channel connection between Heart and Small Intestine) but not palpitations (Heart organ). The Small Intestine and Heart are related as a Yang–Yin pair within the Fire Element, but this connection can be observed more on a channel, rather than an organ level.

On the other hand, the Small Intestine as an organ has an organ relationship with the Spleen, Liver and Bladder. For this reason, some of the Small Intestine symptoms are related to the Spleen (loose stools), some to the Liver (abdominal distension and pain) and some to the Bladder (urinary symptoms) (Fig. 39.1).

Box 39.2 lists the factors that give a 'feel' for Small Intestine pathology.

FULL PATTERNS

Full-Heat in the Small Intestine

Clinical manifestations

Mental restlessness, insomnia, tongue and/or mouth ulcers, pain in the throat, deafness, uncomfortable feeling and heat sensation in the chest, abdominal pain, thirst with desire to drink cold liquids, scanty and dark urine, burning pain on urination, blood in urine (Fig. 39.2).

Tongue: Red with redder and swollen tip, yellow coating.
Pulse: Overflowing-Rapid, especially in the Front position. If there are urinary symptoms the pulse would be Wiry on the Left-Rear position.
Key symptoms: abdominal pain, tongue ulcer, scanty, dark and painful urination.

> **Diagnostic tip**
>
> Abdominal pain, tongue ulcers and scanty, dark painful urination are enough to diagnose Full-Heat in the Small Intestine

- Mental restlessness, insomnia
- Tongue/mouth ulcers, thirst
- Deafness
- Pain in the throat
- Discomfort and heat in the chest
- Abdominal pain
- Scanty-dark urine, pain on urination, blood in urine

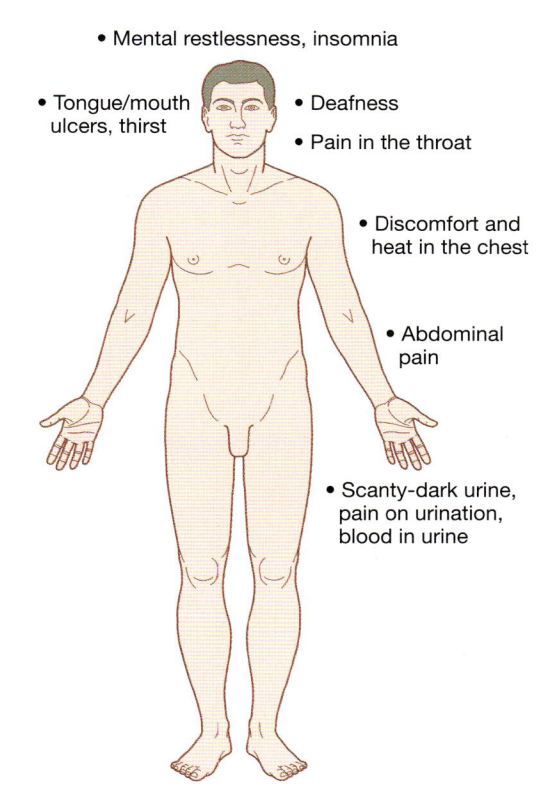

Figure 39.2 Full-Heat in the Small Intestine

Heart-Fire → Full-Heat in the Small Intestine → Heart-Fire

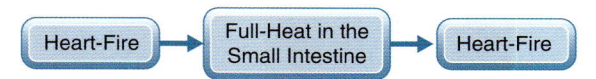

Figure 39.3 Full-Heat in the Small Intestine pattern: precursors and developments

transmitted to the Small Intestine to which the Heart is interiorly– exteriorly related. It interferes with the Small Intestine function of separating fluids in the Lower Burner and burns the fluids, causing scanty and dark urine and pain on urination. In severe cases of Heat, this may cause blood to extravasate, resulting in blood in the urine.

Deafness is caused by obstruction of Fire in the Small Intestine channel (which enters the ear).

The tongue reflects Full-Heat as it is Red with a coating; the tip may be redder and swollen, reflecting Heart-Fire. The pulse is Rapid and Overflowing because of the Heat.

Pathological precursors of pattern

Heart-Fire may lead to Full-Heat in the Small Intestine as the Heart and Small Intestine are related within the Fire Element (Fig. 39.3).

Pathological developments from pattern

Full-Heat in the Small Intestine may lead to Heart-Fire (see Fig 39.3).

Treatment

Principle of treatment: drain Heart-Fire and Small Intestine-Fire.

Acupuncture

Points: S.I.-2 Qiangu, S.I.-5 Yanggu, HE-5 Tongli, HE-8 Shaofu, ST-39 Xiajuxu.

Method: reducing, no moxa.

Explanation
- S.I.-2 clears Small Intestine-Heat
- S.I.-5 also clears Heat in the Small Intestine and it calms the Mind. This point is also very effective in helping the person to gain clarity and to discriminate among choices. It affects the tongue and is used if there are tongue ulcers.
- HE-5 and HE-8 drain Heart-Fire.
- ST-39 is the Lower Sea point for the Small Intestine and it stops abdominal pain.

Aetiology

Diet

The excessive consumption of hot foods (meat, spices, alcohol) can lead to Full-Heat in the Small Intestine. In this case, Heat in the Small Intestine is usually associated with Stomach-Heat.

Emotional strain

Emotional strain resulting from anger, frustration, resentment and worry can all lead to Heat in the Small Intestine. In this case, Heat in the Small Intestine is associated with Heat in the Heart at the channel level, as explained above.

Pathology

This pattern is closely associated with blazing of Heart-Fire and from the Eight-Principle point of view it is a pattern of interior Full-Heat.

Fire in the Heart causes mental restlessness, tongue ulcers, pain in the throat and thirst. Heart-Fire is

Herbal formula

Dao Chi San *Eliminating Redness Powder.*
Dao Chi Qing Xin Tang *Eliminating Redness and Clearing the Heart Decoction.*

Box 39.3 summarizes Full-Heat in the Small Intestine.

Box 39.3 Full-Heat in the Small Intestine

Clinical manifestations

Mental restlessness, insomnia, tongue and/or mouth ulcers, pain in the throat, deafness, uncomfortable feeling and heat sensation in the chest, abdominal pain, thirst with desire to drink cold liquids, scanty and dark urine, burning pain on urination, blood in urine, Red tongue with redder and swollen tip, yellow coating, Overflowing-Rapid pulse especially in the Front position

Treatment

S.I.-2 Qiangu, S.I.-5 Yanggu, HE-5 Tongli, HE-8 Shaofu, ST-39 Xiajuxu

---

Small Intestine-Qi pain

Clinical manifestations

Lower abdominal twisting pain, which may extend to the back, abdominal distension, dislike of pressure on the abdomen, borborygmi, flatulence, abdominal pain relieved by emission of wind, pain in the testis (Fig. 39.4).
Tongue: white coating.
Pulse: Deep-Wiry, especially on the Rear positions.
Key symptoms: lower abdominal twisting pain, borborygmi, Deep-Wiry pulse.

> **Diagnostic tip**
>
> Even just abdominal twisting pain is enough to diagnose Small Intestine-Qi pain

Aetiology

Diet

This pattern can be caused by excessive consumption of cold and raw foods which interferes with the Small Intestine transformation function.

Emotional strain

This pattern can be caused by any factors which induce Liver-Qi stagnation: that is, anger, frustration and resentment.

- Abdominal pain and distension, borborygmi, flatulence
- Pain in testis

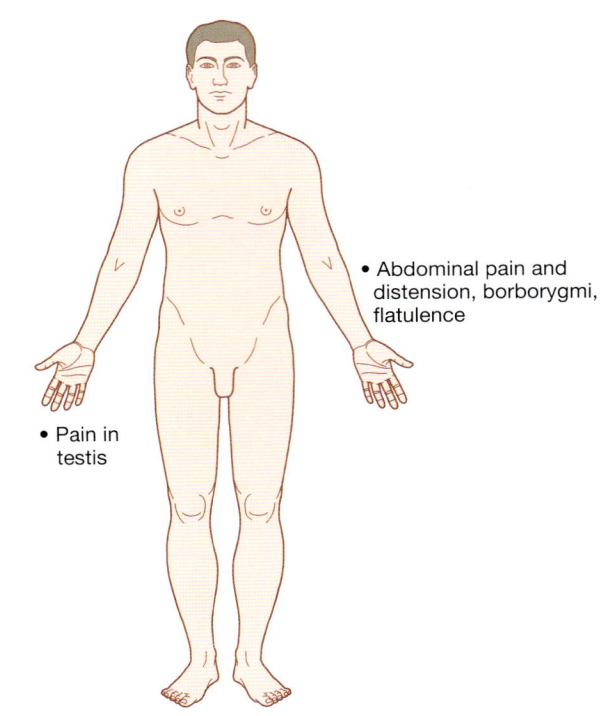

Figure 39.4 Small Intestine-Qi pain

Pathology

This is due to stagnation of Qi in the Small Intestine, and is usually associated with stagnation of Liver-Qi invading the Spleen. It can be an acute or chronic condition. If it is acute, it is a totally Full condition; if it is chronic, it is an Full/Empty condition characterized by Excess of Liver-Qi (stagnation) and Deficiency of Spleen-Qi.

All the symptoms and signs are due to stagnation of Qi in the Small Intestine and Liver, preventing the smooth flow of Liver-Qi and the transformation of fluids by the Small Intestine. Stagnation of Qi causes a distending pain, hence the twisting abdominal pain with distension. The person dislikes pressure on the abdomen as this aggravates the obstruction from stagnation of Qi.

The Deep and Wiry pulse reflects the obstruction of Qi in the Interior.

Pathological precursors of pattern

Liver-Qi stagnation is the most common precursor of this pattern (Fig. 39.5).

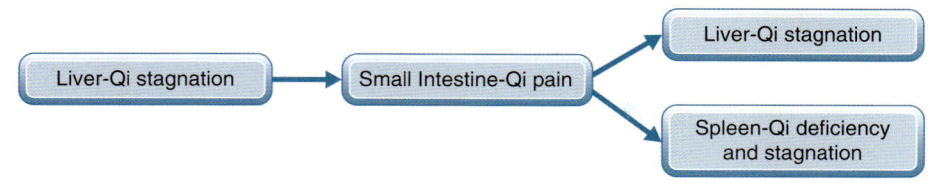

Figure 39.5 Small Intestine-Qi pain pattern: precursors and developments

Pathological developments from pattern

Stagnation of Qi may give rise to Liver-Qi stagnation (if it does not derive from it). Stagnation of Qi in the Small Intestine will also affect the Spleen, leading to both Qi stagnation and Qi deficiency of the Spleen (see Fig. 39.5).

Treatment

Principle of treatment: move Small Intestine-Qi, promote the smooth flow of Liver-Qi.

Acupuncture

Points: Ren-6 Qihai, G.B.-34 Yanglingquan, LIV-13 Zhangmen, ST-27 Daju, ST-29 Guilai, SP-6 Sanyinjiao, LIV-3 Taichong, ST-39 Xiajuxu.

Method: reducing, moxa can be used if there are some Cold signs.

Explanation
- Ren-6 in combination with G.B.-34 moves Qi in the Lower Burner and relieves pain.
- LIV-13 harmonizes the Liver and Spleen. This point would be used particularly in chronic patterns.
- ST-27 and ST-29 move Qi in the lower abdomen, stimulate the Small Intestine functions and stop abdominal pain.
- SP-6 stops abdominal pain.
- LIV-3 relieves stagnation of Liver-Qi
- ST-39 is the Lower Sea point of the Small Intestine and is specific to stop abdominal pain.

Herbal formula

Chai Hu Shu Gan Tang *Bupleurum Soothing the Liver Decoction*.

Box 39.4 summarizes Small Intestine-Qi pain.

Box 39.4   Small Intestine-Qi pain

Clinical manifestations

Lower abdominal twisting pain which may extend to back, abdominal distension, dislike of pressure on abdomen, borborygmi, flatulence, abdominal pain relieved by emission of wind, pain in the testis, white tongue coating. Deep-Wiry pulse, especially on the Rear positions

Treatment

Ren-6 Qihai, G.B.-34 Yanglingquan, LIV-13 Zhangmen, ST-27 Daju, ST-29 Guilai, SP-6 Sanyinjiao, LIV-3 Taichong, ST-39 Xiajuxu

---

Small Intestine-Qi Tied

Clinical manifestations

Severe abdominal pain, dislike of pressure, abdominal distension, constipation, vomiting, borborygmi, flatulence (Fig. 39.6).

- Severe abdominal pain, dislike of pressure, abdominal distension, constipation, vomiting, borborygmi, flatulence

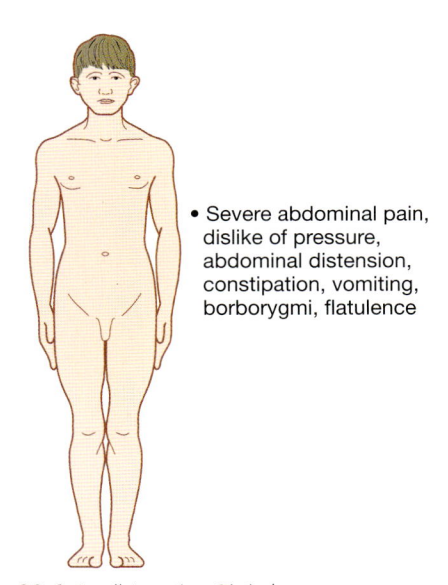

Figure 39.6 Small Intestine-Qi tied

Tongue: thick white coating.
Pulse: Deep, Wiry.
Key symptoms: sudden severe abdominal pain, constipation, vomiting, Deep-Wiry pulse.

> **Diagnostic tip**
>
> Sudden severe abdominal pain, constipation, vomiting and a Deep-Wiry pulse are enough to diagnose Small Intestine-Qi tied

Aetiology

This pattern can be caused by excessive consumption of cold and raw foods which completely blocks the transformation function of the Small Intestine.

Pathology

This pattern is very similar to the previous one and it differs in so far as it is always an acute pattern. It is characterized by obstruction and severe stagnation in the Small Intestine, hence the sudden, severe pain and constipation.

The obstruction in the Small Intestine is such that it interferes with the descending of Stomach-Qi and causes vomiting.

From a Western point of view, it resembles an acute attack of appendicitis. However, it can occur without appendicitis.

Pathological precursors of pattern

Liver-Qi stagnation and Cold in the Intestines may be precursors of this pattern (Fig. 39.7).

Pathological developments from pattern

This pattern may lead to Liver-Qi stagnation (see Fig. 39.7).

Treatment

Principle of treatment: remove obstruction from the Lower Burner, move Qi of Small Intestine.

Acupuncture

Points: ST-39 Xiajuxu, Lanweixue extra point, Ren-6 Qihai, G.B.-34 Yanglingquan, ST-25 Tianshu, SP-6 Sanyinjiao, LIV-3 Taichong.
Method: reducing, electrical stimulation is applicable.
Explanation
- ST-39 stops abdominal pain and moves Small Intestine-Qi.
- Lanweixue is in between Shangjuxu ST-37 and Zusanli ST-36 and corresponds to the appendix. This point is therefore used if it is tender (one selects the most tender spot between ST-36 and ST-37) and appendicitis is suspected.
- Ren-6 and G.B.-34 stop abdominal pain.
- ST-25 stops abdominal pain.
- SP-6 stops abdominal pain.
- LIV-3 stops abdominal pain and spasms and promotes the smooth flow of Liver-Qi.

Herbal formula

Zhi Shi Dao Zhi Wan *Citrus Eliminating Stagnation Pill*.
Tian Tai Wu Yao San *Top-Quality Lindera Powder*.

Box 39.5 summarizes Small Intestine-Qi tied.

Box 39.5 Small Intestine-Qi tied

Clinical manifestations

Severe abdominal pain, dislike of pressure, abdominal distension, constipation, vomiting, borborygmi, flatulence, thick white tongue coating, Deep-Wiry pulse

Treatment

ST-39 Xiajuxu, Lanweixue extra point, Ren-6 Qihai, G.B.-34 Yanglingquan, ST-25 Tianshu, SP-6 Sanyinjiao, LIV-3 Taichong

---

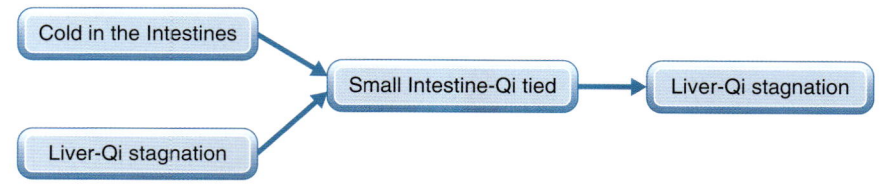

Figure 39.7 Small Intestine-Qi tied pattern: precursors and developments

Infestation of worms in the Small Intestine

Clinical manifestations

(Fig. 39.8)

Abdominal pain and distension, bad taste in mouth, sallow complexion.

Roundworms (ascarid): abdominal pain, vomiting of round worms, cold limbs.
Hookworms: desire to eat strange objects such as soil, wax, uncooked rice or tea leaves.
Pinworms: itchy anus, worse in the evening.
Tapeworms: constant hunger.

Aetiology

The aetiology of this pattern is obviously an external invasion of worms due to the consumption of unclean food.

Pathology

This obviously consists of obstruction of the Small Intestine by worms, which causes abdominal pain, and in the malnourishment following from worm infestation. According to Chinese medicine, infestation by worms is thought to be caused by a Cold condition of the Spleen and Intestines, which allows the worms to thrive.

Pathological precursors of pattern

A Cold condition of Spleen and Intestines deriving from excessive consumption of cold and raw foods is often the precursor of this pattern or, rather, the background that favours the invasion of worms (Fig. 39.9).

Pathological developments from pattern

This pattern may easily lead to deficiency of Spleen-Qi (see Fig. 39.9).

Treatment

Acupuncture is not applicable in this case and herbal treatment is the treatment of choice.

Herbal formula

Li Zhong An Hui Tang *Regulating the Centre and Calming Roundworms Decoction*.
Lian Mei An Hui Tang *Picrorhiza–Mume Calming Roundworms Decoction*.
Hua Chong Wan *Dissolving Parasites Pill*.
Qu Tiao Tang *Expelling Tapeworms Decoction*.

Box 39.6 summarizes infestation of worms in the Small Intestine.

Box 39.6 Infestation of worms in the Small Intestine

Clinical manifestations

Abdominal pain and distension, bad taste in mouth, sallow complexion
Roundworms (ascarid): abdominal pain, vomiting of roundworms, cold limbs
Hookworms: desire to eat strange objects such as soil, wax, uncooked rice or tea leaves
Pinworms: itchy anus, worse in the evening
Tapeworms: constant hunger

Treatment

Herbal formulae:
Li Zhong An Hui Tang *Regulating the Centre and Calming Roundworms Decoction*
Lian Mei An Hui Tang *Picrorhiza–Mume Calming Roundworms Decoction*
Hua Chong Wan *Dissolving Parasites Pill*
Qu Tiao Tang *Expelling Tapeworms Decoction*

Figure 39.8 Infestation of worms in the Small Intestine

- Desire to eat strange objects
- Hunger
- Vomiting of round worms
- Abdominal pain
- Itchy anus
- Cold limbs

Cold in the Intestines → Infestation of worms in the Small Intestine → Spleen-Qi deficiency

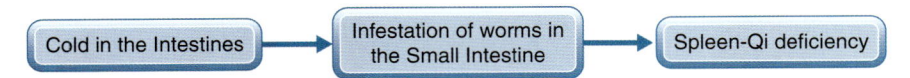

Figure 39.9 Infestation of worms in the Small Intestine pattern: precursors and developments

EMPTY PATTERN

Small Intestine Deficient and Cold

Clinical manifestations

Dull abdominal pain alleviated by pressure, desire for hot drinks, borborygmi, diarrhoea, pale and abundant urination, cold limbs (Fig. 39.10).
Tongue: Pale body, white coating.
Pulse: Deep-Weak-Slow.
Key symptoms: dull abdominal pain, borborygmi, diarrhoea.

> **Diagnostic tip**
>
> Dull abdominal pain, borborygmi and diarrhoea are enough to diagnose Small Intestine Deficient and Cold

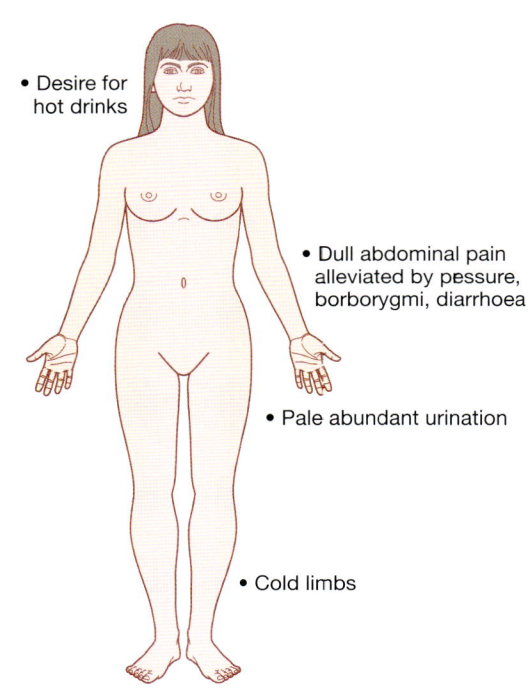

Figure 39.10 Small Intestine Deficient and Cold

Aetiology

The most important aetiological factor is dietary and it consists in the excessive consumption of cold and raw foods.

Pathology

From the Nine-Principle point of view, this is an interior pattern of Deficiency and Cold. It is usually associated with deficiency of Spleen-Yang, and it is often hard to distinguish these two patterns. The main symptom of Small Intestine involvement is borborygmi.

All the other symptoms are due to the presence of Empty-Cold in the Small Intestine, which impairs the separation of food and fluids, resulting in diarrhoea. Cold obstructs the Intestines and causes pain.

Pathological precursors of pattern

Deficiency of Spleen-Yang is nearly always the pathological precursor of this pattern (Fig. 39.11).

Pathological developments from pattern

Although this pattern may derive from a deficiency of Spleen-Yang, it may equally lead to Spleen-Yang deficiency. A long-term condition of Deficiency and Cold in the Small Intestine may also lead to Kidney-Yang deficiency (see Fig. 39.11).

Treatment

Principle of treatment: expel Cold, warm the Intestines, tonify Spleen-Yang.

Acupuncture

Points: Ren-6 Qihai, ST-25 Tianshu, ST-39 Xiajuxu, ST-36 Zusanli, BL-20 Pishu, BL-27 Xiaochangshu.
Method: reinforcing, moxa is applicable.
Explanation
 – Ren-6 with moxa cones on ginger is specific for Empty-Cold in the Intestines.
 – ST-25 stops diarrhoea and alleviates abdominal pain.

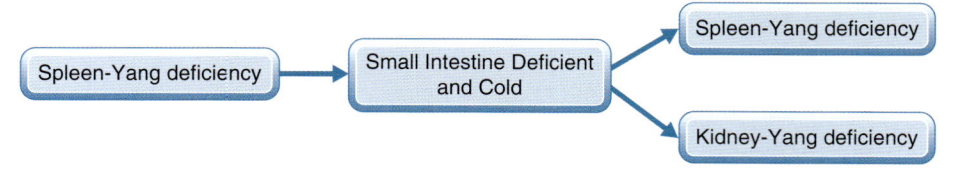

Figure 39.11 Small Intestine Deficient and Cold pattern: precursors and developments

- ST-39, Lower He-Sea point of the Small Intestine, is specific to stop abdominal pain.
- ST-36 with moxa tonifies Yang and expels Cold.
- BL-20 tonifies Spleen-Yang.
- BL-27 is the Back-Transporting point of the Small Intestine and it expels Cold from this organ.

Herbal formula

Xiao Jian Zhong Tang *Small Strengthening the Centre Decoction.*

Shen Ling Bai Zhu San *Ginseng–Poria–Atractylodes Powder.*

Box 39.7 summarizes Small Intestine Deficient and Cold.

Box 39.7 Small Intestine Deficient and Cold

Clinical manifestations

Dull abdominal pain alleviated by pressure, desire for hot drinks, borborygmi, diarrhoea, pale and abundant urination, cold limbs, Pale tongue with white coating, Deep-Weak-Slow pulse

Treatment

Ren-6 Qihai, ST-25 Tianshu, ST-39 Xiajuxu, ST-36 Zusanli, BL-20 Pishu, BL-27 Xiaochangshu

Learning outcomes

In this chapter you will have learned:
- The main functions of the Small Intestine: transforming food and drink and separating the clean from the dirty
- The role of diet and emotional strain in causing Small Intestine pathology
- The importance of understanding Small Intestine pathology in terms of connections made by the channel (with the Heart) and the relation of the organ with other Internal Organs (Spleen, Liver and Bladder)
- How to identify the following Full patterns:
  Full-Heat in the Small Intestine: abdominal pain, tongue ulcers and scanty, dark and painful urine
  Small Intestine-Qi pain: lower abdominal twisting pain, borborygmi and a Deep-Wiry pulse
  Small Intestine-Qi tied: sudden severe abdominal pain, constipation, vomiting, Deep-Wiry pulse
  Infestation of worms in the Small Intestine: abdominal pain and distension, bad taste in mouth, sallow complexion, plus other symptoms, depending on type of worm
- How to identify the following Deficiency pattern:
  Small Intestine Deficient and Cold: dull abdominal pain, borborygmi and diarrhoea

Learning tips

Small Intestine patterns

- In any Small Intestine's intestinal pathology, write 'borborygmi'. There is a great deal of overlap between the Spleen, Liver and Small Intestine in bowel pathology: 'borborygmi' distinguishes a Small Intestine pathology
- Remember that, as a channel, the Small Intestine is related to the Heart, hence mouth and tongue ulcers
- Remember that, as an organ, the Small Intestine is related to the Bladder, hence urinary problems

Small Intestine Heat

- First of all, write general symptoms of Heat: feeling of heat, thirst, Red tongue with yellow coating, Rapid-Overflowing pulse
- Next, remember that, as a channel, the Small Intestine is related to the Heart: tongue ulcers, insomnia, mental restlessness
- Then, add some intestinal symptoms such as abdominal pain
- Finally, remember that, as an organ, the Small Intestine is related to the Bladder: dark urine, burning on urination, blood in the urine

Small Intestine-Qi pain

- Remember a bad case of Liver-Qi stagnation affecting the abdomen: abdominal distension and pain
- Next: adds the two symptoms that should always be added to any bowel pathology related to the Small Intestine: borborygmi and flatulence

Self-assessment questions

1. Complete the following: 'The Small Intestine transforms food in coordination with the _____, whilst it transforms fluids in coordination with the _____ and _____-_____.'
2. Long-term sadness can affect the Small Intestine, causing which particular mental symptoms?
3. Full-Heat in the Small Intestine is usually associated with which pattern?
4. A patient presents with the pattern Small Intestine-Qi pain. What would be their reaction to pressure on their abdomen?
5. What is a likely cause of the pattern Small Intestine Qi tied?
6. What physiological conditions does Chinese medicine suggest favour infestation of the Intestines by worms?
7. A patient has symptoms of Spleen-Yang deficiency and you suspect that the Small Intestine is also Deficient and Cold. Which symptom would confirm this?

See p. 1264 for answers

SECTION 2 PART 6

Large Intestine Patterns

40

> **Key contents**
>
> **General aetiology**
> *Exterior pathogenic factors*
> - Cold
> - Dampness
>
> *Emotional strain*
> - Sadness
> - Worry
> - Anger
>
> *Diet*
>
> **Full patterns**
> Damp-Heat in the Large Intestine
> Heat in the Large Intestine
> Heat obstructing the Large Intestine
> Cold invading the Large Intestine
> Qi stagnation in the Large Intestine
>
> **Empty patterns**
> Large Intestine Dry
> Large Intestine Cold
> Collapse of Large Intestine

The main function of the Large Intestine is to receive food and drink from the Small Intestine. Having reabsorbed some of the fluids, it excretes the stools.

The two main functions of the Large Intestine are (ch. 15):

> - Controls passage and conduction
> - Transforms stools and reabsorb fluids

It is therefore obvious that all the Large Intestine patterns have to do with disturbances of bowel movements.

Before discussing the Large Intestine patterns, I shall discuss the general aetiology as follows:

> - General aetiology
>   - Exterior pathogenic factors
>   - Cold
>   - Dampness
>   - Emotional strain
>   - Sadness
>   - Worry
>   - Anger
>   - Diet

GENERAL AETIOLOGY

Exterior pathogenic factors

Cold

The Large Intestine can be invaded by exterior Cold directly (bypassing the exterior layers of the body). This results from exposure to excessive cold over a prolonged period of time, or to normal seasonal cold but without adequate clothing. Cold-Dampness penetrates from ground level and works its way up to the Lower Burner where it can enter the Large Intestine and cause abdominal pain and diarrhoea. Many cases of lower abdominal pain, especially in children, are due to interior Cold resulting from the invasion of exterior Cold.

Dampness

External dampness may also invade the Large Intestine when the person wears inadequate clothing in cold and damp weather or when the person sits on damp ground.

Emotional strain

Sadness

Sadness affects the Lungs primarily and it may affect the Large Intestine indirectly due to the Lung–Large Intestine relationship within the Metal Element.

Sadness causes a deficiency of Qi in the Lungs and Large Intestine.

Worry

The Large Intestine, being exteriorly–interiorly related to the Lungs, is equally affected by worry. Worry depletes Lung-Qi, which fails to descend and help the Large Intestine in its functions. This results in stagnation of Qi in the Large Intestine, with the ensuing symptoms of abdominal distension and pain and constipation, with bitty stools alternating with diarrhoea.

Anger

Anger, frustration and resentment affect the Large Intestine, causing Qi stagnation in this organ. Such emotions are more likely to affect the Large Intestine when they are experienced after lunch (as, for example, going back to stressful work immediately after lunch).

Diet

Diet obviously affects the Large Intestine directly. Excessive consumption of cold and raw food can give rise to interior Cold and ensuing diarrhoea.

On the other hand, excessive consumption of greasy foods can give rise to Dampness in the Large Intestine. Greasy fried foods may give rise to Damp-Heat in the Large Intestine.

Box 40.1 summarizes the general aetiology of Large Intestine patterns.

The patterns discussed are:

FULL PATTERNS
- Damp-Heat in the Large Intestine
- Heat in the Large Intestine
- Heat obstructing the Large Intestine
- Cold invading the Large Intestine
- Qi stagnation in the Large Intestine

EMPTY PATTERNS
- Large Intestine Dry
- Large Intestine Cold
- Collapse of Large Intestine.

Box 40.2 summarizes factors giving a 'feel' for Large Intestine pathology.

Box 40.1 General aetiology of Large Intestine patterns

- Exterior pathogenic factors
  - Cold
  - Dampness
- Emotional strain
  - Sadness
  - Worry
  - Anger
- Diet

Box 40.2 A 'feel' for Large Intestine pathology

- Bowel problems
- Constipation/diarrhoea

FULL PATTERNS

Damp-Heat in the Large Intestine

Clinical manifestations

Abdominal pain that is not relieved by a bowel movement, abdominal fullness, diarrhoea, mucus and blood in stools, offensive odour of stools, burning in the anus, scanty dark urine, fever, sweating which does not decrease the fever, a feeling of heat, thirst without the desire to drink, a feeling of heaviness of the body and limbs (Fig. 40.1).

Tongue: Red with sticky yellow coating.
Pulse: Slippery-Rapid.
Key symptoms: abdominal pain, diarrhoea with mucus and blood in the stools.

Diagnostic tip

Abdominal pain and diarrhoea with mucus and blood in the stools are enough to diagnose Damp-Heat in the Large Intestine

Aetiology

Diet

This pattern can be caused by excessive consumption of hot and greasy foods, which leads to the formation of Damp-Heat. Alcohol, combined with the consumption of greasy foods, is also often an aetiological factor in this pattern.

Emotional strain

Emotional problems such as anxiety and worry over a long period of time cause interior Heat. In combination

- Thirst with no desire to drink
- Feeling of heat
- Feeling of heaviness
- Abdominal pain and fullness, diarrhoea with mucus and blood, offensive odour, burning in anus
- Scanty dark urine

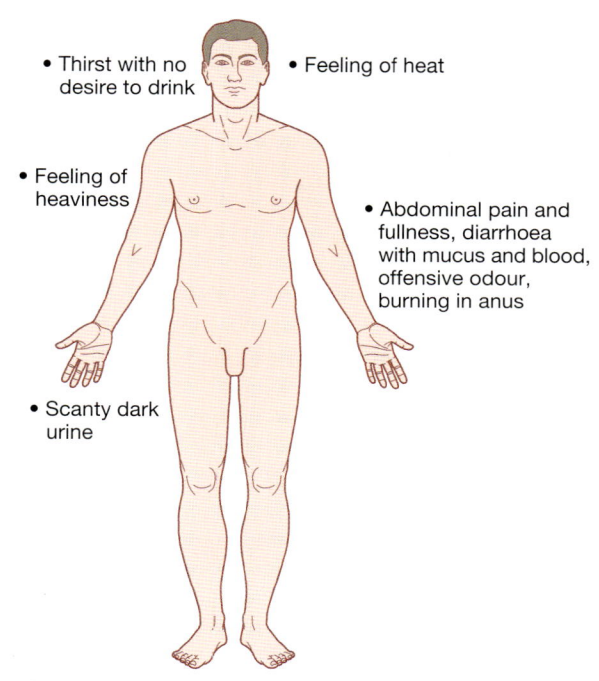

Figure 40.1 Damp-Heat in the Large Intestine

with the above dietary factors, this may lead to the formation of Damp-Heat in the Large Intestine.

Pathology

The retention of Dampness in the Large Intestine interferes with its function of absorbing fluids and excreting stools: hence fluids are not absorbed and diarrhoea results. The mucus in the stools is indicative of Dampness. The blood in the stools is due to Heat in the Large Intestine making the blood come out of the vessels.

Stools with strong odour, burning in the anus, thirst, dark urine, fever, Red tongue and Rapid pulse are all indicative of Heat.

The feeling of heaviness, the feeling of fullness of the abdomen, a sticky tongue coating and Slippery pulse are all indicative of Dampness.

Fever that is not abated by sweating is indicative of Dampness: however, please note that fever would be present only in severe cases. In most cases seen in practice, the patient would have no fever.

The pattern of Damp-Heat may present with many variations in practice depending on whether Heat or Dampness predominates. Also, remember that the Large Intestine may also be affected by Dampness without Heat. In this case, the Heat manifestation will be absent and the stools will have only mucus and not blood.

> **Clinical note**
>
> Remember that the Large Intestine may also be affected by Dampness without Heat. In this case, the Heat manifestation will be absent and the stools will have only mucus and not blood

Although in Western medicine pathologies of the small and large bowel are quite distinct and differentiated, in Chinese medicine an intestinal pathology often involves both the Large and the Small Intestine. For this reason, I find that in Damp-Heat of the Large or Small Intestine, a common pulse finding is that the pulse is equally Slippery or Wiry on both Rear positions (the Small Intestine being on the left-Rear and the Large Intestine on the right-Rear position).

> **Diagnostic tip**
>
> In Damp-Heat of the Large or Small Intestine, a common pulse finding is that the pulse is equally Slippery or Wiry on both Rear positions (the Small Intestine being on the left-Rear and the Large Intestine on the right-Rear side)

> **Clinical note**
>
> Ulcerative colitis and Crohn's disease frequently present with the pattern of Damp-Heat in the Large Intestine

Pathological precursors of pattern

Spleen-Qi deficiency is a very frequent pathological factor of this pattern as it predisposes the patient to the formation of Dampness (Fig. 40.2).

Pathological developments from pattern

First of all, Damp-Heat in the Large Intestine frequently leads to Damp-Heat in the Small Intestine.

The obstruction of the Lower Burner by Dampness may induce a deficiency of Spleen-Qi (see Fig. 40.2).

Treatment

Principle of treatment: clear Heat, resolve Dampness, stop diarrhoea.

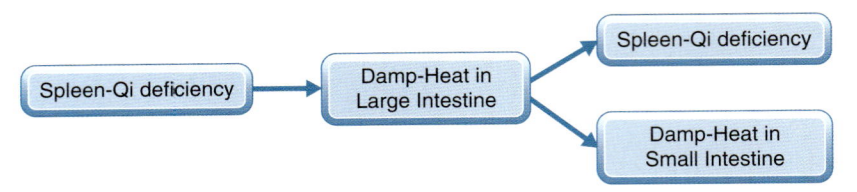

Figure 40.2 Damp-Heat in the Large Intestine pattern: precursors and developments

Acupuncture

Points: SP-9 Yinlingquan, SP-6 Sanyinjiao, Ren-3 Zhongji, BL-22 Sanjiaoshu, ST-25 Tianshu, ST-27 Daju, Ren-6 Qihai, BL-25 Dachangshu, L.I.-11 Quchi, Ren-12 Zhongwan, BL-20 Pishu, ST-37 Shangjuxu, SP-10 Xuehai.

Method: reducing, no moxa.

Explanation
– SP-9 and SP-6 resolve Dampness from the Lower Burner.
– Ren-3 and BL-22 resolve Dampness from the Lower Burner.
– ST-25 is the Front Collecting point of the Large Intestine and stops diarrhoea.
– ST-27 stops abdominal pain.
– Ren-6 moves Qi in the lower abdomen, which will help to resolve Dampness.
– BL-25 clears Heat from the Large Intestine.
– L.I.-11 clears Heat.
– Ren-12 and BL-20 tonify the Spleen to resolve Dampness.
– ST-37, Lower Sea point of the Large Intestine, stops diarrhoea.
– SP-10 stops bleeding.

Herbal formula

Ge Gen Qin Lian Tang *Pueraria–Scutellaria–Coptis Decoction*.
Bai Tou Weng Tang *Pulsatilla Decoction*.
Shao Yao Tang *Paeonia Decoction*.

> **Clinical note**
>
> Bai Tou Weng Tang is my favourite formula (with variations of course) for ulcerative colitis and Crohn's disease

Box 40.3 summarizes Damp-Heat in the Large Intestine.

Box 40.3 Damp-Heat in the Large Intestine

Clinical manifestations

Abdominal pain that is not relieved by a bowel movement, abdominal fullness, diarrhoea, mucus and blood in stools, offensive odour of stools, burning in the anus, scanty dark urine, fever, sweating which does not decrease the fever, a feeling of heat, thirst without desire to drink, feeling of heaviness of the body and limbs, Red tongue with sticky yellow coating, Slippery-Rapid pulse

Treatment

SP-9 Yinlingquan, SP-6 Sanyinjiao, Ren-3 Zhongji, BL-22 Sanjiaoshu, ST-25 Tianshu, ST-27 Daju, Ren-6 Qihai, BL-25 Dachangshu, L.I.-11 Quchi, Ren-12 Zhongwan, ST-37 Shangjuxu, BL-20 Pishu, SP-10 Xuehai

Case history 40.1

A 45-year-old man complained of chronic diarrhoea with mucus in the stools, abdominal pain, flatulence and irritability. His pulse was Wiry, Full and slightly Slippery. His tongue was Red with a sticky yellow coating which was thicker on the root. This condition had been diagnosed as Crohn's disease in Western medical terms.

This is a case of Damp-Heat in the Large Intestine with a background of Liver-Fire (as shown by the Wiry pulse, Red tongue and irritability). This shows how the Yang organ patterns are often accompanied or caused by Yin organ patterns. It also worth noting how there is no direct correspondence between Western medical disease entities and the organ patterns of Chinese medicine. In fact, this condition affected the Small Intestine from a Western medical viewpoint, but the Large Intestine from a Chinese medical viewpoint.

Heat in the Large Intestine

Clinical manifestations

Constipation with dry stools, burning sensation in the mouth, dry tongue, burning and swelling in anus, scanty dark urine (Fig. 40.3).
Tongue: thick yellow (or brown or black) dry coating.
Pulse: Full-Rapid.
Key symptoms: dry stools, burning sensation in anus, thick yellow dry tongue coating.

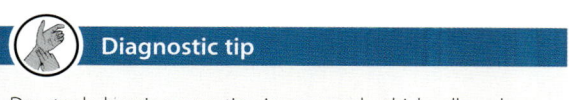

Diagnostic tip

Dry stools, burning sensation in anus and a thick yellow dry tongue coating are enough to diagnose Heat in the Large Intestine

- Burning mouth, dry tongue
- Burning and swelling of anus
- Scanty dark urine
- Constipation, dry stools

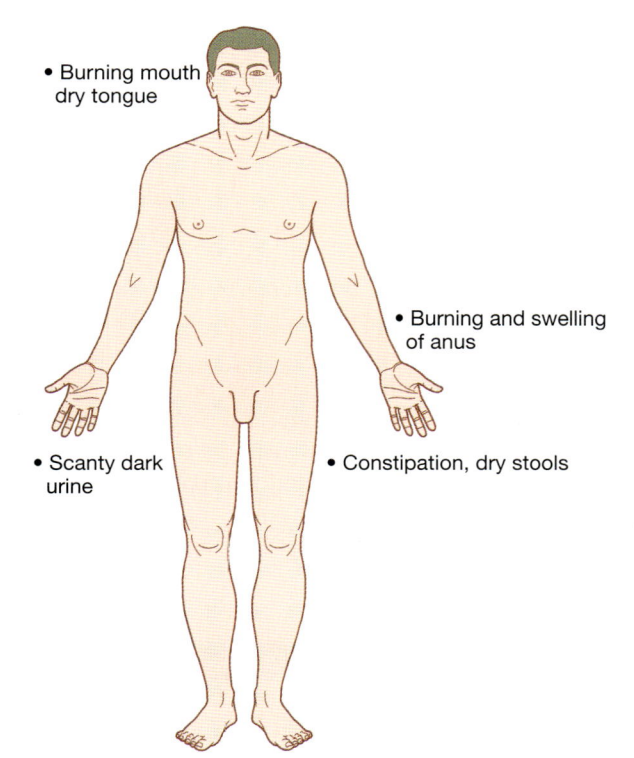

Figure 40.3 Heat in the Large Intestine

Aetiology

This pattern is caused by the excessive consumption of hot foods (such as lamb, beef and alcohol) and 'dry' foods, such as broiled or baked meats.

Pathology

This is an Excess pattern with Full-Heat and Dryness. The Dryness derives not from Deficiency, but is a result of the burning action of Full-Heat on the Body Fluids.

All the symptoms reflect Full-Heat in the Large Intestine: dry stools, burning and swelling of anus, thick yellow dry coating and a Rapid pulse.

The Large Intestine is closely related to the Stomach (within the Bright Yang) and there is also Heat in the Stomach resulting in dry mouth and dry tongue.

The Heat in the Lower Burner makes the urine more concentrated and scanty, hence its dark colour.

Generally speaking, this pattern appears more as an acute condition.

Pathological precursors of pattern

Stomach-Heat may be the pathological precursor of this pattern (Fig. 40.4).

Pathological developments from pattern

Heat in the Large Intestine injures fluids and may lead to Yin deficiency of the Stomach and the Large Intestine (see Fig. 40.4).

Treatment

Principle of treatment: clear Heat in the Large Intestine and Stomach, and promote Body Fluids.

Acupuncture

Points: ST-25 Tianshu, BL-25 Dachangshu, L.I.-11 Quchi, ST-37 Shangjuxu, ST-44 Neiting, L.I.-2 Erjian, SP-6 Sanyinjiao, KI-6 Zhaohai, Ren-12 Zhongwan.
Method: reducing method for points to clear Heat, tonifying method for points to promote fluids (SP-6, Ren-12, KI-6). Positively no moxa.

Stomach-Heat → Heat in Large Intestine → Stomach-Yin deficiency

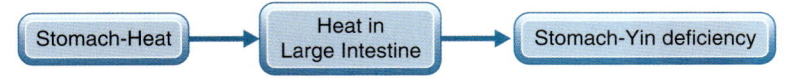

Figure 40.4 Heat in the Large Intestine pattern: precursors and developments

Explanation
- ST-25 and BL-25, Front Collecting and Back Transporting points of the Large Intestine, respectively, clear Heat in the Large Intestine.
- L.I.-11 clears Heat in the Large Intestine.
- ST-37 is the Lower Sea point for the Large Intestine and clears Heat in this organ.
- ST-44 clears Stomach-Heat.
- L.I.-2 clears Heat in Large Intestine.
- SP-6, KI-6 and Ren-12 promote Body Fluids.

Herbal formula

Ma Zi Ren Wan *Cannabis Pill*.

Box 40.4 summarizes Heat in the Large Intestine.

Box 40.4   Heat in the Large Intestine

Clinical manifestations

Constipation with dry stools, burning sensation in the mouth, dry tongue, burning and swelling in anus, scanty dark urine, thick yellow (or brown or black) dry tongue coating, Full-Rapid pulse

Treatment

ST-25 Tianshu, BL-25 Dachangshu, L.I.-11 Quchi, ST-37 Shangjuxu, ST-44 Neiting, L.I.-2 Erjian, SP-6 Sanyinjiao, KI-6 Zhaohai, Ren-12 Zhongwan

---

Heat obstructing the Large Intestine

Clinical manifestations

Constipation, burning in anus, abdominal distension and pain which is worse with pressure, high fever or tidal fever (fever that rises in the afternoon), sweating especially on limbs, vomiting, thirst, delirium (Fig. 40.5).
Tongue: thick dry yellow (or brown-black) coating, Red body.
Pulse: Deep-Full.
Key symptoms: constipation, abdominal pain, fever, thick dry yellow coating.

Diagnostic tip

Constipation, abdominal pain, fever and thick dry yellow coating are enough to diagnose Heat obstructing the Large Intestine

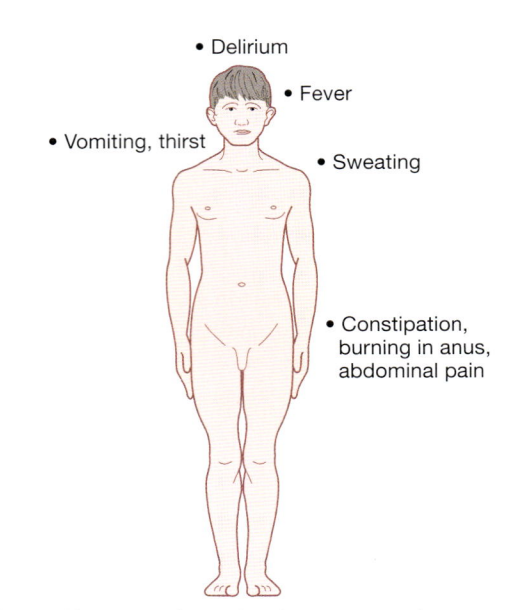

Figure 40.5 Heat obstructing the Large Intestine

Aetiology

This is an acute pattern seen at the middle stage of febrile disease caused by exterior Wind-Cold or Wind-Heat. This pattern occurs when the exterior Wind becomes interior Heat. It is more frequent in children.

Pathology

From the Eight-Principle perspective, this pattern is not different from the previous one, as it is also an interior pattern with Full-Heat. It differs from the previous one in so far as it is an acute pattern appearing during febrile diseases. Therefore, the presence of fever is absolutely essential to diagnose this pattern: if there is no fever, it is not this pattern.

Diagnostic tip

The presence of fever is absolutely essential to diagnose this pattern: if there is no fever, it is not this pattern

---

Heat obstructing the Large Intestine is the pattern of Bright Yang organ pattern seen at the Bright Yang stage of the Six-Stage patterns (ch. 44) or the Intestines Dry-Heat pattern of the Qi Level within the Four-Level patterns (chapter 45) (Figs 40.6 and 40.7).

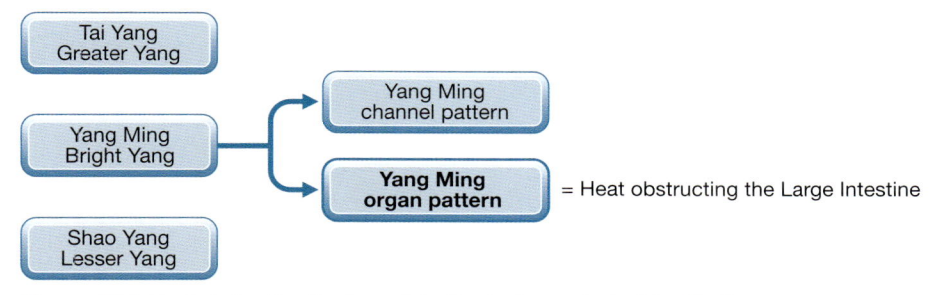

Figure 40.6 Heat obstructing the Large Intestine in the context of the Six Stages

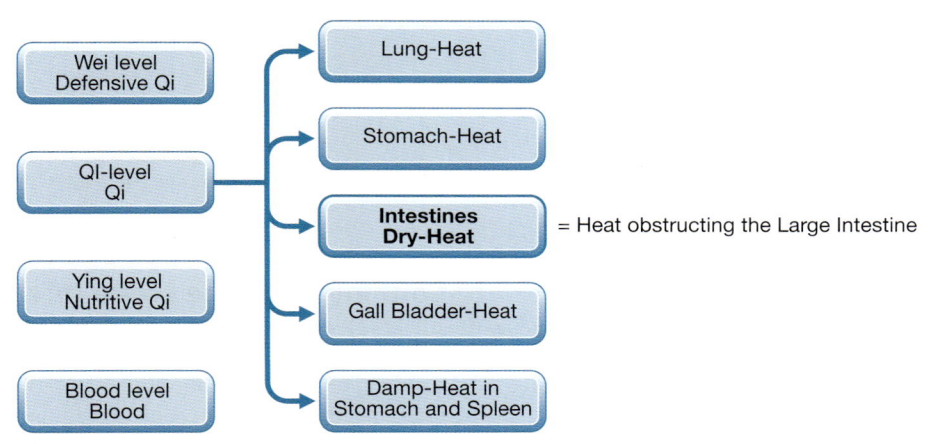

Figure 40.7 Heat obstructing the Large Intestine in the context of the Four Levels

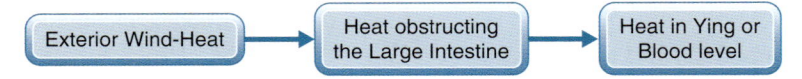

Figure 40.8 Heat obstructing the Large Intestine pattern: precursors and developments

Heat in the Large Intestine causes constipation, abdominal pain and burning in the anus. Heat in the Large Intestine is transmitted to the Stomach and causes thirst and a thick dry yellow coating on the tongue. Constipation and abdominal pain are important symptoms which help to differentiate this pattern from that of Bright Yang channel pattern at the Bright Yang stage of the Six Stages or the Stomach-Heat pattern of the Qi level of the Four Levels (see Figs 40.6 and 40.7).

Heat in the Stomach and Large Intestine vaporizes the Body Fluids and causes profuse sweating. Heat in the Stomach interferes with the Stomach descending function and causes vomiting.

Extreme Heat can mist the Mind and cause delirium. A Full and Deep pulse is typical of interior Heat in Stomach and Intestines. The Deep pulse also helps to differentiate this pattern from that of Bright Yang channel pattern in which the pulse is Big.

Pathological precursors of pattern

As this is the second stage of a febrile disease, it always derives from an invasion of exterior Wind which penetrates in the Interior and turns into Heat (Fig. 40.8).

Pathological developments from pattern

As this pattern occurs during the second stage of an acute febrile disease, there are only three possible outcomes: the patient's body's Qi may react well and he or she recovers completely, the Heat may progress to the next stage, or the patient may appear to recover but there is a residual Heat left in the body.

If this pattern corresponds to the Bright Yang organ pattern of the Bright Yang stage within the Six Stages, it may progress to one of the Yin stages; if it corresponds to the Intestines Dry-Heat pattern at the Qi level within the Four Levels, it may progress to the Nutritive Qi or Blood level (see Fig. 40.7).

Treatment

Principle of treatment: clear Heat in Stomach and Large Intestine, and promote bowel movement.

Acupuncture

Points: L.I.-11 Quchi, L.I.-4 Hegu, SP-15 Daheng, T.B.-6 Zhigou, SP-6 Sanyinjiao, L.I.-2 Erjian, ST-44 Neiting, ST-25 Tianshu, BL-25 Dachangshu.
Method: reducing, no moxa.
Explanation
- L.I.-11 clears Heat in the Large Intestine.
- L.I.-4 clears Large Intestine-Heat and promotes bowel movement.
- SP-15 promotes bowel movement.
- T.B.-6 clears Heat in the Intestines and promotes bowel movement.
- SP-6 nourishes Yin and stops abdominal pain.
- L.I.-2 clears Large Intestine-Heat.
- ST-44 clears Stomach-Heat.
- ST-25 and BL-25 clear Large Intestine-Heat.

Herbal formula

Tiao Wei Cheng Qi Tang *Regulating the Stomach Conducting Qi Decoction.*

Box 40.5 summarizes Heat obstructing the Large Intestine.

Box 40.5 Heat obstructing the Large Intestine

Clinical manifestations

Constipation, burning in anus, abdominal distension and pain which is worse with pressure, high fever or tidal fever (fever that rises in the afternoon), sweating especially on limbs, vomiting, thirst, delirium, thick, dry yellow (or brown-black) tongue coating, Red body, Deep-Full pulse

Treatment

L.I.-11 Quchi, L.I.-4 Hegu, SP-15 Daheng, T.B.-6 Zhigou, SP-6 Sanyinjiao, L.I.-2 Erjian, ST-44 Neiting, ST-25 Tianshu, BL-25 Dachangshu

---

- Feeling cold
- Sudden, cramping abdominal pain, diarrhoea with pain, cold sensation in abdomen

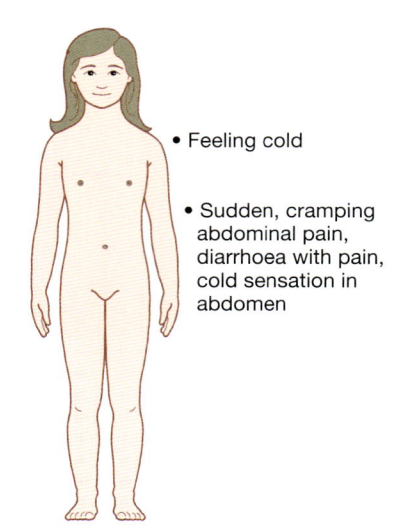

Figure 40.9 Cold invading the Large Intestine

Cold invading the Large Intestine

Clinical manifestations

Sudden, cramping abdominal pain, diarrhoea with pain, feeling of cold, cold sensation in abdomen (Fig. 40.9).
Tongue: thick white coating.
Pulse: Deep-Tight.
Key symptoms: sudden abdominal pain, diarrhoea, feeling of cold.

> **Diagnostic tip**
>
> Sudden abdominal pain, diarrhoea and a feeling of cold are enough to diagnose Cold invading the Large Intestine

Aetiology

This is due to invasion of exterior Cold in the Large Intestine which can take place if the person sits on cold and wet surfaces for prolonged periods or is exposed to very cold weather having the abdomen insufficiently covered.

Pathology

This is an acute pattern caused by invasion of exterior Cold in the Large Intestine. From the Eight-Principle point of view, it is a Full-Cold pattern.

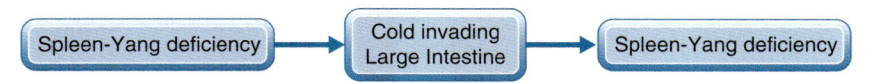

Figure 40.10 Cold invading the Large Intestine pattern: precursors and developments

Even though the Cold is of exterior origin, it invades the Interior immediately, bypassing the skin outer energetics layers and settling in the Large Intestine. The Large Intestine (together with Uterus and Stomach) is one of three organs which can be invaded by exterior Cold directly.

Cold in the Large Intestine interferes with the movement of Qi in the Lower Burner and causes sudden stagnation of Qi, resulting in the sudden pain which is severe and cramping in character as Cold contracts and causes cramps and spasms.

Cold interferes with the Large Intestine function of absorption of fluids, hence the diarrhoea.

The thick tongue coating reflects a sudden invasion of a pathogenic factor and the Deep pulse suggests that the pathogenic factor is in the Interior and Tight suggests that the pathogenic factor is Cold.

Pathogenic precursors of pattern

A deficiency of Yang of the Stomach and Spleen may predispose the patient to invasion of Cold in the Large Intestine (Fig. 40.10).

Pathological developments from pattern

Cold in the Large Intestine may injure Yang and lead to Spleen-Yang deficiency (see Fig. 40.10).

Treatment

Principle of treatment: expel Cold from the Large Intestine, warm the Lower Burner.

Acupuncture

Points: ST-37 Shangjuxu, ST-25 Tianshu, ST-36 Zusanli, SP-6 Sanyinjiao, LIV-3 Taichong, ST-27 Daju.
Method: reducing, moxa is applicable after needling.
Explanation
 – ST-37 is the Lower Sea point of the Large Intestine and it stops diarrhoea and pain.
 – ST-25 is the Front Collecting point of the Large Intestine and it stops diarrhoea and pain.
 – ST-36, with moxa on the needle, can expel Cold from the Large Intestine.

> **Box 40.6 Cold invading the Large Intestine**
>
> **Clinical manifestations**
>
> Sudden, cramping abdominal pain, diarrhoea with pain, feeling of cold, cold sensation in abdomen, thick white tongue coating, Deep-Tight pulse
>
> **Treatment**
>
> ST-37 Shangjuxu, ST-25 Tianshu, ST-36 Zusanli, SP-6 Sanyinjiao, LIV-3 Taichong, ST-27 Daju

 – SP-6 calms abdominal pain.
 – LIV-3 moves Qi in the Lower Burner and calms spasms (in this case of the intestines).
 – ST-27 expels Cold from the Large Intestine.

Herbal formula

Liang Fu Wan *Alpinia Cyperus Pill* plus Zheng Qi Tian Xiang San *Upright Qi Heavenly Fragrance Powder*.

Box 40.6 summarizes Cold invading the Large Intestine.

Qi Stagnation in the Large Intestine

Clinical manifestations

Abdominal distension and pain, constipation with bitty stools, irritability, aggravation of condition according to mood (Fig. 40.11).
Tongue: either normal or slightly Red on the sides.
Pulse: Wiry on both Rear positions.
Key symptoms: abdominal distension and pain, bitty stools.

> **Diagnostic tip**
>
> Abdominal distension and pain with bitty stools are enough to diagnose Qi stagnation in the Large Intestine

Aetiology

Diet

Irregular dietary habits such as eating in a hurry, working while eating, eating standing up, etc., may lead to Qi stagnation in the Large Intestine.

Emotional strain

Frustration, resentment and anger may lead to Qi stagnation: they are more likely to affect the Large Intestine when such emotions are experienced after each lunch.

Pathology

This pattern is characterized by Qi stagnation and distension is the essential symptom of Qi stagnation. The bitty stools and irritability also reflect Qi stagnation.

Pathological precursors of pattern

Liver-Qi stagnation is a frequent precursor of this pattern (Fig. 40.12).

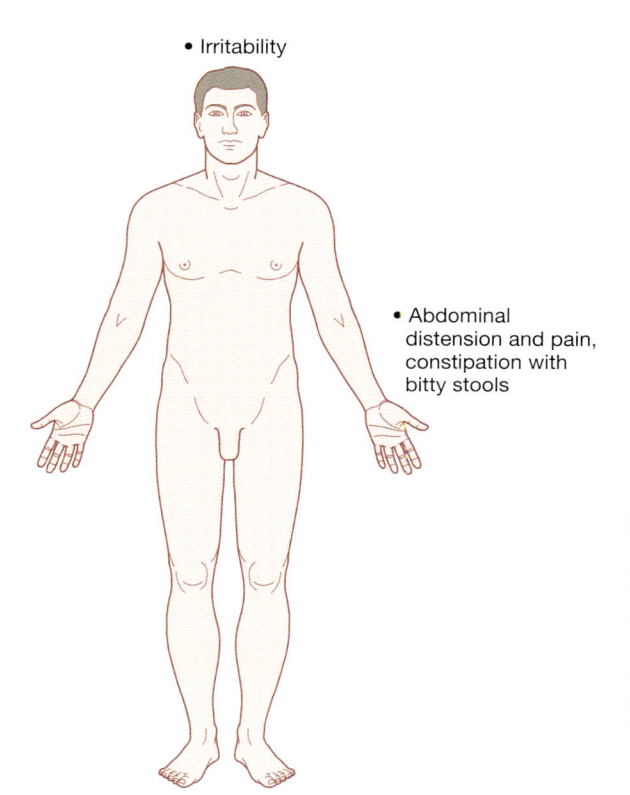

Pathological developments from pattern

If it is not the precursor, Liver-Qi stagnation may derive from this Qi stagnation in the Large Intestine (see Fig. 40.12).

Qi stagnation in the Large Intestine may also lead to the formation of Dampness as the stagnant Qi fails to move and transform fluids.

Treatment

Principle of treatment: move Qi in the Large Intestine.

Acupuncture

Points: Ren-6 Qihai, G.B.-34 Yanglingquan, ST-25 Tianshu, SP-15 Daheng, ST-37 Shangjuxu, SP-6 Sanyinjiao, BL-25 Dachangshu.
Method: reducing.
Explanation
- Ren-6 in combination with G.B.-34 moves Qi in the lower abdomen.
- ST-25 moves Qi in the Large Intestine.
- SP-15 moves Qi in the Large Intestine and promotes the bowel movement.
- ST-37, Lower Sea point of the Large Intestine, regulates Qi of the Large Intestine and is particularly indicated in chronic conditions.
- SP-6 stops abdominal pain.
- BL-25 moves Qi in the Large Intestine.

Herbal formula

Chai Hu Shu Gan Tang *Bupleurum Soothing the Liver Decoction*.

Box 40.7 summarizes Qi stagnation in the Large Intestine.

Box 40.7 Qi stagnation in the Large Intestine

Clinical manifestations

Abdominal distension and pain, constipation with bitty stools, irritability, aggravation of condition according to mood, tongue either normal or slightly Red on the sides, pulse Wiry on both Rear positions

Treatment

Ren-6 Qihai, G.B.-34 Yanglingquan, ST-25 Tianshu, SP-15 Daheng, ST-37 Shangjuxu, SP-6 Sanyinjiao, BL-25 Dachangshu

---

Figure 40.11 Qi stagnation in the Large Intestine

Liver-Qi stagnation → Qi-stagnation in Large Intestine → Liver-Qi stagnation

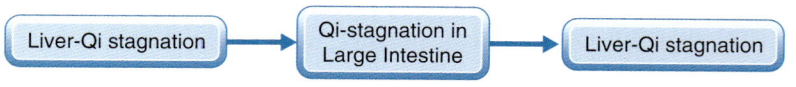

Figure 40.12 Qi stagnation in the Large Intestine pattern: precursors and developments

EMPTY PATTERNS

Large Intestine Dry

Clinical manifestations

Dry stools which are difficult to discharge, dry mouth and throat, thin body, foul breath, dizziness (Fig. 40.13).

Tongue: dry, either Pale or Red body with rootless coating.
Pulse: Fine.
Key symptoms: dry stools which are difficult to discharge, thin body.

> **Diagnostic tip**
>
> Dry stools without other notable symptoms is enough to diagnose Large Intestine Dry

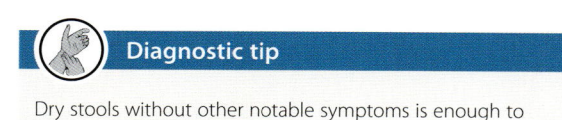

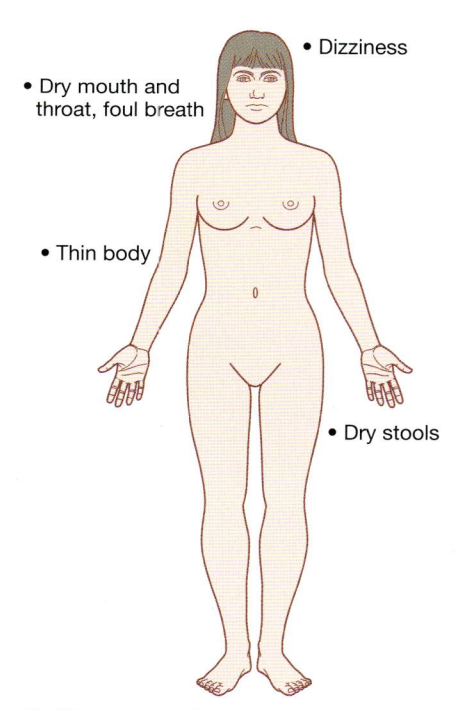

Figure 40.13 Large Intestine Dry
- Dizziness
- Dry mouth and throat, foul breath
- Thin body
- Dry stools

Aetiology

External pathogenic factors

In some countries with very dry and warm weather this pattern may be caused by external Dryness.

Diet

Irregular dietary habits that deplete Yin often lead to Dryness of the Stomach and Intestines. Such habits consist in eating late at night, eating in a hurry, eating irregularly, etc.

Pathology

First of all, this pattern nearly always occurs in combination with Stomach-Yin deficiency. The pattern is simply characterized by a state of Dryness and deficiency of Body Fluids. Dryness is a stage preceding full-blown Yin deficiency.

The foul breath is caused not by Heat but by the retention of Food following constipation.

Pathological precursors of pattern

Usually this pattern is preceded by a deficiency of Qi of the Stomach and the Large Intestine (Fig. 40.14).

Pathological developments from pattern

Yin deficiency of the Stomach and Large Intestine is the common pathological consequence of Dryness (see Fig. 40.14).

Treatment

Principle of treatment: promote fluids in the Large Intestine.

Acupuncture

Points: ST-36 Zusanli, SP-6 Sanyinjiao, Ren-4 Guanyuan, KI-6 Zhaohai, ST-25 Tianshu, SP-15 Daheng.
Method: reinforcing.
Explanation
- ST-36 can promote fluids in Stomach and Large Intestine.
- SP-6 and Ren-4 tonify Yin and promote fluids.

Stomach-Qi deficiency → Large Intestine Dry → Stomach-Yin deficiency

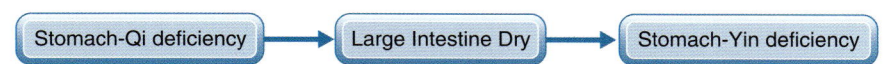

Figure 40.14 Large Intestine Dry pattern: precursors and developments

- KI-6 tonifies Yin and promotes fluids and is particularly indicated to moisten the stools.
- ST-25 moistens the Intestines.
- SP-15 moistens the stool and treats constipation.

Herbal formula

Zeng Ye Tang Increasing Fluids Decoction.
Qing Zao Run Chang Tang Clearing Dryness and Moistening the Intestines Decoction.
Wu Ren Wan Five Seeds Pill.
Tian Di Jian Heaven and Earth Decoction.
Si Wu Ma Zi Ren Wan Four-Substance Cannabis Pill.
Ma Zi Ren Wan Cannabis Pill.

Box 40.8 summarizes Large Intestine Dry.

Box 40.8 Large Intestine Dry

Clinical manifestations

Dry stools which are difficult to discharge, dry mouth and throat, thin body, foul breath, dizziness, dry tongue that is either Pale or Red without rootless coating, Fine pulse

Treatment

ST-36 Zusanli, SP-6 Sanyinjiao, Ren-4 Guanyuan, KI-6 Zhaohai, ST-25 Tianshu, SP-15 Daheng

---

Large Intestine Cold

Clinical manifestations

Loose stools like duck droppings, dull abdominal pain, borborygmi, pale urine, cold limbs (Fig. 40.15).
Tongue: Pale.
Pulse: Deep-Weak.
Key symptoms: loose stools, dull abdominal pain, cold limbs.

> **Diagnostic tip**
>
> Loose stools, dull abdominal pain and cold limbs are enough to diagnose Large Intestine Cold

Aetiology

This pattern can be caused by excessive consumption of cold and raw foods and by chronic exposure to cold weather on the abdomen.

Pathology

This is an interior pattern with Deficient Cold, and it is basically the same as Spleen-Yang deficiency. Please

- Pale urine
- Loose stools, dull abdominal pain, borborygmi
- Cold limbs

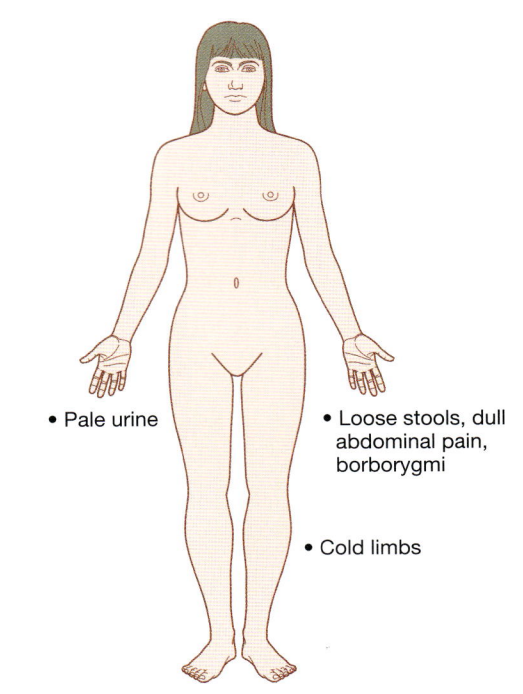

Figure 40.15 Large Intestine Cold

note the difference between this pattern and that of Cold invading the Large Intestine discussed above: the former is characterized by Empty-Cold and is a chronic condition while the latter is characterized by Full-Cold and is an acute condition.

Pathological precursors of pattern

Spleen-Yang deficiency is nearly always the precursor of this pattern (Fig. 40.16).

Pathological developments from pattern

If this pattern does not derive from Spleen-Yang deficiency, it may itself be the precursor of it (see Fig. 40.16).

Treatment

Principle of treatment: tonify and warm Large Intestine and Spleen.

Acupuncture

Points: ST-25 Tianshu, Ren-6 Qihai, ST-36 Zusanli, ST-37 Shangjuxu, BL-25 Dachangshu, BL-20 Pishu.
Method: reinforcing, moxa should be used.

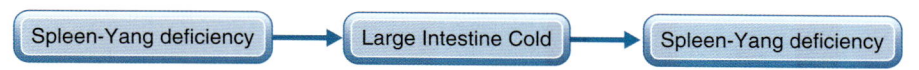

Figure 40.16 Large Intestine Cold pattern: precursors and developments

Explanation
- ST-25 stops diarrhoea and pain.
- Ren-6 tonifies Qi and stops chronic diarrhoea. The warm box can be used on these two points.
- ST-36 tonifies Spleen-Qi.
- ST-37 stops chronic diarrhoea.
- BL-25, Back Transporting point of the Large Intestine, tonifies this organ and stops diarrhoea.
- BL-20 tonifies Spleen-Qi.

Herbal formula

Liang Fu Wan *Alpinia Cyperus Pill*.
Box 40.9 summarizes Large Intestine Cold.

Box 40.9 Large Intestine Cold

Clinical manifestations

Loose stools like duck droppings, dull abdominal pain, borborygmi, pale urine, cold limbs, Pale tongue, Deep-Weak pulse

Treatment

ST-25 Tianshu, Ren-6 Qihai, ST-36 Zusanli, ST-37 Shangjuxu, BL-25 Dachangshu, BL-20 Pishu

---

Collapse of Large Intestine

Clinical manifestations

Chronic diarrhoea, prolapse ani, haemorrhoids, tiredness after bowel movements, cold limbs, no appetite, mental exhaustion, desire to drink warm liquids, desire to have the abdomen massaged (Fig. 40.17).
Tongue: Pale.
Pulse: Deep-Fine-Weak.
Key symptoms: chronic diarrhoea, prolapse ani.

Diagnostic tip

Chronic diarrhoea and prolapse ani are enough to diagnose Collapse of the Large Intestine

Aetiology

This can be caused by any of the causes of Spleen and Stomach deficiency. In particular, excessive physical work is a frequent cause of this pattern.

Pathology

This is due to chronic deficiency of Qi of the Spleen, Stomach and Large Intestine, with sinking of Spleen-Qi.

Sinking of Spleen-Qi causes the prolapse ani and chronic diarrhoea. The deficiency of Stomach and Spleen Qi and Yang causes lack of appetite, cold limbs and desire to drink warm liquids. The desire to have the abdomen massaged and the tiredness after bowel movements indicate a Deficiency pattern.

Pathological precursors of pattern

Sinking of Spleen-Qi is always the precursor of this pattern (Fig. 40.18).

Pathological developments from pattern

Collapse of the Large Intestine may affect other organs in the Lower Burner and particularly the Bladder and it may lead to sinking of Qi affecting the bladder (see Fig. 40.18).

Treatment

Principle of treatment: tonify Stomach and Spleen, raise Qi.
Points: Ren-6 Qihai, ST-25 Tianshu, ST-36 Zusanli, SP-3 Taibai, BL-20 Pishu, BL-21 Weishu, Du-20 Baihui.
Method: reinforcing, moxa is applicable.
Explanation
- Ren-6 tonifies and raises Qi.
- ST-25 tonifies Large Intestine and stops diarrhoea. The warm box could be used on Qihai Ren-6 and Tianshu ST-25.
- ST-36 tonifies Stomach- and Spleen-Qi.
- SP-3 tonifies Spleen-Qi.
- BL-20 and BL-21 tonify Spleen and Stomach.
- Du-20 with direct moxa, raises Qi and is used for prolapse ani.

Herbal formula

Bu Zhong Yi Qi Tang *Tonifying the Centre Benefitting Qi Decoction*.
Box 40.10 summarizes Collapse of Large Intestine.

- Mental exhaustion
- Desire to drink warm liquids
- No appetite
- Desire to have the abdomen massaged
- Chronic diarrhoea, prolapse ani, haemorrhoids, tiredness after bowel movements
- Cold limbs

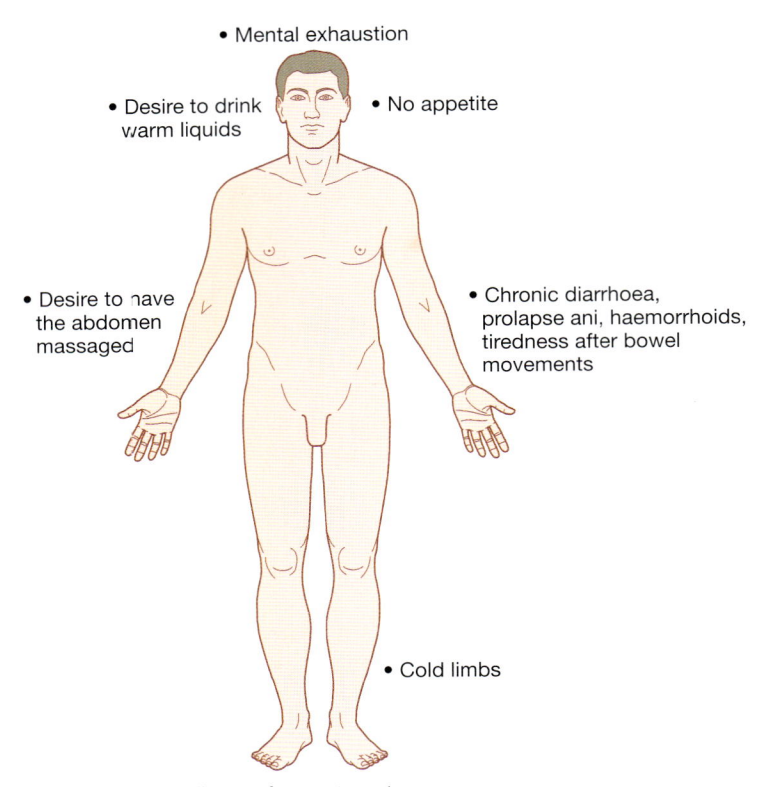

Figure 40.17 Collapse of Large Intestine

Spleen-Qi sinking → Collapse of Large Intestine → Sinking of Bladder-Qi

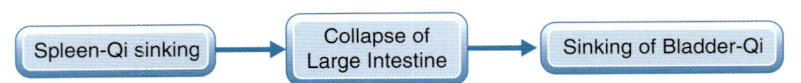

Figure 40.18 Collapse of Large Intestine pattern: precursors and developments

Box 40.10 Collapse of Large Intestine

Clinical manifestations

Chronic diarrhoea, prolapse ani, haemorrhoids, tiredness after bowel movements, cold limbs, no appetite, mental exhaustion, desire to drink warm liquids, desire to have the abdomen massaged
Tongue: Pale
Pulse: Deep-Fine-Weak

Treatment

Ren-6 Qihai, ST-25 Tianshu, ST-36 Zusanli, SP-3 Taibai, BL-20 Pishu, BL-21 Weishu, Du-20 Baihui

Learning outcomes

In this chapter you will have learned:
- The main functions of the Large Intestine: controlling passage and conduction, and transforming stools and reabsorbing fluids
- The role of Exterior Cold and Dampness in causing Large Intestine patterns
- How sadness, worry and anger can adversely affect the Large Intestine
- The role of diet (cold, raw or greasy foods) in causing Large Intestine pathology

- How to identify the following Full patterns:
  Damp-Heat in the Large Intestine: abdominal pain and diarrhoea with mucus and blood in the stools
  Heat in the Large Intestine: dry stools, burning sensation in anus and a thick, yellow, dry tongue coating
  Heat obstructing the Large Intestine: constipation, abdominal pain, fever and thick, dry, yellow tongue coating
  Cold invading the Large Intestine: sudden abdominal pain, diarrhoea and a feeling of cold
  Qi stagnation in the Large Intestine: abdominal distension and pain with bitty stools
- How to identify the following Empty patterns:
  Large Intestine Dry: dry stools which are difficult to discharge, thin body
  Large Intestine Cold: loose stools, dull abdominal pain, cold limbs
  Collapse of Large Intestine: chronic diarrhoea and prolapse ani

Learning tips

Damp-Heat in the Large Intestine

- First, remember the general symptoms of Heat that you should add to any Heat pattern: feeling of heat, thirst, Red tongue with yellow coating, Rapid pulse
- Next, remember the general symptoms of Dampness: abdominal *fullness*, feeling of *heaviness*, *sticky* coating, *mucus* in stools, *Slippery* pulse
- Finally, add the Large Intestine bowel symptoms: diarrhoea (with mucus), abdominal pain

Self-assessment questions

1. What are the two main functions of the Large Intestine?
2. What are the three most common ways the Large Intestine can be directly invaded by exterior Cold and Damp from the environment?
3. Which three emotions can adversely affect the Large Intestine and what affect do they have on Large Intestine-Qi?
4. What is the pathology of diarrhoea in the pattern Damp-Heat in the Large Intestine?
5. Complete the following: 'Heat in the Large Intestine is an _____ pattern with ____ ____ and _____.'
6. How does the pattern Heat obstructing the Large Intestine differ from Heat in the Large Intestine, given that both are interior patterns with Full-Heat?
7. What is the quality of the pain associated with the pattern Cold invading the Large Intestine? Explain the pathology of this pain.
8. What is the most characteristic symptom of Qi stagnation in the Large Intestine?
9. With which pattern is Large Intestine Dry nearly always associated?
10. How does the pattern Large Intestine Cold differ from Cold invading the Large Intestine?
11. Which two pathologies of Qi characterize the pattern Collapse of the Large Intestine?

See p. 1265 for answers

SECTION 2   PART 6

Gall Bladder Patterns — 41

Key contents

General aetiology
Diet
Emotional strain
External pathogenic factors

Full patterns
Dampness in the Gall Bladder
Damp-Heat in the Gall Bladder

Empty patterns
Gall Bladder deficient

Combined patterns
Damp-Heat in the Gall Bladder and Liver

- General aetiology
  - Diet
  - Emotional strain
  - External pathogenic factors

The functions of the Gall Bladder are (ch. 16):

- It stores and excretes bile
- It controls decisiveness
- It controls sinews

The main Gall Bladder function is that of storing bile and its patterns are nearly always very closely related to those of the Liver. The Gall Bladder's job of storing and emptying the bile is dependent on the Liver ensuring the smooth flow of Qi.

The Gall Bladder is easily affected by Dampness deriving from an impairment of the Spleen function of transformation and transportation.

On a mental level, the Gall Bladder is responsible for courage and decisiveness. When the Gall Bladder is deficient, the person lacks courage and finds it difficult to take decisions.

Before discussing the patterns of the Gall Bladder, I shall discuss the general aetiology of Gall Bladder patterns. This is as follows:

GENERAL AETIOLOGY

Diet

An excessive consumption of greasy and fatty foods leads to the formation of Dampness, which can lodge in the Gall Bladder.

Emotional strain

The Gall Bladder, like the Liver, is affected by anger. Anger, frustration and bottled-up resentment can cause stagnation of Liver-Qi, which, in turn, can produce Heat, which affects the Gall Bladder. Pent-up anger over a long period of time implodes to give rise to Heat in Liver and Gall Bladder with symptoms of irritability, bitter taste, thirst, headaches, etc.

From an emotional point of view, the Gall Bladder also affects courage and capacity of taking decisions. A weak Gall Bladder energy may result in timidity and lack of courage. This is also expressed in certain Chinese language expressions such as 'big Gall Bladder' for 'courage' and 'small Gall Bladder' for 'cowardice or timidity'.

External pathogenic factors

Exterior dampness can invade the Gall Bladder, leading to the pattern of Dampness in the Gall Bladder. In hot and humid countries, Dampness and Heat can cause Damp-Heat in the Gall Bladder.

Box 41.1 summarizes the general aetiology of Gall Bladder pathology. Box 41.2 summarizes factors that give a general 'feel' for Gall Bladder patterns.

Box 41.1 General aetiology of Gall Bladder patterns

- Diet
- Emotional strain
- External pathogenic factors

Box 41.2 A 'feel' for Gall Bladder patterns

- Digestive problems
- Hypochondrial pain
- Tendency to obesity
- Difficulty in making decisions

The patterns discussed below are:

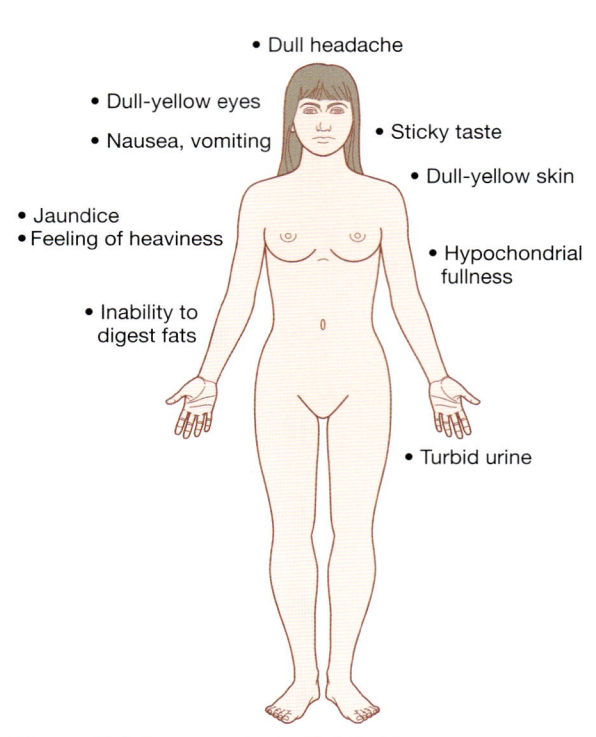

FULL PATTERNS
- Dampness in the Gall Bladder
- Damp-Heat in the Gall Bladder

EMPTY PATTERNS
- Gall Bladder deficient

COMBINED PATTERNS
- Damp-Heat in the Gall Bladder and Liver

FULL PATTERNS

Dampness in the Gall Bladder

Clinical manifestations

Jaundice, dull-yellow eyes and skin, hypochondrial pain, fullness and distension, nausea, vomiting, inability to digest fats, dull-yellow sclera, turbid urine, no thirst, sticky taste, dull headache, feeling of heaviness of the body (Fig. 41.1).
Tongue: thick sticky white coating, either bilateral in two strips or unilateral.
Pulse: Slippery-Wiry.
Key symptoms: hypochondrial fullness, feeling of heaviness, unilateral sticky coating.

Diagnostic tip

Hypochondrial fullness, feeling of heaviness and a unilateral sticky coating are enough to diagnose Dampness in the Gall Bladder

Aetiology

External pathogenic factors

External dampness can invade the Gall Bladder and lead to retention of Dampness in this organ.

Figure 41.1 Dampness in the Gall Bladder

- Dull headache
- Dull-yellow eyes
- Nausea, vomiting
- Sticky taste
- Dull-yellow skin
- Jaundice
- Feeling of heaviness
- Hypochondrial fullness
- Inability to digest fats
- Turbid urine

Diet

The excessive consumption of greasy fatty foods and of dairy foods is the most common cause of this pattern.

Pathology

Dampness in the Gall Bladder causes the typical feeling of fullness in the hypochondrium and a general feeling of heaviness. As Dampness interferes with the smooth flow of Liver-Qi, which stagnates, it may cause hypochondrial distension and pain.

Nausea and vomiting are caused by Dampness obstructing the Middle Burner and preventing Stomach-Qi from descending.

Dampness is 'sticky' and 'turbid' and therefore turbid urine and a sticky taste reflect Dampness. Dampness may lodge in the head to cause a dull headache.

The unilateral sticky tongue coating is typical of a Gall Bladder pathology (Fig. 41.2).

Please note that the clinical manifestations outlined above are taken from Chinese books. The patients I see with Dampness in the Gall Bladder have much milder symptoms even when they have cholecystitis or cholelithiasis. For example, the only symptoms and signs of

Dampness may be a sticky tongue coating, a feeling of heaviness and a Slippery pulse.

Pathological precursors of pattern

Spleen-Qi deficiency may predispose the patient to Dampness and contribute to the development of this pattern. Liver-Qi stagnation in the Middle Burner may also contribute to the formation of Dampness in the Gall Bladder (Fig. 41.3).

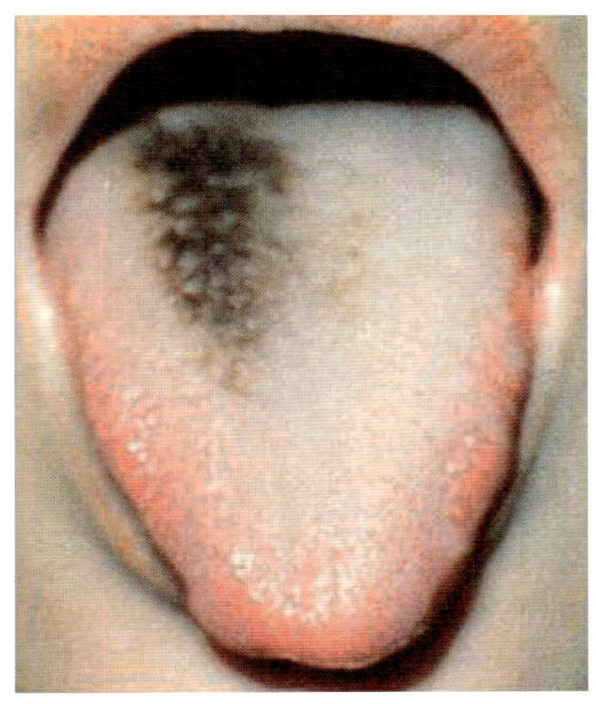

Figure 41.2 Unilateral Gall-Bladder coating

Pathological developments from pattern

First of all, Dampness in the Gall Bladder frequently combines with Heat to form Damp-Heat (described below). Dampness in the Middle Burner obstructs the free flow of Liver-Qi and may lead to Liver-Qi stagnation.

If it combines with Heat, Damp-Heat may lead to Phlegm-Heat (see Fig. 41.3).

Treatment

Principle of treatment: resolve Dampness, clear the Gall Bladder, promote the smooth flow of Liver-Qi.

Acupuncture

Points: G.B.-24 Riyue, LIV-14 Qimen, Ren-12 Zhongwan, G.B.-34 Yanglingquan, extra point Dannangxue, Du-9 Zhiyang, BL-19 Danshu, BL-20 Pishu, T.B.-6 Zhigou, ST-19 Burong.

Method: reducing or even method except BL-20, which should be reinforced if there is a Spleen deficiency. Moxa can be used if there are symptoms of Cold.

Explanation
- G.B.-24, G.B.-34, Du-9 and BL-19 resolve Dampness from the Gall Bladder.
- LIV-14 harmonizes the Liver and Gall Bladder and promotes the smooth flow of Liver-Qi.
- Ren-12 resolves Dampness.
- Dannangxue resolves Dampness from the Gall Bladder.
- BL-20 tonifies the Spleen to resolve Dampness.
- T.B.-6 promotes the smooth flow of Liver-Qi in the hypochondrium.
- ST-19 promotes the descending of Stomach-Qi to relieve obstruction in the Middle Burner and treat nausea and vomiting.

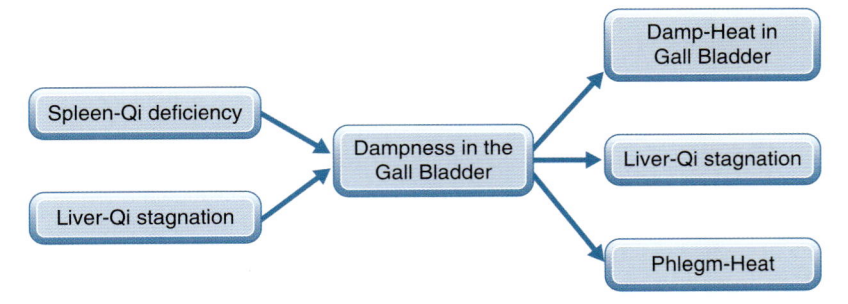

Figure 41.3 Dampness in the Gall Bladder pattern: precursors and developments

Herbal formula

San Ren Tang *Three Seeds Decoction* plus Yin Chen Hao *Herba Artemisiae capillaris*.

Box 41.3 summarizes Dampness in the Gall Bladder.

Box 41.3 Dampness in the Gall Bladder

Clinical manifestations

Jaundice, dull-yellow eyes and skin, hypochondrial pain, fullness and distension, nausea, vomiting, inability to digest fats, dull-yellow sclera, turbid urine, no thirst, sticky taste, dull headache, feeling of heaviness of the body, thick sticky white tongue coating, either bilateral in two strips or unilateral, Slippery-Wiry pulse.

Treatment

G.B.-24 Riyue, LIV-14 Qimen, Ren-12 Zhongwan, G.B.-34 Yanglingquan, extra point Dannangxue, Du-9 Zhiyang, BL-19 Danshu, BL-20 Pishu, T.B.-6 Zhigou, ST-19 Burong

---

Damp-Heat in the Gall Bladder

Clinical manifestations

Hypochondrial pain, fullness and distension, nausea, vomiting, inability to digest fats, yellow complexion, scanty and dark yellow urine, fever, thirst without desire to drink, bitter taste, dizziness, tinnitus, irritability, feeling of heaviness of the body, numbness of the limbs, swelling of the feet, loose stools or constipation, alternation of hot and cold feeling, yellow sclera, feeling of heat (Fig. 41.4).

Tongue: thick sticky yellow coating, either bilateral in two strips or unilateral.
Pulse: Slippery-Wiry-Rapid.
Key symptoms: hypochondrial fullness, bitter taste and thick sticky yellow coating on the right side.

> **Diagnostic tip**
>
> Hypochondrial fullness, bitter taste and thick sticky yellow coating on the right side are enough to diagnose Damp-Heat in the Gall Bladder.

Aetiology

External pathogenic factors

External Dampness can invade the Gall Bladder and lead to retention of Dampness in this organ. Dampness can then easily combine with Heat. In hot and humid countries, Dampness and Heat invade the body to form Damp-Heat.

Diet

The excessive consumption of greasy fatty foods and of dairy foods is the most common cause of this pattern. In particular, this pattern arises if the person consumes greasy and fried foods.

Emotional strain

This pattern is often caused by feelings of anger over a long period of time, causing stagnation of Liver-Qi and implosion of stagnant Qi into Heat.

Pathology

Dampness in the Gall Bladder causes the typical feeling of fullness in the hypochondrium and a general feeling of heaviness. As Dampness interferes with the smooth flow of Liver-Qi, which stagnates, it may cause hypochondrial distension and pain.

Nausea and vomiting are caused by Dampness obstructing the Middle Burner and preventing Stomach-Qi from descending.

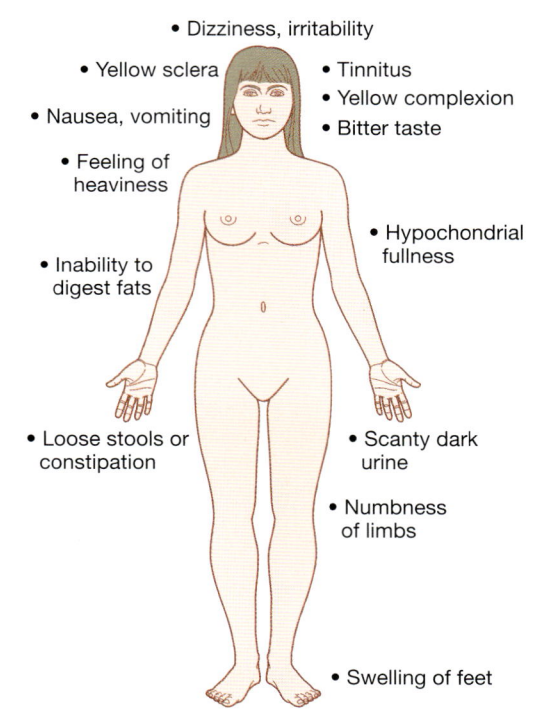

Figure 41.4 Damp-Heat in the Gall Bladder
- Dizziness, irritability
- Yellow sclera
- Nausea, vomiting
- Feeling of heaviness
- Inability to digest fats
- Loose stools or constipation
- Tinnitus
- Yellow complexion
- Bitter taste
- Hypochondrial fullness
- Scanty dark urine
- Numbness of limbs
- Swelling of feet

Dampness is 'sticky' and 'turbid' and therefore turbid urine and a sticky taste reflect Dampness. Dampness may lodge in the head to cause a dull headache.

The unilateral sticky tongue coating is typical of a Gall Bladder pathology.

Bitter taste, fever, dark urine and thirst are all signs of Heat. There is thirst because of the Heat, but no desire to drink because of the presence of Dampness in the Middle Burner.

From a Western point of view, this pattern is often seen in cholelithiasis (stones in the gall bladder). From a Chinese perspective, stones are an extreme form of Dampness and Phlegm in its most substantial state. They are formed over a long period of time from Phlegm under the 'steaming and brewing' action of Heat.

Please note that Chinese books always emphasize Damp-Heat when describing Gall Bladder patterns but many Western patients have Dampness without much Heat.

> **Clinical note**
>
> Gall Bladder stones are an extreme form of Dampness and Phlegm in its most substantial state. They are formed over a long period of time from Phlegm under the 'steaming and brewing' action of Heat

Pathological precursors of pattern

Spleen-Qi deficiency may predispose the patient to Dampness and contribute to the development of this pattern. Liver-Qi stagnation in the Middle Burner may also contribute to the formation of Dampness in the Gall Bladder (Fig. 41.5).

Pathological developments from pattern

Dampness in the Middle Burner obstructs the free flow of Liver-Qi and may lead to Liver-Qi stagnation.

Damp-Heat may lead to Phlegm-Heat (see Fig. 41.5).

Treatment

Principle of treatment: resolve Dampness, clear Heat in Gall Bladder, stimulate the smooth flow of Liver-Qi.

Acupuncture

Points: G.B.-24 Riyue, LIV-14 Qimen, Ren-12 Zhongwan, G.B.-34 Yanglingquan, extra point Dannangxue, Du-9 Zhiyang, BL-19 Danshu, BL-20 Pishu, L.I.-11 Quchi, T.B.-6 Zhigou, ST-19 Burong.

Method: reducing (except on BL-20 which should be reinforced).

Explanation
- G.B.-24 and BL-19 (respectively, Front Collecting and Back Transporting points) clear Heat in Gall Bladder.
- LIV-14 promotes the smooth flow of Liver-Qi.
- Ren-12 and BL-20 resolve Dampness.
- G.B.-34 stimulates the smooth flow of Liver-Qi, resolves Dampness and clears Heat.
- Dannangxue special point (slightly below G.B.-34) has the same functions as G.B.-34 and is only used if it is tender on pressure.
- Du-9 clears Heat in Gall Bladder, stimulates the smooth flow of Liver-Qi and resolves Dampness.
- L.I.-11 clears Heat and resolves Dampness.
- T.B.-6 stimulates the smooth flow of Liver-Qi in the hypochondrium and clears Heat in the Lesser Yang channels.
- ST-19 promotes the descending of Stomach-Qi to relieve obstruction in the Middle Burner and treat nausea and vomiting.

Herbal formula

Yin Chen Hao Tang *Artemisia Capillaris Decoction*.

Box 41.4 summarizes Damp-Heat in the Gall Bladder.

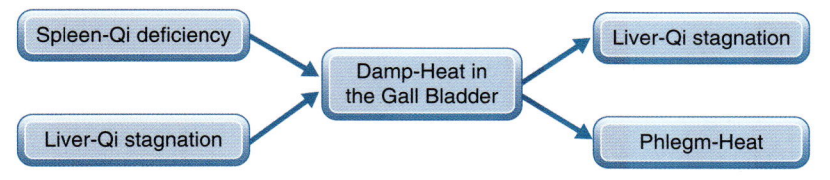

Figure 41.5 Damp-Heat in the Gall Bladder pattern: precursors and developments

Box 41.4 Damp-Heat in the Gall Bladder

Clinical manifestations

Hypochondrial pain, fullness and distension, nausea, vomiting, inability to digest fats, yellow complexion, scanty and dark yellow urine, fever, thirst without desire to drink, bitter taste, dizziness, tinnitus, irritability, feeling of heaviness of the body, numbness of the limbs, swelling of the feet, loose stools or constipation, alternation of hot and cold feeling, yellow sclera, feeling of heat, thick sticky yellow tongue coating, either bilateral in two strips or unilateral, Slippery-Wiry-Rapid pulse

Treatment

G.B.-24 Riyue, LIV-14 Qimen, Ren-12 Zhongwan, G.B.-34 Yanglingquan, extra point Dannangxue, Du-9 Zhiyang, BL-19 Danshu, BL-20 Pishu, L.I.-11 Quchi, T.B.-6 Zhigou, ST-19 Burong

EMPTY PATTERNS

Gall Bladder deficient

Clinical manifestations

Dizziness, blurred vision, floaters, nervousness, timidity, propensity to being easily startled, lack of courage and initiative, indecision, sighing, waking up early in the morning, restless dreams (Fig. 41.6).
Tongue: Pale or normal.
Pulse: Weak.
Key symptoms: timidity, lack of initiative, indecision.

> **Diagnostic tip**
>
> Timidity, lack of initiative and indecision are enough to diagnose Gall Bladder deficient

Aetiology

In this case, there is no 'aetiology' as such as the pattern describes a certain character of the person rather than a set of clinical manifestations. Of course, timidity and lack of courage could also be the result of certain interrelationships within the family during childhood, such as a younger child always 'bullied' by the older brothers or a child who is never encouraged and only reproached. In such a case, one could not 'diagnose' such a pattern of Gall Bladder deficient.

Pathology

More than a 'pattern', this is really the description of a certain character or personality. The key feature of this

- Restless dreams, dizziness
- Blurred vision
- Nervousness, timidity, propensity to be startled, lack of courage, indecision

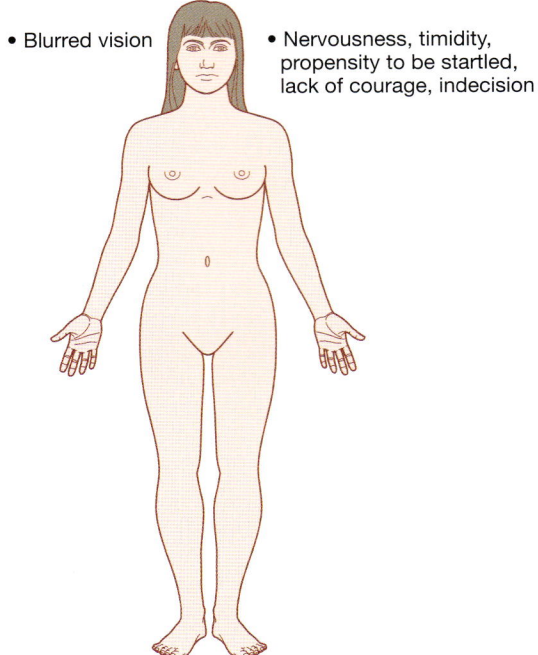

Figure 41.6 Gall Bladder deficient

'pattern' is the character of the person: that is, their lack of courage, timidity and lack of initiative.

The Gall Bladder is the Yang aspect of the Liver, and it is said in Chinese medicine that Liver-Yang can only be in excess, never deficient. However, in this case, this pattern describes a state of deficiency of the Gall Bladder which is usually associated with Liver-Qi deficiency. Although the pattern of Liver-Qi deficiency is not often mentioned, it does exist and its clinical manifestations include some Liver-Blood deficiency symptoms such as dizziness and blurred vision (which are also present in the pattern of Gall Bladder deficient). Essentially, the pattern of Gall Bladder deficient occurs together with that of Liver-Qi deficiency (Fig. 41.7).

In fact, the Gall Bladder represents the Yang aspect of the Liver and, when the Gall Bladder is deficient, Liver-Qi is also deficient, resulting in an indecisive character and depression.

Liver-Qi deficiency usually includes also some Liver-Blood deficiency and this may give rise to fear and lack of courage too (whilst Heat in the Blood may result in

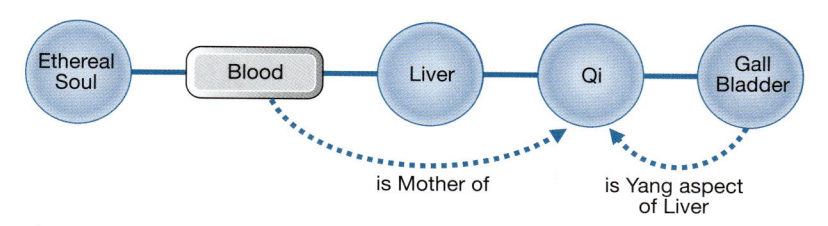

Figure 41.7 Relationship between Liver-Qi and Gall Bladder

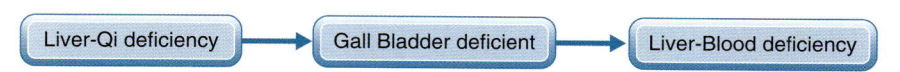

Figure 41.8 Gall Bladder deficient pattern: precursors and developments

anger). Blood is the root of the Ethereal Soul (*Hun*). If Blood is deficient, the Ethereal Soul suffers and this manifests with fear (especially on going to bed at night).

The 'Classic of Categories' (1624) by Zhang Jie Bin says: '*The Liver stores Blood and Blood is the residence of the Ethereal Soul. If the Liver is deficient there is fear, if it is in excess there is anger.*'[1]

Normally, Liver-Blood deficiency gives rise to anxiety and insomnia. However, when it is combined with Liver-Qi deficiency, it gives rise to fear, lack of courage, indecision and often depression. When Liver-Qi is deficient there is not enough 'coming and going' of the Ethereal Soul and the person is timid, shy and depressed (see ch. 7).

Pathological precursors of pattern

Liver-Blood deficiency may cause Liver-Qi deficiency and Gall Bladder deficient (Fig. 41.8).

Pathological developments from pattern

Gall Bladder deficient may give rise to Liver-Blood deficiency (see Fig. 41.8).

Treatment

Principle of treatment: tonify and warm the Gall Bladder and tonify Liver-Qi.

Acupuncture

Points: GB-40 Qiuxu, LIV-8 Ququan, ST-36 Zusanli, SP-6 Sanyinjiao, Ren-4 Guanyuan, BL-18 Ganshu, BL-47 Hunmen.
Method: reinforcing, moxa is applicable.

Explanation
- G.B.-40 is the Source point to tonify the Gall Bladder, and it has a good effect on this particular mental aspect of the Gall Bladder.
- LIV-8, ST-36 and SP-6 tonify Liver-Blood and Liver-Qi.
- Ren-4 tonifies the Liver.
- BL-18 tonifies the Liver and especially Qi and Yang of the Liver.
- BL-47 influences the mental aspect of the Liver and regulates the Ethereal Soul. In this case, it can stimulate its 'coming and going'.

Herbal formula

Wen Dan Tang *Warming the Gall Bladder Decoction*.
An Shen Ding Zhi Wan *Calming the Spirit and Settling the Will-Power Pill*.

NOTE: the formula Wen Dan Tang, originally by Sun Si-Miao, was used for irritability and insomnia deriving from Cold in the Gall Bladder after a severe illness. The original formula omitted Fu Ling and contained Sheng Jiang in a larger dosage (12 g).

Box 41.5 summarizes Gall Bladder deficient.

Box 41.5 Gall Bladder deficient

Clinical manifestations

Dizziness, blurred vision, floaters, nervousness, timidity, propensity to being easily startled, lack of courage and initiative, indecision, sighing, waking up early in the morning, restless dreams, tongue Pale or normal, Weak pulse

Treatment

GB-40 Qiuxu, LIV-8 Ququan, ST-36 Zusanli, SP-6 Sanyinjiao, Ren-4 Guanyuan, BL-18 Ganshu, BL-47 Hunmen

COMBINED PATTERNS

Damp-Heat in the Gall Bladder and Liver

Clinical manifestations

Hypochondrial pain, fullness and distension, nausea, vomiting, inability to digest fats, yellow complexion, scanty and dark yellow urine, fever, thirst without desire to drink, bitter taste, dizziness, yellow sclera, tinnitus, irritability, feeling of heaviness of the body, numbness of the limbs, swelling of the feet, burning on urination, difficulty in urinating, excessive yellow vaginal discharge, loose stools or constipation, alternation of hot and cold feeling, feeling of heat, genital papular skin rashes and itching, swelling and heat of the scrotum (Fig. 41.9).

Tongue: thick sticky yellow coating, either bilateral or only on one side.
Pulse: Slippery-Wiry-Rapid.
Key symptoms: hypochondrial fullness, bitter taste, sticky yellow coating on right side, genital skin rashes and itching.

> **Diagnostic tip**
>
> Hypochondrial fullness, bitter taste, sticky yellow coating on right side, genital skin rashes and itching are enough to diagnose Damp-Heat in the Gall Bladder and Liver

> **Clinical note**
>
> What distinguishes Damp-Heat in the Gall Bladder and Liver from Damp-Heat in the Gall Bladder is the presence of genital symptoms (excessive yellow vaginal discharge, genital papular skin rashes and itching, swelling and heat of the scrotum)

Aetiology

External pathogenic factors

External Dampness can invade the Gall Bladder and Liver and lead to retention of Dampness in these organs. Dampness can then easily combine with Heat. In hot and humid countries, Dampness and Heat invade the body to form Damp-Heat.

Diet

The excessive consumption of greasy fatty foods and of dairy foods is the most common cause of this pattern.

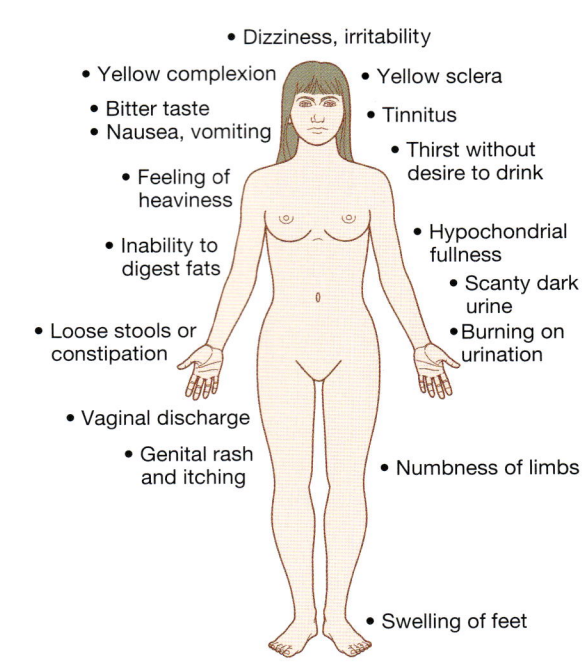

Figure 41.9 Damp-Heat in the Gall Bladder and Liver

In particular, this pattern arises if the person consumes greasy and fried foods.

Emotional strain

This pattern is often caused by feelings of anger over a long period of time, causing stagnation of Liver-Qi and implosion of stagnant Qi into Heat. In case of Damp-Heat in both the Gall Bladder and Liver, emotional strain plays a more important role than it does in Damp-Heat in the Gall Bladder only.

Pathology

The pathology of Damp-Heat in the Gall Bladder has already been discussed above. The involvement of the Liver causes the urinary and genital symptoms: that is, burning on urination, difficulty in urinating, excessive vaginal discharge, genital papular skin rashes and itching, swelling and heat of the scrotum. The involvement of the Liver channels also causes the swelling of the feet.

Pathological precursors of pattern

Damp-Heat in the Gall Bladder is a frequent precursor of this pattern. Long-term stagnation of Liver-Qi,

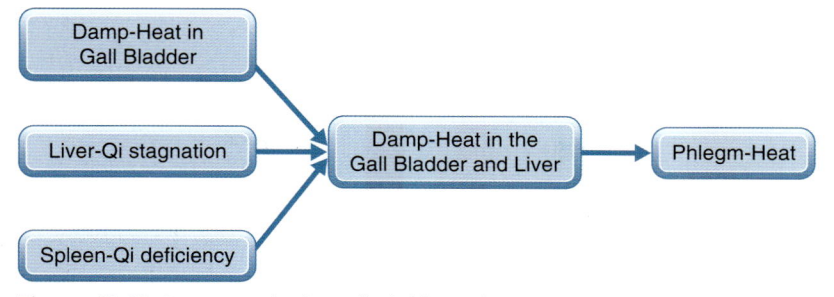

Figure 41.10 Damp-Heat in the Gall Bladder and Liver pattern: precursors and developments

which leads to Dampness and Heat, may also be the precursor of this pattern.

Spleen-Qi deficiency may also be a predisposing factor to this pattern (Fig. 41.10).

Pathological developments from pattern

This pattern may lead to the pattern pathogenic factor Phlegm-Heat (see Fig. 41.10).

Treatment

Principle of treatment: resolve Dampness, clear Heat, clear the Liver and Gall Bladder, and promote the smooth flow of Liver-Qi.

Acupuncture

Points: G.B.-24 Riyue, LIV-14 Qimen, BL-18 Ganshu, Ren-12 Zhongwan, G.B.-34 Yanglingquan, extra point Dannangxue, Du-9 Zhiyang, BL-19 Danshu, BL-20 Pishu, L.I.-11 Quchi, T.B.-6 Zhigou, ST-19 Burong, LIV-3 Taichong, LIV-5 Ligou.

Method: reducing (except BL-20 which should be reinforced), no moxa.

Explanation
– G.B.-24, G.B.-34, Dannangxue, Du-9 and BL-19 resolve Dampness and clear Heat from the Gall Bladder.
– LIV-14 and BL-18 resolve Dampness and clear Heat from the Liver.
– Ren-12 resolves Dampness.
– BL-20 tonifies the Spleen to resolve Dampness.
– L.I.-11 clears Heat.
– T.B.-6 promotes the smooth flow of Liver-Qi in the hypochondrium.
– ST-19 promotes the descending of Stomach-Qi to relieve obstruction in the Middle Burner and treat nausea and vomiting.
– LIV-3 promotes the smooth flow of Liver-Qi.
– LIV-5 promotes the smooth flow of Liver-Qi and resolves Dampness in the urinary and genital areas.

Box 41.6 summarizes Damp-Heat in the Gall Bladder and Liver.

Herbal formula

Long Dan Xie Gan Tang *Gentiana Draining the Liver Decoction*.

Box 41.6 Damp-Heat in the Gall Bladder and Liver

Clinical manifestations

Hypochondrial pain, fullness and distension, nausea, vomiting, inability to digest fats, yellow complexion, scanty and dark yellow urine, fever, thirst without desire to drink, bitter taste, dizziness, yellow sclera, tinnitus, irritability, feeling of heaviness of the body, numbness of the limbs, swelling of the feet, burning on urination, difficulty in urinating, excessive vaginal discharge, loose stools or constipation, alternation of hot and cold feeling, feeling of heat, genital papular skin rashes and itching, swelling and heat of the scrotum, thick sticky yellow tongue coating, either bilateral or only on one side
Pulse: Slippery-Wiry-Rapid.

Treatment

G.B.-24 Riyue, LIV-14 Qimen, BL-18 Ganshu, Ren-12 Zhongwan, G.B.-34 Yanglingquan, extra point Dannangxue, Du-9 Zhiyang, BL-19 Danshu, BL-20 Pishu, L.I.-11 Quchi, T.B.-6 Zhigou, ST-19 Burong, LIV-3 Taichong, LIV-5 Ligou

Learning outcomes

In this chapter you will have learned:
- The importance of the Gall Bladder's function of storing bile
- The close relation of Gall Bladder pathology with that of the Liver
- The susceptibility of the Gall Bladder to be adversely affected by Dampness
- The responsibility of the Gall Bladder on the mental level for courage and decisiveness
- The role of diet (greasy/fatty food), emotional strain (anger) and external Dampness in causing Gall Bladder pathology
- How to identify the following Full patterns:
  Dampness in the Gall Bladder: hypochondrial fullness, feeling of heaviness, unilateral sticky coating
  Damp-Heat in the Gall Bladder: hypochondrial fullness, bitter taste, thick sticky yellow coating on the right side
- How to identify the following Deficiency pattern:
  Gall Bladder deficient: timidity, lack of initiative and indecision
- How to identify the following combined pattern:
  Damp-Heat in the Gall Bladder and Liver: hypochondrial fullness, bitter taste, sticky yellow coating on right side, genital skin rashes and itching

Learning tips

Damp-Heat in the Gall Bladder

- As usual, first write the general symptoms of Heat: feeling of heat, thirst, Red tongue with yellow coating, Rapid pulse
- Then, think of the general symptoms of Dampness: abdominal *fullness*, feeling of *heaviness*, *sticky* tongue coating, *Slippery* pulse
- Remember the area influenced by the Gall Bladder channel, i.e. hypochondrium, hence hypochondrial fullness, distension and pain
- Remember the connection with the Liver channel: irritability
- Finally, remember the important influence of the Gall Bladder channel on the head: dizziness, tinnitus

Self-assessment questions

1. Upon which organ function does the Gall Bladder function of storing and secreting bile depend?
2. Which two aetiological factors can lead to the pattern Dampness in the Gall Bladder?
3. What tongue coating would you expect in the pattern Damp-Heat in the Gall Bladder?
4. Which Western disease is often associated with a diagnosis of Damp-Heat in the Gall Bladder?
5. What is the aetiology of the pattern Gall Bladder deficient?

See p. 1265 for answers

END NOTE

1. Zhang Jie Bin 1982 Classic of Categories (*Lei Jing* 类经), People's Health Publishing House, p. 53. First published in 1624.

SECTION 2 PART 6

Bladder Patterns 42

> **Key contents**
>
> **General aetiology**
> *Exterior pathogenic factors*
> - Cold
> - Dampness
>
> *Emotional strain*
> - Fear
> - Jealousy, suspicion
>
> *Excessive sexual activity*
> *Excessive physical exercise*
>
> **Full patterns**
> *Damp-Heat in the Bladder*
> *Damp-Cold in the Bladder*
>
> **Empty patterns**
> *Bladder Deficient and Cold*
> *Interstitial cystitis*

The function of the Bladder is (ch. 17):

> - It removes water by Qi transformation

The main Bladder function is that of 'Qi transformation': that is, transforming and excreting fluids by the power of Qi. The Bladder receives the Qi for this function from the Kidneys: in disease, therefore, Bladder deficiency often results from Kidney-Yang deficiency. However, the Kidneys do not have Full patterns, so all Full patterns pertaining to the urinary system fall under the category of Bladder patterns. From this point of view, the Bladder patterns are very important, as they fill a gap within the urinary disease patterns.

Physiologically, the Bladder is directly connected to the Small Intestine from which it receives the 'dirty' part of fluids after separation into a dirty and a 'clean' part.

Accumulation of Dampness is the most common pathological factor in Bladder patterns.

Before discussing the Bladder patterns, I shall discuss the general aetiology as follows:

> - General aetiology
>   - Exterior pathogenic factors
>   – Cold
>   – Dampness
>   - Emotional strain
>   – Fear
>   – Jealousy, suspicion
>   - Excessive sexual activity
>   - Excessive physical exercise

GENERAL AETIOLOGY

Exterior pathogenic factors

Climate has an important influence on Bladder conditions. Excessive exposure to cold and damp weather, sitting on damp surfaces or living in damp places can lead to the accumulation of Dampness in the Bladder. This can be manifested as Damp-Cold or Damp-Heat (even if it derives from exterior Cold).

Exposure to Damp-Heat in tropical countries also leads to the accumulation of Damp-Heat in the Bladder directly.

Emotional strain

From an emotional point of view, the Bladder, like the Kidneys, is affected by fear. In particular in children, fear, anxieties or insecurity lead to the sinking of Qi in the Bladder, resulting in nocturnal enuresis.

In adults, Bladder disharmonies are often manifested with feelings of suspicion and jealousy.

Excessive sexual activity

Excessive sexual activity depletes Kidney-Yang and therefore indirectly also the Bladder, as this derives its energy from Kidney-Yang. This can result in frequent and abundant urination, nocturia or incontinence. As explained in the chapter on miscellaneous causes of disease (ch. 22), excessive sexual activity affects men more than women.

Too early sexual activity (in both boys and girls) may injure the Penetrating and Directing Vessels (*Chong* and *Ren Mai*) and cause urinary problems later in life. 'Too early' sexual activity is one that takes place during or even before puberty.

Excessive physical exercise

Excessive physical exercise, especially lifting, may weaken the Bladder and Kidney-Yang and lead to the pattern of Bladder Deficient and Cold.

Box 42.1 summarizes the general aetiology of Bladder patterns.

The patterns discussed below are:

FULL PATTERNS
- Damp-Heat in the Bladder
- Damp-Cold in the Bladder

EMPTY PATTERNS
- Bladder Deficient and Cold

Box 42.2 lists factors giving a 'feel' for Bladder patterns.

Box 42.1 General aetiology of Bladder patterns

- Exterior pathogenic factors
  - Cold
  - Dampness
- Emotional strain
  - Fear
  - Jealousy, suspicion
- Excessive sexual activity
- Excessive physical exercise

Box 42.2 A 'feel' for Bladder patterns

- Urinary problems (discomfort, pain, difficulty, frequency, control)
- Dampness in the Lower Burner (turbid urine, difficulty in urination)
- Sinking of Qi (frequent urination, incontinence)
- Chronic 'cystitis' (often not a real infection but sinking of Qi)
- Thick sticky tongue coating on the root, often with red spots

---

FULL PATTERNS

Damp-Heat in the Bladder

Clinical manifestations

Frequent and urgent urination, burning on urination, difficult urination (stopping in the middle of flow), dark-yellow and/or turbid urine, blood in the urine, fever, thirst with no desire to drink, hypogastric fullness and pain, feeling of heat (Fig. 42.1).

Tongue: thick sticky yellow coating on the root with red spots.
Pulse: Slippery-Rapid and slightly Wiry on the Left-Rear position.
Key symptoms: burning on urination, dark urine, difficult urination.

> **Diagnostic tip**
>
> Burning on urination, dark urine and difficult urination are enough to diagnose Damp-Heat in the Bladder

Aetiology

Exterior pathogenic factors

This pattern can be caused by excessive exposure to Dampness and Cold. Dampness and Cold penetrate the Bladder from below and lead to Dampness in the Bladder, which, in time, can and often does turn into Damp-Heat. Thus, it is important to realize that exterior Cold-Dampness can cause a pattern of Damp-Heat in the Bladder. Indeed, the effect an exterior pathogenic factor has on the body depends also on the person's constitution, and if he or she has a Yang constitution; exterior Dampness can actually give rise to Damp-Heat. In fact, the pattern of Damp-Heat in the Bladder is very common in most countries, including very cold ones.

> **Clinical note**
>
> Exterior Dampness and Cold can and frequently do lead to Damp-Heat in the Bladder

Emotional strain

From an emotional point of view, this pattern can be caused by feelings of suspicion or jealousy bottled up over a long period of time.

- Feeling of heat
- Fever, thirst with no desire to drink
- Feeling of fullness/pain in hypogastrium
- Frequent and urgent urination, difficult burning urination, blood in urine, dark-yellow/turbid urine

Figure 42.1 Damp-Heat in the Bladder

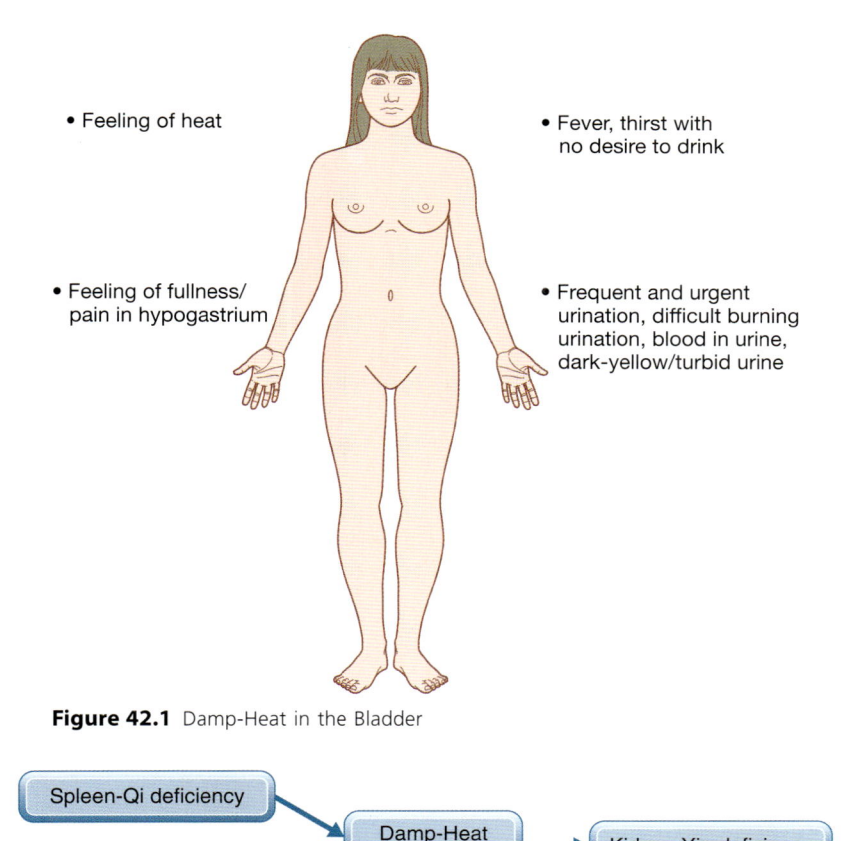

Figure 42.2 Damp-Heat in the Bladder pattern: precursors and developments

Pathology

This pattern is one of interior Full-Heat from the Eight-Principle point of view. It is characterized by the presence of Dampness and Heat in the Bladder.

Dampness obstructs the urinary passages, giving rise to difficult urination, urgent urination and turbid urine. In extreme cases, Dampness can materialize into urinary sand or stones. The sticky tongue coating reflects Dampness.

Heat in the Bladder causes burning on urination, a dark urine, red spots on the root of the tongue and a Rapid pulse.

Pathological precursors of pattern

Dampness in the Bladder (without Heat) frequently turns into Damp-Heat. A deficiency of Spleen-Qi often predisposes the person to the pattern of Dampness in the Bladder. Kidney-Yang deficiency also contributes to the formation of Dampness in the Lower Burner: for this reason, one should not be surprised to see the condition of Damp-Heat in the Bladder (Heat from the Eight-Principle point of view) associated with that of Kidney-Yang deficiency (Empty-Cold from the Eight-Principle point of view) (Fig. 42.2).

Pathological developments from pattern

In chronic conditions, and especially in the elderly, Damp-Heat in the Bladder may lead to Kidney-Yin deficiency (see Fig. 42.2).

Treatment

Principle of treatment: resolve Dampness, clear Heat and open the Water passages of the Lower Burner.

> **Box 42.3 Damp-Heat in the Bladder**
>
> **Clinical manifestations**
>
> Frequent and urgent urination, burning on urination, difficult urination (stopping in the middle of flow), dark-yellow and/or turbid urine, blood in the urine, fever, thirst with no desire to drink, hypogastric fullness and pain, feeling of heat, thick sticky yellow tongue coating on the root with red spots, pulse Slippery-Rapid and slightly Wiry on the Left-Rear position
>
> **Treatment**
>
> SP-9 Yinlingquan, SP-6 Sanyinjiao, BL-22 Sanjiaoshu, BL-28 Pangguangshu, Ren-3 Zhongji, BL-63 Jinmen, BL-66 Tonggu, ST-28 Shuidao.

Acupuncture

Points: SP-9 Yinlingquan, SP-6 Sanyinjiao, BL-22 Sanjiaoshu, BL-28 Pangguangshu, Ren-3 Zhongji, BL-63 Jinmen, BL-66 Tonggu, ST-28 Shuidao.

Method: reducing, no moxa.

Explanation
- SP-9 and SP-6 resolve Dampness from the Lower Burner.
- BL-22 stimulates the transformation of Water in the Lower Burner and opens its Water passages.
- BL-28 is the Back Transporting point of the Bladder and clears Heat from the Bladder.
- Ren-3 is the Front Collecting point of the Bladder and clears Heat from the Bladder.
- BL-63 is the Accumulation point for the Bladder and stops pain on urination, particularly in acute cases.
- BL-66 clears Heat from the Bladder.
- ST-28 promotes the transformation of fluids in the Lower Burner and it therefore contributes to resolving Dampness in the Bladder.

Herbal formula

Ba Zheng San *Eight Upright Powder*.

Box 42.3 summarizes Damp-Heat in the Bladder.

Case history 42.1

A young woman of 30 had been suffering from recurrent and persistent discomfort on urination for 7 years. The problem had started 7 years previously with three acute attacks of burning on urination which were treated with antibiotics even though urine cultures showed no bacterial infections. Ever since then she had been suffering from a constant discomfort in the urethra, sometimes burning on urination, and a sensation of constantly needing to urinate. The colour of the urine varied between dark-yellow and pale. She always felt cold. Her pulse was very Fine, Weak and Deep. Her tongue was Pale, without 'spirit' and with a dirty yellow coating on the root.

The urinary symptoms themselves were obviously due to Damp-Heat obstructing the Bladder (burning on urination, urine sometimes dark, constant discomfort, dirty yellow coating on tongue root). However, this occurred on a background of Kidney-Yang deficiency (very Deep and Fine pulse, very Pale tongue without 'spirit', sometimes pale urine). In treatment, it would be important to clear the Damp-Heat in the Bladder before tonifying and warming Kidney-Yang as a warming method of treatment might aggravate the Damp-Heat of the Bladder.

Case history 42.2

A woman of 73 suffered from persistent burning on urination. The pain was experienced in the urethra and hypogastrium. The urine was dark. Occasionally, there was some hesitancy in urination. Her pulse was Full and Wiry, especially on the Rear position. Her tongue was Deep-Red with a thick sticky yellow coating on the root with red spots on it.

These manifestations indicate retention of Damp-Heat in the Bladder. This is very clearly reflected on the tongue, having a thick yellow coating (indicating Heat) which was sticky (indicating Dampness). The burning on urination was caused by the Heat and the occasional retention of urine by the Dampness obstructing the water passages in the Lower Burner.

Damp-Cold in the Bladder

Clinical manifestations

Frequent and urgent urination, difficult urination (stopping in mid-stream), feeling of heaviness in hypogastrium and urethra, pale and turbid urine (Fig. 42.3).

Tongue: white sticky coating on root.

Pulse: Slippery-Slow and slightly Wiry on Left-Rear position.

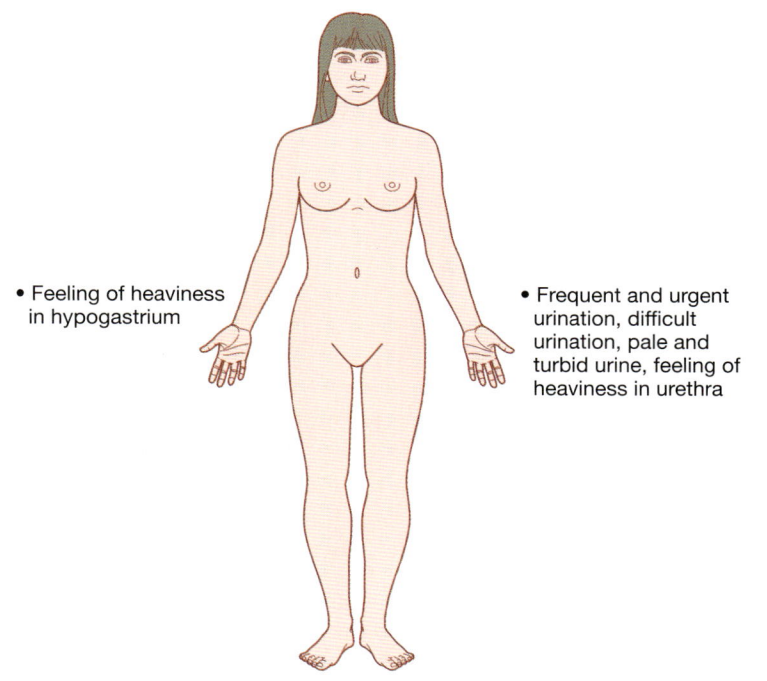

Figure 42.3 Damp-Cold in the Bladder

- Feeling of heaviness in hypogastrium
- Frequent and urgent urination, difficult urination, pale and turbid urine, feeling of heaviness in urethra

Key symptoms: difficult urination, feeling of heaviness, pale turbid urine.

> **Diagnostic tip**
>
> Difficult urination, a feeling of heaviness of the hypogastrium and pale urine are enough to diagnose Damp-Cold in the Bladder

Aetiology

This pattern is caused by excessive exposure to exterior Dampness and Cold.

Pathology

This pattern is characterized by the presence of Dampness and Cold in the Lower Burner. Dampness is heavy, it obstructs the Water passages of the Lower Burner and interferes with the Bladder function of Qi transformation. This causes the urgent and difficult urination and the feeling of heaviness which is typical of Dampness. Dampness is 'dirty' and it causes the urine to be turbid.

The sticky coating and Slippery pulse reflect Dampness.

Pathological precursors of pattern

Spleen-Qi deficiency is often a predisposing factor leading to the formation of Dampness. In urinary problems, Kidney-Yang deficiency is also a frequent predisposing factor leading to the formation of Dampness (Fig. 42.4).

Pathological developments from pattern

Damp-Cold in the Bladder obstructs the Lower Burner and it may lead to Kidney-Yang deficiency (see Fig. 42.4).

Treatment

Principle of treatment: resolve Dampness, expel Cold, and remove obstruction from the Lower Burner's Water passages.

Acupuncture

Points: SP-9 Yinlingquan, SP-6 Sanyinjiao, BL-22 Sanjiaoshu, Ren-3 Zhongji, ST-28 Shuidao, Ren-9 Shuifen, BL-28 Pangguangshu.
Method: reducing, moxa should be used especially if the Cold symptoms are pronounced.

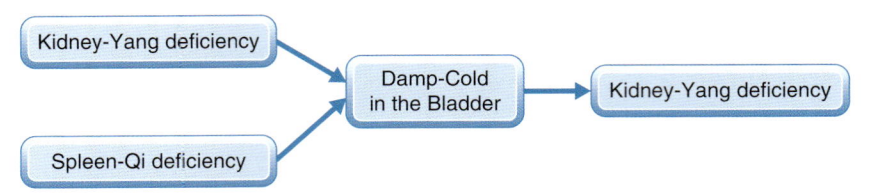

Figure 42.4 Damp-Cold in the Bladder pattern: precursors and developments

Explanation
- SP-9 and SP-6 resolve Dampness from the Lower Burner.
- BL-22 opens the Lower Burner's Water passages.
- Ren-3 and BL-28, Front Collecting and Back Transporting points of the Bladder, respectively, resolve Dampness in the Bladder.
- ST-28 resolves Dampness from the Lower Burner.
- Ren-9 resolves Dampness in general.

Herbal formula

Ba Zheng San *Eight Upright Powder*.
Shi Wei San *Pyrrosia Powder*.

Box 42.4 summarizes Damp-Cold in the Bladder.

Box 42.4 Damp-Cold in the Bladder

Clinical manifestations

Frequent and urgent urination, difficult urination (stopping in mid-stream), feeling of heaviness in hypogastrium and urethra, pale and turbid urine, white sticky tongue coating on root, pulse Slippery-Slow and slightly Wiry on Left-Rear position

Treatment

SP-9 Yinlingquan, SP-6 Sanyinjiao, BL-22 Sanjiaoshu, Ren-3 Zhongji, ST-28 Shuidao, Ren-9 Shuifen, EL-28 Pangguangshu

---

EMPTY PATTERNS

Bladder Deficient and Cold

Clinical manifestations

Frequent pale abundant urination, incontinence, enuresis, lower backache, dizziness, nocturia, white urethral discharge, feeling cold (Fig. 42.5).
Tongue: Pale, wet.
Pulse: Deep-Weak.

Key symptoms: frequent pale abundant urination, Deep-Weak pulse.

> **Diagnostic tip**
>
> Frequent pale and abundant urination and a Deep-Weak pulse are enough to diagnose Bladder Deficient and Cold

Aetiology

Excessive sexual activity

In men, this pattern can be caused by excessive sexual activity that weakens Kidney-Yang. In both men and women, it may also be caused by too early sexual activity (i.e. sexual activity during or even before puberty).

Exterior pathogenic factors

The pattern of Bladder Deficient and Cold can also be caused by excessive exposure to cold or living in cold and damp places. Women are particularly vulnerable to invasion of cold to the Lower Burner, particularly during menstruation.

Excessive physical exercise

Excessive physical exercise and especially lifting may cause the Bladder to become Deficient and Cold.

Pathology

This pattern is similar to those of Kidney-Yang deficiency or Kidney-Qi not Firm but with the emphasis on the pathology of the Bladder rather than Kidneys.

The Bladder derives its Qi from Kidney-Yang to transform fluids and if this is deficient, the Bladder cannot control the fluids which leak out, resulting in frequent abundant and pale urination as well as incontinence, enuresis or nocturia.

Pathological precursors of pattern

Kidney-Yang deficiency is the most frequent pathological precursor of this pattern (Fig. 42.6).

- Dizziness
- Feeling cold
- Lower backache
- Frequent pale abundant urination, incontinence, enuresis, nocturnal urethral discharge

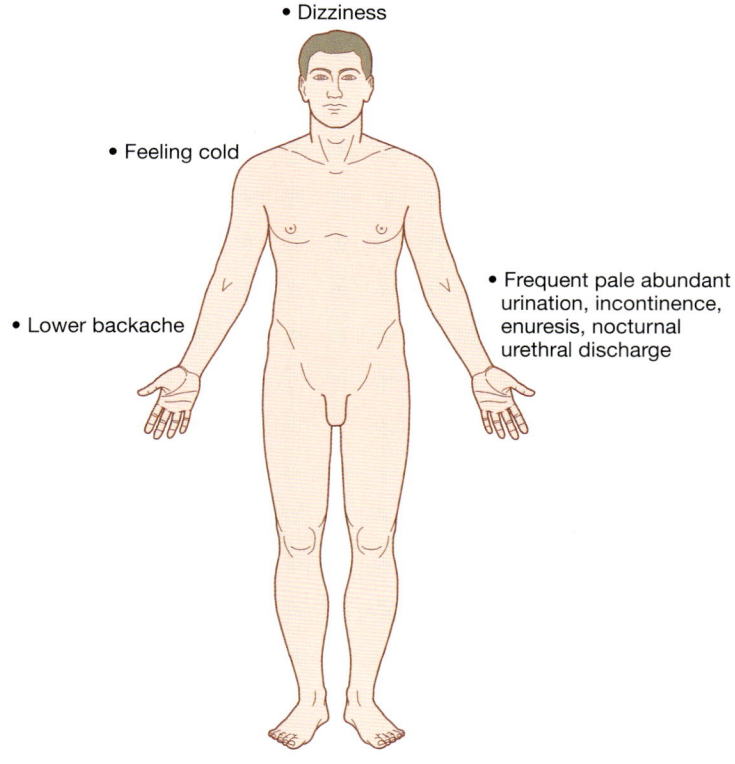

Figure 42.5 Bladder Deficient and Cold

Kidney-Yang deficiency → Bladder Deficient and Cold → Kidney-Yang deficiency

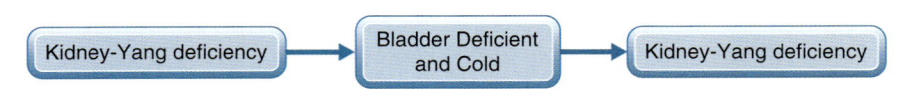

Figure 42.6 Bladder Deficient and Cold pattern: precursors and developments

Pathological developments from pattern

Although Kidney-Yang deficiency may be the precursors of Bladder Deficient and Cold, it may also be the consequence of it (see Fig. 42.6).

Treatment

Principle of treatment: tonify and warm the Bladder and Kidney-Yang.

Acupuncture

Points: BL-23 Shenshu, Du-4 Mingmen, BL-28 Pangguangshu, Ren-4 Guanyuan, Ren-3 Zhongji, Ren-6 Qihai, Du-20 Baihui.
Method: reinforcing, moxa is applicable.

Explanation
- BL-23 and Du-4 with moxa strongly tonify Kidney-Yang and Bladder.
- BL-28 tonifies the Bladder.
- Ren-4 with moxa strengthens Qi and Yang in the Lower Burner.
- Ren-3, Front Collecting point of the Bladder, tonifies the Bladder, Moxa is applicable.
- Ren-6 tonifies Qi in the Lower Burner.
- Du-20 tonifies and lifts Qi and it is particularly indicated if there is enuresis or incontinence.

Herbal formula

Suo Quan Wan *Contracting the Spring Pill*.
Sang Piao Xiao San *Ootheca Mantidis Pill*.

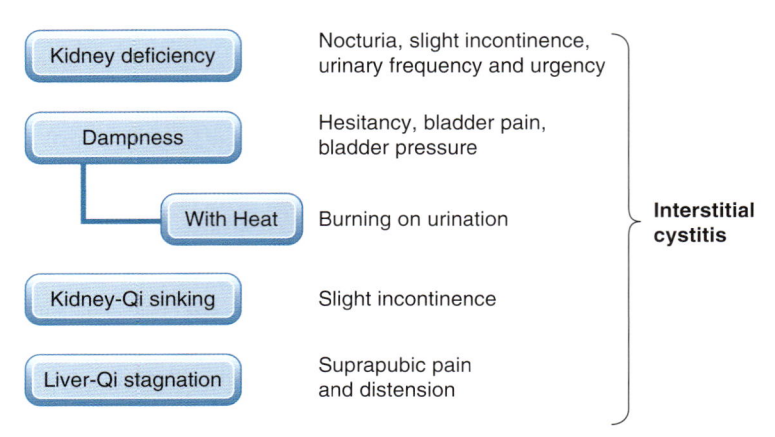

Figure 42.7 Pathology of interstitial cystitis

- Kidney deficiency → Nocturia, slight incontinence, urinary frequency and urgency
- Dampness → Hesitancy, bladder pain, bladder pressure
- With Heat → Burning on urination
- Kidney-Qi sinking → Slight incontinence
- Liver-Qi stagnation → Suprapubic pain and distension

} Interstitial cystitis

Tu Si Zi Wan *Cuscuta Pill*.

Box 42.5 summarizes Bladder Deficient and Cold.

Box 42.5 Bladder Deficient and Cold

Clinical manifestations

Frequent pale and abundant urination, incontinence, enuresis, lower backache, dizziness, nocturia, white urethral discharge, feeling cold, Pale, wet tongue, Deep-Weak pulse

Treatment

BL-23 Shenshu, Du-4 Mingmen, BL-28 Pangguangshu, Ren-4 Guanyuan, Ren-3 Zhongji, Ren-6 Qihai, Du-20 Baihui

---

Interstitial cystitis

Interstitial cystitis is very common, especially in women. The main symptoms are:

- Uncomfortable bladder pressure
- Bladder pain
- Urinary frequency and urgency
- Burning sensation
- Urinary hesitancy
- Suprapubic pain and distension
- Occasionally slight incontinence
- Nocturia

The urine culture is sterile and there is no bacterial infection so antibiotics are ineffective (Fig. 42.7).

From a Chinese perspective, there is usually a Kidney deficiency (nocturia, slight incontinence, urinary frequency and urgency) together with Dampness with or without Heat (uncomfortable bladder pressure, bladder pain, burning sensation, urinary hesitancy).

Often there is also sinking of Kidney-Qi if there is incontinence. In some cases, there may also be Liver-Qi stagnation and this is evidenced by suprapubic pain and distension.

Interestingly, there is usually either significant suprapubic pain with little frequency or a lesser amount of suprapubic pain but with increased urinary frequency. From a Chinese perspective, the former indicates Liver-Qi stagnation and the latter Kidney deficiency.

For interstitial cystitis I usually use variations of Bi Xie Fen Qing Tang *Dioscorea hypoglauca Separating the Clear Decoction*. With acupuncture I use the Directing Vessel (*Ren Mai*) with LU-7 Lieque on the right and KI-6 Zhaohai on the left, plus Ren-3 Zhongji, Du-20 Baihui, SP-9 Yinlingquan, KI-3 Taixi, BL-23 Shenshu and BL-28 Pangguanshu.

Learning outcomes

In this chapter you will have learned:

- The main Bladder function of transforming and excreting fluids
- The concept that the Kidneys do not have Full patterns, and thus all Full patterns of the urinary system are classified as Bladder patterns
- The predisposition of the Bladder to invasion by Dampness, Cold and Damp-Heat
- How fear and anxiety can adversely affect the Bladder
- The association of Bladder disharmonies with feelings of suspicion and jealousy
- How excess sexual activity and excess physical exercise cause Bladder pathology

- How to identify the following Full patterns:
  Damp-Heat in the Bladder: burning on urination, dark urine and difficult urination
  Damp-Cold in the Bladder: difficult urination, feeling of heaviness, pale turbid urine
- How to identify the following Empty pattern:
  Bladder Deficient and Cold: frequent pale abundant urination, Deep-Weak pulse

Learning tips

Damp-Heat in the Bladder

- First, write the general symptoms of Heat: feeling of heat, thirst, Red tongue with yellow coating, Rapid pulse
- Next, think of the general symptoms of Dampness: abdominal *fullness*, feeling of *heaviness*, *sticky* tongue coating, *Slippery* pulse
- Then add the urinary symptoms, remembering that Dampness *obstructs* the urinary passages and causes *turbidity* and Heat concentrates the urine: urinary difficulty and pain, turbid urine, dark urine

Self-assessment questions

1. From which organ does the Bladder receive fluids?
2. How might the Bladder be invaded by Dampness?
3. Why is the pattern of Damp-Heat in the Bladder common even in cold countries?
4. What tongue is associated with the pattern Damp-Heat in the Bladder?
5. What is the pathology of the difficult urination in the pattern Damp-Cold in the Bladder?
6. What is the most frequent pathological precursor to the pattern Bladder Deficient and Cold?

See p. 1265 for answers

SECTION 3

Identification of Patterns according to Pathogenic Factors

INTRODUCTION

Pathogenic factors include external and internal agents of disease. External pathogenic factors are climatic and they include Wind, Cold, Dampness, Dryness, Heat and Fire. Internal pathogenic factors are themselves the result of a disharmony: they then become pathogenic factors. Examples of internal pathogenic factors are Qi stagnation, Blood stasis and Phlegm. In addition, the external climatic pathogenic factors can become internal so that there is corresponding internal pathogenic factor for each external one: for example there is external and internal Dampness.

Section 3 of Part 6 comprises four different methods of identification of patterns:

Chapter 43 Identification of patterns according to pathogenic factors
Chapter 44 Identification of patterns according to the Six Stages
Chapter 45 Identification of patterns according to the Four Levels
Chapter 46 Identification of patterns according to the Three Burners

Identification of patterns according to pathogenic factors

This method of pattern identification is based on the pathological changes occurring when the body is invaded by pathogenic factors such as Wind, Dampness, Cold, Heat, Dryness and Fire. Each of these pathogenic factors may be exterior or interior. This method of identification is discussed in chapter 43.

Identification of patterns according to the Six Stages

This was formulated by Zhang Zhong Jing (born *c.* AD 158) in his 'Discussion on Cold-induced Diseases'. This method of identification is used primarily for the diagnosis and treatment of diseases from exterior Cold, but many of its recommended herbal prescriptions are still used nowadays to treat internal, Hot conditions.

This method of identification has been the bible of Chinese doctors, especially in North China, for about 16 centuries, to be supplanted, especially in South China, by the method of identification of patterns according to the Four Levels and Three Burners. The identification of patterns according to the Six Stages is discussed in chapter 44.

Identification of patterns according to the Four Levels

This was devised by Ye Tian Shi (1667–1746) in his book 'Discussion of Warm Diseases' (*Wen Bing Lun*) and it describes the pathological changes caused by exterior Wind-Heat. It is the most important and most widely used method of identification of patterns for the treatment of febrile infectious diseases that start with invasion of exterior Wind-Heat. I personally find this method of identification of patterns extremely important and useful for the treatment of exterior diseases and their consequences. This method of identification is discussed in chapter 45.

Identification of patterns according to the Three Burners

This was formulated by Wu Ju Tong (1758–1836) in his book 'A Systematic Identification of Febrile Diseases'. This method of identification of patterns is usually combined with the previous one for the diagnosis and treatment of febrile infectious diseases starting with invasion of Wind-Heat. This method of identification is discussed in chapter 46.

Identification of Patterns According to Pathogenic Factors

Pathogenic factors invade the body in various forms: these are Wind, Cold, Dampness, Heat, Dryness and Fire. Each of these can be of exterior or interior origin. They always correspond to a Full pattern according to the Eight Principles. Indeed, from the Eight-Principle point of view, a Full condition is defined as one characterized by the presence of a pathogenic factor while the body's Qi is still relatively intact.

Of course, a pathogenic factor is frequently associated with a Deficiency, in which case the condition is a combined Full–Empty condition. With regard to pathogenic factors, a combined Full–Empty condition can arise in one of two ways: a pathogenic factor can give rise to a Deficiency (e.g. Fire weakens Yin) or a Deficiency can give rise to a pathogenic factor (e.g. Spleen-Qi deficiency gives rise to Dampness).

Generally speaking, pathogenic factors are more relevant as patterns of disharmony than as causes of disease. In chapter 21 they were discussed as causes of disease in relation to climate; we will now discuss them simply as patterns of disease, irrespective of climatic influences.

As was explained previously, the diagnosis of a pathogenic factor is made not on the basis of the patient's history, but on the basis of the pattern of symptoms and signs presented. Of course, when considered as causes of disease, climatic factors have a definite, direct influence on the body and they attack it in a way that corresponds to their nature. For example, a person exposed to a hot, dry climate is likely to develop a pattern of invasion of 'Wind-Dryness'. However, when considered as pathogenic factors, climatic influences are somewhat irrelevant as the diagnosis is made only on the basis of the clinical manifestations. For example, if a person has a runny nose, aversion to cold, sneezing, a headache, a stiff neck, a cough and a Floating pulse, these clinical manifestations denote a pattern of exterior Wind-Cold. It is irrelevant whether this person was exposed to climatic cold or not and it is not usually necessary to ask.

If a patient displays all the symptoms of a particular climatic pathogenic factor (e.g. Wind-Cold), we can diagnose such a pathogenic factor without reference to exposure to that climate (e.g. we do not need to ask whether patient was exposed to wind and cold).

Some internally generated pathogenic factors give rise to similar pathological signs and symptoms as the exterior climatic factors. These will be discussed together with the relevant exterior pathogenic factor.

The pathogenic factors are:

- Wind
- Cold
- Summer-Heat
- Dampness
- Dryness
- Fire

Wind, Summer-Heat, Dryness and Fire are Yang pathogenic factors, which therefore tend to injure Yin. Cold and Dampness are Yin pathogenic factors, which therefore tend to injure Yang. Please note that Dampness is a Yin pathogenic factor even though it may be combined with Heat. Even in such cases, Dampness is obstructive of Yang.

Wind, Cold, Summer-Heat, Dampness and Dryness are seasonal, with the following relationships (the relevant affected organs are in parentheses):

Wind = Spring (Liver)
Cold = Winter (Kidneys)
Summer-Heat = Summer (Heart)
Dampness = Late Summer (Spleen)
Dryness = Autumn (Lungs)

Fire does not have a seasonal association. Of course, the relationship of a particular pathogenic factor with a specific season should not be interpreted too rigidly as each pathogenic factor, though more prevalent in its relevant season, can occur in any season. Summer-Heat is the only pathogenic factor that is strictly seasonal, i.e. it can occur only in the Summer. Also, Summer-Heat is the only pathogenic factor that can be only external: in contrast, all other pathogenic factors can be either externally or internally generated.

Generally Chinese books include also Phlegm and Blood stasis as pathogenic factors. This is because, although Phlegm and Blood stasis are themselves the result of a disharmony, in chronic conditions they become the *cause* of further disharmonies and therefore behave as pathogenic factors. Phlegm and Blood stasis are discussed in chapter 31.

The discussion of the patterns generated by pathogenic factors will be structured under the following headings:

- Wind
  - External Wind
    - Invasion of Wind in the Lung's Defensive Qi portion
      - Wind-Cold
      - Wind-Heat
      - Wind-Dampness
      - Wind-Dryness
      - Wind-Water
    - Invasion of Wind in the channels of the face (facial paralysis)
    - Invasion of Wind in channels and joints (Painful Obstruction Syndrome)
    - Affliction of the Liver channel by external Wind
    - Wind in the skin
  - Internal Wind
- Cold
  - External Cold
    - Invasion of Cold in the Lung's Defensive Qi portion
    - Invasion of channels and joints by Cold (Painful Obstruction Syndrome)
    - Invasion of muscles and sinews by Cold
    - Invasion of external Cold in Stomach, Intestines and Uterus
  - Internal Cold
    - Full-Cold
    - Empty-Cold
- Summer-Heat
- Dampness
  - External Dampness
    - Invasion of Dampness in the Internal Organs
      - External invasion of Dampness in Bladder
      - External invasion of Dampness in Stomach
      - External invasion of Dampness in Intestines
      - External invasion of Dampness in Uterus
      - External invasion of Dampness in Gall Bladder
      - External invasion of Dampness in Spleen
    - Invasion of acute, external Dampness in channels
    - Invasion of external Damp-Heat at Defensive Qi Level
    - External Damp-Heat
    - External Summer-Heat with Dampness
  - Internal Dampness
    Chronic
    - Internal Dampness in Internal Organs
      - Dampness in Stomach and Spleen
      - Dampness in Bladder
      - Dampness in Intestines
      - Dampness in Uterus
      - Dampness in Gall Bladder
      - Dampness in Liver
      - Dampness in Kidneys
    - Chronic Dampness in Channels
    - Internal Dampness in Skin
    Acute
    - Damp-Heat at Qi Level
    - Acute episodes of chronic, internal Dampness
- Dryness
  - External Dryness
  - Internal Dryness
    - Stomach Dryness
    - Lung Dryness
    - Kidney Dryness
- Fire (or Heat)
  - Differences between Heat and Fire
  - General clinical manifestations of Fire
  - Organs affected by Fire
    - Heart
    - Liver
    - Stomach
    - Lungs
    - Intestines
  - Full- versus Empty-Fire
  - Toxic Heat

WIND

Wind is Yang in nature and tends to injure Blood and Yin. Wind is often the vehicle through which other climatic factors invade the body. For example, Cold will often enter the body as Wind-Cold and Heat as Wind-Heat.

The clinical manifestations due to Wind mimic the action of wind itself in Nature: the wind arises quickly and changes rapidly, it moves swiftly, blows intermittently and sways the top of trees. Just as wind in Nature sways the top of trees, Wind causes involuntary movements in the form of tremors or convulsions.

However, Wind can also cause the opposite: that is, paralysis and rigidity. There is a saying that captures this clinical characteristic of Wind: '*Sudden rigidity is due to Wind.*'[1] This refers to the clinical manifestations resulting from both interior and exterior Wind. In fact, interior Wind can cause paralysis (as in Wind-stroke) and exterior Wind can cause facial paralysis or simply stiffness of the neck.

The main clinical manifestations of Wind are:

- Its onset is rapid
- It causes rapid changes in symptoms and signs
- It causes symptoms and signs to move from place to place in the body
- It can cause tremors, convulsions, but also stiffness or paralysis
- It causes numbness and/or tingling
- It affects the top part of the body
- It affects the Lungs first (external Wind)
- It affects the Liver (internal Wind)
- It affects the skin
- It causes itching

These characteristics will be expanded on below.

Wind has a rapid onset

Wind, both exterior and interior, has a rapid onset. For example, an invasion of exterior Wind resulting in a common cold arises quite suddenly; the invasion of Wind in the muscles of the neck results in a stiff neck from one day to the next; Wind-stroke (caused by internal Wind) has a sudden onset.

Wind causes rapid changes

External Wind-Cold may produce quite rapid changes in symptoms from one day to the next or even within a day: this is especially common in children. Another good example of rapid clinical changes are those occurring in skin diseases from Wind.

Wind causes manifestations to move from place to place

The best example of this is the movement of pain from one joint to the other in Wind Painful Obstruction Syndrome (*Bi* Syndrome).

Wind causes convulsions, tremors but also paralysis or stiffness

Wind can produce two opposite manifestations, either involuntary movements, such as tremors, or the lack of movement, for example paralysis or stiffness. All involuntary movements, such as the tremors of Parkinson's disease, tics or convulsions during a febrile disease, are due to internal Wind 'shaking the sinews'.

Wind contracts and can cause the opposite: that is, lack of movement, such as in rigidity, stiffness, paralysis from Wind-stroke or facial paralysis.

Wind causes numbness and/or tingling

Wind often causes numbness and/or tingling, especially unilateral. For example, unilateral numbness of the first three fingers of the hand may herald Wind-stroke. Numbness of the face may be due to invasion of external Wind in the Connecting (*Luo*) channels of the face.

Wind affects the top part of the body

External Wind invading the channels and joints and causing Wind Painful Obstruction Syndrome will typically affect the top part of the body: for example, the neck and shoulders.

Internal Wind may cause headache and vertigo. Skin diseases from Wind will affect the head and hands primarily.

Wind affects the Lungs first (external Wind)

External Wind invading the Exterior of the body affects the Lung's Defensive Qi portion first.

Wind affects the Liver (internal Wind)

Internal Wind always involves a Liver pathology. The symptoms of Wind, such as vertigo, are due to the rising of Liver-Qi to the top of the body. Tremors and convulsions are due to the 'shaking of sinews', which are controlled by the Liver.

Wind affects the skin

Wind can cause a large number of skin diseases characterized by generalized itching, affliction of the top of the body, skin rashes with sudden onset and development.

Wind causes itching

External Wind invasion can cause an itchy throat. Wind in skin diseases is typically characterized by intense itching. Liver-Blood deficiency may give rise to Wind in the skin, causing itching: this is seen, for example, in itching in menopausal women.

All the above manifestations apply to both exterior and interior Wind, except for tremors, convulsions and paralysis, which apply only to interior Wind, and the affliction of the Lungs first, which applies only to external Wind. Only facial paralysis (Bell's palsy) can be caused by exterior Wind.

The subject of Wind will be discussed under the following headings:

> WIND
> - External Wind
>   - Invasion of Wind in the Lung's Defensive Qi portion
>   – Wind-Cold
>   – Wind-Heat
>   – Wind-Dampness
>   – Wind-Dryness
>   – Wind-Water
>   - Invasion of Wind in the channels of the face (facial paralysis)
>   - Invasion of Wind in the channels and joints (Painful Obstruction Syndrome)
>   - Affliction of the Liver channel by external Wind
>   - Wind in the skin
> - Internal Wind

External Wind

External Wind invades the Lung's Defensive Qi portion (the 'Exterior' of the body), causing exterior symptoms such as aversion to cold, fever, occipital stiffness and headache and a Floating pulse. External Wind may be combined with Cold, Heat, Dampness, Dryness and Water.

Exterior Wind can also invade the channels of the face directly and cause deviation of mouth and eyebrows (facial paralysis).

Exterior Wind can also invade any channel, particularly the Yang channels, and settle in the joints, causing stiffness and pain of the joints (Painful Obstruction Syndrome). The pain would typically be 'wandering', moving from one joint to another on different days.

Finally, Wind can also affect some Internal Organs, principally the Liver. Wind pertains to Wood and the Liver according to the Five-Element system of correspondences. This relationship can often be observed when a person prone to migraine headaches is affected by a period of windy weather (particularly an easterly wind) causing a neck ache and headache (Fig. 43.1).

I shall discuss five different types of invasions of external Wind:

> - Invasion of Wind in the Lung's Defensive Qi portion (common cold)
> - Invasion of Wind in the channels of the face (facial paralysis)
> - Invasion of Wind in the channels and joints (Painful Obstruction Syndrome)
> - Affliction of the Liver channel by external Wind
> - Wind in the skin

Invasion of Wind in the Lung's Defensive Qi portion

Exterior Wind penetrates via the skin and interferes with the circulation of Defensive Qi in the space between skin and muscles. Since Defensive Qi warms the muscles, when its circulation is impaired by Wind, the person feels chilly and has aversion to cold. 'Aversion to cold or wind' is a characteristic and essential symptom of invasion of exterior Wind and consists not only of feeling cold and shivering but also of a reluctance to go outside in the cold.

The Lungs control the spreading of Defensive Qi (*Wei Qi*) in the Exterior of the body and also the opening and closing of the pores. The presence of Wind in the space between skin and muscles interferes with the diffusing and descending of Lung-Qi and causes sneezing and possibly coughing. The impairment of the diffusing and descending of Lung-Qi prevents the spreading and descending of Lung fluids, resulting in a runny nose with profuse white discharge.

The fight between the pathogenic Wind and Defensive Qi in the skin and muscles may cause a 'fever' that is not necessarily an actual fever but rather an objective hot feeling of the patient's body on palpation. Wind attacks the most superficial channels first, which are the Greater Yang channels (Small Intestine and

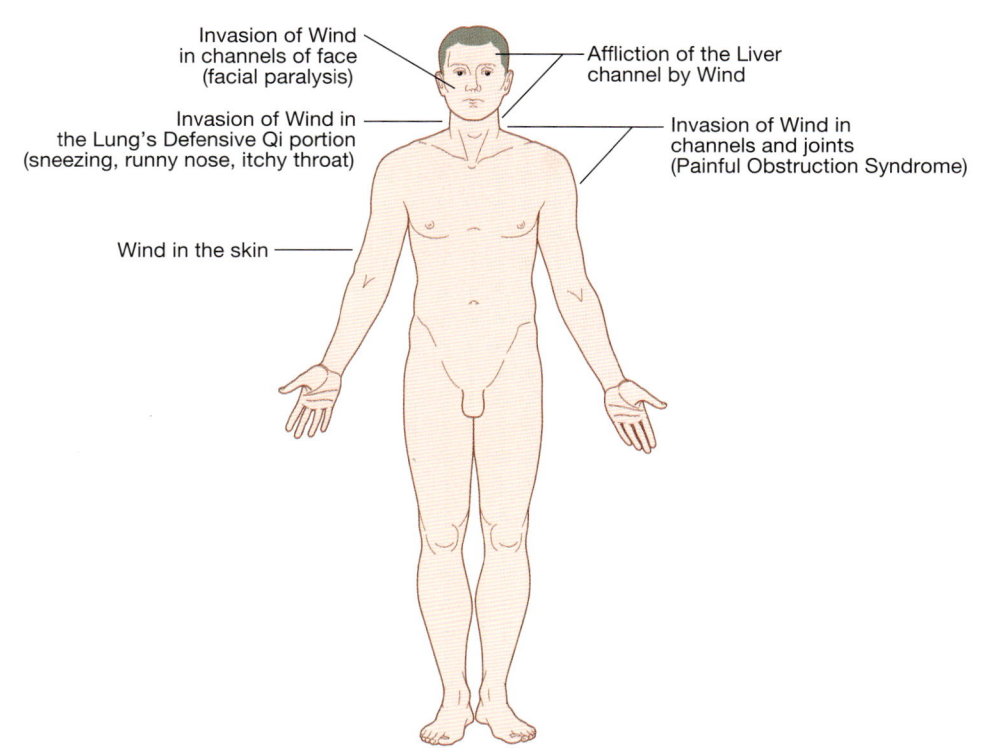

Figure 43.1 Invasions of external Wind

Labels on figure:
- Invasion of Wind in channels of face (facial paralysis)
- Invasion of Wind in the Lung's Defensive Qi portion (sneezing, runny nose, itchy throat)
- Wind in the skin
- Affliction of the Liver channel by Wind
- Invasion of Wind in channels and joints (Painful Obstruction Syndrome)

Bladder), and obstructs the circulation of Defensive Qi within them: this causes stiffness and pain along these channels and particularly in the back of the neck.

Wind attacks the top part of the body and often lodges in the throat, causing an itchy sensation in the throat.

If Wind combines with Cold with a prevalence of the latter, there will be no sweating because Cold contracts the pores. The pulse will be Tight: this corresponds to attack of Cold of the Greater Yang stage within the Six Stages (ch. 44). This is more likely to happen when a person has a relatively strong constitution and a tendency to Excess patterns: then the body's Defensive Qi reacts strongly, the pores will be closed and there will be no sweating. This is an Exterior-Full pattern.

If the Cold is not so prevalent but Wind predominates, the pores are open, the person sweats slightly and the pulse will be slow: this corresponds to the attack of Wind pattern of the Greater Yang stage within the Six Stages (ch. 44). This is more likely to happen to a person with a relatively weak constitution and a tendency to Deficiency patterns: then the Nutritive Qi (*Ying Qi*) is weak, the pores are open and there will be a slight sweating. This is an Exterior-Empty pattern. Please note that although Chinese books describe this pattern as 'Exterior-Empty', they do so only in relation to the invasion of Wind-Cold with the prevalence of Cold that is described as 'Exterior-Full'. But both these patterns are Full patterns from the point of view of the Eight Principles as they are characterized by the presence of a pathogenic factor (Wind).

With the invasion of exterior Wind, Defensive Qi reacts by rushing to the Exterior of the body, and this is reflected on the pulse, which becomes more superficial (Floating pulse).

Thus, to summarize, the symptoms and signs of invasion of exterior Wind are:

- Aversion to cold or wind
- Sneezing, cough
- Runny nose
- 'Fever'
- Occipital stiffness and ache
- Itchy throat
- Sweating or not (depending on whether Wind or Cold is predominant)
- Floating pulse

External Wind combines with other pathogenic factors and primarily Cold, Heat, Dampness and Water. Therefore, I will outline the clinical manifestation of five types of exterior Wind:

- Wind-Cold
- Wind-Heat
- Wind-Dampness
- Wind-Dryness
- Wind-Water

Wind-Cold

Aversion to cold, sneezing, cough, runny nose with white watery mucus, fever, severe occipital stiffness and ache, no sweating, no thirst, Floating-Tight pulse, tongue body colour unchanged, thin white coating.

Explanation

The pathology of invasion of Wind-Cold has already been explained above.

> **Clinical note**
>
> L.I.-4 Hegu, LU-7 Lieque and BL-12 Fengmen (with cupping) are the main points to expel Wind-Cold

Wind-Heat

Aversion to cold, fever, sneezing, cough, runny nose with slightly yellow mucus, occipital stiffness and ache, slight sweating, itchy throat, sore throat, swollen tonsils, thirst, Floating-Rapid pulse, Tongue body colour Red on the tip or sides, thin white coating.

Explanation

The pathology here is the same as in Wind-Cold, except that since Wind is combined with Heat, there are some Heat signs, such as thirst, yellow mucus, more fever, a rapid pulse and a slightly Red tongue body on the tip or sides.

There is aversion to cold in invasions of Wind-Heat because this interferes with the circulation of Defensive Qi in skin and muscles. Since Defensive Qi warms the muscles, an impairment of its circulation leads to aversion to cold in the beginning stages.

The tongue body is Red on the tip or sides because these areas reflect the Exterior of the body, as opposed to the centre of the tongue, which reflects the state of the Interior. The tongue coating is white in the beginning stages as the pathogenic factor is on the Exterior.

> **Clinical note**
>
> L.I.-4 Hegu, LU-7 Lieque, T.B.-5 Waiguan and BL-12 Fengmen (with cupping) are the main points to expel Wind-Heat

Wind-Dampness

Aversion to cold, fever, swollen neck glands, nausea, sweating, occipital stiffness, body aches, muscle ache, feeling of heaviness of the body, swollen joints, Floating-Slippery pulse.

Explanation

This consists in invasion of exterior Wind and Dampness at the beginning stages. Dampness has an obstructive quality: when it obstructs the Connecting channels, it causes swollen glands in the neck; when it obstructs the muscles, it causes muscle ache and feeling of heaviness of the body; when it obstructs the joints, it causes joint ache.

> **Clinical note**
>
> L.I.-4 Hegu, LU-7 Lieque, BL-13 Feishu and Ren-9 Shuifen are the main points to expel Wind-Dampness

Wind-Dryness

Fever, slight aversion to cold, slight sweating, dry skin, nose, mouth and throat, dry cough, sore throat, dry tongue with thin white coating, Floating-Rapid pulse.

Explanation

This is Wind-Heat with Dryness at the Defensive Qi level and, for this reason, there is aversion to cold. Other symptoms are due to Dryness injuring Body Fluids.

The tongue coating is white because the pathogenic factor is on the Exterior.

> **Clinical note**
>
> L.I.-4 Hegu, LU-7 Lieque, LU-9 Taiyuan and BL-12 Fengmen (with cupping) are the main points to expel Wind-Dryness

Wind-Water

Aversion to cold, fever, oedema, especially on the face, swollen face and eyes, cough with profuse white and watery mucus, sweating, no thirst, Floating pulse.

Explanation

In this case, exterior Wind prevents the Lungs from opening the Water passages and diffusing and descending of fluids. Fluids cannot descend, so they overflow under the skin, causing oedema. This would be more prominent in the face as it is caused by a Lung dysfunction which mostly affects the Upper Burner.

The facial oedema that occurs in the beginning stage of acute nephritis would be considered 'Wind-Water'.

Invasion of Wind in the channels of the face (facial paralysis)

As mentioned above, external Wind can invade the body without causing 'exterior symptoms': that is, the aversion to cold and fever that one gets when one catches the common cold or influenza.

In some cases, external Wind can simply invade the channels of the face, causing facial paralysis (Bell's palsy). This is called peripheral facial paralysis in Western medicine (as it involves only the peripheral nerves) to distinguish it from the 'central' facial paralysis caused by a stroke (which involves the central nervous system).

As Wind contracts and stiffens things, an invasion of external Wind in the channels of the face causes facial paralysis: this involves especially the Stomach and Large Intestine channels.

Chinese medicine makes a further distinction in terms of channels affected as, if external Wind affects the main channels of the face, it causes paralysis; if it affects only the Connecting channels of the face, it causes purely numbness.

> **Clinical note**
>
> L.I.-4 Hegu and T.B.-5 Waiguan are the main distal points to use for facial paralysis while ST-7 Xiaguan is the main local point

Invasion of Wind in the channels and joints (Painful Obstruction Syndrome)

Another example of invasion of external Wind without exterior symptoms is that which occurs when external Wind invades the channels and settles in the joints: this is called Painful Obstruction Syndrome (*Bi* Syndrome).

Painful Obstruction Syndrome is usually caused by invasion of Wind, Dampness or Cold but Wind is always present as it acts as a 'spearhead' for Dampness and Cold to invade the joints.

When Wind is the main cause of Painful Obstruction Syndrome, the joint pain is typically 'wandering' (it moves from joint to joint).

Affliction of the Liver channel by external Wind

External Wind may invade the Liver channel in the neck and head, causing a stiff neck (as it also affects the Gall Bladder channel). External Wind may also aggravate a condition of Liver-Yang rising and precipitate a headache: migraine sufferers (when this is caused by Liver-Yang rising) often report that a migraine attack may be precipitated by windy weather.

> **Clinical note**
>
> S.I.-3 Houxi, LIV-3 Taichong, Du-16 Fengfu and G.B.-20 Fengchi are the main points to expel external Wind in the Liver channel

Wind in the skin

Finally, Wind in the skin plays a major role in skin diseases: it is a special type of Wind that is neither external nor internal, or both at the same time. However, it is best categorized and discussed under external Wind. Wind in the skin may be seen as a type of external Wind in so far as many skin diseases may be caused or aggravated by external wind. On the other hand, Wind in the skin may be seen as a type of internal Wind as it may sometimes originate from a Liver disharmony: for example, Liver-Fire or Liver-Blood deficiency.

Box 43.1 summarizes external Wind invasions.

The chief characteristics of Wind in the skin are:

- Intense generalized itching
- Skin rashes that appear suddenly and spread rapidly
- Small, red papules, especially in the top part of the body

> **Clinical note**
>
> L.I.-4 Hegu, L.I.-11 Quchi, T.B.-6 Zhigou, SP-10 Xuehai and BL-12 Fengmen (with cupping) are the main points to expel Wind in the skin

Box 43.1 External Wind invasions

- Invasion of Wind in the Lung's Defensive Qi portion (common cold)
- Invasion of Wind in the channels of the face (facial paralysis)
- Invasion of Wind in the channels and joints (Painful Obstruction Syndrome)
- Affliction of the Liver channel by external Wind (e.g. Liver-Yang headache elicited by external Wind)
- Wind in the skin

Internal Wind

Although some of the clinical manifestations are the same, internal Wind arises from completely different causes than external Wind. Many of its manifestations are also different.

The main clinical manifestations of interior Wind are: tremors, tics, severe dizziness, vertigo and numbness. In severe cases, they are: convulsions, unconsciousness, opisthotonos, hemiplegia and deviation of mouth.

Clinical note

LIV-3 Taichong, Du-16 Fengfu and G.B.-20 Fengchi are the main points to extinguish internal Wind. Other points depend on the underlying condition

Interior Wind is always related to a Liver disharmony. It can arise from several different conditions:

- Extreme Heat can give rise to Liver-Wind. This happens in the late stages of febrile diseases when the Heat enters the Blood portion and generates Wind. This process is like the wind generated by a large forest fire. The clinical manifestations are a high fever, delirium, convulsions, coma and opisthotonos. These signs are frequently seen in meningitis and are due to Wind in the Liver and Heat in the Pericardium.
- Liver-Yang rising can give rise to Liver-Wind in prolonged cases. The clinical manifestations are severe dizziness, vertigo, headache, tremors, tics and irritability.
- Liver-Fire can give rise to Liver-Wind.
- Deficiency of Liver-Blood and/or Liver-Yin can give rise to Liver-Wind. This is due to the deficiency of Blood creating an empty space within the blood vessels which is taken up by interior Wind. This could be compared to the draughts generated sometimes in certain underground (subway) stations. The clinical manifestations are numbness, dizziness, blurred vision, tics and slight tremors (in Chinese called 'chicken feet Wind' as the tremors are like the jerky movements of chicken feet when they scour the ground for food).
- Deficiency of Kidney- and Liver-Yin may also give rise to internal Wind. This is more common in the elderly. The clinical manifestations are dizziness, vertigo, slight tremors.

The patterns caused by internal Wind of the Liver are discussed in greater detail in chapter 34. Box 43.2 summarizes internal Wind.

Box 43.2 Internal Wind

- Extreme Heat (febrile disease)
- Liver-Yang rising
- Liver-Fire
- Liver-Blood and/or Liver-Yin deficiency
- Liver- and Kidney-Yin deficiency

COLD

Cold is a Yin pathogenic factor and, as such, it tends to injure Yang. Cold pertains to Winter but it may invade the body at any time of year. It injures especially the Kidneys. Chapter 74 of the 'Simple Questions' says: 'Cold contracts and it pertains to the Kidneys.'[2]

Cold can be exterior or interior and Full or Empty. Exterior Cold is by definition Full, while interior Cold can be Full or Empty. Interior Full-Cold derives from the invasion of exterior Cold: once it is in the Interior and in the Internal Organs, Cold is interior. Interior Empty-Cold can be formed in one of two ways: either it derives from interior Full-Cold (because after some time Full-Cold damages Yang and therefore becomes Empty-Cold), or it derives from a Yang deficiency (of the Spleen and/or Kidneys) (Figs 43.2 and 43.3).

We can identify five main characteristics of Cold.

Cold injures Yang

Cold, whether exterior or interior, tends to injure Yang: the Spleen and the Kidneys are usually the first organs to be affected by Cold.

Cold congeals Blood

Cold congeals Blood and it is therefore a major cause of Blood stasis. When Blood stagnates, there is intense pain: when the stasis derives from Cold, the pain is accompanied by chilliness, it is aggravated by cold and it is alleviated by the application of heat. Invasion of Cold in the Uterus causing Blood stasis in this organ is a very common example of Cold congealing Blood: it results in painful periods with small, dark clots.

Chapter 39 of the 'Simple Questions' says: '*When Cold invades the channels it retards circulation; outside the channels, it decreases Blood [circulation], inside the channels it impairs the movement of Qi and this results in*

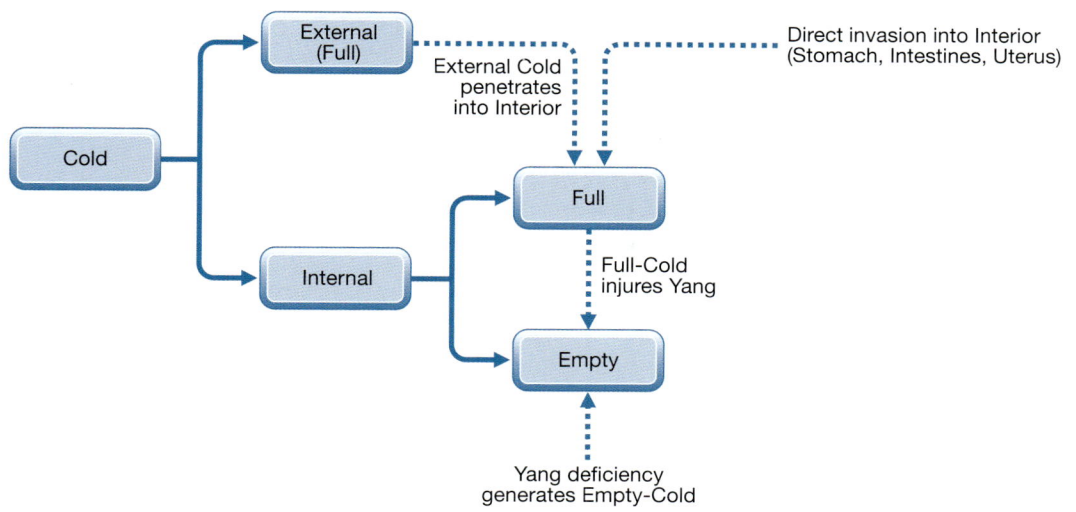

Figure 43.2 External and internal Cold

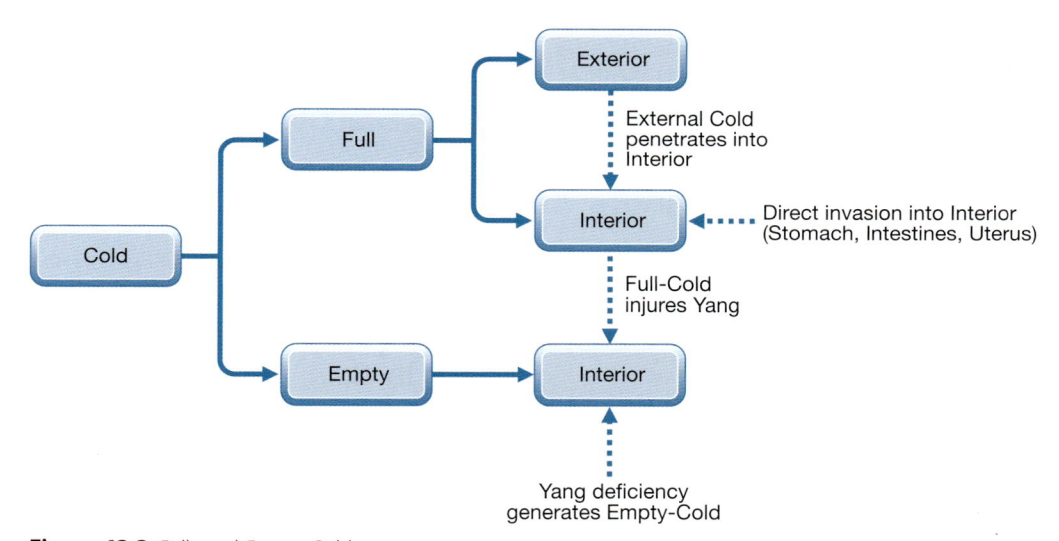

Figure 43.3 Full- and Empty-Cold

pain.'[3] Chapter 43 of the 'Simple Questions' says: 'Cold causes pain.'[4]

> **Clinical note**
>
> Blood stasis deriving from Cold is a very common cause of painful periods in women.

Cold contracts

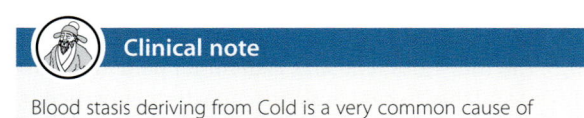

Cold contracts tissues (muscles, sinews, blood vessels, skin). Chapter 39 of the 'Simple Questions' says: '*Cold causes contraction.*'[5] Contraction causes pain and, this, together with Blood stasis discussed above, is another cause of pain from Cold.

For this reason, there is a saying that states '*Retention of Cold causes pain*'.[6]

As cold causes contraction, contraction of muscles and sinews by Cold causes stiffness and pain.

Cold causes clear discharges

Cold is often manifested with thin, watery and clear fluid discharges, such as a clear white discharge from the nose, very pale urine, watery loose stools and clear

> **Box 43.3 Characteristics of Cold**
>
> - Cold is Yin and it injures Yang
> - Cold congeals (Blood)
> - Cold contracts
> - Cold causes clear discharges
> - Cold pertains to the Kidneys

watery vaginal discharges. Another saying clarifies this characteristic of Cold: 'A disease characterized by thin, clear, watery and cool discharges is due to Cold.'[7]

Cold pertains to the Kidneys

In the scheme of correspondences among organs, seasons and climates, Cold pertains to Winter and to the Kidneys. This means that Cold is obviously more prevalent in Winter and that it has a strong tendency to injure the Kidneys (specifically Kidney-Yang). However, it should be pointed out that Cold can occur in any season and that it injures other organs besides the Kidneys (Spleen, Stomach, Heart, Intestines, Uterus).

Box 43.3 summarizes the characteristics of Cold.

The general clinical manifestations of Cold (without distinguishing between Full- or Empty-Cold) are:

- Feeling cold
- Cold limbs
- Thin clear discharges
- Pain (of a spastic or crampy nature)
- Aggravation from cold and alleviation from application of heat
- Desire for warm drinks
- No thirst
- White complexion
- White tongue coating
- Pale tongue body
- Slow pulse

The discussion of Cold will be presented under the following headings:

- External Cold
  - Invasion of Cold in the Lung's Defensive Qi portion
  - Invasion of the channels and joints by Cold (Painful Obstruction Syndrome)
  - Invasion of the muscles and sinews by Cold
  - Invasion of external Cold in Stomach, Intestines and Uterus
- Internal Cold
  - Full-Cold
  - Empty-Cold

External Cold

We can identify four main types of invasion of external Cold (Fig. 43.4):

> 1. Cold, spearheaded by Wind, can invade the Exterior of the body and give rise to symptoms of Wind-Cold, already described above
> 2. Cold can invade the channels and joints directly (without exterior symptoms) and cause Painful Obstruction Syndrome (*Bi* Syndrome), with pain that is often (but not exclusively) in one joint
> 3. Cold can invade the muscles and sinews causing local pain and stiffness
> 4. Cold can invade three organs directly, i.e. the Stomach, Intestines and Uterus

Invasion of Cold in the Lung's Defensive Qi portion

This corresponds to an invasion of Wind-Cold, which has already been discussed above.

Invasion of the channels and joints by Cold (Painful Obstruction Syndrome)

When Cold invades the channels and settles in the joints it causes Cold Painful Obstruction Syndrome (*Bi* Syndrome). This is characterized by intense pain, often in a single joint. The pain is aggravated by exposure to cold and alleviated by the application of heat.

Invasion of the muscles and sinews by Cold

External Cold can invade the muscles and sinews, causing local pain and stiffness. This is a very common occurrence in the muscles of the shoulders and neck. For example, a very stiff, locked neck with a sudden onset is often due to Cold in the muscles of the neck.

Invasion of external Cold in Stomach, Intestines and Uterus

External Cold can invade three organs directly: these are the Stomach (causing epigastric pain and vomiting), the Intestines (causing abdominal pain and diarrhoea) and the Uterus (causing acute dysmenorrhoea). In all these three cases the symptoms are accompanied by chilliness and the pain is aggravated by cold and alleviated by the application of heat.

Please note that although this Cold is of external *origin*, once in these three organs, it is internal Cold.

Box 43.4 summarizes external Cold invasions.

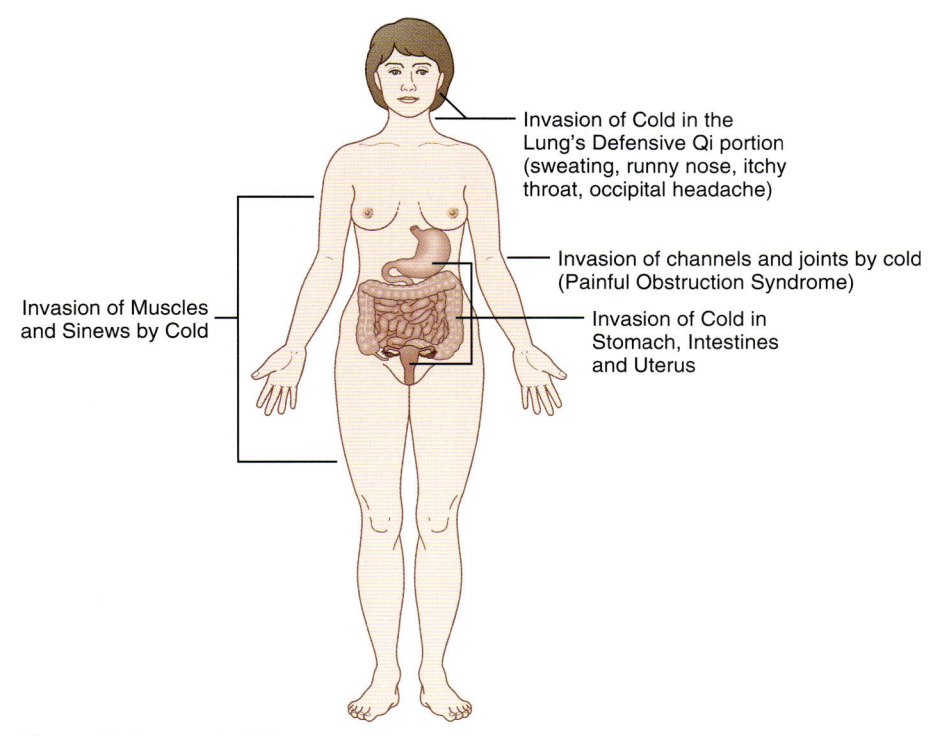

Figure 43.4 External Cold

Labels on figure:
- Invasion of Cold in the Lung's Defensive Qi portion (sweating, runny nose, itchy throat, occipital headache)
- Invasion of channels and joints by cold (Painful Obstruction Syndrome)
- Invasion of Cold in Stomach, Intestines and Uterus
- Invasion of Muscles and Sinews by Cold

Box 43.4 External Cold invasions

- External Cold (with Wind) invasion in the Lung's Defensive Qi portion (common cold)
- Invasion of Cold in the channels and joints (Painful Obstruction Syndrome)
- Invasion of Cold in muscles and sinews (muscle soreness and stiffness)
- Invasion of external Cold in organs directly (Stomach, Intestine and Uterus)
  - Stomach: vomiting and epigastric pain
  - Intestines: diarrhoea and abdominal pain
  - Uterus: acute dysmenorrhoea

Internal Cold

Internal Cold can be Full or Empty (see ch. 30 on the Eight Principles). Interior Full-Cold originates from external Cold, which may be either Wind-Cold or Cold invading certain organs directly. These cases have just been mentioned. In both cases, if the exterior Cold penetrates in the Interior and in the Internal Organs, it becomes interior Full-Cold (Fig. 43.5).

The other two types of invasion of external Cold, i.e. Cold invading channels and joints (Painful Obstruction Syndrome) and Cold invading muscles and sinews, tend to remain external.

Full-Cold

The main clinical manifestations of Full-Cold are:

- Feeling cold
- Cold limbs
- Thin clear discharges
- Severe pain
- Aggravation of pain from pressure
- Aggravation from cold and alleviation from application of heat
- Desire for warm drinks
- No thirst
- Bright white complexion
- Thick, white tongue coating
- Slow-Full-Tight pulse

Generally speaking, interior Full-Cold can last only a relatively short time. After prolonged retention, interior Cold consumes Yang (often of the Spleen first), giving rise to Empty-Cold. Thus a Full-Cold pattern can turn into an Empty-Cold one.

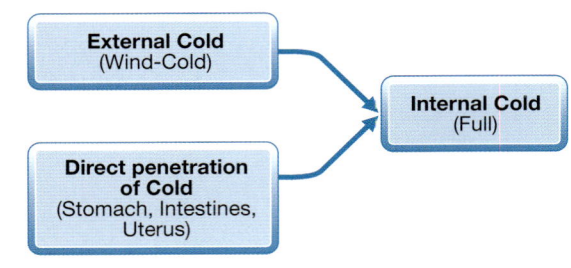

Figure 43.5 Origin of internal Cold

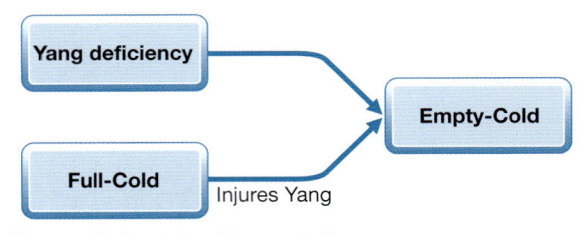

Figure 43.6 Origin of Empty-Cold

The clinical manifestations of Full- and Empty-Cold are very similar as they are the same in nature. The main difference is that Full-Cold is characterized by an acute onset, severe pain and a tongue and pulse of the Excess type: for example, the tongue has a thick white coating and the pulse is Full and Tight.

Empty-Cold

The main clinical manifestations of Empty-Cold are:

- Feeling cold
- Cold limbs
- Thin clear discharges
- Dull pain
- Amelioration of pain from pressure
- Aggravation from cold and alleviation from application of heat
- Desire for warm drinks
- No thirst
- Dull white complexion
- Thin, white tongue coating
- Pale tongue body
- Slow-Weak pulse

Internal Empty-Cold arises from deficiency of Yang, usually of the Spleen, Lungs or Kidneys. In this case the Cold does not come from the exterior, but is interiorly generated by deficiency of Yang (Fig. 43.6).

As mentioned above, Empty-Cold may also derive from the transformation of Full-Cold: in fact, Full-Cold cannot last a long time as Cold injures Yang and therefore after some time it will induce a Yang deficiency. When that happens, Full-Cold changes into Empty-Cold.

Apart from the general manifestations outlined above, other symptoms vary according to which organ is mostly affected. The Heart, Lungs, Spleen, Stomach and Kidneys can suffer from deficiency of Yang and interior Cold.

Table 43.1 Differentiation between Full- and Empty-Cold

	Full-Cold	Empty-Cold
Onset	Acute	Chronic
Pain	Intense, crampy	Dull
Tongue	Thick white coating	Thin white coating, Pale body
Pulse	Full-Tight-Slow	Weak-Deep-Slow

The symptoms of Heart-Yang deficiency (in addition to the above-mentioned general symptoms) with interior Cold are stuffiness and pain in the chest, purple lips and a Knotted pulse.

In Lung-Qi deficiency they are a propensity to catch colds and a cough with white mucus.

In Spleen-Yang deficiency they are diarrhoea or loose stools with some abdominal pain.

In Kidney-Yang deficiency they are frequent, pale and profuse urination, lower backache, cold feet and knees and impotence in men or white leucorrhoea in women.

The manifestations of Yang deficiency of the various organs have been discussed in the chapters on the identification of patterns according to the Internal Organs.

Table 43.1 lists the clinical manifestations of Full- and Empty-Cold.

SUMMER-HEAT

Summer-Heat is a Yang pathogenic factor and, as such, it tends to injure Yin. This pathogenic factor is different from the others in two ways: first, it is definitely related to a specific season since it can only occur in the Summer; secondly, it can be only an external pathogenic factor with no internal equivalent.

The clinical manifestations of Summer-Heat are:

- Fever
- Aversion to cold
- Sweating
- Headache
- A feeling of heaviness
- An uncomfortable sensation in the epigastrium
- Irritability
- Thirst
- Tongue Red in the front or sides with a white sticky coating
- Soggy and Rapid pulse

Summer-Heat invades the Defensive Qi portion of the body (i.e. the Exterior) and that is why there is aversion to cold (even though the exterior Heat is intense). However, it has the strong tendency to move to the Qi level almost from the beginning and that is why there are symptoms of interior Heat such as irritability, thirst, Red tongue and Rapid pulse.

Summer-Heat frequently combines with Dampness and that is why there is a feeling of heaviness and uncomfortable sensation of the epigastrium, a sticky tongue coating and a Soggy pulse. The tongue coating is white because the pathogenic factor is on the Exterior.

To summarize, Summer-Heat includes manifestations of external Wind, Dampness and interior Heat.

In severe cases, Summer-Heat can invade the Pericardium and cause clouding of the mind, manifesting with delirium or unconsciousness.

The characteristics of Summer-Heat may be summarized as follows.

Summer-Heat injures Yin

Summer-Heat is a Yang pathogenic factor and therefore it has a strong tendency to injure Yin (i.e. to injure fluids).

Summer-Heat is a seasonal pathogenic factor

Summer-Heat can occur only in the Summer and it can be only external (i.e. contrary to other external pathogenic factors, there is no internal equivalent).

Summer-Heat invades the top of the body

Summer-Heat invades the top of the body and for this reason there is a headache.

Summer-Heat is scattering

The scattering nature of Summer-Heat causes sweating.

Summer-Heat has some interior Heat

Summer-Heat has a tendency to move into the Interior very quickly and, for this reason, there are some symptoms of interior Heat such as irritability and thirst.

Summer-Heat harbours Dampness

Summer-Heat often harbours Dampness and, for this reason, there is a feeling of heaviness and an uncomfortable sensation of the epigastrium.

Box 43.5 summarizes the characteristics of Summer-Heat.

Box 43.5 Characteristics of Summer-Heat

- Summer-Heat injures Yin
- Summer-Heat is a seasonal pathogenic factor
- Summer-Heat invades the top of the body
- Summer-Heat is scattering
- Summer-Heat has some interior Heat
- Summer-Heat harbours Dampness

DAMPNESS

Dampness is a Yin pathogenic factor and it tends to injure Yang. Climatic Dampness refers not only to damp weather but also to living conditions such as living in a damp house, wearing wet clothes, wading in water, working in damp places or sitting on damp ground.

The characteristics of Dampness are that it is sticky, it is difficult to get rid of, it is heavy, it slows things down, it infuses downwards and it causes repeated attacks. When exterior Dampness invades the body, it tends to invade the lower part first, typically the legs. From the legs, it can flow upwards in the leg channels to settle in any of the pelvic cavity organs. If it settles in the female genital system it causes vaginal discharges, if it settles in the Intestines it will cause loose stools and if it settles in the Bladder it will cause difficulty, frequency and burning of urination.

The 'Simple Questions' in chapter 29 says: *'Wind is a Yang pathogenic factor, Dampness is a Yin pathogenic factor; in invasions of Wind the top part of the body is affected first, in invasions of Dampness the lower part of the body is affected first.'*[8]

> **Box 43.6 General Dampness manifestations**
>
> - Feeling of heaviness
> - Poor appetite
> - Feeling of fullness
> - Sticky taste
> - Urinary difficulty
> - Vaginal discharge
> - Sticky tongue coating
> - Slippery or Soggy pulse

> **Box 43.7 Qualities of Dampness**
>
> - Heaviness
> - Dirtiness
> - Stickiness

The clinical manifestations of Dampness are extremely varied according to its location and nature (hot or cold), but the general ones are a feeling of heaviness of body or head, no appetite, a feeling of fullness of the chest or epigastrium, a sticky taste, urinary difficulty, a white sticky vaginal discharge, a sticky tongue coating and a Slippery or Soggy pulse.

Box 43.6 summarizes the general manifestations of Dampness.

The various clinical manifestations can be correlated to the main characteristics of Dampness as follows.

Dampness is heavy

Dampness is naturally 'heavy': this weighs the body down and causes a feeling of tiredness, heaviness of limbs or head, or a 'muzzy' ('fuzzy') feeling of the head. Since Dampness is heavy, it causes a feeling of fullness and oppression of the chest, epigastrium or abdomen and it tends to settle in the Lower Burner. However, Dampness often affects the head too, causing the above-mentioned symptoms. This happens because it prevents the clear Yang from ascending to the head to brighten the sense orifices and clear the brain.

Dampness is dirty

Dampness is 'dirty' and is reflected in dirty discharges, such as cloudy urine, vaginal discharges or skin diseases characterized by thick and dirty fluids oozing out, such as in certain types of eczema.

Dampness is sticky

Dampness is 'sticky' and this is reflected in a sticky tongue coating, sticky taste and Slippery pulse. The sticky nature of Dampness also accounts for its being very difficult to get rid of. It often becomes chronic, manifesting in frequent, recurrent bouts.

Box 43.7 summarizes the qualities of Dampness.

The clinical manifestations of Dampness can be classified according to its location as follows (Fig. 43.7):

Head: feeling of heaviness and muzziness (fuzziness) of the head
Eyes: red and swollen eyelids, eyes oozing fluid, styes
Mouth: mouth ulcers on gums, swollen red lips
Stomach and Spleen: feeling of fullness of epigastrium, feeling of fullness after eating, sticky taste, loose stools, poor appetite, Soggy pulse
Lower Burner: excessive vaginal discharge, painful periods, infertility, turbid urine, difficult and painful urination, scrotal sweating or eczema, genital eczema, genital itching
Skin: vesicles (Dampness without Heat), papules (Damp-Heat with more Heat), greasy sweat, any oozing skin lesion
Joints: swollen and painful joints (Fixed Painful Obstruction Syndrome from Dampness or also Wandering Painful Obstruction Syndrome if Dampness is mixed with Wind)
Connecting (Luo) channels: numbness and loss of sensation

Dampness can cause a large variety of diseases according to its location which, without distinguishing internal from external Dampness, can be summarized in three locations:

1. Internal organs
2. Channels
3. Skin

The range of diseases according to the location of Dampness is as follows:

Internal Organs

- Stomach and Spleen (epigastric pain and fullness, poor digestion, feeling of fullness, a sticky taste, poor appetite)
- Gall Bladder (hypochondrial fullness and pain)
- Bladder (difficult and painful urination, cloudy urine)
- Uterus (infertility, excessive vaginal discharge, mid-cycle pain and/or bleeding)
- Intestines (loose stools with mucus, abdominal fullness and pain)
- Kidneys (cloudy urine, difficult urination)
- Liver (hypochondrial fullness, distension and pain, jaundice)

Channels

- In the joints (Damp Painful Obstruction Syndrome, achy and swollen joints)
- In the head (feeling of heaviness of the head, dull frontal headache)

Skin

- Dampness is the cause of many skin diseases manifesting with oozing skin lesions, vesicles or papules

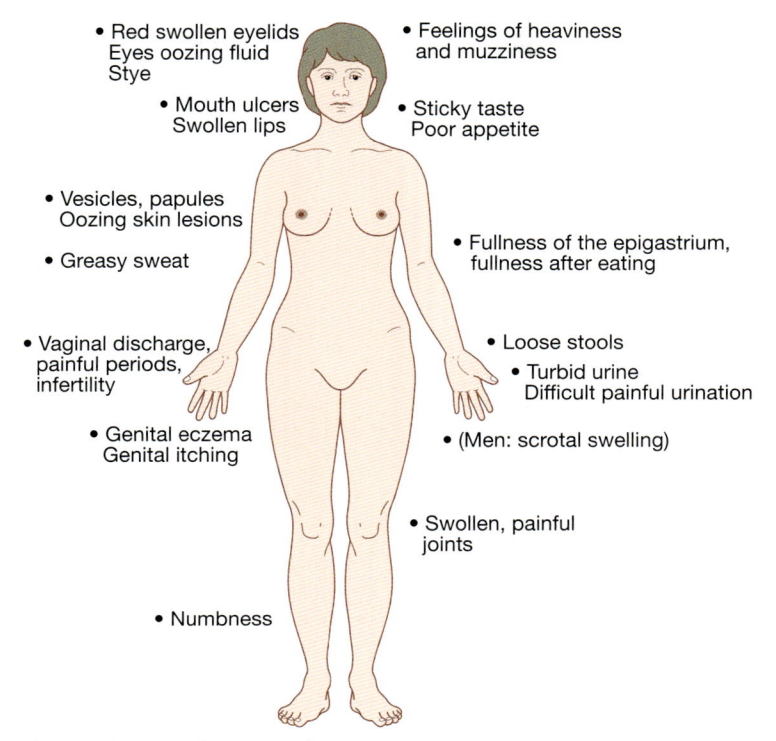

Figure 43.7 Manifestations of Dampness

Labels on figure:
- Red swollen eyelids, Eyes oozing fluid, Stye
- Feelings of heaviness and muzziness
- Mouth ulcers, Swollen lips
- Sticky taste, Poor appetite
- Vesicles, papules, Oozing skin lesions
- Greasy sweat
- Fullness of the epigastrium, fullness after eating
- Vaginal discharge, painful periods, infertility
- Loose stools
- Turbid urine, Difficult painful urination
- Genital eczema, Genital itching
- (Men: scrotal swelling)
- Swollen, painful joints
- Numbness

> **Clinical note**
>
> The main general points to eliminate Dampness are Ren-12 Zhongwan, Ren-9 Shuifen, Ren-5 Shimen, BL-22 Sanjiaoshu, SP-9 Yinlingquan. These are only general points and many other can be used according to type and location of Dampness

The classification of Dampness is quite complex and can be divided into the two broad categories of external or internal Dampness as follows:

EXTERNAL DAMPNESS
- Invasion of Dampness in the Internal Organs
  - External invasion of Dampness in Bladder
  - External invasion of Dampness in Stomach
  - External invasion of Dampness in Intestines
  - External invasion of Dampness in Uterus
  - External invasion of Dampness in Gall Bladder
  - External invasion of Dampness in Spleen
- Invasion of acute, external Dampness in channels
- Invasion of external Damp-Heat at Defensive Qi level
  - External Damp-Heat
  - External Summer-Heat with Dampness

INTERNAL DAMPNESS
- Chronic
  - Internal Dampness in Internal Organs
    - Dampness in Stomach and Spleen
    - Dampness in Bladder
    - Dampness in Intestines
    - Dampness in Uterus
    - Dampness in Gall Bladder
    - Dampness in Liver
    - Dampness in Kidneys
  - Chronic Dampness in channels
  - Internal Dampness in the skin
- Acute
  - Damp-Heat at Qi level
  - Acute episodes of chronic, internal Dampness

Figure 43.8 illustrates the complex classification of Dampness.

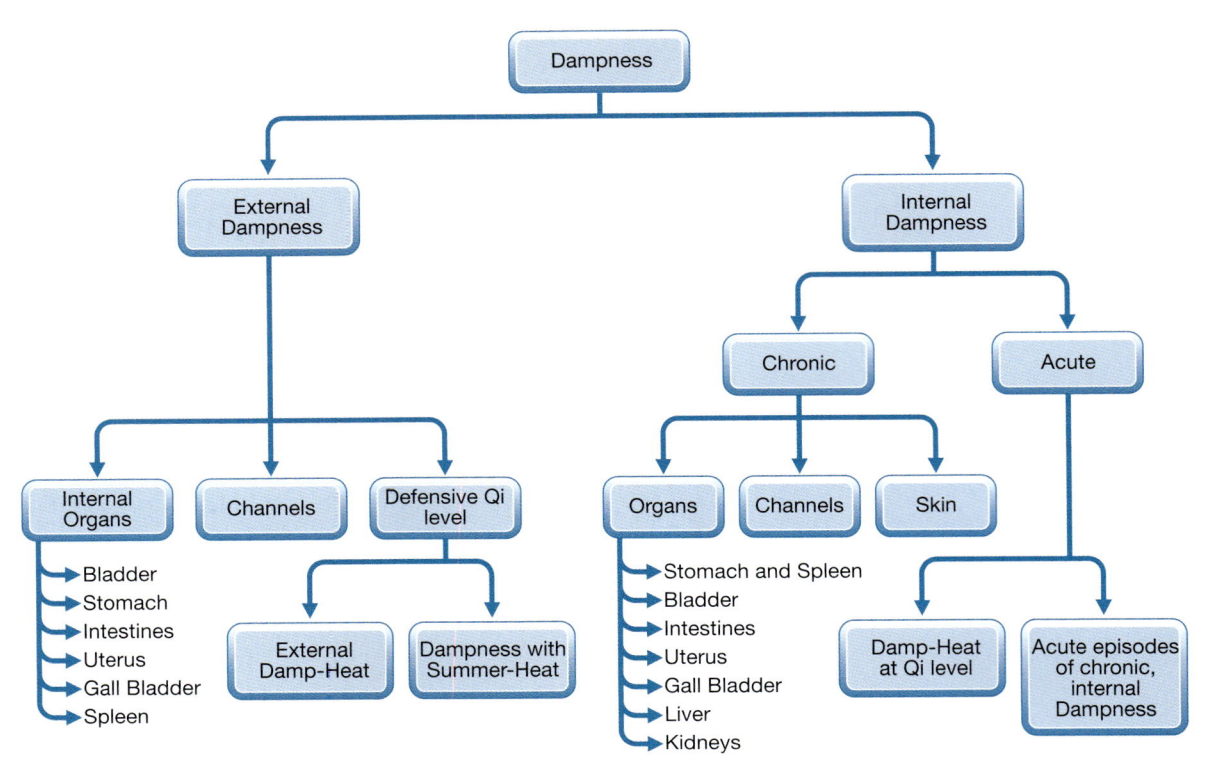

Figure 43.8 Classification of Dampness

External Dampness

There are three possible types of invasions of external Dampness:

1. An invasion of Dampness that may affect the Bladder, Intestines, Stomach, Uterus and Gall Bladder
2. An invasion of Dampness in the channels causing Damp Painful Obstruction Syndrome in its acute stage
3. An invasion of Damp-Heat of the *Warm Disease* type at the Defensive Qi level, manifesting with fever

Invasion of external Dampness in Internal Organs

External Dampness can invade the Bladder, Intestines, Stomach, Uterus and Gall Bladder.

Invasion of external Dampness in Bladder

Difficulty and pain on urination with acute onset, scanty but frequent urination, cloudy urine, feeling of heaviness in the lower abdomen, tongue with a thick sticky coating on the root, pulse perhaps Slippery on the Left-Rear position.

If associated with Heat: burning pain on urination, dark urine, thirst but no desire to drink, yellow tongue coating and a slightly rapid pulse.

Invasion of external Dampness in the Stomach

Acute onset of vomiting and/or watery diarrhoea without smell, epigastric pain, a feeling of stuffiness of the epigastrium, cold limbs, no appetite, white, thick and sticky tongue coating, Slippery pulse.

Invasion of external Dampness in Intestines

Acute onset of watery diarrhoea without smell, abdominal pain, a feeling of heaviness, tongue with a sticky thick white coating, Slippery pulse.

Invasion of external Dampness in Uterus

Acute onset of painful period (as a one-off when periods were not previously painful), excessive vaginal discharge, thick sticky white tongue coating on the root, Slippery pulse.

Invasion of external Dampness in Gall Bladder

Acute onset of hypochondrial pain, a feeling of heaviness, bitter taste, tongue with a sticky yellow coating on one side, Slippery pulse.

Invasion of acute, external Dampness in channels

This is an acute stage of Damp Painful Obstruction Syndrome (*Bi* Syndrome). When one joint only is affected, it is usually Cold-Dampness; when several joints are affected, it is often due to Damp-Heat. The main manifestations are achy and swollen joints with a feeling of heaviness occurring with sudden onset.

Invasion of acute, external Damp-Heat at the Defensive Qi level

This can be external Damp-Heat or Summer-Heat mixed with Dampness.

External Damp-Heat at Defensive Qi level

Aversion to cold, fever, body feels hot to touch, swollen glands, fever higher in the afternoon, headache as if wrapped, a feeling of oppression of the chest and epigastrium, a sticky taste, no thirst, tongue with a white sticky coating (it is white because it is in the beginning stage), pulse Soggy.

External Summer-Heat with Dampness

Fever, slight aversion to cold, sweating, headache, a feeling of heaviness of the body, an uncomfortable sensation of the epigastrium, irritability, thirst, Red tongue with a sticky tongue coating, Soggy-Rapid pulse.

Box 43.8 summarizes external Dampness.

Box 43.8 External Dampness

- External Dampness in organs
  - Bladder: acute urinary difficulty
  - Stomach: acute vomiting
  - Intestines: acute diarrhoea
  - Uterus: acute dysmenorrhoea, vaginal discharge
  - Gall Bladder: acute hypochondrial pain
  - Spleen: acute diarrhoea
- External Dampness in channels/joints: achy and swollen joints
- Damp-Heat at the Defensive Qi level

Internal Dampness

Interior Dampness arises from a deficiency of Spleen and sometimes Kidneys. If the Spleen function of transformation and transportation of Body Fluids fails, these will not be transformed and will accumulate to form Dampness.

There are two possible types of internal Dampness, one chronic, the other acute.

Chronic internal Dampness may involve:

- The Internal Organs
- The channels
- The skin

Acute internal Dampness involves Damp-Heat at the Qi level within the Four-Level identification of patterns acute episodes of a chronic condition.

Chronic Dampness

Chronic Dampness derives either from acute invasion of external Dampness or from dietary causes.

Chronic Dampness in the Internal Organs

Chronic, internal Dampness may be in any of the following organs:

- Stomach and Spleen
- Bladder
- Intestines
- Uterus
- Gall Bladder
- Liver
- Kidneys

The clinical manifestations of chronic internal Dampness in the Internal Organs are indicated below.

Dampness in Stomach and Spleen

Epigastric and abdominal fullness and heaviness, nausea, vomiting, sticky taste, loose stools with mucus, sticky tongue coating, Soggy pulse.

Dampness in Bladder

Urinary difficulty with slight or no pain, cloudy urine, sticky coating on the root of the tongue, Soggy pulse.

Dampness in Intestines

Abdominal fullness and heaviness, loose stools with mucus, sticky coating on the root of the tongue, Soggy pulse.

Dampness in Uterus

Abdominal fullness and heaviness, vaginal discharge, mid-cycle pain and/or bleeding, painful periods, sticky tongue coating on the root, Soggy pulse.

Dampness in Gall Bladder

Hypochondrial fullness and pain, unilateral sticky tongue coating, Soggy pulse.

Dampness in Liver

Urinary difficulty and pain, cloudy urine, hypogastric fullness and distension, vaginal discharge, genital sores and itching, sticky tongue coating on the root, Soggy pulse.

Dampness in Kidneys

Urinary difficulty and pain, cloudy urine, feeling of heaviness of the back, backache, sticky tongue coating on the root, Soggy pulse.

Chronic Dampness in the channels

Chronic retention of Dampness in the channels and joints is, of course, the main cause of Damp Painful Obstruction Syndrome. This manifests with aching, swelling and heaviness of the joints.

Chronic Dampness in the skin

Chronic retention of Dampness in the skin is the main cause of numerous skin diseases, chiefly eczema (atopic or not). Dampness in the skin manifests with vesicles, papules or with skin lesions oozing fluid, and with puffiness of the skin.

Acute Dampness

Generally speaking, acute interior Dampness can be only that seen at the Qi level of the identification of patterns according to the Four Levels (described in ch. 45). This is because acute attacks of Dampness are generally of exterior origin.

Of course, a condition of chronic Dampness can give rise to occasional acute flare-ups: this happens for example in interstitial cystitis (usually due to

---

Box 43.9 Internal Dampness

Chronic

- In the organs
  - Stomach and Spleen
  - Bladder
  - Intestines
  - Uterus
  - Gall Bladder
  - Liver
  - Kidneys
- In the channels/joints
- In the skin

Acute

- Damp-Heat at Qi level
- Acute episode of chronic Dampness

Damp-Heat in the Bladder occurring against a background of Kidney deficiency).

Box 43.9 summarizes internal Dampness.

Case history 43.1

A young woman of 32 suffered from pain in the muscles of neck, shoulders and arms and extreme tiredness. This had started 4 months previously when she fell ill with influenza symptoms, a sore throat, ache in the joints and temperature in May. After 2 weeks she developed more pain in both joints and muscles, the temperature continued at night, she had a feeling of heaviness and she felt hot and cold. This continued for 3 months. The appetite was poor, the sleep was disturbed and she experienced epigastric fullness and distension after eating. The tongue was of a normal colour and had a sticky yellow coating on the root extending towards the centre. The pulse was Soggy.

The sudden attack of fever with ache in the muscles and joints and a feeling of heaviness indicates the invasion of exterior Damp-Heat. The temperature at night also indicates Damp-Heat, which is also confirmed by the sticky yellow coating on the tongue. The long duration of the problem and retention of Dampness have weakened Spleen-Qi, hence the extreme tiredness and Soggy pulse. Her pains in the muscles are still due to the retention of Dampness in the muscles.

Differences between Dampness and Phlegm

Dampness and Phlegm are similar in nature. Both originate from a dysfunction of the Spleen in transforming and transporting fluids. There are, however, some differences between Dampness and Phlegm:

1. Dampness can be of exterior or interior origin, whereas Phlegm can originate only from an interior dysfunction
2. Interior Dampness originates mostly from the impairment of the Spleen in transforming and transporting Body Fluids, whereas the Lungs and Kidneys are also involved in the formation of Phlegm
3. Although Dampness can settle in the head, preventing the clear Yang from ascending, it primarily affects the lower part of the body, while Phlegm primarily affects the middle and upper part of the body. For example, urinary problems are often caused by Dampness in the Lower Burner and Bladder, while intestinal problems manifesting with mucus or blood in the stools are due to Dampness and Heat in the Intestines. Phlegm, on the other hand, mostly affects the chest, causing a feeling of oppression in the chest, the throat, causing some sputum in the throat, or the head, causing a feeling of heaviness, muzziness and dizziness
4. Dampness in the head causes a characteristic feeling of heaviness while Phlegm, contrary to Dampness, also causes dizziness
5. Phlegm can 'mist' the Mind, causing mental problems or sometimes mental retardation in children while Dampness has no such effect
6. Phlegm can be retained in the channels and under the skin, causing swelling and lumps, while Dampness mostly affects the Internal Organs, skin or joints
7. Interior Dampness originates only from a Spleen dysfunction, while Phlegm can also originate from the condensing action of Fire on Body Fluids
8. Dampness affects mostly the Spleen, Stomach, Gall Bladder, Bladder, and Intestines (hence, apart from the Spleen, mostly the Yang organs), while Phlegm affects mostly the Lungs, Heart, Kidney and Stomach (hence, apart from the Stomach, mostly the Yin organs)
9. Although Phlegm has the nature of heaviness, it does not have Dampness's characteristics of being sticky, dirty and flowing downwards
10. Phlegm can associate with various other pathogenic factors giving rise to Cold-Phlegm, Damp-Phlegm, Wind-Phlegm, Dry-Phlegm, Phlegm-Heat and Qi-Phlegm, while Dampness associates with Cold, Heat or Wind
11. Phlegm can assume a very watery and dilute form called Phlegm-Fluids while Dampness only assumes one form
12. From the point of view of pulse diagnosis, both Dampness and Phlegm can manifest with a Slippery pulse. However, Dampness can also manifest with a Soggy pulse, while Phlegm can manifest also with a Wiry pulse
13. From the point of view of tongue diagnosis, both Dampness and Phlegm can manifest with a sticky coating but Phlegm can also manifest with a dry and rough coating. This type of coating is frequently seen inside a central crack in the Stomach area of the tongue, indicating the presence of Phlegm-Heat in the Stomach
14. From the point of view of acupuncture treatment, although there are many similarities in the treatment of Dampness and Phlegm, the Spleen channel is mostly used to eliminate Dampness, while the Stomach channel is mostly used to resolve Phlegm. For example, SP-9 Yinlingquan, SP-6 Sanyinjiao and SP-3 Taibai are the main points to eliminate Dampness, while ST-40 Fenglong is the most important point to resolve Phlegm
15. Dampness can be acute or chronic whereas Phlegm can be only chronic (with the important exception of Phlegm arising in a few days as a result of an invasion of Wind that has become interior and affected the Lungs)
16. Finally, from the point of view of herbal treatment, the herbs used to drain Dampness or resolve Phlegm belong to two entirely different categories with different therapeutic effect

DRYNESS

Dryness is a Yang pathogenic factor and it tends to injure Blood or Yin. It is related to the season of autumn and to the Lungs. It arises in very dry weather, but it can also occur in some artificial conditions such as in very dry, centrally heated buildings.

The clinical manifestations are simply characterized by dryness and they are:

- Dry throat
- Dry lips
- Dry tongue
- Dry mouth
- Dry skin
- Dry stools
- Scanty urination

The discussion of Dryness will be done according to the following headings:

- Dryness
  - External Dryness
  - Internal Dryness
    - Stomach-Dryness
    - Lung-Dryness
    - Kidney-Dryness

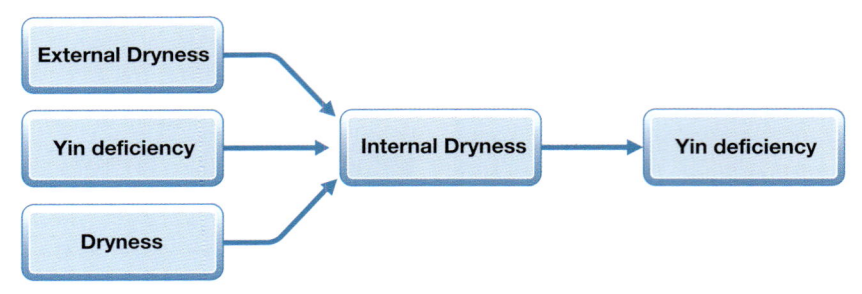

Figure 43.9 Origin of internal Dryness

External Dryness

External Dryness arises from invasion of exterior Wind-Dryness. This occurs when the person suffers an invasion of Wind either in very dry climates or when he or she is exposed to artificial, very dry working conditions.

As this is an invasion of external Wind, there is aversion to cold and fever. Other symptoms are a dry cough, dry mouth, dry throat, dry nose, dry tongue and a Floating pulse.

Internal Dryness

Internal Dryness can arise in one of three ways (Fig. 43.9):

1. It can develop from external Dryness
2. It can derive from deficiency of Yin
3. It can arise by itself internally, usually from dietary causes (in which case it may lead to Yin deficiency)

Internal causes of Dryness include the excessive consumption of drying foods (such as baked foods), irregular eating, which weakens Stomach-Yin, excessive use of the voice (e.g. teachers), which weakens Lung-Yin, excessive sexual activity in men, which weakens Kidney-Yin, chronic menorrhagia in women, which damages Blood and Liver- and Kidney-Yin and smoking, which injures Lung- and Kidney-Yin. It is interesting to note that, from the point of view of Chinese medicine, tobacco has a drying nature and it dries up Blood, Yin and Essence, affecting negatively not only the Lungs but also the Kidneys.

Box 43.10 summarizes internal causes of Dryness.

Tobacco smoking injures Blood, Kidney-Yin and Kidney-Essence. It causes dryness

Box 43.10 Internal causes of Dryness

- Excessive consumption of drying foods (e.g. baked foods)
- Irregular eating, which weakens Stomach-Yin
- Excessive use of the voice (e.g. teachers), which weakens Lung-Yin
- Excessive sexual activity in men, which weakens Kidney-Yin
- Chronic menorrhagia in women, which damages Blood and Liver- and Kidney-Yin
- Tobacco smoking, which injures Lung- and Kidney-Yin

Three organs are particularly affected by Drynes, (namely, the Stomach, Lungs and Kidneys), and the symptoms are the same as for exterior Dryness. As mentioned above, interior Dryness is not always the result of Yin deficiency as it is sometimes the stage preceding it. There is a saying: 'Withering and cracking is due to Dryness.'[9] This describes the dry skin and cracked tongue often seen in Dryness.

Stomach-Dryness

The Stomach is the origin of fluids and if one has an irregular diet, such as eating late at night, eating in a hurry or going back to work straight after eating, the Stomach fluids are depleted and this leads to a state of dryness, which is the precursor of Yin deficiency.

The main clinical manifestations of Stomach-Dryness are a dry mouth, dry tongue, cracks on the tongue.

Clinical note

The main points for Stomach Dryness are Ren-12 Zhongwan, ST-36 Zusanli and SP-6 Sanyinjiao

Box 43.11 summarizes Stomach-Dryness.

Box 43. 11 Stomach-Dryness

Dry mouth, dry tongue, cracks on the tongue

Lung-Dryness

The Lungs like to be kept moist (from the 'vapour' arising from the Kidneys) and dislike Dryness. Excessive use of the voice over many years can cause Dryness in the Lungs, which can be the precursor of Lung-Qi deficiency.

The main clinical manifestations of Lung-Dryness are a dry mouth and throat, dry cough, dry tongue, dry skin and a hoarse voice. Due to the relationship with the Large Intestine, Dryness of the Lungs in severe cases can cause dry stools.

Box 43.12 summarizes Lung-Dryness.

Box 43.12 Lung-Dryness

Dry mouth and throat, dry cough, dry tongue, dry skin and a hoarse voice

Clinical note

The main points for Lung Dryness are Ren-12 Zhongwan, LU-9 Taiyuan and SP-6 Sanyinjiao

Kidney-Dryness

Kidney dryness can arise from excessive sexual activity in men, chronic menorrhagia in women and smoking. The main clinical manifestations of Kidney-Dryness are a dry throat with desire to sip water at night, scanty urination, dry tongue with cracks, dry menstrual blood in women, dry skin.

Box 43.13 summarizes Kidney-Dryness.

Box 43.13 Kidney-Dryness

Dry throat with desire to sip water at night, scanty urination, dry tongue with cracks, dry menstrual blood in women, dry skin

FIRE

'Fire' and 'Heat' are two very common pathogenic factors and the terminology is fraught with difficulties.

Firstly, 'Heat' is generally used with at least two different meanings. On the one hand, 'Heat' is a general term that includes any manifestations characterized by Heat, which may be interior Heat, exterior Wind-Heat, or Fire. In this sense, 'Fire' comes under the general umbrella of 'Heat'.

In a more narrow definition, although Heat and Fire share many common characteristics and the same nature, these two pathogenic factors differ in the degree of intensity (i.e. Fire is more intense than Heat) and their clinical manifestations (and treatment) are somewhat different.

There is another important difference between Heat and Fire. While Heat always denotes pathological Heat, the term 'Fire' can denote either the physiological Fire of the body (the Minister Fire or the Fire of the Gate of Life) or pathological Fire (as in 'Liver-Fire').

In the 'Yellow Emperor's Classic of Internal Medicine', the physiological Fire of the body is sometimes called 'Lesser Fire' (*Shao Huo*) and the pathological Fire 'Exuberant Fire' (*Zhuang Huo*). Chapter 5 of the 'Simple Questions' clearly emphasizes the pathological nature of Exuberant Fire and the physiological one of Lesser Fire: '*Exuberant Fire [zhuang huo] consumes Qi, Lesser Fire [shao huo] makes Qi strong. Exuberant Fire scatters Qi, Lesser Fire generates Qi*'[10] (Fig. 43.10).

Fire is primarily an internal pathogenic factor. The only type of 'external Fire' could be considered that seen in Warm Diseases. Fire can derive from the transformation of other exterior pathogenic factors (e.g. Wind, Cold, Summer-Heat, Dampness), but once it affects the Internal Organs, it is an interior pathogenic factor.

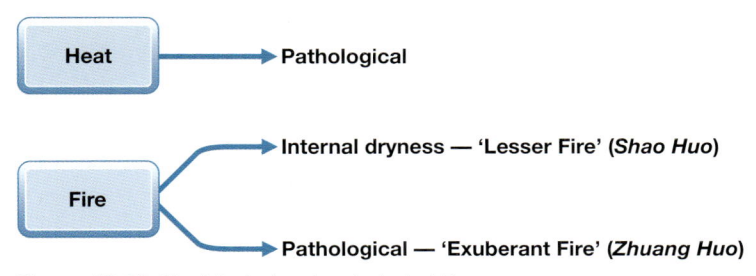

Figure 43.10 Physiological and pathological Fire

- Heat → Pathological
- Fire → Internal dryness — 'Lesser Fire' (*Shao Huo*)
- Fire → Pathological — 'Exuberant Fire' (*Zhuang Huo*)

Other causes of Fire are the excessive consumption of hot foods and alcohol, emotional stress (stagnant Qi turns into Fire) and smoking (Fig. 43.11).

The discussion of Fire will be done according to the following headings:

- Differences between Heat and Fire
- General clinical manifestations of Fire
- Organs affected by Fire
  - Heart
  - Liver
  - Stomach
  - Lungs
  - Intestines
- Full- versus Empty-Fire
- Toxic Heat

Differences between 'Heat' and 'Fire'

As mentioned above, when used in a narrow sense the term 'Heat' denotes a milder form of Fire.

Heat and Fire have obviously the same nature and share similar characteristics; they will both cause thirst, a feeling of heat, some mental restlessness, a Red tongue and a Rapid pulse. However, there are some important differences in the clinical manifestations, possible complications and treatment.

Fire is more 'solid' than Heat, it tends to move and dry out more than Heat and this nature of Fire causes dark scanty urine and dry stools. Fire moves upwards (causing mouth ulcers, for example) or damages the blood vessels (causing bleeding). Also, Fire tends to affect the Mind more than Heat, causing anxiety, mental agitation, insomnia or mental illness.

The nature of Fire therefore is to:

- Rise to the head
- Dry fluids
- Injure Blood and Yin
- Cause bleeding
- Affect the Mind

The differentiation between the Bright Yang channel pattern and Bright Yang organ pattern of the Six-Stage pattern identification illustrates the difference between Heat and Fire well (see ch. 44). The Bright Yang channel pattern is characterized by Heat manifesting with fever, thirst and sweating, but no constipation or abdominal pain. The organ pattern is characterized by similar manifestations, but in addition, there is constipation and abdominal pain.

This is because in the organ pattern the Heat has become 'solid' and has been transformed into Fire, which dries up the faeces in the intestines and causes constipation. In addition, the organ pattern can be characterized by mental changes, such as delirium, as Fire affects the Mind. Exactly the same difference exists between the pattern of Stomach-Heat and that of Intestines Dry-Heat at the Qi level of the Four Levels (see ch. 45).

To give another example, Heat in the Stomach can cause thirst, but Fire in the Stomach will cause bleeding gums, gum ulcers, and haematemesis as Fire moves upwards more than Heat and it agitates the Blood, causing bleeding.

The difference between Liver-Yang rising and Liver-Fire blazing upwards is another appropriate example of the difference between Heat and Fire.

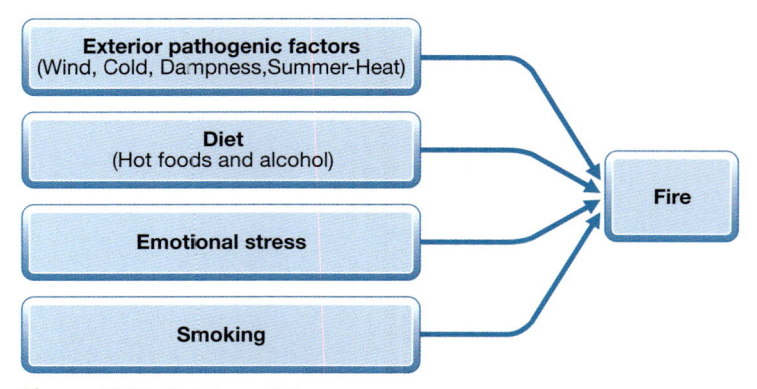

Figure 43.11 Aetiology of Fire

Rising Liver-Yang results from an imbalance between Yin and Yang within the Liver: when Liver-Yang rises upwards excessively it causes dizziness, headaches, a dry throat, irritability and probably a red face. The dry throat, red face and irritability are symptoms of Heat, but not of Fire. If the Liver has excessive Fire, in addition to these symptoms and signs, there will be intense thirst, bitter taste, scanty dark urine, dry stools, pronounced mental restlessness and possibly vomiting of blood or epistaxis.

There is an important difference in the treatment of Heat as opposed to Fire. In Heat patterns, the treatment method consists of 'clearing Heat' (*Xie Re*) with pungent cold herbs to drive Heat outwards (e.g. Bai Hu Tang); in Fire patterns, the treatment method consists in 'draining Fire' (*Xie Huo*) with bitter cold herbs (e.g. Tiao Wei Cheng Qi Tang). Unfortunately, the *pinyin* form of the two above characters *xie* is the same while the characters are different (see Glossary). I render this difference in English using the term 'clearing' for Heat and 'draining' for Fire.

I shall now discuss the clinical manifestations of Fire in more detail.

General clinical manifestations of Fire

Fire is a Yang pathogenic factor and it rises

Fire often causes clinical manifestations in the head because it is in its nature to rise strongly. For example, Liver-Fire may cause redness, swelling and pain of the eyes, Heart-Fire may cause tongue ulcers, Stomach-Fire may cause mouth ulcers.

Fire is very drying

Fire is more drying than Heat and for this reason it causes scanty dark urine and dry stools.

Fire damages Blood and Yin

Because it is drying, Fire may damage Blood and Yin, especially Liver-Blood and Kidney-Yin.

Fire causes bleeding

Fire may cause bleeding from the nose if it affects the Liver, in vomiting if it affects the Stomach and/or Liver, in cough if it affects the Lungs, in the stools if it affects the Intestines, in the urine if it affects the Bladder and/or Liver and under the skin if it affects the Liver.

Fire has the potential to general Wind

In the context of Warm Diseases (ch. 45), Fire at the Qi level may generate Liver-Wind, which would indicate that the disease has progressed to the Blood level bypassing the Nutritive Qi level. This situation is more likely to occur in children.

Fire affects the Mind

Fire affects the Mind more than Heat. It agitates the Mind, causing insomnia, mental restlessness, pronounced irritability, propensity to outbursts of anger (in Liver-Fire) and agitation.

Fire causes ulcers with swelling

Finally, Fire may cause ulcers with a red and swollen rim.

Box 43.14 summarizes the main characteristics of Fire (as opposed to Heat).

Listed below are some of the many sayings that describe the nature and clinical manifestations of Heat or Fire:

'*Diseases manifesting with tympanic sounds are due to Fire.*'[11] This describes the condition of Fire or Heat in the Intestines causing borborygmi and a distended abdomen.

'*Abnormal changes and dark fluids are manifestations of Heat.*'[12] This describes the tendency of Fire to produce rapid changes for the worse in an acute condition. For example, when exterior Wind-Heat invades the Lung-Defensive Qi portion, the Heat can in a few cases rapidly penetrate to the Pericardium, causing a high temperature and coma. This is called 'abnormal transmission'. The second part of the saying refers to dark and concentrated fluids often produced by Fire, such as a dark and scanty urine.

'*Vomiting of sour fluids and sudden down-pouring are manifestations of Heat.*'[13] The first part of this saying

---

Box 43.14 Main characteristics of Fire (as opposed to Heat)

- It blazes upwards
- It is very drying
- It damages Blood and Yin
- It may cause bleeding
- It has the potential to general Wind
- It affects the Mind
- It causes ulcers with swelling

describes a condition of Stomach-Heat causing vomiting and sour regurgitation. The second part of the saying describes the sudden diarrhoea with foul-smelling stools which can occur with Fire in the Intestines.

'*Manic behaviour is a manifestation of Fire.*'[14] Fire can easily affect the Mind, causing restlessness, agitation and in severe cases a manic behaviour (laughing uncontrollably, shouting, hitting people, talking incessantly, etc.). This is a specific characteristic of Fire as opposed to Heat. Chapter 74 of the 'Simple Questions' says: '*Manic behaviour is due to Fire.*'[15]

Organs affected by Fire

Fire can affect the Heart, Liver, Stomach, Lungs and Intestines and its clinical manifestations related to each of these organs have been described in detail in the chapters on the identification of patterns according to the Internal Organs (chs 32–42). Only the essential clinical manifestations will be listed below (Fig. 43.12).

Heart-Fire

Tongue ulcers, insomnia, agitation, mental restlessness, red tip of the tongue.

Liver-Fire

Red, swollen and painful eyes, headaches, bitter taste, irritability, propensity to outbursts of anger, tongue with red sides, Wiry pulse.

Stomach-Fire

Mouth ulcers, thirst, epigastric pain, thick, dry, dark-yellow tongue coating.

Fire in the Lungs

Cough with blood, expectoration of thick yellow sputum.

Fire in the Intestines

Constipation with dry stools, abdominal pain.

Heart-Fire
Mental reslessness, insomnia
Tongue ulcers, red tip of tongue

Stomach-Fire
Mouth ulcers
Thirst
Thick, dry, dark-yellow tongue coating
Epigastric pain

Liver-Fire
Irritability, propensity to angry outbursts
Red, swollen, painful eyes, headache, bitter taste, tongue with red sides

Fire in Lungs
Coughing of blood
Expectoration of thick, yellow sputum

Fire in Intestines
Constipation, dry stools, abdominal pain

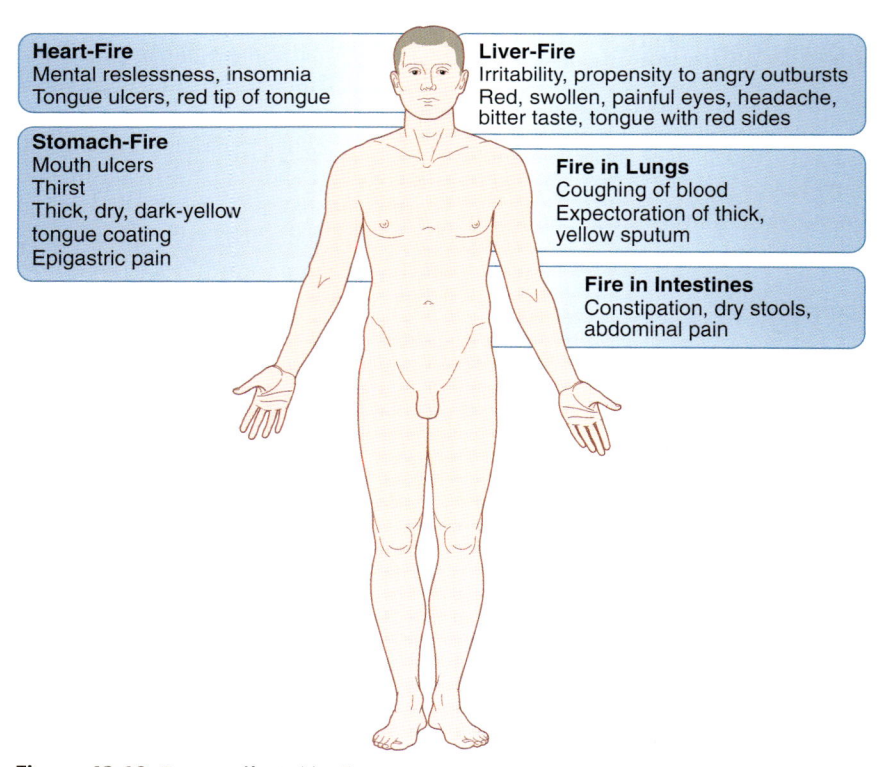

Figure 43.12 Organs affected by Fire

Table 43.2 Differentiation between Full- and Empty-Fire

	Full-Fire	Empty-Fire
Feeling of heat	All the time	In the evening
Thirst	Intense, all the time	In the evening and night (desire to drink in small sips)
Dry mouth	All the time	At night
Bitter taste	Yes	No
Mind	Intense agitation	Vague, mild restlessness in the evening
Tongue	Red with dry dark-yellow coating	Red without coating
Pulse	Full-Deep-Rapid	Floating-Empty, Rapid

Full- versus Empty-Fire

Fire can be of the Excess or Deficient type. The clinical manifestations of Excess Fire are a red face and eyes, a pronounced feeling of heat, a dry mouth, a bitter taste, constipation, scanty dark urine, thirst, mental agitation, a Red tongue with dry yellow coating and a Full-Rapid pulse. When Fire enters the Blood, it may give rise to dark purple spots under the skin (macules) and bleeding.

Deficient Fire (usually called Empty-Heat) arises from deficiency of Yin and is manifested with night sweating, a feeling of heat in the chest, palms and soles, red cheekbones, a dry mouth, afternoon feeling of heat, a Red tongue without coating and a Floating-Empty and Rapid pulse.

Full-Fire is treated by draining Fire with bitter cold herbs while Empty-Fire is treated by nourishing Yin and using herbs that clear Empty-Heat.

Table 43.2 compares and contrasts the clinical manifestations of Full-Fire and Empty-Fire. Box 43.15 summarizes Full- versus Empty-Fire.

Clinical note

The tongue is very important to differentiate Full- from Empty-Heat. In both cases it is Red, but in Full-Heat it has a coating whereas in Empty-Heat it does not

Clinical note

1. Heart-Fire: HE-3 Shaohai
2. Liver-Fire: LIV-2 Xingjian
3. Stomach-Fire: ST-44 Neiting
4. Fire in the Lungs: LU-5 Chize
5. Fire in the Intestines: L.I.-11 Quchi, ST-25 Tianshu

Box 43.15 Full-versus Empty-Fire

Full-Fire

Red face and eyes, a pronounced feeling of heat, a dry mouth, a bitter taste, constipation, scanty dark urine, thirst, mental agitation, dark purple spots under the skin (macules), blood in cough, vomit, urine, stools, epistaxis, Red tongue with dry yellow coating, Full-Rapid pulse

Empty-Fire

Night sweating, a feeling of heat in the chest, palms and soles, red cheekbones, a dry mouth, afternoon feeling of heat, a Red tongue without coating and a Floating-Empty and Rapid pulse

Toxic Heat

Before leaving the discussion of Fire, mention should be made of Toxic Heat (*Re Du*). Toxic Heat is similar in nature to Fire (more than to Heat).

In chronic, interior conditions Toxic Heat develops from Fire and its chief characteristics may be summarized in five words:

- Swelling
- Redness
- Heat
- Pus
- Pain

Toxic Heat is manifested with swelling, for example the swelling of a large boil, a swollen appendix, sometimes a swollen prostate glands, a swollen ulcer, swollen and painful lymph glands, acne with very large and raised pustules, etc.

Toxic Heat is often manifested outwardly with redness and heat, such as a large boil, a carbuncle, acne with large pustules, etc.

Pus in the presence of the above manifestations of swelling, redness and heat also denotes Toxic Heat, for example a large boil and all pustules.

Finally, generally, Toxic Heat causes pain, for example a large boil, a swollen appendix, a swollen prostate gland with pain in the perineum, a carbuncle, etc.

Toxic Heat can also occur as an acute pathogenic factor: in this case, it accompanies Wind-Heat. For example, if a child suffers an invasion of Wind-Heat developing tonsillitis with very swollen tonsils with exudate, this indicates Toxic Heat.

Box 43.16 summarizes Toxic Heat.

Box 43.16 Toxic Heat

- Swelling
- Redness
- Heat
- Pus
- Pain

END NOTES

1. Zhai Ming Yi 1979 Clinical Chinese Medicine (*Zhong Yi Lin Chuang Ji Chu* 中医临床基础) Henan Publishing House, p. 132.
2. 1979 The Yellow Emperor's Classic of Internal Medicine – Simple Questions (*Huang Di Nei Jing Su Wen* 黄帝内经素问). People's Health Publishing House, Beijing, first published c. 100 BC, p. 538.
3. Ibid., p. 218.
4. Ibid., p. 245.
5. Ibid., p. 221.
6. Clinical Chinese Medicine, p. 133
7. Clinical Chinese Medicine, p. 133.
8. Simple Questions, p. 180.
9. Clinical Chinese Medicine, p. 135.
10. Simple Questions, p. 33.
11. Clinical Chinese Medicine, p. 133.
12. Clinical Chinese Medicine, p. 133.
13. Clinical Chinese Medicine, p. 134.
14. Clinical Chinese Medicine, p. 134.
15. Simple Questions, p. 539.

SECTION 3   PART 6

Identification of Patterns According to the Six Stages   44

> **Key contents**
>
> **Greater Yang stage**
> *Channel patterns*
> - Invasion of Wind-Cold with prevalence of Wind
> - Invasion of Wind-Cold with prevalence of Cold
>
> *Organ patterns*
> - Accumulation of Water
> - Accumulation of Blood
>
> **Bright Yang stage**
> *Bright Yang channel pattern*
> *Bright Yang organ pattern*
>
> **Lesser Yang stage**
>
> **Greater Yin stage**
>
> **Lesser Yin stage**
> - Cold transformation
> - Heat transformation
>
> **Terminal Yin stage**

The identification of patterns according to the Six Stages was formulated by Zhang Zhong Jing (AD 150–219) in his celebrated book 'Discussion of Cold-Induced Diseases' 'Shang Han Lun' (c.AD 220). Although the 'Yellow Emperor's Classic of Internal Medicine' deals with the pathology and treatment of diseases of exterior origin in several chapters, the 'Discussion of Cold-Induced Diseases' was the first clinical manual to describe systematically the pathology and treatment of diseases caused by invasion of exterior pathogenic factors. However, the historical and clinical significance of the 'Discussion of Cold-Induced Diseases' goes beyond the mere pathology and treatment of diseases caused by exterior pathogenic factors as many of the herbal formulae from this book are very important and frequently used in the clinic today.

For centuries, the 'Discussion of Cold-Induced Diseases' dominated Chinese medical thinking on diseases of exterior origin and, in consequence, in most cases these were attributed to invasion of Wind with Cold, although the book does describe patterns of Wind-Heat as well. Many centuries later, in the late Ming and especially early Qing dynasty, a new school of thought emerged which emphasized exterior Wind-Heat in the pathology and treatment of exterior diseases and such diseases were called *Wen Bing*, 'Warm Diseases' (see chs 45 and 46). The doctors who described the clinical manifestations and treatment of 'Warm Diseases' are referred to collectively as the 'School of Warm Diseases'.

Although the term 'Warm Disease' (*wen bing*) appears already in the 'Yellow Emperor's Classic of Internal Medicine' and in the 'Discussion of Cold-Induced Diseases' itself, in these books it has a different meaning than the one it has in the School of Warm Diseases. The 'Simple Questions' (*Su Wen*) mentions diseases from exterior Heat in chapters 3, 5, 31, 32, 33, 71 and 74 and the 'Spiritual Axis' (*Ling Shu*) in chapters 23 and 74. Indeed, the 'Simple Questions' itself describes the clinical manifestations of the Six Stages (i.e. Greater Yang, Bright Yang, Lesser Yang, Greater Yin, Lesser Yin and Terminal Yin), although with different symptoms than those in the 'Discussion of Cold-Induced Diseases'. However, as the medical thinking on diseases of exterior origin was dominated by the emphasis of exterior Cold as the main pathogenic factor, even diseases characterized by Heat manifestations (called 'Warm Disease') were explained as a transformation of Cold.

For example, chapter 3 of the 'Simple Questions' says: '*If Cold attacks in Winter it will cause a Warm Disease in Spring*'.[1] Chapter 4 of the 'Simple Questions' says: '*The Essence is the root of the body: if it is stored [in Winter], Warm Diseases will not occur in Spring.*'[2]

The 'Classic of Difficulties' (Nan Jing) says in chapter 58: 'There are five types of injury from Cold: attack of Wind, attack of Cold, Damp-Warmth [shi wen], Heat disease and Warm disease [wen bing].'³

The 'Discussion of Cold-Induced Diseases' became such an authoritative text on the treatment of diseases of exterior origin that a rigid convention developed according to which 'The method should not depart from the Shang Han [Lun]; the prescription should follow Zhong Jing.'⁴

Thus, the term 'Injury from Cold' (Shang Han) has two different meanings. In a broad sense, developed during the centuries following the time of Zhang Zhong Jing until the Song dynasty, shang han does not refer specifically to Cold but to exterior pathogenic factors in general. In a narrow sense, developed in the centuries after the Song dynasty, the term shang han refers to invasions of external Cold and it is a term that is contrasted to the term wen bing, which refers to invasions of external Wind-Heat (Fig. 44.1).

The term shang han has yet another meaning. In the Greater Yang stage of invasion of Wind-Cold there is a further differentiation between prevalence of Cold (no sweating) called shang han, and prevalence of Wind (sweating) called zhong feng (Wind strike).

The concept and nature of 'Wind' as an exterior pathogenic factor has already been discussed in chapters 21 and 43. The 'Discussion on Cold-Induced Diseases' describes two separate types of invasion of exterior pathogenic factors in the beginning stage, that is, an 'attack of Wind' (literally 'Wind-strike' zhong feng)⁵ and an 'attack of Cold' (literally 'injury from Cold' shang han). Essentially these two patterns describe the clinical manifestations arising from an invasion of external Wind with Cold (now called Wind-Cold), the former with the emphasis on Wind, the latter with the emphasis on Cold.

The Six Stages described in the 'Discussion on Cold-Induced Diseases' are (Fig. 44.2):

> Greater Yang stage (Tai Yang)
> - Channel patterns
>   - Invasion of Wind-Cold with prevalence of Wind (Zhong Feng)
>   - Invasion of Wind-Cold with prevalence of Cold (Shang Han)
> - Organ patterns
>   - Accumulation of Water
>   - Accumulation of Blood
>
> Bright Yang stage (Yang Ming)
> - Bright Yang channel pattern
> - Bright Yang organ pattern
>
> Lesser Yang stage (Shao Yang)
>
> Greater Yin stage (Tai Yin)
>
> Lesser Yin stage (Shao Yin)
> - Cold transformation
> - Heat transformation
>
> Terminal Yin stage (Jue Yin)

The first stage, Greater Yang, is the beginning stage and the only exterior stage: at the Greater Yang stage, the exterior Wind is still on the Exterior of the body and the Internal Organs are not affected (although the Greater Yang stage does have two organ patterns as well). All the other stages are characterized by penetration of the pathogenic factor into the Interior, in the Bright Yang stage in the Yang and in the three Yin stages in the Yin. The Lesser Yang stage is somewhat different as it is characterized by the oscillation of the pathogenic factor between the Exterior and the Interior.

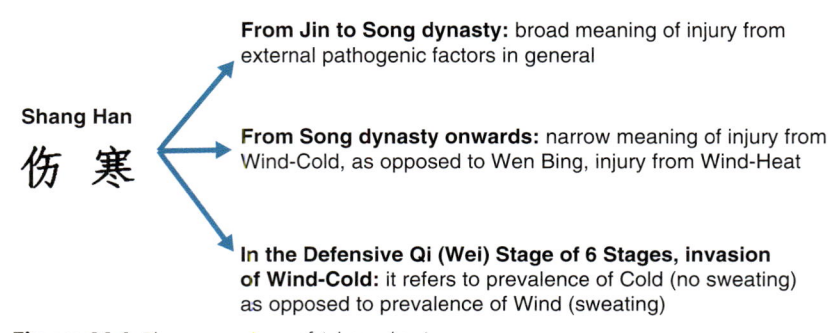

Shang Han
伤 寒

- **From Jin to Song dynasty:** broad meaning of injury from external pathogenic factors in general
- **From Song dynasty onwards:** narrow meaning of injury from Wind-Cold, as opposed to Wen Bing, injury from Wind-Heat
- **In the Defensive Qi (Wei) Stage of 6 Stages, invasion of Wind-Cold:** it refers to prevalence of Cold (no sweating) as opposed to prevalence of Wind (sweating)

Figure 44.1 Three meanings of 'shang han'

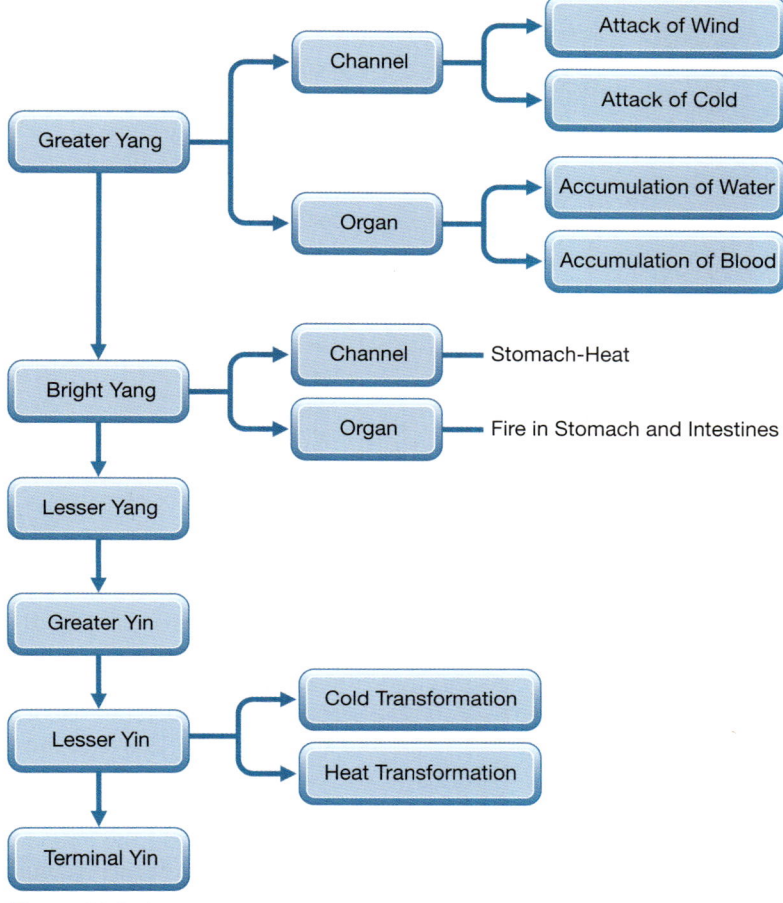

Figure 44.2 The Six Stages

GREATER YANG STAGE

The first stage, Greater Yang, is the beginning stage and the only exterior stage: at the Greater Yang stage, the exterior Wind is still on the Exterior of the body and the Internal Organs are not affected (although the Greater Yang stage does have two organ patterns as well).

There are three essential symptoms of this stage, irrespective of the pattern (Fig. 44.3):

1. Aversion to cold
2. Headache and stiff neck
3. Floating pulse

Aversion to cold

This is caused by obstruction of the space between skin and muscles by exterior Wind and it has already been described above.

Headache and stiff neck

The headache is typically occipital. Wind contracts and stops movement, hence the stiff neck. External Wind obstructs the Greater Yang channels and this causes the typical occipital headache (i.e. along the Greater Yang channels, Small Intestine and Bladder).

Floating pulse

The Floating pulse feels very superficial and, indeed, 'floating' under the finger; it is also relatively large. The

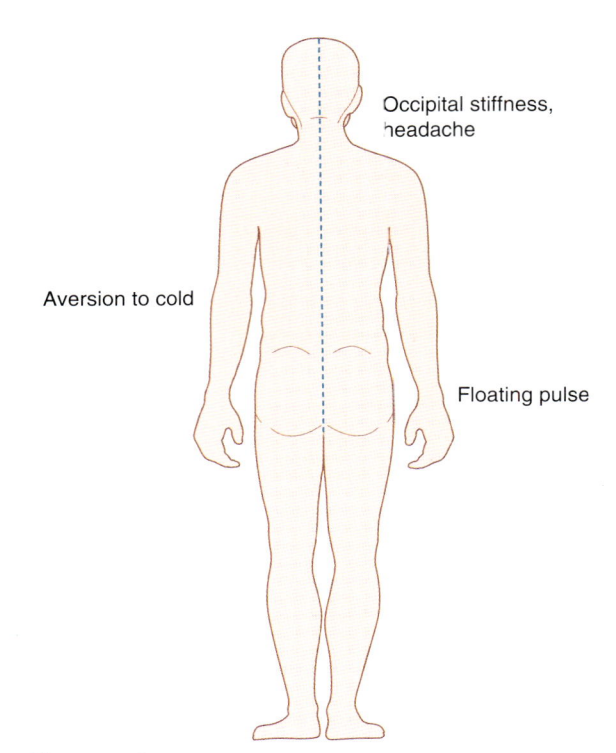

Figure 44.3 Greater Yang stage

Floating pulse reflects the rush of Defensive Qi to the surface of the body to meet and fight the exterior Wind.

> **Clinical note**
>
> The three essential symptoms of external Wind invasion are:
> 1. Aversion to cold
> 2. Occipital headache and stiff neck
> 3. Floating pulse

CHANNEL PATTERNS

Invasion of Wind-Cold with prevalence of Wind (Attack of Wind)

Clinical manifestations

Slight aversion to cold, aversion to wind, slight fever, slight sweating, headache, stiff neck, sneezing, Floating-Slow pulse.

Pathology

This pattern is characterized by two features: there is an emphasis on Wind more than Cold and there is a deficiency of Nutritive Qi (*Ying Qi*) compared to Defensive Qi (*Wei Qi*).

Aversion to cold indicates a subjective feeling of cold experienced by the patient with sudden onset: this cold feeling is typically not alleviated by covering oneself. In fact, in severe cases, the patient may be lying in bed under several blankets and still be shivering. Aversion to cold is caused by the obstruction of the space between the skin and muscles by exterior Wind: this impairs the circulation of Defensive Qi in this space, which therefore cannot warm the muscles. In Attack of Wind (compared to Attack of Cold) the aversion to cold is mild; 'aversion to wind' is the same as 'aversion to cold' but milder.

'Fever' does not refer to an actual fever but to the *objective* hot feeling of the patient's skin to palpation: the simultaneous occurrence of the subjective cold feeling 'aversion to cold' and 'fever' is typical of invasions of exterior Wind. The 'fever' reflects the struggle between the exterior Wind and the body's Qi. What I translate as 'fever' is called *fa re*: that is, 'heat emission' (see Glossary).

In Attack of Wind, the patient is sweating slightly because the deficient Nutritive Qi fails to hold sweat in the space between skin and muscles. The Attack of Wind pattern of the Greater Yang stage is characterized by a relative imbalance between the Defensive Qi and the Nutritive Qi, the former being 'full' and the latter 'empty'. In Chinese, this situation is summarized in the expression 'Defensive [Qi] strong, Nutritive [Qi] weak' (*Wei qiang, Ying ruo*). In this case, the Defensive Qi is 'strong' only in relation to the Nutritive Qi, which is weak.

The occipital headache and stiff neck are caused by the obstruction of Qi in the Greater Yang channels of Small Intestine and Gall Bladder: as Wind naturally invades the upper part of the body, such obstruction manifests itself in the head and neck.

Sneezing is caused by the impairment of the diffusing of Lung-Qi in the nose. The Floating pulse reflects the rush of Defensive Qi towards the surface of the body to fight the external Wind. The pulse is slow because Wind contracts and slows down.

Although both the Attack of Wind and Attack of Cold are Full conditions due to the presence of a pathogenic factor, Attack of Wind is more Empty in relation to the Attack of Cold as in the former the Nutritive Qi is relatively weak.

As for the location of the pathogenic factor, in Attack of Wind this is in the muscles while in Attack of Cold it is in the skin.

Treatment

Treatment principle: release the Exterior, expel Wind and Cold, restore the diffusing of Lung-Qi, harmonize Nutritive and Defensive Qi.

Acupuncture

BL-12 Fengmen with cupping, LU-7 Lieque, L.I.-4 Hegu, G.B.-20 Fengchi, T.B.-5 Waiguan, ST-36 Zusanli, Du-16 Fengfu.

Herbal formula

Gui Zhi Tang *Ramulus Cinnamomi Decoction*.

Box 44.1 summarizes invasion of Wind-Cold with prevalence of Wind.

Box 44.1 Invasion of Wind-Cold with prevalence of Wind (Attack of Wind)

Clinical manifestations

Slight aversion to cold, aversion to wind, slight fever, slight sweating, headache, stiff neck, sneezing, Floating-Slow pulse

Treatment

Acupuncture
BL-12 Fengmen with cupping, LU-7 Lieque, L.I.-4 Hegu, G.B.-20 Fengchi, T.B.-5 Waiguan, ST-36 Zusanli, Du-16 Fengfu
Herbal formula
Gui Zhi Tang *Ramulus Cinnamomi Decoction*

Invasion of Wind-Cold with prevalence of Cold (Attack of Cold)

Clinical manifestations

Aversion to cold, slight fever, no sweating, headache, stiff neck, sneezing, runny nose with white discharge, breathlessness, Floating-Tight pulse.

Pathology

The aversion to cold, fever, headache, stiff neck, sneezing and Floating pulse have already been explained above and the pathology is the same as in Attack of Wind.

A crucial difference between the Attack of Wind and Attack of Cold is that in the former there is a slight sweating while in the latter there is no sweating. The lack of sweating in Attack of Cold reflects a more Full condition than in attack of Wind: that is, both Defensive Qi and Nutritive Qi are in an Excess condition characterized by the invasion of external Wind and by a 'tightness' of the space between the skin and muscles. Cold contracts the pores, which therefore prevents sweating.

The runny nose with white discharge is due to the temporary impairment of the descending of Lung-Qi, which is unable to transform fluids in the Upper Burner and the nose specifically. Breathlessness is also due to the impairment of the descending of Lung-Qi.

The Tight quality of the pulse reflects Cold.

Treatment

Treatment principle: release the Exterior, expel Wind and Cold, restore the diffusing and descending of Lung-Qi.

Acupuncture

BL-12 Fengmen with cupping, LU-7 Lieque, L.I.-4 Hegu, T.B.-5 Waiguan, G.B.-20 Fengchi, Du-16 Fengfu. Moxa is applicable.

Herbal formula

Ma Huang Tang *Ephedra Decoction*.

Table 44.1 differentiates the clinical manifestations of an Attack of Cold from those of an Attack of Wind. Box 44.2 summarizes invasion of Wind-Cold with prevalence of Cold.

Table 44.1 Comparison of Attack of Cold and Attack of Wind in the Greater Yang pattern

	Attack of Cold	Attack of Wind
Sweating	No sweating	Slight sweating
Aches	Pronounced	Slight
Headache	Severe	Mild
Aversion to cold	Pronounced	Slight
Pulse	Floating-Tight	Floating-Slow
Common symptoms	Floating pulse, headache, shivers, aversion to cold	

> **Box 44.2 Invasion of Wind-Cold with prevalence of Cold (Attack of Cold)**
>
> **Clinical manifestations**
>
> Aversion to cold, slight fever, no sweating, headache, stiff neck, sneezing, runny nose with white discharge, breathlessness, Floating-Tight pulse
>
> **Treatment**
>
> *Acupuncture*
> BL-12 Fengmen with cupping, LU-7 Lieque, L.I.-4 Hegu, T.B.-5 Waiguan, G.B.-20 Fengchi. Moxa is applicable, Du-16 Fengfu
> *Herbal formula*
> Ma Huang Tang *Ephedra Decoction*

ORGAN PATTERNS

Accumulation of Water

Clinical manifestations

Aversion to cold, fever, retention of urine, slight thirst, vomiting of fluids soon after drinking, Floating-Rapid pulse.

Pathology

Although the Greater Yang is the beginning stage of an invasion of Wind characterized by the location of the pathogenic factor on the Exterior, it does have two organ patterns in which the pathogenic factors has penetrated in the Interior.

In the case of Accumulation of Water, the pathogenic factor is in the Bladder organ while there are still symptoms of the Wind being on the Exterior: namely, aversion to cold, fever and Floating pulse.

The Bladder's function of Qi transformation is impaired, Water is not transformed and this causes retention of urine, thirst and vomiting after drinking. The thirst is caused by the impairment of the Bladder's separation of fluids and the Bladder's fluids not ascending, not by a deficiency of fluids: for this reason, this thirst is not relieved by drinking and there is vomiting soon after drinking. No matter how much fluids one drinks, these accumulate in the Stomach and they cause vomiting soon after drinking.

Treatment

Treatment principle: release the Exterior, promote the Bladder's function of Qi transformation, promote the excretion of fluids.

Acupuncture

Ren-9 Shuifen, Ren-3 Zhongji, ST-28 Shuidao, LU-7 Lieque, BL-22 Sanjiaoshu, BL-39 Weiyang, BL-64 Jinggu.

Herbal formula

Wu Ling San *Five 'Ling' Powder*.

Box 44.3 summarizes the pattern Accumulation of Water.

> **Box 44.3 Greater Yang organ pattern Accumulation of Water**
>
> **Clinical manifestations**
>
> Aversion to cold, fever, retention of urine, slight thirst, vomiting of fluids soon after drinking, Floating-Rapid pulse
>
> **Treatment**
>
> *Acupuncture*
> Ren-9 Shuifen, Ren-3 Zhongji, ST-28 Shuidao, LU-7 Lieque, BL-22 Sanjiaoshu, BL-39 Weiyang, BL-64 Jinggu
> *Herbal formula*
> Wu Ling San *Five 'Ling' Powder*

Accumulation of Blood

Clinical manifestations

Hypogastric distension, fullness and urgency, blood in urine, mental restlessness, Reddish-Purple tongue without coating, Deep-Fine-Rapid or Deep-Choppy pulse.

Pathology

This pattern is characterized by accumulation of Heat and stasis in the Lower Burner and the Bladder organ. The stasis in the Bladder causes the hypogastric distension, fullness and urgency.

As the Bladder function is affected and the pathogenic factor is at the Blood level, there is blood in the urine.

The Blood is the residence of the Mind: as there is Heat and stasis at the Blood level, there is mental restlessness (what the 'Discussion of Cold-Induced Diseases' literally calls 'manic behaviour' *fa kuang*).

Because of the Blood stasis, the blood vessels are obstructed and for this reason the pulse may be Choppy.

Treatment

Treatment principle: invigorate Blood, eliminate stasis from the Lower Burner, clear Heat from the Bladder.

Table 44.2 Comparison of Accumulation of Water and Accumulation of Blood within the Greater Yang organ pattern

	Accumulation of Water	Accumulation of Blood
Pattern	Heat in the Bladder at Qi level	Heat in the Bladder at Blood level
Symptoms	Urinary retention, no mental changes	Blood in urine, mental changes

Acupuncture

Ren-3 Zhongji, KI-14 Siman, ST-28 Shuidao, BL-39 Weiyang, BL-22 Sanjiaoshu, SP-10 Xuehai, LIV-3 Taichong, SP-6 Sanyinjiao.

Herbal formula

Tao He Cheng Qi Tang *Persica Conducting Qi Decoction*.

Table 44.2 compares the manifestations of Accumulation of Water and Accumulation of Blood of the Greater Yang organ pattern. Box 44.4 summarizes the pattern Accumulation of Blood.

Box 44.4 Greater Yang organ pattern Accumulation of Blood

Clinical manifestations

Hypogastric distension, fullness and urgency, blood in urine, mental restlessness, Reddish-Purple tongue without coating, Deep-Fine-Rapid or Deep-Choppy pulse

Treatment

Acupuncture
Ren-3 Zhongji, KI-14 Siman, ST-28 Shuidao, BL-39 Weiyang, BL-22 Sanjiaoshu, SP-10 Xuehai, LIV-3 Taichong, SP-6 Sanyinjiao

Herbal formula
Tao He Cheng Qi Tang *Persica Conducting Qi Decoction*

BRIGHT YANG STAGE

Bright Yang (*Yang Ming*) channel pattern

Clinical manifestations

High fever, profuse sweating, intense thirst, red face, feeling of heat, irritability, delirium, Red tongue with yellow coating, Overflowing-Rapid or Big-Rapid pulse (Fig. 44.4).

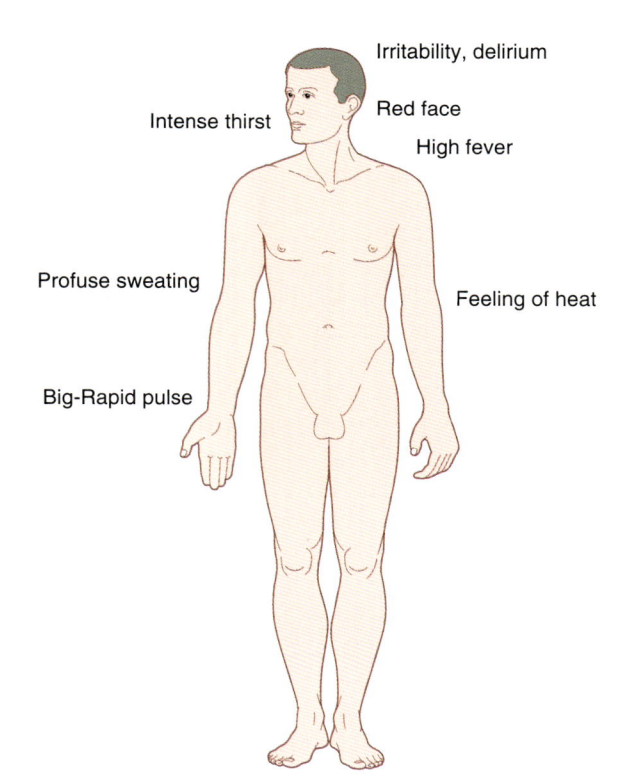

Figure 44.4 Bright Yang channel pattern

Pathology

At the Bright Yang stage, the pathogenic factor has become interior and transformed into Heat. Therefore, from the Eight-Principle point of view, this pattern is interior Full-Hot. This pattern can develop from both the Greater Yang and the Lesser Yang stages.

There are two types of patterns at the Bright Yang stage: one characterized by Heat 'without form' (*wu xing*) and called 'Bright Yang channel pattern', the other characterized by Heat 'with form' (*you xing*) and called 'Bright Yang organ pattern'. One could also say that the channel pattern is characterized by Heat, while the organ pattern is characterized by Fire (see below).

In the channel pattern there is Heat and, although this is interior, it is intense and projected towards the surface of the body: for this reason, it is cleared with *pungent* cold herbs which push the Heat outwards (the pungent taste has an outward, floating movement). I use the term 'clear Heat' (*xie re*) for this action (see Glossary).

This pattern is characterized by what are called the 'four bigs': big thirst, big sweating, big fever and Big pulse. Intense Heat causes the thirst and sweating: the Heat is in the Stomach and, as this is the source of fluids, there is intense thirst. Unlike the Greater Yang stage, in this case, 'fever' does mean an actual fever caused by interior Heat: this is therefore an 'interior fever' while that at the Greater Yang stage is an 'exterior fever'. Besides the fever, there is also a pronounced feeling of heat and definitely no aversion to cold: indeed the disappearance of the aversion to cold and the onset of the aversion to heat heralds the change from the Greater Yang to the Bright Yang stage.

Treatment

Treatment principle: clear Stomach-Heat.

Acupuncture

L.I.-11 Quchi, Du-14 Dazhui, P-3 Quze, ST-44 Neiting, ST-43 Xiangu.

Herbal formula

Bai Hu Tang *White Tiger Decoction*.

Box 44.5 summarizes Bright Yang channel pattern.

Box 44.5 Bright Yang channel pattern

Clinical manifestations

High fever, profuse sweating, intense thirst, red face, feeling of heat, irritability, delirium, Red tongue with yellow coating, Overflowing-Rapid or Big-Rapid pulse

Treatment

Acupuncture
L.I.-11 Quchi, Du-14 Dazhui, P-3 Quze, ST-44 Neiting, ST-43 Xiangu
Herbal formula
Bai Hu Tang *White Tiger Decoction*

Bright Yang (*Yang Ming*) organ pattern

Clinical manifestations

High fever that is worse in the afternoon, profuse sweating, sweating on limbs, abdominal fullness and pain, constipation, dry stools, thirst, dark urine, Red tongue with thick dry yellow coating, Deep-Full-Slippery-Rapid pulse (Fig. 44.5).

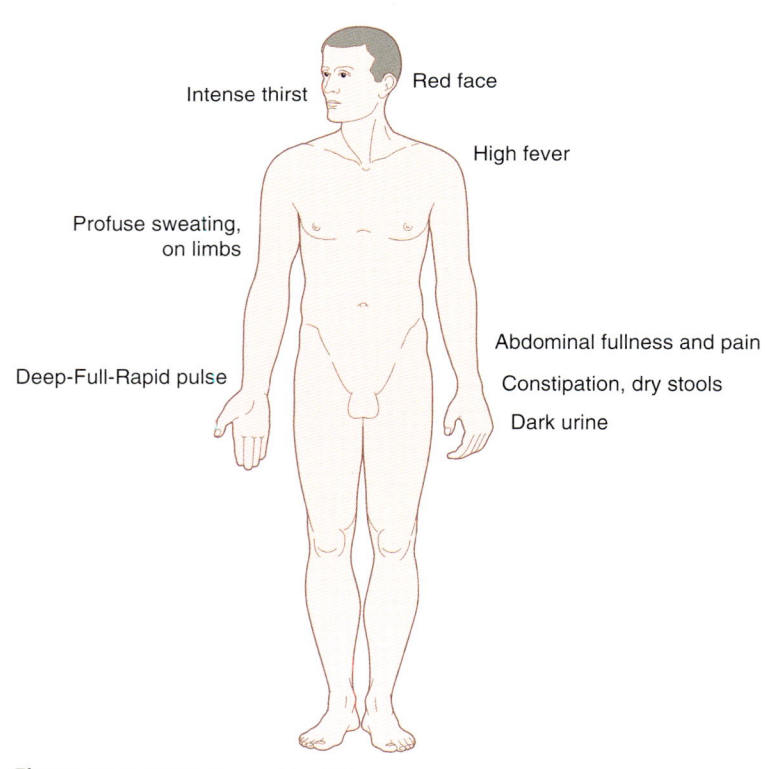

Figure 44.5 Bright Yang organ pattern

Table 44.3 Differences between channel and organ patterns in the Bright Yang pattern of the Six Stages

	Channel pattern	Organ pattern
Common manifestations	Fever, no shivers, feeling of heat, thirst, Red tongue with yellow coating, Rapid pulse	
Differences	Profuse sweating, Overflowing pulse, thin tongue coating	Constipation, abdominal fullness-pain, Deep-Full pulse, thick tongue coating

Pathology

This pattern is also characterized by interior Heat in the Stomach and Intestines. However, the Heat is more intense and it has injured the body fluids, leading to dryness. Some of the clinical manifestations are the same as in the Bright Yang channel pattern: that is, fever, feeling of heat, thirst and sweating.

As Heat (in this case called Fire) has injured the Body Fluids and led to dryness, there are dry stools and constipation: the accumulation of dried-up faeces from constipation causes the abdominal fullness and pain. In this case, not only is Heat more intense (and therefore called Fire) but also it is more drying and at a deeper energetic level than the Heat of the Bright Yang channel pattern. For this reason, it cannot be expelled outward with pungent cold herbs but it must be conducted downwards and expelled through the faeces by stimulating the bowel movement with bitter cold herbs. I call this treatment method 'drain Fire' (*xie huo*, bearing in mind that the '*xie*' here is different than the '*xie*' in 'clear Heat'; see Glossary).

The Deep pulse reflects the deeper location of Fire compared to Heat (in which the pulse was Overflowing or Big).

Treatment

Treatment principle: drain Fire from the Stomach and Intestines, move downward.

Acupuncture

L.I.-11 Quchi, Du-14 Dazhui, P-3 Quze, ST-44 Neiting, ST-43 Xiangu, ST-25 Tianshu, SP-15 Daheng, ST-37 Shangjuxu, SP-6 Sanyinjiao.

Herbal formula

Tiao Wei Cheng Qi Tang *Regulating the Stomach Conducting Qi Decoction.*

Table 44.3 compares the clinical manifestations of the Bright Yang channel pattern with those of Bright Yang organ pattern. Box 44.6 summarizes the Bright Yang organ pattern.

Box 44.6 Bright Yang organ pattern

Clinical manifestations

High fever that is worse in the afternoon, profuse sweating, sweating on limbs, abdominal fullness and pain, constipation, dry stools, thirst, dark urine, Red tongue with thick dry yellow coating, Deep-Full-Slippery-Rapid pulse

Treatment

Acupuncture
L.I.-11 Quchi, Du-14 Dazhui, P-3 Quze, ST-44 Neiting, ST-43 Xiangu, ST-25 Tianshu, SP-15 Daheng, ST-37 Shangjuxu, SP-6 Sanyinjiao
Herbal formula
Tiao Wei Cheng Qi Tang *Regulating the Stomach Conducting Qi Decoction*

LESSER YANG (*SHAO YANG*) STAGE

Clinical manifestations

Alternation of shivers (or cold feeling) and fever (or feeling of heat), bitter taste, dry throat, blurred vision, hypochondrial fullness and distension, no desire to eat or drink, irritability, nausea, vomiting, unilateral thin white coating, Wiry-Fine pulse (Fig. 44.6).

Pathology

In this pattern, the pathogenic factor 'oscillates' between the Greater Yang and the Bright Yang stages: when it goes towards the Greater Yang, the patient has aversion to cold (in the same way as in the Greater Yang stage); when it goes towards the Bright Yang, the patient feels hot or has a fever. For this reason, the Lesser Yang pattern is described as being 'half interior and half exterior': this does not mean that it is half interior and half exterior in character but that the

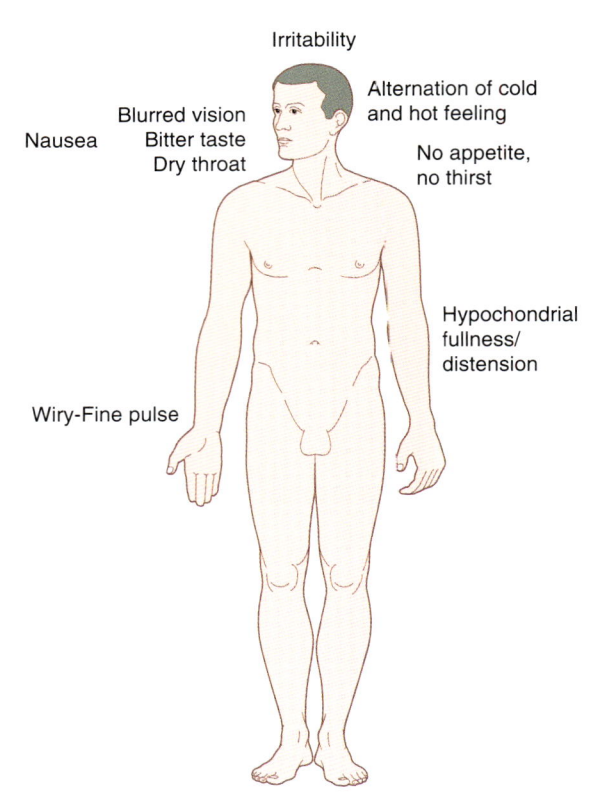

Figure 44.6 Lesser Yang pattern

Box 44.7 Lesser Yang

Clinical manifestations

Alternation of shivers (or cold feeling) and fever (or feeling of heat), bitter taste, dry throat, blurred vision, hypochondrial fullness and distension, no desire to eat or drink, irritability, nausea, vomiting, unilateral thin white coating, Wiry-Fine pulse

Treatment

Acupuncture
T.B.-5 Waiguan, T.B.-6 Zhigou, G.B.-41 Zulinqi, Du-13 Taodao
Herbal formula
Xiao Chai Hu Tang Small Bupleurum Decoction

---

pathogenic factor oscillates (or 'bounces') between the Exterior (Greater Yang) and the Interior (Bright Yang).

It is important to note that the aversion to cold and feeling of heat *alternate* and are not simultaneous as in the Greater Yang pattern. Moreover, if there is no actual fever, the feeling of heat in the Lesser Yang pattern is a *subjective* feeling of heat, while the 'heat emission' of the Greater Yang pattern is an *objective* hot feeling of the patient's body on palpation.

Other symptoms and signs are typical of the Gall Bladder channel: bitter taste, dry throat, blurred vision, hypochondrial fullness and distension, irritability, nausea and vomiting.

Typically, the tongue has a unilateral coating.

Treatment

Treatment principle: harmonize the Lesser Yang.

Acupuncture

T.B.-5 Waiguan, T.B.-6 Zhigou, G.B.-41 Zulinqi, Du-13 Taodao.

Herbal formula

Xiao Chai Hu Tang *Small Bupleurum Decoction*.
Box 44.7 summarizes the Lesser Yang pattern.

GREATER YIN (*TAI YIN*) STAGE

Clinical manifestations

Abdominal fullness, feeling cold, vomiting, no appetite, diarrhoea, no thirst, tiredness, Pale tongue with sticky white coating, Deep-Weak-Slow pulse (Fig. 44.7).

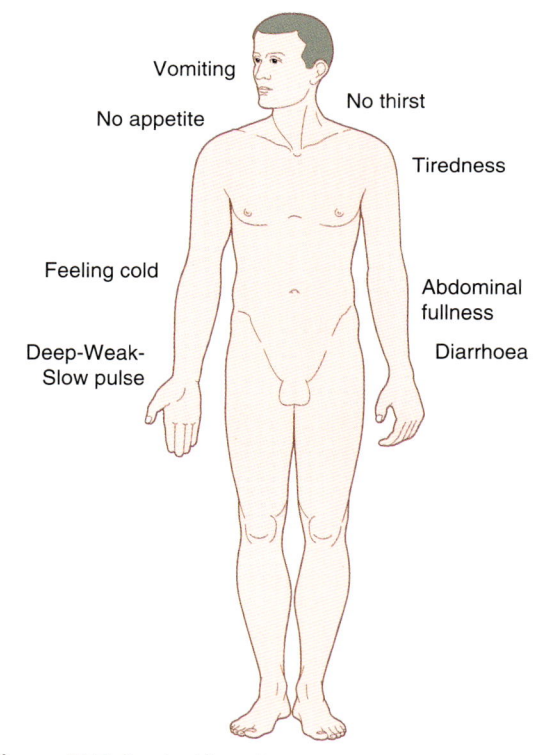

Figure 44.7 Greater Yin pattern

Pathology

The Greater Yin pattern is the first of the Yin patterns. It is characterized by Spleen-Yang deficiency with Cold. The obstruction of Cold in the abdomen causes abdominal fullness and vomiting while the other symptoms are caused by Spleen-Yang deficiency.

From the Eight-Principle point of view, the pattern is interior Empty-Cold.

Treatment

Treatment principle: tonify Spleen-Yang, expel Cold.

Acupuncture

Ren-12 Zhongwan, BL-20 Pishu, ST-36 Zusanli, ST-25 Tianshu, SP-6 Sanyinjiao. Moxa is applicable.

Herbal formula

Li Zhong Tang *Regulating the Centre Decoction*.

Box 44.8 summarizes the Greater Yin pattern.

Box 44.8 Greater Yin

Clinical manifestations

Abdominal fullness, feeling cold, vomiting, no appetite, diarrhoea, no thirst, tiredness, Pale tongue with sticky white coating, Deep-Weak-Slow pulse

Treatment

Acupuncture
Ren-12 Zhongwan, BL-20 Pishu, ST-36 Zusanli, ST-25 Tianshu, SP-6 Sanyinjiao. Moxa is applicable
Herbal formula
Li Zhong Tang *Regulating the Centre Decoction*

LESSER YIN (*SHAO YIN*) STAGE

The Lesser Yin stage has two patterns, called 'Cold transformation' and 'Heat transformation'. These patterns describe, respectively, essentially a deficiency of Kidney-Yang with Empty-Cold and one of Kidney-Yin with Empty-Heat.

Cold transformation

Clinical manifestations

Chills, feeling cold, lying with body curled, listlessness, desire to sleep, cold limbs, diarrhoea, no thirst, frequent pale urination, Pale and wet tongue with white coating, Deep-Weak-Slow pulse (Fig. 44.8).

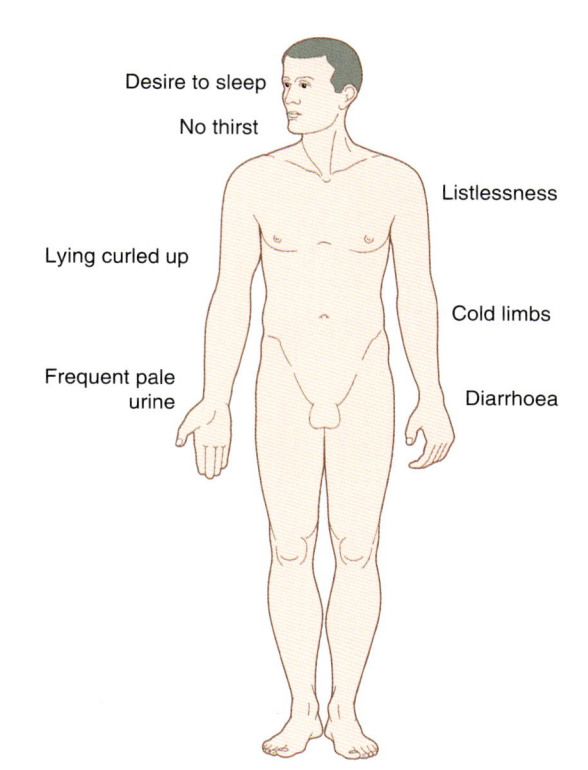

Figure 44.8 Lesser Yin pattern, Cold transformation

Pathology

The pathology of this pattern is essentially Kidney-Yang deficiency with Cold.

Treatment

Treatment principle: tonify Kidney-Yang, expel Cold.

Acupuncture

BL-23 Shenshu, Ren-4 Guanyuan, Ren-6 Qihai, Ren-8 Shenque, KI-7 Fuliu, KI-3 Taixi. Moxa is applicable.

Herbal formula

Si Ni Tang *Four Rebellious Decoction*.

Box 44.9 summarizes the Lesser Yin Cold transformation pattern.

Heat transformation

Clinical manifestations

Feeling of heat, irritability, insomnia, dry mouth and throat at night, dark urine, night sweating, Red tongue without coating, Fine-Rapid pulse (Fig. 44.9).

Box 44.9 Lesser Yin Cold transformation

Clinical manifestations

Chills, feeling cold, lying with body curled, listlessness, desire to sleep, cold limbs, diarrhoea, no thirst, frequent pale urination, Pale and wet tongue with white coating, Deep-Weak-Slow pulse

Treatment

Acupuncture
BL-23 Shenshu, Ren-4 Guanyuan, Ren-6 Qihai, Ren-8 Shenque, KI-7 Fuliu, KI-3 Taixi.
Herbal formula
Si Ni Tang *Four Rebellious Decoction*

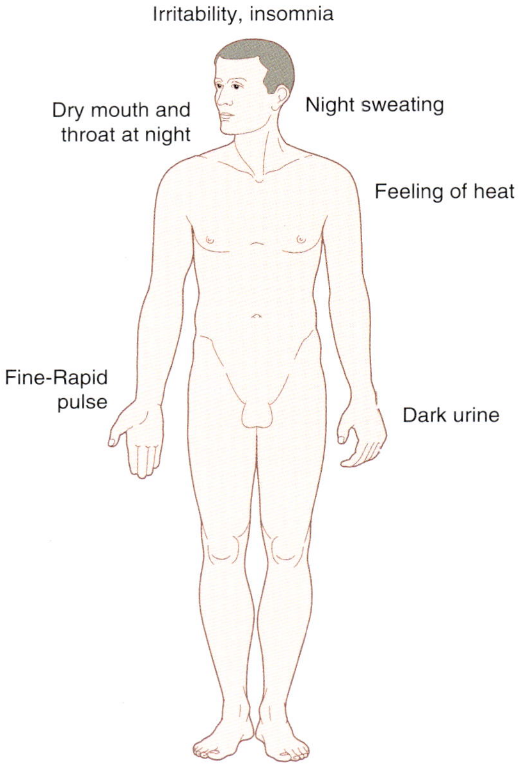

Acupuncture

Ren-4 Guanyuan, Ren-6 Qihai, KI-3 Taixi, KI-6 Zhaohai, SP-6 Sanyinjiao.

Herbal formula

Huang Lian E Jiao Tang *Coptis–Colla Asini Decoction*.

Box 44.10 summarizes the Lesser Yin Heat transformation pattern.

Box 44.10 Lesser Yin Heat transformation

Clinical manifestations

Feeling of heat, irritability, insomnia, dry mouth and throat at night, dark urine, night sweating, Red tongue without coating, Fine-Rapid pulse

Treatment

Acupuncture
Ren-4 Guanyuan, Ren-6 Qihai, KI-3 Taixi, KI-6 Zhaohai, SP-6 Sanyinjiao
Herbal formula
Huang Lian E Jiao Tang *Coptis-Colla Asini Decoction*

TERMINAL YIN (*JUE YIN*) STAGE

Clinical manifestations

Persistent thirst, feeling of energy rising to the chest, pain and heat sensation in heart region, hungry but no desire to eat, cold limbs, diarrhoea, vomiting, vomiting of roundworms, Wiry pulse (Fig. 44.10).

Pathology

This pattern is characterized by Heat above (thirst, feeling of energy rising, pain and heat sensation of heart region, hunger) and Cold below (no desire to eat, cold limbs, vomiting).

In some cases, this pattern is seen in roundworm infestation.

Treatment

Treatment principle: clear Heat above, expel Cold below, harmonize the Liver channel.

Acupuncture

LIV-3 Taichong, L.I.-4 Hegu, SP-4 Gongsun and P-6 Neiguan.

Herbal formula

Wu Mei Wan *Prunus Mume Decoction*.

Box 44.11 sumarizes the Terminal Yin pattern.

Figure 44.9 Lesser Yin pattern, Heat transformation

Pathology

The pathology of this pattern is Kidney-Yin deficiency with Empty-Heat.

Treatment

Treatment principle: nourish Kidney-Yin, clear Empty-Heat.

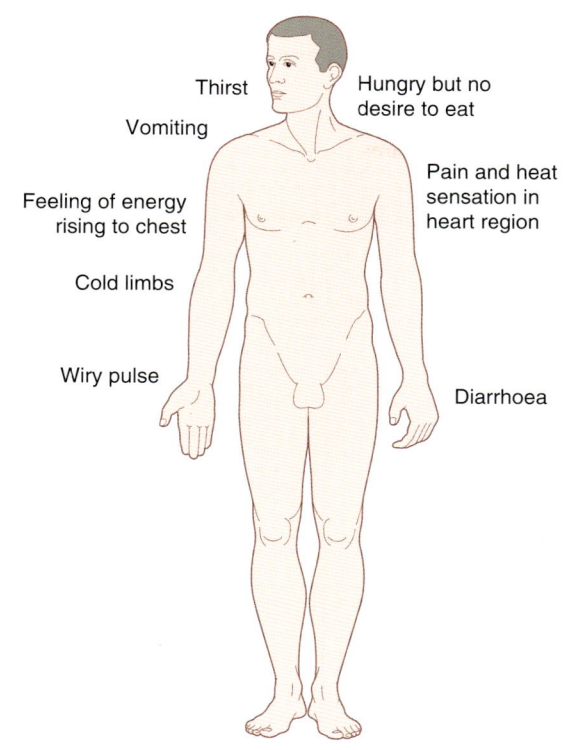

Figure 44.10 Terminal Yin pattern

Labels on figure: Thirst; Vomiting; Feeling of energy rising to chest; Cold limbs; Wiry pulse; Hungry but no desire to eat; Pain and heat sensation in heart region; Diarrhoea

---

Box 44.11 Terminal Yin

Clinical manifestations

Persistent thirst, feeling of energy rising to the chest, pain and heat sensation in heart region, hungry but no desire to eat, cold limbs, diarrhoea, vomiting, vomiting of roundworms, Wiry pulse

Treatment

Acupuncture
LIV-3 Taichong, L.I.-4 Hegu, SP-4 Gongsun and P-6 Neiguan

Herbal formula
Wu Mei Wan *Prunus Mume Decoction*

Learning outcomes

In this chapter you will have learned:
- The historical context for identifying patterns according to the Six Stages (especially Zhang Zhong Jing and his *Shang Han Lun*)
- The three essential symptoms of the Greater Yang stage of external Wind invasion: aversion to cold, headache and stiff neck and a Floating pulse
- How to identify the following Greater Yang stage patterns:

Channel patterns

Invasion of Wind-Cold with a prevalence of Wind: slight sweating, deficiency of Nutritive Qi, mild aversion to cold
Invasion of Wind-Cold with a prevalence of Cold: no sweating, aversion to cold, Floating-Tight pulse

Organ patterns

Accumulation of Water: symptoms of Wind in the Exterior with retention of urine, slight thirst and vomiting after drinking caused by the pathogenic factor in the Bladder
Accumulation of Blood: hypogastric fullness and urgency, blood in urine, and mental restlessness caused by accumulation of Heat and stasis in the Lower Burner and Bladder

- How to identify the following Bright Yang stage patterns:
  Bright Yang channel pattern: characterized by the 'four bigs': big thirst, sweating, fever and pulse
  Bright Yang organ pattern: fever, sweating, thirst, abdominal fullness and constipation caused by more intense Heat at a deeper energetic level than the channel pattern (in Stomach and Intestines)
- How to identify the remaining Six-Stage patterns:
  Lesser Yang: alternation of shivers and fever caused by pathogenic factor oscillating between Greater Yang and Bright Yang stages, with Gall Bladder symptoms
  Greater Yin: characterized by Spleen-Yang deficiency with Cold (abdominal fullness, vomiting and feeling cold)
  Lesser Yin Cold transformation: pathology of Kidney-Yang deficiency with Cold (chills, frequent pale urination, pale and wet tongue with white coat)
  Lesser Yin Heat transformation: pathology of Kidney-Yin deficiency with Empty-Heat (feeling of Heat, dry mouth and throat at night, night sweating, Red tongue without coating)
  Terminal Yin: characterized by Heat above (thirst, feeling of energy rising, pain and heat sensation in heart region, hunger) and Cold below (cold limbs, vomiting)

Self-assessment questions

1. Which text gave the first systematic presentation of the pathology and treatment of diseases caused by invasion of exterior pathogenic factors? Who was the author and in which century was it written?
2. What are the three essential symptoms of a Greater Yang stage invasion?
3. Why is there an occipital headache with an invasion of Wind at the Greater Yang stage?
4. Explain why the invasion of Wind-Cold with prevalence of Wind is characterized by slight sweating?
5. What pulse would you expect to feel in an invasion of Wind-Cold with prevalence of Cold?
6. Explain the pathology of retention of urine, thirst and vomiting after drinking in the organ pattern Accumulation of Water.
7. Why might there be Blood in the urine in the organ pattern Accumulation of Blood?

8. What 'four bigs' characterize the Bright Yang stage channel pattern?
9. How does the pulse differ between the Bright Yang channel and organ patterns?
10. What is the main symptom of the Lesser Yang stage?
11. Which organ pattern does the Greater Yin pattern most resemble?
12. What tongue and pulse would you expect in the Lesser Yin pattern?
13. Give one symptom each of Heat above and Cold below as seen in the Terminal Yin pattern.

See p. 1265 for answers

END NOTES

1. 1979 The Yellow Emperor's Classic of Internal Medicine – Simple Questions (*Huang Di Nei Jing Su Wen* 黄帝内经素问), People's Health Publishing House, Beijing, first published *c.*100 BC, p. 21.
2. Ibid., p. 24.
3. Nanjing College of Traditional Chinese Medicine 1979 A Revised Explanation of the Classic of Difficulties (*Nan Jing Jiao Shi* 难经校释), People's Health Publishing House, Beijing, first published *c.*AD 100, p. 128.
4. Nanjing College of Traditional Chinese Medicine 1978 A Study of Warm Diseases (*Wen Bing Xue* 温病学), Shanghai Scientific Publishing House, Shanghai, p. 12.
5. Not to be confused with the disease of the same name *Zhong Feng* Wind-Stroke.

Identification of Patterns According to the Four Levels

45

Key contents

Nature of Warm Diseases

Relationship between Wind-Heat and Warm Diseases

The Four Levels
Defensive Qi level (Wei)
Qi level (Qi)
Nutritive Qi level (Ying)
Blood level (Xue)

Warm Diseases and skin rashes

Defensive Qi level
Wind-Heat
Summer-Heat
Damp-Heat
Dry-Heat

Qi level
Lung-Heat (Heat in chest and diaphragm)
Stomach-Heat
Intestines Dry-Heat
Gall Bladder-Heat
Damp-Heat in Stomach and Spleen

Nutritive Qi level
Heat in Nutritive Qi level
Heat in the Pericardium

Blood level
Heat victorious moving Blood
Heat victorious stirring Wind
Empty-Wind agitating in the Interior
Collapse of Yin
Collapse of Yang

Latent Heat
Lesser Yang level
Bright Yang level
Lesser Yin level

Relations between the Four Levels, Six Stages and Three Burners

The identification of patterns according to the Four Levels was devised by Ye Tian Shi in his book 'A Discussion on Warm Diseases' (*Wen Bing Lun*, 1746). The identification of patterns according to the Four Levels is clinically the most useful tool to interpret the pathology and establish the treatment of diseases deriving from invasion of Wind-Heat.

As mentioned in chapter 44, the identification of patterns according to the Six Stages, devised by Zhang Zhong Jing in his 'Discussion of Cold-Induced Diseases' (*Shang Han Lun*, AD 220), dominated the thinking on the pathology and treatment of diseases of external origin for 14 centuries. Although many patients clearly suffered from invasion of Wind-Heat during those centuries and some dissenting voices had been heard during the Song and Ming dynasties, it was not until the late Ming and early Qing dynasty (1600s) that a comprehensive theory of diseases from external Wind-Heat was formulated.

In particular, these doctors formulated the theory of 'Warm Diseases' (*Wen Bing*) as a new, distinct disease category different from the diseases from external Wind falling under the umbrella of *Shang Han* diseases (i.e. diseases from invasion of Wind and Cold). As mentioned in the previous chapter, even Warm Diseases were explained as a transformation of Cold pathogen. The doctors who contributed to this theory were collectively referred to as the 'School of Warm Diseases' and the most influential of these were Wu You Ke (1582–1652), author of 'Discussion on Warm Epidemics' (*Wen Yi Lun*), Ye Tian Shi (1677–1746), author of 'Discussion on Warm Diseases' (*Wen Bing Lun*), and Wu Ju Tong (1758–1836), author of 'Systematic Differentiation of Warm Diseases' (*Wen Bing Tiao Bian*). Ye Tian Shi formulated the identification of patterns according to the Four Levels while Wu Ju Tong formulated the identification of patterns according to the Three Burners. Incidentally, Wu Ju Tong formulated the widely used formula for the beginning stage of invasion of Wind-Heat, Yin Qiao San *Forsythia-Lonicera Powder*.

Nature of Warm Diseases

The theory of Warm Diseases represented an important, revolutionary departure in Chinese medicine. All Warm Diseases are by definition caused by external Wind-Heat but they have special characteristics which can be summarized as follows:

- They all manifest with fever
- The pathogenic factor enters through the nose and mouth
- They are infectious
- The pathological developments are rapid
- The pathogenic factor of Warm Diseases has a strong tendency to injure Yin

The second and third characteristics are particularly important and new in Chinese medicine. Until the development of the Warm Diseases School, external pathogenic factors were thought to enter the body through the skin, hence the rationale in sweating as a treatment method in the beginning stages; the Warm Diseases School believes that pathogenic factors enter through the nose and mouth. This is a very perceptive view that accords with that of Western medicine as the bacteria and viruses causing Warm Diseases enter via the mucous membranes of nose and mouth.

Even more important was the discovery of the infectious nature of such diseases. This concept, formulated before the introduction of Western medicine to China, was revolutionary as previously it was thought that the factors determining why a person succumbs to invasions of external pathogenic factors were to be found in the relative imbalance between the external pathogenic factor and the body's Qi. Although such imbalance still plays a role in the development of Warm Diseases, the Warm Diseases School recognized that some of the pathogenic factors causing Warm Diseases can be very strong, indeed 'virulent' to use a Western medical expression, and many people will succumb to them even though their body's Qi may be relatively strong. Moreover, the doctors of the School of Warm Diseases recognized the sometimes epidemic nature of some of these diseases and clearly saw that, on occasions, whole villages or even whole counties would be decimated by an epidemic of an infectious disease.

Relationship between Wind-Heat and Warm Diseases

All Warm Diseases are by definition caused by invasion of Wind-Heat but not every invasion of Wind-Heat is a Warm Disease. By nature, Warm Diseases are more virulent, more infectious, they are characterized by more intense Heat, they develop rapidly and they have a strong tendency to injure Yin.

Examples of 'Warm Diseases' are influenza, measles (*rubeola*), German measles (*rubella*), chicken pox (*varicella*), mononucleosis (glandular fever), mumps (*parotitis*), SARS, meningitis, encephalitis, whooping cough (*pertussis*) and scarlet fever (*scarlatina*).

All Warm Diseases are by definition caused by invasion of Wind-Heat but not every invasion of Wind-Heat is a Warm Disease

Clinical note

Examples of 'warm diseases' are influenza, measles (*rubeola*), German measles (*rubella*), chicken pox (*varicella*), glandular fever (*mononucleosis*), mumps (*parotitis*), SARS, meningitis, encephalitis, whooping cough (*pertussis*) and scarlet fever (*scarlatina*)

The Four Levels

The interpretation of clinical manifestations of Warm Diseases according to the Four Levels was formulated by Ye Tian Shi. This is a brilliant theory that provides the most clinically useful tool to diagnose, interpret and treat diseases caused by external Wind-Heat and their consequences, whether they are Warm Diseases or not.

The theory of the Four Levels is clinically more relevant than that of the Six Stages. For example, one of the most common consequences of an invasion of Wind-Heat is the transformation of external Wind-Heat into interior Phlegm-Heat in the Lungs, causing a chest infection: this situation is contemplated in the Four Levels (corresponding to Lung-Heat, Qi level), while it is not contemplated in the Six Stages.

The Qi level contemplates the pattern of Damp-Heat in Stomach and Spleen as a consequence of an invasion of Wind-Heat: this is a very common clinical situation and yet it is one that is not contemplated in the Six Stages.

The Blood level includes patterns which are characterized by convulsions from the development of internal Wind: these are typical complications of children's diseases such as meningitis but they are not contemplated in the Six Stages.

The Four Levels are the Defensive Qi, Qi, Nutritive Qi and Blood levels (*Wei, Qi, Ying, Xue*): the first level is the only exterior one characterized by the presence of the external Wind-Heat on the energetic surface of the body. The other three levels are all interior and all characterized by interior Heat; however, the brilliance of this theory lies in its identification of three different depths of penetration of interior pathogenic Heat. Each level has its own distinctive pathology and treatment (Fig. 45.1).

Before listing the clinical manifestations of each pattern, I will first discuss the Four Levels in general.

> The three levels Qi, Nutritive Qi and Blood (*Qi, Ying* and *Xue*) are all interior and all characterized by interior Heat but with a difference in energetic depth

Defensive Qi level (*Wei*)

The Defensive Qi level is the beginning stage of invasions of Wind-Heat: it is the only exterior level (i.e. characterized by the presence of the exterior Wind on the Exterior of the body). The Defensive Qi level comprises four different patterns according to the nature of the pathogenic factor: namely, Wind-Heat, Summer-Heat, Damp-Heat and Dry-Heat. Of these four, Wind-Heat is by far the most common one.

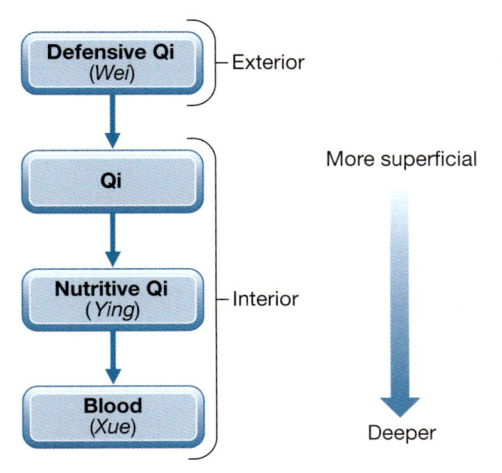

Figure 45.1 The Four Levels

Qi level (*Qi*)

The Qi level is interior, that is, the pathogenic factor has penetrated into the Interior and it has also transformed into Heat. However, the Qi level is the most superficial of the three interior levels. There is a saying about the Qi level stating '*Nobody dies at the Qi level*': this means that, in the context of acute febrile diseases, contrary to the Nutritive Qi and Blood levels, the Qi level is never life-threatening.

The Qi level is characterized by Full Interior Heat with symptoms of fever, thirst, feeling of heat, mental restlessness, Red tongue with thick yellow coating and a Rapid-Full pulse. These are just general symptoms as other manifestations depend on the pattern involved, of which there are five: Lung-Heat (Heat in chest and diaphragm), Stomach-Heat, Intestines Dry-Heat, Gall Bladder-Heat and Damp-Heat in Stomach and Spleen.

With the Qi level, there are actually two types of Heat, one that I call 'Heat' and the other 'Fire'. The pattern of Intestines Dry-Heat is characterized by Fire while the other four are characterized by Heat. Fire has the same nature as Heat but, compared to it, has the following distinguishing features:

- It is more intense (intense thirst, high fever, intense feeling of heat)
- It affects the Mind more (mental restlessness, delirium)
- It dries up more (intense thirst, dry stools, constipation, very dry tongue coating)
- It is at a deeper energetic layer that Heat (Deep pulse compared to Overflowing in Heat)
- It may cause bleeding
- In acute febrile diseases in children it may cause internal Wind quickly

The pattern of Stomach-Heat represents Heat in the Stomach (and it is equivalent to the Bright Yang channel pattern within the Six Stages), while that of Intestines Dry-Heat represents Fire (and it is equivalent to the Bright Yang organ pattern).

Table 45.1 compares the Defensive Qi and Qi levels while Table 45.2 compares Heat and Fire within the Qi level.

Nutritive Qi level (*Ying*)

At the Nutritive Qi level, the Heat has penetrated to a deeper energetic layer and begun to injure the Yin. At this level, Heat is obstructing the Mind and the

Table 45.1 Comparison of Defensive Qi and Qi levels in identification of patterns according to the Four Levels

Level	Eight Principles	Organs	Upright Qi	Location
Defensive Qi	External Heat Full	Not affected	Strong	Exterior (Upright Qi reacts in Exterior: aversion to cold)
Qi	Internal Heat Full	Affected	Strong	Interior (Upright Qi reacts in Interior: no aversion to cold)

Table 45.2 Comparison of Heat and Fire at the Qi level

	Stomach-Heat (Heat)	Intestines Dry-Heat (Fire)
Common manifestations	Fever, feeling of heat, thirst, Red tongue with thick yellow coating, Rapid pulse	
Differences	Profuse sweating, Overflowing pulse, tongue coating not too dry	Constipation, abdominal fullness/pain, mental restlessness, dry mouth, Deep-Full pulse, thick, dry tongue coating

Table 45.3 Comparison of Four Levels

Symptoms	Defensive Qi	Qi	Nutritive Qi/Blood
Fever	Slight fever, aversion to cold	High fever, feeling of heat	Fever at night
Thirst	Slight	Intense, desire to drink cold drinks	Dry mouth, desire to sip liquids
Mental state	Unchanged	May be delirium, generally mind clear	Delirium, fainting, mind confused
Sweating	Slight	Profuse	Night sweating
Tongue	Red sides/front, thin white coating	Red body, thick yellow coating	Red body, no coating
Pulse	Floating-Rapid	Big-Rapid, Deep-Full-Rapid or Slippery-Rapid	Fine-Rapid
Summary	Exterior pattern	Interior pattern, Upright Qi strong	Interior pattern, Upright Qi weak

Pericardium, causing delirium and even coma. Fever at night is a distinctive sign of the Nutritive Qi level.

The tongue appearance at the Nutritive Qi level is an important sign that differentiates this level from the Qi level: at the Nutritive Qi level, the tongue is Deep-Red *without* coating (while at the Qi level, it is Red with a thick coating).

There are two patterns at the Nutritive Qi level: Heat in Nutritive Qi level and Heat in the Pericardium.

Blood level (*Xue*)

The Blood level is the deepest energetic layer, with Heat affecting the Blood. There are several different patterns with varying clinical manifestations but the chief clinical features of the Blood level are as follows:

- There is Yin deficiency
- Heat is affecting the Blood, causing bleeding
- Heat is affecting the Mind, causing delirium or coma
- Heat in the Blood causes bleeding under the skin with the appearance of macules
- Internal Wind develops, causing convulsions and tremors
- Collapse of Yin or Yang may occur

Macules are a definite sign that Heat has reached the Blood level. There are five patterns at the Blood level: Heat victorious moving Blood, Heat victorious stirring Wind, Empty-Wind agitating in the Interior, Collapse of Yin and Collapse of Yang.

Table 45.3 compares the clinical manifestations of the Four levels while Table 45.4 differentiates the Four Levels according to tongue appearance.

Table 45.4 Comparison of tongue appearance in the Four Levels

Tongue	Defensive Qi				Qi	Nutritive Qi	Blood
	Wind-Heat	Summer-Heat	Dry-Heat	Damp-Heat			
Body	Red sides or front	Red	Dry	Red	Red	Deep-Red	Deep-Red
Coating	Thin white or yellow	Thin white	Thin white, dry	White, sticky	Thick, dry, yellow or brown (sticky in Stomach and Spleen Damp-Heat)	No coating	No coating
Remark					Coating more important	Body more important	Body more important

Table 45.5 Comparison of papules, vesicles and macules

Type	Shape	Location	Aftermath
Papule (*Zhen*)	Like small grains, sticking out from skin, red, can be felt on touch	Chest, abdomen, back, face most of all. Seldom on limbs	Leave trace
Vesicle (*Bao*)	Round in shape, white, obvious, like small water vesicles, shaped like grains of rice or pearls, can be felt on touch	Chest, abdomen, axillae, neck, seldom on limbs, never on face	Leave trace
Macule (*Ban*)	Big, circular spots, level with skin, not sticking out, cannot be felt on touch	Chest, abdomen, back, face most of all. Seldom on limbs	Do not leave trace

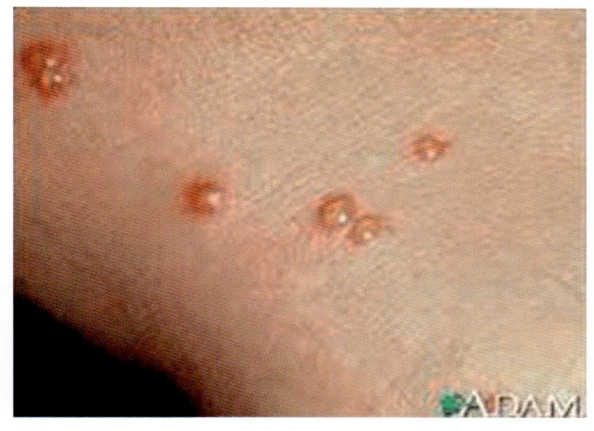

Figure 45.2 Vesicles

Warm Diseases and skin rashes

Many Warm Diseases often manifest with a rash; examples of exanthematous (i.e. manifesting with rash) diseases are measles, German measles and chicken pox. One must distinguish *vesicles*, *papules* and *macules* (Table 45.5).

Vesicles are blister-like spots filled with a clear fluid and they always indicate Dampness (Fig. 45.2). *Papules* are red, solid spots: they generally indicate Heat at

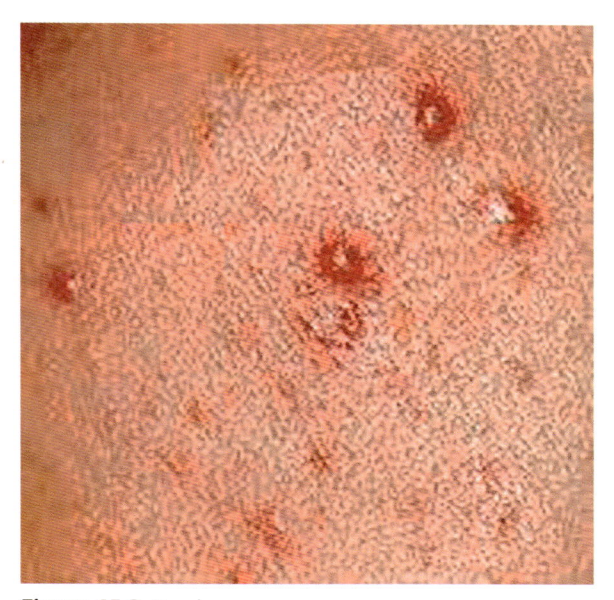

Figure 45.3 Papules

the Qi level, especially in the Lungs and Stomach (Fig. 45.3). *Macules* are spots under the skin, which, unlike vesicles and papules, cannot be felt on palpation: they always indicate Heat at the Nutritive Qi or Blood level (Fig. 45.4).

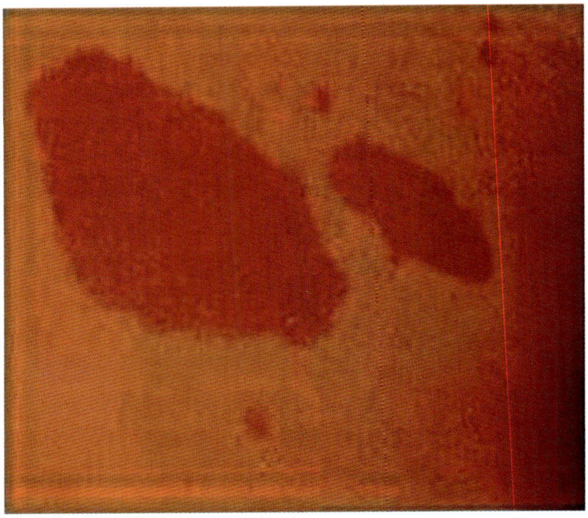

Figure 45.4 Macules

The discussion of the Four Levels will comprise the following topics:

- Defensive Qi level
  - Wind-Heat
  - Summer-Heat
  - Damp-Heat
  - Dry-Heat
- Qi level
  - Lung-Heat (Heat in chest and diaphragm)
  - Stomach-Heat
  - Intestines Dry-Heat
  - Gall Bladder-Heat
  - Damp-Heat in Stomach and Spleen
- Nutritive Qi level
  - Heat in Nutritive Qi level
  - Heat in the Pericardium
- Blood level
  - Heat victorious moving Blood
  - Heat victorious stirring Wind
  - Empty-Wind agitating in the Interior
  - Collapse of Yin
  - Collapse of Yang
- Latent heat
  - Lesser Yang level
  - Bright Yang level
  - Lesser Yin level
- Relations between the Four Levels, Six Stages and Three Burners

DEFENSIVE QI (*WEI*) LEVEL

Wind-Heat

Clinical manifestations

Fever, aversion to cold, headache, sore throat, slight sweating, runny nose with yellow discharge, swollen tonsils, body aches, slight thirst, tongue Red in the front or sides with a thin white coating, Floating-Rapid pulse.

Pathology

The pathology of aversion to cold and 'fever' is the same as for the Greater Yang stage already discussed in chapter 44. Please note that, contrary to what one might think, there *is* aversion to cold in invasions of Wind-Heat because the Wind (whether it is with Cold or Heat) obstructs the Defensive Qi in the space between the skin and muscles so that it cannot warm the body.

In the case of ordinary invasions of Wind-Heat, 'fever' may not be an actual fever but an objective hot feeling of the patient's body on palpation; however, in the case of Warm Diseases, it would be an actual fever.

The headache is caused by the obstruction of the channels of the head by exterior Wind in the same way as for the Greater Yang stage. The body aches, which may be very pronounced, are caused by the obstruction of the muscles by exterior Wind. The tongue coating is white because the pathogenic factor is on the Exterior.

A sore throat is due to invasion of the Wind in the Lung channel in the throat: a sore and red throat is a distinctive sign of invasion of Wind-Heat as compared to Wind-Cold.

Treatment

Treatment principle: release the Exterior, expel Wind-Heat, restore the diffusing and descending of Lung-Qi.

Acupuncture

L.I.-4 Hegu, L.I.-11 Quchi, T.B.-5 Waiguan, Du-14 Dazhui, BL-12 Fengmen (with cupping), LU-11 Shaoshang.

Herbal formula

Yin Qiao San *Lonicera–Forsythia Decoction*.
Sang Ju Yin *Morus–Chrysanthemum Decoction*.

Table 45.6 Comparison of invasion of Wind-Cold (Six Stages) and invasion of Wind-Heat (Four Levels)

	Wind-Cold (Six Stages)	Wind-Heat (Four Levels)
Pathology	Wind-Cold on Exterior obstructing Defensive Qi	Wind-Heat injuring Defensive Qi and impairing descending of Lung-Qi
Penetration route	Through skin	Through nose and mouth
Fever	Slight or absent	Higher
Shivers	Severe	Slight
Aches	Severe	Slight
Headache	Occipital	Deep inside, severe
Sweating	No sweating in prevalence of Cold; sweating only on top part of body in prevalence of Wind	Slight sweating
Thirst	No	Slight
Urine	Clear	Slightly dark
Tongue	Body colour normal, thin white coating	Red sides and/or front, thin white coating
Pulse	Floating-Tight	Floating-Rapid
Treatment	Pungent warm herbs to cause sweating	Pungent cool herbs to release the Exterior

---

Box 45.1 Wind-Heat

Clinical manifestations

Fever, aversion to cold, headache, sore throat, slight sweating, runny nose with yellow discharge, swollen tonsils, body aches, slight thirst, tongue Red in the front or sides with a thin white coating, Floating-Rapid pulse

Treatment

Acupuncture
L.I.-4 Hegu, L.I.-11 Quchi, T.B.-5 Waiguan, Du-14 Dazhui, BL-12 Fengmen (with cupping), LU-11 Shaoshang
Herbal formula
Yin Qiao San *Lonicera–Forsythia Decoction*
Sang Ju Yin *Morus–Chrysanthemum Decoction*

Table 45.6 differentiates the clinical manifestations of invasion of Wind-Cold (Six Stages) and Wind-Heat (Four Levels). Box 45.1 summarizes Wind-Heat.

Clinical note

The formula *Yin Qiao San* (widely available as a patent remedy) is the main treatment for the beginning stage of invasions of Wind-Heat

Summer-Heat

Clinical manifestations

Fever, aversion to cold, sweating, headache, a feeling of heaviness, an uncomfortable sensation in the epigastrium, irritability, thirst, tongue Red in the front or sides with a white sticky coating, Soggy and Rapid pulse.

Pathology

Summer-Heat is a seasonal pathogenic factor: that is, it occurs only in the Summer (while Wind-Heat may occur at any time of year). Summer-Heat invades the Defensive Qi portion of the body (i.e. the Exterior) and that is why there is aversion to cold. However, it has the strong tendency to move to the Qi level almost from the beginning and that is why there are symptoms of interior Heat such as irritability, thirst, Red tongue and Rapid pulse.

Summer-Heat frequently combines with Dampness and that is why there is a feeling of heaviness and uncomfortable sensation of the epigastrium, a sticky tongue coating and a Soggy pulse. The tongue coating is white because the pathogenic factor is on the Exterior.

To summarize, Summer-Heat includes manifestations of external Wind, Dampness and interior Heat.

Treatment

Treatment principle: release the Exterior, expel Summer-Heat, clear Heat, promote fluids.

Acupuncture

L.I.-4 Hegu, L.I.-11 Quchi, T.B.-5 Waiguan, Du-14 Dazhui, Du-26 Renzhong, BL-40 Weizhong, P-9 Zhongchong.

Herbal formula

Qing Luo Yin *Clearing the Connecting Channels Decoction*.

Box 45.2 summarizes Summer-Heat.

Box 45.2 Summer-Heat

Clinical manifestations

Fever, aversion to cold, no sweating, headache, a feeling of heaviness, an uncomfortable sensation in the epigastrium, irritability, thirst, tongue Red in the front or sides with a white sticky coating, Soggy and Rapid pulse

Treatment

Acupuncture
L.I.-4 Hegu, L.I.-11 Quchi, T.B.-5 Waiguan, Du-14 Dazhui, Du-26 Renzhong, BL-40 Weizhong, P-9 Zhongchong
Herbal formula
Qing Luo Yin *Clearing the Connecting Channels Decoction*

Damp-Heat

Clinical manifestations

Fever that is worse in the afternoon, body hot to touch, aversion to cold, swollen glands, headache, a feeling of heaviness, a feeling of oppression of the epigastrium, sticky taste, thirst with no desire to drink, sticky white tongue coating, Soggy pulse.

Pathology

This is Damp-Heat at the Defensive Qi level when Dampness is on the Exterior: for this reason, there is aversion to cold. However, Damp-Heat has a stronger tendency to affect the Qi level than Wind-Heat does. Dampness obstructs the Middle Burner and this causes the feeling of oppression of the epigastrium; as it obstructs the muscles, it causes the typical feeling of heaviness. A sticky taste without desire to drink is typical of Damp-Heat: Heat causes the thirst but as Dampness obstructs the Middle Burner, the person does not feel like drinking. The swollen glands reflect Dampness and are an important distinctive sign for this pattern.

The headache is usually frontal and is due to Dampness in the Stomach channel of the face. The tongue coating is white because the pathogenic factor is on the Exterior.

Treatment

Treatment principle: release the Exterior, resolve Dampness, clear Heat.

Acupuncture

L.I.-4 Hegu, L.I.-11 Quchi, SP-9 Yinlingquan, SP-6 Sanyinjiao, Ren-12 Zhongwan, Ren-9 Shuifen.

Herbal formula

Huo Xiang Zheng Qi San *Agastache Upright Qi Powder*.

Box 45.3 summarizes Damp-Heat.

Box 45.3 Damp-Heat

Clinical manifestations

Fever that is worse in the afternoon, body hot to touch, aversion to cold, swollen glands, headache, a feeling of heaviness, a feeling of oppression of the epigastrium, sticky taste, thirst with no desire to drink, sticky white tongue coating, Soggy pulse

Treatment

Acupuncture
L.I.-4 Hegu, L.I.-11 Quchi, SP-9 Yinlingquan, SP-6 Sanyinjiao, Ren-12 Zhongwan, Ren-9 Shuifen
Herbal formula
Huo Xiang Zheng Qi San *Agastache Upright Qi Powder*

Dry-Heat

Clinical manifestations

Fever, slight aversion to cold, slight sweating, dry skin, nose, mouth and throat, dry cough, sore throat, Dry tongue with thin white coating, Floating-Rapid pulse.

Pathology

This is Dry-Heat at the Defensive Qi level and, for this reason, there is aversion to cold. Other symptoms are due to dryness injuring body fluids.

The tongue coating is white because the pathogenic factor is on the Exterior.

Treatment

Treatment principle: release the Exterior, clear Heat, promote fluids.

Acupuncture

L.I.-4 Hegu, L.I.-11 Quchi, T.B.-5 Waiguan, SP-6 Sanyinjiao, LU-9 Taiyuan, Ren-12 Zhongwan, ST-36 Zusanli.

Herbal formula

Xing Su San *Prunus–Perilla Powder*.
Sang Xing Tang *Morus–Prunus Decoction*.
 Box 45.4 summarizes Dry-Heat.

Box 45.4 Dry-Heat

Clinical manifestations

Fever, slight aversion to cold, slight sweating, dry skin, nose, mouth and throat, dry cough, sore throat, Dry tongue with thin white coating, Floating-Rapid pulse

Treatment

Acupuncture
L.I.-4 Hegu, L.I.-11 Quchi, T.B.-5 Waiguan, SP-6 Sanyinjiao, LU-9 Taiyuan, Ren-12 Zhongwan, ST-36 Zusanli
Herbal formula
Xing Su San *Prunus–Perilla Powder*
Sang Xing Tang *Morus–Prunus Decoction*

QI LEVEL

Lung-Heat (Heat in chest and diaphragm)

Clinical manifestations

High fever, feeling of heat, no aversion to cold, thirst, cough with thin yellow sputum, shortness of breath, sweating, Red tongue with yellow coating, Slippery-Rapid pulse.

Pathology

This is interior Heat at the Qi level in the Lungs. As in all patterns of the Qi level there is fever, a feeling of heat, thirst and sweating.

The descending of Lung-Qi is impaired by the Heat and this causes the cough and shortness of breath.

This pattern may appear also with Phlegm in which case there would be expectoration of profuse sticky yellow sputum.

Treatment

Treatment principle: clear Qi, clear Lung-Heat, resolve Phlegm, restore the descending of Lung-Qi.

Acupuncture

LU-5 Chize, LU-10 Yuji, Du-14 Dazhui, L.I.-11 Quchi, LU-1 Zhongfu, BL-13 Feishu.

Herbal formula

Ma Xing Shi Gan Tang *Ephedra–Prunus–Gypsum–Glycyrrhiza Decoction*.
Xie Bai San *Draining the White Powder*.
Qing Qi Hua Tan Tang *Clearing Qi and Resolving Phlegm Decoction (if there is also Phlegm)*.
Wu Hu Tang *Five Tigers Decoction*.
 Box 45.5 summarizes Lung-Heat.

Box 45.5 Lung-Heat (Heat in chest and diaphragm)

Clinical manifestations

High fever, feeling of heat, no aversion to cold, thirst, cough with thin yellow sputum, shortness of breath, sweating, Red tongue with yellow coating, Slippery-Rapid pulse

Treatment

Acupuncture
LU-5 Chize, LU-10 Yuji, Du-14 Dazhui, L.I.-11 Quchi, LU-1 Zhongfu, BL-13 Feishu
Herbal formula
Ma Xing Shi Gan Tang *Ephedra–Prunus–Gypsum–Glycyrrhiza Decoction*
Xie Bai San *Draining the White Powder*
Qing Qi Hua Tan Tang *Clearing Qi and Resolving Phlegm Decoction (if there is also Phlegm)*
Wu Hu Tang *Five Tigers Decoction*

Stomach-Heat

Clinical manifestations

High fever that is worse in the afternoon, no aversion to cold, feeling of heat, intense thirst, profuse sweating, Red tongue with yellow coating, Overflowing-Rapid pulse.

Pathology

This is interior Heat at the Qi level in the Stomach. As in all patterns of the Qi level there is fever, a feeling of heat, thirst and sweating.

The pathology of this pattern is the same as that for the Bright Yang channel pattern from the Six Stages.

Treatment

Treatment principle: clear Qi, clear Stomach-Heat.

Acupuncture

ST-44 Neiting, ST-34 Liangqiu, ST-21 Liangmen, ST-43 Xiangu, L.I.-11 Quchi, ST-25 Tianshu.

Herbal formula

Bai Hu Tang *White Tiger Decoction*.
  Box 45.6 summarizes Stomach-Heat.

Box 45.6 Stomach-Heat

Clinical manifestations

High fever that is worse in the afternoon, no aversion to cold, feeling of heat, intense thirst, profuse sweating, Red tongue with yellow coating, Overflowing-Rapid pulse

Treatment

Treatment principle: clear Qi, clear Stomach-Heat
Acupuncture
ST-44 Neiting, ST-34 Liangqiu, ST-21 Liangmen, ST-43 Xiangu,
   L.I.-11 Quchi, ST-25 Tianshu
Herbal formula
Bai Hu Tang *White Tiger Decoction*

Intestines Dry-Heat

Clinical manifestations

High fever that is higher in the afternoon, constipation, dry stools, burning in the anus, abdominal fullness and pain, irritability, delirium, Red tongue with thick yellow dry coating, Deep-Full-Rapid pulse.

Pathology

This is Fire (as opposed to Heat) in the Stomach and Intestines. The difference between Heat and Fire has already been described above and the pathology of this pattern is the same as that for the Bright Yang organ stage of the Six Stages.

Treatment

Treatment principle: drain Fire, clear the Stomach and Intestines, move downward.

Acupuncture

L.I.-11 Quchi, ST-25 Tianshu, SP-15 Daheng, ST-37 Shangjuxu, ST-39 Xiajuxu.

Herbal formula

Tiao Wei Cheng Qi Tang *Regulating the Stomach Conducting Qi Decoction*.
  Box 45.7 summarizes Intestines Dry-Heat.

Box 45.7 Intestines Dry-Heat

Clinical manifestations

High fever that is higher in the afternoon, constipation, dry stools, burning in the anus, abdominal fullness and pain, irritability, delirium, Red tongue with thick yellow dry coating, Deep-Full-Rapid pulse

Treatment

Acupuncture
L.I.-11 Quchi, ST-25 Tianshu, SP-15 Daheng, ST-37 Shangjuxu,
   ST-39 Xiajuxu
Herbal formula
Tiao Wei Cheng Qi Tang *Regulating the Stomach Conducting Qi Decoction*

Gall Bladder-Heat

Clinical manifestations

Alternating hot and cold feeling with a prevalence of heat, bitter taste, thirst, dry throat, hypochondrial pain, nausea, a feeling of fullness in the epigastrium, Red tongue with unilateral sticky yellow coating, Wiry-Rapid pulse.

Pathology

This is equivalent to the Lesser Yang pattern of the Six Stages: it occurs when the pathogenic factor oscillates between the Exterior (causing feeling of cold) and the Interior (causing feeling of heat). The main difference between Gall Bladder-Heat of the Four Levels and the Lesser Yang pattern of the Six Stages is that the former is characterized by more Heat and also by some Dampness (hence the sticky tongue coating).

Treatment

Treatment principle: harmonize the Lesser Yang, clear Gall Bladder-Heat.

Acupuncture

G.B.-34 Yanglingquan, G.B.-43 Xiaxi, T.B.-6 Zhigou, T.B.-5 Waiguan.

Herbal formula

Hao Qin Qing Dan Tang *Artemisia–Scutellaria Clearing the Gall Bladder Decoction*.

Box 45.8 summarizes Gall Bladder-Heat.

Box 45.8 Gall Bladder-Heat

Clinical manifestations

Alternating hot and cold feeling with a prevalence of heat, bitter taste, thirst, dry throat, hypochondrial pain, nausea, a feeling of fullness in the epigastrium, Red tongue with unilateral sticky yellow coating, Wiry-Rapid pulse

Treatment

Acupuncture
G.B.-34 Yanglingquan, G.B.-43 Xiaxi, T.B.-6 Zhigou, T.B.-5 Waiguan
Herbal formula
Hao Qin Qing Dan Tang *Artemisia–Scutellaria Clearing the Gall-Bladder Decoction*

Damp-Heat in Stomach and Spleen

Clinical manifestations

Continuous fever which decreases after sweating but soon increases again, a feeling of heaviness of the body and head, a feeling of oppression of the chest and epigastrium, nausea, loose stools, Red tongue with sticky yellow tongue coating, Soggy-Rapid pulse.

Pathology

This is Damp-Heat in the Stomach and Spleen at the Qi level. Dampness obstructs the Middle Burner and this causes a feeling of oppression of the chest and epigastrium and nausea. Dampness impairs the Spleen's transformation and transportation, which causes loose stools. The feeling of heaviness is caused by the obstruction of the muscles by Dampness.

Damp-Heat causes sweating but this does not reduce the fever because sweat comes from the space between skin and muscles and the Dampness is situation in the Interior.

Treatment

Treatment principle: clear Heat in Stomach and Spleen, resolve Dampness.

Acupuncture

Ren-12 Zhongwan, SP-9 Yinlingquan, SP-6 Sanyinjiao, Ren-9 Shuifen, ST-36 Zusanli, L.I.-11 Quchi, Ren-12 Zhongwan, BL-20 Pishu, BL-22 Sanjiaoshu.

Herbal formula

Lian Po Yin *Coptis–Magnolia Decoction*.

Box 45.9 summarizes Damp-Heat in Stomach and Spleen.

Box 45.9 Damp-Heat in Stomach and Spleen

Clinical manifestations

Continuous fever which decreases after sweating but soon increases again, a feeling of heaviness of the body and head, a feeling of oppression of the chest and epigastrium, nausea, loose stools, Red tongue with sticky yellow tongue coating, Soggy-Rapid pulse

Treatment

Acupuncture
Ren-12 Zhongwan, SP-9 Yinlingquan, SP-6 Sanyinjiao, Ren-9 Shuifen, ST-36 Zusanli, L.I.-11 Quchi, Ren-12 Zhongwan, BL-20 Pishu, BL-22 Sanjiaoshu
Herbal formula
Lian Po Yin *Coptis–Magnolia Decoction*

NUTRITIVE QI (*YING*) LEVEL

Heat in Nutritive Qi level

Clinical manifestations

Fever at night, dry mouth with no desire to drink, mental restlessness, insomnia, delirium, incoherent speech or aphasia, macules, Red tongue without coating, Fine-Rapid pulse.

Pathology

At the Nutritive Qi level, Heat affects the Mind and this causes the mental restlessness, delirium and insomnia. Fever at night reflects the penetration of Heat at the Nutritive Qi level.

Heat in the Nutritive Qi level may heat the Blood and cause macules. At this level, Heat has injured Yin and this causes the tongue to have no coating and its redness reflects the Heat.

Treatment

Treatment principle: clear Nutritive Qi Heat, promote fluids.

Acupuncture

P-9 Zhongchong, P-8 Laogong, HE-9 Shaochong, KI-6 Zhaohai, Shixuan extra points.

Herbal formula

Qing Ying Tang *Clearing the Nutritive Qi [Heat] Decoction*.

Box 45.10 summarizes Heat in the Nutritive Qi level.

Box 45.10 Heat in Nutritive Qi level

Clinical manifestations

Fever at night, dry mouth with no desire to drink, mental restlessness, insomnia, delirium, incoherent speech or aphasia, macules, Red tongue without coating, Fine-Rapid pulse.

Treatment

Treatment principle: clear Nutritive Qi Heat, promote fluids
Acupuncture
P-9 Zhongchong, P-8 Laogong, HE-9 Shaochong, KI-6 Zhaohai, Shixuan extra points
Herbal formula
Qing Ying Tang *Clearing the Nutritive Qi [Heat] Decoction*

Heat in the Pericardium

Clinical manifestations

Fever at night, mental confusion, incoherent speech or aphasia, delirium, body hot, hands and feet cold, macules, Red tongue without coating, Fine-Rapid pulse.

Pathology

The pathology of this pattern is essentially the same as the previous one except that there are more mental signs from invasion of the Pericardium by Heat. The cold hands and feet are a sign of False Cold and they are due to the Heat being so intense that it stops the circulation of Qi to the hands.

Treatment

Treatment principle: clear Nutritive Qi Heat, clear Pericardium-Heat, restore consciousness, promote fluids.

Acupuncture

P-9 Zhongchong, P-3 Quze, P-8 Laogong, HE-9 Shaochong, KI-6 Zhaohai, L.I.-11 Quchi, Shixuan extra points.

Herbal formula

Qing Ying Tang *Clearing the Nutritive Qi [Heat] Decoction*.

Box 45.11 summarizes Heat in the Pericardium.

Box 45.11 Heat in the Pericardium

Clinical manifestations

Fever at night, mental confusion, incoherent speech or aphasia, delirium, body hot, hands and feet cold, macules, Red tongue without coating, Fine-Rapid pulse

Treatment

Treatment principle: clear Nutritive Qi Heat, clear Pericardium-Heat, restore consciousness, promote fluids.
Acupuncture
P-9 Zhongchong, P-3 Quze, P-8 Laogong, HE-9 Shaochong, KI-6 Zhaohai, L.I.-11 Quchi, Shixuan extra points
Herbal formula
Qing Ying Tang *Clearing the Nutritive Qi [Heat] Decoction*

BLOOD LEVEL

Heat victorious agitates Blood

Clinical manifestations

High fever, mental restlessness, manic behaviour, dark macules, vomiting of blood, epistaxis, blood in stools, blood in urine, Dark-Red tongue without coating, Wiry-Rapid pulse.

Pathology

Heat has entered the Blood level and it heats the Blood, causing it to spill out of the blood vessels: this causes bleeding at various sites including under the skin (macules). Although macules can appear at the Nutritive Qi level, they are more typical of the Blood level.

Heat in the Blood disturbs the mind and causes mental restlessness and manic behaviour.

Treatment

Treatment principle: clear Blood Heat, stop bleeding.

Acupuncture

BL-17 Geshu, SP-10 Xuehai, LIV-5 Ligou, SP-4 Gongsun, L.I.-11 Quchi, LIV-2 Xingjian, KI-6 Zhaohai, HE-9 Shaochong, Shixuan extra points.

Herbal formula

Xi Jiao Di Huang Tang *Cornus Rhinoceri–Rehmannia Decoction*.

Box 45.12 summarizes Heat victorious agitates Blood.

Box 45.12 Heat victorious agitates Blood

Clinical manifestations

High fever, mental restlessness, manic behaviour, dark macules, vomiting of blood, epistaxis, blood in stools, blood in urine, Dark-Red tongue without coating, Wiry-Rapid pulse

Treatment

Treatment principle: clear Blood Heat, stop bleeding
Acupuncture
BL-17 Geshu, SP-10 Xuehai, LIV-5 Ligou, SP-4 Gongsun, L.I.-11 Quchi, LIV-2 Xingjian, KI-6 Zhaohai, HE-9 Shaochong, Shixuan extra points
Herbal formula
Xi Jiao Di Huang Tang *Cornus Rhinoceri–Rehmannia Decoction*

Heat victorious stirring Wind

Clinical manifestations

High fever, fainting, twitching of limbs, convulsions, rigidity of neck, opisthotonos, eyeballs turning up, clenching of teeth, Dark-Red tongue without coating, Wiry-Rapid pulse.

Pathology

At the Blood level, Heat affects the Liver and this leads to the stirring of internal Wind, much like a forest fire generates strong winds. This is internal Wind of the Full type. Wind causes convulsions, twitching of limbs, rigidity of neck, opisthotonos and clenching of teeth.

Treatment

Treatment principle: clear Blood-Heat, extinguish Wind.

Acupuncture

SP-10 Xuehai, L.I.-11 Quchi, LIV-2 Xingjian, KI-6 Zhaohai, HE-9 Shaochong, LIV-3 Taichong, Du-16 Fengfu, G.B.-20 Fengchi, S.I.-3 Houxi and BL-62 Shenmai in combination, Shixuan extra points.

Herbal formula

Ling Jiao Gou Teng Tang *Cornu Antelopis–Uncaria Decoction*.

Box 45.13 summarizes Heat victorious stirring Wind.

Box 45.13 Heat victorious stirring Wind

Clinical manifestations

High fever, fainting, twitching of limbs, convulsions, rigidity of neck, opisthotonos, eyeballs turning up, clenching of teeth, Dark-Red tongue without coating, Wiry-Rapid pulse

Treatment

Treatment principle: clear Blood-Heat, extinguish Wind
Acupuncture
SP-10 Xuehai, L.I.-11 Quchi, LIV-2 Xingjian, KI-6 Zhaohai, HE-9 Shaochong, LIV-3 Taichong, Du-16 Fengfu, G.B.-20 Fengchi, S.I.-3 Houxi and BL-62 Shenmai in combination, Shixuan extra points
Herbal formula
Ling Jiao Gou Teng Tang *Cornu Antelopis–Uncaria Decoction*

Empty-Wind agitating in the Interior

Clinical manifestations

Low-grade fever, tremor of limbs, twitching, loss of weight, malar flush, listlessness, Dark-Red tongue without coating and Dry, Fine-Rapid pulse.

Pathology

At the Blood level, Heat injures Yin of the Liver and Kidneys and this leads to the stirring of internal Wind: this is internal Wind of an Empty nature. Internal Wind causes the tremor or twitching of limbs.

Treatment

Treatment principle: clear Blood-Heat, nourish Liver- and Kidney-Yin, extinguish Wind.

Acupuncture

LIV-3 Taichong, Du-16 Fengfu, G.B.-20 Fengchi, S.I.-3 Houxi and BL-62 Shenmai in combination, LIV-8 Ququan, KI-6 Zhaohai, KI-3 Taixi, SP-6 Sanyinjiao.

Herbal formula

Zhen Gan Xi Feng Tang *Pacifying the Liver and Extinguishing Wind Decoction.*

Box 45.14 summarizes Empty-Wind agitating in the Interior.

Box 45.14 Empty-Wind agitating in the Interior

Clinical manifestations

Low-grade fever, tremor of limbs, twitching, loss of weight, malar flush, listlessness, Dark-Red tongue without coating and Dry, Fine-Rapid pulse

Treatment

Treatment principle: clear Blood-Heat, nourish Liver- and Kidney-Yin, extinguish Wind
Acupuncture
LIV-3 Taichong, Du-16 Fengfu, G.B.-20 Fengchi, S.I.-3 Houxi and BL-62 Shenmai in combination, LIV-8 Ququan, KI-6 Zhaohai, KI-3 Taixi, SP-6 Sanyinjiao
Herbal formula
Zhen Gan Xi Feng Tang *Pacifying the Liver and Extinguishing Wind Decoction*

Collapse of Yin

Clinical manifestations

Low-grade fever, night sweating, mental restlessness, dry mouth with desire to sip liquids, five-palm heat, malar flush, emaciation, Dark-Red and Dry tongue without coating, Fine-Rapid pulse.

Pathology

Collapse of Yin or of Yang may be the final consequence of Heat at the Blood level. The pathology of Collapse of Yin has already been explained in the chapter on the identification of patterns according to the Eight Principles (ch. 30).

Treatment

Treatment principle: rescue Yin, restore consciousness.

Acupuncture

ST-36 Zusanli, KI-3 Taixi, SP-6 Sanyinjiao, KI-6 Zhaohai, Ren-4 Guanyuan.

Herbal formula

Da Bu Yin Wan *Great Tonifying the Yin Pill.*

Box 45.15 summarizes Collapse of Yin.

Box 45.15 Collapse of Yin

Clinical manifestations

Low-grade fever, night sweating, mental restlessness, dry mouth with desire to sip liquids, five-palm heat, malar flush, emaciation, Dark-Red and Dry tongue without coating, Fine-Rapid pulse

Treatment

Treatment principle: rescue Yin, restore consciousness
Acupuncture
ST-36 Zusanli, KI-3 Taixi, SP-6 Sanyinjiao, KI-6 Zhaohai, Ren-4 Guanyuan
Herbal formula
Da Bu Yin Wan *Great Tonifying the Yin Pill*

Collapse of Yang

Clinical manifestations

Feeling cold, cold limbs, bright-white complexion, profuse sweating on the forehead, listlessness, Pale-Swollen and Short tongue, Hidden, Slow, Scattered pulse.

Pathology

The pathology of Collapse of Yang has already been explained in the chapter on the identification of patterns according to the Eight Principles (ch. 30).

Treatment

Treatment principle: rescue Yang, restore consciousness.

Acupuncture

ST-36 Zusanli, Ren-6 Qihai, Ren-4 Guanyuan, Ren-8 Shenque. Moxa is applicable.

Herbal formula

Shen Fu Tang *Ginseng–Aconitum Decoction.*

Box 45.16 summarizes Collapse of Yang and Box 45.17 summarizes the Four Levels.

Box 45.16 Collapse of Yang

Clinical manifestations

Feeling cold, cold limbs, bright-white complexion, profuse sweating on the forehead, listlessness, Pale-Swollen and Short tongue, Hidden, Slow, Scattered pulse

Treatment

Treatment principle: rescue Yang, restore consciousness
Acupuncture
ST-36 Zusanli, Ren-6 Qihai, Ren-4 Guanyuan, Ren-8 Shenque. Moxa is applicable
Herbal formula
Shen Fu Tang *Ginseng–Aconitum Decoction*

> **Box 45.17 The Four Levels in a nutshell**
>
> - Defensive Qi level: aversion to cold and fever
> - Qi level: no aversion to cold, fever, feeling of heat
> - Nutritive Qi level: mental changes, fever at night
> - Blood level: fever at night, bleeding, macules, internal Wind

LATENT HEAT

The concept of Latent Heat is very old in Chinese medicine, having been mentioned for the first time in the 'Yellow Emperor's Classic of Internal Medicine'. Latent Heat occurs when an external pathogenic factor penetrates the body without causing apparent symptoms at the time; the pathogenic factor penetrates into the Interior, and 'incubates' there, turning into interior Heat. This Heat later emerges with acute symptoms of Heat: when it emerges, it is called Latent Heat.

The reason that an external pathogenic factor invades the body without acute symptoms is usually to be found in a Kidney deficiency: thus, the development of Latent Heat indicates a pre-existing Kidney deficiency, which induces a weakened immune response to the invasion of an external pathogenic factor.

The main clinical manifestations of the emergence of Latent Heat are:

- Acute onset
- Thirst
- Irritability
- Insomnia
- Sudden tiredness and lassitude
- Weary limbs
- Dark urine
- Red tongue
- Rapid pulse

Other symptoms and signs vary according to the type of Latent Heat and these are described below. Please note that the fact that Latent Heat 'emerges' after a period of incubation does not mean that it is being 'expelled' by the body, merely that it is moving outwards and manifesting itself.

Figure 45.5 illustrates the concept of Latent Heat from the 'Yellow Emperor's Classic of Internal Medicine' and Figure 45.6 compares and contrasts the pathology of invasion of Wind-Heat with that of Latent Heat. Figures 45.7, 45.8 and 45.9 illustrate the types of Latent Heat and patterns developing from it.

Table 45.7 compares the clinical manifestations of Wind-Heat and Latent Heat.

Latent Heat can manifest at the Qi or Blood level. There are three main patterns, two at the Qi level and one at the Blood level, as follows:

- Qi level
  - Lesser Yang type
  - Bright Yang type
- Blood level
  - Lesser Yin type

Latent Heat Lesser Yang type

Alternation of chills and fever, bitter taste, hypochondrial pain, red eyes, deafness, vomiting, a feeling of oppression of the diaphragm, Red tongue with unilateral yellow coating, Wiry pulse.

Latent Heat Bright Yang type

Channel pattern

Feeling of heat, thirst, sweating, fever, Big pulse.

Organ pattern

Fever, abdominal fullness and pain, constipation, Red tongue with dry brown coating, Deep-Full pulse.

Winter
- Kidney deficiency not storing Essence (internal cause)
- Cold lurking inside, Cold turns into Heat (external cause)

→ **Spring** (Maturation of conditions for the development of the disease)
- New infection attracts Latent Heat out
- Spring's Yang energy attracts Heat out

→ **Latent Heat**

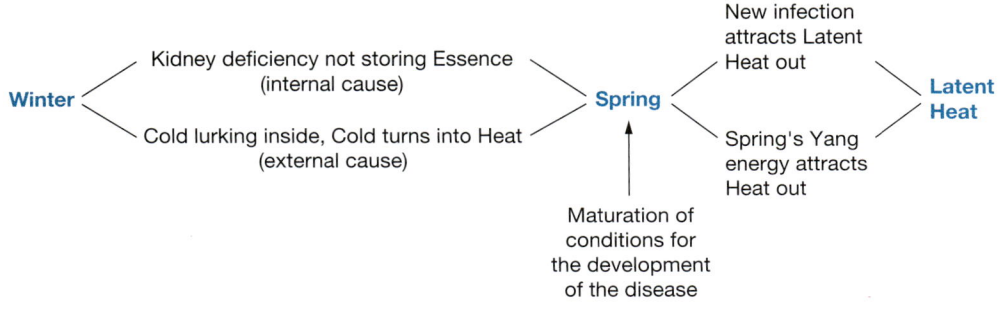

Figure 45.5 Latent Heat

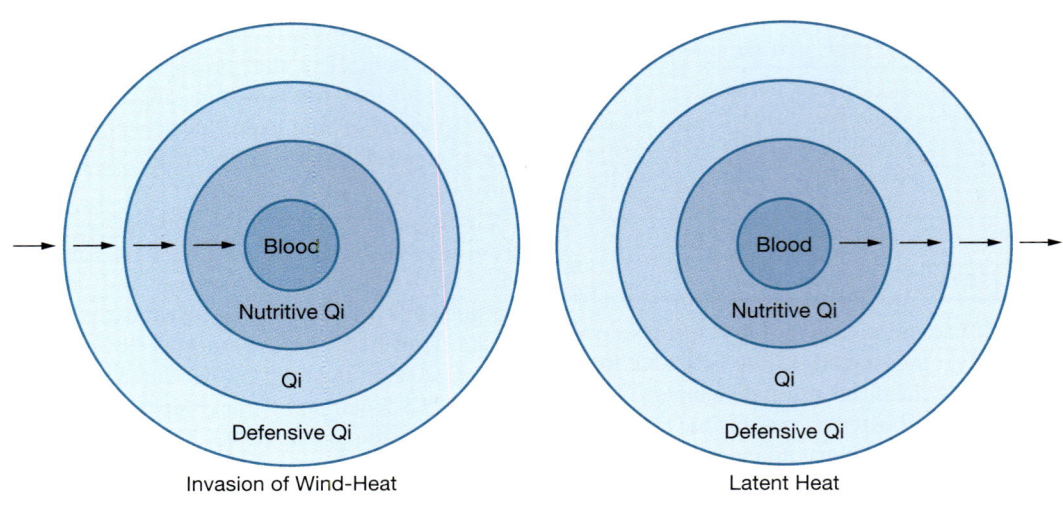

Figure 45.6 Comparison between pathology of Latent Heat and Wind-Heat

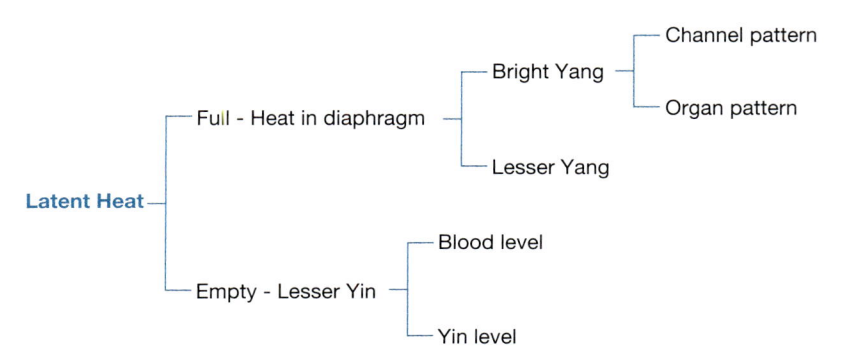

Figure 45.7 Types of Latent Heat

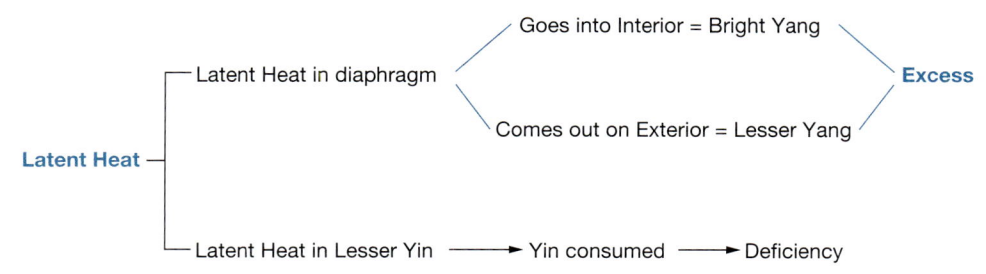

- Latent Heat
  - Full - Heat in diaphragm
    - Bright Yang
      - Channel pattern
      - Organ pattern
    - Lesser Yang
  - Empty - Lesser Yin
    - Blood level
    - Yin level

Figure 45.8 Full and Empty types of Latent Heat

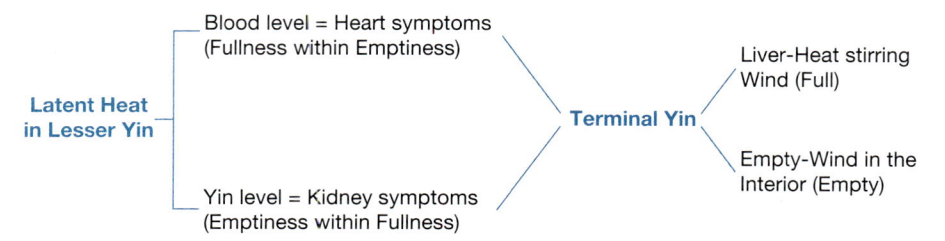

- Latent Heat
  - Latent Heat in diaphragm
    - Goes into Interior = Bright Yang ⎫ Excess
    - Comes out on Exterior = Lesser Yang ⎭
  - Latent Heat in Lesser Yin → Yin consumed → Deficiency

Figure 45.9 Latent Heat in Lesser Yin

- Latent Heat in Lesser Yin
  - Blood level = Heart symptoms (Fullness within Emptiness)
  - Yin level = Kidney symptoms (Emptiness within Fullness)
  - Terminal Yin
    - Liver-Heat stirring Wind (Full)
    - Empty-Wind in the Interior (Empty)

Table 45.7 Comparison of invasion of Wind-Heat and Latent Heat

	Wind-Heat	Latent Heat
Symptoms	Aversion to cold, sweating, fever	No aversion to cold (unless combined with new infection)
Cough	Cough	No cough
Pulse	Floating-Rapid	Rapid, also Wiry or Intermittent
Tongue	Thin white coating	Red tongue from the beginning
Pathology	Easy to have abnormal transmission to Pericardium	Easy to consume Yin and dry up fluids

Table 45.8 Comparison of Qi and Blood level in Latent Heat

	Heat	Thirst	Skin spots	Tongue	Pulse
Qi level	Apparent	Thirst, desire to drink	Papules	Red	Big
Blood level	Not so apparent	Dry mouth, no desire to drink	Macules	Deep-Red	Fine-Rapid

Latent Heat Lesser Yin type

A feeling of weariness of the limbs before the onset of other symptoms, insomnia, irritability, dry mouth and throat, scanty dark urination, headache, backache, tiredness, Red tongue, Rapid pulse.

Nutritive Qi level

Oily beads on forehead, dry mouth and teeth, irritability, delirium, scanty urine, blood in urine, Deep-Red tongue without coating, Fine-Rapid pulse.

Blood level

Delirium, faint feeling, dry limbs, sweating, irritability, macules, blood in urine, epistaxis, Deep-Red tongue without coating, Fine-Rapid pulse.

Table 45.8 compares the manifestations of Latent Heat at the Qi and Blood levels.

RELATIONSHIPS BETWEEN THE FOUR LEVELS, SIX STAGES AND THREE BURNERS

Although the identification of patterns according to the Six Stages dates back to the Han dynasty and those according to the Four Levels and Three Burners to the Qing dynasty, there are many points of contact between the three. First of all, all three of them describe the symptoms of invasion of external Wind when this is on the Exterior in the beginning stages and when it is in the Interior in later stages.

The Greater Yang stage of the Six Stages is similar to the Defensive Qi level within the Four Levels as they both deal with invasions of external Wind, the former Wind-Cold and the latter Wind-Heat.

The two patterns 'Bright Yang channel pattern' and 'Bright Yang organ pattern' of the Bright Yang stage of the Six Stages are practically the same as the patterns 'Heat in Bright Yang' and 'Dry Heat in the Stomach and Intestines' patterns of the Qi level of the Four Levels: indeed the same herbal formulas are applicable. The Lesser Yang stage of the Six Stages is almost the same as the Gall Bladder-Heat of the Qi level, the former being characterized by the predominance of Cold and the latter by that of Heat with some Dampness.

The identification of patterns according to the Three Burners is quite similar to that according to the Four Levels. Many of the patterns are essentially the same as those of the Four Levels, except that they are seen from the perspective of the Three Burners: that is, patterns of the Upper Burner, Middle Burner and Lower Burner. The Middle Burner patterns correspond to the Qi level while those of the Lower Burner correspond to the Nutritive Qi and Blood levels. By contrast, the patterns of the Upper Burner encompass the Defensive Qi, Qi and Nutritive Qi levels.

Further connections among the three methods of pattern identification are highlighted in Figures 45.10–45.12.

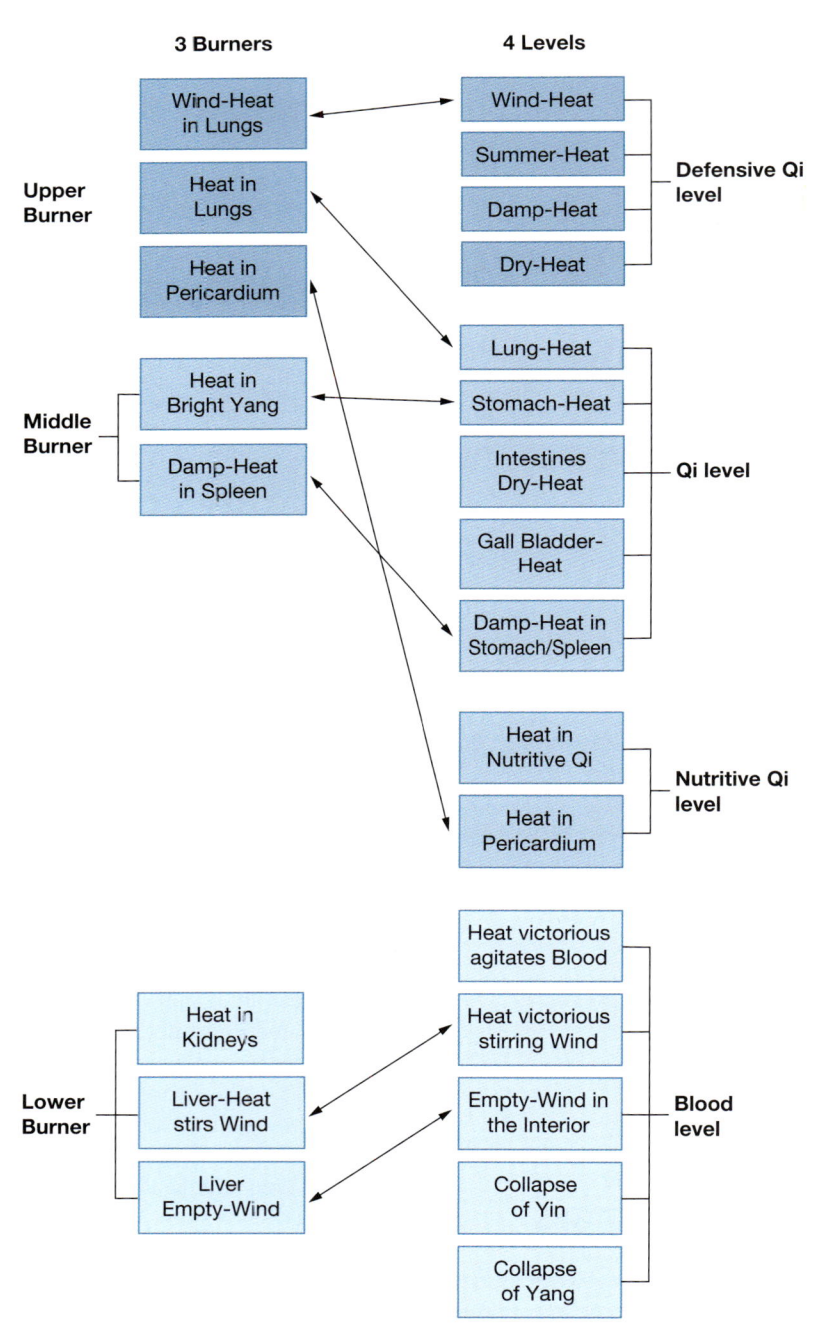

Figure 45.10 Relationship between the Three Burners and the Four Levels

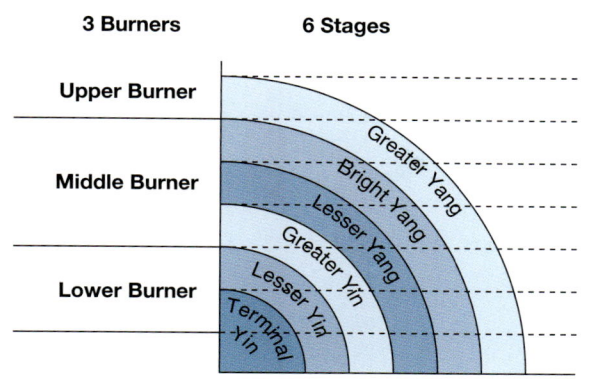

Figure 45.11 Relationship between the Six Stages and the Three Burners

Greater Yang (6 Stages) → Cold in Exterior
Defensive Qi level (4 Levels) → Heat in Exterior → All Exterior patterns
Lung Defensive Qi (3 Burners)
Upper Burner

Bright Yang, channel pattern (6 Stages)
Qi stage, Stomach-Heat (4 Levels) → All the same
Middle Burner, Heat in Bright Yang (3 Burners)

Lesser Yang (6 Stages)
Qi stage, Heat in Gall Bladder (4 Levels) → Both 1/2 interior 1/2 exterior essentially the same (Lesser Yang has prevalence of Cold, Heat in Gall Bladder has prevalence of Heat)

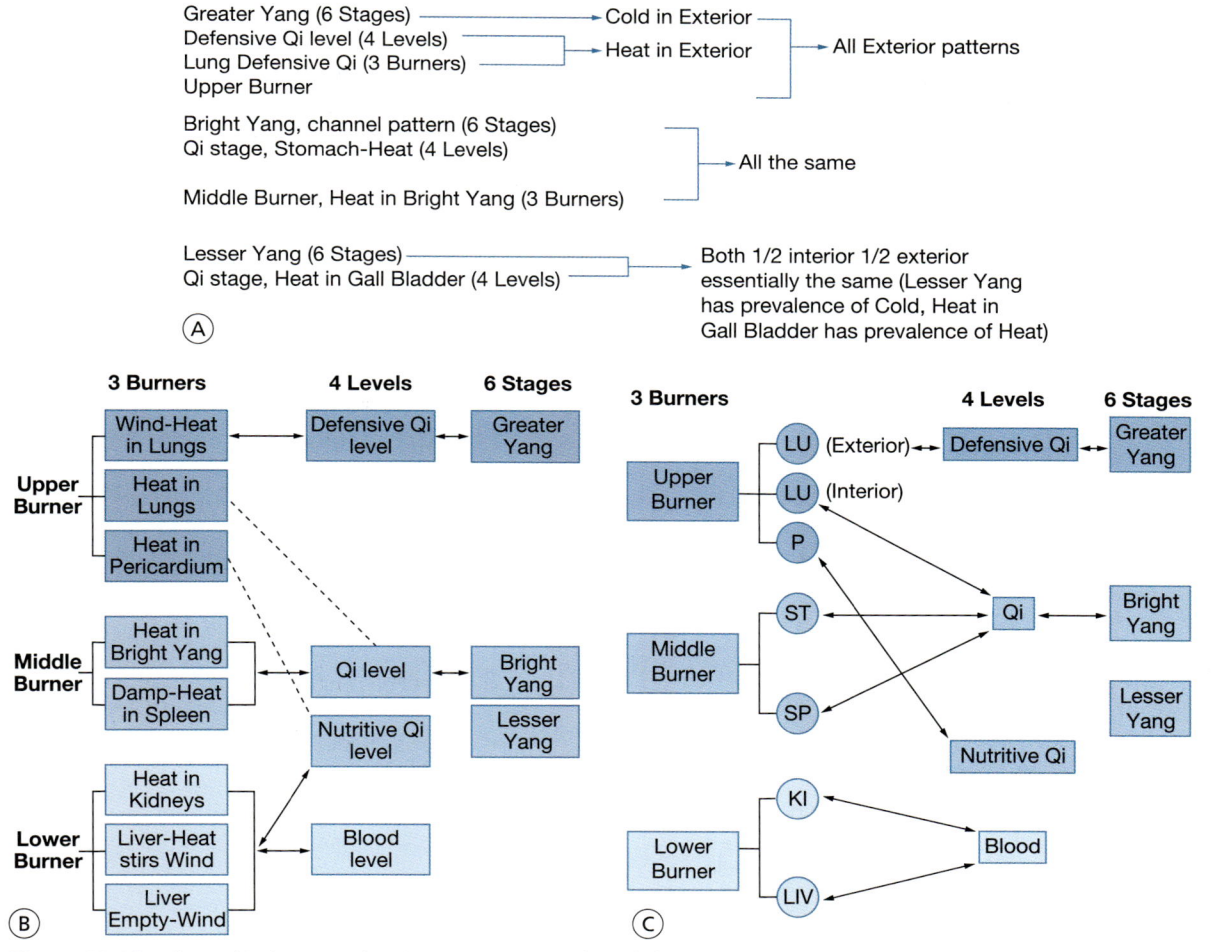

Ⓐ

Figure 45.12 Relationship between the Six Stages, Four Levels and Three Burners

Continued

3 Burners

Upper Burner
- Wind-Heat in Lungs
- Heat in Lungs
- Heat in Pericardium

Middle Burner
- Heat in Bright Yang
- Damp-Heat in Spleen

Lower Burner
- Heat in Kidneys
- Liver-Heat stirs Wind
- Liver Empty-Wind

4 Levels

Defensive Qi level
- Wind-Heat
- Summer-Heat
- Damp-Heat
- Dry-Heat

Qi level
- Lung-Heat
- Stomach-Heat
- Intestines Dry-Heat
- Gall-Bladder Heat
- Damp-Heat in Stomach/Spleen

Nutritive Qi level
- Heat in Nutritive Qi
- Heat in Pericardium

Blood level
- Heat victorious moving Blood
- Heat victorious stirring Wind
- Empty-Wind in the Interior
- Collapse of Yin
- Collapse of Yang

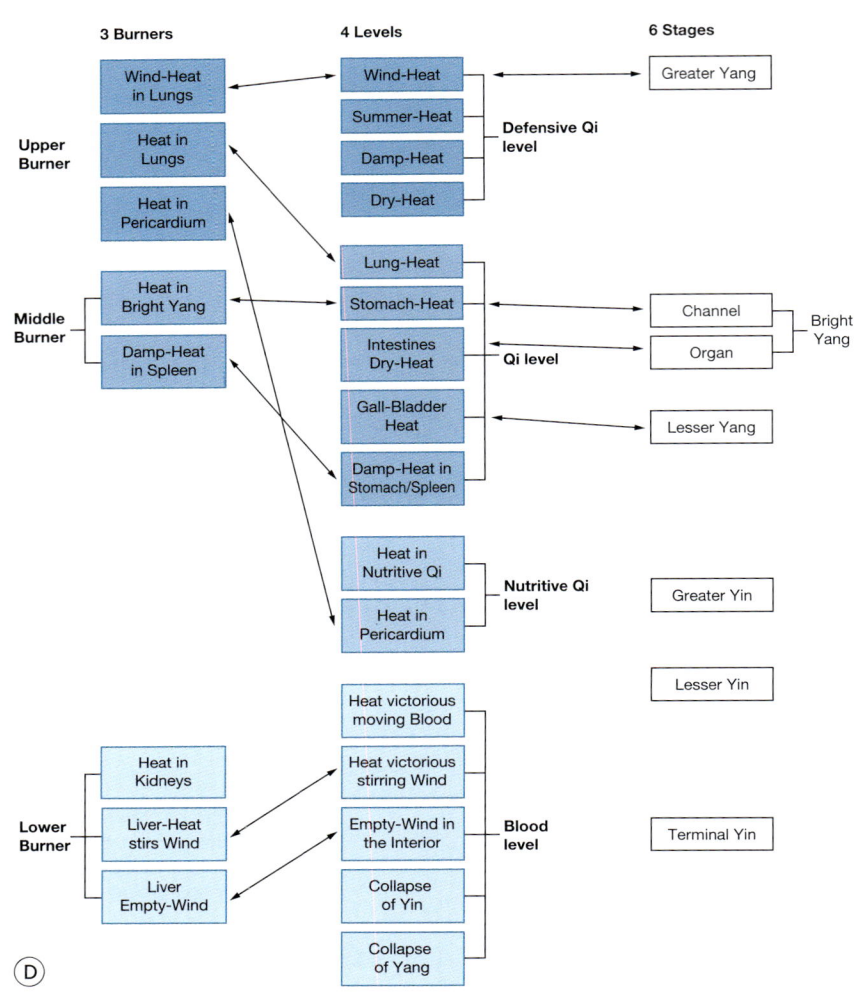

6 Stages

- Greater Yang
- Bright Yang (Channel, Organ)
- Lesser Yang
- Greater Yin
- Lesser Yin
- Terminal Yin

(D)

Figure 45.12 Cont'd

Learning outcomes

In this chapter you will have learned:
- The historical context for identification of patterns according to the Four Levels
- The essential characteristics of Warm Diseases, and how these differed from previously accepted theories
- The theory that Warm Diseases are caused by invasion of Wind-Heat, but that not every invasion of Wind-Heat is a Warm Disease
- The clinical usefulness of the theory of the Four Levels: distinctive pathologies and treatments based on different depths of penetration of pathogenic Heat
- The four different patterns of the Defensive Qi level, where the pathogen is on the Exterior of the body
- The significance of the Qi level, characterized by Full Interior Heat, where the pathogenic factor has penetrated into the Interior and has transformed into Heat
- The characteristics of the Nutritive Qi level, where Heat has penetrated to a deeper energetic level, injures the Yin and obstructs the Mind
- The Blood level as the deepest energetic layer, characterized by Yin deficiency, bleeding, macules, delirium or coma, and symptoms of internal Wind
- The presence of skin rashes as a manifestation of Warm Diseases
- How to identify the following patterns at the Defensive Qi level:
  Wind-Heat: fever, aversion to cold, headache, sore throat, body aches, Floating-Rapid pulse

- *Summer-Heat*: fever, aversion to cold, Soggy and Rapid pulse, with manifestations of external Wind, Dampness and interior Heat
- *Damp-Heat*: aversion to cold, feeling of oppression of epigastrium, feeling of heaviness, thirst without desire to drink, Soggy-Slow pulse
- *Dry-Heat*: fever and aversion to cold with symptoms of dryness injuring Body Fluids

- How to identify the following patterns at the Qi level:
  - *Lung-Heat*: high fever, feeling of heat, thirst, sweating and shortness of breath
  - *Stomach-Heat*: high fever (worse in afternoon), feeling of heat, intense thirst and sweating
  - *Intestines Dry-Heat*: high fever, constipation, burning in anus, abdominal fullness and pain
  - *Gall Bladder-Heat*: alternating hot and cold feeling with prevalence of Heat, hypochondrial pain, nausea, Red tongue with unilateral sticky yellow coating
  - *Damp-Heat in Stomach and Spleen*: continuous fever which decreases after sweating but soon increases again, feeling of heaviness of body and head, feeling of oppression of chest and epigastrium, loose stools, Red tongue with sticky yellow coating

- How to identify the following patterns at the Nutritive Qi level:
  - *Heat in Nutritive Qi level*: fever at night, mental restlessness, insomnia, macules and Red tongue without coating
  - *Heat in the Pericardium*: fever at night, mental confusion, incoherent speech or aphasia, body hot, hands and feet cold

- How to identify the following patterns at the Blood level:
  - *Heat victorious agitates Blood*: high fever, dark macules, vomiting blood, epistaxis, blood in stools and urine and mental restlessness
  - *Heat victorious stirring Wind*: high fever, fainting, twitching of limbs, convulsions, rigidity of neck, opisthotonos and clenching of teeth
  - *Empty-Wind agitating in the Interior*: low-grade fever, tremor of limbs, twitching, malar flush, Dry-Red tongue without coating and Fine-Rapid pulse
  - *Collapse of Yin*: low-grade fever, night sweating, mental restlessness, dry mouth with desire to sip liquids, malar flush and Fine-Rapid pulse
  - *Collapse of Yang*: feeling cold, cold limbs, bright-white complexion, profuse sweating of forehead, Pale, Swollen and Short tongue, Hidden-Slow-Scattered pulse

- How to identify the main clinical manifestations of the emergence of Latent Heat and identify the following patterns:
  - *Latent Heat Lesser Yang type*: alternation of chills and fever, bitter taste, hypochondrial pain, feeling of oppression of the diaphragm, Red tongue with unilateral yellow coating
  - *Latent Heat Bright Yang type (channel pattern)*: feeling of heat, thirst, sweating, fever
  - *Latent Heat Bright Yang type (organ pattern)*: fever, abdominal fullness and pain, constipation, Red tongue with dry brown coating, Deep-Full pulse
  - *Latent Heat Lesser Yin type*: feeling of weariness of the limbs before other symptoms, insomnia, irritability, dry mouth and throat, scanty dark urination, tiredness, Rapid pulse
  - *Latent Heat Lesser Yin type (Ying level)*: oily beads on forehead, dry mouth and teeth, Deep-Red tongue without coating, Fine-Rapid pulse
  - *Latent Heat Lesser Yin type (Blood level)*: delirium, faint feeling, dry limbs, sweating, macules, epistaxis, Deep-Red tongue without coating

- How the theory of the Four Levels relates to that of the Six Stages and Three Burners

Self-assessment questions

1. In which century did Ye Tian Shi formulate and set down the theory of identification of patterns according to the Four Levels in his 'Study of Warm Diseases' (*Wen Bing Lun*)?
2. Give three of the five special characteristics of Warm Diseases.
3. What new perspectives did the Warm Diseases School bring to the theory of external pathogenic factors?
4. Give three general symptoms of a pathogenic factor at the Qi level.
5. Give two general symptoms which differentiate the Nutritive Qi level from the Qi level.
6. Which symptom is a definite sign that Heat has reached the Blood level?
7. Describe a macule.
8. Why is there aversion to cold in invasions of Wind-Heat at the Defensive Qi level?
9. Which three pathogenic factors characterize an invasion of Summer-Heat?
10. You suspect an invasion of Damp-Heat at the Defensive Qi level, and question a patient on their thirst. What is their likely reply?
11. What is the pathology of the cough and shortness of breath in the pattern Lung-Heat at the Qi level?
12. What would be your main treatment principle in the pattern Intestines Dry-Heat?
13. Which Six Stages pattern is associated with Gall Bladder-Heat at the Qi level?
14. Why does sweating not reduce the fever from Damp-Heat in the Stomach and Spleen?
15. How would you expect the tongue to appear in a Nutritive Qi level pattern?
16. What are the three general symptoms which characterize Heat at the Blood level?
17. What is the usual predisposing factor for an external pathogenic factor invading the body without acute symptoms?
18. What are the three main patterns of Latent Heat (and give their levels)?

See p. 1265 for answers

Identification of Patterns According to the Three Burners

46

Key contents

Upper Burner
Wind-Heat in the Lungs' Defensive Qi portion
Heat in the Lungs (Qi level)
Heat in the Pericardium (Nutritive Qi level)

Middle Burner
Heat in Bright Yang
Damp-Heat in the Spleen

Lower Burner
Heat in the Kidneys
Liver-Heat stirs Wind
Liver Empty-Wind

Clinical note

Wu Ju Tong formulated the widely used formula Yin Qiao San *Lonicera–Forsythia Powder*, the formula of choice for the beginning stage of invasions of Wind-Heat

The Three Burner patterns discussed are:

- Upper Burner
  - Wind-Heat in the Lungs' Defensive Qi portion
  - Heat in the Lungs (Qi level)
  - Heat in the Pericardium (Nutritive Qi level)
- Middle Burner
  - Heat in Bright Yang
  - Damp-Heat in the Spleen
- Lower Burner
  - Heat in the Kidneys
  - Liver-Heat stirs Wind
  - Liver Empty-Wind

The identification of patterns according to the Three Burners was formulated by Wu Ju Tong (1758–1836), author of 'Systematic Differentiation of Warm Diseases' (*Wen Bing Tiao Bian*). The identification of patterns according to the Three Burners classifies the clinical manifestations of febrile diseases from invasion of Wind-Heat according to the Three Burners: that is, according to their location rather than their energetic depth as the identification of patterns according to the Four Levels does.

However, the identification of patterns according to the Three Burners has many points in contact with that according to the Four Levels because the patterns of the Middle Burner are essentially the same as some of those of the Qi level and those of the Lower Burner are essentially the same as some of those of the Blood level. By contrast, the patterns of the Upper Burner occur at three levels: Defensive Qi, Qi and Nutritive Qi levels. The connections between the Four Levels, the Three Burners and the Six Stages were highlighted in chapter 45.

UPPER BURNER

Wind-Heat in the Lungs' Defensive Qi portion

Clinical manifestations

Fever, aversion to cold, headache, sore throat, slight sweating, runny nose with yellow discharge, swollen tonsils, body aches, slight thirst, tongue Red in the front or sides with a thin white coating, Floating-Rapid pulse.

Pathology

The pathology of this pattern is the same as that for invasion of Wind-Heat at the Defensive Qi Level of the Four Levels. The tongue coating is white because the pathogenic factor is on the Exterior.

Treatment

Treatment principle: release the Exterior, expel Wind-Heat, restore the diffusing and descending of Lung-Qi.

Acupuncture

L.I.-4 Hegu, L.I.-11 Quchi, T.B.-5 Waiguan, Du-14 Dazhui, BL-12 Fengmen (with cupping), LU-11 Shaoshang.

Herbal formula

Yin Qiao San *Lonicera–Forsythia Powder*.
Sang Ju Yin *Morus–Chrysanthemum Decoction*.

Box 46.1 summarizes Wind-Heat in the Lungs' Defensive Qi portion.

Box 46.1 Wind-Heat in the Lungs' Defensive Qi portion

Clinical manifestations

Fever, aversion to cold, headache, sore throat, slight sweating, runny nose with yellow discharge, swollen tonsils, body aches, slight thirst, tongue Red in the front or sides with a thin white coating, Floating-Rapid pulse

Treatment

Treatment principle: release the Exterior, expel Wind-Heat, restore the diffusing and descending of Lung-Qi
Acupuncture
L.I.-4 Hegu, L.I.-11 Quchi, T.B.-5 Waiguan, Du-14 Dazhui, BL-12 Fengmen (with cupping), LU-11 Shaoshang
Herbal formula
Yin Qiao San *Lonicera–Forsythia Powder*
Sang Ju Yin *Morus–Chrysanthemum Decoction*

Heat in the Lungs (Qi level)

Clinical manifestations

Fever, sweating, cough, breathlessness, thirst, feeling of oppression and pain of the chest, Red tongue with yellow coating, Rapid-Overflowing pulse.

Pathology

The pathology of this pattern is essentially the same as that for the pattern Heat in the Lungs at the Qi Level of the Four Levels.

Treatment

Treatment principle: clear Lung-Heat, resolve Phlegm, restore the descending of Lung-Qi.

Acupuncture

LU-5 Chize, LU-10 Yuji, LU-1 Zhongfu, L.I.-11 Quchi, BL-13 Feishu.

Herbal formula

Ma Xing Shi Gan Tang *Ephedra–Prunus–Gypsum–Glycyrrhiza Decoction*.
Wu Hu Tang *Five Tigers Decoction*.
Xie Bai San *Draining the White Powder*.
Qing Qi Hua Tan Tang *Clearing Qi and Resolving Phlegm Decoction* (if there is also Phlegm).

Box 46.2 summarizes Heat in the Lungs (Qi level).

Box 46.2 Heat in the Lungs (Qi level)

Clinical manifestations

Fever, sweating, cough, breathlessness, thirst, feeling of oppression and pain in the chest, Red tongue with yellow coating, Rapid-Overflowing pulse

Treatment

Treatment principle: clear Lung-Heat, resolve Phlegm, restore the descending of Lung-Qi
Acupuncture
LU-5 Chize, LU-10 Yuji, LU-1 Zhongfu, L.I.-11 Quchi, BL-13 Feishu
Herbal formula
Ma Xing Shi Gan Tang *Ephedra–Prunus–Gypsum–Glycyrrhiza Decoction*
Wu Hu Tang *Five Tigers Decoction*
Xie Bai San *Draining the White Powder*
Qing Qi Hua Tan Tang *Clearing Qi and Resolving Phlegm Decoction* (if there is also Phlegm)

Heat in the Pericardium (Nutritive Qi level)

Clinical manifestations

High fever at night, a burning sensation of the epigastrium, cold limbs, delirium, aphasia, Deep-Red and Stiff tongue without coating, pulse Fine and Rapid.

Pathology

The pathology of this pattern is essentially the same as that for the pattern Heat in the Pericardium at the Nutritive Qi level of the Four Levels.

Treatment

Treatment principle: clear Heat in the Pericardium, restore consciousness, promote fluids.

Acupuncture

P-9 Zhongchong, P-3 Quze, L.I.-11 Quchi, P-8 Laogong, HE-9 Shaochong, KI-6 Zhaohai, Shixuan extra points.

Herbal formula

Qing Ying Tang *Clearing Nutritive Qi Decoction*.

Box 46.3 summarizes Heat in the Pericardium (Nutritive Qi level).

Box 46.3 Heat in the Pericardium (Nutritive Qi level)

Clinical manifestations

High fever at night, a burning sensation of the epigastrium, cold limbs, delirium, aphasia, Deep-Red and Stiff tongue without coating, pulse Fine and Rapid

Treatment

Treatment principle: clear Heat in the Pericardium, restore consciousness, promote fluids
Acupuncture
P-9 Zhongchong, P-3 Quze, L.I.-11 Quchi, P-8 Laogong, HE-9 Shaochong, KI-6 Zhaohai, Shixuan extra points
Herbal formula
Qing Ying Tang *Clearing Nutritive Qi Decoction*

MIDDLE BURNER

Heat in Bright Yang

Clinical manifestations

High fever that is worse in the afternoon, no aversion to cold, feeling of heat, intense thirst, profuse sweating, Red tongue with yellow coating, Overflowing-Rapid pulse.

Pathology

The pathology of this pattern is essentially the same as that for the pattern Stomach-Heat at the Qi level of the Four Levels.

Treatment

Treatment principle: clear Stomach-Heat.

Acupuncture

ST-44 Neiting, ST-34 Liangqiu, ST-21 Liangmen, ST-43 Xiangu, L.I.-11 Quchi, ST-25 Tianshu.

Herbal formula

Bai Hu Tang *White Tiger Decoction*.

Box 46.4 summarizes Heat in Bright Yang.

Box 46.4 Heat in Bright Yang

Clinical manifestations

High fever that is worse in the afternoon, no aversion to cold, feeling of heat, intense thirst, profuse sweating, Red tongue with yellow coating, Overflowing-Rapid pulse

Treatment

Treatment principle: clear Stomach-Heat
Acupuncture
ST-44 Neiting, ST-34 Liangqiu, ST-21 Liangmen, ST-43 Xiangu, L.I.-11 Quchi, ST-25 Tianshu
Herbal formula
Bai Hu Tang *White Tiger Decoction*

Damp-Heat in the Spleen

Clinical manifestations

Fever, epigastric fullness, a feeling of heaviness of the body and head, nausea, vomiting, Red tongue with sticky yellow coating, Soggy and Rapid pulse.

Pathology

The pathology of this pattern is essentially the same as that for the pattern Damp-Heat in Stomach and Spleen from the Qi level of the Four Levels.

Treatment

Treatment principle: clear Heat and resolve Dampness in the Spleen.

Acupuncture

Ren-12 Zhongwan, SP-9 Yinlingquan, SP-6 Sanyinjiao, Ren-9 Shuifen, ST-36 Zusanli, L.I.-11 Quchi, BL-20 Pishu, BL-22 Sanjiaoshu.

Herbal formula

Lian Po Yin *Coptis–Magnolia Decoction*.

Box 46.5 summarizes Damp-Heat in the Spleen.

> **Box 46.5 Damp-Heat in the Spleen**
>
> **Clinical manifestations**
>
> Fever, epigastric fullness, a feeling of heaviness of the body and head, nausea, vomiting, Red tongue with sticky yellow coating, Soggy and Rapid pulse
>
> **Treatment**
>
> *Treatment principle*: clear Heat and resolve Dampness in the Spleen
> *Acupuncture*
> Ren-12 Zhongwan, SP-9 Yinlingquan, SP-6 Sanyinjiao, Ren-9 Shuifen, ST-36 Zusanli, L.I.-11 Quchi, BL-20 Pishu, BL-22 Sanjiaoshu
> *Herbal formula*
> Lian Po Yin *Coptis–Magnolia Decoction*

> **Box 46.6 Heat in the Kidneys**
>
> **Clinical manifestations**
>
> Fever in the afternoon and evening, five-palm heat, dry mouth and throat, night sweating, deafness, lassitude, Deep-Red tongue without coating, Floating-Empty and Rapid pulse
>
> **Treatment**
>
> *Treatment principle*: nourish Kidney-Yin, clear Empty-Heat
> *Acupuncture*
> KI-3 Taixi, KI-6 Zhaohai, SP-6 Sanyinjiao, KI-2 Rangu, L.I.-11 Quchi
> *Herbal formula*
> Huang Lian E Jiao Tang *Coptis–Colla Asini Decoction*
> Xi Jiao Di Huang Tang *Cornus Rhinoceri–Rehmannia Decoction*

LOWER BURNER

Heat in the Kidneys

Clinical manifestations

Fever in the afternoon and evening, five-palm heat, dry mouth and throat, night sweating, deafness, lassitude, Deep-Red tongue without coating, Floating-Empty and Rapid pulse.

Pathology

The pathology of this pattern is essentially the same as that of the pattern Heat transformation from the Lesser Yin stage of the Six Stages.

Treatment

Treatment principle: nourish Kidney-Yin, clear Empty-Heat.

Acupuncture

KI-3 Taixi, KI-6 Zhaohai, SP-6 Sanyinjiao, KI-2 Rangu, L.I.-11 Quchi.

Herbal formula

Huang Lian E Jiao Tang *Coptis–Colla Asini Decoction*.
Xi Jiao Di Huang Tang *Cornus Rhinoceri–Rehmannia Decoction*.
Box 46.6 summarizes Heat in the Kidneys.

Liver-Heat stirs Wind

Clinical manifestations

High fever at night, coma, convulsions, clenched teeth, Deep-Red tongue without coating, Wiry-Fine-Rapid pulse.

Pathology

The pathology of this pattern is essentially the same as that of the pattern Heat victorious stirring Wind from the Blood level of the Four Levels.

Treatment

Treatment principle: clear Heat, extinguish Wind, stop convulsions, restore consciousness.

Acupuncture

LIV-3 Taichong, LIV-2 Xingjian, G.B.-20 Fengchi, Du-16 Fengfu, S.I.-3 Houxi and BL-62 Shenmai in combination, SP-10 Xuehai, L.I.-11 Quchi, KI-6 Zhaohai, HE-9 Shaochong, Shixuan extra points.

Herbal formula

Ling Jiao Gou Teng Tang *Cornu Antelopis–Uncaria Decoction*.
Box 46.7 summarizes Liver-Heat stirs Wind.

> **Box 46.7 Liver-Heat stirs Wind**
>
> **Clinical manifestations**
>
> High fever at night, coma, convulsions, clenched teeth, Deep-Red tongue without coating, Wiry-Fine-Rapid pulse
>
> **Treatment**
>
> *Treatment principle*: clear Heat, extinguish Wind, stop convulsions, restore consciousness
> *Acupuncture*
> LIV-3 Taichong, LIV-2 Xingjian, G.B.-20 Fengchi, Du-16 Fengfu, S.I.-3 Houxi and BL-62 Shenmai in combination, SP-10 Xuehai, L.I.-11 Quchi, KI-6 Zhaohai, HE-9 Shaochong, Shixuan extra points
> *Herbal formula*
> Ling Jiao Gou Teng Tang *Cornu Antelopis–Uncaria Decoction*

> **Box 46.8 Liver Empty-Wind**
>
> **Clinical manifestations**
>
> Low-grade fever, cold limbs, dry and black teeth, dry and cracked lips, convulsions, tremor of limbs, Deep-Red tongue without coating, Deep-Fine-Rapid pulse
>
> **Treatment**
>
> *Treatment principle*: nourish Yin, extinguish Wind, stop convulsions
> *Acupuncture*
> LIV-3 Taichong, LIV-2 Xingjian, G.B.-20 Fengchi, Du-16 Fengfu, S.I.-3 Houxi and BL-62 Shenmai in combination, KI-3 Taixi, KI-6 Zhaohai, SP-6 Sanyinjiao, LIV-8 Ququan
> *Herbal formula*
> Zhen Gan Xi Feng Tang *Pacifying the Liver and Extinguishing Wind Decoction*
> San Jia Fu Mai Tang *Three Carapaces Restoring the Pulse Decoction*
> Da Ding Feng Zhu *Big Stopping Wind Pearl*

Liver Empty-Wind

Clinical manifestations

Low-grade fever, cold limbs, dry and black teeth, dry and cracked lips, convulsions, tremor of limbs, Deep-Red tongue without coating, Deep-Fine-Rapid pulse.

Pathology

The pathology of this pattern is essentially the same as that for the pattern Empty-Wind, agitating the Interior from the Blood level of the Four Levels.

Treatment

Treatment principle: nourish Yin, extinguish Wind, stop convulsions.

Acupuncture

LIV-3 Taichong, LIV-2 Xingjian, G.B.-20 Fengchi, Du-16 Fengfu, S.I.-3 Houxi and BL-62 Shenmai in combination, KI-3 Taixi, KI-6 Zhaohai, SP-6 Sanyinjiao, LIV-8 Ququan.

Herbal formula

Zhen Gan Xi Feng Tang *Pacifying the Liver and Extinguishing Wind Decoction.*
San Jia Fu Mai Tang *Three Carapaces Restoring the Pulse Decoction.*
Da Ding Feng Zhu *Big Stopping Wind Pearl.*
   Box 46.8 summarizes Liver Empty-Wind.

> **Learning outcomes**
>
> In this chapter you will have learned:
> - How identification of patterns according to the Three Burners relates to that of the Four Levels
> - How to identify the following Upper Burner patterns:
>   *Wind-Heat in the Lung Defensive Qi portion*: fever, aversion to cold, headache, sore throat, Floating-Rapid pulse
>   *Heat in the Lungs (Qi level)*: fever, sweating, cough, breathlessness, thirst, Red tongue with yellow coating, Rapid-Overflowing pulse
>   *Heat in the Pericardium (Nutritive Qi level)*: high fever at night, burning sensation in epigastrium, delirium, Deep-Red and Stiff tongue without coating, Fine-Rapid pulse
> - How to identify the following Middle Burner patterns:
>   *Heat in Bright Yang*: high fever worse in the afternoon, no aversion to cold, feeling of heat, intense thirst, profuse sweating, Red tongue with yellow coating, Overflowing-Rapid pulse
>   *Damp-Heat in the Spleen*: fever, epigastric fullness, a feeling of heaviness of the body and head, nausea, Red-tongue with sticky yellow coating, Soggy and Rapid pulse
> - How to identify the following Lower Burner patterns:
>   *Heat in the Kidneys*: fever in afternoon and evening, five-palm heat, dry mouth and throat, night sweating, Deep-Red tongue without coating, Floating-Empty and Rapid pulse
>   *Liver-Heat stirs Wind*: high fever at night, coma, convulsions, clenched teeth, Deep-Red tongue without coating, Wiry-Fine-Rapid pulse
>   *Liver Empty-Wind*: low-grade fever, cold limbs, dry and black teeth, convulsions, tremor of limbs, Deep-Red tongue without coating, Deep-Fine-Rapid pulse

Self-assessment questions

1. How does identification of patterns according to the Three Burners relate to that of the Four Levels?
2. At which of the Four Levels is the pattern Heat in the Lungs?
3. Give three symptoms of the pattern Heat in the Pericardium.
4. You suspect a diagnosis of Heat in the Bright Yang. The patient has a high fever, thirst, feels hot and no aversion to cold. Do these symptoms support your diagnosis?
5. Describe the tongue and pulse for the pattern Heat in the Kidneys.
6. What would be your three primary treatment principles for the pattern Liver Empty-Wind?

See p. 1265 for answers

SECTION 4

Identification of Patterns according to the 12 Channels, Eight Extraordinary Vessels and Five Elements

INTRODUCTION

Identification of patterns according to the 12 channels

This is the oldest of all modes of identification of patterns. Reference to it occurs in the 'Spiritual Axis'.[1] This method of identification of patterns, discussed in chapter 47, describes the symptoms and signs related to each channel, rather than the organ.

This way of identifying patterns comes into its own when an acupuncturist treats a condition which is caused by damage to a channel rather than an Internal Organ or even by damage to an Internal Organ manifesting along its corresponding channel. For this reason, it is not used much for the treatment of internal conditions, as it does not give the doctor enough information to make a diagnosis or formulate a method of treatment. When treating an internal condition (i.e. a disease of an Internal Organ), the identification of patterns according to the Internal Organs is the preferred method.

Identification of patterns according to the Eight Extraordinary Vessels

This method of identification of patterns is based on the interpretation of clinical manifestations arising from a disharmonies of the Eight Extraordinary Vessels. These are discussed in chapter 48 and the pathology of the Eight Extraordinary Vessels is also discussed in chapters 52 and 53.

Identification of patterns according to the Five Elements

This method of identification of patterns is based on the interpretation of clinical manifestations according to the Generating, Overacting and Insulting sequences of the Five Elements. These are described in chapter 49.

END NOTE

1. 1981 Spiritual Axis (*Ling Shu Jing* 灵枢经), People's Health Publishing House, Beijing, first published *c.*100 BC, p. 30–39.

Identification of Patterns According to the 12 Channels

Key contents

Organ versus channel

Lungs

Large Intestine

Stomach

Spleen

Heart

Small Intestine

Bladder

Kidneys

Pericardium

Triple Burner

Gall Bladder

Liver

The pattern identification according to the channels is the oldest of the pattern identification methods. It is found in the 'Spiritual Axis' in chapter 10.[1]

Basically, this method of pattern identification allows us to distinguish symptoms and signs according to the involved channel: it is therefore concerned with the pathological changes occurring in the channel rather than the organ.

After discussing the pathology of organ versus that of channels, I shall list the clinical manifestations of the pathology of Main (*Jing Mai*), Connecting (*Luo Mai*) and Muscle channels (*Jing Jin*).

Organ versus channel

The organs and their relevant channels form an indivisible energetic unit: problems of the Internal Organs can affect the relevant channels and, conversely, problems that start as channel problems can penetrate into the Interior and be transmitted to the organs.

It is important, however, to appreciate both the unity and the separation between the organ and the channel. They form a unity, but they are also energetically separate: the channels pertain to what is called the Exterior, i.e. the superficial energetic layers of the body (including skin and muscles), and the organs pertain to the Interior, i.e. the deep energetic layer of the body, including the organs and bones.

In disease, there can be problems of the channels not affecting the organs and vice versa. It is very important to appreciate (and be able to identify) when a problem is situated in the Exterior and affecting the channels only.

For example, if a person has a pain in the shoulder along the Large Intestine channel without any Large Intestine organ symptoms, one can safely conclude that this is a channel problem only, not affecting the Internal Organs. If, on the contrary, a person suffers from chronic diarrhoea over a long period of time with mucus and blood in the stools and, after some years, develops a pain in the shoulder along the Large Intestine channel, then this channel problem is possibly caused by its corresponding Internal Organ disease. However, even in this case there could be an overlap of an Internal Organ problem with a separate invasion of an exterior pathogenic factor in the channel.

The channels and their relevant Internal Organs can be compared, respectively, to the branches and the roots of a tree (Fig. 47.1). The branches of a tree may be damaged by hail, broken by wind, or wither from excessive heat and dryness but these events will not affect the roots of the tree: this would correspond to a channel problem in the human body. Conversely, if the soil is very poor and the roots do not derive enough nutrients and suffer, this would correspond to a Internal Organ problem in the human body.

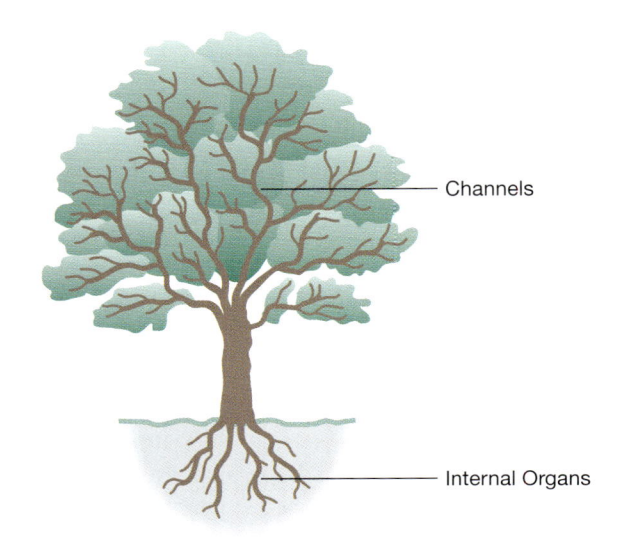

Figure 47.1 Internal Organs and channels

Channel problems can arise from four factors:

First of all, they arise from invasion of exterior pathogenic factors, such as Cold, Wind, or Dampness. These invade the Connecting (*Luo*) channels first, and then the main channels, settling in the joints and causing Painful Obstruction Syndrome (*Bi* Syndrome). This is an extremely frequent cause of channel problems which affects most people at one time or another.

Channel pathology is, in fact, closely related to joint pathology. Joints in Chinese medicine are more than just anatomical entities: they have an important function with regard to the circulation of Qi and Blood, with several implications in pathology.

Joints are places where Qi and Blood concentrate or gather, and they are also the places where Qi goes from the Interior to the Exterior or vice versa. As will be remembered from chapter 4, Qi has complex directions of movement, upwards and downwards and in and out, constituting the ascending/descending and entering/exiting of Qi, respectively. The joints are the places along the channels where Qi enters and exits. It is not by chance that many of the major Transporting (*Shu*) points of the limbs below elbows and knees are situated on joints. As a consequence of this concentration of Qi, the joints are the places where a pathogenic factor easily settles.

When a pathogenic factor invades the joint, it alters the balance of Yin and Yang, upsets the circulation of Qi in the channel and causes Qi and Blood to stagnate: this causes pain and in the long run gives rise to Painful Obstruction Syndrome (*Bi* Syndrome). If the pathogenic factor is associated with Heat, the joint will feel hot; if it is associated with Cold, it will feel cold; if there is Dampness, the joint is swollen; if there is Wind, the pain moves from joint to joint.

Besides being affected by exterior pathogenic factors, joints are affected by general deficiency of Qi and Blood, which may cause their lack of nourishment and hence weakness.

Another frequent cause of channel problems is from overuse of a limb or part of the body, giving rise to local stagnation of Qi. Anyone who, because of their work circumstances, has to constantly repeat the same movements, will be liable to suffer from channel problems, manifesting with local stagnation of Qi. This is a very common cause of repetitive strain injury.

Sports injuries are another frequent cause of channel problems, causing local stagnation of Qi in the channel.

Finally, channel problems can, of course, spring from Internal Organ disharmonies.

The channel pattern identification describes the pathological changes occurring in channels. However, although this is the main aim of this pattern identification, it can be slightly confusing as the symptoms and signs described in the 'Spiritual Axis' also include some from the relevant organ and sometimes even from other organs.

For example, among the Lung channel symptoms and signs are:

- Congested and sore throat, sensation of fullness in the chest, pain in the clavicle and arm, which are due to the Lung channel
- Cough and asthma, which are due to the Lung organ
- Pain in the shoulders and upper back, which is due to the Large Intestine channel, to which the Lung channel is related

Thus channel patterns include some symptoms and signs from the organs themselves. These can safely be ignored, as for organ problems one would much rather use Internal Organ pattern identification. For example, 'cough' and 'asthma' are not sufficiently specific to give an indication of the possible pattern involved. In order to do so, it is necessary to use Internal Organ pattern identification, which gives a more precise account of the picture formed by the pattern. For example, if cough is accompanied by profuse white sputum with a feeling of oppression of the chest and the tongue has a sticky white thick coating, we know that the pattern involved is Damp-Phlegm obstructing the Lungs. If the cough is dry and there is night sweating with a feeling of heat in the chest, soles and palms, we know that the pattern in question is deficiency of Lung-Yin.

However, we must also remember that a channel problem can affect the orifices and sense organs and that such problems are not always related to the Internal Organs. For example, the Kidneys open into the ears but not every ear problem is related to the Kidneys. In fact, Triple Burner channel symptoms include pain in the ear and deafness. By this is obviously meant a pain in the ear and deafness of acute onset, probably from invasion of exterior Wind-Heat, as deafness with a slow onset would most probably be due to a Kidney deficiency. Liver channel symptoms include blurred vision and tinnitus. Thus, not all sense organ problems are related to Internal Organ diseases.

The channel pattern identification is important to identify the affected channel from the symptoms and signs. The clinical manifestations related to the channel itself are therefore more important.

Of course, the channel pattern identification needs to be based on a thorough knowledge of the main channels and their deep pathways.[2]

Apart from this, one must also distinguish Full from Empty conditions of the channels. Full conditions are characterized by intense pain, stiffness, contractions and cramps. Empty conditions are characterized by dull ache, weakness of the muscles, atrophy of the muscles and numbness.

Fullness and Emptiness of the channels can also be differentiated from the colour appearing along the course of the channel and its temperature to the touch. In Full conditions there may be a red colour indicating Heat or a bluish colour, indicating Cold. In the case of Heat, it would also feel hot to the touch. In Empty conditions, there may be a pale streak along the course of the channel and this would feel cold to the touch.

To summarize, if we know the pathway of the channels thoroughly and are able to identify Full or Empty conditions of the channels according to the above guidelines, any clinical manifestation appearing along the channel can be correctly identified.[3]

The following is a list of the channel patterns from chapter 10 of the 'Spiritual Axis'. For the sake of clarity, I have omitted the symptoms and signs of Internal Organ problems, and limited them only to the channel symptoms and signs. In addition to the following clinical manifestations, any pain, numbness, stiffness, tingling or ache along the course of a channel is obviously a channel symptom of the relevant channel.

Lungs

Main channel

Fever, aversion to cold, a feeling of oppression of the chest, pain in the clavicle, shoulders and arms (Fig. 47.2).

Connecting channel

Empty

Yawning, frequent urination, shortness of breath.

Full

Hot palms.

Muscle channel

Pain, contraction and sprain of the muscles along the course of the channel, pain and contraction of the muscles of the chest and shoulder.

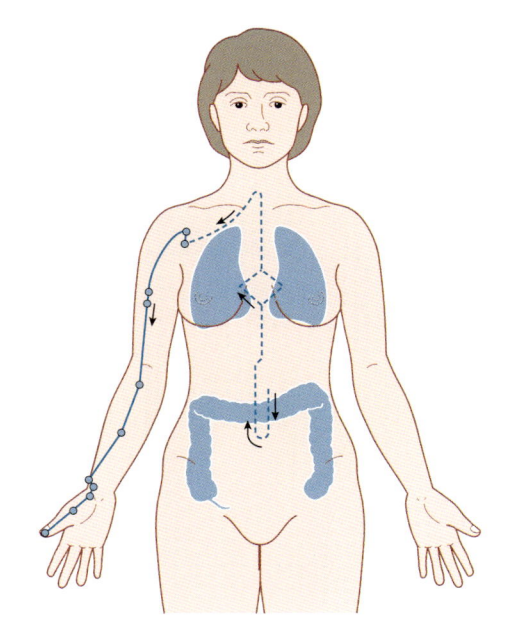

Figure 47.2 Lung main channel

Large Intestine

Main channel

Sore throat, toothache, epistaxis, runny nose, swollen and painful gums, swollen eyes, pain along the course of the channel (Fig. 47.3).

Connecting channel

Empty

Sensation of cold in the teeth, feeling of tightness in diaphragm, loss of sense of smell.

Full

Toothache, deafness, tinnitus, sensation of heat in the centre of the chest, breathlessness.

Muscle channel

Pain, stiffness or sprain of the muscles along the course of the channel, inability to raise the arm, inability to rotate the neck, shoulder ache.

Stomach

Main channel

Pain in the eyes, epistaxis, swelling of neck, facial paralysis, cold legs and feet, pain along the course of the channel (Fig. 47.4).

Connnecting channel

Empty

Flaccidity or atrophy of leg muscles, feeling of cold in the upper teeth.

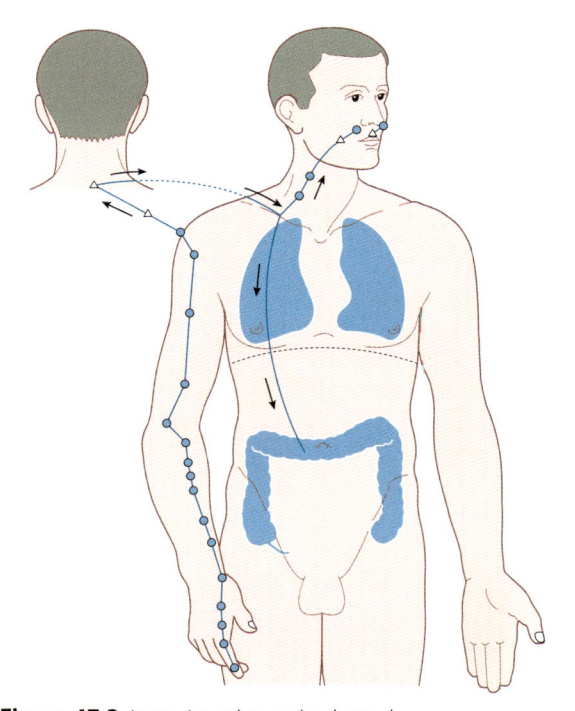

Figure 47.3 Large Intestine main channel

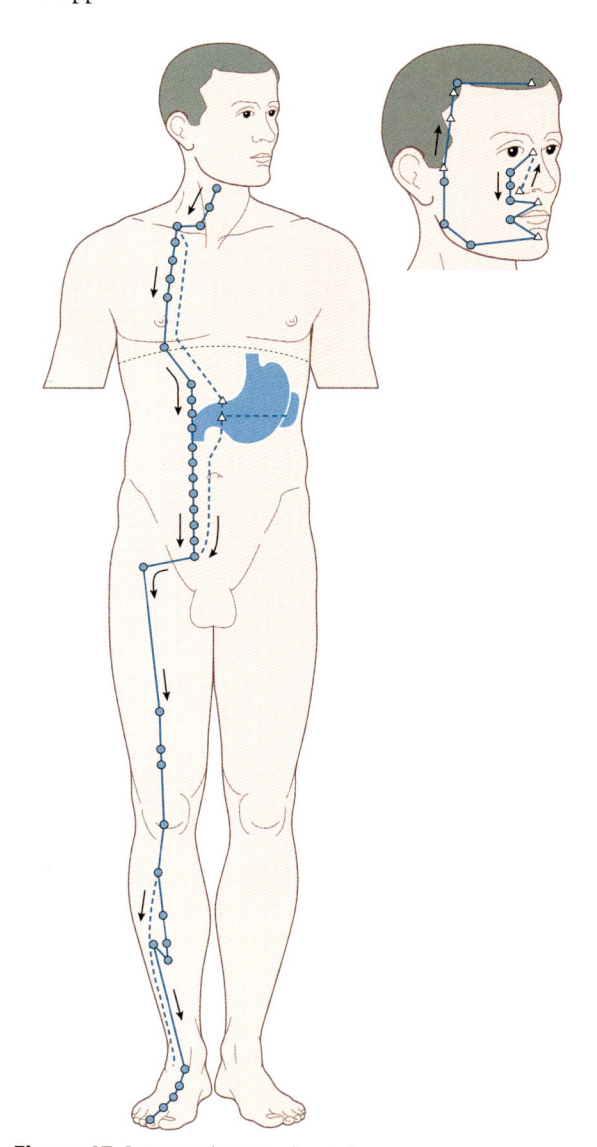

Figure 47.4 Stomach main channel

Full

Epilepsy, manic behaviour or depression, swollen and sore throat, sudden loss of voice, nosebleed.

Great Connnecting channel of the Spleen

Palpitations, feeling of fullness of the chest.

Muscle channel

Sprain of the middle toe, contraction of the muscles of the lower leg and foot, stiffness of the thigh muscles, swelling in the groin, hernia, spasm of abdominal muscles, strained neck and cheek muscles, deviation of eyes and mouth, inability to close the eye due to muscle spasm, inability to open the eyes due to flaccidity of the muscles.

Spleen

Main channel

Vaginal discharge, cold feeling along the channel, weakness of the leg muscles (Fig. 47.5).

Connnecting channel

Empty

Abdominal distension.

Full

Abdominal pain, food poisoning, vomiting, diarrhoea.

Great Connnecting channel of the Spleen

Pain all over the body, weakness and flaccidity of the joints of the four limbs, backache radiating to the abdomen.

Muscle channel

Strain of the big toe, pain in the inner aspect of the ankle, pain in the muscles of the medial aspect of the knee and thigh, strain of the muscles of the groin, strain of the abdominal muscles, pain in the muscles of the chest and middle back.

Heart

Main channel

Pain in the eyes, pain on the inner side of the arm, pain along the scapula (Fig. 47.6).

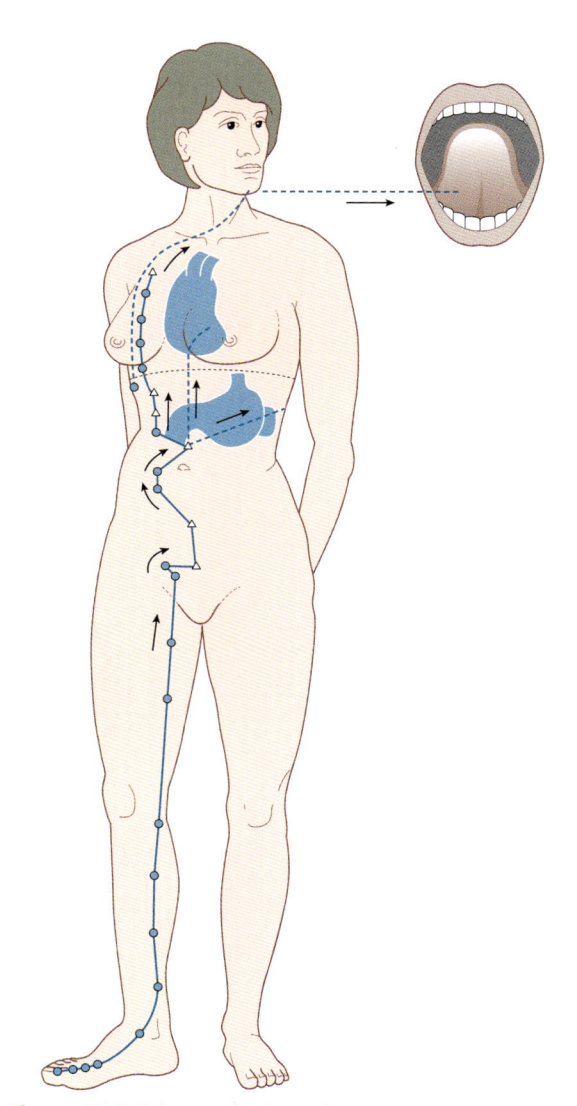

Figure 47.5 Spleen main channel

Connnecting channel

Empty

Aphasia.

Full

Feeling of distension and fullness of the chest and diaphragm.

Muscle channel

Pain, stiffness and sprain of the muscles along the course of the channel.

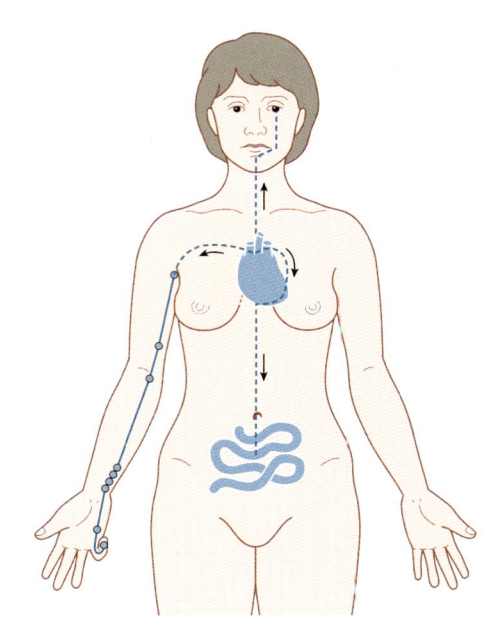

Figure 47.6 Heart main channel

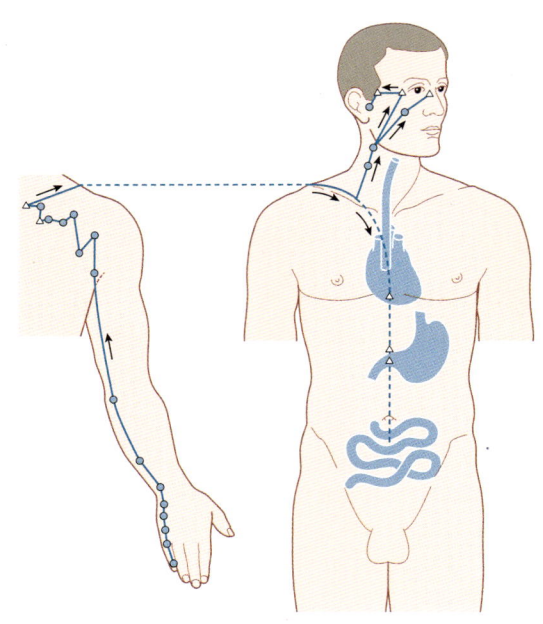

Figure 47.7 Small Intestine main channel

Small Intestine

Main channel

Pain in the neck, pain in the elbow, stiff neck, pain along the lateral side of the arm and scapula (Fig. 47.7).

Connnecting channel

Empty

Scabies, long, finger-shaped warts.

Full

Loose joints of the shoulder, weakness of the muscles of the elbow joint.

Muscle channel

Stiffness and pain of the muscles of the little finger, arm and elbow, sprain and pain of the muscles of the scapula, pain and sprain of the neck muscles, pain from the ear to the mandible, earache radiating to the chin, swelling of the sides of the neck.

Bladder

Main channel

Fever and aversion to cold, headache, stiff neck, pain in the lower back, pain in the eyes, pain behind the leg along the channel (Fig. 47.8).

Connnecting channel

Empty

Runny nose, nosebleed.

Full

Stuffy nose, headache, backache, neck ache, shoulder ache.

Muscle channel

Pain and stiffness of the muscles of the little toe, foot, heel, knee and spine, backache and spasm of the back, stiff neck, inability to raise the shoulder, stiffness of the muscles of the axillary region, inability to twist the waist.

Kidneys

Main channel

Pain in the lower back, pain in the sole of the foot (Fig. 47.9).

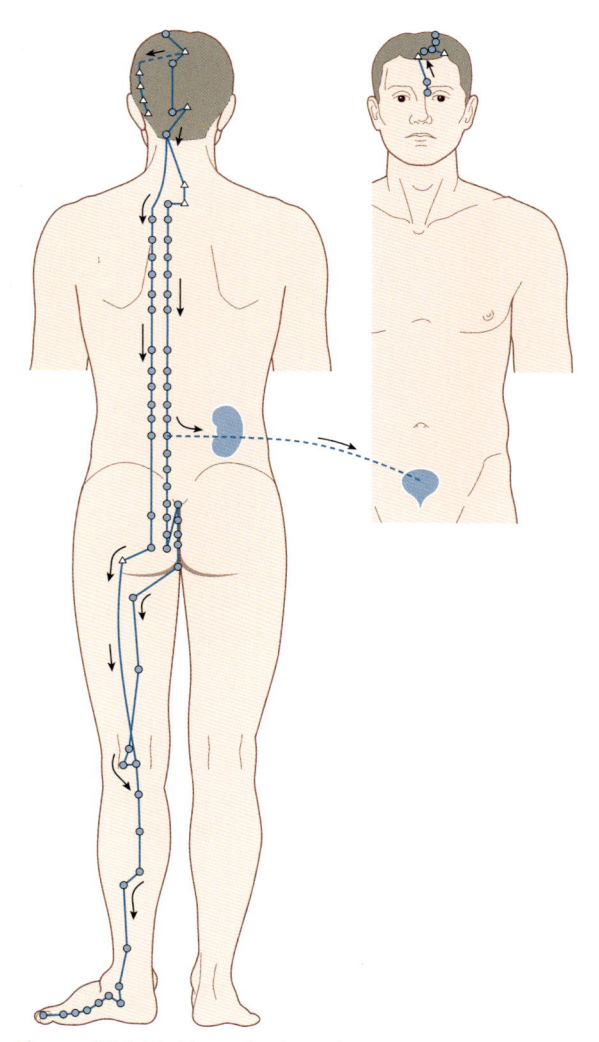

Figure 47.8 Bladder main channel

Connnecting channel

Empty

Lower backache.

Full

Mental restlessness, depression, retention of urine, pain in the heart region, distension and fullness of the chest.

Muscle channel

Pain, stiffness and sprain of the muscles of the toes, foot, inner aspect of the ankle, stiffness of the muscles of the spine and neck, inability to bend forward (if the muscles of the back are affected), inability to bend backwards (if the muscles of the chest are affected, convulsions (arching of the back).

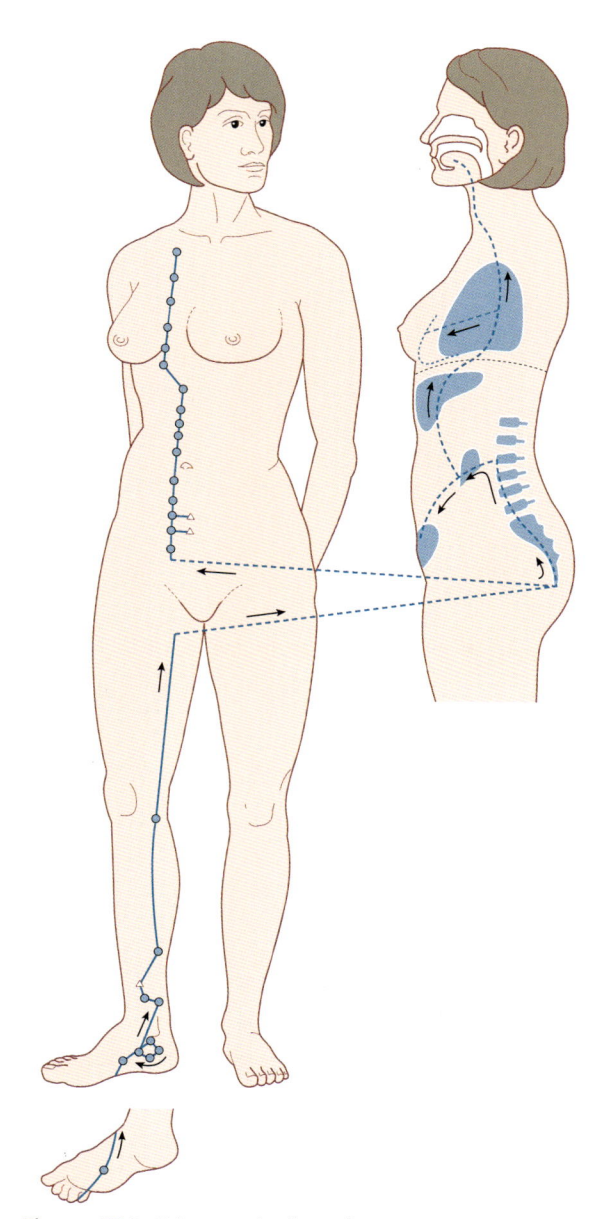

Figure 47.9 Kidneys main channel

Pericardium

Main channel

Stiff neck, pain along the course of the channel, contraction of elbow or hand (Fig. 47.10).

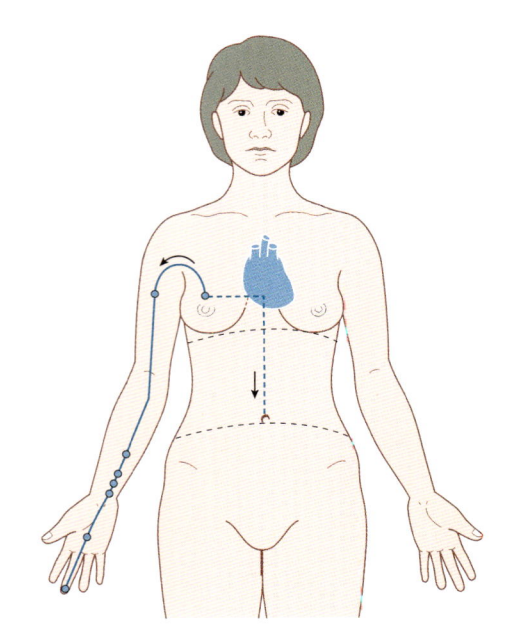

Figure 47.10 Pericardium main channel

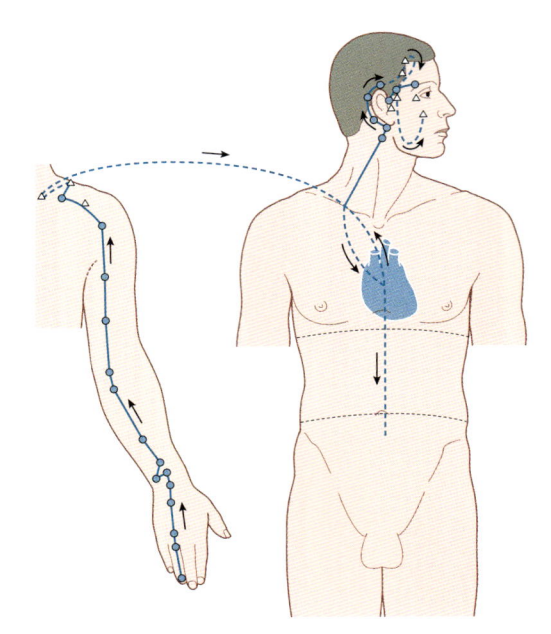

Figure 47.11 Triple Burner main channel

Connnecting channel

Empty

Stiffness of head.

Full

Pain in the heart region, mental restlessness.

Muscle channel

Pain, stiffness and sprain of the muscles of the palms, inner aspect of arm, elbow and axilla, pain in the heart region.

Triple Burner

Main channel

Pain along the course of the channel, pain in the elbow, alternation of chills and fever, deafness, pain and discharge from the ear, pain at the top of the shoulders (Fig. 47.11).

Connnecting channel

Empty

Loosening of elbow joint

Full

Contraction of elbow, swollen and painful throat, dry mouth, pain of the outer aspect of the arm, inability to raise the arm.

Muscle channel

Sprain, stiffness and sprain of the muscles of the ring finger, wrist, elbow, upper arm, shoulder and neck, curling of the tongue.

Gall Bladder

Main channel

Alternation of chills and fever, headache, deafness, pain in the hip and lateral side of legs, pain and distension of breasts (Fig. 47.12).

Connnecting channel

Empty

Weakness and flaccidity of food muscles, cold feet, paralysis of legs, difficulty in standing.

Full

Fainting, hypochondrial pain.

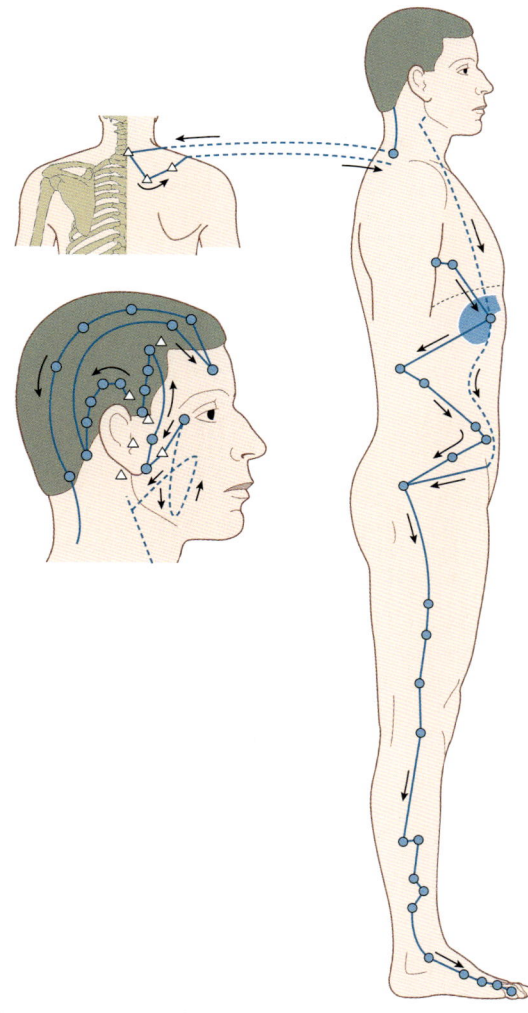

Figure 47.12 Gall Bladder main channel

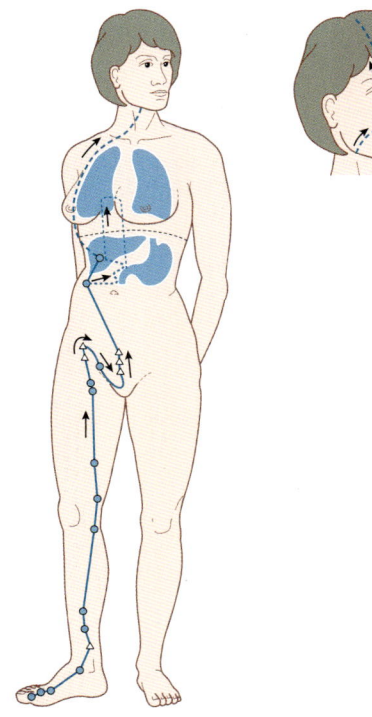

Figure 47.13 Liver main channel

Muscle channel

Pain, stiffness and sprain of the muscles of the fourth toe, external aspect of the ankle, lateral aspect of leg and knee, difficulty in bending knees, paralysis of the legs, chest and hypochondrial pain, inability to open the eyes.

Liver

Main channel

Headache, pain and swelling of the eye, cramps in the legs (Fig. 47.13).

Connecting channel

Empty

Itching of the genital region, impotence.

Full

Swelling and pain of testicle, colic, abnormal erection, hernia.

Muscle channel

Pain, stiffness and sprain of the muscles of the big toe, inner aspect of the ankle and leg, impotence, contraction of the scrotum or vagina, priapism (persistent erection).

As will be realized, some of the symptoms and signs of some of the Yin channels are actually symptoms of the associated Yang channels. For example:

- Lungs: pain in the shoulders (Large Intestine channel)
- Heart: pain in the scapula (Small Intestine channel)
- Pericardium: pain in the neck (Triple Burner channel)

6

Learning outcomes

In this chapter you will have learned:
- The relationship between the channels and the organs in disease
- How channel problems are caused: exterior invasion, overuse of a part of the body, injury and Internal Organ disharmony
- The importance of differentiating between Fullness and Emptiness in channel problems
- How to identify the following channel patterns:
  - *Lungs*: fever, aversion to cold, oppression of chest, pain in clavicle, shoulders and arms
    Connecting: yawning, frequent urination, shortness of breath (Empty); hot palms (Full)
    Muscle: pain, contraction of muscles along channel, chest and shoulder
  - *Large Intestine*: sore throat, toothache, epistaxis, runny nose, swollen and painful gums
    Connecting: sensation of cold in teeth, tightness in diaphragm, loss of smell (Empty); toothache, deafness, tinnitus, sensation of heat in centre of chest (Full)
    Muscle: pain, stiffness along channel, inability to raise arm or rotate neck
  - *Stomach*: pain in eyes, epistaxis, swelling of neck, facial paralysis, cold legs and feet
    Connecting: flaccidity/atrophy of leg muscles, feeling cold in upper teeth (Empty); epilepsy, mania/depression, sore throat, nosebleed (Full); palpitations, feeling of fullness of chest (Great Connecting channel of Spleen)
    Muscle: sprain of middle toe, contraction of leg/feet muscles, swelling in groin, hernia, strained neck/cheek muscles, deviation of eye/mouth, eye muscle problems
  - *Spleen*: vaginal discharge, cold feeling along channel, weakness of leg muscles
    Connecting: abdominal distension (Empty); abdominal pain, food poisoning, vomiting, diarrhoea (Full); pain all over body, weakness/flaccidity of joints, backache radiating to abdomen (Great Connecting channel of Spleen)
    Muscle: strain of big toe, pain in inner ankle, muscles of medial thigh/knee, strain of groin/abdomen, pain in muscles of chest/middle back
  - *Heart*: pain in eyes, inner side of arm, along scapula
    Connecting: aphasia (Empty); distension/fullness of chest/diaphragm (Full)
    Muscle: pain/stiffness/sprain along muscles of channel
  - *Small Intestine*: pain in neck, elbow, lateral side of arm and scapula, stiff neck
    Connecting: scabies, long, finger-shaped warts (Empty); loose joints of shoulder, weakness of muscles of elbow (Full)
    Muscle: stiffness/pain along little finger, arm, elbow, scapula, neck, ear, earache
  - *Bladder*: fever/aversion to cold, headache, stiff neck, lower back pain, pain in eyes
    Connecting: runny nose, nosebleed (Empty); stuffy nose, back/neck/shoulder ache (Full)
    Muscle: pain/stiffness along little toe, foot, heel, knee, spine, neck, axilla
  - *Kidneys*: pain in lower back, sole of foot
    Connecting: lower backache (Empty); mental restlessness, depression, retention of urine, pain in heart region, distension/fullness of chest (Full)
    Muscle: pain/stiffness in toes, foot, inner ankle, spine, neck, inability to bend back or forward
  - *Pericardium*: stiff neck, contraction of elbow or hand
    Connecting: stiffness of head (Empty), pain in heart region, mental restlessness (Full)
    Muscle: pain/stiffness in palms, inner arm, elbow, axilla, pain in heart region
  - *Triple Burner*: pain in elbow, top of shoulders, alternating chills/fever, deafness, ear pain
    Connecting: loose elbow joint (Empty); contraction of elbow, swollen/painful throat, dry mouth, inability to raise arm
    Muscle: stiffness/sprain of ring finger, wrist, elbow, shoulder, neck, curling of tongue
  - *Gall Bladder*: alternating chills/fever, headache, deafness, pain in hip, lateral leg, breasts
    Connecting: weakness/flaccidity of foot muscles, cold feet, paralysis of legs (Empty); fainting, hypochondrial pain (Full)
    Muscle: pain/stiffness of fourth toe, external ankle, lateral leg/knee, chest, difficulty bending knees, inability to open eyes
  - *Liver*: headache, pain/swelling of eye, leg cramps
    Connecting: genital itching, impotence (Empty); swelling/pain of testicle, colic, abnormal erection, hernia (Full)
    Muscle: pain, stiffness of big toe, inner ankle/leg, impotence, priapism, contraction of scrotum or vagina

Self-assessment questions

1. Describe the relative energetic location of the channels and organs.
2. Give four ways in which channel problems can be caused.
3. Describe the energetic functioning of joints.
4. How might you differentiate Full from Empty by colour appearing along a channel?
5. What is the main symptom of Fullness in the Lung Connecting channel?
6. What mouth symptom might there be with Emptiness of the Large Intestine Connecting channel?
7. What muscular symptom would implicate the main channel of the Spleen?
8. Which main channel would you suspect was involved if there was pain in the lower back and sole of the foot?

9. If a patient has alternation of chills and fever and pain and discharge from their ear, which channel do you think is involved?
10. Give any symptoms of the genital region which can be problems in the Liver channels.

See p. 1265 for answers

END NOTES

1. 1981 Spiritual Axis (*Ling Shu Jing* 灵枢经), People's Health Publishing House, Beijing, first published *c*.100 BC, p. 30–38.
2. For a description of the main channels and their deep pathways see Maciocia, 'The Channels of Acupuncture', Elsevier, Edinburgh, 2006.
3. Bensky D-O'Connor J 1981 'Acupuncture, a Comprehensive Text', Eastland Press, Seattle.

Identification of Patterns According to the Eight Extraordinary Vessels

SECTION 4   PART 6

48

The following patterns will be discussed:

- Governing Vessel (*Du Mai*)
- Directing Vessel (*Ren Mai*)
- Penetrating Vessel (*Chong Mai*)
- Combined Directing and Penetrating Vessel patterns
  - Directing and Penetrating Vessels empty
  - Directing and Penetrating Vessels unstable
  - Directing and Penetrating Vessels deficient and cold
  - Blood stasis in the Directing and Penetrating Vessels
  - Blood stasis and Dampness in the Directing and Penetrating Vessels
  - Full-Heat in the Directing and Penetrating Vessels
  - Empty-Heat in the Directing and Penetrating Vessels
  - Damp-Heat in the Directing and Penetrating Vessels
  - Stagnant Heat in the Directing and Penetrating Vessels
  - Full-Cold in the Directing and Penetrating Vessels
  - Uterus deficient and cold
  - Dampness and Phlegm in the Uterus
  - Stagnant Cold in the Uterus
  - Fetus Heat
  - Fetus Cold
  - Blood rebelling upwards after childbirth
- Girdle Vessel (*Dai Mai*)
- Yin Stepping Vessel (*Yin Qiao Mai*)
- Yang Stepping Vessel (*Yang Qiao Mai*)
- Yin Linking Vessel (*Yin Wei Mai*)
- Yang Linking Vessel (*Yang Wei Mai*)

For each extraordinary vessel, the applicable prescriptions will be listed: the formulae indicated are general ones from Li Shi Zhen's 'A Study of the Extraordinary Vessels'[1] while the ones for the combined patterns of the Directing and Penetrating Vessels are formulae specific to each pattern and are taken from 'Diagnosis, Patterns and Treatment in Chinese Medicine'.[2] The pulse pictures are also taken from Li Shi Zhen's 'A Study of the Extraordinary Vessels'. As for acupuncture, given the wide variety of symptoms pertaining to each extraordinary vessel, only the opening points for each will be mentioned.

GOVERNING VESSEL (*DU MAI*)

Clinical manifestations

Stiffness and pain of the spine, backache, weak back, arching of the back, headache, tremors, convulsions, epilepsy, prolapse of the anus, blood in the stools, incontinence of urine, painful urination, nocturnal emissions, impotence, irregular periods, infertility, dry throat, poor memory, dizziness, tinnitus, depression, chills and fever, manic behaviour.

Pulse: Floating and Long on all three positions of the left side (Fig. 48.1).

Connecting channel

Stiffness of the back, feeling of heaviness of the head, tremor of the head.

Treatment

Acupuncture

S.I.-3 Houxi and BL-62 Shenmai.

Herbs[3]

Spine, Marrow, Brain

Lu Rong *Cornu Cervi parvum*
Lu Jiao *Cornu Cervi*
Lu Jiao Shuang *Cornu Cervi degelatinatum*
Marrow of beef and goat

Yang channels, Bladder, Gall Bladder

Fu Zi *Radix Aconiti carmichaeli praeparata*
Qiang Huo *Radix et Rhizome Notopterygii*
Rou Gui *Cortex Cinnamomi cassiae*
Du Huo *Radix Angelicae pubescentis*
Fang Feng *Radix Ledebouriellae sesloidis*
Jing Jie *Herba seu Flos Schizonepetae tenuifoliae*
Xi Xin *Herba Asari cum radice*
Gao Ben *Rhizoma et Radix Ligustici sinensis*

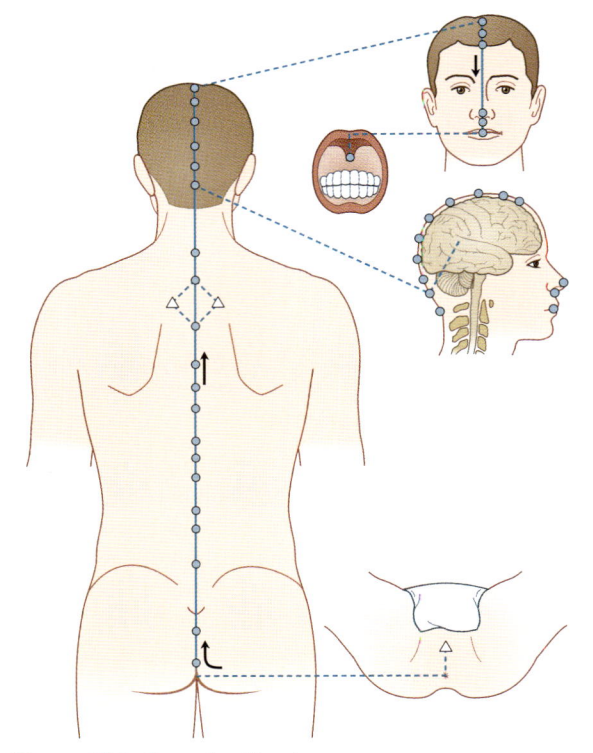

Figure 48.1 Governing Vessel

Cang Er Zi *Fructus Xanthii*
Gan Jiang *Rhizoma Zingiberis officinalis*
Chuan Jiao *Pericarpium Zanthoxyli bungeani*
Gui Zhi *Ramulus Cinnamomi cassiae*
Fu Zi *Radix Aconiti carmichaeli praeparata*
Wu Tou *Radix Aconiti carmichaeli*

Prescription
None given by Li Shi Zhen but any Kidney-Yang tonic prescription containing the above herbs will strengthen the Governing Vessel.

DIRECTING VESSEL (*REN MAI*)

Clinical manifestations

Nocturnal emissions, incontinence of urine, retention of urine, vaginal discharge, irregular periods, infertility, pain in the genital region, epigastric and abdominal pain, abdominal masses, menopausal symptoms (night sweating, hot flushes), problems during pregnancy, amenorrhoea, oedema.
Pulse: Fine-Tight-Long on both Front positions (Fig. 48.2).

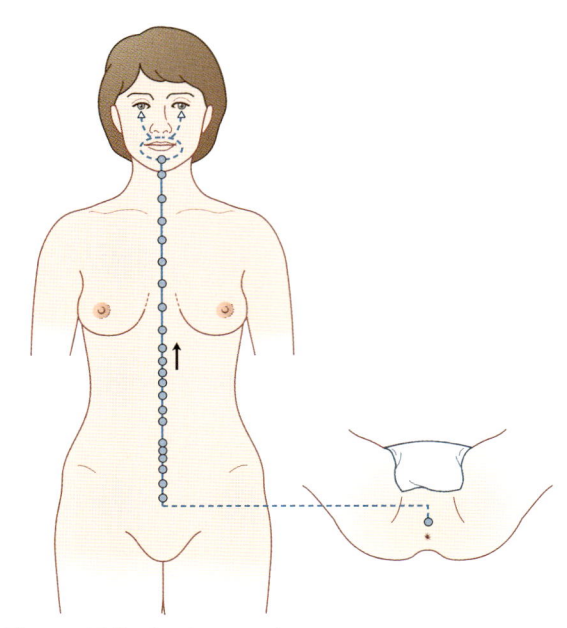

Figure 48.2 Directing Vessel

Connecting channel
Pain and itching of the abdomen.

Treatment
Acupuncture
LU-7 Lieque and KI-6 Zhaohai.

Herbs
Uterus and Blood tonics

Gui Ban *Plastrum Testudinis*
Gui Ban Jiao *Colla Plastri Testudinis*
Bie Jia *Carapacis Amydae sinensis*
E Jiao *Gelatinum Corii Asini*
Zi He Che *Placenta hominis*
Zi Shi Ying *Fluoritum*
Ai Ye *Folium Artemisiae Argyi*

Nourishing Yin and clearing Empty-Heat

Zhi Mu *Radix Anemarrhenae*
Huang Bo *Cortex Phellodendri*
Xuan Shen *Radix Scrophulariae ningpoensis*
Sheng Di Huang *Radix Rehmanniae glutinosae*
Gou Qi Zi *Fructus Lycii*

Prescription
Da Bu Yin Wan *Great Tonifying the Yin Pill*.

PENETRATING VESSEL (*CHONG MAI*)

Clinical manifestations

Irregular periods, infertility, painful periods, vomiting and nausea, feeling of anxiety (*Li Ji*, 'internal urgency'), breathlessness, abdominal pain and distension, feeling of energy rising from the abdomen to the chest, feeling of tightness and pain of the epigastrium and chest, palpitations, a feeling of obstruction in the throat, a feeling of heat in the face, cold and numb feet with purple colour, umbilical pain, premenstrual tension, breast distension, breast nodules, menopausal symptoms (hot flushes, anxiety, palpitations), morning sickness, spontaneous bruising, nosebleed, fungal infections of the big toe (Fig. 48.3).

Pulse: Deep and Firm on all three positions of either side or Deep and Firm on both Middle positions or Wiry on both Middle positions.

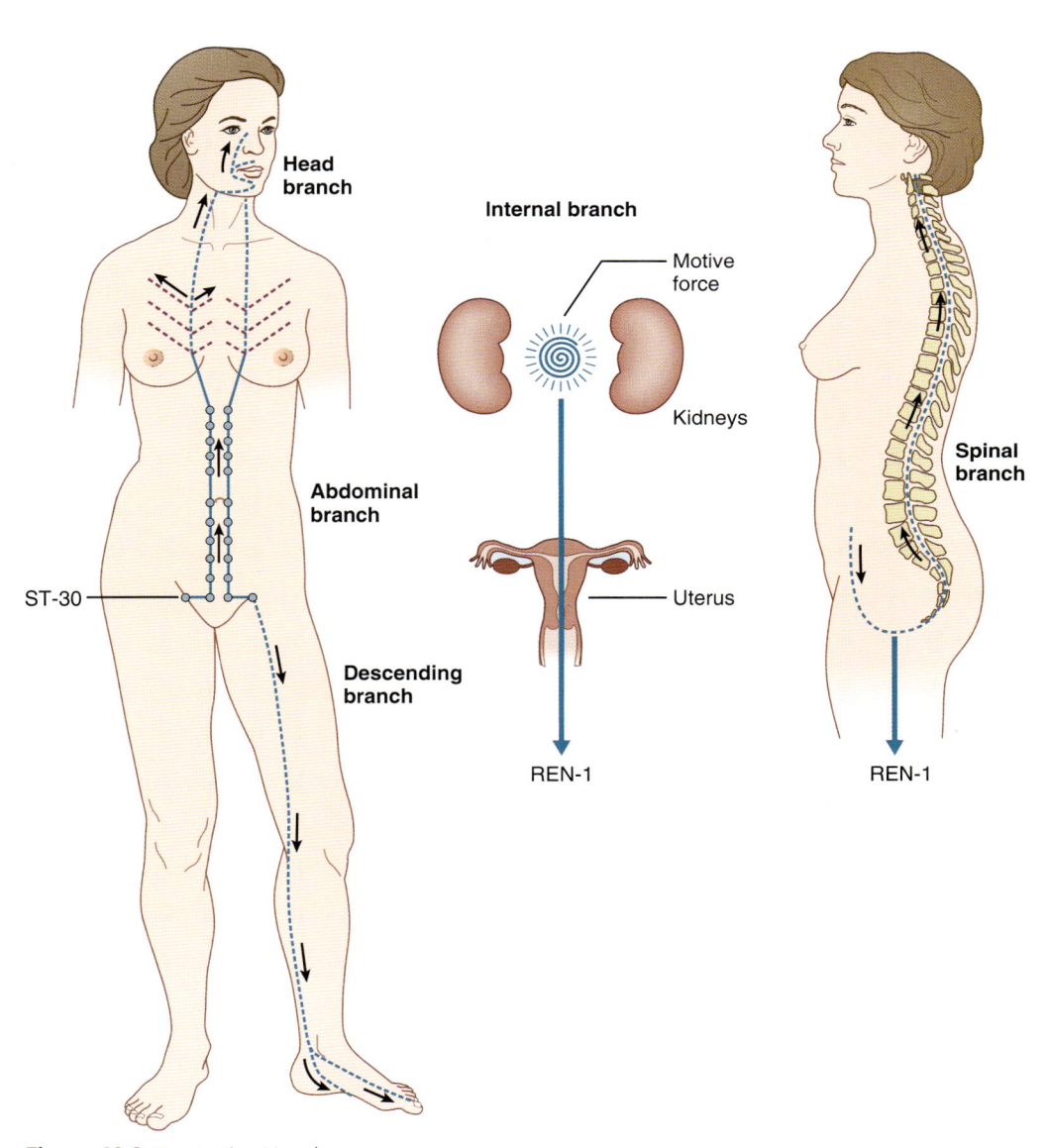

Figure 48.3 Penetrating Vessel

Treatment

Acupuncture

SP-4 Gongsun and P-6 Neiguan.

Herbs

Uterus tonics

Gui Ban *Plastrum Testudinis*
Bie Jia *Carapacis Amydae sinensis*
E Jiao *Gelatinum Corii Asini*
Zi He Che *Placenta hominis*

Rebellious Qi

Yan Hu Suo *Rhizoma Corydalis Yanhusuo*
Chuan Lian Zi *Fructus Meliae toosendan*
Xiang Fu *Rhizoma Cyperi rotundi*
Yu Jin *Tuber Curcumae*
Chen Xiang *Lignum Aquilariae*
Tao Ren *Semen Persicae*
Dang Gui *Radix Angelicae sinensis*
Qing Pi *Pericarpium Citri reticulatae viridae*
Wu Zhu Yu *Fructus Evodiae rutaecarpae*
Cong Bai *Herba Allii fistulosi*
Xiao Hui Xiang *Fructus Foeniculi vulgaris*
Chong Wei Zi *Semen Leonurus heterophylli*
Wu Yao *Radix Linderae Strychnifoliae*

Prescription

None given by Li Shi Zhen.

Women's Treasure remedy

Penetrating Vessel

COMBINED DIRECTING AND PENETRATING VESSEL PATTERNS

Directing and Penetrating Vessels empty

Gynaecological manifestations

Delayed cycle, scanty periods, amenorrhoea, infertility.

Other manifestations

Dull, pale complexion, dizziness, blurred vision, tiredness, depression, backache, weakness of the back and knees, decreased libido.
Tongue: Pale.
Pulse: Deep and Weak, especially on both Rear positions.

Treatment

Acupuncture

LU-7 Lieque on the right and KI-6 Zhaohai on the left, Ren-4 Guanyuan, KI-13 Qixue, BL-23 Shenshu. Moxa is applicable.

Prescription

Da Bu Yuan Jian *Great Tonifying the Origin Decoction*
Gui Shen Wan *Tonifying the Kidneys Pill*
Shou Tai Wan *Fetus Longevity Pill*

Women's Treasure remedy

Unicorn Pearl

Directing and Penetrating Vessels unstable

Gynaecological manifestations

Early periods, shortened cycle, heavy periods, irregular periods, persistent, chronic vaginal discharge, miscarriage, persistent lochial discharge after childbirth.

Other manifestations

Dull-pale complexion, depression, backache, weak knees, bearing down feeling, frequency of urination, incontinence of urine, urination at night.
Tongue: Pale.
Pulse: Deep and Weak, especially on both Rear positions.

Treatment

Acupuncture

LU-7 Lieque on the right and KI-6 Zhaohai on the left, Ren-4 Guanyuan, KI-13 Qixue, BL-23 Shenshu, Du-20 Baihui, Ren-6 Qihai, extra point Zigong. Moxa is applicable.

Prescription

Gu Chong Tang *Consolidating the Penetrating Vessel Decoction*
An Chong Tang *Calming the Penetrating Vessel Decoction*
Yi Qi Gu Chong Tang *Benefitting Qi and Consolidating the Penetrating Vessel Decoction*
Bu Shen Gu Chong Wan *Tonifying the Kidneys and Consolidating the Penetrating Vessel Pill*
Lu Jiao Tu Si Zi Wan *Cornus Cervi–Cuscuta Pill*

Directing and Penetrating Vessels deficient and cold

Gynaecological manifestations

Early or late periods, abdominal pain, amenorrhoea, infertility, dull abdominal pain after childbirth, prolonged trickling after the period, pale and dilute menstrual blood.

Other manifestations

Dull abdominal pain alleviated by pressure and application of heat, cold limbs, feeling of cold, pronounced feeling of cold during the period, decreased libido.
Tongue: Pale and wet.
Pulse: Deep, Weak and Slow.

Treatment

Acupuncture

LU-7 Lieque on the right and KI-6 Zhaohai on the left, Ren-4 Guanyuan, KI-13 Qixue, BL-23 Shenshu, extra point Zigong. Moxa must be used.

Prescription

Wen Jing Tang *Warming the Menses Decoction*
Dang Gui Jian Zhong Tang *Angelica Warming the Centre Decoction*
Wen Shen Tiao Qi Tang *Warming the Kidneys and Regulating Qi Decoction*
Yu Yun Tang *Promoting Pregnancy Decoction*
Bu Shen Yang Xue Tang *Tonifying the Kidneys and Nourishing Blood Decoction*

Women's Treasure remedy

Unicorn Pearl.

Blood stasis in the Directing and Penetrating Vessels

Gynaecological manifestations

Irregular cycle, brown spotting before the period, painful periods with dark blood and clots, amenorrhoea (from blood stasis), infertility, retention of lochia after childbirth.

Other manifestations

Lower abdominal pain, umbilical pain, pain and distension of the breasts, anxiety, irritability, mental restlessness, tendency to worry, breast lumps, abdominal masses.
Tongue: Purple.
Pulse: Wiry or Choppy.

Treatment

Acupuncture

SP-4 Gongsun on the right and P-6 Neiguan on the left, KI-14 Siman, ST-29 Guilai, SP-6 Sanyinjiao, LIV-3 Taichong, KI-5 Shuiquan.

Prescription

Xiao Yao San *Free and Easy Wanderer Powder*
Yue Ju Wan *Ligusticum–Gardenia Pill*
Wu Yao San *Lindera Powder*
Ge Xia Zhu Yu Tang *Eliminating Stasis below the Diaphragm Decoction*
Gui Zhi Fu Ling Wan *Ramulus–Cinnamomi–Poria Pill*
Xiang Leng Wan *Aucklandia–Sparganium Pill*

Women's Treasure remedy

Stir Field of Elixir
Harmonizing the Moon

Blood stasis and Dampness in the Directing and Penetrating Vessels

Gynaecological manifestations

Irregular cycle, heavy periods, dark menstrual blood with clots, brown spotting before the period, painful periods, chronic vaginal discharge, abdominal masses, ovarian cysts, endometriosis, infertility.

Other manifestations

Lower abdominal pain, a feeling of heaviness of the abdomen.
Tongue: Purple, Swollen with sticky coating.
Pulse: Wiry and Slippery.

Treatment

Acupuncture

SP-4 Gongsun on the right and P-6 Neiguan on the left, KI-14 Siman, ST-29 Guilai, SP-6 Sanyinjiao, LIV-3 Taichong, KI-5 Shuiquan, SP-9 Yinlingquan, ST-28 Shuidao, Ren-3 Zhongji, BL-22 Sanjiaoshu.

Prescription

Tao Hong Si Wu Tang *Prunus–Carthamus Four Substances Decoction*
Shao Fu Zhu Yu Tang *Lower Abdomen Eliminating Stasis Decoction*
San Miao Hong Teng Tang *Three Wonderful Sargentodoxa Decoction*
Qing Re Tiao Xue Tang *Clearing Heat and Regulating Blood Decoction*
Cang Fu Dao Tan Wan *Atracylodes–Cyperus Conducting Phlegm Pill*
Yin Jia Wan *Lonicera–Amyda Pill*

Women's Treasure remedy

Stir Field of Elixir plus Clear the Palace

Full-Heat in the Directing and Penetrating Vessels

Gynaecological manifestations

Early cycle, heavy periods, menstrual blood bright-red or dark-red, flooding and trickling, mid-cycle bleeding, nosebleed during the period, profuse lochial discharge after childbirth, fever after childbirth.

Other manifestations

Red face, feeling of heat, thirst, irritability, insomnia.
Tongue: Red with yellow coating.
Pulse: Rapid-Overflowing, Full at the middle level.

Treatment

Acupuncture

LU-7 Lieque on the right and KI-6 Zhaohai on the left, LI-11 Quchi, SP-10 Xuehai, Ren-3 Zhongji, LIV-3 Taichong, SP-6 Sanyinjiao.

Prescription

Qing Jing Tang *Clearing the Menses Powder*
Bao Yin Jian *Protecting the Yin Decoction*
Qing Re Gu Jing Tang *Clearing Heart and Consolidating the Menses Decoction*
Qing Gan Yin Jing Tang *Clearing the Liver and Guiding the Period Decoction*
Jie Du Huo Xue Tang *Expelling Poison and Invigorating Blood Decoction*
Jing Fang Si Wu Tang *Schizonepeta–Ledebouriella Four Substances Decoction*

Women's Treasure remedy

Drain Redness

Empty-Heat in the Directing and Penetrating Vessels

Gynaecological manifestations

Early cycle, long periods, trickling after the period, mid-cycle bleeding, scanty or heavy periods.

Other manifestations

Feeling of heat in the afternoon, malar flush, night sweating, five-palm heat, insomnia, mental restlessness, dry throat at night.
Tongue: Red without coating.
Pulse: Floating-Empty or Fine and Rapid.

Treatment

Acupuncture

LU-7 Lieque on the right and KI-6 Zhaohai on the left, Ren-4 Guanyuan, KI-2 Rangu, SP-6 Sanyinjiao.

Prescription

Liang Di Tang *Two 'Di' Decoction*
Yi Yin Jian *One Yin Decoction*

Women's Treasure remedy

Clear Empty-Heat and Cool the Menses

Damp-Heat in the Directing and Penetrating Vessels

Gynaecological manifestations

Excessive yellow or red sticky vaginal discharge with offensive odour, mid-cycle bleeding and/or pain, heavy periods, painful periods, long periods.

Other manifestations

Abdominal pain, feeling of heaviness in the abdomen, pain on urination, mucus in the stools, feeling of heat, low-grade fever, cloudy urine.
Tongue: sticky-yellow coating.
Pulse: Slippery and Rapid.

Treatment

Acupuncture

LU-7 Lieque on the right and KI-6 Zhaohai on the left, Ren-3 Zhongji, ST-28 Shuidao, Ren-9 Shuifen, SP-9

Yinlingquan, SP-6 Sanyinjiao, L.I.-11 Quchi, BL-22 Sanjiaoshu.

Prescription

Zhi Dai Wan *Stopping Vaginal Discharge Pill*
Long Dan Xie Gan Tang *Gentiana Draining the Liver Decoction*

Women's Treasure remedy

Drain Redness

Stagnant Heat in the Directing and Penetrating Vessels

Gynaecological manifestations

Early cycle, scanty or heavy periods, premenstrual tension, periods stopping and starting, red clots.

Other manifestations

Abdominal distension, breast distension, irritability, propensity to outbursts of anger, feeling of heat, dry throat.
Tongue: Red sides.
Pulse: Wiry.
 This is Heat deriving from long-term stagnation of Qi.

Treatment

Acupuncture

LU-7 Lieque on the right and KI-6 Zhaohai on the left if the pulse is Wiry, or SP-4 Gongsun on the right and P-6 Neiguan on the left if the pulse is Firm, LIV-3 Taichong, Ren-6 Qihai, KI-14 Siman, LIV-2 Xingjian, LIV-14 Qimen.

Prescription

Dan Zhi Xiao Yao San *Moutan–Gardenia Free and Easy Wanderer Powder*
Hua Gan Jian *Transforming the Liver Decoction*

Three Treasures remedy

Freeing the Sun

Full-Cold in the Directing and Penetrating Vessels

Gynaecological manifestations

Delayed cycle, painful periods with severe cramping pain and a pronounced feeling of cold during the period, bright-red blood with small dark clots, infertility, abdominal pain after childbirth.

Other manifestations

Abdominal pain that is aggravated by pressure and alleviated by the application of heat, feeling cold, cold limbs, bright-white complexion.
Tongue: Pale or Bluish-Purple.
Pulse: Deep, Slow, Tight.

Treatment

Acupuncture

LU-7 Lieque on the right and KI-6 Zhaohai on the left, Ren-4 Guanyuan, Ren-3 Zhongji, ST-28 Shuidao, KI-14 Siman, Extra Point Zigong, ST-36 Zusanli, SP-6 Sanyinjiao, KI-5 Shuiquan. Moxa must be used.

Prescription

Shao Fu Zhu Yu Tang *Lower Abdomen Eliminating Stasis Decoction*
Wen Jing Tang *Warming the Menses Decoction*
Suo Gong Zhu Yu Tang *Contracting the Uterus and Eliminating Stasis Decoction*

Women's Treasure remedy

Warm the Menses

Uterus deficient and cold

Gynaecological manifestations

Irregular cycle, scanty period, painful period with dull pain that is alleviated by the application of heat, excessive vaginal discharge, infertility, miscarriage, threatened miscarriage, abdominal pain during childbirth, retention of lochia after childbirth.

Other manifestations

Chronic dull, lower abdominal pain that is alleviated by pressure and the application of heat, abdomen feels soft on palpation, feeling cold, cold limbs, loose stools, frequent and pale urination.
Tongue: Pale.
Pulse: Deep and Weak.

Treatment

Acupuncture

LU-7 Lieque on the right and KI-6 Zhaohai on the left, Ren-4 Guanyuan, KI-13 Qixue, BL-23 Shenshu, extra point Zigong. Moxa must be used.

Prescription

Ai Fu Nuan Gong Wan *Artemisia–Cyperus Warming the Uterus Pill*
Wen Jing Tang *Warming the Menses Decoction*
Nei Bu Wan *Inner Tonification Pill*
Sheng Hua Tang *Generating and Resolving Decoction*

Women's Treasure remedy

Warm the Menses

Dampness and Phlegm in the Uterus

Gynaecological manifestations

Delayed cycle, amenorrhoea, scanty or heavy periods, excessive vaginal discharge, infertility, ovarian cysts, myomas, polycystic ovary syndrome, phantom pregnancy.

Other manifestations

Abdominal pain, feeling of heaviness in the abdomen, a feeling of oppression of the chest, sputum in the throat, a feeling of heaviness of the body, weariness, loose stools, dull-pale complexion, overweight.
Tongue: Swollen with a sticky coating.
Pulse: Slippery.

Treatment

Acupuncture

LU-7 Lieque on the right and KI-6 Zhaihai on the left, Ren-3 Zhongji, ST-28 Shuidao, extra point Zigong, Ren-9 Shuifen, SP-9 Yinlingquan, SP-6 Sanyinjiao, BL-22 Sanjiaoshu.

Prescription

Cang Fu Dao Tan Wan *Atractylodes–Cyperus Conducting Phlegm Pill*
Wei Ling Tang *Stomach 'Ling' Decoction*
Wan Dai Tang *Ending Vaginal Discharge Decoction*
Qi Gong Wan *Arousing the Uterus Pill*
Tiao Zheng San *Regulating the Upright Powder*

Women's Treasure remedy

Clear the Palace

Stagnant Cold in the Uterus

Gynaecological manifestations

Delayed cycle, painful periods with severe cramps, dark menstrual blood with clots, brown spotting before the period, periods stopping and starting, abdominal pain after childbirth, retention of lochia after childbirth, white vaginal discharge, feeling of cold in the vagina, infertility.

Other manifestations

Abdominal pain that is aggravated by pressure and alleviated by the application of heat, feeling of cold in the abdomen, feeling cold, cold limbs, purple lips.
Tongue: Bluish-Purple and wet.
Pulse: Deep-Wiry-Slow or Deep-Choppy-Slow.

Treatment

Acupuncture

LU-7 Lieque on the right and KI-6 Zhaohai on the left if the pulse is Choppy or SP-4 Gongsun on the right and P-6 Neiguan on the left if the pulse is Wiry, KI-14 Siman, ST-29 Guilai, Ren-6 Qihai, SP-10 Xuehai, ST-36 Zusanli, SP-6 Sanyinjiao, LIV-3 Taichong. Moxa should be used.

Prescription

Wen Jing Tang *Warming the Menses Decoction*
Shao Fu Zhu Yu Tang *Lower Abdomen Eliminating Stasis Decoction*
Sheng Hua Tang *Generating and Resolving Decoction*
Ai Fu Nuan Gong Wan *Artemisia–Cyperus Warming the Uterus Pill*
Hei Shen San *Black [Bean] Spirit Powder*

Women's Treasure remedy

Warm the Menses plus Stir Field of Elixir

Foetus Heat

Gynaecological manifestations

Vaginal bleeding during pregnancy, threatened miscarriage, mental restlessness during pregnancy, history of miscarriages.

Other manifestations

Red face, feeling of heat, thirst, abdominal pain, insomnia, mental restlessness, mouth ulcers.
Tongue: Red with yellow coating.
Pulse: Rapid and Overflowing.

Treatment
Acupuncture

LU-7 on the right, KI-6 on the left, L.I.-11 Quchi, SP-10 Xuehai, KI-2 Rangu, LIV-2 Xingjian, P-7 Daling, P-3 Quze.

Prescription

Bao Yin Jian *Protecting Yin Decoction*
Gu Tai Jian *Consolidating the Fetus Decoction*
Qing Hai Wan *Clearing the Sea Pill*
Qing Re An Tai Yin *Clearing Heat and Calming the Fetus Decoction*

Foetus Cold
Gynaecological manifestations
Threatened miscarriage, fetus not growing, miscarriage, history of miscarriages.

Other manifestations
Feeling cold, cold limbs, sour regurgitation, nausea, vomiting, abdominal pain, loose stools.
Tongue: Pale.
Pulse: Deep and Slow.

Treatment
Acupuncture

LU-7 on the right, KI-6 on the left, ST-36 Zusanli, BL-23 Shenshu, KI-9 Zhubin. Moxa must be used.

Prescription

Li Yin Jian *Regulating Yin Decoction*
Chang Tai Bai Zhu San *Long [Life] Fetus Atractylodes Powder*
Bu Shen Gu Chong Wan *Tonifying the Kidneys and Consolidating the Penetrating Vessel Pill*
Bu Shen An Tai Yin *Tonifying the Kidneys and Calming the Fetus Decoction*

Women's Treasure remedy

Planting Seeds

Blood rebelling upwards after childbirth
Gynaecological manifestations
Retention of lochia or scanty lochia after childbirth.

Other manifestations
Mental restlessness, manic behaviour, nosebleed, vomiting of blood, red face, coughing of blood, abdominal pain, dark complexion, stiff joints, clenched teeth.
Tongue: Purple.
Pulse: Wiry.

Treatment
Acupuncture

SP-4 Gongsun on the right and P-6 Neiguan on the left, KI-14 Siman, SP-10 Xuehai, ST-29 Guilai, LIV-3 Taichong, SP-6 Sanyinjiao, Ren-3 Zhongji, LIV-1 Dadun, SP-1 Yinbai, P-7 Daling.

Prescription

Duo Ming San *Seizing Life Powder*
Sheng Hua Tang *Generating and Resolving Decoction*
Wu Zhi San *Five Citrus Powder*
Di Sheng Tang *Supporting the Sage Decoction*
Fo Shou San *Buddha's Hand Powder*

GIRDLE VESSEL (*DAI MAI*)
Clinical manifestations
Feeling of cold and pain of the middle and lower back, mid-back pain radiating to the abdomen, abdominal pain radiating to the mid-back, flaccidity and weakness of the lower back, abdominal distension, chronic vaginal discharge, prolapse of the uterus, weakness and atrophy of the lower limbs, miscarriage, cold feet, amenorrhoea, irregular periods, feeling of cold in the genital area, infertility, nocturnal emissions, umbilical pain, painful periods (from Dampness), a feeling of fullness of the abdomen, back feeling as if sitting in water, a feeling of heaviness of the body, a feeling of heaviness of the abdomen as if wearing a belt 'carrying 5000 coins', hernia.
Pulse: Wiry on both Middle positions (Fig. 48.4).

Treatment
Acupuncture

G.B.-41 Zulinqi and T.B.-5 Waiguan.

Herbs

Astringent herbs which infuse to the Lower Burner

Wu Wei Zi *Fructus Schisandrae chinensis*
Shan Yao *Radix Dioscoreae oppositae*

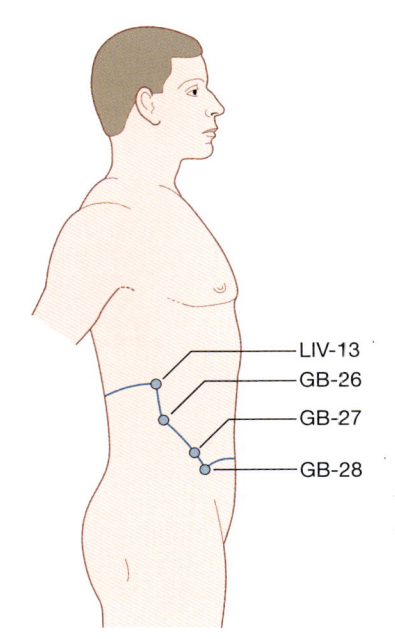

Figure 48.4 Girdle Vessel

Qian Shi *Semen Euryales ferocis*
Fu Pen Zi *Fructus Rubi*
Sang Piao *Xiao Ootheca mantidis*

Herbs which consolidate the Uterus and lift Qi

Dang Gui *Radix Angelicae sinensis*
Bai Shao *Radix Paeoniae albae*
Xu Duan *Radix Dipsaci*
Long Gu *Os Draconis*
Ai Ye *Folium Artemisiae*
Sheng Ma *Rhizoma Camicifugae*
Gan Cao *Radix Glycyrrhizae uralensis*

Prescription

Gan Jiang Ling Zhu Tang *Glycyrrhiza–Zingiberis–Poria–Atractylodes Decoction*
Dang Gui Shao Yao San *Angelica–Paeonia Powder*
Liang Shou Tang *Two Receiving Decoction*
Variation of Bu Zhong Yi Qi Tang *Tonifying the Centre and Benefiting Qi Decoction* plus Ba Ji Tian *Radix Morindae officinalis*, Du Zhong *Cortex Eucommiae ulmoidis*, Gou Ji *Rhizoma Cibotii Barometz*, Xu Duan *Radix Dipsaci Asperi*, Wu Wei Zi *Fructus Schisandrae chinensis*
Shou Tai Wan *Fetus Longevity Pill*

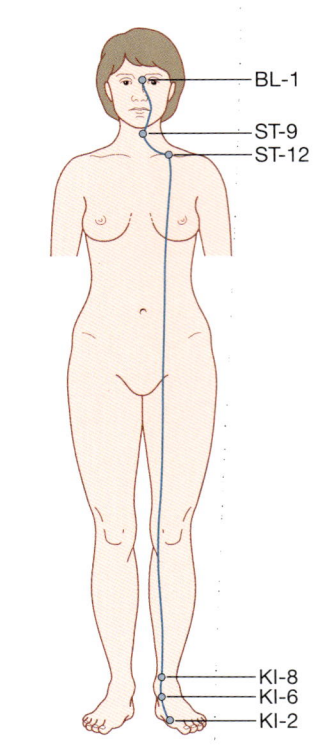

Figure 48.5 Yin Stepping Vessel

YIN STEPPING VESSEL (*YIN QIAO MAI*)

Clinical manifestations

Sleepiness, epilepsy (seizures at night), pain in the back and hip radiating to the groin and genitals, hypogastric pain, tremors of the legs, foot turning inwards, abdominal pain, tightness of the muscles of the inner aspect of the leg and flaccidity of those of the outer aspect, abdominal masses, myomas, difficult delivery, retention of placenta (Fig. 48.5).
Pulse: Wiry on both Rear positions.

Treatment

Acupuncture

KI-6 Zhaohai and LU-7 Lieque.

Herbs

Yan Hu Suo *Rhizoma Corydalis yanhusuo*
Gua Lou *Fructus Trichosanthis*
Ban Xia *Rhizoma Pinelliae ternatae*
Dan Nan Xing *Rhizoma Arisaematis praeparata*
Zhi Mu *Radix Anemarrhenae asphodeloidis*

Huang Bo *Cortex Phellodendri*
Yuan Zhi *Radix Polygalea tenufoliae*
Suan Zao Ren *Semen Ziziphi spinosae*
Shi Chang Pu *Rhizoma Acori graminea*

Prescription

Si Wu Tang *Four Substances Decoction*
Ban Xia Tang *Pinellia Decoction*

YANG STEPPING VESSEL (*YANG QIAO MAI*)

Clinical manifestations

Insomnia, epilepsy (seizures during the day), pain and redness of the inner corner of the eye, backache, sciatica with pain along the lateral aspect of the leg, tremor of the legs, foot turning outwards, tightness of the muscles of the outer aspect of the leg and flaccidity of those of the inner aspect, Wind-stroke, hemiplegia, aphasia, facial paralysis, severe dizziness, chills and fever, headache, stiff neck, manic behaviour, manic depression, fright, 'seeing ghosts', inability to raise the leg when lying down (Fig. 48.6).

Pulse: Wiry on both Front positions.

Treatment

Acupuncture

BL-62 Shenmai and S.I.-3 Houxi.

Herbs

Ma Huang *Herba Ephedrae*
Fang Feng *Radix Ledebouriellae sesloidis*
Cang Zhu *Rhizoma Atractylodis lanceae*
Zhi Gan Cao *Radix Glycyrrhizae uralensis praeparata*
Fang Ji *Radix Stephaniae tetrandae*

Prescription

Sheng Yang Tang *Raising the Yang Decoction*

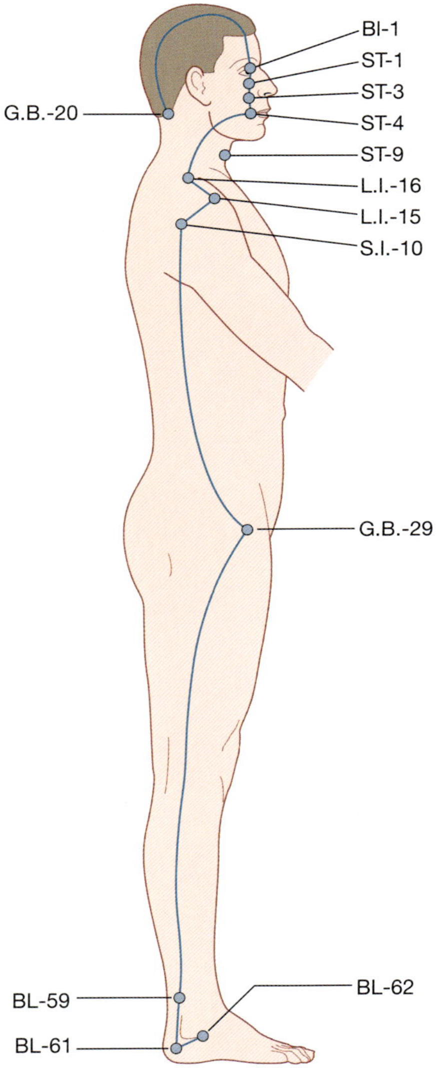

YIN LINKING VESSEL (*YIN WEI MAI*)

Clinical manifestations

Pain in the heart region, fullness and pain of the chest and hypochondrium, pain in the kidney region, dryness of the throat, anxiety, insomnia, pensiveness, obsessive thoughts, lack of will-power, loss of self-control, depression, sadness, a feeling of knot in the chest which feels tight and full on palpation, melancholy, crying, forgetfulness, mental cloudiness, palpitations, shock (Fig. 48.7).

Pulse: Wiry on the lateral side of the Rear position extending towards the medial side of the front position.

Treatment

Acupuncture

P-6 Neiguan and SP-4 Gongsun.

Figure 48.6 Yang Stepping Vessel

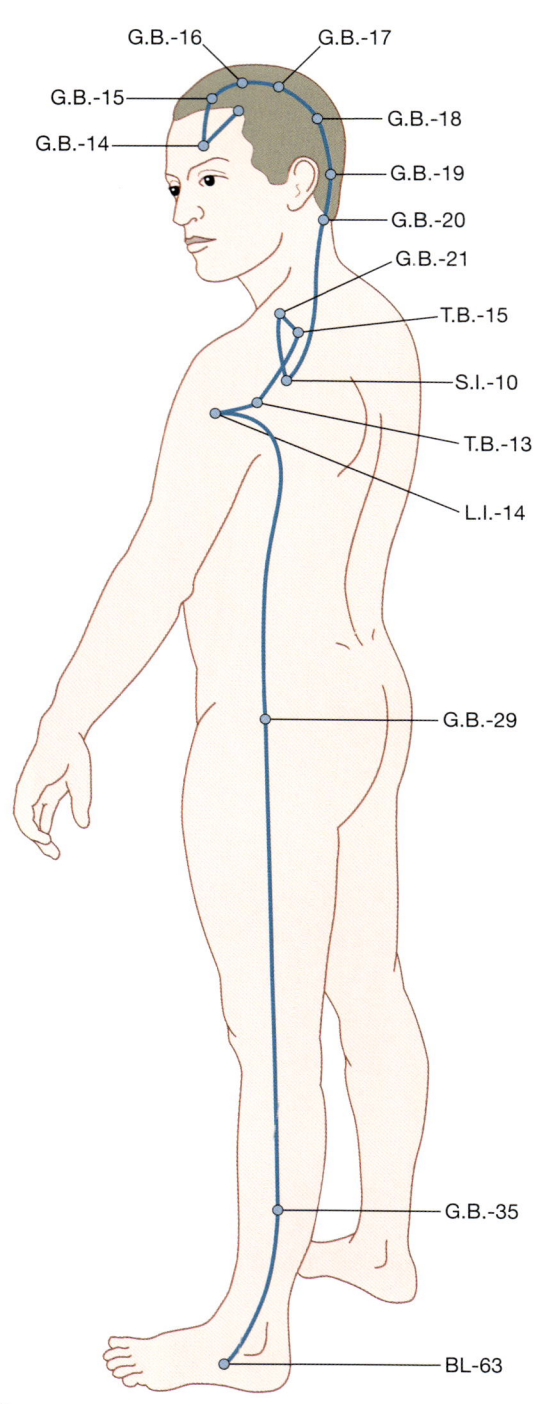

Figure 48.7 Yang Linking Vessel

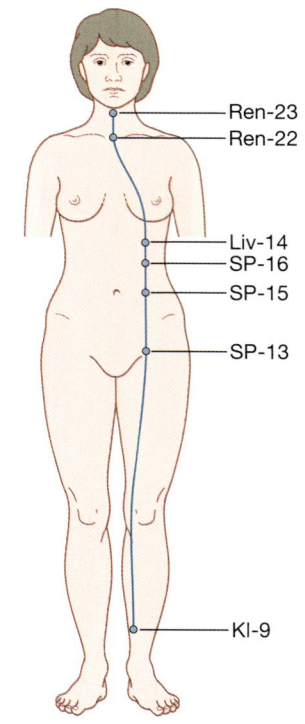

Figure 48.8 Yin Linking Vessel

Herbs

Dang Gui *Radix Angelicae sinensis*
Chuan Xiong *Radix Ligustici Chuanxiong*

Prescription

Dang Gui Si Ni Tang *Angelica Four Rebellious Decoction*
Wu Zhu Yu Tang *Evodia Decoction*
Si Ni Tang *Four Rebellious Decoction*
Li Zhong Tang *Regulating the Centre Decoction*

YANG LINKING VESSEL (*YANG WEI MAI*)

Clinical manifestations

Alternations of chills and fevers, weakness of the limbs, dizziness on eye movement, earache, stiff neck, hypochondrial pain, pain in the lateral side of the leg, tinnitus, deafness, sweating.

Pulse: Wiry on the medial side of the Rear position extending towards the lateral side of the Front position (Fig. 48.8).

Treatment

Acupuncture
T.B.-5 Waiguan and G.B.-41 Zulinqi.

Herbs
Gui Zhi *Ramulus Cinnamomi cassiae*
Bai Shao *Radix Paeoniae lactiflorae*
Huang Qi *Radix Astragali membranacei*

Prescription
Dang Gui Gui Zhi Tang *Angelica–Ramulus–Cinnamomi Decoction*

END NOTES

1. Wang Luo Zhen 1985 A Compilation of the Study of the Eight Extraordinary Vessels (*Qi Jing Ba Mai Kao Jiao Zhu* 奇经八脉考校注), Shanghai Science Publishing House, Shanghai. The Study of the Eight Extraordinary Vessels (*Qi Jing Ba Mai Kao* 奇经八脉考) by Li Shi Zhen was published in 1578.
2. Cheng Shao En 1994 Diagnosis, Patterns and Treatment in Chinese Medicine (*Zhong Yi Zheng Hou Zhen Duan Zhi Liao Xue* 中醫证候诊断治疗学), Beijing Science Publishing House, Beijing, p. 241–278.
3. The herbs and prescriptions are from a Qing dynasty book called The Materia Medica of Proper Combinations (*De Pei Ben Cao*), reported in Wang Luo Zhen 1985 A Compilation of the Study of the Eight Extraordinary Vessels (*Qi Jing Ba Mai Kao Jiao Zhu* 奇经八脉考校注), Shanghai Science Publishing House, Shanghai, p. 129–131.

SECTION 4 PART 6

Identification of Patterns According to the Five Elements

49

Key contents

Generating sequence patterns
Wood not generating Fire
Fire not generating Earth
Earth not generating Metal
Metal not generating Water
Water not generating Wood

Overacting sequence patterns
Wood overacting on Earth
Earth overacting on Water
Water overacting on Fire
Fire overacting on Metal
Metal overacting on Wood

Insulting sequence patterns
Wood insulting Metal
Metal insulting Fire
Fire insulting Water
Water insulting Earth
Earth insulting Wood

We can distinguish the Five-Element patterns according to the Generating, Overacting and Insulting sequences.

The patterns discussed are:

- Generating sequence patterns
  - Wood not generating Fire
  - Fire not generating Earth
  - Earth not generating Metal
  - Metal not generating Water
  - Water not generating Wood
- Overacting sequence patterns
  - Wood overacting on Earth
  - Earth overacting on Water
  - Water overacting on Fire
  - Fire overacting on Metal
  - Metal overacting on Wood
- Insulting sequence patterns
  - Wood insulting Metal
  - Metal insulting Fire
  - Fire insulting Water
  - Water insulting Earth
  - Earth insulting Wood

The identification of patterns according to the Five Elements is based on the pathological changes occurring in dysfunctions of the Generating, Overacting and Insulting sequences of the Five Elements.

These patterns are not of primary importance in practice as most of them describe clinical conditions which are better expressed by the Internal Organ patterns. In certain cases, however, some Five-Element patterns can describe conditions which fall outside the scope of the Internal Organ patterns. An example of this is the pattern of Deficient Qi of Wood (manifesting with timidity and indecision) which is not included among the Internal Organ patterns.

GENERATING SEQUENCE PATTERNS

These patterns describe conditions of deficiency of each organ when this is induced by its Mother Element.

Wood not generating Fire

The clinical manifestations are timidity, a lack of courage, indecision, palpitations and insomnia (in particular, waking up in the early hours of the morning).

This pattern is sometimes also described as a pattern of Deficient Gall Bladder. It is an unusual pattern in so far as, according to the theory of the Internal Organs, Liver-Qi or the Gall Bladder can hardly ever be deficient. This pattern describes such a situation. More than a pattern, it really describes a certain character and personality, and its salient feature is the lack of courage and timidity. It corresponds to the Internal Organ pattern of Deficient Gall Bladder.

In fact, Liver-Qi may be deficient and this deficiency manifests primarily on a psychological level with the above-mentioned timidity, lack of resolve and difficulty in making decisions. It corresponds to a situation when the Ethereal Soul (*Hun*) does not 'come and go' enough; it does not provide enough 'movement' to the Mind (*Shen*).

Fire not generating Earth

The clinical manifestations are loose stools, chilliness and weakness of the limbs.

This pattern basically describes a condition of Spleen-Yang deficiency due to failure of the physiological Fire of the body in providing Heat to the Spleen to transform and transport. According to the theory of the Internal Organs, however, the Spleen derives the warmth necessary to its functions not from the Heart, but from Kidney-Yang. This is because, even though the Kidneys pertain to the Water Element, they also are the source of physiological Fire in the body. The relationship between Kidney-Yang and the Spleen is clinically more relevant than that between the Fire of the Heart and the Spleen.

Earth not generating Metal

The clinical manifestations are phlegm in the chest, cough and tiredness.

This pattern describes the situation when a Spleen deficiency (causing the tiredness) leads to the formation of Phlegm, which obstructs the Lungs.

Metal not generating Water

The clinical manifestations are cough, breathlessness, loss of voice and asthma.

This pattern corresponds to the Internal Organ pattern of Kidneys not receiving Qi.

Water not generating Wood

The clinical manifestations are dizziness, blurred vision, headaches and vertigo.

This pattern is the same as the Internal Organ pattern of Kidney- and Liver-Yin deficiency.

OVERACTING SEQUENCE PATTERNS

Wood overacting on Earth

The clinical manifestations are hypochondriac and epigastric pain, a feeling of distension, irritability, loose stools, poor appetite and greenish face.

When the clinical manifestations pertain to one Element and the face colour pertains to the Element which overacts on it, the face colour usually shows the origin of the disharmony. In this case, loose stools and poor appetite are symptoms of deficiency of Earth (Spleen) but the face is greenish: this indicates that the root of the problem is in Wood, i.e. Wood overacting on Earth. This same principle applies to all the following cases of disharmony of the Overacting sequence.

The pattern of Wood overacting on Earth is very common and it is exactly the same as the pattern of 'Liver invading the Spleen' already discussed (ch. 34).

Earth overacting on Water

The main clinical manifestations are oedema, difficult urination and a yellow face.

This pattern occurs when a deficient Spleen fails to transform and transport fluids which accumulate and obstruct the Kidney function of transformation and excretion of fluids.

Water overacting on Fire

The clinical manifestations are oedema of the ankles, backache, feeling cold, dizziness, expectoration of thin watery sputum, palpitations.

This pattern corresponds to the pattern of Kidney-Yang deficient Water overflowing to the Heart.

Fire overacting on Metal

The clinical manifestations are cough with profuse yellow sputum, a feeling of heat and a red face.

This pattern corresponds to Full-Heat in the Lungs.

Metal overacting on Wood

The clinical manifestations are tiredness, irritability, a feeling of distension, cough and a white face.

This pattern corresponds to a situation when the lack of descending of Lung-Qi impairs the free flow of Liver-Qi.

INSULTING SEQUENCE PATTERNS

Wood insulting Metal

The clinical manifestations are cough, asthma and a feeling of distension of chest and hypochondrium.

The Liver channel influences the chest and stagnant Liver-Qi or Liver-Fire can obstruct the chest and prevent Lung-Qi from descending.

Metal insulting Fire

The clinical manifestations are palpitations, insomnia and breathlessness.

This pattern basically describes a condition of both Lung- and Heart-Qi deficiency.

Fire insulting Water

The clinical manifestations are a malar flush, dry mouth at night, insomnia, dizziness, lower backache and night sweating.

This pattern is identical to the Internal Organ pattern of 'Kidney and Heart not harmonized', i.e. Kidney-Yin deficiency giving rise to Heart Empty-Heat.

Water insulting Earth

The clinical manifestations are loose stools, oedema, tiredness and weakness of the limbs.

This pattern corresponds to Spleen- and Kidney-Yang deficiency.

Earth insulting Wood

The clinical manifestations are jaundice and hypochondriac pain and distension.

This pattern is caused by a failure of the Spleen in transforming fluids, leading to Dampness. Dampness accumulates and obstructs the smooth flow of Liver-Qi, impeding the free flow of bile.

Learning outcomes

In this chapter you will have learned:
- How to identify the following Generating sequence patterns:
  Wood not generating Fire: timidity, lack of courage, indecision, palpitations, insomnia
  Fire not generating Earth: loose stools, chilliness, weakness of the limbs
  Earth not generating Metal: phlegm in the chest, cough, tiredness
  Metal not generating Water: cough, breathlessness, loss of voice, asthma
  Water not generating Wood: dizziness, blurred vision, headaches, vertigo
- How to identify the following Overacting sequence patterns:
  Wood overacting on Earth: hypochondriac/epigastric pain, a feeling of distension, irritability, loose stools, poor appetite, greenish face
  Earth overacting on Water: oedema, difficult urination, yellow face
  Water overacting on Fire: oedema of the ankles, backache, feeling cold, dizziness, expectoration of thin watery sputum, palpitations
  Fire overacting on Metal: cough with profuse yellow sputum, feeling of heat, red face
  Metal overacting on Wood: tiredness, irritability, feeling of distension, cough, white face
- How to identify the following Insulting sequence patterns:
  Wood insulting Metal: cough, asthma and a feeling of distension of chest and hypochondrium
  Metal insulting Fire: palpitations, insomnia, breathlessness
  Fire insulting Water: malar flush, dry mouth at night, insomnia, dizziness, lower backache, night sweating
  Water insulting Earth: loose stools, oedema, tiredness, weakness of the limbs
  Earth insulting Wood: jaundice, hypochondriac pain and distension

Self-assessment questions

1. Which organ pattern corresponds to the pattern of Wood not generating Fire?
2. Describe the symptoms and their pathology caused when Earth does not generate Metal.
3. Identify the following clinical manifestations in terms of their Five-Element sequence pattern: dizziness, blurred vision, headaches and vertigo.
4. If a patient has multiple symptoms involving the Lungs, but has a yellow face, where do you suspect lies the origin of the disharmony?
5. Which Internal Organ pattern corresponds to the pattern of Fire insulting Water?

See p. 1266 for answers

PART 7

The Acupuncture Points

INTRODUCTION

Part 7 will discuss the functions of the acupuncture points and the principles governing their combinations.

Section 1 discusses the functions of the acupuncture points according to the category they fall into, for example Source (*Yuan*) points, Five Transporting (*Shu*) points, etc.

Section 2 describes the actions and functions of the main points of each channel and of some extra points.

Part 7 is divided into the following parts:

Section 1: Categories of points
    Chapter 50   The Five Transporting points
    Chapter 51   Other categories of points
        Source points
        Connecting points
        Back Transporting points
        Front Collecting points
        Accumulation points
        Gathering points
        Points of the Four Seas
        Window of Heaven points
        12 Heavenly Star points of Ma Dan Yang
        Sun Si Miao's 13 Ghost points
        Points of the Eye System (*Mu Xi*)
        Five Command points
    Chapter 52   The Eight Extraordinary Vessels – Introduction
    Chapter 53   The Eight Extraordinary Vessels

Section 2: The function of the points
    Chapter 54   Lung channel
    Chapter 55   Large Intestine channel
    Chapter 56   Stomach channel
    Chapter 57   Spleen channel
    Chapter 58   Heart channel
    Chapter 59   Small Intestine channel
    Chapter 60   Bladder channel
    Chapter 61   Kidney channel
    Chapter 62   Pericardium channel
    Chapter 63   Triple Burner channel
    Chapter 64   Gall Bladder channel
    Chapter 65   Liver channel
    Chapter 66   Directing Vessel
    Chapter 67   Governing Vessel
    Chapter 68   Extra points

SECTION 1

Categories of points

INTRODUCTION

Before discussing the functions of the points individually, it is important to discuss the general functions of certain categories of points. Although each point has specific functions peculiar to its nature and location, functions of the points can also be discussed according to the category they fall into. For example, LIV-2 has many functions specific to its nature and location but, as a Fire and Spring point, it shares certain common characteristics and functions with other Fire and Spring points. This inevitably involves making some generalizations, but it is nevertheless useful to grasp the nature and functions of points by categories.

Section 1 discusses the functions of the points in the context of the categories they fall into as follows:

> Chapter 50   The Five Transporting points
> Chapter 51   The functions of specific categories of points
>   Source points
>   Connecting points
>   Back Transporting points
>   Front Collecting points
>   Accumulation points
>   Gathering points
>   Points of the Four Seas
>   Window of Heaven points
>   12 Heavenly Star points of Ma Dan Yang
>   Sun Si Miao's 13 Ghost points
>   Points of the Eye System (*Mu Xi*)
>   Five Command points
> Chapter 52   The Eight Extraordinary Vessels – Introduction
> Chapter 53   The Eight Extraordinary Vessels

The Five Transporting Points (*Shu* Points)

SECTION 1 PART 7 50

> **Key contents**
>
> **Energetic actions of the Five Transporting points**
> Well point
> Spring point
> Stream point
> River point
> Sea point
>
> **Actions of the Five Transporting points from the classics**
> According to the 'Classic of Difficulties'
> According to the 'Spiritual Axis'
> - Chapter 44
> - Chapter 4
> - Chapter 6
>
> According to the seasons
> According to the Five Elements
>
> **Summary**

The Five Transporting points (*Shu* points) are the points that lie between the fingers and elbows or between the toes and knees. They are assigned to the Five Elements so that they are mostly known in the West as 'Element points' or sometimes 'command points'. In France they are known as 'antique points'.

The Chinese name for these points is '*Shu*' 输, which is nearly the same character as for the Back Transporting points, meaning 'transporting'. In order to illustrate the nature of these points, the ancient Chinese compared the section of channel between fingers/toes and elbows/knees to a river, starting from a 'well' point at the tips of the fingers or toes, getting gradually larger and deeper and ending in 'sea' point at the elbows or knees. Thus from fingers/toes to elbows/knees there is a progression in the size and depth of the channel: it is narrowest and most superficial at the fingers/toes and widest and deepest at the elbows/knees.

It is important to note that this progression of size and depth of the channel is *irrespective* of the direction of flow of the channel, i.e. it applies equally to Yin or Yang channels of both arms and legs. Even though the Yin channels of the hand flow downwards towards the fingers, and the Yang channels of the hand flow upwards towards the chest, the comparison of the channel to a river, with its springhead at the fingers and its delta at the elbows, applies equally to both. Exactly the same applies to the leg channels (Figs 50.1 and 50.2).

The implication of this is that the section of channel between fingers/toes and elbows/knees is more superficial than the rest, and this is one of the reasons for the importance of the points lying along its path. The energetic action of the points situated along this section of a channel is more dynamic than other points and this explains their frequent use in clinical practice. Indeed, one could conceivably practice acupuncture using only these points. As one may have experienced many times, the effect of, say, LIV-3 Taichong is far more dynamic than, say, LIV-10 Wuli or LIV-11 Yinlian (situated on the thigh).

The other implication of the fact that the section of channel between fingers/toes and elbows/knees is more superficial is that this section represents the connection between the body and the environment. It is the section of channel which is influenced most promptly and directly by climate and exterior pathogenic factors. For this reason the points along this section of channel are more directly related to the seasons and can be used according to their cycle. For the same reason, the points along this section of channel are the points of entry of exterior pathogenic factors such as Cold, Dampness and Wind.

Another reason for the dynamism of the points in this section of the channel is that at the fingertips and toes the energy changes polarity, from Yin to Yang or

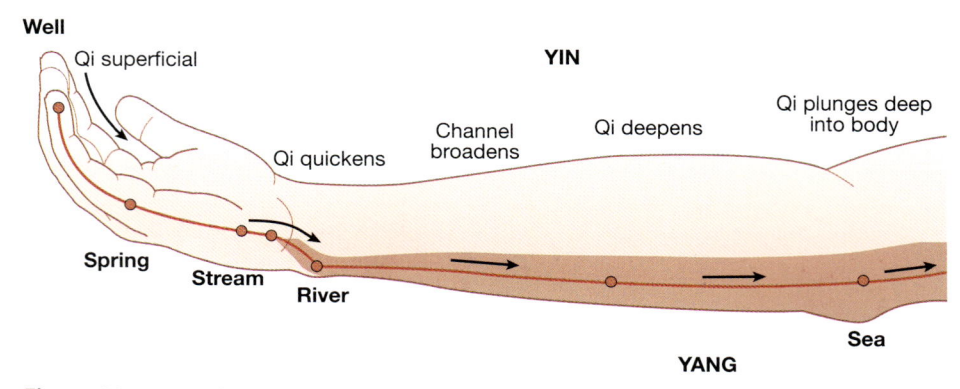

Figure 50.1 Flow of Qi in the Five Transporting points

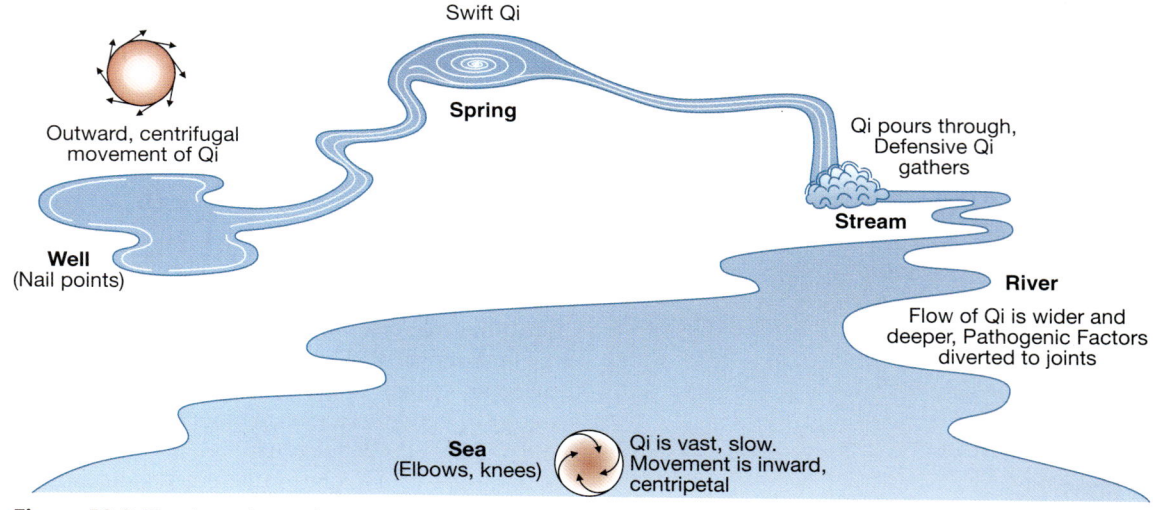

Figure 50.2 The channel as a river

vice versa. Due to this change of polarity, the Qi of the channel is more unstable and therefore more easily influenced (Fig. 50.3).

Even though we normally say that this change of polarity takes place at the fingers and toes, it cannot take place immediately at one single point and the inertia from one channel at its end carries on to a certain extent through the next channel up to the elbow or knee.

For example, the Lung channel ends at the tip of the thumb where the polarity changes to Yang and the energy flows into the Large Intestine channel. However, this change from Yin to Yang polarity cannot take place instantly in one point at the fingertips, but the inertia from the Lung channel is, to a certain extent, carried through to the initial section of the Large Intestine channel.

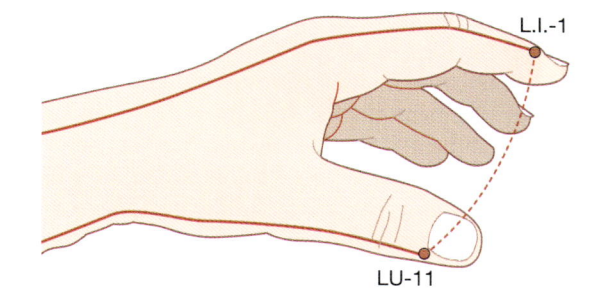

Figure 50.3 Change from Yin to Yang at fingertips

This can be compared to the meeting of two rivers: when two wide rivers meet, they do not just merge at the point of junction, but often the current from one river carries on flowing independently within the second river for some time. The progression of the

Five-Element points along the channel is probably in relation to this change of polarity, as the second point belongs to Fire in Yin channels and Water in Yang channels. This might be because the second point represents the point at which the inertia of the incoming channel is felt most and manifests itself (Fig. 50.4).

For example, the Lung channel inertial movement continues into the Large Intestine channel, particularly at the second point along the channel, which therefore belongs to Water, reflecting the Yin character of the Lung channel. Similarly, the second point of Yin channels belongs to Fire, reflecting the inertia of the incoming Yang channels.

Thus, the second point along the channel represents the point of maximum inertia from the previous channel, after which the inertia becomes less and less, disappearing totally at the fifth point along the channel. This explains the particularly unstable state of the energy in the end/beginning section of a channel at the fingertips and toes. This instability is another reason accounting for the dynamism of the points along it and is made use of in practice.

Three reasons for the dynamism of points at the end/beginning of a channel:
1. Channel is more superficial
2. Change from Yin to Yang (and vice versa)
3. Second point is in contrast with polarity of channel (Water for Yang and Fire for Yin channels)

Five of the points situated along this section of channel are particularly important, and they are called the Five Transporting (*Shu*) points: they also coincide with what we call the Element points. However, the dynamics of these points is irrespective of their Five-Element character.

Each of the five points occupying the same location along the channel has a name. The names I will use are:

- Well point (*Jing*): the point at the tips of fingers or toes
- Spring point (*Ying*): the second point of the five (in all cases it is the second point along the channel)
- Stream point (*Shu*): the third point of the five (in all cases it is the third point along the channel, except for the Gall Bladder channel where it is the fourth)
- River point (*Jing*): the fourth point of the five, not always the fourth point along the channel
- Sea point (*He*): the fifth point of the five (in all cases it is the point at the elbows and knees)

These names do not represent literal translations of the Chinese names, but I have preferred them to the literal translations as these might have created some confusion. The use of the above names is also justified by the analogy of these points with stages in the course of a river found in chapter 1 of the 'Spiritual Axis', where it says that '*at the Well points Qi flows out, at the Spring points it slips and glides, at the Stream points it pours, at the River points it moves, at the Sea points it enters.*'[1] The 'Classic of Difficulties' gives the same description in chapter 69.[2]

The actual meanings of their names are:

Jing = well
Ying = spring (of water), pool (of water)
Shu = to transport
Jing = to pass through
He = to unite, join

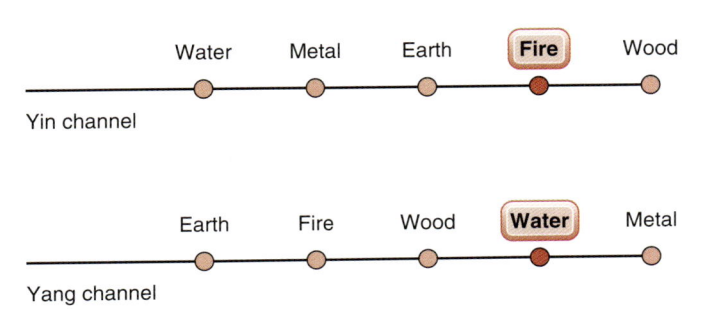

Figure 50.4 Spring-Ying points of Yin and Yang channels

These names are in relation to the energetic action of these points, which will be discussed below:

- Energetic actions of the Five Transporting points
  - Well point
  - Spring point
  - Stream point
  - River point
  - Sea point
- Actions of the Five Transporting points from the Classics
  - According to chapter 68 of the 'Classic of Difficulties'
  - According to the 'Spiritual Axis', chapters 4, 6 and 44
  - According to the seasons, as in chapter 61 of 'Simple Questions' and chapter 44 of 'Spiritual Axis'
  - According to the Five-Element character of the points, as in chapters 64 and 69 of the 'Classic of Difficulties'
- Summary

ENERGETIC ACTIONS OF THE FIVE TRANSPORTING POINTS

Each of the Five Transporting points has a specific energetic action within the channel dynamics that explains the meaning of their names.

Well point

This is the point of departure of Qi (in the sense outlined above and therefore applying to both Yin and Yang channels of arm and leg). At this point the channel is at its most superficial and thinnest and the energy changes polarity from Yin to Yang or vice versa. Because the energy is more superficial and changes polarity, the Well point has a particularly dynamic effect when needled (Fig. 50.5).

The energy is at its most unstable state here, so that it can be easily and readily influenced and changed. This explains the use of these points in acute situations, as the Well points tend to be used to eliminate pathogenic factors quickly in acute conditions. For example, they are used to extinguish internal Wind in the acute stage of Wind-stroke.

According to the 'Classic of Difficulties', these points have an 'outward' movement: that is, the energy of the channel tends to go outwards in a centrifugal movement at these points.[3] The outward, centrifugal tendency of the Well points is exploited to eliminate pathogenic factors quickly as they pass through these points.

Several examples can be cited, such as the use of LU-11 Shaoshang for fainting, P-9 Zhongchong for fainting and heat-stroke, HE-9 Shaochong and S.I.-1 Shaoze for loss of consciousness, SP-1 Yinbai for convulsions, KI-1 Yongchuan for loss of consciousness and infantile convulsions and L.I.-1 Shangyang for loss of consciousness. The extra points Shixuan situated at the fingertips have actions which are equivalent to those of the Well points: the Shixuan points are used to extinguish internal Wind in acute conditions (e.g. acute state of Wind-stroke).

Box 50.1 summarizes the Well points.

> **Box 50.1 Well (*Jing*) points**
>
> - Point of departure of Qi
> - At fingertips and toe ends (except KI-1)
> - Channel is most superficial and thinnest
> - Change of polarity (Yin to Yang or vice versa)
> - Dynamic
> - Used to expel pathogenic factors
> - Centrifugal movement

Spring point

At this point the Qi of the channel is very powerful and full of potential energy ready to manifest, like the swirling movement of water in a mountain spring. Hence the 'Spiritual Axis' says that at this point the Qi 'slips' or 'glides', i.e. it is swift. Because of this nature, the Spring points are also very dynamic and powerful points which can quickly change situations: they all have a particularly strong action and are generally used to eliminate pathogenic factors (whether interior or exterior), and in particular to clear Heat.

Because of their dynamism, these points are to be used sparingly. The Spring points of the feet are more powerful than those of the hands and, if there is a choice, those of the hands are to be chosen first (see also ch. 70). For example, in deciding on a distal point to affect the temples in migraine headaches due to

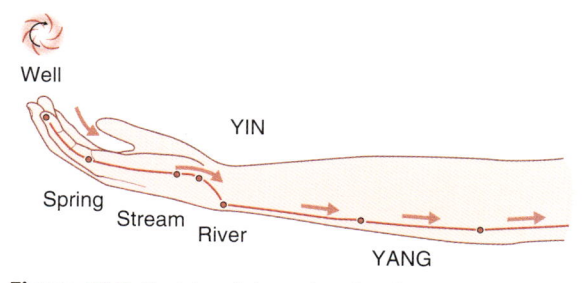

Figure 50.5 Centripetal dynamics of Well-Jing points

rising of Liver-Yang, one might have a choice between using the Gall Bladder or Triple Burner channel Spring point (G.B.-43 Xiaxi or T.B.-2 Yemen, respectively): the Triple Burner Spring point is slightly less powerful and dynamic than that of the Gall Bladder channel and therefore it might be preferred, especially in case of first treatment. Of course, this does not mean that the Spring point of a hand channel is always to be preferred to that of a foot channel as, in many cases, one does not have a choice, or one might deliberately want to have a particularly strong effect.

Box 50.2 summarizes the Spring points.

> **Box 50.2 Spring (*Ying*) points**
> - Second point from fingers or toes
> - Dynamic
> - Like the swirling movement of a mountain spring at its source
> - Clear Heat
> - Fire points in Yin channels and Water points in Yang channels

Stream point

At this point the Qi of the channel 'pours' through, it swirls and the flow starts to be bigger and slightly deeper within the channel. At this point, the flow of Qi is rapid and large enough to carry other things with it, hence its name 'transporting'.[4] At these points, exterior pathogenic factors can be 'transported' into the Interior and penetrate deeper in the channels. On the other hand, at these points Defensive Qi gathers.

Box 50.3 summarizes the Stream points.

> **Box 50.3 Stream (*Shu*) points**
> - Third point along channel (except G.B.-41)
> - Qi 'pours', flow becomes bigger and deeper
> - Pathogenic factors enter through this point
> - Defensive Qi concentrates at this point

River point

At this point the Qi of the channel is much bigger, wider and also deeper. The Qi flows like a large current after coming a long distance from its source. At these points, exterior pathogenic factors are deviated towards joints, bones and sinews: this is probably why the points are called *Jing*, which, in this case, means 'to pass through'.

Box 50.4 summarizes the River points.

> **Box 50.4 River (*Jing*) points**
> - Qi of channel much bigger and deeper
> - Qi flows like a current
> - Pathogenic factors are deviated towards joints and sinews at these points

Sea point

At this point the Qi of the channel is vast and deep; it collects, comes together and joins the general circulation of the body, like a large river flowing into the sea. According to chapter 65 of the 'Classic of Difficulties' at this point, the Qi has an inward, centripetal movement (as opposed to the outward, centrifugal movement of the Well point).[5]

Compared to and contrasted with the Well points, the Sea points are much less dynamic and their effect is less quick and dramatic. This is due to the fact that, at the Sea points, Qi flows much slower and it flows inwards and deeper so that it is not so unstable and cannot be quickly and easily affected.

Box 50.5 summarizes the Sea points.
Table 50.1 summarizes the names and functions of the Five Transporting points.

> **Box 50.5 Sea (*He*) points**
> - Qi of the channel is vast and deep
> - Qi of channel goes deep in the body and joins general Qi circulation
> - Centripetal movement
> - Less dynamic than other Transporting points

Table 50.1 Names and functions of the Five Transporting points

Pinyin	Chinese	Literal meaning	My terminology
Jing	井	Well	Well
Ying	荥	Spring, pool	Spring
Shu	输	To transport	Stream
Jing	经	To pass through	River
He	合	To unite, to join	Sea

ACTIONS OF THE FIVE TRANSPORTING POINTS FROM THE CLASSICS

We can discuss the clinical use of the Five Transporting points from four different viewpoints:

1. According to chapter 68 of the 'Classic of Difficulties'
2. According to the 'Spiritual Axis', chapters 4, 6 and 44
3. According to the seasons, as in chapter 61 of 'Simple Questions' and chapter 44 of 'Spiritual Axis'
4. According to the Five-Element character of the points as in chapter 64 and 69 of the 'Classic of Difficulties'

Box 50.6 summarizes the Five Transporting points.

According to the 'Classic of Difficulties'

Chapter 68 of the 'Classic of Difficulties' deals with the use of the Five Transporting points and gives guidelines which are still valid and widely followed today. These are:

- Well points: used for *'fullness under the heart'*
- Spring points: used for *'hot sensations of the body'*
- Stream points: used for *'feeling of heaviness and joint pain'*
- River points: used for *'breathlessness, cough and hot and cold sensations'*
- Sea points: used for *'rebellious Qi and diarrhoea'*.[6]

Box 50.6 The Five Transporting points

1. All Five Transporting points are situated between the fingers and elbows and the toes and knees
2. The Five Transporting points are related to each of the Five Elements
3. The section of channel where the Five Transporting points are situated is like a river, starting at the fingers and toes and ending at the elbows and knees
4. There is a progression of depth and size of channels from the fingers/toes to elbows/knees, i.e. thinnest and most superficial at the fingers/toes and thickest and deepest at the elbows/knees
5. The channel changes polarity at the fingers and toes, i.e. from Yin to Yang and vice versa
6. The change in polarity and superficiality of the channel at the extremities accounts for the particularly dynamic action of the points at the fingertips and toes
7. The Five Transporting points are called Well (*Jing*), Spring (*Ying*), Stream (*Shu*), River (*Jing*) and Sea (*He*)
8. The first point (Well) has a centrifugal movement and the last point (Sea) a centripetal one

We can expand on the clinical use of these points as follows:

Well points

The Well points (*Jing*) are used for irritability, mental restlessness and anxiety. This applies to both Yin and Yang channels. The Well points have a particularly strong effect on the mental state and quickly change the mood. Examples of Well points used in this way are P-9 Zhongchong (irritability, insomnia), HE-9 Shaochong (mental disorders, anxiety, manic depression), SP-1 Yinbai (hysteria, insomnia), ST-45 Lidui (insomnia, mental confusion) and KI-1 Yongquan (anxiety).

Spring points

The Spring points (*Ying*) are used for febrile diseases or to clear Heat. The Spring points are very widely used to clear Heat and practically all of them do. It is important to note that their Heat-clearing action is irrespective of their Five-Element character.

For example, HE-8 Shaofu is a Fire point and ST-44 Neiting is a Water point, but they both clear Heat by virtue of being the Spring points. Virtually all Spring points clear Heat in their respective channel and organ. Examples of widely used points are HE-8 Shaofu and P-8 Laogong to drain Heart-Fire, LIV-2 Xingjian to drain Liver-Fire, ST-44 Neiting to clear Stomach-Heat, KI-2 Rangu to clear Kidney Empty-Heat, LU-10 Shaoshang to clear Lung-Heat or to expel Wind-Heat.

Stream points

The Stream points (*Shu*) are used for Painful Obstruction Syndrome (*Bi* Syndrome), especially if from Dampness. This applies to Yang channels more than Yin ones. Examples are: L.I.-3 Sanjian, T.B.-3 Zhongzhu and S.I.-3 Houxi for Painful Obstruction Syndrome of the fingers and ST-43 Xiangu for the toes.

These points can be used not only as local points for Painful Obstruction Syndrome of fingers and toes but also as distal points to clear Wind and Dampness from the channels. For example, ST-43 Xiangu is an important distal point to clear Wind-Dampness and Heat from the channels; S.I.-3 Houxi, T.B.-3 Zhongzhu and L.I.-3 Sanjian can all be used as distal points to clear obstructions from Dampness and Cold from the respective channels.

River points

The River points (*Jing*) are used for cough, asthma and upper respiratory diseases. This applies more to Yin than Yang channels, and among the Yang channels it applies more to the Bright Yang channels. Examples are: LU-8 Jingqu for cough and asthma, SP-5 Shangqiu for dry cough and ST-41 Jiexi and L.I.-5 Yangxi for sore throat of an Excess nature. The River point P-5 Jianshi is used for hot and cold sensations.

Sea points

The Sea points (*He*) are used for all stomach and intestinal diseases. This applies mostly to Yang channels, but also to Yin ones. Obvious examples of Sea points of Yang channels treating stomach and intestinal problems are ST-36 Zusanli and G.B.-34 Yanglingquan. The Sea points of the Yin channels of the leg also treat problems of the Yang organs as SP-9 Yinlingquan, KI-10 Yingu and LIV-8 Ququan can all clear Damp-Heat in Bladder or Intestines. Finally, the Sea points of the Pericardium channel P-3 Quze can also clear Heat in the Intestines. Other digestive indications of the Sea points are indicated below in the section on Chapter 44 of the 'Spiritual Axis'.

In addition to these Sea points, the Yang channels of the arm also have a so-called Lower Sea point. These are:

- ST-37 Shangjuxu for the Large Intestine
- ST-39 Xiajuxu for the Small Intestine
- BL-39 Weiyang for the Triple Burner

These three points are directly connected to their respective organs and function like Sea points, i.e. they treat problems of the Yang organs. In particular, ST-37 Shangjuxu is used for chronic diarrhoea and Damp-Heat of the Large Intestine, ST-39 Xiajuxu for intestinal pain and BL-39 Weiyang for enuresis (if reinforced when the Lower Burner is deficient) or retention of urine and oedema (if reduced when the Lower Burner is in Excess).

The 'Spiritual Axis' deals with the use of BL-39 Weiyang in chapter 2: '*Weiyang [BL-39] receives the Lower Burner, if it is in Excess there is retention of urine, if it is deficient there is enuresis or incontinence. The point is to be reduced in the former case and reinforced in the latter.*'[7]

The 'Spiritual Axis' lists all the Sea points in chapter 4 and it gives ST-37 Shangjuxu for the Large Intestine, ST-39 Xiajuxu for the Small Intestine and BL-39 Weiyang for the Triple Burner.[8]

These three points therefore function as Sea points for the Large Intestine, Small Intestine and Triple Burner and their upper Sea points (L.I.-11 Quchi, S.I.-8 Xiaohai and T.B.-10 Tianjing) mostly treat channel problems of the neck, shoulders and face (but not exclusively).

Box 50.7 summarizes the Five transporting points according to the 'Classic of Difficulties'.

> The Yang channels of the arm (Small Intestine, Large Intestine and Triple Burner) have two sets of Sea points:
> 1. The Upper Sea points (S.I.-8, L.I.-11, T.B.-10) used mostly for problems of the neck, shoulders, face, head
> 2. The Lower Sea points (ST-39, ST-37 and BL-39) used mostly for problems of the relevant organs (Small Intestine, Large Intestine, Bladder and Triple Burner)

According to the 'Spiritual Axis'

Chapter 44

The 'Spiritual Axis' says in chapter 44: '*Yin organs correspond to Winter, use Well points; colour corresponds to Spring, use Spring points; seasons correspond to Summer, use the Stream points; sounds correspond to Late Summer, use the River points; flavours correspond to Autumn, use the Sea points … When the Yin organs are affected use the Well points; when the disease effects a change in the complexion colour, use the Spring points; when the disease manifests intermittently, use the Stream points; when the disease affects the voice and there is stagnation of Qi and Blood in the channels, use the River points; when the Stomach is affected and there are digestive disorders, use the Sea points.*'[9]

> **Box 50.7 The Five Transporting points according to the 'Classic of Difficulties'**
>
> 1. *Well points*: 'fullness under the heart' (irritability, mental restlessness, insomnia)
> 2. *Spring points*: 'hot sensations of the body' (clear Heat)
> 3. *Stream points*: 'feeling of heaviness and joint pain' (Painful Obstruction Syndrome from Dampness)
> 4. *River points*: 'breathlessness, cough, hot and cold sensations' (cough, asthma)
> 5. *Sea points*: 'rebellious Qi and diarrhoea' (digestive disorders)

These rules are fairly straightforward and have some points in common with those from chapter 68 of the 'Classic of Difficulties'. The 'Spiritual Axis' recommends the use of the Well points in Yin organs diseases: this is similar to the 'Classic of Difficulties' recommendation of these points in mental restlessness and irritability, particularly if deriving from a Heart pattern.

The 'Spiritual Axis' use of the River points for problems of the voice coincides with the 'Classic of Difficulties' use for problems of the throat. The use of the Sea points is also practically the same in the two classics. However, the 'Spiritual Axis' recommendations are much less followed in clinical practice than those from the 'Classic of Difficulties' as they are of lesser practical significance.

The particular use of the Five Transporting points recommended in chapter 44 of the 'Spiritual Axis' does not have an important clinical relevance. For example, the use of the Well points for problems of the Yin organs is not generally followed and, in fact, it contradicts chapter 6 of the same book, which recommends using the Spring and Stream points for problems of the Yin organs. The suggested use of the Spring points when there is a change in the complexion colour and of the Stream points when the disease is intermittent are also not of great clinical relevance.

The use of the River points when the voice is affected is confirmed by their indications:

> *L.I.-5 Yangxi*: raving, laughter
> *ST-41 Jiexi*: raving
> *P-5 Jianshi*: loss of voice, halting speech
> *SP-5 Shangqiu*: impaired speech, laughter, sighing
> *HE-4 Lingdao*: loss of voice
> *KI-7 Fuliu*: curled tongue with inability to speak
> *T.B.-6 Zhigou*: sudden loss of voice
> *LIV-4 Zhongfeng*: sighing

The use of the Sea points for digestive disorders is common and there are many examples of such points:

> *LU-5 Chize*: vomiting, diarrhoea, abdominal distension
> *L.I.-11 Quchi*: abdominal distension and pain
> *ST-36 Zusanli*: all digestive disorders
> *SP-9 Yinlingquan*: diarrhoea
> *HE-3 Shaohai*: vomiting with foamy saliva
> *BL-40 Weizhong*: vomiting, diarrhoea
> *KI-7 Fuliu*: diarrhoea, abdominal distension, borborygmi
> *P3-Quze*: diarrhoea, vomiting due to Summer-Heat
> *T.B.-10 Tianjing*: vomiting pus and blood
> *G.B.-34 Yanglingquan*: vomiting
> *LIV-8 Ququan*: diarrhoea

Box 50.8 summarizes the Five Transporting points according to chapter 44 of the 'Spiritual Axis'.

> **Box 50.8 Chapter 44 of 'Spiritual Axis'**
>
> 1. *Well points*: for Yin organs
> 2. *Spring points*: when there is a change in complexion colour
> 3. *Stream points*: intermittent symptoms
> 4. *River points*: when voice is affected
> 5. *Sea points*: Stomach diseases

Chapter 4

The 'Spiritual Axis' gives other guidelines concerning use of the Five Transporting points, some of which are in contradiction with other chapters of the same book. It says in chapter 4: '*The divergent branches of the Yang channels reach into the Interior and connect with the Yang organs ... the Spring and Stream points [together, Tr.] treat channel problems, the Sea points treat organ problems*'.[10]

It then goes on to list the Sea points of the Yang channels, listing only the Lower Sea points for the Yang channels of the arm, Large Intestine, Small Intestine and Triple Burner: that is, ST-37 Shangjuxu, ST-39 Xiajuxu and BL-39 Weiyang.

The Spring and Stream points of the Yang channels are frequently used in the treatment of Painful Obstruction Syndrome (*Bi* Syndrome) as the Stream point is a point of concentration of Defensive Qi and the Spring point is a powerful point which can be used to move the Qi of the channel and to expel pathogenic factors, in particular Heat.

The use of the Yang Sea points is in agreement with the use of these points according to the 'Classic of Difficulties' and to chapter 44 of the 'Spiritual Axis' itself: that is, to treat problems of the Yang organ themselves. This method is frequently applied in clinical practice and examples have been given above.

Box 50.9 summarizes the Five Transporting points according to chapter 4 of the 'Spiritual Axis'.

> **Box 50.9 Chapter 4 of 'Spiritual Axis'**
>
> - *Spring and Stream points (of Yang channels) together*: for channel problems
> - *Sea (Lower) points*: internal (Yang) organ problems

Chapter 6

Chapter 6 of the 'Spiritual Axis' gives yet different recommendations for the clinical use of the Five Transporting points. It says: *'In the Interior there are 5 Yin and 6 Yang organs, in the Exterior there are bones, sinews and skin. Both in the Interior and Exterior there is Yin and Yang. Within the Interior, the 5 Yin organs pertain to Yin and the 6 Yang organs pertain to Yang; within the Exterior sinews and bones pertain to Yin and the skin pertains to Yang. For diseases of Yin within Yin [i.e. Yin organs], use the Spring and Stream points of the Yin channels together. For diseases of Yang within Yang [i.e. the skin], use the Sea points of the Yang channels. For diseases of Yin within Yang [i.e. sinews and bones], use the River points of the Yin channels. For diseases of Yang within Yin [i.e. the Yang organs], use the Connecting points.'*[11]

To summarize (Fig. 50.6):

> *Yin within Yin* = Yin Organs = use Spring and Stream points of Yin channels in combination (e.g. LIV-2 Xingjian and LIV-3 Taichong)
> *Yang within Yang* = Skin = use the Sea points of Yang channels (e.g. L.I.-11 Quchi)
> *Yin within Yang* = Sinews and bones = use the River points of Yin channels (e.g. SP-5 Shangqiu)
> *Yang within Yin* = Yang organs = use the Connecting (*Luo*) points of Yang channels

These recommendations are only partially applied in clinical practice. The Spring and Stream points are frequently used together to clear Heat from the Yin organs; sometimes the Spring point can be reduced to clear Heat, and the Stream point tonified to nourish the Yin of the channel. A good example is the use of LIV-2 Xingjian (reduced to clear Liver-Fire) and LIV-3 Taichong (reinforced to nourish Liver-Yin). This technique can be used to nourish Liver-Yin and subdue Liver-Yang in headaches, or to nourish Liver-Yin and clear Liver-Fire in urinary diseases caused by Liver-Fire and Bladder-Heat.

The Sea points of the Yang channels, especially the upper Sea points (such as L.I.-11 Quchi, S.I.-8 Xiaohai and T.B.-10 Tianjing) are frequently used to treat the 'skin': that is, release the Exterior in invasions of exterior pathogenic factors. In particular, L.I.-11 and T.B.-10 are used to release the Exterior and expel Wind-Heat. L.I.-11 Quchi is an important point for skin diseases as it cools Blood. The following are examples of indications of these points for skin diseases:

> *L.I.-11 Quchi*: erysipelas, urticaria, dry scaly skin, itchiness, herpes zoster
> *BL-40 Weizhong*: sores, erysipelas, eczema, urticaria
> *T.B.-10 Tianjing*: urticaria

The River points of the Yin channels are frequently used to treat problems of sinews and bones (in Painful Obstruction Syndrome). This is also because the Qi at these points is diverted to sinews, bones and joints. The following are examples of indications related to joint and sinew problems in River points of the Yin channels:

> *SP-5 Shangqiu*: pain and contraction of sinews, Bone Painful Obstruction Syndrome (*Bi* Syndrome), feeling of heaviness with joint ache
> *HE-4 Lingdao*: spasms
> *KI-7 Fuliu*: atrophy of the legs
> *LIV-4 Zhongfeng*: contracted sinews, lumbar pain

Of course, the River points of the Yang channels also treat joint and sinew problems and the chief example among them is ST-41 Jiexi.

The rule of using the Connecting points to treat problems of the Yang organs is not widely followed as the Lower Sea points would be preferred in this case.

Box 50.10 summarizes the Five Transporting points according to chapter 6 of the 'Spiritual Axis'.

> **Box 50.10 Chapter 6 of 'Spiritual Axis'**
>
> - *Spring and Stream points (of Yin channels) together*: for Yin organ problems
> - *River points (of Yin channels)*: for sinews and bones
> - *Sea points (of Yang channels)*: for skin problems
> - *Connecting (Luo) points (of Yang channels)*: for the Yang organs

Yang within Yang = Skin = Sea points of Yang channels

Yin within Yang = Sinews/Bones = River points of Yin channels

Yang within Yin = Yang organs = Connecting points

Yin within Yin = Yin organs = Spring and Stream points of Yin channels

Figure 50.6 Use of the Five Transporting points according to chapter 6 of the 'Spiritual Axis'

According to the seasons

Chapter 44 of the 'Spiritual Axis' gives guidelines as to the use of the Five Transporting points according to the seasons. It says: '*In Winter use the Well points, in Spring use the Spring points, in Summer use the Stream points, in Late Summer use the River points, in Autumn use the Sea points*'.[12]

These rules find only limited application in clinical practice as it is not always possible to choose points according to the cycle of seasons, as this choice might conflict with the requirements of treatment according to the actual condition of the patient. However, these guidelines may be followed more when giving preventive seasonal treatments to patients who seek treatment to keep well rather than for specific conditions.

Chapter 61 of the 'Simple Questions' discusses the use of the Five Transporting points according to the seasons: '*In Autumn, use the River points to drain Yin pathogenic factors and the Sea points to drain Yang pathogenic factors ... In Winter, use the Well points to subdue rebellious Yin Qi and the Spring points to strengthen Yang Qi*'.[13] These instructions, in contradiction with those from chapter 44 of the 'Spiritual Axis', are not widely followed.

Box 50.11 summarizes the Five Transporting Points according to the seasons.

Box 50.11 Five Transporting points according to seasons

1. *Well points*: in Winter
2. *Spring points*: in Spring
3. *Stream points*: in Summer
4. *River points*: in Late Summer
5. *Sea points*: in Autumn

According to the Five Elements

The Five Transporting points are also used according to their Five-Element character. This was established in the 'Classic of Difficulties' for the first time. In chapter 64 it says that the Yin channels' Well point belongs to Wood and the Yang channels' Well point belongs to Metal.[14]

The use of the Five Transporting points according to their Five-Element character is discussed in chapter 69 of the 'Classic of Difficulties', with the terse advice: '*In case of Deficiency tonify the Mother, in case of Excess drain the Child.*'[15]

Following this principle and keeping in mind the Generating Cycle of the Five Elements, in case of Deficiency of a channel we can choose the point on that channel corresponding to the 'Mother' Element in order to tonify it. In case of Excess, we would choose the point corresponding to the 'Child' Element in order to drain it. For example, if the Liver is deficient, the Liver belongs to Wood, Water is the Mother of Wood, we therefore select (and reinforce) the point LIV-8 Ququan, which corresponds to Water. If the Liver were in Excess, we would choose (and reduce) the point LIV-2 Xingjian corresponding to Fire, as Fire is the Child of Wood. Table 50.2 lists the tonification and drainage points according to the Mother–Child relationship in the Five Elements.

In accordance with this theory, therefore, every channel has a tonification and drainage point corresponding to its Mother and Child Element, respectively. It must be stressed, however, that the needle technique is all important when tonifying or draining (i.e. reinforcing method to tonify and reducing method to drain); in other words we cannot rely only on the tonification or drainage character of a point, in order to tonify or drain.

Table 50.2 Tonification and drainage points according to the Five Elements

Channel	Tonification (Mother)	Drainage (Child)
Lungs	LU-9 Taiyuan	LU-5 Chize
Large Intestine	L.I.-11 Quchi	L.I.-2 Erjian
Stomach	ST-41 Jiexi	ST-45 Lidui
Spleen	SP-2 Dadu	SP-5 Shangqiu
Heart	HE-9 Shaochong	HE-7 Shenmen
Small Intestine	S.I.-3 Houxi	S.I.-8 Xiaohai
Bladder	BL-67 Zhiyin	BL-65 Shugu
Kidneys	KI-7 Fuliu	KI-1 Yongquan
Pericardium	P-9 Zhongchong	P-7 Daling
Triple Burner	T.B.-3 Zhongzhu	T.B.-10 Tianjing
Gall Bladder	G.B.-43 Xiaxi	G.B.-38 Yangfu
Liver	LIV-8 Ququan	LIV-2 Xingjian

Furthermore, the tonification or drainage character of a point is very often overridden by its other characteristics, so that the rule of tonifying and draining according to tonification and drainage points suffers many exceptions.

For example, HE-9 Shaochong and P-9 Zhongchong are tonification points but are more often used for draining instead in acute cases, by virtue of their being the Well points. HE-7 Shenmen is the drainage point but is more often used to tonify Heart-Blood to nourish the Mind. L.I.-11 Quchi is the tonification point, but it also cools Blood and releases the Exterior and is by its very nature a draining point. SP-2 Dadu is the tonification point, but would not be the most indicated point to tonify the Spleen, as SP-3 Taibai, Ren-12 Zhongwan, ST-36 Zusanli or BL-20 Pishu would be much better for this purpose. SP-2, on the contrary, is often used in febrile diseases to clear Heat and promote sweating. BL-67 Zhiyin is the tonification point but, again, owing to its being a Well point, is often used to drain in acute cases, or also to subdue rising Qi which is causing headaches.

Apart from being applied in the theory of tonification and drainage points, the Five-Element points are also used in another very common way to eliminate pathogenic factors.

There is a correspondence between the Five Elements and pathogenic factors:

- Wood corresponds to Wind
- Fire corresponds to Heat or Fire
- Earth corresponds to Dampness
- Metal corresponds to Dryness
- Water corresponds to Cold

In accordance with this correspondence, the Five-Element points can be used to expel the relevant pathogenic factors (whether exterior or interior). The only exception is the Metal point, which is not used to eliminate Dryness. The reason for this lies in the very nature of Dryness. While Heat, Fire, Wind, Dampness and Cold are pathogenic factors that manifest as an Excess pattern, Dryness manifests as a deficiency of Body Fluids, and the way to correct this is by nourishing fluids rather than by 'expelling' Dryness.

The application of this correspondence between the Five Elements and pathogenic factors is mostly used in Excess patterns to eliminate the relevant pathogenic factor (Table 50.3). It also applies rather more to Yin than Yang channels, but not exclusively.

This method of using the Element points to expel the relevant pathogenic factors can be applied to some of the points of Yang channels too. In particular, some of the Wood points are used to subdue Interior Wind, such as S.I.-3 Houxi, other Wood Yang points are used to expel exterior Wind in Painful Obstruction Syndrome and some of the Fire points are used to clear Heat, such as L.I.-5 Yangxi and ST-41 Jiexi.

Table 50.3 lists all the Yin channel Transporting points with their clinical use in the elimination of the pathogenic factors related to the Five Elements.

Table 50.4 summarizes the actions and functions of the Five Transporting points according to the various viewpoints discussed above.

Box 50.12 summarizes the Five Transporting points according to the Five Elements and Box 50.13 summarizes the Five Transporting points to expel pathogenic factors.

SUMMARY

We can now summarize the actions of the Five Transporting points according to the various perspectives explored above.

Well points

'Classic of Difficulties'

For '*fullness under the heart*', mental restlessness, anxiety.

Chapter 44 of 'Spiritual Axis'

To treat Yin organs.

According to seasons

In Winter.

According to pathogenic factors and Five Elements

Expel Wind.

Spring points

'Classic of Difficulties'

For '*hot sensations of the body*', to clear Heat.

Chapter 44 of 'Spiritual Axis'

When there is a change in the complexion.

Table 50.3 Correlation between Element points and pathogenic factors

Element	Point	Pathogenic factor	Use
Wood	Yin channels Wood points	Wind	Extinguish Internal Wind (acute stage of Wind-stroke)
	Yang channels Wood points		Expel exterior Wind in Painful Obstruction Syndrome
Fire	HE-8 Shaofu	Heat or Fire	Expels Summer-Heat or drains Heart-Fire
	LU-10 Yuji		Expels Wind-Heat or clears Lung-Heat
	P-8 Laogong		Expels Summer-Heat or drains Heart-Fire
	LIV-2 Xingjian		Drains Liver-Fire
	SP-2 Dadu		Clears Heat in febrile diseases
	KI-2 Rangu		Clears Empty-Heat, cools Blood
	L.I.-5 Yangxi		Clears Heat in Large Intestine and Damp-Heat in Painful Obstruction Syndrome
	S.I.-5 Yanggu		Resolves Damp-Heat in Painful Obstruction Syndrome
	ST-41 Jiexi		Clears Stomach Heat and Damp-Heat in Painful Obstruction Syndrome
Earth	HE-7 Shenmen	Dampness Phlegm	Not used to resolve Phlegm
	P-7 Daling		Resolves Phlegm from Heart
	LU-9 Taiyuan		Resolves Phlegm from Lung
	SP-3 Taibai		Resolves Dampness
	LIV-3 Taichong		Resolves Dampness
	KI-3 Taixi		Not used to resolve Phlegm
	ST-36 Zusanli		Resolves Dampness
	G.B.-34 Yanglingquan		Resolves Dampness
	BL-40 Weizhong		Resolves Dampness
	L.I.-11 Quchi		Resolves Damp-Heat
	S.I.-8 Xiaohai		Resolves Dampness in Upper Burner
	T.B.-10 Tianjing		Resolves Dampness in Upper Burner
Water	HE-3 Shaohai	Cold	Not used to expel Cold
	P-3 Quze		Not used to expel Cold
	LU-5 Chize		Expels Cold from Lungs
	LIV-8 Ququan		Expels Damp-Cold from Lower Burner
	SP-9 Yinlingquan		Expels Damp-Cold from Lower Burner
	KI-10 Yingu		Expels Damp-Cold from Lower Burner

Chapter 4 of the 'Spiritual Axis'

For channel problems (together with Stream point).

Chapter 6 of the 'Spiritual Axis'

For Yin organ problems (together with Stream point). Spring point of Yin channels.

According to seasons

In Spring.

According to pathogenic factors and Five Elements

Clear Heat.

Stream points

'Classic of Difficulties'

For *'feeling of heaviness and joint pain'*, to resolve Dampness, Painful Obstruction Syndrome.

Chapter 44 of 'Spiritual Axis'

When there are intermittent symptoms.

Chapter 4 of the 'Spiritual Axis'

For channel problems (together with Spring point).

Chapter 6 of the 'Spiritual Axis'

For Yin organ problems (together with Spring point). Stream points of Yin channels.

Table 50.4 Characteristics and functions of the Five Transporting points

Description	Well	Spring	Stream	River	Sea
'Spiritual Axis' ch. 1	Qi goes out	Qi is swift, slips	Qi pours	Qi moves, goes	Qi enters
Other descriptions	Like spring-head; Qi of channel comes out; Qi is small, superficial	Minute trickle from a spring; Qi begins to flow; Qi flows swiftly	Like water flowing from surface to depth; Qi irrigates the body	Like water freely flowing in a river; Qi flowing in the channels; Qi is bigger	Like many river streams returning to the sea; Qi of channel comes to an end, Qi is vast and deep, it comes together
'Spiritual Axis' ch. 2 and ch. 6	Point of departure of Qi	Point of convergence	Point of entry of pathogenic factors	Concentration point	Qi joins body circulation
'Classic of Difficulties' ch. 68	Fullness under heart; mental irritation	Hot sensation, Heat diseases	Heaviness of body, painful joints, Painful Obstruction Syndrome	Breathlessness, coughing, feeling hot and cold; Lung diseases	Rebellious Qi, diarrhoea, digestion; diseases of Yang organs
'Spiritual Axis' ch. 44	When Yin organs are affected	When illness manifests on the complexion	When illness is characterized by amelioration and aggravation	When illness reflects in the voice	For Stomach diseases
'Spiritual Axis' ch. 4		Exterior diseases (Yang channels)	Exterior diseases (Yang channels)		Interior diseases (Yang organs)
'Spiritual Axis' ch. 6		For Yin organs (Yin channels)	For Yin organs (Yin channels)	For sinews and bones	For skin and muscles

---

Box 50.12 Five Transporting points according to the Five Elements

- Tonification and drainage points according to Mother–Child relationships
- Use of Element points to expel relevant pathogenic factors

Box 50.13 Five Transporting points to expel pathogenic factors

- *Wood*: Wind
- *Fire*: Heat or Fire
- *Earth*: Dampness
- *Metal*: none
- *Water*: Cold

According to seasons

In Summer.

According to pathogenic factors and Five Elements

Resolve Dampness or Phlegm.

River points

'Classic of Difficulties'

Fog, '*breathlessness, cough and hot and cold sensations*', cough, asthma.

Chapter 44 of 'Spiritual Axis'

When voice is affected.

Chapter 6 of the 'Spiritual Axis'

For sinews and bones. River points of the Yin channels.

According to seasons

In Late Summer.

Sea points

'Classic of Difficulties'

For '*rebellious Qi and diarrhoea*', digestive disorders.

Chapter 44 of 'Spiritual Axis'

For Stomach diseases.

Chapter 4 of the 'Spiritual Axis'

For Internal (Yang) organ problems.

Chapter 6 of the 'Spiritual Axis'

For skin problems. Sea points of Yang channels.

According to seasons

In Autumn.

According to pathogenic factors and Five Elements

Expel Cold.

Learning outcomes

In this chapter you will have learned:
- How the Qi of the channels between the fingers/toes and elbows/knees resembles stages along the flow of a river, beginning at a springhead, and ending at the sea
- The importance of the Transporting points in clinical practice due to their particularly dynamic effect
- The connection between the superficial section of channel between fingers/ toes and elbows/knees and the environment, seasons and climate
- The reasons for the dynamism of points at the end and beginning of a channel (channel is more superficial, change from Yin to Yang, inertia of flow of previous channel)
- The specific energetic action of the Well points: superficial and dynamic, used in acute conditions, outward centrifugal movement eliminates pathogenic factors
- The nature of the Spring points: dynamic and powerful, clear Heat
- The action of the Stream points: flow becomes bigger and deeper, point where pathogenic factors enter the Interior and Defensive Qi concentrates
- The nature of the River points: where Qi flows deeper and wider, where pathogenic factors are deviated towards joints, bones and sinews
- The action of the Sea points: where the Qi is deeper and slower and joins the rest of the body, points have inward centripetal movement and the Qi is more stable
- The actions of the Well points according to the following perspectives:
  'Classic of Difficulties': 'fullness under the heart', mental restlessness, anxiety
  Chapter 44 of 'Spiritual Axis': to treat Yin organs
  According to seasons: in Winter
  According to pathogenic factors and Five Elements: expel Wind
- The actions of the Spring points according to the following perspectives:
  'Classic of Difficulties': 'hot sensations of the body', clear Heat
  Chapter 44 of 'Spiritual Axis': when there is a change in the complexion
  Chapter 4 of the 'Spiritual Axis': channel problems (together with Stream point)
  Chapter 6 of the 'Spiritual Axis': Yin organs problems (together with Stream point). Spring point of Yin channels
  According to seasons: in Spring
  According to pathogenic factors and Five Elements: clear Heat
- The actions of the Stream points according to the following perspectives:
  'Classic of Difficulties': 'feeling of heaviness and joint pain', resolve Dampness, Painful Obstruction Syndrome
  Chapter 44 of 'Spiritual Axis': intermittent symptoms
  Chapter 4 of the 'Spiritual Axis': channel problems (together with Spring point)
  Chapter 6 of the 'Spiritual Axis': Yin organ problems (together with Spring point), Stream points of Yin channels
  According to seasons: in Summer
  According to pathogenic factors and Five Elements: resolve Dampness or Phlegm
- The actions of the River points according to the following perspectives:
  'Classic of Difficulties': 'breathlessness, cough and hot and cold sensations', cough, asthma
  Chapter 44 of 'Spiritual Axis': when voice is affected
  Chapter 6 of the 'Spiritual Axis': sinews and bones. River points of the Yin channels
  According to seasons: in Late Summer
- The actions of the Sea points according to the following perspectives:
  'Classic of Difficulties': 'rebellious Qi and diarrhoea', digestive disorders
  Chapter 44 of 'Spiritual Axis': Stomach diseases
  Chapter 4 of the 'Spiritual Axis': Internal (Yang) Organ problems
  Chapter 6 of the 'Spiritual Axis': skin problems. Sea points of Yang channels
  According to seasons: in Autumn
  According to pathogenic factors and Five Elements: expel Cold

Self-assessment questions

1. The Stream point is the third point on all channels apart from which channel?
2. Describe the state of the Qi at the Well points.
3. What kind of Qi is said to gather at the Stream points?
4. Which set of points are often used for irritability, mental restlessness and anxiety?
5. Which points are often used for Painful Obstruction Syndrome?
6. What are the Lower Sea points for the Large and Small Intestines and Triple Burner?
7. Complete the following: 'The ___ points of the ____ channels are often used to treat skin diseases.'
8. When might you think of using the Five Transporting points according to the seasons?
9. Complete the following: 'If a channel is deficient we can choose the point on that channel corresponding to the _____ Element in order to tonify it.'

10. According to the theory of correspondence between the Five-Element points and pathogenic factors, which points would you use to clear Dampness and Wind?

See p. 1266 for answers

END NOTES

1. 1981 Spiritual Axis (*Ling Shu Jing* 灵枢经), People's Health Publishing House, Beijing, first published *c.*100 BC, p. 3.
2. Nanjing College of Traditional Chinese Medicine 1979 A Revised Explanation of the Classic of Difficulties (*Nan Jing Jiao Shi* 难经校释), People's Health Publishing House, Beijing, first published *c.* AD 100, p. 148.
3. Classic of Difficulties, p. 142.
4. Shanghai College of Traditional Medicine (translated by Dan Bensky and John O'Connor), Acupuncture – a Comprehensive Text, Eastland Press, Chicago, 1975, p. 126.
5. Classic of Difficulties, p. 142.
6. Classic of Difficulties, p. 148.
7. Spiritual Axis, p. 7.
8. Spiritual Axis, p. 14.
9. Spiritual Axis, p. 86.
10. Spiritual Axis, p. 14.
11. Spiritual Axis, p. 18–19.
12. Spiritual Axis, p. 86.
13. 1979 The Yellow Emperor's Classic of Internal Medicine – Simple Questions (*Huang Di Nei Jing Su Wen* 黄帝内经素问), People's Health Publishing House, Beijing, first published *c.*100 BC, p. 330.
14. Classic of Difficulties, p. 139.
15. Classic of Difficulties, p. 151.

The Functions of Specific Categories of Points

Key contents

Source (*Yuan*) points

Connecting (*Luo*) points

Back Transporting (*Shu*) points

Front Collecting (*Mu*) points

Accumulation (*Xi*) points

Gathering (*Hui*) points

Points of the Four Seas

Window of Heaven points

12 Heavenly Star points of Ma Dan Yang

Sun Si Miao's 13 Ghost points

Points of the Eye System (*Mu Xi*)

Five Command points

The categories of points discussed in the chapters are:

- Source (*Yuan*) points
- Connecting (*Luo*) points
- Back Transporting (*Shu*) points
- Front Collecting (*Mu*) points
- Accumulation (*Xi*) points
- Gathering (*Hui*) points
- Points of the Four Seas
- Window of Heaven points
- 12 Heavenly Star points of Ma Dan Yang
- Sun Si Miao's 13 Ghost points
- Points of the Eye System (*Mu Xi*)
- Five Command points

SOURCE (*YUAN*) POINTS

The nature and use of the Source points is dealt with in the first chapter of the 'Spiritual Axis' and chapter 66 of the 'Classic of Difficulties'. In order to understand the use of the Source points, it is worth looking at these two chapters closely.

The Source (*Yuan*) points are:

- LU-9 Taiyuan
- L.I.-4 Hegu
- ST-42 Chongyang
- SP-3 Taibai
- HE-7 Shenmen
- S.I.-4 Wangu
- BL-64 Jinggu
- KI-3 Taixi
- P-7 Daling
- T.B.-4 Yangchi
- G.B.-40 Qiuxu
- LIV-3 Taichong

Chapter 1 of the 'Spiritual Axis'

This chapter makes two statements in connection with the Source points, one regarding their use in diagnosis, the other in treatment.

The first statement says: '*Select the Source points when the 5 Yin organs are diseased.*'[1] This clearly indicates that the Source points directly affect the Yin organs.

The other statement says: '*If the 5 Yin organs are diseased, abnormal reactions will appear at the 12 Source points. If we know the correspondence of Source points to the relevant Yin organ, we can diagnose when a Yin organ is diseased.*'[2] This statement clearly indicates that the Source points are in relationship with the Original Qi (*Yuan Qi*) and that changes on the skin over the Source points indicate abnormalities in the Yin organs' function and can therefore be used for diagnosis.

Abnormalities that can be observed on the Source points include swellings, redness, congested blood vessels (common on KI-3 Taixi), varicose veins, a deep sunken dip around the point (also commonly seen on KI-3), whiteness, a bluish colour or very flaccid skin.

When the 'Spiritual Axis' proceeds to list the Source points, however, it gives different points from the ones we usually consider. The 'Spiritual Axis' lists the Source points as:

LU-9 Taiyuan for the Lungs	2 points
P-7 Daling for the Heart	2 points
SP-3 Taibai for the Spleen	2 points
LIV-3 Taichong for the Liver	2 points
KI-3 Taixi for the Kidneys	2 points
Total	10 points
Ren-15 Jiuwei, Source point for Fat tissue (*Gao*)	1 point
Ren-6 Qihai, Source point for Membranes (*Huang*)	1 point
Grand total	12 points

Regarding these last two points, the 'Spiritual Axis' says: '*The Original Qi of Fat tissues [Gao] gathers at Jiuwei [Ren-15], the Original Qi of Membranes [Huang] gathers at Qihai [Ren-6].*'[3] Although the book uses a different name for Ren-6 (Boyang), this is the old name for Qihai, i.e. Ren-6 (Fig. 51.1).

Ren-15 and Ren-6 are also considered the Source points for the chest and abdomen, respectively, as well as the Source points for all the Yin and all the Yang organs, respectively. 'Gao' may also indicate the area below the heart (controlled by Ren-15) and 'Huang' the area above the diaphragm (controlled by Ren-6).

Ren-15 is used for mental–emotional problems arising from disharmonies of the Yin organs (e.g. Heart-Yin deficiency), such as anxiety, mental restlessness or insomnia, and is an extremely useful point to calm the Mind. Ren-6 is used in Deficiency conditions of the Yang organs as it strongly tonifies Yang Qi.

The surprising element in this chapter is that the 'Spiritual Axis' mentions Source points only for the Yin organs. This is because the Qi of the Source points stems from the Original Qi, which is related to the Yin organs and the Kidneys in particular. The Source points are therefore used mostly to tonify the Yin organs. However, it should be said that chapter 2 of the 'Spiritual Axis' itself does mention the Source points of the Yang channels as we know them today.[4]

In contrast, the Source points of the Yang organs do not have a similar function and do not tonify the Yang organs in the same way as the Yin Source points tonify the Yin organs. The Yang Source points are mostly used in Excess patterns to expel pathogenic factors.

For example, L.I.-4 Hegu is used to release the Exterior and expel Wind, S.I.-4 Yanggu can be used to move stagnant Liver-Qi and stop pain in the costal region, BL-64 Jinggu can be used to expel Damp-Heat from the Lower Burner, G.B.-40 Qiuxu can be used for stagnation of Liver-Qi, ST-42 Chongyang can be used to expel Wind from the face in facial paralysis and T.B.-4 Yangchi can be used to clear Gall Bladder-Heat causing deafness or to regulate the Lesser Yang.

Of course, the Source points of the Yang channels *can* also be used to tonify the relevant Yang organs (as ch. 66 of the 'Classic of Difficulties' says), but this is not their main use, and they would not be the best points to do that. To tonify the Yang organs, the best points would be the Lower Sea points.

However, one exception springs to mind and that is that of T.B.-4 Yangchi. As we will see below, chapter 66 of the 'Classic of Difficulties' says that the Original Qi springs forth from between the Kidneys through the intermediary of the Triple Burner. Therefore, the Triple Burner is like the emissary of the Original Qi; as the Source points are in direct contact with the Original Qi, T.B.-4 can therefore be used to strengthen the Original Qi and this point is used in this way particularly in Japanese acupuncture. It is interesting to note, however, that none of the indications from old Chinese

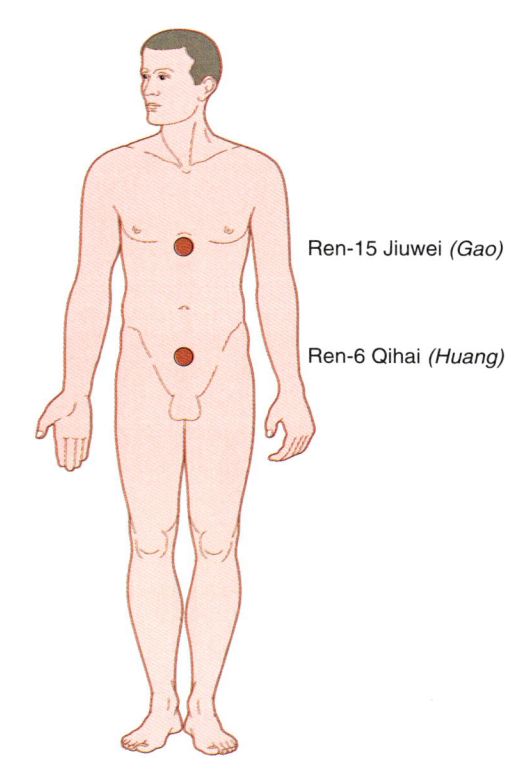

Figure 51.1 Yuan points of *Gao* and *Huang* according to the 'Spiritual Axis'

texts refer to a tonifying action of this point on the Original Qi.

The other surprising statement in this chapter is the mention of P-7 Daling as the Source point of the Heart. This is because in the times when the 'Spiritual Axis' was written the Heart and Pericardium were considered as a single organ, hence the constant reference to '5 Yin and 6 Yang organs'. It was only later that the Pericardium and Heart were split into two separate organs to preserve the symmetry of 12 organs and 12 channels.

In the Yin channels, the Source points coincide with the Stream points, that is, the third point from the distal end of the channel; in the Yang channels, the Source point follows the Stream point (*Shu*) and is therefore the fourth point from the distal end of the channel (except for the Gall Bladder channel in which the Source point is the fifth from the distal end).

To summarize, the functions of the Source points as from the 'Spiritual Axis' are:

- The Source points are in a relationship with the Original Qi
- They can be used in diagnosis as they reflect the state of the Original Qi of each Yin organ
- They are used in treatment mostly to tonify the Yin organs
- The Source points of the Yin organs are more important than those of the Yang organs

Box 51.1 summarizes the functions of the Source points in chapter 1 of the 'Spiritual Axis'.

Box 51.1 Source points: 'Spiritual Axis'

- The Source points are in relationship with the Original Qi
- They can be used in diagnosis as they reflect the state of the Original Qi of each Yin organ
- They are used in treatment mostly to tonify the Yin organs
- The Source points of the Yin organs are more important than those of the Yang organs

Chapter 66 of the 'Classic of Difficulties'

This chapter of the 'Classic of Difficulties' lists the 12 Source points as we know them: that is, one for each of the six Yin and six Yang organs. The only difference with the Source points as normally known nowadays is that it lists both P-7 and HE-7 as Source points for the Heart.[5] This is due again to the fact that in those times the Heart and Pericardium were considered as one organ, and the Pericardium could not therefore have a Source point.

The rest of this short chapter clarifies the relation between Original Qi, Triple Burner and Source points. It says: '*The Original Qi is the Motive Force [Dong Qi] situated between the two kidneys, it is life-giving and is the root of the 12 channels. The Triple Burner causes the Original Qi to differentiate [for its different uses around the body]; the Original Qi passes through the Three Burners and then spreads to the 5 Yin and 6 Yang organs and their channels. The places where the Original Qi stays are the Source [Yuan] points.*'[6]

This chapter therefore confirms that the Source points are in relationship with the Original Qi. In contrast to chapter 1 of the 'Spiritual Axis', the 'Classic of Difficulties' says that the Source points can be used to tonify both Yin and Yang organs (Fig. 51.2).

In particular, the role of the Triple Burner as the 'ambassador' or 'avenue', through which the Original Qi arises from in between the two Kidneys and differentiates into its various forms to spread to the five Yin and six Yang organs, explains a particular use of the Source point of the Triple Burner channel, T.B.-4 Yangchi. As mentioned above, this point can be used to tonify Original Qi directly and activate its circulation in the channels. Combined with the Source point of the Stomach, ST-42 Chongyang, T.B.-4 tonifies Qi and the Original Qi.

Box 51.2 summarizes the Source points according to the 'Classic of Difficulties'.

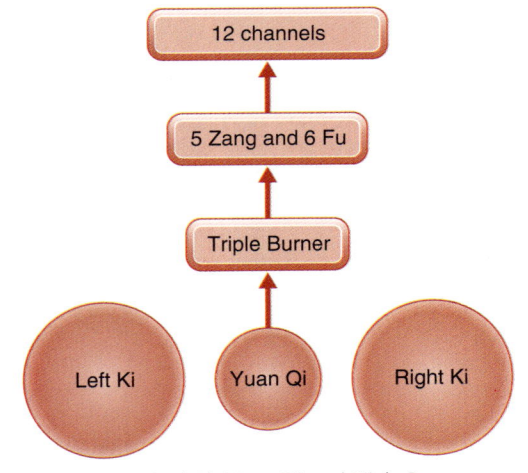

Figure 51.2 Original Qi (*Yuan Qi*) and Triple Burner

Box 51.2 Source (*Yuan*) points: 'Classic of Difficulties'

- The Source points are in a relationship with the Original Qi
- Original Qi reaches the Internal Organs, 12 channels and finally the 12 Source points through the intermediary of the Triple Burner
- The Source points tonify both Yin and Yang organs

CONNECTING (*LUO*) POINTS

There are 16 Connecting channels, one for each of the 12 main channels, one each for the Directing and Governing Vessels (*Ren* and *Du Mai*), one 'Great Connecting Channel' for the Spleen and one 'Great Connecting Channel' for the Stomach.[7] However, there are only 15 Connecting points as no mention is made of a Connecting point for the Great Connecting channel of the Stomach.

The Connecting points are:

- LU-7 Lieque
- L.I.-6 Pianli
- ST-40 Fenglong
- SP-4 Gongsun
- HE-5 Tongli
- S.I.-7 Zhizheng
- BL-58 Feiyang
- KI-4 Dazhong
- P-6 Neiguan
- T.B.-5 Waiguan
- G.B.-37 Guangming
- LIV-5 Ligou
- Du-1 Changqiang for the Governing Vessel (*Du Mai*)
- Ren-15 Jiuwei for the Directing Vessel (*Ren Mai*)
- SP-21 Dabao Great Connecting channel of the Spleen

For a detailed description of the pathways of the Connecting channels, see Maciocia 'The Channels of Acupuncture'. The pathways of the Connecting channels in broad lines are as follows:

- *Lung Connecting channel*: from LU-7 Lieque to the thenar eminence
- *Large Intestine Connecting channel*: from L.I.-6 Pianli to the teeth and ears
- *Stomach Connecting channel*: from ST-40 Fenglong to the neck
- *Spleen Connecting channel*: from SP-4 Gongsun to the stomach and intestines
- *Heart Connecting channel*: from HE-5 Tongli to the tongue and eyes
- *Small Intestine Connecting channel*: from S.I.-7 Zhizheng to the shoulder
- *Bladder Connecting channel*: from BL-58 Feiyang to the Kidney channel on the leg
- *Kidney Connecting channel*: from KI-4 Dazhong to the pericardium
- *Pericardium Connecting channel*: from P-7 Daling to the heart
- *Triple Burner Connecting channel*: from T.B.-5 Waiguan to the pericardium in the chest
- *Gall Bladder Connecting channel*: from G.B.-37 Guangming to dorsum of foot
- *Liver Connecting channel*: from LIV-5 Ligou to the external genitalia
- *Governing Vessel Connecting channel*: from Du-1 Changqiang to the spine and occiput
- *Directing Vessel Connecting channel*: from Ren-15 Jiuwei to the abdomen
- *Great Connecting channel of the Spleen*: from SP-21 Dabao to the chest and ribs

Each of the 12 Connecting channels related to the main channels departs from its relevant Connecting point and branches out, travelling upwards along a separate trajectory.

There are three ways of using the Connecting points. The Connecting point can be used in conjunction with the Source point of its interiorly–exteriorly related channel; it can be used on its own, according to the symptomatology of the Connecting channels themselves; or it can be used to affect the area influenced by the Connecting channel.

Before discussing these three ways of using the Connecting points, we must briefly describe the nature and characteristics of the Connecting channels themselves. When we say 'Connecting channel' we can refer to two separate entities: one is the Connecting channel itself which departs from the Connecting point and travels upwards in the pathways briefly described above; the other is the whole area of the body that lies between the main channel and the skin. In the latter case, the Connecting channel would be more appropriately described as the 'Connecting channels area' because it does not denote an actual channel but a whole part of the body that is irrigated by the Connecting channels (Figs 51.3–51.5).

The Connecting channels are called *Luo Mai*: *Luo* implies the meaning of 'network'. The main channels are called *Jing Mai* and *Jing* implies the meaning of

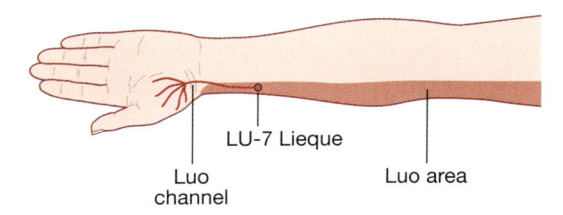

Figure 51.3 Connecting channel and Connecting channels area

Cou Li-Wei level	Superficial Luo
Wei level	Luo channel
Qi level	Main channel
Blood level	Deep Luo channel

Figure 51.4 Connecting and main channels areas

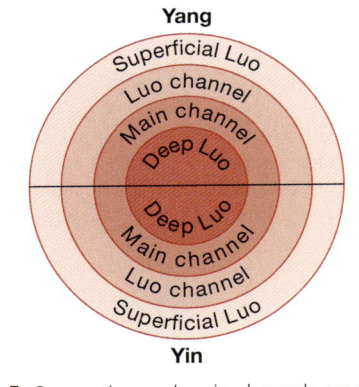

Figure 51.5 Connecting and main channels areas in section

The Connecting channels are more superficial than the main channels and they run in all directions, horizontally rather than vertically, like a net. In particular, they fill the space between skin and muscles: that is, the *Cou Li* space.

The 12 main channels are situated between the Yang and Yin Connecting channels. It is through the Yin and Yang Connecting channels that Nutritive and Defensive Qi and Qi and Blood of the main channels spread in all directions, permeate and irrigate the Internal Organs. It is also through the Connecting channels that the essence of the Internal Organs is transported to the main channels and, through them, to the whole body.

The Connecting channels cannot penetrate the big joints of the body (as the main channels do) and they are therefore restricted to the spaces in between the deep pathway of the main channels and the surface of the body: for this reason, they are very prone to stagnation of Qi and/or Blood.

> The Connecting channels cannot penetrate the big joints of the body (as the main channels do) and they are therefore restricted to the spaces in between the deep pathway of the main channels and the surface of the body: for this reason, they are very prone to stagnation of Qi and/or Blood

Chapter 10 of the 'Spiritual Axis' says: '*The Connecting channels cannot course through the large joints; in order to [enter and] exit they must move by alternate routes. They then enter and come together again under the skin and therefore they can be seen from the outside. To needle the Connecting channel one must needle above the accumulation where Blood is concentrated. Even if there is no blood accumulation, one must prick to cause bleeding quickly to drain the pathogenic factors out: if this is not done, Bi syndrome may develop.*'[9]

Thus, the Connecting channels occupy the space between the main channels and the skin; however, within this space, there are also degrees of depth. On the superficial layers just below the skin there are smaller Connecting channels called Minute and Superficial Connecting channels.

The main branches of the Connecting channels are called *Bie* ('divergent'; this is the same word as that used for Divergent channels). The Minute Connecting

'line', 'route', or 'way'. Chapter 17 of the 'Spiritual Axis' confirms that the Connecting channels are 'horizontal' or 'crosswise': '*The Main channels are in the Interior, their branches and horizontal [or crosswise] forming the Connecting channels.*'[8]

> The '*Connecting channel*' is the pathway of Qi departing from each Connecting point
> The '*Connecting channels area*' is the area of the body crisscrossed by the Connecting channels between the main channels and the skin

channels are called *Sun*, while the Superficial ones are called are called *Fu*.

Chapter 17 of the ' Spiritual Axis' says: '*The Main channels are in the Interior, their branches and horizontal [or crosswise] forming the Connecting channels: branching out from these are the Minute Connecting channels.*'[10] Chapter 10 of the 'Spiritual Axis' says: '*The more superficial branches of the channels which can be seen are the Connecting channels.*'[11]

However, the Connecting channels also have a deeper layer beyond the main channels: these can be called the deep Connecting channels and they are connected to the blood vessels and Blood in general. One can distinguish three layers in the channel network related to Wei, Qi and Blood:

1. *An outside*: the superficial Connecting channels = Defensive Qi (*Wei*) level
2. *A centre*: the Connecting channels = Qi and Nutritive Qi (*Ying*) level
3. *An inside*: the deep, Blood Connecting channels = Blood level

These three levels could be related to the Four Levels of Defensive Qi, Qi, Nutritive Qi and Blood.

Let us now discuss these three ways of using the Connecting points.

Use of the Connecting points in conjunction with the Source points

Since each Connecting channel joins with its interiorly–exteriorly related channel (e.g. Lungs–Large Intestine), the Connecting point can treat not only the channel to which it belongs but also its interiorly–exteriorly related channel. In other words, when we use LU-7 Lieque we affect not only the Lung channel but also the Large Intestine channel. In fact, in this example, it is precisely for this reason that LU-7 affects the head and face (i.e. through the Large Intestine channel). In fact, the Connecting channel that departs from LU-7 goes to the thenar eminence and this could not explain the effect of this point on the head.

When a Source point is used to tonify a given channel/organ, the Connecting point of its interiorly–exteriorly related channel can be used to strengthen the treatment. The Connecting point is thus chosen as a secondary point to reinforce the action of the Source point, chosen as the main point to treat the primarily affected channel.

For example, in case of Lung-Qi deficiency we may choose to use the Lung channel Source point (i.e. LU-9 Taiyuan) and reinforce its action by using the Connecting point of its interiorly–exteriorly related channel (i.e. L.I.-6 Pianli).

This technique finds its rationale in the pathway of the Connecting channels as these join up with their interiorly–exteriorly related channels. This is also reflected in the fact that the symptomatology of each Connecting channel often includes symptoms of its interiorly–exteriorly related channel.

The 'Great Compendium of Acupuncture' (*Zhen Jiu Da Cheng*, 1601) discusses the combination of Source point with associated Connecting point and calls this combination the Guest–Host method, the Source point being the Host and the Luo point the Guest. It should be noted that the Source point is the main point, that is, the choice of points is determined by the pathology of the Host (i.e. the Source point of the diseased channel). The symptoms are as follows, listing the Host (Source point) first and Guest (Connecting point) second:

- *LU-9 Taiyuan and L.I.-6 Pianli*: feeling of oppression of the chest, hot palms, cough, swelling of the throat, dry throat, sweating, shoulder pain, pain in the breasts, expectoration of phlegm, breathlessness
- *L.I.-4 Hegu and LU-7 Lieque*: toothache, swollen gums, yellow eyes, dry mouth, runny nose, epistaxis, swollen throat, shoulder pain
- *SP-3 Taibai and ST-40 Fenglong*: stiff tongue, acid reflux, vomiting, abdominal distension, feeling of heaviness, constipation, weakness, swelling of lower limbs
- *ST-42 Chongyang and SP-4 Gongsun*: abdominal distension and fullness, feeling of oppression of the chest, epistaxis, phlegm, foot pain, ankle pain
- *HE-7 Shenmen and S.I.-7 Zhizheng*: heart pain, dry throat, thirst, yellow eyes, dry mouth, hot palms, palpitations, vomiting of blood, fright
- *S.I.-4 Wangu and HE-5 Tongli*: stiff neck, swelling and pain of throat, shoulder pain, deafness, yellow eyes, pain of lateral side of upper arms
- *KI-3 Taixi and BL-58 Feiyang*: dark complexion, no thirst, desire to lie down, decreased vision, feeling of heat, backache, weakness of lower limbs, shortness of breath, timidity (literally 'Heart and Gall Bladder shivering and dithering')
- *BL-64 Jinggu and KI-4 Dazhong*: eye pain, neck ache, pain from neck to back to lower limbs, mania, epilepsy, opisthotonos, pain eyebrow region, epistaxis, yellow eyes, contraction of tendons, prolapse ani
- *T.B.-4 Yangchi and P-6 Neiguan*: tinnitus, deafness, swelling of throat, dry throat, swelling of eyes, ear ache, sweating, pain

- between scapulae, elbow pain, constipation, incontinence of urine, retention of urine
- P-7 Daling and T.B.-5: contracture of palms, arm pain, inability to extend arm, fullness of chest, swelling of axilla, palpitations, red face, yellow eyes, laughing and crying without reason, mental restlessness, heart pain, hot palms
- LIV-3 Taichong and G.B.-37 Guangming: abdominal distension and hypogastric swelling in women, chest fullness, vomiting, hernia, urinary retention or incontinence
- G.B.-40 Qiuxu and LIV-5 Ligou: dull complexion, headache, eye pain, swelling of neck, goitre, hypochondrial pain, swelling and sweating of axilla

The combinations I personally use most are described below with the relevant symptoms:

- L.I.-4 Hegu and LU-7 Lieque: restore the descending of Lung-Qi, expel Wind, treat headaches
- T.B.-4 Yangchi and P-6 Neiguan: regulate the Triple Burner, move Liver-Qi, calm the Mind
- SP-3 Taibai and ST-40 Fenglong: tonify the Spleen and resolve Phlegm
- LIV-3 Taichong and G.B.-37 Guangming: brighten the eyes in Liver patterns
- BL-64 Jinggu and KI-4 Dazhong: treat sciatica (BL-64 on affected side, KI-4 on opposite one)

Box 51.3 summarizes the combination of Source (*Yuan*) and Connecting (*Luo*) points.

Box 51.3 Combination of Source (*Yuan*) and Connecting (*Luo*) points

- Mentioned in the 'Great Compendium of Acupuncture, 1601' as 'Guest–Host' combination
- Source point is taken as main point to treat affected channel, e.g. LU-9 Taiyuan
- Connecting point of interiorly–exteriorly related channel is added to reinforce treatment, e.g. L.I.-6 Pianli

Use of the Connecting points on their own according to chapter 10 of the 'Spiritual Axis'

The use of the Connecting points by themselves is based on the Full or Empty symptomatology of each Connecting channel. The Full and Empty symptoms of the Connecting channels are described in chapter 10 of the 'Spiritual Axis'.[12] They are listed in Table 51.1.

The indications of the Connecting points according to the Full and Empty symptoms from chapter 10 of the Spiritual Axis do not have the same clinical relevance for all points. For example, the indications for L.I.-6 Pianli ('sensation of cold in teeth, fullness and congestion in the chest') are not of great clinical significance.

The indications with greater clinical significance are as follows:

- ST-40 Fenglong: insanity (Full)
- SP-4 Gongsun: abdominal pain (Full), abdominal distension (Empty)
- HE-5 Tongli: aphasia (Empty)
- KI-4 Dazhong: backache (Empty)
- P-6 Neiguan: chest pain (Full)
- LIV-5 Ligou: genitalia problems (Full), itching genitals (Empty)

Box 51.4 summarizes the use of the Connecting points on their own according to chapter 10 of the 'Spiritual Axis'.

Box 51.4 Use of the Connecting points on their own according to chapter 10 of the 'Spiritual Axis'

- Connecting points used on their own
- Connecting points chosen according to Full or Empty state of the Connecting channel

Use of the Connecting points according to their energetic influence

Use of the Connecting points to affect the superficial areas of a channel in tendinomuscular problems

This is probably the most important use of the Connecting channels and points. Each channel has a 'Connecting area' that is like a network of small channels in the superficial part of the body between the main channels and the skin along the pathway of the whole channel (see Figs 51.4 and 51.5). The pathology of this area, and therefore of the Connecting channels, consists primarily of invasions of external pathogenic factors causing tendinomuscular problems. Therefore, the Connecting points are extremely important to affect the superficial areas of the channels and particularly the joints, sinews, muscles and skin in tendinomuscular problems.

For example, in case of tendinitis of the elbow along the Large Intestine channel, the Connecting point

Table 51.1 Full and Empty symptoms of the Connecting channels

Channel	Full		Empty
Lung (LU-7 Lieque)	Hot palms and wrists		Yawning, frequent urination, incontinence of urine
Large Intestine (L.I.-6 Pianli)	Toothache, deafness		Sensation of cold in teeth, fullness and congestion in the chest
Stomach (ST-40 Fenglong)	Full: insanity (*Kuang*)	Rebellious: throat obstruction, loss of voice	Flaccid or atrophied muscles of legs
Spleen (SP-4 Gongsun)	Full: abdominal pain	Rebellious Qi: food poisoning (*Huo Luan*)	Abdominal distension
Heart (HE-5 Tongli)	Fullness and oppression of chest		Aphasia
Small Intestine (S.I.-7 Zhizheng)	Loose joints, atrophy of arm muscles, stiff elbow		Long, finger-shaped warts, itching scabs
Bladder (BL-58 Feiyang)	Nasal congestion, headache, backache		Clear nasal discharge, nosebleed
Kidneys (KI-4 Dazhong)	Full: retention of urine	Rebellious: irritability, depression, oppression of chest	Lower backache
Pericardium (P-6 Neiguan)	Chest pain		Stiffness of the head and neck
Triple Burner (T.B.-5 Waiguan)	Spasm of the elbow		Flaccid arm muscles
Gall Bladder (G.B.-37 Guangming)	Fainting		Weak and flaccid foot muscles, difficult to stand from sitting position
Liver (LIV-5 Ligou)	Full: swelling of testicle, hernia-like disorders (*Shan*)	Rebellious: abnormal erection	Itching of pubic region
Ren Mai (Ren-15 Jiuwei)	Pain in the skin of abdomen		Itching of the skin of abdomen
Du Mai (Du-1 Changqiang)	Stiffness of spine		Heaviness of the head, tremor of head
Great Luo of Spleen (SP-21 Dabao)	Ache and pain all over body		Weak limb muscles
Great Luo of Stomach (*Xu Li*)	Rapid breathing, irregular breathing, sensation of knot in chest		

L.I.-6 Pianli will affect the Connecting channel area, i.e. the sinews and muscles situated between the main channels and the skin, which is where the pathology of tendinitis is situated.

When they are used for channel problems, the Connecting points are sometimes chosen on the opposite side to where the problem is, on the same channel in acute cases and on the interiorly–exteriorly related channel. For example, if there is an acute pain in the right shoulder along the Large Intestine channel and some local points on the Large Intestine are used on the right side, L.I.-6 Pianli can be added on the left side to reinforce the treatment. In a chronic case, LU-7 Lieque would be used on the left side.

Use of the Connecting points to treat stagnation

The Connecting channels (and therefore points) are not used only for superficial tendinomuscular problems. As discussed above, the Connecting channels occupy the area between the main channels and the skin, they are 'horizontal', forming a network of small channels, and they cannot penetrate through the large joints as the main channels do. This means that the Connecting channels in this area are very prone to stagnation of Qi and stasis of Blood. Indeed, it could be said that most stagnation symptoms in the body occur in the Connecting channels area. For example, breast distension from Qi stagnation in women occurs in the Connecting channels area of the breast; a myoma (fibroid) in the Uterus is due to Blood stasis in the Blood Connecting channels of the Uterus; a feeling of lump in the throat is due to Qi stagnation in the Connecting channels of the throat, and so on.

Therefore the Connecting points have a very important use in moving Qi and Blood in the channels when these are affected by Qi stagnation or Blood stasis.

Use of the Connecting points according to manifestations on the skin

The 'Spiritual Axis' also says in chapter 10 that *'When the Connecting channels are Full they can be seen, when they are Empty they cannot be seen.'*[13] This is due to the fact that the Connecting channels are more superficial than the main channels and branch out into the smaller branches of the Superficial and Minute channels.

In Full patterns, the Connecting channels and their smaller branches are congested and can therefore be seen. A greenish coloration suggests stagnation in these channels, a bluish colour indicates Cold, a reddish coloration suggests Heat, and a purple colour indicates Blood stasis.

The channel pathway areas should also be palpated and they can feel cold or hot to the touch. This, together with the coloration, indicates retention of Cold or Heat in the Connecting channels and their branches: that is, an Excess condition.

In Deficiency patterns, the Connecting channels and their branches are void of Qi, so nothing can be observed outwardly in terms of colour, but in chronic severe cases, a flaccidity of the muscles can be observed.

In Excess conditions of the Connecting channels the Connecting point must be reduced, and in Deficiency conditions it must be reinforced. In case of venule and capillary congestion manifesting with macules on a Connecting channel, these blood vessels can be pricked and bled.

Box 51.5 summarizes the use of the Connecting points according to their energetic influence.

Box 51.5 Use of the Connecting points according to their energetic influence

- Use of the Connecting points to affect the superficial areas of a channel in tendinomuscular problems
- Use of the Connecting points to eliminate stagnation of Qi and/or Blood in the Connecting channels areas
- Use of the Connecting points to drain or tonify the superficial Connecting channels according to manifestations on the skin

Obviously, apart from the above uses, the Connecting points are also often used in practice according to their specific action, irrespective of their being Connecting points. For example, ST-40 Fenglong is very much used to resolve Phlegm, irrespective of it being the Connecting point of the Stomach channel. T.B.-5 Waiguan is often used to expel Wind-Heat, P-6 Neiguan is very much used for chest problems and emotional problems, LU-7 Lieque can be used to affect the head, and so on.

In conclusion, the Connecting points can basically be used in six different ways, summarized in Box 51.6.

Box 51.6 Six ways of using Connecting points

1. In conjunction with the Source point of the primarily affected channel to reinforce its action
2. According to the Full–Empty symptomatology from chapter 10 of the 'Spiritual Axis'
3. According to their range of action in terms of energetic layers, i.e. to affect the superficial layers in channel problems
4. For stagnation of Qi and stasis of Blood in the Connecting channels areas
5. To drain or tonify the Connecting channels according to manifestations on the skin
6. According to their specific action, irrespective of their being Connecting points (e.g. ST-40 Fenglong to resolve Phlegm)

BACK TRANSPORTING (*SHU*) POINTS

The importance of the Back Transporting points in treatment cannot be overemphasized. They are particularly important for the treatment of chronic diseases and, indeed, one may go so far as to say that a chronic disease cannot be treated without using these points at some time during the course of treatment (Fig. 51.6).

The Chinese character (*Shu* 俞) denoting these points means 'to transport', indicating that they transport Qi

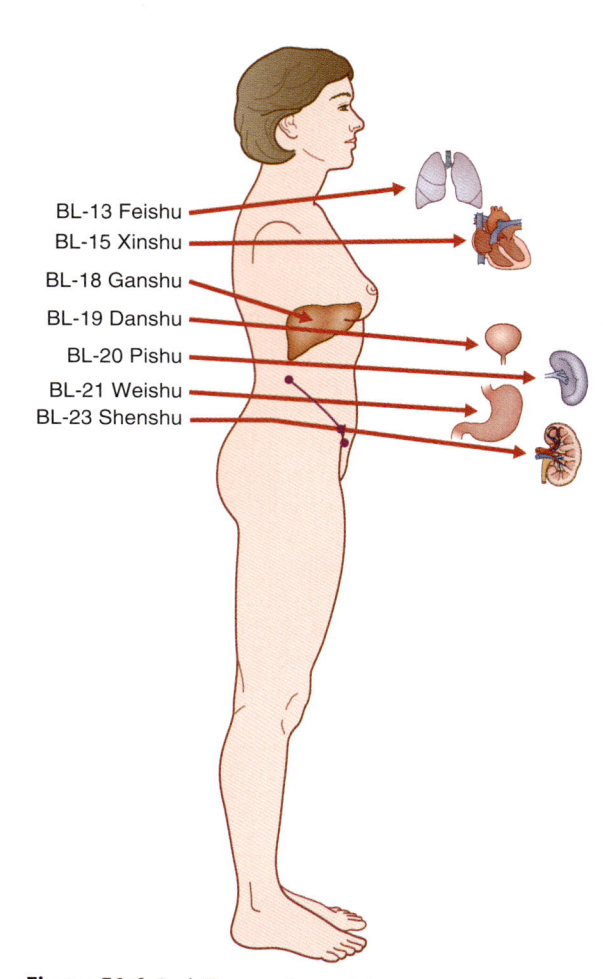

- BL-13 Feishu
- BL-15 Xinshu
- BL-18 Ganshu
- BL-19 Danshu
- BL-20 Pishu
- BL-21 Weishu
- BL-23 Shenshu

Figure 51.6 Back Transporting points

to the inner organs. Each point takes its name from the corresponding organ. For example, '*Xin*' means 'Heart' and '*Xinshu*' is the Back Transporting for the Heart.

There is a Back Transporting point for each of the Yin and Yang organs. They are located on the back, on the Bladder channel, one and a half *cun* from the midline, level with an intervertebral space. The Back Transporting points are:

- *Lungs*: BL-13 Feishu
- *Pericardium*: BL-14 Jueyinshu
- *Heart*: BL-15 Xinshu
- *Liver*: BL-18 Ganshu
- *Gall Bladder*: BL-19 Danshu
- *Spleen*: BL-20 Pishu
- *Stomach*: BL-21 Weishu
- *Triple Burner*: BL-22 Sanjiaoshu

- *Kidneys*: BL-23 Shenshu
- *Large Intestine*: BL-25 Dachangshu
- *Small Intestine*: BL-27 Xiaochangshu
- *Bladder*: BL-28 Pangguangshu

In addition to these points, there are a few others which are situated on the Bladder channel very close to the Back Transporting points but are not related to organs. They are related to parts of the body or channels. These are:

- *Governing Vessel*: BL-16 Dushu
- *Diaphragm*: BL-17 Geshu
- *Sea of Qi*: BL-24 Qihaishu
- *Lower back and Uterus*: BL-26 Guanyuanshu
- *Sacrum*: BL-29 Zhonglushu
- *Anus*: BL-30 Baihuanshu

The Back Transporting points affect the organs directly and are therefore used in Interior diseases of the Yin or Yang organs. This is a very important aspect of the clinical effect of these points. They act in quite a different way than all the other points. When treating the Internal Organs, other points work by stimulating the Qi of the channel, which then flows along the channel like a wave, eventually reaching the Internal Organs. In my experience, when we needle the Back Transporting points, Qi goes *directly* to the relevant organ, not through the intermediary of its channel. For this reason, I usually retain the needle in these points a shorter time than for other body points (usually no longer than 10 minutes when used to tonify in an adult).

Clinical note

The Back Transporting points act in quite a different way than all the other points. When treating the Internal Organs, other body points work by stimulating the Qi of the channel, which then flows along the channel like a wave, eventually reaching the Internal Organs. In my experience, when we needle the Back Transporting points, Qi goes *directly* to the relevant organ, not through the intermediary of its channel

The Back Transporting points can be used in both acute or chronic conditions, but are more frequently used in chronic ones.

The Back Transporting points are Yang in character and are especially used to tonify the Yang. However, they can be used for deficiency of Yin as well. Chapter 67 of the 'Classic of Difficulties' says: '*Yin diseases move to the Yang [area]; Yang diseases move to the Yin [area]. The Front-Collecting [Mu] points are situated on the Yin surface [and therefore treat Yang diseases]; the Back-Transporting [Shu] points are situated on the Yang surface [and therefore treat Yin diseases].*'[14] According to this statement, the Back Transporting points would be used to treat 'Yin diseases' and the Front Collecting points 'Yang diseases'. 'Yin diseases' can mean either diseases of the Yin organs or diseases characterized by Cold: this would therefore mean that the Back Transporting points would be used to tonify the Yin organs and to warm. Conversely, 'Yang diseases' can mean either diseases of the Yang organs or diseases characterized by Heat: this would therefore mean that the Front Collecting points would be used to nourish Yin or to clear Heat. These guidelines are certainly valid but they should not be adhered to too rigidly; in other words, the Back Transporting points can also be used to tonify the Yin organs and clear Heat and, conversely, the Front Collecting points can be used also to tonify the Yang and to warm.

Yet another interpretation of 'Yin' or 'Yang diseases' could be that of chronic and acute diseases, respectively: in this interpretation, the Back Transporting points would be used for 'Yin diseases' (i.e. chronic diseases), and the Front Collecting points for 'Yang diseases' (i.e. acute diseases). Although this rule should not be interpreted rigidly, it is certainly a valid rule which finds a widespread clinical application: that is, using the Back Transporting points for chronic and the Front Collecting points for acute diseases. The various uses of the Back Transporting and Front Collecting points are summarized in Table 51.2.

Another characteristic of these points is that they are used to affect the sense organ of the corresponding organ. For example, BL-18 Ganshu is the Back Transporting point of the Liver and can be used for eye diseases.

In practice, the Back Transporting points tend to produce a stronger effect than the Front Collecting points. They are therefore very useful when the patient feels very tired, exhausted or depressed. In these cases, if the Stomach and Spleen are deficient, for example, the use of BL-20 Pishu and BL-21 Weishu will produce a strong tonifying effect.

The use of BL-17 Geshu and BL-19 Danshu (in Chinese called the 'Four Flowers'), also has a strong tonifying effect on Qi and Blood. The point BL-23 Shenshu should be used in any deficiency of the Kidneys, particularly Kidney-Yang, as it strongly tonifies the Kidneys.

Although the Back Transporting points are mostly used to tonify the organs, they can also be used in Excess patterns to expel pathogenic factors. In particular, they can be used to subdue rebellious Qi and clear Heat. For example, the point BL-21 Weishu can be used to subdue rebellious Stomach-Qi in case of belching, nausea or vomiting. The point BL-18 Ganshu can be used to move stagnant Liver-Qi. BL-15 Xinshu can be used to clear Heart-Fire and BL-13 Feishu to stimulate the diffusing and descending of Lung-Qi and release the Exterior.

The Back Transporting points can also be used for diagnostic purposes as they become tender on pressure or even spontaneously tender when the corresponding organ is diseased.

The 'Spiritual Axis' discusses this and other aspects of the Back Transporting points in chapter 51: '*The Back-Transporting point for the centre of the thorax is below the tip of the big vertebra (Du-14 Dazhui), that for the Lungs is below the 3rd vertebra, that for the Heart below the 5th vertebra, that for the diaphragm below the*

Table 51.2 Clinical use of Back Transporting and Front Collecting points

	Back Transporting points	**Front Collecting points**
Chapter 67 of the 'Classic of Difficulties'	For 'Yin diseases'	For 'Yang diseases'
Organs	Diseases of Yin organs	Diseases of Yang organs
Heat/Cold	Cold syndromes (warm the organs)	Heat syndromes (clear Heat)
Duration of disease	Chronic diseases	Acute diseases

7th vertebra, that for the Liver below the 9th vertebra, that for the Spleen below the 11th vertebra, that for the Kidneys below the 14th vertebra, all of them are situated 1.5 cun from the spine. Soreness is relieved on pressing on these points. Moxa is applied on these points, never needling. In order to tonify them one lets the moxa cones burn out on the skin slowly, in order to sedate them one blows on the moxa cones and then puts them out quickly.'15

This passage establishes the use of the Back Transporting points in diagnosis when they become tender on pressure. The last statement could seem surprising as it forbids the needling of these points, which are needled so frequently in practice. The prevalent view is that prohibiting the needling of these points was an over-cautious attitude so that they would not be needled too deeply. In fact, these points, and especially those on the upper part, should not be needled deeply because of possible injury to the lungs. They should be needled quite superficially (but not just under the skin) and obliquely towards the midline.

Another point of interest in this passage is the mention of a method of moxibustion for drainage, contrary to the prevalent idea that moxibustion is generally used for tonification only.

In addition to the above line of Back Transporting points along the Bladder channel, there are also six other points on the outer line of the Bladder channel on the back which are particularly important. These are:

- *BL-42 Pohu*: 'Door of the Corporeal Soul' (level with BL-13 Feishu, Lungs)
- *BL-43 Gaohuangshu*: '*Gaohuang* Transporting point' (level with BL-14 Jueyinshu)
- *BL-44 Shentang*: 'Hall of the Mind' (level with BL-15 Xinshu, Heart)
- *BL-47 Hunmen*: 'Door of the Ethereal Soul' (level with BL-18 Ganshu, Liver)
- *BL-49 Yishe*: 'House of the Mind' (level with BL-20 Pishu, Spleen)
- *BL-52 Zhishi*: 'Room of Will-Power' (level with BL-23 Shenshu, Kidneys)

With the exception of BL-43 Gaohuangshu, the other five points exert a special effect on the corresponding mental aspect of each of the five Yin ogans: that is, the Corporeal Soul (*Po*) of the Lungs, Mind (*Shen*) of the Heart, Ethereal Soul (*Hun*) of the Liver, Intellect (*Yi*) of the Spleen and Will-power (*Zhi*) of the Kidneys. The 'Explanation of the Acupuncture Points' says that these points are like a 'window', 'door' or 'gate'; it says that *the 5 Yin Organs are stored [or hidden] but these can be seen from the outside [at these points].*'16

These points can therefore be used in emotional and psychological problems of the relevant Yin organs. It is strange that, in spite of their names linking these points to spiritual aspects of the five Yin Organs, the old texts do not report many mental–emotional indications for these points. However, in my experience, these points do have a profound mental–emotional effect, as indicated below.

BL-42 Pohu can be used for deep emotional problems related to sadness or grief affecting the Lungs. BL-44 Shentang can be used for emotional problems related to the Heart causing anxiety and insomnia, in particular if due to Heart-Fire or Heart Empty-Heat. BL-47 Hunmen can be used to help a person find a sense of direction in life. It is very useful in certain cases of depression when the person feels confused and unable to plan his or her life. This point is also effective to treat other emotional problems related to the Liver manifesting with mood swings, a feeling of frustration, resentment and anger. This point can both stimulate (when the person is depressed) or restrain (when the person is 'manic') the movement of the Ethereal Soul.

BL-49 Yishe can be used in patients who exceed in mental work or who are prone to pensiveness. BL-52 Zhishi can be used for Kidney deficiency manifesting with great exhaustion, depression, lack of will-power and a feeling of powerlessness and hopelessness.

The action of these points is stronger if they are combined with the relevant Back Transporting points of the corresponding Yin organ: for example, BL-23 Shenshu and BL-52 Zhishi for the Kidneys.

The point BL-43 Gaohuangshu is the Back Transporting point for the area between the heart and the diaphragm (which is called '*Gaohuang*'). However, its use can only be understood by referring to the other meaning of '*Gaohuang*'. In a broader sense, '*Gaohuang*' also indicates the site of any disease which is chronic and very difficult, if not impossible, to treat. This point is therefore used in very chronic diseases, particularly of the Lungs, and especially Lung-Yin deficiency. Historically, it was used for tuberculosis of the Lungs.

I personally use the Back Transporting points after using and retaining the needles in the front of the body. I would usually retain the body points approximately 20 minutes (in an adult), withdraw them, ask the patient to turn over, and then use the Back

Transporting points. I generally leave these points in a shorter time, i.e. no longer than 10 minutes (in an adult), whether I am tonifying or draining. In order to drain pathogenic factors through these points, I use needling; to tonify the relevant organs through these points I use needling to nourish Blood and Yin and direct moxa cones to tonify Qi and Yang.

Box 51.7 summarizes the Back Transporting (*Shu*) points.

Box 51.7 Back Transporting (*Shu*) points

- All situated on the Bladder channel in the back
- One for each Internal Organ
- Affect the Internal Organs directly (rather than through their channels)
- They are particularly important to tonify the Yin organs
- Often used to warm the Internal Organs
- For chronic diseases
- Affect relevant sense organs (e.g. BL-18 Ganshu for eyes)
- Used for diagnosis (tenderness on pressure)

FRONT COLLECTING (*MU*) POINTS

The Front Collecting points are all (with one exception) located on the chest or abdomen. The Chinese character *Mu* (募) literally means 'to raise, collect, enlist, recruit'. In this context it has the meaning of 'collecting': that is, the points where the energy of the relevant organs collects or gathers.

These points are used both in diagnosis and treatment. They are used in diagnosis because they become tender, either on pressure or spontaneously, when their relevant organ becomes diseased. From the diagnostic point of view, they are more important than the Back Transporting points.

In treatment, they are used either to tonify the Internal Organs or to expel pathogenic factors, often clearing Heat. The Front Collecting points are Yin in character and are more often used in acute diseases; however, they can also be used in chronic ones. In fact, this is another possible interpretation of the statement from chapter 67 of the 'Classic of Difficulties' according to which the Front Collecting points (on a Yin surface) are used for 'diseases of Yang' (and vice versa for the Back Transporting points). 'Diseases of Yang' can be interpreted as acute diseases, for which the Front Collecting points are used and 'diseases of Yin' can be interpreted as chronic diseases, for which the Back Transporting points are used. However, as above, this rule should not be adhered to too rigidly as the Front Collecting points can indeed be used for chronic diseases and, conversely, the Back Transporting points for acute diseases.

The combination of the Front Collecting points with the Back Transporting points enhances the therapeutic results and provides a particularly strong treatment. If a patient is seen at rather infrequent intervals (2 weeks or more), the combination of Front Collecting and Back Transporting points is effective in providing more lasting therapeutic results. If a patient is seen at frequent intervals (twice a week or more), it is better to alternate the use of the Front Collecting points with that of the Back Transporting points in each treatment session.

The Front Collecting points are (in order of anatomical location from top to bottom):

- *Lungs*: LU-1 Zhongfu
- *Pericardium*: Ren-17 Shanzhong
- *Heart*: Ren-14 Juque
- *Liver*: LIV-14 Qimen
- *Gall Bladder*: G.B.-24 Riyue
- *Spleen*: LIV-13 Zhangmen
- *Stomach*: Ren-12 Zhongwan
- *Triple Burner*: Ren-5 Shimen
- *Kidney*: G.B.-25 Jingmen
- *Large Intestine*: ST-25 Tianshu
- *Small Intestine*: Ren-4 Guanyuan
- *Bladder*: Ren-3 Zhongji

The main therapeutic uses of these points are as follows:

- *LU-1 Zhongfu*: used in acute Excess patterns of the Lungs, to clear Lung-Heat
- *Ren-17 Shanzhong*: used to tonify and/or move Qi in the chest
- *Ren-14 Juque*: used in Heart patterns with anxiety to calm the Mind
- *LIV-14 Qimen*: used to move Liver-Qi when it stagnates in the hypochondrium. It harmonizes Liver and Stomach
- *G.B.-24 Riyue*: used to clear Gall Bladder Damp-Heat in acute Excess patterns of Liver and Gall Bladder
- *LIV-13 Zhangmen*: used to move Liver-Qi when it stagnates in the epigastrium or lower abdomen causing Spleen deficiency. It harmonizes Liver and Spleen
- *Ren-12 Zhongwan*: widely used to tonify Stomach-Qi or Stomach-Yin and Spleen-Qi to resolve Phlegm and Dampness
- *Ren-5 Shimen*: used in Excess patterns of the Lower Burner, such as Damp-Heat accumulating in the Lower Burner

- *G.B.-25 Jingmen*: used in acute Excess patterns of the Bladder, to clear Heat and Dampness
- *ST-25 Tianshu*: used to regulate the Intestines and stop diarrhoea and pain
- *Ren-4 Guanyuan*: used to regulate the Small Intestine. However, this point is not much used in this capacity as it has many other important functions such as tonifying the Kidneys and Original Qi
- *Ren-3 Zhongji*: used in acute Excess patterns of the Bladder, such as Damp-Heat

It should be noted that only three Front Collecting points are located on the channel relevant to the corresponding organ: that is, LIV-14 Qimen for the Liver, G.B.-24 Riyue for the Gall Bladder and LU-1 Zhongfu for the Lungs. All the others are located on channels not corresponding to their organs: for example, the Front Collecting point of the Small Intestine is Ren-4, while that for the Spleen is LIV-13. It follows, therefore, that with the exception of the three above-mentioned points, the Front Collecting points treat disorders of the Internal Organs but not those of their respective channels. For example, Ren-4 will treat disorders of the Small Intestine but not problems of the Small Intestine channel.

A more detailed account of the actions of these points is given in the chapters on the functions of points (chs 53–64). Box 51.8 summarizes the use of the Front Collecting (*Mu*) points.

Box 51.8 Front Collecting (*Mu*) points

- All situated on chest or abdomen
- Often used in diagnosis (tenderness on pressure or sometimes spontaneous tenderness)
- Used especially (but not only) in acute diseases
- Often used to clear Heat
- Often combined with the Back Transporting point to achieve a stronger treatment effect

ACCUMULATION (*XI*) POINTS

The Accumulation points are all located between the fingers/toes and elbows/knees, with the exception of ST-34 Liangqiu, which is above the knee. The term *Xi* means 'crevices' and this refers to the fact that the Accumulation points are located in 'crevices' where the Qi of the channels gathers and concentrates to plunge deeper from the superficial layers of the channel.

They are points where the Qi of the channel gathers and are used mostly in acute patterns, especially when there is pain. They are therefore primarily indicated for channel problems and are usually reduced, as they are mostly used for Excess patterns. Another characteristic of these points is that they can be used to stop bleeding, especially in acute cases and especially for the Yin channels.

The Accumulation points are:

- *Lungs*: LU-6 Kongzui
- *Large Intestine*: L.I.-7 Wenliu
- *Stomach*: ST-34 Liangqiu
- *Spleen*: SP-8 Diji
- *Heart*: HE-6 Yinxi
- *Small Intestine*: S.I.-6 Yanglao
- *Bladder*: BL-63 Jinmen
- *Kidneys*: KI-5 Shuiquan
- *Pericardium*: P-4 Ximen
- *Triple Burner*: T.B.-7 Huizong
- *Gall Bladder*: G.B.-36 Waiqiu
- *Liver*: LIV-6 Zhongdu

For example, LU-6 Kongzui is frequently used for an acute attack of asthma, ST-34 Liangqiu can be used for acute epigastric pain, SP-8 Diji for acute dysmenorrhoea, BL-63 Jinmen and LIV-6 Zhongdu for acute cystitits.

The clinical application of the Accumulation points is briefly as follows:

- *LU-6 Kongzui*: important point for acute asthma and coughing of blood
- *L.I.-7 Wenliu*: for acute or painful syndromes of Large Intestine channel
- *ST-34 Liangqiu*: acute and/or painful syndromes of the breast, knee pain, acute epigastric pain
- *SP-8 Diji*: acute painful period, excessive menstrual bleeding
- *HE-6 Yinxi*: severe heart pain (acute), bleeding
- *S.I.-6 Yanglao*: severe pain of shoulder and scapula, eye diseases with pain
- *BL-63 Jinmen*: painful hernia-like disorders, acute cystitis
- *KI-5 Shuiquan*: blood in the urine, painful periods
- *P-4 Ximen*: severe chest pain, nosebleed, vomiting of blood, coughing of blood
- *T.B.-7 Huizong*: pain in the arm (useful in postviral fatigue syndrome)
- *G.B.-36 Waiqiu*: pain along the Gall Bladder channel
- *LIV-6 Zhongdu*: painful periods, excessive menstrual bleeding, painful urination

In addition, there are four Accumulation points for four of the extraordinary vessels (i.e. the Yang and Yin

Stepping Vessels and the Yang and Yin Linking Vessels). These are:

- BL-59 Fuyang for the Yang Stepping Vessel
- KI-8 Jiaoxin for the Yin Stepping Vessel
- G.B.-35 Yangjiao for the Yang Linking Vessel
- KI-9 Zhubin for the Yin Linking Vessel

The Qi of the extraordinary vessels accumulates at these points, which makes them particularly powerful points to activate the Qi of these vessels. They can be used in combination with the opening points of the extraordinary vessels. For example, the point BL-59 Fuyang is used for sciatica on the lateral side of the leg in combination with BL-62 Shenmai when there is pronounced stiffness and inability to walk properly.

Box 51.9 summarizes the Accumulation (*Xi*) points.

Box 51.9 Accumulation (*Xi*) points

- All located between the elbows and fingers and between the knees and toes
- Used for acute conditions
- Used to stop pain
- Used to stop bleeding (especially Yin channels)

GATHERING (*HUI*) POINTS

The Gathering (*Hui*) points are points that have a special influence on certain tissues, organs, energy or Blood. The Chinese character (*Hui* 会) denoting these points means 'to gather' or 'to meet' and to 'collect'. Various types of energies or tissues 'gather' or 'concentrate' at these points. The Gathering points are:

- LIV-13 Zhangmen for the Yin organs
- Ren-12 Zhongwan for the Yang organs
- Ren-17 Shanzhong for Qi
- BL-17 Geshu for Blood
- G.B.-34 Yanglingquan for sinews
- LU-9 Taiyuan for blood vessels
- BL-11 Dashu for bones
- G.B.-39 Xuanzhong for Marrow

Each of these points has a special influence on the above tissues, organs, energy or Blood.

LIV-13 Zhangmen is used to affect all the Yin organs, but in particular the Spleen and is used for Spleen deficiency, especially if accompanied by stagnation of Liver-Qi.

Ren-12 Zhongwan is very frequently used to tonify Stomach and Spleen, thus influencing all the Yang organs, especially in digestive diseases.

Ren-17 Shanzhong is used to tonify the Lungs and Heart and the Gathering Qi (*Zong Qi*): it is often combined with other points to tonify Qi. Ren-17 is also a point of the Sea of Qi, which is an added reason for its strong connection with Qi and particularly the Gathering Qi (*Zong Qi*). It can also be used to move Qi in the chest, especially in emotional problems, particularly worry and anxiety.

BL-17 Geshu is used to either tonify Blood if used only with moxa, or to move Blood if used with needle. It is also useful to move Blood locally to relieve upper backache.

G.B.-34 Yanglingquan is used for weakness or stiffness of joints and Painful Obstruction Syndrome (*Bi Syndrome*). It is the main point to influence all sinews: for example, in contracture, stiffness or weakness of the sinews.

LU-9 Taiyuan is used to tonify Lung-Qi, particularly when all the pulses are deep and thin. It also stimulates the circulation as it influences the arteries and veins.

BL-11 Dashu can be used for chronic arthritis to affect the bones, and for all bone diseases. It is an important point for Bone Painful Obstruction Syndrome (*Bi Syndrome*).

G.B.-39 Xuanzhong is used to nourish Marrow and Yin in case of Wind-stroke. It is also used with moxa to prevent Wind-stroke.

The above-mentioned functions of these points are only those related to their particular characteristic as Gathering points. Each of them has several other actions which may be unrelated to this particular characteristic. Other actions of these points are discussed in the relevant chapters on the actions of the points (chs 53–67).

Box 51.10 summarizes the Gathering (*Hui*) points.

Box 51.10 Gathering (*Hui*) points

- Points that influence certain organs, types of Qi and tissues
- The Qi of organs and tissues 'gathers' at these points

POINTS OF THE FOUR SEAS

The Four Seas are mentioned in chapter 33 of the 'Spiritual Axis'. It says: *'The human body has 4 Seas and 12 water channels. The water channels pour into the Seas of* which there is one in the East, one in the West, one in the North and one in the South, making the 4 Seas ... there is the Sea of Marrow, Sea of Blood, Sea of Qi and Sea of Food [literally 'Water and Grain'].'[17]

The symptoms and points of the Four Seas mentioned in this chapter are as follows:

Sea of Food

Excess: abdominal fullness.
Deficiency: hunger but no desire to eat.
Points: ST-30 Qichong (upper), ST-36 Zusanli (lower).

Sea of Qi

Excess: feeling of fullness of the chest, breathlessness, red face.
Deficiency: shortness of breath, no desire to speak.
Points: Ren-17 Shanzhong, Du-15 Yamen, Du-14 Dazhui, ST-9 Renying.

Sea of Blood

Excess: feeling of body getting larger, feeling unwell without being able to pinpoint the trouble.
Deficiency: feeling of the body getting smaller, unable to pinpoint trouble.
Points: BL-11 Dashu (upper), ST-37 Shangjuxu and ST-39 Xiajuxu (lower).

Sea of Marrow

Excess: full of vigour, great physical strength.
Deficiency: dizziness, tinnitus, weak legs, blurred vision, desire to lie down.
Points: Du-20 Baihui (upper), Du-16 Fengfu (lower).

Box 51.11 summarizes the points of the Four Seas.

Box 51.11 Points of the Four Seas

- *Sea of Food*: ST-30 Qichong (upper), ST-36 Zusanli (lower)
- *Sea of Qi*: Ren-17 Shanzhong, Du-15 Yamen, Du-14 Dazhui, ST-9 Renying
- *Sea of Blood*: BL-11 Dashu (upper), ST-37 Shangjuxu and ST-39 Xiajuxu (lower)
- *Sea of Marrow*: Du-20 Baihui (upper), Du-16 Fengfu (lower)

WINDOW OF HEAVEN POINTS

Although these points clearly form a group or 'category' of points, they are actually not explicitly mentioned in the ancient text as a category of points. For example, modern Chinese acupuncture dictionaries have no entries for 'Window of Heaven points'. However, chapter 21 of the 'Spiritual Axis' clearly lists some of the Window of Heaven points as a group of points with common characteristics. This chapter says: '*ST-9 Renying is located on the artery on the side of the neck. ST-9 pertains to the Bright Yang channel of foot [Stomach] and is situated in front of the muscle on the side of the neck. The point L.I.-18 Futu is on the Bright Yang channel of the hand [Large Intestine] is located behind the muscle on the side of the neck. Next to it there is T.B.-16 Tianyou pertaining to the Lesser Yang channel of hand [Triple Burner]; still next to it is BL-10 Tianzhu of the Greater Yang channel of foot [Bladder]. The channel [or blood vessel] below the axilla belongs to the Greater Yin of hand [Lungs] and the point is called LU-3 Tianfu.*'[18]

The same chapter then lists the symptoms for which each of these points is used: '*For headache from rebellious Yang and fullness of the chest with breathlessness, use ST-9 Renying. For sudden loss of voice, use L.I.-18 Futu and bleed the root of the tongue. For sudden deafness with excess Qi, blurred vision and diminished hearing, use T.B.-16 Tianyou. For sudden twitching, epilepsy and dizziness with inability of the legs to support the body, use BL-10 Tianzhu. For sudden, severe thirst, rebellious Qi, Liver and Lungs struggling against each other, and bleeding from mouth and nose, use LU-3 Tianfu. These are the 5 Regions of the Windows of Heaven.*'[19]

Thus, this chapter of the 'Spiritual Axis' mentions only five Window of Heaven points. Chapter 2 of the same book adds another five to make a total of 10 as follows:

- ST-9 Renying
- L.I.-18 Futu
- T.B.-16 Tianyou
- BL-10 Tianzhu
- LU-3 Tianfu
- Ren-22 Tiantu
- S.I.-16 Tianchuang
- S.I.-17 Tianrong (or G.B.-9 Tianchong)
- Du-16 Fengfu
- P-1 Tianchi

Some doctors thought that S.I.-17 Tianrong should in fact be G.B.-9 Tianchong. This would be more logical since each of the six Yang channels would then be represented (Fig. 51.7A, B). With the exception of LU-3 Tianfu and P-1 Tianchi, all the points are on the neck

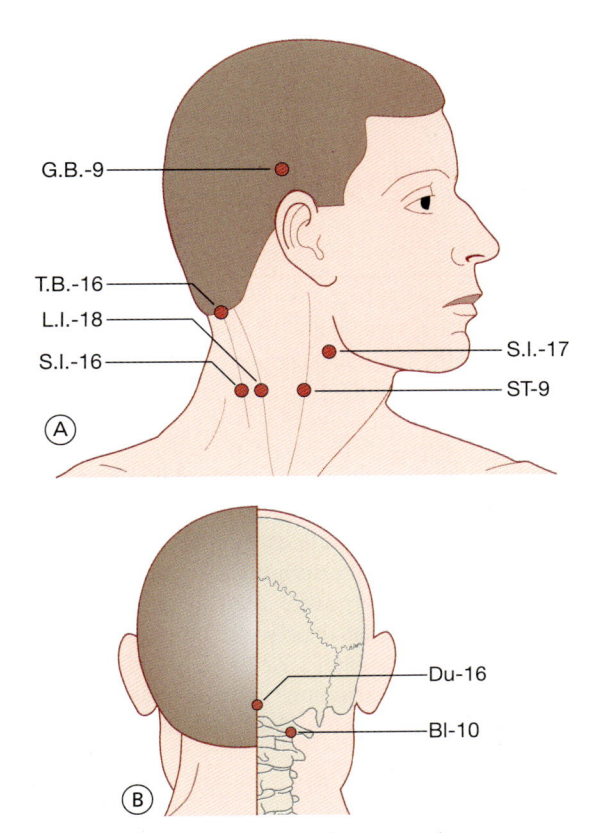

Figure 51.7A and B Window of Heaven points

brief list of the indications of the Window of Heaven points related to subduing rebellious Qi:

- *ST-9 Renying*: rebellious Lung-Qi (fullness of chest, breathlessness), rebellious Stomach-Qi (vomiting), rebellious Liver-Qi (headache, dizziness)
- *L.I.-18 Futu*: rebellious Lung-Qi (cough, wheezing)
- *T.B.-16 Tianyou*: rebellious Liver-Qi (headache, dizziness)
- *BL-10 Tianzhu*: rebellious Liver-Qi (headache, dizziness)
- *LU-3 Tianfu*: rebellious Lung-Qi (cough, wheezing, breathlessness)
- *Ren-22 Tiantu*: rebellious Lung-Qi (cough, fullness of chest, breathlessness), rebellious Stomach-Qi (vomiting)
- *S.I.-16 Tianchuang*: rebellious Liver-Qi (headache)
- *S.I.-17 Tianrong*: rebellious Lung-Qi (cough, wheezing, breathlessness), rebellious Stomach-Qi (vomiting)
- *Du-16 Fengfu*: rebellious Lung-Qi (breathlessness), rebellious Stomach-Qi (vomiting), rebellious Liver-Qi (headache, dizziness, head Wind)
- *P-1 Tianchi*: rebellious Lung-Qi (cough, fullness of chest, breathlessness), rebellious Liver-Qi (headache)

By virtue of their capacity to subdue rebellious Qi from the head, many of the Window of Heaven points have a mental–emotional effect especially in anxiety, insomnia and mental restlessness deriving from rushing upwards of Qi: for example, in Liver-Yang rising, Liver-Fire, Heart-Fire, Kidney Empty-Heat, etc.

As they regulate the ascending and descending of Qi to and from the head, these points can also do the opposite: that is, promote the rising of clear Yang to the head. The rising of clear Yang to the head will brighten the sense orifices (ears, eyes, nose, mouth) and the Mind's orifices. They can therefore be used to open the Mind's orifices in people with slightly manic behaviour, obsessions, confused thinking, confusion about life's issues, etc.

For more information on the nature and functions of the Window of Heaven points, see Maciocia 'The Channels of Acupuncture'.[20]

Box 51.12 summarizes the Window of Heaven points.

Box 51.12 Window of Heaven points

- All bar two situated on the neck
- Regulate the ascending and descending of Qi to and from the neck
- Used for imbalances of Qi between the head and the body
- Subdue rebellious Qi from the head
- Calm the Mind by subduing rebellious Qi
- They can also promote the rising of clear Qi to the head

which confirms the nature of these points as 'gateways' of Qi between the head and the body.

Seven out of these 10 points contains the word 'Heaven' (*Tian*) in their name. The Window of Heaven points have certain common characteristics and actions. The main common action is that of regulating the ascending and descending of Qi to and from the head. All the Window of Heaven points except two (P-1 and LU-3) are situated on the neck, which is the strategic crossroads of Qi between the head and the torso. These points can therefore be used when there is an imbalance of Qi between the head and the body with too much Qi or too little Qi in the head. Too much Qi in the head is generally due to rebellious Qi rushing upwards and these points are widely used to subdue rebellious Qi from the head. ST-9 Renying is probably the best example of this action.

Most of the Window of Heaven points subdue rebellious Qi from the head, which can manifest as Lung-Qi, Stomach-Qi and Liver-Qi especially. The following is a

12 HEAVENLY STAR POINTS OF MA DAN YANG

The 12 Heavenly Star points were listed by Ma Dan Yang (1123–1183) during the Jin dynasty. He considered these 12 points to be the most important points of the body capable of treating most diseases and all parts of the body. They certainly are important points, all of which are widely used in practice (perhaps with the exception of BL-57 Chengshan). The 12 Heavenly Star points are:

- ST-36 Zusanli
- ST-44 Neiting
- L.I.-11 Quchi
- L.I.-4 Hegu
- BL-40 Weizhong
- BL-57 Chengshan
- LIV-3 Taichong
- BL-60 Kunlun
- G.B.-30 Huantiao
- G.B.-34 Yanglingquan
- HE-5 Tongli
- LU-7 Lieque

Ma Dan Yang lists these points as pairs, as follows:

- ST-36 and ST-44
- L.I.-11 and L.I.-4
- BL-40 and BL-57
- LIV-3 and BL-60
- G.B.-30 and G.B.-34
- HE-5 and LU-7

Ma Dan Yang says about the combination of these pairs of points: '*When appropriate, combine the points in pairs [e.g. ST-36 and ST-44]; when appropriate, to block [pathogenic factors] use one.*'[21]

SUN SI MIAO'S 13 GHOST POINTS

These points were formulated by Sun Si Miao in his '1000 Golden Ducats Prescriptions' (*Qian Jin Yao Fang*, AD 652). These points were used for severe mental illness such as manic depression or psychosis. The points are listed in Table 51.3.

Sun Si Miao's instructions were to needle the left side first in men and the right side first in women

Table 51.3 Sun Si Miao's 13 Ghost points

Point	Name	Alternative name	Translation	Chinese
Du-26	Renzhong	Gui Gong	G. Palace	鬼宫
LU-11	Shaoshang	Gui Xin	G. True (Believe)	鬼信
SP-1	Yinbai	Gui Yan	G. Eye	鬼眼
P-7	Daling	Gui Xin	G. Heart	鬼心
BL-62	Shenmai	Gui Lu	G. Road	鬼路
Du-16	Fengfu	Gui Zhen	G. Pillow	鬼枕
ST-6	Jiache	Gui Chuang	G. Bed	鬼床
Ren-24	Chengjiang	Gui Shi	G. Market	鬼市
P-8	Laogong	Gui Ku	G. Cave	鬼窟
Du-23	Shangxing	Gui Tang	G. Hall	鬼堂
Ren-1	Huiyin	Gui Cang	G. Hidden	鬼藏
Extra	Yu Men	Gui Cang	G. Hidden	鬼藏
L.I.-11	Quchi	Gui Chen	G. Minister	鬼臣
Extra	Hai Quan	Gui Feng	G. Seal	鬼封

and withdraw them in the reverse order. Use one point at a time in succession. The points Ren-1 and Yu Men are not needled but direct moxa cones are applied to them.

POINTS OF THE EYE SYSTEM (*MU XI*)

The Eye System (*Mu Xi*) is described in chapter 80 of the 'Spiritual Axis' which says: '*The Essence and Qi of the 5 Yin and 6 Yang Organs ascends to the eyes to give clarity of vision ... it communicates with many channels constituting an 'Eye System' which ascends to the vertex and enters the brain, to then surface at the occiput. Therefore, when pathogenic factors enter the occiput (due to a deficiency of Blood), they penetrate this pathway to the Eye System into the Brain. This causes the brain to 'revolve' and a tightness of the Eye System*'[22] (Fig. 51.8).

The Eye System is closely connected to the Yang channels of the face: indeed, four Yang channels begin or end around the orbit of the eye: the Bladder, Stomach, Triple Burner and Gall Bladder. Through the Eye System, these four Yang channels enter the brain, even though the main channels are not described as entering the brain. Indeed, many modern Chinese books translate 'Eye System' as 'optic nerve'. Although this is a reductionist view of the Eye System, it certainly influences the optic nerve; an important implication of this is that treatment of these four Yang channels is essential to treat pathologies of the optic nerve.

Another implication of the Eye System is that the beginning and end points of these four Yang channels (i.e. BL-1 Jingming, ST-1 Chengqi, T.B.-23 Sizhukong, and G.B.-1 Tongziliao) all influence the brain, the hypothalamus and the pituitary gland. The connection between these points and the brain explains their use in various pathologies, such as dizziness, tinnitus and mental–emotional problems.

Three groups of points, all from Yang channels, influence the Eye System and they are as follows (Figs 51.9–51.11):

1. *Periorbital*: BL-1 Jingming, BL-2 Zanzhu, GB-1 Tonziliao, TB-23 Sizhukong, ST-1 Chengqi, Yuyao (extra point in the middle of the eyebrow)
2. *Temporal*: GB-4 Hanyan, G.B.-5 Xuanlu, G.B.-6 Xuanli, G.B.-7 Qubin. (GB-5 is the most important as it is in direct connection with the brain), ST-8 Touwei
3. *Occipital*: Du-16 Fengfu, BL-10 Tianzhu and G.B.-20 Fengchi

Since it is at these points that the Eye System enters the Brain, they can be used for brain disorders, neurological disorders and mental illness (such as epilepsy, convulsions, mental illness).

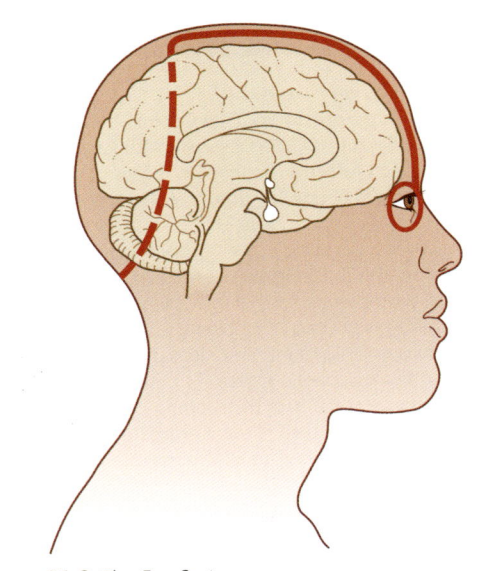

Figure 51.8 The Eye System

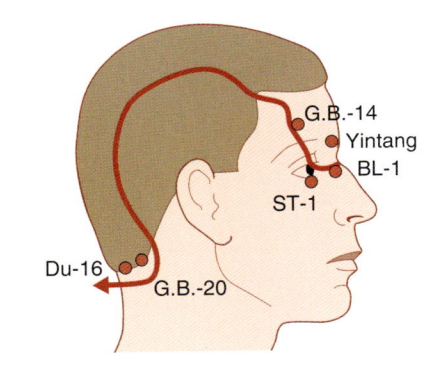

Figure 51.9 Periorbital points of Eye System

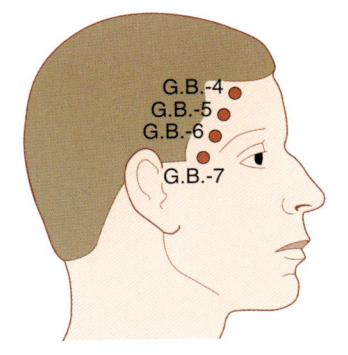

Figure 51.10 Temporal points of Eye System

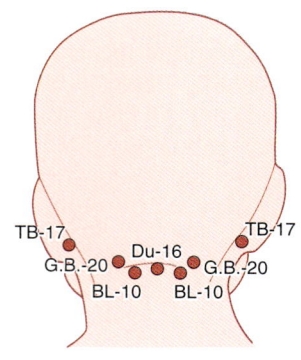

Figure 51.11 Occipital points of Eye System

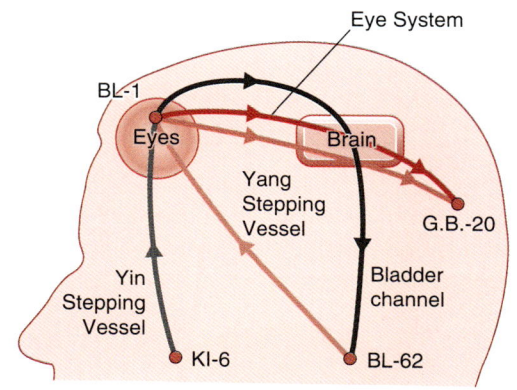

Figure 51.12 Eye System and Yin and Yang Stepping Vessels (*Yin* and *Yang Qiao Mai*)

Box 51.13 The Eye System

- Starts from the eye
- It is connected to the channels of Bladder, Stomach, Triple Burner, Gall Bladder around the eye
- Communicates with the Brain
- Emerges at the occiput
- It crosses three Yang channels, i.e. the Governing Vessel, Bladder and Gall Bladder, on the occiput
- Is connected to the extraordinary vessels (Governing Vessel, Yin and Yang Stepping Vessels and the Yang Linking Vessel)
- Its points are used for neurological, brain and mental disorders

The Eight Extraordinary Vessels, especially the Governing Vessel, Yin and Yang Stepping Vessels and the Yang Linking Vessel, enter the Brain and connect with the Eye System (Fig. 51.12).

Boxes 51.13 and 51.14 summarize the Eye System and the points of the Eye System.

Box 51.14 Points of the Eye System

- BL-1 Jingming
- BL-2 Zanzhu
- GB-1 Tongziliao
- TB-23 Sizhukong
- ST-1 Chengqi
- Yuyao (extra point in the middle of the eyebrow)
- GB-4 Hanyan
- G.B.-5 Xuanlu
- G.B.-6 Xuanli
- G.B.-7 Qubin (GB-5 is the most important as it is in direct connection with brain)
- ST-8 Touwei
- Du-16 Fengfu
- BL-10 Tianzhu
- G.B.-20 Fengchi

FIVE COMMAND POINTS

The Five Command points are those points that have the strongest and most general influence on a specific area. The Five Command points are as summarized in Box 51.15.

Box 51.15 The Five Command points

- ST-36 Zusanli for the abdomen
- BL-40 Weizhong for the back
- LU-7 Lieque for the head
- L.I.-4 Hegu for the face
- P-6 Neiguan for the chest

Learning outcomes

In this chapter you will have learned:
- The importance of the Source (*Yuan*) points: their relation to the Original Qi (*Yuan Qi*), diagnostic significance and tonifying effect, particularly on the Yin organs
- The nature of the Connecting (*Luo*) channels and their pathways
- The various ways of using of the Connecting points: in conjunction with the Source points; according to the Full–Empty symptomatology of the channel; to treat the superficial layers in channel problems; for stagnation of Qi and Blood; according to manifestations on the skin; according to their specific actions
- The importance of the Back Transporting (*Shu*) points, which connect directly with their relevant organ: to tonify the Yin organs, for chronic disease, to affect the sense organs and for diagnosis
- The functions of the Front Collecting (*Mu*) points: their use in diagnosis, for clearing Heat and in combination with the Back Transporting points for a stronger effect

- The role of the Accumulation (*Xi*) points: for channel problems, acute and Excess patterns, and to stop pain and bleeding
- The use of the Gathering points (*Hui*), which have a special influence on the tissues, organs, energy and Blood
- The functions of the points of the Four Seas (Food, Qi, Blood and Marrow)
- The role of the Window of Heaven points, which regulate the ascending and descending of Qi between head and body and have mental–emotional effects
- The recommendations of specific points by Ma Dan Yang and Sun Si Miao
- The points of the Eye System and their use in neurological, brain and mental disorders
- The use of the Five Command points, which have a strong, general influence on specific areas

Self-assessment questions

1. The Source (*Yuan*) points are used particularly to tonify which organs?
2. What type of Qi is accessed when needling the Source points?
3. Describe the two possible meanings of the term 'Connecting Channel' (*Luo*)?
4. To which pathology are the Connecting channels particularly susceptible?
5. Which outer Bladder channel point can be used to help a person find a sense of direction in life if they are confused and depressed?
6. Which Front Collecting (*Mu*) point might you use to treat an acute Excess pattern of the Bladder?
7. What are the Gathering points (*Hui*) for the Yin and Yang organs, respectively?
8. Which of the Four Seas might you treat if a patient has dizziness, tinnitus, blurred vision and weak legs (and which points would you needle)?
9. On which part of the body do most of the Window of Heaven points lie?
10. Which four channels are the main influences on the Eye System?

See p. 1266 for answers

END NOTES

1. 1981 Spiritual Axis (*Ling Shu Jing* 灵枢经), People's Health Publishing House, Beijing, first published *c*.100 BC, p. 3.
2. Ibid., p. 3.
3. Ibid., p. 4.
4. Ibid., p. 4–8.
5. Nanjing College of Traditional Chinese Medicine 1979 A Revised Explanation of the Classic of Difficulties (*Nan Jing Jiao Shi* 难经校释), People's Health Publishing House, Beijing, first published *c*. AD 100, p. 143.
6. Ibid., p. 144.
7. For a detailed description of the Connecting channels pathways, see Maciocia G 'The Channels of Acupuncture', Elsevier, Edinburgh, 2006.
8. Spiritual Axis (*Ling Shu Jing*), p. 50.
9. Ibid., p. 37.
10. Ibid., p. 50.
11. Ibid., p. 37.
12. Ibid., p. 37–39.
13. Ibid., p. 39.
14. Classic of Difficulties, p. 146.
15. Spiritual Axis, p. 100.
16. Yue Han Zhen 1654 An Explanation of Acupuncture Points (*Jing Xue Jie* 经穴解), People's Health Publishing House, Beijing (1990), p. 211.
17. Spiritual Axis, p. 73.
18. Ibid., p. 56.
19. Ibid., p. 56.
20. 'The Channels of Acupuncture', p. 171–173.
21. Cheng Bao Shu 1988 Great Dictionary of Acupuncture (*Zhen Jiu Da Ci Dian* 针灸大辞典), Beijing Science Publishing House, Beijing, p. 162.
22. Spiritual Axis, p. 151.

SECTION 1 PART 7

The Eight Extraordinary Vessels – Introduction

52

Key contents

Introduction

Functions of the extraordinary vessels
The extraordinary vessels as reservoirs of Qi
The extraordinary vessels and the Kidney-Essence
The extraordinary vessels and Defensive Qi
The extraordinary vessels and the life cycles
The extraordinary vessels and the Six Extraordinary Yang Organs
The extraordinary vessels and the Four Seas
The extraordinary vessels and the orifices
The extraordinary vessels' regulating, balancing and integrating function

Energetic dynamics of the extraordinary vessels
Governing, Directing and Penetrating Vessels (Du, Ren and Chong Mai)
Yin and Yang Stepping Vessels (Yin and Yang Qiao Mai)
Yin and Yang Linking Vessels (Yin and Yang Wei Mai)
Girdle Vessel (Dai Mai)

Clinical use of the extraordinary vessels
Points to open the extraordinary vessels
Opening points versus points on the extraordinary vessels
- Using the opening and coupled points
  - Using the opening and coupled points reaches the area governed by that vessel
  - Using the opening and coupled points brings into play the role of extraordinary vessels as reservoirs
- Using a point on the vessel

When to use an extraordinary vessel
- Problems of several channels simultaneously
- Complicated conditions
- Involvement of an organ and a different channel
- Confusing situations of Heat–Cold and Deficiency–Excess
- Some mental–emotional problems
- Some neurological problems
- When the pulse has the same quality in several positions

In order to discuss the function and clinical use of the extraordinary vessel points, it is necessary to discuss the nature and functions of the vessels themselves. The main source of knowledge for the extraordinary vessels derives from the following classics:

- The 'Spiritual Axis', chapters 17, 21, 41, 44 and 62
- The 'Classic of Difficulties', chapters 27, 28 and 29
- The 'Study of the Eight Extraordinary Vessels' (*Qi Jing Ba Mai Kao*) by Li Shi Zhen, 1578
- The 'Compendium of Acupuncture' (*Zhen Jiu Da Cheng*) by Yang Ji Zhou, 1601

The discussion of the extraordinary vessels will be conducted according to the following headings:

- Introduction
- Functions of the extraordinary vessels
  - The extraordinary vessels as reservoirs of Qi
  - The extraordinary vessels and the Kidney-Essence
  - The extraordinary vessels and Defensive Qi
  - The extraordinary vessels and the life cycles
  - The extraordinary vessels and the Six Extraordinary Yang Organs
  - The extraordinary vessels and the Four Seas
  - The extraordinary vessels and the orifices
  - The extraordinary vessels' regulating, balancing and integrating function
- Energetic dynamics of the extraordinary vessels
  - Governing, Directing and Penetrating Vessels (*Du, Ren* and *Chong Mai*)
  - Yin and Yang Stepping Vessels (*Yin* and *Yang Qiao Mai*)
  - Yin and Yang Linking Vessels (*Yin* and *Yang Wei Mai*)
  - Girdle Vessel (*Dai Mai*)
- Clinical use of the extraordinary vessels
  - Points to open the extraordinary vessels

- Opening points versus points on the extraordinary vessels
  - Using the opening and coupled points
    - Using the opening and coupled points reaches the area governed by that vessel
    - Using the opening and coupled points brings into play the role of extraordinary vessels as reservoirs
  - Using a point on the vessel
- When to use an extraordinary vessel
  - Problems of several channels simultaneously
  - Complicated conditions
  - Involvement of an organ and a different channel
  - Confusing situations of Heat–Cold and Deficiency–Excess
  - Some mental–emotional problems
  - Some neurological problems
  - When the pulse has the same quality in several positions

INTRODUCTION

Opinions as to why the extraordinary vessels are called 'extraordinary' (*qi*) vary. The 'Classic of Difficulties' says that they are 'extraordinary' because they are not 'restrained' by the main channels system. Li Shi Zhen says that they are 'extraordinary' because they do not pertain to the main channel system and do not have exterior–interior relationships. Modern textbooks say that 'extraordinary' means 'odd, a little extra, surplus', meaning that the extraordinary vessels are separate and different from the main channels. This implies that they *add* something to the main channel system.

> **Clinical note**
>
> The extraordinary vessels are called 'extraordinary' because:
> - They do not belong to the main channels system
> - They do not have exterior–interior relationships
> - They add something to the channel system

The extraordinary vessels do not have exterior–interior relationships and are not each directly related to an Internal Organ in the way the main channels are.

The Eight Extraordinary Vessels and their opening points are:

- Directing Vessel (*Ren Mai*) LU-7
- Governing Vessel (*Du Mai*) S.I.-3
- Penetrating Vessel (*Chong Mai*) SP-4
- Girdle Vessel (*Dai Mai*) G.B.-41
- Yin Linking Vessel (*Yin Wei Mai*) P-6
- Yang Linking Vessel (*Yang Wei Mai*) T.B.-5
- Yin Stepping Vessel (*Yin Qiao Mai*) KI-6
- Yang Stepping Vessel (*Yang Qiao Mai*) BL-62

With the exception of the Governing and Directing Vessels, the extraordinary vessels do not have their own points as the main channels do, but they flow through points of various main channels. Therefore each extraordinary vessel influences more than one main channel: as we will see shortly, this is an important characteristic and accounts for their clinical use. As the Governing and Directing Vessels have their own points, they have the dual quality of a main channel and an extraordinary vessel: for this reason, the main channels are sometimes counted as 14 rather than 12. As we shall see shortly, this accounts for an important difference in the use of the points of these two vessels compared to the other six.

For a more detailed discussion of these points see Maciocia 'The Channels of Acupuncture'.[1]

FUNCTIONS OF THE EXTRAORDINARY VESSELS

It is difficult to generalize about the main functions of the extraordinary vessels as each of them has its own individual characteristics. However, the main functions can be summarized as follows:

The extraordinary vessels as reservoirs of Qi

The extraordinary vessels act as reservoirs of energy in relation to the main channels, which are compared to rivers (Fig. 52.1). This idea comes from the 'Classic of Difficulties' in chapters 27 and 28.[2]

Chapter 27 of the 'Classic of Difficulties' says: '*The sages built ditches and reservoirs and they kept the waterways open in order to be prepared for above-normal situations [i.e. floods]. When there are heavy rains, ditches and reservoirs are full to the brim ... in the human body, when the channels are over-filled they cannot absorb the excess [and this overflow from the main channels is absorbed by the extraordinary vessels].*'[3]

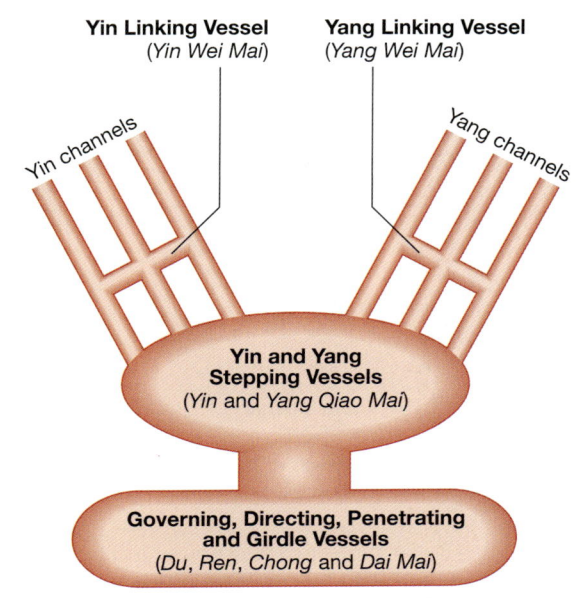

Figure 52.1 Extraordinary vessels as reservoirs

[Labels in figure: Yin Linking Vessel (Yin Wei Mai); Yang Linking Vessel (Yang Wei Mai); Yin channels; Yang channels; Yin and Yang Stepping Vessels (Yin and Yang Qiao Mai); Governing, Directing, Penetrating and Girdle Vessels (Du, Ren, Chong and Dai Mai)]

The 'Classic of Difficulties' repeats and expands on the previous chapter: '*The sages built ditches and reservoirs; when these are full they overflow into deep lakes … in the human body, when the channels are over-filled, they overflow into the 8 extraordinary vessels where they are no longer part of the general circulation.*'[4]

The 'Study of the Eight Extraordinary Vessels' by Li Shi Zhen says, in a similar way: '*when the Qi of the channels overflows, it flows into the extraordinary vessels where it is turned into irrigation, warming the organs internally and irrigating the space between skin and muscles externally.*'[5] The influence of the extraordinary vessels on the space between skin and muscles implies their important role in protection from pathogenic factors.

The extraordinary vessels are like reservoirs absorbing the overflow of excess Qi from the main channels (which are like canals)

As we shall see shortly, the Yin and Yang Stepping Vessels are the first in line to perform this function: this is a further reason why their pathology consists primarily in Excess of Yin or Yang.

As the extraordinary vessels have many intersections with the main channels, they integrate and regulate the channel system and absorb overflows from the main channels. The Yin and Yang Linking Vessels and the Yin and Yang Stepping Vessels are particularly good examples of this. To take the Yang Stepping Vessel as an example, this vessel connects with many channels. It starts from the Bladder channel, and connects with the Gall Bladder, Small Intestine, Large Intestine, Stomach, Triple Burner and Bladder channels and with the Directing and Yin Stepping Vessels.

This means that the extraordinary vessels can both absorb energy from the main channels and transfer energy to them when needed. This happens in cases of shock, for example.

Box 52.1 summarizes the extraordinary vessels as reservoirs of Qi.

> **Box 52.1 The extraordinary vessels as reservoirs of Qi**
>
> - Reservoirs of Qi absorbing excess Qi from main channels
> - Qi in reservoirs warms the organs internally and irrigates the space between skin and muscles externally
> - The extraordinary vessels can both absorb Qi from main vessels and transfer Qi to them

The extraordinary vessels and the Kidney-Essence

The extraordinary vessels all derive directly or indirectly from the Kidneys and they all contain the Essence (*Jing*), which is stored in the Kidneys. They circulate the Essence around the body, thus contributing to integrating the circulation of Nutritive Qi and Defensive Qi with that of the Essence. The three main extraordinary vessels, the Governing, Directing and Penetrating Vessels, all start in the Lower Burner, in the space between the kidneys where the lower *Dan Tian* is located.

Chapter 65 of the 'Spiritual Axis' says: '*The Directing and Penetrating Vessels originate from the Lower Dan Tian [literally 'Bao'].*'[6] The actual term used by the 'Spiritual Axis' is '*Bao*', which is often translated as 'uterus'. However, while the term '*Zi Bao*' refers to the Uterus, the word '*Bao*' indicates a structure that is common to both men and women: in women, it is the Uterus; in men, it is the 'Room of Sperm'. Both these structures reside in the Lower *Dan Tian* and store Essence and, as the extraordinary vessels originate from here, they are closely connected to Essence.

We mentioned above that the overflow Qi that runs into the extraordinary vessels '*irrigates the space between skin and muscles*': as the extraordinary vessels originate from the space between the Kidneys and relate to the Essence, we can see that, through the extraordinary vessels, the Kidney-Essence plays a role in the defence from exterior pathogenic factors in the space between the skin and muscles.

> The overflow Qi that runs into the extraordinary vessels '*irrigates the space between skin and muscles*': as the extraordinary vessels originate from the space between the Kidneys and relate to the Essence, through the extraordinary vessels, the Kidney-Essence plays a role in the defence from exterior pathogenic factors in the space between the skin and muscles

For this reason, the extraordinary vessels are the link between the Pre-Heaven and the Post-Heaven Qi in so far as they are connected to the main channels and circulate the Essence all over the body. The extraordinary vessels are sometimes called the 'root of the Great Avenue of Pre-Heaven'. Li Shi Zhen says: '*The extraordinary vessels are the root of the Great Avenue of Pre-Heaven, the Governing, Directing and Penetrating Vessels [Du-Ren-Chong Mai] are the Source of Creation.*' The expression 'Source of Creation' is interesting as it probably refers to the role of the Governing, Directing and Penetrating Vessels in embryology as energetic blueprints along which the channels are formed.

The extraordinary vessels therefore represent a deeper level of treatment related to the Pre-Heaven Qi and the basic constitution of an individual: this applies particularly to the Governing, Directing and Penetrating Vessels.

Box 52.2 summarizes the extraordinary vessels and the Kidney-Essence.

The extraordinary vessels and Defensive Qi (*Wei Qi*)

We mentioned above that the overflow Qi that runs into the extraordinary vessels '*irrigates the space between skin and muscles*': as the space between skin and muscles is the space where the Defensive Qi circulates, protecting the body from invasion of external pathogenic

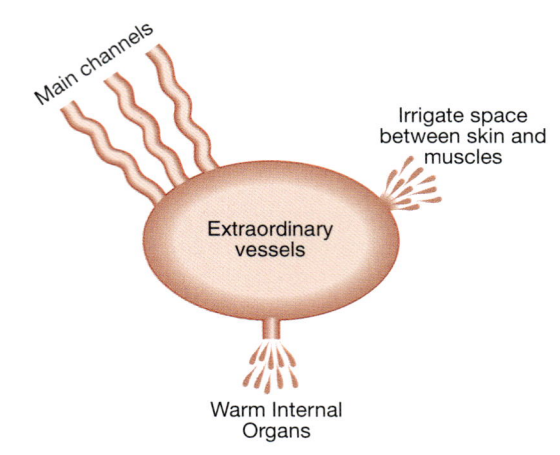

Figure 52.2 Relation between extraordinary vessels and space between skin and muscles

---

Box 52.2 The extraordinary vessels and the Kidney-Essence

- They all derive from space between Kidneys
- They circulate Essence, especially Governing, Directing and Penetrating Vessels
- They bring Essence into play in protecting the body from exterior pathogenic factors
- They link between Pre-Heaven and Post-Heaven Essence

---

factors, the extraordinary vessels play a role in the circulation of Defensive Qi (Fig. 52.2).

The extraordinary vessels circulate Defensive Qi over the thorax, abdomen and back. This is a function which is performed especially by the Penetrating, Directing and Governing Vessels. In fact, the Governing Vessel obviously influences Defensive Qi as it governs all Yang energies and moreover controls all the Yang channels in the back, which have a protective function. The Penetrating Vessel, being the Sea of the 12 channels, controls all channels and in particular all Connecting channels which flow in the superficial layers of the body with the Defensive Qi.

The extraordinary vessels' role in the circulation of Defensive Qi is another way in which these vessels integrate various types of Qi which would otherwise not be integrated. The extraordinary vessels originate from the space between the Kidneys and relate to the Essence, and, as we have seen, they irrigate the space between the skin and muscles where Defensive Qi circulates:

therefore, we can see that, through the extraordinary vessels, the Kidney-Essence plays a role in the defence from exterior pathogenic factors in the space between the skin and muscles.

The Defensive Qi is a Yang type of Qi and, as such, it is dependent on Kidney-Yang. Although it is mainly the Lungs that diffuse Defensive Qi, this type of Qi actually originates from the Kidneys. As discussed in chapter 3, Defensive Qi originates from the Essence and Original Qi and is transformed from Kidney-Yang. Defensive Qi has its root in the Lower Burner (Kidneys), it is nourished by the Middle Burner (Stomach and Spleen), and it spreads outwards in the Upper Burner (Lungs). Chapter 18 of the 'Spiritual Axis' says: *'Nutritive Qi comes out from the Middle Burner and the Defensive Qi comes out from the Lower Burner.'*[7]

Since the extraordinary vessels circulate Defensive Qi, which protects the body from exterior pathogenic factors, they also play a role in the body's resistance to pathogenic factors. As all extraordinary vessels derive from the Kidneys, this also explains the important role played by the Kidneys in the resistance to pathogenic factors and the connection between the Kidneys, the Kidney-Essence and Defensive Qi.

Box 52.3 summarizes the extraordinary vessels and Defensive Qi, and Box 52.4 summarizes the extraordinary vessels and life cycles (see below).

Box 52.3 The extraordinary vessels and Defensive Qi

- Qi overflowing into extraordinary vessels irrigates the space between skin and muscles where Defensive Qi circulates
- Extraordinary vessels circulate Defensive Qi in abdomen, chest and back
- The extraordinary vessels play a role in protection from exterior pathogenic factors

---

Box 52.4 The extraordinary vessels and life cycles

- Govern 7- and 8-year life cycles in women and men, respectively
- Life cycles dependent on the extraordinary vessels' storing of Essence
- *Tian Gui* is a transformation of Kidney-Essence through the agency of the extraordinary vessels: it is menstrual blood in women and sperm in men

---

The extraordinary vessels and the life cycles

The Governing, Directing and Penetrating Vessels regulate the 7- and 8-year cycles of, respectively, women's and men's lives. These life cycles are described in the 'Simple Questions' in Chapter 1.[8] These basically describe the ebb and flow of Essence as the basis for sexual maturation and decline and obviously correspond to the hormonal life changes in Western medicine. For example the 'Simple Questions' says that *'at 14 (in a girl) the Tian Gui arrives, the Directing Vessel circulates well, the Penetrating Vessel is flourishing, she begins her periods and she can therefore bear children ... at the age of 49 the Directing Vessel begins to become empty, the Penetrating begins to decline ... menstruation stops ... and she cannot bear children any longer'*.[9] Similarly for men. *Tian Gui* refers to the precious essence that forms menstrual blood in women and sperm in men: this precious essence is a direct transformation of the Kidney-Essence.

Thus, the extraordinary vessels, and in particular the Governing, Directing and Penetrating Vessels, are the vehicles through which the Kidney-Essence is transformed into *Tian Gui*, which is responsible for sexual maturation and decline.

The extraordinary vessels and the Six Extraordinary Yang Organs

The extraordinary vessels integrate the Six Extraordinary Yang Organs (Brain, Uterus, Blood Vessels, Gall Bladder, Marrow and Bones) with the Internal Organs and main channels (see also ch. 19). The word '*qi*' in '*Qi Guai Zhi Fu*' (Extraordinary Yang Organs) is the same as in '*Qi Jing Ba Mai*' (extraordinary vessels).

The Kidneys are the connection between the extraordinary vessels and Internal Organs and also between extraordinary Yang organs and Internal Organs. Hence the extraordinary vessels are a vehicle through which the extraordinary Yang organs are connected and integrated with the Internal Organs in the body's physiology.

Thus the extraordinary vessels *are* connected to the Internal Organs via the extraordinary Yang organs; otherwise they would be like 'water without a source' or 'wood without a root'. We can therefore see a closed circle of relationships (Fig. 52.3).

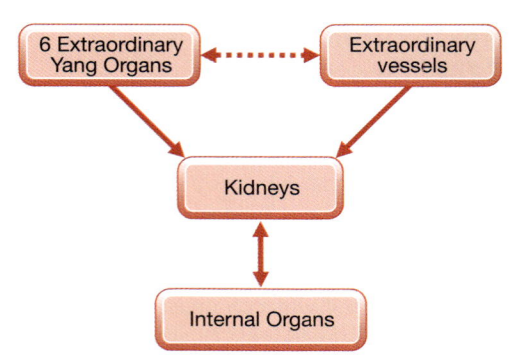

Figure 52.3 Relationship between extraordinary vessels, extraordinary Yang organs and Internal Organs

Specifically, the correspondence between extraordinary vessels and extraordinary Yang organs is as follows:

> *Brain* = Governing Vessel (*Du Mai*), Yin–Yang Stepping Vessels (*Yin* and *Yang Qiao Mai*)
> *Uterus* = Penetrating and Directing Vessels (*Chong* and *Ren Mai*)
> *Blood Vessels* = Penetrating Vessel (*Chong Mai*)
> *Gall Bladder* = Girdle Vessel (*Dai Mai*)
> *Marrow* = Penetrating and Governing Vessel (*Chong* and *Du Mai*)
> *Bones* = Penetrating, Governing and Directing Vessels (*Chong*, *Du* and *Ren Mai*)

Box 52.5 summarizes the extraordinary vessels and the Six Extraordinary Yang Organs.

The extraordinary vessels and the Four Seas

The extraordinary vessels are also related to the Four Seas (ch. 19):

> *Sea of Marrow (Brain)*: Governing Vessel and Yin–Yang Stepping Vessels. *Points*: Du-20 Baihui, Du-16 Fengfu
> *Sea of Qi (chest)*: Directing Vessel. *Points*: ST-9 Renying, Ren-17 Shanzhong
> *Sea of Food (Stomach)*: Penetrating Vessel. *Points*: ST-30 Qichong and ST-36 Zusanli
> *Sea of Blood*: Penetrating Vessel. *Points*: BL-11 Dashu, ST-37 Shangjuxu, ST-39 Xiajuxu

The fact that the Penetrating Vessel corresponds to the Sea of Food confirms that this vessel is closely linked to the Stomach and it therefore links the Pre-Heaven with the Post-Heaven Qi.

Box 52.5 The extraordinary vessels and the Six Extraordinary Yang organs

- The extraordinary vessels integrate the Six Extraordinary Yang Organs with the Internal Organs
- *Brain*: Governing Vessel, Yin–Yang Stepping Vessels
- *Uterus*: Penetrating and Directing Vessels
- *Blood Vessels*: Penetrating Vessel
- *Gall Bladder*: Girdle Vessel
- *Marrow*: Penetrating and Directing Vessels
- *Bones*: Penetrating, Governing and Directing Vessels

Box 52.6 summarizes the extraordinary vessels and the Four Seas.

The extraordinary vessels and the orifices

Pathogenic factors in the extraordinary vessels show in the orifices, as listed below and summarized in Box 52.7:

- Yin–Yang Stepping Vessels: eyes
- Governing Vessel: nose and Mind
- Directing Vessel: mouth
- Yang Linking Vessel: ears
- Directing and Penetrating Vessels: urethra and anus
- Yin Linking Vessel: Mind

The extraordinary vessels' regulating, balancing and integrating function

The extraordinary vessels have a very important balancing and regulating function in the body: words such as 'regulate', 'balance' and 'integrate' describe the functions and nature of the extraordinary vessels (Fig. 52.4).

For example, the extraordinary vessels (the 'reservoirs' or 'lakes') regulate the flow of Qi from the main channels (the 'rivers' or 'canals') to absorb excesses of Yang or Yin, or vice versa to supplement Yang or Yin. As mentioned, the Yin and Yang Stepping Vessels (*Yin* and *Yang Qiao Mai*) are the first line of reservoirs to perform this function.

'Regulating', however, also implies regulation of Qi among the Yin and Yang channels and this function is performed primarily by the Yin and Yang Linking Vessels (*Yin* and *Yang Wei Mai*), which 'link' the Yin and Yang channels, respectively, and also by the Governing and Directing Vessels (*Du* and *Ren Mai*), which govern and direct all the Yang and Yin channels, respectively.

Box 52.6 The extraordinary vessels and the Four Seas

- The extraordinary vessels integrate the Four Seas with the Internal Organs
- *Sea of Blood*: Penetrating Vessel
- *Sea of Qi*: Directing Vessel
- *Sea of Marrow*: Governing Vessel and Yin–Yang Stepping Vessels
- *Sea of Food*: Penetrating Vessel

Box 52.7 The extraordinary vessels and the orifices

- Pathogenic factors in the extraordinary vessels show in the orifices
- *Eyes*: Yin–Yang Stepping Vessels
- *Nose and Mind*: Governing Vessel
- *Mouth*: Directing Vessel
- *Ears*: Yang Linking Vessel
- *Urethra and anus*: Directing and Penetrating Vessels
- *Mind*: Yin Linking Vessel

8 Extraordinary Vessels

- **Regulating**: Yin and Yang Linking Vessels link Yin and Yang. Governing and Directing Vessels govern all Yang and all Yin
- **Balancing**: Yin and Yang Stepping Vessels balance Yin and Yang. Extraordinary Vessels balance Yin–Yang in the trunk
- **Integrating**: Exraordinary Vessels integrate Zangfu with eight extra Fu and with the Four Seas

Figure 52.4 Regulating, balancing and integrating function of the Eight Extraordinary Vessels

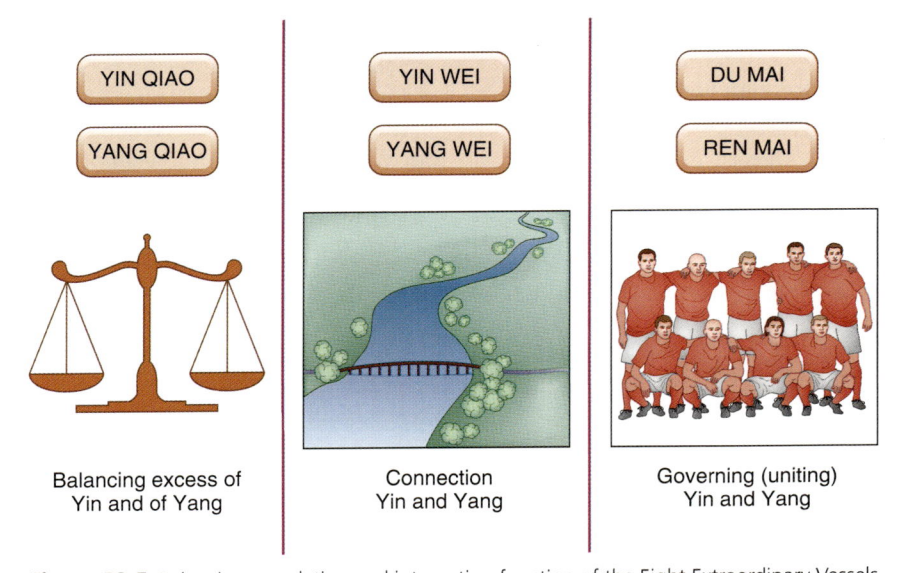

YIN QIAO / YANG QIAO	YIN WEI / YANG WEI	DU MAI / REN MAI
Balancing excess of Yin and of Yang	Connection Yin and Yang	Governing (uniting) Yin and Yang

Figure 52.5 Balancing, regulating and integrating function of the Eight Extraordinary Vessels

As for 'balancing', the extraordinary vessels perform an important function in balancing Yin and Yang in the trunk and also the head. They are part of a sophisticated balancing mechanism whereby the Connecting (*Luo*) channels balance Yin and Yang in the limbs, the extraordinary vessels balance Yin and Yang in the trunk and head, and the Divergent channels (*Jing Bie*) balance Yin and Yang in the head.

The function of balancing Yin and Yang is performed especially by the Yin and Yang Stepping Vessels (*Yin* and *Yang Qiao Mai*) (Fig. 52.5).

Due to the energetic vortex created by them, the extraordinary vessels balance Left and Right, Above and Below, Front and Back, and Interior and Exterior.

'Integrating' means that the extraordinary vessels have the important function of integrating various structures and organs with the Internal Organs and the main channel system, structures that would otherwise not be integrated.

For example, the extraordinary vessels integrate the Six Extraordinary Yang Organs (especially Brain and Uterus) and the Four Seas with the Internal Organs, they integrate the Yin and Yang channels among themselves, and they integrate the Fat Tissue (*Gao*) and Membranes (*Huang*) with the Internal Organs.

Box 52.8 summarizes the extraordinary vessels' regulating, balancing and integrating functions.

Beyond the above functions, it is impossible to generalize as each of the extraordinary vessels has special characteristics of its own.

Box 52.9 summarizes the general functions of the extraordinary vessels.

> **Box 52.9 Functions of the extraordinary vessels**
>
> - Reservoirs of Qi
> - Related to Kidneys
> - Related to Defensive Qi
> - Control life cycles
> - Integrate the Six Extraordinary Yang Organs
> - Integrate the Four Seas
> - Control the orifices
> - Regulating, balancing and integrating function

ENERGETIC DYNAMICS OF THE EXTRAORDINARY VESSELS

The extraordinary vessels can be grouped according to their opening points as shown in Table 52.1.

As can be seen from the table, the opening point of one channel (e.g. SP-4 Gongsun for the Penetrating Vessel) is the coupled point of another channel within a pair (e.g. Yin Linking Vessel), and vice versa for the coupled point. In fact, P-6 Neiguan is the opening point of the Yin Linking Vessel and coupled point of the Penetrating Vessel.

When paired like this, the two points, when used together, influence a certain area of the body, as shown in Table 52.2 and Figures 52.6–52.9. The clinical use of these points will be discussed below.

The extraordinary vessels can be grouped in a different way that takes into account their nature rather than their opening points. From this point of view, they can be grouped as follows:

- Directing, Governing and Penetrating Vessels
- Yin and Yang Stepping Vessels
- Yin and Yang Linking Vessels
- Girdle Vessel

> **Box 52.8 The extraordinary vessels' regulating, balancing and integrating functions**
>
> - Regulate flow from main channels
> - Regulate excess of Yang or of Yin
> - Link the Yin channels and the Yang channels
> - Balance Yin and Yang in trunk and head
> - Balance Left–Right, Above–Below, Interior–Exterior and Back–Front
> - Integrate various structures into channel system and Internal Organs, e.g. Six Extraordinary Yang Organs, Four Seas, Fat Tissue (*Gao*) and Membranes (*Huang*)

Table 52.1 Opening and associated points of the extraordinary vessels

Extraordinary vessel	Opening point	Associated point
Directing Vessel Yin Stepping Vessel	LU-7 Lieque KI-6 Zhaohai	KI-6 Zhaohai LU-7 Lieque
Governing Vessel Yang Stepping Vessel	S.I.-3 Houxi BL-62 Shenmai	BL-62 Shenmai S.I.-3 Houxi
Penetrating Vessel Yin Linking Vessel	SP-4 Gongsun P-6 Neiguan	P-6 Neiguan SP-4 Gongsun
Girdle Vessel Yang Linking Vessel	G.B.-41 Zulinqi T.B.-5 Waiguan	T.B.-5 Waiguan G.B.-41 Zulinqi

Table 52.2 Areas influenced by the extraordinary vessels

	Main area	Diseases	Combined area	Points
Directing Vessel	Chest–abdomen	Hernia, abdominal masses, Yin Excess, eyes closed	Lungs, throat, chest, diaphragm, abdomen	LU-7 Lieque
Yin Stepping Vessel	Inner aspect of leg, eyes			KI-6 Zhaohai
Governing Vessel	Back, spine	Stiffness or weakness of spine, Yang Excess, eyes open	Inner canthus, neck, scapula, spine/back/brain	S.I.-3 Houxi
Yang Stepping Vessel	Outer aspect lower limb, eyes			BL-62 Shenmai
Penetrating Vessel	Abdomen–chest	Rebellious Qi, internal urgency, heart pain	Heart, chest, stomach, abdomen, inner aspect of legs	SP-4 Gongsun
Yin Linking Vessel	Abdomen–sides of body			P-6 Neiguan
Girdle Vessel	Waist	Fullness abdomen, 'sitting in water', hot–cold	Ear, cheek, outer canthus, shoulder, neck, occiput	G.B.-41 Zulinqi
Yang Linking Vessel	Head			T.B.-5 Waiguan

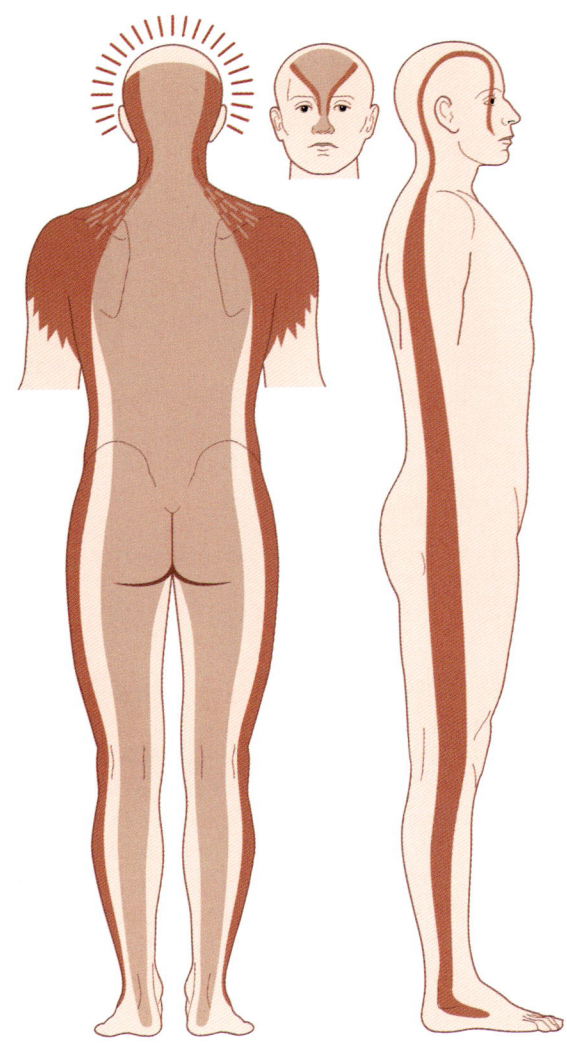

Figure 52.6 Common area of Governing Vessel and Yang Stepping Vessel

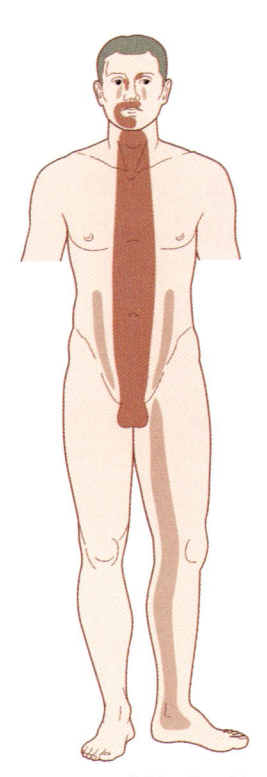

Figure 52.7 Common area of Directing Vessel and Yin Stepping Vessel

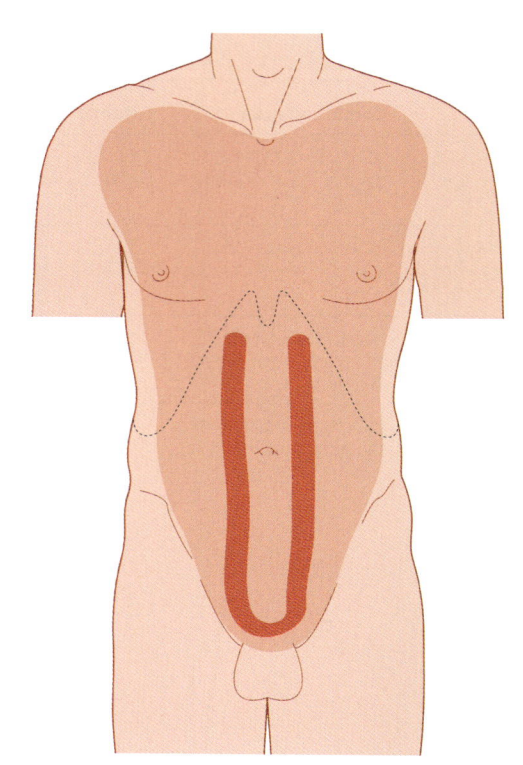

Figure 52.8 Common area of Penetrating Vessel and Yin Linking Vessel

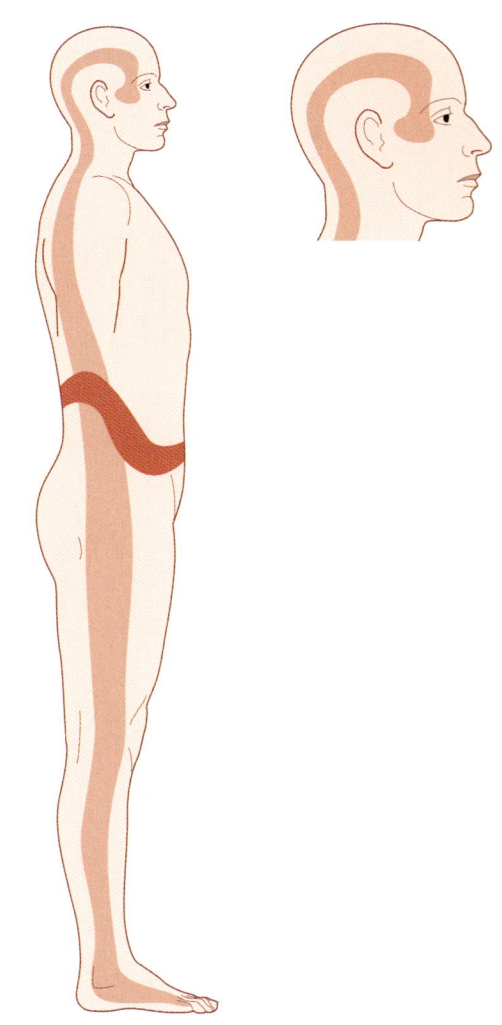

Figure 52.9 Common area of Girdle Vessel and Yang Linking Vessel

Governing, Directing and Penetrating Vessels (*Du*, *Ren* and *Chong Mai*)

These three vessels can be considered as three branches of the same vessel. The 'Mirror of Medicine Abstracted by Master Luo' says: '*The Penetrating, Directing and Governing vessels are three branches from the same source. The Penetrating Vessel is the Sea of Blood, the Directing Vessel governs all Yin channels and the Governing Vessel governs all Yang channels.*'[10]

All these three vessels originate directly from the space between the Kidneys and flow down to the perineum (at Ren-1 Huiyin) from where they take different pathways: the Directing Vessel flows up the abdomen along the midline, the Governing Vessel up the back, and the Penetrating vessel up the abdomen along the Kidney channel (Fig. 52.10). These three vessels can be seen as the source of all the other extraordinary vessels as they originate directly from the Kidneys and are therefore connected to the Essence. They, more than the other extraordinary vessels, can be used in clinical practice to affect the patient's energy at a deep constitutional level.

The 'Classic of Categories' (*Lei Jing*, 1624) by Zhang Jing Yue says: '*The Directing Vessel [Ren Mai] starts at Zhongji … Zhongji is the name of a point of the Directing Vessel that is 1 cun above the pubic bone, underneath this point is the Uterus. The Directing, Penetrating and Governing Vessels [Ren, Chong and Du Mai] all start from the Uterus and emerge at Ren-1 Huiyin. From Ren-1 Huiyin the Directing Vessel [Ren Mai] flows up the abdomen, the Governing Vessel [Du Mai] up the back and the Penetrating Vessel [Chong Mai] connects with the Kidney channel and*

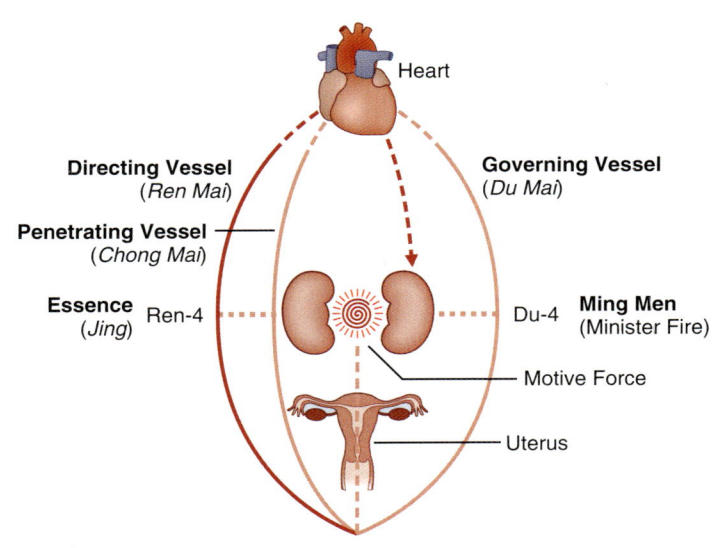

Figure 52.10 Common origin of Governing, Directing and Penetrating Vessels

disperses in the chest. The Penetrating Vessel flows up from the pubic bone to Ren-4 Guanyuan, up inside the abdomen, to the throat and into the eyes, following the Directing Vessel pathway.'[11]

Box 52.10 summarizes the Governing, Directing and Penetrating Vessels.

Box 52.10 Governing, Directing and Penetrating Vessels

- All three originate from same place (space between Kidneys)
- Three branches of same vessel

Yin and Yang Stepping Vessels (*Yin* and *Yang Qiao Mai*)

These two vessels are directly complementary: the Yin Stepping Vessel starts at KI-6 Zhaohai and flows up to the eye, carrying Yin Qi to it; the Yang Stepping Vessel starts at BL-62 Shenmai and flows up to the eye, carrying Yang Qi to it. Thus when Qi is in excess in the Yin Stepping Vessel, the person will be constantly sleepy and the eyes will want to close, while when Qi is in excess in the Yang Stepping Vessel, the person is awake and the eyes are open.[12]

The two Stepping Vessels also control the state of the muscles of the legs. When the Yin Stepping Vessel is diseased, the Yin is tight and the Yang is relaxed (i.e. the muscles of the inner aspect of the leg are tight, and those of the outer aspect too relaxed). When the Yang Stepping Vessel is diseased, the Yang is tight and the Yin relaxed (i.e. the muscles of the inner aspect of the leg are relaxed and those of the outer aspect tight).[13]

The two Stepping Vessels harmonize Left and Right and Medial–Lateral structures of the Yin and Yang, respectively, and can therefore be used to correct structural imbalances in the body, such as one leg shorter than the other, one scapula higher than the other, unilateral sweating, or the muscles on one side being tighter than the other. For example, one of the indications for KI-2 Rangu (beginning point of the Yin Stepping Vessel) is 'one foot hot and the other cold'.

Box 52.11 summarizes the Yin and Yang Stepping Vessels.

Box 52.11 Yin and Yang Stepping Vessels

- Yin Stepping Vessel is offshoot of Kidney channel; Yang Stepping Vessel is offshoot of Bladder channel
- Balance Left and Right and Medial–Lateral

Yin and Yang Linking Vessels (*Yin* and *Yang Wei Mai*)

The two Linking Vessels complement each other in so far as they link the Yin and Yang channels. In addition, their opening points belong to the Lesser Yang and

Terminal Yin channels, that is, the Triple Burner and Pericardium, respectively, which are internally–externally related.

The two Linking vessels harmonize Interior–Exterior and Nutritive Qi–Defensive Qi.

Box 52.12 summarizes the Yin and Yang Linking Vessels.

> **Box 52.12 Yin and Yang Linking Vessels**
> - Yin Linking Vessel links all the Yin channels; Yang Linking Vessel links all the Yang channels
> - Balance Interior–Exterior
> - Balance Nutritive and Defensive Qi

Girdle Vessel (*Dai Mai*)

The Girdle Vessel stands on its own as it is the only horizontal channel in the body. It encircles the main channels and, because of this, it exerts an influence on the circulation of Qi to the legs.

Dividing the body in two halves, it harmonizes Above and Below.

Box 52.13 summarizes the Girdle Vessel and Box 52.14 summarizes the energetics of the extraordinary vessels.

Thus the extraordinary vessels form an energetic vortex of the whole body which develops from the Kidneys in much the same way as the embryo develops along a central axis. The moment a sperm enters the ovum it determines a ventral and a dorsal surface (the Directing and Governing Vessels, respectively). When the cell first divides it determines a Left and Right side (the Yin and Yang Stepping Vessels), an Above and Below (Penetrating and Girdle Vessels), an Interior and Exterior (Yin and Yang Linking Vessels) and a Front and Back (Directing and Governing Vessels). Thus, far from being 'secondary' vessels, the extraordinary vessels are the primary energetic forces along which the whole body and all the other channels are formed. It is for this reason that Li Shi Zhen called them the 'Source of Creation' (Fig. 52.11).

The extraordinary vessels form a vortex of energy emanating from the centre of the body, from the space between the Kidneys, where the Motive Force (*Dong Qi*) resides.

The Penetrating Vessel is at the centre of this energetic vortex, as it is also the 'Sea of the Five Yin and Six Yang Organs', the 'Sea of Blood' and 'Sea of the 12 channels' (the meaning of which will be explained in ch. 53), and it starts from between the Kidneys. The Qi and Blood of the Penetrating Vessel are then distributed all over the body in small channels at the Defensive Qi energetic level. When its Qi reaches KI-6 Zhaohai, KI-9 Zhubin, BL-62 Shenmai, BL-63 Jinmen and GB-26 Daimai, it gives rise to the Yin Stepping Vessel, Yin Linking Vessel, Yang Stepping Vessel, Yang Linking Vessel, and Girdle Vessel, respectively. Thus the Penetrating Vessel can be seen as the origin of these five extraordinary vessels.

The Directing and Governing Vessels determine and define the coronal plane of the body, the Girdle Vessel defines the transverse plane, while the Yang Stepping and Linking Vessels define the sagittal plane (Fig. 52.12).

In ancient texts, the extraordinary vessels were often compared to a family nucleus, as follows (taken from the 'Great Compendium of Acupuncture', 1601):[14]

> **Box 52.13 Girdle Vessel**
> - Only horizontal channel
> - Divides the body in two halves
> - Harmonizes Above and Below

> **Box 52.14 Energetics of the extraordinary vessels**
> - *Governing, Directing and Penetrating Vessels*: three branches with same origin from the space between the Kidneys
> - *Penetrating Vessel*: centre of vortex
> - *Governing and Directing Vessel*: define Back and Front
> - *Yin and Yang Stepping Vessels*: define Left and Right (of Yin and Yang)
> - *Yin and Yang Linking Vessels*: define Interior and Exterior
> - *Girdle Vessel*: defines Above and Below

> - *Father*: Penetrating Vessel (*Chong Mai*)
> - *Mother*: Yin Linking Vessel (*Yin Wei Mai*)
> - *Husband*: Governing Vessel (*Du Mai*)
> - *Wife*: Yang Stepping Vessel (*Yang Qiao Mai*)
> - *Son*: Yang Linking Vessel (*Yang Wei Mai*)
> - *Daughter*: Girdle Vessel (*Dai Mai*)
> - *Host*: Directing Vessel (*Ren Mai*)
> - *Guest*: Yin Stepping Vessel (*Yin Qiao Mai*)

Bearing in mind the Confucian social customs prevalent in China at the time, being the father, the Penetrating Vessel is the centre of this family nucleus, therefore

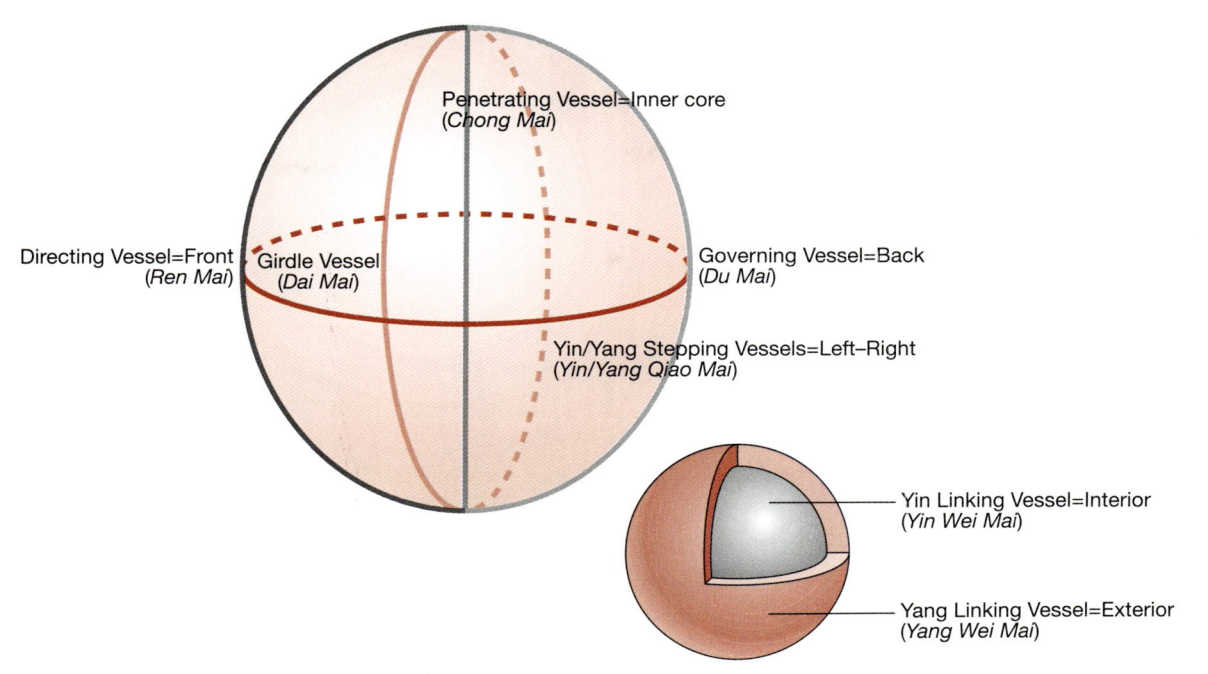

Figure 52.11 Vortex of extraordinary vessels

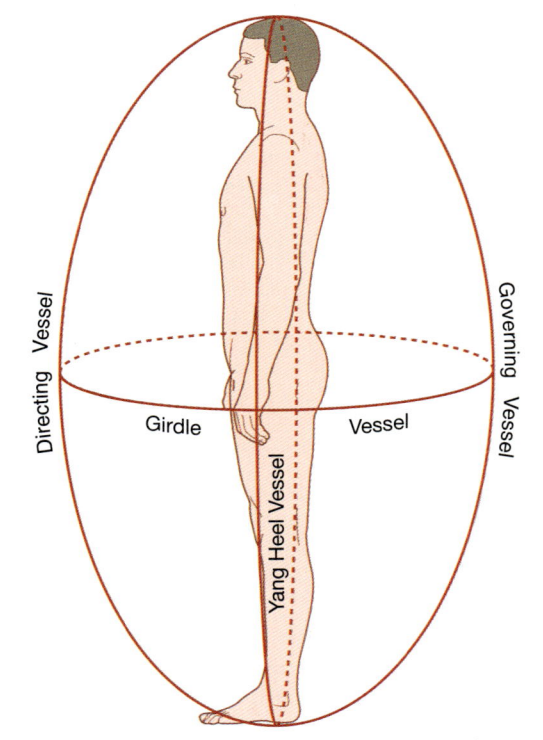

Figure 52.12 Planes defined by extraordinary vessels

the most important of the Eight Extraordinary Vessels. Indeed, in the 'vortex' of Qi created by the Eight Extraordinary Vessels, the Penetrating Vessel is at the centre of it.

Thus the extraordinary vessels regulate the following structures:

- *Governing–Directing Vessels*: Back and Front
- *Penetrating–Girdle Vessels*: Vertical and Horizontal
- *Yin–Yang Stepping Vessels*: Medial and Lateral and Left–Right (one of the Yin, the other of the Yang)
- *Yin–Yang Linking Vessels*: Interior and Exterior, Yin and Yang, Nutritive Qi and Defensive Qi

The 'Study of the Extraordinary Vessels' by Li Shi Zhen says that:

- Yang Linking Vessel controls the Exterior = Heaven
- Yin Linking Vessel controls the Interior = Earth
- Yang Stepping Vessel controls Left–Right of Yang = East
- Yin Stepping Vessel controls Left–Right of Yin = West
- Governing Vessel controls Back-Yang = South
- Directing/Penetrating Vessels control Front-Yin = North
- Girdle Vessel binds (Fig. 52.13)

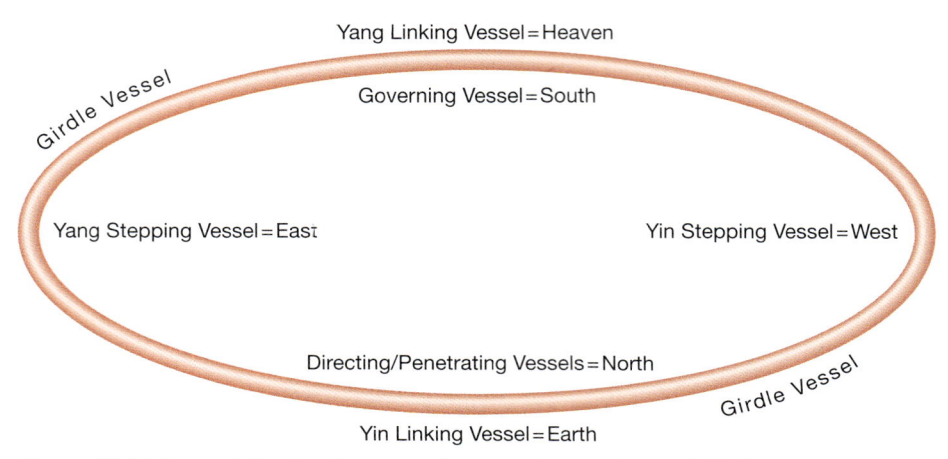

Figure 52.13 Planes defined by the extraordinary vessels according to Li Shi Zhen

- Yang Linking Vessel = Heaven
- Governing Vessel = South
- Girdle Vessel
- Yang Stepping Vessel = East
- Yin Stepping Vessel = West
- Directing/Penetrating Vessels = North
- Girdle Vessel
- Yin Linking Vessel = Earth

Bearing in mind the above-mentioned energetic vortex of the extraordinary vessels, in treatment one can relate the extraordinary vessels to body areas and physical imbalances. For example, 'harmonizing Left and Right' means that the Yang Stepping Vessel can be used for structural imbalances between left and right side of the body on the lateral (Yang) side: for example, one leg longer than the other, one scapula higher than the other, etc.

CLINICAL USE OF THE EXTRAORDINARY VESSELS

The extraordinary vessels can be grouped in two different ways described above. According to their opening and coupled points, they can be arranged into four pairs of vessels of the same polarity (both Yin or both Yang) sharing similar pathways; i.e.

- Directing Vessel and Yin Stepping Vessel (*Ren Mai* and *Yin Qiao Mai*): LU-7 and KI-6
- Governing Vessel and Yang Stepping Vessel (*Du Mai* and *Yang Stepping Vessel*): S.I.-3 and BL-62
- Penetrating Vessel and Yin Linking Vessel (*Chong Mai* and *Yin Wei Mai*): SP-4 and P-6
- Girdle Vessel and Yang Linking Vessel (*Dai Mai* and *Yang Wei Mai*): G.B.-41 and T.B.-5

In this arrangement in pairs, the opening point of one vessel is the coupled point of its paired channel and vice versa.

Points to open the extraordinary vessels

The opening points of the extraordinary vessels can be used in different ways and there is no general consensus on this question. Taking the Directing Vessel (*Ren Mai*) as an example, the points could be used in four different ways:

1. Only the opening point bilaterally, e.g. LU-7 Lieque bilaterally
2. Opening and coupled point bilaterally, e.g. LU-7 Lieque and KI-6 Zhaohai bilaterally. This method is suitable for a wide range of problems
3. Opening and coupled point unilaterally and crossed over, e.g. LU-7 Lieque on one side and KI-6 Zhaohai on the other. This method is suitable for problems of the head and face and of the Internal Organs. This technique is especially suitable for children, old people, weak body condition, anxiety. One must not use too many other needles, otherwise the needles on one limb cannot move Qi well (especially if there are scars or boils with pus)
4. Opening and coupled point unilaterally on the same side, e.g. LU-7 Lieque and KI-6 Zhaohai on the same side. This method is suitable for unilateral problems of back and limbs, or unilateral backache, unilateral sprains, Painful Obstruction Syndrome, Wind-stroke sequelae. Needle only affected side

I personally use the third and fourth techniques (primarily the third). Because of this arrangement in pairs, the opening point of one vessel is usually used in conjunction with the opening point of the paired vessel. As I see it, it is like a door that requires two keys to be opened. This technique, called 'host–guest', was indicated for the very first time in the 'Guide to Acupuncture Channels' (1295, *Zhen Jiu Jing Zhi Nan*) and later expanded in the 'Great Compendium of Acupuncture' (1601, *Zhen Jiu Da Cheng*). This latter text mentions the extraordinary vessels' points as pairs in many passages, clearly implying that they are used as a couple. For example, it says: '*Neiguan ought to go with Gongsun; Waiguan is put together with Zulinqi; Lieque is coupled with Zhaohai; Houxi mutually follows Shenmai.*'[15]

For example, when using the Directing Vessel, one would needle LU-7 Lieque and KI-6 Zhaohai *in this order*. I personally needle these two points on opposite sides. The needles are withdrawn in reverse order. I personally use the opening and coupled points of a vessel according to sex: that is, in a man I use the opening point on the left and the coupled point on the right, and vice versa in a woman. For example, to open the Directing Vessel in a man, I needle LU-7 Lieque on the left, followed by KI-6 on the right *in this order*; in a woman, I would use LU-7 Lieque on the right followed by KI-6 on the left.

> **Clinical note**
>
> I use the opening and coupled points of the extraordinary vessels unilaterally and crossed over, e.g. for the Directing Vessel, LU-7 on the right and KI-6 on the left, inserted in this order. I leave them in 15 or 20 minutes and then withdraw them in reverse order. I often use other points with the opening and coupled points of an extraordinary vessel

Although this method of unilateral and crossed-over needling is not in the 'Great Compendium of Acupuncture', this book does advise to needle the opening point of the chosen vessel first, followed by that of its coupled vessel (e.g. LU-7 and KI-6). The 'Compendium of Acupuncture' calls this method the 'host–guest' technique, in which the opening point of the vessel we want to open is the 'host' and its coupled point (which is also the opening point of the coupled vessel) is the 'guest'. For example, if we want to open the Girdle Vessel, G.B.-41 Zulinqi is needled first and is the 'host' point and T.B.-5 Waiguan is needled second and is the 'guest' point.[16]

Other classics also confirm that the pair of points are both used and that they are inserted in a specific order.

For example, the 'Guide to Acupuncture Channels' (1295) lists the opening point of each extraordinary vessel, specifically indicating its combination with its coupled point. For example, for the Penetrating Vessel, it says: '*SP-4 Gongsun, two points, on the Spleen channel … combine with P-6 Neiguan.*'

The 'Great Compendium of Acupuncture' (Zhen Jiu Da Chen) says: '*Neiguan ought to go with Gongsun; Waiguan is put together with Zulinqi; Lieque is coupled with Zhaohai; Houxi mutually follows Shenmai.*'

The 'Gatherings from Eminent Acupuncturists' (Zhen Jiu Ju Ying, 1529) also clearly recommends using the opening points of the extraordinary vessels in pairs. For example, when it gives the symptomatology of each extraordinary vessel (under the heading of its opening point), it always ends the passage by citing a pair of points; for example, saying for SP-4: '*Needle SP-4 Gongsun first and then follow with P-6 Neiguan.*'

The 'Great Treatise of Acupuncture' (Zhen Jiu Da Quan) says: '*SP-4 Gongsun is paired with P-6 Neiguan, LU-7 Lieque can be coupled with KI-6 Zhaohai, G.B.-41 Zulinqi and T.B.-5 can act as host and guest, S.I.-3 Houxi and BL-62 respond to each other.*'

When used in such pairs, the extraordinary vessel points also harmonize Above and Below as the paired points are always one from the arm and one from the leg. Using these pairs one transcends the action of the individual points, bringing into play the energy of the extraordinary vessels.

Opening points versus points on the extraordinary vessels

Having discussed the question as to whether one need to use only the opening point or combine it with its coupled point to open a given extraordinary vessel, the next question that arises is: What is the difference between using the opening and coupled point of an extraordinary vessel (e.g. LU-7 and KI-6 for the Directing Vessel) and using a point on the vessel itself (e.g. Ren-4 Guanyuan)?

An extraordinary vessel may be used in two possible ways:

- Using the opening points (together with coupled point)
- Using a point on the vessel

Let us look at these two treatments in turn.

Using the opening and coupled points

Using the opening and coupled points achieves two results:

- It reaches the area governed by that vessel (e.g. the Directing Vessel, LU-7 and KI-6 to reach the mouth and gums)
- It brings into play the extraordinary vessels' role of reservoirs of Qi, i.e. to absorb and regulate excesses and stagnation. This is particularly necessary when the pulse has the same quality in different positions

Let us look at these two effects in detail.

Using the opening and coupled points reaches the area governed by that vessel

Let us start with an example. A man complains of a patch of dry eczema below his nose and an itchy anus. These two problems are apparently unrelated and diagnosing according to patterns one would say that the eczema below the nose is due to Wind-Heat while the itchiness of the anus is due to Damp-Heat in the Lower Burner. However, there is one factor that unites these two symptoms and that is the Governing Vessel (*Du Mai*): these two symptoms occur in the area influenced by the Governing Vessel. Therefore, treating the Governing Vessel will treat *both* these symptoms simultaneously, whatever the patterns causing them (of course, treatment of the Governing Vessel can be combined with treatment of the patterns). However, in this case, 'treating' the Governing Vessel means using its opening and coupled points, i.e. S.I.-3 Houxi and BL-62 Shenmai (needled in this order and on opposite sides). It is *only* by using these two points in combination that we affect the *whole* area influenced by the Governing Vessel. If we used any point on the Governing Vessel itself (e.g. Du-26 Renzhong or Du-3 Yaoyanguan), it would not affect the *whole* tract of the vessel.

Another example will clarify this concept (Fig. 52.14). Let us say a woman suffers from bleeding gums and excessive vaginal discharge. Again, we can diagnose these two symptoms separately and the bleeding gums might be due to Stomach-Heat and the excessive vaginal discharge to Damp-Heat in the Lower Burner. However, these two symptoms are connected by the fact that they are both on the area influenced by the Directing Vessel: we can influence the *whole* area of this vessel (both the gums and the genital system) by using the opening and coupled points, i.e. LU-7 Lieque and

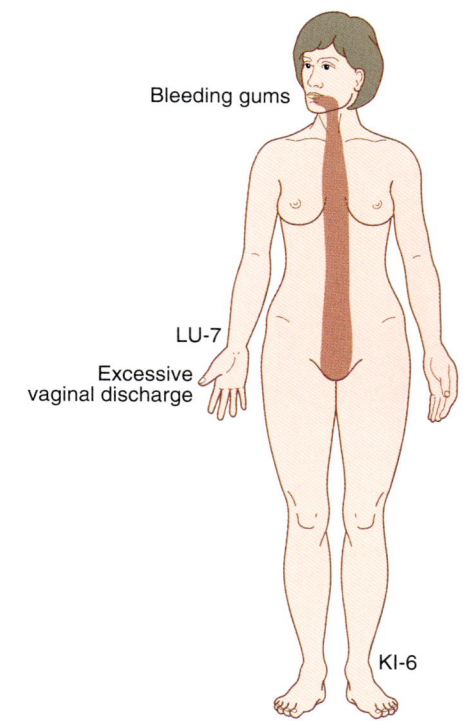

Figure 52.14 LU-7 and KI-6 influence the whole area of the Directing Vessel

KI-6 Zhaohai (needled in this order and on opposite sides). As in the previous example, these two points may be combined with others treating the appropriate patterns; however, the point is that these two points will have an effect of those two symptoms irrespective of the patterns.

Using the opening and coupled points to bring into play the role of extraordinary vessels as reservoirs

As we have discussed above, the extraordinary vessels function like reservoirs to absorb excesses or imbalances of Qi from the main channels in the same way reservoirs absorb excess rain from rivers. In many cases, the extraordinary vessels are used therefore to absorb excesses of Qi or remove stagnation of Qi and/or Blood. In such situations, the pulse will reflect a pathology of the extraordinary vessels by having the same pulse quality and intensity in more than one position.

Why should this be? If the main channels are like rivers (reflected in 12 individual positions on the pulse) and the extraordinary vessels like reservoirs absorbing

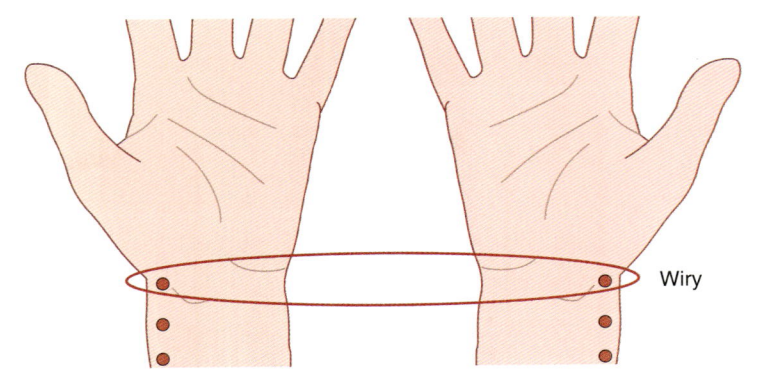

Figure 52.15 Yang Stepping Vessel pulse

Qi from more than one main channel, the 'reservoir pathology' will be reflected on the pulse by having the same quality and intensity in more than one position.

For example, in Blood stasis in the Penetrating Vessel (*Chong Mai*), the pulse will feel Firm on both Middle positions of right and left or Firm in all three positions of the left (Fig. 52.15). The same quality and intensity of a pulse in more than one position reflects the 'flooding' and 'overflowing' of the main channels into the extraordinary vessels. It is in such situations that we want to 'bring into play the role of the extraordinary vessels as reservoirs'. To regulate such stasis and absorb the excess, only the opening and coupled points (SP-4 and P-6) will do and a point on the vessel itself (e.g. KI-14 Siman) would not have the effect of bringing into play the role of extraordinary vessels as reservoirs.

Another example could be a pulse that is Wiry on both Front positions of right and left: this reflects a pathology of Excess of Yang in the Yang Stepping Vessel (*Yang Qiao Mai*) in the head (Fig. 52.16). Again, in this case, to bring into play the role of the Yang Stepping Vessel to absorb Excess Yang Qi in the head, we need to use the opening and coupled points, i.e. BL-62 Shenmai and S.I.-3 Houxi.

Therefore, especially in Full conditions of the extraordinary vessels it is necessary to use the opening and coupled point of the vessel in order to bring into play its role of reservoir. Of course, these points are frequently combined with points on the vessel. For example, in case of Blood stasis in the Penetrating Vessel (*Chong Mai*), we use SP-4 and P-6 to bring into play its role as reservoir and we can add a point on the vessel itself such as KI-14 Siman, which has the effect of moving Blood.

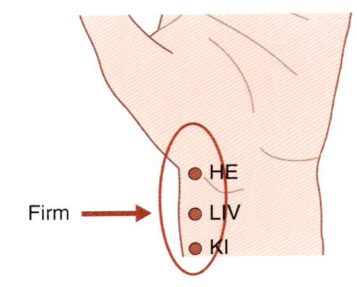

Figure 52.16 Penetrating Vessel pulse

Using the opening points of the extraordinary vessels is particularly necessary also because they do not have their own points but meander from one channel to the other. The Yang Stepping Vessel (*Yang Qiao Mai*) is a particularly good example of this (Fig. 52.17). Therefore it is only by using the opening points that we can influence the whole channel. Of course, the Directing and Governing Vessels are an exception because they do have their own points.

Using a point on the vessel

What is the effect of using a point on the course of an extraordinary vessel? There is no general answer to this question as we must distinguish between the Governing/Directing Vessels and the other vessels.

The Governing and Directing Vessels (*Du Mai* and *Ren Mai*) have their own points and, from this point of view, they are like the main channels. Using a point on the vessel itself will strengthen, tonify or move the Qi of that particular vessel. For example, Ren-4 Guanyuan will strengthen and 'consolidate' the Directing Vessel; Ren-6 Qihai can move Qi in the Directing Vessel.

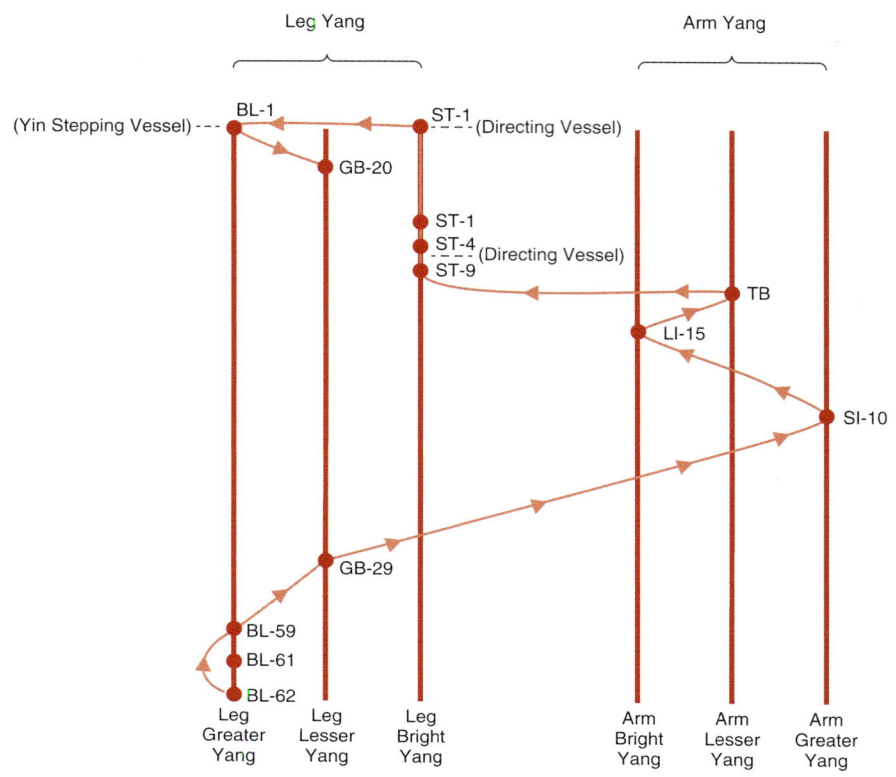

Figure 52.17 Pathway of the Yang Stepping Vessel

Often, such points on the vessel are combined with the opening and coupled points of that vessel. For example, it is very common to use LU-7 Lieque and KI-6 Zhaohai to open the Directing Vessel (*Ren Mai*), together with Ren-4 Guanyuan to strengthen and consolidate the vessel. The same applies to the Governing Vessel.

For other vessels, the effect of using a point on a vessel is different and it is much less powerful. As the other vessels do not have their own points, the effect of using a point on the vessel itself is very limited and it is used mainly to direct the treatment to a local area.

For example, if we used S.I.-10 Naohu on its own (the Yang Stepping Vessel *Yang Qiao Mai* goes through this point), we would have very little effect on this vessel. This point could merely be used in conjunction with the opening and coupled points (in this case BL-62 and S.I.-3) to direct the effect of the treatment to the local area of the scapula. Using BL-62 and S.I.-3 would open the Yang Stepping Vessel to perform its function of absorbing excess of Yang energy in the top part of the body, whereas using S.I.-10 would have no such effect.

Finally, the Penetrating Vessel (*Chong Mai*) is yet a different case that is placed in between the two above cases. Although the Penetrating Vessel does not have its own points as the Governing and Directing Vessels do, it does go through all the Kidney channel points. Therefore some of these points on the Kidney channel do have a powerful effect on the Penetrating Vessel in a way that points on other vessels (such as S.I.-10 mentioned above for the Yang Stepping Vessel) would not have. For example, KI-13 Qixue strengthens and consolidates the Penetrating Vessel.

Clinical note

- Using a point on the Governing, Directing or Penetrating Vessels (without their opening and coupled points) can tonify or move Qi and Blood in that channel
- Using a point on the other extraordinary vessels (without their opening and coupled points) has little effect on that vessel apart from a purely local effect
- Points on the extraordinary vessels are often combined with their opening and coupled points

When to use an extraordinary vessel

What guidelines can be given for choosing to use the extraordinary vessels in practice? In other words, when do we choose to use an extraordinary vessel instead of a main channel?

Let us start by defining when we use a main channel. We use a main channel basically either in problems of the Internal Organs or in channel problems. For example, if a patient suffers from Liver-Qi stagnation, we can use points on the Liver main channel and we do not need to use an extraordinary vessel. Similarly, if a patient suffers from a straightforward channel problem along a particular channel, we use a main channel.

However, there are many situations when an extraordinary vessel is indicated and these are summarized below:

- Problems of several channels simultaneously
- Complicated conditions
- Involvement of an Internal Organ with a different channel
- Confusing situations of Heat–Cold and Deficiency–Excess
- Some mental–emotional problems
- Some neurological problems
- When the pulse has the same quality in several positions

Let us consider examples.

Problems of several channels simultaneously

In channel problems, if the pathology affects clearly only one channel, then we use that main channel. However, if the channel problem affects more than one channel simultaneously, this indicates the use of an extraordinary vessel. Why should that be? This is also due to the nature of the extraordinary vessels as 'reservoirs' of Qi. As they are reservoirs, they receive the inflow from many different channels: therefore, when many channels are involved, using the 'reservoir' (i.e. an extraordinary vessel) will affect all of them.

A good example is that of sciatica. If a patient suffers from sciatica that is clearly along the Bladder channel, we need use only the Bladder main channel with distal and local points. However, very often, sciatic pain starts on the Bladder channel in the buttock; it then travels down the Gall Bladder channel on the thigh and then down the Stomach channel on the leg. In order to affect all three channels, we can use the Yang Stepping Vessel's (*Yang Qiao Mai*) opening and coupled points (i.e. BL-62 Shenmai and S.I.-3 Houxi).

This approach is used not only in channel problems but also in Internal Organs problems. For example, we also use this approach every time we use the Directing Vessel (*Ren Mai*) in gynaecological problems because this vessel strongly influences the Liver, Kidney and Spleen channels in the Lower Burner, which are the source of most gynaecological pathologies.

Complicated conditions

The extraordinary vessels are often very useful in complicated conditions. By 'complicated', I mean chronic conditions characterized by multiple, confusing patterns and many different symptoms in different body systems.

For example, let us consider a patient suffering from symptoms in various body systems, such as chronic asthma, some digestive problems, some gynaecological problems, allergies, etc. The combination of these symptoms suggest the use of the Directing Vessel (*Ren Mai*) because this vessel treats the Lungs, it nourishes Yin, it can treat digestive complaints and, most of all, gynaecological diseases. Therefore using the opening and coupled points of the Directing Vessel (i.e. LU-7 and KI-6) may have an influence on all the patient's conditions.

Another good example of the use of an extraordinary vessels in complicated conditions is that of rebellious Qi of the Penetrating Vessel (*Chong Mai*), which will be explained in more detail in chapter 53. Suffice to say here that when the Qi of the Penetrating Vessel rebels upwards it causes many different symptoms starting from the lower abdomen and ending in the head. If we analysed these symptoms one by one, we would diagnose many different patterns of various organs with Fullness and Emptiness and Heat and Cold. However, when seen in their totality, it becomes clear that they are due to rebellious Qi of the Penetrating Vessel (*Chong Mai*) and they are caused by the fact that this vessel influences many different channels. Therefore the use of its opening and coupled points (i.e. SP-4 and P-6) will treat all the symptoms caused by such a complicated condition.

Involvement of an organ and a different channel

In most cases, if a pathology of an Internal Organ affects a channel, it will affect its related channel: for example, a Liver pattern may affect the Liver channel. Frequently, however, a pathology of an Internal Organ may affect a different channel: for example, a Liver pattern affecting the Bladder channel.

Frequently, an extraordinary vessel will address this situation. For example, Liver-Yang rising will normally cause headaches along the Gall Bladder channel on the head (the Gall Bladder channel is interiorly–exteriorly related to the Liver channel). In some cases, however, Liver-Yang rising may produce headaches along the Bladder channel on the occiput. In such a situation, we can use an extraordinary vessel and, in this case, the Yang Stepping Vessel (*Yang Qiao Mai*), as this channel absorbs excesses of Qi in the top of the head. We therefore use the opening and coupled points of this vessel (i.e. BL-62 Shenmai and S.I.-3 Houxi). Of course, these two points may be combined with other points that subdue Liver-Yang such as LIV-3 Taichong.

Confusing situations of Heat–Cold and Deficiency–Excess

The extraordinary vessels are particularly useful also in situations characterized by complex conditions with simultaneous occurrence of Heat and Cold and Fullness and Emptiness. Again, this capacity of the extraordinary vessels is linked to their nature as 'reservoirs' of Qi. Being reservoirs of Qi, they tend to regulate and balance the flow of Qi among the channels, thus making them suitable in conditions of both Deficiency and Excess and Cold and Heat.

Some mental–emotional problems

Some of the extraordinary vessels are particularly indicated for mental–emotional problems, probably due to their regulating, integrating and balancing function, which was discussed above.

For example, one of the indications of the Directing Vessel (*Ren Mai*) is mania after labour. One of the major symptoms of the Penetrating Vessel (*Chong Mai*) is mental restlessness and anxiety associated with rebellious Qi.

The Governing Vessel affects three organs which have a profound influence on the mind: that is, the Kidneys (and therefore Will-power, *Zhi*); the Heart (and therefore the Mind, *Shen*); and the Brain (and therefore the Mind, *Shen*). For this reason, the Governing Vessel can be used to strengthen Will-power and nourish the Heart in depression.

For example, the Yin Linking Vessel (*Yin Wei Mai*) is used to nourish Blood, strengthen the Heart and calm the Mind; the Yang Stepping Vessel (*Yang Qiao Mai*) is used to absorb excesses of Yang in the head when they cause mental agitation and restlessness.

Some neurological problems

Some of the extraordinary vessels can be used for neurological problems such as multiple sclerosis. In particular, the Governing Vessel and the Girdle Vessel can be used to stimulate the circulation of Qi in the legs and spine in neurological problems.

When the pulse has the same quality in several positions

This aspect has already been mentioned above. As the extraordinary vessels are 'reservoirs', their Qi overflows from the main channels and this is reflected in the pulse having the same quality and strength in more than one position. For example, a Floating pulse on all three positions of the left indicates the Governing Vessel.

Box 52.15 summarizes the clinical use of the extraordinary vessels.

Box 52.15 Clinical use of the extraordinary vessels

- Points to open the extraordinary vessels: e.g. LU-7 and KI-6 (unilateral, crossed-over) for the Directing Vessel
- Opening points versus points on the vessels
  - Using the opening and coupled points, e.g. LU-7 and KI-6, for the Directing Vessel
    – The opening and coupled points reach the whole area of the vessel
    – The opening and coupled points bring into play the role of the extraordinary vessels as reservoirs
  - Using a point on the vessel
- When to use an extraordinary vessel
  - Problems of several channels simultaneously
  - Complicated conditions
  - Involvement of an organ and a different channel
  - Confusing situations of Heat–Cold and Full–Empty
  - Some mental–emotional problems
  - Some neurological problems
  - When the pulse has the same quality in different positions

Learning outcomes

In this chapter you will have learned:
- The various theories as to why the extraordinary vessels are called 'extraordinary'
- The function of the extraordinary vessels as reservoirs of Qi
- The function of the extraordinary vessels as deriving from and circulating Essence
- The role of the extraordinary vessels in circulating Defensive Qi
- The function of the extraordinary vessels in regulating the life cycles
- The role of the extraordinary vessels in integrating the Six Extraordinary Yang Organs with the other Internal Organs and main channels
- The relationship between the extraordinary vessels and the Four Seas
- How pathogenic factors in the extraordinary vessels show up in the orifices
- The significance of the regulating, balancing and integrating functions of the extraordinary vessels
- The close energetic relationship between the Governing, Directing and Penetrating channels, three branches with the same origin (the space in between the Kidneys)
- The dynamics of the Yin and Yang Stepping Vessels, which define left and right (of Yin and Yang), and can be used to correct structural imbalances in the legs
- The dynamics of the Yin and Yang Linking Vessels, which link all the Yin and Yang channels, balance Interior–Exterior and balance Nutritive and Defensive Qi
- The functions of the Girdle Vessel, the only horizontal channel, which divides the body in two halves and can be used to harmonize Above and Below
- The idea, rooted in the theory of the energetic formation of an embryo, that the extraordinary vessels form an energetic vortex of the whole body emanating from the space between the Kidneys
- The different ways that opening and coupled points can be used to open the Vessels
- How to use the Vessels in different ways: either to reach the area governed by the channel, or to utilize their role as reservoirs to move stagnation and absorb excess
- The effects of using points on the extraordinary vessels themselves
- When to use the extraordinary vessels: with problems involving several channels; in complicated conditions; where an organ affects a different channel; with mental and neurological problems; when the pulse has the same quality in several positions

Self-assessment questions

1. Give two theories as to why the extraordinary vessels are called 'extraordinary'.
2. Explain how the extraordinary vessels are involved in mediating the Kidneys' role of defence from exterior pathogenic factors.
3. Complete the following: 'The extraordinary vessels _____ the Six Extraordinary Yang Organs with the Internal Organs.'
4. With which orifice are the Yin and Yang Stepping Vessels (*Yin* and *Yang Qiao Mai*) associated?
5. Which vessels are the first in line to absorb excesses of Yang or Yin in the main channels?
6. The Yin Stepping Vessel is the offshoot of which channel?
7. Complete the following: 'The two Linking Vessels (*Yin Wei Mai*) link the ____ and ____ channels and harmonize _____–_____ and _____ Qi–Defensive Qi.'
8. What is the main function of the Girdle Vessel (*Dai Mai*)?
9. Which extraordinary vessel is seen to be the origin of the Stepping, Linking and Girdle vessels, and was seen as the 'Father' of the 'family' of vessels?
10. Which points would you needle (and in which order) to open the Directing Vessel (*Ren Mai*)?

See p. 1266 for answers

END NOTES

1. Maciocia G 2006 The Channels of Acupuncture, Elsevier, Edinburgh, p. 371–642.
2. Nanjing College of Traditional Chinese Medicine 1979 An Explanation of the 'Classic of Difficulties' (*Nan Jing Jiao Shi* 难经校释), People's Health Publishing House, Beijing, p. 68–69. The 'Classic of Difficulties' itself was published *c.* AD 100.
3. Explanation of the 'Classic of Difficulties', p. 68–69.
4. Classic of Difficulties, p. 71.
5. Wang Luo Zhen 1985 A Compilation of the 'Study of the Eight Extraordinary Vessels' (*Qi Jing Ba Mai Kao Jiao Zhu* 奇经八脉考校注), Shanghai Science Publishing House, Shanghai, p. 1. The 'Study of the Eight Extraordinary Vessels' itself was written by Li Shi Zhen and published in 1578.
6. 1981 Spiritual Axis (*Ling Shu Jing* 灵枢经), People's Health Publishing House, Beijing, first published *c.*100 BC, p. 120.
7. Spiritual Axis, p. 52.
8. Simple Questions, p. 4–6.
9. Ibid. p. 4.
10. Luo Guo Gang 1789 Mirror of Medicine Abstracted by Master Luo (*Meng Shi Hui Yue Yi Jing* 罗氏会约医镜), cited in Zhang Qi Wen 1995 Menstrual Diseases (*Yue Jing Bing Zheng* 月经病证), People's Hygiene Publishing House, Beijing, p. 15.
11. Zhang Jie Bin (also called Zhang Jing Yue) 1982 Classic of Categories (*Lei Jing* 类经), People's Health Publishing House, Beijing, first published in 1624, p. 280.
12. Spiritual Axis, p. 50.
13. Classic of Difficulties, p. 73.
14. Yang Ji Zhou 1980 Compendium of Acupuncture (*Zhen Jiu Da Cheng* 针灸大成), People's Health Publishing House, Beijing, first published in 1601, p. 643–644.
15. Compendium of Acupuncture, p. 647.
16. Compendium of Acupuncture, p. 650.

SECTION 1 PART 7

The Eight Extraordinary Vessels

53

Key contents

Governing Vessel (*Du Mai*)
Pathway
Clinical applications
- Tonify Kidney-Yang
- Strengthen the back
- Nourish the Brain and Marrow
- Strengthen the Mind (*Shen*)
- Expel exterior Wind
- Extinguish interior Wind

Classical indications
Herbal therapy
- Herbs
- Formulae

Directing Vessel (*Ren Mai*)
Pathway
Clinical applications
- Nourish Yin
- Regulate the Uterus and Blood
- Move Qi in the Lower Burner and Uterus
- Promote the descending of Lung-Qi and the Kidney's receiving of Qi
- Promote the transformation, transportation and excretion of fluids
- Activate the Triple Burner
- Control the Fat Tissue and Membranes (*Gao* and *Huang*)
- Combination of Governing and Directing Vessels' points

Classical indications
Herbal therapy
- Herbs
- Formulae

Penetrating Vessel (*Chong Mai*)
Pathway
Clinical applications
- Clinical significance of the five branches of the Penetrating Vessel
  - Internal branch
  - Abdominal branch
  - Head branch
  - Spinal branch
  - Descending branch
- Clinical significance of the various names of the Penetrating Vessel
  - Sea of Blood
  - Sea of the 12 Channels
  - Sea of the Five Yin and Six Yang Organs
- Rebellious Qi of the Penetrating Vessel
- Blood stasis in gynaecology
- The Penetrating Vessel and the Membranes (*Huang*)
- The Penetrating Vessel and the female breast
- The Penetrating Vessel and the Heart
- The Penetrating Vessel and the Stomach
- The Penetrating Vessel and Qi circulation in the feet
- The Penetrating Vessel and the ancestral muscles (*zong jin*)
- Comparison and differentiation between the Directing and Penetrating Vessels

Classical indications
Herbal therapy
- Herbs
- Formulae

Girdle Vessel (Dai Mai)
Pathway
Clinical applications
- Harmonize the Liver and Gall Bladder
- Resolve Dampness in the Lower Burner
- Regulate circulation of Qi in the legs
- Affect Qi of Stomach channel in the legs

Classical indications
Herbal therapy
- Herbs
- Formulae

Yin Stepping Vessel (Yin Qiao Mai)
Pathway
Clinical applications
- The Yin Stepping Vessel and sleep
- The Yin Stepping Vessel and Atrophy Syndrome (*Wei* Syndrome)
- Abdominal pain

Classical indications
Herbal therapy
- Herbs
- Formulae

Yang Stepping Vessel (Yang Qiao Mai)
Pathway
Clinical applications
- Absorb Excess Yang from the head
- The Yang Stepping Vessel and the eyes
- The Yang Stepping Vessel in mental problems
- The Yang Stepping Vessel in backache and sciatica
- The Yang Stepping Vessel and the hip

Classical indications
Herbal therapy
- Herbs
- Formulae

Combined Yin and Yang Stepping Vessels pathology

Yin Linking Vessel (Yin Wei Mai)
Pathway
Clinical applications
- Nourish Blood and Yin
- Mental–emotional problems
- Headaches

Classical indications
Herbal therapy
- Herbs
- Formulae

Yang Linking Vessel (Yang Wei Mai)
Pathway
Clinical applications
- Intermittent fevers
- Sides of the body
- Ear problems

Classical indications
Herbal therapy
- Herbs
- Formulae

Combined Yin and Yang Linking Vessels pathology
The Yin and Yang Linking Vessels and the waist
Yang and Yin Linking Vessels influence head and abdomen, respectively
Harmonization of Nutritive and Defensive Qi

In this chapter I shall discuss the clinical use of the extraordinary vessels in detail. The discussion will be carried out under the following headings:

- Governing Vessel (*Du Mai*)
  - Pathway
  - Clinical applications
    - Tonifies Kidney-Yang
    - Strengthens the back
    - Nourishes the Brain and Marrow
    - Strengthens the Mind (*Shen*)
    - Expels exterior Wind
    - Extinguishes interior Wind
  - Classical indications
  - Herbal therapy
    - Herbs
    - Formulae
- Directing Vessel (*Ren Mai*)
  - Pathway
  - Clinical applications
    - Nourishes Yin
    - Regulates the Uterus and Blood
    - Moves Qi in the Lower Burner and Uterus
    - Promotes the descending of Lung-Qi and the Kidney's receiving of Qi
    - Promotes the transformation, transportation and excretion of fluids

- Activates the Triple Burner
- Controls the Fat Tissue and Membranes (*Gao* and *Huang*)
- Combination of Governing and Directing Vessels' points
  - Classical indications
  - Herbal therapy
    - Herbs
    - Formulae
- Penetrating Vessel (*Chong Mai*)
  - Pathway
  - Clinical applications
    - Clinical significance of the five branches of the Penetrating Vessel
      - Internal branch
      - Abdominal branch
      - Head branch
      - Spinal branch
      - Descending branch
    - Clinical significance of the various names of the Penetrating Vessel
      - Sea of Blood
      - Sea of the 12 Channels
      - Sea of the five Yin and six Yang Organs
    - Rebellious Qi of the Penetrating Vessel
    - Blood stasis in gynaecology
    - The Penetrating Vessel and the Membranes (*Huang*)
    - The Penetrating Vessel and the female breast
    - The Penetrating Vessel and the Heart
    - The Penetrating Vessel and the Stomach
    - The Penetrating Vessel and Qi circulation in the feet
    - The Penetrating Vessel and the ancestral muscles (*zong jin*)
    - Comparison and differentiation between the Directing and Penetrating Vessels
  - Classical indications
  - Herbal therapy
    - Herbs
    - Formulae
- Girdle Vessel (*Dai Mai*)
  - Pathway
  - Clinical applications
    - Harmonizes the Liver and Gall Bladder
    - Resolves Dampness in the Lower Burner
    - Regulates circulation of Qi in the legs
    - Affects Qi of Stomach channel in the legs
  - Classical indications
  - Herbal therapy
    - Herbs
    - Formulae
- Yin Stepping Vessel (*Yin Qiao Mai*)
  - Pathway
  - Clinical applications
    - The Yin Stepping Vessel and sleep
    - The Yin Stepping Vessel and Atrophy Syndrome (*Wei* Syndrome)
    - Abdominal pain
  - Classical indications
  - Herbal therapy
    - Herbs
    - Formulae
- Yang Stepping Vessel (*Yang Qiao Mai*)
  - Pathway
  - Clinical applications
    - Absorb Excess Yang from the head
    - The Yang Stepping Vessel and the eyes
    - The Yang Stepping Vessel in mental problems
    - The Yang Stepping Vessel in backache and sciatica
    - The Yang Stepping Vessel and the hip
  - Classical indications
  - Herbal therapy
    - Herbs
    - Formulae
- Combined Yin and Yang Stepping Vessel pathology
- Yin Linking Vessel (*Yin Wei Mai*)
  - Pathway
  - Clinical applications
    - Nourishes Blood and Yin
    - Mental–emotional problems
    - Headaches
  - Classical indications
  - Herbal therapy
    - Herbs
    - Formulae
- Yang Linking Vessel (*Yang Wei Mai*)
  - Pathway
  - Clinical applications
    - Intermittent fevers
    - Sides of the body
    - Ear problems
  - Classical indications
  - Herbal therapy
    - Herbs
    - Formulae

- Combined Yin and Yang Linking Vessel pathology
  - The Yin and Yang Linking Vessels and the waist
  - Yang and Yin Linking Vessels influence head and abdomen, respectively
  - Harmonization of Nutritive and Defensive Qi

GOVERNING VESSEL (*DU MAI*)

Opening point: S.I.-3 Houxi.
Coupled point: BL-62 Shenmai.
Starting point: Du-1 Changqiang.
Connecting point: Du-1 Changqiang.
Area of body influenced: external genitalia, anus, back, spine, back of neck and head.

Pathway

The internal pathway of the Governing Vessel is more complex than the mere line arising from the perineum and flowing along the spine to the head and upper lip. First of all, it originates in between the two kidneys (together with the Directing and Penetrating Vessels); it then flows downwards to the perineum and emerges at Ren-1 Huiyin. From here it goes to Du-1 Changqiang and all along the spine to the head, down to the upper lip (Fig. 53.1).

Chapter 28 of the 'Classic of Difficulties' describes the pathway of the Governing Vessel simply as: '*The Governing Vessel starts from a point at the lowest end of the body [perineum], it ascends inside the spine, reaches the point Du-16 Fengfu and from here it enters the brain.*'[1]

The 'Golden Mirror of Medicine' (Yi Zong Jin Jian, 1742) says: '*The Governing vessel arises within the lower abdomen, externally in the abdomen, internally in the "Bao" ["Uterus"] ... also called Dan Tian in both men and women: in women it is the uterus, in men it is the Room of Sperm.*'[2]

Chapter 60 of the 'Simple Questions' has the following pathway for the Governing Vessel: '*It starts in the lower abdomen, goes down to the pubic bone, in women to the vagina. Its Connecting channel goes around the vagina, passes to the perineum, then the buttocks, down to meet the Kidney and Bladder channels inside the upper thighs; it then rises up the spine and wraps around the kidneys ... in men it goes around the penis and then the perineum ... the main vessel starts in the lower abdomen, goes up to the umbilicus, past the heart, throat, chin, around lips and reaches the eyes.*'[3]

The description of this pathway of the Governing Vessel is important as it highlights certain aspects of it that are not often mentioned. For example, it is interesting that the Governing Vessel in women goes to the vagina as this is an area that would be normally be connected only with the Directing Vessel (*Ren Mai*).

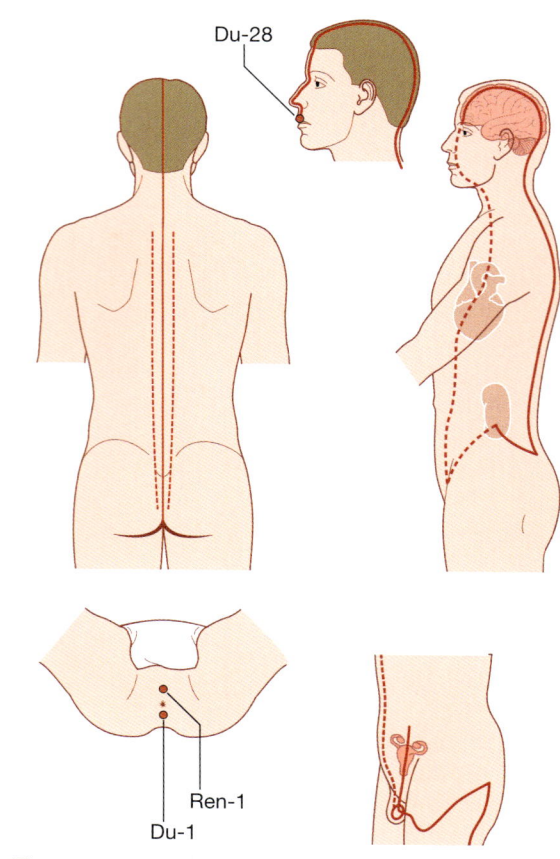

Figure 53.1 The Governing Vessel

The second interesting aspect of the description of the Governing Vessel's pathway in chapter 60 of the 'Simple Questions' is the mention of a 'main vessel' that *rises* from the lower abdomen in the centre of the abdomen to end in the eyes. This, of course, sounds very much like the Directing Vessel's pathway. This poses the questions as to whether this pathway is indeed a branch of the Governing Vessel or the Directing Vessel itself.

Some see this 'main vessel' as being the Directing Vessel. In fact, paradoxically, in clinical practice, it does not matter too much whether such a pathway is a branch of the Governing Vessel or the Directing Vessel itself. Indeed, the Governing and Directing Vessels are almost like two branches of the same vessel, one Yang and one Yin, intersecting inside.

Li Shi Zhen says (reporting the opinion of Hua Bo Ren): '*The Directing and Governing Vessels are two branches* from the same source, one in the front of the body, the other in the back. Just as the human body has the Directing and Governing Vessels, nature has midnight and midday: these two vessels are separate but also joined. When we try to divide these, we see that Yin and Yang are inseparable; when we try to see them as one, we see that it is an indivisible whole. They are one but two, they are two but one.'[4]

The 'main vessel' of the Governing Vessel in the abdomen mentioned in chapter 60 of the 'Simple Questions' is called 'Connecting channel' by Li Shi Zhen who gives the same pathway. Li Shi Zhen also says that once it reaches the eyes, this part of the Governing Vessel continues its ascent *'from BL-1 Jingming to the top of the head where it joins the Liver channel and it enters the brain. It then descends along the occiput, it joins the Bladder channel at BL-11 Dashu and then descends inside the spine and reaches the Kidneys.'*[5] Therefore, it would appear that, according to this passage, the Governing Vessel also a branch that *descends* rather than ascends the back and the spine.

In fact, chapter 16 of the 'Spiritual Axis' also has the Governing Vessel running *down* the spine. This chapter describes the circulation of Qi in all the 14 channels and, after describing the pathway of the first 11 channels, it comes to the Liver and it says: '*[The Liver channel] reaches the vertex, moves down in the occiput, down the spine to enter the sacrum: this is the Governing Vessel.*'[6]

The Connecting channel of the Governing Vessel ascends the back from Du-1 Changqiang in parallel lines.

Box 53.1 summarizes the pathway of the Governing Vessel.

Box 53.1 Governing Vessel – summary of pathway

- It starts inside the lower abdomen between the kidneys, it goes to the uterus and the pubic bone. In women, it flows around the vagina and passes to the perineum; in men, it flows around the penis and goes to the perineum
- From here, it goes to the buttocks where it connects with the Kidney and Bladder channels in the upper thighs
- From the perineum it rises in the spine
- It reaches Du-16 Fengfu where it enters the Brain
- It ascends to the vertex and down along the forehead and nose to end at Du-28 Yinjiao
- The abdominal branch of the Governing Vessel starts in the perineum, flows up the abdomen (in the midline), up to the umbilicus, past the heart, throat, chin, around the lips and reaches the eyes
- The Connecting channel of the Governing Vessel ascends the back from Du-1 Changqiang in parallel lines

---

Clinical applications

The Governing Vessel is called the 'Sea of Yang channels' as it exerts an influence on all the Yang channels and it can be used to strengthen the Yang of the body. It can strengthen the spine and tonify Kidney-Yang.

The Governing Vessel also nourishes the spine and brain as the inner pathway of the vessel enters the brain. In this sense, it can be used to strengthen the Kidney function of nourishing Marrow and Brain, for such symptoms as dizziness and poor memory.

Tonifies Kidney-Yang

Being the governor of all Yang of the body, the Governing Vessel can be used to tonify Yang and in particular Kidney-Yang in both men and women. The main point that tonifies Kidney-Yang is Du-4 Mingmen used with moxa. When direct moxa cones are applied to this point, it constitutes a powerful tonification of Yang. This point is combined with the opening and coupled points of the Governing Vessel so that we use three points: S.I.-3 Houxi on one side, BL.-62 Shenmai on the other and Du-4 Mingmen, in this order.

In women, the Governing Vessel can be used to tonify Kidney-Yang in gynaecological problems. We could say that, in gynaecology, we can use the Governing Vessel in any case when we might use the Directing Vessel but there is a pronounced Kidney-Yang deficiency. Bearing in mind that a branch of the Governing Vessel also goes to the vagina, this vessel can be used also for chronic, excessive vaginal discharge occurring against a background of pronounced Kidney-Yang deficiency.

Strengthens the back

The Governing Vessel is extremely useful in all cases of chronic lower backache due to Kidney deficiency, especially (but not exclusively) when the pain is on the midline of the back. The use of the opening and coupled points can strengthen the back and actually straighten the spine. In men the Governing Vessel can be used on its own, and in women it is best combined with the Directing Vessel, crossing over the opening and coupled points.

Thus in a woman, one could use S.I.-3 Houxi on the right, BL-62 Shenmai on the left, LU-7 Lieque on the left and KI-6 Zhaohai on the right, the needles being inserted in this order and taken out in the reverse order.

When used for lower backache, the Governing Vessel opening and coupled points are used first and left in for about 10–15 minutes. This has the effect of opening the Governing Vessel, making it more receptive to further treatment with local points. It also has the effect of actually straightening the spine. After withdrawing the opening and coupled point needles, local points can be used, particularly Du-3 Yaoyangguan or the extra point Shiqizhuixia situated on the midline below the tip of L-5 lumbar vertebra.

Nourishes the Brain and Marrow

The Kidney-Essence produces Marrow, which fills the spine and the Brain. Flowing inside the spine and into the brain, the Governing Vessel has a deep influence on the nourishment of the brain. In particular, the Governing Vessel balances Yin and Yang in the head and brain as it carries Kidney-Essence but is Yang in nature. The Governing Vessel connects with the Brain upwards and the Kidneys downwards: it is therefore the channel connection between Kidneys and Brain. The Kidneys store Essence and the Brain is filled by Marrow: to nourish the Essence and fill Marrow one can use the Governing Vessel.

Cheng Xing Gan says: '*When Marrow is full thinking is clear. Too much thinking leads to Heart-Fire which burns the brain causing dizziness, blurred vision, tinnitus ... The Marrow is rooted in the Essence and connects downwards with the Governing Vessel: when the Gate of Life warms and nourishes, the Marrow is full.*' Hence Heart, Brain and Kidneys are all related to the Governing Vessel with a relation of mutual nourishment and influence.

Tonifying the Governing Vessel therefore can nourish the Marrow and the brain for such symptoms as dizziness, tinnitus, weak legs, blurred vision and desire to lie down. These are actually symptoms of deficiency of the Sea of Marrow. The points that affect the Sea of Marrow are, in fact, on the Governing Vessel and they are Du-20 Baihui (upper), Du-16 Fengfu (lower). It will remembered from the discussion of the pathway of this vessel that the Governing Vessel meets the Liver channel on the vertex where it enters the brain, proceeding then downwards (Li Shi Zhen), but it also enters the brain at Du-16 Fengfu, from where it proceeds upwards (chapter 28 of the 'Classic of Difficulties').

To nourish the Marrow and brain, the two points Du-20 and Du-16 can be combined with the opening and coupled points of the Governing Vessel: that is, S.I.-3 Houxi on one side and BL-62 Shenmai on the other.

Strengthens the Mind (*Shen*)

The Mind (*Shen*) is closely related to the Kidney-Essence. As we saw in chapter 3, the 'Spiritual Axis' in chapter 8 says: '*Life comes about through the Essence; when the two Essences [of mother and father] unite, they form the Mind*'.[7] Zhang Jie Bin says: '*The two Essences, one Yin, one Yang, unit. ... to form life; the Essences of mother and father unite to form the Mind.*'[8] Therefore the Mind comes into being originally from the Prenatal Essence, which is stored in the Kidneys. Of course, after birth, it is supplemented by the Postnatal Essence (Fig. 53.2).

Therefore, although the Mind (*Shen*) is housed in the Heart, its basic biological foundation is in the Kidney-Essence. As the Kidney-Essence produces Marrow, which fills the Brain, there were, over the centuries, Chinese doctors who attributed mental functions and consciousness to the Brain rather than the Heart. This is the meaning of Li Shi Zhen's reference to the Brain being the residence of the *Yuan Shen* (Original Mind): that is, the Brain is formed from Marrow and Kidneys, which store the Prenatal Essence that is the origin of

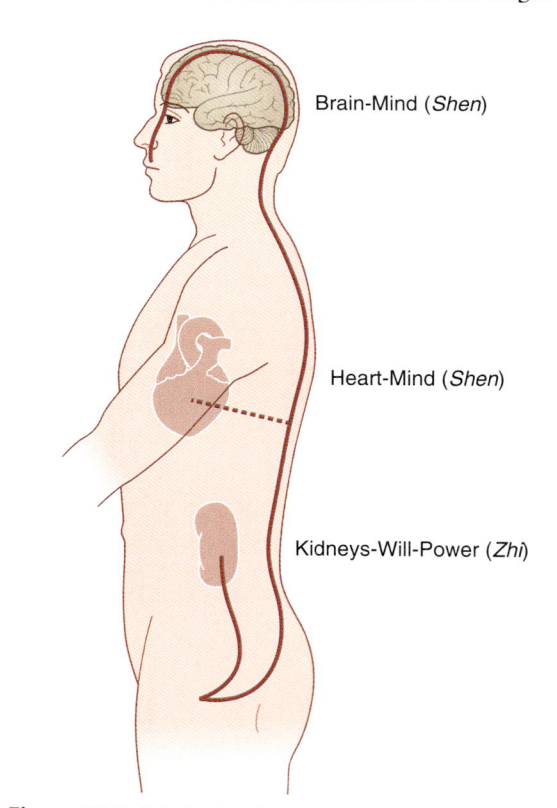

Figure 53.2 Relationship between the Governing Vessel, Will-power and Mind

the Mind. Of course, this ability to accommodate two opposing realities as both 'true' is in the very nature and essence of Chinese medicine. The Mind is indeed housed in the Heart and it depends on Heart-Blood for its nourishment, but it also resides in the Brain and originates from the Prenatal Essence. It follows, therefore, that in order to 'strengthen' the Mind, it is necessary to treat both the Heart and the Kidneys. For example, in depression, it is often necessary to tonify both the Kidneys and the Heart.

By its very nature and because of its pathway (its ascending branch flowing '*past the heart*'), the Governing Vessel can strengthen the Mind by strengthening the three structures which affect the Mind, i.e. the Kidneys (and therefore Will-power), the Heart and the Brain. Cheng Xing Gan says: '*When Marrow is full thinking is clear. Too much thinking leads to Heart-Fire which burns the brain causing dizziness, blurred vision, tinnitus ... The Marrow is rooted in the Essence and connects downwards with the Governing Vessel: when the Gate of Vitality warms and nourishes, the Marrow is full.*'

> **Clinical note**
>
> Du-14 Dazhui with direct moxa tonifies both Kidney- and Heart-Yang and therefore strengthens the Will-power (*Zhi*) and the Mind (*Shen*)

Thus, the *Du Mai* has a strong influence on the mental–emotional state because it is the channel connection between the Kidneys, Heart and Brain: one could therefore say that it influences the Mind in two ways (Western and Chinese): through the Kidneys (the Essence as the basis of the Three Treasures), the Heart (residence of the Mind) and Brain (residence of the Mind according to some ancient Chinese doctors, notably Li Shi Zhen and Wang Qing Ren).

Due to its relation with the Kidneys, Heart and Brain, the Governing Vessel is clinically often used for depression and I certainly use it in this way. The most frequently used points for depression are (in combination with the opening and coupled points, i.e. S.I.-3 and BL-62):

- *Du-24*: calms the Mind and stimulates memory
- *Du-20*: lifts mood, stimulates memory and opens the Mind's orifices
- *Du-14*: lifts mood, tonifies the Heart, stimulates the rising of clear Qi

I use these points often in conjunction with Directing Vessel's points (to balance Yin–Yang) such as:

- *Ren-15*: calms the Mind, relaxes the chest, settles the Corporeal Soul, and is a very useful point for most emotional problems

Finally, many Governing Vessel's points have mental–emotional indications, which are reported below. Please note that I translate '*dian-kuang*' as 'manic depression', a modern term. *Dian Kuang* indicates a mental illness characterized by two alternating states of depression and almost stupor and manic behaviour.

- *Du-27 Duiduan*: manic depression
- *Du-26 Renzhong*: manic depression, inappropriate laughter, unexpected laughter or crying
- *Du-24 Shenting*: manic depression, ascends to high places and sings, discards clothing and runs around
- *Du-23 Shangxing*: manic depression
- *Du-22 Xinhui*: somnolence, fright palpitations
- *Du-20 Baihui*: agitation and oppression, fright palpitations, disorientation, crying, sadness and crying with desire to die, mania
- *Du-19 Houding*: mad walking, insomnia
- *Du-18 Qiangjian*: mad walking, insomnia, manic depression
- *Du-17 Naohu*: mania
- *Du-16 Fengfu*: mania, incessant talking, mad walking, desire to commit suicide, sadness, fear with palpitations
- *Du-13 Taodao*: unhappiness, disorientation
- *Du-12 Shenzhu*: mad walking, delirious raving, seeing ghosts, rage with desire to kill people
- *Du-11 Shendao*: sadness, anxiety, fright palpitations, disorientation, timidity
- *Du-8 Jinsuo*: mania, mad walking, incessant talking, anger injuring the Liver
- *Du-4 Mingmen*: fear, fright
- *Du-1 Changqiang*: mania, mad walking

Expels exterior Wind

In attacks of exterior Wind, the Governing Vessel can be used to release the Exterior and expel Wind at the Greater Yang stage of the Six Stages. It is therefore used for such symptoms as aversion to cold, fever, runny nose, headache, stiff neck and a Floating pulse. The points to use are the opening and coupled points (S.I.-3 and BL.-62) and Du-16 Fengfu.

The Governing Vessel can also be used to treat intermittent fevers and cases of residual Heat where the pathogenic factors are not completely expelled. A typical example of this condition is postviral fatigue syndrome. In these cases, the points Du-13 Taodao and Du-14 Dazhui are indicated.

Extinguishes interior Wind

In conditions of interior Wind, the Governing Vessel can be used to extinguish interior Wind, for such symptoms as dizziness, tremors, convulsions, epilepsy, or for the sequelae of Wind-stroke. The points to use are the opening and coupled points (S.I.-3 and BL-62) together with Du-16 Fengfu and Du-20 Baihui.

Box 53.2 summarizes the clinical applications of the Governing Vessel.

Box 53.2 Clinical applications of the Governing Vessel

- Tonify Kidney-Yang
- Strengthen the back
- Nourish the Brain and Marrow
- Strengthen the Mind
- Expel exterior Wind
- Extinguish interior Wind

Classical indications

Chapter 60 of the 'Simple Questions' gives the following symptoms for the Governing Vessel: '*Qi rises from the lower abdomen causing heart pain, retention of urine and faeces and hernia. In women, it causes infertility, haemorrhoids, incontinence of urine and a dry throat.*'[9] This passage is interesting as it relates abdominal symptoms to the Governing rather than the Directing or Penetrating Vessel: such symptoms are obviously related to the abdominal branch of the Governing Vessel described above.

The 'Classic of Difficulties' says: '*When the Governing Vessel is diseased there is stiffness of the spine and fainting.*'[10] Li Shi Zhen says: '*When the Governing Vessel is full there is rigidity of the back which is bent backwards ... when it is empty there is a feeling of heaviness of the head and shaking of the head.*'[11] This passage from Li Shi Zhen clearly refers to a condition of internal Wind of the Governing Vessel.

The 'Golden Mirror of Medicine' (Yi Zong Jin Jian, 1742) gives the following clinical manifestations for the Governing Vessel: '*Contraction of the hands and feet, tremors of limbs, aphasia from Wind-stroke, epilepsy, headache, eye swelling with discharge, chronic backache and knee ache, occipital stiffness from unresolved invasion of Wind-Cold, toothache, numbness of limbs, night-sweating.*'[12]

According to the 'Pulse Classic', diseases of the Governing Vessel include mania in adults and epilepsy in children, for which one must moxa Du-20 Baihui. It says: '*If the pulse is floating on all three positions and beating straight up and down, it indicates [a pathology of] the Governing Vessel. In this case there is stiffness and pain of the back with inability to bend forwards or backwards. In adults there is mania, in children epilepsy.*'[13]

Box 53.3 summarizes classical indications for the Governing Vessel.

Box 53.3 Classical indications for the Governing Vessel

- *Simple Questions*: heart pain, retention of urine and faeces and hernia, infertility, haemorrhoids, incontinence of urine and a dry throat
- *Classic of Difficulties*: stiffness of the spine and fainting
- *Li Shi Zhen*: when full there is rigidity of the back, which is bent backwards; when empty there is a feeling of heaviness of the head and shaking of the head
- *Golden Mirror of Medicine*: contraction of the hands and feet, tremors of limbs, aphasia from Wind-stroke, epilepsy, headache, eye swelling with discharge, chronic backache and knee ache, occipital stiffness from unresolved invasion of Wind-Cold, toothache, numbness of limbs, night sweating
- *Pulse Classic*: stiffness and pain of the back with inability to bend forwards or backwards. In adults there is mania, in children epilepsy

---

Herbal therapy

Herbs

Lu Rong *Cornu Cervi parvum* enters the Governing Vessel, generates Essence, nourishes Marrow and Blood, benefits Yang and strengthens sinews and bones. Also the marrow of goat and beef strengthens the Governing Vessel (Li Shi Zhen also includes dog meat as strengthening the Governing Vessel).

Qiang Huo *Radix et Rhizoma Notopterygii*, Du Huo *Radix Angelicae pubescentis*, Fang Feng *Radix Ledebouriellae sesloidis*, Jing Jie *Herba seu Flos Schizonepetae tenuifoliae*, Xi Xin *Herba Asari cum radice*, Gao Ben *Rhizoma et Radix Ligustici sinensis*, Cang Er Zi *Fructus Xanthii*, Huang Lian *Rhizoma Coptidis*, Da Huang *Rhizoma Rhei*, Fu Zi *Radix Aconiti carmichaeli praeparata*, Wu Tou *Radix Aconiti carmichaeli*.

Formulae

Not given by Li Shi Zhen but any Kidney-Yang tonic containing one or more of the above herbs enters the Governing Vessel.

DIRECTING VESSEL (REN MAI)

Opening point: LU-7 Lieque.
Coupled point: KI-6 Zhaohai.
Starting point: Ren-1 Huiyin.
Connecting point: Ren-15 Jiuwei.
Area of body influenced: genitals, abdomen, thorax, lungs, throat, face.

The Directing vessel is called the 'Sea of the Yin channels' as it exerts an influence on all the Yin channels of the body. It originates from the space between the Kidneys (like the Governing and Penetrating Vessels) and flows through the uterus down to Ren-1 Huiyin, where the superficial pathway starts. The Directing Vessel is of paramount importance for the reproductive system of both men and women, but particularly women, as it regulates puberty, menstruation, fertility, conception, pregnancy, childbirth and menopause (Fig. 53.3).

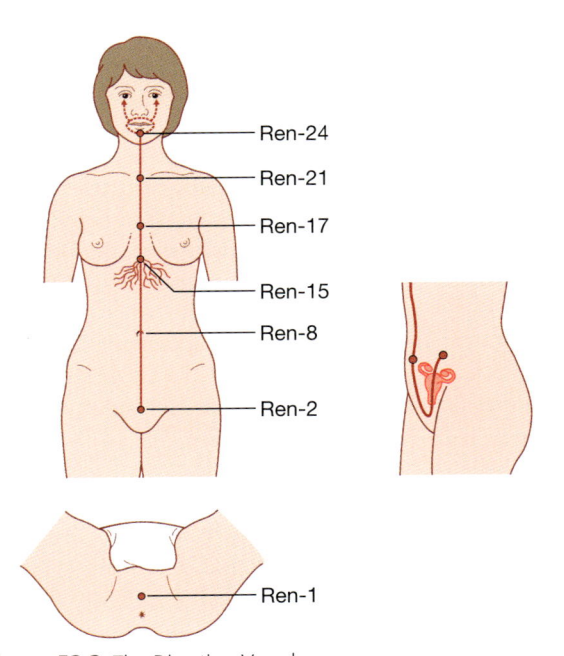

Figure 53.3 The Directing Vessel

Pathway

Chapter 60 of the 'Simple Questions' describes the pathway of the Directing Vessel (Ren Mai): *'The Directing Vessel starts below the point Ren-3 Zhongji. It then comes up to edge of the hair (superior edge of pubic bone), it enters the abdomen and reaches Ren-4 Guanyuan. It then goes up to the throat, circles around the chin, reaches the face and enters the eyes.'*[14]

It is worth reporting the more detailed pathway described by Li Shi Zhen: *'The Directing Vessel starts inside the abdomen below Ren-3 Zhongji, it rises up and comes to the surface at Ren-2 Qugu, up towards the edge of the hair at Ren-3 Zhongji, it moves in the abdomen connecting with Liver, Spleen and Kidneys [channels], then up to Ren-4 Guanyuan and to Ren-5 Shimen and Ren-6 Qihai. It then meets the Liver and Penetrating Vessel at Ren-7 Yinjiao. Then it reaches Ren-8 Shenque, Ren-9 Shuifen and Ren-10 Xiawan where it connects with the Spleen channel. It rises up to Ren-11 Jianli and Ren-12 Zhongwan where it meets the Small Intestine, Triple Burner and Stomach channels. Then it goes to Ren-13 Shangwan, Ren-14 Juque, Ren-15 Jiuwei, Ren-17 Shanzhong, Ren-22 Tiantu and Ren-23 Lianquan where it meets the Yin Linking Vessel (Yin Wei Mai). Then it travels up to the chin to Ren-24 Chengjiang where it meets the Governing Vessel and the Stomach and Large Intestine channel. Then it circles around the lips and inside the mouth, it divides and goes up to ST-1 Chengqi where it ends.'*[15]

The same passage from Li Shi Zhen describes the pathway of the Connecting channel of the Directing Vessel: *'The Connecting channel of the Directing Vessel separates from Ren-15 Jiuwei and it spreads over the abdomen.'*[16]

Box 53.4 summarizes the pathway of the Directing Vessel.

> **Box 53.4 Directing Vessel – summary of pathway**
>
> - It starts inside the lower abdomen between the kidneys, it flows through the uterus and emerges at the perineum
> - From the perineum, it rises up the abdomen on the midline
> - It connects with the Penetrating Vessel at Ren-4 Guanyuan and Ren-7 Yinjiao
> - It travels up the centre of the chest, throat, chin and face
> - It circles around the lips and inside the mouth, it divides and it enters the eyes ending at ST-1 Chengqi
> - The Connecting channel of the Directing Vessel separates from Ren-15 Jiuwei and it spreads over the abdomen

Clinical applications

Nourishes Yin

The Directing Vessel can be used to nourish all the Yin of the body. Its name establishes a correspondence and symmetry with the Governing Vessel as the latter 'governs' all the Yang and the former 'directs' all the Yin.

In this context it is particularly useful to nourish Yin in women after menopause as the Directing Vessel controls the Uterus and determines the 7-year life cycles of women. It can therefore regulate the energy of the reproductive system and, after the menopause, nourish Blood and Yin to reduce the effects of Empty-Heat symptoms deriving from Yin deficiency.

It can therefore be used for such symptoms as night sweating, hot flushes, feeling of heat, mental restlessness, anxiety, dry mouth at night, dizziness, tinnitus or insomnia, all symptoms of Kidney-Yin deficiency with Empty-Heat. When used in this way, the opening and coupled points (LU-7 Lieque and KI-6 Zhaohai) are best combined with Ren-4 Guanyuan.

Regulates the Uterus and Blood

The Directing Vessel regulates the Uterus and Blood in women, so that it is responsible for puberty, menstruation, fertility, conception, pregnancy, childbirth and menopause. It can be used for infertility to promote the supply of Blood to the Uterus and in many menstrual disorders such as amenorrhoea, menorrhagia, metrorrhagia and irregular periods.

Moves Qi in the Lower Burner and Uterus

The Directing Vessel moves Qi in the Lower Burner and Uterus so that it can be used for abdominal masses but especially those deriving from Qi stagnation rather than Blood stasis. In men, it is used for hernia. Chapter 29 the 'Classic of Difficulties' says: *'The Directing Vessel's diseases consist in internal stagnation which, in men, can give rise to the 7 kinds of hernia*[17] *and, in women, to abdominal masses [from Qi stagnation, i.e. jia and ju].'*[18]

In general, the Directing Vessel is used in cases of gynaecological problems due to stagnation of Qi. In these cases one must use the opening and coupled points to move Qi (LU-7 and KI-6). The Qi-moving action of these two points is also due to their intrinsic nature as LU-7 Lieque promotes the downward flow of Lung-Qi towards the Kidneys. This point provides a powerful stimulation and movement of Qi, which in turn moves Blood. The coupled point KI-6 Zhaohai tonifies the Yin and has a strong upward-flowing movement; hence the use of both points sets the Qi in motion like a wheel and resolves stagnation, especially when they are used unilaterally and crossed over.

Promotes the descending of Lung-Qi and the Kidneys' receiving of Qi

The sphere of action of the Directing Vessel extends not only to the Lower Burner but also the Middle and Upper Burner. It can in fact also be used to stimulate the descending of Lung-Qi and the Kidneys' receiving of Qi. For this reason, it is used for chronic asthma with its opening and coupled points (LU-7 and KI-6) together with Ren-17 Shanzhong.

Promotes the transformation, transportation and excretion of fluids

The Directing Vessel is very important for the correct distribution of fluids in the abdomen; hence it can be used in oedema and urinary problems. Oedema is usually caused by:

- The Lungs not descending Qi and transforming fluids.
- Spleen-Yang not moving fluids.
- Kidney-Yang not moving, transforming and excreting fluids.

By using the Directing Vessel we can send the Qi down by using LU-7 Lieque and stimulate the Kidneys by using KI-6 Zhaohai, together with points such as Ren-9 Shuifen and Ren-5 Shimen.

The use of LU-7 Lieque in the context of the Directing Vessel also stimulates the Bladder to excrete fluids. This reflects the very close relationship between the Lungs and the Bladder. For this reason, the Directing Vessel is frequently used for urinary problems in women from stagnation in the Lower Burner or Qi sinking. To affect urination, use the opening and coupled points of the Directing Vessel (LU-7 and KI-6) together Ren-3 Zhongji coupled with Du-20 Baihui for sinking of Qi or Du-26 Renzhong for Qi stagnation.

Activates the Triple Burner

Many points on the Directing Vessel can be used to activate the Triple Burner: Ren-17 Shanzhong for the Upper Burner, Ren-12 Zhongwan and Ren-9 Shuifen for the Middle Burner and Ren-6 Qihai, Ren-5 Shimen and Ren-3 Zhongji for the Lower Burner.

The points of the Directing Vessel are also important to regulate the metabolism of fluids and the entering/exiting and ascending/descending of Qi.

Controls Fat Tissue and Membranes (*Gao* and *Huang*)

Some of the Directing Vessel's points are related to Fat Tissue (*Gao*) and Membranes (*Huang*). Chapter 1 of the 'Spiritual Axis' mentions the Source points as being the following:

- P-7 Daling for the Heart
- LU-9 Taiyuan for the Lungs
- KI-3 Taixi for the Kidneys
- SP-3 Taibai for the Spleen
- LIV-3 Taichong for the Liver
- Ren-15 Jiuwei for Fat Tissue (*Gao*)
- Ren-6 Qihai for Membranes (*Huang*)

The 'Spiritual Axis' says literally: '*The Source of Gao comes out at Jiuwei, one point. The Source of Huang comes out at Boyang, one point.*'[19] All Chinese books and dictionaries say that *Boyang* is Ren-6 Qihai, but some think it is Ren-8 Shenque. However, note that an alternative name for Ren-6 Qihai is 'Xia Huang' (i.e. 'Lower Membranes').

'*Gao*' literally means 'fat' and some people say it refers to adipose tissue. '*Huang*' literally means 'membranes' and some people say it refers to other types of connective tissues such as the fascia (superficial and deep), the mesenterium and omentum and the stroma encapsulating the organs.

Thus, *Gao* and *Huang* represent a whole range of connective tissue, including adipose tissue, superficial and deep fascia, peritoneum, mesentery, omentum, stroma, etc. They cover the whole body with a layer immediately below the skin and an inner layer wrapping and anchoring the organs, muscles and bones.

In particular, the Membranes have three functions: they *anchor* the organs, they *connect* the organ among themselves and they *wrap* the organs. The 'Classic of Categories' says: '*The Membranes [Huang] are in between the abdominal cavities and the muscle patterns [Li as in Cou Li], they extend up and down in the crevices.*'[20] In this statement, the term *Li* is the same as in *Cou Li*, the former indicating the body cavities, the latter meaning 'patterns': in this case, 'muscle patterns' (*rou li*) simply indicates the muscle fibres.

With reference to the two points Ren-15 and Ren-6 (or Ren-8), these are the Source points of Fat Tissue and Membranes, which means that these points and the whole Directing Vessel on the abdomen are embryologically related to the development of connective tissue. Using these points can therefore act at a deep energetic level to regulate and equalize tensions and weaknesses in the 'membranes' of the abdomen and thorax.

Bearing in mind that the superficial fascia are thinnest on the Yang surfaces and extremities and thickest on Yin surfaces, the Membranes acquire particular importance in the abdomen: the Directing Vessel gives us a way to act on the deeper fascia of abdomen and thorax, while the Five Transporting (*Shu*) points in arms and legs act more on the head, neck and limbs themselves. In other words, again, the extraordinary vessels perform a function of *integration* of various structures into the channel system.[21]

Thus, from this point of view, the extraordinary vessels present an additional component to Chinese medical anatomy integrating the vast structure of connective tissue with the Internal Organs and channels. We are used to considering Chinese medicine, with its concept of Qi, as emphasizing function to the detriment of structure, and we are used to thinking of channels through which Qi flow to organs. The system seen in this way is rather theoretical and unrealistic and excessively abstract. The ancient Chinese did consider structure as well as function and they did not overlook the vast network and connections provided by the connective tissue in between organs. From this point of view, this confirms the extraordinary vessels' function of *regulating* and *integrating* various structures and energies with the channels and Internal Organs system.

Box 53.5 summarizes the Membranes (*Huang*).

Box 53.5 The Membranes (*Huang*)

- The Membranes *anchor* the organs, *connect* the organs and *wrap* the organs
- They fill the spaces, especially in the abdominal cavity, between the organs and the muscles
- They correspond to the connective tissues of the abdomen, e.g. fascia, mesenterium, omentum, stroma
- Ren-6 Qihai is the Source point of the Membranes
- The Directing and Penetrating Vessels influence the Membranes
- Membranes are subject to stagnation, manifesting often in a Penetrating Vessel's pathology

Combination of Governing and Directing Vessels' points

As discussed above, the Governing and Directing Vessels are like two branches of one channel, one Yang the other Yin, both originating from the same place and both flowing to the Heart. They could really be seen as one channel. Therefore, balancing points from the Governing and Directing Vessels is a very important aspect of Yin–Yang and Back–Front balancing and a very effective treatment in practice.

Finally, as these two vessels both flow upwards to the head and the Governing Vessel flows into the brain, combining their points also has a very powerful and important mental effect that can be either excitatory or calming.

The following are examples of combination of points from the Governing and Directing Vessels:

- *Du-19 Houding* and *Ren-15 Jiuwei* to calm the Mind. Du-19 calms the Mind and extinguishes (internal) Wind while Ren-15 calms the Mind and nourishes the Heart. This combination has a powerful calming effect as Ren-15 nourishes and Du-19 calms. Ren-15 will also relieve anxiety manifesting with a feeling of oppression in the chest
- *Du-20 Baihui* and *Ren-15 Jiuwei* to calm the Mind and lift mood. This combination can simultaneously calm the Mind with Ren-15 and improve the mood and lift depression with Du-20. It is an excellent combination for mental depression with anxiety
- *Du-14 Dazhui* and *Ren-4 Guanyuan*, both with direct moxa cones, to tonify and warm Yang. Du-14, with moxa, warms all the Yang channels and the Bladder, while Ren-4, with moxa, tonifies and warms Kidney-Yang which is the foundation for all the Yang energies of the body. Thus this combination tonifies the Bladder and Kidney-Yang and Yang Qi in general
- *Du-16 Fengfu* and *Ren-24 Chengjiang* to treat occipital headache[22]
- *Du-20 Baihui* and *Ren-12 Zhongwan* to tonify the Stomach and Spleen and lift mood. This combination is good to lift depression occurring against a background of deficiency of Stomach and Spleen
- *Du-24 Shenting* and *Ren-4 Guanyuan* to nourish the Kidneys, strengthen the Original Qi and calm the Mind. This combination calms the Mind by nourishing Kidney-Yin and strengthening the Original Qi. It is suitable for severe anxiety occurring against a background of Kidney-Yin deficiency. It is particularly indicated for anxiety as it roots Qi in the Lower Burner and draws it downwards away from the head and the Heart where it harasses the Mind
- *Yintang* and *Ren-4 Guanyuan* to calm the Mind and nourish the Kidneys: this combination is similar to the previous one as it roots Qi in the Lower Burner by nourishing the Kidneys and strengthening the Original Qi. Whilst the previous combination is better for anxiety and worrying, this one is better for insomnia
- *Du-20 Baihui* and *Ren-4 Guanyuan* to calm the Mind, nourish the Kidneys, strengthen the Original Qi and lift mood. This combination lifts mood and relieves depression by nourishing Kidney-Yin and strengthening the Original Qi. It is suitable for depression and anxiety occurring against a background of Kidney-Yin deficiency
- *Du-20 Baihui* and *Ren-6 Qihai* to tonify and raise Qi. Ren-6 tonifies Qi in general while Du-20 raises Qi: the combination of these two points is excellent to tonify and raise Qi in case of prolapses or simply sinking of Qi. However, its use need not be confined to such conditions; it also has a powerful mood-lifting effect in depression

Box 53.6 summarizes clinical applications of the Directing Vessel.

Box 53.6 Clinical applications of the Directing Vessel

- Nourish Yin
- Regulate the Uterus
- Move Qi in the Lower Burner and Uterus
- Promote the descending of Lung-Qi and the Kidney's receiving of Qi
- Promote the transformation, transportation and excretion of fluids
- Activate the Triple Burner
- Control Fat Tissue and Membranes
- Combination of Directing and Governing Vessels' points

Classical indications

Chapter 29 of the 'Classic of Difficulties' says: '*The Directing Vessel's diseases consist in internal stagnation which, in men, can give rise to the 7 kinds of hernia*[23] *and, in women, to abdominal masses [from Qi stagnation, i.e. jia and ju].*'[24]

Chapter 60 of the 'Simple Questions' says similarly: '*Diseases of the Directing Vessel cause the 7 kinds of* hernia-type disorders [Shan] in men and abdominal masses [from Qi stagnation] in women [Jia and Ju].'[25]

The 'Pulse Classic' says: 'If both Front-position pulses feel like small pellets, this is a Directing Vessel's pulse. This causes finger-shaped accumulations of Qi in the abdomen which may surge up towards the heart. There will be inability to bend the body and rigidity. If the pulse feels Tight, Fine, Full and Long up to the Middle Position, it is a Directing Vessel's pulse. There will be umbilical pain radiating downwards to the pubic bone and a severe pain in the genitals.'[26]

The 'Golden Mirror of Medicine' (Yi Zong Jin Jian, 1742) gives the following clinical manifestations for the Directing Vessel: 'Haemorrhoids, swelling of the anus, dysentery, coughing of sputum with blood, toothache, swollen throat, difficult urination, chest and abdominal pain, difficulty in swallowing with choking sensation, aphasia after labour, backache, cold abdomen, dead fetus that cannot be expelled with Qi rising to the diaphragm.'[27]

Li Shi Zhen gives the indications of the Connecting channel of the Directing Vessel: 'When the Connecting channel of the Directing Vessel is full there is pain on the skin of the abdomen; when it is empty there is itching over the abdomen.'[28]

The 'Classic of Categories' says: 'Diseases of the Directing Vessel include the 7 types of hernial disorders in men [shan] and leukorrhoea and abdominal masses [from Qi stagnation, i.e. jia ju] in women ... it is white-red leukorrhoea. These are abdominal masses of the jia type [as in zheng-jia] and of the ju type [as in ji ju].'[29] Zhang Jing Yue therefore clarifies specifically that the abdominal masses in a Directing Vessel's pathology are of the non-substantial type from Qi stagnation. In fact, there are two terms to indicate 'abdominal masses', Zheng-Jia and Ji-Ju, in which 'zheng' and 'ji' indicate actual, fixed masses (from Blood stasis, which I call 'Blood Masses'), and 'jia' and 'ju' indicate non-substantial abdominal masses that come and go (from Qi stagnation, which I call 'Qi Masses'). Generally, Zheng-Jia refers to abdominal masses in gynaecological conditions, whereas Ji-Ju occur in both men and women.

Box 53.7 summarizes classical indications for the Directing Vessel.

Herbal therapy

Herbs

Gui Ban *Plastrum Testudinis*. Ye Tian Shi mentions: Bie Jia *Carapax Trionycis*, E Jiao *Gelatinum Corii Asini*, Zhi Mu *Radix Anemarrhenae asphodeloidis*, Huang Bo *Cortex Phellodendri*, Xuan Shen *Radix Scrophulariae ningpoensis* and Sheng Di *Radix Rehmanniae glutinosae* (i.e. herbs which subdue Empty-Heat).

Formulae

Da Bu Yin Wan *Great Tonifying Yin Pill*.

Case history 53.1

A man of 37 suffered from chronic asthma characterized by difficulty in inhalation. There was no sputum and he felt very tired generally. His voice was low and his complexion pale, he also had a lower backache and felt cold. His pulse was Deep and Weak and his tongue was Pale. These manifestations clearly point to deficient Kidney-Yang being unable to hold Qi, resulting in asthma. Besides this, there was also a Lung-Qi deficiency as evidenced by the low voice and pale complexion.

The opening and coupled points of the Directing Vessel (LU-7 Lieque on the left and KI-6 Zhaohai on the right) were used to tonify the Lungs and to stimulate the descending of Lung-Qi and the Kidney function of reception of Qi.

Box 53.7 Classical indications for the Directing Vessel

- *Classic of Difficulties*: internal stagnation, which, in men, can give rise to the seven kinds of hernia and, in women, to abdominal masses (from Qi stagnation, i.e. jia and ju)
- *Simple Questions*: seven kinds of hernia-type disorders (Shan) in men and abdominal masses (from Qi stagnation) in women
- *Pulse Classic*: finger-shaped accumulations of Qi in the abdomen which may surge up towards the heart, inability to bend the body and rigidity, umbilical pain radiating downwards to the pubic bone and severe pain in the genitals
- *Golden Mirror of Medicine*: haemorrhoids, swelling of the anus, dysentery, coughing of sputum with blood, toothache, swollen throat, difficult urination, chest and abdominal pain, difficulty in swallowing with choking sensation, aphasia after labour, backache, cold abdomen, dead fetus that cannot be expelled with Qi rising to the diaphragm
- *Classic of Categories*: seven types of hernial disorders in men (Shan) and leukorrhoea and abdominal masses in women, white-red leukorrhoea.

Case history 53.2

A woman of 41 had a large fibroid in the uterus for several years. Her periods were very heavy and painful and the menstrual blood was dark. Her lower abdomen was extremely hard and the fibroid was clearly felt on palpation.

She was treated several times using the opening and coupled points of the Directing Vessel, producing a complete normalization of her periods and a very marked softening of her lower abdomen. The size of the abdominal swelling was also markedly reduced. Obviously a fibroid of that size cannot be dissolved, but the use of the Directing Vessel at least normalized her periods, took the menstrual pain away and made her lower abdomen much more comfortable.

PENETRATING VESSEL (*CHONG MAI*)

Opening point: SP-4 Gongsun.
Coupled point: P-6 Neiguan.
Starting point: Ren-1 Huiyin.
Area of body influenced: feet, medial aspect of legs, uterus, lumbar spine, abdomen, chest, heart, throat, face, head.

The Penetrating Vessel is very complex as it has many different functions at different levels. In a way, it could be considered to be the origin of the other extraordinary vessels (excluding Governing and Directing Vessels) as it originates in between the Kidneys and spreads its Qi all over the abdomen and chest and all over the body at the Defensive Qi level. When this energy arrives at the relevant starting points, it gives rise to the Yin and Yang Linking Vessels, the Yin and Yang Stepping Vessels and the Girdle Vessel.

In modern Chinese, the word '*chong*' means to 'infuse', 'charge, rush, dash' but also 'thoroughfare, important place'. Chinese books say that, in the context of the *Chong Mai*, *chong* has also the meaning of *jie* ('streets'), *dong* ('activity, movement'), *xing* ('movement') and *tong* ('free passage'). All these words and the attributes they represent apply to the Penetrating Vessel and it is difficult to choose a single English name for it. I chose the word 'penetrating' as it combines the idea of 'rushing' with that of 'streets, channels' that 'penetrate' the body. The idea of 'penetrating' is also related to the penetration of Membranes (*Huang*) and channels by the Penetrating Vessel.

The Penetrating Vessel is described as the 'Sea of the five Yin and six Yang Organs', the 'Sea of the 12 channels' and the 'Sea of Blood'. It is described as the Sea of the five Yin and six Yang Organs as it is a fundamental vessel which connects the Pre-Heaven and the Post-Heaven Qi, due to its connection with Kidneys and Stomach. It is connected to the Kidneys as it originates in that area and it distributes Essence all over the body; it is connected to the Stomach as it passes through the point ST-30 Qichong which is a point for the Sea of Food.

Furthermore, the Penetrating Vessel is connected to the Spleen, Liver and Kidney channels along which it flows on the inner aspect of the leg, down to the big toe.

It is called the 'Sea of the 12 channels' because it branches out in many small capillary-like vessels that circulate Defensive Qi over the abdomen and chest. It is called the 'Sea of Blood' because it is related to the Blood in the Uterus and because it controls all the Blood Connecting channels (see below).

Bearing in mind the comparison of the Eight Extraordinary Vessels to a family group, discussed above, the Penetrating Vessel is the 'father' within this group and therefore the most important member, the centre of the family nucleus and the beginning of the family (Fig. 53.4).

Pathway

Chapter 60 of the 'Simple Questions' describes the pathway of the Penetrating Vessel briefly: '*The Penetrating Vessel starts at ST-30 Qichong [in this text called its alternative name of Qijie], close to the Kidney channel, it goes up both sides of the umbilicus to disperse into the chest.*'[30] Chapter 39 of the 'Simple Questions' says: '*The Penetrating Vessel starts at Ren-4 Guanyuan.*'[31]

Chapter 28 of the 'Classic of Difficulties' describes the pathway of the Penetrating Vessel briefly as: '*The Penetrating Vessel starts at ST-30 Qichong [here called with its alternative name of Qijie] and rises parallel to the Stomach channel, surrounds the umbilicus and then disperses inside the chest.*'[32]

Chapter 38 of the 'Spiritual Axis' has a more detailed description of the Penetrating Vessel's pathway: '*The Penetrating Vessel is the Sea of the five Yin and six Yang Organs, it rises up to the neck and chin oozing into the Yang and irrigating the Essence. Then it goes down pouring into the Great Connecting channel of the Kidneys, exits at*

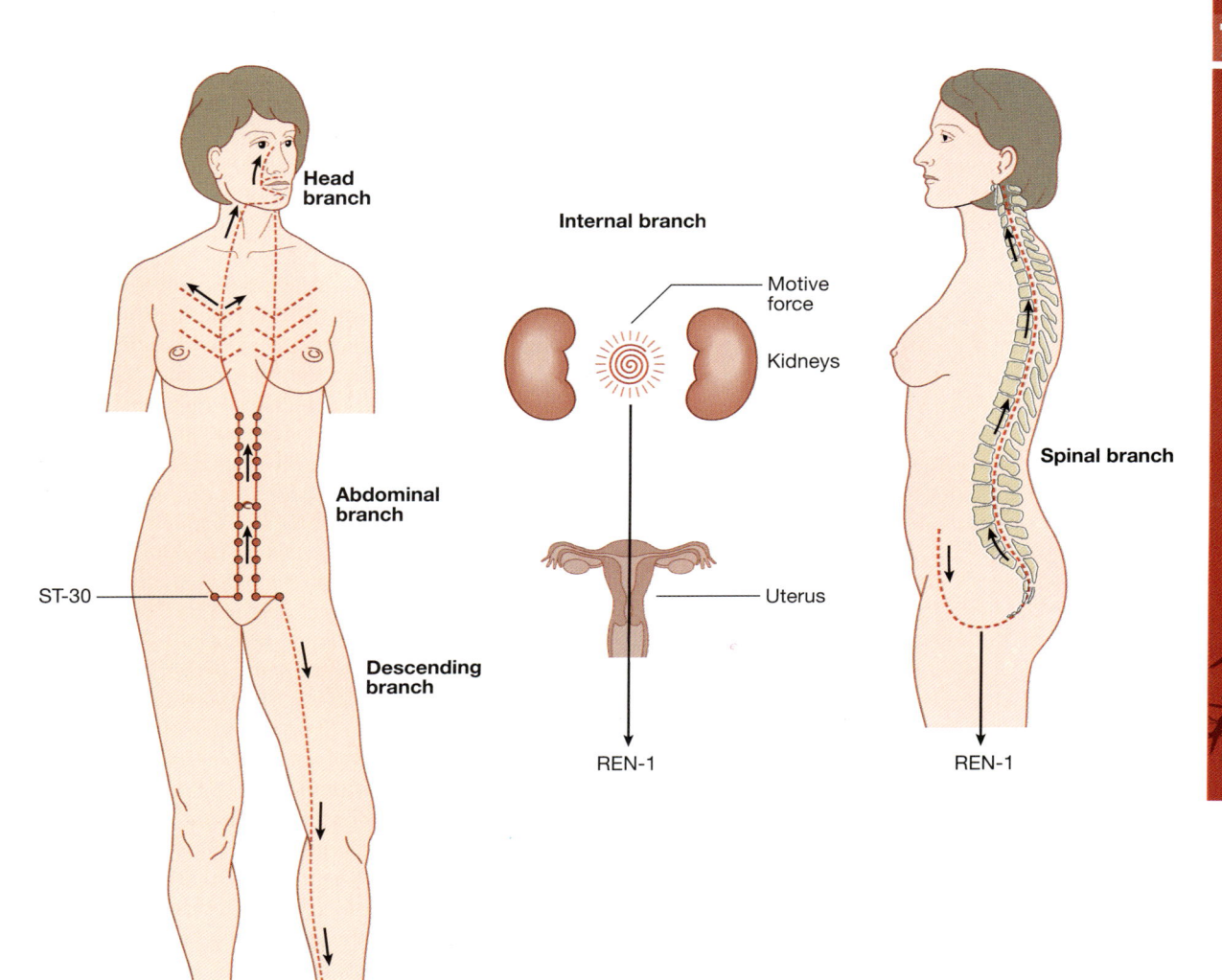

Figure 53.4 The Penetrating Vessel

ST-30 Qichong [in this text called with its alternative name of Qijie]. It goes down the thigh, entering behind the knee, then down along the bone of the leg on the medial side to reach the internal malleolus where it separates. One branch runs alongside the Kidney channel oozing into the three Yin; another branch comes up the dorsum of the foot and then down to the space between the first and second toe oozing into the Connecting channels and warming the muscles.'[33]

The 'Classic of Categories' confirms that Qijie is indeed ST-30 Qichong: *'The Penetrating Vessel starts at Qijie, it connects with the Kidney channel, it rises up the abdomen either side of the umbilicus, it reaches the chest where it disperses. "Starts" indicates that the vessel emerges towards the surface at this point, not that it originates from that point. Qijie is Qichong [ST-30], a point of the Stomach channel on either side of the pubic bone. It goes to KI-11 Henggu, KI-12 Dahe, etc. in total [along] 11 points [therefore up to KI-21 Youmen].'*[34]

Chapter 62 of the 'Spiritual Axis' gives a similar and slightly abbreviated pathway: *'The Penetrating Vessel is the Sea of the 12 Channels and the Great Connecting* channel of the Kidneys. It originates below the kidneys and surfaces at ST-30 Qichong. It then goes down the inside of the thigh to behind the knee, down inside the lower leg bone along the Kidney channel to reach the internal malleolus where it divides. One branch goes down to the Kidney channel, the other to the dorsum of the foot and then down to the area between the first and second toe, where it pours in the Connecting channels keeping the lower leg warm.'[35]

The 'Classic of Categories' gives a more detailed description of the descending branch of the Penetrating Vessel: '*Another branch descends connecting with the Great Connecting channel of the Kidneys, it emerges at ST-30 Qichong, it descends along the inner thigh, enters the back of the knee, it goes down along the inner aspect of the tibia, to reach the internal malleolus where it divides. One branch goes down to connect with the Kidney channel, pouring into the three Yin; another branch goes to the arch of the foot and then to the space in between the big toe, pouring into the Connecting channels and warming the muscles. When the Connecting channels [in the foot] stagnate, the arch [of the foot] cannot be lifted and it becomes cold.*'[36]

Although the texts do not specifically name the point between the first and second toe, it is generally accepted that this is LIV-3 Taichong. Indeed, the *chong* in the name for LIV-3 *Taichong* is the same character as *chong* in *Chong Mai*. This is also confirmed by the statement in chapter 1 of the 'Spiritual Axis' that describes the 7- and 8-year life cycles of men and women. Where it says that at 14 in girls the 'Penetrating Vessel is flourishing', the actual expression used is not 'Penetrating Vessel' but '*Taichong Vessel*': that is, the 'LIV-3 Vessel'.

Chapter 65 of the 'Spiritual Axis' describes the spinal branch of the Penetrating Vessel: '*The Penetrating and Directing Vessels originate inside the uterus, a branch rises up the front of the spine making the Sea of the Channels. The branch that runs up the surface of the abdomen rises only up the right side and then reunites [with the Directing Vessel] at the throat; then it separates and circles around the lips.*' This passage is important as it mentions the spinal branch of the Penetrating Vessel in the lumbar spine. It is, however, also an intriguing passage as it is the only one that mentions an abdominal branch of the Penetrating Vessel that rises up only on the right side.

The 'ABC of Acupuncture' (*Zhen Jiu Jia Yi Jing*, AD 282) says: '*The Penetrating Vessel starts at ST-30 Qichong and joins the Kidney channel to flow up to the umbilicus and then to the chest where it disperses.*'[37] In another passage it says: '*The Penetrating and Directing Vessels start from the uterus, rise up inside the spine, they are the Sea of the Channels. [The Penetrating Vessel] rises up the surface of the abdomen, reaches the throat and then encircles the mouth.*'[38] This passage seems to imply that both the Penetrating and Directing Vessels rise up inside the spine.

The 'Elucidation of the Yellow's Emperor's Classic of Internal Medicine' (*Huang Di Nei Jing Tai Su*) by Yang Shang Shan of the Sui dynasty (581-618) highlights the connection between the Penetrating Vessel, the Motive Force (*Dong Qi*) in the Lower *Dan Tian* and the Sea of Blood: '*Below the umbilicus and in between the kidneys is the Moving Qi [or Motive Force, Dong Qi] which is the source of human life: it is the root of the 12 channels. The Sea of Blood is the Penetrating Vessel which is [also] the Sea of the five Yin and six Yang Organs and the Sea of the 12 Channels: it oozes into the Yang and irrigates the Essence and it therefore reaches all the Yin and Yang Organs. The Moving Qi below the umbilicus is in the Uterus. The Penetrating Vessel starts in the Uterus and it is the Sea of the Channels. We therefore know that the Penetrating Vessel creates life through the Moving Qi. The Penetrating Vessel moves up and down and, in its downward movement it connects with the Great Connecting channel of the Kidneys: therefore this downward movement [of Kidney-Qi] is not the Kidney channel.*' As we can see, this commentary reiterates very clearly that the Qi of the Kidneys descends to the legs not through the Kidney channel but through the Penetrating Vessel.

When describing the pathway of the Penetrating Vessel, Li Shi Zhen specifies the points it goes through: '*The Penetrating Vessel is the Sea of the Channels and the Sea of Blood. It originates in the lower abdomen and inside the uterus together with the Directing Vessel. It then emerges at ST-30 Qichong between the Stomach and Kidney channel. It then flows up to KI-11 Henggu bilaterally and 5 fen from the midline. It then flow to KI-12 Dahe, KI-13 Qixue, KI-14 Siman, KI-15 Zhongzhu, KI-16 Huangshu, KI-17 Shangqu, KI-18 Shiguan, KI-19 Yindu, KI-20 Tonggu and KI-21 Youmen. It then disperses in the chest: in total 24 points.*'[39] This passage clearly implies that the Penetrating Vessel flows through the points of the Kidney channel only up to KI-21 Youmen, whereas some authors have it flow through all the Kidney channel points up to KI-27 Shufu.

Chapter 33 of the 'Spiritual Axis' discusses the Four Seas: the Sea of Food, Sea of Marrow, Sea of Qi and Sea of Blood. The Sea of Blood is identified with the Penetrating Vessel but confusingly in this passage it is called the 'Sea of the 12 Channels': *'The Penetrating Vessel is the Sea of the 12 Channels: its upper point is BL-11 Dashu and its lower points ST-37 Shanjuxu and ST-39 Xiajuxu.'*[40]

The 'Classic of Categories' has an interesting summary of the energetic sphere of action of the Penetrating Vessel and explains more in depth the meaning of this vessel's being the 'Sea of the 12 Channels': *'The Penetrating Vessel is the Sea of the 12 Channels, it goes upwards to connect with Bl-11 Dashu and downwards to connect with ST-37 Shangjuxu and ST-39 Xiajuxu. The Penetrating Vessel goes down to ST-30 Qichong and up to connect with the Kidney channel. It goes up the eyes and head and down to the feet; it goes to the back [in the lumbar spine] and to the front in the abdomen. It goes into the Interior in the rivers and valleys [the big and small muscles of the abdomen] and into Exterior in the skin and muscles. It therefore connects with both Yin and Yang and both Interior and Exterior...100 diseases originate from the Penetrating Vessel because it is the most 'penetrating' [of the channels]. It controls the Qi and Blood of the 12 Channels which nourish the whole body and for this reason it is called the Sea of the 5 Yin and 6 Yang Organs.'*[41]

Boxes 53.8 and 53.9 summarize, respectively, the pathway and the points of the Penetrating Vessel.

We can identify five distinct branches of the Penetrating Vessel's pathway, which I shall call:

1. Internal branch
2. Abdominal branch
3. Head branch
4. Spinal branch
5. Descending branch

The pathways of these branches therefore are as follows:

- *The internal branch*: originating inside the abdomen, flowing through the uterus, emerging at Ren-1 Huiyin. It descends to this point through the 'Great Connecting channel of the Kidneys', which is probably the Uterus Channel (*Bao Luo*) that connects the Uterus to the Kidneys
- *The abdominal branch*: emerging at ST-30 Qichong and flowing through all Kidney points up to KI-21 Youmen and dispersing in the chest
- *The head branch*: flowing over the throat, around the chin and into the eyes
- *The spinal branch*: ascending inside the lumbar spine from Ren-1 Huiyin
- *The descending branch:* descending from ST-30-Qichong along the inner aspect of the leg down to the big toe area

Box 53.8 Penetrating Vessel – summary of pathway

- *Internal branch*: originates inside the lower abdomen, flows through the uterus and emerges at the perineum at Ren-1 Huiyin
- *Abdominal branch*: it emerges at ST-30 Qichong, connects with the Kidney channel at KI-11 Henggu and ascends through the Kidney channel to KI-21 Youmen, then disperses in the chest and breasts
- *Head branch*: ascends alongside the throat, chin, curves around the lips and terminates below the eyes
- *Spinal branch*: emerges from Ren-1 Huiyin and ascends inside the lumbar spine to the level of BL-23 Shenshu
- *Descending branch*: emerges from ST-30 Qichong, it descends along the inner aspect of the thigh and lower leg to the internal malleolus. On the foot, at the heel it separates, one branch going to the arch to connect with the Kidney channel and another branch going to the big toe to connect with the Liver channel

Box 53.9 Points of the Penetrating Vessel

- Ren-1 Huiyin
- ST-30 Qichong
- All Kidney points from KI-11 Henggu to KI-21 Youmen

Clinical applications

The clinical applications of the Penetrating Vessel can be discussed from many different angles. I shall start by explaining briefly the clinical significance of its five branches, then that of its various names, and finally, its clinical applications according to patterns and diseases.

Clinical significance of the five branches of the Penetrating Vessel

The internal branch

The two most important aspects of this branch are that it arises inside the abdomen in between the Kidneys and that it flows through the Uterus. This means that the Penetrating Vessel is functionally related to the Kidneys and the Uterus very closely. For this reason, it is a very important vessel in gynaecological problems. Although the classics always say that this vessel flows through the Uterus, it could be postulated that in men it flows through the prostate.

Arising from the space between the Kidneys, the Penetrating Vessel (together with the Governing and Directing Vessels) determines the 7- and 8-year life cycles of women and men, respectively and is closely involved in the transformation of the Kidney-Essence into *Tian Gui* (i.e. menstrual blood in women and sperm in men).

All the points of the Penetrating Vessel on the lower abdomen (which are on the Kidney channel apart from ST-30 Qichong), therefore affect the Kidneys and the Uterus.

The abdominal branch

The Penetrating Vessel flows through the Kidney points on the abdomen up to KI-21 Youmen to then disperse in the chest. The 'chest' indicated in the ancient texts includes the breast.

The pathology of rebellious Qi of the Penetrating Vessel (see below) affects the abdominal branch of this vessel, causing a variety of different symptoms from the lower abdomen to the chest, breasts, throat and face.

The abdominal branch of the Penetrating Vessel penetrates the Membranes (*Huang*) of the abdomen and some of the symptoms of rebellious Qi of the Penetrating Vessel are due to tension and tightness of the Membranes (fullness, distension and pain of the abdomen).

The head branch

As it flows over the throat, rebellious Qi of the Penetrating Vessel often causes a feeling of lump in the throat (which therefore is not always related to Liver-Qi stagnation). According to chapter 65 of the 'Spiritual Axis', the Penetrating Vessel brings Qi and Blood to the chin area and, in women, losing some Blood with menstruation, the Penetrating Vessel has relatively less Blood than Qi in this area compared to men. The lack of Blood in this area is the reason why women do not have a beard; as men have relatively more Blood in the head branch of the Penetrating Vessel, this Blood promotes the growth of hair on the face. Interestingly, facial hair increases after the menopause as, due to the stoppage of the menses, this branch of the Penetrating Vessel has relatively more Blood than before and this promotes the growth of hair.[42]

The head branch of the Penetrating Vessel is responsible for the contradictory feeling of heat of the face in rebellious Qi of this vessel (contradictory because it associated with cold feet).

The spinal branch

The spinal branch of the Penetrating Vessel starts from Ren-1 Huiyin and flows inside the lumbar spine. This branch accounts for menstrual pain that is sometimes felt in the lower back.

The descending branch

The descending branch of the Penetrating Vessel flows from ST-30 Qichong down the inner aspect of the leg to the internal malleolus and the foot. On the foot, it separates, one branch joining the Kidney channel, the other the Liver channel and ending at LIV-3 Taichong.

The descending branch of the Penetrating Vessel is significant in practice for several reasons:

Firstly, through the descending branch of the Penetrating Vessel, the Kidneys bring Yin Qi down to the legs. The passage from chapter 38 of the 'Spiritual Axis' quoted above is actually preceded by a question from the Yellow Emperor wondering why the Yin Leg channels flow from the feet to the abdomen/chest except for the Kidney channel that descends. The answer clarifies that it is not the Kidney channel, but the descending branch of the Penetrating Vessel that descends. This implies that the Penetrating Vessel has the important function of ensuring the descending of Yin to the legs: this means that it is the vessel to treat whenever there is a deficiency of Yin in the legs, as, for example, in restless legs syndrome.

The descending branch of the Penetrating Vessel is therefore an important way in which Kidney-Qi descends to the legs.

Secondly, through its descending branch, the Penetrating Vessel influences all three Yin channels of the leg and it strengthens the interaction between the Liver, Spleen and Kidney channels. It is probably also because of the Penetrating Vessel that SP-6 Sanyinjiao is a meeting point of the three Yin channels of the leg. This means that a pathology of the Penetrating Vessel may affect the Liver, Spleen and Kidney channels on the leg. Vice versa, whenever we use the three Yin channels of the leg (especially in combination), we are affecting the Penetrating Vessel as well. Therefore, Penetrating Vessel points such as KI-11 Henggu, KI-12 Dahe and KI-13 Qixue affect the circulation of Qi in the three Yin channels of the leg.

Thirdly, the descending branch of the Penetrating Vessel brings Qi to the feet, warming them. Therefore, cold feet could be a pathology of the Penetrating Vessel (i.e. its Qi failing to descend).

Fourthly, the descending branch of the Penetrating Vessel ends at LIV-3 Taichong: this means that this point acts on the Penetrating Vessel. Every time we use LIV-3, we are activating the Penetrating Vessel. It is also for its connection with the Penetrating Vessel (which is the Sea of Blood) that this point is such an important point to move Blood in the Uterus.

Fifthly, it is probably because of the connection with the Penetrating Vessel and its integration of the three Yin of the leg that SP-6 Sanyinjiao affects the Uterus and is effective in many gynaecological conditions.

Sixthly, fungal infections of the big toe may be a symptom of a Penetrating Vessel pathology.

Clinical significance of the various names of the Penetrating Vessel

The Penetrating Vessel is variously called the 'Sea of Blood', 'Sea of the five Yin and six Yang Organs' and 'Sea of the 12 Channels'.

Sea of Blood

Chapter 33 of the 'Spiritual Axis', as mentioned above, says that the Penetrating Vessel is the Sea of Blood and its upper point is BL-11 Dashu and its lower points ST-37 Shangjuxu and ST-39 Xiajuxu. Regarding the symptoms of a pathology of the Sea of Blood, the same chapter says: *'When the Seas function harmoniously there is life; when they function against the normal flow there is disease ... When the Sea of Blood is in excess, the person has the feeling of the body getting bigger and the person is unable to pin-point the trouble; when the Sea of Blood is deficient, the person has the feeling of the body getting smaller and is unable to pin-point the trouble.'*[43]

The above symptoms of Fullness and Emptiness of the Sea of Blood are rather rare and not clinically important and it is not clear how the above points are connected to the Penetrating Vessel or why they are points of the Sea of Blood. The most important aspect of the Penetrating Vessels being the Sea of Blood is in gynaecology.

The Penetrating Vessel has a deep influence on the gynaecological system because it originates from between the Kidneys, it is responsible for the 7-year cycles of women and for the transformation of Kidney-Essence into menstrual blood, and it flows through the Uterus. In addition to these factors, being the Sea of Blood means that the Penetrating Vessel affects many Blood pathologies which are extremely common in gynaecological diseases. In particular, the Penetrating Vessel is involved in all cases of Blood stasis in gynaecological disorders.

To invigorate Blood of the Penetrating Vessel in gynaecology, one needs to use the opening and coupled points, SP-4 Gongsun and P-6 Neiguan, together with KI-14 Siman and LIV-3 Taichong.

The Penetrating Vessel's control of all the Blood Connecting channels (see immediately below) explains the connection between disharmony of Blood in the Uterus and the development of muscular pains, something which often occurs after childbirth. It also explains why women often suffer external invasions during menstruation: the depletion of Blood in the Penetrating Vessel induces an emptiness of the Blood Connecting channels and therefore the space between skin and muscles becomes empty and prone to invasion of external pathogenic factors.

Apart from the gynaecological system, the Blood of the whole body relies for its movement and circulation on the Penetrating Vessel. Being the Sea of Blood and Sea of the 12 Channels (see below), the Penetrating Vessel controls all the Blood Connecting channels. The Blood Connecting channels are the deep level of the Connecting (*Luo*) channels, a level that is connected with Blood and blood vessels. The Penetrating Vessel, through its opening and coupled points (SP-4 and P-6) affects all the Blood Connecting channels. As these channels are involved in Blood stasis, the Penetrating Vessel can be used to treat Blood stasis not only in the gynaecological system but anywhere in the body.

Another aspect of the Penetrating Vessel being the Sea of Blood is that it is related to body hair. When Blood of the Penetrating Vessel is abundant it moistens the skin and promotes the growth of body hair; if the Blood of the Penetrating Vessel is deficient, the skin is dry and the body hair brittle. Chapter 65 of the Spiritual Axis says: *'The Penetrating and Directing Vessels go to the throat, lips and mouth. If both Qi and Blood are abundant the skin is filled and the muscles warmed, if only Blood is abundant, it will penetrate into the skin and a beard grows. Women have more Qi than Blood because they lose some of the latter with the periods, hence the Penetrating and Directing Vessels carry less Blood to chin and lips and therefore no beard grows.'*[44]

Finally, another aspect of the Penetrating Vessel being the Sea of Blood is in relation to Blood and Heart. The Penetrating Vessel is related to the Heart in two ways: firstly because it disperses in the chest, secondly because it is the Sea of Blood and the Heart governs Blood. Because of this connection, the Penetrating Vessel can be used for palpitations and anxiety during the menopause, symptoms which are themselves caused by the decline of the Blood of the Penetrating Vessel with consequent rebellious Qi escaping upwards along the vessel. In the ancient texts, one of the indications of the Penetrating Vessel is the 'nine kinds of heart pain'.

The Penetrating Vessel can also be used for irregularities of the heart rhythm.

Box 53.10 summarizes the Penetrating Vessel as the 'Sea of Blood'.

Box 53.10 The Penetrating Vessel – 'Sea of Blood'

- Controls Blood of the Uterus and transformation of Kidney-Essence into *Tian Gui* (menstrual blood)
- Controls all Blood Connecting channels
- Upper point of Sea of Blood: BL-11 Dashu; lower points of Sea of Blood: ST-37 Shangjuxu and ST-39 Xiajuxu
- Blood stasis central pathology of Penetrating Vessel
- Blood of Penetrating Vessel promotes the growth of beard in men
- Influences Heart-Blood (palpitations, anxiety) and the heart rhythm

---

Sea of the 12 Channels

The Penetrating Vessel is also called the 'Sea of the 12 channels'. *Chong* has also the meaning of *jie* ('streets'), *dong* ('activity, movement'), *xing* ('movement') and *tong* ('free passage'), all terms that refer to the flow of Qi in the channels which are compared to 'streets', 'avenues' or 'crossroads'.

Since it is both the Sea of Blood and Sea of the 12 Channels, the Penetrating Vessel influences the movement of Qi and Blood in the whole body. Yang Shang Shan says: '*Under the umbilicus is the Motive Force in between the two kidneys which governs human life and is the root of the 12 channels: this is the Sea of Blood of the Penetrating Vessel, the Sea of the five Yin and six Yang Organs and of the 12 channels. It oozes into the Yang, irrigates the Essence ... it is the Motive Force below the umbilicus and in the uterus. It moves upwards and downwards, it is the Penetrating Vessel.*'45 Hence here *Chong* means *Dong* ('motive').

It is the Sea of the 12 channels also because it affects channels nearly all over the body, except the arms, and because it controls all the secondary channels over the abdomen and chest. The Penetrating Vessel is the Sea of the 12 Channels also because it controls all the Blood Connecting channels.

The concept of 'streets', 'avenues' or 'crossroads' (*jie*) with regard to the Penetrating Vessel is worth exploring. Chapter 52 of the 'Spiritual Axis' says: '*In the chest Qi has streets; in the abdomen Qi has streets; in the head Qi has streets; in the lower legs Qi has streets. Therefore if [there is a problem with] Qi in the head, stop it at the brain; if [there is a problem with] Qi in the chest, stop it at the front of the chest and at the Back-Transporting points; if [there is a problem with] Qi in the abdomen, stop it at the Back-Transporting points and at the Penetrating Vessel on the right and left of the umbilicus which is the Moving Qi [or Motive Force, Dong Qi]; if [there is a problem with] Qi in the lower legs, stop it at ST-30 Qichong [here called Qijie] and at BL-57 Chengshan.*'46

From this passage, it is apparent that the Penetrating Vessel controls all the channels ('streets') of the abdomen and the alternative name of ST-30, 'Avenues of Qi' (*Qijie*) is significant. In fact, the Qi of the Penetrating Vessel emerges from the deep abdomen at this point which has a powerful dynamic effect on the circulation of Qi in the channels of the abdomen.

Box 53.11 summarizes the Penetrating Vessel as the Sea of the 12 Channels.

Box 53.11 Penetrating Vessel – 'Sea of the 12 Channels'

- Controls all channels of the abdomen
- Controls circulation of Qi and Blood in all channels (except in the arms)
- Controls all Connecting channels

Sea of the Five Yin and Six Yang Organs

The Penetrating Vessel is the 'Sea of the five Yin and six Yang Organs' because it is the extraordinary vessel at the centre of the energetic vortex created by them (see ch. 52, Fig. 52.11). It is the 'father' of the other extraordinary vessels. The Penetrating Vessel is the link between the Pre-Heaven Qi (Kidneys) and the Post-Heaven Qi (Stomach).

Due to its complex pathway, the Penetrating Vessel influences many organs directly. As we have seen, it is directly related to the three Yin channels of the leg, Kidneys, Liver, and Spleen. It is closely connected to the Stomach (emerging at ST-30) and the Heart. Therefore, it is related to the Kidney (Pre-Heaven Qi), Stomach (Post-Heaven Qi) and the Heart (the Emperor), which are the *Three Treasures* of Essence, Qi and Mind.

Box 53.12 summarizes the Penetrating Vessel as the Sea of the five Yin and six Yang Organs.

> **Box 53.12 Penetrating Vessel – 'Sea of the Five Yin and Six Yang Organs'**
>
> - Root of Pre-Heaven Qi (through Kidney connection) and Post-Heaven Qi (through Stomach connection)
> - Influences the three Yin channels of the leg (Liver, Kidneys and Spleen)
> - Affects the Heart
> - At the centre of energetic vortex of extraordinary vessels

Rebellious Qi of the Penetrating Vessel

One of the most common pathologies of the Penetrating Vessel is rebellious Qi and 'internal urgency' (*Li Ji*): this has been recognized since the times of the 'Classic of Difficulties' (*Nan Jing*). Chapter 29 of the 'Classic of Difficulties' says: '*The pathology of the Penetrating Vessel is rebellious Qi with internal urgency [li ji].*'[47] 'Internal urgency' indicates a feeling of vague anxiety and restlessness. It may also be interpreted on a physical level as an uncomfortable, tight sensation from the lower abdomen upwards towards the heart. Modern Chinese books say that 'internal urgency' may also indicate pain, constipation, retention of urine, hernia, anxiety, dizziness and nausea, especially with an emotional background.

Li Shi Zhen said: '*When Qi rebels upwards, there is internal urgency and feeling of heat: this is rebellious Qi of the Penetrating Vessel.*'[48]

Rebellious Qi of the Penetrating Vessel causes various symptoms at different levels of abdomen and chest. It causes primarily fullness, distension or pain in these areas. By plotting the pathway of the Penetrating Vessel, we can list the possible symptoms of rebellious Qi of the Penetrating Vessel starting from the bottom (Figs 53.5 and 53.6):

- Cold feet
- Fullness/distension/pain of the lower abdomen
- Hypogastric fullness/distension/pain
- Painful periods, irregular periods
- Fullness/distension/pain of the umbilical area
- Fullness/distension/pain of the epigastrium
- Feeling of tightness below the xiphoid process
- Feeling of tightness of the chest
- Palpitations
- Feeling of distension of the breasts in women
- Slight breathlessness
- Sighing
- Feeling of lump in the throat
- Feeling of heat of the face
- Headache
- Anxiety, mental restlessness, 'internal urgency' (*li ji*)

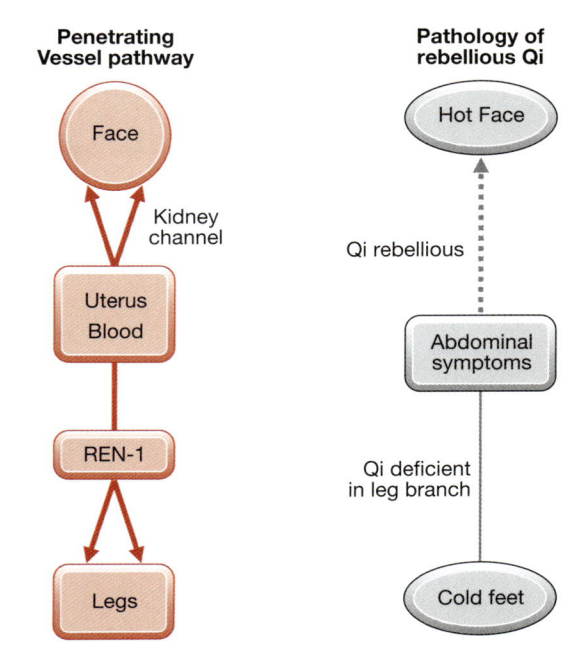

Figure 53.5 Schematic representation of rebellious Qi of the Penetrating Vessel

Obviously, not all these symptoms need occur simultaneously to diagnose rebellious Qi of the Penetrating Vessel but it is necessary to have at least three to four symptoms at different levels (e.g. lower abdomen, epigastrium, chest, throat). For example, if someone had fullness, distension or pain of the lower abdomen, that would not be enough to diagnose the condition of rebellious Qi of the Penetrating Vessel. A feeling of energy rising from the lower abdomen up towards the throat would be a strong indication of rebellious Qi of the Penetrating Vessel.

What makes the Qi of the Penetrating Vessel rebel upwards? In my experience, this may happen for two reasons manifesting with two conditions, one Full, the other mixed Full/Empty. Firstly, the Qi of the Penetrating Vessel can rebel upwards by itself from emotional stress that makes Qi rise or stagnate, such as anger, repressed anger, worry, frustration, resentment, etc. In this case, Qi rebels upwards by itself and the condition is Full and I call this 'primary' rebellious Qi of the Penetrating Vessel.

Qi of the Penetrating Vessel may rebel upwards also as a consequence of a Deficiency in this vessel in the lower abdomen: in such cases, Qi of the lower *Dan Tian*

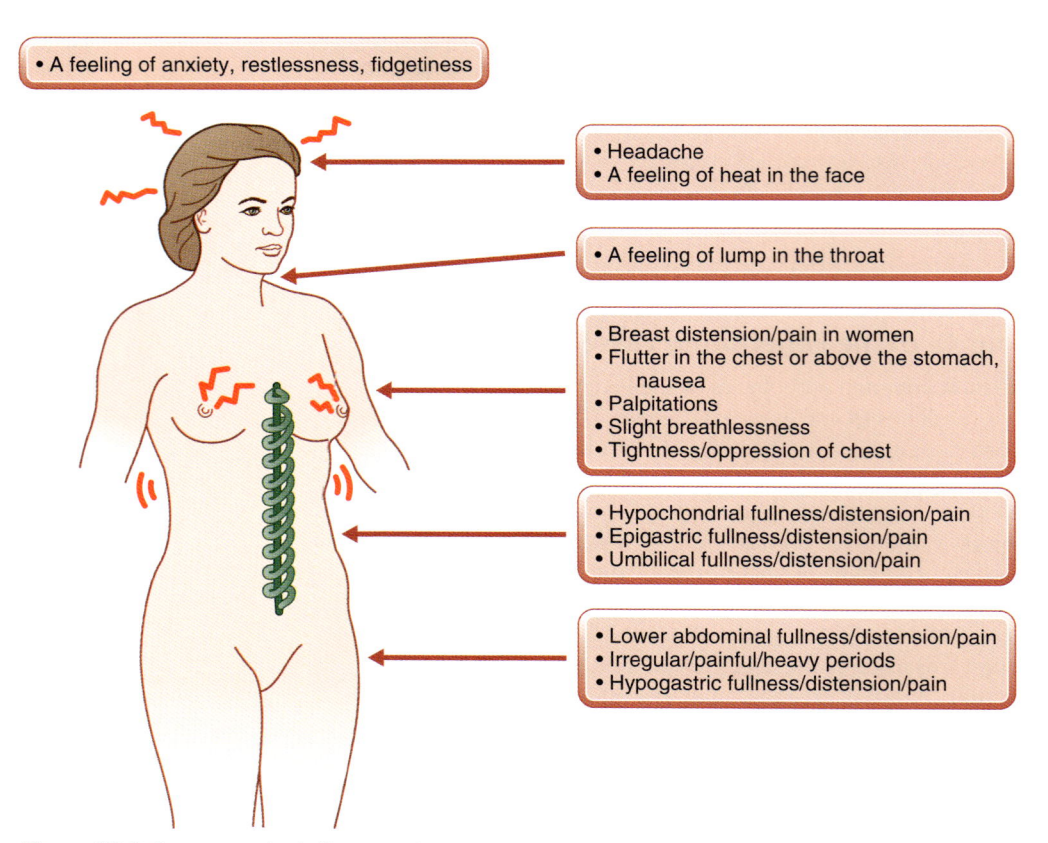

Figure 53.6 Symptoms of rebellious Qi of the Penetrating Vessel

Labels on figure:
- A feeling of anxiety, restlessness, fidgetiness
- Headache
- A feeling of heat in the face
- A feeling of lump in the throat
- Breast distension/pain in women
- Flutter in the chest or above the stomach, nausea
- Palpitations
- Slight breathlessness
- Tightness/oppression of chest
- Hypochondrial fullness/distension/pain
- Epigastric fullness/distension/pain
- Umbilical fullness/distension/pain
- Lower abdominal fullness/distension/pain
- Irregular/painful/heavy periods
- Hypogastric fullness/distension/pain

is weak and the Qi of the Penetrating Vessel 'escapes' upwards: this is therefore a mixed Full/Empty condition and I call this 'secondary' rebellious Qi of the Penetrating Vessel. The Empty condition is deficiency of Blood and/or deficiency of the Kidneys (which may be Yin or Yang). This second condition is more common in women.

Li Shi Zhen mentions the possibility of this pattern when he says: *'When there is Blood deficiency leading to internal urgency, use Dang Gui.'*[49] The 'Classic of Categories' also hints to Blood deficiency as a background for rebellious Qi of the Penetrating Vessel: *'The Qi of the Penetrating Vessel rises up to the chest, Qi is not regulated and therefore it rebels in the diaphragm, Blood is deficient and therefore there is internal urgency in the abdomen and chest.'*[50]

Clinical note

- *'Primary' rebellious Qi of the Penetrating Vessel*: the Qi of the Penetrating Vessel rebels upwards by itself from emotional stress that makes Qi rise or stagnate. Full condition
- *'Secondary' rebellious Qi of the Penetrating Vessel*: Qi of the Penetrating Vessel rebels upwards as a consequence of a Deficiency (of Blood and Kidneys) in this vessel in the lower abdomen. Full/Empty condition

A particular feature of the syndrome of rebellious Qi of the Penetrating Vessel is that it is characterized by a feeling of heat in the face and cold feet. This is due to the fact, as Qi rebels upwards towards the face, it causes a feeling of heat there; on the other hand, as it rebels upwards, there is proportionately less Qi in the descending branch of the Penetrating Vessel, which causes cold feet. In fact, as have seen above, the old texts specifically say that the descending branch of the Penetrating Vessel warms the feet.

An example of treatment of what I call 'primary' rebellious Qi of the Penetrating Vessel (i.e. of the Full type) in a woman is: SP-4 Gongsun on the right, P-6 Neiguan on the left, L.I.-4 Hegu on the right, LIV-3 Taichong on the left, KI-14 Siman bilaterally and KI-21 Youmen bilaterally.

An example of treatment of what I call 'secondary' rebellious Qi of the Penetrating Vessel (i.e. of the Full/Empty type) against a background of Blood and Kidney deficiency in a woman is: SP-4 Gongsun on the right, P-6 Neiguan on the left, L.I.-4 Hegu on the right, LIV-3 Taichong on the left, KI-13 Qixue bilaterally, Ren-4 Guanyuan and KI-21 Youmen bilaterally.

Rebellious Qi of the Penetrating Vessel may also cause dizziness, for which one can use Du-20 Baihui, BL-11 Dashu, ST-37 Shangjuxu and ST-39 Xiajuxu.

Rebellious Qi of the Penetrating Vessel may also cause nausea, in which case one can use BL-11 Dashu, ST-37 Shangjuxu, ST-39 Xiajuxu and ST-30 Qichong.

Blood stasis in gynaecology

The Penetrating Vessel is the Sea of Blood and its pathology is at the root of many gynaecological problems. The three Blood pathologies that affect the Penetrating Vessel are Blood deficiency, Blood-Heat and Blood stasis. When there is Blood deficiency, the woman may suffer from amenorrhoea or scanty periods. When there is Blood-Heat, the periods may be very heavy; when there is Blood stasis, the periods will be painful and the menstrual blood will be dark with clots.

The Penetrating Vessel is used particularly to invigorate Blood when there is Blood stasis in the Uterus: indeed, this is *the* pathology of the Penetrating Vessel. Therefore we can use this vessel in any case of Blood stasis in the Uterus. The points to use are the opening and coupled points (SP-4 and P-6) plus KI-14 Siman and SP-10 Xuehai.

> **Clinical note**
>
> The Penetrating Vessel is *the* vessel to use for Blood stasis in gynaecological diseases. Use SP-4 on the right, P-6 on the left, KI-14 and SP-10

The Penetrating Vessel and the Membranes (*Huang*)

The nature and function of the Membranes have already been discussed above under the Directing Vessel. The Penetrating Vessel also influences the Membranes in the abdomen and chest and, indeed, its syndrome of Qi rebellious involves the Membranes: that is, Qi stagnates in the Membranes and rebels upwards, causing the various abdominal and chest symptoms.

The Penetrating Vessel and the female breast

The Penetrating Vessel disperses in the chest and the breasts, and therefore its Qi has a deep influence on the breasts. Moreover, being the 'Sea of the 12 Channels', the Penetrating Vessel influences all channels including the Connecting channels; being the 'Sea of Blood', the Penetrating Vessel influences all Blood Connecting channels (Fig. 53.7).

As the female breast is richly irrigated by Connecting channels, a pathology of Qi stagnation in the Penetrating Vessel affects the breasts, causing breast distension and/or pain and, in the long run, breast lumps.

Another way in which the Penetrating Vessel affects the female breast is through the Membranes (*Huang*). The Penetrating Vessel, together with the Directing Vessel, controls the Membranes in the abdomen and chest. The connective tissue within the female breast is part of the Membranes and Qi stagnation in the Penetrating Vessel always affects the Membranes and therefore the breasts.

As the Penetrating Vessel arises from the Uterus (which stores menstrual blood) and by virtue of its being the Sea of Blood and controlling the Blood connecting channels, the Penetrating Vessel is responsible for the production of breast milk after childbirth. Breast milk is a direct transformation of menstrual blood into milk (the Chinese say 'Blood turns white'): as the periods cease after childbirth, menstrual Blood turns into milk and flows up to the breasts via the Penetrating Vessel.

If the Qi of the Penetrating Vessel stagnates after childbirth, the breast milk may not come out: this is a Full condition of agalactia, i.e. the milk is there but it is difficult to express because of the Qi stagnation. On the other hand, if the Blood of the Penetrating Vessel is deficient, the breast milk may be lacking because

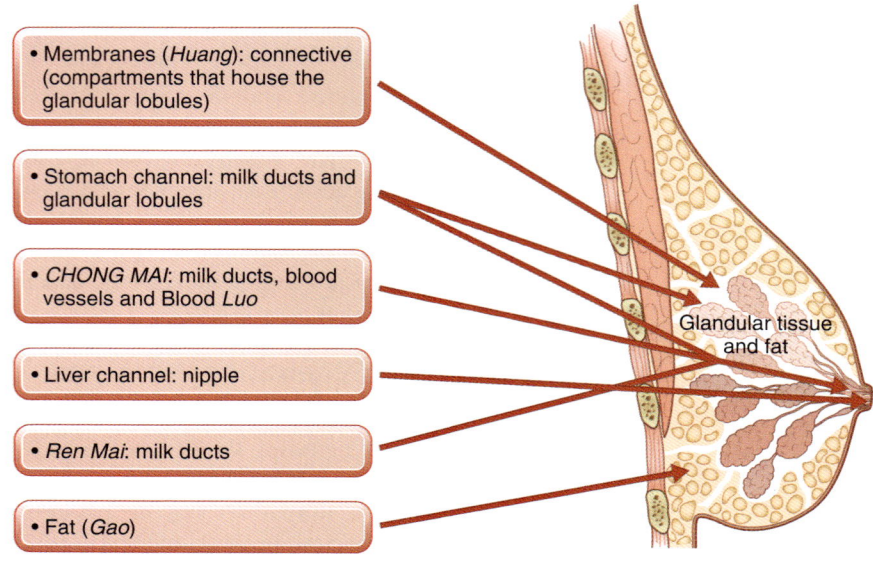

- Membranes (*Huang*): connective (compartments that house the glandular lobules)
- Stomach channel: milk ducts and glandular lobules
- *CHONG MAI*: milk ducts, blood vessels and Blood *Luo*
- Liver channel: nipple
- *Ren Mai*: milk ducts
- Fat (*Gao*)

Figure 53.7 The Penetrating Vessel and the female breast

there is not enough Blood to be transformed into milk: this is an Empty cause of agalactia.

The Penetrating Vessel and the Heart

The Penetrating Vessel has a deep influence on the Heart as it flows around the heart. Indeed, in the various passages quoted above mentioning the 'Great Connecting channel of the Kidneys' in connection with the descending branch of the Penetrating Vessel, the Chinese expression is actually 'the Great Connecting channel of the Lesser Yin' and some authors think it might refer to a Great Connecting channel of the Heart rather than that of the Kidneys.

As mentioned in chapter 19, the Heart is connected to the Uterus via the Uterus Vessel (*Bao Mai*). There is a debate as to whether this 'Uterus Vessel' (*Bao Mai*) is part of the Penetrating Vessel or whether it is a separate channel: I rather tend to think the former. Heart-Qi and Heart-Blood descend towards the Uterus, promoting the discharge of menstrual blood during the bleeding phase and the discharge of the eggs during ovulation, which are under the control of the Penetrating Vessel.

Apart from gynaecology, the Penetrating Vessel influences the heart rhythm and can be used for arrhythmia.

The Penetrating Vessel and the Stomach

The Penetrating Vessel emerges from the point ST-30 Qichong, which is the upper point of the Sea of Food. Therefore, the Penetrating Vessel is closely connected to the Stomach via this point. The Kidneys are the Gate of the Stomach: hence the Penetrating Vessel, originating from the Kidneys, treats both.

There are two clinical implications in the connection between the Penetrating Vessel and the Stomach. Firstly, this vessel can be used for any Stomach disorder, but particularly those of a Full nature, for example stagnation of Qi in the Stomach, Stomach-Qi not descending, Blood stasis in the Stomach, Stomach-Heat, etc. The points to use are the opening and coupled points of the Penetrating Vessel (SP-4 and P-6) plus KI-21 Youmen and ST-19 Burong.

Secondly, the Penetrating Vessel affects the Stomach channel's connection with the Heart. The Great Connecting of the Stomach is called *Xu Li* and the beating of the heart in the left ventricle represents, from the Chinese point of view, the beating of *Xu Li*. This means that the Stomach channel can be used to treat heart problems and particularly problems of arrhythmia. However, the Stomach influences the Heart also via the Penetrating Vessel as this vessel connects with Stomach and Heart.

The relationship of the Penetrating Vessel with both the Uterus and the Stomach explains morning sickness in pregnancy: this is due to rebellious Qi in the Penetrating Vessel deriving from the profound changes taking place in the Uterus in the first 3 months of pregnancy. In women who suffer very severe morning sickness and vomiting for longer than 3 months, there is usually a pre-existing condition of rebellious Qi in the Penetrating Vessel.

Due to the relationship between the Stomach and the Penetrating Vessel, the herb Ban Xia *Rhizoma Pinelliae* (which enters the Stomach) is sometimes used to regulate the Penetrating Vessel: for example, this is the rationale for the inclusion of Ban Xia *Rhizoma Pinelliae* in the formula Wen Jing Tang *Warming the Menses Decoction* (for Cold in the Uterus).

The Penetrating Vessel and Qi circulation to the feet

As the Penetrating Vessel's descending branch goes to the dorsum of the foot and big toe, and as this vessel influences all Connecting channels, problems of circulation to the feet with coldness, numbness, tingling, purple colour, etc., may be related to this vessel. In these cases treat SP-4 Gongsun and P-6 Neiguan, together with some abdominal points such as KI-13 Qixue.

Some doctors say that, due to the Penetrating Vessel's toe branch, a fungal infection of the big toe can affect the Heart (due to the connection between this vessel and the Heart).

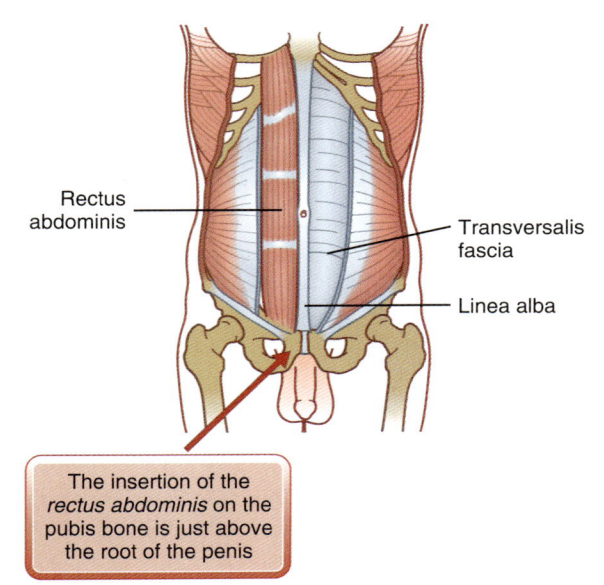

The Penetrating Vessel and the 'ancestral muscles' (*Zong Jin*)

The meaning of the term *Zong Jin* (literally 'ancestors' muscles') is the subject of varying interpretations. The two main ones are that this term refers to the *rectus abdominis* muscles (the muscles than run either side of the midline) or that it refers to the penis. There are passages in the old text that would support both views (Fig. 53.8).

The *rectus abdominis* muscles are muscles than run vertically in the abdomen, either side of the midline, attached to the lower ribs above and the symphysis pubis (pubic bone) below. Chapter 44 of the 'Simple Questions' mentions the ancestral muscles: 'The Penetrating Vessel is the Sea of the Channels, it irrigates the rivers and valleys and it connects with the Bright Yang [Stomach channel] in the ancestral muscles. Thus, Yin and Yang meet in the ancestral muscles and connect with the avenues of the abdomen which are under the control of the Stomach: they are all restrained by the Girdle Vessel [Dai Mai] and connect with the Governing Vessel [Du Mai].'[51]

In the above passage, 'rivers and valleys' refers to 'large and small meeting points of the muscles'; '*Yin and Yang*' refer to the Penetrating Vessel and the Stomach channel, respectively. As the Penetrating Vessel runs along all the Kidney points, which are 0.5 *cun* from the midline, and the Stomach channel points are 2 *cun* from the midline, they more or less enclose the *rectus abdominis* muscles in between them. In fact, the Kidney channel lies on the medial border of the *rectus abdominis* and the Stomach channel lies on the muscle itself but towards its lateral border.

The Penetrating Vessel is related to the state of the ancestral muscles of the abdomen: if the Penetrating Vessel is not flourishing, the ancestral muscles are slack. A slackness of the ancestral muscles may cause prolapses of the uterus in women and some kinds of atrophy of the legs.

If we take the 'ancestral muscle' (*zong jin*) to mean the penis, then the Penetrating Vessel influences the penis and, in particular, the *corpus spongiosum* and *corpus cavernosum*. As erection depends on these two structures filling with Blood, the Penetrating Vessel, being the Sea of Blood and influencing the *zong jin*,

Figure 53.8 The Penetrating Vessel and the ancestral muscles (*Zong Jin*)

The insertion of the *rectus abdominis* on the pubis bone is just above the root of the penis plays a role in erection and therefore erectile dysfunctions (impotence or priapism).

Comparison and differentiation between the Directing and Penetrating Vessels

The Directing Vessel corresponds to Qi, the Penetrating Vessel to Blood. The Directing Vessel is therefore used in problems due to deficiency or stagnation of Qi, whereas the Penetrating Vessel is used more in problems due to stasis of Blood but also the rebellious Qi, which is a typical pathology of this vessel. This does not mean, however, that the Directing Vessel is not used in Blood problems, since they are often due to Qi problems.

Some doctors say that the Directing Vessel is responsible for pregnancy and the Penetrating Vessel for problems *not* to do with pregnancy.

The Directing Vessel corresponds to the Lungs (= Qi) and the Penetrating Vessel corresponds to the Heart and Spleen (= Blood). One would therefore use the Directing Vessel more for Lung problems and the Penetrating Vessel for Heart and Spleen problems.

The Directing Vessel is more used in cases of deficiency of Qi or stagnation of Qi, whereas the Penetrating Vessel is more used when there is an actual material accumulation (of Blood stasis, Food or Phlegm), but also the typical rebellious Qi.

I personally choose the Directing Vessel more when the pulse is Weak, Short or Fine (all signs of Qi deficiency), and the Penetrating Vessel when the pulse is Slippery, Full, Long, Wiry, Firm (all signs of Excess).

The Directing Vessel has more of a circular action on the median plane of the body, whilst the Penetrating Vessel has more of a dispersing action. What is meant by this is that the Directing Vessel is more used in cases of stagnant or deficient Qi in the centre line of the body (in any of the Three Burners). It thus acts on the central Qi (i.e. the Qi of the median line) by stimulating the circulation along the centre, like a wheel. The Penetrating Vessel is more used in cases of stagnant Qi and/or Blood spreading horizontally and creating obstruction in the chest and abdomen.

In abdominal pain (from gynaecological or intestinal origin), the Directing Vessel controls the *Xiao Fu* area (the central-lower abdominal area), while the Penetrating Vessel controls the *Shao Fu* area (the lower-lateral abdominal area).

To use asthma as an example, both vessels are effective in this condition. The Directing Vessel is used when the asthma is due to Lung and Kidney deficiency (the person is often thin), while the Penetrating Vessel is more used when the asthma is due to rebellious Qi but also stagnation of Phlegm (and therefore presents with copious expectoration, a Slippery pulse and a thick tongue coating, and the person is often overweight or robust) (Figs 53.9 and 53.10).

The area where the differences between the Directing and Penetrating Vessels is most blurred is that of gynaecological problems, particularly menstrual disorders. The choice is made clear if we refer to the above points. In particular one would use the Directing Vessel when the menstrual problems are caused by a disorder of Qi, and the Penetrating Vessel when they are caused by a disorder of Blood: also, the Directing Vessel more for conception, fertility, pregnancy, menarche and menopause, and the Penetrating Vessel more for menstruation and in particular painful periods. The Penetrating Vessel is *the* vessel to use in painful periods.

Box 53.13 summarizes the clinical applications of the Penetrating Vessel.

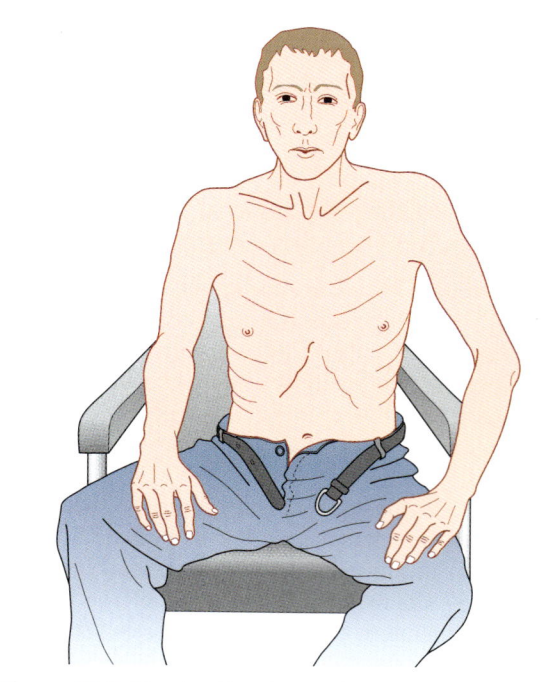

Figure 53.9 Directing Vessel type of asthma patient

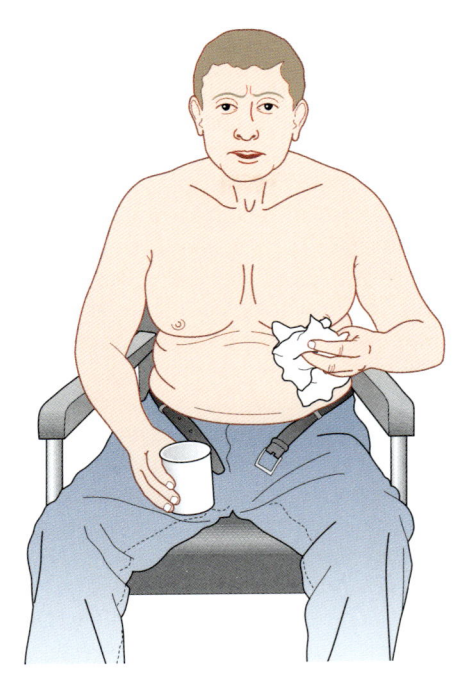

Figure 53.10 Penetrating Vessel type of asthma patient

Box 53.13 Clinical Applications of the Penetrating Vessel

- Clinical significance of the five branches of the Penetrating Vessel
  - Internal branch
  - Abdominal branch
  - Head branch
  - Spinal branch
  - Descending branch
- Clinical significance of the names of the Penetrating Vessel
  - Sea of Blood
  - Sea of the 12 Channels
  - Sea of the five Yin and six Yang Organs
- Rebellious Qi of the Penetrating Vessel
- Blood stasis in gynaecology
- Membranes
- Female breast
- Heart
- Stomach
- Circulation of Qi to feet
- Ancestral muscles

Classical indications

Chapter 29 of the 'Classic of Difficulties' says: '*The pathology of the Penetrating Vessel is rebellious Qi with internal urgency [li ji].*'[52]

The 'Pulse Classic' says: '*When the pulse is hard and full at the middle level of [both] Middle positions, it indicates [a pathology of] the Penetrating Vessel. This causes abdominal pain which harasses the Heart upwards, abdominal masses, hernial swellings, infertility, urinary incontinence and hypochondrial fullness with irritability.*'[53]

The 'Golden Mirror of Medicine' (Yi Zong Jin Jian, 1742) lists the following symptoms for the Penetrating Vessel: '*Nine kinds of heart pain, tightness of the chest, regurgitation of food, abdominal masses from excessive drinking [of alcohol] and eating, borborygmi, epigastric pain in the region of the diaphragm, malaria, blood in the stools, retention of placenta with stagnant Blood causing fainting.*'[54]

Li Shi Zhen quotes Li Dong Yuan: '*In Autumn and Winter Stomach-Qi rebels upwards in the Penetrating Vessel, there is movement under the hypochondrium, this is called Jue Ni (Terminal Rebellious Qi). When Qi rebels upwards, the person cannot breathe, there is a wheezing sound and he or she cannot lie down.*'[55]

Li Shi Zhen quotes Sun Si Miao: '*When Qi rises from the lower abdomen to chest and throat, hands and feet are cold, there is a feeling of heat in the face, dysuria, the Front pulse position is Deep and the Rear pulse position Scattered: use Fu Ling Wu Wei Zi Tang (Fu Ling, Wu Wei Zi, Rou Gui, Gan Cao). If there is a feeling of fullness in the chest eliminate Rou Gui.*'[56]

Li Shi Zhen said: '*When Qi rebels upwards, there is internal urgency and feeling of heat: this is rebellious Qi of the Penetrating Vessel.*'[57]

Chapter 39 of the 'Simple Questions' says: '*When Cold invades the Penetrating Vessel, as this vessel originates from Ren-4 Guanyuan and rises straight up the abdomen, the vessel will be obstructed and Qi will stagnate: this will cause breathlessness when the abdomen is palpated.*'[58]

Box 53.14 summarizes classical indications for the Penetrating Vessel.

Herbal therapy

Herbs

Ye Tian Shi said that diseases of the Penetrating Vessel are characterized by Connecting channel pathology, which causes distension, and Qi stagnation, which causes pain. One must therefore use pungent aromatic herbs, which enter the Connecting channels, and bitter herbs, which open and make Qi descend.

> **Box 53.14 Classical indications for the Penetrating Vessel**
>
> - *Classic of Difficulties*: rebellious Qi with internal urgency (*li ji*)
> - *Pulse Classic*: abdominal pain which harasses the Heart upwards, abdominal masses, hernial swellings, infertility, urinary incontinence and hypochondrial fullness with irritability
> - *Golden Mirror of Medicine*: nine kinds of heart pain, tightness of the chest, regurgitation of food, abdominal masses from excessive drinking (of alcohol) and eating, borborygmi, epigastric pain in the region of the diaphragm, malaria, blood in the stools, retention of placenta with stagnant Blood causing fainting
> - *Li Shi Zhen*: movement under the hypochondrium, the person cannot breathe, there is a wheezing sound and he or she cannot lie down
> - *Li Shi Zhen*: cold hands and feet, feeling of heat in the face, dysuria, Front pulse Deep, Rear pulse Scattered
> - *Simple Questions*: breathlessness when the abdomen is palpated

The main substance that nourishes the Penetrating Vessel is Gui Ban *Plastrum Testudinis*. The herbs used to subdue rebellious Qi of the Penetrating Vessel are Yan Hu Suo *Rhizoma Corydalis yanhusuo*, Chuan Lian Zi *Fructus Meliae toosendan*, Xiang Fu *Rhizoma Cyperi rotundi*, Yu Jin *Tuber Curcumae*, Chen Xiang *Lignum Aquilariae*, Tao Ren *Semen Persicae*, Dang Gui *Radix Angelicae sinensis*, Qing Pi *Pericarpium Citri reticulatae viride*, Wu Zhu Yu *Fructus Evodiae rutaecarpae*, Cong Bai *Herba Allii fistulosi*, Xiao Hui Xiang *Fructus Foeniculi vulgaris*.

Formulae

None given by Li Shi Zhen. The *Women's Treasure* formula *Penetrating Vessel* nourishes Blood of the Penetrating Vessel, tonifies the Kidneys and subdues rebellious Qi.

Case history 53.3

A man of 45 suffered from chronic indigestion with a sensation of fullness of the epigastrium, belching and nausea. His pulse was Full and Tight especially in the Middle position, and his tongue had a thick white coating. The clinical manifestations point to retention of food in the Middle Burner. The opening and coupled points of the Penetrating Vessel (SP-4 Gongsun and P-6 Neiguan) were used, producing a complete recovery after several treatments.

Case history 53.4

A 45-year-old woman had been suffering from tiredness, blurred vision, palpitations, a panicky, anxious feeling in the chest with a feeling of energy rising, insomnia, headaches during the periods, premenstrual tension with abdominal distension, a feeling of heat in the face but cold hands and feet. Her tongue was Pale-Purple and her pulse was Fine but also slightly Firm in all three positions of the left side.

Most of her symptoms are due to rebellious Qi in the Penetrating Vessel against a background of Blood deficiency (Fine pulse, Pale tongue, tiredness, blurred vision, insomnia). All the other symptoms are due to rebellious Qi in the Penetrating Vessel and the contradiction between the hot feeling of the face and cold limbs is typical of this pattern and occurs frequently in women.

The points used were:

- *SP-4* Gongsun on the right and *P-6* Neiguan on the left to open the Penetrating Vessel.
- *Ren-4* Guanyuan to tonify Blood in the Penetrating Vessel: this will also have the effect of subduing rebellious Qi by rooting it downwards (Ren-4, a point of the Directing Vessel affects also the Penetrating Vessel).
- *KI-13* Qixue to strengthen the Kidneys and consolidate the root of the Penetrating Vessel.
- *SP-6* Sanyinjiao to nourish Liver and Kidneys and strengthen the root.
- *L.I.-4* Hegu and *LIV-3* Taichong to harmonize the ascending and descending of Qi and calm the Mind.

Case history 53.5

A 59-year-old woman suffered from a pain in the chest accompanied by an anxiety feeling, abdominal distension and pain. Her pulse was slightly Wiry and her tongue was slightly Purple.

This is also due to rebellious Qi in the Penetrating Vessel affecting the chest. The points used were:

- *SP-4* Gongsun on the right and *P-6* Neiguan on the left to open the Penetrating Vessel. P-6 would also open the chest and relieve pain there.
- *Ren-4* Guanyuan to tonify the Kidneys and the Uterus and root Qi of the Penetrating Vessel.
- *L.I.-4* Hegu on the right and *ST-40* Fenglong on the left to harmonize the rising and descending

of Qi and thus subdue rebellious Qi. These two points will also indirectly affect the Penetrating Vessel as they belong to Bright Yang, to which the vessel is related. This is another way in which they will help to subdue rebellious Qi. In addition, ST-40 also opens and relaxes the chest.

Case history 53.6

A 13-year-old boy had been suffering from asthma since childhood. He complained of wheezing, breathlessness, tightness of the chest, inability to lie down and a distinctive sensation of energy rising from the stomach to the chest and face. He also suffered from a cough with expectoration of thick yellow sputum. His tongue was Red with a yellow coating and his pulse was Slippery.

This is another example of rebellious Qi in the Penetrating Vessel, obstructing the chest and forcing Phlegm-Heat towards the lungs. The points used were:
- *SP-4* Gongsun on the left and *P-6* Neiguan on the right to open the Penetrating Vessel. P-6 will also open the chest and help breathing.
- *BL-11* Dashu bled, to clear Heat in the Sea of Blood and subdue rebellious Qi in the Penetrating Vessel.
- *ST-37* Shangjuxu and *ST-39* Xiajuxu to clear Heat from the Sea of Blood downwards and relieve the chest.
- *LU-5* Chize to clear Phlegm-Heat from the Lungs and restore the descending of Lung-Qi.

Case history 53.7

A 23-year-old woman suffered from painful periods. The pain occurred during the period and was very intense and cramp-like. It was relieved by the application of a hot-water bottle.

This is an example of obstruction of the Penetrating Vessel by cold. The points used (with needles and moxa) were:
- *SP-4* Gongsun on the right and *P-6* Neiguan on the left to open the Penetrating Vessel.
- *Ren-4* Guanyuan and *KI-16* Huangshu to strengthen the Penetrating Vessel and expel Cold from the Uterus.

Case history 53.8

A 54-year-old man suffered from pain and numbness of the second and third toes of his right foot. The toes looked purple and felt cold.

This is due to stasis of Cold in the Connecting channels of the Penetrating Vessel, which irrigates and warms the toes. The points used were:
- *ST-30* Qichong to open the circulation of the Penetrating Vessel to the toes. The Bright Yang is in relation with the Penetrating Vessel.
- *ST-39* Xiajuxu, connected to the lower Sea of Blood of the Penetrating Vessel, stimulates the circulation of Blood to the legs.
- *LIV-3* Taichong is a point of the Penetrating Vessel.

Case history 53.9

A 65-year-old woman complained of hot flushes every 50 minutes after a total hysterectomy 10 years previously. She could not have HRT as she had developed breast cancer (mastectomy) 2 years previously. With the hot flushes, she also experienced a suffocating feeling, with anxiety. She also suffered from night sweating and insomnia. Her urination was frequent and pale and her feet were generally cold. Her pulse was Deep, slightly Slippery on the right side and slightly Wiry on the left. Her tongue was of a normal colour, Swollen, with a yellow coating and Stomach cracks.

This is an example of rebellious Qi in the Penetrating Vessel causing the feeling of heat and anxiety. It is not a typical Empty-Heat pattern as the tongue is not Red. The cold feet are due to the derangement of Qi in the Penetrating Vessel, rebelling upwards and failing to warm the legs.

I used:
- *SP-4* Gongsun on the right and *P-6* Neiguan on the left to open the Penetrating Vessel.
- *L.I.-4* Hegu on the right and *ST-40* Fenglong on the left to harmonize the ascending and descending of Qi, thus helping to subdue rebellious Qi and regulate the Bright Yang, to which the Penetrating Vessel is related.
- *Ren-4* Guanyuan to nourish the Uterus, consolidate the root and strengthen the Penetrating Vessel.

GIRDLE VESSEL (*DAI MAI*)

Opening point: G.B.-41 Zulinqi.
Coupled point: T.B.-5 Waiguan.
Starting point: G.B.-26 Daimai.
Area of body influenced: genitals, waist, hips.

The Girdle Vessel is the only horizontal vessel of the body and it encircles the channels in the abdomen and back like a belt. It divides the body into two halves. It is closely related to the Liver and Gall Bladder and it connects with the Kidney Divergent channel. Because of this, the Girdle vessel 'guides and supports' the Qi of the Uterus and the Essence.

Because the Girdle Vessel connects with LIV-13 (Spleen) and BL-23 (Kidneys), it connects the Post-Heaven with the Pre-Heaven Qi (in a similar way to the Penetrating Vessel).

Thus, the Girdle Vessel interrelates with and restrains the Liver's smooth flow of Qi when this is pathological (through LIV-13), and harmonizes the ascending of Spleen-Qi and the descending of Kidney-Qi.

Hence the Kidney's nourishment of the Essence, the Spleen's raising of Qi and the Liver's smooth flow of Qi all rely on the Girdle Vessel's being 'relaxed and stretched' (Fig. 53.11).

Pathway

The Girdle Vessel flows through LIV-13 Zhangmen, G.B.-26 Daimai, G.B.-27 Wushu and G.B.-28 Weidao. In the back, it connects with the Kidney Divergent channel at the height of BL-23 Shenshu.

The 'Classic of Difficulties' says: '*The Girdle Vessel originates from the hypochondrium and it encircles the body.*'[59] Li Shi Zhen says: '*The Girdle Vessel originates in the hypochondrium at the point LIV-13 Zhangmen and it then connects with G.B.-26 Daimai, G.B.-27 Wushu and G.B.-28 Weidao.*'[60]

Chapter 11 of the 'Spiritual Axis' says: '*The Kidney Divergent channel goes behind the knee and it connects with the Bladder channel. It then goes up to the kidneys area level with the 14th vertebra where it exits into the Girdle Vessel.*'[61]

Boxes 53.15 and 53.16 summarize, respectively, the pathway and points of the Girdle Vessel.

Clinical applications

Harmonizes the Liver and Gall Bladder

It can be used to harmonize the Liver and Gall Bladder, particularly in Excess patterns of the Liver, when the Gall Bladder pulse is Full and Wiry, for such symptoms as temporal headaches.

Resolves Dampness in the Lower Burner

The Girdle Vessel is like a belt encircling the leg channels in the abdomen and back: the tension of this belt regulates the circulation of Qi to and from the legs. If the belt is too loose, the leg channels are not 'restrained' and Dampness infuses into the Lower Burner.

Box 53.15 Girdle Vessel – summary of pathway

- Originates in the hypochondrium at the point LIV-13 Zhangmen and it then connects with G.B.-26 Daimai, G.B.-27 Wushu and G.B.-28 Weidao encircling the waist like a belt
- In the back, at the level of BL-23 Shenshu, it connects with the Kidney Divergent channel

---

Box 53.16 Points of the Girdle Vessel

- LIV-13 Zhangmen
- G.B.-26 Daimai
- G.B.-27 Wushu
- G.B.-28 Weidao

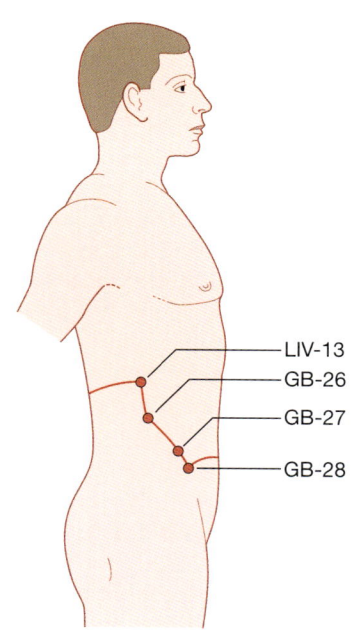

Figure 53.11 The Girdle Vessel

The Girdle Vessel can therefore be used to resolve Dampness in the Lower Burner, which causes such symptoms as burning on urination, difficulty in urination and, especially, excessive vaginal discharge.

Regulates circulation of Qi in the legs

The Girdle Vessel encircles the leg channels and it affects their circulation. Disorders of this channel can therefore impair the circulation of Qi in the leg channels, resulting in such symptoms as cold legs and feet ('like sitting in cold water'), purple feet or tense outer leg muscles (due to Liver-Blood not moistening the sinews).

Affects Qi of Stomach channel in the legs

The Girdle Vessel particularly affects the circulation of Qi in the Stomach channel and can cause weakness of the leg muscles, and in severe cases, atrophy. In these cases the opening and coupled point of the Girdle Vessel can be used to ease the vessel and tonify the Stomach and Spleen channels.

Chapter 44 of the 'Simple Questions' mentions the ancestral muscles: *'The Penetrating Vessel is the Sea of the Channels, it irrigates the rivers and valleys and it connects with the Bright Yang [Stomach channel] in the ancestral muscles. Thus, Yin and Yang meet in the ancestral muscles and connect with the avenues of the abdomen which are under the control of the Stomach: they are all restrained by the Girdle Vessel [Dai Mai] and connect with the Governing Vessel [Du Mai]. So when Bright Yang is empty, the ancestral muscles become slack as the Girdle Vessel fails to tighten them, the legs [muscles] become weak and atrophied and there may be paralysis.'*[62]

As explained above, the 'ancestral muscles' are the *rectus abdominis* muscles and this passage is saying that the Girdle Vessel 'pulls' or 'binds' the other channels: when it is slack, the Qi of the leg channels cannot flow to the legs and these become weak. The most important channel to treat is the Stomach because of its connection with the Penetrating Vessel at ST-30 Qichong and also because it controls the ancestral muscles. When needling G.B.-26 Daimai, G.B.-27 Wushu and G.B.-28 Weidao, the needling sensation should radiate down towards ST-30 Qichong (Fig. 53.12).

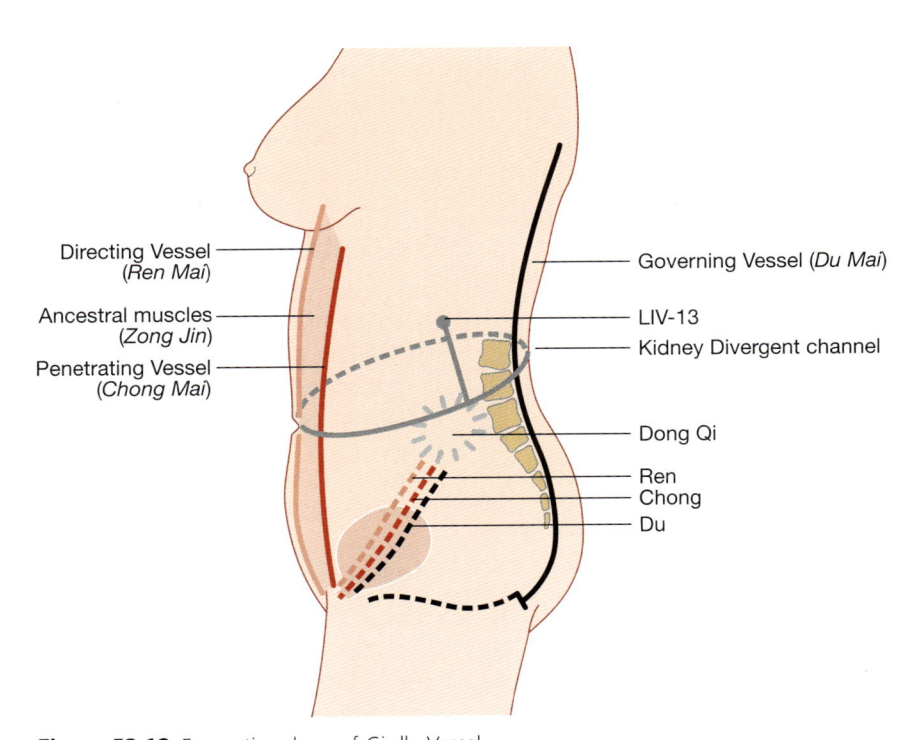

Figure 53.12 Energetic sphere of Girdle Vessel

The Girdle Vessel and abdominal pain

Another symptom of the Girdle vessel is abdominal pain that radiates to the lower back or, in the opposite direction, backache that radiates to the lower abdomen.

The Girdle Vessel in gynaecology

The Girdle Vessel is quite important in some gynaecological complaints and particularly excessive vaginal discharge. In gynaecology, some authors say that the Girdle Vessel's Deficiency pathology is secondary to a deficiency of the Directing Vessel, while its Excess pathology is secondary to an excess in the Penetrating Vessel.

Fullness and Emptiness of the Girdle Vessel

The Girdle Vessel's pathology can be classified as Full or Empty.

Full

The Full pathology of the Girdle Vessel consists in it 'not being harmonized', due to this vessel being too 'tight'. The main symptoms are:

- Fullness of the abdomen, back feels as if sitting in water. This is due to invasion of Damp-Cold in the Spleen channel
- Backache radiating to lower abdomen
- Feelings of heaviness of the body, coldness of the back, as if sitting in water, or of heaviness of the abdomen as if carrying 5000 coins. This is due to exposure to dampness and rain

The Full pathology of the Girdle Vessel is related to the Penetrating Vessel.

Empty

The Empty pathology of the Girdle Vessel is due to Qi deficiency and to this vessel being too slack. It is related to Kidney and Liver deficiency, the Girdle Vessel not restraining the Essence, Spleen-Qi sinking, and the Girdle Vessel not propping up the Post-Heaven Qi, so that Directing, Governing and Penetrating vessels become deficient.

When the Girdle Vessel is slack, Qi cannot rise, the organs sag, hernias develop, Atrophy Syndrome (*Wei* Syndrome) develops, there may be miscarriages, and prolapses occur. This is due to long-term Qi deficiency, Post- and Prenatal Qi deficiency, clear Qi descending (rather than ascending), and the Girdle Vessel being too slack.

The treatment principle is to tonify Pre- and Post-Heaven Qi, raise the clear Qi and consolidate the Girdle Vessel.

The fetus depends on the Kidneys and the Directing Vessel, but also on the Girdle Vessel. If the Girdle Vessel is slack, Qi cannot rise, the fetus is not stabilized, and the mother may miscarry.

The Empty pathology of the Girdle Vessel is related to the Directing Vessel.

Box 53.17 summarizes Full and Empty conditions in the Girdle Vessel.

Box 53.17 Girdle Vessel

Full

Vessel too 'tight'. Full pathology is related to the Penetrating Vessel

- Fullness of the abdomen, back feels as if sitting in water
- Backache radiating to lower abdomen
- Feelings of heaviness of the body, coldness of the back, as if sitting in water, or of heaviness of the abdomen as if carrying 5000 coins

Empty

Vessel too slack. Empty pathology is related to the Directing Vessel

- Hernia
- Atrophy Syndrome (*Wei* Syndrome)
- Miscarriage
- Prolapses

The Girdle Vessel and the hips

The Girdle Vessel flows through the waist and influences the hip. It can therefore be used for hip pain, particularly when there is a condition of deficiency of Liver-Blood and excess of Liver-Yang, with Liver-Blood deficiency leading to malnourishment of sinews and joints.

Box 53.18 summarizes clinical applications of the Girdle Vessel.

Classical indications

Chapter 29 of the 'Classic of Difficulties' says: '*When the Girdle Vessel is diseased, there is abdominal fullness and the back feels swollen as if sitting in water.*'

Li Shi Zhen says: '*The back and abdomen feel swollen like a balloon filled with water. In women there is lateral-lower*

> **Box 53.18 Clinical applications of the Girdle Vessel**
>
> - Harmonize the Liver and Gall Bladder
> - Resolve Dampness from Lower Burner
> - Regulate circulation of Qi to legs
> - Affect Stomach-Qi in legs
> - Abdominal pain
> - Leukorrhoea
> - Fullness and Emptiness of the Girdle Vessel
> - Hips

> **Box 53.19 Classical indications for the Girdle Vessel**
>
> - *Classic of Difficulties*: abdominal fullness and the back feels swollen as if sitting in water
> - *Li Shi Zhen*: back and abdomen feel swollen like a balloon filled with water. In women there is lateral-lower abdominal pain, internal urgency, irregular periods and white-red vaginal discharge
> - *Simple Questions*: backache radiating to the lower abdomen and difficulty in breathing in
> - *Simple Questions*: ancestral muscles slack, leg muscles weak and atrophied, paralysis
> - *Pulse Classic*: backache and abdominal pain radiating to the leg
> - *Golden Mirror of Medicine*: difficulty in lifting and moving arms and legs after Wind-stroke, numbness and contraction of limbs, head Wind pain, swelling from the back of the neck to chin, red and painful eyes with dizziness, toothache, deafness, swelling of throat, 'floating Wind' itching, contraction of sinews, pain in the thigh, hypochondrial distension, pain in the limbs

abdominal pain, internal urgency, irregular periods and white-red vaginal discharge.'[63]

Chapter 63 of the 'Simple Questions' says: 'When pathogenic factors enter the Greater Yin Connecting channels there is backache radiating to the lower abdomen and difficulty in breathing in.'[64]

Chapter 44 of the 'Simple Questions' says: 'When Bright Yang is empty, the ancestral muscles become slack as the Girdle Vessel fails to tighten them, the legs [muscles] become weak and atrophied and there may be paralysis.'[65]

The 'Pulse Classic' says: 'If the pulse is Wiry on both left and right side, it indicates a Girdle Vessel pathology with backache and abdominal pain radiating to the leg.'[66]

The 'Golden Mirror of Medicine' says: 'Difficulty in lifting and moving arms and legs after Wind-stroke, numbness and contraction of limbs, head Wind pain, swelling from the back of the neck to chin, red and painful eyes with dizziness, toothache, deafness, swelling of throat, "floating Wind" itching, contraction of sinews, pain in the thigh, hypochondrial distension, pain in the limbs.'[67]

Box 53.19 summarizes the classical indications for the Girdle Vessel.

Herbal therapy

Herbs

Herbs that affect the Girdle Vessel include those that infuse to the Lower Burner, consolidate and have an astringent property. Some of the herbs (such as Sheng Ma *Rhizoma Cimicifugae*) have an ascending movement and may be used to treat pathological conditions of the Girdle Vessel characterized by the 'belt' being too slack and Qi sinking. The astringent quality of some of these herbs would treat persistent vaginal discharges, which are a major symptom of this vessel.

Herbs that enter the Girdle Vessel include: Wu Wei Zi *Fructus Schisandrae chinensis*, Shan Yao *Radix Dioscoreae oppositae*, Qian Shi *Semen Euryales ferocis*, Fu Pen Zi *Fructus Rubi chingii*, Sang Piao Xiao *Ootheca Mantidis*, Dang Gui *Radix Angelicae sinensis*, Bai Shao *Radix Paeoniae lactiflorae*, Xu Duan *Radix Dipsaci asperi*, Long Gu *Os Draconis*, Ai Ye *Folium Artemisiae argyi*, Sheng Ma *Rhizoma Cimicifugae*, Gan Cao *Radix Glycyrrhizae uralensis*.

Formulae

In case of a Girdle Vessel disharmony with a prolapsed uterus, one can use Liang Shou Tang *Two Receiving Decoction*. This is because tonifying the Governing and Directing vessels to correct a prolapse is not enough, as one must also tonify the 'umbilical area' by tightening the Girdle vessel.

For the same purpose one can also use Bu Zhong Yi Qi Tang *Tonifying the Centre and Benefiting Qi Decoction* plus Ba Ji Tian *Radix Morindae officinalis*, Du Zhong *Cortex Eucommiae ulmoidis*, Gou Ji *Rhizoma Cibotii barometz*, Xu Duan *Radix Dipsaci asperi* and Wu Wei Zi *Fructus Schisandrae chinensis* to tonify the extraordinary vessels, consolidate the Girdle vessel and raise clear Qi.

The fetus depends on the Kidneys and the Directing Vessel, but also on the Girdle Vessel. If the Girdle Vessel is slack, Qi cannot rise, the fetus is not stabilized, and the mother may miscarry. In such a case, one should tonify the Girdle vessel with Shou Tai Wan *Fetus Longevity Pill*.

If there is a Girdle Vessel disharmony with Dampness infusing down to the genital system one can use Gan Jiang Ling Zhu Tang *Glycyrrhiza–Zingiberis–Poria–Atractylodes Decoction*, which warms the Spleen, resolves Dampness, opens the Girdle Vessel and strengthens the back.

For backache radiating to the abdomen some doctors use pungent herbs to scatter and sweet ones to moderate urgency such as Yan Hu Suo *Rhizoma Corydalis yanhusuo*, Dang Gui *Radix Angelicae sinensis*, Sang Ji Sheng *Ramulus Sangjisheng*, Gou Qi Zi *Fructus Lycii chinensis* and Xiao Hui Xiang *Fructus Foeniculi vulgaris*. Dang Gui enters both the Penetrating and Girdle vessels.

Dang Gui Shao Yao San *Angelica–Paeonia Powder* treats the Girdle Vessel, for such symptoms as abdominal pain, irregular periods, oedema and leukorrhoea. It contains a high proportion of Bai Shao, which treats abdominal pain from the Girdle Vessel's disorder, and Chuan Xiong, which moves Qi of the Penetrating Vessel.

Case history 53.10

A woman of 45 suffered from chronic migraine headaches characterized by a severe throbbing ache on the temple. Her pulse was Wiry and Full and her tongue was Red with a yellow coating. The headaches were clearly due to the rising of Liver-Yang and the Girdle Vessel opening and coupled points (G.B.-41 Zulinqi and T.B.-5 Waiguan) were used several times in successive treatments, producing a complete cure.

Case history 53.11

A woman of 72 suffered from chronic cystitis characterized by severe burning on urination and dark and scanty urine. She also experienced a severe distending sensation in the hypogastrium. Her pulse was Full, Rapid and very Wiry, particularly in the Middle position. Her tongue was Deep-Red and had a yellow coating which was thicker on the root. The root of the tongue also had red spots. This problem was caused by the downward infusion of Liver-Fire and Damp-Heat affecting the Bladder. The opening and coupled points of the Girdle Vessel were used several times in succession, together with other points to clear Liver- and Bladder-Heat, producing a nearly complete cure.

YIN STEPPING VESSEL (*YIN QIAO MAI*)

Opening point: KI-6 Zhaohai.
Coupled point: LU-7 Lieque.
Starting point: KI-6 Zhaohai.
Accumulation point: KI-8 Jiaoxin.
Area of body influenced: inner side of legs, abdomen (only unilateral symptoms), eyes.

I originally called the *Yin Qiao Mai* and *Yang Qiao Mai* 'Yin Heel Vessel' and 'Yang Heel Vessel', respectively, because they both originate from the heels (although '*qiao*' does not mean 'heel'). As the word *qiao* conveys the idea of 'raising the foot to step',[68] I have chosen to call the *Yin* and *Yang Qiao Mai* 'Yin Stepping Vessel' and 'Yang Stepping Vessel', respectively.

As mentioned in the introduction to this chapter, the Eight Extraordinary Vessels function as reservoirs to absorb excesses of Qi from the main channel. The Yin and Yang Stepping Vessels represent the 'first line' of reservoirs which absorb excesses of Yin or Yang, respectively. However, they do not perform this function in the same part of the body: the Yin Stepping Vessel absorbs excesses of Yin in the abdomen while the Yang Stepping Vessel absorbs excesses of Yang in the head.

The Yin and Yang Stepping Vessels are closely related, especially in their relationship with the eyes. They both flow up to the eyes, the Yin Stepping Vessel bringing them Yin energy, the Yang Stepping Vessel bringing them Yang energy. When the Yin Stepping Vessel is diseased, the eyes cannot stay open and tend to close all the time: that is, the person feels constantly sleepy. When the Yang Stepping Vessel is diseased, the eyes cannot close and tend to stay open all the time (i.e. the person cannot sleep).

The Yin and Yang Stepping Vessels also exert an influence on the tone of the leg muscles. When the Yin Stepping Vessel is in Excess, the inner leg muscles are tight, and the outer leg muscles loose: when the Yang Stepping Vessel is in Excess, the inner leg muscles are loose and the outer ones tight.

The Yin Stepping Vessel is an offshoot of the Kidney channel, while the Yang Stepping Vessel is an offshoot of the Bladder channel (Fig. 53.13).

Pathway

Chapter 28 of the 'Classic of Difficulties' says: '*The Yin Stepping Vessel starts from inside the heel, goes around the internal malleolus and rises up to the throat going past the Penetrating Vessel.*'[69]

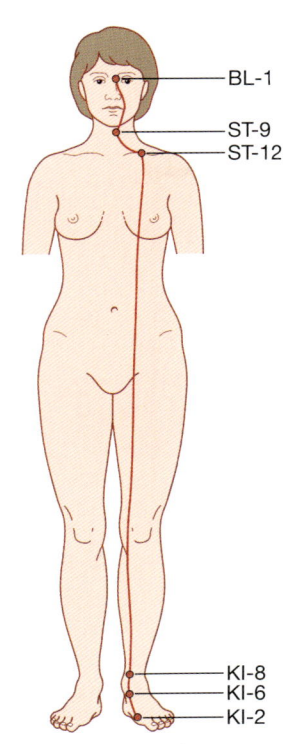

Figure 53.13 Yin Stepping Vessel

Chapter 17 of the 'Spiritual Axis' describes the pathway of the Yin Stepping Vessel as follows: '*The [Yin] Stepping Vessel separates from the Kidney channel and originates from behind KI-2 Rangu and flows up to the internal malleolus. It rises on the inner thigh to the genitals. Then it rises inside the chest and joins with ST-12 Quepen coming to the area in front of ST-9 Renying entering the cheekbone and reaching BL-1 Jingming.*'[70]

Chapter 21 of the 'Spiritual Axis' describes another aspect of the pathway of the Yin Stepping Vessel in relation to that of the Yang Stepping Vessel: '*The Bladder channel passes through the occiput and enters the brain: it belongs to the root of the eyes and it is called Eye System ... In the brain, it divides into two vessels that become the Yin and Yang Stepping Vessels. The Yin and Yang Stepping Vessels cross over each other, the Yang entering the Yin and the Yin coming out into the Yang, crossing at the inner corner of the eye.*'[71]

Li Shi Zhen describes the pathway of the Yin Stepping Vessel in greater detail: '*The Yin Stepping Vessel starts inside the heel behind KI-2 Rangu, goes to KI-6 Zhaohai, up to the internal malleolus and then 2 cun up to KI-8 Jiaoxin which is its Accumulation point [Xi-Cleft point). It then ascends along the inside of the leg and enters the genitals. It proceeds upwards and enters inside the chest, it connects with ST-12 Quepen, it emerges in front of ST-9 Renying, reaches the throat where it crosses with the Penetrating Vessel, it then reaches the inner corner of the eye.*'[72]

Citing Zhang Zi Yang (Song dynasty), Li Shi Zhen gives another detail on the Yin Stepping Vessel's pathway: '*The Yin Stepping Vessel reaches the area in front of the coccyx and below the scrotum [i.e. perineum].*'[73]

Boxes 53.20 and 53.21 summarize the pathway and points of the Yin Stepping Vessel.

Clinical applications

The Yin Stepping Vessel and sleep

Because of its relation with the eyes, the Yin Stepping Vessel can be used in disturbances of sleep, whether insomnia or somnolence. In this context, it is often used in conjunction with the Yang Stepping Vessel. In cases of insomnia, the Yin Stepping Vessel is tonified (by tonifying KI-6 Zhaohai) and the Yang Stepping Vessel drained (by reducing BL-62 Shenmai). In cases of somnolence, the Yin Stepping Vessel is drained (by reducing KI-6 Zhaohai) and the Yang Stepping Vessel is tonified (by reinforcing BL-62 Shenmai). In both cases, the point BL-1 Jingming can be added to establish a connection between the Yin and Yang Stepping

---

Box 53.20 Yin Stepping Vessel – summary of pathway

- Originates inside the heel on the medial side, goes to KI-2 Rangu, ascends to the internal malleolous and then to KI-8 Jiaoxin
- It rises on the inner leg and thigh to reach the genitals
- It ascends the abdomen and chest and connects with ST-12 Quepen
- It goes up to the throat connecting with ST-9 Renying and then to the eye at BL-1 Jingming where it meets the Yang Stepping Vessel

---

Box 53.21 Points of the Yin Stepping Vessel

- KI-2 Rangu
- KI-6 Zhaohai
- KI-8 Jiaoxin (Accumulation point)
- ST-12 Quepen
- ST-9 Renying
- BL-1 Jingming

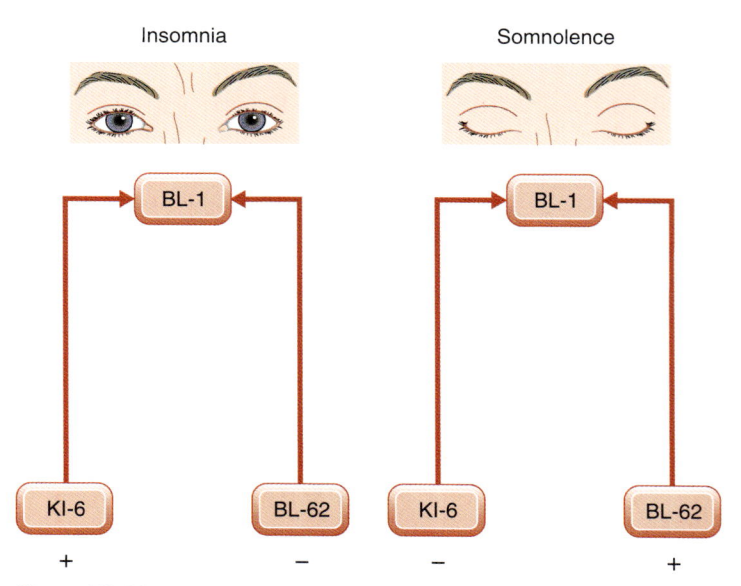

Figure 53.14 Yin Stepping Vessel and sleep

Vessels, so that Yin and Yang energy in the eyes can be balanced (Fig. 53.14).

The 'Spiritual Axis' also suggests KI-6 Zhaohai for painful red eye.

The Yin Stepping Vessel and Atrophy Syndrome (*Wei* Syndrome)

The Yin Stepping Vessel can be used in certain cases of Atrophy Syndrome (*Wei* Syndrome), when the muscles of the inner aspect of the legs are tight and those of the outer aspect loose and the foot turns inwards. This makes walking very difficult and the person prone to tripping. The Yin Stepping Vessel's opening and coupled points can be used to balance the tension of the inner and outer leg muscles.

Abdominal pain

The Yin Stepping Vessel extends its range of action to the abdomen and can be used in Excess patterns of the Lower Burner in women for such symptoms as abdominal distention, abdominal masses, difficult delivery or retention of placenta, all of which arise from stagnation. However, the Yin Stepping Vessel is chosen only when the abdominal symptoms are unilateral. In my experience, the Yin Stepping Vessel can be used to treat adhesions following surgery.

Box 53.22 summarizes the clinical applications of the Yin Stepping Vessel.

Box 53.22 Clinical applications of the Yin Stepping Vessel

- Sleep
- Atrophy Syndrome (*Wei* Syndrome)
- Abdominal pain

Classical indications

Chapter 17 of the 'Spiritual Axis' says: '*The Qi of the Yin and Yang Stepping Vessels reaches the eyes, moistening them. If Qi does not nourish them, the eyes will be unable to close.*'[74]

Chapter 29 of the 'Classic of Difficulties' says: '*When the Yin Stepping Vessel is diseased, the Yang is slack and the Yin tense.*'[75] This statement is generally thought to refer to the state of the leg muscles: that is, '*Yang is slack*' means that the muscles of the lateral side of the leg are slack and '*Yin is tense*' means that the muscles of the medial side of the legs are tight. Although this interpretation is correct, it should not restrict a broader interpretation of the above statement. In fact, 'Yang' and 'Yin' above could also refer to back and front, head and abdomen, etc. Moreover, they can also be interpreted in a broad sense of Excess of Yin (*Yin is tense*) and Deficiency of Yang (*Yang is slack*).

Chapter 21 of the 'Spiritual Axis' says: '*If the Yang Stepping Vessel is in Excess, the eyes stay open; if the Yin Stepping Vessel is in Excess, the eyes want to close.*'[76]

The 'Golden Mirror of Medicine' lists the following symptoms for the Yin Stepping Vessel: '*Obstruction of the throat, difficult urination, chest distension, painful urination, borborygmi, abdominal masses from excessive consumption of alcohol, abdominal pain, vomiting, diarrhoea, regurgitation of food, breast abscess, dry stools, difficult labour causing fainting, wind and blood from anus, discomfort in the diaphragm, feeling of lump in the throat.*'[77]

Box 53.23 summarizes classical indications for the Yin Stepping Vessel.

Box 53.23 Classical indications for the Yin Stepping Vessel

- *Classic of Difficulties*: Yang is slack and the Yin tense
- *Spiritual Axis*: eyes want to close
- *Golden Mirror of Medicine*: obstruction of the throat, difficult urination, chest distension, painful urination, borborygmi, abdominal masses from excessive consumption of alcohol, abdominal pain, vomiting, diarrhoea, regurgitation of food, breast abscess, dry stools, difficult labour causing fainting, wind and blood from anus, discomfort in the diaphragm, feeling of lump in the throat

---

Herbal therapy

Herbs

The herbs that affect the Yin Stepping Vessel are: Yan Hu Suo *Rhizoma Corydalis yanhusuo*, Gua Lou *Fructus Trichosanthis*, Ban Xia *Rhizoma Pinelliae ternatae*, Dan Nan Xing *Pulvis Arisaemae cum felle bovis*, Zhi Mu *Radix Anemarrhenae asphodeloidis*, Huang Bo *Cortex Phellodendri*, Yuan Zhi *Radix Polygalae tenuifoliae*, Suan Zao Ren *Semen Ziziphi spinosae* and Shi Chang Pu *Rhizoma Acori graminei*.

Formulae

Formulae that affect the Yin Stepping Vessel include Si Wu Tang *Four Substances Decoction* and Ban Xia Tang *Pinellia Decoction* (which is composed only of Ban Xia *Rhizoma Pinelliae ternatae* and Shu Mi, husked sorghum).

Case history 53.12

A man of 28 suffered from continuous somnolence. This followed a car accident during which he suffered a fracture of the skull. He came for treatment as he was studying hard for an exam and could not keep awake.

The point BL-62 Shenmai on the left side was reinforced to stimulate the Yang Stepping Vessel, KI-6 Zhaohai on the right side was reduced to drain the Yin Stepping Vessel, and the point BL-1 Jingming was used bilaterally with even method. After only one treatment the somnolence completely disappeared and he could not actually sleep for 2 days!

YANG STEPPING VESSEL (*YANG QIAO MAI*)

Opening point: BL-62 Shenmai.
Coupled point: S.I.-3 Houxi.
Starting point: BL-62 Shenmai.
Accumulation point: BL-59 Fuyang.
Area of body influenced: lateral aspect of leg, back, neck, head, eyes.

The Yang Stepping Vessel is the first line of defence in the system of reservoirs to absorb excesses of Yang in the head.

The Yang Stepping Vessel is an offshoot of the Bladder channel and it brings Yang energy up to the eyes. Its influence on the eyes and the muscle tone of the lateral side of the legs has already been mentioned in the discussion of the Yin Stepping Vessel.

Although the Yin and Yang Stepping Vessels are somewhat symmetrical in their functions, there are some differences in their practical use.

Whilst the Yin Stepping Vessel's sphere of influence is mostly in the lower abdomen and genitals (apart from its action on the eyes), the Yang Stepping Vessel's sphere of action is mostly in the head, absorbing excess Yang or stagnation in the head area. For this reason, it is used for Wind-stroke, hemiplegia, aphasia and facial paralysis (Fig. 53.15).

Pathway

Chapter 28 of the 'Classic of Difficulties' describes the pathway of the Yang Stepping Vessel briefly: '*The Yang Stepping Vessel originates inside the heel, it goes up to the external malleolus and rises up to join with G.B.-20 Fengchi.*'[78]

Li Shi Zhen gives a more detailed pathway as follows: '*The Yang Stepping Vessel is an offshoot of the Bladder channel. It starts inside the heel, it goes up to the external malleolus to BL-62 Shenmai and then to BL-61 Pushe. It then rises 3 cun to BL-59 Fuyang, which is its Accumulation point. It then rises along the external surface of the leg,*

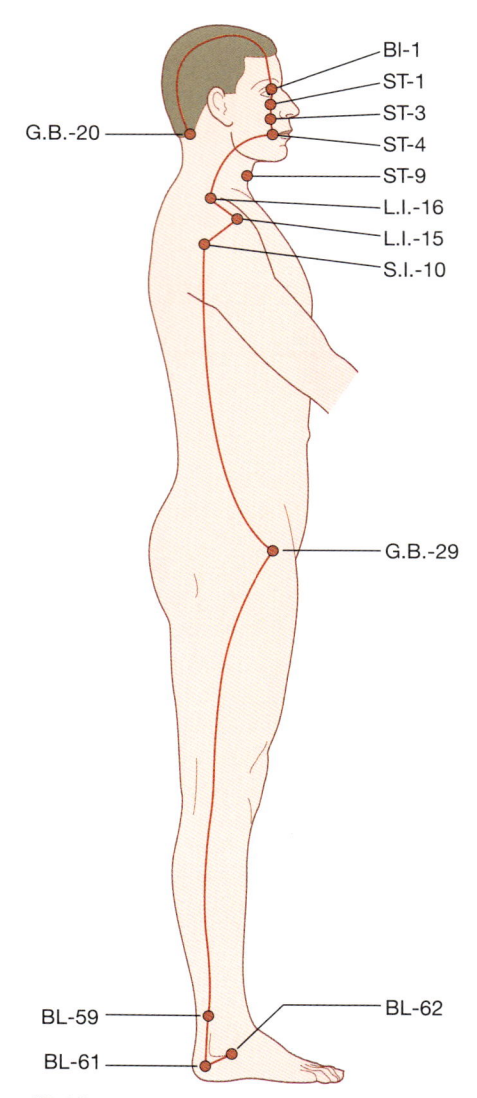

Figure 53.15 Yang Stepping Vessel

Box 53.24 Yang Stepping Vessel – summary of pathway

- Originates inside the heel on the lateral side, goes to the external malleolus and BL-62 Shenmai
- It ascends on the lateral side of the leg and connects with BL-61 Pushe and BL-59 Fuyang
- It ascends on the lateral side of the upper thigh and hip and connects with G.B.-29 Juliao
- It goes to S.I.-10 Naoshu where it connects with the Small Intestine channel and the Yang Linking Vessel. It rises outside the shoulder and connects with the Large Intestine channel at L.I.-16 Jugu and with the Large Intestine and Triple Burner channels at L.I.-15 Jianyu
- It rises to ST-9 Renying and it connects with the Large Intestine and Stomach channels and the Directing Vessel at ST-4 Dicang. It goes up to the Stomach channel to ST-3 Juliao and then rejoins the Directing Vessel at ST-1 Chengqi
- It then goes to the inner corner of the eye where it connects with the Small Intestine, Bladder and Stomach channels and with the Yin Stepping Vessel at BL-1 Jingming. From here, it continues over the skull, passes behind the ear and enters G.B.-20 Fengchi, where it ends

Box 53.25 Points of the Yang Stepping Vessel

- BL-62 Shenmai
- BL-61 Pushe
- BL-59 Fuyang (Accumulation point)
- G.B.-29 Juliao
- S.I.-10 Naoshu
- L.I.-15 Jianyu
- L.I.-16 Jugu
- ST-9 Renying
- ST-4 Dicang
- ST-3 Juliao
- ST-1 Chengqi
- BL-1 Jingming

behind the hypochondrium, then up to the scapula where it connects with the Small Intestine channel and the Yang Linking Vessel at S.I.-10 Naoshu. It rises outside the shoulder and connects with the Large Intestine channel at L.I.-16 Jugu and with the Large Intestine and Triple Burner channels at L.I.-15 Jianyu. It rises to ST-9 Renying and it connects with the Large Intestine and Stomach channels and the Directing Vessel at ST-4 Dicang. It goes up to the Stomach channel to ST-3 Juliao and then rejoins the Directing Vessel at ST-1 Chengqi. It then goes to the inner corner of the eye where it connects with the Small Intestine, Bladder and Stomach channels and with the Yin Stepping Vessel at BL-1 Jingming. From here, it continues over the skull, passes behind the ear and enters G.B.-20 Fengchi where it ends. In total 23 points.'[79]

Boxes 53.24 and 53.25 summarize the pathway and points of the Yang Stepping Vessel.

Clinical applications

Absorbs Excess Yang from the head

As mentioned above, the Yang Stepping Vessel is the first line of reservoirs to absorb excesses of Yang, but it does so primarily in the head. 'Excess of Yang in the head' can manifest in a variety of ways: for example, Liver-Fire or Liver-Yang rising affecting the head,

Liver-Wind, etc. Absorbing Excess Yang from the head also has a mental implication as the Yang Stepping Vessel is used for mental symptoms such as mania, agitation, etc.

Absorbing Excess Yang from the head also implies extinguishing internal Wind and the Yang Stepping Vessel is used for such conditions as Wind-stroke, facial paralysis, aphasia, numbness or epilepsy.

It may also be used to expel exterior Wind from the head for symptoms of aversion to cold, fever, sneezing, headache, stiff neck, runny nose and Floating pulse. It is particularly indicated if the exterior attack is accompanied by severe headache and stiff neck.

The Yang Stepping Vessel and the eyes

As mentioned above, the Yang Stepping Vessel brings Yang Qi to the eyes (the Yin Stepping Vessel brings Yin Qi to the eyes). When the Yang Stepping Vessel is Full, there is too much Yang Qi in the eyes and they cannot close, so that the person suffers from insomnia. To correct this, one can drain the Yang Stepping Vessel by reducing BL-62 Shenmai, tonify the Yin Stepping Vessel by reinforcing KI-6 Zhaohai and insert BL-1 Jingming to establish a communication between these two vessels at the level of the eyes so that Excess Yang is drained away and Yin is transported to them.

The Yang Stepping Vessel in mental problems

As mentioned above, 'Excess of Yang in the head' has also an implication on a mental level and the Yang Stepping Vessel can be used for symptoms such as mania, agitation, or insomnia.

A particular indication for the use of the Yang Stepping Vessel in these mental conditions is a pulse that is Full and Wiry on both Front positions of left and right.

In ancient texts, it is indicated in cases of 'attraction to ghosts and demons' and 'missing a dead relative excessively'.[80]

The '1000 Golden Ducat Prescriptions' indicates the Yang Stepping Vessel for 'fright', 'seeing ghosts' and manic depression (*dian-kuang*).[81]

The Yang Stepping Vessel in backache and sciatica

The Yang Stepping Vessel is very useful to treat unilateral backache and sciatica. As mentioned in the introduction, in channel problems, the extraordinary vessels are particularly indicated when the symptoms overlap several channels. For example, the Yang Stepping Vessel is particularly indicated in sciatica when the pain affects the Bladder, Gall Bladder and Stomach channels (or also just the first two).

In such cases, I needle BL-62 Shenmai on the affected side and S.I.-3 on the opposite side. If there is a pronounced stiffness, I add the Accumulation point of the Yang Stepping Vessel (i.e. BL-59 Fuyang). After leaving these needles in for 15 minutes, I then ask the patient to turn over and I treat the local points on the back.

Again, the Yang Stepping Vessel is particularly indicated in back problems occurring against a background of a Full condition and the pulse is Full and Wiry. I do not use the Yang Stepping Vessel when the backache is bilateral.

> **Clinical note**
>
> The Yang Stepping Vessel is excellent to treat sciatica when the pain overlaps among the Bladder, Gall Bladder and Stomach channels. Use BL-62 Shenmai on the affected side and S.I.-3 on the opposite side. Leave in for 15 minutes and then use local points

The Yang Stepping Vessel and the hip

As the Yang Stepping Vessel flows through the point G.B.-29 Juliao, this vessel affects both the Bladder and Gall Bladder channels in the hip area: for this reason, I often use the Yang Stepping Vessel to treat hip pain. In such cases, I use BL-62 Shenmai on the affected side and S.I.-3 on the opposite side. After retaining these points for 15 minutes, I ask the patient to lie on the opposite side so that I can needle G.B.-30 Huantiao.

Box 53.26 summarizes clinical applications of the Yang Stepping Vessel.

> **Box 53.26 Clinical applications of the Yang Stepping Vessel**
>
> - Absorb Excess Yang from head
> - Eyes
> - Mental problems
> - Backache and sciatica
> - Hip

Classical indications

Chapter 29 of the 'Classic of Difficulties' says: '*When the Yang Stepping Vessel is diseased, the Yin is slack and the Yang tense*'.[82] This statement is generally thought to refer to the state of the leg muscles: that is, '*Yin is slack*' means that the muscles of the medial side of the leg are slack and '*Yang is tense*' means that the muscles of the lateral side of the legs are tight. Although this interpretation is correct, it should not restrict a broader interpretation of the above statement. In fact, 'Yang' and 'Yin' above could also refer to back and front, head and abdomen, etc. Moreover, they can also be interpreted in a broad sense of Excess of Yang (*Yang is tense*) and Deficiency of Yin (*Yin is slack*).

Chapter 63 of the 'Simple Questions' suggests using the Yang Stepping Vessel for eye pain: '*When pathogenic factors are in the Yang Stepping Vessel, it will cause eye pain in the inner corner: needle the point half a cun below the external malleolus [BL-62 Shenmai] twice. Needle the right side when the left eye is affected and the left side when the right eye is affected. The condition will be cured in the time it takes to walk 10 Li (Chinese mile) [5.76 km or 3.57 miles]*'.[83] This statement is interesting as it recommends contralateral needling: that is, needling the right side for afflictions of the left eye and vice versa. This is presumably due to the fact that the Yin and Yang Stepping Vessels cross over the other side when they rise to the head: this is somewhat in convergence with Western medicine as the nerve tracts from one side of the body enter the opposite side of the brain.

Chapter 21 of the 'Spiritual Axis' says: '*When the Yang Stepping Vessel is in Excess, the eyes stay open.*'[84]

Citing Wang Shu He, Li Shi Zhen says: '*When the pulse of the Front position of both left and right side is Wiry, it indicates a disease of the Yang Stepping Vessel. This causes backache, epilepsy, apoplexy, crying like a sheep, aversion to wind, hemiplegia and tightness of the body.*'[85] He also says: '*In epilepsy, treat the Stepping Vessels: the Yang in men and the Yin in women.*'[86]

The 'Golden Mirror of Medicine' gives the following indications for the Yang Stepping Vessel: '*Stiff back and spine, Wind in ankles and feet, aversion to wind, sweating, headache, numbness of hands and feet, upper arm cold, thunder headache, red eyes, breast abscess, deafness, epistaxis, epilepsy, limb pain, unilateral fullness, swelling and sweating of the body, dribbling of urination.*'[87]

Citing Zhang Jie Gu, Li Shi Zhen says: '*When the Yang Stepping Vessel is diseased, the Yang is tense, there is mad walking [mania] and the eyes cannot close.*'[88] It is interesting to note that in manic patients, one of the characteristic symptoms is staying awake at night, not from insomnia but from deliberately staying up to do things.

Box 53.27 summarizes the classical indications for the Yang Stepping Vessel.

Box 53.27 Classical indications for the Yang Stepping Vessel

- *Classic of Difficulties*: Yin is slack and the Yang tense
- *Simple Questions*: eye pain in the inner corner
- *Spiritual Axis*: eyes stay open
- *Li Shi Zhen*: backache, epilepsy, apoplexy, crying like a sheep, aversion to wind, hemiplegia and tightness of the body
- *Golden Mirror of Medicine*: stiff back and spine, Wind in ankles and feet, aversion to wind, sweating, headache, numbness of hands and feet, upper arm cold, thunder headache, red eyes, breast abscess, deafness, epistaxis, epilepsy, limb pain, unilateral fullness, swelling and sweating of the body, dribbling of urination
- *Li Shi Zhen*: mad walking (mania) and the eyes cannot close

---

Herbal therapy

Herbs

Herbs that enter the Yang Stepping Vessel include: Ma Huang *Herba Ephedrae*, Fang Feng *Radix Ledebouriellae divaricatae*, Cang Zhu *Rhizoma Atractylodis lanceae*, Zhi Gan Cao *Radix Glycyrrhizae uralensis praeparata* and Fang Ji *Radix Stephaniae tetrandae*.

Formulae

None given by Li Shi Zhen.

Case history 53.13

A man of 43 suffered from giddiness and an ache on the lateral side of the legs. His blood pressure was high. His face was red and the muscles on the lateral side of the legs were very tight. He appeared very tense. His pulse was Full, Rapid and Wiry and his tongue was Red.

The Yang Stepping Vessel was chosen to calm the Yang, relax the muscles on the lateral side of the legs, subdue interior Wind (manifested by the giddiness) and calm the Mind. The successive use of its opening and coupled points (BL-62 Shenmai on the left and S.I.-3 Houxi on the right) produced a marked improvement.

COMBINED YIN AND YANG STEPPING VESSEL PATHOLOGY

As mentioned above, there is a symmetry between the Yang and Yin Stepping Vessels from various points of view as follows:

- The Yin Stepping Vessel absorbs excesses of Yin Qi; the Yang Stepping Vessel absorbs excesses of Yang Qi
- The Yin Stepping Vessel brings Yin Qi to the eyes; the Yang Stepping Vessel brings Yang Qi to the eyes
- The Yin and Yang Stepping Vessels control the left and right side of the body, the former for the Yin and the latter for the Yang channels
- Defensive Qi flows in the Yin Stepping Vessel at night and in the Yang Stepping Vessel in the daytime
- The Yin and Yang Stepping Vessels control the tension of the leg muscles, the former in the medial and the latter in the lateral side
- The Yin Stepping Vessel branches out of the Kidney channel, the Yang Stepping Vessel out of the Bladder channel
- The Yin and Yang Stepping Vessels cross over each other, the Yang entering the Yin and the Yin coming out into the Yang, crossing at the inner corner of the eye.

The Yin and Yang Stepping Vessels are very important for the circulation and balance of Yin and Yang Qi in the head and eyes; they perform a very important role also in the circulation of Defensive Qi in the head and neck.

The Yin Stepping Vessel is an offshoot of the Kidney channel, which flows from the feet up to the head (to the root of the tongue); the Yang Stepping Vessel is an offshoot of the Bladder channel, which flows from the head down to the feet. All the extraordinary vessels flow from the lower part of the body towards the top: therefore the Yin Stepping Vessel flows upwards in the same way as the Kidney channel. With regard to the flow of Yang, there is an apparent contradiction as the Yang Stepping Vessel is an offshoot of the Bladder channel but it flows from the lower part of the body towards the head, while the Bladder channel flows from the head to the feet. As we shall see shortly, this is not really a contradiction but an important way in which the channel system keeps the balance of Yin and Yang in the head.

It is worth repeating here the statement from chapter 21 of the 'Spiritual Axis': *'The Bladder channel passes through the occiput and enters the brain: it belongs to the root of the eyes and it is called Eye System ... In the brain, it divides into two vessels that become the Yin and Yang Stepping Vessels. The Yin and Yang Stepping Vessels cross over each other, the Yang entering the Yin and the Yin coming out into the Yang, crossing at the inner corner of the eye.'*[89]

The Eye System (Mu Xi) is described in chapter 80 of the 'Spiritual Axis': *'The Essence and Qi of the five Zang and six Fu ascend to the eyes to give vision ... They communicate with many channels constituting an Eye System (Mu Xi), which ascends to the vertex, enters the brain and then surfaces at the occiput.'*[90] The Eye System intersects with the extraordinary vessels as follows (Fig. 53.16):

- *Governing Vessel*: Yintang
- *Directing Vessel*: ST-1 Chengqi
- *Yang Stepping Vessel*: ST-1 Chengqi, BL-1 Jingming, G.B.-20 Fengchi
- *Yin Stepping Vessel*: BL-1 Jingming
- *Yang Linking Vessel*: G.B.-14 Yangbai, G.B.-20 Fengchi, Du-16 Fengfu

In particular, the Governing Vessel has four areas of convergence with the Eye System, as follows:

1. Du-16 Fengfu: including BL-10 Tianzhu, G.B.-20 Fengfu and TB-17 Yifeng. The Governing Vessel enters the brain from here. The Yang Stepping Vessel connects with G.B.-20 from where it enters the brain and connects with Eye System
2. Du-20 Baihui: including Sishencong, Du-21 Qianding and BL-7 Tongtian. Du-20 Baihui is a point of the Sea of Marrow
3. Bijiao: including Yintang and Du-24 Shenting. Bijiao is an extra point situated on the Governing Vessel, on the bridge of the nose level with the centre of the pupils
4. Du-26 Renzhong and Du-25 Suliao: connect with the brain indirectly through the Eye System

Furthermore, the Gall Bladder Muscle channel in the head plays a role in the regulation of Yin and Yang in

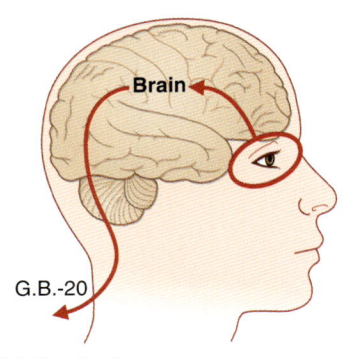

Figure 53.16 The Eye System

the head. Chapter 13 of the 'Spiritual Axis', describing the pathways of all the Muscle channels, says of the Gall Bladder Muscle channel: *'When there is contraction of the muscles of the neck from the left towards the right, the right eye will be unable to open because the [Gall Bladder] Muscle channel passes through the right angle of the forehead moving hand in hand with the Stepping Vessels. As the left [side] affects the right [side], an impairment of the Muscle channel on the left angle of the forehead will cause paralysis of the right foot: this is called 'mutual intersection of the Muscle channels.'*[91]

Bearing in mind the above, the Yin and Yang Stepping Vessels perform an important role in regulating the ascending and descending of Defensive Qi in the head and eyes and, in so doing, balancing Yin and Yang in the head and eyes. The Yin Stepping Vessel brings Yin Qi up to the eyes; it meets the Yang Stepping Vessel at BL-1 Jingming from where Yang Qi descends away from the eyes: this ensures the balance of Yin and Yang in the head and eyes (Fig. 53.17).

With regard to Defensive Qi, in the daytime it flows in the Yang and in the night in the Yin. The flow of Defensive Qi to and away from the eyes in the 24 hours determines our states of wakefulness and sleep. When Defensive Qi arrives in the eyes in the morning (emerging from the Yin), it makes the eyes open and we wake up; when Defensive Qi moves away from the eyes at night (leaving the Yang), the eyes want to close and we fall asleep. Therefore, in pathology, a deficiency and failure of ascending of the Defensive Qi in the daytime will make us sleepy and it will make it difficult to wake up; if the Defensive Qi fails to descend from the eyes at night, the eyes want to stay open and we cannot fall asleep (Fig. 53.18).

The Yin and Yang Stepping Vessels play an important role in the ascending and descending of the Defensive Qi to and from the eyes in the daytime and at night, respectively. Citing the above statement from chapter 21 of the 'Spiritual Axis', *'The Yin and Yang Stepping Vessels cross over each other, the Yang entering the Yin and the Yin coming out into the Yang, crossing at the inner corner of the eye'*: this ensures the proper ascending and descending of the Defensive Qi to and from the eyes.

Therefore, although the Yang Stepping Vessel *ascends* towards the head to BL-1 Jingming, the Bladder channel from which it derives *descends* from the head and the eyes: this allows the Yang Stepping Vessel to bring Yang Qi away from the eyes when appropriate: that is, coordinate with the Yin Stepping Vessel to regulate and balance Yin and Yang Qi in the head and eyes.

Moreover, the descending movement of the Yang Stepping Vessel in relation to Defensive Qi is also related to the Eye System as, in this system, there is a movement of Qi from the eyes into the brain and out at the occiput in the region of G.B.-20 Fengchi, which is where the Yang Stepping Vessel ends.

Therefore, as it ascends from the feet towards the eyes, the Yang Stepping Vessel brings necessary Yang Qi to the eyes; equally, due its relation with the Bladder channel (which descends from the head), the Eye System and the Gall Bladder Muscle channel mentioned above, the Yang Stepping Vessel brings Yang Qi and Defensive Qi *away* from the eyes when appropriate (i.e. at night). This resolves the apparent contradiction that the Yang Stepping Vessel both brings and takes away Yang Qi from the eyes.

Citing the 'ABC of Acupuncture', Li Shi Zhen says: *'When the eyes want to close and cannot stay open, it is due to the Defensive Qi staying in the Yin and not moving into the Yang: as it stays in the Yin, Yin Qi is in excess and when this is in excess the Yin Stepping Vessel is full. Its Qi cannot enter the Yang, which becomes empty and this causes the eyes to want to close. When the eyes cannot close and stay open, it is due to the Defensive Qi staying in the Yang and not moving into the Yin: as it stays in the Yang, Yang Qi is in excess and when this is in excess the Yang Stepping Vessel*

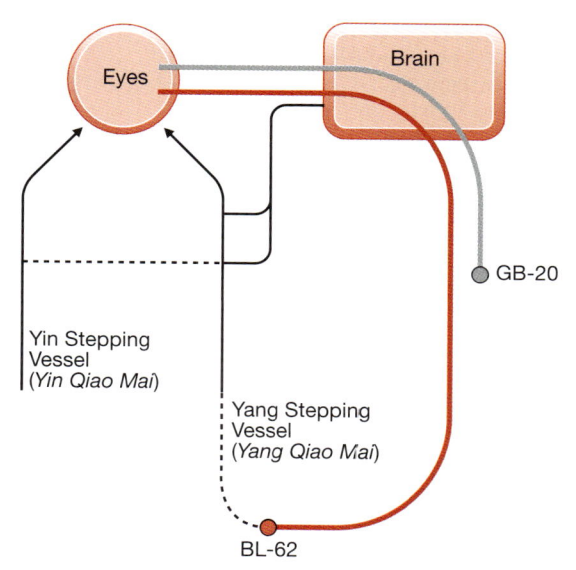

Figure 53.17 Relationship between Yin–Yang Stepping Vessels, brain and eyes

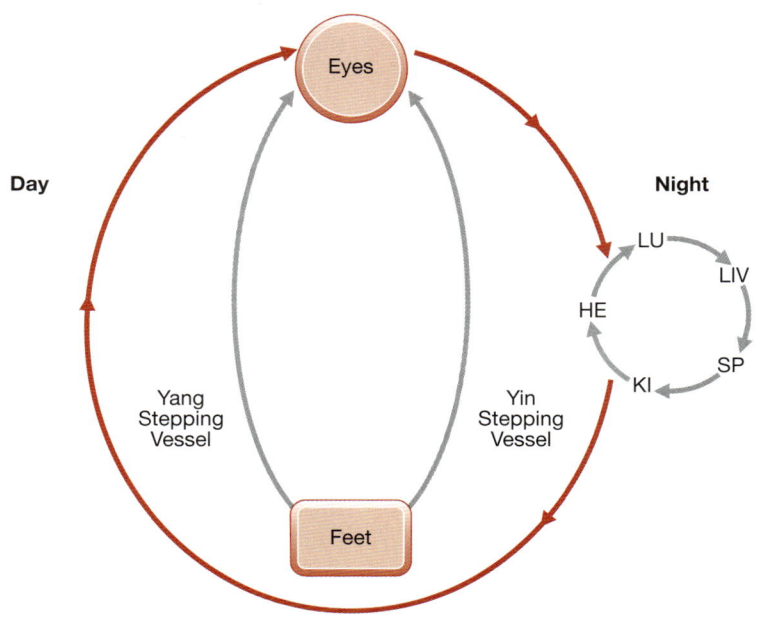

Figure 53.18 Yin and Yang Stepping Vessels and Defensive Qi circadian rhythm

is full. Its Qi cannot enter the Yin, which becomes empty and this causes the eyes to want to stay open.'[92]

The 'ABC of Acupuncture' has an interesting comment on the nature of the Yin and Yang Stepping Vessel in relation to channels differentiating between men and women. It says: 'Of the Stepping Vessels, one is Yang and the other Yin but which is counted? In men, the Yang is counted; in women the Yin is counted. The one that is counted in is [taken to be] a channel; the one that is not counted is [taken to be] a Connecting channel.'

The commentary explains that the total length of the 14 channels is 16 *zhang* and 2 *chi*: this length is arrived at counting the Yang Stepping Vessel in men and Yin Stepping Vessel in women. Therefore, in men, the Yang Stepping Vessel is like a channel while the Yin Stepping Vessel is like a Connecting channel; vice versa in women. This passage is interesting because it differentiates the anatomy of channels according to sex.

Box 53.28 summarizes the pathology of the combined Yin and Yang Stepping Vessels.

YIN LINKING VESSEL (*YIN WEI MAI*)

Opening point: P-6 Neiguan.
Coupled point: SP-4 Gongsun.
Starting point: KI-9 Zhubin.

Box 53.28 Combined Yin and Yang Stepping Vessels pathology

- The Yin Stepping Vessel absorbs excesses of Yin Qi; the Yang Stepping Vessel absorbs excesses of Yang Qi
- The Yin Stepping Vessel brings Yin Qi to the eyes; the Yang Stepping Vessel brings Yang Qi to the eyes
- The Yin and Yang Stepping Vessels control the left and right side of the body, the former for the Yin and the latter for the Yang channels
- Defensive Qi flows in the Yin Stepping Vessel at night and in the Yang Stepping Vessel in the daytime
- The Yin and Yang Stepping Vessels control the tension of the leg muscles, the former in the medial and the latter in the lateral side
- The Yin Stepping Vessel branches out of the Kidney channel, the Yang Stepping Vessel out of the Bladder channel
- The Yin and Yang Stepping Vessels cross over each other, the Yang entering the Yin and the Yin coming out into the Yang, crossing at the inner corner of the eye

Accumulation point: KI-9 Zhubin.
Area of body influenced: chest, heart.

The Yin Linking Vessel connects all the Yin channels. This is partly due to the fact that its opening point is P-6 Neiguan, pertaining to the Terminal Yin, which is the 'hinge' of the Yin channels (Fig. 53.19).

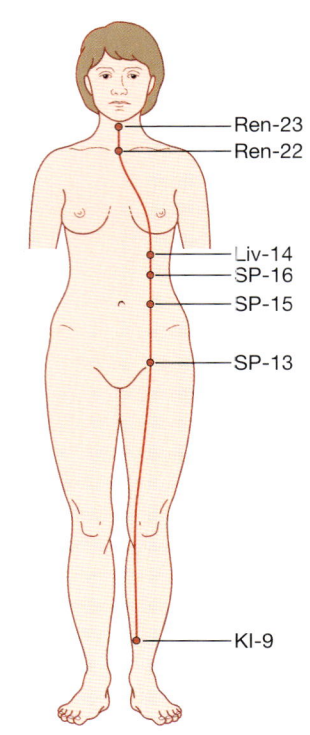

Figure 53.19 The Yin Linking Vessel

Box 53.29 Yin Linking Vessel – summary of pathway

- Starts from KI-9 Zhubin, and goes to the centre of the muscle
- It rises along the inner side of the leg to the lower-central abdomen (*Xiao Fu*) where it connects with the Spleen, Liver, Kidney and Stomach channels at SP-13 Fushe
- It then rises and connects with the Spleen channel at SP-15 Daheng and SP-16 Fuai
- It goes up to the hypochondrium where it connects with the Liver channel at LIV-14 Qimen
- It goes up to the chest, diaphragm and throat where it connects with the Directing Vessel at the point Ren-22 Tiantu and Ren-23 Lianquan, then rising to the forehead where it ends

Box 53.30 Points of the Yin Linking Vessel

- KI-9 Zhubin (Accumulation point)
- SP-6 Sanyinjiao (possibly)
- SP-13 Fushe
- SP-15 Daheng
- SP-16 Fuai
- LIV-14 Qimen
- Ren-22 Tiantu
- Ren-23 Lianquan

Pathway

Chapter 28 of the 'Classic of Difficulties' says only that: '*The Yin Linking Vessel starts from a point where all the Yin [channels] intersect.*'[93] The area where the Yin Linking Vessel starts is considered now to be KI-9 Zhubin. However, the 'Elucidation of the Yellow Emperor's Classic of Internal Medicine' thinks that this point is SP-6 Sanyinjiao (which means 'meeting of the three Yin'.[94]

This statement is preceded by a description of the function of both Yin and Yang Linking Vessels: '*The Yang and Yin Linking Vessels link like a network around the body to absorb the overflowing Qi that cannot flow into the Main channels.*'[95]

Li Shi Zhen describes the pathway of the Yin Linking Vessel as follows: '*The Yin Linking Vessel starts at the point where all the Yin [channels] intersect, it originates from KI-9 Zhubin which is its Accumulation point 5 cun above the internal malleolus and it goes to the centre of the muscle. It then rises along the inner side of the leg to the lower-central abdomen [Xiao Fu] where it connects with the Spleen, Liver, Kidney and Stomach channels at SP-13 Fushe. It then rises and connects with the Spleen channel at SP-15 Daheng and SP-16 Fuai. It goes up to the hypochondrium where it connects with the Liver channel at LIV-14 Qimen. It goes up to the chest, diaphragm and throat where it connects with the Directing Vessel at the point Ren-22 Tiantu and Ren-23 Lianquan, then rising to the forehead where it ends. In total 14 points.*'[96]

Boxes 53.29 and 53.30 summarize the pathway and points of the Yin Linking Vessel.

Clinical applications

Nourish Blood and Yin

Since it connects all the Yin channels, the Yin Linking Vessel can be used for deficiency of Blood and/or Yin, especially if accompanied by psychological symptoms such as insomnia, anxiety, mental restlessness, thinking too much, obsession, loss of will-power and lack of self-control. In this context, it has a remarkable effect in calming the mind, especially in women and is especially effective combined with its starting and Accumulation point, KI-9 Zhubin.

Mental–emotional problems

Since the Yin Linking Vessel nourishes Blood, it has a tonifying action on the Heart and can be used for such symptoms as chest pain or a feeling of stuffiness, oppression or tightness of the chest, anxiety, apprehension, depression or nightmares. The association of the Yin Linking Vessel with the mental state is very old and is mentioned in chapter 41 of the 'Simple Questions' quoted below.

The 'Great Compendium of Acupuncture' lists among many other symptoms:

- Knot in the chest which feels tight and full on palpation (P-6 Neiguan, P-7 Daling, Ren-12 Zhongwan, SP-6 Sanyinjiao)
- Stagnant Qi, easily losing control, too much thinking, melancholy, sadness, pain in the heart and abdomen (P-6 Neiguan, BL-12 Fengmen, Ren-17 Shanzhong, P-8 Laogong, ST-36 Zusanli)
- Sadness and crying (P-6 Neiguan, HE-5 Tongli, S.I.-3 Houxi, HE-7 Shenmen, KI-4 Dazhong)
- Forgetfulness, mental cloudiness (P-6 Neiguan, BL-15 Xinshu, HE-5 Tongli, HE-9 Shaochong)
- Anxiety (P-6 Neiguan, ST-18 Rugen, HE-5 Tongli, BL-15 Xinshu, BL-19 Danshu)
- Heart and Gall Bladder deficient, shock, palpitations (P-6 Neiguan, BL-19 Danshu, HE-5 Tongli, G.B.-41 Zulinqi)[97]

Clinical note

The Yin Linking Vessel is excellent to treat depression and sadness in women occurring against a background of Blood deficiency. Needle P-6 on the right, SP-4 on the left, Ren-15 Jiuwei and KI-9 bilaterally

Headaches

The Yin Linking Vessel is effective in treating headaches from deficiency of Blood, especially if they are at the back of the neck. This is due to the fact that it nourishes Blood and its opening point P-6 Neiguan, being also the connecting point of the Pericardium channel, affects the Triple Burner channel area on the neck.

Box 53.31 summarizes the clinical applications of the Yin Linking Vessel.

Classical indications

Chapter 41 of the 'Simple Questions' says: '*In backache caused by the Feiyang channel, the pain travels upwards*

Box 53.31 Clinical applications of the Yin Linking Vessel

- Nourish Blood and Yin
- Mental–emotional problems
- Headaches

gradually with a feeling of sadness; if the pain becomes severe the patient has a feeling of fear. To treat this pain use the Feiyang channel and needle the point 5 cun above the internal malleolus, which connects with the Yin Linking Vessel [i.e. KI-9 Zhubin]'.[98]

Chapter 29 of the 'Classic of Difficulties' says: '*When the Yin Linking Vessel is diseased, there is heart pain and depression.*'[99] The same chapter says: '*The Yang Linking Vessels links all the Yang, the Yin Linking Vessel links all the Yin. When Yin and Yang cannot link with each other, there will be pensiveness, obsession, loss of will power and lack of self-control.*'[100]

The 'Golden Mirror of Medicine' lists the following symptoms for the Yin Linking Vessel: '*Feeling of fullness, stuffiness and distension of the chest, borborygmi, diarrhoea, anal prolapse, difficulty in swallowing, diaphragm stagnation from excessive consumption of alcohol, hard lumps to the side of the hypochondrium, hypochondrial and heart pain in women, internal urgency, abdominal pain, unresolved attack of Wind-Cold that leaves a tightness in the chest, malaria.*'[101]

Box 53.32 summarizes the classical indications for the Yin Linking Vessel.

Box 53.32 Classical indications for the Yin Linking Vessel

- *Simple Questions*: backache with pain travelling upwards gradually with a feeling of sadness; if the pain becomes severe the patient has a feeling of fear
- *Classic of Difficulties*: heart pain and depression, pensiveness, obsession, loss of will-power and lack of self-control
- *Golden Mirror of Medicine*: feeling of fullness, stuffiness and distension of the chest, borborygmi, diarrhoea, anal prolapse, difficulty in swallowing, diaphragm stagnation from excessive consumption of alcohol, hard lumps to the side of the hypochondrium, hypochondrial and heart pain in women, internal urgency, abdominal pain, unresolved attack of Wind-Cold that leaves a tightness in the chest, malaria

Herbal therapy

Herbs

The herbs that affect this vessel are Dang Gui *Radix Angelicae sinensis* and Chuan Xiong *Radix Ligustici Chuanxiong*.

Some herbs affect both the Yang and Yin Linking Vessels. These include: Lu Jiao Shuang *Cornu Cervi degelatinatum*, Xiao Hui Xiang *Fructus Foeniculi vulgaris*, Dang Gui *Radix Angelicae sinensis*, Gui Zhi *Ramulus Cinnamomi cassiae*, Bai Shao *Radix Paeoniae lactiflorae*, Huang Qi *Radix Astragali membranacei*.

Formulae

Dang Gui Si Ni Tang *Angelica Four Rebellious Decoction* (for the Liver), Wu Zhu Yu Tang *Evodia Decoction* (for the Liver), Si Ni Tang *Four Rebellious Decoction* (for the Kidneys), and Li Zhong Tang *Regulating the Centre Decoction* (for the Spleen).

Case history 53.14

A woman of 54 suffered from severe anxiety and claustrophobia. She was afraid to go to the theatre, church or in the underground. She was anxious when alone at home and felt a tight gripping sensation in the chest. Her pulse was Choppy and her tongue pale, but with a red tip. The clinical manifestations were due to deficiency of Blood, depriving the mind of its residence and resulting in severe anxiety. Due to the deficiency of Blood and the typical sensation of tightness in the chest, the Yin Linking Vessel was used (P-6 Neiguan on the right and SP-4 Gongsun on the left), producing excellent results.

YANG LINKING VESSEL (*YANG WEI MAI*)

Opening point: T.B.-5 Waiguan.
Coupled point: G.B.-41 Zulinqi.
Starting point: BL-63 Jinmen.
Accumulation point: G.B.-35 Yangjiao.
Area of body influenced: lateral aspect of leg, sides of body, lateral aspect of neck and head, ears.

The Yang Linking Vessel connects all the Yang channels (Fig. 53.20).

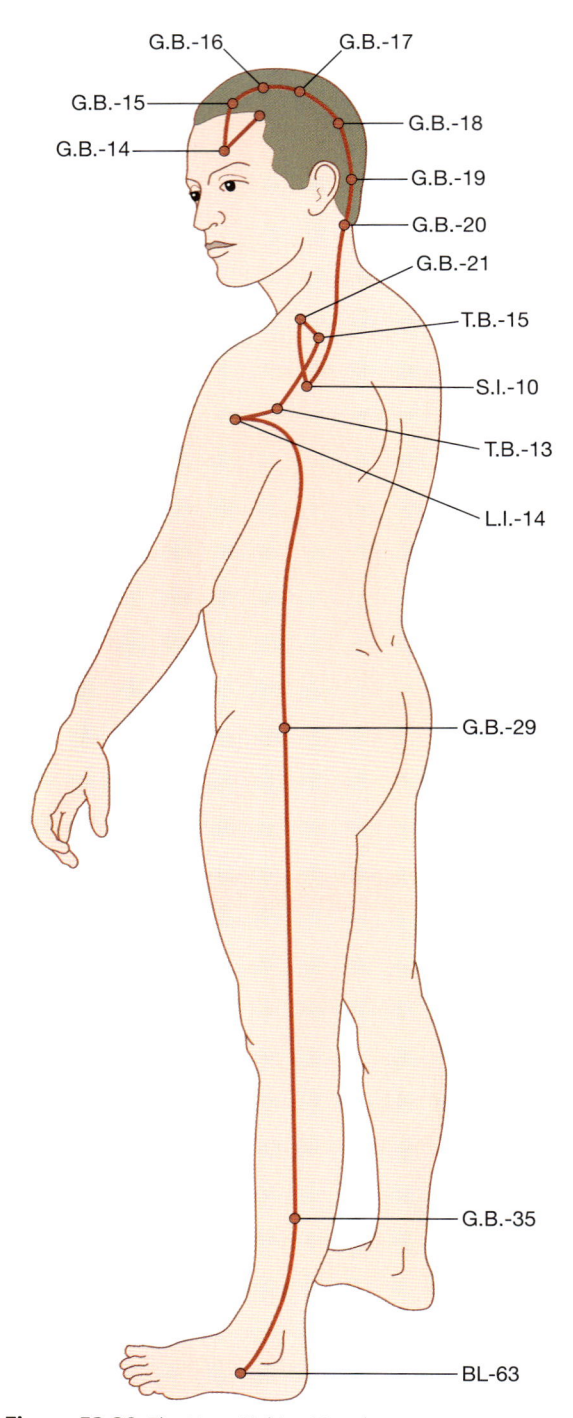

Figure 53.20 The Yang Linking Vessel

Pathway

Chapter 28 of the 'Classic of Difficulties' says: '*The Yang Linking Vessel starts at the point where the Yang channels intersect.*'[102] The 'Elucidation of the Yellow Emperor's Classic of Internal Medicine' says that this point is G.B.-35 Yangjiao (which means 'meeting of the Yang').[103]

Li Shi Zhen gives a detailed pathway for the Yang Linking Vessel: '*The Yang Linking Vessel starts at the point where the Yang channels intersect, at BL-63 Jinmen, which is 1.5 cun below the external malleolus. It goes up 7 cun to G.B.-35 Yangjiao, which is its Accumulation point. It travels up the thigh to G.B.-29 Juliao. It then rises up the hypochondrium to the shoulder at L.I.-14 Binao where it connects with the Large Intestine, Small Intestine and Bladder channels, then ascends to T.B.-13 Naohui and T.B.-15 Tianliao. It then goes to G.B.-21 where it connects with the Triple Burner, Gall Bladder and Stomach channels. It goes to the back of the shoulder to S.I.-10 Naoshu where it connects with the Small Intestine channel and the Yang Stepping Vessel. It rises up behind the ear to reach G.B.-20 Fengchi where it intersects with the Triple Burner and Gall Bladder channels. Then it goes to G.B.-19 Naokong, G.B.-18 Chengling, G.B.-17 Zhengying, G.B.-16 Muchuang, G.B.-15 Linqi and to the forehead to G.B.-14 Yangbai where it connects with the Gall Bladder, Triple Burner, Large Intestine and Stomach channels. It then proceeds to the forehead, enters the eye and ascends to G.B.-13 Benshen. In total 32 points.*'[104]

Boxes 53.33 and 53.34 summarize the pathway and points of the Yang Linking Vessel.

Clinical applications

Intermittent fevers

The Yang Linking Vessel is used for intermittent fevers and alternation of chills and fever. These are symptoms of affection of the Lesser Yang stage in the Six-Stage patterns of penetration of exterior pathogenic factor (see ch. 44). The chief symptom at this stage is alternation of chills and fever because the pathogenic factor is lodged half in the Interior and half in the Exterior.

Some doctors say that all the Yang channels are linked by the Yang Linking Vessel at G.B.-20 Fengchi. They say that this point's action of expelling external Wind is due to its relation with the Yang Linking Vessel, *not* the Gall Bladder. On the other hand, its action of extinguishing internal Wind is, on the contrary, due to its relation with the Gall Bladder.

Box 53.33 Yang Linking Vessel – summary of pathway

- Starts at BL-63 Jinmen, and goes up to G.B.-35 Yangjiao, which is its Accumulation point
- It travels up the thigh to G.B.-29 Juliao, rises up the hypochondrium and to the shoulder at L.I.-14 Binao where it connects with the Large Intestine, Small Intestine and Bladder channels, then ascends to T.B.-13 Naohui and T.B.-15 Tianliao
- It then goes to G.B.-21 where it connects with the Triple Burner, Gall Bladder and Stomach channels, goes to the back of the shoulder to S.I.-10 Naoshu where it connects with the Small Intestine channel and the Yang Stepping Vessel
- It rises up behind the ear to reach G.B.-20 Fengchi where it intersects with the Triple Burner and Gall Bladder channels, goes to G.B.-19 Naokong, G.B.-18 Chengling, G.B.-17 Zhengying, G.B.-16 Muchuang, G.B.-15 Linqi and to the forehead to G.B.-14 Yangbai where it connects with the Gall Bladder, Triple Burner, Large Intestine and Stomach channels
- It then proceeds to the forehead, enters the eye and ascends to G.B.-13 Benshen

---

Box 53.34 Points of the Yang Linking Vessel

- BL-63 Jinmen
- G.B.-35 Yangjiao
- G.B.-29 Juliao
- L.I.-14 Binao
- T.B.-13 Naohui
- T.B.-15 Tianliao
- G.B.-21 Jianjing
- S.I.-10 Naoshu
- G.B.-20 Fengchi
- G.B.-19 Naokong
- G.B.-18 Chengling
- G.B.-17 Zhengying
- G.B.-16 Muchuang
- G.B.-15 Linqi
- G.B.-14 Yangbai
- G.B.-13 Benshen

Sides of the body

The Yang Linking Vessel exerts its influence on the sides of the body and is used for such symptoms as hypochondrial pain, pain in the lateral aspect of the leg (such as sciatica along the Gall Bladder channel) and pain in the lateral side of the neck.

Ear problems

The Yang Linking Vessel affects the ears and can be used for ear problems due to the rising of Liver-Fire, such as tinnitus and deafness. It can also be used in any

> **Box 53.35 Clinical applications of the Yang Linking Vessel**
>
> - Intermittent fevers
> - Sides of body
> - Ear problems

ear diseases caused by a Gall Bladder disharmony such as ear discharge from Damp-Heat in the Gall Bladder.

Box 53.35 summarizes clinical applications of the Yang Linking Vessel.

Classical indications

Chapter 29 of the 'Classic of Difficulties' says: '*When the Yang Linking Vessel is diseased there is [alternation of feeling of] heat and [feeling of] cold and irritability.*'[105]

Chapter 41 of the 'Simple Questions' says: '*The Yang Linking Vessel causes backache with sudden swelling. Needle the point on the dividing muscle of the calf on the Bladder channel 1 foot above the ground.*'[106] This point is probably BL-57 Chengshan.

Li Shi Zhen says: '*When there is sweating, aversion to cold, fever and the pulse is Floating on the Front and Weak on the Rear position, it indicates a disease of the Yang Linking Vessel.*'[107]

The 'Golden Mirror of Medicine' lists the following symptoms for the Yang Linking Vessel: '*Swelling and pain of the limbs, cold knees, paralysis or limbs, Wind headache, bone and muscles problems of the back and loins, ache in the head, neck and around eyebrows, hot limbs, numbness of limbs, night sweating, red and swollen eyes, spontaneous sweating during an invasion of Wind-Cold, feeling of heat superficially.*'[108]

Box 53.36 summarizes the classical indications for the Yang Linking Vessel.

Herbal therapy

Herbs

Herbs that affect this vessel are those that harmonize Nutritive and Defensive Qi: that is, Gui Zhi *Ramulus Cinnamomi cassiae*, Bai Shao *Radix Paeoniae lactiflorae* and Huang Qi *Radix Astragali membranacei*.

Some herbs affect both the Yang and Yin Linking Vessels. These include: Lu Jiao Shuang *Cornu Cervi degelatinatum*, Xiao Hui Xiang *Fructus Foeniculi vulgaris*, Dang Gui *Radix Angelicae sinensis*, Gui Zhi *Ramulus Cinnamomi cassiae*, Bai Shao *Radix Paeoniae lactiflorae*, Huang Qi *Radix Astragali membranacei*.

> **Box 53.36 Classical indications for the Yang Linking Vessel**
>
> - *Classic of Difficulties*: alternation of feeling of heat and feeling of cold and irritability
> - *Simple Questions*: backache with sudden swelling
> - *Li Shi Zhen*: sweating, aversion to cold, fever, pulse Floating on the Front and Weak on the Rear position
> - *Golden Mirror of Medicine*: swelling and pain of the limbs, cold knees, paralysis of limbs, Wind headache, bone and muscles problems of the back and loins, ache in the head, neck and around eyebrows, hot limbs, numbness of limbs, night sweating, red and swollen eyes, spontaneous sweating during and invasion of Wind-Cold, feeling of heat superficially

Formulae

Gui Zhi Tang *Ramulus Cinnamomi Decoction*.

Case history 53.15

A boy of 12 had a middle-ear infection and the Yang Linking Vessel was used (T.B.-5 Waiguan on the left and G.B.-41 Zulinqi on the right), producing a complete cure.

COMBINED YIN AND YANG LINKING VESSEL PATHOLOGY

The Yin and Yang Linking Vessels and the waist

The Yang and Yin Linking Vessels link all the Yang and Yin channels and when they are overfull one cannot turn the waist.

Yang and Yin Linking Vessels influence head and abdomen, respectively

Defensive Qi is Yang and controls the Exterior. The Yang Linking Vessel unites the three Yang channels at the level of the head, and when pathogenic factors enter this vessel there is alternation of hot and cold feeling and headache. This explains the use of T.B.-5 Waiguan both for invasions of Wind and for headache.

Nutritive Qi is Yin and controls the Interior. The Yin Linking Vessel unites the three Yin channels at the level of the abdomen; dysfunction or invasion of pathogenic factors causes abdominal and chest pain.

Harmonization of Nutritive and Defensive Qi

When Yin and Yang link up, Nutritive and Defensive Qi are harmonized: when these are not harmonized the person feels sorry, thinks too much, is depressed, may have obsessive thoughts, loss of will-power and lack of self-control.

Citing Zhang Jie Gu, Li Shi Zhen says: '*Defensive Qi is Yang and is on the Exterior, when the Yang Linking Vessel is invaded by pathogenic factors the disease is on the Exterior and there is alternation of feeling of cold and feeling of heat with irritability. Nutritive Qi is Yin and is in the Interior, when the Yin Linking Vessel is attacked by pathogenic factors the disease is in the Interior and there is heart pain with depression. When Yin and Yang are mutually linked, the Nutritive and Defensive Qi are harmonized. When Nutritive and Defensive Qi are not harmonized there is pensiveness, obsession, loss of will power and lack of self-control. When there is spontaneous sweating it indicates that the Nutritive and Defensive Qi are not harmonized in which case use Gui Zhi Tang Ramulus Cinnamomi Decoction.*'[109]

In sweating from Defensive Qi not being harmonized with the Nutritive Qi use Du-16 Fengfu and G.B.-20 Fengchi. Needle these two points first to release the Exterior (sweating, headache, Floating pulse). This approach can also be used for 'chronic Wind' in the muscles of Greater and Lesser Yang areas causing muscle ache and stiffness.

Box 53.37 summarizes the areas of pathology of the combined Yin and Yang Linking Vessels.

Box 53.37 Yin and Yang Linking Vessel combined pathology

- Waist
- Head and abdomen
- Harmonize Nutritive and Defensive Qi

Learning outcomes

In this chapter you will have learned:

- The opening and coupled points of the Governing Vessel (S.I.-3 Houxi and BL-62 Shenmai), theories of its pathway and the areas of the body it influences
- The clinical applications of the Governing Vessel: tonify Kidney-Yang; strengthen the back; nourish the Brain and Marrow; strengthen the Mind; expel exterior Wind; extinguish interior Wind
- The opening and coupled points of the Directing Vessel (LU-7 Lieque and KI-6 Zhaohai), its pathway and sphere of influence
- The clinical applications of the Directing Vessel: nourish Yin; regulate the Uterus and Blood; move Qi in the Lower Burner and Uterus; promote descending of Lung-Qi and the Kidney's receiving of Qi; promote transformation, transportation and excretion of fluids; activate the Triple Burner; control Fat Tissue and Membranes; the combination of Governing and Directing Vessel points
- The opening and coupled points of the Penetrating Vessel (SP-4 Gongsun and P-6 Neiguan), theories of its pathway and the areas of the body it influences
- The clinical significance of the five branches of the Penetrating Vessel (internal, abdominal, head, spinal and descending)
- The significance of the various names of the Penetrating Vessel (Sea of Blood, Sea of the Five Yin and Six Yang Organs and Sea of the 12 Channels)
- The clinical significance of rebellious Qi and Blood stasis in the Penetrating Vessel
- The influence of the Penetrating Vessel on the Membranes, female breast, Heart, Stomach, feet and 'ancestral muscles'
- The similarities and differences between the use of the Directing and Penetrating Vessels
- The opening and coupled points of the Girdle Vessel (G.B.-41 Zulinqi and T.B.-5 Waiguan), its pathway and sphere of influence
- The clinical applications of the Girdle Vessel: harmonize Liver and Gall Bladder; resolve Dampness in the Lower Burner; regulate circulation of Qi in the legs; affect Qi of the Stomach channel in the legs; abdominal pain; gynaecological complaints; symptoms of Fullness and Emptiness of the Girdle Vessel; influence the hip
- The opening and coupled points of the Yin Stepping Vessel (KI-6 Zhaohai and LU-7 Lieque), its pathway and the areas of the body it influences
- The clinical applications of the Yin Stepping Vessel: sleep disturbance; atrophy syndrome; abdominal pain
- The opening and coupled points of the Yang Stepping Vessel (BL-62 Shenmai and S.I.-3 Houxi), its pathway and the areas of the body it influences
- The clinical applications of the Yang Stepping Vessel: absorb excess Yang from head; insomnia; mental problems; backache and sciatica; hip pain
- The symmetry of the functions of the Yin and Yang Stepping Vessels: absorb excess Yin/Yang Qi; bring Yin/Yang Qi to eyes; control left/right side of body; Defensive Qi in Yin at night/Yang in day; tension of medial/lateral leg muscles; branch out of Kidney/Bladder channel; crossing over each other at inner corner of eye
- The intersections made by the Eye System with the extraordinary vessels
- The opening and coupled points of the Yin Linking Vessel (P-6 Neiguan and SP-4 Gongsun), its pathway and the areas of the body it influences

- The clinical applications of the Yin Linking Vessel: nourish Blood and Yin; Mental–emotional problems; headaches (plus classical indications and herbal therapy)
- The opening and coupled points of the Yang Linking Vessel (T.B.-5 Waiguan and G.B.-41 Zulinqi), its pathway and the areas of the body it influences
- The clinical applications of the Yang Linking Vessel: intermittent fevers; sides of the body; ear problems
- How the Yin and Yang Linking Vessels are combined in Pathology: the waist; influence head and abdomen, respectively; harmonizing Nutritive and Defensive Qi

Self-assessment questions

1. Describe the internal pathway of the Governing Vessel.
2. Complete the following: 'The Governing vessel is called the "___ of ____ channels" as it exerts an influence on all the ____ channels and it can be used to strengthen the ____ of the body'.
3. Which extraordinary vessel would be best to use to treat the menopausal symptoms of night sweating, hot flushes, feeling of heat and mental restlessness?
4. Complete the following: the Penetrating Vessel is described as the 'Sea of the five ___ and six '___ organs'[5], the 'Sea of the __ _____s'[6] and the 'Sea of _____'.
5. Which Penetrating Vessel points are on the lower abdomen, and which two organs do they especially influence?
6. The Penetrating Vessel is known as the 'Sea of Blood'. Why does it have such a deep influence on the gynaecological system?
7. What extraordinary vessel pathology is indicated by a feeling of energy rising from the lower abdomen up towards the throat?
8. Which point connects the Penetrating Vessel and the Stomach?
9. Complete the following: 'The Directing Vessel corresponds to __, the Penetrating Vessel to _____'.
10. Apart from Liver and Gall Bladder channels, with which channel does the Girdle Vessel connect?
11. What is the opening point of the Yin Stepping Vessel?
12. Complete the following: 'In cases of insomnia, the ____ Stepping Vessel is tonified and the ____ Stepping Vessel is drained'.
13. How does opening the Yang Stepping Vessel help treat mental problems?
14. Give two of the three main clinical applications of the Yin Linking Vessel.
15. Which general area of the body is the main area of influence of the Yang Linking Vessel?

See p. 1266 for answers

END NOTES

1. Nanjing College of Traditional Chinese Medicine 1979 A Revised Explanation of the Classic of Difficulties (*Nan Jing Jiao Shi* 难经校释), People's Health Publishing House, Beijing, first published *c.* AD 100, p. 70.
2. Wu Qian 1977 Golden Mirror of Medicine (*Yi Zong Jin Jian* 医宗金鉴), People's Health Publishing House, Beijing, p. 129. First published in 1742.
3. 1979 The Yellow Emperor's Classic of Internal Medicine – Simple Questions (*Huang Di Nei Jing Su Wen* 黄帝内经素问), People's Health Publishing House, Beijing, first published *c.*100 BC, p. 320.
4. Wang Luo Zhen 1985 A Compilation of the 'Study of the Eight Extraordinary Vessels' (*Qi Jing Ba Mai Kao Jiao Zhu* 奇经八脉考校注), Shanghai Science Publishing House, Shanghai. The 'Study of the Eight Extraordinary Vessels' (*Qi Jing Ba Mai Kao* 奇经八脉考) by Li Shi Zhen was published in 1578. Study of the Eight Extraordinary Vessels, p. 81.
5. Study of the Eight Extraordinary Vessels, p. 81.
6. 1981 Spiritual Axis (*Ling Shu Jing* 灵枢经, People's Health Publishing House, Beijing, first published *c.*100 BC, p. 49.
7. Spiritual Axis, p. 23.
8. Zhang Jie Bin (also called Zhang Jing Yue) 1982 Classic of Categories (*Lei Jing* 类经), People's Health Publishing House, Beijing, first published in 1624, p. 49.
9. Simple Questions, p. 321.
10. Classic of Difficulties, p. 74. I translate the word *jue* in this passage as 'fainting'. Unschuld translates it as 'the spine is bent backwards'. Matsumoto translates it as 'rebellious'.
11. Study of the Eight Extraordinary Vessels, p. 89.
12. Golden Mirror of Medicine, p. 2106.
13. Wang Shu He 1984 'The Pulse Classic' (*Mai Jing* 脉经), People's Health Publishing House, Beijing. First published *c.* AD 280, p. 91.
14. Simple Questions, p. 319.
15. Study of the Eight Extraordinary Vessels, p. 71.
16. Study of the Eight Extraordinary Vessels, p. 71.
17. Please note that I translate the Chinese term 'Shan' (疝) as 'hernia' for simplicity although the term *Shan* encompasses a wider range of disorders which involve pain and/or swelling of the abdomen or scrotum, some of which may not be hernia.
18. Classic of Difficulties, p. 74.
19. Spiritual Axis, p. 4.
20. Classic of Categories, p. 561.
21. My clinical experience has actually led me to conclude that the points on the limbs act in quite a different way, or rather in a different medium, than those on the abdomen. I have noticed over and over again in practice that the insertion of a point on a limb (e.g. P-6 Neiguan) frequently causes a strong needling sensation with immediate propagation down the limb like an electric current. Thus, Qi travels very fast down the channel. With points in the abdomen, the needling sensation is never quite so strong nor does it often travel down the channel. In some cases, it does propagate but often horizontally and only after the needles have been in place for some time. I therefore think that the needling sensation in the abdomen travels along the Membranes of the abdomen, which accounts for its slower movement compared to that in the limbs.
22. Wang Guo Rui 1329 The Jade Dragon Classic of Spiritual Acupuncture from Bian Que (*Bian Que Shen Ying Zhen Jiu Yu Long Jing*), cited in Chinese Acupuncture Therapy, p. 216.
23. Please note that I translate the Chinese term 'Shan' (疝) as 'hernia' for simplicity although the term *Shan* encompasses a wider range of disorders which involve pain and/or swelling of the abdomen or scrotum, some of which may not be hernia.
24. Classic of Difficulties, p. 74.
25. Simple Questions, p. 320.
26. Pulse Classic, p. 92.
27. Golden Mirror of Medicine, p. 2107.
28. Study of the Eight Extraordinary Vessels, p. 71.
29. Classic of Categories, p. 281.
30. Simple Questions, p. 319.
31. Simple Questions, p. 219–220.
32. Classic of Difficulties, p. 70.
33. Spiritual Axis, p. 79–80.

34. Classic of Categories, p. 281.
35. Spiritual Axis, p. 112–113.
36. Classic of Categories, p. 281.
37. Huang Fu Mi 282 'The ABC of Acupuncture' (*Zhen Jiu Jia Yi Jing* 针 灸 甲 乙 经), People's Health Publishing House, Beijing, 1979, p. 257.
38. ABC of Acupuncture, p. 255–256.
39. Study of the Eight Extraordinary Vessels, p. 52.
40. Spiritual Axis, p. 73.
41. Classic of Categories, p. 281.
42. Spiritual Axis, p. 120.
43. Spiritual Axis, p. 73.
44. Spiritual Axis, p. 120.
45. Study of the Eight Extraordinary Vessels, p. 65.
46. Spiritual Axis, p. 101.
47. Classic of Difficulties, p. 73–74.
48. Study of the Eight Extraordinary Vessels, p. 60.
49. Study of the Eight Extraordinary Vessels, p. 61.
50. Classic of Categories, p. 281.
51. Simple Questions, p. 249.
52. Classic of Difficulties, p. 73–74.
53. Pulse Classic, p. 92.
54. Golden Mirror of Medicine, p. 2104.
55. Study of the Eight Extraordinary Vessels, p. 60.
56. Ibid., p. 61.
57. Ibid., p. 60.
58. Simple Questions, p. 219–220.
59. Classic of Difficulties, p. 70.
60. Study of the Eight Extraordinary Vessels, p. 99.
61. Spiritual Axis, p. 39–40.
62. Simple Questions, p. 249.
63. Study of the Eight Extraordinary Vessels, p. 102.
64. Simple Questions, p. 344.
65. Simple Questions, p. 249.
66. Pulse Classic, p. 90.
67. Golden Mirror of Medicine, p. 2105.
68. Study of the Eight Extraordinary Vessels (commentary), p. 30.
69. Classic of Difficulties, p. 70.
70. Spiritual Axis, p. 50.
71. Spiritual Axis, p. 56.
72. Study of the Eight Extraordinary Vessels, p. 29.
73. Ibid., p. 29.
74. Spiritual Axis, p. 50.
75. Classic of Difficulties, p. 73.
76. Spiritual Axis, p. 56.
77. Golden Mirror of Medicine, p. 2108.
78. Classic of Difficulties, p. 70.
79. Study of the Eight Extraordinary Vessels, p. 35.
80. Ibid., p. 48.
81. Ibid., p. 49.
82. Classic of Difficulties, p. 73.
83. Simple Questions, p. 346–347.
84. Spiritual Axis, p. 56.
85. Study of the Eight Extraordinary Vessels, p. 40.
86. Ibid., p. 40.
87. Golden Mirror of Medicine, p. 2107.
88. Study of the Eight Extraordinary Vessels, p. 41.
89. Spiritual Axis, p. 56.
90. Spiritual Axis, p. 151.
91. Spiritual Axis, p. 43.
92. Study of the Eight Extraordinary Vessels, p. 42.
93. Classic of Difficulties, p. 70–71.
94. Elucidation of the Yellow Emperor's Classic of Internal Medicine, p. 155.
95. Classic of Difficulties, p. 70.
96. Study of the Eight Extraordinary Vessels, p. 9.
97. Heilongjiang Province National Medical Research Group 1984 An Explanation of the Great Compendium of Acupuncture (*Zhen Jiu Da Cheng Jiao Shi* 针 灸 大 成 校 释), People's Health Publishing House, Beijing, p. 670. The 'Great Compendium of Acupuncture' itself was first published in 1601.
98. Simple Questions, p. 231.
99. Classic of Difficulties, p. 73.
100. Ibid., p. 73.
101. Golden Mirror of Medicine, p. 2105.
102. Classic of Difficulties, p. 70.
103. Elucidation of the Yellow Emperor's Classic of Internal Medicine, p. 155.
104. Study of the Eight Extraordinary Vessels, p. 13.
105. Classic of Difficulties, p. 73.
106. Simple Questions, p. 230.
107. Study of the Eight Extraordinary Vessels, p. 18.
108. Golden Mirror of Medicine, p. 2106.
109. Study of the Eight Extraordinary Vessels, p. 18.

SECTION 2

The functions of the points

INTRODUCTION

Acupuncture points can be classified into various categories according to their common energetic actions. For example, all Accumulation (*Xi*) points can be said to have an action on the Qi of the channel and be able to treat acute and painful conditions. Likewise, all Back Transporting points can treat chronic problems, while all Source (*Yuan*) points tonify the Yin organs directly. Therefore, we can attribute a certain function to a point by reference to the function of the category it belongs to. For example, it is possible to say that LU-6 Kongzui treats acute cough by virtue of its being an Accumulation point as all such points treat acute conditions.

The problem with any classification of points is that it always suffers from many exceptions because not all points within a given category have necessarily the same function. This is due to the fact that most theories of Chinese medicine, and the theory of the function of points in particular, probably resulted from a combination of the inductive with the deductive method. For example, if a point such as LIV-2 Xingjian was found from experience to eliminate Liver-Fire, after a process of further experimentation, the theory might have been formulated that all Fire points eliminate Heat. Thus, one might say that LIV-2 eliminates Liver-Fire not because it is the Fire point, but it is the Fire point *because*, according to many centuries' experience, it drains Liver-Fire. It is not clear whether the practical experience of LIV-2 clearing Liver-Fire preceded the generalization according to which Fire points drain Fire.

The implication of this is that each point has certain energetic functions, discovered over centuries of accumulated clinical experience, which may or may not be related to their 'classification'.

Having discussed the energetic action of the various categories of points in chapter 48, we can now add the energetic action of each point. By 'action' of a point, I mean the definition of a point's effect in terms of general actions, for example 'moving Qi', 'expelling Wind', 'nourishing Blood', etc. By contrast, a point's 'indications' are the symptoms for which it is effective, for example cough, nausea, tiredness, etc.

Box P7-S2.1 summarizes actions and indications of points.

There is no contradiction between the 'actions' and the 'indications' of a point as the actions are nothing but a summarization and generalization of a point's effects: such actions are necessarily derived from an analysis of the indications. For example, if a point is indicated for cough and breathlessness, we can deduce that that point's action is to 'restore the descending of Lung-Qi'.

> **Box P7-S2.1   Actions and indications of points**
>
> The 'action' of a point is the definition of a point's effect in terms of general actions, e.g. 'moving Qi', 'expelling Wind', 'nourishing Blood', etc. By contrast, a point's 'indications' are the symptoms for which it is effective, e.g. cough, nausea, tiredness, etc.

> There is no contradiction between the 'actions' and the 'indications' of a point as the actions are nothing but a summarization and generalization of a point's effects: such actions are necessarily derived from an analysis of the indications

Although a systematic exposition of the points' actions has been done only relatively recently in the history of Chinese medicine, elements of such actions have appeared in Chinese medicine texts from very early times. For example, when the 'Classic of Difficulties' says that all the Spring (*Ying*) points are used for 'hot sensations of the body', this is nothing but an expression of the general 'action' of the Spring points (i.e. to 'clear Heat').

> **Clinical note**
>
> When the 'Classic of Difficulties' says that all the Spring (*Ying*) points are used for 'hot sensations of the body', this is nothing but an expression of the general 'action' of the Spring points, i.e. to 'clear Heat'

Some think that the 'actions' of the points have been worked out only recently by modern, post-1949 Chinese doctors and that the 'actions' of the points represent a 'herbalization' of acupuncture. I tend to disagree with this view. Indeed, I think that the actions of the points are simply implicit in the indications. If the indications of a point are listed in a random way, it is difficult to see the 'actions' of a point but if we order the indications in groups, the actions of a point become apparent.

For example, let us take BL-7 Tongtian as an example. Among the indications are nasal congestion and discharge, headache, dizziness, anosmia, deviation of mouth, sudden collapse, unconsciousness. We can easily identify two groups of symptoms:

1. Nasal congestion and discharge, anosmia
2. Headache, dizziness, deviation of mouth, sudden collapse, unconsciousness

We can therefore identify two 'actions':

1. Clear the nose
2. Extinguish internal Wind and subdue Yang

Thus, the actions are implicit in the indications and they are nothing but a description of the indications themselves.

When considering the actions of the points, we should not, however, be too rigid or too reductive about their interpretation. In other words, the actions of the points are useful summarizations and generalizations about the effect of a point and should not become a way to reduce the effects of a point to narrow categorizations. For example, one of the most important and most frequently quoted actions of the point ST-40 Fenglong is to 'resolve Phlegm'; although this is important, we should not forget the wide range of other actions that this point has.

There is another important reason why we should not reduce the nature of a point to its 'actions'. There are five basic ways of looking at a point:

1. Its indications as they were listed in the texts of Chinese medicine, e.g. 'cough'
2. Its 'actions', e.g. 'restores the descending of Lung-Qi'
3. The area influenced by the point
4. The nature of the point according to its classification within a given group of points, e.g. LU-6 Kongzui as Accumulation point
5. The energetic action of the point within the channel system

Indications

Any point can be used simply according to the classical indications. In general, one would never use a point only according to its indications, firstly, because for common indications, there may be scores of points with that particular indication and secondly, because choosing a point only according to its indication may lead us to treat entirely the wrong channel. For example, if we are treating a patient suffering from chronic cough due to Phlegm in the Lungs, LU-5 Chize would be an obvious point to use because it is on the Lung channel, it resolves Phlegm, it has cough as an indication and it restores the descending of Lung-Qi. If we simply looked at the indications of a point without regard to channel and pattern involved, we might wrongly use P-1 Tianchi simply because it has cough among its indications.

Although I personally never use a point only according to its indications, it is important to keep these in mind when choosing a point. For example, when we are deciding on a point combination, there may be two or three points with a similar action to choose from: in such cases, an awareness of the indications can help us to choose the most appropriate point both according to its action and its indications.

For example, supposing a patient suffers from slurred speech after Wind-stroke and also depression. We decide to treat the Heart channel as it reaches the tongue and affects the mental state. Practically every Heart point would have these two effects. However, if we look at the indications of the Heart channel points, we see that HE-5 Tongli would be the best to use as it has 'stiff tongue, loss of voice and inability to speak' among its indications.

There is another reason why a knowledge of the indications of a point is important. Supposing we want to use a point on the Lung channel in a patient suffering from chronic cough. We would therefore choose a point whose action is to 'restore the descending of Lung-Qi' and whose indications include cough. Practically every point on the Lung channel is indicated for cough, for example LU-5 Chize, LU-7 Lieque, etc. In particular, these two points also strongly restore the descending of Lung-Qi. However, if the patient suffers from other symptoms (as all patients do) and we find such symptoms in the indications of a particular Lung channel point, this would be a strong reason for choosing that point (providing it does restore the descending of Lung-Qi and it has cough among its indications). For example, if this patient also suffered from headaches, LU-7 Lieque would be the better point to use as it affects the head and treats headaches, a function that LU-5 Chize does not have.

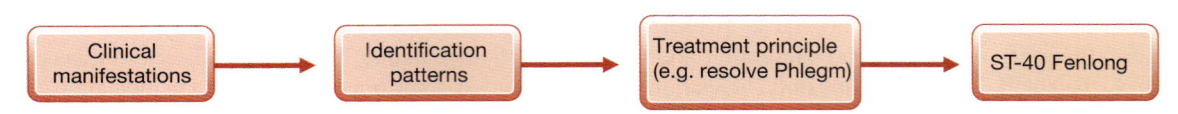

Figure P7-S2.1 Relationship between identification of patterns, treatment principle and point selection

Clinical manifestations → Identification patterns → Treatment principle (e.g. resolve Phlegm) → ST-40 Fenlong

Actions

I always try to choose a point according to its action because there is a logical connection between our diagnosis, identification of pattern, treatment principle and choice of points (Fig. P7-S2.1). For example, a patient presents with chronic cough and we diagnose the pattern of Damp-Phlegm in the Lungs occurring against a background of Spleen-Qi deficiency. As the disease is chronic, we choose to treat both the Root (*Ben*), that is, tonify Spleen-Qi, and the Manifestation (*Biao*), that is, resolve Damp-Phlegm from the Lungs. In order to do the latter we need to resolve Phlegm and restore the descending of Lung-Qi.

We can therefore choose some points according to their actions which correspond to the treatment principle formulated. For example, we would choose BL-20 Pishu to tonify the Spleen, ST-40 Fenlong to resolve Phlegm, and LU-7 Lieque to restore the descending of Lung-Qi. However, LU-5 Chize also restores the descending of Lung-Qi and, in addition, it resolves Phlegm from the Lungs and therefore, according to its action of resolving Phlegm, might be a better choice.

The area influenced by the point

Each point in a channel influences a certain area. This is determined by general and empirical factors. There is a general rule that there is a correspondence between the two extremities of a channel, that is, a point at one extremity of a channel influences its other end; a point further up from the extremity influences the area further down from the opposite extremity (see Fig. 70.8 in ch. 70).

The nature of the point according to its classification within a given group of points

When choosing a point it is always necessary to keep in mind the nature of a point by virtue of it belonging to a specific category of points. For example, we may want to choose a point to tonify the Stomach; if the patient has a general deficiency of Yang and digestive symptoms, it may be advantageous to choose Ren-12 Zhongwan to tonify the Stomach (rather than BL-21 Weishu, for example) because Ren-12 is the Gathering point (*Hui*) of all Yang Organs.

The energetic action of the point within the channel system

Finally, a point should be chosen also within the context of a point combination that takes into account the ascending/descending and entering/exiting of Qi within the channel system in order to harmonize Above–Below, Left–Right, Front–Back and Yin–Yang. For this reason, we should not reduce the effect of a point merely to its 'action'. For example, it would be wrong to reduce the effect of ST-40 Fenglong simply to that of 'resolving Phlegm'. We should use ST-40 also in the context of a point combination that takes into account the dynamics of the channel system. In case of Phlegm in the chest, ST-40 could be needled on one side and LU-7 Lieque on the opposite side to harmonize Left–Right, Above–Below and Yin–Yang: this will achieve a more dynamic result. When points are balanced in this way, the combination itself moves Qi powerfully without the need for a very vigorous needle manipulation.

Stressing the importance of a vigorous needle manipulation (to drain pathogenic factors) is based on a view of a point in isolation; when we take the channel system into account we can formulate balanced combinations according to the above-mentioned parameters. To go back to the above example of Phlegm in the chest, if we reduce ST-40's effect to that of 'resolving Phlegm' we would needle it with a vigorous reducing technique to eliminate a pathogenic factor (i.e. Phlegm). However, if we used a combination that balances Above–Below, Left–Right and Yin–Yang, we exploit the dynamism of the channel system to eliminate pathogenic factors. An example of such a combination might be LU-7 Lieque on the left, ST-40 Fenglong on the right, L.I.-4 Hegu on the right, KI-7 Fuliu on the left, Ren-12 Zhongwan, and Ren-9 Shuifen (Fig. P7-S2.2).

Box P7-S2.2 summarizes the five ways of looking at points.

I will discuss not all the points, but only the most commonly used ones. This information has been drawn from various different sources, some ancient and some modern. The main sources are:

'The Spiritual Axis' (*Ling Shu* c.100 BC)[1]
'The Simple Questions' (*Su Wen* c.100 BC)[2]
'The Classic of Difficulties' (*Nan Jing* c.100 BC)[3]
'The Compendium of Acupuncture' (*Zhen Jiu Da Cheng*, 1601)[4]
'Clinical Application of Frequently Used Acupuncture Points' (*Chang Yong Shu Xue Lin Chuang Fa*, 1985)[5]
'Selection of Acupuncture Point Combinations from the "Discussion on Cold-induced Diseases"' (*Shang Han Lun Zhen Jiu Pei Xue Xuan Zhu*, 1984)[6]
'Clinical Records of *Tai Yi Shen* Acupuncture' (*Tai Yi Shen Zhen Jiu Ling Zheng Lu*, 1984)[7]
'Great Treatise of Chinese Acupuncture' (*Zhong Guo Zhen Jiu Da Quan*, 1988)[8]
Liu Han Yin 1988 Practical Treatise of Acupuncture (*Shi Yong Zhen Jiu Da Quan*), Beijing Publishing House, Beijing.[9]
Jiao Shun Fa 1987 An Enquiry into Chinese Acupuncture (*Zhong Guo Zhen Jiu Qiu Zhen*), Shanxi Science Publishing House.[10]
Zhang Sheng Xing 1984 A Compilation of Explanations of the Meaning of the Acupuncture Points Names (*Jing Xue Shi Yi Hui Jie*), Shanghai Science Publishing House, Shanghai.[11]
Yu Zhong Quan 1988 A Practical Study of the Differentiation of Acupuncture Points (*Jing Xue Bian Zheng Yun Yong Xue*), Sichuan Science Publishing House, Chengdu.[12]
Liu Guan Jun 1990 Acupuncture Theory and Clinical Patterns (*Zhen Jiu Ming Li Yu Lin Zheng*), People's Health Publishing House, Beijing.[13]
Yue Han Zhen 1990 An Explanation of the Acupuncture Points (*Jing Xue Jie*), People's Health Publishing House, Beijing. Originally published in 1654.[14]
Notes from the First Advanced International Acupuncture Course at the Nanjing College of Traditional Chinese Medicine, 1981.
Notes from Dr J.H.F. Shen's Seminars, 1978, 1979 and 1981.
Personal communications from Dr Su Xin Ming of the Nanjing College of Traditional Chinese Medicine.
Personal communications from Dr Chen Jing Hua of the Beijing Friendship Hospital.
Personal communications from Dr J.H.F. Shen.

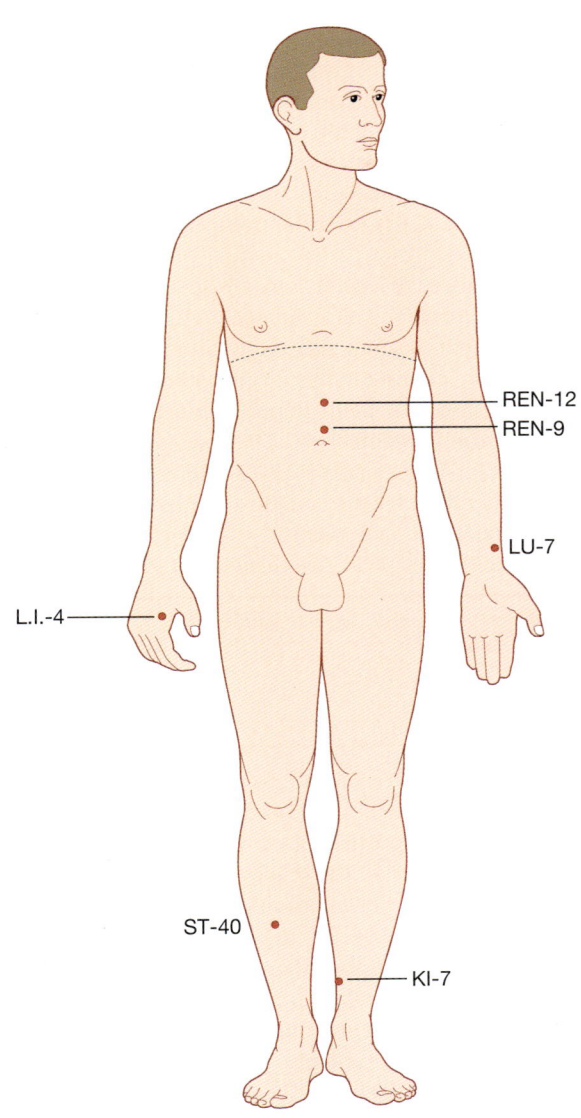

Figure P7-S2.2 Example of point combination

In addition to the above sources, the action of certain points has also been drawn from the author's own experience. Whenever this is so, this is made clear in the text with the expression '*in my experience*'.

When discussing the energetic action of each point it is usually implied that different actions require different needle manipulations. All points that expel pathogenic factors should be needled with a reducing method, while all points that tonify the body's Qi

Box P7-S2.2 Five ways of looking at a point

1. Its indications as they were listed in the texts of Chinese medicine, e.g. 'cough'
2. Its 'actions', e.g. 'restores the descending of Lung-Qi'
3. The area influenced by the point
4. The nature of the point according to its classification within a given group of points, e.g. LU-6 Kongzui as Accumulation point
5. The energetic action of the point within the channel system

should be needled with a reinforcing method. For example, if a certain point 'eliminates exterior Wind', it is implied that in order to do that, it should be needled with reducing method. Likewise, if a certain point 'nourishes Blood', it is implied that it should be reinforced.

For the sake of clarity, the following is a list of the main energetic actions mentioned together with their corresponding manipulation method.

Reinforcing method	Reducing method
Tonify Qi or Yang	Expel exterior Wind Extinguish interior Wind
Nourish Blood, Yin or Essence	Drain Fire or Clear Heat
Tonify Original Qi	Resolve Dampness
Promote Fluids	Expel interior Cold
Warm Yang	Resolve Phlegm
Lift the Mind	Open the orifices Promote resuscitation Stop pain Move Qi Invigorate Blood Remove obstructions from the channels

In some cases, either the reinforcing or reducing method is applicable, according to the nature of the pattern, i.e. whether it is a Deficiency or Excess pattern. These are:

- Benefit the sinews
- Benefit the eyes or ears
- Calm the Mind

The usual condition applies whereby in certain cases the reducing method, although indicated, should not be applied.

These are:

- When the condition is chronic (over 6 months' duration)
- When the patient is very old
- When the patient is very weak

In all these cases the reducing method should be replaced by the even method.[15]

Finally, in giving the actions of each point I have tried to tread a middle way between giving as detailed information as possible, and giving the essential actions for each point. Giving too little information on a point may miss some important action, but giving too much information may make it impossible for the reader to form an idea of the essential nature and functions of the point.

For example, the point Ren-13 Shangwan, besides subduing rebellious Stomach-Qi (which is its most essential action), may also tonify Stomach-Qi. I have omitted the latter action as it is not frequently used in this way since the point Ren-12 Zhongwan is much better to tonify Stomach-Qi. There would be no point in using Ren-13 instead of Ren-12 to tonify Stomach-Qi. I have therefore tried to capture the essential nature and functions of each point.

For each point, I will give the following information:

1. Name in Chinese (*pinyin*) with translation
2. Nature of point
3. Actions
4. Indications
5. Comments

Given the nature of the present textbook, I have omitted to give the location and needling instructions of the points as these belong to an acupuncture manual rather than a text on the theory of Chinese medicine. For the best source of information on the location and needling instructions for the points in English the reader is referred to the 'Manual of Acupuncture' by Deadman and Al Khafaji.[16]

Section 2 on the Functions of the Points is divided into the following chapters:

Chapter 54	Lung channel
Chapter 55	Large Intestine channel
Chapter 56	Stomach channel
Chapter 57	Spleen channel
Chapter 58	Heart channel
Chapter 59	Small Intestine channel
Chapter 60	Bladder channel
Chapter 61	Kidney channel
Chapter 62	Pericardium channel
Chapter 63	Triple Burner channel
Chapter 64	Gall Bladder channel
Chapter 65	Liver channel
Chapter 66	Directing Vessel
Chapter 67	Governing Vessel
Chapter 68	Extra points

END NOTES

1. 1981 Spiritual Axis (*Ling Shu Jing* 灵枢经), People's Health Publishing House, Beijing, first published *c*.100 BC.
2. 1979 The Yellow Emperor's Classic of Internal Medicine-Simple Questions (*Huang Di Nei Jing Su Wen* 黄帝内经素问), People's Health Publishing House, Beijing, first published *c*.100 BC.
3. Nanjing College of Traditional Chinese Medicine 1979 A Revised Explanation of the Classic of Difficulties (*Nan Jing Jiao Shi* 难经校释), People's Health Publishing House, Beijing, first published *c*.AD 100.
4. Yang Ji Zhou 1980 Compendium of Acupuncture (*Zhen Jiu Da Cheng* 针灸大成), People's Health Publishing House, Beijing, first published in 1601.
5. Li Shi Zhen 1985 Clinical Application of Frequently Used Acupuncture Points (*Chang Yong Shu Xue Lin Chuang Fa Hui* 常用腧穴临床发挥), Beijing.
6. Shan Yu Dang 1984 Selection of Acupuncture Point Combinations from the Discussion of Cold-induced Diseases (*Shang Han Lun Zhen Jiu Pei Xue Xuan Zhu* 伤寒论针灸配穴选注), Beijing.
7. Ji Jie Yin 1984 Clinical Records of *Tai Yi Shen* Acupuncture (*Tai Yin Shen Zhen Jiu Lin Zheng Lu* 太乙神针灸临证录), Shanxi Province Scientific Publishing House.
8. Wang Xue Tai 1988 Great Treatise of Chinese Acupuncture (*Zhong Guo Zhen Jiu Da Quan* 中国针灸大全), Henan Science Publishing House.
9. Liu Han Yin 1988 Practical Treatise of Acupuncture (*Shi Yong Zhen Jiu Da Quan* 实用针灸大全), Beijing Publishing House, Beijing.
10. Jiao Shun Fa 1987 An Enquiry into Chinese Acupuncture (*Zhong Guo Zhen Jiu Qiu Zhen* 中国针灸求真), Shanxi Science Publishing House.
11. Zhang Cheng Xing 1984 A Compilation of Explanations of the Meaning of the Acupuncture Points Names (*Jing Xue Shi Yi Hui Jie* 经穴释义汇解), Shanghai Science Publishing House, Shanghai.
12. Yu Zhong Quan 1988 A Practical Study of the Differentiation of Acupuncture Points (*Jing Xue Bian Zheng Yun Yong Xue* 经穴辨证运用学), Sichuan Science Publishing House, Chengdu.
13. Liu Guan Jun 1990 Acupuncture Theory and Clinical Patterns (*Zhen Jiu Ming Li Yu Lin Zheng* 针灸明理与临证), People's Health Publishing House, Beijing.
14. Yue Han Zhen 1990 An Explanation of the Acupuncture Points (*Jing Xue Jie* 经穴解), People's Health Publishing House, Beijing. Originally published in 1654.
15. There are many different reducing needling techniques. The two main ones are according to rotation or lift and thrust. According to rotation, the needle is rotated back and forth rapidly and with large amplitude; according to lift and thrust, the needle is lifted rapidly and vigorously and thrust slowly and gently. In both cases the manipulation may be repeated a few times during the time of retention of the needle. The even needling method consists in obtaining *deqi*, rotating the needle back and forth fairly vigorously for a few rotations and then leaving it in without further manipulation. As a general rule, a gentle needling manipulation is reinforcing while a vigorous one is reducing.
16. Deadman P, Al-Khafaji M 1998 A Manual of Acupuncture, Journal of Chinese Medicine Publications, Hove, England.

SECTION 2   PART 7

Lung Channel   54

Main channel pathway

The Lung channel originates from the Middle Burner and runs down to connect with the large intestine. It then ascends to the stomach, passes the diaphragm and enters the lung. From here it ascends to the throat and then emerges at LU-1 Zhongfu. From here, it descends along the medial aspect of the arm and reaches the styloid process of the radius. It then goes to the thenar eminence and ends at the medial side of the tip of the thumb (Fig. 54.1).

Connecting channel pathway

After separating from the main channel at LU-7 Lieque, the Lung Connecting channel connects with the Large Intestine channel. From LU-7 Lieque a branch flows to the thenar eminence where it scatters (Fig. 54.2).

Box 54.1 gives an overview of the Lung points.

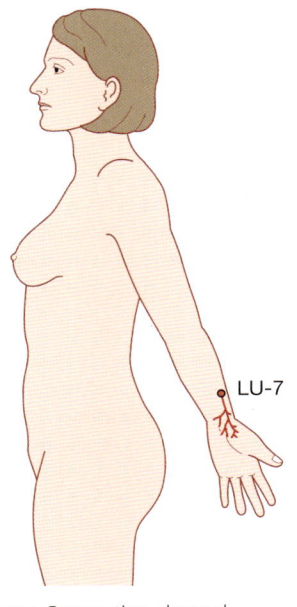

Figure 54.2 Lung Connecting channel

Box 54.1 Overview of Lung points

- Affect the chest and throat
- All stimulate the descending of Lung-Qi and treat cough and asthma
- Expel exterior Wind

LU-1 ZHONGFU *CENTRAL PALACE*

Location

On the lateral chest, 1 *cun* below LU-2 Yunmen, in the first intercostal space, 6 *cun* lateral to the midline.

Nature

Front Collecting (*Mu*) point of the Lungs.
Meeting point of Greater Yin (Lungs-Spleen).

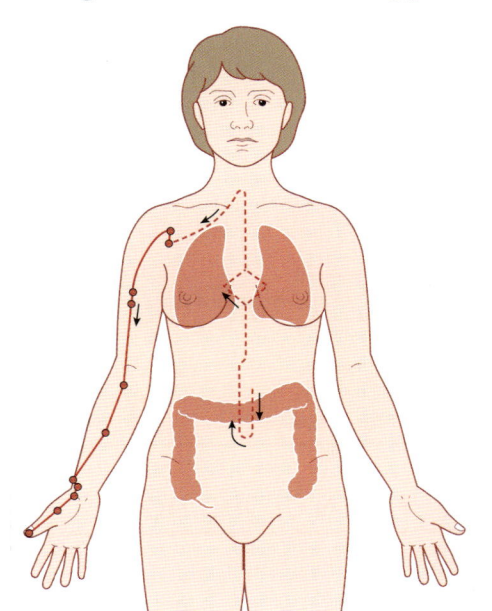

Figure 54.1 Lung main channel

Actions

Promotes the descending of Lung-Qi and stops cough.
Resolves Phlegm from the Lungs.
Disperses fullness from the chest and stops chest pain.

Indications

Cough, wheezing, breathlessness, coughing of blood.
Coughing phlegm, feeling of oppression of the chest.
Chest fullness and pain, shoulder pain, upper backache.

Comments

This point is mostly used in acute Excess patterns of the Lungs to disperse fullness from the chest, resolve Phlegm from the Lungs and clear Lung-Heat. Thus it would be commonly used in the later stages of invasion of the Lungs by an exterior pathogenic factor, when this has penetrated into the Interior. In particular, it is very well indicated for cough caused by retention of Phlegm in the Lungs.

According to 'An Explanation of Acupuncture Points' (*Jing Xue Jie*, 1654), LU-1 is a point where the Qi of the Lungs gathers as the Qi of the channel emerges from the Interior.[1] By virtue of this nature, this point can be used to disperse accumulation of Lung-Qi in the chest causing chest fullness and pain.

This point is not usually used when the pathogenic factor is still on the Exterior. This explains why this point is not indicated for sore throat from invasion of exterior Wind-Heat. However, since it has a good effect on making Lung-Qi descend and stopping cough, it can be used in the early stages of invasion from an exterior pathogenic factor if cough is a prominent symptom. In these cases, LU-1 would be needled as a secondary point together with points to release the Exterior, such as LU-7 Lieque and L.I.-4 Hegu.

LU-1 is an important point for the treatment of whooping cough during its second stage (i.e. Lung-Heat stage).

It is also effective in treating chest pain deriving from Heart-Blood stasis or retention of Phlegm in the chest. In the first case, LU-1 moves Lung-Qi and therefore helps to move Blood in the chest, particularly if combined with P-6 Neiguan. Combined with ST-40 Fenglong it can resolve Phlegm retained in the chest by moving Qi in the chest.

LU-1 is effective in treating shoulder or upper back pain deriving from a Lung channel dysfunction, such as in Lung-Heat, Damp-Phlegm or Phlegm-Heat obstructing the Lungs. The 'Simple Questions' in chapter 22 says: *'When the Lungs are diseased, Qi rebels upwards causing breathlessness and there is pain in the shoulders or [upper] back'*.[2]

LU-1 can be combined with BL-13 Feishu to tonify the Lungs or to eliminate pathogenic factors in both acute and chronic cases. However, the combination of both front and back points is rather powerful and, in most cases, is not necessary. Generally speaking, the Front Collecting (*Mu*) point LU-1 would be chosen more for Excess and acute conditions, and the Back Transporting (*Shu*) point BL-13 Feishu more for Deficiency and chronic conditions.

Combined with ST-36 Zusanli and SP-3 Taibai, LU-1 can be used to tonify the Spleen and Lungs. This combination of points is based on the nature of LU-1 as a meeting point of the Lung and Spleen channel. In Five-Element terms, this combination is called 'Filling Earth to generate Metal'.

It is useful to compare the functions of the Front Collecting point of the Lungs LU-1 Zhongfu with those of the Back Transporting point BL-13 Feishu:

LU-1 (Front Collecting point)	BL-13 (Back Transporting point)
Mostly for Excess patterns	Mostly for Deficiency patterns
Mostly to treat the Manifestation	Mostly to treat the Root
Better for acute cases	Better for chronic cases
Treats pain in the chest	Treats pain in the upper back

Box 54.2 summarizes the functions of LU-1.

Box 54.2 LU-1 – summary of functions

- Mostly for Excess patterns
- Disperse chest fullness, resolve Phlegm, clear Heat
- Invigorates Blood in the chest with P-6 Neiguan
- Upper shoulder and back pain

LU-2 YUNMEN *CLOUD DOOR*

Location

On anterior-lateral chest, below the clavicle, 6 *cun* lateral to the midline.

Nature

None.

Actions

Disperses fullness in the chest.
Promotes the descending of Lung-Qi and stops cough.

Indications

Chest pain, feeling of oppression of the chest, feeling of heat in the chest, shoulder pain.
Cough, wheezing, breathlessness.

Comments

The energetic actions of this point are similar to those of LU-1 Zhongfu, but less strong. In addition to these, it can be used for local channel problems such as Painful Obstruction Syndrome of the shoulder, when the person cannot adduct the arm (i.e. bring the arm over close to the body towards the opposite side).

Box 54.3 summarizes the functions of LU-2.

Box 54.3 LU-2 – summary of functions

- Similar to LU-1 Zhongfu
- Painful Obstruction Syndrome of the shoulder (difficulty in adducting arm)

LU-3 TIANFU *HEAVENLY PALACE*

Location

On the anterior arm, 3 *cun* below the anterior axillary fold, 6 *cun* above LU-5 Chize.

Nature

Window of Heaven point.

Actions

Promotes the descending of Lung-Qi.
Regulates the ascending and descending of Qi.
Stops bleeding.
Opens the Mind's orifices and soothes the Corporeal Soul (*Po*).

Indications

Cough, wheezing, breathlessness.
Somnolence, insomnia, sadness, weeping, forgetfulness, goitre.
Epistaxis, coughing of blood.
'Talking to ghosts'.

Comments

The actions and indications of this point are closely related to its being a Window of Heaven point. As explained in chapter 51, one of the characteristics of these points is that they regulate the ascending and descending of Qi from the body to and from the head: they do so in the crucial neck area (the gateway between the body and the head). Therefore, they can both subdue rebellious Qi and promote the ascending of clear Qi to the head (Fig. 54.3).

The first group of indications clearly refer to the effect of this point in promoting the descending of Lung-Qi.

The second group of indications refer to the mental–emotional effect of this point in regulating the ascending and descending of Qi to and from the head. In fact, insomnia is due to Qi ascending too much to the head (or not descending from it) while somnolence and forgetfulness are due to clear Qi not ascending to the head.

The 'Explanation of the Acupuncture Points' says that LU-3 can make Qi rise to treat forgetfulness, sadness and weeping due to Qi not rising to head.[3] Forgetfulness is an important indication for this point: this is forgetfulness due to clear Qi not rising to the head. According to the 'Explanation of the Acupuncture Points', this point treats forgetfulness by stimulating the ascending of Qi of both Lungs and Heart.[4]

The sign of goitre is also related to the ascending and descending of Qi to and from the head in the area of the neck. As the neck is the crucial crossroads of Qi on its way to and from the head, it is prone to stagnation of Qi, which, in time, may give rise to some Phlegm in the neck manifesting with a goitre.

The regulation of the ascending and descending of Qi by this point makes it also apt to stop bleeding: however, this is only bleeding 'upwards' such as in epistaxis and haemoptysis: this point stops this type of bleeding by subduing rebellious Qi.

Finally, 'talking to ghosts' features heavily in this point's indications. Generally speaking, when ancient books mention such symptoms as talking to or seeing ghosts among the indications of a point, it means that the point is indicated for relatively serious mental–emotional problems and, in particular, when the Mind is obstructed. Obstruction of the Mind can potentially

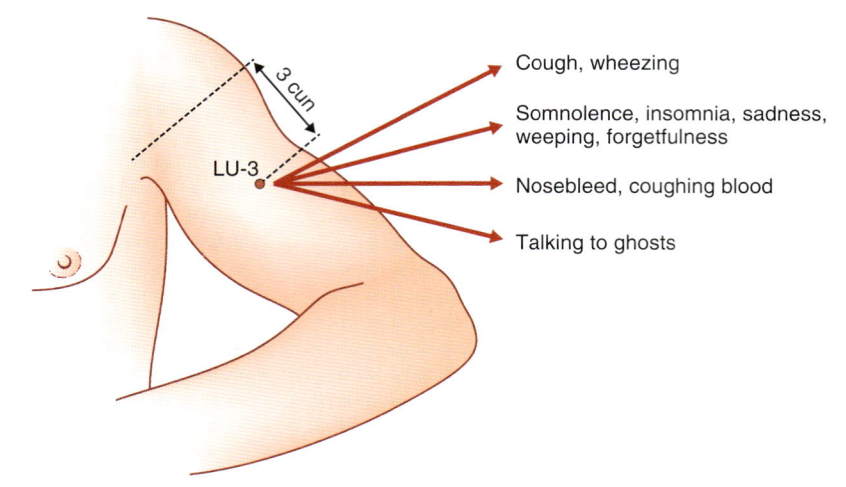

Figure 54.3 LU-3 Tianfu

- Cough, wheezing
- Somnolence, insomnia, sadness, weeping, forgetfulness
- Nosebleed, coughing blood
- Talking to ghosts

cause serious mental problems such as manic depression or psychosis. Again, this point can open the Mind's orifices, i.e. de-obstruct the Mind by regulating the ascending and descending of Qi to and from the head: it opens the Mind's orifices by promoting the descending of turbid Qi from the head and the ascending of clear Qi to the head. This is a general function of the Window of Heaven points.

It is interesting to compare the names of LU-3 Tianfu and LU-1 Zhongfu and their implications. 'Fu' means 'palace': this usually confers importance to a point, indicating that it is at the centre of an important directing and governing structure as a palace is. LU-1 is a 'central' palace while LU-3 is a 'heavenly' palace. LU-1 is a central palace because, although it is located in the upper chest, the Lung channel originates from the Middle Burner and emerges at this point: for this reason, this point can also promote the descending of Stomach-Qi, it has a certain effect on the Middle Burner and it does not have an effect on the head. By contrast, LU-3 is a 'heavenly' palace, which means that its sphere of action is very much the head, as indicated above.

Box 54.4 summarizes the functions of LU-3.

Box 54.4 LU-3 – summary of functions

- Regulate ascending and descending of Qi to and from head
- Mental–emotional effect as Window of Heaven point
- Goitre
- Stop bleeding (upwards)

LU-5 CHIZE *FOOT MARSH*

Location
In the crease of the elbow on the radial side of the biceps.

Nature
Sea (*He*) point.
Water point.
Drainage point.

Actions
Clears Lung-Heat.
Promotes the descending of Lung-Qi.
Resolves Phlegm from the Lungs.
Regulates the Water passages and benefits the Bladder.
Relaxes the sinews.

Indications
Tidal fever, dry mouth and tongue, agitation and fullness of the chest.
Cough, wheezing, breathlessness.
Cough with expectoration of profuse phlegm.
Oedema of limbs, enuresis, frequent urination, retention of urine.
Pain in the upper arm and shoulder, inability to raise the arm, Wind Painful Obstruction Syndrome of the elbow, stiffness and pain of the elbow, swelling and pain of the knee.

Comments

This point is mostly used for interior patterns of an Excess nature characterized by Heat in the Lungs with such symptoms as cough, fever, yellow sputum and thirst. This point would be applicable at the Qi level (second stage) of the Four-Level pattern identification characterized by Full Interior-Heat in the Lungs.

It can also be used in chronic conditions characterized by retention of Phlegm and Heat in the Lungs, such as may happen in chronic bronchitis. In this case it would be combined with ST-40 Fenglong and other points to resolve Phlegm.

In cases when Lung-Heat has injured the Body Fluids, LU-5 can be combined with KI-6 Zhaohai to clear the Lungs and nourish Yin. In connection with fluids, the 'Explanation of the Acupuncture Points' says that LU-5 can be used for 'sadness and crying deriving from dryness of the Lungs' and this point can treat these symptoms by reinforcing the point to promote Water.[5]

It is also an important point to use in the second stage of whooping cough characterized by Phlegm and Heat in the Lung, combined with LU-10 Yuji and ST-40 Fenglong.

However, in my experience, LU-5 can also be used for interior patterns of an Excess-Cold nature, with retention of Cold-Phlegm in the Lungs, manifesting with such symptoms as cough with profuse white sticky sputum and chilliness. In all these cases, this point would be needled with reducing method.

LU-5 also has an effect on the Bladder in opening the Water passages and facilitating urination. It is therefore used for enuresis or frequent urination. The 'Explanation of the Acupuncture Points' says that this point should be reinforced to affect the Bladder and Kidneys in cases of enuresis.[6] However, in my experience, this point can also be used for retention of urine caused by obstruction of the Lungs by Damp-Phlegm preventing Lung-Qi from descending and from opening the Water passages in the Lower Burner. In this case, LU-5 would be reduced and would be combined with such points as SP-9 Yinlingquan and Ren-3 Zhongji.

Finally, LU-5 relaxes the sinews of the arm along the Lung channel and can be used in Painful Obstruction Syndrome or paralysis of the arm and/or shoulder when the patient is unable to raise the arm. The 'ABC of Acupuncture' (AD 259) states: '*When the arm cannot be raised to the head, or there is pain in the elbow, use LU-5.*'[7]

The 'Illustrated Manual of Acupuncture Points as Shown on the Bronze Man' (AD 1026) says: '*LU-5 can treat Wind-Painful Obstruction Syndrome of the elbow and inability to raise the arm.*'[8]

Box 54.5 summarizes the functions of LU-5.

Box 54.5 LU-5 – summary of functions

- Mostly for Excess patterns
- Resolves Phlegm and clears Heat from Lungs
- Opens Water passages and benefits Bladder
- Relaxes the sinews of arm and shoulder

LU-6 KONGZUI CONVERGENCE HOLE

Location

On the anterior forearm, 7 *cun* above LU-9 Taiyuan.

Nature

Accumulation (*Xi*) point.

Actions

Regulates Lung-Qi in the channel.
Promotes the descending of Lung-Qi.
Clears Heat.
Stops bleeding.

Indications

Chest pain, swelling and pain of the throat, pain in the elbow and upper arm, inability to raise the arm, difficulty in flexing and extending fingers.
Cough, wheezing, breathlessness.
Heat syndromes of the Lungs without sweating.
Coughing of blood, vomiting of blood.

Comments

This point is mostly used in acute Excess patterns of the Lungs, especially for an acute attack of asthma. It also stops bleeding, which is a property of all Accumulation points.

Like all Accumulation points, it treats pain and channel problems: for this reason, it is an important point for pain along the Lung channel in the elbow and upper arm.

Box 54.6 summarizes the functions of LU-6.

> **Box 54.6 LU-6 – summary of functions**
>
> - As Accumulation point, it stops pain and is used in acute conditions
> - Acute asthma
> - Clears Lung-Heat
> - Stops bleeding

LU-7 LIEQUE *BRANCHING CLEFT*

Location

On the radial aspect of the forearm, 1.5 *cun* above the crease of the wrist between the tendons of brachioradialis and abductor pollicis longus.

Nature

Connecting (*Luo*) point.
Opening point of the Directing Vessel (*Ren Mai*).
One of the 12 Heavenly Star points of Ma Dan Yang.

Actions

Promotes the descending and diffusing of Lung-Qi.
Releases the Exterior and expels exterior Wind.
Opens the Directing Vessel.
Benefits the Bladder and opens Water passages.
Benefits the head and neck.
Regulates the ascending and descending of Qi in the head.
Opens the nose.
Communicates with the Large Intestine channel.

Indications

Cough, wheezing, breathlessness, sneezing.
Aversion to cold and fever.
Retention of lochiae, retention of dead fetus, postpartum aphasia, pain in the penis, pain in the external genitalia, nocturnal emissions.
Blood in the urine, painful urination, difficult urination.
Headache, stiffness and pain of the neck, deviation of eye and mouth, toothache.
Poor memory, palpitations, propensity to (inappropriate) laughter, frequent yawning.
Nasal polyps, nasal congestion and discharge.

Comments

This is an extremely important point. It is a major point to release the Exterior in invasions of exterior Wind-Cold or Wind-Heat. This point contributes to the elimination of the pathogenic factor by stimulating the descending and diffusing of Lung-Qi, thus releasing the Lung-Defensive Qi portion and stimulating sweating. The Lungs control the space between the skin and muscles where Defensive Qi circulates, and spread fluids all over the skin. The use of this point (with reducing method) will stimulate the circulation of the Defensive Qi and open the pores to cause sweating (Fig. 54.4).

LU-7 is therefore used in the beginning stages of the common cold or influenza, with sneezing, stiff neck, headache, aversion to cold, fever and a Floating pulse. In treating exterior invasions of Wind-Cold or Wind-Heat it is often combined with L.I.-4 Hegu, as they both release the Exterior. This combination is called 'Guest–Host' as the Connecting channel of the Lungs (the 'Guest') joins with the Large Intestine channel (the 'Host').

Because of the Lung's connection with the nose, LU-7 is used to treat sneezing, nasal obstruction, runny nose and loss of the sense of smell. In all these cases, it would be combined with L.I.-20 Yingxiang. As this point promotes the diffusing of Lung-Qi and opens the nose, it is also an important point in the treatment of allergic rhinitis.

Far from being used only in exterior patterns, LU-7 Lieque has a very wide-ranging energetic action in interior patterns too. It is the best point on the Lung channel to stimulate the descending of Lung-Qi and it

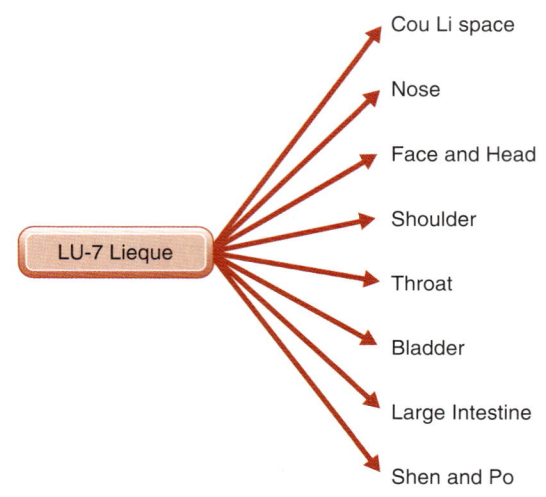

Figure 54.4 Areas affected by LU-7 Lieque

LU-7 Lieque → Cou Li space, Nose, Face and Head, Shoulder, Throat, Bladder, Large Intestine, Shen and Po

is therefore a very important point to use in all types of cough or asthma, whether acute or chronic.

LU-7 is also one of the best points to affect the face and head and can be used in combination with other points to direct the effect of the treatment to face and head. Because of this, it is very frequently used in headaches.

In my experience, LU-7 is a very important point from the psychological and emotional point of view, and can be used in emotional problems caused by worry, grief or sadness. LU-7 is particularly indicated in cases in which the person bears his or her problems in silence and keeps them inside. LU-7 tends to stimulate a beneficial outpouring of repressed emotions. Weeping is the sound associated with the Lungs according to the Five Elements, and those who have been suppressing their emotions may burst out crying when this point is used or shortly after. 'Tendency to crying' is listed as a prominent indication for LU-7 in the 'Explanation of the Acupuncture Points'.[9]

The Lungs are the residence of the Corporeal Soul (*Po*) and this point will release the emotional tensions of the Corporeal Soul, manifesting on a physical level with tense shoulders, shallow breathing and a feeling of oppression in the chest. These symptoms are often due to excessive worrying over a long period of time, preventing the free breathing of the Corporeal Soul and constraining the Lung energy. LU-7 will calm the Mind, settle the Corporeal Soul, open the chest and release tension.

Being the Connecting point, it is very useful and effective in channel problems of the Large Intestine and Lung channels. It is often used as a distal point for Painful Obstruction Syndrome of the shoulder, if the problem is along the Large Intestine channel. In these cases, LU-7 is often used on the opposite side to where the problem is.

As LU-7 opens the Directing Vessel (*Ren Mai*), some of its indications are for problems following labour and problems of the external genitalia. Its effect in promoting the expulsion of lochia or of a dead fetus is also related to its action of stimulating the descending of Qi. However, as indicated in chapter 52, to open the extraordinary vessels, I use both the opening and coupled points (in the case of the Directing Vessel, LU-7 Lieque and KI-6 Zhaohai).

In conjunction with KI-6 Zhaohai, it opens the Directing Vessel, stimulates the descending of Lung-Qi and the Kidney function of receiving Qi. Because of this, it is beneficial in chronic asthma from Lung and Kidney deficiency. The combination of LU-7 and KI-6 nourishes Yin, regulates the uterus and the menstrual function, benefits the throat and moistens the eyes. It is excellent for a dry and sore throat deriving from Yin deficiency.

The Lungs are indirectly related to the Bladder and control the Water passages. LU-7 is the main point on the Lung channel to affect the Lung function of opening the Water passages. It therefore can be used in oedema of the face or urinary retention in Excess patterns, when an exterior pathogenic factor obstructs the descending of Lung-Qi: this results in Lung-Qi being unable to open the Water passages and connect with the Bladder. In this case, it is needled with reducing method.

LU-7 is also effective in urinary retention of the Empty type, when deficient Lung-Qi fails to descend and communicate with the Bladder. This gives rise to urinary retention of the Deficient type and is particularly common in the elderly. In this case it is needled with reinforcing method.

Interestingly, although this point is very much used to promote the descending of Lung-Qi, it may also promote the ascending of clear Qi to the Heart and head: for this reason, it is used for poor memory, palpitations, propensity to (inappropriate) laughter, crying and frequent yawning due to the failure of the clear Qi to rise to the Heart and head so that the Mind and Corporeal Soul suffer. The 'Explanation of the Acupuncture Points' specifically says: '*In forgetfulness due to insufficient rising of Qi, reinforce LU-7 Lieque to promote the ascending of Qi.*'[10]

Lung-Qi also communicates with the Large Intestine and, in my experience, it provides the Qi necessary for the act of defecation. When Lung-Qi is weak, it may fail to communicate with the Large Intestine and constipation ensues. This constipation is of the Deficient type and is common in old people. It is characterized by difficulty in passing stools, or passing them with great strain and feeling exhausted afterwards. In these cases, LU-7 will tonify Lung-Qi and help it to reach the Large Intestine to give it strength for the act of defecation.

I use the combination of LU-7 Lieque and ST-40 Fenglong frequently, often on opposite sides, for example LU-7 on the left and ST-40 on the right or vice versa. This combination can resolve Phlegm from the Lungs as both these points affect the chest, LU-7 regulates the Water passages and resolves Phlegm by making Qi descend, while ST-40 opens the chest and resolves Phlegm in general. I use this combination also simply to open the chest when there is stagnation of Qi from emotional stress.

I have changed the translation of the name of this point from *Broken Sequence* to *Branching Cleft* in accordance with Zhang Sheng Xing's 'A Compilation of Explanations of the Meaning of the Acupuncture Points Names'.[11] According to Dr Zhang, '*lie*' has the meaning of 'coming apart' and '*que*' that of 'cleft, opening'. 'Branching cleft' therefore refers to the fact that LU-7 is located in a cleft of the bone and at this point the channel branches outwards toward the Large Intestine channel. This interpretation of this point's name is also found in the 'Explanation of the Acupuncture Points' which says: '*The Lung channel deviates towards the Large Intestine channel at LU-7: here there is a cleft from which the Connecting [Luo] channel of the Lungs goes towards the Large Intestine channel.*'[12]

Box 54.7 summarizes the functions of LU-7.

Box 54.7 LU-7 – summary of functions

- Releases the Exterior to expel exterior Wind
- Sneezing in allergic rhinitis
- Affects the head: headache
- Treats the effects of worry, sadness and grief
- Affects menstruation (with KI-6)
- Affects the Bladder and opens Water passages (urinary retention)
- It may make Qi rise to the head to treat sadness and poor memory
- Affects the Large Intestine and defecation (constipation in the elderly)

LU-8 JINGQU RIVER [POINT] DITCH

Location

1 *cun* above the crease of the wrist, just lateral to the radial artery.

Nature

River (*Jing*) point.
Metal point.

Actions

Promotes the descending of Lung-Qi.

Indications

Cough, wheezing, breathlessness.
Distension and pain in the chest.
Febrile disease without sweating.

Comments

This point is effective in treating problems of the throat and lungs, and such symptoms as cough and asthma, fitting into the category of River point indications according to chapter 68 of the 'Classic of Difficulties'. It is often added to other points to treat chronic throat problems.

I have changed the translation of this point's name because the word '*Jing*' in its name refers not to 'channel' but to the 'River' point of the Five Transporting points (*Jing, Ying, Shu, Jing* and *He*, i.e. Well, Spring, Stream, River and Sea). It therefore indicates a 'ditch' of the 'river' [point]. It is a ditch because at this point the Qi of the channel deviates towards joints.

Box 54.8 summarizes the functions of LU-8.

Box 54.8 LU-8 – summary of functions

- Problems of throat

LU-9 TAIYUAN SUPREME ABYSS

Location

In the crease of the wrist, just lateral to the radial artery.

Nature

Source (*Yuan*) and Stream (*Shu*) point.
Earth point.
Gathering (*Hui*) point for arteries and veins.
Tonification point.

Actions

Resolves Phlegm.
Promotes the descending of Lung-Qi and stops cough.
Tonifies Lung-Qi and Lung-Yin.
Tonifies Gathering Qi (*Zong Qi*).
Promotes the circulation of blood and influences the pulse.
Clears Lungs and Liver-Heat.

Indications

Cough with expectoration of sputum, feeling of oppression of the chest.
Cough, wheezing, breathlessness.
Absence of pulse or very feeble pulse.

Comments

This is another major point of the Lung channel. It is the main point to tonify Lung-Qi and Lung-Yin, especially in chronic conditions. Being the Source and tonification point, it is eminently suited to tonify the Lungs in Deficiency conditions.

I personally use it is more frequently in Deficiency rather than Excess patterns, and for interior rather than exterior conditions. However, as its indications show, it can be used also for Excess patterns.

I use it to resolve Phlegm obstructing the Lungs but in chronic more than acute cases with such symptoms as chronic cough with sticky sputum.

The chest is the seat of Gathering Qi (*Zong Qi*), which is closely related to Lungs and Heart. LU-9 tonifies the Gathering Qi of the chest and can be used in patients who are particularly Qi deficient, suffer from cold hands and have a weak voice. These last two are signs of deficiency of Gathering Qi. When tonifying Gathering Qi, LU-9 is often combined with Ren-17 Shanzhong.

LU-9 is also indicated when all the pulses are extremely Weak and Deep and nearly impossible to feel, an indication that is related to its function of controlling all blood vessels described below.

LU-9 is the Gathering (*Hui*) point of all the blood vessels. The 'Classic of Difficulties' in chapter 1 says: '*The Inch Mouth [the Front position of the pulse corresponding to LU-9] is the great meeting place of all the blood vessels, and the Lungs give impetus to the pulse.*'[13] The Front position of the pulse is considered the convergence point of all the blood vessels of the body and for this reason the acupuncture point on its site, LU-9, is said to influence all the blood vessels and the pulse. It is because of this nature that we feel the pulse on the radial artery which overlies the Lung channel.

It is not by chance that this position was chosen as the best place to feel the pulse. It is because the Lungs govern Qi and one can therefore feel the movement of Qi within the Blood at this position. LU-9 can therefore influence all blood vessels and can be used for poor circulation, cold hands and feet, chilblains and varicose veins. The Lungs' influence on the blood vessels is a further expression of the close relationship existing between the Lungs and Heart. The Lungs govern Qi, the Heart controls Blood and they mutually affect each other. LU-9 tonifies Lung-Qi and stimulates the circulation of Heart Qi and Blood in the chest: it is therefore also used to tonify Heart Qi and Blood indirectly in such symptoms as breathlessness on exertion, listlessness and palpitations.

Finally, LU-9 can be used to clear Lung- and Liver-Heat in cases when Liver-Fire overflows towards the chest, obstructing the descending of Lung-Qi.

It is useful to compare the actions of LU-9 with those of LU-7:

LU-7 Lieque	LU-9 Taiyuan
For Exterior problems	For Interior problems
For Excess patterns	For Deficiency patterns
Has an outward movement	Has an inward movement
Affects Qi	Affects Qi and Blood
For channel problems	Not so much for channel problems
Better for emotional problems	Not so much for emotional problems
Good for acute conditions	More for chronic conditions
Opens Water passages	Does not open Water passages
Affects Bladder	Does not affect Bladder

Box 54.9 summarizes the functions of LU-9.

Box 54.9 LU-9 – summary of functions

- Tonifies Lung-Qi and Lung-Yin
- Resolves Phlegm from the Lungs in chronic cases
- Tonifies Gathering Qi (*Zong Qi*) and therefore Lungs and Heart
- Affects all blood vessels

LU-10 YUJI *FISH BORDER*

Location

On the thenar eminence, medial to the first metacarpal bone and in its mid-point.

Nature

Spring (*Ying*) point.
Fire point.

Actions

Clears Lung-Heat.
Promotes the descending of Lung-Qi and stops cough.
Benefits the throat.
Calms the Mind.

Indications

Feeling of heat, dry throat.
Cough, breathlessness.
Painful obstruction of the throat, sore throat, dry throat.
Sadness, fear, mental restlessness, anger, manic behaviour, fright.

Comments

This is the main point to clear Lung-Heat and it can be used for both Full- or Empty-Heat. LU-5 Chize also clears Lung-Heat, but more when Heat is combined with Phlegm obstructing the chest. LU-10, on the contrary, clears Lung-Heat especially in acute situations: for example, at the Qi level of the Four-Level pattern identification.

LU-10 also clears Heat from the throat, and is therefore used in sore throat from Heat or from Wind-Heat. It is not used for sore throat from Yin deficiency, except when combined with other points such as KI-6 Zhaohai.

As it clears Heat, it also clears Heat from the Heart and treats mental–emotional symptoms deriving from Heart-Heat such as fear, mental restlessness, anger, manic behaviour, fright.

Box 54.10 summarizes the functions of LU-10.

> **Box 54.10 LU-10 – summary of functions**
> - Expels Wind-Heat and benefits the throat: acute sore throat and tonsillitis
> - Extinguishes interior Wind and promotes resuscitation

LU-11 SHAOSHANG *LESSER METAL*

Location

On the lateral corner of the thumbnail.

Nature

Well (*Jing*) point.
Wood point.

Actions

Expels exterior Wind.
Stimulates the diffusing and descending of Lung-Qi.
Benefits the throat.
Extinguishes interior Wind, opens the orifices and promotes resuscitation.

Indications

Aversion to cold, fever.
Cough, breathlessness.
Sore throat, painful obstruction of the throat, swollen tonsils, mumps.
Loss of consciousness from Wind-stroke.

Comments

This point expels exterior Wind and especially Wind-Heat and is often used for sore throat and swollen tonsils from attack of Wind-Heat: in this case it is bled. It is usually used only for acute sore throat from exterior Wind-Heat.

It is also effective for interior Wind, and is used in conjunction with the other Well points of the hand in apoplexy and loss of consciousness from Wind-stroke to open the orifices and promote resuscitation.

I have translated the name of this point as 'Lesser Metal' instead of the usual 'Lesser Merchant', as the word '*Shang*' in this context indicates one of the traditional five sounds that was related to Metal in the Five Elements. This particular sound is the sound of metal when struck.[14] The Lungs pertain to Metal and the Well point is where the channel is at its smallest and most superficial, hence 'Lesser Metal'.

It is useful to compare the functions of five major points of the Lung channel:

> - LU-5 Chize clears Lung-Heat, resolves Phlegm
> - LU-7 Lieque releases the Exterior, circulates Defensive Qi, stimulates the diffusing and descending of Lung-Qi
> - LU-9 Taiyuan tonifies the Lungs
> - LU-10 Yuji clears Lung-Heat, benefits the throat
> - LU-11 Shaoshang expels Wind-Heat, stimulates the diffusing and descending of Lung-Qi, benefits the throat

Fig. 54.5 illustrates the target areas influenced by the Lung points.

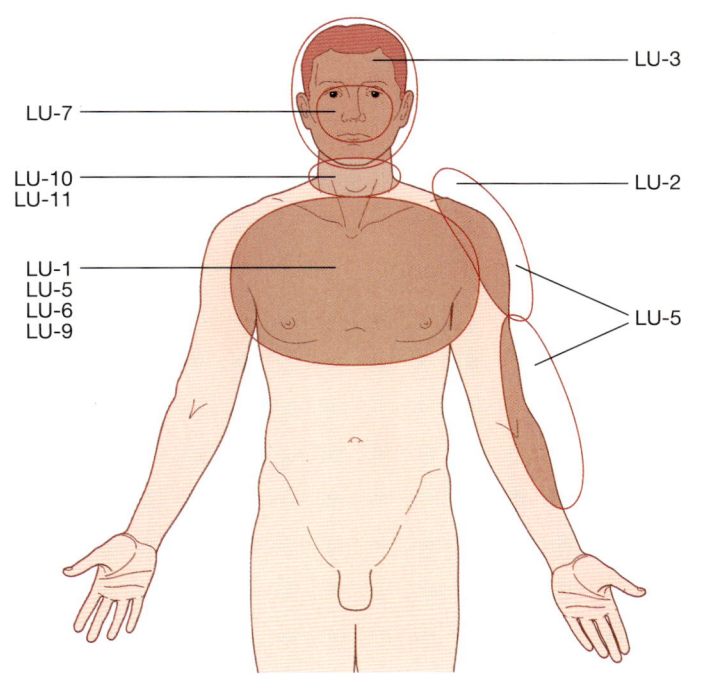

Figure 54.5 Target areas of Lung points

END NOTES

1. Yue Han Zhen 1990 An Explanation of the Acupuncture Points (*Jing Xue Jie* 经 穴 解), People's Health Publishing House, Beijing. Originally published in 1654, p. 24.
2. 1979 The Yellow Emperor's Classic of Internal Medicine – Simple Questions (*Huang Di Nei Jing Su Wen* 黄 帝 内 经 素 问), People's Health Publishing House, Beijing, first published *c.*100 BC, p. 145.
3. An Explanation of the Acupuncture Points, p. 26–27.
4. Ibid., p. 27.
5. Ibid., p. 29.
6. Ibid., p. 29.
7. Huang Fu Mi AD 259 The ABC of Acupuncture. In: Clinical Application of Frequently Used Acupuncture Points, p. 41.
8. Wang Wei Yi 1026 Illustrated Manual of Acupuncture Points as Shown on the Bronze Man (*Tong Ren Shu Xue Zhen Jiu Tu Jing* 铜 人 腧 穴 针 灸 图 经). In: Li Shi Zhen 1985 Clinical Application of Frequently Used Acupuncture Points (*Chang Yong Shu Xue Lin Chuang Fa Hui* 常 用 腧 穴 临 床 发 挥), People's Health Publishing House, Beijing, p. 41.
9. An Explanation of the Acupuncture Points, p. 31.
10. Ibid., p. 32.
11. Zhang Sheng Xing 1984 A Compilation of Explanations of the Meaning of the Acupuncture Points Names (*Jing Xue Shi Yi Hui Jie* 经 穴 释 义 汇 解), Shanghai Science Publishing House, Shanghai, p. 19.
12. An Explanation of the Acupuncture Points, p. 31.
13. Nanjing College of Traditional Chinese Medicine 1979 A Revised Explanation of the Classic of Difficulties (*Nan Jing Jiao Shi* 难 经 校 释), People's Health Publishing House, Beijing, first published *c.* AD 100, p. 2.
14. A Compilation of Explanations of the Meaning of the Acupuncture Points Names, p. 24.

SECTION 2 PART 7

Large Intestine Channel 55

Main channel pathway

The Large Intestine channel starts from the tip of the index finger. It then runs along the radial side of the index finger and up the lateral-anterior aspect of the arm. It then reaches the shoulder at the point L.I.-15 Jianyu. From here, it connects with Du-14 Dazhui and descends to the supraclavicular fossa to enter the lung. From the supraclavicular fossa it ascends along the sternocleidomastoid muscle to the cheek and enters the gums of the lower teeth. It then curves around the philtrum and crosses over to end at the side of the nose where it links with the Stomach channel (Fig. 55.1).

Connecting channel pathway

The Connecting channel starts at L.I.-6 Pianli from where a branch connects with the Lung channel. From L.I.-6 a branch runs along the main channel on the arm to the shoulder, jaw and teeth. From the jaw, another branch enters the ear (Fig. 55.2).

Box 55.1 gives an overview of the Large Intestine points.

> **Box 55.1 Overview of Large Intestine points**
>
> - Affect the arm, shoulder, neck and head
> - Expel exterior Wind
> - Treat the face and sinuses
> - Many points dissipate nodules and treat goitre

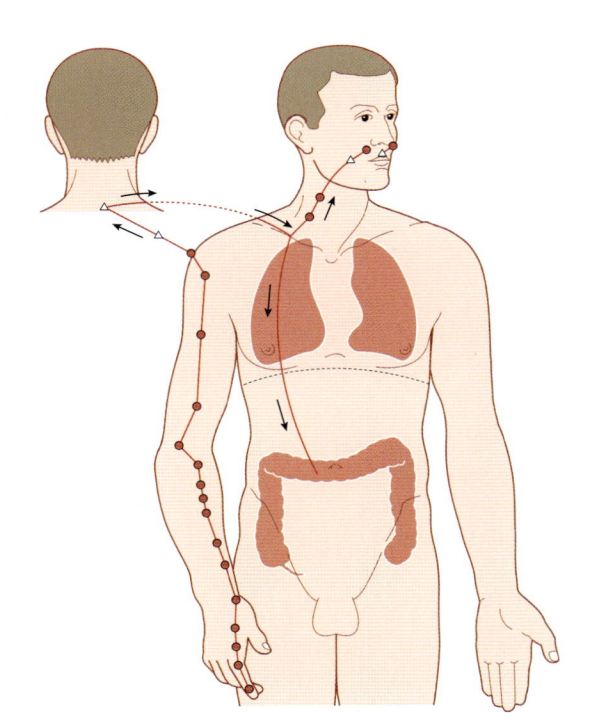

Figure 55.1 Large Intestine main channel

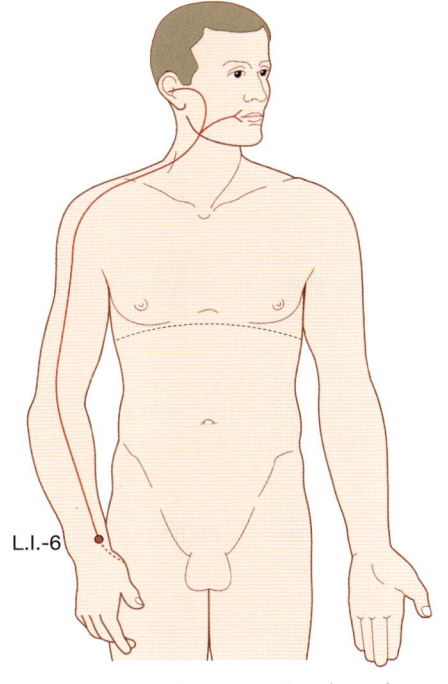

Figure 55.2 Large Intestine Connecting channel

L.I.-1 SHANGYANG *METAL YANG*

Location

At the lateral corner of the nail of the index finger.

Nature

Well (*Jing*) point.
Metal point.

Actions

Clears Heat.
Brightens the eyes.
Benefits the ears.
Benefits the throat.
Expels Wind and scatters Cold.
Extinguishes interior Wind and promotes resuscitation.
Removes obstructions from the channel.

Indications

Heat syndromes without sweating.
Blurred vision.
Tinnitus, deafness.
Sore throat, painful obstruction of the throat.
Aversion to cold, fever.
Loss of consciousness from Wind-stroke.
Pain in the shoulder and back that radiates to the supraclavicular fossa, numbness and heat of the fingers.

Comments

As a Well point, this point is effective in Excess patterns to remove obstructions quickly. Hence its use in the acute stage of Wind-stroke, combined with all the other Well points of the hands, to subdue interior Wind.

This point clears both interior and exterior Heat, so that it can be used in exterior attacks of Wind-Heat invading the Lung's Defensive Qi portion especially with sore throat, as well as in case of interior Heat in the Large Intestine.

Its action on the eyes is limited to cases of exterior Wind-Heat invading the eyes, such as in acute conjunctivitis. The 'Explanation of Acupuncture Points' recommends contralateral needling of L.I.-1 for eye problems.[1] The same text says that L.I.-1 also benefits the ears and treats tinnitus and deafness.[2]

Besides clearing Heat, this point can also expel Wind and Cold from the channel for the treatment of Painful Obstruction Syndrome of the shoulder. It can be used in this way as a distal point to clear the channel. If the problem is caused by Wind and Cold, moxa cones can be used instead of needling.

As for LU-11 Shaoshang, and for the same reasons, I have translated the word '*Shang*' as 'Metal'. The Large Intestine also pertains to Metal. L.I.-1 is the first point of the Metal Yang channel, hence the name 'Metal Yang'.[3]

Box 55.2 summarizes the functions of L.I.-1.

> **Box 55.2 L.I.-1 – summary of functions**
> - Large Intestine-Heat
> - Eye and ear problems
> - Extinguish interior Wind and promote resuscitation
> - Remove obstructions from the channel, elbow and shoulder pain

L.I.-2 ERJIAN *SECOND INTERVAL*

Location

On the lateral border of the index finger in front of the metacarpophalangeal joint.

Nature

Spring (*Ying*) point.
Water point.
Drainage point.

Actions

Clears Heat.
Expels Wind-Heat.
Removes obstructions from the channel.

Indications

Febrile diseases.
Aversion to cold, fever.
Pain and stiffness of the shoulder.

Comments

As a Spring point, this point clears Heat in the Large Intestine and is used in cases of interior Heat, with symptoms of constipation, dry stools, fever and abdominal pain.

It also expels Wind-Heat in acute invasions of exterior Wind.

Box 55.3 summarizes the functions of L.I.-2.

> **Box 55.3 L.I.-2 – summary of functions**
> - Clears Heat in the Large Intestine
> - It expels Wind-Heat in acute invasions of exterior Wind

L.I.-3 SANJIAN THIRD INTERVAL

Location
On the lateral border of the index finger behind the metacarpophalangeal joint.

Nature
Stream (*Shu*) point.
Wood point.

Actions
Expels exterior Wind.
Brightens the eyes.
Benefits the throat.
Regulates the Intestines.
Expels Wind and Cold from the channel.

Indications
Aversion to cold, fever, sneezing.
Acute eye pain.
Painful obstruction of the throat.
Diarrhoea from Cold and Dampness, borborygmi.

Comments
This point expels Wind and Cold from the channel in Painful Obstruction Syndrome of the hand, for which it is a widely used point. This action is partly due to its being the Stream point as these points are indicated in aches of the joints.

L.I.-3 can also be used to expel Wind-Heat in exterior invasions and it is mostly in this context that it brightens the eyes and benefits the throat.

Box 55.4 summarizes the functions of L.I.-3.

> **Box 55.4 L.I.-3 – summary of functions**
> - Expels Wind and Cold from the channel in Painful Obstruction Syndrome of the hand
> - Expels Wind-Heat in exterior invasions

L.I.-4 HEGU ENCLOSED VALLEY

Location
On the dorsum of the hand, between the first and second metacarpal bone (index and thumb) at the midpoint of the second metacarpal bone, close to its radial border.

Nature
Source (*Yuan*) point.
Ma Dan Yang's Heavenly Star point.

Actions
Expels exterior Wind and releases the Exterior.
Promotes the diffusing of Lung-Qi, regulates the Defensive Qi and sweating.
Stops pain.
Removes obstructions from the channel.
Tonifies Qi and consolidates the Exterior.
Harmonizes the ascending and descending of Qi.
Benefits the eyes, nose, ears and mouth.
Promotes labour.
Calms the Mind.

Indications
Aversion to cold, fever, sneezing, headache, sweating.
Sweating, absence of sweating.
Toothache, painful obstruction of throat, swelling of face, deviation of eye and mouth, lockjaw.
Painful Obstruction Syndrome (*Bi* Syndrome), hemiplegia, pain in the arm, contraction of fingers.
Tinnitus, deafness, redness, swelling and pain of the eye, blurred vision, nosebleed, nasal congestion and discharge, sneezing, mouth ulcers, lips not closing, tightness of lips.
Amenorrhoea, prolonged labour, delayed labour, retention of dead fetus.

Comments
L.I.-4 Hegu is the main point to expel Wind-Heat and to release the Exterior. L.I.-4 also has a strong direct sphere of influence on the face, so that, in exterior invasions, it is used to relieve nasal congestion, sneezing, burning eyes, etc. L.I.-4 regulates sweating and Defensive Qi in the space between skin and muscles so that it can be used both to stop and to promote sweating in exterior invasions of Wind. To promote sweating, L.I.-4 is tonified and KI-7 Fuliu drained: vice versa to stop sweating.

L.I.-4 also stimulates the diffusing of Lung-Qi, which explains its strong action in releasing the Exterior and expelling exterior Wind, so that it would be used for such symptoms and signs as nasal congestion, sneezing, cough, stiff neck, aversion to cold and a Floating pulse: that is, the beginning stages of a common cold, influenza or many other exterior diseases. As this point stimulates the diffusing of Lung-Qi, it makes it useful to relieve the symptoms of allergic rhinitis.

L.I.-4 has a powerful calming and antispasmodic action, so that it can be used in many painful conditions, both in the channels and in the organs and especially the Stomach, Intestines and Uterus.

It is also widely used as a distal point in Painful Obstruction Syndrome of the arm or shoulder, since it removes obstructions from the channel.

Since it has a strong direct influence on face and eyes, ears, nose and mouth, it is often used as a distal point when treating problems of the face, including mouth, nose, ears and eyes, such as allergic rhinitis, conjunctivitis, mouth ulcers, styes, sinusitis, epistaxis, toothache, trigeminal neuralgia, facial paralysis and frontal headaches. There is a saying in Chinese medicine: 'The face and mouth are reached by L.I.-4' (this rhymes in Chinese, '*Mian kou Hegu shou*'). L.I.-4 is an important distal point for facial problems such as deviation of eye and mouth following Wind-stroke, peripheral facial paralysis and trigeminal neuralgia.

Clinical note

L.I.-4 Hegu is an important distal point for all diseases of the face

It is sometimes combined with LIV-3 Taichong (this combination is called the 'Four Gates'), to expel interior or exterior Wind from the head and to stop pain. Although the combination of the Four Gates (L.I.-4 and LIV-3) is widely used in the West to calm the Mind, Chinese books actually do not mention this action. However, in my experience, L.I.-4 does have an influence on the Mind and can be used to soothe the Mind and allay anxiety, particularly if combined with LIV-3 Taichong and with Du-24 Shenting and G.B.-13 Benshen.

Although it is not often used in this way, L.I.-4 can also be used as a tonifying point rather than in its more common use as a draining one. Combined with other points, it can tonify Qi and consolidate the Exterior (i.e. strengthen the Defensive Qi). In order to do this, it would be combined with ST-36 Zusanli and Ren-6 Qihai. This treatment could be used for chronic allergic rhinitis owing to deficiency of Lung-Qi and weakness of the Exterior energetic layers (i.e. Defensive Qi), which make the person prone to chronic attacks of Wind. This treatment would only be suitable in between the attacks to strengthen Qi and the Exterior in order to reinforce the Defensive Qi to repel Wind.

L.I.-4 can harmonize the ascending of Yang and descending of Yin. This means that it can be used to subdue ascending rebellious Qi (such as ascending Stomach-Qi, Lung-Qi or Liver-Qi) or to raise Qi when it is sinking (such as sinking Spleen-Qi). Thus, in the former case, it can be used to subdue Stomach-Qi in epigastric pain, Liver-Yang rising in migraine (especially combined with LIV-3 Taichong) or Lung-Qi in asthma. In the latter case, it could be used to raise Spleen-Qi, especially in combination with Ren-6 Qihai. However, this last use is not common.

Finally, L.I.-4 is an empirical point to promote delivery during labour, hence its contraindication in pregnancy.

Box 55.5 summarizes the functions of L.I.-4.

Box 55.5 L.I.-4 – summary of functions

- Expels exterior Wind: colds, upper respiratory infections and influenza beginning stages
- Regulates sweating
- Benefits eyes, ears, nose and mouth
- Distal point for all problems of the face
- Combined with LIV-3 Taichong (the 'Four Gates') to expel exterior Wind, extinguish interior Wind and calm the Mind
- Regulates ascending/descending of Qi, hence subdues rebellious Qi in the head
- Good for allergic rhinitis
- Empirical point to promote labour
- Calms the Mind
- Forbidden in pregnancy

L.I.-5 YANGXI *YANG STREAM*

Location

On the radial side of the wrist, in the depression between the tendons of extensor pollicis longus and brevis.

Nature

River (*Jing*) point.
Fire point.

Actions

Expels Wind and releases the Exterior.
Stops pain.
Clears Heat.
Calms the Mind and opens the Mind's orifices.
Benefits nose, ears and eyes.

Indications

Aversion to cold, fever, sneezing.
Wrist pain, contraction of fingers, difficulty in raising elbow.
Febrile diseases.
Manic behaviour, propensity to (inappropriate) laughter, 'seeing ghosts', fright.
Sneezing, nosebleed, tinnitus, deafness, ear pain, redness, swelling and pain of the eye, lacrimation, toothache.

Comments

This point has similar functions to L.I.-4 Hegu in releasing the Exterior and expelling Wind-Heat in the beginning stages of exterior invasions. However, in these situations, L.I.-4 would be preferred as it is stronger in its action of releasing the Exterior.

L.I.-5 clears Heat in the Large Intestine and is used in febrile diseases. In connection with this function, this point calms the Mind and opens the Mind's orifices when there is Fire in the Bright Yang causing manic behaviour, propensity to (inappropriate) laughter and fright.

Similarly to L.I.-4, L.I.-5 benefits eyes, ears and nose and is used for sneezing, nosebleed, tinnitus, deafness, ear pain, redness, swelling and pain of the eye, lacrimation, toothache.

L.I.-5 is frequently used for Painful Obstruction Syndrome of hand and wrist.

Box 55.6 summarizes the functions of L.I.-5.

Box 55.6   L.I.-5 – summary of functions

- Releases the Exterior and expels Wind
- Clears Heat in the Large Intestine
- It calms the Mind and opens the Mind's orifices by draining Fire in Bright Yang
- Benefits eyes, ears and nose
- Frequently used for Painful Obstruction Syndrome (*Bi* Syndrome) of the wrist and hand

---

L.I.-6 PIANLI *LATERAL PASSAGE*

Location

On the lateral side of the forearm, 3 *cun* proximal to L.I.-5 Yangxi on the line connecting L.I.-5 and L.I.-11 Quchi, 3 *cun* above the wrist crease.

Nature

Connecting (*Luo*) point.

Actions

Regulates the Lung's Water passages.
Removes obstructions from the channel.

Indications

Difficult urination, oedema, ascites, borborygmi with abdominal oedema.
Toothache, tinnitus, deafness, redness and pain of the eye, blurred vision, sneezing, nosebleed, deviation of mouth.

Comments

L.I.-6 Pianli is an important point to regulate Lungs' Water passages (i.e. whenever the Lung function of controlling Water passages is impaired). This can happen when an exterior pathogenic factor obstructs the circulation of Defensive Qi in the space between skin and muscles, giving rise to oedema of the face and hands. This can also happen in chronic conditions of Lung-Qi deficiency.

Box 55.7 summarizes the functions of L.I.-6.

Box 55.7   L.I.-6 – summary of functions

- Important point to regulate the Lung's Water passages and therefore the movement and transformation of fluids in the Upper Burner

---

L.I.-7 WENLIU *WARM GATHERING*

Location

On the lateral side of the forearm, on the line connecting L.I.-5 and L.I.-11 Quchi, 5 *cun* above the wrist crease.

Nature

Accumulation (*Xi*) point.

Actions

Clears Heat.
Regulates the Intestines.
Opens the Mind's orifices.
Removes obstructions from the channel.

Indications

Mouth ulcers, hot tongue, tonsillitis.
Borborygmi with abdominal pain, abdominal distension.
Inappropriate laughter, manic behaviour, 'seeing ghosts'.
Headache, deviation of eye and mouth, redness and swelling of the eye, facial pain, furuncles of face, toothache, pain in the arm and shoulder with difficulty in raising the arm.

Comments

L.I.-7 Wenliu, like most Accumulation points, stops pain and removes obstructions from the channel and is particularly useful in acute situations. It is widely used in Painful Obstruction Syndrome of the channel and also Heat conditions of the mouth and face.

L.I.-7 opens the Mind's orifices in mental–emotional conditions occurring against a background of Heat in Bright Yang. As mentioned before, whenever ancient books mention 'seeing ghosts' or 'talking to ghosts', it usually means that the point is indicated in serious mental conditions such as psychosis.

I have changed the translation of this point's name in accordance with the 'Compilation of Explanations of the Meaning of the Acupuncture Points Names'.[4] This book explains that the character for *liu* means 'to flow' with the radical for 'water' on its left, but, without it, its meaning is equivalent to *liu*, i.e. 'to remain, to stay'; for this reason, this book translates this point's name as 'Warm Remaining' and I have preferred 'Warm Gathering'. The energetic explanation of this name is that this point is on the Large Intestine channel, which is part of the Bright Yang. The Bright Yang has 'much Qi and much Blood' and it is therefore the strongest Yang; Yang equals warmth, which accumulates at this point.

However, other books do not concur with this interpretation and say that the character *liu* means to 'flow' and cannot be interpreted as 'to stay, to remain'.[5]

Box 55.8 summarizes the functions of L.I.-7.

Box 55.8 L.I.-7 – summary of functions

- As Accumulation point, it is used for painful and acute conditions of the channel
- It clears Heat in the face (swollen tonsils, facial furuncles, etc.)
- It opens the Mind's orifices

L.I.-10 SHOUSANLI *ARM THREE MILES*

Location

On the radial side of the forearm, on the line connecting L.I.-5 and L.I.-11 Quchi, 2 *cun* below the transverse cubital crease.

Nature

None.

Actions

Removes obstructions from the channel.
Regulates the Intestines.
Tonifies Qi.

Indications

Pain and rigidity of the arm and shoulder, paralysis of the arm, numbness of the arm, atrophy of the arms, contraction and rigidity of the elbow.
Abdominal pain, vomiting, diarrhoea, feeling of cold in the intestines.
Tiredness.

Comments

This is a very important and widely used point for all channel problems of the Large Intestine channel. It is a very important point in the treatment of Painful Obstruction Syndrome, Atrophy Syndrome and sequelae of Wind-stroke affecting the arm. It is also a major point for the treatment of any channel problem affecting the forearm and hands.

L.I.-10 has also some tonifying property and is considered by some as a 'ST-36 Zusanli' of the arm (hence its name '*San Li*'): that is, a powerful Qi and Blood tonic.

Box 55.9 summarizes the functions of L.I.-10.

> **Box 55.9 L.I.-10 – summary of functions**
>
> - Very important point for channel problems of the Large Intestine, sequelae of Wind-stroke, Atrophy (*Wei*) Syndrome and Painful Obstruction Syndrome (*Bi* Syndrome)
> - Regulates the Intestines (abdominal pain, diarrhoea)
> - Has general tonic properties similar to those of ST-36 Zusanli

L.I.-11 QUCHI *POOL ON BEND*

Location

On the lateral end of the transverse cubital crease, at midpoint between LU-5 Chize and the lateral epicondyle of the humerus.

Nature

Sea (*He*) point.
Earth point.
Tonification point.
Ma Dan Yang's Heavenly Star point.

Actions

Clears Heat and cools Blood.
Removes obstructions and Heat from the channel.
Resolves Dampness.
Regulates the Intestines.
Benefits the sinews and joints.

Indications

High fever, thirst, hot skin.
Toothache, redness and pain of the eye, lacrimation, pain in front of the ear.
Abdominal distension and pain, vomiting, diarrhoea.
Erysipelas, urticaria, dry and scaly skin, itching, shingles.
Numbness of upper arm, Painful Obstruction Syndrome (*Bi* Syndrome) of arms and shoulder, hemiplegia, contraction of the arm, pain and rigidity of elbow and shoulder, atrophy of arm.

Comments

L.I.-11 Quchi point has an extremely wide-ranging action in many different types of conditions.

Firstly, it clears Heat. Although some modern Chinese books say it expels Wind-Heat,[6] most books say that it clears interior Heat; in the context of febrile diseases of exterior origin, therefore, this point is best to clear Heat in the Interior, i.e. Heat at the Qi Level within the Four-Level identification of patterns.

L.I.-11 also clears Heat in general in interior chronic conditions and can be used in interior Heat patterns of virtually any organ. It is very frequently used in Liver-Fire patterns.

L.I.-11 also cools the Blood and is therefore widely used in skin diseases due to Heat in the Blood, such as urticaria, psoriasis and eczema. It has an ancient history of use for skin diseases for which it is a very important point. It treats skin diseases also by virtue of being a Sea point of a Yang channel. In fact, chapter 6 of the 'Spiritual Axis' says: '*In diseases of Yang within Yang [i.e. skin], use the Sea points of the Yang channels.*'[7] Although not all Sea points of the Yang channels are indicated in skin diseases, two important ones stand out: namely, L.I.-11 Quchi and BL-40 Weizhong.

L.I.-11 resolves Dampness, particularly Damp-Heat, and can therefore be used in such patterns occurring in any part of the body. This point's action in clearing Heat and resolving Dampness also makes it very important for skin diseases characterized by Damp-Heat, such as papular or vesicular skin eruptions or acne.

It also treats Damp-Heat in the Spleen and Intestines with digestive symptoms such as diarrhoea.

Finally, L.I.-11 benefits the sinews and joints, which means that it can be used in Painful Obstruction Syndrome, Atrophy Syndrome and Wind-stroke paralysis, particularly of the arms and shoulders.

I have changed the name of this point to '*Pool on Bend*' from '*Crooked Pond*'. 'Pool' refers to the nature of this Sea point, i.e. the point where the channel joins the general circulation of Qi like a river joins the sea. 'Bend' refers to the bend of the elbow where the point is located (and the point is indeed located and needled with the elbow bent). Therefore it is not the pool (or pond) that is crooked but rather the pool is situated on a bend.

Box 55.10 summarizes the functions of L.I.-11.

> **Box 55.10 L.I.-11 – summary of functions**
>
> - Very important point for skin diseases both from Blood-Heat and Damp-Heat
> - Important point to clear Heat in general
> - Frequently used for channel and joint problems of the arm in Painful Obstruction Syndrome (*Bi* Syndrome), sequelae of Wind-stroke and Atrophy (*Wei*) Syndrome

L.I.-12 ZHOULIAO *ELBOW CREVICE*

Location
On the lateral side of the arm, on the border of the humerus, 1 *cun* above and 1 *cun* lateral to L.I.-11.

Nature
None.

Actions
Removes obstructions from the channel.

Indications
Contraction, numbness and rigidity of the upper arm, pain and rigidity of the elbow.

Comments
This is a secondary point, but it is worth mentioning here because it is very useful to treat tendinitis of the elbow ('tennis elbow'), provided the main problem is along the Large Intestine channel.
Box 55.11 summarizes the functions of L.I.-12.

Box 55.11 L.I.-12 – summary of functions

- Useful local point in the treatment of tendinitis of the elbow ('tennis elbow')

L.I.-14 BINAO *UPPER ARM*

Location
On the lateral side of the arm, in a depression between the insertion of deltoid muscle and the brachialis muscle, 3/5th of the distance of the line between L.I.-11 Quchi and L.I.-15 Jianyu.

Nature
Meeting point of the Large Intestine, Small Intestine and Bladder channels.
Point of the Yang Linking Vessel (*Yang Wei Mai*).

Actions
Removes obstructions from the channel.
Brightens the eyes.
Resolves Phlegm and dissipates nodules.

Indications
Pain and numbness of the upper arm and shoulder, Painful Obstruction Syndrome (*Bi* Syndrome) of the upper arm and shoulder, atrophy of the upper arm, inability to raise the arm, contraction and stiffness of the neck.
Redness, swelling and pain of the eye.
Scrofula, goitre.

Comments
This is not a major point, but still rather important and frequently used. Firstly, it is very much used in Painful Obstruction Syndrome of the arm and shoulder to remove obstructions from the channel (i.e. obstructions caused by Wind, Cold and Dampness).
It also has an action on the eyes in so far as it clears and enhances vision. In this case the needle should be slanted upwards.
L.I.-14 also resolves Phlegm and dissipates Phlegm masses, and is therefore used for goitre and nodules.
Box 55.12 summarizes the functions of L.I.-14.

Box 55.12 L.I.-14 – summary of functions

- Important local point for Painful Obstruction Syndrome (*Bi* Syndrome) of the upper arm and shoulder
- Affects the eyes and brightens vision
- It dissipates nodules and goitre

L.I.-15 JIANYU *SHOULDER BONE*

Location
With the arm abducted, in the depression anterior and inferior to the acromion, at the origin of the deltoid muscle.

Nature
Point of the Yang Stepping Vessel (*Yang Qiao Mai*).

Actions
Removes obstructions from the channel.
Expels Wind and Dampness.
Resolves Phlegm and dissipates nodules.

Indications
Shoulder pain, weakness of shoulder, Painful Obstruction Syndrome (*Bi* Syndrome) of the

shoulder from Wind and Dampness, inability to raise (abduct) the arm, contraction and numbness of the arm, hemiplegia, paralysis, sequelae of Wind-stroke, atrophy of arm.
Urticaria from Wind.
Scrofula, goitre.

Comments

This is a major point for the treatment of Painful Obstruction Syndrome of the shoulder as it benefits sinews and removes obstructions from the channel. It is also a major and frequently used point for Atrophy Syndrome and paralysis of the arm from Wind-stroke.

Like L.I.-14, it dissipates nodules and goitre.

Box 55.13 summarizes the functions of L.I.-15.

Box 55.13 L.I.-15 – summary of functions

- Very important point for channel problems of the shoulder and arm, Painful Obstruction Syndrome (*Bi* Syndrome), Atrophy (*Wei*) Syndrome and sequelae of Wind-stroke
- Dissipates nodules and goitre

L.I.-16 JUGU *GREAT BONE*

Location

On the upper aspect of the shoulder, in the depression between the acromial extremity of the clavicle and the scapular spine.

Nature

Point of the Yang Stepping Vessel (*Yang Qiao Mai*).

Actions

Removes obstructions from the channel.
Dissipates nodules.

Indications

Pain of the shoulder and upper back, difficulty in raising the arm, pain of upper arm.
Scrofula, goitre.

Comments

L.I.-16 point is frequently used in conjunction with L.I.-15 for channel problems of the shoulder. Its association with the Yang Stepping Vessel means that it has a particularly moving action on Qi and Yang in the shoulder and upper arm.

Box 55.14 summarizes the functions of L.I.-16.

Box 55.14 L.I.-16 – summary of functions

- Useful local point for shoulder and upper arm problems

L.I.-17 TIANDING *HEAVEN'S TRIPOD*

Location

On the lateral side of the neck, on the posterior border of the sternocleidomastoid muscle, 1 *cun* below L.I.-18 Futu.

Nature

None.

Actions

Benefits the throat and voice.
Dissipates nodules.

Indications

Sudden loss of voice, painful obstruction of throat.
Goitre, scrofula.

Comments

L.I.-17 is mentioned here primarily because it is an important local point for goitre and thyroid problems.

Box 55.15 summarizes the functions of L.I.-17.

Box 55.15 L.I.-17 – summary of functions

- Important local point for goitre and thyroid problems

L.I.-18 FUTU *SUPPORT THE PROTUBERANCE*

Location

On the lateral side of the neck, level with the tip of the Adam's apple, between the sternal head and clavicular head of the sternocleidomastoid muscle.

Nature

Window of Heaven point.

Actions

Benefits the throat and voice.
Subdues rebellious Qi and relieves cough and wheezing.
Resolves Phlegm and dissipates nodules.

Indications

Swelling and pain of the throat, sudden loss of voice, rattling sound in throat, difficulty in swallowing.
Cough, wheezing, breathlessness.
Goitre, scrofula.

Comments

L.I.-18 is widely used as a local point for throat problems, such as tonsillitis, mumps, laryngitis, aphasia, hoarse voice.

This is also an important local point for nodules in this area such as nodules on the vocal cords and goitre. It is also a local point for thyroid problems.

As a Window of Heaven point, it harmonizes the ascending and descending of Qi to and from the head. Its action in relieving cough, wheezing and breathlessness is related to its being a Window of Heaven point: that is, subduing rebellious Qi in the throat and regulating the ascending and descending of Qi to and from the head. The 'Explanation of Acupuncture Points' says that L.I.-18 is used for rebellious Qi.[8]

The 'protuberance' to which the point's name refers is the hyoid bone (Adam's apple).

Box 55.16 summarizes the functions of L.I.-18.

Box 55.16 L.I.-18 – summary of functions

- Important local point for throat and voice problems
- Important local point for goitre and thyroid problems

L.I.-20 YINGXIANG *WELCOME FRAGRANCE*

Location

In the nasolabial groove, at the midpoint lateral to the border of the ala nasi.

Nature

Meeting point of Stomach and Large Intestine.

Actions

Expels exterior Wind.
Opens the nose.
Removes obstructions from the channel.

Indications

Aversion to cold, fever, sneezing.
Nasal congestion and discharge, sneezing, loss of sense of smell, nasal polyps, nasal sores, nosebleed.
Deviation of eye and mouth, swelling and itching of face, red-hot eyes.

Comments

L.I.-20 is an important local point for nose problems of any kind such as sneezing, loss of the sense of smell, epistaxis, sinusitis, runny nose, stuffed nose, allergic rhinitis and nasal polyps.

It also expels exterior Wind and is used as a local point in invasions of Wind-Cold or Wind-Heat when there is sneezing, stuffed nose and runny nose. As it expels exterior Wind, it is also widely used as a local point in facial paralysis, trigeminal neuralgia and tic.

> **Clinical note**
>
> For nasal polyps, sinusitis and loss of sense of smell, I personally find the extra point *Bitong* more effective than L.I.-20 Yingxiang. The latter is better at expelling Wind from the face

Box 55.17 summarizes the functions of L.I.-20.
Figure 55.3 illustrates the target areas of the Large Intestine channel points.

Box 55.17 L.I.-20 – summary of functions

- Important local point for any nose problem
- Expels exterior Wind and is used when there is pronounced sneezing
- Expels Wind from the face in facial paralysis, trigeminal neuralgia and tics

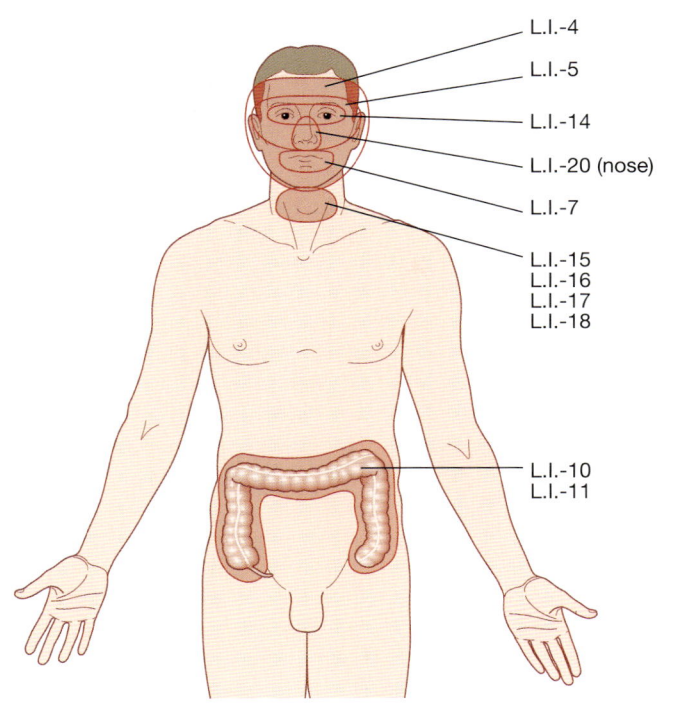

Figure 55.3 Target areas of Large Intestine points

END NOTES

1. Yue Han Zhen 1990 An Explanation of the Acupuncture Points (*Jing Xue Jie* 经 穴 解), People's Health Publishing House, Beijing. Originally published in 1654, p. 45.
2. Ibid., p. 45.
3. Zhang Sheng Xing 1984 A Compilation of Explanations of the Meaning of the Acupuncture Points Names (*Jing Xue Shi Yi Hui Jie* 经 穴 释 义 汇 解), Shanghai Science Publishing House, Shanghai, p. 27.
4. Ibid., p. 31.
5. Wang Xue Tai 1988 Great Treatise of Chinese Acupuncture (*Zhong Guo Zhen Jiu Da Quan* 中 国 针 灸 大 全), Henan Science Publishing House, p. 247.
6. Li Shi Zhen 1985 Clinical Application of Frequently Used Acupuncture Points (*Chang Yong Shu Xue Lin Chuang Fa Hui* 常 用 腧 穴 临 床 发 挥). People's Health Publishing House, Beijing, p. 93.
7. 1981 Spiritual Axis (*Ling Shu Jing* 灵 枢 经). People's Health Publishing House, Beijing, first published c.100 BC, p. 18.
8. An Explanation of the Acupuncture Points, p. 60.

SECTION 2 | PART 7

Stomach Channel | 56

Main channel pathway

The Stomach channel starts from the lateral side of the ala nasi (at L.I.-20 Yingxiang). It ascends along the nose and meets the Bladder channel at BL-1 Jingming. It then enters the upper gums. It curves around the lips and links with the Directing Vessel at Ren-24 Chengjiang. It then runs along the lower jaw and ascends in front of the ear to reach the forehead. From ST-5 Daying a branch goes down to the throat and the supraclavicular fossa. It then passes through the diaphragm, enters the stomach and the spleen.

From the supraclavicular fossa, a branch follows the superficial channel down to the breast and abdomen to pass through ST-30 Qichong. Another branch from the stomach connects with the point ST-30. From this point it follows the superficial channel to run along the anterior aspect of the upper leg and the anterior border of the tibia to end at the second toe. A branch from ST-42 Chongyang links with the Spleen channel (Fig. 56.1).

Connecting channel pathway

The Connecting channel starts at ST-40 Fenglong and connects with the Spleen channel. Another branch runs along the anterior border of the tibia up to the thigh and abdomen to the top of the head where it converges with the other Yang channels. A branch separates from the neck and goes forward to the throat (Fig. 56.2).

Box 56.1 gives an overview of the Stomach points.

Box 56.1 Overview of Stomach points

- Affect leg, abdomen, chest, throat, face
- Treat the limbs and Painful Obstruction Syndrome (*Bi* Syndrome)
- Treat all abdominal symptoms
- Strengthen Qi and Blood and resistance to pathogenic factors
- Resolve Phlegm
- Treat problems of the face and sinuses

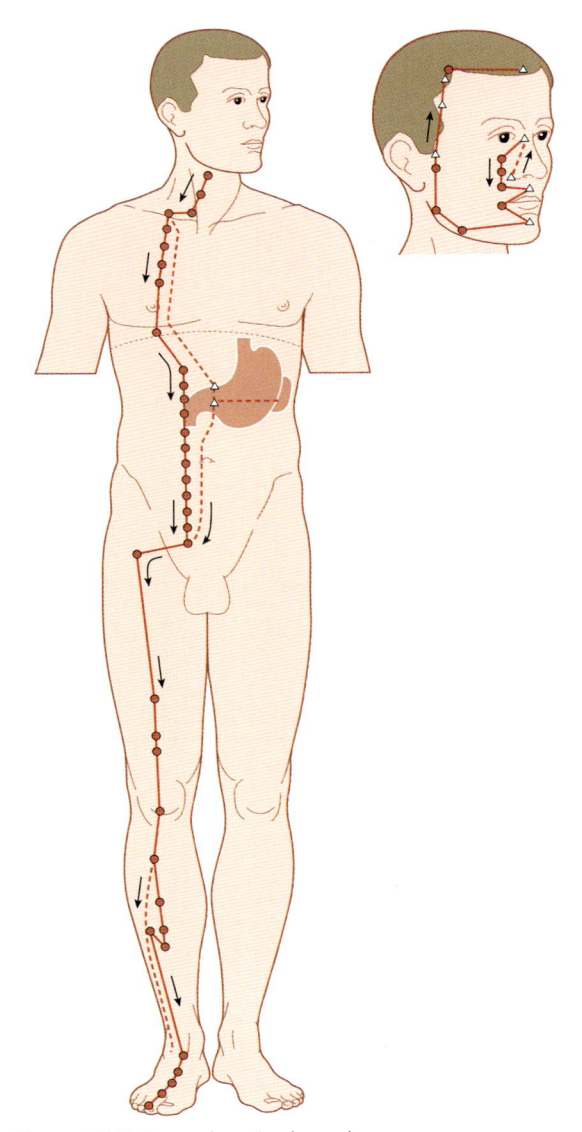

Figure 56.1 Stomach main channel

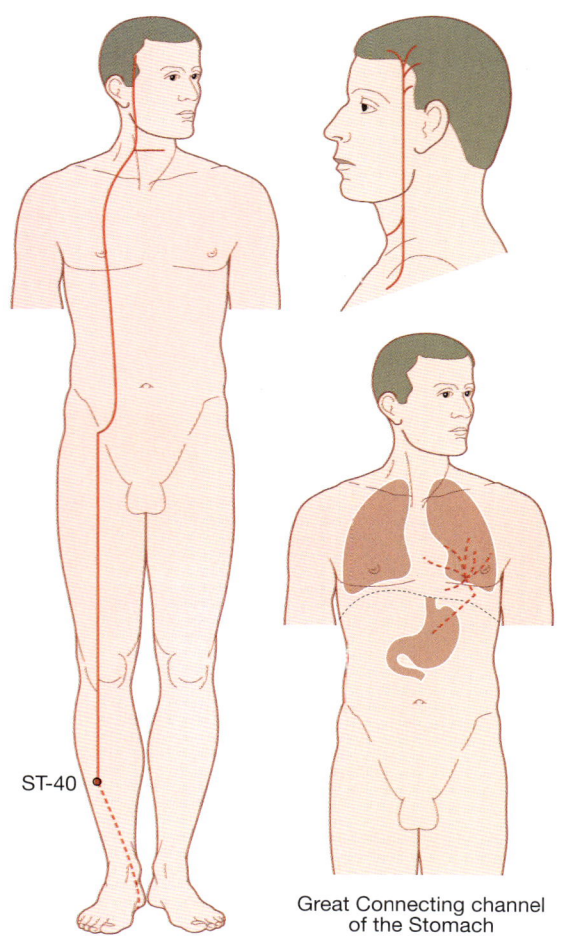

Figure 56.2 Stomach Connecting channel

ST-1 CHENGQI *CONTAINING TEARS*

Location
Directly below the pupil (when looking straight ahead), between the eyeball and the infraorbital ridge.

Nature
Point of the Yang Stepping Vessel (*Yang Qiao Mai*).
Point of the Directing Vessel (*Ren Mai*).

Actions
Expels Wind.
Brightens the eyes.
Clears Heat.

Indications
Deviation of eye and mouth, inability to speak, tinnitus, deafness.
Redness, swelling and pain of the eye, lacrimation on exposure to wind, blurred vision, myopia, diminished night vision, itchy eyes, twitching of eyelids.

Comments
This point is used mostly for eye problems and has a very wide range of indications such as acute and chronic conjunctivitis, myopia, astigmatism, squint, colour blindness, night blindness, glaucoma, atrophy of the optic nerve, cataract, keratitis and retinitis.

As it expels Wind (both interior and exterior) it is used for eye problems deriving from exterior Wind-Heat (such as swelling, pain and lacrimation and paralysis of the eyelid), as well as those deriving from interior Wind (such as tic of the eyelid).

Box 56.2 summarizes the functions of ST-1.

Box 56.2 ST-1 – summary of functions

- All eye problems from Heat, and from exterior and interior Wind
- Expels Wind from the face (facial paralysis, tic of eyelids)

ST-2 SIBAI *FOUR WHITES*

Location
Directly below the pupil (when looking straight ahead), in the depression at the infraorbital foramen.

Nature
Point of Yang Stepping Vessel (*Yang Qiao Mai*).

Actions
Expels Wind.
Brightens the eyes.
Clears Heat.

Indications
Deviation of eye and mouth, twitching of eyelids.

Redness and pain of the eye, blurred vision, itchy eyes, spontaneous lacrimation.
Roundworms in the bile duct.

Comments

This point is also used mostly for eye problems with the same range of indications as ST-1 Chengqi. It is similarly used to expel exterior Wind (swelling of eyes, allergic rhinitis or facial paralysis) and interior Wind (twitch of the eyelid). In particular, it is frequently used as a local point for the treatment of facial paralysis and trigeminal neuralgia.

A curious and seemingly inexplicable empirical use of this point is for biliary ascariasis.

Box 56.3 summarizes the functions of ST-2.

> **Box 56.3 ST-2 – summary of functions**
> - Local point for eye problems
> - Local point for Wind in the face (both external and internal)

ST-3 JULIAO *GREAT CREVICE*

Location

Directly below the pupil (when looking straight ahead), level with the lower border of the ala nasi, on the lateral side of the nasolabial groove.

Nature

Point of Yang Stepping Vessel (*Yang Qiao Mai*).

Actions

Expels Wind.
Removes obstructions from the channel.
Relieves swellings.

Indications

Aversion to cold, excessive lacrimation.
Toothache, epistaxis.
Pain and swelling of the nose and cheek, swelling and pain of lips, swelling of knee.

Comments

This point is used to expel exterior and interior Wind in exactly the same manner as ST-1 Chengqi and ST-2 Sibai. In particular, it is frequently used for facial paralysis and trigeminal neuralgia.

This point differs from ST-1 Chengqi and ST-2 Sibai in so far as its range of action extends not only to the eye but also to the nose; hence its use in the treatment of epistaxis and nasal obstruction.

Box 56.4 summarizes the functions of ST-3.

> **Box 56.4 ST-3 – summary of functions**
> - Eye problems
> - Local point for nose problems

ST-4 DICANG *EARTH GRANARY*

Location

0.4 *cun* lateral to the corner of the mouth.

Nature

Meeting point of Stomach and Large Intestine channels.
Point of Yang Stepping Vessel (*Yang Qiao Mai*).
Point of the Directing Vessel (*Ren Mai*).

Actions

Expels Wind.
Removes obstructions from the channel.

Indications

Deviation of eye and mouth, trigeminal neuralgia, drooling, numbness of the lips and face, contraction of facial muscles, movement of eyeball, twitching of eyelids, itchy eyes, blurred vision, inability to close the eye.
Cheek pain, toothache.

Comments

This point eliminates exterior Wind and is a major local point for the treatment of facial paralysis for which it is nearly always used if the mouth is deviated. As can be seen from the above indications, this point is also an important local point for internal Wind causing facial paralysis after Wind-stroke with deviation of eye and mouth, drooling from mouth and inability to close eye completely.

It also has an effect on the muscles of the face and is therefore used in aphasia.

Box 56.5 summarizes the functions of ST-4.

> **Box 56.5 ST-4 – summary of functions**
>
> - Expels Wind (deviation of eye and mouth, trigeminal neuralgia, drooling, numbness of the lips and face, contraction of facial muscles, movement of eyeball, twitching of eyelids, itchy eyes, blurred vision, inability to close the eye)
> - Removes obstructions from the channel (cheek pain, toothache)
> - Affects muscles of face and can be used for aphasia

ST-6 JIACHE *JAW CHARIOT*

Location

In the depression one finger-breadth anterior and superior to the lower angle of the mandible, at the prominence of the masseter muscle when the teeth are clenched.

Nature

One of Sun Si Miao's ghost points.

Actions

Expels Wind.
Removes obstructions from the channel.

Indications

Deviation of eye and mouth, lockjaw, inability to open the mouth after Wind-stroke.
Swelling of cheek, toothache, tension and pain of the jaw.

Comments

This is another major local point to expel exterior Wind affecting the face and it is nearly always used as a local point in facial paralysis combined with L.I.-4 Hegu. It is also used for mumps and spasm of the masseter muscle. It is also a local point to extinguish internal Wind in the face for facial paralysis following Wind-stroke.

It is combined with L.I.-4 Hegu for problems of the lower jaw including toothache.

Box 56.6 summarizes the functions of ST-6.

ST-7 XIAGUAN *LOWER GATE*

Location

At the lower border of the zygomatic arch in the depression anterior to the condyloid process of the mandible.

> **Box 56.6 ST-6 – summary of functions**
>
> - This is a major local point to expel exterior Wind affecting the face
> - Important local point for facial paralysis combined with L.I.-4 Hegu
> - Mumps and spasm of the masseter muscle
> - Local point to extinguish internal Wind in the face for facial paralysis following Wind-stroke
> - Combined with L.I.-4 Hegu for problems of the lower jaw including toothache

Nature

Meeting point of Stomach and Gall Bladder channels.

Actions

Removes obstructions from the channel.
Benefits the ear.
Expels Wind.

Indications

Lockjaw, dislocation of jaw, toothache, swelling and pain of lower gums, pain in the cheeks, swelling of cheeks.
Tinnitus, deafness, itchy ears, purulent discharge from the ears.
Deviation of eye and mouth, trigeminal neuralgia.

Comments

This point is also frequently used in facial paralysis and trigeminal neuralgia but it extends its influence to the ear too: hence its use also for otitis, deafness and earache. It is a major local point for trigeminal neuralgia and many doctors consider it to be the main one, affecting all three branches of the trigeminal nerve. It is therefore used as the main point for every branch combined with other appropriate local points according to the branch affected. For example, a doctor uses ST-7 as the main local point for trigeminal neuralgia combined with Yuyao for the upper branch, ST-2 Sibai for the middle branch and Ren-24 Chengjiang for the lower branch.[1]

It is combined with ST-44 Neiting for problems of the upper jaw and toothache.

Box 56.7 summarizes the functions of ST-7.

Box 56.7 ST-7 – summary of functions

- An important local point for Wind in the face (both internal and external)
- Important local point for trigeminal neuralgia
- Important point for jaw problems

Box 56.8 ST-8 – summary of functions

- A major point to resolve Phlegm from the head (dizziness, blurred vision, feeling of muzziness and heaviness of the head)
- Major local point for headaches from Phlegm
- Eye problems

ST-8 TOUWEI *HEAD CORNER*

Location

At the corner of the forehead, 4.5 *cun* lateral to Du-24 Shenting and 05. *cun* within the anterior hairline.

Nature

Point of Yang Linking Vessel (*Yang Wei Mai*).
Meeting point of Stomach and Gall Bladder channels.

Actions

Expels Wind and stops pain.
Brightens the eyes.

Indications

Splitting headache as if head were cracked open, dizziness, eye pain, lacrimation on exposure to wind, twitching of eyelids.
Blurred vision.

Comments

This is a major local point for dizziness deriving from Dampness and Phlegm retained in the head and preventing the clear Yang from rising upwards to brighten the orifices. It is therefore frequently used for dizziness (only if deriving from Phlegm), 'muzziness' of the head and a feeling of cloudiness or heaviness of the head.

It is also an important local point for frontal headaches deriving from Dampness or Phlegm preventing the clear Yang from reaching the head.

It can also be used for eye problems and excessive lacrimation deriving from invasions of exterior Wind.

Box 56.8 summarizes the functions of ST-8.

ST-9 RENYING *PERSON'S WELCOME*

Location

Level with the tip and 1.5. *cun* lateral to the Adam's apple between the anterior border of the sternocleidomastoid muscle and the lateral border of the thyroid cartilage. The point is between the carotid artery and the lateral border of the cartilage.

Nature

Point of the Sea of Qi.
Meeting point of the Stomach and Gall Bladder channels.
Window of Heaven point.

Actions

Regulates the ascending and descending of Qi to and from head.
Subdues rebellious Qi.
Dissipates nodules.

Indications

Headache, dizziness, blurred vision, red face, fullness of chest, shortness of breath, wheezing.
Goitre, scrofula.

Comments

ST-9 is used to remove obstructions from the head and to subdue rebellious Qi. This function is due to its nature of Window of Heaven point as these points regulate the ascending and descending of Qi to and from the head. ST-9 is therefore often used in Excess patterns characterized by excess Qi on the top part of the body.

It also dissipates nodules, with such symptoms as adenitis, nodules on the vocal cords and swelling of the thyroid.

According to chapter 33 of the 'Spiritual Axis', this point is a point of the Sea of Qi (together with Ren-17 Shanzhong, Du-15 Yamen and Du-14 Dazhui).[2] It can therefore be used to tonify Qi, although it is more often used to regulate Qi and eliminate imbalances in the distribution of Qi resulting in Excess above and Deficiency below.

Box 56.9 summarizes the functions of ST-9.

> **Box 56.9 ST-9 – summary of functions**
>
> - Used to remove obstructions from the head and to subdue rebellious Qi
> - ST-9 is often used in Excess patterns characterized by excess Qi on the top part of the body
> - It dissipates nodules, with such symptoms as adenitis, nodules on vocal cords and swelling of the thyroid
> - Point of the Sea of Qi. Used to regulate Qi and eliminate imbalances in the distribution of Qi resulting in Excess above and Deficiency below

ST-12 QUEPEN *EMPTY BASIN*

Location

Above the clavicle at its midpoint, 4 *cun* lateral to the midline, on the mamillary line (in men). In women, one cannot rely on the mamillary line as a point of reference.

Nature

Meeting point of Stomach, Large Intestine, Small Intestine, Triple Burner and Gall Bladder channels.

Actions

Subdues rebellious Qi.
Removes obstructions from the channel.

Indications

Cough, breathlessness, fullness of the chest.
Pain of the supraclavicular fossa, pain in the shoulder radiating to the neck, pain in the upper limbs, inability to raise the arm.

Comments

ST-12 point is useful in Excess patterns characterized by rebellious Stomach-Qi and Lung-Qi causing such symptoms as breathlessness and asthma.

This point is an important convergence point for all Yang channels except the Bladder channel. In reality, it affects the Bladder channel as well, as the Bladder muscle channel goes through the supraclavicular fossa. In subduing rebellious Qi, it can affect most of the Yang channels and it therefore has a powerful effect.

In my experience, it also has a calming effect on the Mind, by virtue of its sending Qi downwards. It is therefore used for anxiety, nervousness and insomnia due to a Stomach disharmony.

Box 56.10 summarizes the functions of ST-12.

> **Box 56.10 ST-12 – summary of functions**
>
> - Excess patterns characterized by rebellious Stomach-Qi and Lung-Qi causing such symptoms as breathlessness and asthma
> - Important convergence point for all Yang channels
> - Calming effect on the Mind, by virtue of its sending Qi downwards

ST-18 RUGEN *BREAST ROOT*

Location

Directly below the nipple (in men), in the fifth intercostal space. In women, one cannot rely on the nipple as a point of reference and the point is 4 *cun* from the midline.

Nature

None.

Actions

Benefits the breasts and reduces swelling.
Moves Qi in the chest and stops cough.

Indications

Breast abscess, breast pain, swelling and distension, agalactia.
Cough, breathlessness, feeling of oppression of the chest, difficulty in swallowing.

Comments

This point is mostly used as a local point for breast problems in women. First of all, it regulates Stomach-Qi in relation to the breast and can be used in mastitis, premenstrual swelling of breast and lumps in the breast.

It regulates lactation in nursing mothers: that is, it will either promote or reduce it as the situation demands.

Box 56.11 summarizes the functions of ST-18.

> **Box 56.11 ST-18 – summary of functions**
> - Local point for breast problems in women
> - Regulates lactation in nursing mothers

ST-19 BURONG *FULL*

Location

On the abdomen, 2 *cun* lateral to the midline, 6 *cun* above the umbilicus, level with Ren-14 Juque.

Nature

None.

Actions

Harmonizes the Middle Burner and subdues rebellious Stomach-Qi.
Subdues rebellious Lung-Qi.

Indications

Feeling of fullness in the epigastrium, sour regurgitation, nausea, epigastric distension and pain, vomiting, lack of appetite.
Cough, breathlessness.

Comments

ST-19 is an important local point for epigastric fullness and Full patterns of the Stomach. It may be used for Stomach-Qi stagnation, rebellious Stomach-Qi, Dampness in the Stomach and Retention of Food.

I have translated the name of this point simply as '*Full*' as its name means exactly that, i.e. that the Stomach is full and cannot take any more food. In fact, *Bu* means 'cannot' and *Rong* means 'to contain, to hold' (i.e. the Stomach cannot contain any more food).

A feeling of fullness is an important sign for the use of this point. Its energetic action is also linked to its being level and in proximity with KI-21 Youmen, which is the last point of the Penetrating Vessel. At this point, the Penetrating Vessel goes deeper into the chest and KI-21 is a point that is used to subdue rebellious Qi in digestive problems.

ST-19 is an important point for nausea and vomiting deriving from Full Stomach patterns.

Box 56.12 summarizes the functions of ST-19.

> **Box 56.12 ST-19 – summary of functions**
> - Important local point for epigastric fullness and Full patterns of the Stomach
> - A feeling of fullness is an important sign for the use of this point
> - Linked to KI-21 Youmen, the last point of the Penetrating Vessel, which subdues rebellious Qi in digestive problems
> - Important point for nausea and vomiting deriving from Full Stomach patterns

ST-20 CHENGMAN *SUPPORTING FULLNESS*

Location

On the abdomen, 2 *cun* lateral to the midline, 5 *cun* above the umbilicus, level with Ren-13 Shangwan.

Nature

None.

Actions

Harmonizes the Middle Burner and subdues rebellious Stomach-Qi.
Subdues rebellious Lung-Qi.

Indications

Feeling of fullness in the epigastrium, sour regurgitation, nausea, epigastric distension and pain, hiccup, vomiting, lack of appetite.
Cough, breathlessness.

Comments

This point has functions and actions that are very similar to those of ST-19 Burong. ST-20 is also used for Full Stomach patterns with a feeling of fullness and nausea.

Box 56.13 summarizes the functions of ST-20.

> **Box 56.13 ST-20 – summary of functions**
> - For Full Stomach patterns with a feeling of fullness and nausea

ST-21 LIANGMEN *BEAM DOOR*

Location

On the abdomen, 2 *cun* lateral to the midline, 4 *cun* above the umbilicus, level with Ren-12 Zhongwan.

Nature

None.

Actions

Moves Stomach-Qi and stops pain.
Clears Stomach-Heat.
Raises Qi and stops diarrhoea.

Indications

Epigastric pain and distension.
Chronic diarrhoea.

Comments

This is an important local point for Stomach problems, particularly of an Excess nature. As a rule of thumb, the epigastric points on the Directing Vessel (such as Ren-12) are used more in Deficiency patterns, whereas the points on the Stomach channel (such as ST-21) are used more in Excess patterns. ST-21, in particular, is very frequently used for Excess patterns of the Stomach, with Stomach-Qi rebelling upwards and causing nausea or vomiting.

It also clears Stomach-Heat and is used for thirst and a burning sensation in the epigastrium, especially combined with Neiting ST-44.

It is also used in acute painful patterns with epigastric pain, especially in combination with Liangqiu ST-34.

Box 56.14 summarizes the functions of ST-21.

Box 56.14 ST-21 – summary of functions

- Important local point for Stomach problems, particularly of an Excess nature
- Clears Stomach-Heat (thirst, burning sensation in the epigastrium), combined with ST-44 Neiting
- Acute painful patterns with epigastric pain, combined with ST-34 Liangqiu

---

ST-22 GUANMEN *PASS GATE*

Location

On the abdomen, 2 *cun* lateral to the midline, 3 *cun* above the umbilicus, level with Ren-11 Jianli.

Nature

None.

Actions

Moves Stomach-Qi.
Regulates the Water passages.
Regulates the Intestine and urination.

Indications

Epigastric and abdominal distension and pain, feeling of fullness in the epigastrium.
Constipation, borborygmi, oedema, enuresis.

Comments

Apart from its action in moving Qi in the epigastrium which practically all Stomach abdominal points have, the importance of this point lies in its action in regulating the Water passages of the Middle Burner. It is therefore an important point for Dampness in the Middle and/or Lower Burner or oedema. For this purpose, it is frequently combined with Ren-9 Shuifen and Ren-11 Jianli.

Another characteristic that distinguishes this point from ST-19, ST-20 and ST-21 is that its influence extends to the lower abdomen as well as the epigastrium.

Box 56.15 summarizes the functions of ST-22.

Box 56.15 ST-22 – summary of functions

- Moves Qi in the epigastrium and abdomen
- Regulates the Water passages of the Middle Burner
- It is an important point for Dampness in the Middle and/or Lower Burner or oedema. Frequently combined with Ren-9 Shuifen and Ren-11 Jianli

---

ST-25 TIANSHU *HEAVENLY PIVOT*

Location

On the abdomen, 2 *cun* lateral to the umbilicus.

Nature

Front Collecting point of the Large Intestine channel.

Actions

Regulates the Intestines.
Regulates Stomach and Spleen.
Moves Qi and invigorates Blood.
Resolves Dampness.
Clears Heat in the Stomach and Intestines.
Calms the Mind and opens the Mind's orifices.

Indications

Abdominal distension and pain, umbilical pain, borborygmi, constipation.
Chronic diarrhoea from Spleen deficiency, undigested food in stools.
Abdominal masses in women (*Zheng Jia*), period pain, irregular menstruation, infertility.
Leukorrhoea, oedema, swelling of face, turbid urine.

Comments

This is a very frequently used point. It can be used in all Excess patterns of the Stomach giving rise to abdominal (rather than epigastric) problems such as abdominal distension and pain. It is particularly indicated to stop diarrhoea from Spleen deficiency.

As a Front Collecting point, it is especially indicated in acute patterns of the Large Intestine.

When used with direct moxibustion, it tonifies and warms the Spleen and the Intestines, and is a special point for chronic diarrhoea arising from Spleen-Yang deficiency. In this case, it is combined with Ren-6 Qihai and ST-37 Shangjuxu.

In the context of diseases from invasion of exterior Wind-Heat, it is an important point to use in the Bright Yang stage of the Six-Channel pattern identification, or the Qi level of the Four-Level pattern identification. In these cases, it is combined with L.I.-11 Quchi.

From a psychological point of view, it is effective in mental irritation, anxiety, schizophrenia and mania, when these are due to a Stomach disharmony, particularly Excess patterns of the Stomach such as Phlegm-Fire in the Stomach.

An important characteristic of this point, compared to the ones above, is that it affects the uterus and menstruation and it is frequently used for painful periods to move Qi and Blood.

Furthermore, this point resolves Dampness in the Intestines and oedema. As it resolves Dampness, it may also treat diarrhoea from Dampness. ST-25 is therefore a very important point for diarrhoea as it can treat both that from Spleen deficiency and that from Dampness.

I consider this point essential to treat all bowel problems: for these diseases, I combine it with BL-25 Dachangshu, ST-37 Shangjuxu and ST-39 Xiajuxu.

Box 56.16 summarizes the functions of ST-25.

> **Box 56.16 ST-25 – summary of functions**
>
> - Used in all Excess patterns of the Stomach giving rise to abdominal (rather than epigastric) problems
> - Stops diarrhoea from Spleen deficiency
> - Especially indicated in acute patterns of the Stomach and Intestines
> - Important point to use in the Bright Yang stage of the Six-Channel pattern identification, or the Qi level of the Four-Level pattern identification to clear interior Heat in Stomach and Intestines
> - From a psychological point of view, it is effective in mental irritation, anxiety and agitation due a Stomach disharmony, particularly Excess patterns of the Stomach such as Phlegm-Fire in the Stomach
> - It affects the uterus and menstruation and it is frequently used for painful periods to move Qi and Blood
> - Resolves Dampness in the Intestines and oedema

Clinical note

Although ST-25 is obviously on the Stomach channel, it is more important as a point for the Intestines (it is the Front Collecting *Mu* point for the Large Intestine). It also affects the Uterus

ST-27 DAJU BIG GREATNESS

Location

On the abdomen, 2 *cun* lateral to the midline, 2 *cun* inferior to the umbilicus, level with Ren-5 Shimen.

Nature

None.

Actions

Regulates the Intestines.
Resolves Dampness and benefits urination.
Firms the Essence.

Indications

Abdominal distension, fullness and pain.
Difficult urination, retention of urine.
Premature ejaculation, seminal emissions.

Comments

This point is frequently used in Excess patterns of the Stomach giving rise to lateral abdominal pain. It moves Qi in cases of stagnant Qi in the lower abdomen.

Box 56.17 summarizes the functions of ST-27.

> **Box 56.17 ST-27 – summary of functions**
>
> - Important point for abdominal disorders from a Full condition
> - Resolves Dampness and benefits urination
> - Firms the Essence

ST-28 SHUIDAO WATER PASSAGES

Location
On the abdomen, 2 *cun* lateral to the midline, 3 *cun* inferior to the umbilicus, level with Ren-4 Guanyuan.

Nature
None.

Actions
Moves Qi in the Lower Burner.
Opens the Water passages and benefits urination.
Regulates menstruation.

Indications
Abdominal distension, fullness and pain.
Retention of urine, oedema.
Hypogastric pain in women, painful periods, infertility, abdominal masses in women (*Zheng Jia*), retention of dead fetus, retention of placenta.

Comments
The ST-28 point has several different actions. Firstly, it opens the Water passages of the Lower Burner and stimulates its excretion of fluids. It is therefore used in oedema, difficult urination and retention of urine, if caused by an Excess pattern. This point is a major point to stimulate the transformation, transportation and excretion of fluids, specifically in the Lower Burner.

It is one of three points performing this function in relation to fluids, all of them containing the word '*shui*' ('water') in their names:

> - Du-26 Shuigou ('Water Ditch', also called Renzhong) for the Upper Burner
> - Ren-9 Shuifen ('Water Separation') for the Middle Burner
> - ST-28 Shuidao ('Water Passages') for the Lower Burner

ST-28 also moves Qi and Blood in the lower abdomen, and can be used to regulate the menses in any menstrual problem caused by stagnation of Qi and Blood. This point has an ancient history of use for infertility and it is the most important point to use in infertility caused by obstruction of the Uterus by Damp-Phlegm. I use this point in every case of polycystic ovary syndrome.

Box 56.18 summarizes the functions of ST-28.

> **Box 56.18 ST-28 – summary of functions**
>
> - A very important point to open the Water passages of the Lower Burner and stimulates its excretion of fluids (oedema, difficult urination and retention of urine)
> - Moves Qi and Blood in the lower abdomen
> - Regulate the menses in any menstrual problem caused by stagnation of Qi and Blood, particularly painful periods
> - Ancient history of use for infertility – it is the most important point to use in infertility caused by obstruction of the Uterus by Damp-Phlegm (e.g. polycystic ovary syndrome)

ST-29 GUILAI RETURN

Location
On the abdomen, 2 *cun* lateral to the midline, 4 *cun* inferior to the umbilicus, level with Ren-3 Zhongji.

Nature
None.

Actions
Invigorates Blood in the Uterus and Lower Burner.
Lifts Qi and firms the Essence.

Indications
Amenorrhoea (from Blood stasis), painful periods, irregular periods, abdominal masses, infertility, retraction of testicles.
Prolapse of uterus, seminal emissions, impotence, nocturia.

Comments
This is an important point to eliminate stasis of Blood in the Uterus and regulate the menses. It is very much used in all menstrual problems related to stasis of Blood, particularly for dysmenorrhoea with dark

clotted blood. It can also be used to treat amenorrhoea, but only if caused by stasis of Blood. Some think that its name is due to its action in bringing on the 'return' of the menses.

Although this point is used primarily in Excess patterns with stasis of Blood, it can also be used to tonify and raise Qi in case of prolapse of the uterus. In this case, ST-29 is tonified in combination with Ren-6 Qihai, ST-36 Zusanli and Du-20 Baihui (this last point with direct moxibustion).

Box 56.19 summarizes the functions of ST-29.

Box 56.19 ST-29 – summary of functions

- An important point to eliminate stasis of Blood in the Uterus and regulate the menses (painful periods, amenorrhoea from Blood stasis)
- It can also be used to tonify and raise Qi in case of prolapse of the uterus
- Firms the Essence (seminal emission, impotence)

ST-30 QICHONG *PENETRATING QI*

Location
On the lower abdomen, 2 *cun* lateral to the midline, level with the superior border of the symphysis pubis, level with Ren-2 Qugu.

Nature
Point of the Penetrating Vessel (*Chong Mai*),
Point of the Sea of Food.

Actions
Regulates Qi in the Lower Burner,
Regulates the Penetrating Vessel,
Subdues rebellious Qi,
Tonifies the Sea of Food,
Invigorates Blood in the Uterus.

Indications
Hypogastric pain, abdominal fullness and distension, twisting pain in the abdomen, heat in the body with abdominal pain, hardness below the umbilicus.
Abdominal fullness and pain with feeling of energy rising to the chest and Heart, Qi of fetus rushing upwards to harass the Heart.
Irregular menstruation, amenorrhoea (from Blood stasis), excessive uterine bleeding, painful periods, infertility, retention of placenta, difficult lactation.
Swelling and pain of vagina, swelling and pain of penis, testicle pain, retraction of testicles, impotence.

Comments
This is a powerful point with many different actions. Most of its actions are due to it being a point of the Penetrating Vessel (*Chong Mai*) and the *chong* in its name refers to the *Chong Mai*. Indeed, it is a very dynamic point because it is the point from which the Penetrating Vessel emerges from the Interior.

First of all, it moves Qi and Blood in the lower abdomen, Uterus and genitals and is therefore indicated in many abdominal and genital problems of an Excess nature, such as abdominal pain, abdominal masses, hernia, painful periods, swelling of penis, retention of placenta and swelling of prostate.

ST-30 is on the Penetrating Vessel and since this vessel is the Sea of Blood, this point strongly invigorates Blood. Being a point on the Penetrating Vessel, it can be combined with its opening and coupled points (SP-4 Gongsun and P-6 Neiguan) to enhance its action and direct the therapeutic effect to the lower abdomen and genitals.

It is an important point to subdue rebellious Qi of the Penetrating Vessel (see ch. 53) in conjunction with its opening and coupled points SP-4 Gongsun and P-6 Neiguan.

Being the point of the Sea of Food means that it stimulates the Stomach function of rotting and ripening and the Spleen function of transformation, thus generally revitalizing the digestive system and tonifying Qi.

Finally, since it is simultaneously a major point of the Penetrating Vessel and the Sea of Food, it is the link between the Root of the Pre-Heaven Qi (Kidneys) and the Root of the Post-Heaven Qi (Stomach). Because of this connection, it can be used to tonify strongly Pre- and Post-Heaven Qi.

In many of the classics this point is also called *Qijie*, i.e. 'Streets of Qi', which was also a name for the *Chong Mai* and a reference to the Penetrating Vessel influence on all channels of the abdomen.

Box 56.20 summarizes the functions of ST-30.

> **Box 56.20 ST-30 – summary of functions**
>
> - Moves Qi and Blood in the lower abdomen, Uterus and genitals and is therefore indicated in many abdominal and genital problems from Qi stagnation and Blood stasis
> - It invigorates Blood in the Uterus
> - An important point to subdue rebellious Qi of the Penetrating Vessel SP-4 Gongsun and P-6 Neiguan
> - As a point of the Sea of Food, it stimulates the Stomach function of rotting and ripening and the Spleen function of transformation
> - As a point of the Penetrating Vessel (which is the Sea of Blood) and of the Sea of Food, it is the link between the Root of the Pre-Heaven Qi (Kidneys) and the Root of the Post-Heaven Qi (Stomach)

ST-31 BIGUAN *THIGH GATE*

Location

On the anterior aspect of the thigh, at the junction of a vertical line downward from the anterior superior iliac spine and a horizontal line level with the lower border of the symphysis pubis, in the depression lateral to the sartorius muscle.

Nature

None.

Actions

Removes obstructions from the channel.
Expels Wind and Dampness.

Indications

Atrophy of legs, Painful Obstruction Syndrome (*Bi* Syndrome) of the legs, hemiplegia, numbness of the legs, hip pain, pain in the thigh, contraction of thigh muscles, Cold Painful Obstruction Syndrome of the knees, rigidity of knee joint.

Comments

This point is frequently used as a local point in Atrophy (*Wei*) Syndrome, Painful Obstruction Syndrome and sequelae of Wind-stroke. It strengthens the leg, facilitates its movement and, in particular, it facilitates the raising of the leg, an important factor, especially in Atrophy Syndrome, when the leg is often dragged. It is an important point in multiple sclerosis, which is a form of Atrophy Syndrome.

When needling this point to affect the whole leg, it is desirable to obtain the needling sensation to propagate all the way down the leg, or at least past the knee.

Box 56.21 summarizes the functions of ST-31.

> **Box 56.21 ST-31 – summary of functions**
>
> - Frequently used as a local point in Atrophy (*Wei*) Syndrome, Painful Obstruction Syndrome (*Bi* Syndrome) and sequelae of Wind-stroke. It is an important point in multiple sclerosis

ST-32 FUTU *CROUCHING RABBIT*

Location

On the thigh, on a line drawn between the lateral border of the patella and the anterior superior iliac spine, in a depression 6 *cun* above the superior border of the patella.

Nature

None.

Actions

Removes obstructions from the channel.
Expels Wind and Dampness.

Indications

Painful Obstruction Syndrome (*Bi* Syndrome) and Atrophy (*Wei*) Syndrome of the legs, paralysis from Wind-stroke, numbness, contraction and pain of the thighs, knee pain.

Comments

This is another local point for leg problems similar in effect to ST-31 Biguan, but not with such a strong action in lifting the leg.

Box 56.22 summarizes the functions of ST-32.

> **Box 56.22 ST-32 – summary of functions**
>
> - Frequently used as a local point in Atrophy (*Wei*) Syndrome, Painful Obstruction Syndrome (*Bi* Syndrome) and sequelae of Wind-stroke

ST-34 LIANGQIU BEAM MOUND

Location
On the thigh, on a line drawn between the lateral border of the patella and the anterior superior iliac spine, in a depression 2 *cun* above the superior border of the patella.

Nature
Accumulation (*Xi*) point.

Actions
Subdues rebellious Stomach-Qi.
Removes obstructions from the channel.
Expels Dampness and Wind.

Indications
Epigastric pain, sour regurgitation.
Swelling and pain of the knee, rigidity of the knee, pain in the leg, numbness of lower leg, Cold Painful Obstruction Syndrome (*Bi* Syndrome) of the knee.

Comments
As an Accumulation point, ST-34 point is used for acute, Excess and painful patterns of the Stomach. It subdues rebellious Stomach-Qi causing such symptoms as hiccup, nausea, vomiting and belching.

It is frequently used in the treatment of Painful Obstruction Syndrome of the knee to expel exterior Dampness, Wind and Cold from the knee joint.

Box 56.23 summarizes the functions of ST-34.

Box 56.23 ST-34 – summary of functions

- As an Accumulation point, ST-34 is used for acute, Excess and painful patterns of the Stomach. It subdues rebellious Stomach-Qi (hiccup, nausea, vomiting and belching)
- Frequently used in the treatment of Painful Obstruction Syndrome of the knee to expel exterior Dampness, Wind and Cold from the knee joint

---

ST-35 DUBI CALF NOSE

Location
On the knee, in the hollow when the knee is flexed immediately below the patella and lateral to the patellar ligament.

Nature
None.

Actions
Removes obstructions from the channel.
Relieves swelling.

Indications
Swelling and pain of knee joint, difficulty in flexing and extending the knee, weak knees, numbness of the knees, numbness of lower leg.

Comments
This is an important point for the treatment of Painful Obstruction Syndrome of the knee for which it is nearly always used to expel Dampness and Cold. It is particularly effective when moxa is burned on the needle. This method of treatment should obviously not be used for Hot-Painful Obstruction Syndrome.

This point, together with the corresponding point on the medial side of the knee, is also known as Xiyan *Knee Eye*, an extra point (see ch. 67).

Box 56.24 summarizes the functions of ST-35.

Box 56.24 ST-35 – summary of functions

- An important point for the treatment of Painful Obstruction Syndrome (*Bi* Syndrome) of the knee for which it is nearly always used to expel Dampness and Cold. It is particularly effective when moxa is burned on the needle

---

ST-36 ZUSANLI THREE MILES OF THE FOOT

Location
Below the knee, 3 *cun* below ST 35 Dubi, one fingerbreadth lateral to the anterior crest of the tibia.

Nature
Sea (*He*) point.
Earth point.
Point of the Sea of Food.
Ma Dan Yang's Heavenly Star point.

Actions
Benefits Stomach and Spleen.
Tonifies Qi and Blood.

Tonifies the Original Qi.
Brightens the eyes.
Regulates Nutritive and Defensive Qi.
Regulates the Intestines.
Raises Yang.
Expels Wind and Damp.
Expels Cold.
Resolves oedema.
Rescues Yang and promotes resuscitation.

Indications

Epigastric pain, nausea, vomiting, hiccup, belching, poor appetite, difficult digestion.
Deficiency of Qi, deficiency of Blood and Yin, shortness of breath, tiredness, dizziness, postpartum dizziness, blurred vision, palpitations.
Eye diseases.
Aversion to cold, fever, febrile disease with heavy head.
Manic depression, manic singing, raving and laughing, inappropriate laughter.
Borborygmi, abdominal distension and pain, flatulence, diarrhoea, undigested food in the stools.
Pain in the knee and leg.
Oedema, lower abdominal swelling with retention of urine.

Comments

This is of course a major point to tonify Qi and Blood in Deficiency patterns. It is the main point to tonify the Root of Post-Heaven Qi (i.e. Stomach and Spleen). Although it is on the Stomach channel, ST-36 Zusanli strongly tonifies Spleen-Qi as well as Stomach-Qi. It is used in all cases of Deficiency of Stomach and Spleen, and to strengthen the body and mind in very debilitated persons, or after a chronic disease.

Since it tonifies Upright Qi (*Zheng Qi*), it also strengthens the resistance to attack from exterior pathogenic factors. It can therefore be used for prevention of attacks from exterior climatic factors. When used for prevention, moxa only is applied to this point. Some doctors recommend the use of this point with direct moxibustion every 5–7 days for about 10 minutes each time, to strengthen the Upright Qi and the resistance to disease. However, this use of ST-36 is not considered suitable for those under 30 years of age.

Li Dong Yuan (1180–1251), author of the celebrated 'Discussion on Stomach and Spleen' (*Pi Wei Lun*), said: '*For old people with deficiency of Qi, use ST-36 Zusanli and Ren-6 Qihai frequently with 50–60 moxa cones each time.*'[3]

ST-36 can tonify not only Qi, Yang, Blood and Yin but also the Original Qi (*Yuan Qi*). Although the Original Qi resides in the Kidneys and it is related to the Pre-Heaven Qi, it relies on the Stomach and Spleen for its supplementation.

ST-36 is also indicated in all Deficiency patterns of the Stomach, with dull epigastric pain, no appetite, etc. It also regulates the Intestines, treating abdominal distension and pain and constipation of a Deficient nature.

It brightens the eyes and can be used for blurred vision and declining eyesight in old age.

It is also used in attacks of exterior Wind-Cold, with prevalence of Wind (Greater-Yang Wind pattern of the Six-Stage pattern identification), to regulate Nutritive and Defensive Qi. In this case, the exterior Wind-Cold invades the skin and interferes with the circulation of Defensive Qi: the pores are open and the person sweats slightly. This situation is characterized by a weakness of Nutritive Qi, which causes the person to sweat. Needling ST-36 regulates and harmonizes Nutritive and Defensive Qi so that tonifying the former stops sweating and moving the latter expels the pathogenic factors. When used in this way, ST-36 is needled not with reinforcing, but even method.

The 'Discussion on Cold-induced Diseases' in clause 8 says: '*At the Greater-Yang stage, if a headache persists for more than seven days, it is because the pathogenic factor has circulated through the Greater Yang channel. If the pathogenic factor tends to be transmitted to the next channel [Bright Yang channel], needling points on the Stomach channel will stop this transmission.*'[4]

Since it regulates Nutritive and Defensive Qi, it is also used in all cases of oedema, when the Defensive Qi is weak in the space between skin and muscles and fluids overflow from the channels to invade the space under the skin. ST-36 resolves oedema by consolidating the space between skin and muscles.

Used with direct moxibustion, ST-36 raises Yang and is used for prolapses in combination with Ren-6 Qihai and Du-20 Baihui.

ST-36 is not only used as a tonifying point, but it can also be used with even or reducing method to eliminate Dampness or Cold. As can be seen from the indications, it also moves Qi in the Stomach and Intestines. However, it is much more frequently used to tonify.

ST-36 can also expel Wind and Dampness from the channels in Painful Obstruction Syndrome (*Bi*

Syndrome). In my experience, besides its obvious action on Painful Obstruction Syndrome of the knee, for which it acts also as a local point, it also has an influence as a distal point for Painful Obstruction Syndrome of the wrist.

Box 56.25 summarizes the functions of ST-36.

> **Box 56.25 ST-36 – summary of functions**
>
> - Major point to tonify Qi, Blood, Yang, Yin and the Original Qi
> - Very important in all Deficiency patterns of Stomach and Intestines
> - Strengthens the Upright Qi (*Zheng Qi*) and resistance to exterior pathogenic factors
> - Brightens the eyes – for chronic eye diseases
> - Harmonizes Nutritive and Defensive Qi in exterior invasions of Wind to regulate the space between the skin and muscles
> - Resolves oedema
> - Raises Yang – for prolapses
> - Expels Cold (with moxibustion)
> - Expels Wind and Dampness in Painful Obstruction Syndrome (*Bi* Syndrome)

ST-37 SHANGJUXU *UPPER GREAT EMPTINESS*

Location

On the lower leg, 3 *cun* inferior to ST-36 Zusanli, one finger-breadth lateral to the anterior crest of the tibia.

Nature

Lower Sea point of the Large Intestine channel. Point of the Sea of Blood.

Actions

Regulates the Stomach and Intestines and resolves retention of Food.
Eliminates Damp-Heat.
Subdues rebellious Qi.

Indications

Borborygmi, diarrhoea, abdominal pain and distension, umbilical pain.
Shortness of breath, breathlessness, Qi rushing up the chest, fullness of the chest.

Comments

The most important aspect of this point is related to its character as Lower Sea point for the Large Intestine channel. As such, it serves the same function for the Large Intestine channel as ST-36 Zusanli does for the Stomach channel. It can therefore be used to affect the Large Intestine directly to treat a wide range of intestinal symptoms. It is especially indicated for chronic diarrhoea, and for Damp-Heat patterns of the Large Intestine with loose, offensive stools with mucus and blood.

ST-37 also opens the chest and subdues rebellious Qi, which makes it applicable in the treatment of asthma and breathlessness.

According to the 'Spiritual Axis' (ch. 33), this point, together with ST-39 Xiajuxu and BL-11 Dashu, is a point of the Sea of Blood and it can therefore be used to tonify Blood (see also ch. 51).[5]

Box 56.26 summarizes the functions of ST-37.

> **Box 56.26 ST-37 – summary of functions**
>
> - Regulates the Stomach and Intestines and resolves retention of Food (borborygmi, diarrhoea, abdominal pain and distension, umbilical pain)
> - Eliminates Damp-Heat (shortness of breath, breathlessness, Qi rushing up the chest, fullness of the chest)
> - Subdues rebellious Qi
> - Important point to stop chronic diarrhoea

Clinical note

I personally use this point as a set of points for bowel diseases. These are: ST-25 Tianshu, ST-37 Shangjuxu, ST-39 Xiajuxu and BL-25 Dachangshu.

ST-38 TIAOKOU *NARROW OPENING*

Location

On the anterior aspect of the lower leg, 8 *cun* below ST-35 Dubi, one finger-breadth from the anterior crest of the tibia.

Nature

None.

Actions

Expels Wind and Dampness.
Removes obstruction from the channel.

Indications

Atrophy of leg, Painful Obstruction Syndrome (*Bi* Syndrome) of legs, Damp Painful Obstruction Syndrome, numbness, coldness and swelling of leg, inability to stand for long.
Shoulder pain, inability to raise the shoulder.

Comments

This point is mostly used as an empirical distal point for pain and stiffness of the shoulder joint. It is usually needled first with reducing method while the patient gently rotates the shoulder, and then local points are used.

Box 56.27 summarizes the functions of ST-38.

> **Box 56.27 ST-38 – summary of functions**
>
> - Important as a distal point for inability to raise the shoulder

ST-39 XIAJUXU *LOWER GREAT EMPTINESS*

Location

On the lower leg, 3 *cun* inferior to ST-37 Shangjuxu, one finger-breadth lateral to the anterior crest of the tibia.

Nature

Lower Sea (*He*) point of the Small Intestine channel.
Point of the Sea of Blood.

Actions

Regulates the Small Intestine.
Eliminates Damp-Heat.
Eliminates Wind-Damp.

Indications

Lower abdominal pain, diarrhoea.
Painful Obstruction Syndrome (*Bi* Syndrome) and Atrophy (*Wei*) syndrome of the leg, paralysis of leg.

Comments

Being the Lower Sea point for the Small Intestine, this point is used for all patterns of this Yang organ. In particular, it is used for lower abdominal pain with borborygmi and flatulence.

It is also used to resolve Damp-Heat in the Small Intestine with such symptoms as cloudy dark urine and stools with mucus. In combination with ST-37 Shangjuxu, it is used for pain in the legs caused by Wind and Dampness.

As a point for the Sea of Blood, it can be used to tonify Blood together with BL-37 Shangjuxu and BL-11 Dashu.

In my experience, the three points ST-36, ST-37 and ST-39 can treat restless legs.

Box 56.28 summarizes the functions of ST-39.

> **Box 56.28 ST-39 – summary of functions**
>
> - Being the Lower Sea point for the Small Intestine, this point is used for all patterns of this Yang organ. In particular, it is used for lower abdominal pain with borborygmi and flatulence
> - Resolves Damp-Heat in the Small Intestine (cloudy dark urine and stools with mucus)
> - In combination with ST-37 Shangjuxu, it is used for pain in the legs caused by Wind and Dampness
> - As a point for the Sea of Blood, it can be used to tonify Blood together with BL-37 Shangjuxu and BL-11 Dashu

ST-40 FENGLONG *ABUNDANT BULGE*

Location

On the anterior aspect of the lower leg, 8 *cun* superior to the external malleolus, lateral to ST-38 Tiaokou, two finger-breadths from the anterior crest of the tibia.

Nature

Connecting (*Luo*) point.

Actions

Resolves Phlegm and Dampness.
Opens the chest and subdues rebellious Qi.
Promotes the descending of Lung-Qi and stops cough.
Calms the Mind and opens the Mind's orifices.

Indications

Feeling of oppression of the chest, profuse sputum, swelling of the face, dizziness, headache, swelling of the throat, feeling of heaviness of the body.
Cough with sputum, breathlessness, wheezing.
Manic depression, inappropriate laughter, inappropriate elation, desire to ascend to high places and sing, undress and run around, mental restlessness, seeing 'ghosts'.

Comments

This is a very important point since it is the point to resolve Phlegm in all its manifestations and in all parts of the body. It eliminates substantial Phlegm, such as profuse expectoration from the chest, Phlegm in the form of lumps, such as lumps under the skin, thyroid lumps and uterus lumps, and non-substantial Phlegm, such as the one that clouds the Mind and obstructs the Mind's orifices causing mental disturbances or simply headache, dizziness and muzziness of the head. In all these cases this point should be needled with reducing method to resolve Phlegm.

Owing to its Phlegm-eliminating action, it is very much used in the treatment of asthma as it also has the effect of opening the chest and soothing breathing.

Another action of this point is to calm the Mind, on which it has a profound effect. It can be used in all cases of anxiety, fears and phobias, not only if they are caused by misting of the Mind by Phlegm but also if they are caused by rebellious Qi.

The Phlegm-resolving of this point should not be overemphasized, overlooking its other functions. Apart from its use in resolving Phlegm, ST-40 can also be used to subdue rebellious Qi of the Stomach and Lungs when the person is very anxious, and the anxiety reflects on the Stomach function, with such symptoms as tightness of the epigastrium, a feeling of knot in the Stomach or, as some people say, a feeling of 'butterflies in the stomach'.

Finally, this point also has an action on the chest and it is used to open and relax the chest when it is painful or there is a feeling of oppression: it may be used after bruising of the chest and ribcage. In these cases, it may be used in combination with P-6 Neiguan, normally unilaterally and crossed over (Fig. 56.3).

Box 56.29 summarizes the functions of ST-40.

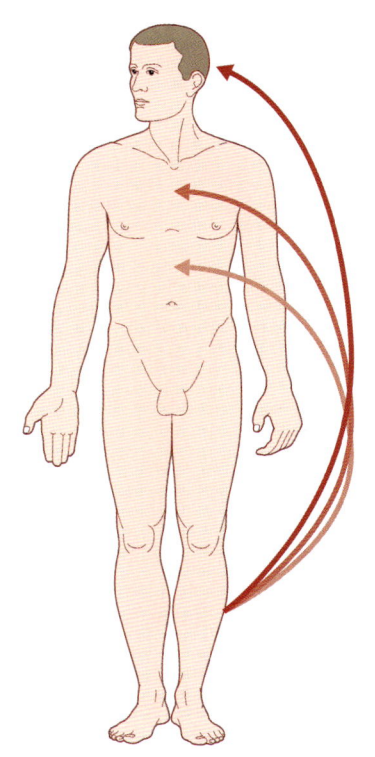

Figure 56.3 Actions of ST-40 Fenglong

Box 56.29 ST-40 – summary of functions

- A major point to resolve Phlegm in all its manifestations and in all parts of the body, e.g. substantial Phlegm (profuse expectoration from the chest), Phlegm in the form of lumps (lipomas, goitre, fibroids), and nonsubstantial Phlegm such as the one that clouds the Mind and obstructs the Mind's orifices causing mental disturbances or simply headache, dizziness and muzziness of the head
- It is used for asthma as it opens the chest and subdues rebellious Qi
- Calms the Mind (anxiety, fears and phobias)
- Subdues rebellious Qi of the Stomach and Lungs when the person is very anxious, and the anxiety reflects on the Stomach function, with such symptoms as tightness of the epigastrium, a feeling of knot in the Stomach
- Opens the chest

Clinical note

In my experience, the Phlegm-resolving effect of ST-40 is overemphasized. ST-40 has many other functions:
- Subdues rebellious Stomach-Qi
- All Full conditions of the Stomach
- Opens the chest (with LU-7 or P-6)
- Calms the Mind
- Regulates the Heart

ST-41 JIEXI *DISPERSING STREAM*

Location

On the ankle, level with the prominence of the lateral malleolus in a depression between the tendons of the extensor hallucis longus and extensor digitorum communis.

Nature

River (*Jing*) point.
Fire point.
Tonification point.

Actions

Clears Heat.
Calms the Mind.
Removes obstructions from the channel.

Indications

Swelling of the face, frontal headache, red face and eyes, dizziness.
Abdominal distension, belching, abdominal fullness, hunger with inability to eat, constipation.
Febrile diseases.
Manic behaviour, agitation, weeping, fright, 'seeing ghosts'.
Swelling and pain of the ankle, drop foot, feeling of heaviness of the knee, sciatica, Sinew Painful Obstruction Syndrome (*Bi* Syndrome), Dampness Painful Obstruction Syndrome.

Comments

This point is frequently used in Painful Obstruction Syndrome of the foot to expel Cold and Dampness. As a River point it particularly affects joints and is frequently used for problems of the ankle. ST-41 is important to use in multiple sclerosis when the foot drops and makes walking difficult. In such cases, ST-41 inserted deeply has the effect of lifting the foot.

It clears Stomach-Heat and is used for burning epigastric pain and thirst. It is also effective for headache or sore throat due to Stomach-Heat.

It also calms the Mind and conducts Heat downwards away from the head.

Box 56.30 summarizes the functions of ST-41.

Box 56.30 ST-41 – summary of functions

- Frequently used in Painful Obstruction Syndrome of the foot to expel Cold and Dampness
- Clears Stomach-Heat and is used for burning epigastric pain and thirst
- Also effective for headache or sore throat due to Stomach-Heat
- Calms the Mind and conducts Heat downwards away from the head

ST-42 CHONGYANG *PENETRATING YANG*

Location

At the highest point of the dorsum of the foot, between the tendons of the extensor hallucis longus and digitorum longus, where the dorsal artery of the foot pulsates.

Nature

Source (*Yuan*) point.

Actions

Regulates the Intestines.
Tonifies Stomach and Spleen.
Opens the Mind's orifices.
Removes obstructions from the channel.

Indications

Abdominal distension, epigastric pain.
Manic depression, desire to ascend to high places and sing, discard clothes and run around.
Deviation of eye and mouth, swelling and pain of face, toothache, pain inside the mouth.
Swelling and pain of dorsum of foot, atrophy of foot.

Comments

This point can tonify the Stomach and the Spleen as it is the Source point. Combined with T.B.-4 Yangchi, it powerfully tonifies the Middle Burner and dispels Cold from the joints and is used for Painful Obstruction Syndrome from Cold.

This point also opens the Mind's orifices and is used for mental illness.

Box 56.31 summarizes the functions of ST-42.

Box 56.31 ST-42 – summary of functions

- As Source point, it tonifies the Stomach
- It opens the Mind's orifices
- It removes obstructions from the channel

ST-43 XIANGU *SINKING VALLEY*

Location

On the dorsum of the foot, in the depression distal to the junction of the second and third metatarsal bones, 1 *cun* above ST-44 Neiting.

Nature

Stream (*Shu*) point.
Wood point.

Actions

Expels Wind and clears Heat.
Removes obstruction from the channel.
Regulates the Intestines.
Resolves oedema.

Indications

Swelling and pain of the dorsum of the foot, rigidity of the toes, Heat Painful Obstruction Syndrome (*Bi* Syndrome).
Abdominal distension, fullness and pain, borborygmi, belching.
Oedema of face, swelling of eyes.

Comments

This point is mostly used as a general point to expel Wind and Heat from the joints in Painful Obstruction Syndrome. It also resolves oedema from the face.

Box 56.32 summarizes the functions of ST-43.

> **Box 56.32 ST-43 – summary of functions**
> - General point for Painful Obstruction Syndrome (*Bi* Syndrome) from Wind and Heat
> - Resolve oedema from the face

ST-44 NEITING *INNER COURTYARD*

Location

On the dorsum of the foot, between the second and third toes, 05. *cun* proximal to the margin of the web.

Nature

Spring (*Ying*) point.
Water point.

Actions

Clears Heat.
Regulates the Intestines and resolves Damp-Heat.
Calms the Mind.
Expels Wind from the face.

Indications

Febrile disease, feeling of heat, thirst.
Abdominal distension and pain, borborygmi, diarrhoea, blood in stools, constipation.
Aversion to the sound of people talking, desire for silence.
Pain in the eye, toothache, facial pain, deviation of eye and mouth.

Comments

This is a very important point of the Stomach channel. First of all, it clears Heat from the Stomach channel, and can be used for bleeding gums and any Stomach complaint with Heat. It is mostly used for Excess patterns.

In the context of diseases from exterior pathogenic factors, it is used in febrile diseases at the Bright Yang stage of the Six Channels, or the Qi level of the Four Levels.

It is very effective to stop pain along the Stomach channel, particularly the lower jaw.

Often combined with L.I.-4 Hegu, it eliminates Wind from the face, and is therefore used in facial paralysis and trigeminal neuralgia.

Box 56.33 summarizes the functions of ST-44.

> **Box 56.33 ST-44 – summary of functions**
> - Important point to clear Stomach-Heat
> - Used in febrile diseases at the Bright Yang stage of the Six Channels, or the Qi level of the Four Levels to clear Stomach-Heat
> - Effective to stop pain along the Stomach channel, particularly the lower jaw
> - Often combined with L.I.-4 Hegu, it eliminates Wind from the face, and is therefore used in facial paralysis and trigeminal neuralgia

ST-45 LIDUI *SICK MOUTH*

Location

On the lateral corner of the nail of the second toe.

Nature

Well (*Jing*) point.
Metal point.
Drainage point.

Actions

Clears Stomach-Heat.
Clears Heat from Stomach channel.
Calms the Mind and opens the Mind's orifices.
Promotes resuscitation.
Resolves retention of Food.

Indications

Excessive hunger, febrile disease.
Swelling of the face, feeling of heat in the face, nosebleed, yellow nasal discharge, toothache, cracked lips.
Excessive dreaming, fright, insomnia, dizziness, manic depression, desire to ascend high places, sing, discard clothes and run around.
Loss of consciousness.

Comments

This point is frequently used to calm the Mind, when this is disturbed in the context of a Stomach pattern, usually from an Excess pattern, such as Stomach-Fire being transmitted to the Heart and giving rise to Heart-Fire. The use of this point can, at the same time, sedate the Stomach and calm the Mind. It is often used for insomnia in this context.

One particular use of this point is to clear Heart-Fire, in which case it is used with direct moxa cones.

Box 56.34 summarizes the functions of ST-45.

Figure 56.4 illustrates the target areas of the Stomach channel points.

Box 56.34 ST-45 – summary of functions

- Clears Stomach-Heat
- Clears Heat in the Stomach channel in the face
- Calms the Mind and drains Heart-Fire

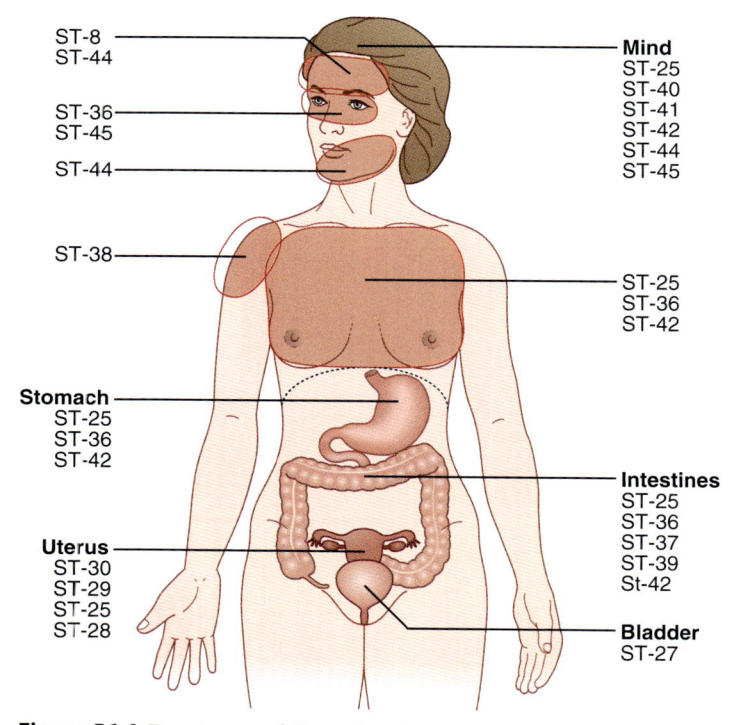

Figure 56.4 Target areas of Stomach points

END NOTES

1. Acupuncture and Moxibustion, no. 7, 1998, p. 425.
2. 1981 Spiritual Axis (*Ling Shu Jing* 灵枢经), People's Health Publishing House, Beijing, first published *c.*100 BC, p. 73.
3. Li Dong Yuan 1249 Discussion on Stomach and Spleen. In: Li Shi Zhen 1985 Clinical Application of Frequently Used Acupuncture Points (*Chang Yong Shu Xue Lin Chuang Fa Hui* 常用腧穴临床发挥), People's Health Publishing House, Beijing, p. 195.
4. Nanjing College of Traditional Chinese Medicine, Shang Han Lun Research Group 1980 Discussion on Cold-induced Diseases (*Shang Han Lun* 伤寒论) by Zhang Zhong Jing, Shanghai Scientific Publishing House, Shanghai, first published *c.* AD 220, p. 369.
5. Spiritual Axis, p. 73.

SECTION 2 PART 7

Spleen Channel | 57

Main channel pathway

The Spleen channel starts from the tip of the big toe and runs along the medial aspect of the foot to ascend the medial malleolus. It then follows the posterior aspect of the tibia, passes the knee and thigh to enter the abdomen. It enters the spleen and stomach from where it ascends, traversing the diaphragm and reaching the oesophagus. It ends at the centre of the tongue.

From the stomach, a branch goes through the diaphragm and links with the heart (Fig. 57.1).

Connecting channel pathway

From the point SP-4 Gongsun, the Connecting channel links with the Stomach channel. Another branch enters the abdomen and connects with the large intestine and stomach (Fig. 57.2.).

Box 57.1 gives an overview of the Spleen points.

Box 57.1 Overview of Spleen points

- Affect inner aspect of leg, abdomen
- Affect the Uterus
- Affect Blood (stop bleeding, cool Blood, invigorate Blood and nourish Blood)
- Nourish Yin

SP-1 YINBAI *HIDDEN WHITE*

Location

On the lateral angle of the nail of the big toe.

Nature

Well (*Jing*) point.
Wood point.
One of Sun Si Miao's Ghost points.

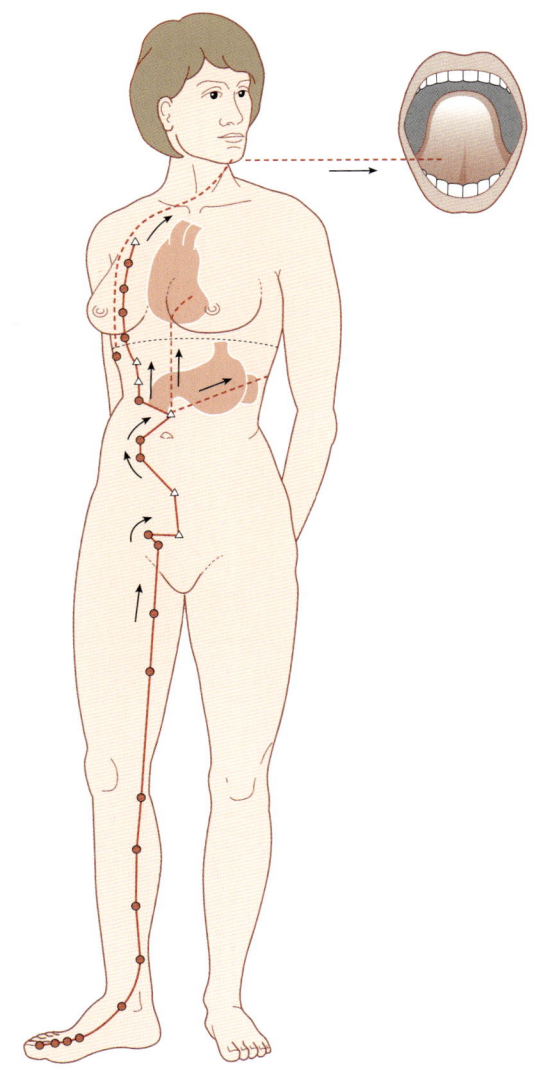

Figure 57.1 Spleen main channel

Uterine bleeding, blood in the urine, blood in the stools, vomiting blood, nosebleed, febrile disease with nosebleed.
Agitations, sighing, sadness, manic depression, excessive dreaming, insomnia.

Comments

SP-1 is normally used in Excess patterns of the Spleen. A special use of this point is with direct moxa to stop bleeding from any part of the body and particularly from the uterus. It stops bleeding by strengthening the Spleen's function of holding Blood. It can therefore also be used for bleeding from the nose, stomach, bladder or intestines.

Another use of this point is in cases of mental restlessness and depression in Excess patterns resulting from stasis of Blood. In such conditions it calms the Mind and stops excessive dreaming.

Box 57.2 summarizes the functions of SP-1.

Box 57.2 SP-1 – summary of functions

- SP-1 is normally used in Excess patterns of the Spleen
- With direct moxibustion, stops bleeding from any part of the body and particularly from the uterus
- Mental restlessness and depression in Excess patterns resulting from stasis of Blood

---

SP-2 DADU *BIG CAPITAL*

Location

On the medial aspect of the foot, in the depression anterior and inferior to the proximal metatarsophalangeal joint.

Nature

Spring (*Ying*) point.
Fire point.
Tonification point.

Actions

Regulates the Spleen.
Resolves Dampness.
Clears Heat.
Calms the Mind.

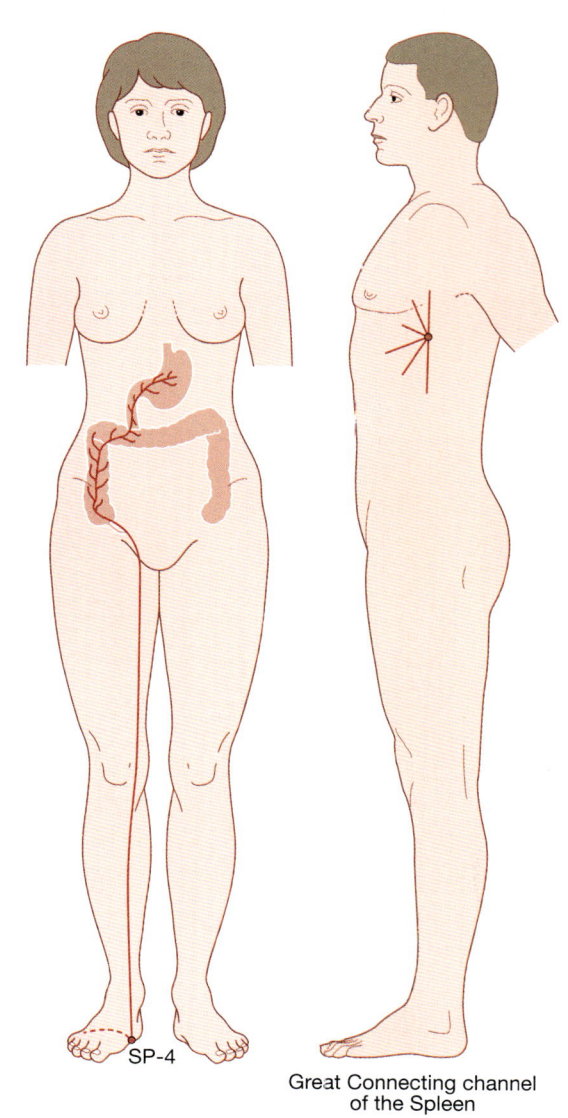

Figure 57.2 Spleen Connecting channel and Great Connecting channel

Actions

Regulates the Spleen.
Stops bleeding.
Calms the Mind.

Indications

Abdominal distension, diarrhoea, vomiting, no desire to eat.

Indications

Abdominal distension, epigastric pain, vomiting, diarrhoea, constipation.
Sudden swelling of limbs, feeling of heaviness of the body, feeling of oppression of the chest.
Febrile disease without sweating.
Agitation, insomnia.

Comments

Although this is the 'tonification' point of the Spleen according to the Five Elements, it is seldom used to tonify the Spleen, as it is more frequently used to clear Heat in Excess patterns. In particular, it is used in the course of a febrile disease from exterior Heat, at its beginning stage to cause sweating and clear Heat.

It also calms the Mind and it is used when the Mind is unsettled against a background of Heat in the Spleen and Stomach.

Box 57.3 summarizes the functions of SP-2.

Box 57.3 SP-2 – summary of functions

- Clears Heat in Excess patterns
- Febrile diseases from exterior Heat
- Calms the Mind: Mind is unsettled against a background of Heat in the Spleen and Stomach

---

SP-3 TAIBAI *SUPREME WHITE*

Location

On the medial aspect of the foot, in the depression posterior and inferior to the proximal metatarsophalangeal joint of the big toe.

Nature

Stream (*Shu*) and Source (*Yuan*) point.
Earth point.

Actions

Strengthens the Spleen.
Stimulates Intellect (*Yi*).
Resolves Dampness.
Regulates the Intestines.
Strengthens the spinal muscles.

Indications

Deficiency of Spleen and Stomach, tiredness, poor appetite.
Poor memory, confused thinking, muzziness of the head, difficulty in concentrating.
Feeling of heaviness of the body and the four limbs, feeling of heaviness and muzziness of the head, dull frontal headache.
Borborygmi, diarrhoea, undigested food in the stools, constipation, abdominal pain and distension, epigastric distension and pain.
Chronic backache against a background of Spleen and Kidney deficiency.

Comments

SP-3 is a major point to tonify the Spleen, as it is the Source point of the channel and also the Earth point of an Earth channel: as the Spleen belongs to Earth, which is at the centre of the Five Elements, the Source point of the Spleen is the 'centre of the centre'. It is very frequently used to tonify the Spleen in any of its deficiency patterns.

In my experience, SP-3 stimulates the mental faculties pertaining to the Intellect (*Yi*), which are associated with the Spleen, and it can be used in cases when Spleen-Qi has been weakened by excessive mental work. The use of SP-3 can then stimulate the brain, promote memory and induce mental clarity. This point is useful to stimulate mental powers in patients suffering from postviral, chronic fatigue syndrome.

Another important function of this point is to resolve Dampness, for which it is a major point. It is used in any Dampness pattern in the Upper, Middle or Lower Burner. When used to resolve Dampness, it should be needled with reducing method. Examples of symptoms and signs of Dampness are: confused thinking, feeling of heaviness and muzziness (fuzziness) of the head, feeling of fullness of the epigastrium, no appetite, feeling of heaviness of the body and sticky tongue coating. In my experience, SP-3 is particularly useful to resolve Dampness from the head, where it causes a feeling of heaviness and muzziness of the head and a dull frontal headache.

SP-3 is also frequently used in chronic retention of Phlegm in the Lungs. Phlegm is retained in the Lungs, but it originates from the Spleen due to the impairment of its function of transportation and transformation.

> **Box 57.4 SP-3 – summary of functions**
>
> - Major point to tonify the Spleen
> - Stimulates the Intellect (*Yi*) and mental faculties
> - Regulates the Intestines (abdominal distension and pain, diarrhoea)
> - Resolves Dampness, particularly from the head
> - Resolves Phlegm and strengthens the Lungs
> - Strengthens the spinal muscles

Reinforcing SP-3 can at the same time tonify the Spleen to strengthen the Lungs (strengthening the Earth to nourish Metal) and resolve Phlegm.

A more unusual use of this point is to strengthen the spine. According to chapter 4 of the 'Simple Questions', the Spleen controls the spine.[1] In my experience, SP-3 is a very useful point to strengthen and straighten the spine in cases of chronic backache.

Box 57.4 summarizes the functions of SP-3.

SP-3 can straighten the spine

SP-4 GONGSUN *MINUTE CONNECTING CHANNELS*

Location

On the medial aspect of the foot, in the depression distal and inferior to the base of the first metatarsal bone.

Nature

Connecting (*Luo*) point.
Opening point of Penetrating Vessel.

Actions

Harmonizes the Middle Burner.
Regulates the Intestines.
Regulates the Penetrating Vessel.
Calms the Mind and opens the Mind's orifices.
Stops bleeding.
Regulates menstruation.
Benefits feet and toes.

Indications

Epigastric fullness, distension and pain, oesophageal constriction.
Abdominal fullness, distension and pain, borborygmi, diarrhoea, undigested food in the stools.
Manic depression, anxiety, insomnia, mental restlessness, chest pain.
Blood in the stools, uterine bleeding.
Painful periods, irregular periods, retention of placenta, retention of lochia.
Pain in the heel, numbness of feet, cold feet, hot soles, pain in arch of foot, pain in the big toe, fungal infection of the big toe.

Comments

This is a complex point with a very wide sphere of action. SP-4 is used for Excess patterns of the Stomach and Spleen such as retention of Dampness in the epigastrium, stasis of Blood in the Stomach, Stomach-Heat and Stomach-Qi rebelling upwards. It is therefore used to dispel fullness of the epigastrium and to stop epigastric or abdominal pain.

Its other functions derive from its relation with the Penetrating Vessel (*Chong Mai*). This vessel is the 'Sea of the 12 Channels' as well as the 'Sea of Blood'; it enters the Uterus and regulates menstruation. SP-4, by activating and regulating the Penetrating Vessel, regulates menstruation and stops excessive bleeding, also by reinforcing the Spleen function of holding Blood.

The Penetrating Vessel goes through the heart and its syndrome of rebellious Qi affects the Heart and Mind: for this reason, this point can be used for anxiety, mental restlessness, chest tightness and pain and insomnia.

All Connecting (*Luo*) points of the Yin channels stop bleeding in the appropriate channels. SP-4 therefore stops bleeding from the digestive system. However, by its connection with the Penetrating Vessel (which is the Sea of Blood), it can stop bleeding from any part of the body (the Penetrating Vessel also controls all the Blood Connecting channels).

The Penetrating Vessel's descending branch goes to the arch and sole of the foot and then the big toe. For this reason, SP-4 can treat pain, coldness and numbness of the feet and problems of the big toe.

The Chinese name of this point is usually translated as 'grandfather grandson', which is what the two

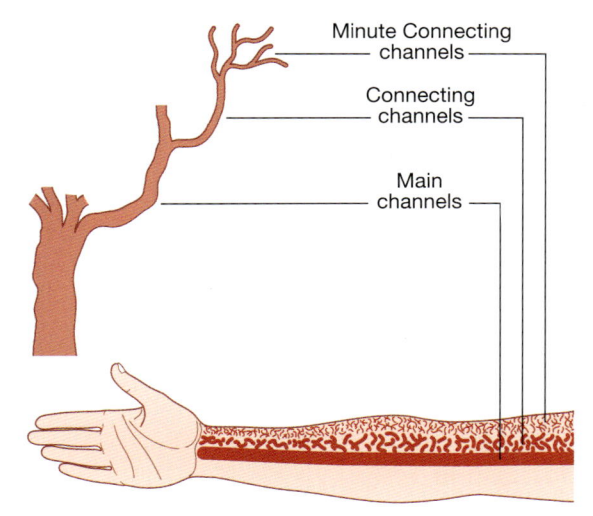

Figure 57.3 Minute Connecting channels

characters can mean, but they can also have the entirely different meaning of 'general Minute Connecting channels'. In fact, the character '*gong*' means 'general' and '*sun*' can mean 'second growth of plants' and is the same character as that indicating the Minute Connecting channels. Therefore the second growth of plants would be an evocative image for the Minute Connecting channels: in fact, they 'sprout' from the Connecting channels like the second growth of plants.

The Minute Connecting channels are capillary-like channels distributed superficially throughout the body and they are branches of the Connecting channels themselves (Fig. 57.3). This name would be quite plausible as the Penetrating Vessel (of which this point is the opening point) controls the network of Minute Connecting channels all over the body. In addition, the Spleen itself controls these secondary channels through its point SP-21 Dabao.

The book 'An Explanation of the Acupuncture Points' has an unusual interpretation of this point's name. It says that SP-1 pertains to Wood, SP-2 to Fire and SP-3 to Earth. Wood generates Fire, which generates Earth: this can be compared to three generations of grandparent, parent, son or daughter, in which SP-1 would be a grandparent, SP-2 a parent and SP-3 a son/daughter; therefore SP-4 would be the grandchild.[2] However, following this logic, all fourth points along a Yin channel could be called the 'grandchild' and the text fails to explain why only the Spleen channel's fourth point takes that name!

Finally, Gong Sun was also the name of the Yellow Emperor so that this point's name could also be translated as 'Yellow Emperor'. This could be a reference to the position of the Penetrating Vessel as the central, most important of the Eight Extraordinary Vessels, for which reason it was compared to the father within a family.

Box 57.5 summarizes the functions of SP-4.

Box 57.5 SP-4 – summary of functions

- Important point for Excess patterns of the Middle Burner. Fullness and pain
- Important point to regulate the Intestines, for Excess patterns. Fullness and pain
- Opening point of the Penetrating Vessel
- Calms the Mind and opens the Mind's orifices (anxiety, mental restlessness, chest pain and tightness)
- Stops bleeding, especially from Intestines and Uterus
- Regulates menstruation, especially painful periods
- Benefits feet and toes (cold feet, numbness of feet, pain in foot, fungal infection of big toe)

SP-5 SHANGQIU *METAL MOUND*

Location

On the depression below and in front of the medial malleolus, midpoint between the tuberosity of the navicular bone and the tip of the medial malleolus.

Nature

River (*Jing*) point.
Metal point.
Sedation point.

Actions

Strengthens the Spleen.
Regulates the Intestines.
Resolves Dampness.
Benefits sinews and joints.
Calms the Mind and opens the Mind's orifices.

Indications

Spleen deficiency, tiredness, lassitude, somnolence, lethargy, desire to lie down.

Abdominal distension, borborygmi, diarrhoea, undigested food in stools, constipation.
Pain and contraction of sinews, ankle pain, pain in the inner thigh, Bone Painful Obstruction Syndrome (*Bi* Syndrome), feeling of heaviness of the body with painful joints.
Manic depression, agitation, excessive pensiveness, inappropriate laughter, nightmares, melancholy.

Comments

SP-5 is an important point for sinews and joints. Being the River point, it is the point where the Qi of the channel is diverted to bones and joints. This point is in fact very much used for chronic Painful Obstruction Syndrome from Dampness, especially of the knee or ankle. In fact, it can also be used as a general River point for every channel's Painful Obstruction Syndrome from Dampness.

I have translated this point's name as '*metal mound*' instead of the usual '*merchant mound*', as the first character, in this context, can mean 'metal', in a Five-Element sense (in the same way as LU-11 Shaoshang and L.I.-1 Shangyang).[3]

Box 57.6 summarizes the functions of SP-5.

Box 57.6 SP-5 – summary of functions

- Important point to affect all sinews and joints in Painful Obstruction Syndrome (*Bi* Syndrome)
- Strengthens the Spleen in Spleen deficiency (tiredness, lassitude, desire to lie down)
- Regulates the Intestines
- Calms the Mind and opens the Mind's orifices

SP-6 SANYINJIAO *THREE YIN MEETING*

Location

On the medial side of the lower leg, 3 *cun* superior to the prominence of the medial malleolus, in a depression close to the medial crest of the tibia.

Nature

Meeting point of three Yin of the leg.

Actions

Strengthens the Spleen.
Resolves Dampness.
Promotes the function of the Liver and the smooth flow of Liver-Qi.
Tonifies the Kidneys.
Nourishes Blood and Yin.
Benefits urination.
Regulates the uterus and menstruation.
Moves Blood and eliminates stasis.
Cools Blood.
Stops pain.
Calms the Mind.

Indications

Spleen and Stomach deficiency.
Feeling of heaviness, oedema, abdominal fullness.
Abdominal distension, cold abdomen, umbilical pain.
Dizziness, blurred vision, tinnitus.
Irregular menstruation, infertility, excessive uterine bleeding, painful periods.
Abdominal masses, painful periods, retention of lochia, retention of dead fetus.
Difficult urination, enuresis, turbid urine.
Seminal emissions, impotence, sexual hyperactivity, pain in penis, contracted testicles.
Palpitations, insomnia, Gall Bladder deficiency timidity.

Comments

This is one of the most important points of all, with a very wide range of action.

First of all, it tonifies the Spleen and can be used in all Spleen deficiency patterns, with poor appetite, loose stools and tiredness. In particular, combined with ST-36 Zusanli, it strongly tonifies the Middle Burner Qi and is extremely effective in tonifying Qi and Blood to relieve chronic tiredness.

Besides tonifying Qi, SP-6 is one of the main points to resolve Dampness, whether it is associated with Cold or Heat, particularly in the Lower Burner. In this context it is a major point to use in all Lower Burner patterns caused by Damp-Cold or Damp-Heat, with symptoms of vaginal discharge, mucus in the stools, cloudy urine and itchiness of the scrotum or vagina.

SP-6 also has a specific action on the urinary function in connection with obstruction of Dampness in the Lower Burner. It is therefore indicated in urinary symptoms caused by Dampness in the Lower Burner, such as difficult urination, painful urination with cloudy urine or retention of urine. This point has a marvellous action in 'smoothing out' obstructions and relieving pain.

SP-6 is the crossing point of the Spleen, Liver and Kidney channels, and it therefore has an action on those two channels also. In particular, it can be used to promote the smooth flow of Liver-Qi when this is stagnant, particularly in the Lower Burner, with such symptoms as abdominal pain and distension, constipation with small bitty stools and painful periods.

Being the crossing point of the Spleen, Liver and Kidney channels also means that it can be used to nourish Yin and, indeed, this is a very important action of this point.

From the emotional point of view, it helps to smooth Liver-Qi to calm the Mind and allay irritability.

Being the meeting point of the Kidney channel, as well, it tonifies the Kidneys, in particular Kidney-Yin, and is therefore used in cases of dizziness, tinnitus, night sweating, feeling of heat, dry mouth and other Kidney-Yin deficiency symptoms.

SP-6 has a deep influence on Blood. First of all, it can nourish Blood and Yin, and is very frequently used in both Blood or Yin deficiency, often combined with ST-36 Zusanli.

It can also eliminate stasis of Blood, especially in relation to the Uterus, and is therefore used to move Blood in the Lower Burner, for such symptoms as dysmenorrhoea with clotted blood or bleeding in the stools with dark blood.

It can also cool Blood and is therefore used in cases of Blood-Heat, either in the context of exterior Heat diseases at the Blood stage, or simply in chronic cases of Blood-Heat, such as in certain types of skin diseases.

It stops bleeding both by tonifying the Spleen and by cooling and invigorating Blood: it is especially effective for bleeding from the bowel or Uterus.

SP-6 also has the function of stopping pain, particularly in the lower abdomen, and it can be used to stop lower abdominal pain, whatever its cause. This function in stopping pain is obviously related to its action in smoothing out Liver-Qi, eliminating Dampness and tonifying the Spleen, all of which would help to regulate Qi in the lower abdomen.

SP-6 is a major point to use in any gynaecological complaint, as it regulates the Uterus and menstruation, stops pain and resolves Dampness from the genital system. It is used to regulate the period if the cycle is irregular, for leukorrhoea, menorrhagia and dysmenorrhoea. It is an essential point to use in many gynaecological conditions.

Finally, SP-6 has a strong calming action on the Mind, and is often used for insomnia, particularly if from Blood or Yin deficiency. In particular, it is used for Spleen- and Heart-Blood deficiency, when the Spleen is not making enough Blood, the Heart is not supplied with enough Blood and the Mind lacks residence and floats at night, so that insomnia ensues. SP-6 is the point to use in this case as it will simultaneously tonify the Spleen, nourish Blood and calm the Mind.

Box 57.7 summarizes the functions of SP-6.

Box 57.7 SP-6 – summary of functions

- Major point to tonify the Spleen in Spleen deficiency (with ST-36 Zusanli)
- Very important to resolve Dampness in the Lower Burner (gynaecological and urinary problems)
- Moves Liver-Qi and pacifies the Liver
- Lower abdominal pain
- Nourishes Yin
- Nourishes Blood (with ST-36 Zusanli and LIV-8 Ququan)
- Invigorates Blood and eliminates stasis
- Stops bleeding
- Cools Blood in febrile diseases or chronic Blood-Heat (skin diseases)
- Major point for many gynaecological problems
- Calms the Mind

SP-8 DIJI *EARTH PIVOT*

Location

On the medial side of the lower leg, 3 *cun* inferior to SP-9 Yinlingquan, in a depression just posterior to the medial crest of the tibia.

Nature

Accumulation (*Xi*) point.

Actions

Harmonizes the Spleen and resolves Dampness.
Regulates Qi and Blood.
Regulates the Uterus.

Removes obstructions from the channel.
Stops pain.
Stops bleeding.

Indications

Abdominal distension and pain, poor appetite.
Irregular menstruation, painful periods, abdominal masses in women (*Zheng Jia*).
Excessive menstrual bleeding, blood in the stools.

Comments

Like all Accumulation points, SP-8 removes obstructions and stops pain, particularly in acute, Excess patterns. It is very much used in acute cases of dysmenorrhoea to stop pain. It is also used as part of a treatment strategy for chronic dysmenorrhoea, when this point would be used just before the period to move Qi and invigorate Blood (usually with reducing method), and other points would be used (usually with reinforcing method) to treat the root of the condition.

SP-8 regulates the Uterus and stops pain by invigorating Blood (i.e. removing stasis of Blood). Like all Accumulation points, this point can also stop acute bleeding and it is used to stop excessive menstrual bleeding and bleeding from the bowel.

I have translated the character *ji* in the point's name as 'pivot'. It should be pointed out that this *ji* is the same as in *Qi Ji* which means 'Qi Mechanism' (see ch. 4). Therefore the name of this point could also be translated as 'Earth Mechanism', which would imply that this point regulates the Qi Mechanism: that is, it harmonizes the ascending/descending and entering/exiting of Qi.

Box 57.8 summarizes the functions of SP-8.

Box 57.8 SP-8 – summary of functions

- As Accumulation point, it treats acute pain
- Frequently used to stop menstrual pain
- Stops excessive menstrual bleeding

SP-9 YINLINGQUAN *YIN MOUND SPRING*

Location

On the medial side of the lower leg, in a depression in the angle formed by the medial condyle of the tibia and the posterior border of the tibia.

Nature

Sea (*He*) point.
Water point.

Actions

Regulates the Spleen.
Resolves Dampness.
Opens the Water passages.
Benefits the Lower Burner.
Benefits urination.

Indications

Abdominal distension and pain, poor appetite, diarrhoea.
Oedema, swelling of legs.
Difficult urination, retention of urine, enuresis, painful urination.
Swelling of knees, Painful Obstruction Syndrome (*Bi* Syndrome) of legs.

Comments

SP-9 is a major point to resolve Dampness from the Lower Burner. It is very much used in all conditions caused by obstruction of Dampness in the Lower Burner, whether it is Damp-Cold or Damp-Heat. It is therefore used for such symptoms as difficult urination, retention of urine, painful urination, cloudy urine, vaginal discharge, diarrhoea with foul-smelling stools, mucus in the stools and oedema of the legs or abdomen. In all these cases the point should be reduced to eliminate Dampness.

SP-9 is also much used for Painful Obstruction Syndrome of the knee, particularly if from Dampness (in which case the knee is swollen), as it removes obstructions and resolves Dampness.

Box 57.9 summarizes the functions of SP-9.

Box 57.9 SP-9 – summary of functions

- Major point to resolve Dampness in the Lower Burner
- Resolves oedema in the Lower Burner
- Resolves Dampness in urinary problems
- Painful Obstruction Syndrome (*Bi* Syndrome) of the knee with swelling

SP-10 XUEHAI *SEA OF BLOOD*

Location

2 *cun* proximal to the superior border of the patella, in the depression on the bulge of the vastus medialis muscle, directly above SP-9 Yinlingquan (Fig. 57.4).

Nature

None.

Actions

Cools Blood.
Invigorates Blood and eliminates stasis.
Stops bleeding.
Regulates menstruation.
Nourishes Blood.
Subdues rebellious Qi.

Indications

Urticaria, eczema, erysipelas, herpes zoster, hot sores, ulcers and itching of scrotum, itching of genitals.
Irregular menstruation, painful periods, amenorrhoea, uterine bleeding, sudden uterine bleeding after childbirth.

Comments

SP-10 is traditionally the subject of controversy with regard to its action on Blood: some are adamant that it only invigorates Blood, others that it cools Blood, yet others that it can nourish Blood. The fact is that this point can do all of those things.

It certainly cools Blood but especially in relation to the skin as its indications show: urticaria and skin rashes. It is also obvious from the indications that it can stop uterine bleeding and also invigorate Blood in the Uterus (painful periods). However, does it stop uterine bleeding by cooling Blood or by tonifying the Spleen's function of holding blood in the vessels? Again, the answer is 'both'.

Needled with reinforcing method, it can also nourish the Blood, but it is not frequently used in this way, as SP-6 would be better.

Perhaps the best source to understand the functions of SP-10 is the text 'An Explanation of the Acupuncture Points' (1654).[4] This books says that SP-10 can be used for uterine bleeding of the *lou* type (i.e. trickling of blood) or of the *beng* type (i.e. flooding) due to irregular diet, overwork, or Qi deficiency: in such cases, seven moxa cones should be applied to this point. This clearly shows that SP-10 can be used to stop bleeding.

The same book also interestingly says that SP-10 can be used for Qi that rebels upwards due to a Blood deficiency causing abdominal distension. The book says: *'When Blood is empty, Qi rebels upwards causing abdominal distension: use this point with reducing method to subdue rebellious Qi and with reinforcing method to nourish Blood.'*[5] This passage clearly shows that SP-10 can be used to nourish Blood.

The 'Great Dictionary of Chinese Acupuncture' lists the following indications for SP-10: irregular menstruation, painful periods, amenorrhoea, menorrhagia,

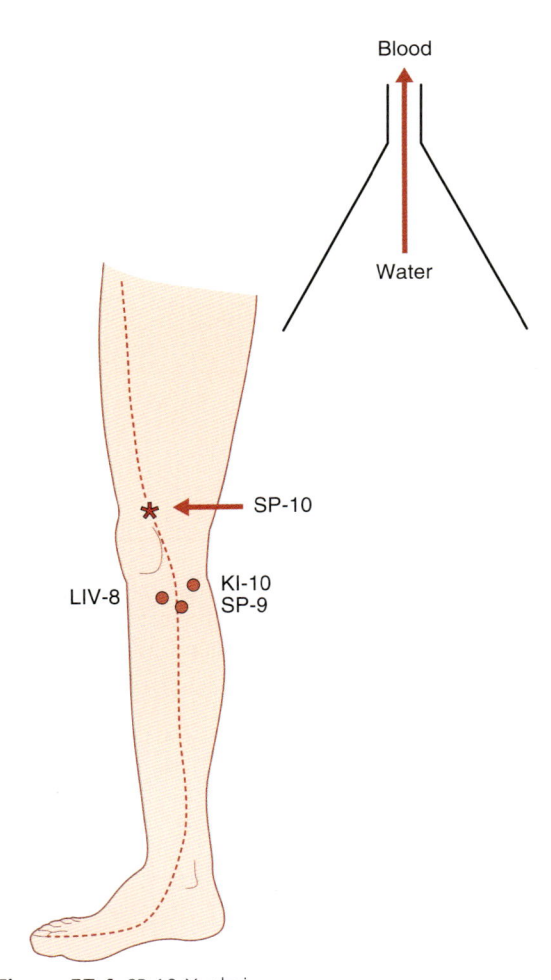

Figure 57.4 SP-10 Xuehai

skin eruptions, itching, Painful Urination Syndrome (*Lin*), Qi rebelling in abdomen. The dictionary says that this point invigorates Blood of the Spleen and treats abdominal distension.[6]

SP-10 pertains to the Spleen channel: the Spleen is the Postnatal source of Blood and gathers Blood (i.e. holds Blood in the vessels). The Heart governs Blood, the Liver stores Blood and the Kidneys play a role in making Blood.

The points KI-10 Yingu, LIV-8 Ququan and SP-9 Yinlingquan (all Water points) create like a tide of Yin, which then passes through the Blood Connecting channels at the point SP-10. Thus, SP-10 is like an Accumulation (*Xi*) point of Blood (another name for SP-10 is *Xuexi*, i.e. 'Blood Accumulation point') that holds Blood and stops bleeding by making Blood return to the channels.

In conclusion, SP-10 has a wide-ranging action on Blood as it can nourish Blood (with reinforcing method or moxa), hold Blood (in bleeding, reinforcing method), regulate Blood, cool Blood and invigorate Blood (the last three with reducing method). Hence SP-10 affects the channels of Spleen, Liver and Kidneys.

Box 57.10 summarizes the functions of SP-10.

Box 57.10   SP-10 – summary of functions

- Nourishes Blood
- Cools Blood in skin diseases
- Invigorates Blood in the Uterus
- Stops bleeding

SP-12 CHONGMEN PENETRATING DOOR

Location

On the lateral side of the femoral artery, 3.5. *cun* lateral to Ren-2 Qugu.

Nature

Meeting point of Spleen and Liver.
Point of the Yin Linking Vessel (*Yin Wei Mai*).

Actions

Moves Qi and invigorates Blood.
Subdues rebellious Qi of the Penetrating Vessel.
Resolves Dampness and benefits urination.

Indications

Abdominal fullness and pain, abdominal masses (*Ji Ju*), haemorrhoids, fetus Qi rushes upwards to harass the Heart, difficult lactation.
Difficult urination, retention of urine, painful urination, excessive vaginal discharge.

Comments

SP-12 moves Qi and invigorates Blood. This action and the above indications related to it, are related to this point's connection with the Penetrating Vessel. In fact, the character *chong* in the point's name is the same as in *Chong Mai*, Penetrating Vessel. For example, the symptom of fetus Qi rushing upwards to harass the Heart is a symptom of rebellious Qi of the Penetrating Vessel.

SP-12 is also useful as a local point for Painful Obstruction Syndrome (*Bi* Syndrome) of the hip, when the pain extends to the groin.

Box 57.11 summarizes the functions of SP-12.

Box 57.11   SP-12 – summary of functions

- Moves Qi and invigorates Blood
- Subdues rebellious Qi of the Penetrating Vessel
- Resolves Dampness in the Bladder

SP-15 DAHENG BIG HORIZONTAL STROKE

Location

On the abdomen, level with the umbilicus, on the lateral border of the rectus abdominis muscle.

Nature

Point of Yin Linking Vessel (*Yin Wei Mai*).

Actions

Strengthens the Spleen.
Strengthens the limbs.
Regulates Qi.

Resolves Dampness.
Benefits the Large Intestine.

Indications

Sighing, sadness, tiredness, poor appetite.
Inability to raise and move the four limbs, weakness of the limbs.
Abdominal pain, cold lower abdomen.
Chronic diarrhoea with mucus in stools.
Constipation.

Comments

This is quite an important point for abdominal complaints. First of all, it strengthens the function of the Spleen and promotes the Spleen transformation and transportation, especially in relation to bowel movements. This point is therefore often used in chronic constipation of the deficiency type: that is, when Spleen-Qi is deficient and fails to promote the function of the Large Intestine in moving the stools.

By strengthening the Spleen, it particularly strengthens the limbs as it stimulates the Spleen to transport food essences to the limbs. It can be used for cold and weak limbs.

This point can also resolve Dampness in the Intestines and is therefore used in chronic diarrhoea with mucus in the stools.

SP-15 also regulates Qi in the abdomen and promotes its smooth flow of Liver-Qi, so that it can be used to stop abdominal pain from stagnation of Liver-Qi.

This point's name requires an explanation: '*heng*' means '*horizontal*', but it is also the horizontal stroke in Chinese writing. The 'stroke' in this case is the line drawn across the umbilicus encompassing Ren-8 Shenque, KI-16 Huangshu, ST-25 Tianshu and SP-15 Daheng.

Box 57.12 summarizes the functions of SP-15.

Box 57.12 SP-15 – summary of functions

- Regulates Qi in the abdomen (abdominal pain)
- Strengthens the Spleen (tiredness, sadness)
- Benefits the limbs (weak limbs)
- Resolves Dampness (mucus in stools)
- Benefits the Large Intestine (constipation of the Deficient type)

SP-21 DABAO *GENERAL CONTROL*

Location

On the midaxillary line, in the seventh intercostal space.

Nature

Connecting point of the Great Connecting channel of the Spleen.

Actions

Invigorates Blood in the Blood Connecting channels.
Benefits the sinews.
Regulates Qi in the chest.

Indications

Pain in the whole body.
Weak limbs, flaccidity of limbs, weak joints.
Cough, breathlessness, chest pain, pain in the ribs, hypochondrial distension.

Comments

SP-21 controls all the Blood Connecting channels throughout the body. It is used in generalized pains due to stasis of Blood in the Connecting channels, the main symptoms being muscular pain moving throughout the body.

SP-21 is the point of departure of the Great Connecting channel of the Spleen, which, from this point, disperses in the chest and ribs.

This point's name is translated as 'general control', as the word '*bao*' (which normally would mean 'envelop') here has the meaning of 'controlling', 'taking upon oneself'. The name therefore refers to the general controlling action of this point on all the Blood Connecting channels.[7]

Box 57.13 summarizes the functions of SP-21.

Figure 57.5 illustrates the target areas of points of the Spleen channel.

Box 57.13 SP-21 – summary of functions

- Invigorates Blood in all Blood Connecting channels (pain in the whole body)
- Benefits the sinews
- Regulates Qi in the chest

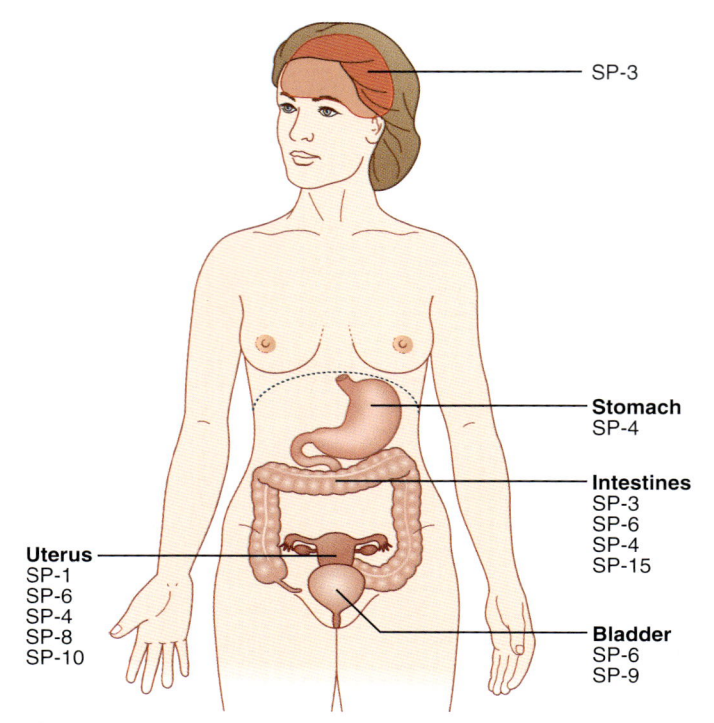

Figure 57.5 Target areas of Spleen channel points

Labels on figure:
- SP-3 (head)
- Stomach: SP-4
- Intestines: SP-3, SP-6, SP-4, SP-15
- Uterus: SP-1, SP-6, SP-4, SP-8, SP-10
- Bladder: SP-6, SP-9

END NOTES

1. 1979 The Yellow Emperor's Classic of Internal Medicine – Simple Questions (*Huang Di Nei Jing Su Wen* 黄帝内经素问), People's Health Publishing House, Beijing, first published c.100 BC, p. 23.
2. Yue Han Zhen 1990 An Explanation of the Acupuncture Points (*Jing Xue Jie* 经穴解), People's Health Publishing House, Beijing, originally published in 1654, p. 117.
3. Zhang Sheng Xing 1984 A Compilation of Explanations of the Meaning of the Acupuncture Points Names (*Jing Xue Shi Yi Hui Jie* 经穴释义汇解), Shanghai Science Publishing House, Shanghai, p. 89–90.
4. An Explanation of the Acupuncture Points, p. 125.
5. Ibid., p. 125.
6. Cheng Bao Shu 1988 Great Dictionary of Acupucture (*Zhen Jiu Da Ci Dian* 针灸大辞典), Beijing Science Publishing House, Beijing, p. 314.
7. A Compilation of Explanations of the Meaning of the Acupuncture Points Names, p. 102.

SECTION 2 | PART 7

Heart Channel | 58

Main channel pathway

The Heart channel originates from the heart. It then emerges, passes through the diaphragm and connects with the small intestine. A branch from the heart ascends to the throat and eye.

Another branch from the heart enters the lung and emerges at the axilla, from where it joins the superficial channel running along the medial aspect of the arm to end at the medial side of the tip of the little finger (Fig. 58.1).

Connecting channel pathway

From HE-5 Tongli, the Connecting channel links with the Small Intestine channel. Another branch follows the main channel, enters the heart and ascends to the tip of the tongue and eye (Fig. 58.2).

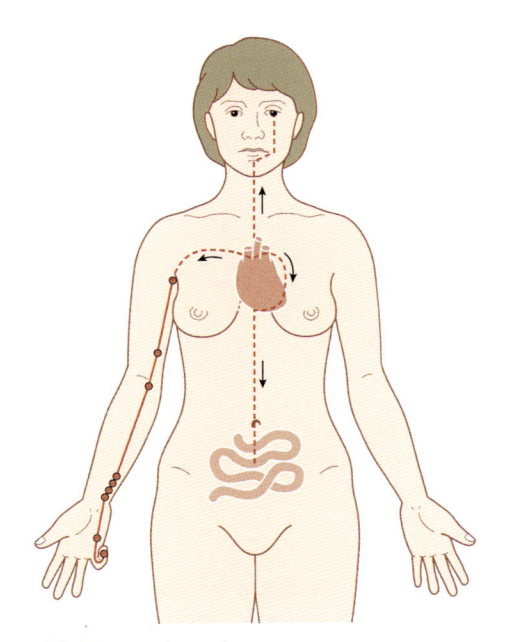

Figure 58.1 Heart channel

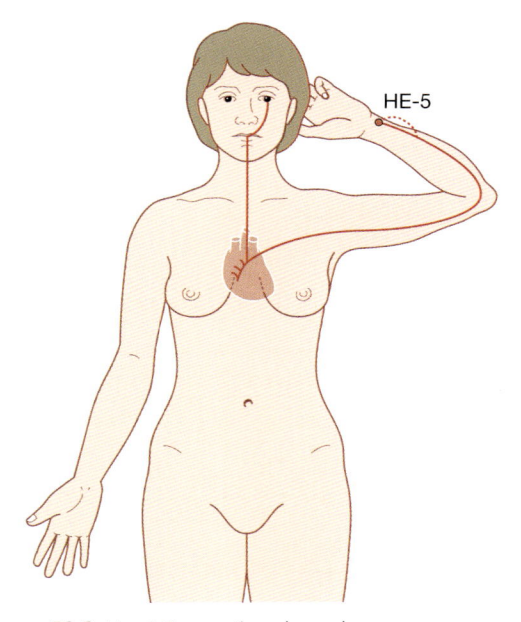

Figure 58.2 Heart Connecting channel

> **Box 58.1 Overview of Heart points**
> - Treat the Mind
> - Affect the inner aspect of arm, chest and eye

Box 58.1 gives an overview of Heart channel points.

HE-1 JIQUAN *SUPREME SPRING*

Location

At the apex of the axillary fossa, where the axillary artery pulsates.

Nature

None.

Actions

Nourishes Heart-Yin and clears Empty-Heat.
Calms the Mind.
Removes obstructions from the channel.

Indications

Heart pain, chest pain, distension and fullness of hypochondrium.
Sadness, anxiety, palpitation.
Thirst, dry throat.
Inability to raise the shoulder, pain in the axilla.

Comments

This point can be used to nourish Heart-Yin and clear Heart Empty-Heat with such symptoms as dry mouth, night sweating, mental restlessness and insomnia.

It is also used in the sequelae of Wind-stroke for paralysis of the arm.

Box 58.2 summarizes the functions of HE-1.

Box 58.2 HE-1 – summary of functions

- Nourishes Heart-Yin and clears Empty-Heat (thirst, dry throat)
- Calms the Mind (sadness, anxiety, palpitation)
- Removes obstructions from the channel (heart pain, chest pain, distension and fullness of hypochondrium, inability to raise the shoulder, pain in the axilla)

HE-3 SHAOHAI *LESSER-YIN SEA*

Location

Midway between P-3 Quze and the medial epicondyle of the humerus, at the medial end of the transverse cubital crease when the elbow is flexed.

Nature

Sea (*He*) point.
Water point.

Actions

Removes obstructions from the channel.
Calms the Mind.
Clears Heat.

Indications

Heart pain, fullness of the chest, pain in the axilla, pain in the elbow.
Manic behaviour, inappropriate laughter, mental restlessness, anxiety.
Red eyes.

Comments

This point is used mostly to drain Heart-Fire or clear Heart Empty-Heat. It has an important calming action on the mental level (by clearing Heart-Fire), and is indicated for anxiety and mental restlessness.

It is also used as a local point to remove obstructions from the Heart channel in Painful Obstruction Syndrome, Atrophy Syndrome or sequelae of Wind-stroke.

I have translated its name as 'Lesser-Yin Sea' instead of 'Lesser Sea', as the '*Shao*' here clearly refers to '*Shao Yin*': that is, Lesser Yin, to which the Heart belongs. It is for this reason that the character '*Shao*' recurs in the points HE-8 Shaofu and HE-9 Shaochong.

Box 58.3 summarizes the functions of HE-3.

Box 58.3 HE-3 – summary of functions

- Removes obstructions from the channel (heart pain, fullness of the chest, pain in the axilla, pain in the elbow)
- Calms the Mind (manic behaviour, inappropriate laughter, mental restlessness, anxiety)
- Clears Heat (red eyes)

HE-4 LINGDAO *SPIRIT PATH*

Location

On the radial side of the tendon of the flexor carpi ulnaris muscle, 1.5 *cun* above the transverse crease of the wrist.

Nature

River (*Jing*) point.
Metal point.

Actions

Calms the Mind.
Subdues rebellious Qi.
Relaxes the sinews.

Indications

Sadness, fear, anxiety, mental restlessness.
Retching, redness and swelling of the eyes.
Contraction of the elbow and arm.

Comments

This point is mostly used in channel problems, also because, as a River point, it has a special action on joints and bones. It is therefore used for spasm and neuralgia of the forearm and Painful Obstruction Syndrome (*Bi* Syndrome) of elbow and wrist, if the obstruction is along the Heart and Small Intestine channels.

As it subdues rebellious Qi, HE-4 can also be used for nausea, as this symptom is often related to ascending of Heart-Qi rather than Stomach-Qi.

Box 58.4 summarizes the functions of HE-4.

Box 58.4 HE-4 – summary of functions

- Calms the Mind (sadness, fear, anxiety, mental restlessness)
- Subdues rebellious Qi (retching, redness and swelling of the eyes)
- Relaxes the sinews (contraction of the elbow and arm)

HE-5 TONGLI *INNER COMMUNICATION*

Location

On the radial side of the tendon of the flexor carpi ulnaris muscle, 1 *cun* above the transverse crease of the wrist.

Nature

Connecting (*Luo*) point.

Actions

Calms the Mind.
Tonifies Heart-Qi.
Benefits the tongue.
Benefits eyes and head.
Regulates the Uterus.
Benefits the Bladder.

Indications

Sadness, mental restlessness, anger, fright, depression, agitation.
Palpitations, weak Heart-Qi.
Loss of voice, aphasia, stuttering, stiff tongue.
Red eyes, eye pain, red face, headache, dizziness.
Excessive menstrual bleeding.
Enuresis.

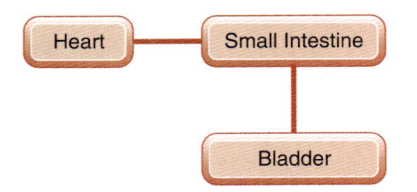

Figure 58.3 Connections between Heart, Small Intestine and Bladder

Comments

HE-5 is one of the main points to tonify Heart-Qi, and, in my experience, is the point of choice out of all the Heart channel points for this purpose. It is indicated in all symptoms of Heart-Qi deficiency and, in particular, it has a marked effect on the tongue, and is the point of choice for aphasia.

Being the Connecting point, HE-5 Tongli connects with the Small Intestine channel; this, in turn, connects with the Bladder channel within the Greater Yang. It is through this route that the Heart channel can influence the Bladder and urination. This connection manifests itself when Heart-Fire is transmitted to the Small Intestine and from this to the Bladder, giving rise to Bladder-Heat (Fig. 58.3).

The main manifestations are thirst, bitter taste, insomnia, tongue ulcers, burning on urination and haematuria. This point is indicated also for enuresis.

As the Connecting channel goes to the eyes, this point is indicated for Heat in the eyes deriving from Heart-Heat. Heart-Qi rises to the head and may cause headache and dizziness for which this point can be used.

The Heart is connected to the Uterus via the Uterus Vessel (*Bao Mai*) and HE-5 is the main point to affect such a vessel in such problems as excessive uterine bleeding (Fig. 58.4).

Box 58.5 summarizes the functions of HE-5.

Box 58.5 HE-5 – summary of functions

- Calms the Mind (sadness, mental restlessness, anger, fright, depression, agitation)
- Tonifies Heart-Qi (palpitations, weak Heart-Qi)
- Benefits the tongue (loss of voice, aphasia, stuttering, stiff tongue)
- Benefits eyes and head (red eyes, eye pain, red face, headache, dizziness)
- Regulates the Uterus (excessive menstrual bleeding)
- Benefits the Bladder (enuresis)

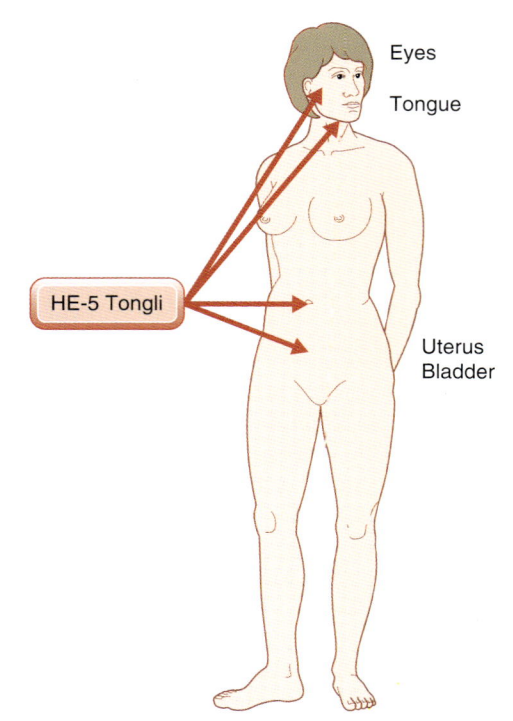

Figure 58.4 Target areas of HE-5 Tongli

HE-6 YINXI *YIN CREVICE*

Location

On the radial side of the tendon of the flexor carpi ulnaris muscle, 0.5 *cun* above the transverse crease of the wrist.

Nature

Accumulation (*Xi*) point.

Actions

Invigorates Heart-Blood.
Subdues rebellious Qi.
Nourishes Heart-Yin and clears Empty-Heat of the Heart.
Stops sweating.
Calms the Mind.

Indications

Heart pain, stabbing pain in the chest, fullness of the chest, palpitations.
Nosebleed, vomiting of blood.
Night sweating, 'steaming bones' (night sweating from Yin deficiency).

Comments

This point is frequently used to nourish Heart-Yin with symptoms of night sweating, dry mouth, insomnia, etc. In particular, in combination with KI-7 Fuliu, it is the point of choice to stop night sweating from Heart-Yin deficiency.

It also clears Heart Empty-Heat and is therefore useful for mental restlessness and a feeling of heat deriving from Empty-Heat.

As an Accumulation point, it strongly moves Qi and Blood in the channel and it can be used for Blood stasis in the chest causing a stabbing chest pain.

HE-6 also subdues rebellious Qi and it stops bleeding upwards (caused by rebellious Qi) such as from the nose or in vomit.

Box 58.6 summarizes the functions of HE-6.

Box 58.6 HE-6 – summary of functions

- Invigorates Heart-Blood (heart pain, stabbing pain in the chest, fullness of the chest, palpitations)
- Subdues rebellious Qi (nosebleed, vomiting of blood)
- Nourishes Heart-Yin and clears Empty-Heat of the Heart (night sweating, 'steaming bones')
- Stops sweating
- Calms the Mind

HE-7 SHENMEN *MIND DOOR*

Location

On the wrist, at the ulnar end of the transverse crease of the wrist, in the depression at the proximal border of the pisiform bone.

Nature

Source (*Yuan*) and Stream (*Shu*) point.
Drainage point.

Actions

Calms the Mind and opens the Mind's orifices.
Nourishes Heart-Blood.

Indications

Insomnia, poor memory, manic depression, inappropriate laughter, shouting at people, sadness, fear, mental restlessness, agitation, palpitations.

Comments

This is the most important point on the Heart channel and one of the major points of the body. It can be used in virtually any Heart pattern in order to calm the Mind, which is its main action. However, it primarily nourishes Heart-Blood and is the point of choice for Heart-Blood deficiency causing the Mind to be deprived of its 'residence', resulting in anxiety, insomnia, poor memory, palpitations and a Pale tongue.

In my experience, it is a 'gentle' point and therefore not the choice point in Excess patterns of the Heart, characterized by Heart-Fire or Heart Phlegm-Fire, for which other points would be better indicated (such as P-5 Jianshi, or HE-8 Shaofu). It is, however, the best point to calm the Mind when there is anxiety, and worrying under stressful situations.

As the Heart is the residence for the Mind, which in Chinese medicine includes mental activity, thinking, memory and consciousness, this point has an effect not only on emotional problems such as anxiety but also on memory and mental capacity. In fact, this point can be used for mental retardation in children.[1]

The Heart is connected to the Kidneys within the Lesser Yin and, in my experience, Heart points have an effect on some Kidney functions and especially the menstrual function in women and the urinary and sexual functions in both men and women. With regard to menstruation, HE-7 nourishes Heart-Blood and this influences the Uterus (via the Uterus Vessel, *Bao Mai*) in a similar way to Liver-Blood. In my experience, HE-7 can be used to nourish Blood in menstrual problems such as amenorrhoea or scanty periods.

Due to the connection between Heart and Kidneys, HE-7 can be used in my experience for impotence in men and lack of sexual desire in women.

The Heart channel also has an anti-itching effect and I find HE-7 and HE-8 the two best points to achieve this effect. Therefore, HE-7 is very useful in skin diseases such as eczema to stop itching.

In my experience, HE-7 has also an antispasmodic effect and I use it frequently for this purpose in chronic backache from a Kidney deficiency, especially in men when there is a pronounced stiffness of the back. A very effective combination is that of S.I.-3 on the left and BL-62 on the right to open the Governing Vessel (*Du Mai*), HE-7 on the right and KI-4 Dazhong on the left (Fig. 58.5). After retaining these points, I then use

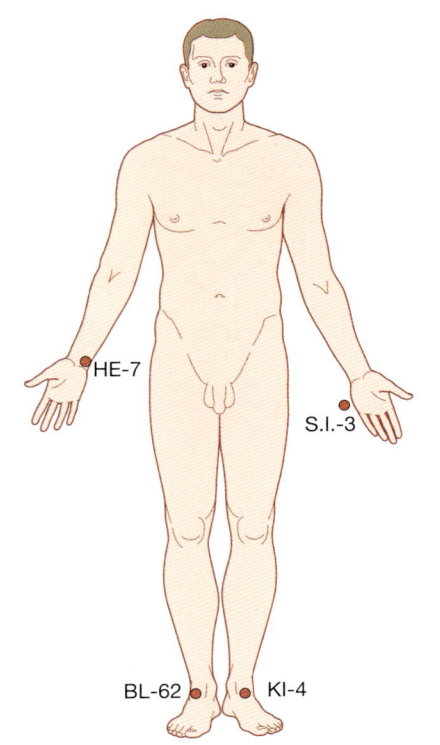

Figure 58.5 Governing Vessel and Heart point combination for backache

BL-23 Shenshu, BL-26 Guanyuanshu and the extra point Shiqizhuixia (below the tip of the fifth lumbar vertebra).

With regard to the antispasmodic effect of HE-7, I find this point also very useful to treat tremors of the arm, as in Parkinson's disease.

HE-7 is a good point to use in the syndrome of Gall Bladder Qi deficiency manifesting with timidity, fearfulness, indecision and depression: for this syndrome I use HE-7 with G.B.-40 Qiuxu (Fig. 58.6).

Interestingly, the ancient classics do not always stress the use of this point for emotional or mental problems. For example, the 'ABC of Acupuncture' (AD 282) by Huang Fu Mi says only that this point is used for cold hands, vomiting of blood and rebellious Qi.[2] The 'Thousand Ducat Prescriptions' (AD 652) by Sun Si Miao says that this point can be used for contraction of the arm.[3]

A comparison between the functions of HE-7 and P-7 Daling is given under the latter point in chapter 62.

Box 58.7 summarizes the functions of HE-7.

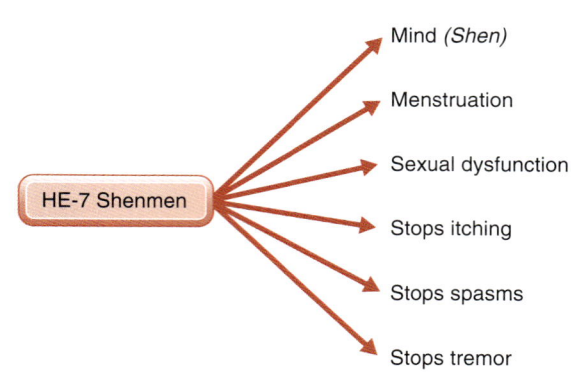

Figure 58.6 Therapeutic range of HE-7 Shenmen

HE-7 Shenmen → Mind (Shen), Menstruation, Sexual dysfunction, Stops itching, Stops spasms, Stops tremor

---

Box 58.7 HE-7 – summary of functions

- Calms the Mind and opens the Mind's orifices (insomnia, poor memory, manic depression, inappropriate laughter, shouting at people, sadness, fear, mental restlessness, agitation, palpitations)
- Most important point to nourish Heart-Blood
- Can treat impotence in men and lack of libido in women
- Stops itching in skin diseases
- Has an antispasmodic effect, good for backache in men and good for tremors of the arm (Parkinson's disease)
- With G.B.-40, strengthens the Mind and promotes decisiveness

---

HE-8 SHAOFU *LESSER-YIN MANSION*

Location

On the palm, between the fourth and fifth metacarpal bones where the tip of the little finger rests when a fist is made.

Nature

Spring (*Ying*) point.
Fire point.

Actions

Clears Heart-Fire, Heart Empty-Heat and Heart Phlegm-Fire.
Calms the Mind.
Benefits the Bladder.
Regulates the Uterus and lifts sinking Qi.

Indications

Palpitations, sadness, worry, chest pain, agitation, mental restlessness.
Itching of genitals, difficult urination, enuresis.
Prolapse of uterus.

Comments

HE-8 Shaofu is a stronger point than HE-7 Shenmen. Its main action is to clear Heat in the Heart, whether it is Full-Heat, Empty-Heat or Heat with Phlegm. Its main range of action is therefore in Excess patterns of the Heart. The main symptoms would be insomnia with restless dreams, thirst, bitter taste, mental restlessness or hypomania, dark urine, tongue ulcers, and a Red tongue with redder tip and yellow coating.

HE-8 also calms the Mind, but mostly in the context of Excess patterns with Heat in the Heart.

HE-8 influences the Bladder via the Small Intestine to which the Bladder is connected within the Greater Yang. For this reason, it affects urination and can be used for difficult urination and enuresis.

As the Heart is connected to the Kidneys via the Lesser Yin, the Heart channel may influence the Kidney channel in the genital area and, for this reason, this point can treat itching of the genitals from Heat. The 'Explanation of the Acupuncture Points' says that HE-8 is reduced to drain Fire in urinary problems.[4]

As the Heart is connected to the Uterus through the Uterus Vessel (*Bao Mai*), HE-8 can be used to lift sinking Qi causing prolapse of the uterus. The text 'An Explanation of the Acupuncture Points' says that, in order to lift sinking Qi in prolapse of the uterus, this point should be reinforced.[5]

Box 58.8 summarizes the functions of HE-8.

Box 58.8 HE-8 – summary of functions

- Clears Heart-Fire, Heart Empty-Heat and Heart Phlegm-Fire
- Calms the Mind (palpitations, sadness, worry, chest pain, agitation, mental restlessness)
- Benefits the Bladder (difficult urination, enuresis)
- Regulates the Uterus and lifts sinking Qi (prolapse of uterus)

HE-9 SHAOCHONG *LESSER-YIN PENETRATING*

Location

At the medial corner of the nail of the little finger.

Nature

Well (*Jing*) point.
Wood point.
Tonification point.

Actions

Clears Heat.
Calms the Mind.
Opens the Mind's orifices.
Extinguishes Wind.
Promotes resuscitation.
Benefits the tongue and eyes.

Indications

Palpitations, heart pain, thirst, feeling of heat.
Loss of consciousness from Wind-stroke.
Manic depression, fright, sadness, agitation, mental restlessness.
Pain at the root of the tongue, swollen tongue, eye pain, red eyes.

Comments

HE-9 Shaochong is mostly used in Excess patterns with Heat in the Heart. It is similar in action to HE-8 Shaofu in so far as it clears Heat, but, like all Well points, it also extinguishes internal Wind and can therefore be used for Wind-stroke. In this context, it is used to restore consciousness as it opens the Mind's orifices when these are obstructed by internal Wind.

In accordance with the general action of Well points indicated in the 'Classic of Difficulties', this point relieves a feeling of fullness in the heart region.

Box 58.9 summarizes the functions of HE-9.

As all Heart channel points 'calm the Mind', the differences between the various points are illustrated in tabular form (Table 58.1).

Fig. 58.7 illustrates the target area of the Heart channel points.

Box 58.9 HE-9 – summary of functions

- Clears Heat
- Calms the Mind (palpitations, heart pain, thirst, feeling of heat)
- Opens the Mind's orifices (manic depression, fright, sadness, agitation, mental restlessness)
- Extinguishes Wind (loss of consciousness from Wind-stroke)
- Promotes resuscitation
- Benefits the tongue and eyes (pain at the root of the tongue, swollen tongue, eye pain, red eyes)

Table 58.1 Comparison of Heart channel points

Point	Action	Action on Mind
HE-3	Clears Full-Heat	For severe mental symptoms such as hypomania and severe depression
HE-5	Tonifies Heart-Qi	To lift the Mind, in mild depression and sadness
HE-6	Nourishes Heart-Yin	For the typical mental restlessness of Yin deficiency, i.e. vague and indefinable restlessness and anxiety, fidgeting, with feeling of heat in the face
HE-7	Nourishes Heart-Blood	The main point for insomnia and anxiety from Heart-Blood deficiency
HE-8	Drains Heart-Fire	For severe mental disturbances in Excess patterns with Full-Heat, such as hypomania, excessive dreaming and psychosis
HE-9	Clears Heat, extinguishes internal Wind	To open the 'Heart orifices' and restore consciousness, severe anxiety, hypomania

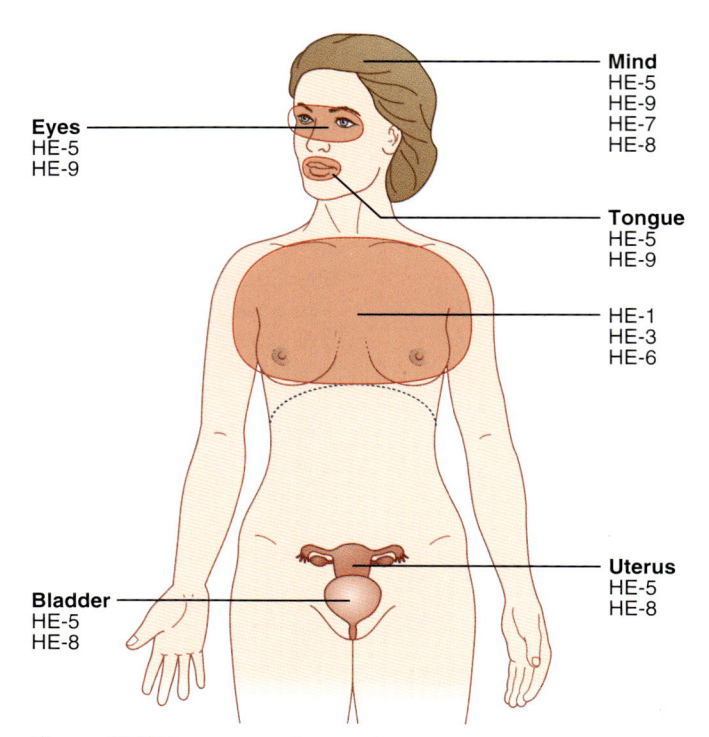

Figure 58.7 Target areas of Heart channel points

Labels on figure:
- **Mind**: HE-5, HE-9, HE-7, HE-8
- **Eyes**: HE-5, HE-9
- **Tongue**: HE-5, HE-9
- HE-1, HE-3, HE-6 (chest)
- **Uterus**: HE-5, HE-8
- **Bladder**: HE-5, HE-8

END NOTES

1. Ji Jie Yin 1984 Clinical Records of Tai Yi Shen Acupuncture (*Tai Yi Shen Zhen Jiu Lin Zheng Lu* 太乙神针灸临证录), Shanxi Province Scientific Publishing House, Shanxi, p. 23.
2. Zhang Shan Chen 1982 Essential Collection of Acupuncture Points from the ABC of Acupuncture (*Zhen Jiu Jia Yi Jing Shu Xue Zhong Ji* 针灸甲乙经腧穴重辑), Shandong Scientific Publishing House, Shandong, first published AD 282, p. 112.
3. Sun Si Miao AD 652 Thousand Ducat Prescriptions, cited in Anwei College of Traditional Chinese Medicine – Shanghai College of Traditional Chinese Medicine 1987 Dictionary of Acupuncture (*Zhen Jiu Xue Ci Dian* 针灸大辞典), Shanghai Scientific Publishing House, Shangai, p. 477.
4. Yue Han Zhen 1990 An Explanation of the Acupuncture Points (*Jing Xue Jie* 经穴解), People's Health Publishing House, Beijing, originally published in 1654, p. 143.
5. Ibid., p. 143.

SECTION 2 PART 7

Small Intestine Channel | 59

Main channel pathway

The Small Intestine channel starts at the ulnar side of the tip of the little finger. Following the ulnar side of the dorsum of the hand, it reaches the wrist and ascends along the posterior aspect of the arm to the shoulder joint. Circling around the scapula, it connects with Du-14 Dazhui and goes forward to the supraclavicular fossa to connect with the heart. From here it descends to the oesophagus and connects with the small intestine.

The superficial pathway of the channel from the supraclavicular fossa ascends to the neck and the cheek to enter the ear. From the cheek, a branch goes to the infraorbital region to link with the Bladder channel at the inner canthus (BL-1 Jingming) (Fig. 59.1).

Connecting channel pathway

From S.I.-7 Zhizheng the Small Intestine Connecting channel links with the Heart channel. Another branch goes up the arm and elbow and joins with the shoulder (Fig. 59.2).

Box 59.1 gives an overview of Small Intestine points.

Box 59.1 Overview of Small Intestine points

- Affect the arm, shoulder and neck
- Expel Wind
- Affect eye and ear

Figure 59.1 Small Intestine channel

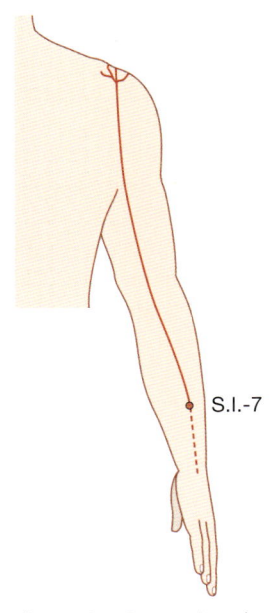

Figure 59.2 Small Intestine Connecting channel

S.I.-1 SHAOZE *LESSER MARSH*

Location
At the lateral corner of the nail of the little finger.

Nature
Well (*Jing*) point.
Metal point.

Actions
Expels Wind-Heat.
Extinguishes Wind and promotes resuscitation.
Removes obstructions from the channel.
Clears Heat.
Subdues rebellious Qi.
Promotes lactation.

Indications
Aversion to cold, fever, febrile disease.
Loss of consciousness from Wind-stroke.
Cold sensation below the heart, feeling of oppression and pain of the chest, pain in the ribs, stiff neck, pain in the back of the shoulder, pain in arm and elbow.
Headache, dizziness, red eyes, nosebleed, deafness, tinnitus, stiff tongue, thirst, mouth ulcers.
Agalactia.

Comments
Like most of the Well points, S.I.-1 is used for Excess patterns to eliminate pathogenic factors. S.I.-1 expels Wind-Heat in exterior attacks, especially when the symptoms affect the head and neck, causing stiff neck and headache. It is also good to treat acute tonsillitis from invasion of exterior Wind-Heat.

It also extinguishes internal Wind and promotes resuscitation in cases of internal Wind and Phlegm blocking the orifices and causing sudden unconsciousness, as in Wind-stroke.

Apart from its role in exterior patterns, it can also be used as a distal point for channel problems of the neck, such as chronic stiff neck or acute torticollis.

Finally, it is an empirical point to promote lactation after childbirth, mostly in Excess patterns: that is, when lactation is inhibited by the presence of some pathogenic factor or stagnation (such as stagnant Liver-Qi).

Box 59.2 summarizes the functions of S.I.-1.

> **Box 59.2 S.I.-1 – summary of functions**
> - Expels Wind-Heat (aversion to cold, fever, febrile disease)
> - Extinguishes Wind and promotes resuscitation (loss of consciousness from Wind-stroke)
> - Removes obstructions from the channel (cold sensation below the heart, feeling of oppression and pain of the chest, pain in the ribs, stiff neck, pain in the back of the shoulder, pain in arm and elbow)
> - Clears Heat (red eyes, nosebleed, thirst, mouth ulcers)
> - Subdues rebellious Qi (headache, dizziness, deafness, tinnitus, stiff tongue)
> - Promotes lactation (agalactia)

S.I.-2 QIANGU *FRONT VALLEY*

Location
On the ulnar border of the little finger just distal to the metacarpophalangeal joint.

Nature
Spring (*Ying*) point.
Water point.

Actions
Expels Wind-Heat.
Benefits eyes, nose and ears.
Removes obstructions from the channel.

Indications
Mumps, aversion to cold, fever, febrile disease, cough.
Blurred vision, eye pain, red eyes, nasal congestion, nosebleed, tinnitus.
Stiff neck and upper back, pain in the scapula, pain in the arm, pain in the wrist, pain in the little finger.

Comments
Like all Spring points, S.I.-2 Qiangu clears Heat, both interior and exterior. It can therefore be used to expel exterior Wind-Heat, especially if it affects neck and eyes, and also to clear interior Heat from the Small Intestine channel, but mostly in acute febrile diseases.

In my experience, owing to its relationship with the Bladder within the Greater Yang, it can also be used to clear Bladder-Heat when this causes burning on urination.

Box 59.3 summarizes the functions of S.I.-2.

> **Box 59.3 S.I.-2 – summary of functions**
>
> - Expels Wind-Heat (mumps, aversion to cold, fever, febrile disease, cough)
> - Benefits eyes, nose and ears (blurred vision, eye pain, red eyes, nasal congestion, nosebleed, tinnitus)
> - Removes obstructions from the channel (stiff neck and upper back, pain in the scapula, pain in the arm, pain in the wrist, pain in the little finger)

S.I.-3 HOUXI *BACK STREAM*

Location

On the ulnar border of the hand, proximal to the head of the fifth metacarpophalangeal joint.

Nature

Stream (*Shu*) point.
Wood point.
Opening point of Governing Vessel (*Du Mai*).
Tonification point.

Actions

Regulates the Governing Vessel and extinguishes interior Wind.
Expels exterior Wind.
Benefits sinews.
Benefits eyes, nose and ears.

Indications

Epilepsy, headache, dizziness, vertigo.
Stiff neck (on occiput), occipital headache, difficulty in turning neck, pain in the upper back and shoulder, lower backache.
Malaria, aversion to cold, fever, febrile disease.
Deafness, tinnitus, blurred vision, redness and pain of the eyes, swelling of eyes, nosebleed.

Comments

S.I.-3 has a wide range of actions. Firstly, it is the opening point of the Governing Vessel (*Du Mai*), and is therefore needled for all symptoms of this extraordinary vessel. Many of its indications relate to the Governing Vessel. In particular, it extinguishes interior Wind from the Governing Vessel. Symptoms and signs of interior Wind in this vessel include convulsions, tremors, epilepsy, stiff neck, giddiness and headache.

S.I.-3 also expels exterior Wind and is widely used in attacks of exterior Wind-Cold or Wind-Heat whenever there are pronounced symptoms affecting neck and head, such as stiff neck, occipital headache, and aches down the spine and back.

This point has also a deep effect on the muscles and sinews along the course of the Governing Vessel, Small Intestine and Bladder channel. It is therefore widely used for any channel problem along these three channels, in particular in the occipital region. It affects the upper more than lower back area along the Small Intestine and Bladder channel although it does have lower backache among its indications principally due to its relationship with the Governing Vessel. It is more effective in acute rather than chronic cases.

In combination with BL-62 Shenmai, it activates the Governing Vessel and can be used to affect the whole spine and back (upper and lower) in both acute and chronic cases of backache. This combination is indicated only if the backache is either on the spine itself or across the lower back on both sides, but not if the pain is only on one side of the lower back. In men, I often use S.I.-3 on the left, BL-62 on the right, HE-7 Shenmen on the right and KI-4 Dazhong on the left (Fig. 59.3).

The treatment is also different according to sex. In men, it is sufficient to treat only the Governing Vessel by using S.I.-3 and BL-62. In women, it is better to treat the Governing and Directing Vessels simultaneously by using S.I.-3, BL-62, LU-7 Lieque and KI-6 Zhaohai. The order and laterality of needling in a woman would be as follows: S.I.-3 on the right, BL-62 on the left, LU-7 on the left and KI-6 on the right. The needles should be withdrawn in the reverse order. This combination of distal points is extremely effective for chronic lower backache in women. These points would be used first to remove obstructions from the Governing Vessel, and the local points would be used afterwards (see Fig. 59.3).

Also in combination with BL-62, S.I.-3 activates the Governing Vessel and it tonifies the Kidneys as this extraordinary vessel emerges from the Kidneys. The use of S.I.-3 and BL-62 to tonify the Kidneys is more appropriate in men than in women.

Finally, in my experience, S.I.-3 has an effect on the Mind, in so far as it affects the brain, through the Governing Vessel. It 'clears the Mind' in the sense that it helps the person to gain mental strength, to lift

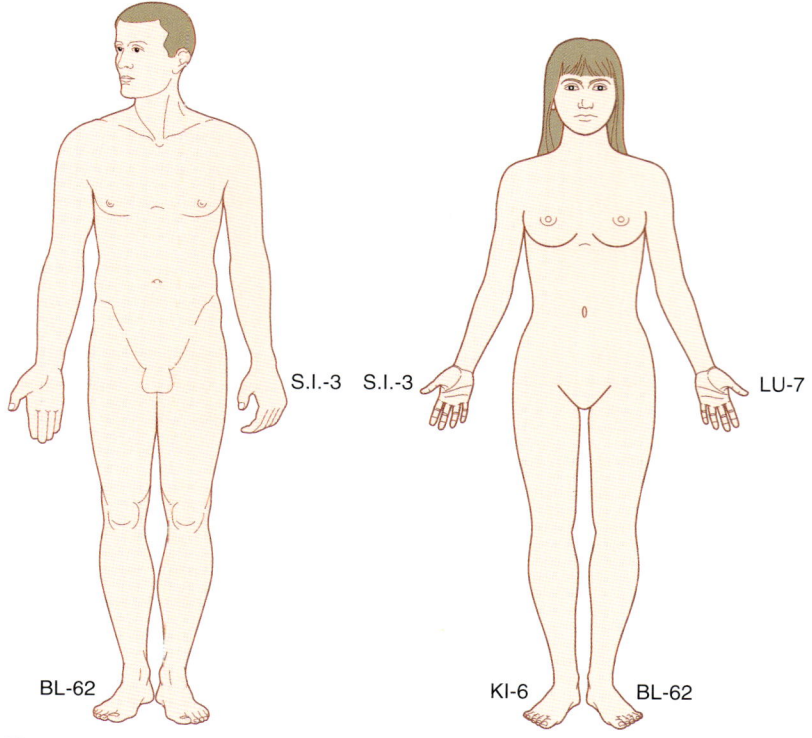

Figure 59.3 Opening points of the Governing Vessel in men and women

depression and to gain clarity of mind. Just as S.I.-3 strengthens the spine on a physical level, it can also strengthen the Mind and give the person the strength to face difficulties.

Box 59.4 summarizes the functions of S.I.-3.

Box 59.4 S.I.-3 – summary of functions

- Regulates the Governing Vessel and extinguishes interior Wind (epilepsy, headache, dizziness, vertigo)
- Expels exterior Wind (malaria, aversion to cold, fever, febrile disease)
- Benefits sinews (stiff neck (on occiput), occipital headache, difficulty in turning neck, pain in the upper back and shoulder, lower backache)
- Benefits eyes, nose and ears (deafness, tinnitus, blurred vision, redness and pain of the eyes, swelling of eyes, nosebleed)
- S.I.-3 and BL-62 used for chronic backache in men (combined with LU-7 and KI-6 for chronic backache in women)
- S.I.-3 and BL-62 tonify the Kidneys
- S.I.-3 and BL-62 clear the Mind and lift depression

S.I.-4 WANGU *WRIST BONE*

Location

On the ulnar border of the hand, between the base of the fifth metacarpal bone and the triquetral bone.

Nature

Source (*Yuan*) point.

Actions

Removes obstructions from the channel.
Resolves Damp-Heat.

Indications

Contraction of fingers, wrist pain, contraction of arm and elbow, stiff neck, pain in the shoulder, headache, pain in the lateral ribs.
Jaundice, febrile disease.

Comments

S.I.-4 is mostly used for channel problems of the Small Intestine, extending its influence to the wrist, elbow and neck. It is therefore used for Painful Obstruction Syndrome of the wrist or elbow.

In spite of its being the Source point, this point is not much used for internal problems of the Small Intestine, for which the Lower Sea (ST-39 Xiajuxu), Front Collecting (Ren-4 Guanyuan) or Back Transporting (BL-27 Xiaochangshu) points would be preferred.

An empirical use of this point is for hypochondrial pain, cholecystitis, and jaundice from Damp-Heat obstructing the Gall Bladder.

Box 59.5 summarizes the functions of S.I.-4.

> **Box 59.5 S.I.-4 – summary of functions**
> - Removes obstructions from the channel (contraction of fingers, wrist pain, contraction of arm and elbow, stiff neck, pain in the shoulder, headache, pain in the lateral ribs)
> - Resolves Damp-Heat (jaundice, febrile disease)

S.I.-5 YANGGU *YANG VALLEY*

Location

On the ulnar aspect of the wrist, in the depression between the head of the ulna and the triquetral bone.

Nature

River (*Jing*) point.
Fire point.

Actions

Clears Heat.
Calms the Mind.
Benefits ears and eyes.

Indications

Manic behaviour.
Tinnitus, deafness, blurred vision, redness, swelling and pain of the eyes.

Comments

In my experience, S.I.-5 is very useful for its mental effect: it 'clears the Mind' in the sense that it helps the person to gain mental clarity and distinguish the right choice to make among several. It can help a person at difficult times to distinguish what is right to do at a particular moment in life.

S.I.-5 can be used in a similar way to S.I.-4 Wangu for channel problems, and in my experience, it also helps to eliminate Dampness from the knees when they are swollen and hot.

Box 59.6 summarizes the functions of S.I.-5.

> **Box 59.6 S.I.-5 – summary of functions**
> - Clears Heat
> - Calms the Mind (manic behaviour)
> - Benefits ears and eyes (tinnitus, deafness, blurred vision, redness, swelling and pain of the eyes)
> - In my experience, it helps to discriminate between issues

S.I.-6 YANGLAO *NOURISHING THE ELDERLY*

Location

On the dorsal ulnar aspect of the forearm, in the depression on the radial side of the styloid process of the ulna.

Nature

Accumulation (*Xi*) point.

Actions

Brightens the eyes.
Benefits sinews.
Removes obstructions from the channel.

Indications

Blurred vision, eye pain.
Severe shoulder pain, severe pain of upper arm, redness and swelling of elbow, contracture of sinews, Painful Obstruction Syndrome (*Bi* Syndrome) of the feet.

Comments

As an Accumulation point, S.I.-6 is used for any channel problems of the Small Intestine, particularly acute cases with tightness of the sinews causing stiff neck and shoulders. Its effect on the feet is due to its relationship with the Bladder channel within the Greater Yang.

S.I.-6 also benefits the eyesight but only in patterns related to Heart or Small Intestine.

Box 59.7 summarizes the functions of S.I.-6.

> **Box 59.7 S.I.-6 – summary of functions**
> - Brightens the eyes (blurred vision, eye pain)
> - Benefits sinews
> - Removes obstructions from the channel (severe shoulder pain, severe pain of upper arm, redness and swelling of elbow, contracture of sinews, Painful Obstruction Syndrome (*Bi* Syndrome) of the feet)

> **Box 59.8 S.I.-7 – summary of functions**
> - Expels Wind-Heat (aversion to cold, fever, febrile disease, fever with neck pain)
> - Subdues rebellious Qi (headache, dizziness, blurred vision)
> - Removes obstructions from the channel (stiff neck, contracture of elbow, pain in the fingers)
> - Calms the Mind (manic depression, fright, sadness, anxiety, mental restlessness)

S.I.-7 ZHIZHENG *BRANCH TO HEART CHANNEL*

Location
On the dorsal ulnar aspect of the forearm, 5 *cun* above the transverse crease of the wrist, on the line connecting S.I.-5 Yanggu and S.I.-8 Xiaohai.

Nature
Connecting (*Luo*) point.

Actions
Expels Wind-Heat.
Subdues rebellious Qi.
Removes obstructions from the channel.
Calms the Mind.

Indications
Aversion to cold, fever, febrile disease, fever with neck pain.
Headache, dizziness, blurred vision.
Stiff neck, contracture of elbow, pain in the fingers.
Manic depression, fright, sadness, anxiety, mental restlessness.

Comments
S.I.-7 can treat any channel problem, as all Connecting points do. It is particularly good for elbow problems.

Being the Connecting point, it connects with the Heart channel, and because of this connection, it can be used to calm the Mind in severe anxiety and mental restlessness.

In my experience, this point helps to resolve thyroid Phlegm swellings when combined with L.I.-6 Pianli.

I have translated this point's name as 'Branch to Heart Channel', because '*Zheng*' in this case means 'chief' or 'ruler': that is, the Heart, which is the 'Monarch' of all the other organs.

Box 59.8 summarizes the functions of S.I.-7.

S.I.-8 XIAOHAI *SMALL INTESTINE SEA*

Location
On the medial aspect of the elbow, in the depression between the olecranon of the ulna and the medial epicondyle of the humerus.

Nature
Sea (*He*) point.
Earth point.
Drainage point.

Actions
Resolves Damp-Heat.
Removes obstructions from the channel.

Indications
Swelling and pain of the neck, swelling of cheek and gums, yellow eyes.
Pain in the neck, pain in the scapula, pain of the shoulder, pain in upper arm and elbow.

Comments
S.I.-8 resolves Damp-Heat (as all the Sea points of the three arm Yang channels do) and is therefore effective in treating acute swelling of the glands of the neck and parotitis.

It also removes obstructions from the channel and is used in Painful Obstruction Syndrome of the elbow and neck.

I have translated this point's name as 'Small Intestine Sea' rather than 'Small Sea', as the character '*Xiao*' here indicates '*Xiao Chang*': that is, the Chinese name for 'Small Intestine'.

Box 59.9 summarizes the functions of S.I.-8.

> **Box 59.9 S.I.-8 – summary of functions**
>
> - Resolves Damp-Heat (swelling and pain of the neck, swelling of cheek and gums, yellow eyes)
> - Removes obstructions from the channel (pain in the neck, pain in the scapula, pain of the shoulder, pain in upper arm and elbow)

S.I.-9 JIANZHEN UPRIGHT SHOULDER

Location

Posterior and inferior to the shoulder joint, when the arm is adducted, the point is 1 *cun* above the posterior end of the axillary fossa.

Nature

None.

Actions

Removes obstructions from the channel.

Indications

Pain in the shoulder and upper arm, inability to raise the arm, pain in the scapula, Wind Painful Obstruction Syndrome (*Bi* Syndrome).

Comments

S.I.-9 is not a major point, but it is worth remembering as it is one of several important local points for shoulder problems. S.I.-9 is one of the points that should always be checked for tenderness when selecting local points for Painful Obstruction Syndrome of the shoulder.

Box 59.10 summarizes the functions of S.I.-9.

> **Box 59.10 S.I.-9 – summary of functions**
>
> - Removes obstructions from the channel (pain in the shoulder and upper arm, inability to raise the arm, pain in the scapula, Wind Painful Obstruction Syndrome (*Bi* Syndrome))
> - Important local point for shoulder problems that should always be checked for tenderness

S.I.-10 NAOSHU HUMERUS TRANSPORTING POINT

Location

On the shoulder, directly above the posterior end of the axillary fossa, in the depression inferior to the scapular spine.

Nature

Meeting point of Small Intestine and Bladder channel.
Point of Yang Stepping Vessel (*Yang Qiao Mai*).
Point of Yang Linking Vessel (*Yang Wei Mai*).

Actions

Removes obstructions from the channel.

Indications

Pain of the shoulder and scapula, pain in the arm, inability to raise the shoulder.

Comments

S.I.-10 is another important point for Painful Obstruction Syndrome of the shoulder, and one always to be checked for tenderness when selecting local points. In particular, this point is situated both on the Yang Stepping and Yang Linking Vessels' trajectory and it especially increases the mobility of the shoulder whenever its joint movement is limited (as in 'frozen shoulder').

Box 59.11 summarizes the functions of S.I.-10.

> **Box 59.11 S.I.-10 – summary of functions**
>
> - Removes obstructions from the channel (pain of the shoulder and scapula, pain in the arm, inability to raise the shoulder)
> - Important local point for shoulder problems that should always be checked for tenderness
> - Point of the Yang Stepping and Yang Linking Vessels

S.I.-11 TIANZONG HEAVENLY ATTRIBUTION

Location

On the scapula, in the depression in the centre of the subscapular fossa, one third of the distance from the midpoint of the inferior border of the scapular spine to the inferior angle of the scapula.

Nature

None.

Actions

Removes obstructions from the channel.
Opens the chest.
Benefits the breast.

Indications

Pain in the shoulder, pain in the scapula, pain in the elbow.
Feeling of fullness of the chest and lateral ribs.
Swelling and pain of the breast, breast abscess, insufficient lactation.

Comments

Like S.I.-9 and S.I.-10, S.I.-11 is an important local point for shoulder and scapula problems that should always be checked for tenderness. It is more frequently used than S.I.-9 and S.I.-10 and, in my experience, it is nearly always tender on pressure in Painful Obstruction Syndrome of the shoulder. In my experience, it gives particularly good results in this condition when chosen as one of the local points. After obtaining the needling sensation, a reducing technique should be applied, which should then be followed by application of moxa to the needle. It is best to needle this point with the patient sitting up.

Another characteristic of S.I.-11, which distinguishes it from the other Small Intestine points on the scapula, is that it affects the front of the torso, relieving pain and fullness of the chest and lateral ribs. Yet another distinguishing feature is that it affects the breast in women, treating pain and swelling of the breast, breast lumps and lactation problems.

Box 59.12 summarizes the functions of S.I.-11.

Box 59.12 S.I.-11 – summary of functions

- Removes obstructions from the channel (pain in the shoulder, pain in the scapula, pain in the elbow)
- Opens the chest (feeling of fullness of the chest and lateral ribs)
- Benefits the breast (swelling and pain of the breast, breast abscess, insufficient lactation)
- It is usually the most tender point on pressure in shoulder problems

---

S.I.-12 BINGFENG *WATCHING WIND*

Location

On the scapula, in the centre of the suprascapular fossa, directly above S.I.-11 Tianzong, in the depression when the arm is lifted.

Nature

Meeting point of Small Intestine, Gall Bladder, Triple Burner and Large Intestine channels.

Actions

Removes obstructions from the channel.

Indications

Pain of the shoulder and scapula, inability to raise the arm, stiff neck, inability to turn head, pain in the arm.

Comments

S.I.-12 is another important local point for shoulder problems that should always be checked for tenderness on palpation.

Box 59.13 summarizes the functions of S.I.-12.

Box 59.13 S.I.-12 – summary of functions

- Removes obstructions from the channel (pain of the shoulder and scapula, inability to raise the arm, stiff neck, inability to turn head, pain in the arm)

S.I.-13 QUYUAN *BENT WALL*

Location

In the region of the scapula, on the medial extremity of the suprascapular fossa, midway between S.I.-10 and the spinous process of T2.

Nature

None.

Actions

Expels Wind.
Removes obstructions from the channel.

Indications

Painful Obstruction Syndrome (*Bi* Syndrome).
Pain of the shoulder and scapula, inability to raise arm.

Comments

S.I.-13 is another important local point for shoulder problems that should always be checked for tenderness on palpation. Similar to S.I.-11 Tianzong, this point should also be reduced and moxa applied to the needle afterwards. It is best to needle this point with the patient sitting up.

A distinguishing characteristic of this point, however, is that it can expel Wind from the joints in general and it is therefore used as a general point for Wind Painful Obstruction Syndrome (*Bi* Syndrome).

Box 59.14 summarizes the functions of S.I.-13.

Box 59.14 S.I.-13 – summary of functions

- Expels Wind (Painful Obstruction Syndrome (*Bi* Syndrome))
- Removes obstructions from the channel (pain of the shoulder and scapula, inability to raise arm)

Clinical note

S.I.-9, S.I.-10, S.I.-11, S.I.-12 and S.I.-13 are important points to treat problems of the shoulder joint and 'frozen shoulder', usually in combination with L.I.-15 Jianyu and/or T.B.-14 Jianliao. These two points affect the acromioclavicular articulation but problems of the shoulders involve also the scapulohumeral articulation, which is affected by the above Small Intestine point

---

S.I.-14 JIANWAISHU *TRANSPORTING POINT OF THE OUTSIDE OF THE SHOULDER*

Location

On the back, 3 *cun* lateral to the lower border of the spinous process of T1.

Nature

None.

Actions

Expels Wind.
Removes obstructions from the channel.

Indications

Wind Painful Obstruction Syndrome (*Bi* Syndrome).
Pain of the shoulder and scapula, pain in the arm and elbow, stiff neck.

Comments

S.I.-14 is another local point that should always be checked for tenderness on pressure in shoulder problems.

S.I.-14 is also used for generalized Wind Painful Obstruction Syndrome (*Bi* Syndrome).

Box 59.15 summarizes the functions of S.I.-14.

Box 59.15 S.I.-14 – summary of functions

- Expels Wind (Wind Painful Obstruction Syndrome (*Bi* Syndrome))
- Removes obstructions from the channel (pain of the shoulder and scapula, pain in the arm and elbow, stiff neck)

S.I.-15 JIANZHONGSHU *TRANSPORTING POINT OF THE CENTRE OF THE SHOULDER*

Location

On the back, 2 *cun* lateral to the lower border of the spinous process of C7.

Nature

None.

Actions

Promotes the descending of Lung-Qi.
Removes obstructions from the channel.

Indications

Cough, coughing of blood.
Pain in the shoulder and scapula.

Comments

The indications for this point are the same as for the previous two points. However, this point is slightly less important as a local point and is less often tender on pressure.

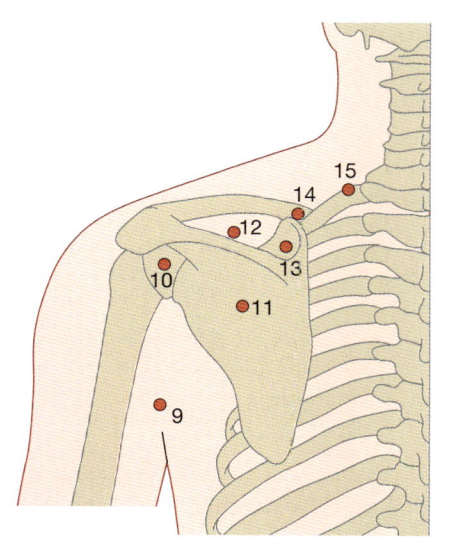

Figure 59.4 Small Intestine points on the scapula

Box 59.16 S.I.-15 – summary of functions

- Promotes the descending of Lung-Qi (cough, coughing of blood)
- Removes obstructions from the channel (pain in the shoulder and scapula)

Figure 59.4 illustrates the location of the Small Intestine points on the scapula. Box 59.16 summarizes the functions of S.I.-15.

S.I.-16 TIANCHUANG *HEAVENLY WINDOW*

Location

On the posterior border of the sternocleidomastoid muscle, posterior to L.I.-18 Futu, level with the Adam's apple.

Nature

Window of Heaven point.

Actions

Subdues rebellious Qi.
Extinguishes internal Wind.
Calms the Mind.
Benefits ears.

Indications

Feeling of heat in the face, cheek pain.
Loss of voice from Wind-stroke, clenched teeth, headache.
Manic behaviour, manic depression, 'talking with ghosts'.
Deafness, tinnitus, ear pain.

Comments

S.I.-16 is one of the Window of Heaven points: as such, it subdues rebellious Qi from the head, it regulates the ascending and descending of Qi to and from the head and it calms the Mind.

In my experience, this point has an important mental effect related partly to its being a Small Intestine point and partly to its being a Window of Heaven point. The psychic equivalent of the Small Intestine's physical action of separating clear from turbid fluids is the capacity to discriminate between issues with clarity. As we have seen, S.I.-5 has this particular effect of stimulating the capacity to discriminate between issues. S.I.-16 has the same effect but in an even stronger way due to its nature as Window of Heaven point. I therefore use this point when the person is confused about life's issues, unable to distinguish the right path and depressed.

Box 59.17 summarizes the functions of S.I.-16.

Box 59.17 S.I.-16 – summary of functions

- Subdues rebellious Qi (feeling of heat in the face, cheek pain)
- Extinguishes internal Wind (loss of voice from Wind-stroke, clenched teeth, headache)
- Calms the Mind (manic behaviour, manic depression, 'talking with ghosts')
- Benefits ears (deafness, tinnitus, ear pain)
- Facilitates the Mind's capacity of discriminating between issues

---

S.I.-17 TIANRONG *HEAVENLY APPEARANCE*

Location

On the lateral aspect of the neck, posterior to the angle of the mandible, in the depression on the anterior border of the sternocleidomastoid muscle.

Nature

Window of Heaven point.

Actions

Subdues rebellious Qi.
Resolves Dampness.
Expels Toxic Heat.
Benefits the ears.

Indications

Breathlessness, wheezing, cough, vomiting.
Goitre, scrofula of neck, swelling and pain of the neck.
Mumps, tonsillitis.
Tinnitus, deafness.

Comments

S.I.-17 resolves exterior or interior Dampness and is indicated in the treatment of swelling of the cervical glands and goitre. It also resolves Toxic Heat in parotitis (mumps) and tonsillitis.
Box 59.18 summarizes the functions of S.I.-17.

Box 59.18 S.I.-17 – summary of functions

- Subdues rebellious Qi (breathlessness, wheezing, cough, vomiting)
- Resolves Dampness (goitre, scrofula of neck, swelling and pain of neck)
- Expels Toxic Heat (mumps, tonsillitis)
- Benefits the ears (tinnitus, deafness)

S.I.-18 QUANLIAO *ZYGOMA CREVICE*

Location

On the face, directly below the outer canthus of the eye, in the depression on the lower border of the zygomatic bone.

Nature

Meeting point of Small Intestine and Triple Burner channels.

Meeting point of the three Yang Muscle channels of the leg.

Actions

Expels Wind.
Clears Heat and resolves swelling.

Indications

Deviation of eye and mouth, twitching of eyelids.
Facial pain, swelling of cheek, abscess of lip, red face.

Comments

S.I.-18 is an important local point in the treatment of facial paralysis, tic or trigeminal neuralgia and all manifestations of Wind in the face.
Box 59.19 summarizes the functions of S.I.-18.

Box 59.19 S.I.-18 – summary of functions

- Expels Wind (deviation of eye and mouth, twitching of eyelids)
- Clears Heat and resolves swelling (facial pain, swelling of cheek, abscess of lid, red face)

S.I.-19 TINGGONG *LISTENING PALACE*

Location

On the region of the face, anterior to the tragus and posterior to the condyloid process of the mandible, in the depression formed when the mouth is open.

Nature

Meeting point of Small Intestine, Gall Bladder and Triple Burner channels.

Action

Benefits the ears.

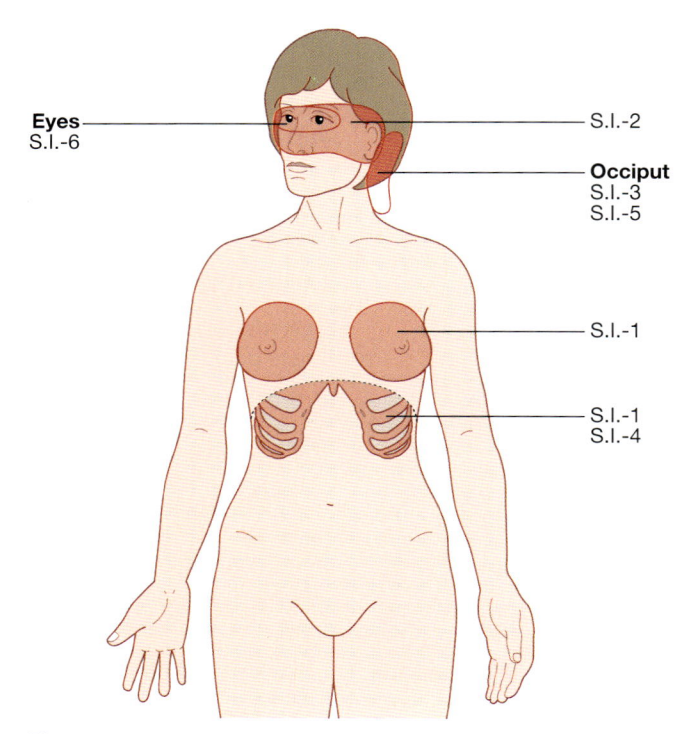

Figure 59.5 Target areas of Small Intestine channel points

Indications

Tinnitus, deafness, ear discharge, ear pain, itching inside the ears.

Comments

S.I.-19 is an important and frequently used local point for tinnitus and deafness. It is particularly indicated for Deficiency types of tinnitus and deafness, especially if associated with a Lung and Heart-Qi deficiency. It is frequently combined with T.B.-17 Yifeng to combine one point in front and the other behind the ear in order to stimulate the movement of Qi in the ear.

Box 59.20 summarizes the functions of S.I.-19.

Figure 59.5 illustrates the target areas of the Small Intestine points.

Box 59.20 S.I.-19 – summary of functions

- Benefits the ears (tinnitus, deafness, ear discharge, ear pain, itching inside the ears)

SECTION 2　PART 7

Bladder Channel　60

Main channel pathway

The Bladder channel starts at the inner canthus of the eye. It ascends the forehead and joins the Governing Vessel (*Du Mai*) at the point Du-20 Baihui. From here a branch goes to the temple. From the vertex, the channel enters the brain to re-emerge at the nape of the neck. From here, it flows down the occiput and all the way down the back. From the lumbar area, it enters the kidney and bladder.

Another branch from the occiput runs down the back along the medial aspect of the scapula, down the back to the gluteus and the popliteal fossa. Here it meets the previous branch and runs along the posterior aspect of the leg to end at the lateral aspect of the fifth toe where it links with the Kidney channel (Fig. 60.1).

Connecting channel pathway

The Bladder Connecting channel separates at BL-58 Feiyang on the leg and flows down to connect with the Kidney channel (Fig. 60.2).

Box 60.1 provides an overview of the Bladder points.

BL-1 JINGMING *EYE BRIGHTNESS*

Location

On the face, in the depression superior to the inner canthus near the medial border of the orbit.

Nature

Point of Yin and Yang Stepping Vessels (*Yin* and *Yang Stepping Vessels*).
Meeting point of Bladder, Small Intestine, Stomach, Gall Bladder and Triple Burner.

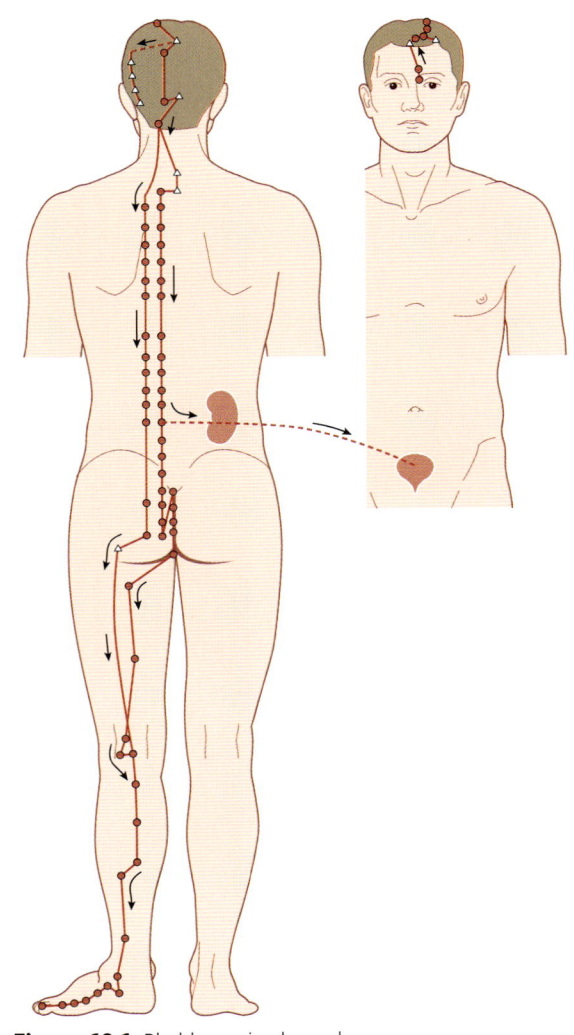

Figure 60.1 Bladder main channel

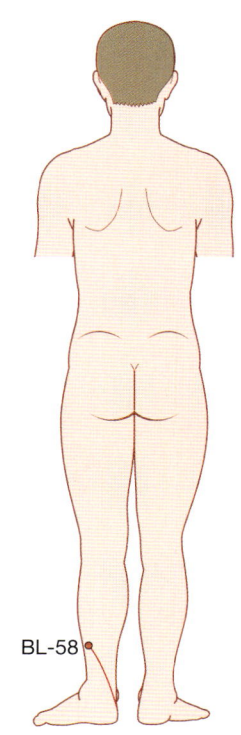

Figure 60.2 Bladder Connecting channel

Box 60.1 Overview of Bladder points

- Affect back of leg, anus, back, bladder, neck, head, brain
- Treat backache
- Affect the eye
- Expel exterior Wind
- Extinguish interior Wind
- Affect all Internal Organs through the Back Transporting points

---

Actions

Expels Wind.
Clears Heat.
Stops itching.
Brightens the eyes.

Indications

Lacrimation on exposure to wind, aversion to cold fever, headache.
Redness, swelling and pain of the eyes, redness and itching of the inner corner of the eyes.
Blurred vision, diminished night vision, myopia, Childhood Nutritional Impairment eye diseases.

Comments

BL-1 is obviously used mostly for eye diseases, of both interior and exterior character.

It can expel exterior Wind and clear Heat, which means that it can treat eye problems from Wind-Heat, such as conjunctivitis and runny eyes. It can also clear interior Heat and therefore help eye problems deriving from Liver-Fire, such as red, painful, swollen and dry eyes. It stops pain and itching of the eyes deriving from Heat.

BL-1 is a point where Qi goes into the Yin at night and comes out in the morning: this is connected to the circulation of Defensive Qi (*Wei Qi*) in the 24 hours, circulating in the three Yang organs (Greater Yang, Lesser Yang, Bright Yang) in the day and in the five Yin organs (Kidney, Heart, Lungs, Liver, Spleen) at night. Therefore this point has the function of a passage or gate between Yin and Yang and, as such, it is a dynamic point. Because of its role as a gate between Yin and Yang in the circadian circulation of Defensive Qi, this point can be used for either insomnia or somnolence. BL-1 can therefore be used in conjunction with the opening points of both the Yin and Yang Stepping Vessels (*Yin Qiao Mai* and *Yang Qiao Mai*) for the treatment of insomnia.

As explained in chapter 52, the Yin Stepping Vessel transports Yin Qi to the eye, whilst the Yang Stepping Vessel transports Yang Qi to it. If Yang is in excess, the eyes will stay open and the person finds it difficult to fall asleep. In this case one can reinforce KI-6 Zhaohai to stimulate the Yin Stepping Vessel, reduce BL-62 Shenmai to drain the Yang Stepping Vessel and needle BL-1 with even method. The needling of BL-1 closes the circle between the Yin and Yang Stepping Vessels and allows the balance of Yin and Yang Qi in the eyes to be re-established. For somnolence, reduce KI-6 Zhaohai, reinforce BL-62 Shenmai and use BL-1 Jingming with even method. The regulation and exchange of Yin and Yang at this point takes place via the Yin and Yang Stepping Vessels, both of which converge at this point (see Fig. 53.14 in ch. 53).

As this point is the convergence of many Yang channels (in fact, all of them except the Large Intestine channel), similarly to Du-14 Dazhui, it can be used to clear Heat in a wide variety of eye diseases (such as red, swollen and painful eyes) or to promote the rising of Clear Yang to the eyes to treat such symptoms as blurred vision.

Box 60.2 summarizes the functions of BL-1.

> **Box 60.2 BL-1 – summary of functions**
> - Expels Wind (lacrimation on exposure to wind, aversion to cold fever, headache)
> - Clears Heat (redness, swelling and pain of the eyes, redness and itching of the inner corner of the eyes)
> - Stops itching
> - Brightens the eyes (blurred vision, diminished night vision, myopia)

> **Box 60.3 BL-2 – summary of functions**
> - Expels Wind (redness, swelling and pain of the eye, itching of the eyes, epilepsy, twitching of eyelids, excessive lacrimation, haemorrhoid pain)
> - Clears Heat
> - Brightens the eyes (blurred vision, dizziness, diminished night vision, eye nebula)
> - Subdues Liver-Qi (headache, dizziness, pain in the eyebrow, nosebleed, facial pain, cheek pain)

BL-2 ZANZHU (OR CUANZHU) GATHERED BAMBOO

Location

Superior to the inner canthus in a depression on the eyebrow, close to the medial end.

Nature

None.

Actions

Expels Wind.
Clears Heat.
Brightens the eyes.
Subdues Liver-Yang.

Indications

Redness, swelling and pain of the eye, itching of the eyes, epilepsy, twitching of eyelids, excessive lacrimation, haemorrhoid pain.
Blurred vision, dizziness, diminished night vision, eye nebula.
Headache, dizziness, pain in the eyebrow, nosebleed, facial pain, cheek pain.

Comments

This is an important local point for the eye. First of all, it expels exterior Wind from the face and removes obstructions from the channel: this means that it can be used to treat facial paralysis, facial tics and trigeminal neuralgia, all problems caused by Wind affecting the channels of the face.

It brightens the eyes and subdues Liver-Qi, but only locally in relation to the Liver function of nourishing the eyes and in relation to headaches. It can therefore be used in any Liver pattern affecting the eyes, such as 'floaters' in the eyes, red eyes, blurred vision and persistent headaches around or 'behind' the eyes.

Box 60.3 summarizes the functions of BL-2.

BL-5 WUCHU FIVE PLACES

Location

0.5 *cun* directly posterior to BL-4 Quhai, 1 *cun* within the anterior hairline and 1.5 *cun* lateral to Du-23 Shangxing.

Nature

None.

Actions

Extinguishes interior Wind and subdues Liver-Qi.

Indications

Rigidity of spine, opisthotonos, epilepsy, tetany, vertigo, headache, dizziness, pain in the eye.

Comments

BL-5 is a local point to extinguish interior Wind affecting the Governing Vessel. It is used for the treatment of epilepsy, convulsions or rigidity of the spine in children during a febrile disease.

It is used as a local point in the treatment of headaches from Liver-Yang rising.

Box 60.4 summarizes the functions of BL-5.

> **Box 60.4 BL-5 – summary of functions**
> - Extinguishes interior Wind and subdues Liver-Qi (rigidity of spine, opisthotonos, epilepsy, tetany, vertigo, headache, dizziness, pain in the eye)

BL-7 TONGTIAN PENETRATING HEAVEN

Location

1.5 *cun* posterior to BL-6 Chengguang and 4 *cun* within the anterior hairline, 1.5. *cun* lateral to the midline.

Nature

None.

Actions

Extinguishes Wind and subdues Liver-Yang.
Benefits the nose.

Indications

Headache, deviation of eye and mouth, stiff neck, feeling of heaviness of the head, loss of consciousness.
Nasal congestion and discharge, loss of sense of smell, nosebleed, nasal sores.

Comments

BL-7 is an important local point that extinguishes interior Wind from the head. It can be used for severe headache or facial paralysis, as well as for dizziness and vertigo. It is particularly important as a local point for headaches on the vertex deriving from Liver-Yang or Liver-Wind rising, as well as from Liver-Blood deficiency.

It is also used as a local point to subdue interior Wind, which may result in convulsions and unconsciousness.

This point also has an effect on the nose, and can be used in rhinitis to clear the nose.

Box 60.5 summarizes the functions of BL-7.

> **Box 60.5 BL-7 – summary of functions**
>
> - Extinguishes Wind and subdues Liver-Yang (headache, deviation of eye and mouth, stiff neck, feeling of heaviness of the head, loss of consciousness)
> - Benefits the nose (nasal congestion and discharge, loss of sense of smell, nosebleed, nasal sores)

BL-9 YUZHEN *JADE PILLOW*

Location

On the posterior aspect of the head, 2.5 *cun* superior to the posterior hairline, 1.3 *cun* lateral to the midline, level with the superior border of the external occipital protuberance.

Nature

None.

Actions

Subdues Liver-Yang.
Brightens the eyes.
Expels exterior Wind.
Extinguishes interior Wind.
Opens the Mind's orifices.

Indications

Occipital headache, dizziness, neck pain with inability to turn the head, feeling of heaviness of the head, red face.
Eye pain, myopia.
Aversion to cold, fever, body aches.
Epilepsy, loss of consciousness.
Manic behaviour.

Comments

BL-9 is an important local point for the treatment of headaches from Liver-Yang rising especially when, besides causing a headache, it causes a pronounced stiffness and ache of the neck.

Box 60.6 summarizes the functions of BL-9.

> **Box 60.6 BL-9 – summary of functions**
>
> - Subdues Liver-Yang (occipital headache, dizziness, neck pain with inability to turn the head, feeling of heaviness of the head, red face)
> - Brightens the eyes (eye pain, myopia)
> - Expels exterior Wind (aversion to cold, fever, body aches)
> - Extinguishes interior Wind (epilepsy, loss of consciousness)
> - Opens the Mind's orifices (manic behaviour)

BL-10 TIANZHU *HEAVEN PILLAR*

Location

On the lateral aspect of the trapezius muscle, 1.3 *cun* lateral to Du-15 Yamen.

Nature

Window of Heaven point.

Actions

Extinguishes Wind and subdues Liver-Yang.
Expels exterior Wind.
Strengthens the Greater Yang channels.
Clears the brain.
Opens the sense orifices.

Removes obstructions from the channel.
Opens the Mind's orifices.

Indications

Dizziness, muscle cramps, stiffness of the neck with inability to turn the head, headache, feeling of heaviness of the head, epilepsy.
Aversion to cold, fever, body aches.
Inability of the legs to support the body, soft legs, weak legs that cannot sustain the body.
Mental confusion, difficulty in concentrating and poor memory.
Eye pain, red eyes, blurred vision, lacrimation, difficulty in speaking, nasal congestion, loss of sense of smell.
Pain in the body, pain in the shoulder and back.
Manic behaviour, incessant talking, 'seeing ghosts'.

Comments

Small Intestine and Bladder pertain to Greater Yang, which opens on to the Exterior. Of the three Yang, the Greater Yang channels are the most Yang or 'most exterior'; in addition, the area on the top of the body, like the occiput, is even more Yang in relation, for example, to the inferior part of the Bladder channel. This has two main implications. On the one hand, it means that the points in this area are Yang in nature and can therefore be used either to tonify Yang ('inability to support the body') or to expel Yang pathogenic factors such as Wind (epilepsy, stiff neck).

On the other hand, being Yang and being at the top of the body, this area suffers from rebellious Qi flowing up and points in this area can be used to subdue rebellious Qi (dizziness, headache). Being Yang in nature, due to its channel polarity and position, BL-10 treats excess of Yang causing mental problems ('incessant talking, seeing ghosts, manic behaviour'). Being situated on the hinge of the occiput and being like a gate of Yang Qi, BL-10 re-establishes the balance in the flow of Yang to and from the head and can be used when there is excess Yang above and deficient Yang below ('soft legs, weak legs that cannot sustain the body').

BL-10 is an important point to expel both interior and exterior Wind from the head and is a major local point for occipital or vertical headache from any origin. It can be used to expel exterior Wind in the case of stiff neck and headache deriving from invasions of Wind-Cold.

It can extinguish interior Wind and is used in this way mostly for occipital headaches deriving from Liver-Wind rising. However, it can be used for virtually any type of occipital headache.

As BL-10 is situated at the point where the Bladder channel and the Eye System emerge from the brain, this point can be used to clear the brain and stimulate memory and concentration.

It has a special effect on the eyes and is used to increase vision, especially if the eyesight is diminished from Kidney deficiency.

Finally, it can be used as a distal point for bilateral acute lower backache. This point is usually needled first with reducing method while the patient (in a standing position) gently bends forwards and backwards. After a few minutes of this, the patient is made to lie down and local points are used on the lower back.

As a Window of Heaven point, BL-10 regulates the ascending and descending of Qi to and from the head and subdues rebellious Qi: this is another reason why this is a major point for the treatment of headaches from Liver-Yang rising and mental–emotional problems.

Box 60.7 summarizes the functions of BL-10.

Box 60.7 BL-10 – summary of functions

- Extinguishes Wind and subdues Liver-Yang (dizziness, muscle cramps, stiffness of the neck with inability to turn the head, headache, feeling of heaviness of the head, epilepsy)
- Expels exterior Wind (aversion to cold, fever, body aches)
- Strengthens the Greater Yang channels (inability of the legs to support the body, soft legs, weak legs that cannot sustain the body)
- Clears the brain (mental confusion, difficulty in concentrating and poor memory)
- Opens the sense orifices (eye pain, red eyes, blurred vision, lacrimation, difficulty in speaking, nasal congestion, loss of sense of smell)
- Removes obstructions from the channel (pain in the body, pain in the shoulder and back)
- Opens the Mind's orifices (manic behaviour, incessant talking, 'seeing ghosts')

BL-11 DAZHU *BIG SHUTTLE*

Location

On the back, 1.5 *cun* lateral to the lower border of the spinous process of the first thoracic vertebra.

Nature

Point of the Sea of Blood.
Gathering (*Hui*) point for Bones.

Meeting point of Bladder, Small Intestine, Triple Burner and Gall Bladder channels.

Actions

Nourishes Blood.
Expels exterior Wind.
Subdues Liver-Yang.
Strengthens bones.
Restores the descending of Lung-Qi.

Indications

Blood diseases, anaemia.
Aversion to cold, fever, invasions of Wind, chronic rhinitis, propensity to catching colds.
Headache, dizziness, blurred vision.
Bone diseases, rigidity of the neck and spine, pain in the back and scapula, lower backache, collapse, inability to stand for long periods.
Cough, feeling of fullness of the chest, breathlessness.

Comments

BL-11 has three main areas of influence. Firstly, it is a point of the Sea of Blood and it can be used to nourish Blood, but not in a general sense. It mostly tonifies Blood on the surface of the body and particularly in the space between skin and muscles (*cou li*). Therefore, besides expelling Wind (see below), it can be used to prevent invasions of Wind by 'firming' the space between skin and muscles, which it does by tonifying Blood in that area. Because of this action, this point can also be used to treat allergies such as allergic rhinitis.

From this point of view, the action of this point is similar to the formula Gui Zhi Tang (*Ramulus Cinnamomi Decoction*): that is, it strengthens the Nutritive Qi and it expels Wind. To tonify Blood, BL-11 should be needled with reinforcing method or direct moxa cones should be applied. Another use of this particular function is for generalized muscular ache (Painful Obstruction Syndrome from Wind). This point helps by nourishing Blood and therefore strengthening the Nutritive Qi to throw off the pathogenic factor.

In relation to this point being the Sea of Blood, BL-11 is also related to the Penetrating Vessel (*Chong Mai*) because this vessel is the Sea of Blood. In fact, chapter 33 of the 'Spiritual Axis' says that: '*The Penetrating Vessel is the Sea of Blood and its upper point is BL-11 Dazhu and its lower points are ST-37 Shangjuxu and ST-39 Xiajuxu.*'[1] From this point of view, this point can be used to affect the Sea of Blood of the Penetrating Vessel and it specifically treats Blood in the outer parts ('chronic rhinitis, propensity to catching colds') and the upper parts of the body ('dizziness, blurred vision').

Secondly, as BL-11 is close to BL-12 Fengmen (which expels Wind), it also has an outward movement and expels external Wind; this action is also partly related to the fact that the Governing Vessel extends a branch to this point. Therefore BL-11 releases the Exterior and expels exterior Wind, in a similar way to BL-12 Fengmen, and can be used in the beginning stages of attacks of exterior Wind-Cold or Wind-Heat. In this case it should be needled with reducing method or cupped.

Thirdly, it is a Gathering point for Bones, and it can nourish the bones. It is therefore used either to promote bone formation in children and prevent bone degeneration in the elderly, or to treat bone deformities in chronic arthritis (Bone Painful Obstruction Syndrome, *Bi* Syndrome).

BL-11 can also be used to stimulate the descending of Qi and particularly Lung-Qi, especially in the beginning stages of invasion of Wind when the pathogenic factor is on the Exterior.

'Shuttle' is a reference to the spine, resembling the shuttle of a loom. An alternative name for this point is *Dashu*, 'shu' being the same character as in the Back *Shu* (Back Transporting) points. From this point of view, therefore, the name of this point could be translated as 'big Back Transporting point' and this is a reference to the fact that this point is the first and the highest of the Back Transporting points. This name may also be a reference to the fact that this point influences all the five Yin and six Yang organs, also by virtue of its being the Gathering point of Bones and the point of the Sea of Blood. Another name is *Beishu* (i.e. Back Transporting point); yet another is *Bailao* (i.e. '100 fatigues'), a reference to its being a point of the Sea of Blood and Gathering point for bones and its use in diseases from exhaustion.

The alternative names of the point hint to some of its functions. The fact that is called *Beishu*, i.e. *Shu* (Back Transporting) point of the back, indicates that it controls all the Back Transporting points of the back and strengthens the back ('bone diseases'). From this point of view, BL-11, controlling Blood and Bones, is like the structure of the body, the armour.

The other name, *Bailao* ('100 fatigues'), indicates the tonifying use of this point in chronic deficiency of

> **Box 60.8 BL-11 – summary of functions**
>
> - Nourishes Blood (blood diseases, anaemia)
> - Nourishes Blood in the outer parts ('chronic rhinitis, propensity to catching colds') and the upper parts of the body ('dizziness, blurred vision')
> - Expels exterior Wind (aversion to cold, fever, invasions of Wind)
> - Subdues Liver-Yang (headache, dizziness, blurred vision)
> - Strengthens bones (bone diseases, rigidity of the neck and spine, pain in the back and scapula, lower backache)
> - Restores the descending of Lung-Qi (cough, feeling of fullness of the chest, breathlessness)

Blood or Yin especially characterized by Deficiency below ('dizziness, blurred vision, collapse, inability to stand for long').

Box 60.8 summarizes the functions of BL-11.

FENGMEN BL-12 *WIND DOOR*

Location

1.5 *cun* lateral to the lower border of the spinous process of T-2.

Nature

Meeting point of Bladder channel with Governing Vessel.

Actions

Expels external Wind.
Regulates Nutritive (*Ying*) and Defensive (*Wei*) Qi and consolidates the space between skin and muscles.
Stimulates the diffusing and descending of Lung-Qi.
Strengthens the back.
Benefits the nose.

Indications

Aversion to cold, fever, occipital headache and stiffness of the neck from invasion of Wind.
Too relaxed state of the space between the skin and muscles, propensity to catching colds, clear watery nasal discharge.
Cough, coughing blood, breathlessness, sneezing, allergic rhinitis.
Lumbar pain, stiff neck.
Urticaria on back, carbuncles on back.
Abundant nasal discharge, nasal congestion, nosebleed.

Comments

BL-12 is the main point to use in the very beginning stages of invasions of exterior Wind-Cold or Wind-Heat; reducing this point will release the Exterior, relieve the exterior symptoms (stuffy nose, sneezing, aversion to cold, body aches and headache) and expel Wind. It is extremely effective, especially if it is cupped. When reduced or cupped in these cases, it acts by stimulating the diffusing of Lung-Qi: that is, spreading the Defensive Qi all over the space between the skin and muscles to fight off the pathogenic factor.

It can also be used with even needling to regulate Nutritive and Defensive Qi: that is, in invasions of exterior Wind-Cold with the prevalence of Wind resulting in slight sweating (see ch. 44).

For the same reason, BL-12 consolidates the space between the skin and muscles when this is a too 'relaxed' state, i.e. the pores are open, Defensive Qi is weak and therefore the person is prone to invasion of external Wind.

As this point stimulates the diffusing of Lung-Qi, benefits the nose and expels Wind, it is often used in chronic allergic rhinitis with sneezing and profuse clear watery nasal discharge. In both the above cases, BL-12 is combined with points that tonify Qi such as BL-13 Feishu, ST-36 Zusanli and Ren-6 Qihai, all needled with reinforcing method.

One particular use of this point is for skin diseases in the back. This function is a result of its two actions of affecting the back and expelling Wind.

Box 60.9 summarizes the functions of BL-12.

> **Box 60.9 BL-12 – summary of functions**
>
> - Expels external Wind (aversion to cold, fever, occipital headache and stiffness of the neck from invasion of Wind)
> - Regulates Nutritive and Defensive Qi and consolidates the space between skin and muscles (too relaxed state of the space between the skin and muscles, propensity to catching colds, clear and watery nasal discharge)
> - Stimulates the diffusing and descending of Lung-Qi (cough, coughing blood, breathlessness, sneezing, allergic rhinitis)
> - Strengthens the back (lumbar pain, stiff neck)
> - Benefits the nose (abundant nasal discharge, nasal congestion, nosebleed)
> - Best point to expel exterior Wind when used with cupping

BL-13 FEISHU *LUNG BACK TRANSPORTING POINT*

Location
1.5 *cun* lateral to the lower border of the spinous process of T-3.

Nature
Back Transporting point of the Lungs.

Actions
Stimulates the diffusing and descending of Lung-Qi.
Expels external Wind.
Regulates Nutritive and Defensive Qi.
Tonifies Lung-Qi and nourishes Lung-Yin.
Clears Heat.
Calms the Mind.

Indications
Cough, wheezing, breathlessness, fullness of the chest, persistent cough in children, chest pain (from Lung patterns), expectoration of phlegm.
Aversion to cold, fever, cough, sneezing.
Lung-Qi deficiency, consumption, 'steaming bones', night sweating, fever from Yin deficiency, dry mouth and throat.
Lung abscess, rapid pulse, fever.
Manic behaviour, desire to commit suicide.

Comments
BL-13 point can be used in both exterior and interior patterns of the Lungs. In exterior patterns, it releases the Exterior by stimulating the diffusing and descending of Lung-Qi, and thus helps to expel Wind-Cold or Wind-Heat. In particular, it is indicated if the exterior attack is accompanied by cough. In invasions of exterior Wind-Cold with the prevalence of Wind (manifested with sweating), it can regulate Nutritive and Defensive Qi in the same way as BL-12 Fengmen.

In interior patterns, it restores the descending of Lung-Qi and is therefore used for cough, wheezing and breathlessness.

BL-13 also clears interior Heat from the Lungs, and is therefore used in acute conditions of the Lungs characterized by Heat at the Qi level (of the Four-Level pattern identification), as may happen in acute bronchitis following an invasion of Wind. The symptoms at this stage are a high fever, thirst, a cough with sticky yellow sputum, breathlessness, restlessness, a Rapid pulse and a Red tongue body with a thick yellow dry coating.

Needled with reinforcing method, or direct moxa, it tonifies Lung-Qi and is effective for chronic deficiency of Lung-Qi, especially if combined with Du-12 Shenzhu. When needled in this way, it also consolidates the space between the skin and muscles when this is too 'relaxed', making the person prone to invasions of external Wind.

BL-13 also nourishes Lung-Yin and, for this purpose, it is frequently combined with BL-43 Gaohuangshu.

The indication 'desire to commit suicide' must be seen in the context of the Corporeal Soul (*Po*), which is housed in the Lungs. The Corporeal Soul is a physical soul with a centripetal movement, constantly materializing and constantly separating into different constituent aspects. The Corporeal Soul is in a relationship with *gui*, i.e. ghosts or spirits (of dead people).

Confucius said: '*Qi is the fullness of the Mind (Shen); the Corporeal Soul (Po) is the fullness of Gui*'. He Shang Gong said: '*The turbid and humid five flavours from bones, flesh, blood, vessels and the six passions ... this Gui is called Corporeal Soul [Po]. This is Yin in character and enters and exits through the mouth and communicates with Earth.*' The centripetal forces of *Gui* within the Corporeal Soul, constantly fragmenting, are, eventually, the germ of death. With regard to fragmenting, there is a resonance between *Gui* 鬼 and *kuai* 塊 (*gui* with 'earth' in front), which means 'pieces'.

Because of the connection between the Corporeal Soul and death, points associated with the Corporeal Soul (such as BL-13 Feishu) are indicated for suicidal thoughts. As we shall see below, the point BL-42 Pohu (which is on the outer Bladder line level with BL-13 Feishu) is also indicated for suicidal thoughts.

Box 60.10 summarizes the functions of BL-13.

Box 60.10 BL-13 – summary of functions

- Stimulates the diffusing and descending of Lung-Qi (cough, wheezing, breathlessness, fullness of the chest, persistent cough in children, chest pain (from Lung patterns), expectoration of phlegm)
- Expels external Wind (aversion to cold, fever, cough, sneezing)
- Regulates Nutritive and Defensive Qi
- Tonifies Lung-Qi and nourishes Lung-Yin (Lung-Qi deficiency, consumption, 'steaming bones', night sweating, fever from Yin deficiency, dry mouth and throat)
- Clears Heat (lung abscess, rapid pulse, fever)
- Calms the Mind (manic behaviour, desire to commit suicide)

BL-14 JUEYINSHU *TERMINAL YIN BACK TRANSPORTING POINT*

Location
1.5 *cun* lateral to the lower border of the spinous process of T-4.

Nature
Back Transporting point for the Pericardium.

Actions
Regulates the Heart.
Opens the chest.
Stops pain.

Indications
Heart pain, palpitations, agitation, mental restlessness.
Cough, breathlessness, feeling of fullness of the chest, chest pain.

Comments
BL-14 is frequently used in heart conditions, such as arrhythmia, tachycardia, angina pectoris and coronary heart disease. In particular, it has a pronounced effect on the chest and in relieving pain.

The 'Explanation of the Acupuncture Points' says: '*When the Heart is not settled, the Pericardium channel is affected and there is chest pain: BL-14 should be reduced. The chest is the residence of the Heart, Lungs and Pericardium.*'[2]

This point also strongly moves Qi and invigorates Blood. The same text says: '*When there is accumulation, Qi cannot circulate properly and it stagnates causing stasis of Blood. The Pericardium controls Blood and draining this point will eliminate the stagnation and the mental restlessness.*'[3]

Box 60.11 summarizes the functions of BL-14.

Box 60.11 BL-14 – summary of functions

- Regulates the Heart (heart pain, palpitations, agitation, mental restlessness)
- Opens the chest (cough, breathlessness, feeling of fullness of the chest, chest pain)
- Stops pain

BL-15 XINSHU *HEART BACK TRANSPORTING POINT*

Location
1.5 *cun* lateral to the lower border of the spinous process of T-5.

Nature
Back Transporting point for the Heart.

Actions
Calms the Mind.
Nourishes the Heart.
Stimulates the Brain.
Clears Heat.
Regulates Heart-Qi and invigorates Blood.

Indications
Anxiety, weeping, fright, insomnia, excessive dreaming, manic depression.
Disorientation, delayed speech development, poor memory, poor concentration, mental confusion, Heart-Qi deficiency in children.
Heart pain, fullness of the chest, chest pain, palpitations, irregular pulse.

Comments
BL-15 is a very important point for many Heart patterns. Firstly, it calms the Mind and can be used for nervous anxiety and insomnia mostly deriving from Excess conditions of the Heart, such as Heart-Fire or Heart Empty-Heat. In these cases it is needled with reducing method.

It also calms the Mind by nourishing the Heart and, for this reason, it is used for poor memory and insomnia. At the same time as calming the Mind, it also stimulates the brain if used with reinforcing method or with direct moxibustion. In particular, used with direct moxibustion, it has a good effect in stimulating the brain and is effective for depression, mental confusion and poor concentration in adults and slow development in children.

BL-15 also moves Qi and invigorates Blood and is therefore used for pain in the chest deriving from stasis of Blood.

Box 60.12 summarizes the functions of BL-15.

> **Box 60.12 BL-15 – summary of functions**
>
> - Calms the Mind (anxiety, weeping, fright, insomnia, excessive dreaming, manic depression)
> - Nourishes the Heart (disorientation, delayed speech development, poor memory, poor concentration, mental confusion, Heart-Qi deficiency in children)
> - Stimulates the Brain
> - Clears Heat
> - Regulates Heart-Qi and invigorates Blood (heart pain, fullness of the chest, chest pain, palpitations, irregular pulse)

BL-16 DUSHU *GOVERNING VESSEL BACK TRANSPORTING POINT*

Location

1.5 *cun* lateral to the lower border of the spinous process of T-6.

Nature

Back Transporting point for the Governing Vessel.

Actions

Regulates the Heart.
Moves Qi and invigorates Blood.

Indications

Heart pain.
Epigastric pain, abdominal distension, breast abscess.

Comments

BL-16 is used mostly for stasis of Blood of the Heart causing heart and chest pain.
Box 60.13 summarizes the functions of BL-16.

> **Box 60.13 BL-16 – summary of functions**
>
> - Regulates the Heart (heart pain)
> - Moves Qi and invigorates Blood (epigastric pain, abdominal distension, breast abscess)

BL-17 GESHU *DIAPHRAGM BACK TRANSPORTING POINT*

Location

1.5 *cun* lateral to the lower border of the spinous process of T-7.

Nature

Back Transporting Point for the diaphragm.
Gathering (*Hui*) point for Blood.

Actions

Invigorates Blood.
Cools Blood.
Stops bleeding.
Nourishes Blood.
Opens the chest and diaphragm.
Subdues rebellious Qi.
Benefits the sinews.
Tonifies Qi and Blood.

Indications

Heart pain, stabbing chest pain.
Coughing of blood, vomiting of blood, nosebleed.
Epigastric pain, vomiting, hiccup, difficult digestion, sour regurgitation.
Painful Obstruction Syndrome (*Bi* Syndrome) of the whole body, pain in the whole body, swelling, distension and pain of the body.

Comments

BL-17 is an important point with many functions. First of all, it has a multifaceted effect on Blood as it can invigorate, cool and nourish Blood and stop bleeding. Its primary function is to invigorate Blood and stop bleeding. An interesting passage in the 'Explanation of Acupuncture Points' correlates the multiple functions of this point in relation to Blood to its location in between BL-15 Xinshu and BL-18 Ganshu: '*BL-17 Geshu communicates with BL-15 Xinshu above and BL-18 Ganshu below: the Heart generates Blood and the Liver stores Blood, hence this point affects Blood.*'[4]

Firstly, BL-17 invigorates Blood, i.e. removes stasis of Blood from any organ, but only if needed (no moxa) with either reducing or even method. It is used as a general point to remove stasis of Blood in any organ and from any part of the body, but especially the upper part. It can be combined with the Back Transporting points to eliminate stasis of Blood of the relevant organs. For example, combined with BL-18 Ganshu it removes stasis of Liver-Blood whilst combined with BL-15 Xinshu it removes stasis of Heart-Blood. As BL-17 invigorates Blood especially in the upper part and SP-10 Xuehai in the lower part of the body, these two points are frequently combined to invigorate Blood and eliminate stasis in any part of the body.

> **Clinical note**
>
> As BL-17 invigorates Blood especially in the upper part and SP-10 Xuehai in the lower part of the body, these two points are frequently combined to invigorate Blood and eliminate stasis in any part of the body

Secondly, BL-17 cools Blood and stops bleeding but primarily bleeding upwards: that is, coughing of blood, vomiting of blood and epistaxis. This action in stopping bleeding upward is also connected to its action in subduing rebellious Qi, a pathology that is often present in bleeding upwards.

Thirdly, although the ancient texts seldom stress this function, BL-17 can nourish Blood if used with direct moxibustion: it is therefore used for Deficiency of Blood of any organ. It is usually combined with the Back Transporting points to nourish the Blood of the relevant organs. For example, it is combined with BL-18 Ganshu to nourish Liver-Blood, with BL-15 Xinshu to nourish Heart-Blood and with BL-20 Pishu to promote the Spleen function of producing Blood.

Fourthly, BL-17 moves Qi in the diaphragm and chest and is used for feeling of oppression and pain of the chest and fullness in the epigastrium.

Fifthly, BL-17 pacifies Stomach-Qi and it subdues rebellious Stomach-Qi, which is Stomach-Qi going upwards instead of downwards. It therefore treats such symptoms as hiccup, belching, nausea and vomiting.

Sixthly, BL-17 has a general tonification effect on all Qi and Blood of the whole body, if used with direct moxibustion. To this effect, it is usually combined with BL-19 Danshu, and the combination of these two points is called the 'Four Flowers'.[5]

Another combination to tonify Qi and Blood in general is with BL-18 Ganshu and BL-20 Pishu, with direct moxibustion. This combination is called the 'Magnificent Six' (counting each point bilaterally).

Box 60.14 summarizes the functions of BL-17.

BL-18 GANSHU *LIVER BACK TRANSPORTING POINT*

Location

1.5 *cun* lateral to the lower border of the spinous process of T-9.

Box 60.14 BL-17 – summary of functions

- Invigorates Blood (heart pain, stabbing chest pain)
- Cools Blood
- Stops bleeding (coughing of blood, vomiting of blood, nosebleed)
- Nourishes Blood (with direct moxa)
- Opens the chest and diaphragm
- Subdues rebellious Qi (epigastric pain, vomiting, hiccup, difficult digestion, sour regurgitation)
- Benefits the sinews (Painful Obstruction Syndrome (*Bi* Syndrome) of the whole body, pain in the whole body, swelling, distension and pain of the body)
- Tonifies Qi and Blood (with BL-19 Danshu)

Nature

Back Transporting point for the Liver.

Actions

Resolves Damp-Heat.
Clears Heat.
Moves Liver-Qi and eliminates stagnation.
Brightens the eyes.
Benefits the sinews.
Extinguishes Wind.
Nourishes Liver-Blood.
Invigorates Liver-Blood.
Stops bleeding.

Indications

Jaundice.
Distension and pain of the hypochondrium, epigastric pain, abdominal pain, hypogastric pain.
Blurred vision, red eyes, diminished night vision, excessive lacrimation, redness, pain and itching of the eyes, pain in upper orbit.
Lumbar pain, pain in the neck and shoulders, muscle cramps, pain in the sinews.
Rigidity of neck and spine, lockjaw, opisthotonos, tetany.
Dizziness, blurred vision.
Abdominal masses (*Ji Ju*).
Coughing blood, vomiting blood, nosebleed.

Comments

BL-18 can be used in most Liver patterns, such as for stagnation of Liver-Qi, retention of Damp-Heat in Liver and Gall Bladder, Liver-Fire, Blood stasis in the Liver, Liver-Blood deficiency. It is frequently used to move stagnant Liver-Qi causing distension of the epigastrium and hypochondrium, sour regurgitation, nausea, etc. In resolving Damp-Heat it can be used for jaundice and cholecystitis.

As it invigorates Blood, it can be used for abdominal masses (*Ji Ju*) from Blood stasis (*Ji*). However, BL-18 can also be used for Liver Deficiency patterns, such as deficiency of Liver-Blood; in this case it should be needled with reinforcing method, or only direct moxibustion should be applied. When used to nourish Liver-Blood, it can be combined with BL-17 Geshu.

When needled with reducing method, BL-18 can be used to extinguish interior Wind. Finally, BL-18 can be used to promote vision in all eye disorders related to a Liver disharmony, such as poor night vision, blurred vision, floaters in the eyes, red and painful and swollen eyes.

Box 60.15 summarizes the functions of BL-18.

> **Box 60.15 BL-18 – summary of functions**
>
> - Resolves Damp-Heat (jaundice)
> - Clears Heat
> - Moves Liver-Qi and eliminates stagnation (distension and pain of the hypochondrium, epigastric pain, abdominal pain, hypogastric pain)
> - Brightens the eyes (blurred vision, red eyes, diminished night vision, excessive lacrimation, redness, pain and itching of the eyes, pain in upper orbit)
> - Benefits the sinews (lumbar pain, pain in the neck and shoulders, muscle cramps, pain in the sinews)
> - Extinguishes Wind (rigidity of neck and spine, lockjaw, opisthotonos, tetany)
> - Nourishes Liver-Blood (dizziness, blurred vision)
> - Invigorates Liver-Blood (abdominal masses (*Ji Ju*))
> - Stops bleeding (coughing blood, vomiting blood, nosebleed)

BL-19 DANSHU *GALL BLADDER BACK TRANSPORTING POINT*

Location

1.5 *cun* lateral to the lower border of the spinous process of T-10.

Nature

Back Transporting point for the Gall Bladder.

Actions

Resolves Damp-Heat in Liver and Gall Bladder.
Subdues rebellious Qi.
Tonifies Gall Bladder Qi.
Regulates the Lesser Yang.
Tonifies Deficiency.

Indications

Jaundice, yellow sclera, bitter taste.
Distension and pain of the chest and hypochondrium, vomiting, difficulty in swallowing, retching.
Timidity, dithering, depression, palpitations.
Alternation of feeling of heat and feeling of cold, dry throat, blurred vision, hypochondrial distension.
'Steaming bones', night sweating, fever from Yin deficiency, dry throat.

Comments

BL-19 is an important point to resolve Damp-Heat from the Liver and Gall Bladder and is therefore used in cholecystitis and jaundice.

It pacifies the Stomach and subdues rebellious Stomach-Qi, which makes it useful to treat belching, nausea and vomiting.

Similar to BL-17 Geshu, it relaxes the diaphragm, and is used for hiccup and a feeling of fullness under the diaphragm, usually caused by stagnation of Liver-Qi.

The Gall Bladder pertains to the Lesser Yang and BL-19 is an important point to eliminate pathogenic factors from the Lesser Yang in the Lesser Yang Pattern within the Six Stages (ch. 44) or the pattern of Gall Bladder Heat within the Four Levels (ch. 45).

Box 60.16 summarizes the functions of BL-19.

> **Box 60.16 BL-19 – summary of functions**
>
> - Resolves Damp-Heat in Liver and Gall Bladder (jaundice, yellow sclera, bitter taste)
> - Subdues rebellious Qi (distension and pain of the chest and hypochondrium, vomiting, difficulty in swallowing, retching)
> - Tonifies Gall Bladder Qi (timidity, dithering, depression, palpitations)
> - Regulates the Lesser Yang (alternation of feeling of heat and feeling of cold, dry throat, blurred vision, hypochondrial distension)
> - Tonifies Deficiency ('Steaming bones', night sweating, fever from Yin deficiency, dry throat)

BL-20 PISHU *SPLEEN BACK TRANSPORTING POINT*

Location
1.5 *cun* lateral to the lower border of the spinous process of T-11.

Nature
Back Transporting point for the Spleen.

Actions
Tonifies Spleen and Stomach.
Resolves Dampness.
Regulates the Intestines.
Lifts Spleen-Qi and stops bleeding.
Nourishes Blood.

Indications
Poor appetite, tiredness, loose stools, weak limbs, abdominal distension.
Feeling of fullness, feeling of heaviness, sticky taste, jaundice, feeling of heaviness of the limbs.
Abdominal distension and pain, borborygmi, diarrhoea, undigested food in stools.
Prolapse of stomach or uterus, bearing-down feeling in the lower abdomen.

Comments
BL-20 is a very important point among all the Back Transporting points. It is a major point to tonify the Spleen and Stomach and invigorate the Spleen function of transformation and transportation. It is used in any Spleen-Qi deficiency pattern with symptoms of tiredness, loose stools, no appetite, abdominal distension. Combined with BL-21 Weishu, it provides a powerful tonification of the Root of Post-Heaven Qi, i.e. Stomach and Spleen, and is used to tonify Qi and Blood when a person is physically and mentally exhausted over a long period of time.

By tonifying Spleen-Qi, this point also resolves Dampness and Phlegm, which derive from the dysfunction of the Spleen activity of transformation and transportation of fluids. BL-20 is therefore used in practically every condition with chronic Dampness or Phlegm.

By tonifying Spleen-Qi, BL-20 also nourishes Blood as the Spleen is the origin of Blood. This point is therefore very much used to nourish Blood, often in combination with BL-23 Shenshu. In this case the point should be tonified or direct moxa applied.

As it tonifies Spleen-Qi, it strengthens two other aspects of Spleen-Qi. It lifts Spleen-Qi when this is sinking and causing a prolapse or simply a bearing-down feeling in the lower abdomen. By tonifying Spleen-Qi, it stops bleeding caused by deficient Spleen-Qi not holding the Blood in the vessels. When it is used for excessive menstrual bleeding, it is combined with BL-23 Shenshu.

In conclusion, BL-20 is a very important point to be reinforced in nearly all chronic diseases when the person is very depleted in energy.

Box 60.17 summarizes the functions of BL-20.

Box 60.17 BL-20 – summary of functions

- Tonifies Spleen and Stomach (poor appetite, tiredness, loose stools, weak limbs, abdominal distension)
- Resolves Dampness (feeling of fullness, feeling of heaviness, sticky taste, jaundice, feeling of heaviness of the limbs)
- Regulates the Intestines (abdominal distension and pain, borborygmi, diarrhoea, undigested food in stools)
- Lifts Spleen-Qi and stops bleeding (prolapse of stomach or uterus, bearing-down feeling in the lower abdomen)
- Nourishes Blood
- Very important tonifying point

BL-21 WEISHU *STOMACH BACK TRANSPORTING POINT*

Location
1.5 *cun* lateral to the lower border of the spinous process of T-12.

Nature
Back Transporting point for the Stomach.

Actions
Subdues rebellious Stomach-Qi.
Tonifies the Stomach.
Resolves Dampness.

Indications
Epigastric pain, epigastric distension and fullness, vomiting, sour regurgitation.
Thin body, lack of appetite, tiredness, weak limbs.
Oedema, jaundice.

Comments

BL-21, like BL-20 Pishu, is a major point to tonify Stomach- and Spleen-Qi. It tonifies both Stomach-Qi and Spleen-Qi, and is often combined with BL-20 Pishu to tonify Qi and Blood in general. The main difference with BL-20 is in the direction of Qi stimulated by the point: BL-21 stimulates the descending of Stomach-Qi, whereas BL-20 stimulates the ascending of Spleen-Qi. Hence the use of BL-21 to subdue ascending Stomach-Qi when this causes belching, hiccup, nausea and vomiting.

BL-21 also resolves Dampness, by tonifying Spleen-Qi and promoting the Spleen function of transformation and transportation of fluids.

Finally, when needled with reducing method, BL-21 stimulates the descending of Stomach-Qi and relieves retention of food in the Stomach, the cause of fullness of the epigastrium, sour regurgitation and belching.

Box 60.18 summarizes the functions of BL-21.

Box 60.18 BL-21 – summary of functions

- Subdues rebellious Stomach-Qi (epigastric pain, epigastric distension and fullness, vomiting, sour regurgitation)
- Tonifies the Stomach (thin body, lack of appetite, tiredness, weak limbs)
- Resolves Dampness (oedema, jaundice)

BL-22 SANJIAOSHU *TRIPLE BURNER BACK TRANSPORTING POINT*

Location

1.5 *cun* lateral to the lower border of the spinous process of L-1.

Nature

Back Transporting point for the Triple Burner.

Actions

Resolves Dampness.
Opens the Water passages in the Lower Burner.
Invigorates Blood.
Regulates the Lesser Yang.

Indications

Oedema, difficult urination, turbid urine, blood in the urine.
Abdominal masses (both *Zheng Jia* and *Ji Ju*).
Alternation of feeling of heat and feeling of cold, headaches, dizziness, bitter taste.

Comments

BL-22 is a major point to stimulate the transformation, transportation and excretion of fluids in the Lower Burner. The Lower Burner keeps the Water passages open so that 'dirty' fluids may be excreted. This point regulates this particular function of the Lower Burner and thus ensures that the Water passages are open, fluids are properly transformed and dirty fluids excreted.

By stimulating the transformation and excretion of fluids, it resolves Dampness in the Lower Burner and treats such symptoms as urinary retention, painful urination, oedema of the legs, and any other manifestation of Dampness in the Lower Burner.

BL-22 invigorates Blood and does so primarily by promoting the transformation and excretion of fluids in the Lower Burner: from this point of view, its function is similar to that of the herb Ze Lan *Herba Lycopi lucidi*.

The effect of this point on the Lesser Yang channels and Lesser Yang pattern requires an explanation. As we have seen in chapter 3, the Triple Burner is like the 'envoy' of the Original Qi (*Yuan Qi*) emerging from the space between the kidneys; put differently, the Triple Burner helps the Original Qi to 'differentiate' into its different aspects in different parts of the body. Chapter 66 of the 'Classic of Difficulties' discusses the connection between the Original Qi (in this chapter called *Dong Qi*, 'Motive Force') and the Triple Burner. It says: '*The Original Qi is the Motive Force [Dong Qi] situated between the two kidneys, it is life-giving and it is the root of the 12 channels. The Triple Burner causes the Original Qi to differentiate [for its different uses around the body]; the Original Qi passes through the Three Burners and then spreads to the five Yin and six Yang organs and their channels.*'[6]

BL-22 is just above BL-23, Back Transporting point of the Kidneys, so this is the area from where the Triple Burner helps the Original Qi to emerge from the Kidneys and spread to the Internal Organs (Fig. 60.3). Because of its connection with the Triple Burner, this point can be used for the Lesser Yang Pattern.

Moreover, the point 1.5 *cun* lateral to BL-22 is BL-51 Huangmen, which, although situated in the Lower Burner, has an upward 'movement' and it affects the breast and the area below the heart (*Huang*). For this

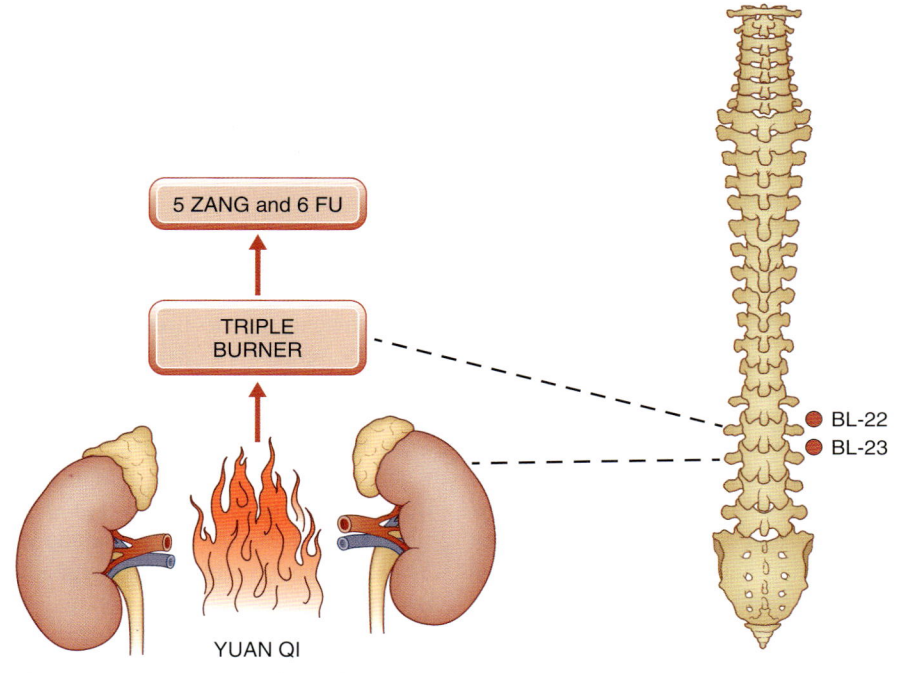

Figure 60.3 BL-22 Sanjiaoshu and the Original Qi

reason too, although BL-22 affects the Lower Burner, it also has an upward 'movement' and it can be used for headache and dizziness.

Box 60.19 summarizes the functions of BL-22.

Box 60.19 BL-22 – summary of functions

- Resolves Dampness
- Opens the Water passages in the Lower Burner (oedema, difficult urination, turbid urine, blood in the urine)
- Invigorates Blood (abdominal masses (both *Zheng Jia* and *Ji Ju*))
- Regulates the Lesser Yang (alternation of feeling of heat and feeling of cold, headaches, dizziness, bitter taste)

BL-23 SHENSHU *KIDNEY BACK TRANSPORTING POINT*

Location

1.5 *cun* lateral to the lower border of the spinous process of L-2.

Nature

Back Transporting point for the Kidneys.

Actions

Tonifies the Kidneys and nourishes the Kidney-Essence.
Consolidates Kidney-Qi.
Strengthens the lower back.
Nourishes Blood.
Benefits bones and Marrow.
Resolves Dampness and benefits urination.
Strengthens the Kidney function of reception of Qi.
Strengthens the Uterus and the Directing, Governing and Penetrating Vessels.
Brightens the eyes.
Benefits the ears.

Indications

Tiredness, exhaustion, lack of will-power, depression, impotence, lack of sexual desire.
Seminal emissions, nocturnal emissions, premature ejaculation.
Lower backache, feeling of cold in the back, weak and cold knees.
Blood deficiency, blurred vision, dizziness, tiredness, scanty periods.

Bone diseases, weak bones, osteoporosis, poor memory, poor concentration, dizziness.
Oedema, difficult urination, turbid urine, nocturnal enuresis, incontinence of urine, frequent urination, nocturia, dripping of urine, blood in urine.
Chronic asthma from Kidney deficiency.
Amenorrhoea, scanty periods, irregular periods, infertility, Cold in the Uterus, heavy periods (from Deficiency).
Blurred vision, dry eyes, diminished vision in the elderly, glaucoma, diminished night vision.
Tinnitus, deafness.

Comments

BL-23 is one of the major points of the body and the main point to tonify the Kidneys. This point must be used (obviously with reinforcing method) in any chronic Kidney deficiency. Being on the back (a Yang surface) it is slightly better to tonify Kidney-Yang, but it can also be used to nourish Kidney-Yin. The main difference between its use for tonifying Kidney-Yang or Kidney-Yin is in the use of moxa: this would be used to tonify Kidney-Yang, but not to tonify Kidney-Yin. This point can therefore be used in the treatment of any Kidney deficiency whether Yin or Yang. It strengthens all aspects of the Kidneys: Kidney-Yin, Kidney-Yang, Kidney-Essence, Kidney-Qi and the Kidney's receiving of Qi from the Lungs.

It is also one of the main points to nourish the Kidney-Essence (the other is Ren-4 Guanyuan) and is used for impotence, nocturnal emissions, infertility, spermatorrhoea and lack of sexual desire. It is also very frequently used for chronic asthma with Kidney deficiency to stimulate the Kidney function of receiving Qi.

The Kidneys store Essence and are the foundation of life. Essence is the material foundation for the Mind. If Essence is strong and flourishing, the Mind will be happy and positive. If Essence is weak, the body is always weak and exhausted, and the Mind also will suffer, with a lack of will-power, negativity, a lack of initiative and depression. In all these cases, BL-23 is a powerful tonic for the Kidneys and their mental aspect: it will stimulate the Mind, strengthen the will-power, stimulate the spirit of initiative and lift depression. This effect is particularly strong if BL-23 is combined with BL-52 Zhishi.

As the Kidneys influence the lower back, this point is very frequently used to strengthen the lower back in chronic backache. Indeed, it is a point which should be always employed for the treatment of chronic lower backache.

As the Kidneys play a role in the formation of Blood, this point is frequently used in combination with BL-20 Pishu to promote the formation of Blood in Blood deficiency.

As the Kidneys control the bones and produce Marrow, this point is also used in any bone pathology (such as arthritic bone deformities, osteoporosis and osteomalacia) and to nourish Marrow in a Chinese medicine sense. It is therefore used in symptoms of deficiency of the Sea of Marrow: that is, dizziness, poor memory, tinnitus, weak legs, blurred vision, fatigue and a constant desire to sleep.[7]

This point also resolves Dampness from the Lower Burner. It is commonly said that the Kidney cannot have Excess patterns: this is not entirely true, as they can suffer from retention of Dampness in conjunction with the Bladder. In these cases, BL-23 can be needled with reducing method together with BL-28 Pangguangshu and SP-9 Yinlingquan to resolve Dampness from the Lower Burner. In this connection, it is used for the treatment of acute urinary stones.

BL-23 is also an important point to strengthen the Uterus and regulate menstruation due to the connection between the Uterus and the Kidneys (via the Uterus Channel *Bao Luo*). This point therefore strengthens the Directing, Governing and Penetrating Vessels but only in relation to the Uterus and menstruation. In particular, it is an important point to consolidate the Governing, Directing and Penetrating Vessels in excessive menstrual bleeding from a Spleen and Kidney deficiency (in combination with BL-20 Pishu).

The Kidneys open into the ears, and this point can treat all chronic ear problems related to Kidney deficiency, mostly tinnitus and deafness. It is not indicated for the treatment of acute ear problems (such as otitis or ear infections) as these would be treated more via the Triple Burner and Gall Bladder channels.

Finally, the Kidneys also influence the eyes and vision. Kidney-Yin nourishes and moistens the eyes and promotes good sight. Many chronic eye disorders, such as poor vision and dry eyes in the elderly, are the result of a deficiency of Kidney-Yin failing to nourish and moisten the eyes. BL-23 is the main point to affect the eyes in these cases.

Box 60.20 summarizes the functions of BL-23.

> **Box 60.20 BL-23 – summary of functions**
>
> - Tonifies the Kidneys and nourishes the Kidney-Essence (tiredness, exhaustion, lack of will-power, depression, impotence, lack of sexual desire)
> - Consolidates Kidney-Qi (seminal emissions, nocturnal emissions, premature ejaculation)
> - Strengthens the lower back (lower backache, feeling of cold in the back, weak and cold knees)
> - Nourishes Blood (blood deficiency, blurred vision, dizziness, tiredness, scanty periods)
> - Benefits bones and Marrow (bone diseases, weak bones, osteoporosis, poor memory, poor concentration, dizziness)
> - Resolves Dampness and benefits urination (oedema, difficult urination, turbid urine, nocturnal enuresis, incontinence of urine, frequent urination, nocturia, dripping of urine, blood in urine)
> - Strengthens the Kidney function of reception of Qi (chronic asthma from Kidney deficiency)
> - Strengthens the Uterus and the Directing, Governing and Penetrating Vessels (amenorrhoea, scanty periods, irregular periods, infertility, Cold in the Uterus, heavy periods (from Deficiency))
> - Brightens the eyes (blurred vision, dry eyes, diminished vision in the elderly, glaucoma, diminished night vision)
> - Benefits the ears (tinnitus, deafness)

BL-24 QIHAISHU *SEA OF QI BACK TRANSPORTING POINT*

Location

1.5 *cun* lateral to the lower border of the spinous process of L-3.

Nature

None.

Actions

Strengthens the lower back.
Regulates menstruation.
Invigorates Blood.

Indications

Lower backache, stiffness of the lower back, Painful Obstruction Syndrome (*Bi* Syndrome) of the legs.
Painful periods, irregular periods, leukorrhoea.
Haemorrhoids, bleeding haemorrhoids, blood in the stools.

Comments

BL-24 is not a major point in terms of its energetic action, but it is frequently used as a local point in chronic or acute lower backache.

Apart from this, it also invigorates Blood and eliminates stasis in the Lower Burner, and is therefore used for uterine bleeding and irregular menstruation.

Box 60.21 summarizes the functions of BL-24.

> **Box 60.21 BL-24 – summary of functions**
>
> - Strengthens the lower back (lower backache, stiffness of the lower back, Painful Obstruction Syndrome (*Bi* Syndrome) of the legs)
> - Regulates menstruation (painful periods, irregular periods, leukorrhoea)
> - Invigorates Blood (haemorrhoids, bleeding haemorrhoids, blood in the stools)

BL-25 DACHANGSHU *LARGE INTESTINE BACK TRANSPORTING POINT*

Location

1.5 *cun* lateral to the lower border of the spinous process of L-4.

Nature

Back Transporting point for the Large Intestine.

Actions

Promotes the function of the Large Intestine.
Strengthens the lower back.

Indications

Borborygmi, diarrhoea, undigested food in the stools, blood in the stools, difficult bowel evacuation, constipation, prolapse of rectum, abdominal distension and pain, hypogastric pain, umbilical pain.
Lower backache, stiffness of lower back, Painful Obstruction Syndrome (*Bi* Syndrome) of the legs.

Comments

First of all, BL-25 point promotes the excreting function of the Large Intestine and can be used to treat both constipation and diarrhoea: for the latter, it is often used in combination with BL-20 Pishu. Being the Back

Transporting point, it is especially indicated for any chronic disease of the Large Intestine.

BL-25 is also indicated in Excess patterns of the Large Intestine to relieve abdominal fullness and distension.

It is also frequently used as a local point for both chronic or acute lower backache. In acute backache, this point is often tender on pressure and, if so, it should be needled with reducing method.

Box 60.22 summarizes the functions of BL-25.

> **Box 60.22 BL-25 – summary of functions**
> - Promotes the function of the Large Intestine (borborygmi, diarrhoea, undigested food in the stools, blood in the stools, difficult bowel evacuation, constipation, prolapse of rectum, abdominal distension and pain, hypogastric pain, umbilical pain)
> - Strengthens the lower back (lower backache, stiffness of lower back, Painful Obstruction Syndrome (*Bi* Syndrome) of the legs)

BL-26 GUANYUANSHU ORIGIN GATE BACK TRANSPORTING POINT

Location
1.5 *cun* lateral to the lower border of the spinous process of L-5.

Nature
None.

Actions
Strengthens the lower back.
Moves Qi and Blood in the Lower Burner.
Benefits urination.

Indications
Lower backache, sciatica, pain in the buttocks, weakness or stiffness of the lower back, difficulty in bending the back.
Abdominal distension and pain, abdominal masses (*Ji Ju*).
Enuresis, frequent urination, difficult urination.

Comments
BL-26 is very frequently used as a local point in chronic lower backache and should always be used if tender on pressure. In my experience, this is the most effective point for lower backache (both bilateral and unilateral) and it is nearly always tender on pressure. It is very close to the sacroiliac joint, which is often involved in lower backache. I use BL-26 nearly always in conjunction with BL-23 Shenshu and with the extra point Shiqizhuixia, which is on the Governing Vessel below the tip of L-5.

Box 60.23 summarizes the functions of BL-26.

> **Box 60.23 BL-26 – summary of functions**
> - Strengthens the lower back (lower backache, sciatica, pain in the buttocks, weakness or stiffness of the lower back, difficulty in bending the back)
> - Moves Qi and Blood in the Lower Burner (abdominal distension and pain, abdominal masses (*Ji Ju*))
> - Benefits urination (enuresis, frequent urination, difficult urination)

BL-27 XIAOCHANGSHU SMALL INTESTINE BACK TRANSPORTING POINT

Location
1.5 *cun* lateral to the midline at the level of the first sacral foramen.

Nature
Back Transporting Point for the Small Intestine.

Actions
Promotes the function of the Small Intestine.
Resolves Dampness.
Benefits urination.

Indications
Diarrhoea, blood and mucus in the stools, constipation, difficult bowel evacuation, abdominal pain.
Dark urine, enuresis, retention of urine, difficult urination, blood in the urine.

Comments
BL-27 point stimulates the Small Intestine function of receiving and separating, and can be used in any Small Intestine pattern, with such symptoms as borborygmi, abdominal pain and mucus in the stools. BL-27 also

eliminates Damp-Heat from the Lower Burner and benefits urination, so that it can be used to treat such symptoms as cloudy urine, difficult urination and burning on urination. This point's effect on the urinary function is due partly to the relationship between the Small Intestine and Bladder within the Greater Yang channels and partly to the functional relationship between these two organs. In fact, the Small Intestine separates the fluids it receives from the Stomach into a 'clean' part, which goes to the Bladder for excretion as urine, and a 'dirty' part, which goes to the Large Intestine partly for reabsorption and partly for excretion in the stools (see Fig. 14.2 in ch. 14).

Box 60.24 summarizes the functions of BL-27.

Box 60.24 BL-27 – summary of functions

- Promotes the function of the Small Intestine (diarrhoea, blood and mucus in the stools, constipation, difficult bowel evacuation, abdominal pain)
- Resolves Dampness
- Benefits urination (dark urine, enuresis, retention of urine, difficult urination, blood in the urine)

BL-28 PANGGUANGSHU *BLADDER BACK TRANSPORTING POINT*

Location

1.5 *cun* lateral to the midline at the level of the second sacral foramen.

Nature

Back Transporting point for the Bladder.

Actions

Regulates the Bladder.
Resolves Dampness in Lower Burner.
Eliminates stagnation and dissolves masses.
Opens the Water passages in the Lower Burner.
Strengthens the lower back.

Indications

Difficult urination, dark urine, retention of urine, enuresis, turbid urine.
Swelling of external genitalia, ulcers on genitals, itching in genitals, swelling and pain of the vagina, swelling of penis.
Abdominal pain, abdominal masses (*Ji Ju*), constipation.
Stiffness and pain of the sacrum, lower backache, stiffness of the lower back, pain in buttocks, numbness of legs, sciatica.

Comments

BL-28 is very much used in urinary disorders. Firstly, it expels Dampness from the Bladder and the Lower Burner and it can therefore treat retention of urine, difficult urination and cloudy urine. It also clears Heat from the Bladder and can be used for painful and burning urination. Combined with BL-23 Shenshu and SP-9 Yinlingquan, it is used to expel renal stones.

BL-28 also generally opens the Water passages of the Lower Burner and ensures that the dirty fluids are transformed and excreted. It is a point that is often combined with BL-20 Pishu to transform fluids in the Lower Burner and promote diuresis.

Combined with BL-23 Shenshu, it strengthens the lower back and it is especially used for pain in the buttocks and sciatica.

Box 60.25 summarizes the functions of BL-28.

Box 60.25 BL-28 – summary of functions

- Regulates the Bladder (difficult urination, dark urine, retention of urine, enuresis, turbid urine)
- Resolves Dampness in Lower Burner (swelling of external genitalia, ulcers on genitals, itching in genitals, swelling and pain of the vagina, swelling of penis)
- Eliminates stagnation and dissolves masses (abdominal pain, abdominal masses (*Ji Ju*), constipation)
- Opens the Water passages in the Lower Burner
- Strengthens the lower back (stiffness and pain of the sacrum, lower backache, stiffness of the lower back, pain in buttocks, numbness of legs, sciatica)

BL-30 BAIHUANSHU *WHITE RING TRANSPORTING POINT*

Location

1.5 *cun* lateral to the midline at the level of the fourth sacral foramen.

Nature

None.

Actions

Benefits the anus.
Strengthens the lower back and legs.
Regulates menstruation.
Firms Qi.

Indications

Itchy anus, prolapse of anus and/or rectum, haemorrhoids, difficult defecation.
Pain in the lower back and sacrum.
Irregular periods, painful periods, heavy periods.
Seminal emissions, leukorrhoea.

Comments

BL-30 has an effect on the anus, and is mostly used for anal problems, such as haemorrhoids, prolapse of anus, spasm of anus and incontinence of faeces.

'White Ring' in its name refers to the anus.
Box 60.26 summarizes the functions of BL-30.

Box 60.26 BL-30 – summary of functions

- Benefits the anus (itchy anus, prolapse of anus and/or rectum, haemorrhoids, difficult defecation)
- Strengthens the lower back and legs (pain in the lower back and sacrum)
- Regulates menstruation (irregular periods, painful periods, heavy periods)
- Firms Qi (seminal emissions, leukorrhoea)

BL-32 CILIAO *SECOND CREVICE*

Location

Over the second sacral foramen.

Nature

None.

Actions

Benefits urination and defecation.
Regulates menstruation and resolves Dampness.
Strengthens the lower back.

Indications

Painful urination, dark urine, retention of urine, enuresis, difficulty in urination and defecation, constipation, borborygmi, diarrhoea.
Leukorrhoea, painful periods, irregular periods, infertility, labour pain.
Lower backache, sacral pain, numbness of lower back, lower backache radiating to genitals, sciatica.

Comments

The four points BL-31, BL-32, BL-33 and BL-34 are called the *Four Crevices* because the word 'liao' means 'crevice'. They are called that because the points lie in the four sacral foramina. For this reason, BL-31 Shangliao is called 'Upper crevice', BL-32 Ciliao 'Second crevice', BL-33 Zhongliao 'Middle crevice' and BL-34 Xialiao 'Lower crevice'.

However, BL-32 Ciliao is the most important of these four points, with the broadest indications and the one which is most tonifying to the Kidneys and the Essence. BL-32 is an important point to use for the treatment of infertility in women. It is used for painful periods when the pain is on the sacrum.

In addition, this point is also used to stimulate the ascending of Qi in prolapse of the anus or uterus.

BL-36 CHENGFU *RECEIVING SUPPORT*

Location

On the posterior aspect of the thigh, in the middle of the transverse gluteal fold.

Nature

None.

Actions

Removes obstructions from the channel.
Treats haemorrhoids.

Indications

Sciatica, lower backache, sacral pain.
Chronic haemorrhoids, bleeding haemorrhoids.

Comments

This point is mostly used as a local point for lower backache with pain radiating down the back of the leg (sciatica). When needled, one should try and obtain the radiation of the needling sensation down the leg.

Although it has an effect on haemorrhoids, the two points BL-57 Chengshan and BL-58 Feiyang are more frequently used for this purpose.

Box 60.27 summarizes the functions of BL-36.

> **Box 60.27 BL-36 – summary of functions**
>
> - Removes obstructions from the channel (sciatica, lower backache, sacral pain)
> - Treats haemorrhoids (chronic haemorrhoids, bleeding haemorrhoids)

BL-37 YINMEN *HUGE GATE*

Location

On the posterior aspect of the thigh, 6 *cun* below BL-36 Chengfu, on the line connecting BL-36 and BL-40 Weizhong.

Nature

None.

Actions

Benefits the lower back.

Indications

Lower backache, sacral pain, sciatica.

Comments

BL-37 is also frequently used as a local point for pain radiating down the back of the leg. It is particularly effective if it is gently heated with a moxa stick.

Box 60.28 summarizes the functions of BL-37.

> **Box 60.28 BL-37 – summary of functions**
>
> - Benefits the lower back (lower backache, sacral pain, sciatica)

BL-39 WEIYANG *SUPPORTING YANG*

Location

At the lateral end of the popliteal transverse crease, on the medial side of the tendon of the biceps femoris muscle.

Nature

Lower Sea point for the Lower Burner.

Actions

Opens the Water passages in the Lower Burner.
Stimulates the transformation and excretion of fluids in the Lower Burner.
Benefits the Bladder.

Indications

Oedema in the lower part of the body.
Difficult urination, retention of urine, painful urination, enuresis.

Comments

BL-39 is an important point to stimulate the transformation and excretion of fluids in the Lower Burner. It ensures that the Water passages of the Lower Burner are unobstructed so that dirty fluids can be excreted properly. It is therefore used in all Excess patterns of the Lower Burner characterized by the accumulation of fluids in the form of Dampness or oedema: this could manifest with urinary retention, burning on urination, difficult urination or oedema of the ankles.

In particular, when the Lower Burner is in Excess, i.e. its Water passages are obstructed (manifested with retention of urine), this point should be reduced so as to open the Water passages and stimulate the excretion of fluids. If the Lower Burner is Deficient, i.e. the Water passages are in a relaxed state and fluids are not contained (manifested with incontinence of urine or enuresis), this point should be reinforced so as to strengthen Qi in the Lower Burner and 'tighten' the Water passages so that fluids can be contained.

Box 60.29 summarizes the functions of BL-39.

> **Box 60.29 BL-39 – summary of functions**
>
> - Opens the Water passages in the Lower Burner (oedema in the lower part of the body)
> - Stimulates the transformation and excretion of fluids in the Lower Burner
> - Benefits the Bladder (difficult urination, retention of urine, painful urination, enuresis)

BL-40 WEIZHONG *SUPPORTING MIDDLE*

Location

On the midpoint of the transverse crease of the popliteal fossa, between the tendons of the biceps femoris and semitendinosus muscles.

Nature

Sea (*He*) Point.
Earth point.
Ma Dan Yang's 12 Heavenly Star point.

Actions

Clears Heat and cools Blood.
Removes obstructions from the channel.
Clears Summer-Heat.

Indications

Lower backache, sciatica, stiffness of the lower back, knee pain.
Injury by Summer-Heat, fever, aversion to cold, sweating, headache, a feeling of heaviness, an uncomfortable sensation in the epigastrium, irritability, thirst.

Comments

BL-40 is a point with a wide range of actions. Firstly, it can clear Heat and resolve Dampness from the Bladder, and it can therefore be used for the symptom of burning during urination.

It relaxes the sinews and benefits the back and it is one of the most important distal points for lower backache. It can be used for any kind of lower backache, whether chronic or acute, and of the Excess or Deficiency type. However, it is best used in acute rather than chronic and Excess rather than Deficient type of lower backache. In fact, in very weak patients with pronounced Deficient and Cold symptoms, this point should not be used as it tends to have a reducing effect and to cool Blood. In these cases, it can be replaced by BL-60 Kunlun. As far as the location of the backache is concerned, it is best used when the ache is either bilateral or unilateral, but not on the midline (i.e. on the spine itself).

BL-40 also cools Blood and it is frequently used in skin diseases characterized by Heat in the Blood.

Finally, BL-40 clears Summer-Heat and is used in acute attacks of Heat in summertime causing fever, delirium and a red skin rash.

Box 60.30 summarizes the functions of BL-40.

Box 60.30 BL-40 – summary of functions

- Clears Heat and cools Blood
- Removes obstructions from the channel (lower backache, sciatica, stiffness of the lower back, knee pain)
- Clears Summer-Heat (injury by Summer-Heat, fever, aversion to cold, sweating, headache, a feeling of heaviness, an uncomfortable sensation in the epigastrium, irritability, thirst)

BL-42 POHU DOOR OF THE CORPOREAL SOUL

Location

3 *cun* lateral to the midline, level with the lower border of the spinous process of T-3 and level with BL-13 Feishu.

Nature

This is the point on the outer Bladder line corresponding to BL-13 Feishu, the Back Transporting point for the Lungs.

Actions

Tonifies the Lungs.
Soothes the Corporeal Soul (*Po*).
Stimulates the descending of Lung-Qi.

Indications

Consumption, dry cough.
Sadness, grief, feeling of oppression of the chest, depression, suicidal thoughts, 'three corpses flowing'.
Cough, wheezing, breathlessness.

Comments

BL-42 has two main actions, on a physical and psychological level. On a physical level, it can be used to regulate and send Lung-Qi downwards in the treatment of cough and asthma.

It is also frequently used for Painful Obstruction Syndrome of the upper back and shoulders and is frequently tender on pressure. Needling this point can greatly relieve pain and stiffness of the upper back or scapula area.

On a psychological level, it is related to the Corporeal Soul ('*Po*'), which is the mental–spiritual aspect residing in the Lungs (see ch. 8). It strengthens and roots the Corporeal Soul in the Lungs. It frees breathing when the Corporeal Soul is constricted by worry, sadness or grief. It calms the Mind and settles the Corporeal Soul to make the person turn inwards and be comfortable with oneself.

It is used for emotional problems related to the Lungs, particularly sadness, grief and worry. It has a very soothing effect on the spirit and it nourishes Qi when this is dispersed by a prolonged period of sadness or grief.

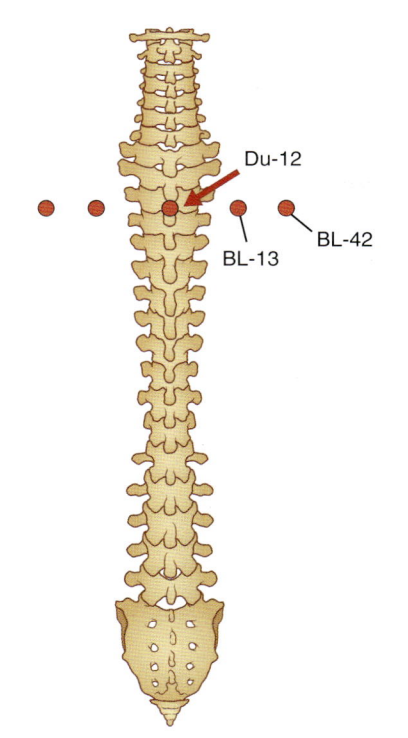

Figure 60.4 Location of BL-13 Feishu, Du-12 Shenzhu and BL-42 Pohu

The 'Explanation of the Acupuncture Points' reports the interesting indication 'three corpses flowing' for this point.[8] The association with corpses and death should be interpreted in the way that this point is indicated for suicidal thought. As we have seen above when discussing the indications of BL-13 Feishu, the Corporeal Soul is associated with *Gui* (ghosts, spirits) and with a centripetal movement eventually ending in death. For this reason, these two points are indicated for suicidal thoughts. In fact, all three Lung-related points, BL-13 Feishu, Du-12 Shenzhu and BL-42 Pohu (all on the same level), have indications to do with death (Fig. 60.4). These are:

- BL-13 Feishu: 'desire to commit suicide'
- Du-12 Shenzhu: 'desire to kill people'
- BL-42 Pohu: 'three corpses flowing'

Box 60.31 summarizes the functions of BL-42.

Box 60.31 BL-42 – summary of functions

- Tonifies the Lungs (consumption, dry cough)
- Soothes the Corporeal Soul (*Po*) (sadness, grief, feeling of oppression of the chest, depression, suicidal thoughts, 'three corpses flowing')
- Stimulates the descending of Lung-Qi (cough, wheezing, breathlessness)

BL-43 GAOHUANGSHU (or GAOHUANG) *TRANSPORTING POINT OF GAOHUANG*

Location

3 *cun* lateral to the midline, level with the lower border of the spinous process of T-4 and level with BL-14 Jueyinhsu.

Nature

This is the point on the outer Bladder line corresponding to BL-14 Jueyinshu, the Back Transporting point for the Pericardium.

Actions

Nourishes Lung-Yin.
Nourishes the Heart.
Nourishes the Essence.
Tonifies the Stomach and Spleen.

Indications

Dry cough, wheezing, coughing of blood, exhaustion, night sweating, consumption, weight loss.
Poor memory, palpitations, insomnia, dizziness.
Seminal emissions, nocturnal emissions, impotence.
Deficiency of Stomach and Spleen, undigested food in the stools, weak limbs.

Comments

BL-43 is an intriguing point. It has a very old history and is mentioned in one of the earliest references to acupuncture.[9] Its name is very difficult to translate. The two combined characters '*Gaohuang*' indicate the space between the heart and diaphragm. This is supposed to be the location of all chronic and nearly incurable diseases: hence the use of this point in very chronic diseases with great debility.

This point tonifies the Qi of the whole body and is used when the person is very debilitated after a chronic illness. In these cases, it is usually treated with direct moxibustion with moxa cones.

It nourishes the Essence, and can be used for Kidney deficiency manifesting with nocturnal emissions, low sexual energy or poor memory.

It nourishes Lung-Yin and is used to tonify the Lungs and promote the Yin after a chronic lung disease that has injured the Yin and left the person with a chronic dry cough and debility. In this case it is needled only and moxa is not used.

Finally, it invigorates the Mind, by promoting the Essence function of nourishing the brain and by nourishing the Heart. It therefore stimulates memory and lifts the spirit, especially after a long-standing disease.

Box 60.32 summarizes the functions of BL-43.

> **Box 60.32 BL-43 – summary of functions**
> - Nourishes Lung-Yin (dry cough, wheezing, coughing of blood, exhaustion, night sweating, consumption, weight loss)
> - Nourishes the Heart (poor memory, palpitations, insomnia, dizziness)
> - Nourishes the Essence (seminal emissions, nocturnal emissions, impotence)
> - Tonifies the Stomach and Spleen (deficiency of Stomach and Spleen, undigested food in the stools, weak limbs)

BL-44 SHENTANG *MIND HALL*

Location

3 *cun* lateral to the midline, level with the lower border of the spinous process of T-5 and level with BL-15 Xinshu.

Nature

This point is on the outer Bladder line in correspondence with BL-15 Xinshu, the Back Transporting point for the Heart.

Actions

Calms the Mind.
Subdues rebellious Qi.

Indications

Depression, insomnia, anxiety, mental restlessness, sadness, grief, worry.

Cough, wheezing, breathlessness, difficulty in swallowing, fullness of the chest.

Comments

BL-44 is mostly used for emotional and psychological problems related to the Heart. It is best used in conjunction with BL-15 Xinshu, for anxiety, insomnia and depression. BL-44 strengthens and calms the Mind. It stimulates the Mind's clarity and intelligence. If left in a long time (over 15 minutes) it calms the Mind and clears Heart-Fire.

Box 60.33 summarizes the functions of BL-44.

> **Box 60.33 BL-44 – summary of functions**
> - Calms the Mind (depression, insomnia, anxiety, mental restlessness, sadness, grief, worry)
> - Subdues rebellious Qi (cough, wheezing, breathlessness, difficulty in swallowing, fullness of the chest)

BL-47 HUNMEN *DOOR OF THE ETHEREAL SOUL*

Location

3 *cun* lateral to the midline, level with the lower border of the spinous process of T-9 and level with BL-18 Ganshu.

Nature

This point is on the outer Bladder line in correspondence with BL-18 Ganshu, the Back Transporting point for the Liver.

Actions

Regulates Liver-Qi and benefits the sinews.
Roots the Ethereal Soul (*Hun*).

Indications

Costal pain, hypochondrial pain, fullness of the chest, contracture of sinews.
Fear, depression, insomnia, excessive dreaming, lack of sense of direction in life, 'possession by corpse'.[10]

Comments

BL-47 is used for emotional problems related to the Liver, such as depression, frustration and resentment over a long period of time. This point settles and roots the Ethereal Soul in the Liver. It strengthens the Ethereal Soul's capacity of planning, sense of aim in life, life-dreams, and projects. It is a 'door', so this point regulates the 'coming and going' of the Ethereal Soul and Mind: that is, relationships with other people and the world in general. It has an outward movement which could be compared and contrasted with the inward movement of BL-42 Pohu.

The 'Explanation of Acupuncture Points' (1654) confirms that, due to this point's nature of 'window', 'gate' or 'door', the Ethereal Soul goes in and out through it. This confirms the dynamic nature of this point in stimulating the movement of the Ethereal Soul and Mind; however, it can also work the other way: that is, to calm down the excessive movement of the Ethereal Soul.

In my experience, when used in conjunction with BL-18 Ganshu, it has a profound influence on a person's capacity of planning his or her life by rooting and steadying the Ethereal Soul. It can help a person find a sense of direction and purpose in life. This point will also help to lift mental depression associated with such difficulties.

Because it roots the Ethereal Soul, it can be used for a vague feeling of fear occurring at night in persons suffering from severe deficiency of Yin. When used to calm down the excessive movement of the Ethereal Soul, this point can be used for slightly manic behaviour and mental confusion.

On a physical level, this point is very useful in treating stagnant Liver-Qi insulting the Lungs (as it happens in some types of asthma).

Box 60.34 summarizes the functions of BL-47.

BL-49 YISHE *INTELLECT ABODE*

Location

3 *cun* lateral to the midline, level with the lower border of the spinous process of T-11 and level with BL-20 Pishu.

Nature

This point is on the outer Bladder line in correspondence with BL-20 Pishu, the Back Transporting point for the Spleen.

Actions

Resolves Damp-Heat.
Benefits the Intellect (*Yi*).

Indications

Abdominal fullness, hypochondrial distension, diarrhoea, vomiting, feeling of heat, yellow sclera and complexion.
Poor memory, poor concentration, worry, pensiveness, obsessive thinking.

Comments

BL-49 strengthens the Intellect (*Yi*), clears the Mind (*Shen*) and stimulates memory and concentration. It also relieves the Mind and Intellect of obsessive thoughts, brooding, worry and pensiveness. It can also be used for obsessive thoughts, which are often related to a Spleen deficiency and are like the pathological correspondent of this organ's mental activity of memorization and concentration.

On a physical level, this point can be used with direct moxa to dry the Spleen of Dampness and also to tonify the Lungs (according to the principle of strengthening Earth to tonify Metal). 'An Explanation of the Acupuncture Points' says: '*The Spleen loathes Dampness and likes Dryness: moxa this point with many moxa cones.*'[11]

Box 60.35 summarizes the functions of BL-49.

Box 60.34 BL-47 – summary of functions

- Regulates Liver-Qi and benefits the sinews (costal pain, hypochondrial pain, fullness of the chest, contracture of sinews)
- Roots the Ethereal Soul (*Hun*) (fear, depression, insomnia, excessive dreaming, lack of sense of direction in life, 'possession by corpse')
- In my experience, this point can regulate the 'coming and going' of the Ethereal Soul and help a person develop a sense of direction and purpose in life

---

Box 60.35 BL-49 – summary of functions

- Resolves Damp-Heat (abdominal fullness, hypochondrial distension, diarrhoea, vomiting, feeling of heat, yellow sclera and complexion)
- Benefits the Intellect (*Yi*) (poor memory, poor concentration, worry, pensiveness, obsessive thinking)

BL-51 HUANGMEN *DOOR OF GAOHUANG*

Location

3 *cun* lateral to the midline, level with the lower border of the spinous process of L-1 and level with BL-22 Sanjiaoshu.

Nature

This point is on the outer Bladder line in correspondence with BL-22 Sanjiaoshu, the Back Transporting point for the Triple Burner.

Actions

Regulates the Triple Burner.
Ensures the smooth spread of the Triple Burner Qi to the heart region.
Benefits the breasts.

Indications

Fullness and hardness below the heart.
Breast diseases, fullness, distension and pain of the breasts, breast lumps.

Comments

BL-51 is another intriguing point, and in order to understand its functions, we have to recollect one of the Triple Burner functions. As was mentioned in the chapter on the functions of the Yang organs, one of the Triple Burner's functions is that of being the 'ambassador', 'envoy' or the 'avenue' through which the Original Qi comes out of the Kidneys and spreads to the Internal Organs and the 12 channels. The Triple Burner also ensures the smooth flow of Qi in the region between the heart and diaphragm, i.e. the '*Gaohuang*' region, as mentioned in connection with point BL-43 Gaohuangshu. Hence the name of this point: '*Huang*' indicates the '*Gaohuang*' region (i.e. below the heart and above the diaphragm) and '*men*' indicates '*door*' to describe the Triple Burner's function as an entrance or outlet for Qi in this region.

However, there is another possible interpretation of this point's name. *Huang* here could refer to the *Huang* Membranes rather than to *Gaohuang* (i.e. the space below the heart and above the diaphragm). If we take *Huang* to refer to the Membranes, this would explain the effect of this point on women's breasts as these are rich in Membranes (the connective tissue of the breast).

Both interpretations are possible as the indication of this point for 'hardness below the heart' clearly refers to the *Gaohuang* region below the heart and above the diaphragm.

This point's name should be seen in conjunction with that of point BL-53 '*Baohuang*', on the outer Bladder line in correspondence with BL-28 Pangguangshu, the Back Transporting point for the Bladder. The 'Acupuncture Textbook by Hui Yuan' says that the Triple Burner penetrates upwards to the '*Gaohuang*' region, and downwards to the '*Baohuang*' region: that is, the uterus and bladder.[12] Thus, this point regulates the movement of the Triple Burner upwards to the diaphragm region, whilst the point '*Baohuang*' BL-53 regulates the movement of the Triple Burner downwards to the uterus, genitals and urinary system.

In fact, the 'Illustrated Classic of Acupuncture points as found on the Bronze Model' says that BL-51 is indicated for a feeling of tightness below the heart and diseases of the breast in women.[13] It is interesting that this point, which is in correspondence with BL-22 Sanjiaoshu, the Back Transporting point for the Lower Burner, is not indicated for diseases of the Lower Burner but for those of the Upper Burner (although it does also stimulate the transformation and excretion of fluids in the Lower Burner).

Box 60.36 summarizes the functions of BL-51.

Box 60.36 BL-51 – summary of functions

- Regulates the Triple Burner
- Ensures the smooth spread of the Triple Burner Qi to the heart region (fullness and hardness below the heart)
- Benefits the breasts (breast diseases, fullness, distension and pain of the breasts, breast lumps)

BL-52 ZHISHI *ROOM OF WILL-POWER*

Location

3 *cun* lateral to the midline, level with the lower border of the spinous process of L-2 and level with BL-23 Shenshu.

Nature

This point is on the outer Bladder line in correspondence with BL-23 Shenshu, the Back Transporting point for the Kidneys.

Actions

Tonifies the Kidneys and the Essence.
Benefits urination.
Strengthens the back.
Strengthens will-power.

Indications

Exhaustion, dizziness, tinnitus, backache, weak sexual function, impotence, infertility, premature ejaculation, nocturnal emissions.
Difficult urination, dribbling urination.
Chronic lower backache, sciatica.
Depression, lack of motivation, lack of drive, lack of will-power.

- BL-23 Shenshu, BL-52 Zhishi and BL-47 Hunmen to strengthen will-power and drive, and to instil a sense of direction and aim in one's life. This combination is excellent to treat the mental exhaustion, lack of drive and aimlessness and confusion which is typical of chronic depression
- BL-23 Shenshu, BL-52 Zhishi and BL-49 Yishe to strengthen will-power and drive and empty the Mind (*Shen*) and Intellect (*Yi*) of obsessive thoughts, worries and confused thinking
- BL-23 Shenshu, BL-52 Zhishi and BL-42 Pohu to strengthen will-power and drive, settle the Corporeal Soul (*Po*) and release emotions constrained in the chest and diaphragm
- BL-23 Shenshu, BL-52 Zhishi and BL-44 Shentang to strengthen will-power and drive, calm the mind and relieve anxiety, depression, mental restlessness and insomnia. This combination harmonizes Kidneys and Heart (and therefore Will-power and Mind) on a mental–emotional level

Comments

BL-52 is outside BL-23 Shenshu, the Back Transporting point for the Kidneys. Similar to BL-23 Shenshu, it has a tonifying effect on the Kidneys and, combined with it, reinforces its effect.

BL-52 can be used in chronic lower backache, especially if the point is tender on pressure, as it strengthens the back by tonifying the Kidneys.

This point also nourishes the Essence and can be used in male sexual problems such as impotence, lack of sexual desire and premature ejaculation; in women, it is an important point for the treatment of infertility from a Kidney deficiency.

Finally, this point strengthens will-power and determination, which are the mental–spiritual phenomena pertaining to the Kidneys. It is a very useful point in the treatment of certain types of depression, when the person lacks motivation and drive and lacks the will-power and mental strength to make an effort to get out of the spiral of depression. Needling this point with reinforcing method, especially if combined with BL-23, will stimulate the will-power and lift the spirit.

BL-52 strengthens will-power, drive, determination, the capacity of pursuing one's goals with single-mindedness, spirit of initiative and steadfastness. I often use this point if there is a Kidney deficiency, in combination with one of the other four points affecting the Spiritual Aspects of the Yin organs: that is, BL-42 Pohu, BL-44 Shentang, BL-47 Hunmen and BL-49 Yishe, as a solid mental–emotional foundation for the other aspects of the psyche. The following are some examples of such combinations:

If we analyse the names of the above five points (BL-42, BL-44, BL-47, BL-49 and BL-52), we can detect a pattern as the points correspond to a house – an image for the psyche – with the Mind (*Shen*), Will-power (*Zhi*) and Intellect (*Yi*) corresponding to 'hall', 'room' and 'abode', respectively, and the Ethereal Soul (*Hun*) and Corporeal Soul (*Po*) corresponding to a 'door' and 'window', respectively. The images of door and window fit well the nature of the Ethereal Soul and Corporeal Soul, which provide movement to the psyche, the former providing the 'coming and going of the Mind' and the latter the 'entering and exiting of the Essence'. The correspondence of the Heart to a hall also fits in with old Chinese customs according to which the hall is the most important room of the house as it is the one that gives the first impression to visitors: for this reason, it was always kept scrupulously clean. The 'Explanation of the Acupuncture Points' confirms the image of a house in the names of these five points (although it makes reference to a 'gate' that is not in these points' names and not to the 'hall'): '*There is a door, a gate, a window, an abode and a room: the image of a house.*'[14]

Box 60.37 summarizes the functions of BL-52.

BL-53 BAOHUANG *BLADDER VITALS*

Location

3 *cun* lateral to the midline, level with the lower border of the second sacral vertebra.

> **Box 60.37 BL-52 – summary of functions**
>
> - Tonifies the Kidneys and the Essence (exhaustion, dizziness, tinnitus, backache, weak sexual function, impotence, infertility, premature ejaculation, nocturnal emissions)
> - Benefits urination (difficult urination, dribbling urination)
> - Strengthens the back (chronic lower backache, sciatica)
> - Strengthens will-power (depression, lack of motivation, lack of drive, lack of will-power)
> - I often use BL-52 in conjunction with one of the other points of the outer Bladder line (BL-42, BL-44, BL-47 and BL-49)

Nature

None.

Actions

Opens the Water passages in the Lower Burner.
Stimulates the transformation and excretion of fluids and benefits the Bladder.

Indications

Hardness and fullness of the hypogastrium, retention of urine, dribbling urination, oedema.

Comments

BL-53 has a similar action to BL-22 Sanjiaoshu, in so far as it stimulates the transformation and excretion of dirty fluids in the Lower Burner. It is mostly used for urinary problems such as retention of urine, difficult urination and burning urination.

The name of this point should be seen in conjunction with BL-51 Huangmen, in so far as BL-51 controls the spread of the Triple Burner's Qi in the Upper Burner, and BL-53 controls the spread of the Triple Burner's Qi in the Lower Burner.

The actions of BL-51 and BL-53 should also be seen in the context of the Membranes (*Huang*). BL-51 affects the Membranes in the upper part of the body (hence its effect on the breasts) while BL-53 affects the Membranes in the lower part of the body (hence its effect on the Bladder).

Some authors think that '*Bao*' here could refer also to the Uterus, in which case this point can be used for menstrual problems and affects the Membranes in the lower abdomen.

Box 60.38 summarizes the functions of BL-53.

> **Box 60.38 BL-53 – summary of functions**
>
> - Opens the Water passages in the Lower Burner
> - Stimulates the transformation and excretion of fluids and benefits the Bladder (hardness and fullness of the hypogastrium, retention of urine, dribbling urination, oedema)

BL-54 ZHIBIAN *LOWERMOST EDGE*

Location

On the buttock, 3 *cun* lateral to the sacrococcygeal hiatus.

Nature

None.

Actions

Benefits the lower back.
Benefits urination.
Treats haemorrhoids.

Indications

Lower backache, pain in the buttocks, sciatica, Painful Obstruction Syndrome (*Bi* Syndrome) of the legs.
Difficult urination, retention of urine, dark urine.
Haemorrhoids.

Comments

BL-54 is not remarkable for its energetic action, but it is a very important local point for the treatment of lower backache radiating to buttocks and legs. It must always be checked for tenderness when treating ache extending to the buttocks and the back of the legs (along the Bladder channel). If it is tender, it should be needled with a long needle (i.e. at least 5 cm/2 in) and a good needling sensation obtained, preferably to radiate downwards some way towards the leg. If the needling sensation radiates all the way down to the foot, it may not be necessary to use any other point. If the buttock and leg ache is due to obstruction by Cold and Damp, moxibustion with a moxa stick is very effective and should always be used in conjunction with needling.

Box 60.39 summarizes the functions of BL-54.

> **Box 60.39 BL-54 – summary of functions**
> - Benefits the lower back (lower backache, pain in the buttocks, sciatica, Painful Obstruction Syndrome (*Bi* Syndrome) of the legs)
> - Benefits urination (difficult urination, retention of urine, dark urine)
> - Treats haemorrhoids (haemorrhoids)

> **Box 60.40 BL-57 – summary of functions**
> - Relaxes the sinews and removes obstructions from the channel (pain and stiffness of the lower back, sciatica, difficulty in sitting and standing, inability to stand for a long time, contracture of sinews)
> - Treats haemorrhoids (haemorrhoids, bleeding haemorrhoids, swollen and painful haemorrhoids, prolapse of rectum)

BL-57 CHENGSHAN
SUPPORTING MOUNTAIN

Location

On the posterior midline of the lower leg between BL-40 Weizhong and BL-60 Kunlun, below the gastrocnemius muscle in the apex of the depression.

Nature

One of Ma Dan Yang's Heavenly Star points.

Actions

Relaxes the sinews and removes obstructions from the channel.
Treats haemorrhoids.

Indications

Pain and stiffness of the lower back, sciatica, difficulty in sitting and standing, inability to stand for a long time, contracture of sinews.
Haemorrhoids, bleeding haemorrhoids, swollen and painful haemorrhoids, prolapse of rectum.

Comments

BL-57 is used as a distal point for the treatment of lower backache and sciatica, with similar effect and range of action as BL-40 Weizhong. It is also frequently used as an empirical distal point for the treatment of haemorrhoids.

As a local point it relaxes the muscles and tendons of the lower leg and is therefore used in cramps of the gastrocnemius.

Box 60.40 summarizes the functions of BL-57.

BL-58 FEIYANG *FLYING UP*

Location

On the posterior aspect of the lower leg, behind the external malleolus, 7 *cun* directly above BL-60 Kunlun, 1 *cun* inferior and lateral to BL-57 Chengshan.

Nature

Connecting (*Luo*) point.

Actions

Removes obstructions from the channel.
Subdues rebellious Qi from the head.
Strengthens the Kidneys.
Treats haemorrhoids.

Indications

Lower backache, sciatica, inability to stand, atrophy of legs.
Headache, dizziness, neck ache, occipital headache, nosebleed.
Lower backache, tinnitus, dizziness.
Haemorrhoids, swollen and painful haemorrhoids, bleeding haemorrhoids.

Comments

BL-58 is used as a distal point in the treatment of lower backache and sciatica. A particular function of this point is to treat sciatica when the pain is somewhat in between the Bladder and Gall Bladder channel in the leg.

Being the Connecting point, BL-58 communicates with the Kidneys and it can be used to strengthen the Kidneys in conjunction with the Kidney's Source point, KI-3 Taixi. In particular, this point can simultaneously strengthen the Kidneys and subdue rebellious Qi in the head causing headache, dizziness and stiff neck.

> **Box 60.41 BL-58 – summary of functions**
> - Removes obstructions from the channel (lower backache, sciatica, inability to stand, atrophy of legs)
> - Subdues rebellious Qi from the head (headache, dizziness, neck ache, occipital headache, nosebleed)
> - Strengthens the Kidneys (lower backache, tinnitus, dizziness)
> - Treats haemorrhoids (haemorrhoids, swollen and painful haemorrhoids, bleeding haemorrhoids)

> **Box 60.42 BL-59 – summary of functions**
> - Removes obstructions from the channel (thigh pain, Wind Painful Obstruction Syndrome (*Bi* Syndrome) of legs, atrophy of legs, inability to raise leg, feeling of heaviness of the legs, sciatica, ulcers on legs, redness and swelling of lateral malleolus)
> - Invigorates the Yang Stepping Vessel
> - Benefits the back (lower backache with pronounced stiffness)

This point is therefore ideal to treat headaches from Liver-Yang rising but occurring on the Bladder channel against a background of Kidney deficiency.

It is also an empirical distal point for the treatment of haemorrhoids. This point's (and BL-57's) effect on haemorrhoids is explained by the pathway of the Bladder Divergent channel which goes to the anus.

Box 60.41 summarizes the functions of BL-58.

BL-59 FUYANG *INSTEP YANG*

Location
On the lower leg, 3 *cun* directly above BL-60 Kunlun.

Nature
Point of the Yang Stepping Vessel (*Yang Qiao Mai*).
Accumulation (*Xi*) point of the Yang Stepping Vessel.

Actions
Removes obstructions from the channel.
Invigorates the Yang Stepping Vessel.
Benefits the back.

Indications
Thigh pain, Wind Painful Obstruction Syndrome (*Bi* Syndrome) of legs, atrophy of legs, inability to raise leg, feeling of heaviness of the legs, sciatica, ulcers on legs, redness and swelling of lateral malleolus.
Lower backache with pronounced stiffness.

Comments
BL-59 is a frequently used distal point in the treatment of lower backache, particularly in chronic cases with weakness of the leg and back. This point strengthens the muscles and makes movement of the leg easier. The Yang Stepping Vessel promotes movement and agility and this point is its Accumulation point: hence its effect in stimulating movement of the leg and back. It is effective only for unilateral backache.

Box 60.42 summarizes the functions of BL-59.

BL-60 KUNLUN *KUNLUN (MOUNTAINS)*

Location
Behind the ankle joint, between the prominence of the lateral malleolus and the Achilles tendon.

Nature
River (*Jing*) point.
Fire point.

Actions
Clears Heat.
Extinguishes interior Wind and subdues rebellious Qi from the head.
Removes obstructions from the channel.
Strengthens the back.
Invigorates Blood and promotes labour.

Indications
Feeling of heat in the head, redness, pain and swelling of the eye, bursting eye pain, nosebleed.
Epilepsy, lockjaw, headache, dizziness.
Stiff neck, backache, upper backache, sciatica.
Chronic lower backache.
Difficult labour, retention of placenta.

Comments
BL-60 has a wide range of action. Firstly, it is very much used as a distal point in the treatment of backache. It differs from BL-40 Weizhong in so far as it is better for chronic rather than acute backache, and better for backache of Deficiency rather than Excess type.

Furthermore, its sphere of influence extends to the shoulders, neck and occiput (unlike BL-40), and is therefore much used for Painful Obstruction Syndrome of the shoulder, neck and head. This is also due to its effect in eliminating Wind (exterior or interior), which normally attacks the top part of the body. It also extinguishes internal Wind and treats tremors of the legs.

Owing to its sphere of action being on the occiput and head, it is very much used as a distal point for headaches deriving from Kidney deficiency, particularly deficiency of Kidney-Yang.

BL-60 is also effective to clear internal Heat from the Bladder channel affecting the eyes and nose.

The empirical use of BL-60 for difficult labour is well established and this means that it is a point forbidden during pregnancy.

Its name is probably because the Kunlun mountains in Sichuan are where the source of the Yangtze river is located. The Bladder channel is the longest channel of the body (just like the Yangtze river is the longest in China), and the point is near the prominence of the external malleolus, which could be compared to the Kunlun mountains.

Box 60.43 summarizes the functions of BL-60.

Box 60.43 BL-60 – summary of functions

- Clears Heat (feeling of heat in the head, redness, pain and swelling of the eye, bursting eye pain, nosebleed)
- Extinguishes interior Wind and subdues rebellious Qi from the head (epilepsy, lockjaw, headache, dizziness)
- Removes obstructions from the channel (stiff neck, backache, upper backache, sciatica)
- Strengthens the back (chronic lower backache)
- Invigorates Blood and promotes labour (difficult labour, retention of placenta)

BL-62 SHENMAI *NINTH CHANNEL*

Location

On the lateral side of the foot, 0.5 *cun* inferior to the inferior border of the lateral malleolus, posterior to the peroneal tendon.

Nature

Opening and beginning point of the Yang Stepping Vessel (*Yang Qiao Mai*).

Actions

Removes obstructions from the channel.
Benefits the eyes.
Opens the Yang Stepping Vessel and harmonizes left and right in the Yang Stepping Vessel.
Extinguishes interior Wind.
Subdues rebellious Qi from the head.
Expels exterior Wind.
Calms the Mind.

Indications

Stiff neck, occipital headache, stiff back, Cold Painful Obstruction Syndrome (*Bi* Syndrome) of the back, pain in the legs.
Insomnia, somnolence, red eyes, eye pain.
Imbalances between left and right (one leg longer than the other, one scapula higher than the other, sweating on one side of the body, hemiplegia, etc.), excess of Yang in the head.
Epilepsy (attacks in daytime), opisthotonos, lockjaw, tremors, Wind-stroke, deviation of eye and mouth.
Headache, dizziness.
Aversion to cold, fever, occipital headache and stiffness.
Manic behaviour, insomnia.

Comments

BL-62's action is mostly due to its being the opening and beginning point of the Yang Stepping Vessel. This vessel controls movement and agility, and this point can be used in chronic backache in a similar way to BL-59 Fuyang.

BL-62 Shenmai also relaxes the tendons and muscles of the outer leg, and is used when the muscles of the outer leg are tense, and those of the inner aspect of the leg are relaxed.

The Yang Stepping Vessel flows up to the eye and meets the Yin Stepping Vessel at BL-1 Jingming. The Yang Stepping Vessel brings Yang energy and the Yin Stepping Vessel brings Yin energy to the eyes. The 'Spiritual Axis' in chapter 17 says: '*The Yin Stepping Vessel branches off from the Kidney channel [at Rangu KI-2], it travels upwards … reaching the inner canthus of the eye. Here it meets the Yang Stepping Vessel. When the Yin and Yang Stepping Vessels are harmonized, the eyes will be moistened. When the energy of the Yin Stepping Vessel is deficient, the eyes will not be able to close.*'[15]

As was mentioned before, BL-62 can be used in combination with KI-6 Zhaohai for the treatment of insomnia, in which case, BL-62 is reduced and KI-6 reinforced; and vice versa for somnolence.

Besides its effect on the eye, BL-62 influences the spine and brain and eliminates interior Wind, and is therefore used in the treatment of epilepsy, but only if the attacks occur mostly in the daytime (if the attacks occur at night, KI-6 would be used).

As the Yin and Yang Stepping Vessels harmonize left and right (of the Yin and Yang channels, respectively), BL-62 can be used to harmonize left and right of the Yang channels such as in one leg longer than the other, one scapula higher than the other, sweating on one side of the body, hemiplegia, etc.

The 'Shen' character in the point's name indicates the Ninth Earthly Branch, which is the time corresponding to the Bladder: hence the translation as 'Ninth channel'.

Box 60.44 summarizes the functions of BL-62.

> **Box 60.44 BL-62 – summary of functions**
>
> - Removes obstructions from the channel (stiff neck, occipital headache, stiff back, Cold Painful Obstruction Syndrome (*Bi* Syndrome) of the back, pain in the legs)
> - Benefits the eyes (insomnia, somnolence, red eyes, eye pain)
> - Opens the Yang Stepping Vessel and harmonizes left and right in the Yang Stepping Vessel (imbalances between left and right (one leg longer than the other, one scapula higher than the other, sweating on one side of the body, hemiplegia, etc.), excess of Yang in the head)
> - Extinguishes interior Wind (epilepsy (attacks in daytime), opisthotonos, lockjaw, tremors, Wind-stroke, deviation of eye and mouth)
> - Subdues rebellious Qi from the head (headache, dizziness)
> - Expels exterior Wind (aversion to cold, fever, occipital headache and stiffness)
> - Calms the Mind (manic behaviour, insomnia)

BL-63 JINMEN *GOLDEN DOOR*

Location

On the lateral side of the foot, posterior to the tuberosity of the fifth metatarsal bone.

Nature

Accumulation (*Xi*) point.
Beginning point of Yang Linking Vessel (*Yang Wei Mai*).

Actions

Removes obstructions from the channel.

Indications

Lower backache, knee pain, Painful Obstruction Syndrome (*Bi* Syndrome) of the legs, pain in the legs, pain on the external malleolus.

Comments

Like all Accumulation points, BL-63 is used in acute cases to stop pain. Judging from the indications, this effect of this Accumulation point is limited to channel problems and, surprisingly, this point does not have any urinary indications.

However, in my experience, it can be used in acute Bladder patterns to clear Heat and stop pain, for such symptoms as frequent and burning urination.

Box 60.45 summarizes the functions of BL-63.

> **Box 60.45 BL-63 – summary of functions**
>
> - Removes obstructions from the channel (lower backache, knee pain, Painful Obstruction Syndrome (*Bi* Syndrome) of the legs, pain in the legs, pain on the external malleolus)
> - In my experience, this point can relieve urinary pain in acute urinary problems

BL-64 JINGGU *CAPITAL BONE*

Location

On the lateral side of the foot, anterior and inferior to the tuberosity of the fifth metatarsal bone.

Nature

Source (*Yuan*) point.

Actions

Subdues rebellious Qi from the head.
Extinguishes interior Wind.
Calms the Mind.

Indications

Headache, dizziness, redness of inner canthus of eye.
Tremor of the head, epilepsy.
Palpitations, insomnia, manic depression, fright.

Comments

BL-64 is the Source point of the Bladder: like many Source points of the Yang channels (in contrast to those of the Yin channels), it is not usually used to tonify the relevant organ.

BL-64 is a useful point to subdue rebellious Qi from the head causing headaches and dizziness and Liver-Wind causing tremor of the head, when both occur against a background of Kidney deficiency.

In my experience, BL-64 can stimulate the Water passages of the Lower Burner when used in conjunction with T.B.-4 Yangchi.

Box 60.46 summarizes the functions of BL-64.

It clears Heat from the Bladder channel in the head and eyes: however, in my experience, it can be used in acute cystitis to clear Heat from the Bladder.

It expels exterior Wind and is frequently used in the beginning stages of an attack of Wind-Cold (Greater Yang stage) with pronounced headache and stiff neck.

Box 60.47 summarizes the functions of BL-65.

> **Box 60.46 BL-64 – summary of functions**
>
> - Subdues rebellious Qi from the head (headache, dizziness, redness of inner canthus of eye)
> - Extinguishes interior Wind (tremor of the head, epilepsy)
> - Calms the Mind (palpitations, insomnia, manic depression, fright)
> - In my experience, this point can stimulate the Water passages of the Lower Burner when combined with T.B.-4 Yangchi

> **Box 60.47 BL-65 – summary of functions**
>
> - Subdues rebellious Qi from the head (headache, dizziness, occipital headache)
> - Clears Heat (redness and pain of the eye, redness of inner canthus of eye, yellow sclera)
> - Expels exterior Wind (aversion to cold, fever, occipital stiffness and ache)

BL-65 SHUGU *BINDING BONE*

Location

On the lateral side of the foot, posterior and inferior to the head of the fifth metatarsal bone.

Nature

Stream (*Shu*) point.
Wood point.
Drainage point.

Actions

Subdues rebellious Qi from the head.
Clears Heat.
Expels exterior Wind.

Indications

Headache, dizziness, occipital headache.
Redness and pain of the eye, redness of inner canthus of eye, yellow sclera.
Aversion to cold, fever, occipital stiffness and ache.

Comments

BL-65 can be used as a distal point for any problems along the Bladder channel, particularly if they affect the head. It is therefore used for Painful Obstruction Syndrome of the neck, for which it is particularly useful.

BL-66 TONGGU *PASSING VALLEY*

Location

On the lateral side of the foot, anterior and inferior to the fifth metatarsal joint.

Nature

Spring (*Ying*) point.
Water point.

Actions

Clears Heat.
Promotes the rising of clear Qi to the head.

Indications

Difficult urination, burning pain on urination, scanty dark urine, redness of eyes, nosebleed.
Feeling of heaviness of the head, dizziness.

Comments

Like all Spring points, BL-66 clears Heat and is particularly useful to clear Bladder-Heat in acute cases of cystitis as it is more dynamic and powerful than other Bladder points in its clearing Heat action. It also clears Heat from the Bladder channel, especially in relation to the eyes and nose.

BL-66 can stimulate the rising of clear Qi to the head to dispel Dampness in the head that is causing a feeling of heaviness and muzziness of the head.

Box 60.48 summarizes the functions of BL-66.

> **Box 60.48 BL-66 – summary of functions**
>
> - Clears Heat (difficult urination, burning pain on urination, scanty dark urine, redness of eyes, nosebleed)
> - Promotes the rising of clear Qi to the head (feeling of heaviness of the head, dizziness)

> **Box 60.49 BL-67 – summary of functions**
>
> - Subdues rebellious Qi from the head (headache, dizziness, occipital headache, neck ache)
> - Clears Heat (red eyes, eye pain)
> - Resolves Damp-Heat (difficult urination, painful urination)
> - Promotes labour (retention of placenta, malposition of fetus, delayed labour, prolonged or difficult labour)

BL-67 ZHIYIN *REACHING YIN*

Location
On the dorsal aspect of the little toe at the lateral angle of the nail of the little toe.

Nature
Well (*Jing*) point.
Metal point.
Tonification point.

Actions
Subdues rebellious Qi from the head.
Clears Heat.
Resolves Damp-Heat.
Promotes labour.

Indications
Headache, dizziness, occipital headache, neck ache.
Red eyes, eye pain.
Difficult urination, painful urination.
Retention of placenta, malposition of fetus, delayed labour, prolonged or difficult labour.

Comments
As a Well point, BL-67 eliminates Wind (both interior and exterior) and is frequently used for headache from exterior or interior Wind.

Being the end point of the channel, it can be used to affect the opposite end, and it is therefore used to clear the eyes, for such symptoms as blurred vision or pain in the eye (usually from Wind).

It is used empirically for malposition of the fetus. This is normally done in the eighth month of pregnancy, burning five moxa cones on each side, once a day for 10 days.

Box 60.49 summarizes the functions of BL-67.

The target areas of the Bladder channel points are illustrated in Figure 60.5.

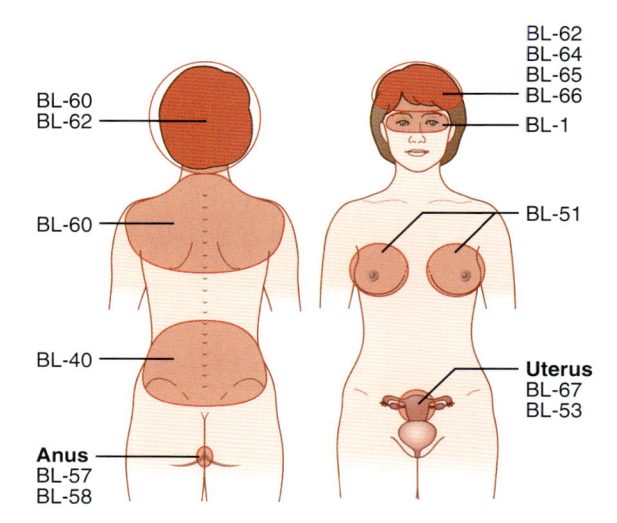

Figure 60.5 Target areas of Bladder channel points

END NOTES

1. 1981 Spiritual Axis (*Ling Shu Jing* 灵枢经), People's Health Publishing House, Beijing, first published *c*.100 BC, p. 73.
2. Yue Han Zhen 1990 An Explanation of the Acupuncture Points (*Jing Xue Jie* 经穴解), People's Health Publishing House, Beijing, originally published in 1654, p. 183.
3. Ibid., p. 183.
4. Ibid., p. 186.
5. This combination of points was first mentiond in the 'Gatherings of Eminent Acupuncturists' (*Zhen Jiu Ju Ying* 针灸聚英) by Gao Wu, AD 1529.
6. Ibid., p. 144.
7. Spiritual Axis, p. 73.
8. An Explanation of the Acupuncture Points, p. 207.
9. The name '*Gaohuang*' is mentioned in the *Zuo Chuan*, historical annals from the Spring and Autumn Period (770–476 BC). This is also the first historical mention of acupuncture. The annals report that a certain prince of Jin was severely ill and a famous doctor was sent for. The text then reports the conversation of two demons inside the prince's body deciding what would be the best place to hide in order to escape the doctor's subtle diagnostic skills. They decide to hide in the region of *Gaohuang* between the heart and diaphragm so that no therapeutic method, whether acupuncture or herbs, could possibly reach them. Ever since then, the name *Gaohuang* indicates a chronic disease which is very difficult to cure. A complete account of this reference can be found in Needham J-Lu G D 1980 Celestial Lancets, Cambridge University Press, Cambridge, p. 78.

10. An Explanation of the Acupuncture Points, p. 211.
11. Ibid., p. 213.
12. Jiao Hui Yuan, Acupuncture Textbook by Hui Yuan (*Hui Yuan Zhen Jiu Xue* 会 元 针 灸 学). In: An Explanation of the Meaning of Acupuncture Points Names, p. 167.
13. The Illustrated Classic of Acupuncture Points as Found on the Bronze Model. In: An Explanation of the Meaning of Acupuncture Points Names, p. 167.
14. An Explanation of the Acupuncture Points, p. 211.
15. Spiritual Axis, p. 50.

SECTION 2 PART 7

Kidney Channel 61

Main channel pathway

The Kidney channel starts under the fifth toe and runs to the sole of the foot (at KI-1 Yongquan). Running under the navicular bone and behind the medial malleolus, it ascends the medial side of the leg up to the inner aspect of the thigh. It then goes towards the sacrum (at Du-1 Changqiang), ascends along the lumbar spine and enters the kidney and urinary bladder. It then goes forwards to enter the liver, passes through the diaphragm and enters the lung. From here it ascends to the throat and terminates at the root of the tongue.

From the lung, a branch joins the heart and flows to the chest to connect with the Pericardium channel (Fig. 61.1).

Connecting channel pathway

The Kidney Connecting channel starts at KI-4 Dazhong from where a branch connects with the Bladder channel. A branch runs along the main Kidney channel to the perineum and ascends through the lumbar spine (Fig. 61.2).

Box 61.1 gives an overview of Kidney points.

> **Box 61.1 Overview of Kidney points**
>
> - Affect the inner aspect of leg, genitals, urinary system, abdomen, chest, throat
> - Affect the Uterus and menstruation
> - Important points to tonify the Original Qi (*Yuan Qi*) and the Essence (*Jing*)
> - Strengthen the Kidney's receiving of Qi (chronic asthma)
> - Strengthen the lower back

KI-1 YONGQUAN *BUBBLING SPRING*

Location

On the sole, in the depression when the foot is in plantarflexion, approximately at the anterior third

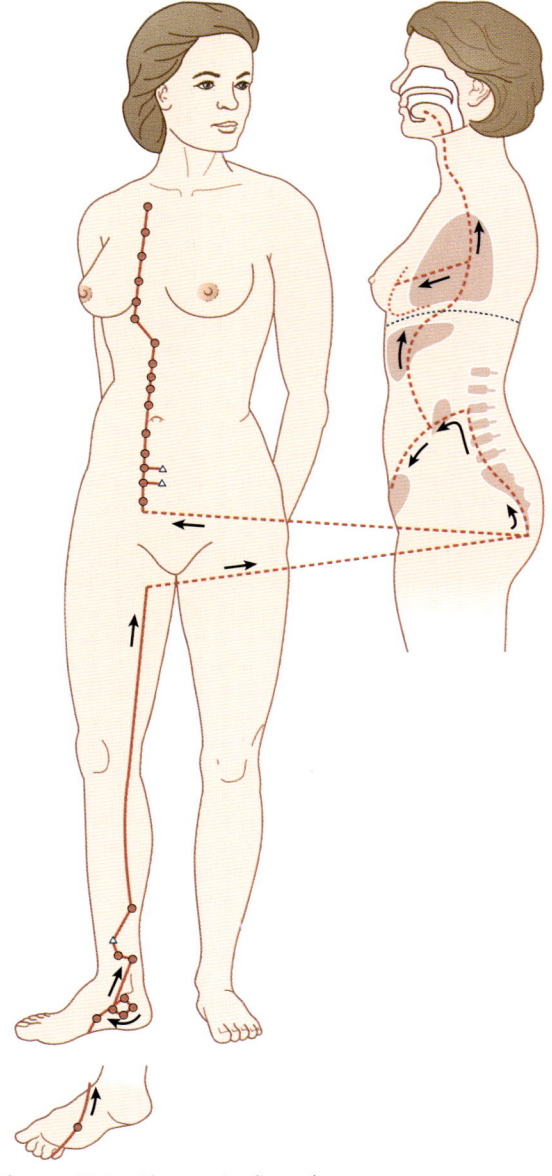

Figure 61.1 Kidney main channel

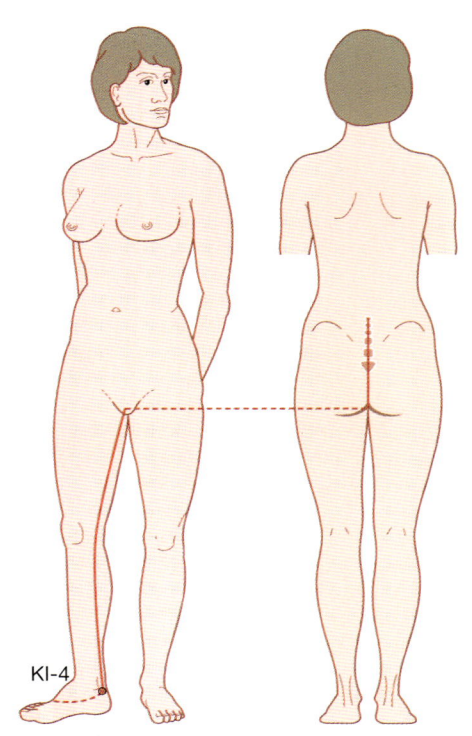

Figure 61.2 Kidney Connecting channel

and the posterior two-thirds of the line from the web between the second and third toes to the back of the heel.

Nature

Well (*Jing*) point.
Wood point.
Drainage point.

Actions

Nourishes Yin and clears Empty-Heat.
Regulates the Lower Burner
Extinguishes interior Wind
Calms the Mind
Restores consciousness.

Indications

Dry tongue, dry throat, dizziness, tinnitus, night sweating.
Constipation, difficult defecation, difficult urination, abdominal pain in pregnancy with urinary retention, abdominal fullness, umbilical pain, infertility, impotence.
Epilepsy, headache, vertigo.
Agitation, insomnia, poor memory, fear, rage with desire to kill people, manic behaviour.
Unconsciousness from Wind-stroke.

Comments

KI-1 has a marked reducing effect on the body's Qi and is used in Excess patterns.

Firstly, it tonifies Yin and clears Empty-Heat deriving from Yin deficiency. Since it nourishes Yin and clears Empty-Heat, it is frequently used for the pattern of Yin deficiency with Empty-Heat in the Heart (Heart and Kidney not harmonized).

KI-1 also extinguishes internal Wind: hence its use for epilepsy and to promote resuscitation. It can be used in acute situations when the person is unconscious, to restore consciousness and clear the brain.

It has a very strong calming effect on the Mind, and is used in severe anxiety or mental illness such as hypomania.

Being on the sole of the foot, it has a strong sinking action: that is, it eliminates pathogenic factors (such as Wind or Empty-Heat) from the head and it brings down rebellious ascending Qi (particularly Liver-Yang or Liver-Wind).

Box 61.2 summarizes the functions of KI-1.

Box 61.2 KI-1 – summary of functions

- Nourishes Yin and clears Empty-Heat (dry tongue, dry throat, dizziness, tinnitus, night sweating)
- Regulates the Lower Burner (constipation, difficult defecation, difficult urination, abdominal pain in pregnancy with urinary retention, abdominal fullness, umbilical pain, infertility, impotence)
- Extinguishes interior Wind (epilepsy, headache, vertigo)
- Calms the Mind (agitation, insomnia, poor memory, fear, rage with desire to kill people, manic behaviour)
- Restores consciousness (unconsciousness from Wind-stroke)

KI-2 RANGU *BLAZING VALLEY*

Location

On the medial aspect of the foot, below the tuberosity of the navicular bone, at the junction of the red and white skin.

Nature

Spring (*Ying*) point.
Fire point.
Beginning point of Yin Stepping Vessel (*Yin Qiao Mai*).

Actions

Clears Empty-Heat and cools Blood.
Invigorates the Yin Stepping Vessel (*Yin Qiao Mai*).

Indications

Dry throat, night sweating, feeling of heat in the evening, five-palm heat, malar flush.
Itching of genitals, infertility, irregular menstruation, difficult urination, unilateral abdominal pain, abdominal masses.

Comments

KI-2 is the main point to clear Empty-Heat from the Kidneys. It is very much used in such symptoms as red cheekbones, five-palm heat, feeling of heat in the evening, mental restlessness, thirst without desire to drink and dry throat and mouth at night. It can be combined with LU-10 Yuji to clear Empty-Heat from the Lungs, or with HE-6 Yinxi to clear Empty-Heat from the Heart.

Being the Spring point, it is a very dynamic point and more used in Excess patterns.

Being the beginning point of the Yin Stepping Vessel, it can be used to move Qi and Blood in this vessel. In this context, it is especially used for unilateral abdominal pain and abdominal masses.

Box 61.3 summarizes the functions of KI-2.

Box 61.3 KI-2 – summary of functions

- Clears Empty-Heat and cools Blood (dry throat, night sweating, feeling of heat in the evening, five-palm heat, malar flush)
- Invigorates the Yin Stepping Vessel (itching of genitals, infertility, irregular menstruation, difficult urination, unilateral abdominal pain, abdominal masses)

KI-3 TAIXI *GREATER STREAM*

Location

On the medial aspect of the foot, posterior to the medial malleolus, in the depression between the tip of the medial malleolus and Achilles tendon.

Nature

Stream (*Shu*) and Source (*Yuan*) point.
Earth point.

Actions

Tonifies the Kidneys (both Yin and Yang).
Strengthens the Kidney's receiving of Qi.
Calms the Mind.
Benefits Essence.
Strengthens the lower back and knees.
Regulates the uterus.

Indications

Backache, dizziness, tinnitus, exhaustion, feeling cold, frequent urination, cold and weak knees, dry throat, night sweating, hot palms.
Cough, wheezing, breathlessness.
Insomnia, excessive dreaming, poor memory.
Seminal emissions, nocturnal emissions, impotence, premature ejaculation, weakened sexual function.
Lower backache, weak knees, achy knees, cold legs.
Irregular periods, infertility, scanty or heavy periods.

Comments

KI-3 is an extremely important point used to tonify the Kidneys in any deficiency pattern of Kidney-Yin or Kidney-Yang. It tonifies every aspect of the Kidneys (i.e. Kidney-Yin, Kidney-Yang, Kidney-Qi, Kidney-Essence and the Kidney's receiving of Qi from the Lungs). Being the Source point, it is in contact with the Original Qi (*Yuan Qi*) of the Kidney channel, and since the Kidneys are the foundation of all the Qi of the body and the seat of the Original Qi, this point goes straight to the core of the Original Qi.

As the Kidneys also store Essence, this point can tonify the Essence, the bones and Marrow. The main difference in the tonification of Kidney-Yin or Kidney-Yang is in the use of moxa: moxa is used to tonify Kidney-Yang.

KI-3 is one of the main points to tonify the Kidneys together with BL-23 Shenshu and Ren-4 Guanyuan.

Essence nourishes the uterus and this point can regulate the function of the uterus: it is therefore used in such symptoms as irregular periods, amenorrhoea and excessive bleeding.

Finally, the Kidneys rule the lower back and KI-3 can be used to treat any type of chronic ache of the lower back.

Box 61.4 summarizes the functions of KI-3.

> **Box 61.4 KI-3 – summary of functions**
>
> - Tonifies the Kidneys (both Yin and Yang) (backache, dizziness, tinnitus, exhaustion, feeling cold, frequent urination, cold and weak knees, dry throat, night sweating, hot palms)
> - Strengthens the Kidney's receiving of Qi (cough, wheezing, breathlessness)
> - Calms the Mind (insomnia, excessive dreaming, poor memory)
> - Benefits Essence (seminal emissions, nocturnal emissions, impotence, premature ejaculation, weakened sexual function)
> - Strengthens the lower back and knees (lower backache, weak knees, achy knees, cold legs)
> - Regulates the uterus (irregular periods, infertility, scanty or heavy periods)

KI-4 DAZHONG *BIG BELL*

Location

On the medial aspect of the foot, 0.5 *cun* posterior to the midpoint of the line drawn between KI-3 Taixi and KI-5 Shuiquan on the anterior border of the Achilles tendon.

Nature

Connecting (*Luo*) point.

Actions

Strengthens the Kidney's receiving of Qi.
Calms and lifts the Mind.
Benefits urination.
Strengthens the back.

Indications

Cough, coughing of blood, wheezing, breathlessness, rattling sound in throat, feeling of oppression of the chest.
Palpitations, agitation, mental retardation, manic behaviour, propensity to anger, somnolence, fright, unhappiness, desire to close doors and remain at home.
Difficult urination, dribbling of urine, retention of urine.
Lower backache.

Comments

Being the Connecting point, KI-4 connects with the Bladder channel and is therefore very useful to treat chronic backache from Kidney deficiency. I often use it in conjunction with the Governing Vessel as follows (in a man):

> - S.I.-3 on the left and BL-62 on the right
> - HE-7 on the right and KI-4 on the left

KI-4, in common with other Yin Connecting points, also has a marked effect on the Mind and can be used both to calm the Mind and to 'lift' the spirit when the person is exhausted and depressed from a chronic Kidney deficiency.

Box 61.5 summarizes the functions of KI-4.

> **Box 61.5 KI-4 – summary of functions**
>
> - Strengthens the Kidney's receiving of Qi (cough, coughing of blood, wheezing, breathlessness, rattling sound in throat, feeling of oppression of the chest)
> - Calms and lifts the Mind (palpitations, agitation, mental retardation, manic behaviour, propensity to anger, somnolence, fright, unhappiness, desire to close doors and remain at home)
> - Benefits urination (difficult urination, dribbling of urine, retention of urine)
> - Strengthens the back (lower backache)

KI-5 SHUIQUAN *WATER SPRING*

Location

1 *cun* below KI-3 Taixi anterior and superior to the calcaneus tuberosity.

Nature

Accumulation (*Xi*) point.

Actions

Benefits urination.
Regulates the uterus and menstruation.

Indications

Difficult urination, dribbling of urine.
Scanty periods, amenorrhoea, irregular menstruation, painful periods, prolapse of uterus.

Comments

Being the Accumulation point, KI-5 can be used in acute conditions to stop pain, and is therefore used in acute cystitis or urethritis.

It also stops abdominal pain around the umbilicus and it regulates Blood in the uterus. In particular, it is used for amenorrhoea from Kidney deficiency.

Box 61.6 summarizes the functions of KI-5.

> **Box 61.6 KI-5 – summary of functions**
>
> - Benefits urination (difficult urination, dribbling of urine)
> - Regulates the uterus and menstruation (scanty periods, amenorrhoea, irregular menstruation, painful periods, prolapse of uterus)

KI-6 ZHAOHAI *SHINING SEA*

Location

On the medial aspect of the foot, in the depression 1 *cun* below the tip of the medial malleolus in the groove formed by two ligamentous bundles.

Nature

Opening point of Yin Stepping Vessel (*Yin Qiao Mai*).

Actions

Nourishes Kidney-Yin.
Benefits the eyes.
Calms the Mind.
Invigorates the Yin Stepping Vessel.
Benefits the throat.
Regulates the uterus and menstruation.

Indications

Dizziness, tinnitus, night sweating, backache.
Dry eyes, blurred vision, red eyes, floaters, insomnia, somnolence.
Insomnia, epilepsy (night-time attacks), sadness, fright, nightmares.
Itching of genitals, involuntary erection, hypogastric pain, abdominal pain, tightness and contraction of the muscles of the inner aspect of the legs, cramps of feet, hemiplegia.
Dry throat, dry cough.
Irregular periods, amenorrhoea, painful periods, infertility from Cold in the Uterus, difficult labour, postpartum umbilical pain.

Comments

KI-6 is a major point with many different functions. First of all, it is the best point on the Kidney channel to nourish Kidney-Yin and is widely used in Yin deficiency. It is also very useful to nourish fluids and moisten dryness, for such symptoms as dry throat and dry eyes.

As was mentioned before, the Yin Stepping Vessel carries Yin energy to the eyes to nourish and moisten them, so this point can stimulate the Qi of the Yin Stepping Vessel to flow up to the eyes. It is a very important point to use in all chronic eye diseases, particularly in old people with deficiency of Yin.

By nourishing Yin, KI-6 also calms the Mind, in cases of anxiety and restlessness deriving from Yin deficiency. Furthermore, it is used to treat insomnia, as its use brings Yin energy to the eyes and makes them close at night.

By tonifying the Yin and promoting fluids, KI-6 also cools the Blood and is therefore used for skin diseases characterized by Heat in the Blood.

By carrying Yin energy upwards, KI-6 moistens and benefits the throat, and it is an important point to use for chronic dryness or soreness of the throat deriving from Yin deficiency.

KI-6 also influences the uterus and can be used for amenorrhoea from Kidney deficiency and prolapse of the uterus.

Some of this point's functions are due to its being the beginning and opening point of the Yin Stepping Vessel, causing symptoms such as hypogastric pain, abdominal pain, tightness and contraction of the muscles of the inner aspect of the legs, cramps of the feet, hemiplegia.

Box 61.7 summarizes the functions of KI-6.

> **Box 61.7 KI-6 – summary of functions**
>
> - Nourishes Kidney-Yin (dizziness, tinnitus, night sweating, backache)
> - Benefits the eyes (dry eyes, blurred vision, red eyes, floaters, insomnia, somnolence)
> - Calms the Mind (insomnia, epilepsy (night-time attacks), sadness, fright, nightmares)
> - Invigorates the Yin Stepping Vessel (itching of genitals, involuntary erection, hypogastric pain, abdominal pain, tightness and contraction of the muscles of the inner aspect of the legs, cramps of feet, hemiplegia)
> - Benefits the throat (dry throat, dry cough)
> - Regulates the uterus and menstruation (irregular periods, amenorrhoea, painful periods, infertility from Cold in the Uterus, difficult labour, postpartum umbilical pain)

KI-7 FULIU *RETURNING CURRENT*

Location
On the medial aspect of the lower leg, 2 *cun* directly above KI-3, on the anterior border of the Achilles tendon.

Nature
River (*Jing*) point.
Metal point.
Tonification point.

Actions
Tonifies the Kidneys.
Resolves Dampness.
Opens the Water Passages of the Lower Burner and resolves oedema.
Strengthens the lower back.
Regulates sweating.

Indications
Backache, dizziness, tinnitus, weak knees, tiredness.
Diarrhoea, abdominal fullness, mucus and blood in the stools, borborygmi, feeling of heaviness in the rectum.
Oedema, difficult urination, retention of urine, painful urination, turbid urine, blood in the urine.
Backache, ache in the knees, cold knees.
Sweating, night sweating.

Comments
KI-7 tonifies the Kidneys in a similar way to KI-3, the only difference being that KI-7 is better to tonify Kidney-Yang.

KI-7 is an important point to resolve Dampness in the Lower Burner causing urinary or intestinal symptoms and to eliminate oedema in the legs.

It can either promote or stop sweating: it is frequently used in combination with L.I.-4 Hegu to cause sweating in attacks of exterior Wind-Cold, and with HE-6 Yinxi to stop sweating from Kidney-Yin deficiency. To promote sweating, KI-7 is reduced, while to stop sweating it is reinforced.

There is an ongoing debate as to whether KI-7 'tonifies Kidney-Yang or Kidney-Yin': some argue the former, some the latter. In my experience, it is better to tonify Kidney-Yang: its indications in eliminating oedema would seem to support that as one needs to tonify Yang to eliminate oedema (a Yin pathogenic factor).

When I use KI-7 to tonify Kidney-Yang I generally use moxa on the needle to strengthen its Yang-tonifying action. However, that does not mean that KI-7 would aggravate a Kidney-Yin deficiency: indeed, among its classical indications there is 'dry tongue and parched mouth'.

Acupuncture works differently than herbal medicine and nearly every point can be used to tonify Yang or Yin depending on whether one uses moxa or not. Ren-4 Guanyuan is also a very good example of this as it is an excellent Yin tonic point, but, with direct moxa cones, it can tonify Kidney-Yang.

Box 61.8 summarizes the functions of KI-7.

Box 61.8 KI-7 – summary of functions

- Tonifies the Kidneys (backache, dizziness, tinnitus, weak knees, tiredness)
- Resolves Dampness (diarrhoea, abdominal fullness, mucus and blood in the stools, borborygmi, feeling of heaviness in the rectum)
- Opens the Water Passages of the Lower Burner and resolves oedema (oedema, difficult urination, retention of urine, painful urination, turbid urine, blood in the urine)
- Strengthens the lower back (backache, ache in the knees, cold knees)
- Regulates sweating (sweating, night sweating)

KI-8 JIAOXIN *MEETING THE SPLEEN CHANNEL*

Location
On the medial aspect of the lower leg, 2 *cun* directly above KI-3 Taixi, 0.5 *cun* anterior to KI-7, posterior to the medial border of the tibia.

Nature
Accumulation (*Xi*) point of the Yin Stepping Vessel (*Yin Qiao Mai*).

Actions
Benefits the Uterus and regulates menstruation.
Resolves Dampness.
Removes obstructions from the channel.

Indications
Painful periods, heavy periods, irregular periods, amenorrhoea.

Abdominal fullness, diarrhoea, retention of urine, painful urination, turbid urine, difficult urination, swelling and pain of testicles, itching of genitals.
Unilateral abdominal pain, abdominal masses.

Comments

Being the accumulation point of the Yin Stepping Vessel, KI-8 can invigorate this vessel and is particularly good to eliminate obstructions along the vessel and dissolve abdominal masses, especially abdominal masses in women (*Zheng Jia*). The Yin Stepping Vessel can move Qi, eliminate Yin excesses and dissolve masses. This point is therefore important for abdominal pain deriving from obstruction and stagnation in the Yin Stepping Vessel.

KI-8 is also important to regulate menstruation, particularly for menstrual problems deriving from stasis of Blood.

Box 61.9 summarizes the functions of KI-8.

Box 61.9 KI-8 – summary of functions

- Benefits the Uterus and regulates menstruation (painful periods, heavy periods, irregular periods, amenorrhoea)
- Resolves Dampness (abdominal fullness, diarrhoea, retention of urine, painful urination, turbid urine, difficult urination, swelling and pain of testicles, itching of genitals)
- Removes obstructions from the channel (unilateral abdominal pain, abdominal masses)

KI-9 ZHUBIN *GUEST HOUSE*

Location

On the medial aspect of the lower leg, 5 *cun* above KI-3 Taixi on the line drawn between KI-3 and KI-10 Yingu, 1 *cun* posterior to the medial border of the tibia.

Nature

Accumulation (*Xi*) point of Yin Linking Vessel (*Yin Wei Mai*).

Actions

Calms the Mind and opens the Mind's orifices.
Tonifies Kidney-Yin.
Opens the chest.
Regulates the Yin Linking Vessel.

Indications

Anxiety, insomnia, palpitations, manic behaviour, vomiting of phlegm.
Backache, dizziness, tinnitus, night sweating, dry throat.
Feeling of stuffiness under the xiphoid process, feeling of oppression of the chest.

Comments

KI-9 is an excellent point to calm the Mind in cases of deep anxiety and mental restlessness deriving from Kidney-Yin deficiency. It has a profound calming effect and it tonifies Kidney-Yin at the same time.

It also relaxes any tension or feeling of oppression felt in the chest, often with palpitations. Because it tonifies Kidney-Yin, calms the Mind and treats palpitations, this point is particularly indicated in the pattern of 'Heart and Kidneys not harmonized'.

I often use this point, the Accumulation and starting point of the Yin Linking Vessel, with the opening points of this vessel (i.e. P-6 Neiguan and SP-4 Gongsun).

The name of the point refers to a 'guest': the guest is the Heart and the host the Kidneys. The name highlights the fact that this point promotes the communication between Heart and Kidneys. I personally use this point in emotional problems and anxiety affecting the Heart and occurring against a background of Kidney deficiency.

Box 61.10 summarizes the functions of KI-9.

Box 61.10 KI-9 – summary of functions

- Calms the Mind and opens the Mind's orifices (anxiety, insomnia, palpitations, manic behaviour, vomiting of phlegm)
- Tonifies Kidney-Yin (backache, dizziness, tinnitus, night sweating, dry throat)
- Opens the chest (feeling of stuffiness under the xiphoid process, feeling of oppression of the chest)
- Regulates the Yin Linking Vessel

KI-10 YINGU *YIN VALLEY*

Location

At the medial end of the popliteal crease, between the semitendinosus and semimembranosus tendons, located with the knee slightly flexed.

Nature

Sea (*He*) point.
Water point.

Actions

Resolves Dampness from the Lower Burner.
Tonifies Kidney-Yin.

Indications

Hypogastric pain and fullness, abdominal distension and pain, difficult urination, turbid urine, painful urination.
Backache, tinnitus, deafness, night sweating, dark urine, dry throat.

Comments

KI-10 has two main uses. First of all, in common with the other two Yin Sea points around the knee, SP-9 Yinlingquan and LIV-8 Ququan, it resolves Dampness from the Lower Burner, and is therefore used for urinary symptoms such as difficulty, pain, and frequency of urination.

Secondly, this point can also be used to nourish Kidney-Yin. In this respect, it differs from KI-6 Zhaohai in so far as the latter does not only nourish Kidney-Yin but it specifically sends Yin up especially to the throat and eyes: it is therefore the best point to use to nourish Kidney-Yin when there is a dry throat and eyes. KI-9 Zhubin also nourishes Kidney-Yin and it is better than KI-10 when there are mental–emotional problems such as anxiety and insomnia.

Box 61.11 summarizes the functions of KI-10.

Box 61.11 KI-10 – summary of functions

- Resolves Dampness from the Lower Burner (hypogastric pain and fullness, abdominal distension and pain, difficult urination, turbid urine, painful urination)
- Tonifies Kidney-Yin (backache, tinnitus, deafness, night sweating, dark urine, dry throat)

KI-11 HENGGU *PUBIC BONE*

Location

On the lower abdomen, 5 *cun* below the centre of the umbilicus, 0.5 *cun* lateral to the anterior midline.

Nature

Point of the Penetrating Vessel (*Chong Mai*).

Actions

Resolves Dampness.
Moves Qi and Blood in the Lower Burner.
Clears Heat.

Indications

Difficulty in urination, retention of urine, hypogastric fullness.
Genital pain, lower abdominal pain.
Inner canthus or eyes red and painful.

Comments

KI-11 (like all abdominal points of the Kidney channel up to KI-21), is a point of the Penetrating Vessel and some of its indications can be explained as a pathology of this vessel: these are genital pain and lower abdominal pain. The Penetrating Vessel is the Sea of Blood and one of its chief pathologies is Blood stasis. On the other hand, the Penetrating Vessel is also the 'Sea of the 12 Channels' and 'Sea of the Avenues of the Abdomen' and it is prone to Qi stagnation in the abdomen.

KI-11, like many of the other Kidney points on the abdomen, affect the eyes ('inner canthus of eyes red and painful'): this is due to the Penetrating Vessel's pathway, which reaches the eyes.

KI-11 is the first of the Kidney points on the Penetrating Vessel after it emerges at the point ST-30 Qichong: for this reason, KI-11, like ST-30, is a dynamic point that can move Qi and Blood forcefully.

Box 61.12 summarizes the functions of KI-11.

Box 61.12 KI-11 – summary of functions

- Resolves Dampness (difficulty in urination, retention of urine, hypogastric fullness)
- Moves Qi and Blood in the Lower Burner (genital pain, lower abdominal pain)
- Clears Heat (inner canthus or eyes red and painful)

KI-12 DAHE *BIG GLORY*

Location

On the lower abdomen, 4 *cun* below the centre of the umbilicus, 0.5 *cun* lateral to the anterior midline.

Nature

Point of the Penetrating Vessel (*Chong Mai*).

Actions

Tonifies the Kidneys.
Benefits the Essence.
Regulates the Uterus and menstruation.
Clears Heat.

Indications

Backache, tinnitus, deafness, night sweating, dry throat and eyes.
Impotence, seminal emissions.
Prolapse of uterus, irregular periods, painful periods, infertility.
Inner corner of the eyes red.

Comments

KI-12 is a point where the Essence concentrates: it tonifies the Kidneys and primarily Kidney-Yin. The '*he*' in its name means 'glory', 'flourishing', 'bright', 'luminous': this refers to the fact that the Essence (*Jing*) concentrates at this point and also to the fact that, according to ancient Chinese views, it is at this point that the first enlargement of the uterus manifests in pregnancy.

KI-12 has an important influence on the Uterus and menstruation, which is partly due to its being a point of the Penetrating Vessel. In gynaecology, it is used mostly to tonify the Kidneys, strengthen the Uterus and consolidate the Penetrating and Directing Vessels.

This point is also used to promote ovulation when used at the beginning of the third phase of the menstrual cycle (i.e. starting 1 week after the end of bleeding). When used to promote ovulation, KI-12 is combined with Ren-3 Zhongji and SP-6 Sanyinjiao.

Box 61.13 summarizes the functions of KI-12.

Box 61.13 KI-12 – summary of functions

- Tonifies the Kidneys (backache, tinnitus, deafness, night sweating, dry throat and eyes)
- Benefits the Essence (impotence, seminal emissions)
- Regulates the Uterus and menstruation (prolapse of uterus, irregular periods, painful periods, infertility)
- Clears Heat (inner corner of the eyes red)
- Promotes ovulation.

KI-13 QIXUE *QI HOLE*

Location

On the lower abdomen, 3 *cun* below the centre of the umbilicus, 0.5 *cun* lateral to the anterior midline.

Nature

Point of the Penetrating Vessel (*Chong Mai*).
Meeting point of the Liver and Spleen channels.[1]

Actions

Tonifies the Kidneys and Essence.
Strengthens the Uterus and consolidates the Penetrating and Directing Vessels (*Chong* and *Ren Mai*).
Moves Qi and Blood.
Regulates the two lower orifices (urethra and anus).
Clears Heat.

Indications

Backache, tinnitus, deafness, weak knees.
Amenorrhoea, irregular periods, excessive menstrual bleeding, infertility, impotence.
Abdominal pain, Running Piglet Syndrome,[2] backache radiating up and down.
Urinary difficulty, diarrhoea, turbid urine.
Inner corner of the eyes red.

Comments

KI-13 has a dual function, one to tonify and one to reduce. First of all, it can be used as a powerful tonification of the Kidneys and the Kidney-Essence (it is level with Ren-4 Guanyuan, which tonifies the Kidneys and Essence). This is due also to its being a point of the Penetrating Vessel which circulates the Kidney-Essence.

On the other hand, the Penetrating Vessel is responsible for circulation of Qi and Blood in the abdomen. This point can therefore be used for Excess patterns characterized by abdominal fullness and rebellious Qi in the Penetrating Vessel. The pattern of rebellious Qi in the Penetrating Vessel is a type of Running Piglet Syndrome; this is characterized by a feeling of surging of Qi from the lower abdomen to the chest and throat, accompanied by lower abdominal fullness and pain, often painful periods, a feeling of tightness in the chest, palpitations, a feeling of lump in the throat and anxiety (see ch. 53).

Although KI-13, like most other Kidney points on the lower abdomen, can be used for Excess patterns with stagnation of Qi and Blood in the abdomen, I personally use this point primarily to tonify the Kidneys, strengthen the Uterus and consolidate the Penetrating and Directing Vessels.

KI-13 is an important point to strengthen the Uterus and consolidate the Penetrating and Directing Vessels. It is frequently used for menstrual irregularities and especially excessive menstrual bleeding.

KI-13 is an important point to strengthen the Kidney's receiving of Qi in chronic asthma, in which case I use this point in combination with Ren-4 Guanyuan.

Box 61.14 summarizes the functions of KI-13.

Box 61.14 KI-13 – summary of functions

- Tonifies the Kidneys and Essence (backache, tinnitus, deafness, weak knees)
- Strengthens the Uterus and consolidates the Penetrating and Directing Vessels (*Chong* and *Ren Mai*) (amenorrhoea, irregular periods, excessive menstrual bleeding, infertility, impotence)
- Moves Qi and Blood (abdominal pain, Running Piglet Syndrome, backache radiating up and down)
- Regulates the two lower orifices (urethra and anus) (urinary difficulty, diarrhoea, turbid urine)
- Clears Heat (inner corner of the eyes red)

KI-14 SIMAN *FOUR FULLNESSES*

Location

On the lower abdomen, 2 *cun* below the centre of the umbilicus, 0.5 *cun* lateral to the anterior midline.

Nature

Point of the Penetrating Vessel (*Chong Mai*).

Actions

Moves Qi and Blood in the lower abdomen.
Regulates the Uterus and menstruation.
Nourishes Essence and Marrow.

Indications

Lower abdominal pain, umbilical pain, constipation, Running Piglet Syndrome.
Painful periods, excessive menstrual bleeding, irregular periods, retention of lochia, excessive vaginal discharge, infertility.

Comments

KI-14 is the most important point of the Penetrating Vessel to move Qi and invigorate Blood in the lower abdomen and Uterus. The Penetrating Vessel is the Sea of Blood and Blood stasis is one of its most common pathologies: KI-14 is the main point to invigorate Blood in the Penetrating Vessel. Although its classical indications do not include abdominal masses, I frequently use this point in myomas together with ST-28 Shuidao. KI-14 is also a very important point to invigorate Blood in endometriosis (which is always characterized by Blood stasis), in which case I combine it with ST-29 Guilai.

I also use KI-14 for rebellious Qi of the Penetrating Vessel in combination with its opening points (i.e. SP-4 Gongsun and P-6 Neiguan).

Although I personally use KI-14 primarily in Excess patterns with Blood stasis, it does have a nourishing function and it specifically nourishes the Essence and the Marrow. In fact, its alternative names include *Suifu*, which means the '*Fu* of Marrow', and *Suizhong*, which means 'Central Marrow'. According to some, 'Fullness' in this point's name refers to the 'filling up' of Marrow in the lower abdomen near KI-14.

There are many interpretations of the significance of this point's name. 'Four' may refer to the four fullnesses of Qi, Blood, Food and Dampness. Another interpretation is that 'Four' refers to a feeling of fullness in the lower abdomen radiating in four directions. According to yet another interpretation, 'Four' refers to stagnation in four organs: that is, the Small Intestine, Large Intestine, Bladder and Uterus.[3] 'Four' also refers to the fact that KI-14 is the fourth point from KI-11.

Box 61.15 summarizes the functions of KI-14.

Box 61.15 KI-14 – summary of functions

- Moves Qi and Blood in the lower abdomen (lower abdominal pain, umbilical pain, constipation, Running Piglet Syndrome)
- Regulates the Uterus and menstruation (painful periods, excessive menstrual bleeding, irregular periods, retention of lochia, excessive vaginal discharge, infertility)
- Nourishes Essence and Marrow

KI-16 HUANGSHU *TRANSPORTING POINT OF 'HUANG'*

Location

On the abdomen, 0.5 *cun* lateral to the centre of the umbilicus.

Nature

Point of the Penetrating Vessel (*Chong Mai*).

Actions

Tonifies the Kidneys.
Benefits the Membranes (*Huang*).
Benefits the Heart.
Moves Qi and Blood in the abdomen.
Regulates the Intestines.

Indications

Backache, tinnitus, deafness, tiredness, weak knees.
Abdominal distension and pain, umbilical pain.
Constipation, diarrhoea, Cold in the Large Intestine.

Comments

KI-16 is related to '*Gaohuang*', which is the space between the heart and the diaphragm. Kidney-Qi goes through this point to connect upwards with the diaphragm and the Heart: hence the name of this point (*Gaohuang* refers to the space between and the heart and the diaphragm). According to the 'Explanation of the Acupuncture Points', KI-16 Huangshu should be seen in connection with BL-17 Geshu.[4]

BL-17, Back Transporting point of the diaphragm, influences the *Gaohuang* region, which is above the diaphragm. BL-17 is situated either side of the Governing Vessel (*Du Mai*), which governs all Yang, and KI-16 is either side of the Directing Vessel (*Ren Mai*), which governs all Yin (Fig. 61.3). It is because of the connection between KI-16 and the diaphragm that it can affect both Heart and Lungs. I use KI-16 to calm the Heart and relieve anxiety deriving from rebellious Qi of the Penetrating Vessel.

It is worth noting that KI-16 is called '*Huangshu*', which means 'Transporting point for Huang'. '*Shu*' is a character that refers usually to points on the back of the body, such as in the Back Transporting (*Shu*) points. The fact that KI-16 is called a *Shu* point would seem to confirm the idea that it is in relationship with BL-17 on the back.

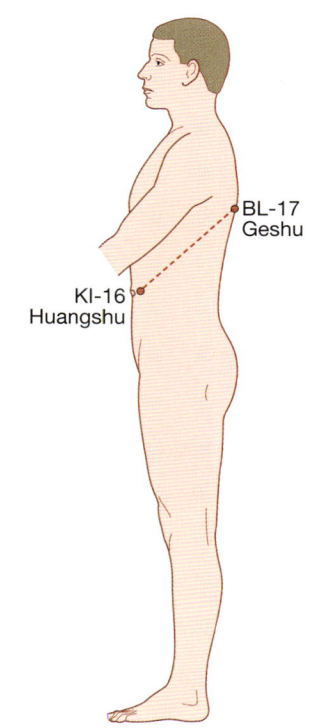

Figure 61.3 Relationship between KI-16 and BL-17

'*Huang*' in the name of this point refers also to the Membranes (*Huang*). The membranes run inside the abdomen (corresponding to the superficial and deep fascia, mesenterium and omentum) and penetrate upwards in the chest and diaphragm. KI-16, being near the umbilicus, controls the origin of Membranes. Because of its connection with the Membranes, I use KI-16 to subdue rebellious Qi of the Penetrating Vessel. Being in the centre of the abdomen, this point is in connection with the Membranes extending to the Kidneys below and to the Heart above: because of this, this point can be used to harmonize Kidneys and Heart.

This means that this point can be used to tonify the Kidneys, and, at the same time, tonify the Heart and calm the Mind. It is therefore useful when Kidney-Yin is deficient and fails to nourish the Heart.

Box 61.16 summarizes the functions of KI-16.

KI-17 SHANGQU *BENT METAL*

Location

On the upper abdomen, 2 *cun* above the umbilicus, 0.5 *cun* lateral to the midline.

Box 61.16 KI-16 – summary of functions

- Tonifies the Kidneys (backache, tinnitus, deafness, tiredness, weak knees)
- Benefits the Membranes (*Huang*) (abdominal distension and pain, umbilical pain)
- Benefits the Heart
- Moves Qi and Blood in the abdomen
- Regulates the Intestines (constipation, diarrhoea, Cold in the Large Intestine)

Nature

Point of the Penetrating Vessel (*Chong Mai*).

Actions

Regulates the Spleen, harmonizes the Stomach and dissolves accumulation.

Indications

Constipation, diarrhoea, abdominal masses (*Ji Ju*), abdominal fullness and pain, difficulty in swallowing, nausea and vomiting.

Comments

KI-17 affects the large bowel. '*Shang*' refers to the Metal element, in this case the Large Intestine, in the same way as in L.I.-1 Shangyang. 'Bend' in this point's name refers to the bend between the ascending and the transverse colon. For this reason, KI-17 is used as a local point to stimulate the function of the Large Intestine, especially in constipation and abdominal pain.

Box 61.17 summarizes the functions of KI-17.

Box 61.17 KI-17 – summary of functions

- Regulates the Spleen, harmonizes the Stomach and dissolves accumulation (constipation, diarrhoea, abdominal masses (*Ji Ju*), abdominal fullness and pain, difficulty in swallowing, nausea and vomiting)

KI-21 YOUMEN *DOOR OF DARKNESS*

Location

On the upper abdomen, 6 *cun* above the umbilicus, 0.5 *cun* lateral to the midline.

Nature

Point of the Penetrating Vessel (*Chong Mai*).

Actions

Harmonizes the Stomach.
Subdues rebellious Qi and stops vomiting.
Benefits the breasts.
Moves Qi in the chest.

Indications

Vomiting of foamy saliva, hiccup, sour regurgitation, retching, nausea and vomiting in pregnancy, epigastric fullness, poor appetite, feeling of fullness below the xiphoid process, difficulty in swallowing.
Breast distension and pain, breast milk not flowing.
Chest pain, hypochondrial distension, cough, pain in the centre of the chest in women.

Comments

KI-21 is the point where the Penetrating Vessel leaves its superficial pathway and penetrates into the interior to disperse in the chest and breasts: this explains its name in which 'darkness' refers to the interior of the chest. As with most points with the word 'door' (*men*) in their names, KI-21 regulates the entering and exiting of Qi. It does so in the epigastric region, in particular the stomach, and it subdues rebellious Stomach-Qi: for this reason it is a very important local point for nausea and vomiting, in which case I use it in combination with ST-19 Burong.

I use KI-21 also to subdue rebellious Qi of the Penetrating Vessel, usually in combination with its opening points (SP-4 Gongsun and P-6 Neiguan) and with KI-14 Siman or KI-13 Qixue, depending on whether the condition is Full or Full–Empty.

KI-21 is an important point also to move Qi in the chest and breasts.

Box 61.18 summarizes the functions of KI-21.

Box 61.18 KI-21 – summary of functions

- Harmonizes the Stomach (vomiting of foamy saliva, hiccup, sour regurgitation, retching, nausea and vomiting in pregnancy, epigastric fullness, poor appetite, feeling of fullness below the xiphoid process, difficulty in swallowing)
- Subdues rebellious Qi and stops vomiting
- Benefits the breasts (breast distension and pain, breast milk not flowing)
- Moves Qi in the chest (chest pain, hypochondrial distension, cough, pain in the centre of the chest in women)

KI-23 SHENFENG *MIND SEAL*

Location

In the fourth intercostal space, 2 *cun* lateral to the midline.

Nature

None.

Actions

Opens the chest and stops cough.
Harmonizes the Stomach and subdues rebellious Qi.
Benefits the breasts.

Indications

Feeling of tightness of the chest, cough, wheezing, breathlessness, hypochondrial distension and fullness.
Nausea, vomiting, difficulty in swallowing, poor appetite.
Breast distension and pain, breast abscess.

Comments

KI-23 is mostly used as a local point in breathing problems to harmonize the Lungs and Kidneys: that is, to promote the descending of Lung-Qi and the Kidney's receiving of Qi.

It is also used as a local point for rebellious Stomach-Qi causing nausea and vomiting.

Box 61.19 summarizes the functions of KI-23.

Box 61.19 KI-23 – summary of functions

- Opens the chest and stops cough (feeling of tightness of the chest, cough, wheezing, breathlessness, hypochondrial distension and fullness)
- Harmonizes the Stomach and subdues rebellious Qi (nausea, vomiting, difficulty in swallowing, poor appetite)
- Benefits the breasts (breast distension and pain, breast abscess)

KI-24 LINGXU *SPIRIT BURIAL GROUND*

Location

In the third intercostal space, 2 *cun* lateral to the midline.

Nature

None.

Actions

Promotes the free flow of Liver-Qi.
Opens the chest and promotes the descending of Lung-Qi.

Indications

Distension and pain of the hypochondrium.
Cough, wheezing, breathlessness.

Comments

KI-24, like KI-23, is used as a local point in breathing problems to harmonize the Lungs and Kidneys: that is, to promote the descending of Lung-Qi and the Kidney's receiving of Qi. In addition, it moves Liver-Qi in the chest and hypochondrium.

Box 61.20 summarizes the functions of KI-24.

Box 61.20 KI-24 – summary of functions

- Promotes the free flow of Liver-Qi (distension and pain of the hypochondrium)
- Opens the chest and promotes the descending of Lung-Qi (cough, wheezing, breathlessness)

KI-25 SHENCANG *MIND STORAGE*

Location

In the second intercostal space, 2 *cun* lateral to the midline.

Nature

None.

Actions

Opens the chest and promotes the descending of Lung-Qi.
Subdues rebellious Stomach-Qi.

Indications

Cough, wheezing, breathlessness, chest pain.
Nausea, vomiting, difficulty in swallowing, poor appetite.

Comments

KI-25, like KI-23 and KI-24, is used as a local point in breathing problems to harmonize the Lungs and Kidneys: that is, to promote the descending of Lung-Qi and the Kidney's receiving of Qi. In addition, this point subdues rebellious Stomach-Qi and treats nausea and vomiting.

Box 61.21 summarizes the functions of KI-25.

> **Box 61.21 KI-25 – summary of functions**
> - Opens the chest and promotes the descending of Lung-Qi (cough, wheezing, breathlessness, chest pain)
> - Subdues rebellious Stomach-Qi (nausea, vomiting, difficulty in swallowing, poor appetite)

KI-27 SHUFU *TRANSPORTING POINT MANSION*

Location

On the lower border of the clavicle, 2 *cun* lateral to the midline.

Nature

None.

Actions

Promotes the descending of Lung-Qi and stops cough.
Harmonizes the Stomach and stops vomiting.

Indications

Cough, wheezing, breathlessness, chest pain.
Nausea, vomiting, poor appetite.

Comments

KI-27 is an important local point for the treatment of asthma from Kidney deficiency. It promotes the Kidney's receiving of Qi and the descending of Lung-Qi.

Box 61.22 summarizes the functions of KI-27. Figure 61.4 illustrates the target areas of the Kidney channel points.

> **Box 61.22 KI-27 – summary of functions**
> - Promotes the descending of Lung-Qi and stops cough (cough, wheezing, breathlessness, chest pain)
> - Harmonizes the Stomach and stops vomiting (nausea, vomiting, poor appetite)

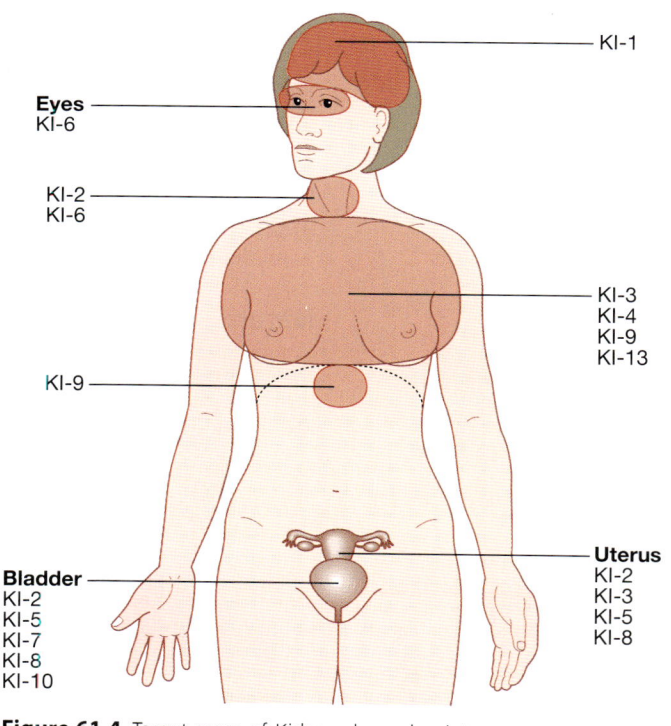

Figure 61.4 Target areas of Kidney channel points

END NOTES

1. Yue Han Zhen 1990 An Explanation of the Acupuncture Points (*Jing Xue Jie* 经 穴 解), People's Health Publishing House, Beijing, originally published in 1654, p. 264.
2. The 'Running Piglet Syndrome' indicates a pattern characterized by an uncomfortable sensation of energy rising from the lower abdomen to the chest and throat, accompanied by abdominal pain, a feeling of fullness of the chest, palpitations and anxiety. The Running Piglet Syndrome is related to rebellious Qi in the Kidney and Liver channels. Rebellious Qi in the Penetrating Vessel is a form of Running Piglet Syndrome.
3. An Explanation of the Acupuncture Points, p. 265.
4. Ibid., p. 266.

SECTION 2   PART 7

Pericardium Channel 62

Main channel pathway

The Pericardium channel originates from the chest and enters the pericardium. It then descends through the diaphragm to the abdomen to communicate with the Upper, Middle and Lower Burner.

A branch from the centre of the chest emerges laterally from the nipple to run along the superficial channel to the axilla and down the medial aspect of the arm to end at the medial side of the middle finger.

A branch from P-8 Laogong links with the Triple Burner channel at the point T.B.-1 Guanchong (Fig. 62.1).

Connecting channel pathway

The Connecting channel starts from the point P-6 Neiguan and flows up to the chest to the pericardium and heart (Fig. 62.2).

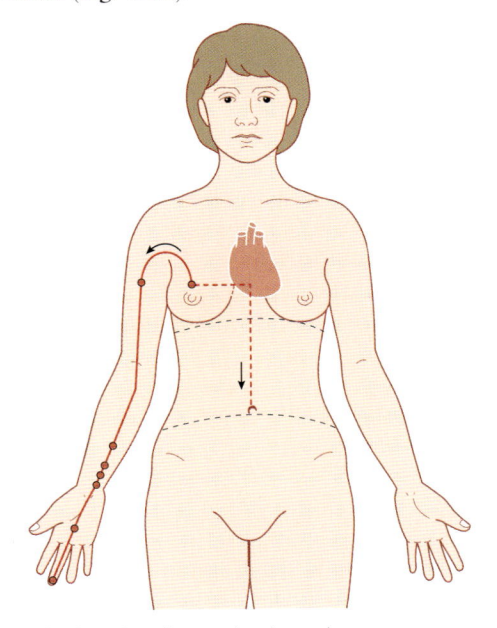

Figure 62.1 Pericardium main channel

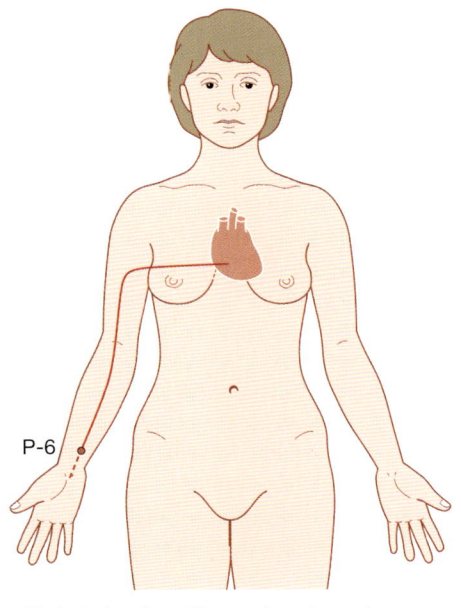

Figure 62.2 Pericardium Connecting channel

Box 62.1   Overview of Pericardium points

- Cool Blood
- Clear Heat and cool Blood at Nutritive Qi (*Ying*) and Blood levels in late stages of febrile diseases (Triple Burner channel is for Defensive Qi and Qi levels)
- Open the Mind's orifices
- In connection with Uterus
- Affect chest

Box 62.1 gives an overview of the Pericardium points.

P-1 TIANCHI *HEAVENLY POOL*

Location

1 *cun* lateral and slightly superior to the nipple, in the fourth intercostal space.

Nature

Meeting point of Pericardium, Liver, Gall Bladder and Triple Burner channels.
Window of Heaven point.

Actions

Opens the chest, promotes the descending of Qi and resolves Phlegm.
Dissipates nodules.
Benefits the breasts.

Indications

Cough with profuse sputum, rattling sound in the throat, feeling of oppression of the chest, breathlessness.
Swelling in the axilla, scrofula of neck.
Breast diseases, breast abscess, insufficient lactation.

Comments

P-1 can be used as a local point for distension and pain of the breast caused by stagnation of Liver-Qi. However, it is hardly ever used for this purpose as it would be very inconvenient to needle in women, especially when the breasts are tender and distended.

It is also used for Phlegm obstructing the Lungs.
Box 62.2 summarizes the functions of P-1.

Box 62.2 P-1 – summary of functions

- Opens the chest, promotes the descending of Qi and resolves Phlegm (cough with profuse sputum, rattling sound in the throat, feeling of oppression of the chest, breathlessness)
- Dissipates nodules (swelling in the axilla, scrofula of neck)
- Benefits the breasts (breast diseases, breast abscess, insufficient lactation)

P-3 QUZE *MARSH ON BEND*

Location

On the transverse crease of the elbow, on the ulnar side of the tendon biceps brachii muscle.

Nature

Sea (*He*) point.
Water point.

Actions

Clears Heat and cools Blood.
Harmonizes the Stomach and subdues rebellious Qi.
Moves Qi and Blood in the chest.
Calms the Mind.
Extinguishes interior Wind.
Invigorates Blood and eliminates stasis.

Indications

Febrile disease at the Nutritive Qi (*Ying*) or Blood level, agitation, mental restlessness, delirium, cold hands, fever at night, dry mouth, coughing or vomiting of blood, macules.
Vomiting, nausea, epigastric pain.
Heart pain, palpitations, feeling of tightness below the heart.
Fright, anxiety, mental restlessness.
Tremor of hands or head, paralysis of arm.

Comments

P-3 clears Heat at the Nutritive Qi and Blood levels (of the Four-Level pattern identification) in the late stages of febrile diseases with a macular rash and convulsions. Its cooling Blood action makes this point useful for skin diseases from Blood-Heat.

P-3 stimulates the descending of Stomach-Qi and is used to subdue rebellious Stomach-Qi manifesting with nausea and vomiting.

Besides cooling Blood, it also invigorates Blood and eliminates stasis. It is therefore useful in chronic conditions of Blood-Heat, when the Heat over a long period of time congeals the Blood and causes stasis. It is used for Blood stasis primarily in the chest.

Finally, P-3 can also be used to calm the Mind, when there is severe anxiety caused by Heart-Fire.

Box 62.3 summarizes the functions of P-3.

Box 62.3 P-3 – summary of functions

- Clears Heat and cools Blood (febrile disease at the Nutritive Qi or Blood level, agitation, mental restlessness, delirium, cold hands, fever at night, dry mouth, coughing or vomiting of blood, macules)
- Harmonizes the Stomach and subdues rebellious Qi (vomiting, nausea, epigastric pain)
- Moves Qi and Blood in the chest (heart pain, palpitations, feeling of tightness below the heart)
- Calms the Mind (fright, anxiety, mental restlessness)
- Extinguishes interior Wind (tremor of hands or head, paralysis of arm)
- Invigorates Blood and eliminates stasis

P-4 XIMEN *CLEFT DOOR*

Location
On the palmar aspect of the forearm, 5 *cun* above the transverse crease of the wrist, on the line connecting P-3 Quze and P-7 Daling.

Nature
Accumulation (*Xi*) point.

Actions
Invigorates Blood and eliminates stasis.
Cools Blood and stops bleeding.
Calms the Mind.
Removes obstructions from the channel and stops pain.

Indications
Chest pain, heart pain.
Coughing of blood, vomiting of blood, nosebleed.
Agitation, anxiety, insomnia, mental restlessness, depression, fright.

Comments
P-4 is an important point of the Pericardium channel and, being the Accumulation point, it is used in acute conditions particularly to stop pain. It has an influence on the chest and stops chest pain. Being the Accumulation point, it is the best point to use for painful and especially acute painful conditions of the channel.

P-4 has a special action in calming the Heart and regulating its rhythm, so it is the point of choice to use for arrhythmia and palpitations.

It also invigorates Blood and eliminates stasis, especially in the chest, so that it is a very important point to use for chest pain due to stasis of Heart-Blood.

It also cools Blood and can be used for skin diseases caused by Blood-Heat.

Finally, P-4 strengthens the Mind in cases of Heart deficiency, which may give rise to fear, anxiety, insomnia and depression.

Box 62.4 summarizes the functions of P-4.

Box 62.4 P-4 – summary of functions

- Invigorates Blood and eliminates stasis (chest pain, heart pain)
- Cools Blood and stops bleeding (coughing of blood, vomiting of blood, nosebleed)
- Calms the Mind (agitation, anxiety, insomnia, mental restlessness, depression, fright)
- Removes obstructions from the channel and stops pain

P-5 JIANSHI *INTERMEDIARY*

Location
On the medial side of the forearm, 3 *cun* proximal to P-7 Daling, between the tendons of the palmaris longus and flexor carpi radialis.

Nature
River (*Jing*) point.
Metal point.
Meeting of the three Yin channels of the arm.

Actions
Calms the Mind, opens the Mind's orifices and resolves Phlegm in the Heart.
Harmonizes the Stomach and subdues rebellious Qi.
Invigorates Blood and regulates menstruation.

Indications
Palpitations, agitation, feeling of oppression of the chest, manic behaviour, fright, mental restlessness, poor memory, 'seeing ghosts'.
Epigastric pain, vomiting, nausea.
Irregular menstruation, painful periods, clotted menstrual blood, retention of lochia.

Comments
P-5 is a very important point to resolve Phlegm obstructing the Mind's orifices. This is the non-substantial Phlegm obstructing the Heart and 'misting' the mental faculties, resulting in acute cases in delirium, aphasia and coma. In acute cases, this happens at the Blood level (of the Four-Level pattern identification) of febrile diseases.

In chronic cases, Phlegm obstructing the Heart can cause mental illness such as manic depression, in which periods of deep depression alternate with periods of manic behaviour with incessant talking, uncontrolled activity and reckless behaviour.

In other cases, the same pathology of Phlegm obstructing the Heart can cause epilepsy, with the person losing consciousness during the epileptic fit and foaming heavily from the mouth (which is indicative of Phlegm).

P-5 has an effect on the Stomach, mostly in subduing rebellious Stomach-Qi causing nausea and vomiting.

P-5 has an important Blood-invigorating action and it influences menstruation. The influence of several Pericardium points on menstruation is partly due to its relationship with the Liver within the Terminal Yin (*Jue Yin*).

Finally, it is an empirical point for malaria.

Box 62.5 summarizes the functions of P-5.

> **Box 62.5   P-5 – summary of functions**
>
> - Calms the Mind, opens the Mind's orifices and resolves Phlegm in the Heart (palpitations, agitation, feeling of oppression of the chest, manic behaviour, fright, mental restlessness, poor memory, 'seeing ghosts')
> - Harmonizes the Stomach and subdues rebellious Qi (epigastric pain, vomiting, nausea)
> - Invigorates Blood and regulates menstruation (irregular menstruation, painful periods, clotted menstrual blood, retention of lochia)

P-6 NEIGUAN *INNER GATE*

Location

On the medial side of the forearm, 2 *cun* proximal to P-7 Daling, between the tendons of the palmaris longus and flexor carpi radialis.

Nature

Connecting (*Luo*) point.
Opening point of the Yin Linking Vessel (*Yin Wei Mai*).

Actions

Opens the chest and moves Qi and Blood.
Calms the Mind.
Moves Liver-Qi.
Harmonizes the Stomach.

Indications

Chest pain, palpitations, feeling of tightness of the chest.
Insomnia, manic behaviour, poor memory, anxiety, fright, sadness, depression.
Hypochondrial distension and pain.
Nausea, vomiting, hiccup, belching, epigastric distension and pain.
Irregular and painful periods.

Comments

P-6 is one of the most important points of acupuncture, with a great number of different functions.

It has a specific action on the chest, and can therefore be used for any chest problems. More specifically it moves Qi and Blood in the chest and is the point of choice for discomfort or pain of the chest due to stagnation of Qi or Blood.

It has a powerful calming action on the Mind and can be used in anxiety caused by any of the Heart patterns. It also calms the Mind by its indirect action on the Liver (to which the Pericardium is related within the Terminal Yin). It can therefore be used for irritability due to stagnation of Liver-Qi, particularly if combined with anxiety from a Heart pattern.

It is particularly effective in women and is most useful to calm the Mind in women suffering from premenstrual depression and irritability. It also promotes sleep.

In addition to its action on the Heart and Liver, it is a major point to affect the Stomach, particularly the upper and middle part of the Stomach. It subdues rebellious Stomach-Qi and is the point of choice to treat nausea and vomiting. It can also be used in most Excess Stomach patterns characterized by epigastric pain, acid regurgitation, hiccup and belching.

As it is the Connecting point of the Pericardium channel, it connects with the Triple Burner channel and, in my experience, it is effective in treating neck ache on the occiput, especially in women. Women often suffer from neck ache after a hysterectomy and this point is very effective in treating it. Indeed, the 'Explanation of the Acupuncture Points' says: '*When the Pericardium is empty there is stiffness of the head.*'[1]

Finally, owing to its relationship with the Liver and its action of invigorating Blood, this point indirectly connects with the Blood of the Uterus, and can be used to regulate irregular or painful periods. The Pericardium influences the Uterus also, due to the connection between the Heart and Uterus through the Uterus Vessel (*Bao Mai*) (Fig. 62.3).

It is interesting to explore the meaning of the name of this point, '*Nei Guan*'. '*Nei*' means 'inner' and there is no disagreement about this. By contrast, the second half of the name, '*Guan*', can have different interpretations. In ordinary, everyday language, '*guan*' means to 'shut', 'close', 'turn off' or 'lock up'. If we go to a shop and we find it closed, one would say that the shop '*guan le*': that is, it is shut or 'it shut' (in the past). If we interpret '*guan*' in this sense, then P-6 is an 'inner closure', an 'inner stop cock' or something similar. Could it be

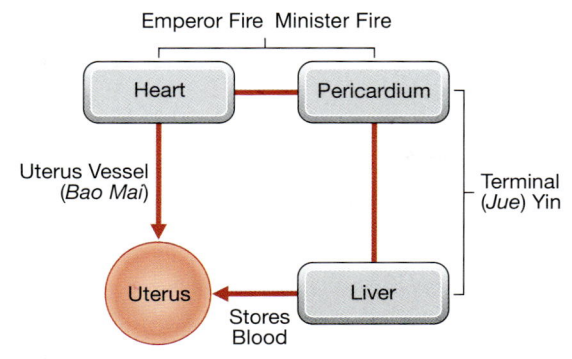

Figure 62.3 Relationship between Pericardium, Heart, Liver and Uterus

interpreted in this way? Yes, it could, and in this sense, P-6 would be the point that closes the Yin in the Interior and this should be seen in relation to and analogous to T.B.-5 Waiguan, the 'outer closure': that is, the point that closes the Yang on the outside.

However, the nature of P-6 is such that it is a very dynamic point and this does not fit in with its translation as 'inner closure' because 'closure' implies to stop something, as, for example, when one closes a tap (faucet) to stop the flow of water.

If we look up the other meanings of '*guan*' (in Chinese one word can have multiple meanings), we find that it also means 'mountain pass', 'critical juncture', 'customs house' or 'barrier' (of a customs house). According to 'Analysis of Chinese Characters', '*guan*' is a crossbar of a gate, to shut or bar the gate, a custom house barrier.[2] The character is composed of the radical '*Men*' (door). Inside the 'door' there is '*guan*', which means to pass threads through a web with a shuttle.

The script represents the warp of a textile. The downstrokes in the lower part represent a shuttle carrying the thread through to form a woof. By extension, it means to fix transversely. The crossbar of the gate passes through the slots and iron loops like a shuttle passing through the warp.

Translating '*guan*' in this way, would change the meaning of '*Nei Guan*' entirely. The point would then be an 'inner critical juncture' or an 'inner barrier' (of a customs house). Notice that it is the barrier of a customs house that is open to let goods through.

This would change the nature of the point entirely, making it a dynamic point that is a critical juncture and that lets things through. In my opinion, this reflects the nature and functions of P-6 more accurately. The reference to 'fixing transversely' is also interesting as it would be an allusion to the flow of the *Luo* channels flowing 'transversely' in relation to the main channels that flow 'vertically' (P-6 is of course the *Luo* point of the Pericardium channel).

Box 62.6 summarizes the functions of P-6.

Box 62.6 P-6 – summary of functions

- Opens the chest and moves Qi and Blood (chest pain, palpitations, feeling of tightness of the chest)
- Calms the Mind (insomnia, manic behaviour, poor memory, anxiety, fright, sadness, depression)
- Moves Liver-Qi (hypochondrial distension and pain)
- Harmonizes the Stomach (nausea, vomiting, hiccup, belching, epigastric distension and pain)
- Invigorates Blood and regulates menstruation (irregular periods, painful periods)

P-7 DALING *GREAT HILL*

Location

At the wrist joint, between the tendons of palmaris longus and flexor carpi radialis, level with HE-7 Shenmen.

Nature

Source (*Yuan*) and Stream (*Shu*) point.
Earth point.
Drainage point.

Actions

Calms the Mind and opens the Mind's orifices.
Clears Heat and Toxic Heat.
Harmonizes the Stomach.

Indications

Insomnia, manic behaviour, palpitations, agitation, mental restlessness, sadness, fright.
Febrile disease, red eyes, thirst, eczema of hands, carbuncles, furuncles.
Epigastric pain, vomiting.

Comments

P-7's most important function is that of calming the Mind. In this respect, it has all the same functions as

HE-7 Shenmen. As a matter of fact, historically, P-7 Daling was used as the Source point of the Heart channel. The first chapter of the 'Spiritual Axis' lists P-7 as the Source point of the Heart.[3]

In my experience, P-7 is more effective in women and HE-7 more effective in men to calm the Mind. P-7 is also better to deal with the emotional consequences of the breaking up of relationships.

P-7 also clears Heart-Fire and is particularly important to use when Heart-Fire causes mental problems such as great anxiety and mental restlessness or even manic behaviour.

Box 62.7 summarizes the functions of P-7.

Table 62.1 compares and contrasts the actions of HE-7 Shenmen and P-7 Daling.

Box 62.7 P-7 – summary of functions

- Calms the Mind and opens the Mind's orifices (insomnia, manic behaviour, palpitations, agitation, mental restlessness, sadness, fright)
- Clears Heat and Toxic Heat (febrile disease, red eyes, thirst, eczema of hands, carbuncles, furuncles)
- Harmonizes the Stomach (epigastric pain, vomiting)

P-8 LAOGONG *LABOUR PALACE*

Location

Between the second and third metacarpal bones, proximal to the metacarpophalangeal joint, at the radial side of the third metacarpal bone.

Nature

Spring (*Ying*) point.
Fire point.
One of Sun Si Miao 13 Ghost points.

Actions

Drains Heart-Fire.
Calms the Mind.
Clears Heat, cools Blood and promotes resuscitation.

Indications

Heart pain, tongue ulcers, thirst, insomnia, agitation.
Manic behaviour, fright, anxiety, mental restlessness.
Febrile disease at the Nutritive Qi or Blood levels, loss of consciousness, agitation, mental restlessness, delirium, cold hands, fever at night, dry mouth, coughing or vomiting of blood, macules.

Comments

P-8 is the most effective point on the Pericardium channel to clear Heart-Fire. Being the Spring point, it is a particularly dynamic point to clear Heat. In particular, it has a specific effect in clearing tongue ulcers deriving from Heart-Fire.

In acute febrile diseases, P-8 clears Heat and cools Blood and is used for high fever at night and delirium.

Box 62.8 summarizes the functions of P-8.

Table 62.1 A comparison of HE-7 Shenmen and P-7 Daling

HE-7 Shenmen	P-7 Daling
Both can nourish Heart-Blood and calm the Mind	
More for Deficiency patterns	More for Excess patterns
Not for Warm diseases	Important for Warm diseases, Heat in Pericardium (Nutritive Qi level)
Gentle action in calming Mind	Better for severe anxiety and mania
Not so strong in opening the Mind's orifices	Opens Mind's orifices
Better for men	Better for women
	Especially indicated for emotional upsets deriving from the breaking of relationships

Box 62.8 P-8 – summary of functions

- Drains Heart-Fire (heart pain, tongue ulcers, thirst, insomnia, agitation)
- Calms the Mind (manic behaviour, fright, anxiety, mental restlessness)
- Clears Heat, cools Blood and promotes resuscitation (febrile disease at the Nutritive Qi or Blood levels, loss of consciousness, agitation, mental restlessness, delirium, cold hands, fever at night, dry mouth, coughing or vomiting of blood, macules)

P-9 ZHONGCHONG *CENTRE RUSH*

Location

In the centre of the tip of the distal phalanx of the middle finger.

Nature

Well (*Jing*) point.
Wood point.
Tonification point.

Actions

Clears Heat and restores consciousness.
Extinguishes interior Wind.
Calms the Mind.

Indications

Fever, loss of consciousness.
Wind-stroke.
Agitation, anxiety, palpitations, insomnia.

Comments

P-9 is mostly used to clear Heat, either in chronic conditions with mental symptoms, or in acute cases of Heat at the Nutritive Qi level.

It also extinguishes interior Wind and restores consciousness and is used in acute Wind-stroke, together with all the other Well points of the hands.

Box 62.9 summarizes the functions of P-9.

Box 62.9 P-9 – summary of functions

- Clears Heat and restores consciousness (fever, loss of consciousness)
- Extinguishes interior Wind (Wind-stroke)
- Calms the Mind (agitation, anxiety, palpitations, insomnia)

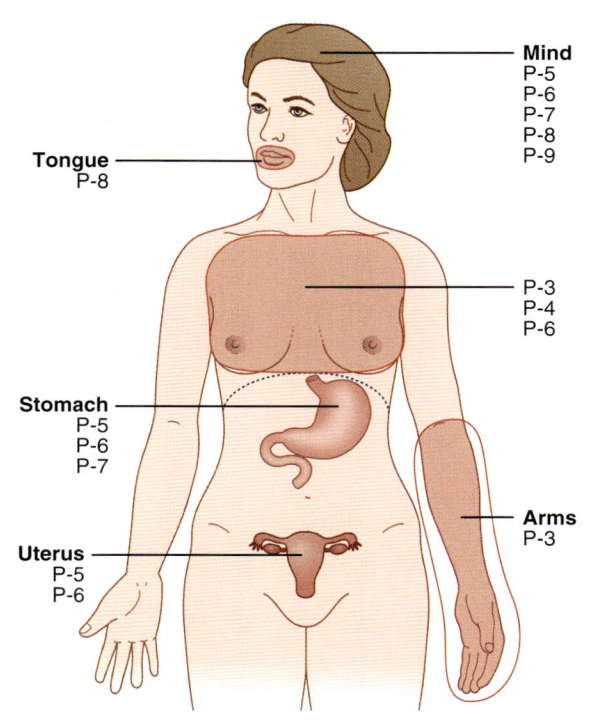

Figure 62.4 Target areas of Pericardium channel points

The following is a comparison between P-3 Quze, P-4 Ximen, P-5 Jianshi, P-6 Neiguan and P-7 Daling. They can all calm the Mind:

- P-3 clears Heat and cools Blood. Its functions of regulating the Intestines and cooling Blood are important
- P-4 regulates the Pericardium and stops pain in acute conditions. Its use in acute conditions with pain is the most important one
- P-5 resolves Phlegm from the Heart, for symptoms of Phlegm misting the Heart
- P-6 opens the chest, calms the Mind and regulates Liver-Qi. Its most important aspects are those of relieving tightness of the chest associated with a Heart pattern, calming anxiety, particularly in women, and indirectly moving Liver-Qi and its resulting emotional irritability and depression
- P-7 calms the Mind, particularly for emotional problems deriving from difficult relationships. More often used for women than men

Fig. 62.4 illustrates the target areas of the Pericardium channel points.

END NOTES

1. Yue Han Zhen 1990 An Explanation of the Acupuncture Points (*Jing Xue Jie* 经 穴 解), People's Health Publishing House, Beijing, originally published in 1654, p. 286.
2. G.D. Wilder and J.H. Ingram, Analysis of Chinese Characters, AMA Publications, 1922, p. 38.
3. 1981 Spiritual Axis (*Ling Shu Jing* 灵 枢 经), People's Health Publishing House, Beijing, first published c.100 BC, p. 3.

SECTION 2   PART 7

Triple Burner Channel 63

Main channel pathway

The Triple Burner channel starts at the tip of the ring finger. Running between the fourth and fifth metacarpal bones, it flows to the wrist and up the lateral aspect of the arm between the radius and ulna. It then reaches the shoulder joint and the supraclavicular fossa from where it goes down to the chest to connect with the pericardium. It then descends through the diaphragm to the abdomen to join the Middle and Lower Burners.

From the chest, a branch goes up to the supraclavicular fossa from where it ascends to the neck and the region behind the ear. It then turns downwards to the cheek and terminates in the infraorbital region.

From behind the ear, a branch enters the ear, re-emerges in front of the ear and links with the Gall Bladder channel (Fig. 63.1).

Connecting channel pathway

The Connecting channel starts at T.B.-5 Waiguan and flows up the arm along the main channel to the shoulder and chest where it links with the Pericardium channel (Fig. 63.2).

Box 63.1 provides an overview of Triple Burner points.

> **Box 63.1   Overview of Triple Burner points**
>
> - Clear Heat at Defensive Qi (*Wei*) and Qi levels in febrile diseases
> - Affect arms, shoulders, neck, head
> - Used for ear problems related to Heat or Damp-Heat
> - Regulate the Lesser Yang
> - Move Qi and regulate the Qi Mechanism

Figure 63.1 Triple Burner main channel

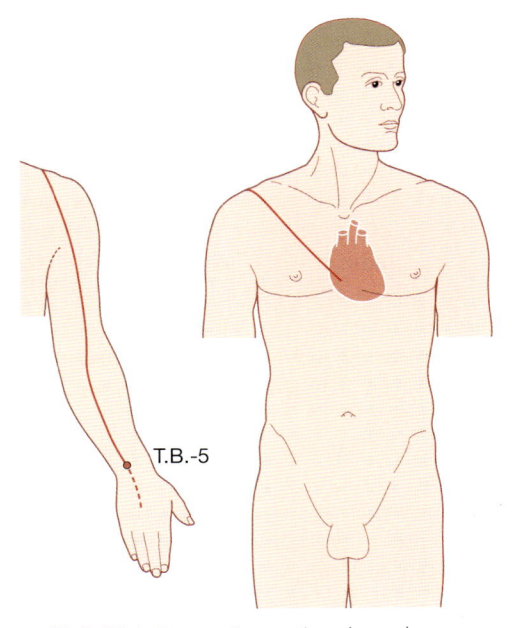

Figure 63.2 Triple Burner Connecting channel

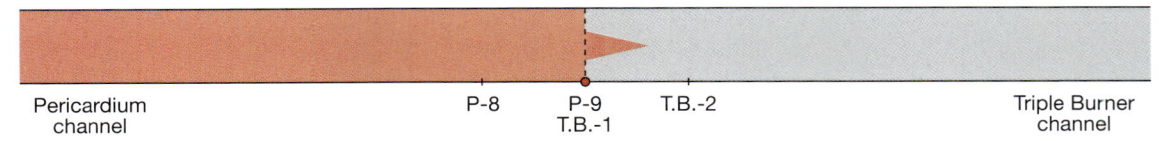

Figure 63.3 Connection between Pericardium and Triple Burner channel at the fingertips

T.B.-1 GUANCHONG *PENETRATING THE GATE*

Location

At the lateral angle of the nail of the fourth finger.

Nature

Well (*Jing*) point.
Metal point.

Actions

Clears Heat.
Expels exterior Wind.
Clears Pericardium-Heat.
Benefits the ears.

Indications

Red eyes, dry mouth, thirst, bitter taste.
Febrile disease, aversion to cold, fever, alternation of feeling of cold and feeling of heat.
Heart pain, stiff tongue, curled tongue, pain at the root of the tongue, cracked tongue.
Tinnitus, deafness, earache.

Comments

T.B.-1 is used in exterior patterns of invasion of exterior Wind-Heat causing fever, sore throat or earache. In invasions of Wind-Heat, it is the presence of earache that indicates the use of the Triple Burner channel.

This point can be used for both the Greater Yang and the Lesser Yang stage of the Six-Stage pattern identification. However, it is particularly important for the Lesser Yang stage.

T.B.-1 also affects the Pericardium and can clear Pericardium-Heat: this explains the many indications for tongue problems. Its effect on the Pericardium channel is due to the influence of the Qi of the Pericardium channel, which ends at the fingertips. This phenomenon can be compared to that of a tributary of a river flowing into another river: where the waters of the two rivers meet, the flow from the first river can still be seen as a separate current before the two rivers merge completely. In a similar way, when the Pericardium channel ends and merges into the Triple Burner channel at the fingertips, the influence of the Pericardium-Qi persists for a little way into the Triple Burner channel: for this reason, T.B.-1 has many indications related to tongue problems which stem from Heat in the Pericardium (Fig. 63.3).

The above is actually a general principle that applies to all the channels that *start* at the fingertips or toes (i.e. the Yang channels of the hand and the Yin channels of the foot): their first point (Well) receives the influence of the Qi deriving from the related channel that ends at the fingers or toes (e.g. Triple Burner from Pericardium, Large Intestine from Lungs, Kidneys from Bladder, Spleen from Stomach, etc.).

Like many other Triple Burner points, T.B.-1 benefits the ears; as we have seen, many Kidney channel points also 'benefit the ears' and it is therefore important to clarify the different actions of the Triple Burner and Kidney channels on the ears. The Kidneys nourish the ears in the sense that they send Qi and Essence up to the ears to promote good hearing. Therefore, a Kidney pathology causes mostly slow-onset, chronic ear problems such as slow-onset tinnitus and deafness. The Triple Burner influences the ears through its channel and also through its related channel within the Lesser Yang: that is, the Gall Bladder channel. A pathology of the Triple Burner (or Gall Bladder) channel causes mostly acute ear problems, infective ear problems and ear problems connected to invasions of exterior Wind-Heat: examples are earache, ear discharge, otitis, an acute earache with invasion of Wind-Heat in children, itching in the ear, eczema in the ears, etc.

Finally, T.B.-1 can also be used as a distal point to remove obstructions from the channel. In my experience, it is very effective as a distal point for shoulder problems occurring on the Triple Burner channel. In such cases, it is combined with T.B.-14 Jianliao.

Box 63.2 summarizes the functions of T.B.-1.

> **Box 63.2 T.B.-1 – summary of functions**
>
> - Clears Heat (red eyes, dry mouth, thirst, bitter taste)
> - Expels exterior Wind (febrile disease, aversion to cold, fever, alternation of feeling of cold and feeling of heat)
> - Clears Pericardium-Heat (heart pain, stiff tongue, curled tongue, pain at the root of the tongue, cracked tongue)
> - Benefits the ears (tinnitus, deafness, earache)

T.B.-2 YEMEN *FLUID DOOR*

Location

On the dorsum of the hand, proximal to the margin of the web between the fourth and fifth fingers.

Nature

Spring (*Ying*) point.
Water point.

Actions

Clears Heat in the head.
Regulates the Lesser Yang.
Benefits the ear.
Removes obstructions from the channel.

Indications

Red eyes, red face, dry eyes, swelling and pain of the throat, toothache, bleeding gums, pain in the gums.
Alternation of feeling of cold and feeling of heat, malaria.
Earache, tinnitus, deafness, sudden deafness.
Pain in the arm, inability to raise the arm, redness and swelling on dorsum of hand, contraction of fingers, neck ache, wrist ache.

Comments

Some of the actions of T.B.-2 in relation to invasions of exterior Wind-Heat are the same as those of T.B.-1 Guanchong. In particular, T.B.-2 has a pronounced action on the Lesser Yang pattern characterized by alternation of feeling of cold and feeling of heat.

T.B.-2 is an important distal point for ear problems and is used in cases of earache due to infection of the middle ear (which could accompany invasions of exterior Wind-Heat). It is also effective in treating tinnitus.

It clears interior Heat from the Triple Burner and Gall Bladder channel, especially in relation to the head, with many symptoms that are related to Heat affecting the eyes. It is suitable also to treat eye problems from Heat deriving from Liver-Fire.

This point is also widely used for Painful Obstruction Syndrome of the fingers and of the arm.

Box 63.3 summarizes the functions of T.B.-2.

> **Box 63.3 T.B.-2 – summary of functions**
>
> - Clears Heat in the head (red eyes, red face, dry eyes, swelling and pain of the throat, toothache, bleeding gums, pain in the gums)
> - Regulates the Lesser Yang (alternation of feeling of cold and feeling of heat, malaria)
> - Benefits the ear (earache, tinnitus, deafness, sudden deafness)
> - Removes obstructions from the channel (pain in the arm, inability to raise the arm, redness and swelling on dorsum of hand, contraction of fingers, neck ache, wrist ache)

T.B.-3 ZHONGZHU *MIDDLE ISLET*

Location

On the dorsum of the hand, proximal to the fourth and fifth metacarpophalangeal joints.

Nature

Stream (*Shu*) point.
Wood point.
Tonification point.

Actions

Clears Heat in the head.
Regulates the Lesser Yang.
Benefits the ear.
Subdues Liver-Yang.
Removes obstructions from the channel.

Indications

Redness and pain of the eyes, itchy face, red face.
Febrile disease, alternation of feeling of cold and feeling of heat, malaria.
Tinnitus, deafness, earache.
Headache, dizziness, headache on temple.
Inability to flex or extend fingers, redness and swelling of the arm.

Comments

Some of the actions of T.B.-3 are basically the same as those of T.B.-2 Yemen: that is, in clearing Heat from the head, benefiting the ears, treating the Lesser Yang patterns and removing obstructions from the channel. T.B.-3, however, has some additional functions and, in particular, it subdues Liver-Yang: it can therefore be used in Liver-Yang rising headaches, especially when the headache is on the temple.

In my experience, T.B.-3 moves Qi and eliminates stagnation. Due to its relationship with the Gall Bladder (within the Lesser Yang) and between this latter organ and the Liver, T.B.-3 indirectly affects the Liver, so that it can be used to eliminate stagnation of Liver-Qi manifesting with hypochondrial pain, depression and mood swings. On a psychological level, it moves Qi and lifts depression deriving from stagnation of Liver-Qi, particularly in combination with Du-20 Baihui. It is extremely effective in lifting the Mind when a person is depressed.

Box 63.4 summarizes the functions of T.B.-3.

Box 63.4 T.B.-3 – summary of functions

- Clears Heat in the head (redness and pain of the eyes, itchy face, red face)
- Regulates the Lesser Yang (febrile disease, alternation of feeling of cold and feeling of heat, malaria)
- Benefits the ear (tinnitus, deafness, earache)
- Subdues Liver-Yang (headache, dizziness, headache on temple)
- Removes obstructions from the channel (inability to flex or extend fingers, redness and swelling of the arm)

T.B.-4 YANGCHI *YANG POND*

Location

On the dorsum of the wrist, between the tendons of the extensor digitorum communis and extensor digiti minimi.

Nature

Source (*Yuan*) point.

Actions

Removes obstructions from the channel.
Benefits the ears.
Regulates the Lesser Yang.
Promotes fluids transformation.
Benefits Original Qi (*Yuan Qi*).
Tonifies Penetrating and Directing Vessels (*Chong Mai* and *Ren Mai*).

Indications

Wrist pain, neck ache, pain in the shoulder and arm, redness and swelling of wrist.
Tinnitus, deafness, earache.
Febrile disease, alternation of feeling of cold and feeling of heat, malaria.
Swelling of the legs, urinary difficulty, urinary retention, oedema of the legs.
Tiredness, poor appetite, backache, weak knees.
Irregular periods, amenorrhoea.

Comments

T.B.-4 has many different functions. Firstly, it relaxes sinews and removes obstructions from the channel, which means that it can be used to treat Painful Obstruction Syndrome of the arm and shoulder. It is also very effective for headaches of the occiput deriving from exterior invasion of Wind.

The Triple Burner, and particularly the Lower Burner, is in charge of the transformation of fluids, and, in my experience, this point can stimulate this function whenever fluids are not being transformed properly and Dampness accumulates in the Lower Burner. T.B.-4 is particularly effective in this connection combined with BL-64 Jinggu: the combination of these two points stimulates the transformation and excretion of fluids in the Lower Burner very effectively. The word 'Pool' in this point's name confirms its effect on Body Fluids.

In my experience, T.B.-4 regulates the function of the Stomach and tonifies the Stomach, especially in conjunction with ST-42 Chongyang. The combination of these two points is very effective in tonifying Stomach and Spleen and giving energy if the person is very tired.

As explained in chapter 51 dealing with the functions of the Source points, these points are in a relationship with the Original Qi. In particular, according to the 'Classic of Difficulties', Original Qi arises between the Kidneys and spreads to the Internal Organs via the Triple Burner, so that the Triple Burner is like the 'ambassador' or 'intermediary' for the Original Qi.[1] This point is therefore not just a Source point, but the Source point of the Triple Burner, which is the intermediary for the Original Qi. T.B.-4 can thus be used to tonify Original Qi in all chronic diseases when the Kidneys have become deficient and the person's energy is greatly weakened.

Because of its connection with Original Qi, this point is also connected with the Penetrating and Directing Vessels and can be used to regulate their Qi and Blood. It is therefore used in irregular or painful periods and amenorrhoea.

These last two functions are derived from the Japanese tradition of acupuncture, as Chinese texts do not make any mention of a connection between T.B.-4 and the Original Qi and the Penetrating and Directing Vessels.

In my experience, T.B.-64 regulates the Water passages of the Lower Burner when used in conjunction with BL-64 Jinggu.

Box 63.5 summarizes the functions of T.B.-4.

Box 63.5 T.B.-4 – summary of functions

- Removes obstructions from the channel (wrist pain, neck ache, pain in the shoulder and arm, redness and swelling of wrist)
- Benefits the ears (tinnitus, deafness, earache)
- Regulates the Lesser Yang (febrile disease, alternation of feeling of cold and feeling of heat, malaria)
- Promotes fluids transformation (swelling of the legs, urinary difficulty, urinary retention, oedema of the legs)
- Benefits Original Qi (tiredness, poor appetite, backache, weak knees)
- Tonifies Penetrating and Directing Vessels (irregular periods, amenorrhoea)

T.B.-5 WAIGUAN *OUTER GATE*

Location

2 *cun* proximal to T.B.-4 Yangchi, between the radius and the ulna, on the radial side of the extensor digitorum communis tendons.

Nature

Connecting (*Luo*) point.
Opening point of the Yang Linking Vessel (*Yang Wei Mai*).

Actions

Expels Wind-Heat.
Benefits the ears.
Clears Heat in the head.
Subdues Liver-Yang.
Removes obstructions from the channel.

Indications

Febrile disease, aversion to cold, fever, earache, alternation of aversion to cold and aversion to heat.
Tinnitus, deafness, earache, itching of ears, redness, pain and swelling of the ear.
Redness, pain and swelling of the eyes, stiffness of the tongue, mouth ulcers, cracked lips, nosebleed, mumps.
Headache, dizziness, one-sided headache, vertical headache, neck ache.
Pain of the shoulder and neck, stiff neck, arm pain, contraction of elbow, elbow and wrist pain, paralysis of arm, swelling and redness of arm, pain in the fingers with inability to grasp, tremor of hand.

Comments

T.B.-5 is a major point to release the Exterior and expel Wind-Heat. It must nearly always be used to expel Wind-Heat when there are such symptoms as fever, sore throat, slight sweating, aversion to cold and a Floating-Rapid pulse. It is especially indicated in invasions of external Wind-Heat when there is an earache. It can be used for the Greater Yang stage of the Six Stages (Wind-Heat type), or the Defensive Qi level of the Four Levels and also for the Lesser Yang pattern within the Six-Stage pattern identification or the Gall Bladder-Heat pattern of the Four-Level pattern identification.

It is the main point to regulate the Lesser Yang, when the pathogenic factor is half in the Exterior and half in the Interior, with such symptoms as alternation of chills and fever, irritability, hypochondrial pain, bitter taste, blurred vision and a Wiry pulse. According to some sources, this point can actually expel all six pathogenic factors: that is, Wind, Heat, Cold, Dampness Dryness and Fire.[2]

This point is also a major point for the treatment of Painful Obstruction Syndrome of the arm, shoulder and neck and is, indeed, a general point for Painful Obstruction Syndrome from Wind. As it is the Connecting point, it affects the whole area irrigated by the Connecting channel and the muscles and sinews along the channel.

T.B.-5 benefits the ears and can be used whenever there is an ear infection from an invasion of exterior Wind-Heat or tinnitus and deafness from Liver-Fire or Liver-Yang rising.

Finally, T.B.-5 indirectly subdues Liver-Yang rising (because of the Triple Burner connection with the Gall Bladder within the Lesser Yang), and is very much used as a distal point to treat migraine headaches on the temples from rising of Liver-Yang.

Box 63.6 summarizes the functions of T.B.-5.

Box 63.6 T.B.-5 – summary of functions

- Expels Wind-Heat (febrile disease, aversion to cold, fever, earache, alternation of aversion to cold and aversion to heat)
- Benefits the ears (tinnitus, deafness, earache, itching of ears, redness, pain and swelling of the ear)
- Clears Heat in the head (redness, pain and swelling of the eyes, stiffness of the tongue, mouth ulcers, cracked lips, nosebleed, mumps)
- Subdues Liver-Yang (headache, dizziness, one-sided headache, vertical headache, neck ache)
- Removes obstructions from the channel (pain of the shoulder and neck, stiff neck, arm pain, contraction of elbow, elbow and wrist pain, paralysis or arm, swelling and redness of arm, pain in the fingers with inability to grasp, tremor of hand)

T.B.-6 ZHIGOU *BRANCHING DITCH*

Location

3 *cun* proximal to T.B.-4 Yangchi, between the radius and the ulna, on the radial side of the extensor digitorum communis muscle.

Nature

River (*Jing*) point.
Fire point.

Actions

Regulates Qi and benefits the chest and costal region.
Clears Heat in the head.
Benefits the Large Intestine.
Removes obstructions from the channel.
Expels Wind.
Regulates the Directing Vessel (*Ren Mai*).

Indications

Pain in the costal region on the lateral side, abdominal pain, chest pain, feeling of oppression of the chest.
Redness and heat of the face, febrile disease, sudden loss of voice, redness, swelling and pain of the eyes, swelling and pain of the throat.
Constipation.
Pain in the axilla, pain in the shoulder and arm, Painful Obstruction Syndrome (*Bi Syndrome*) of the elbow, tremor of hand, paralysis of arm, numbness of hand.
Skin rashes from Wind and Heat.

Comments

T.B.-6 point regulates Qi in the Three Burners and removes stagnation of Liver-Qi, especially when combined with G.B.-34 Yanglingquan. Its area of action is on the lateral costal region (see below, Fig. 63.4). However, its Qi-moving action extends to other areas than just the costal region. Indeed, T.B.-6 moves and unblocks Qi in the Three Burners themselves. As we have seen in chapter 18, the Triple Burner controls the ascending/descending and entering/exiting of Qi in the Qi Mechanism. The Triple Burner is responsible for the transformation and penetration of Qi in all the cavities and in all organs. This whole process is called 'Qi Transformation by the Triple Burner': the result of the Qi transformation is the production of Nutritive Qi (*Ying Qi*), Defensive Qi (*Wei Qi*), Blood and Body Fluids. That is also why the Triple Burner is said to control 'all kinds of Qi'.

Chapter 38 of the 'Classic of Difficulties' confirms that the Triple Burner exerts its influence on all types of Qi: '*The Triple Burner is the place where the Original Qi is separated: it supports all of the Qi.*'[3] Chapter 31 confirms the influence of the Triple Burner on the movement of Qi in all parts of the body: '*The Qi of the Triple Burner gathers in the avenues of Qi [Qi Jie].*'[4] This means that the Triple Burner is responsible for the free passage of Qi in all channels but also all structures (such as cavities) of the body.

T.B.-6 is the best point of the Triple Burner channel to stimulate the transformation and penetration of Qi in all three Burners: this transformation and penetration of Qi is important also for the movement, transformation and excretion of fluids in the Three Burners.

The Triple Burner's transformation and penetration of Qi affects also the Uterus and menstruation. The 'Explanation of the Acupuncture Points' says: '*When the Qi of the Triple Burner stagnates, the Directing Vessel [Ren Mai] is obstructed; T.B.-6 should be reduced to* unblock Qi; when Qi moves, Blood moves [and the Directing Vessel will be unblocked].'⁵

> **Clinical note**
>
> T.B.-6 Zhigou is the best point to stimulate the Triple Burner's function of transportation and penetration of Qi

T.B.-6 clears Heat and can be used at the Qi level of invasions of Heat when there is constipation and abdominal pain. It promotes the bowel movement mostly in the context of febrile diseases of Heat patterns.

This point also clears Heat from the head in a similar way to T.B.-2, T.B.-3 and T.B.-5 and it affects the eyes.

It expels Wind-Heat in the skin and is widely used in skin diseases from Wind characterized by red rashes and hives that come and go or move quickly, such as in urticaria. In this case, it is combined with G.B.-31 Fengshi.

Because of its action in expelling Wind-Heat, it is a major point for the treatment of herpes zoster when combined with G.B.-31 Fengshi, especially if the skin eruptions are on the lateral costal region.

It is interesting that T.B.-6 affects the chest due to its connection with the Pericardium channel more than the point T.B.-5 Waiguan (as it would have been logical to think given that T.B.-5 is the Connecting point). The 'Explanation of the Acupuncture Points' says: '*The Triple Burner channels go to the centre of the chest, when there is stagnation, there is a feeling of oppression of the chest and the point T.B.-6 should be reduced to relieve the feeling of oppression. When there is heart pain, the Pericardium channel's Qi rebels upwards and this point should be reduced.*'⁶

Box 63.7 summarizes the functions of T.B.-6.

Box 63.7   T.B.-6 – summary of functions

- Regulates Qi and benefits the chest and costal region (pain in the costal region on the lateral side, abdominal pain, chest pain, feeling of oppression of the chest)
- Clears Heat in the head (redness and heat of the face, febrile disease, sudden loss of voice, redness, swelling and pain of the eyes, swelling and pain of the throat)
- Benefits the Large Intestine (constipation)
- Removes obstructions from the channel (pain in the axilla, pain in the shoulder and arm, Painful Obstruction Syndrome (*Bi* Syndrome) of the elbow, tremor of hand, paralysis of arm, numbness of hand)
- Expels Wind (skin rashes from Wind and Heat)
- Regulates the Directing Vessel

T.B.-7 HUIZONG *CONVERGING CHANNELS*

Location

3 *cun* proximal to T.B.-4 Yangchi, level with and on the ulnar side of T.B.-6 Zhigou, between the ulna and the extensor digitorum communis muscle.

Nature

Accumulation (*Xi*) point.

Actions

Removes obstructions from the channel.
Benefits the ears.

Indications

Pain in the arm and shoulder, pain in the elbow, pain and contraction of the fingers.
Tinnitus, deafness, earache.

Comments

Like all Accumulation points, T.B.-7 can be used in acute Excess patterns to stop pain. Its areas of action are the ears, temples and eyebrows. It is also effective for muscle ache in the arms in postviral fatigue syndrome.

Box 63.8 summarizes the functions of T.B.-7.

Box 63.8   T.B.-7 – summary of functions

- Removes obstructions from the channel (pain in the arm and shoulder, pain in the elbow, pain and contraction of the fingers)
- Benefits the ears (tinnitus, deafness, earache)

T.B.-8 SANYANGLUO *CONNECTING THREE YANG*

Location

On the dorsal aspect of the forearm, on the line connecting T.B.-4 Yangchi and the tip of the elbow, 4 *cun* above the transverse crease of the wrist between the ulna and radius.

Nature

Meeting point of the three Yang channels of the arm.

Actions

Removes obstructions from the channel.
Benefits the throat and voice.

Indications

Pain in the arm and shoulder, pain in the elbow, pain and contraction of the fingers.
Sudden loss of voice.

Comments

T.B.-8 is mostly used for Painful Obstruction Syndrome of the arm, neck, shoulders and occiput. As it is the meeting point of the three Yang channels of the arm, it is particularly effective when the area of pain involves more than one channel on the Yang surface of arm and shoulders. It relaxes the sinews and relieves pain and stiffness.

Box 63.9 summarizes the functions of T.B.-8.

Box 63.9 T.B.-8 – summary of functions

- Removes obstructions from the channel (pain in the arm and shoulder, pain in the elbow, pain and contraction of the fingers)
- Benefits the throat and voice (sudden loss of voice)

T.B.-10 TIANJING *HEAVENLY WELL*

Location

On the lateral aspect of the arm, when the elbow is flexed, the point is in the depression 1 *cun* directly above the tip of the elbow.

Nature

Sea (*He*) point.
Earth point.
Drainage point.

Actions

Resolves Phlegm and dissipates nodules.
Subdues rebellious Qi.
Calms the Mind.

Indications

Scrofula, coughing of phlegm.
Chest pain, cough, pain in the lateral costal region.
Manic behaviour, sadness, fright, palpitations.

Comments

First of all, this point is used in the treatment of Painful Obstruction Syndrome along the course of the channel. It relaxes the sinews and will stop pain and relieve stiffness, particularly of the elbow.

It resolves Dampness and Phlegm and is used particularly for external invasions of Damp-Heat manifesting with such symptoms as swelling of glands and tonsils.

It dissipates nodules, which is another aspect of its action in resolving Dampness and Phlegm, and is used to treat swellings of the lymph glands.

It can be used in invasions of exterior Wind-Cold with prevalence of Wind to regulate Nutritive and Defensive Qi, stop sweating and release the Exterior.

Finally, it can be used in a similar way to T.B.-3 Zhongzhu to relieve stagnation of Liver-Qi and allay depression and mood swings.

Box 63.10 summarizes the functions of T.B.-10.

Box 63.10 T.B.-10 – summary of functions

- Resolves Phlegm and dissipates nodules (scrofula, coughing of phlegm)
- Subdues rebellious Qi (chest pain, cough, pain in the lateral costal region)
- Calms the Mind (manic behaviour, sadness, fright, palpitations)

T.B.-13 NAOHUI *SHOULDER CONVERGENCE*

Location

On the lateral aspect of the arm, on the line connecting the olecranon and T.B.-4 Yangchi, 3 *cun* below T.B.-14 Jianliao, on the posterior and inferior border of the deltoid muscle.

Nature

Point of the Yang Linking Vessel (*Yang Wei Mai*).

Actions

Dissipates nodules.
Removes obstructions from the channel.

Indications

Goitre, scrofula.
Pain in the arm and shoulder, inability to raise the arm.

Comments

T.B.-13 is not an important point energetically but it is important as a local point for pain in the upper arm and shoulder, and one that should always be tested for tenderness.

Box 63.11 summarizes the functions of T.B.-13.

Box 63.11 T.B.-13 – summary of functions

- Dissipates nodules (goitre, scrofula)
- Removes obstructions from the channel (pain in the arm and shoulder, inability to raise the arm)

T.B.-14 JIANLIAO SHOULDER CREVICE

Location

At the origin of the deltoid muscle, posterior and inferior to the lateral extremity of the acromion.

Nature

None.

Actions

Removes obstructions from the channel.

Indications

Pain in the arm and shoulder, inability to raise the arm, numbness in the arm, feeling of heaviness of the shoulder.

Comments

T.B.-14 is an important local point for pain and arthritis of the shoulder joint, and should also always be tested for tenderness when choosing between this point and L.I.-15 Jianyu.

Box 63.12 summarizes the functions of T.B.-14.

Box 63.12 T.B.-14 – summary of functions

- Removes obstructions from the channel (pain in the arm and shoulder, inability to raise the arm, numbness in the arm, feeling of heaviness of the shoulder)
- This point should always be checked for tenderness in shoulder problems

---

T.B.-15 TIANLIAO HEAVENLY CREVICE

Location

In the suprascapular fossa, midway between G.B.-21 Jianjing and T.B.-13 Quyuan.

Nature

Point of the Yang Linking Vessel (*Yang Wei Mai*).
Meeting point of Triple Burner and Gall Bladder channels.

Actions

Removes obstructions from the channel.
Opens the chest and regulates Qi.
Clears Heat.

Indications

Pain of the shoulder and arm, stiffness and pain of the neck, pain in the clavicle.
Feeling of oppression of the chest, feeling of heat of the chest, feeling of heat, febrile disease.

Comments

T.B.-15 is an important local point for pain in the shoulder and should always be tested for tenderness. It is nearly always tender in cases of pain and stiffness of the shoulders and it gives very good results when needled with moxa.

Box 63.13 summarizes the functions of T.B.-15.

Box 63.13 T.B.-15 – summary of functions

- Removes obstructions from the channel (pain of the shoulder and arm, stiffness and pain of the neck, pain in the clavicle)
- Opens the chest and regulates Qi (feeling of oppression of the chest, feeling of heat of the chest, feeling of heat, febrile disease)
- Clears Heat

T.B.-16 TIANYOU *WINDOW OF HEAVEN*

Location

On the posterior border of the sternocleidomastoid muscle, 1 *cun* inferior to G.B.-12 Wangu, on a line drawn between BL-10 Tianzhu and T.B.-17 Tianrong.

Nature

Window of Heaven point.

Actions

Regulates the ascending and descending of Qi and subdues rebellious Qi.
Brightens the sense orifices.

Indications

Headache, dizziness, swollen face, scrofula.
Sudden deafness, blurred vision, excessive lacrimation, sneezing, nosebleed, loss of sense of smell.

Comments

T.B.-16 is a Window of Heaven point and all its actions and indications reflect this nature. As explained in chapter 51, one of the main characteristics of the these points is that they regulate the ascending and descending of Qi to and from the head. They can therefore both subdue rebellious Qi from the head and promote the ascending of clear Qi to the head.

The first action is reflected in this point's function in treating headache and dizziness from Liver-Yang rising. The second action is reflected in this point's ability to brighten the sense orifices by promoting the ascending of clear Qi to them.

Box 63.14 summarizes the functions of T.B.-16.

Box 63.14 T.B.-16 – summary of functions

- Regulates the ascending and descending of Qi and subdues rebellious Qi (headache, dizziness, swollen face, scrofula)
- Brightens the sense orifices (sudden deafness, blurred vision, excessive lacrimation, sneezing, nosebleed, loss of sense of smell)

T.B.-17 YIFENG *WIND SCREEN*

Location

Posterior to the lobe of the ear, in the depression between the angle of the mandible and the mastoid process.

Nature

Meeting point of Triple Burner and Gall Bladder channels.

Actions

Expels Wind.
Benefits the ears.

Indications

Deviation of eye and mouth, tetany.
Tinnitus, deafness, ear discharge, itching inside the ear, redness, swelling and pain of the ear.

Comments

This is a major local point for ear problems. It can be used in all ear problems of exterior or interior origin. It is used in ear infections from exterior Wind-Heat, or for deafness and tinnitus from Liver-Yang rising, Liver-Fire or Kidney deficiency.

As it expels Wind from the face, it is also used in other problems caused by exterior Wind, such as trigeminal neuralgia and facial paralysis. According to some doctors, needling this point fairly deeply (at least an inch) and obtaining a good needling sensation is an effective treatment for facial paralysis. In such disease it should always be needled if there is tenderness on pressure on the mastoid area.

Box 63.15 summarizes the functions of T.B.-17.

T.B.-21 ERMEN *EAR DOOR*

Location

On the face, in the depression anterior to the supratragus notch and on the posterior border of the condyloid process of the mandible.

Nature

None.

Actions

Benefits the ears.
Expels Wind.

> **Box 63.15 T.B.-17 – summary of functions**
>
> - Expels Wind (deviation of eye and mouth, tetany)
> - Benefits the ears (tinnitus, deafness, ear discharge, itching inside the ear, redness, swelling and pain of the ear)

Indications

Tinnitus, deafness, ear discharge, redness and swelling of the ear.
Deviation of eye and mouth, toothache, gum pain, stiff lips, stiff neck.

Comments

T.B.-21 is used mostly as a local point for ear problems (mostly tinnitus and deafness), especially if deriving from rising of Liver-Yang.

Box 63.16 summarizes the functions of T.B.-21.

> **Box 63.16 T.B.-21 – summary of functions**
>
> - Benefits the ears (tinnitus, deafness, ear discharge, redness and swelling of the ear)
> - Expels Wind (deviation of eye and mouth)

T.B.-23 SIZHUKONG *SILK BAMBOO HOLE*

Location

On the face, in the depression at the lateral end of the eyebrow.

Nature

None.

Actions

Extinguishes interior Wind.
Brightens the eyes.

Indications

Headache, dizziness, tetany, epilepsy.
Deviation of eye, blurred vision, red eyes, twitching of eyelids.

Comments

T.B.-23 is used as a local point for eye problems and particularly headache around the outer corner of the eyebrow, especially if due to rising of Liver-Yang. When used for ear problems, it is frequently combined with a point in front of the ear such as S.I.-19 Tinggong.

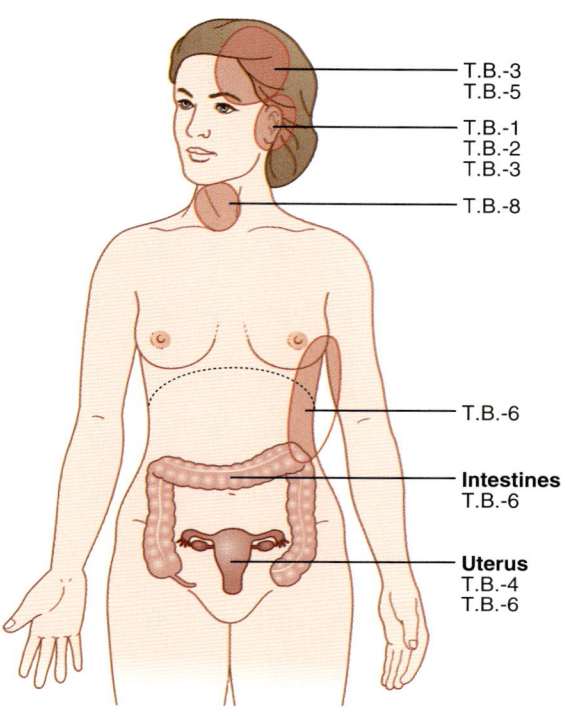

Figure 63.4 Target areas of Triple Burner channel points

> **Box 63.17 T.B.-23 – summary of functions**
>
> - Extinguishes interior Wind (headache, dizziness, tetany, epilepsy)
> - Brightens the eyes (deviation of eye, blurred vision, red eyes, twitching of eyelids)

Box 63.17 summarizes the functions of T.B.-23.

It is also used as a local point in facial paralysis, if there is inability to raise the outer corner of the eyebrow.

Fig. 63.4 illustrates the target areas of the Triple Burner channel points.

END NOTES

1. Nanjing College of Traditional Chinese Medicine 1979 A Revised Explanation of the Classic of Difficulties (*Nan Jing Jiao Shi* 难经校释), People's Health Publishing House, Beijing, first published c. AD 100, p. 144.
2. Ji Jie Yin 1984 Clinical Records of Tai Yi Shen Acupuncture (*Tai Yi Shen Zhen Jiu Lin Zheng Lu* 太乙神针灸临证录), Shanxi Province Scientific Publishing House, Shanxi, p. 46.
3. Classic of Difficulties, p. 94.
4. Ibid., p. 80.
5. Yue Han Zhen 1990 An Explanation of the Acupuncture Points (*Jing Xue Jie* 经穴解), People's Health Publishing House, Beijing, originally published in 1654, p. 301.
6. Ibid., p. 301.

SECTION 2 PART 7

Gall Bladder Channel 64

Main channel pathway

The Gall Bladder channel starts at the outer canthus of the eye. It ascends the forehead and curves downwards to the region behind the ear (at G.B.-20 Fengchi). From here it runs down the neck to the supraclavicular fossa.

A branch from the region behind the ear enters the ear. Another branch from the outer canthus meets the Triple Burner channel in the infraorbital region. It then descends to the neck and the supraclavicular fossa where it meets the main branch. From here, it descends to the chest and, passing through the diaphragm, it enters the liver and Gall Bladder. It then runs down the hypochondrial region and the lateral side of the abdomen to reach the point G.B.-30 Huantiao.

The main portion of the channel from the supraclavicular fossa goes to the axilla and the lateral side of the chest to the ribs and hip where it meets the previous branch. It then descends along the lateral aspect of the thigh and leg to end at the lateral side of the fourth toe.

From G.B.-41 Zulinqi, a branch goes to LIV-1 Dadun (Fig. 64.1).

Connecting channel pathway

The Connecting channel starts at G.B.-37 Guangming and connects with the Liver channel. Another branch proceeds downwards and scatters over the dorsum of the foot (Fig. 64.2).

Box 64.1 gives an overview of Gall Bladder points.

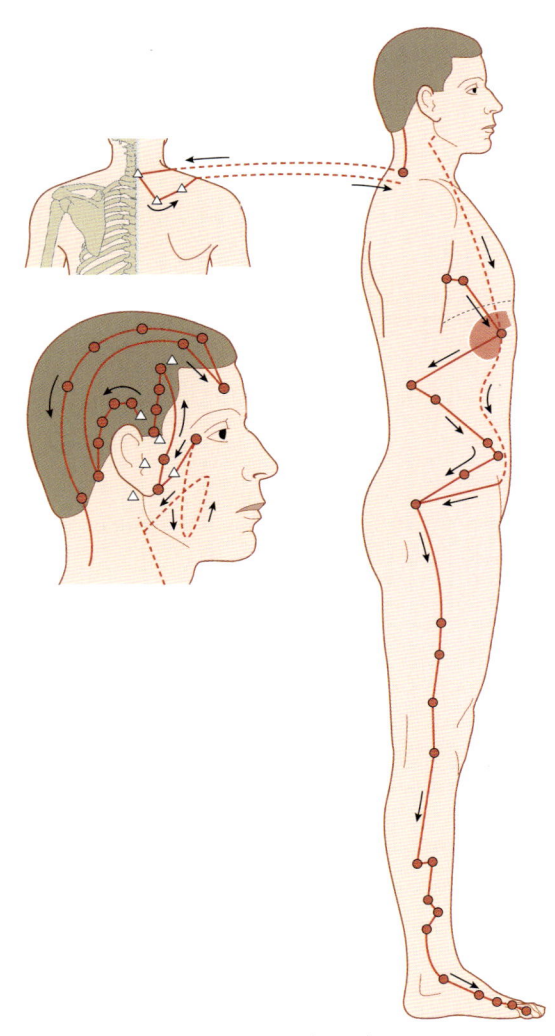

Figure 64.1 Gall Bladder main channel

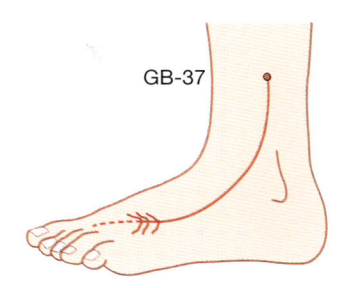

Figure 64.2 Gall Bladder Connecting channel

Box 64.1 Overview of Gall Bladder points

- Affect the lateral side of the leg, hypochondrium, shoulder, neck, head
- Important points (both local and distal) to treat headaches
- Enter the brain
- Affect the sinews
- Several important points of the Eye System
- Several points open the Mind's orifices
- Closely related to the Yang Linking Vessel (*Yang Wei Mai*) and Girdle Vessel (*Dai Mai*)

G.B.-1 TONGZILIAO PUPIL CREVICE

Location
Lateral to the outer canthus of the lateral side of the orbit.

Nature
Meeting point of Small Intestine, Gall Bladder and Triple Burner channels.
Point of the Eye System.

Actions
Expels Wind.
Clears Heat.
Brightens the eyes.
Subdues Liver-Yang.

Indications
Eye pain, itchy eyes, redness, swelling and pain of the eye, lacrimation on exposure to wind, redness and itching of the outer canthus of the eye, myopia, blurred vision, diminished night vision, deviation of eye.
Headache, dizziness.

Comments
G.B.-1 is an important local point for a wide range of eye problems. It expels Wind-Heat and is used for conjunctivitis from an exterior attack of Wind-Heat.

It clears Heat and is therefore used as a local point for eye problems caused by Liver-Fire, such as red, dry and painful eyes, which may occur with iritis, keratitis or conjunctivitis.

It is also widely used as a local point for migraine headaches around the temple and outer corner of the eye due to rising of Liver-Fire or Liver-Yang.

Its ability in treating headaches is also due to its being a point of the Eye System (periorbital group, see ch. 51). The Eye System starts from the convergence of channels around the orbit of the eye and it enters the brain.

Box 64.2 summarizes the functions of G.B.-1.

Box 64.2 G.B.-1 – summary of functions

- Expels Wind
- Clears Heat
- Brightens the eyes (eye pain, itchy eyes, redness, swelling and pain of the eye, lacrimation on exposure to wind, redness and itching of the outer canthus of the eye, myopia, blurred vision, diminished night vision, deviation of eye)
- Subdues Liver-Yang (headache, dizziness)

G.B.-2 TINGHUI HEARING CONVERGENCE

Location
Anterior to the intratragus notch, at the posterior border of the condyloid process of the mandible.

Nature
None.

Actions
Removes obstructions from the channel.
Expels exterior Wind.
Benefits the ears.

Indications
Mumps, toothache, deviation of eye and mouth, jaw pain.
Tinnitus, deafness, earache, ear discharge, redness and swelling of ear, itching of ear.

Comments

G.B.-2 is an important local point for ear problems. It is very much used as a local point for tinnitus and deafness caused by rising of Liver-Yang or Liver-Fire.

As it expels exterior Wind, in particular Wind-Heat, it is also an important local point for the treatment of otitis media from exterior Wind-Heat.

Box 64.3 summarizes the functions of G.B.-2.

Box 64.3 G.B.-2 – summary of functions

- Removes obstructions from the channel (mumps, toothache, deviation of eye and mouth, jaw pain)
- Expels exterior Wind
- Benefits the ears (tinnitus, deafness, earache, ear discharge, redness and swelling of ear, itching of ear)

G.B.-4 HANYAN *JAW SERENITY*

Location

In front of the ear, directly above ST-7, in the depression on the upper border of the zygomatic arch.

Nature

Meeting point of Gall Bladder, Triple Burner and Stomach channels.
Point of the Eye System.

Actions

Subdues Liver-Yang.
Extinguishes interior Wind.

Indications

Headache, dizziness, blurred vision.
Convulsions, lockjaw, epilepsy, deviation of eye and mouth.

Comments

G.B.-4 is an important local point for headaches from Liver-Yang rising. It treats headaches also by virtue of its being a point of the Eye System. It should be needled horizontally (i.e. at a 15-degree angle) towards the back of the head.

Box 64.4 summarizes the functions of G.B.-4.

Box 64.4 G.B.-4 – summary of functions

- Subdues Liver-Yang (headache, dizziness, blurred vision)
- Extinguishes interior Wind (convulsions, lockjaw, epilepsy, deviation of eye and mouth)

G.B.-5 XUANLU *HANGING SKULL*

Location

Within the hairline of the temporal region, at the midpoint of the arc connecting ST-8 Touwei and G.B.-7 Qubin.

Nature

Meeting point of the Gall Bladder, Stomach, Triple Burner and Large Intestine channels.
Point of the Eye System.

Actions

Subdues Liver-Yang.
Extinguishes interior Wind.

Indications

Headaches, dizziness, blurred vision.
Convulsions, lockjaw, aphasia.

Comments

G.B.-5 is used for interior Wind causing convulsions, spasticity and aphasia.[1] Apart from this, it is an important local point for temporal headaches from Liver-Yang rising.

G.B.-5 belongs to the temporal group of points of the Eye System and it is the most important of this group as it is in direct communication with the brain. It should be needled horizontally (i.e. at a 15-degree angle) towards the back of the head.

Box 64.5 summarizes the functions of G.B.-5.

Box 64.5 G.B.-5 – summary of functions

- Subdues Liver-Yang (headache, dizziness, blurred vision)
- Extinguishes interior Wind (convulsions, lockjaw, aphasia)

G.B.-6 XUANLI *DEVIATION FROM HANGING SKULL*

Location

Within the hairline of the temporal region, at the junction of the upper three-quarters and lower quarter of the arc connecting ST-8 Touwei and G.B.-7 Qubin.

Nature

Meeting point of Gall Bladder, Triple Burner, Stomach and Large Intestine channels.

Actions

Subdues Liver-Yang.
Opens the Mind's orifices.

Indications

Headache, dizziness, blurred vision.
Disturbance of will-power, lack of motivation and speech difficulties.

Comments

G.B.-6 is an important local point for the treatment of migraine headaches on the side of the head due to rising of Liver-Yang, Liver-Fire or Liver-Wind. It should be needled horizontally (i.e. at a 15-degree angle) towards the back of the head.

It can also be used for ear problems with pain extending to the side of the head, along the Gall Bladder channel.

This point is also used in psychiatric practice for disturbance of will-power, lack of motivation and speech difficulties.[2]

Box 64.6 summarizes the functions of G.B.-6.

Box 64.6 G.B.-6 – summary of functions

- Subdues Liver-Yang (headache, dizziness, blurred vision)
- Opens the Mind's orifices (disturbance of will-power, lack of motivation and speech difficulties)

G.B.-8 SHUAIGU *LEADING VALLEY*

Location

On the head, directly above the apex of the auricle and T.B.-20 Jiaosun, 1.5 *cun* within the hairline.

Nature

Meeting point of Gall Bladder and Bladder channels.

Actions

Subdues Liver-Yang.
Extinguishes interior Wind.
Harmonizes the Stomach and subdues rebellious Stomach-Qi.

Indications

Headache, dizziness, blurred vision, feeling of heaviness of the head.
Deviation of eye and mouth.
Vomiting, inability to eat, injury by alcohol.

Comments

G.B.-8 is widely used as a local point for headaches from Liver-Yang rising.

Box 64.7 summarizes the functions of G.B.-8.

Box 64.7 G.B.-8 – summary of functions

- Subdues Liver-Yang (headache, dizziness, blurred vision, feeling of heaviness of the head)
- Extinguishes interior Wind (deviation of eye and mouth)
- Harmonizes the Stomach and subdues rebellious Stomach-Qi (vomiting, inability to eat, injury by alcohol)

G.B.-9 TIANCHONG *PENETRATING HEAVEN*

Location

On the head, directly above the posterior border of the auricle, 2 *cun* within the hairline, 0.5 *cun* posterior to G.B.-8 Shuaigu.

Nature

Meeting of the Gall Bladder and Bladder channels.

Actions

Subdues Liver-Yang.
Extinguishes interior Wind.
Calms the Mind.
Resolves Dampness and clears Heat in the head.

Indications

Headache, tinnitus, dizziness.
Epilepsy, tetany, convulsions.
Fright, fear, palpitations, manic behaviour.
Itchy ears, toothache, swelling and pain of gums, goitre.

Comments

G.B.-9 is a very important local point of the Gall Bladder channel. First of all, it is very much used as a local point for migraine headaches on the side of the head from rising of Liver-Yang, Liver-Fire or Liver-Wind. This point helps to subdue the rising of rebellious Qi and conducts it downwards.

Another important function of this point is that of eliminating interior Wind and its manifestations, especially convulsions, epilepsy or contraction of muscles.

G.B.-9 has a powerful mental effect, and is used to calm the Mind. In serious mental disorders such as hypomania, it is an important adjuvant to the treatment with distal points.

This point is also used for disturbance of movement (such as ataxia) and speech originating from a central nervous system disease. When used in this way it is combined with G.B.-5 Xuanlu, L.I.-11 Quchi and G.B.-34 Yanglingquan.[3]

It is interesting to note that, judging from the name and the indications, this point should be a Window of Heaven point but it is not mentioned as one. Its actions include two important actions of the Window of Heaven points: that is, subduing rebellious Qi from the head and calming the Mind.

Box 64.8 summarizes the functions of G.B.-9.

Box 64.8 G.B.-9 – summary of functions

- Subdues Liver-Yang (headache, tinnitus, dizziness)
- Extinguishes interior Wind (epilepsy, tetany, convulsions)
- Calms the Mind (fright, fear, palpitations, manic behaviour)
- Resolves Dampness and clears Heat in the head (itchy ears, toothache, swelling and pain of gums, goitre)

G.B.-11 TOUQIAOYIN *(HEAD) YIN ORIFICES*

Location

On the head, posterior to the auricle, posterior and superior to the mastoid process, at the junction of the middle third and lower third of the arc connecting G.B.-9 Tianchong and G.B.-12 Wangu.

Nature

Meeting point of the Gall Bladder, Bladder, Small Intestine and Triple Burner channels.

Actions

Subdues Liver-Yang.
Brightens the sense orifices.

Indications

Headache, dizziness, pain behind ear, stiff neck.
Eye pain, ear pain, tinnitus, deafness, stiff tongue, bleeding tongue, bitter taste.

Comments

G.B.-11 is used as a local point for headaches from Liver-Yang rising or from Liver-Fire, especially when the pain is behind the ear.

Its name indicates that it brightens the orifices related to the Yin organs (although its indications do not include nose problems).

Box 64.9 summarizes the functions of G.B.-11.

Box 64.9 G.B.-11 – summary of functions

- Subdues Liver-Yang (headache, dizziness, pain behind ear, stiff neck)
- Brightens the sense orifices (eye pain, ear pain, tinnitus, deafness, stiff tongue, bleeding tongue, bitter taste)

G.B.-12 WANGU *WHOLE BONE*

Location

On the head, posterior to the auricle, in the depression posterior and inferior to the mastoid process.

Nature

Meeting point of Gall Bladder and Bladder channels.

Actions

Subdues Liver-Yang.
Extinguishes interior Wind.
Calms the Mind.

Indications

Headache, dizziness.
Tremor of head, hemiplegia, deviation of eye and mouth, clenched jaw, contraction of muscles around the mouth, epilepsy.
Manic behaviour, agitation, insomnia.

Comments

G.B.-12 can be used as a local point both to subdue Liver-Yang (causing headaches) and to extinguish interior Wind (such as in epilepsy).

This point is frequently used for insomnia from rising of Liver-Yang or Liver-Fire combined with BL-18 Ganshu and BL-19 Danshu.

Box 64.10 summarizes the functions of G.B.-12.

> **Box 64.10 G.B.-12 – summary of functions**
> - Subdues Liver-Yang (headache, dizziness)
> - Extinguishes interior Wind (tremor of head, hemiplegia, deviation of eye and mouth, clenched jaw, contraction of muscles around the mouth, epilepsy)
> - Calms the Mind (manic behaviour, agitation, insomnia)

G.B.-13 BENSHEN *MIND ROOT*

Location

On the head, 0.5 *cun* within the anterior hairline of the forehead, 3 *cun* lateral to Du-24 Shenting, at the junction of the medial two-thirds and the lateral third of the line connecting Du-24 and ST-8 Touwei.

Nature

Point of the Yang Linking Vessel (*Yang Wei Mai*).
Meeting point of the three Yang Muscle channels of the arm.

Actions

Calms the Mind (*Shen*).
Subdues Liver-Yang.
Extinguishes Wind.
Resolves Phlegm.
Gathers Essence (*Jing*) to the head.
Clears the brain.

Indications

Manic behaviour, fright.
Headache, dizziness.
Epilepsy, hemiplegia, convulsions.
Vomiting of foamy saliva, epilepsy with foaming at the mouth.

Comments

G.B.-13 is a very important point for mental and emotional problems. This point, combined with HE-5 Tongli and G.B.-38 Yangfu, is very much used in psychiatric practice of the Nanjing Traditional Chinese Medicine Hospital for Schizophrenia and Split Personality.[4] It is also indicated when the person has persistent and unreasonable feelings of jealousy and suspicion.

Apart from these mental traits, it has a powerful effect in calming the Mind and relieving anxiety deriving from constant worry and fixed thoughts. Its effect is enhanced if it is combined with Du-24 Shenting.

Its deep mental and emotional effect is also due to its action of 'gathering' Essence to the head. The Kidney-Essence is the root of our Pre-Heaven Qi and is the foundation for our mental and emotional life. A strong Essence is the fundamental prerequisite for a clear Mind (*Shen*) and a balanced emotional life. This is the meaning of this point's name, 'Root of the Mind': that is, this point gathers the Essence which is the root of the Mind (*Shen*). The Kidney-Essence is the source of Marrow that fills up the Brain (called Sea of Marrow): G.B.-13 is a point where Essence and Marrow 'gather'. The 'Great Dictionary of Acupuncture' says that this point '*makes the Mind [Shen] return to its root*':[5] the 'root' of the Mind is the Essence: hence this point 'gathers' the Essence to the Brain and affects the Mind. As it connects the Mind and the Essence, it also treats both the Heart and the Kidneys and therefore the Mind (*Shen*) and Will-power (*Zhi*): for this reason, it is an important point in the treatment of depression.

When combined with other points to nourish Essence (such as Ren-4 Guanyuan), G.B.-13 attracts Essence towards the head with the effect of calming the Mind and strengthening clarity of mind, memory and will-power. The connection between G.B.-13 and the Essence is confirmed by the text 'An Enquiry into Chinese Acupuncture', which has among the indications of this point: '*excessive menstrual bleeding, impotence and seminal emissions.*'[6]

G.B.-13 also subdues Liver-Yang and it can therefore be used as a local point in chronic headaches from Liver-Yang rising. It also extinguishes internal Wind and is effective for Wind-stroke and epilepsy. Finally, it resolves Phlegm in the context of mental–emotional disorders or epilepsy: that is, it opens the Mind's orifices when these are clouded by Phlegm. The 'Explanation of the Acupuncture Points' says: '*The indications of G.B.-13 show that it eliminates the three pathogenic factors of Wind, Fire and Phlegm from the Lesser Yang, in which cases this point should be reduced.*'[7]

Box 64.11 summarizes the functions of G.B.-13.

> **Box 64.11 G.B.-13 – summary of functions**
> - Calms the Mind (manic behaviour, fright)
> - Subdues Liver-Yang (headache, dizziness)
> - Extinguishes Wind (epilepsy, hemiplegia, convulsions)
> - Resolves Phlegm (vomiting of foamy saliva, epilepsy with foaming at the mouth)
> - Gathers Essence to the head
> - Clears the brain

> **Box 64.12 G.B.-14 – summary of functions**
> - Subdues Liver-Yang (headache, dizziness)
> - Extinguishes interior Wind (opisthotonos, deviation of eye and mouth, drooping of eyelid, twitching of eyelid)
> - Brightens the eyes (itching of eyelid, eye pain, lacrimation on exposure to wind, diminished night vision, myopia)

G.B.-14 YANGBAI *YANG WHITE*

Location
On the forehead, directly above the pupil of the eye, 1 *cun* above the eyebrow.

Nature
Point of the Yang Linking Vessel (*Yang Wei Mai*).
Meeting point of the Gall Bladder, Triple Burner, Stomach and Large Intestine channels.

Actions
Subdues Liver-Yang.
Extinguishes interior Wind.
Brightens the eyes.

Indications
Headache, dizziness.
Opisthotonos, deviation of eye and mouth, drooping of eyelid, twitching of eyelid.
Itching of eyelid, eye pain, lacrimation on exposure to wind, diminished night vision, myopia.

Comments
G.B.-14 is an important and frequently used point to eliminate Wind from the face, especially in the treatment of facial paralysis. When treating facial paralysis, the choice of local points is made according to the area of paralysis, and this is determined by asking the patient to perform certain actions with the facial muscles. If the patient cannot form ridges on the forehead by raising the eyebrows, this point should be used on the affected side. It is needled horizontally downwards.

G.B.-14 is also an important local point for unilateral frontal headaches on the Gall Bladder channel deriving from Liver-Yang rising.

Finally, G.B.-14 is used as a local point for eye problems related to the Gall Bladder and Liver channels.

Box 64.12 summarizes the functions of G.B.-14.

G.B.-15 LINQI *FALLING TEARS*

Location
On the head, directly above the pupil of the eye, 0.5 *cun* within the anterior hairline, at the midpoint of the line connecting Du-24 Shenting and ST-8 Touwei.

Nature
Point of the Yang Linking Vessel (*Yang Wei Mai*).
Meeting point of Gall Bladder and Bladder channels.

Actions
Subdues Liver-Yang.
Extinguishes interior Wind.
Brightens the eyes.
Calms the Mind.

Indications
Headache, dizziness.
Wind-stroke, epilepsy, loss of consciousness.
Redness and pain of the eyes, blurred vision, lacrimation on exposure to wind, pain in the outer canthus, pain above eyebrows.
Obsessive thoughts, pensiveness, oscillation of moods.

Comments
G.B.-15 has a deep effect on the emotional life and is particularly indicated to balance the moods when the person oscillates between periods of low spirits and periods of elation.[8] In my experience, this point is effective to stop obsessive thoughts and pensiveness.

G.B.-15 is used as a local point for headaches from Liver-Yang rising and it has a special effect on the eyes.

Box 64.13 summarizes the functions of G.B.-15.

> **Box 64.13 G.B.-15 – summary of functions**
>
> - Subdues Liver-Yang (headache, dizziness)
> - Extinguishes interior Wind (Wind-stroke, epilepsy, loss of consciousness)
> - Brightens the eyes (redness and pain of the eyes, blurred vision, lacrimation on exposure to wind, pain in the outer canthus, pain above eyebrows)
> - Calms the Mind (obsessive thoughts, pensiveness, oscillation of moods)

G.B.-17 ZHENGYING *TOP CONVERGENCE*

Location

On the head, 2.25 *cun* posterior to the anterior hairline, 2.25 *cun* lateral to the midline of the head.

Nature

Point of the Yang Linking Vessel (*Yang Wei Mai*).

Actions

Subdues Liver-Yang.
Resolves Phlegm and opens the Mind's orifices.

Indications

Headache, dizziness, blurred vision.
Blurred vision from Phlegm, nausea, vomiting, obsessive thoughts, pensiveness, manic behaviour.

Comments

G.B.-17 has a strong mental–emotional effect in opening the Mind's orifices and resolving Phlegm. In my experience, it is effective to eliminate Phlegm from the head when this obstructs the Mind causing obsessive thoughts, pensiveness and mild manic behaviour.

According to the 'An Enquiry into Chinese Acupuncture', G.B.-17 can be used for schizophrenia and hysteria.[9]

Box 64.14 summarizes the functions of G.B.-17.

> **Box 64.14 G.B.-17 – summary of functions**
>
> - Subdues Liver-Yang (headache, dizziness, blurred vision)
> - Resolves Phlegm and opens the Mind's orifices (blurred vision from Phlegm, nausea, vomiting, obsessive thoughts, pensiveness, manic behaviour)

G.B.-18 CHENGLING *SPIRIT RECEIVER*

Location

On the head, 4 *cun* posterior to the anterior hairline, 2.25 *cun* lateral to the midline of the head.

Nature

Point of the Yang Linking Vessel (*Yang Wei Mai*).

Actions

Subdues Liver-Yang.
Calms the Mind and opens the Mind's orifices.
Benefits the nose and stimulates the diffusing and descending of Lung-Qi.

Indications

Headache, dizziness.
Obsessive thoughts, pensiveness.
Sneezing, nosebleed, nasal congestion, breathlessness, aversion to cold.

Comments

G.B.-18 has a deep effect on mental problems such as obsessional thoughts and dementia.[10] Like nearly all Gall Bladder points on the head, it subdues Liver-Yang and is used as a local point for headaches from Liver-Yang rising.

According to the 'An Enquiry into Chinese Acupuncture', G.B.-18 can be used for diseases of the blood vessels of the brain and traumas to the skull.[11]

Box 64.15 summarizes the functions of G.B.-18.

> **Box 64.15 G.B.-18 – summary of functions**
>
> - Subdues Liver-Yang (headache, dizziness)
> - Calms the Mind and opens the Mind's orifices (obsessive thoughts, pensiveness)
> - Benefits the nose and stimulates the diffusing and descending of Lung-Qi (sneezing, nosebleed, nasal congestion, breathlessness, aversion to cold)

G.B.-19 NAOKONG *BRAIN CAVITY*

Location

On the region of the head, on the lateral side of the superior border of the external occipital protuberance, 2.25 *cun* lateral to the midline of the head.

Nature

Point of the Yang Linking Vessel (*Yang Wei Mai*).

Actions

Subdues Liver-Yang.
Clear Gall Bladder channel Heat.
Brightens the eyes and benefits ears and nose.
Calms the Mind.

Indications

Headache, dizziness.
Blurred vision, redness, swelling and pain of the eyes, tinnitus, deafness, nose ache, nasal congestion, nosebleed.
Manic depression, fright, palpitations.

Comments

G.B.-19 is another local point for headaches from Liver-Yang rising. Compared to other Gall Bladder points on the skull, G.B.-19 has a stronger Heat-clearing action.

Like other Gall Bladder points on the skull, G.B.-19 benefits the sense orifices. Its name implies that, at this point, the Gall Bladder channel is in communication with the brain.

Box 64.16 summarizes the functions of G.B.-19.

Box 64.16 G.B.-19 – summary of functions

- Subdues Liver-Yang (headache, dizziness)
- Clear Gall Bladder channel Heat
- Brightens the eyes and benefits ears and nose (blurred vision, redness, swelling and pain of the eyes, tinnitus, deafness, nose ache, nasal congestion, nosebleed)
- Calms the Mind (manic depression, fright, palpitations)

G.B.-20 FENGCHI *WIND POOL*

Location

On the nape, below the occiput, at the level of Du-16 Fengfu, in the depression between the upper portion of sternocleidomastoid and trapezius muscles.

Nature

Point of the Yang Linking Vessel (*Yang Wei Mai*).
Meeting point of the Gall Bladder and Triple Burner channels.

Actions

Expels exterior Wind.
Extinguishes interior Wind.
Subdues Liver-Yang.
Brightens the eyes.
Benefits the ears.
Clears Heat.
Nourishes Marrow and clears the Brain.

Indications

Aversion cold, fever, body aches, occipital stiffness and ache.
Vertigo, Wind-stroke, hemiplegia, lockjaw, deviation of eye and mouth, epilepsy.
Headache, dizziness, blurred vision.
Blurred vision, diminished night vision, redness and pain of the eyes, redness and pain of the outer canthus, excessive lacrimation.
Tinnitus, deafness, blocked ears.

Comments

G.B.-20 is a major point with many different actions. Firstly, as its name implies, it eliminates both interior and exterior Wind. It is very much used to eliminate exterior Wind-Cold or Wind-Heat, particularly if the headache and stiff neck that are normally caused by exterior Wind are very pronounced. It is combined with LU-7 Lieque to expel Wind-Cold, and L.I.-4 Hegu and T.B.-5 Waiguan to expel Wind-Heat.

G.B.-20 extinguishes interior Wind and is used for such symptoms as dizziness and vertigo. It is the point of choice to use for dizziness and vertigo from internal Wind or from rising of Liver-Yang or Liver-Fire. In all these cases, it is needled with reducing method.

Some authors say that G.B.-20 expels exterior Wind by virtue of it being a point of the Yang Linking Vessel (*Yang Wei Mai*), while it extinguishes interior Wind by virtue of it being a Gall Bladder channel point.

G.B.-20 point subdues Liver-Yang or Liver-Fire and is therefore used for headaches deriving from rising of Liver-Yang.

It is a major point for eye problems, particularly if associated with a Liver disharmony. This action is also partly due to its being a point of the Eye System (occipital group): in fact, the Eye System emerges from the brain at the occiput. G.B.-20 can be used for blurred vision, cataract, iritis and optic nerve atrophy. It is particularly indicated for eye problems deriving from

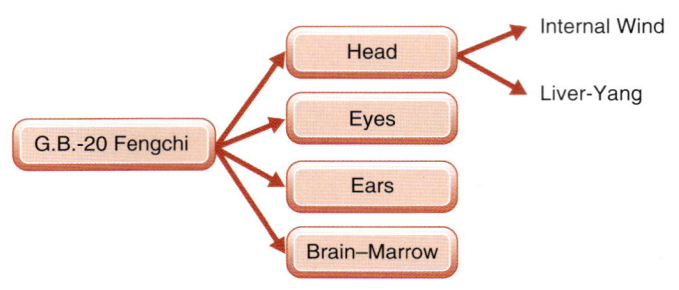

Figure 64.3 Areas of influence of G.B.-20 Fengchi

Box 64.17 G.B.-20 – summary of functions

- Expels exterior Wind (aversion cold, fever, body aches, occipital stiffness and ache)
- Extinguishes interior Wind (vertigo, Wind-stroke, hemiplegia, lockjaw, deviation of eye and mouth, epilepsy)
- Subdues Liver-Yang (headache, dizziness, blurred vision)
- Brightens the eyes (blurred vision, diminished night vision, redness and pain of the eyes, redness and pain of the outer canthus, excessive lacrimation)
- Benefits the ears (tinnitus, deafness, blocked ears)
- Clears Heat
- Nourishes Marrow and clears the Brain

Liver-Fire, in which case it is needled with reducing method. However, it can also be used with reinforcing method to improve vision and clear the eyes when these are not nourished by deficient Liver-Blood.

It also has an effect on the ears, and can be used for tinnitus and deafness deriving from the rising of Liver-Yang.

Used with reinforcing method, it tonifies Marrow and nourishes the brain, so that it can be used for deficiency of the Sea of Marrow, with such symptoms as poor memory, dizziness and vertigo. Its action on the Brain and Marrow is also due to its being a point of the Eye System (Fig. 64.3).

When used to affect the eyes, G.B.-20 should be needled obliquely towards the eye of the same side; when used to eliminate Wind, it should be needled angled towards the opposite eye.

Box 64.17 summarizes the functions of G.B.-20.

G.B.-20's two major functions are:
1. Eliminate Wind (exterior and interior)
2. Brighten the eyes

G.B.-21 JIANJING *SHOULDER WELL*

Location

On the shoulder, directly above the nipple, at the midpoint of the line connecting Du-14 Dazhui and the acromion.

Nature

Meeting point of Gall Bladder and Triple Burner channels.
Point of the Yang Linking Vessel (*Yang Wei Mai*).

Actions

Relaxes sinews.
Benefits the breasts and promotes lactation.
Stimulates the descending of Qi and promotes delivery.
Stimulates the descending of Lung-Qi.

Indications

Stiffness and pain of the neck and top of shoulders.
Breast pain, breast abscess, breast milk not flowing.
Difficult or prolonged labour, retention of placenta.
Cough, breathlessness, red face.

Comments

G.B.-21 has three main functions. Firstly, it is used as a local point for the treatment of Painful Obstruction Syndrome (*Bi Syndrome*) of the shoulders and neck. It relaxes the sinews and relieves stiffness, and is nearly always tender on pressure.

Secondly, it is an empirical point to promote lactation in nursing mothers. Thirdly, it is an empirical point to use for many problems of childbirth such as retention of placenta, postpartum haemorrhage or threatened miscarriage. It does so because it promotes the

> **Box 64.18 G.B.-21 – summary of functions**
>
> - Relaxes sinews (stiffness and pain of the neck and top of shoulders)
> - Benefits the breasts and promotes lactation (breast pain, breast abscess, breast milk not flowing)
> - Stimulates the descending of Qi and promotes delivery (difficult or prolonged labour, retention of placenta)
> - Stimulates the descending of Lung-Qi (cough, breathlessness, red face)

descending of Qi and, for this reason, it is forbidden in pregnancy.

Box 64.18 summarizes the functions of G.B.-21.

G.B.-22 YUANYE AXILLA ABYSS

Location

On the lateral side of the chest, when the arm is raised, the point is on the mid-axillary line, 3 *cun* below the axilla, in the fourth intercostal space.

Nature

Meeting point of the three Yin Muscle channels of the arm.

Actions

Promotes the descending of Lung-Qi and opens the chest.

Indications

Cough, fullness of the chest, pain in the lateral costal region.

Comments

G.B.-22 is the meeting point of the three Yin Muscle channels of the arm: that is, Lungs, Pericardium and Heart. Being a meeting point of Muscle channels, G.B.-22 can be used for muscular ache and stiffness of the chest and costal regions where the Muscle channels of the above three channels run.

Box 64.19 summarizes the functions of G.B.-22.

> **Box 64.19 G.B.-22 – summary of functions**
>
> - Promotes the descending of Lung-Qi and opens the chest (cough, fullness of the chest, pain in the lateral costal region)

G.B.-24 RIYUE SUN AND MOON

Location

In the seventh intercostal space, on the mamillary line (4 *cun* lateral to the anterior midline).

Nature

Front Collecting (*Mu*) point of the Gall Bladder.
Meeting point of the Gall Bladder and Spleen channels.
Point of the Yang Linking Vessel (*Yang Wei Mai*).

Actions

Resolves Damp-Heat.
Moves Liver-Qi.
Harmonizes the Middle Burner and subdues rebellious Qi.

Indications

Hypochondrial fullness, bitter taste, feeling of heaviness, sticky taste, inability to digest fats.
Hypochondrial distension, pain in the ribs, epigastric pain, abdominal distension.
Vomiting, acid regurgitation, hiccup, belching.

Comments

G.B.-24 is an important point to resolve Damp-Heat affecting the Gall Bladder and Liver, manifesting with such symptoms and signs as jaundice, hypochondrial pain, a feeling of heaviness, nausea and a sticky yellow tongue coating. In severe cases, it gives rise to the formation of gallstones. To resolve Damp-Heat this point is often combined with G.B.-34 Yanglingquan and L.I.-11 Quchi.

It also promotes the free flow of Liver-Qi and is commonly used in the treatment of hypochondrial pain and distension.

Box 64.20 summarizes the functions of G.B.-24.

> **Box 64.20 G.B.-24 – summary of functions**
>
> - Resolves Damp-Heat (hypochondrial fullness, bitter taste, feeling of heaviness, sticky taste, inability to digest fats)
> - Moves Liver-Qi (hypochondrial distension, pain in the ribs, epigastric pain, abdominal distension)
> - Harmonizes the Middle Burner and subdues rebellious Qi (vomiting, acid regurgitation, hiccup, belching)

G.B.-25 JINGMEN *CAPITAL DOOR*

Location

On the lateral side of the abdomen, 1.8 *cun* posterior to LIV-13 Zhangmen, on the lower border of the free end of the 12th floating rib.

Nature

Front Collecting (*Mu*) point of the Kidneys.

Actions

Regulates the Water Passages of the Lower Burner.
Regulates the Spleen and the Intestines.
Strengthens the lower back.

Indications

Difficult urination, dark urine.
Borborygmi, diarrhoea, abdominal distension and pain.
Lower backache, inability to stand for long, pain in the lateral costal region and back, hip pain.

Comments

Although this is the Front Collecting point for the Kidney, it is used more for diagnosis than treatment of Kidney problems.

Box 64.21 summarizes the functions of G.B.-25.

Box 64.21 G.B.-25 – summary of functions

- Regulates the Water Passages of the Lower Burner (difficult urination, dark urine)
- Regulates the Spleen and the Intestines (borborygmi, diarrhoea, abdominal distension and pain)
- Strengthens the lower back (lower backache, inability to stand for long, pain in the lateral costal region and back, hip pain)

G.B.-26 DAIMAI *GIRDLE VESSEL*

Location

On the lateral side of the abdomen, 1.8 *cun* below LIV-13 Zhangmen, where the vertical line of the free end of the 11th rib and the horizontal line of the umbilicus intersect.

Nature

Beginning point of the Girdle Vessel (*Dai Mai*).

Actions

Resolves Dampness in the Lower Burner.
Regulates the Girdle Vessel and the Uterus.

Indications

Leukorrhoea.
Irregular periods, painful periods, amenorrhoea, infertility, prolapse of uterus, hypogastric fullness in women, lower abdominal pain in women.

Comments

G.B.-26 is an important point for gynaecological problems. It regulates the Uterus and menstruation and can be used for irregular periods and dysmenorrhoea. It acts on the Uterus and menstruation by regulating the Girdle Vessel, which harmonizes the Liver and Gall Bladder. I usually use this point in conjunction with the opening points of the Girdle Vessel: that is, G.B.-41 and T.B.-5.

The Girdle Vessel encircles the leg channels and its dysfunction can lead to impaired circulation in these channels and to the infusing of Dampness in the Lower Burner. This point can therefore be used to treat chronic vaginal discharges and vaginal prolapse.

The points G.B.-27 Wushu and G.B.-28 Weidao have similar indications and actions to G.B.-26 Daimai.

Box 64.22 summarizes the functions of G.B.-26.

Box 64.22 G.B.-26 – summary of functions

- Resolves Dampness in the Lower Burner (leukorrhoea)
- Regulates the Girdle Vessel and the Uterus (irregular periods, painful periods, amenorrhoea, infertility, prolapse of uterus, hypogastric fullness in women, lower abdominal pain in women)

G.B.-29 JULIAO *SQUATTING CREVICE*

Location

On the region of the hip, at the midpoint of the line connecting the anterior iliac spine and the greater trochanter of the femur.

Nature

Point of the Yang Stepping Vessel (*Yang Qiao Mai*).

Actions

Removes obstructions from the channel.

Indications

Hip pain, pain in the back/side of the leg, pain in the lateral side of the buttocks, pain radiating to the groin, sciatica.

Comments

G.B.-29 is mostly used as a local point for Painful Obstruction Syndrome of the hip. It is often tender on pressure and is very effective in combination with G.B.-30 Huantiao.

Box 64.23 summarizes the functions of G.B.-29.

> **Box 64.23 G.B.-29 – summary of functions**
>
> - Removes obstructions from the channel (hip pain, pain in the back/side of the leg, pain in the lateral side of the buttocks, pain radiating to the groin, sciatica)

G.B.-30 HUANTIAO *JUMPING CIRCLE*

Location

On the lateral side of the buttocks, when the patient is in the lateral recumbent position and the thigh is flexed, this point is at the junction of the lateral third and medial third of the line connecting the greater trochanter and the hiatus of the sacrum.

Nature

Meeting point of Gall Bladder and Bladder channels. Ma Dan Yang's Heavenly Star point.

Actions

Removes obstructions from the channel.
Resolves Dampness and expels Wind.
Tonifies Qi and Blood.

Indications

Hip pain, pain in the buttocks, pain in the lateral side of the leg, sciatica, hemiplegia, atrophy of leg, numbness of leg, rigidity of knee.
Urticaria, eczema.
Tiredness, poor appetite, loose stools, blurred vision.

Comments

G.B.-30 is an important point with different functions extending beyond its obvious use as a local point for the hip joint. It is, of course, an important point for Painful Obstruction Syndrome (*Bi* Syndrome) of the hip and should always be needled in these cases at least 2 inches (5 cm) deep. This point should be needled with the patient lying on his or her side and with the leg slightly bent.

G.B.-30 is also an important point in the treatment of Atrophy Syndrome and sequelae of Wind-stroke: the use of G.B.-30 Huantiao can stimulate the circulation of Qi and Blood to the whole leg and strengthen the sinews.

It is also widely used in the treatment of sciatica with pain extending down the lateral side of the leg. In these cases, G.B.-30 should be needled, trying to obtain the radiation of the needling sensation all the way down to the foot. If this is so, then no other point need be used. If the needling sensation extends only part of the way down the leg, other points may be used as a kind of 'shuttle', such as G.B.-31 Fengshi or G.B.-34 Yanglingquan, depending on how far the needling sensation from G.B.-30 has reached.

Apart from resolving Dampness and expelling Wind in the context of Painful Obstruction Syndrome (*Bi* Syndrome), G.B.-30 also does so in the context of skin diseases. As we will see shortly, in this respect, it is similar to G.B.-31 Fengshi: this latter point, however, has a stronger effect on expelling Wind in skin diseases.

Apart from the above, this point also has a general tonifying effect on Qi and Blood of the whole body. This effect is almost as strong as that of ST-36 Zusanli.

Finally, G.B.-30 also resolves Damp-Heat in the Lower Burner and can be used to affect the anus or genitals, depending on the direction of the needle. By resolving Damp-Heat, G.B.-30 can be used to treat such symptoms as itchy anus or groin, vaginal discharge and urethritis.

Box 64.24 summarizes the functions of G.B.-30.

> **Box 64.24 G.B.-30 – summary of functions**
>
> - Removes obstructions from the channel (hip pain, pain in the buttocks, pain in the lateral side of the leg, sciatica, hemiplegia, atrophy of leg, numbness of leg, rigidity of knee)
> - Resolves Dampness and expels Wind (urticaria, eczema)
> - Tonifies Qi and Blood (tiredness, poor appetite, loose stools, blurred vision)
> - Can be used for Damp-Heat in the anus, urethra and vagina

G.B.-31 FENGSHI *WIND MARKET*

Location
On the midline of the lateral aspect of the thigh, 7 *cun* above the transverse popliteal crease.

Nature
None.

Actions
Expels Wind.
Relieves itching.
Removes obstructions from the channel.

Indications
Skin diseases from Wind, itching, herpes zoster. Sciatica, hemiplegia, atrophy of leg, numbness of leg, rigidity of knee.

Comments
G.B.-31 is an important point for the treatment of skin diseases due to Wind-Heat moving in the Blood. These would be manifested with the sudden appearance of red rashes which move from place to place, such as in urticaria. It is also used to expel Wind-Heat in herpes zoster, usually combined with T.B.-6 Zhigou.

Apart from this, it is widely used for the treatment of Atrophy Syndrome and sequelae of Wind-stroke to relax the sinews and invigorate the circulation of Qi and Blood to the legs.

Box 64.25 summarizes the functions of G.B.-31.

Box 64.25 G.B.-31 – summary of functions

- Expels Wind (skin diseases from Wind, itching, herpes zoster)
- Relieves itching
- Removes obstructions from the channel (sciatica, hemiplegia, atrophy of leg, numbness of leg, rigidity of knee)

G.B.-33 XIYANGGUAN *KNEE YANG GATE*

Location
On the lateral aspect of the thigh, 3 *cun* above G.B.-34 Yanglingquan, in the depression anterior to the lateral epicondyle of the femur.

Nature
None.

Actions
Resolves Dampness and expels Wind.
Removes obstructions from the channel.

Indications
Redness, swelling and pain of the lateral side of the knee, rigidity of knee, Wind and Dampness Painful Obstruction Syndrome (*Bi* Syndrome) of the knee, numbness.

Comments
G.B.-33 is mostly used as a local point for Painful Obstruction Syndrome of the knee, especially when there is great stiffness and the pain is on the lateral side of the knee. It is particularly indicated for problems of the ligaments and tendons of the knee, as the Liver and Gall Bladder control sinews.

Box 64.26 summarizes the functions of G.B.-33.

Box 64.26 G.B.-33 – summary of functions

- Resolves Dampness and expels Wind
- Removes obstructions from the channel (redness, swelling and pain of the lateral side of the knee, rigidity of knee, Wind and Dampness Painful Obstruction Syndrome (*Bi* Syndrome) of the knee, numbness)

G.B.-34 YANGLINGQUAN *YANG HILL SPRING*

Location
On the lateral aspect of the lower leg, in the depression anterior and inferior to the head of the fibula.

Nature
Sea (*He*) point.
Earth point.
Gathering (*Hui*) point for sinews.

Actions
Promotes the smooth flow of Liver-Qi.
Resolves Damp-Heat in Liver and Gall Bladder.
Benefits the sinews.
Removes obstruction from the channel.

Indications
Hypochondrial, epigastric and abdominal distension, irritability, moodiness, depression, sighing.

Bitter taste, hypochondrial fullness, inability to digest fats, feeling of heaviness.
Contracture of sinews, stiff neck and shoulders, pain in the elbow, hip pain, sciatica.
Pain in the calf muscles, Painful Obstruction Syndrome (*Bi* Syndrome) and Atrophy (*Wei*) Syndrome of the lower leg, swelling, pain and redness of the knee, rigidity of knee, Cold Painful Obstruction Syndrome of the knee.

Comments

G.B.-34 is one of the major points of the body. First of all, it is an extremely important point to promote the smooth flow of Liver-Qi. It is used whenever there is stagnation of Liver-Qi, especially in the hypochondrial area. When combined with other points, it can also affect stagnation of Liver-Qi in other areas, such as the epigastrium (combined with Ren-12 Zhongwan) or the lower abdomen (combined with Ren-6 Qihai).

By regulating Liver-Qi, it helps to make Stomach-Qi descend and can be used for such symptoms of ascending Stomach-Qi as nausea and vomiting.

G.B.-34 resolves Damp-Heat in Liver and Gall Bladder, usually combined with G.B.-24 Riyue.

It is an important point to relax the sinews whenever there are contractions of the muscles, cramps or spasms. As its indications show, it affects the sinews of all joints.

G.B.-34 is an important point in the treatment of Painful Obstruction Syndrome, Atrophy Syndrome and sequelae of Wind-stroke to invigorate the circulation of Qi and Blood in the legs and relax the tendons. This action is partly due to its being the Gathering (*Hui*) point for sinews.

Box 64.27 summarizes the functions of G.B.-34.

Box 64.27 G.B.-34 – summary of functions

- Promotes the smooth flow of Liver-Qi (hypochondrial, epigastric and abdominal distension, irritability, moodiness, depression, sighing)
- Resolves Damp-Heat in Liver and Gall Bladder (bitter taste, hypochondrial fullness, inability to digest fats, feeling of heaviness)
- Benefits the sinews (contracture of sinews, stiff neck and shoulders, pain in the elbow, hip pain, sciatica)
- Removes obstruction from the channel (pain in the calf muscles, Painful Obstruction Syndrome (*Bi* Syndrome) and Atrophy (*Wei*) Syndrome of the lower leg, swelling, pain and redness of the knee, rigidity of knee, Cold Painful Obstruction Syndrome of the knee)

G.B.-35 YANGJIAO *YANG CROSSING*

Location

On the lateral aspect of the lower leg, 7 *cun* above the tip of the external malleolus, on the posterior border of the fibula.

Nature

Meeting point of the three Yang channels of the leg.
Accumulation (*Xi*) point of the Yang Linking Vessel (*Yang Wei Mai*).

Actions

Removes obstructions from the channel.

Indications

Swelling and pain of the knee, Painful Obstruction Syndrome (*Bi* Syndrome) and Atrophy (*Wei*) Syndrome of the lower leg, cold Painful Obstruction Syndrome, fullness and distension of the hypochondrium and lateral costal region.

Comments

G.B.-35 is mostly used in acute pain along the Gall Bladder channel with stiffness and cramp of the leg muscles. As the Accumulation (*Xi*) point of the Yang Linking Vessel, it affects the Yang channels of the leg.

Box 64.28 summarizes the functions of G.B.-35.

Box 64.28 G.B.-35 – summary of functions

- Removes obstructions from the channel (swelling and pain of the knee, Painful Obstruction Syndrome (*Bi* Syndrome) and Atrophy (*Wei*) Syndrome of the lower leg, cold Painful Obstruction Syndrome, fullness and distension of the hypochondrium and lateral costal region)

G.B.-36 WAIQIU *OUTER MOUND*

Location

On the lateral aspect of the lower leg, 7 *cun* above the tip of the external malleolus, on the anterior border of the fibula, at the level of G.B.-35 Yangjiao.

Nature

Accumulation (*Xi*) point of the Gall Bladder channel.

Actions

Removes obstruction from the channel.

Indications

Hypochondrial distension, Painful Obstruction Syndrome (*Bi* Syndrome) and Atrophy (*Wei*) Syndrome of the lower leg.

Comments

Being the Accumulation point, G.B.-36 is used in all painful conditions of the channel or organ.
Box 64.29 summarizes the functions of G.B.-36.

Box 64.29 G.B.-36 – summary of functions

- Removes obstruction from the channel (hypochondrial distension, Painful Obstruction Syndrome (*Bi* Syndrome) and Atrophy (*Wei*) Syndrome of the lower leg)

G.B.-37 GUANGMING *BRIGHTNESS*

Location

On the lateral aspect of the lower leg, 5 *cun* above the tip of the external malleolus, on the anterior border of the fibula.

Nature

Connecting (*Luo*) point.

Actions

Brightens the eyes.
Conducts Fire downwards.

Indications

Eye pain, diminished night vision, itching of eyes, myopia, blurred vision.
Red, swollen and painful eyes, headache, bitter taste.

Comments

The most important function of G.B.-37 is that of benefiting the eyes, improving eyesight and eliminating 'floaters' in the eyes. It is particularly effective for eye problems due to Liver-Fire as it conducts Fire downwards.
Box 64.30 summarizes the functions of G.B.-37.

Box 64.30 G.B.-37 – summary of functions

- Brightens the eyes (eye pain, diminished night vision, itching of eyes, myopia, blurred vision)
- Conducts Fire downwards (red, swollen and painful eyes, headache, bitter taste)

G.B.-38 YANGFU *YANG AID*

Location

On the lateral aspect of the lower leg, 4 *cun* above the tip of the external malleolus, slightly anterior to the anterior border of the fibula.

Nature

River (*Jing*) point.
Fire point.
Drainage point.

Actions

Subdues Liver-Yang.
Clears Heat.

Indications

Headache, pain on the outer canthus of the eye.
Bitter taste, sighing, hypochondrial pain, feeling of heat.

Comments

This point can be used to clear Liver-Fire and to subdue Liver-Yang. In this connection, it is an important distal point for chronic migraine headaches from rising of Liver-Yang or Liver-Fire.
Box 64.31 summarizes the functions of G.B.-38.

Box 64.31 G.B.-38 – summary of functions

- Subdues Liver-Yang (headache, pain on the outer canthus of the eye)
- Clears Heat (bitter taste, sighing, hypochondrial pain, feeling of heat)

G.B.-39 XUANZHONG *HANGING BELL*

Location

On the lateral aspect of the lower leg, 3 *cun* above the tip of the external malleolus, on the anterior border of the fibula.

Nature

Gathering (*Hui*) point for Marrow.

Actions

Subdues Liver-Yang.
Expels Wind.
Nourishes Marrow and bone marrow.

Indications

Headache, dizziness, stiff neck.
Stiff and painful neck, inability to turn head, Painful Obstruction Syndrome (*Bi* Syndrome) of the neck.

Comments

The most important function of G.B.-39 is that of nourishing the Marrow. However, judging by the indications of this point, it seems to affect the bone marrow more than the Marrow and the Brain. It is indicated in chronic Bone Painful Obstruction Syndrome (*Bi* Syndrome), which is characterized by a deficiency of the Liver and Kidney and of the sinews and bones. This point nourishes the bones by nourishing the bone marrow. The regular use of this point in old people is said to help to prevent Wind-stroke.

Apart from this, it is an important point to remove obstructions from the Lesser Yang (*Shao Yang*) channels from the lateral side of the neck, especially when the neck is very stiff and the person cannot turn the neck from side to side. In such cases, the needle is reduced quite vigorously while the patient is asked to gently turn the head from side to side.

However, in my practice, I use G.B.-39 in its capacity of Gathering point of Marrow. To treat the neck, I prefer an extra point that is near G.B.-39 on the Gall Bladder channel. This point is called *Juegu*, which means 'disappearing bone'. It is called thus because the point is located by palpating the fibula starting from below G.B.-39: the point Juegu is situated at the hollow where the fibula is not felt any longer as it 'disappears' below the overlying muscle. The point is usually higher than G.B.-39.

Box 64.32 summarizes the functions of G.B.-39.

Box 64.32 G.B.-39 – summary of functions

- Subdues Liver-Yang (headache, dizziness, stiff neck)
- Expels Wind (stiff and painful neck, inability to turn head, Painful Obstruction Syndrome (*Bi* Syndrome) of the neck)
- Nourishes Marrow and bone marrow

G.B.-40 QIUXU *MOUND RUINS*

Location

On the foot, anterior and inferior to the external malleolus, in the depression on the lateral side of the tendon of the extensor digitorum longus.

Nature

Source (*Yuan*) point.

Actions

Promotes the smooth flow of Liver-Qi.
Clears Gall Bladder-Heat.

Indications

Hypochondrial distension, sighing, depression, moodiness.
Swelling, redness and pain of the eye, headache, bitter taste.

Comments

G.B.-40 can be used to promote the smooth flow of Liver-Qi whenever Liver-Qi is stagnant, causing hypochondrial pain and distension and sighing.

In my experience, this point can be used to strengthen the Gall Bladder mental aspect: that is, the strength of character which allows one to take difficult decisions. It is also the best point to use to strengthen the Gall Bladder and Heart in the syndrome of 'deficiency of the Gall Bladder' characterized by timidity, lack of initiative, difficult in making decisions and depression.

On a mental level, the Gall Bladder channel can be used to stimulate the 'coming and going' of the

Ethereal Soul when the person is depressed and lacks a sense of direction and purpose in life. In my experience, G.B.-40 is the best point to stimulate this aspect of the Gall Bladder.

Box 64.33 summarizes the functions of G.B.-40.

Box 64.33 G.B.-40 – summary of functions

- Promotes the smooth flow of Liver-Qi (hypochondrial distension, sighing, depression, moodiness)
- Clears Gall Bladder-Heat (swelling, redness and pain of the eye, headache, bitter taste)
- Stimulates the 'coming and going' of the Ethereal Soul when the person is depressed

---

G.B.-41 ZULINQI (FOOT) FALLING TEARS

Location

On the lateral side of the dorsum of the foot, proximal to the fourth metatarsophalangeal joint, in the depression lateral to the tendon of the extensor digiti minimi.

Nature

Stream (*Shu*) point.
Wood point.
Opening point of the Girdle Vessel (*Dai Mai*).

Actions

Subdues Liver-Yang.
Promotes the smooth flow of Liver-Qi.
Clears Heat in the Gall Bladder channel.
Benefits the breasts.
Resolves Damp-Heat and regulates the Girdle Vessel.

Indications

Headache, dizziness, blurred vision.
Hypochondrial distension and pain, fullness of the chest.
Red, swollen and painful eyes, pain in the outer canthus, dry eyes.
Breast distension and pain, breast lumps, breast abscess.
Leukorrhoea.

Comments

G.B.-41 resolves Damp-Heat in the genital region, with such symptoms as chronic vaginal discharge, cystitis and urethritis. It does so by virtue of being the opening point of the Girdle Vessel (*Dai Mai*).

It promotes the smooth flow of Liver-Qi in the hypochondrium and it subdues Liver-Yang, which makes it suitable to treat headaches.

G.B.-41 has an influence in Painful Obstruction Syndrome from Dampness, particularly of the knee and hip.

This point influences the female breast and, in my experience, it is an important point to affect the breasts in breast distension and pain and in breast lumps.

Box 64.34 summarizes the functions of G.B.-41.

Box 64.34 G.B.-41 – summary of functions

- Subdues Liver-Yang (headache, dizziness, blurred vision)
- Promotes the smooth flow of Liver-Qi (hypochondrial distension and pain, fullness of the chest)
- Clears Heat in the Gall Bladder channel (red, swollen and painful eyes, pain in the outer canthus, dry eyes)
- Benefits the breasts (breast distension and pain, breast lumps, breast abscess)
- Resolves Damp-Heat and regulates the Girdle Vessel (leukorrhoea)

G.B.-43 XIAXI STREAM INSERTION

Location

On the lateral side of the dorsum of the foot, proximal to the margin of the web between the fourth and fifth toes.

Nature

Spring (*Ying*) point.
Water point.
Tonification point.

Actions

Subdues Liver-Yang.
Benefits the ears.
Resolves Damp-Heat.

Indications

Headache, dizziness, blurred vision.
Tinnitus, deafness, itchy ears, earache.
Hypochondrial fullness, breast abscess, swelling of limbs, redness, swelling and pain of the dorsum of the foot.

Comments

G.B.-43 is effective in treating temporal headaches from rising of Liver-Yang. It is frequently used as a distal point for migraine headaches affecting the Gall Bladder channel on the temples.

It is also effective for ear problems such as tinnitus from Liver-Yang rising or otitis media from exterior Damp-Heat.

Box 64.35 summarizes the functions of G.B.-43.

Box 64.35 G.B.-43 – summary of functions

- Subdues Liver-Yang (headache, dizziness, blurred vision)
- Benefits the ears (tinnitus, deafness, itchy ears, earache)
- Resolves Damp-Heat (hypochondrial fullness, breast abscess, swelling of limbs, redness, swelling and pain of the dorsum of the foot)

G.B.-44 ZUQIAOYIN (FOOT) YIN ORIFICE

Location

On the foot, on the lateral side of the end of the fourth toe, 0.1 *cun* from the corner of the nail.

Nature

Well (*Jing*) point.
Metal point.

Actions

Subdues Liver-Yang.
Clears Heat and brightens the eyes.
Calms the Mind.

Indications

Headache, dizziness, blurred vision, stabbing pain in the head.
Pain in the outer canthus, redness, swelling and pain of the eye.
Insomnia, nightmares, somnolence, agitation, anxiety.

Comments

G.B.-44 is used for migraine headaches around the eyes from rising of Liver-Yang. It has an influence on the eyes, and is used for red and painful eyes from the flaring up of Liver-Fire.

It also calms the Mind, in cases of insomnia and agitation deriving from Liver-Fire.

Box 64.36 summarizes the functions of G.B.-44.

Figure 64.4 illustrates the target areas of the Gall Bladder channel points. It will be useful to compare the action of the main Gall Bladder points together with two of the Triple Burner points, as there is some overlap in the area influenced by these two channels (Table 64.1 and see Fig. 64.3).

Box 64.36 G.B.-44 – summary of functions

- Subdues Liver-Yang (headache, dizziness, blurred vision, stabbing pain in the head)
- Clears Heat and brightens the eyes (pain in the outer canthus, redness, swelling and pain of the eye)
- Calms the Mind (insomnia, nightmares, somnolence, agitation, anxiety)

Table 64.1 Comparison of Yanglingquan G.B.-34, Qiuxu G.B.-40, Zulinqi G.B.-41, Xiaxi G.B.-43, Zuqiaoyin G.B.-44, Zhigou T.B.-6. and Waiguan T.B.-5

Point	Action	Area Affected
G.B.-34	Promotes the smooth flow of Liver-Qi	Hypochondrium
G.B.-40	Promotes the mental strength related to a strong Gall Bladder	Ears, temples, head
G.B.-41	Resolves Damp-Heat	Genital area and breast
G.B.-43	Subdues Liver-Yang	Temples and ears
G.B.-44	Calms the Mind	Eyes
T.B.-6	Moves Liver-Qi	Lateral costal region
T.B.-5	Expels Wind-Heat	Temples, ears

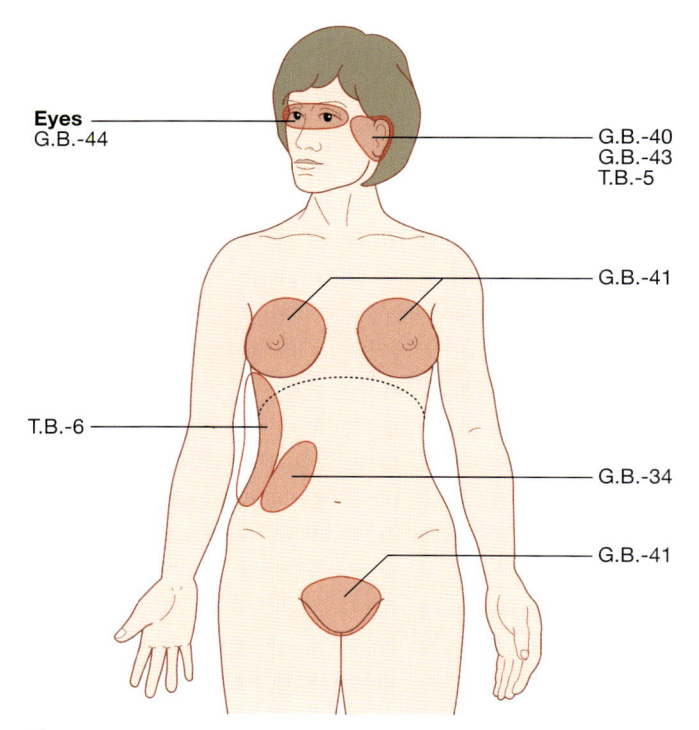

Figure 64.4 Target areas of Gall Bladder channel points

END NOTES

1. Dr Zhang Ming Jiu, personal communication, Nanjing, 1982.
2. Dr Zhang Ming Jiu, personal communication, Nanjing, 1982.
3. Dr Zhang Ming Jiu, personal communication, Nanjing, 1982.
4. Dr Zhang Ming Jiu, personal communication, Nanjing, 1982.
5. Cheng Bao Shu 1988 Great Dictionary of Acupuncture (*Zhen Jiu Da Ci Dian* 针 灸 大 辞 典), Beijing Science Publishing House, Beijing, p. 11.
6. Jiao Shun Fa 1987 An Enquiry into Chinese Acupuncture (*Zhong Guo Zhen Jiu Qiu Zhen* 中 国 针 灸 求 真), Shanxi Science Publishing House, p. 52.
7. Yue Han Zhen 1990 An Explanation of the Acupuncture Points (*Jing Xue Jie* 经 穴 解), People's Health Publishing House, Beijing, originally published in 1654, p. 334.
8. Dr Zhang Ming Jiu, personal communication, Nanjing, 1982.
9. An Enquiry into Chinese Acupuncture, p. 52.
10. Dr Zhang Ming Jiu, personal communication, Nanjing, 1982.
11. An Enquiry into Chinese Acupuncture, p. 52.

SECTION 2   PART 7

Liver Channel 65

Main channel pathway

The Liver channel starts on the big toe and runs upwards on the dorsum of the foot and medial malleolus and then up the medial aspect of the leg. It then reaches the genital region, curves around the genitalia and goes up to the lower abdomen. Proceeding further up, it curves around the stomach and enters the liver and gall bladder. It then continues to ascend, passes through the diaphragm and branches out in the hypochondrial and costal region. From here, it ascends to the throat and reaches the eye. Running further upwards it goes to the top of the head to meet the Governing Vessel (Fig. 65.1).

Connecting channel pathway

The Liver Connecting channel starts at LIV-5 Ligou and connects with the Gall Bladder channel. Another branch flows upwards on the medial aspect of the leg and thigh to the genitals (Fig. 65.2).

Box 65.1 gives an overview of the Liver points.

> **Box 65.1   Overview of Liver points**
> - Affect the inner aspect of the leg, abdomen, hypochondrium, throat and head
> - Important distal points for headaches from Liver-Yang rising
> - Invigorate Blood, especially in the Uterus
> - Several important points for urinary problems
> - Several important points for genital problems

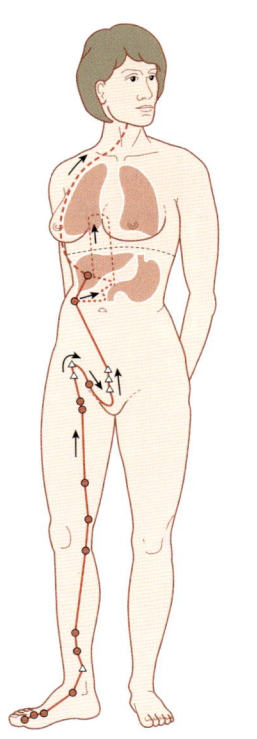

Figure 65.1 Liver main channel

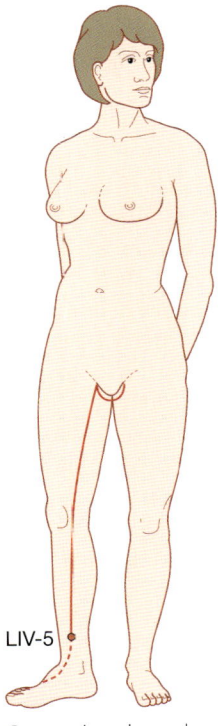

Figure 65.2 Liver Connecting channel

LIV-1 DADUN BIG MOUND

Location

On the foot, on the lateral side of the end of the big toe, 0.1 *cun* from the corner of the nail.

Nature

Well (*Jing*) point.
Wood point.

Actions

Regulates menstruation.
Resolves Damp-Heat in the genitourinary system.
Promotes resuscitation.

Indications

Irregular periods, excessive uterine bleeding, prolapse of uterus.
Swelling and pain of the genitalia, pain in the penis, retraction of genitals, swelling of testicles, swelling and redness of vulva, retention of urine, blood in urine, painful urination, frequent urination, difficulty in urination, turbid urine.
Loss of consciousness, epilepsy.

Comments

This point has a marked action on the Lower Burner. First of all, it stops uterine bleeding from Heat in the Blood (it would not be indicated in uterine bleeding from Qi deficiency).

It resolves Damp-Heat in the Lower Burner in the two main areas of urinary function and external genitalia. The Liver channel has an important influence on the external genitalia and such diseases are part of the broad group of diseases falling under the category of Hernial and Genitourinary Disorders (*shan* diseases).

LIV-1, in particular, is a major point to use for Hernial and Genitourinary Disorders (*shan*). '*Shan*' is a general term for a wide variety of disorders. Traditionally, seven types of *shan* disorders were listed: these can be broadly differentiated into three general categories. The 'Concise Dictionary of Chinese Medicine' lists these three groups as follows:

> 1. Hernial-type diseases characterized by a protrusion of an organ or tissue out of the abdominal cavity
> 2. Diseases of the external genitalia in men and women
> 3. Severe abdominal pain accompanied by constipation and retention of urine or difficulty in urination[1]

> **Box 65.2 LIV-1 – summary of functions**
> - Regulates menstruation (irregular periods, excessive uterine bleeding, prolapse of uterus)
> - Resolves Damp-Heat (swelling and pain of the genitalia, pain in the penis, retraction of genitals, swelling of testicles, swelling and redness of vulva, retention of urine, blood in urine, painful urination, frequent urination, difficulty in urination, turbid urine)
> - Promotes resuscitation (loss of consciousness, epilepsy)

Diseases of the external genitalia mentioned among the indications above are part of Hernial and Genitourinary Disorders (*shan*) and LIV-1 can be used for enlarged scrotum, itchy scrotum, redness and swelling of the vulva, pruritus vulvae, etc.

LIV-1 resolves Damp-Heat from the urinary system and benefits urination so that it can be used for such symptoms as difficult urination, retention of urine, turbid urine and painful urination.

Finally, LIV-1 restores consciousness (as many Well points do) and is used in the acute stage of Wind-stroke.

Box 65.2 summarizes the functions of LIV-1.

LIV-2 XINGJIAN TEMPORARY IN-BETWEEN

Location

On the dorsum of the foot, proximal to the margin of the web between the first and second toes.

Nature

Spring (*Ying*) point.
Fire point.
Drainage point.

Actions

Drains Liver-Fire and subdues Liver-Yang.
Extinguishes interior Wind.
Cools Blood and stops bleeding.
Calms the Mind.
Resolves Damp-Heat in the genitourinary system.

Indications

Bitter taste, headache, thirst, dark urine, dry stools, irritability, propensity to outbursts of anger, red eyes, dizziness, tinnitus, eye pain, feeling of heat.

Wind-stroke, deviation of eye and mouth, tetany, epilepsy, loss of consciousness.
Excessive menstrual bleeding, coughing of blood, vomiting of blood.
Propensity to outbursts of anger, sadness, fright, 'seeing ghosts', manic behaviour, insomnia, palpitations.
Pain and itching of genitals, pain in the penis, Hernial and Genitourinary Disorders (*shan*), painful urination, retention of urine, difficult urination, turbid urine, excessive vaginal discharge, constipation, abdominal distension.

Comments

LIV-2 is *the* point to drain Liver-Fire. It is a point which is only used to drain the Liver in Excess patterns, mostly to drain Liver-Fire, but also to subdue Liver-Yang and extinguish Liver-Wind.

Since it drains Liver-Fire, it is used for bitter taste, thirst, a red face, headaches, dream-disturbed sleep, scanty dark urine, constipation, red eyes, a Red tongue with thick yellow coating and a Rapid-Wiry pulse. Since it subdues Liver-Yang, it is widely used to treat migraine headaches from rising Liver-Yang. As it expels interior Wind, LIV-2 is used for epilepsy and children's convulsions.

LIV-2 has an important Blood-cooling action which is used to stop bleeding from Blood-Heat. The Blood-cooling action is related to its Fire-draining action. As the Liver stores Blood, when the Liver has Fire, this is transferred to the Blood heating it. Blood-Heat is a major cause of bleeding. Indeed, bleeding is an important potential consequence of Liver-Fire, which helps to distinguish it from Liver-Heat or Liver-Yang rising (which do not cause bleeding).

LIV-2 is also the main point to clear Liver-Fire when this causes cough (from Liver insulting the Lungs in the Insulting cycle of the Five Elements). The 'Simple Questions' in chapter 38 says: '*Each of the five Yin and six Yang organs can cause cough ... cough caused by the Liver is accompanied by pain below the ribs; in severe cases the person is unable to turn the body and has a sensation of swelling and fullness below the ribs.*'[2]

In these cases, Liver-Fire 'insults' the Lungs and obstructs the chest, causing cough and breathlessness. This is frequently accompanied by Phlegm, which combines with the Fire of the Liver to ascend to the chest.

Box 65.3 summarizes the functions of LIV-2.

> **Box 65.3 LIV-2 – summary of functions**
>
> - Drains Liver-Fire and subdues Liver-Yang (bitter taste, headache, thirst, dark urine, dry stools, irritability, propensity to outbursts of anger, red eyes, dizziness, tinnitus, eye pain, feeling of heat)
> - Extinguishes interior Wind (Wind-stroke, deviation of eye and mouth, tetany, epilepsy, loss of consciousness)
> - Cools Blood and stops bleeding (excessive menstrual bleeding, coughing of blood, vomiting of blood)
> - Calms the Mind (propensity to outbursts of anger, sadness, fright, 'seeing ghosts', manic behaviour, insomnia, palpitations)
> - Resolves Damp-Heat in genitourinary system (pain and itching of genitals, pain in the penis, Hernial and Genitourinary Disorders (*shan*), painful urination, retention of urine, difficult urination, turbid urine, excessive vaginal discharge, constipation, abdominal distension)

LIV-3 TAICHONG *BIGGER PENETRATING*

Location

On the dorsum of the foot, in the depression distal to the junction between the first and second metatarsal bones.

Nature

Source (*Yuan*) and Stream (*Shu*) point.
Earth point.
Ma Dan Yang's Heavenly Star point.

Actions

Subdues Liver-Yang.
Extinguishes interior Wind.
Promotes the smooth flow of Liver-Qi.
Resolves Dampness.
Invigorates Blood and regulates menstruation.
Calms the Mind.
Calms spasms.

Indications

Headache, dizziness, blurred vision, numbness of head.
Opisthotonos, epilepsy, deviation of eye and mouth.
Hypochondrial distension, irritability, epigastric and abdominal distension, sighing, breast distension, nausea, constipation, borborygmi.
Hypogastric fullness, Hernial and Genitourinary Disorders (*shan*), swollen testicles, pain in genitalia, retracted testicles, swollen vulva, difficult urination, retention of urine, jaundice.

Amenorrhoea, irregular periods, painful periods, excessive menstrual bleeding, prolapse of uterus.
Propensity to outbursts of anger, irritability, insomnia, worrying.
Cramps, stiffness of the lower back with inability to bend, contracture of sinews.

Comments

LIV-3 is a major point. It is an extremely important point of the Liver channel used mostly to drain the Liver in Excess patterns, although it can also be used with reinforcing method to nourish Liver-Blood.

LIV-3's main action is that of subduing Liver-Yang, and it is very frequently used in migraine headaches from rising of Liver-Yang. It is somewhat gentler than LIV-2 Xingjian.

It also extinguishes interior Wind and it has a specific action in calming spasms, contraction and cramps of the muscles. Combined with L.I.-4 Hegu, it expels Wind from the face, and is used for such symptoms as facial paralysis and tic. This combination is called the 'Four Gates' and it also calms the Mind, regulates the ascending and descending of Qi and subdues rebellious Qi.

LIV-3 has a profound calming effect on the Mind, and is effective in calming very tense people who are prone to short temper or experience feelings of deep frustration and repressed anger. However, its calming action is not limited to its action on feelings of anger, which are typical of a Liver disharmony, as it is also effective in general irritability and tendency to worry from emotional stress. Its calming action is enhanced when combined with L.I.-4 Hegu (the 'Four Gates').

LIV-3 is a very important gynaecological point as it activates the Penetrating Vessel (*Chong Mai*). Indeed, the name of this point is related to the Penetrating Vessel as the character *chong* in this point's name is the same as in *Chong Mai*. In fact, when the first chapter of the 'Simple Questions' refers to the Penetrating Vessel being 'flourishing' at 14 in girls (and 16 in boys), it calls this vessel not the *Chong Mai* but the *Taichong Vessel*: that is, the 'LIV-3 Vessel'. Therefore, whenever we use LIV-3 we activate the Penetrating Vessel and, in particular, we invigorate Blood in the Uterus. For this reason, LIV-3 is a major point for Blood stasis and painful periods. This effect is due also to its spasm-calming effect: LIV-3 calms spasms, resolves contraction and stops pain.

LIV-3 resolves Dampness primarily from the genitourinary system but also from the Liver and Gall Bladder (as the indication 'jaundice' shows). In this context, it is used for Hernial and Genitourinary Disorders (*shan*) in a similar way to LIV-1 Dadun.

Needled with reducing method and followed by moxibustion, it can expel Cold from the Liver channel, and treat genital swelling and orchitis in men, or chronic white vaginal discharge in women.

Box 65.4 summarizes the functions of LIV-3.

It is useful to compare the nature and action of LIV-2 Xingjian and LIV-3 Taichong (Table 65.1).

Box 65.4 LIV-3 – summary of functions

- Subdues Liver-Yang (headache, dizziness, blurred vision, numbness of head)
- Extinguishes interior Wind (opisthotonos, epilepsy, deviation of eye and mouth)
- Promotes the smooth flow of Liver-Qi (hypochondrial distension, irritability, epigastric and abdominal distension, sighing, breast distension, nausea, constipation, borborygmi)
- Resolves Dampness (hypogastric fullness, Hernial and Genitourinary Disorders (*shan*), swollen testicles, pain in genitalia, retracted testicles, swollen vulva, difficult urination, retention of urine, jaundice)
- Invigorates Blood and regulates menstruation (amenorrhoea, irregular periods, painful periods, excessive menstrual bleeding, prolapse of uterus)
- Calms the Mind (propensity to outbursts of anger, irritability, insomnia, worrying)
- Calms spasms (cramps, stiffness of the lower back with inability to bend, contracture of sinews)

Table 65.1 A comparison of LIV-2 Xingjian and LIV-3 Taichong

LIV-2	LIV-3
Specific to drain Liver-Fire	Not so much for Liver-Fire, more to subdue Liver-Yang
No strong mental effect	Strong mental calming effect
Used only to drain	Can be used to nourish Liver-Blood
No specific effect on spasms	Specific effect on spasms
Quite a harsh point	Gentler point
Mostly to subdue rebellious Qi	To subdue rebellious Qi but also to promote the smooth flow of Qi when it stagnates horizontally (e.g. in epigastrium or hypochondrium)
Area affected is mostly head, secondarily genitals	Areas affected are head, epigastrium, hypochondrium, abdomen

LIV-4 ZHONGFENG *MIDDLE SEAL*

Location
Anterior to the prominence of the medial malleolus, in the depression just medial to the tendon of the tibialis anterior when the ankle is extended.

Nature
River (*Jing*) point.
Metal point.

Action
Promotes the smooth flow of Liver-Qi in the Lower Burner.
Resolves Dampness in the genitourinary system.

Indications
Hypogastric and abdominal distension, umbilical pain. Pain and retraction of genitals, Hernial and Genitourinary Disorders (*shan*), difficult urination, painful urination, turbid urine, retention of urine, swelling of lower abdomen.

Comments
LIV-4 is mostly used to promote the smooth flow of Liver-Qi in the Lower Burner and, more specifically, in the genital and urinary region. It is thus used for urinary symptoms with a feeling of distension in the hypogastrium deriving from stagnation of Liver-Qi.

It also resolves Dampness and treats Hernial and Genitourinary Disorders (*shan*) in a similar way to LIV-1 and LIV-3.

Box 65.5 summarizes the functions of LIV-4.

Box 65.5 LIV-4 – summary of functions

- Promotes the smooth flow of Liver-Qi in the Lower Burner (hypogastric and abdominal distension, umbilical pain)
- Resolves Dampness in the genitourinary system (pain and retraction of genitals, Hernial and Genitourinary Disorders (*shan*), difficult urination, painful urination, turbid urine, retention of urine, swelling of lower abdomen)

LIV-5 LIGOU *GOURD DITCH*

Location
5 *cun* above the prominence of the medial malleolus, posterior to the medial crest of the tibia, between this and the gastrocnemius muscle.

Nature
Connecting (*Luo*) point.

Actions
Promotes the smooth flow of Liver-Qi.
Resolves Damp-Heat in the genitourinary system.

Indications
Hypogastric distension, abdominal distension.
Hernial and Genitourinary Disorders (*shan*), itching, swelling and pain of genitals, swelling and pain of testicles or vulva, priapism (persistent erection), abdominal fullness, difficult urination, retention of urine.

Comments
LIV-5 has a specific affinity for the genital and urinary area. The Liver Connecting (*Luo*) channel departs from this point and flows up the inner aspect of the thigh to encircle the genitals. This point can therefore be used for any urinary symptom deriving from stagnation of Liver-Qi, such as distension of the hypogastrium, distension and pain before urination and retention of urine.

It resolves Dampness in this area and is therefore used for Hernial and Genitourinary Disorders (*shan*) with such symptoms as vaginal discharge, cloudy urine, swelling and pain of the vulva, pain in the scrotum, etc.

Besides influencing the genital area, this point also affects the throat and is used for stagnation of Liver-Qi in the throat causing the typical sensation of lump in the throat and of being unable to swallow. This sensation is related to emotional tension and it comes and goes according to the emotional state. It is called 'Plum-Stone Syndrome' in Chinese medicine, as the person feels as if he or she has an obstruction in the throat.

Box 65.6 summarizes the functions of LIV-5.

Box 65.6 LIV-5 – summary of functions

- Promotes the smooth flow of Liver-Qi (hypogastric distension, abdominal distension)
- Resolves Damp-Heat in the genitourinary system (Hernial and Genitourinary Disorders (*shan*), itching, swelling and pain of genitals, swelling and pain of testicles or vulva, priapism (persistent erection), abdominal fullness, difficult urination, retention of urine)

LIV-6 ZHONGDU *MIDDLE CAPITAL*

Location
5 *cun* above the prominence of the medial malleolus, posterior to the medial crest of the tibia, between this and the gastrocnemius muscle.

Nature
Accumulation (*Xi*) point.

Actions
Removes obstructions from the channel.

Indications
Lower abdominal pain, hypogastric pain, cold lower leg, pain in the inner aspect of the leg.

Comments
LIV-6, like LIV-5, also has an affinity with the genital and urinary area and has a similar action to LIV-4 Zhongfeng and LIV-5 Ligou, the only difference being that it is the Accumulation (*Xi*) point and is therefore useful in Excess patterns and acute cases to stop pain. For example, it is a very useful point for acute urinary pain (such as in cystitis) deriving from Damp-Heat and stagnation of Liver-Qi.

Box 65.7 summarizes the functions of LIV-6.

> **Box 65.7 LIV-6 – summary of functions**
> - Removes obstructions from the channel (lower abdominal pain, hypogastric pain, cold lower leg, pain in the inner aspect of the leg)

LIV-7 XIGUAN *KNEE GATE*

Location
Posterior and inferior to the medial condyle of the tibia, 1 *cun* posterior to SP-9 Yinlingquan.

Nature
None.

Actions
Resolves Dampness and expels Wind.
Benefits the knee.

Indications
Swelling and pain of the knee, pain of the inner aspect of the knee, Painful Obstruction Syndrome (*Bi* Syndrome) of the knee, rigidity of the knee.

Comments
This is used as a local point for Painful Obstruction Syndrome of the knee, particularly if from Wind and when the pain is on the inner aspect of the knee.

Box 65.8 summarizes the functions of LIV-7.

> **Box 65.8 LIV-7 – summary of functions**
> - Resolves Dampness and expels Wind (swelling and pain of the knee, pain of the inner aspect of knee, Painful Obstruction Syndrome (*Bi* Syndrome) of the knee, rigidity of the knee)
> - Benefits the knee

LIV-8 QUQUAN *SPRING ON BEND*

Location
Superior to the medial end of the popliteal crease, anterior to the tendons of the semitendinosus and semimembranosus muscles, 1 *cun* in front of KI-10 Yingu.

Nature
Sea (*He*) point.
Water point.
Tonification point.

Actions
Benefits the Bladder and genitals.
Resolves Dampness from the Lower Burner.
Invigorates Blood and regulates menstruation.
Nourishes Liver-Blood.

Indications
Swelling and itching of genitals, pain in the genitals, pain in the penis, impotence, difficult urination, retention of urine.
Abdominal masses in women (*Zheng Jia*), painful periods, amenorrhoea, infertility from Blood stasis, umbilical pain.

Comments
LIV-8's main function is to eliminate Dampness obstructing the Lower Burner for such symptoms as

urinary retention, cloudy urine, burning urination, vaginal discharge, pruritus vulvae. It is effective for both Damp-Heat and Damp-Cold.

LIV-8 also invigorates Blood in the Uterus and it is used for painful periods and abdominal masses.

Used with reinforcing method, it can also nourish Liver-Blood.

Box 65.9 summarizes the functions of LIV-8.

> **Clinical note**
>
> To nourish Liver-Blood, I generally use LIV-8 Ququan, ST-36 Zusanli, SP-6 Sanyinjiao and Ren-4 Guanyuan

---

Box 65.9 LIV-8 – summary of functions

- Benefits the Bladder and genitals
- Resolves Dampness from the Lower Burner (swelling and itching of genitals, pain in the genitals, pain in the penis, impotence, difficult urination, retention of urine)
- Invigorates Blood and regulates menstruation (abdominal masses in women (*Zheng Jia*), painful periods, amenorrhoea, infertility from Blood stasis, umbilical pain)
- Nourishes Liver-Blood

LIV-13 ZHANGMEN
COMPLETION GATE

Location

Anterior and inferior to the free end of the 11th rib.

Nature

Front Collecting (*Mu*) point of the Spleen.
Gathering (*Hui*) point for the five Yin organs.
Meeting point of the Liver and Gall Bladder channels.

Actions

Promotes the smooth flow of Liver-Qi and harmonizes Liver and Spleen.

Indications

Hypochondrial distension, pain in the ribs, abdominal distension and pain, diarrhoea, undigested food in the stools, borborygmi, constipation.

Comments

LIV-13 is very much used whenever Liver-Qi stagnates and invades the Stomach and Spleen, preventing Spleen-Qi from ascending (resulting in loose stools, diarrhoea and abdominal distension) and Stomach-Qi from descending (resulting in retention of food, belching and fullness in the epigastrium). The use of this point will promote the smooth flow of Liver-Qi and eliminate stagnation, as well as strengthen the Spleen. It is therefore the main point to use whenever Liver and Spleen are not harmonized. Typically, the pulse is Wiry on the left and Weak on the right.

Needled with reinforcing method, this point can also be used to tonify Stomach and Spleen. If moxa is used in addition, it can tonify and warm the Spleen in deficiency of Spleen-Yang.[3]

Box 65.10 summarizes the functions of LIV-13.

Box 65.10 LIV-13 – summary of functions

- Promotes the smooth flow of Liver-Qi and harmonizes Liver and Spleen (hypochondrial distension, pain in the ribs, abdominal distension and pain, diarrhoea, undigested food in the stools, borborygmi, constipation)
- Tonifies Stomach and Spleen. If moxa is used in addition, it can tonify and warm the Spleen-Yang

---

LIV-14 QIMEN *CYCLIC GATE*

Location

In line with the mamillary line, in the sixth intercostal space, 4 *cun* lateral to the midline.

Nature

Front Collecting (*Mu*) point of the Liver.
Point of the Yin Linking Vessel (*Yin Wei Mai*).
Meeting point of Spleen and Liver channels.

Actions

Promotes the smooth flow of Liver-Qi and harmonizes Liver and Stomach.

Indications

Hypochondrial distension, sighing, breast distension, epigastric distension and pain, hiccup, belching, vomiting, hardness of epigastrium.

Comments

LIV-14 has a similar function to that of LIV-13 Zhangmen, the main difference being that this point affects mostly the Stomach, whilst LIV-13 affects more the Spleen.

Please note that there is an alternative location for LIV-14 at the lower edge of the ribcage in line with the nipple (or, in women, 4 *cun* from the midline) (Fig. 65.3). In fact, one could look upon these as two separate points. The one in the intercostal space is used more for channel problems, while the one at the lower edge of the ribcage is used more for organ problems.

This point is frequently used whenever Liver-Qi stagnates and invades the Stomach, causing belching, nausea, vomiting and hypochondrial distension and pain. It harmonizes Liver- and Stomach-Qi. The pulse is typically Wiry on both Middle positions.

Box 65.11 summarizes the functions of LIV-14.

Figure 65.4 illustrates the different areas influenced by various Liver channel points in treatment.

> **Box 65.11 LIV-14 – summary of functions**
>
> - Promotes the smooth flow of Liver-Qi and harmonizes Liver and Stomach (hypochondrial distension, sighing, breast distension, epigastric distension and pain, hiccup, belching, vomiting, hardness of epigastrium)

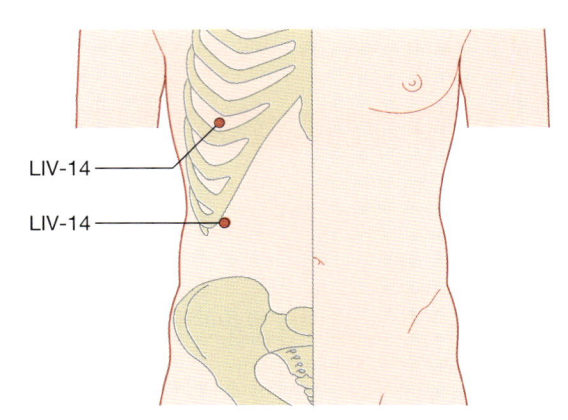

Figure 65.3 Alternative locations of LIV-14 Qimen

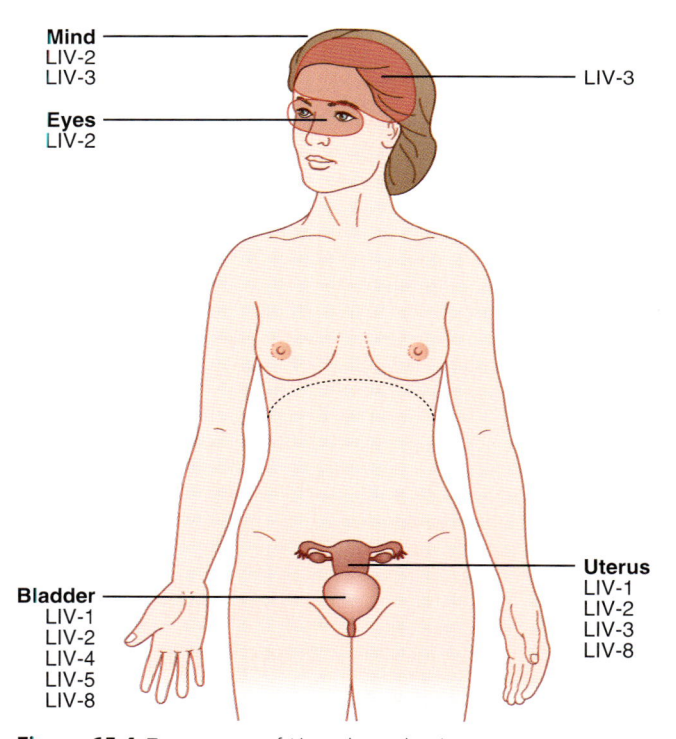

Mind
LIV-2
LIV-3

Eyes
LIV-2

LIV-3

Bladder
LIV-1
LIV-2
LIV-4
LIV-5
LIV-8

Uterus
LIV-1
LIV-2
LIV-3
LIV-8

Figure 65.4 Target areas of Liver channel points

END NOTES

1. 1980 Concise Dictionary of Chinese Medicine (*Jian Ming Zhong Yi Ci Dian* 简明中医辞典), People's Health Publishing House, Beijing, p. 569.
2. 1979 The Yellow Emperor's Classic of Internal Medicine – Simple Questions (*Huang Di Nei Jing Su Wen* 黄帝内经素问), People's Health Publishing House, Beijing, first published *c*.100 BC, p. 215.
3. Li Shi Zhen 1985 Clinical Application of Frequently Used Acupuncture Points (*Chang Yong Shu Xue Lin Chuang Fa Hui* 常用腧穴临床发挥), People's Health Publishing House, Beijing, p. 742.

SECTION 2 PART 7

Directing Vessel (*Ren Mai*) 66

Main channel pathway

The Directing Vessel originates from the uterus (or deep in the lower abdomen in men) and emerges at the perineum. It runs anteriorly to the pubic region and all the way up to the throat along the midline of the body. From the throat it ascends to curve around the lips and up to the eyes to meet the Stomach channel at the point ST-1 Chengqi (Fig. 66.1).

Connecting channel pathway

This channel starts at the tip of the xiphoid process from the point Ren-15 Jiuwei and spreads over the abdomen (Fig. 66.2).

Box 66.1 provides an overview of Directing Vessel points.

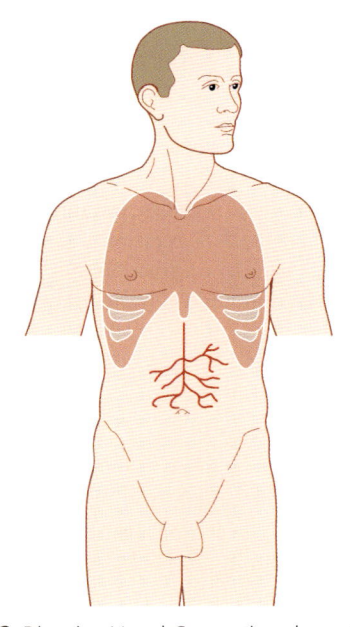

Figure 66.2 Directing Vessel Connecting channel

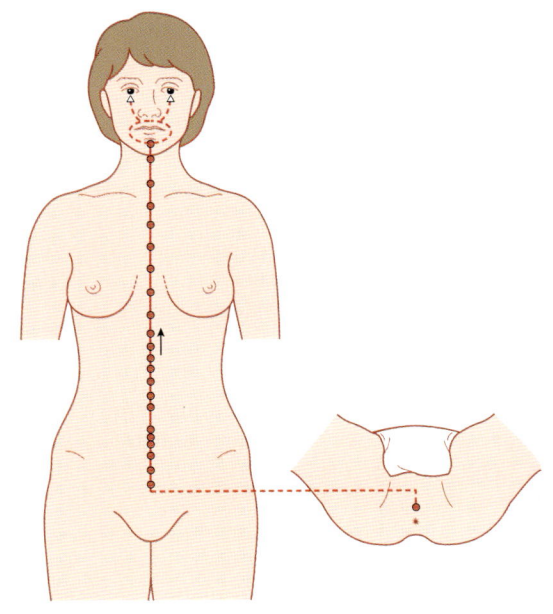

Figure 66.1 Directing Vessel

Box 66.1 Overview of Directing Vessel points

- Cannot treat gynaecological problems without points of the Directing Vessel
- Affects genitals, abdomen, throat, face
- Nourish Yin
- Establish communication between Lungs and Kidneys
- Regulate the Triple Burner
- Affect the Membranes (*Huang*)

REN-1 HUIYIN *MEETING OF YIN*

Location

In the perineum, midway between the anus and the scrotum in men, and the anus and the posterior labial commissure in women.

Nature

Beginning point of Directing, Penetrating and Governing Vessels (*Ren Mai, Chong Mai, Du Mai*).
One of Sun Si Miao's Ghost points.

Actions

Regulates the two lower orifices and genitalia and resolves Dampness.
Promotes resuscitation.
Calms the Mind and opens the Mind's orifices.
Nourishes Yin.

Indications

Difficult urination and defecation, enuresis, impotence, pain in penis, sweating of genitals, swelling of testicles, swelling of vulva and vagina, prolapse of rectum, haemorrhoids, pain in anus, pain in urethra, itching and pain of perineum, Hernial and Genitourinary Disorders (*shan*).
Coma, unconsciousness from drowning.
Manic depression.

Comments

Ren-1 is the point where the three extraordinary vessels, Directing, Governing and Penetrating Vessels (*Ren Mai, Du Mai* and *Chong Mai*), emerge from the interior: for this reason, it is a dynamic point with a powerful action in moving Qi and Blood and also in subduing rebellious Qi (as in mental problems). Some of its indications (epilepsy, manic depression, haemorrhoids, prolapse of anus) reflect a Governing Vessel pathology.

Ren-1 resolves Dampness in the genital area and in the urethra and anus: it can be used for vaginal discharge, pruritus vulvae or itching of scrotum, urinary difficulty, difficulty in defecation, etc.

As one of Sun Si Miao's Ghost points, it calms the Mind and opens the Mind's orifices and it can be used in manic depression.

This point also nourishes Yin and benefits the Kidney-Essence: it is used for incontinence, enuresis and nocturnal emissions deriving from Yin deficiency.

It is an empirical point to promote resuscitation after drowning.

Box 66.2 summarizes the functions of Ren-1.

Box 66.2 Ren-1 – summary of functions

- Regulates the two lower orifices and genitalia and resolves Dampness (difficult urination and defecation, enuresis, impotence, pain in penis, sweating of genitals, swelling of testicles, swelling of vulva and vagina, prolapse of rectum, haemorrhoids, pain in anus, pain in urethra, itching and pain of perineum, Hernial and Genitourinary Disorders)
- Promotes resuscitation (coma, unconsciousness from drowning)
- Calms the Mind and opens the Mind's orifices (manic depression)
- Nourishes Yin

REN-2 QUGU *CURVED BONE*

Location

On the midline in the lower abdomen, at the superior border of the pubic symphysis, 5 *cun* below the umbilicus.

Nature

Meeting point of Directing Vessel and Liver channels.

Actions

Benefits the Bladder and regulates urination.
Consolidates the Essence.
Strengthens the Kidneys and the Essence.

Indications

Dribbling of urine, difficult urination, retention of urine, enuresis, itchy scrotum, contraction of penis, pain in genitalia, vaginal itching, Hernial and Genitourinary Disorders (*shan*)
Seminal emissions, premature ejaculation, chronic vaginal discharge, impotence.
Exhaustion of the five Yin organs.

Comments

Ren-2 has a dual function. On the one hand, it resolves Dampness in the urinary system and treats Hernial and Genitourinary Disorders (*shan*) in a similar way to Ren-1.

On the other hand, this point has a 'firming' and consolidating action on the Essence, treating seminal emissions and premature ejaculation in men and chronic vaginal discharge in women. It also tonifies the

Kidneys and the Essence, as the indication 'Exhaustion of the five Yin organs' shows.

Ren-2 is a good alternative to the use of Ren-1 to treat urination, resolve Dampness and firm the Essence.

Box 66.3 summarizes the functions of Ren-2.

Box 66.3 Ren-2 – summary of functions

- Benefits the Bladder and regulates urination (dribbling of urine, difficult urination, retention of urine, enuresis, itchy scrotum, contraction of penis, pain in genitalia, vaginal itching, Hernial and Genitourinary Disorders (*shan*))
- Consolidates the Essence (seminal emissions, premature ejaculation, chronic vaginal discharge, impotence)
- Strengthens the Kidneys and the Essence (exhaustion of the five Yin organs)

REN-3 ZHONGJI *MIDDLE POLE*

Location

On the midline of the lower abdomen, 4 *cun* below the umbilicus, 1 *cun* superior to the pubic symphysis.

Nature

Front Collecting (*Mu*) point of the Bladder.
Meeting point of Directing Vessel, Spleen, Liver and Kidneys channels.
Meeting point of the three Yin Muscle channels of the leg.

Actions

Resolves Dampness from the Lower Burner.
Promotes the Bladder function of Qi transformation.
Benefits the Uterus and regulates menstruation.
Strengthens the Kidneys and nourishes the Essence.

Indications

Genital itching, pain in the genitals, excessive vaginal discharge, Hernial and Genitourinary Disorders (*shan*).
Retention of urine, frequent urination, dark urine, pain on urination.
Infertility, irregular periods, amenorrhoea, excessive uterine bleeding, abdominal masses in women (*Zheng Jia*), retention of placenta, retention of lochia, persistent lochial discharge.
Lower backache, dizziness, tinnitus, weak knees, deficiency of Original Qi (*Yuan Qi*).

Comments

Ren-3 is a very important point for genitourinary problems. It is the main point to affect the Bladder and its function of Qi transformation. It can therefore be used for any urinary problem, particularly acute ones. It is more frequently used with reducing method in Excess patterns. However, it can also be used with reinforcing method to strengthen the Bladder.

This point is specific to resolve Damp-Heat from the Bladder and is used for such symptoms as pain and burning on urination and interrupted flow of urine. It clears Heat from the Bladder and is usually combined with some distal points for such symptoms as fever, burning on urination and blood in the urine. To treat these problems, it is often combined with SP-6 Sanyinjiao, SP-9 Yinlingquan or LIV-5 Ligou, depending on the presenting pattern.

Ren-3 also affects the Uterus and menstruation and it can be used in many menstrual irregularities both to consolidate and strengthen the Directing Vessel and to invigorate Blood in the Uterus for such problems as painful periods, retention of placenta, abdominal masses, etc.

Finally, Ren-3 has also a general tonic effect on the Kidneys and the Original Qi: however, I personally use this point for Excess rather than Deficiency patterns and more to invigorate Blood and resolve Dampness than to nourish Blood. For Deficiency patterns, I tend to prefer Ren-4 Guanyuan.

Box 66.4 summarizes the functions of Ren-3.

Box 66.4 Ren-3 – summary of functions

- Resolves Dampness from the Lower Burner (genital itching, pain in the genitals, excessive vaginal discharge, Hernial and Genitourinary Disorders (*shan*))
- Promotes the Bladder function of Qi transformation (retention of urine, frequent urination, dark urine, pain on urination)
- Benefits the Uterus and regulates menstruation (infertility, irregular periods, amenorrhoea, excessive uterine bleeding, abdominal masses in women (*Zheng Jia*), retention of placenta, retention of lochia, persistent lochial discharge)
- Strengthens the Kidneys and nourishes the Essence (lower backache, dizziness, tinnitus, weak knees, deficiency of Original Qi (*Yuan Qi*))

REN-4 GUANYUAN *GATE TO THE ORIGINAL QI*

Location

On the midline of the lower abdomen, 3 *cun* below the umbilicus, 2 *cun* superior to the pubic symphysis.

Nature

Front Collecting (*Mu*) point of the Small Intestine.
Meeting point of Directing Vessel, Spleen, Liver and Kidneys channels.
Meeting point of the Directing and Penetrating Vessels.

Actions

Nourishes Blood and Yin.
Strengthens the Kidneys.
Strengthens the Uterus and regulates menstruation.
Benefits Original Qi (*Yuan Qi*).
Benefits the Bladder.
Subdues rebellious Qi in the Penetrating Vessel.
Regulates the Small Intestine.
Strengthens the Kidney's receiving of Qi.
Roots the Mind (*Shen*) and the Ethereal Soul (*Hun*).

Indications

Lower backache, weak knees, dizziness, tinnitus, feeling of cold in the back, dark face, frequent urination, impotence.
Infertility, cold sensation in the vagina, amenorrhoea, bleeding in pregnancy, persistent lochial discharge.
Retention of urine, dark urine, painful urination, blood in the urine.
Feeling of cold in the lower abdomen, Running Piglet Syndrome, abdominal fullness, umbilical pain.
Diarrhoea, undigested food in the stools, incontinence of stools in the elderly.
Cough, coughing of blood, breathlessness.
Fear, fright, insomnia.

Comments

Ren-4 is an extremely important point. It is one of the most powerful points to tonify Qi and Blood and strengthen the body and mind.

First of all, it can be used to tonify Blood and Yin in any pattern of deficiency of Blood and/or Yin. It nourishes Yin firstly because the Directing Vessel controls all the Yin channels and, secondly, because Ren-4 is the meeting point of the Directing Vessel with the Liver, Spleen and Kidney channels. 'Dark face' in the above indications is a sign of Kidney-Yin deficiency.

Besides this, Ren-4 also strengthens the Yang, when used with direct moxibustion and can be used in this way to rescue the Yang in the acute stages of Wind-stroke due to collapse of Yang. It can therefore be used in any pattern from deficiency of Yang, particularly Kidney-Yang.

Ren-4 is probably the main point to affect the Uterus and menstruation, so that it is used for most menstrual disorders such as amenorrhoea, scanty periods, irregular periods or heavy periods. Ren-4 also has a long history of use for infertility. In menstrual problems, and in gynaecological problems in general, I usually use Ren-4 in combination with the opening points of the Directing Vessel: that is, LU-7 Lieque and KI-6 Zhaohai.

It tonifies the Kidneys and Original Qi (*Yuan Qi*) and is a very powerful point to strengthen the general level of energy and the Kidneys. It is thus an important point to treat chronic diseases or patients with a poor constitution. Ren-4 can tonify both Kidney-Yang (with direct moxibustion) and Kidney-Yin.

Ren-4 point can calm the Mind (*Shen*) and settle the Ethereal Soul (*Hun*) by nourishing Blood and Yin. It can strengthen the Lower Burner in persons who are very anxious, especially if such anxiety derives from Yin deficiency. This point tonifies the Qi of the Lower Burner, thus rooting Qi downwards and subduing the rising of Qi to the head, which happens in severe anxiety. In this way it has a powerful calming effect.

Ren-4 can root the Ethereal Soul and can be used for a vague feeling of fear at night, which is said to be due to the floating of the Ethereal Soul.

Its Kidney tonic action extends also to that of strengthening the Kidney's receiving of Qi so that Ren-4 is an important point to tonify the Kidneys in chronic asthma. In such cases, it is often combined with KI-13 Qixue.

Some of the indications for Ren-4 pertain to the Penetrating Vessel as this vessel goes through this point. Penetrating Vessel indications for Ren-4 are a feeling of cold in the lower abdomen, Running Piglet

Table 66.1 Comparison between Ren-3 Zhongji and Ren-4 Guanyuan

Ren-3	Ren-4
Affects the Bladder	Affects the Uterus
Mostly to reduce in Excess patterns	Mostly to tonify in Deficiency patterns
Mild general tonic effect	Strong general tonic effect
No effect on the Mind	Powerful calming effect on the Mind
No effect on Original Qi	Tonifies Original Qi
Resolves Dampness	Does not resolve Dampness
Clears Heat	Can tonify Yang

Box 66.5 Ren-4 – summary of functions

- Nourishes Blood and Yin
- Strengthens the Kidneys (lower backache, weak knees, dizziness, tinnitus, feeling of cold in the back, dark face, frequent urination, impotence)
- Strengthens the Uterus and regulates menstruation (infertility, cold sensation in the vagina, amenorrhoea, bleeding in pregnancy, persistent lochial discharge)
- Benefits Original Qi
- Benefits the Bladder (retention of urine, dark urine, painful urination, blood in the urine)
- Subdues rebellious Qi in the Penetrating Vessel (feeling of cold in the lower abdomen, Running Piglet Syndrome, abdominal fullness, umbilical pain)
- Regulates the Small Intestine (diarrhoea, undigested food in the stools, incontinence of stools in the elderly)
- Strengthens the Kidney's receiving of Qi (cough, coughing of blood, breathlessness)
- Roots the Mind (*Shen*) and the Ethereal Soul (*Hun*) (fear, fright, insomnia)

Syndrome, abdominal fullness and umbilical pain. When used to subdue rebellious Qi in the Penetrating Vessel, I combine this point with the opening points of the Penetrating Vessel (i.e. SP-4 Gongsun and P-6 Neiguan).

Finally, Ren-4 also affects the Bladder and is used for similar problems as those indicated under Ren-3. However, although both Ren-3 and Ren-4 affect both Bladder and Uterus, I personally use Ren-3 more for Bladder problems and Ren-4 more for the Uterus.

To summarize, Ren-4 is probably the most important tonic point of the body as it tonifies all forms of Qi, as follows:

- Qi
- Yang
- Blood
- Yin
- Essence (*Jing*)
- Original Qi (*Yuan Qi*)
- Kidney-Yin and Kidney-Yang
- The Directing Vessel and the Penetrating Vessel (*Ren Mai* and *Chong Mai*)
- Defensive Qi (*Wei Qi*)
- Nutritive Qi (*Ying Qi*)

It is useful to compare the actions of Ren-3 Zhongji and Ren-4 Guanyuan (Table 66.1).
Box 66.5 summarizes the functions of Ren-4.

REN-5 SHIMEN *STONE DOOR*

Location

On the midline of the lower abdomen, 2 *cun* below the umbilicus, 3 *cun* superior to the pubic symphysis.

Nature

Front Collecting (*Mu*) point of the Triple Burner.

Actions

Opens the Water passages and promotes the transformation and excretion of fluids in the Lower Burner.
Regulates Qi in the Lower Burner.
Regulates the Uterus.
Strengthens Original Qi.

Indications

Difficult urination, retention of urine, painful urination, dark urine, oedema, diarrhoea, genital itching, swelling of scrotum, swelling of vulva, swelling of penis.
Twisting pain in the lower abdomen, Hernial and Genitourinary Disorders (*shan*), umbilical pain, retraction of testicles, Running Piglet Syndrome.

Persistent lochial discharge, abdominal masses, heavy periods, stone-like hardness of lower abdomen.
Exhaustion.

Comments

In order to understand the function of this point, one must recall the role of the Triple Burner in relation to Original Qi (*Yuan Qi*). As was discussed in chapter 3, the Original Qi arises from between the Kidneys and spreads to the five Yin and six Yang organs via the intermediary of the Triple Burner. Ren-5 is the Front Collecting (*Mu*) point of the Triple Burner and rouses the Original Qi to circulate to all the organs and channels. It can therefore be used to tonify Original Qi in persons with Kidney deficiency and a poor constitution.

Another important function of the Triple Burner (and specifically the Lower Burner) is to transform and excrete fluids, and to ensure that the Water passages of the Lower Burner are open. Ren-5 stimulates this function of the Triple Burner, and specifically the Lower Burner: its use is therefore indicated for oedema of the abdomen, urinary retention, difficult urination, diarrhoea or vaginal discharge.

The Triple Burner relies on the smooth movement of Qi and ascending/descending and entering/exiting of Qi in all cavities of the body: from this point of view, its function is similar to that of the Liver in relation to the smooth flow of Liver-Qi. Ren-5 stimulates the free flow of Qi and the entering/exiting of Qi in the lower abdomen: when this function is impaired there may be pain in the lower abdomen, Hernial and Genitourinary Disorders (*shan*), umbilical pain, and Running Piglet Syndrome, for which this point is indicated. It is worth noting the presence of the word '*men*' (i.e. 'door') in the point's name: generally, all points with 'door' in their name promote the entering and exiting of Qi. It is also said that Ren-5 is like a 'door' through which the Qi of the Directing Vessel goes in and out.

Ren-5 is used for menstrual disorders but its action is not so strong and general as that of Ren-4 Guanyuan. With regard to menstrual disorders, the main difference between these two points is that Ren-5 is better when there is Dampness in the Lower Burner or Phlegm in the Uterus.

Box 66.6 summarizes the functions of Ren-5.

Box 66.6 Ren-5 – summary of functions

- Opens the Water passages and promotes the transformation and excretion of fluids in the Lower Burner (difficult urination, retention of urine, painful urination, dark urine, oedema, diarrhoea, genital itching, swelling of scrotum, swelling of vulva, swelling of penis)
- Regulates Qi in the Lower Burner (twisting pain in the lower abdomen, Hernial and Genitourinary Disorders (*shan*), umbilical pain, retraction of testicles, Running Piglet Syndrome)
- Regulates the Uterus (persistent lochial discharge, abdominal masses, heavy periods, stone-like hardness of lower abdomen)
- Strengthens Original Qi (exhaustion)

REN-6 QIHAI *SEA OF QI*

Location

On the midline of the lower abdomen, 1.5 *cun* below the umbilicus, 3.5 *cun* superior to the pubic symphysis.

Nature

Source point for Membranes (*Huang*).

Actions

Tonifies Qi and Yang.
Raises sinking Qi.
Tonifies Original Qi (*Yuan Qi*).
Regulates Qi in the Lower Burner.

Indications

Qi deficiency, Original Qi deficiency, collapse of Yang, tiredness, cold limbs, loose stools, weak voice.
Prolapse of uterus, profuse menstrual bleeding from Qi deficiency, chronic and persistent vaginal discharge, frequent urination, incontinence of urine, a feeling of bearing down.
Hernial and Genitourinary Disorders (*shan*), umbilical pain, abdominal pain.

Comments

Ren-6 is a major point of the body. First of all, it has a powerful tonifying effect on Qi and Yang, especially if used with direct moxibustion. It can be used for extreme physical and mental exhaustion and depression. It tonifies Kidney-Yang and the Original Qi and this point is especially effective when treated with direct moxa

Table 66.2 Comparison between Ren-6 Qihai and Ren-4 Guanyuan

Ren-4	Ren-6
Nourishes Blood and Yin	Tonifies Qi and Yang
No effect in moving Qi	Moves Qi and eliminates stagnation
Affects Uterus	Affects Intestines
Tonifies the Kidneys	Tonifies the Spleen

cones and can therefore be used for such symptoms as chilliness, loose stools, profuse pale urination, physical weakness, mental depression and lack of will-power.

Ren-6 also raises sinking Qi and is used in all cases of sinking of Qi in the lower abdomen causing prolapse of uterus, profuse menstrual bleeding from Qi deficiency, chronic and persistent vaginal discharge, frequent urination, incontinence of urine and a feeling of bearing down.

Besides tonifying Qi, Ren-6 also moves Qi and eliminates stagnation in the Lower Burner. It can therefore be used for lower abdominal pain deriving from stagnation of Qi. Combined with G.B.-34 Yanglingquan, it moves stagnant Qi in the lower abdomen and relieves pain and distension in this area.

It will be useful to compare the actions of Ren-6 Qihai with those of Ren-4 Guanyuan (Table 66.2).

Box 66.7 summarizes the functions of Ren-6.

Box 66.7 Ren-6 – summary of functions

- Tonifies Qi and Yang (Qi deficiency, Original Qi deficiency, collapse of Yang, tiredness, cold limbs, loose stools, weak voice)
- Raises sinking Qi (prolapse of uterus, profuse menstrual bleeding from Qi deficiency, chronic and persistent vaginal discharge, frequent urination, incontinence of urine, a feeling of bearing down)
- Tonifies Original Qi (Yuan Qi)
- Regulates Qi in the Lower Burner (hernial and Genitourinary Disorders (shan), umbilical pain, abdominal pain)

REN-7 YINJIAO *YIN CROSSING*

Location

On the midline of the lower abdomen, 1 *cun* below the umbilicus, 4 *cun* superior to the pubic symphysis.

Nature

Meeting point of Directing Vessel and Kidney channels.
Meeting point of Directing and Penetrating Vessels.

Actions

Regulates the Uterus and menstruation.
Regulates the Penetrating Vessel.
Resolves Dampness from the Lower Burner.
Nourishes Yin.

Indications

Heavy periods, painful periods, irregular periods, amenorrhoea, infertility.
Hardness and pain of the abdomen, Running Piglet Syndrome, chest pain, hypogastric pain, umbilical pain.
Hernial and Genitourinary Disorders (*shan*), retraction of testicles, itching of genitals from Dampness, retention of urine and faeces.
Menopausal hot flushes.

Comments

Ren-7 regulates the Uterus and menstruation in two ways. Firstly, it influences the Uterus and menstruation as a Directing Vessel's point and, from this point of view, it is used for irregular periods, heavy periods and infertility. Secondly, it is a meeting point with the Penetrating Vessel and it is therefore used to invigorate Blood in the Penetrating Vessel to treat painful periods.

Ren-7 resolves Dampness in the Lower Burner and can be used for a wide range of Hernial and Genitourinary Disorders (*shan*) of the Bladder and genitalia such as retraction of testicles, itching of genitals from Dampness and retention of urine.

In my experience, Ren-7 can be used to nourish Kidney-Yin and I use it frequently to do that in menopausal problems. Its name 'Yin Crossing' indicates that it is a concentration of Yin Qi as it is the meeting point of the Directing and Penetrating Vessels and of the Liver and Kidney channel. According to the 'A Study of Acupuncture', at this point the Qi of the Original Yang intersects with Yin.[1] In fact, it is here that the essence of *Tian Gui* (menstrual blood in women and sperm in men) meets Yin Qi; the Water separates upwards and mixes with the essence of the Directing Vessel while Yang Qi descends. The Original Yin infuses into the

Lower *Dan Tian*, and Water and Fire cross: hence the name 'Yin Crossing'.

It is this crossing of Original Yang and Original Yin at this point that explains its dual functions in nourishing Yin and in tonifying Yang to resolve Dampness.

Box 66.8 summarizes the functions of Ren-7.

Box 66.8 Ren-7 – summary of functions

- Regulates the Uterus and menstruation (heavy periods, painful periods, irregular periods, amenorrhoea, infertility)
- Regulates the Penetrating Vessel (hardness and pain of the abdomen, Running Piglet Syndrome, chest pain, hypogastric pain, umbilical pain)
- Resolves Dampness from the Lower Burner (Hernial and Genitourinary Disorders (*shan*), retraction of testicles, itching of genitals from Dampness, retention of urine and faeces)
- Nourishes Yin (menopausal hot flushes)

REN-8 SHENQUE *SPIRIT PALACE*

Location

In the centre of the umbilicus.

Nature

None.

Actions

Rescues Yang.
Strengthens the Spleen.
Tonifies Original Qi (*Yuan Qi*).

Indications

Loss of consciousness from Wind-stroke, collapse of Yang.
Cold in the abdomen, diarrhoea, borborygmi, diarrhoea in the elderly and children, prolapse of rectum.
Infertility.

Comments

Ren-8 strongly tonifies Yang. It is used to rescue Yang in the acute stage of Wind-stroke of the flaccid type characterized by collapse of Yang.

In other situations it can be used for severe deficiency of Kidney-Yang and of the Original Qi with internal Cold and extreme weakness. This point is not needled but used with indirect moxibustion with moxa cones after filling the navel with salt.

Ren-8 also strengthens Spleen-Yang and is particularly used for chronic diarrhoea from Spleen-Yang deficiency.

I have translated the word *Shen* as 'Spirit' rather than 'Mind' as, in this case, *Shen* refers not to the *shen* of the Heart (which I translate as 'Mind') but to the sum total of Mind (*Shen*), Ethereal Soul (*Hun*), Corporeal Soul (*Po*), Intellect (*Yi*) and Will-power (*Zhi*). This is confirmed by the fact that there is an extra point 1 *cun* from Ren-8 that is called *Hun She*: that is, 'Abode of the Ethereal Soul'.

It is worth exploring the meaning of this point's name as it sheds lights on its nature and functions. The 'Great Dictionary of Chinese Acupuncture' reports an explanation of the meaning of this point from an old text: '*Ren-8 is the Abode of the Spirit [Shen She]. Heaven is above, Earth is below, Person is in the Middle; on both sides there is KI-13 Qixue and KI-16 Huangshu. Above there is Ren-9 Shuifen and Ren-10 Xiawan; below there is Ren-4 Guanyuan [here called Bao Men] and Ren-3 Zhongji. The umbilicus is in the centre like an opening of a door through which the Spirit communicates with the Pre-Heaven Essence. When mother and father unite, a fetus is formed, the umbilical cord is formed linking the fetus to the mother's Gate of Life [Ming Men] like a lotus stem. The Pre-Heaven Essence generates Water and the Kidneys: like an unopened lotus flower, the five Elements come into being and the mother's Qi is transferred. In 10 months to the fetus is fully formed, the Spirit infuses through the centre of the umbilicus and forms a new human being.*'[2]

According to this image, Ren-8 is at the centre of an energetic vortex with three levels: Heaven above (Ren-9 and Ren-10), Earth below (Ren-4 and Ren-7) and Person in the centre (Ren-8), with KI-13 and KI-16 on either side like watchtowers guarding the entrance to the Imperial Palace (Fig. 66.3). I translated the word *que* in this point's name as 'Palace' (rather than 'gate' or 'gateway' as most authors do) to indicate the energetic importance of this point: i.e. like an Imperial Palace that is the residence of the Spirit) (Fig. 66.4).

The word *que* also implies the idea of an open space, something empty: this is the space through which the fetus was connected to the mother's Gate of Life (*Ming Men*), the space through which the Spirit entered the fetus and was nourished by the mother (Fig. 66.5). Because of this association, Ren-8 is the point that most affects out Pre-Heaven Qi. However, this 'space' is not like a 'gate' (*guan*) or 'door' (*men*) through which Qi moves in and out and this point therefore does not

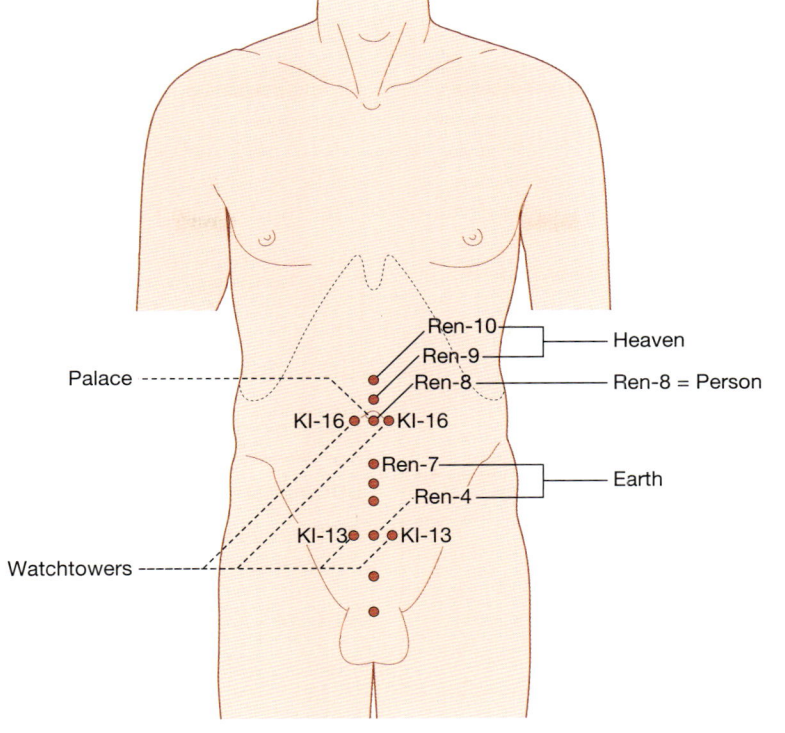

Figure 66.3 Heaven, Earth and Person in Ren-8 Shenque

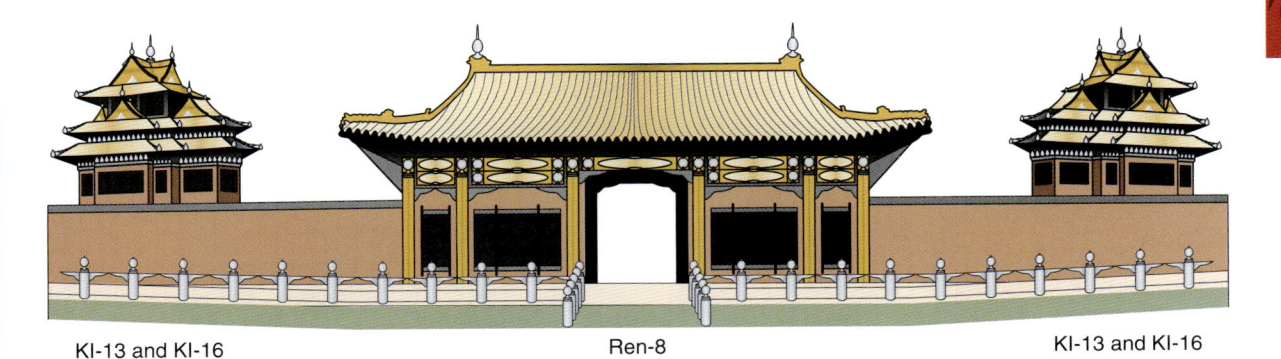

Figure 66.4 KI-13 and KI-16 as watchtowers for Ren-8, imperial gate

Fetus connected to mother's *Ming Men* through umbilical cord

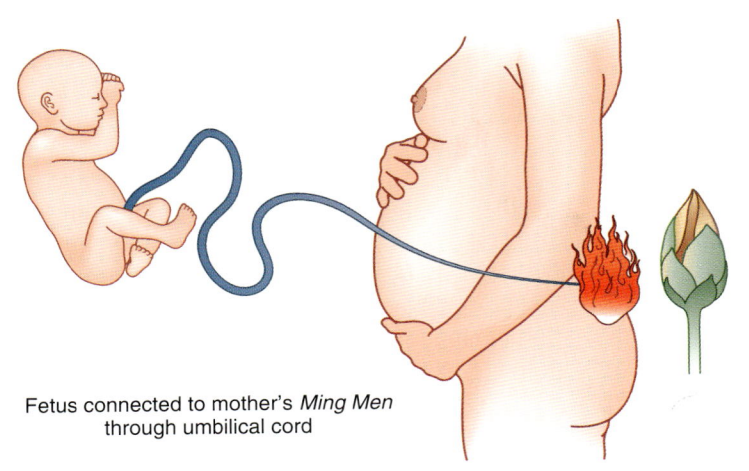

Figure 66.5 Umbilical cord connection with mother's *Ming Men*

have the function that most points with *guan* or *men* in their name have, i.e. that of promoting the movement and entering/exiting of Qi: this 'space' is rather like the entrance to a palace, a 'space' that is the residence of the Spirit, and that is why I translate the word *que* in this point's name as 'palace'.

The connection between the fetus and the mother through Ren-8 is also shown by one of the many alternative names for this point, *Ming Di*, which means 'Life's Stem', the 'stem' being the umbilical cord and 'Life' referring to the mother's Gate of Life (*Ming Men*).

Box 66.9 summarizes the functions of Ren-8.

Box 66.9 Ren-8 – summary of functions

- Rescues Yang (loss of consciousness from Wind-stroke, Collapse of Yang)
- Strengthens the Spleen (cold in the abdomen, diarrhoea, borborygmi, diarrhoea in the elderly and children, prolapse of rectum)
- Tonifies Original Qi (infertility)

REN-9 SHUIFEN *WATER SEPARATION*

Location

On the midline of the abdomen, 1 *cun* above the umbilicus, 7 *cun* below the sternocostal angle.

Nature

None.

Actions

Opens the Water passages and promotes the transformation of fluids.

Indications

Oedema.

Comments

Ren-9 is a very important point to promote the transportation, transformation and excretion of fluids in all parts of the body. It is used whenever there is a Water pathology in the form of Dampness, Phlegm or oedema. In particular, it promotes the separation of clear from turbid fluids in the Small Intestine and their distribution to the Bladder and Large Intestine, respectively. Ren-9 is especially indicated for ascites (abdominal oedema). A particular combination for promoting the transformation and transportation of fluids in the Middle Burner is Ren-9 with Ren-11 Jianli and ST-22 Guanmen.

Its name is a clear reference to its action of promoting the separation of clear from turbid fluids.

Box 66.10 summarizes the functions of Ren-9.

Box 66.10 Ren-9 – summary of functions

- Opens the Water passages and promotes the transformation of fluids (oedema)

REN-10 XIAWAN *LOWER EPIGASTRIUM*

Location

On the midline of the abdomen, 2 *cun* above the umbilicus, 6 *cun* below the sternocostal angle.

Nature

Meeting of Directing Vessel and Spleen channels.

Actions

Promotes the descending of Stomach-Qi.
Resolves stagnation of food.

Indications

Abdominal and epigastric fullness, abdominal hardness, epigastric pain, nausea, undigested food in the stools.

Comments

Ren-10 is a useful point that promotes the descending of Stomach-Qi. By promoting the descending of Stomach-Qi it is used for retention of food in the Stomach, with such symptoms as abdominal distension, feeling of fullness after eating and sour regurgitation.

It also promotes the passage of food from the Stomach to the Intestines and removes obstructions.

This is one of three points that are in control of the three parts of the epigastrium. If one divides the epigastric area in three equal parts, Ren-13 Shangwan controls the upper part, Ren-12 Zhongwan the middle part, and Ren-10 Xiawan the lower part. From a Western anatomical point of view one can say that Ren-13 controls the *fundus* (upper part) of the stomach and oesophagus, Ren-12 the *body* (middle part) of the stomach, and Ren-10 the *pylorus* (lower part) of the stomach and the duodenum (Fig. 66.6).

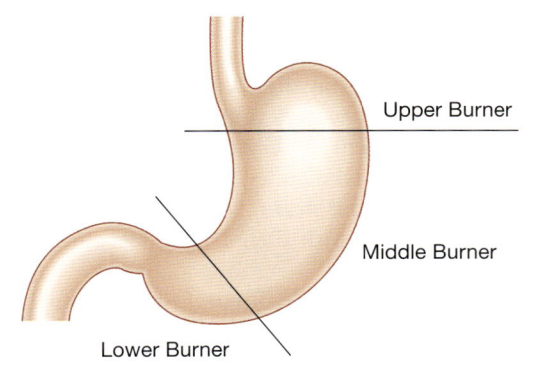

Figure 66.6 Threefold division of the Stomach and Directing Vessel's points

Each of these three points can be used to affect the relevant part of the stomach with their related disorders. Thus Ren-10 is effective in stimulating the descending of Stomach-Qi: that is, in promoting the movement of food down the pylorus and duodenum. Ren-12 affects the stomach digestion itself, and Ren-13 affects the oesophagus and stops hiccups, nausea and belching by subduing rebellious Stomach-Qi.

Box 66.11 summarizes the functions of Ren-10.

Box 66.11 Ren-10 – summary of functions

- Promotes the descending of Stomach-Qi
- Resolves stagnation of food (abdominal and epigastric fullness, abdominal hardness, epigastric pain, nausea, undigested food in the stools)

REN-11 JIANLI *BUILDING MILE*

Location
On the midline of the abdomen, 3 *cun* above the umbilicus, 5 *cun* below the sternocostal angle.

Nature
None.

Actions
Promotes the Stomach's rotting and ripening of food.
Promotes the descending of Stomach-Qi.

Indications
Epigastric and abdominal distension, abdominal pain, vomiting.

Comments
Ren-11 is widely used for Stomach problems to promote digestion and stimulate the descending of Stomach-Qi. It is therefore used for a feeling of fullness and distension in the epigastrium, nausea, vomiting and epigastric pain. It is better for Excess patterns.

Box 66.12 summarizes the functions of Ren-11.

Box 66.12 Ren-11 – summary of functions

- Promotes the Stomach's rotting and ripening of food (epigastric and abdominal distension, abdominal pain, vomiting)
- Promotes the descending of Stomach-Qi

REN-12 ZHONGWAN *MIDDLE OF EPIGASTRIUM*

Location
On the midline of the abdomen, 4 *cun* above the umbilicus, 4 *cun* below the sternocostal angle.

Nature
Front Collecting (*Mu*) point of the Stomach.
Gathering (*Hui*) point for the Yang organs.
Front Collecting (*Mu*) point of the Middle Burner.
Meeting point of Directing Vessel, Small Intestine, Triple Burner and Stomach channels.

Actions
Tonifies Stomach and Spleen.
Resolves Dampness and Phlegm.
Regulates Stomach-Qi.
Calms the Mind.

Indications
Tiredness, loose stools, poor appetite, weak limbs, desire to lie down.
Abdominal fullness, a sticky taste, a feeling of heaviness, nausea.
All diseases of Stomach and Spleen, epigastric pain, poor digestion, easily full, sour regurgitation, nausea, vomiting, epigastric distension.
Worry, anxiety, pensiveness.

Comments
Ren-12 is a major point for many Stomach problems. Although its indications clearly show that it can be

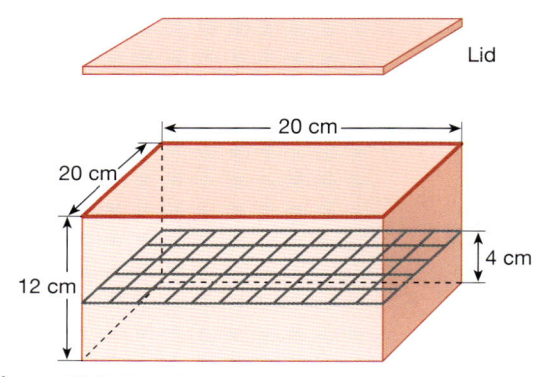

Figure 66.7 Moxa box

used to harmonize the Stomach and promote the descending of Stomach-Qi in Full conditions, I personally use it primarily to tonify Stomach- and Spleen-Qi in Deficiency patterns (as opposed to Ren-11 Jianli and Ren-13 Shangwan, which are better for Excess patterns).

Firstly, it tonifies Stomach- and Spleen-Qi, especially if combined with ST-36 Zusanli. It has a gentle action and is not a strong tonifying point. It can be used in any Deficiency pattern of Stomach and Spleen, with such symptoms and signs as lack of appetite, tiredness and dull epigastric pain relieved by eating.

It is the best point to use, particularly with moxa, for Empty-Cold patterns of the Stomach and Spleen. This could be used directly on the point with moxa cones, or the point can be heated with a moxa stick, or a 'moxa box' can be applied on the area around the point. The moxa box is a wooden box without bottom with a metal griddle about a third of the way down from the upper edge. Loose moxa is placed on the metal griddle and lit and a loose lid is placed over the box. This method of moxibustion is excellent for Empty-Cold conditions of Stomach and Spleen (Fig. 66.7).

Ren-12 can also nourish Stomach- and Spleen-Yin and I use this point whenever the tongue lacks a coating (which indicates a deficiency of Stomach-Yin) or when the tongue has a Stomach crack, even in the absence of any digestive symptoms. When I use it to nourish Stomach-Yin, I combine Ren-12 with ST-36 Zusanli and SP-6 Sanyinjiao.

Ren-12 has a general tonifying effect also because it is the Gathering (*Hui*) point of all the Yang organs.

Another important use of Ren-12 is to resolve Dampness and Phlegm. It does so by tonifying the Spleen's function of transportation and transformation of fluids. It is very widely used in any pattern involving Dampness or Phlegm in any part of the body.

It is interesting that the traditional indications for this point include 'worry, anxiety and pensiveness'. I personally find Ren-12 very effective in calming the Mind in patients who suffer from digestive problems caused by emotional strain. For this action, I usually combine Ren-12 with Ren-15 Jiuwei and Du-24 Shenting.

Finally, Ren-12 also subdues rebellious Stomach-Qi (i.e. Stomach-Qi ascending instead of descending), but I personally use Ren-13 Shangwan for this function.

Box 66.13 summarizes the functions of Ren-12.

Box 66.13 Ren-12 – summary of functions

- Tonifies Stomach and Spleen (tiredness, loose stools, poor appetite, weak limbs, desire to lie down)
- Resolves Dampness and Phlegm (abdominal fullness, a sticky taste, a feeling of heaviness, nausea)
- Regulates Stomach-Qi (all diseases of Stomach and Spleen, epigastric pain, poor digestion, easily full, nausea, sour regurgitation, nausea, vomiting, epigastric distension)
- Calms the Mind (worry, anxiety, pensiveness)

REN-13 SHANGWAN *UPPER EPIGASTRIUM*

Location

On the midline of the abdomen, 5 *cun* above the umbilicus, 3 *cun* below the sternocostal angle.

Nature

Meeting point of the Directing Vessel, Stomach and Small Intestine channels.

Actions

Subdues rebellious Stomach-Qi.

Indications

Nausea, vomiting, vomiting of blood, difficulty in swallowing, sour regurgitation, epigastric distension and fullness.

Comments

Ren-13 is the best point to subdue rebellious Stomach-Qi, causing such symptoms as hiccup, belching, nausea, vomiting and a feeling of fullness in the upper epigastrium. It is used mostly in Excess patterns of the Stomach.

It is useful to compare and contrast the actions of Ren-13 and Ren-10 Xiawan. The former, pertaining to the upper part of the Stomach, 'subdues rebellious Stomach-Qi' while the latter, pertaining to the lower part of the Stomach, 'promotes the descending of Stomach-Qi': although similar, these two actions are not exactly the same.

Ren-13 actively subdues rebellious Stomach-Qi when this causes strong nausea, vomiting, belching and hiccups. When Stomach-Qi fails to descend, it will also cause some nausea but this will be slight and probably it will be confined to nausea without vomiting. When Stomach-Qi fails to descend, moreover, there will be symptoms in the lower abdomen as Stomach-Qi is not going down to the Intestines effectively: Ren-10 is the point to promote the descending of Stomach-Qi in this context. By contrast, when Stomach-Qi rebels upwards, there will be symptoms only in the Upper Burner (i.e. hiccups, reflux, belching, nausea and vomiting): Ren-13 is the point to subdue rebellious Stomach-Qi.

I often use Ren-13 for morning sickness in pregnancy with ST-36 Zusanli and P-6 Neiguan.

Box 66.14 summarizes the functions of Ren-13.

Box 66.14 Ren-13 – summary of functions

- Subdues rebellious Stomach-Qi (nausea, vomiting, vomiting of blood, difficulty in swallowing, sour regurgitation, epigastric distension and fullness)
- Used for morning sickness with P-6 Neiguan and ST-36 Zusanli

Clinical note

Ren-13 Shangwan subdues rebellious Stomach-Qi while Ren-10 Xiawan promotes the descending of Stomach-Qi. Please note that these two actions are not the same. 'Subduing rebellious Stomach-Qi' means that it is used in Full conditions with rebellious Stomach-Qi (nausea, vomiting, acid reflux, belching). 'Promoting the descending of Stomach-Qi' means that it is used in Empty conditions when Stomach-Qi is not descending because it is Empty

REN-14 JUQUE GREAT PALACE

Location

On the midline of the abdomen, 6 *cun* above the umbilicus, 2 *cun* below the sternocostal angle.

Nature

Front Collecting (*Mu*) point of the Heart.

Actions

Regulates Heart-Qi.
Calms the Mind and opens the Mind's orifices.
Subdues rebellious Stomach-Qi.

Indications

Heart pain, chest pain, phlegm in the chest, fullness of the chest.
Anxiety, insomnia, manic depression, shouting, anger, disorientation, agitation.
Epigastric distension, difficulty in swallowing, nausea, vomiting, sour regurgitation.

Comments

Ren-14 acts on the Stomach and on the Heart. It subdues rebellious Stomach-Qi in the same way as Ren-13 Shangwan, and it is ideally indicated for digestive problems with rebellious Stomach-Qi of an emotional origin, as it treats both Stomach and Heart. However, there is an important difference between these two points. Nausea and vomiting are not always due to rebellious Stomach-Qi as they may also be due to rebellious Heart-Qi: this happens especially in cases in which nausea and vomiting occur against a background of emotional stress. Ren-14 is particularly indicated for nausea and vomiting from rebellious Heart-Qi.

Ren-14 calms the Mind and is frequently used for the pattern of Phlegm-Heat misting the Heart and leading to mental symptoms, or for the pattern of Heart-Fire leading to insomnia, agitation and anxiety. However, this does not mean that Ren-14 cannot be used for mental–emotional symptoms occurring against a background of Heart deficiency. However, in this latter case, I personally tend to use more Ren-15 Jiuwei.

The character *que* in this point's name is the same as that in *Shen Que* for Ren-8: for this reason, I have translated it as 'Palace' in accordance with 'Spirit Palace' of Ren-8. There is therefore a correspondence between these two points. The Spirit (*Shen*) relies on the Essence of the Kidneys as its foundation (see ch. 3). Therefore, Ren-8 affects the Spirit through the Essence and Ren-14 through the Mind (*Shen*) of the Heart (Fig. 66.8).

Box 66.15 summarizes the functions of Ren-14.

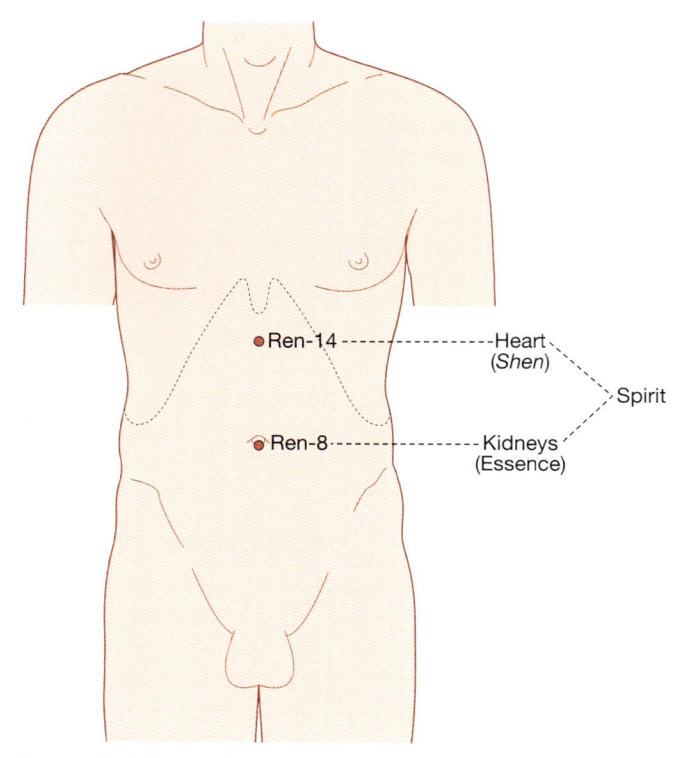

Figure 66.8 Relationship between Ren-14 and Ren-8

Box 66.15 Ren-14 – summary of functions

- Regulates Heart-Qi (heart pain, chest pain, phlegm in the chest, fullness of the chest)
- Calms the Mind and opens the Mind's orifices (anxiety, insomnia, manic depression, shouting, anger, disorientation, agitation)
- Subdues rebellious Stomach-Qi (epigastric distension, difficulty in swallowing, nausea, vomiting, sour regurgitation)

REN-15 JIUWEI *DOVE TAIL*

Location

On the midline of the abdomen, 7 *cun* above the umbilicus, 1 *cun* below the sternocostal angle.

Nature

Connecting (*Luo*) point of the Directing Vessel.
Source (*Yuan*) point of the five Yin organs (ch. 1 of the 'Spiritual Axis').
Source (*Yuan*) of Fat Tissue (*Gao*) (ch. 1 of the 'Spiritual Axis').

Actions

Calms the Mind and opens the Mind's orifices.
Opens the chest and promotes the descending of Qi.

Indications

Manic depression, palpitations, anxiety, insomnia. Fullness and pain of the chest, wheezing, breathlessness, a feeling of oppression of the chest, sighing, cough.

Comments

Ren-15 is a very important and powerful point to calm the Mind. According to chapter 1 of the 'Spiritual Axis', it is the source point of all the Yin organs, which means that it affects the Original Qi (*Yuan Qi*) of all Yin organs.[3]

This point nourishes all Yin organs and it calms the Mind, particularly in Deficiency of Yin and/or Blood. It has a very powerful calming action in severe anxiety, worry, emotional upsets, fears or obsessions. Although its indications show that it can be used to open the Mind's orifices in serious mental conditions from a

Full condition, I personally use this point in mental–emotional states occurring against a background of deficiency of Blood or Yin.

Ren-15 has an important influence on the chest: it opens the chest and promotes the descending of Qi. A useful aspect of this action is that Ren-15 promotes the descending of both Lung-Qi (cough, wheezing, breathlessness) and Heart-Qi (anxiety, sighing, feeling of oppression of the chest).

The Connecting (*Luo*) channel of the Directing Vessel starts at this point, which controls it. From this point, the Connecting Vessel branches out in numerous small branches fanning out over the abdomen. When the Connecting Vessel is empty there is itching of the abdomen; when it is in Excess there is pain of the abdomen. Ren-15 can be used for Empty or Full conditions of the Connecting channel.

This point is located at the tip of the xiphoid process, which is commonly known as 'dove-tail' in China: hence the name of the point.

Box 66.16 summarizes the functions of Ren-15.

Box 66.16 Ren-15 – summary of functions

- Calms the Mind and opens the Mind's orifices (manic depression, palpitations, anxiety, insomnia)
- Opens the chest and promotes the descending of Qi (fullness and pain of the chest, wheezing, breathlessness, a feeling of oppression of the chest, sighing, cough)

REN-17 SHANZHONG (OR TANZHONG) *MIDDLE OF CHEST*

Location

On the midline of the sternum, level with the junction of the fourth intercostal space and the sternum.

Nature

Front Collecting (*Mu*) point of the Pericardium.
Front Collecting (*Mu*) point of the Upper Burner.
Gathering (*Hui*) point for Qi.
Point of the Sea of Qi.
Meeting point of the Directing Vessel, Spleen, Kidney, Small Intestine and Triple Burner channels.

Actions

Tonifies Qi and strengthens the Gathering Qi (*Zong Qi*).
Opens the chest, regulates Qi and promotes the descending of Qi.
Benefits the breasts and promotes lactation.

Indications

Weak voice, tiredness, propensity to catching colds, spontaneous sweating.
Chest pain, wheezing, breathlessness, cough, fullness and oppression of the chest.
Insufficient lactation, breast abscess, breast distension.

Comments

Ren-17 is a very important point to tonify Qi: it is both the Gathering (*Hui*) point for Qi and a point of the Sea of Qi. It tonifies the Qi of the chest and the Gathering Qi (*Zong Qi*), which is related to Heart and Lungs. Thus, this point is used to tonify Qi, but only in relation to Lung-Qi not so much Spleen- or Kidney-Qi. If the deficiency of Qi is due to weakness of the Stomach or Spleen, this point alone would not be enough to tonify Qi, but other points would have to be used, such as ST-36 Zusanli, Ren-12 Zhongwan and Ren-6 Qihai.

Besides tonifying Qi, it also moves Qi and eliminates stagnation of Qi in the chest. It is therefore used in any condition of stagnation of Qi in the chest, with such symptoms as a feeling of constriction, tightness, oppression or pain in the chest.

Ren-17 dispels fullness from the chest, promotes the descending of Lung-Qi and helps breathing. It is therefore used for breathlessness from any origin, whether it is from Lung-Qi or Heart-Qi deficiency or from obstruction of the chest by Phlegm.

Finally, it benefits the breasts and can be used to treat insufficient lactation both from deficiency of Qi and Blood and from Qi stagnation. When used for the breasts, Ren-17 is inserted towards the affected breast. When used for Qi, it is inserted horizontally downwards.

Box 66.17 summarizes the functions of Ren-17.

Box 66.17 Ren-17 – summary of functions

- Tonifies Qi and strengthens the Gathering Qi (*Zong Qi*) (weak voice, tiredness, propensity to catching colds, spontaneous sweating)
- Opens the chest, regulates Qi and promotes the descending of Qi (chest pain, wheezing, breathlessness, cough, fullness and oppression of the chest)
- Benefits the breasts and promotes lactation (insufficient lactation, breast abscess, breast distension)

REN-22 TIANTU *HEAVEN PROJECTION*

Location

On the midline, in the centre of the suprasternal fossa, 0.5 *cun* above the suprasternal notch.

Nature

Point of the Yin Linking Vessel (*Yin Wei Mai*).
Window of Heaven point.

Actions

Stimulates the descending of Lung-Qi.
Resolves Phlegm.
Benefits the throat and voice.

Indications

Cough, wheezing, breathlessness, rattling sound in the throat.
Phlegm in the throat.
Feeling of obstruction in the throat, throat ulcers, swelling of throat, dry throat, hoarse voice, sudden loss of voice, goitre.

Comments

Ren-22 stimulates the descending of Lung-Qi and is widely used in both acute and chronic cough and asthma.

It resolves Phlegm in the throat and Lungs and promotes the expelling of sputum. It is used in acute situations such as acute bronchitis with profuse sputum, or chronic retention of Phlegm in the throat.

Ren-22 is an important local point for problems of the throat and voice.

Box 66.18 summarizes the functions of Ren-22.

Box 66.18 Ren-22 – summary of functions

- Stimulates the descending of Lung-Qi (cough, wheezing, breathlessness, rattling sound in the throat)
- Resolves Phlegm (phlegm in the throat)
- Benefits the throat and voice (feeling of obstruction in the throat, throat ulcers, swelling of throat, dry throat, hoarse voice, sudden loss of voice, goitre)

REN-23 LIANQUAN *CORNER SPRING*

Location

On the anterior midline of the neck, in the depression above the hyoid bone.

Nature

Point of Yin Linking Vessel (*Yin Wei Mai*).

Actions

Benefits the tongue and speech.
Subdues rebellious Qi.

Indications

Swelling below the tongue, difficulty in speaking, sudden loss of voice, aphasia after Wind-stroke, contraction of the root of the tongue, protrusion of tongue, dry throat, mouth ulcers, tongue ulcers.
Cough, wheezing, breathlessness, vomiting of foamy saliva.

Comments

Ren-23 is mostly used for aphasia or slurred speech following Wind-stroke. It affects the tongue directly and can be used in conjunction with HE-5 Tongli for speech difficulties or aphasia. It is also used for local throat problems such as nodules on the vocal cords.

Box 66.19 summarizes the functions of Ren-23.

Box 66.19 Ren-23 – summary of functions

- Benefits the tongue and speech (swelling below the tongue, difficulty in speaking, sudden loss of voice, aphasia after Wind-stroke, contraction of the root of the tongue, protrusion of tongue, dry throat, mouth ulcers, tongue ulcers)
- Subdues rebellious Qi (cough, wheezing, breathlessness, vomiting of foamy saliva)

REN-24 CHENGJIANG *SALIVA RECEIVER*

Location

On the midline, in the centre of the mentolabial groove.

Nature

Meeting point of the Directing Vessel, Governing Vessel, Large Intestine and Stomach channels.
One of Sun Si Miao's Ghost points.

Actions

Extinguishes interior Wind.
Removes obstructions from the channel in the face.

Mind
Ren-1

Lungs
Ren-17
Ren-22

Heart
Ren-14
Ren-15

Stomach
Ren-12
Ren-22

Intestines
Ren-10
Ren-11

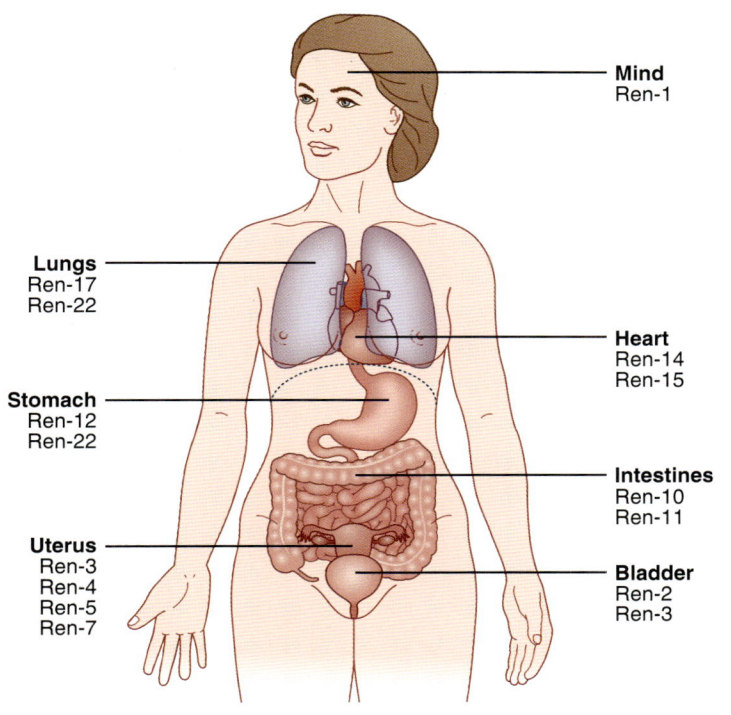

Uterus
Ren-3
Ren-4
Ren-5
Ren-7

Bladder
Ren-2
Ren-3

Figure 66.9 Target areas of Directing Vessel points

Indications

Hemiplegia, deviation of mouth, lockjaw, epilepsy, tetany.
Pain and numbness of the face, swelling of face, toothache, gum pain, sudden loss of voice, purple lips.

Comments

Ren-24 is mostly used as a local point for Wind invading the face and causing facial paralysis. It is used for paralysis of the mouth.

Its indications clearly reflect the pathway of the Directing Vessel on the face circling around the mouth and reaching the eyes.

Figure 66.9 illustrates the target areas of the Directing Vessel points.

Box 66.20 summarizes the functions of Ren-24.

Box 66.20 Ren-24 – summary of functions

- Extinguishes interior Wind (hemiplegia, deviation of mouth, lockjaw, epilepsy, tetany)
- Removes obstructions from the channel in the face (pain and numbness of the face, swelling of face, toothache, gum pain, sudden loss of voice, purple lips)

END NOTES

1. Yang Jia San 1989 A Study of Acupuncture (*Zhen Jiu Xue* 针灸学), Beijing Science Publishing House, Beijing, p. 402.
2. Yang Jia San 1988 Great Dictionary of Chinese Acupuncture (*Zhong Guo Zhen Jiu Da Ci Dian* 中国针灸大辞典), Beijing Sports College Publishing House, Beijing, p. 739.
3. 1981 Spiritual Axis (*Ling Shu Jing* 灵枢经), People's Health Publishing House, Beijing, first published c.100 BC, p. 3.

SECTION 2 PART 7

Governing Vessel 67

Main channel pathway

The Governing Vessel originates from the uterus (or deep inside the lower abdomen in men) and goes to the perineum, where it emerges. It then ascends on the midline all the way up the back and neck to Du-16 Fengfu, from where it enters the brain. It then ascends to the vertex and down the front of the face to the upper lip (Fig. 67.1).

Connecting channel pathway

After separating from the point Du-1 Changqiang, the Connecting channel flows upwards along both sides of the spine to the occiput, from where it scatters over the top of the head. At the scapulae, a branch joins the Bladder channel and the upper spine (Fig. 67.2).

Box 67.1 gives an overview of the Governing Vessel points.

Box 67.1 Overview of Governing Vessel points
- Affect genitals, back, head, brain
- Important mental effect
- Tonify the Kidneys
- Extinguish internal Wind

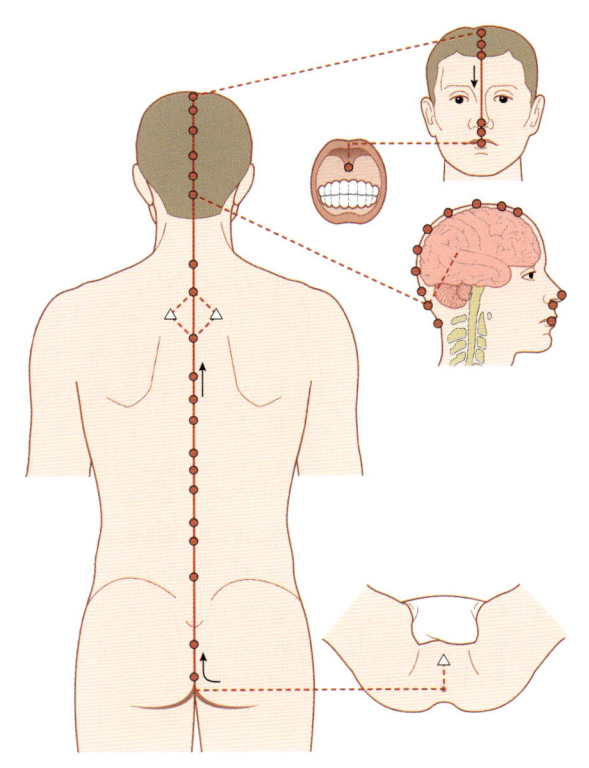

Figure 67.1 Governing Vessel

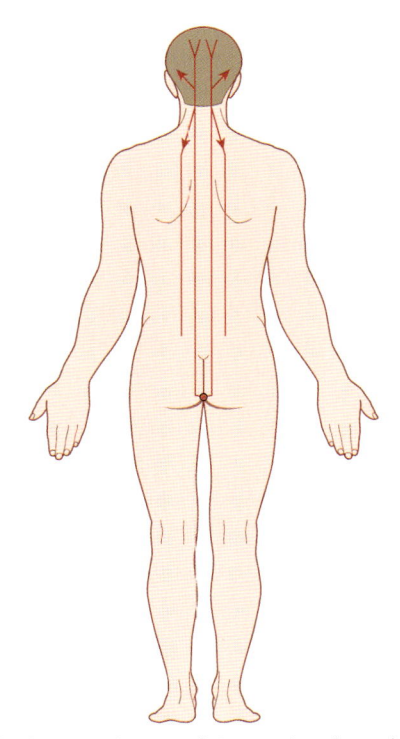

Figure 67.2 Governing Vessel Connecting channel

DU-1 CHANGQIANG *LONG STRENGTH*

Location
Below the tip of the coccyx, at the midpoint between the tip of the coccyx and the anus.

Nature
Connecting (*Luo*) point of the Governing Vessel.

Actions
Regulates Governing and Directing Vessels.
Resolves Dampness.
Regulates the two lower orifices.
Calms the Mind and opens the Mind's orifices.
Extinguishes interior Wind.

Indications
Painful urination, difficult urination, retention of urine, dark urine, haemorrhoids, difficult defecation, diarrhoea, prolapse of rectum.
Manic depression.
Opisthotonos, tetany, epilepsy, tremor of head.

Comments
Du-1 is the beginning and Connecting point of the Governing Vessel. Being the Connecting point, it connects with the Directing Vessel. It can therefore be used to eliminate obstructions from both the Directing and the Governing Vessel. For this reason, it affects both lower orifices.

Du-1 is very much used as a local point for prolapse of the anus. It also resolves Damp-Heat in the anus and is therefore used for haemorrhoids.

Being at the lowermost end of the Governing Vessel, Du-1 can be used to affect the top part (i.e. the brain). It is therefore used to calm the Mind and open the Mind's orifices in mental diseases characterized by agitation and hypomania.

Box 67.2 summarizes the functions of Du-1.

Box 67.2 Du-1 – summary of functions

- Regulates Governing and Directing Vessels
- Resolves Dampness
- Regulates the two lower orifices (painful urination, difficult urination, retention of urine, dark urine, haemorrhoids, difficult defecation, diarrhoea, prolapse of rectum)
- Calms the Mind and opens the Mind's orifices (manic depression)
- Extinguishes interior Wind (opisthotonos, tetany, epilepsy, tremor of head)

DU-2 YAOSHU *TRANSPORTING POINT OF LOWER BACK*

Location
On the sacrum, on the posterior median line in the hiatus of the sacrum.

Nature
None.

Actions
Extinguishes interior Wind.
Strengthens the lower back.

Indications
Epilepsy.
Pain in the sacrum, lower backache, stiffness of the lower back.

Comments
This is an important point to eliminate interior Wind and its manifestations, particularly spasms and convulsions. For this reason, this is a major point to use to treat epilepsy. When used for epilepsy, it should be needled obliquely upwards, trying to obtain the needling sensation to travel upwards as far as possible.

Besides this, it can be used as a local point in chronic sacral backache from Kidney-Yang deficiency.

Box 67.3 summarizes the functions of Du-2.

Box 67.3 Du-2 – summary of functions

- Extinguishes interior Wind (epilepsy)
- Strengthens the lower back (pain in the sacrum, lower backache, stiffness of the lower back

---

DU-3 YAOYANGGUAN *LUMBAR YANG GATE*

Location
On the lumbar region, on the posterior median line, in the depression below the spinous process of L-4.

Nature
None.

> **Box 67.4 Du-3 – summary of functions**
> - Strengthens the lower back and legs (lower backache, sciatica, stiffness of lumbar region)
> - Tonifies Yang (impotence, white leukorrhoea)

Actions
Strengthens the lower back and legs.
Tonifies Yang.

Indications
Lower backache, sciatica, stiffness of lumbar region.
Impotence, white leukorrhoea.

Comments
Du-3 is very frequently used as a local point in lower backache, particularly if due to Kidney-Yang deficiency. It is also especially indicated when the backache radiates to the legs. Besides strengthening the lower back by tonifying Kidney-Yang, it also strengthens the legs, and is an important point to use for weakness of the legs in Atrophy Syndrome.

Box 67.4 summarizes the functions of Du-3.

DU-4 MINGMEN *GATE OF LIFE*

Location
On the lumbar region, on the posterior median line, in the depression below the spinous process of L-2.

Nature
None.

Actions
Tonifies Kidney-Yang and warms the Gate of Life (*Ming Men*).
Tonifies the Original Qi (*Yuan Qi*).
Expels Cold.
Strengthens the Governing Vessel.
Strengthens the lower back.
Benefits Essence (*Jing*).
Clears the Mind (*Shen*).
Clears Heat.
Extinguishes interior Wind.

Indications
Backache, dizziness, tinnitus, cold knees, feeling of cold in the lower back, frequent pale urination, tiredness.
Chilliness, cold knees and back, cold feet, pain from Cold.
Lower backache from Kidney deficiency.
Seminal emissions.
Depression, lack of will-power, mental confusion.
Heat in the body.
Tremor of head, opisthotonos, epilepsy.

Comments
The Fire of the Gate of Life (*Ming Men*) is closely linked to the Pre-Heaven Essence. Situated in between the Kidneys, the Fire of the Gate of Life is the physiological Fire of the body which provides the warmth that is essential for all physiological processes of the body and for all the Internal Organs. The Fire of the Gate of Life is already present from birth and, indeed, from conception. The Pre-Heaven Essence is also present from conception and birth but it then 'matures' into the Kidney-Essence (with the help of the warmth of the Fire of the Gate of Life) at puberty when it generates menstrual blood and eggs in women and sperm in men.

Thus, the Fire of the Gate of Life can be said to represent the Yang aspect of the Pre-Heaven Essence, while the Pre-Heaven Essence proper (transforming into Kidney-Essence at puberty) represents the Yin aspect (see Fig. 3.3 in ch. 3). Du-4's alternative name, '*Jing Gong*', which is 'Palace of Essence (*Jing*)', clearly shows the connection of the Gate of Life with the Essence (i.e. it is the Yang aspect of the Essence).

The Fire of the Gate of Life accumulates at the point Du-4 Mingmen on the spine at conception, while the Pre-Heaven Essence concentrates at the point Ren-4 Guanyuan, also at conception (see Fig. 3.4 in ch. 3). This correlates with the Uterus (where menstrual blood is stored) in women and with the Room of Sperm in men.[1] Chapter 36 of the 'Classic of Difficulties' says: '*The Gate of Life is the residence of the Mind and Essence and it is connected to the Original Qi [Yuan Qi]: in men it houses the Sperm; in women the Uterus.*'[2]

Du-4 is the most powerful point to strengthen Kidney-Yang and all the Yang energies in general, especially if used with moxa. It tonifies and warms the Fire of the Gate of Life. It is therefore used for Kidney-Yang deficiency with such symptoms as chilliness, abundant clear urination, tiredness, lack of vitality, depression, weak knees and legs, a Pale tongue and a Deep-Weak pulse. If this point is used with moxa, caution must be exercised, as it is a very warming point. One must therefore make sure not only that there is indeed a deficiency of Kidney-Yang but also that there is internal Cold. A person may suffer from deficiency of Kidney-Yang, but also have some internal Heat somewhere else in the body (e.g. Damp-Heat in the Intestines). In such a case, this point would not be indicated as it would aggravate the Heat condition.

Original Qi is related to the Pre-Heaven Qi and to the person's constitution and basic vitality. This point strengthens Original Qi and is therefore indicated for chronic weakness on a physical and mental level.

Du-4 also benefits the Yang aspect of the Kidney-Essence and is indicated in all sexual disorders due to weakness of Essence, such as impotence, premature ejaculation or nocturnal emissions.

Du-4 is very effective in strengthening the lower back and knees and is indicated in chronic lower backache deriving from deficiency of Kidney-Yang.

Du-4 is specific to eliminate interior Cold deriving from Yang deficiency. This could be in the Spleen, manifesting with chronic diarrhoea, in the Bladder, manifesting with profuse clear urination, incontinence or enuresis, in the Intestines, manifesting with abdominal pain, or in the Uterus, manifesting with dysmenorrhoea or infertility.

The Governing Vessel has a strong influence on the Mind (*Shen*) because it affects it in three different ways. Firstly, the Governing Vessel emanates from the space between the Kidneys and is related to the Essence (in particular, the Yang aspect of the Essence). The Essence (*Jing*) is the foundation of Qi and Mind (*Shen*) and the residence of Will-power (*Zhi*): a strong Essence, therefore, will create the basis for a strong Mind and Will-power. Secondly, the Governing Vessel flows through the heart and it therefore affects the Mind through the Heart. Thirdly, the Governing Vessel enters the Brain, which, according to some doctors, is the residence of the Mind (*Shen*). For these reasons, the Governing Vessel, and in particular Du-4, affects the Mind: it clears the Mind and lifts moods and it is an important point to treat depression occurring against a background of Kidney-Yang deficiency.

> **Box 67.5 Du-4 – summary of functions**
>
> - Tonifies Kidney-Yang and warms the Gate of Life (*Ming Men*) (backache, dizziness, tinnitus, cold knees, feeling of cold in the lower back, frequent pale urination, tiredness)
> - Tonifies the Original Qi (*Yuan Qi*)
> - Expels Cold (chilliness, cold knees and back, cold feet, pain from Cold)
> - Strengthens the Governing Vessel
> - Strengthens the lower back (lower backache from Kidney deficiency)
> - Benefits Essence (seminal emissions)
> - Clears the Mind (depression, lack of will-power, mental confusion)
> - Clears Heat (heat in the body)
> - Extinguishes interior Wind (tremor of head, opisthotonos, epilepsy)

Interestingly, although Du-4 is a warming point, it can be used also to clear Heat; however, I personally do not use this point in this way.

Box 67.5 summarizes the functions of Du-4.

DU-8 JINSUO *TENDON SPASM*

Location

On the back, on the posterior median line, in the depression below the spinous process of T-9.

Nature

None.

Actions

Extinguishes interior Wind and relaxes the sinews.

Indications

Opisthotonos, spasms, epilepsy, stiffness and contraction of spine.

Comments

As the name clearly implies, Du-8 extinguishes interior Wind and its manifestations (i.e. convulsions, muscle spasms, tremor or epilepsy). It can also be used simply to relieve spasms and contracture of the sinews in the absence of interior Wind.

Box 67.6 summarizes the functions of Du-8.

> **Box 67.6 Du-8 – summary of functions**
>
> - Extinguishes interior Wind and relaxes the sinews (opisthotonos, spasms, epilepsy, stiffness and contraction of spine)

> **Box 67.7 Du-9 – summary of functions**
> - Regulates Liver and Gall Bladder
> - Resolves Damp-Heat (jaundice, feeling of heaviness, bitter taste, hypochondrial fullness, epigastric fullness)
> - Opens the chest and diaphragm (chest fullness)

DU-9 ZHIYANG *REACHING YANG*

Location
On the back, on the posterior median line, in the depression below the spinous process of T-7.

Nature
None.

Actions
Regulates Liver and Gall Bladder.
Resolves Damp-Heat.
Opens the chest and diaphragm.

Indications
Jaundice, feeling of heaviness, bitter taste, hypochondrial fullness, epigastric fullness.
Chest fullness.

Comments
Du-9 is related to the Liver and Gall Bladder and resolves Dampness in these two organs. It is a major point for jaundice and it is used for hypochondrial fullness.

It affects the chest and diaphragm and resolves stagnation of Qi in these areas, which gives rise to a feeling of distension or oppression, hiccups and sighing.

Box 67.7 summarizes the functions of Du-9.

DU-11 SHENDAO *MIND WAY*

Location
On the back, on the posterior median line, in the depression below the spinous process of T-5.

Nature
None.

Actions
Strengthens the Heart and calms the Mind.
Clears Heat.
Extinguishes interior Wind.

> **Box 67.8 Du-11 – summary of functions**
> - Strengthens the Heart and calms the Mind (sadness, anxiety, poor memory, palpitations, disorientation, timidity)
> - Clears Heat (fever, feeling of heat)
> - Extinguishes interior Wind (epilepsy in children, lockjaw)

Indications
Sadness, anxiety, poor memory, palpitations, disorientation, timidity.
Fever, feeling of heat.
Epilepsy in children, lockjaw.

Comments
Du-11 is on the same level as BL-15 Xinshu, the Back Transporting point of the Heart, and its action mostly extends to the Heart. It nourishes the Heart and calms the Mind, and therefore treats depression, sadness, or anxiety.

However, Du-11 also clears Heat and can therefore be used to clear Heart-Heat or drain Heart-Fire.

Box 67.8 summarizes the functions of Du-11.

DU-12 SHENZHU *BODY PILLAR*

Location
On the back, on the posterior median line, in the depression below the spinous process of T-3.

Nature
None.

Actions
Clears Lung-Heat.
Extinguishes interior Wind.
Calms the Mind and opens the Mind's orifices.
Tonifies Lung-Qi.

Indications
Heat in the chest, cough, feeling of heat, breathlessness, thirst, agitation.
Epilepsy in children, opisthotonos.
Manic behaviour, 'seeing ghosts', rage with desire to kill people.
Tiredness, weak voice, propensity to catch cold, allergic rhinitis, asthma.

Comments
Du-12 has two distinct functions according to whether it is reduced or reinforced. When used with reducing

method it eliminates interior Wind and calms spasms, convulsions and tremors. It is also used for epilepsy. With reducing method, it also clears Lung-Heat.

When used with reinforcing method, it tonifies Lung-Qi (it is at the same level as the Back Transporting point of the Lungs BL-13 Feishu) and generally strengthens the body. It is used to tonify the Lungs and to strengthen the body after a debilitating chronic illness. In my experience, Du-12 is also an important point to strengthen the Lungs in allergic rhinitis and asthma: I use it to treat the Root (*Ben*) in these two diseases to strengthen the Lungs and prevent recurrence. For example, I use it in the autumn to prevent the occurrence of seasonal allergic rhinitis in the spring. When I use Du-12 to strengthen the Lungs I always combine it with BL-13 Feishu.

The indication 'desire to kill people' for this point is interesting. As discussed in chapter 60 under the points BL-13 Feishu and BL-42 Pohu, the indication 'desire to commit suicide' for BL-13 Feishu must be seen in the context of the Corporeal Soul (*Po*), which is housed in the Lungs. The Corporeal Soul is a physical soul with a centripetal movement, constantly materializing and constantly separating into different constituent aspects. The Corporeal Soul is in relationship with *gui*: that is, ghosts or spirits (of dead people). The centripetal forces of *gui* within the Corporeal Soul, constantly fragmenting, are, eventually, the germ of death. It is therefore interesting that the three points related to the Lungs (which house the Corporeal Soul), all aligned on the back, are indicated either for desire to commit suicide or desire to kill: that is, they are related to thoughts of death. The indications are as follows:

- BL-13 Feishu: 'desire to commit suicide'
- BL-42 Pohu: 'three corpses flowing'
- Du-12 Shenzhu: 'desire to kill people'

Box 67.9 summarizes the functions of Du-12.

Box 67.9 Du-12 – summary of functions

- Clears Lung-Heat (heat in the chest, cough, feeling of heat, breathlessness, thirst, agitation)
- Extinguishes interior Wind (epilepsy in children, opisthotonos)
- Calms the Mind and opens the Mind's orifices (manic behaviour, 'seeing ghosts', rage with desire to kill people)
- Tonifies Lung-Qi (tiredness, weak voice, propensity to catching cold, allergic rhinitis, asthma)

DU-13 TAODAO *KILN WAY*

Location

On the back, on the posterior median line, in the depression below the spinous process of T-1.

Nature

Meeting point of Governing Vessel and Bladder channels.

Actions

Regulates the Lesser Yang.

Indications

Malaria, alternation of feeling of cold and feeling of heat.

Comments

Du-13 is effective to eliminate Heat at the Lesser Yang stage of the Six-Stage pattern identification, the cardinal sign of which is the alternation of feeling of cold and feeling of heat.

Du-13 is also effective in clearing lingering residual Heat in postviral fatigue syndrome.

Box 67.10 summarizes the functions of Du-13.

Box 67.10 Du-13 – summary of functions

- Regulates the Lesser Yang (malaria, alternation of feeling of cold and feeling of heat)
- Good to clear residual Heat

DU-14 DAZHUI *BIG VERTEBRA*

Location

On the posterior median line, in the depression below the spinous process of C7.

Nature

Meeting point of Governing Vessel with all Yang channels.
Point of the Sea of Qi.

Actions

Clears Heat.
Releases the Exterior and expels exterior Wind.
Regulates Nutritive and Defensive Qi.

Extinguishes interior Wind.
Clears the Mind.
Tonifies Yang.

Indications

Fever, feeling of heat.
Aversion to cold, fever, body aches, occipital headache and stiffness.
Invasion of external Wind, aversion to cold, fever, slight sweating.
Epilepsy.
Depression, tiredness, poor memory, poor concentration.
Chilliness, profuse pale urination.

Comments

Du-14 can have opposite effects according to the needling method used. When used with a reducing method it releases the Exterior and is used in exterior attacks of Wind-Heat: this point will release the Exterior and eliminate Wind-Heat. It is specifically used for invasions of Wind-Heat as opposed to Wind-Cold. It also regulates Nutritive and Defensive Qi when the person has been attacked by exterior Wind and is sweating.

When needled with reducing method, Du-14 also extinguishes interior Wind and clears interior Heat, and can be used in virtually any pattern of interior Heat.

If used with reinforcing method and, in particular, with direct moxa, Du-14 tonifies the Yang and can be used in any interior pattern of Yang deficiency. In particular, it tonifies Heart- and Kidney-Yang.

Since it is also the meeting point of all the Yang channels, which transport clear Yang upwards to the head, it is a point of the Sea of Qi, and the Governing Vessel enters the brain, Du-14 can also clear the Mind and stimulate the brain when the person is depressed and confused.

Box 67.11 summarizes the functions of Du-14.

> **Box 67.11 Du-14 – summary of functions**
>
> - Clears Heat (fever, feeling of heat)
> - Releases the Exterior and expels exterior Wind (aversion to cold, fever, body aches, occipital headache and stiffness)
> - Regulates Nutritive and Defensive Qi (invasion of external Wind, aversion to cold, fever, slight sweating)
> - Extinguishes interior Wind (epilepsy)
> - Clears the Mind (depression, tiredness, poor memory, poor concentration)
> - Tonifies Yang (chilliness, profuse pale urination)

DU-15 YAMEN *DOOR TO DUMBNESS*

Location

On the back of the neck, 0.5 *cun* directly above the midpoint of the posterior hairline, below the spinous process of C1.

Nature

Point of the Yang Linking Vessel (*Yang Wei Mai*).
Point of the Sea of Qi.

Actions

Extinguishes interior Wind.
Benefits the tongue and stimulates speech.
Clears the Mind.

Indications

Loss of consciousness from Wind-stroke, epilepsy.
Stiffness of tongue, inability to speak, loss of voice, flaccidity of tongue.
Feeling of heaviness of the head, poor memory, poor concentration.

Comments

Du-15's main action is that of stimulating speech. It is used to promote the faculty of speech in children with speech difficulties or adults after a Wind-stroke. Many extraordinary claims were made during the Cultural Revolution in China regarding the effect of this point in treating deaf-mute children. Chinese doctors are now admitting that most of these claims were exaggerated if not outright false.

Used with reinforcing method, Du-15 nourishes the brain and clears the Mind by promoting the rising of clear Yang to the head also by virtue of being a point of the Sea of Qi.

Box 67.12 summarizes the functions of Du-15.

> **Box 67.12 Du-15 – summary of functions**
>
> - Extinguishes interior Wind (loss of consciousness from Wind-stroke, epilepsy)
> - Benefits the tongue and stimulates speech (stiffness of tongue, inability to speak, loss of voice, flaccidity of tongue)
> - Clears the Mind (feeling of heaviness of the head, poor memory, poor concentration)

DU-16 FENGFU *WIND PALACE*

Location

On the back of the neck, 1 *cun* directly above the midpoint of the posterior hairline, directly below the external occipital protuberance, in the depression between the trapezius muscle of both sides.

Nature

Point of the Yang Linking Vessel (*Yang Wei Mai*).
Point of the Sea of Marrow.
Window of Heaven point.
One of Sun Si Miao's Ghost points.
Point of the Eye System.

Actions

Extinguishes interior Wind.
Expels exterior Wind.
Nourishes Marrow and benefits the Brain.
Calms the Mind and opens the Mind's orifices.

Indications

Opisthotonos, aphasia from Wind-stroke, Wind-stroke, hemiplegia.
Aversion to cold, fever, body aches, occipital stiffness and headache.
Headache, dizziness, tinnitus, blurred vision.
Manic behaviour, desire to commit suicide, sadness, fear.

Comments

Du-16 eliminates both exterior and interior Wind. It can therefore be used for exterior attacks of Wind-Cold or Wind-Heat, as well as for patterns of interior Wind, such as in Wind-stroke, epilepsy or severe giddiness.

Its capacity in eliminating Wind in general makes it a very important point to relieve headaches from Liver-Yang rising, Liver-Wind, Liver-Fire and acute headaches from exterior Wind. Its action in treating headaches is also partly due to this point's being a point of the Eye System which emerges from the Brain at Du-16 Fengfu.

Du-16 is a point of the Sea of Marrow. Marrow fills up the brain, and this point can clear the Mind and stimulate the brain.

Box 67.13 summarizes the functions of Du-16.

Box 67.13 Du-16 – summary of functions

- Extinguishes interior Wind (opisthotonos, aphasia from Wind-stroke, Wind-stroke, hemiplegia)
- Expels exterior Wind (aversion to cold, fever, body aches, occipital stiffness and headache)
- Nourishes Marrow and benefits the Brain (headache, dizziness, tinnitus, blurred vision)
- Calms the Mind and opens the Mind's orifices (manic behaviour, desire to commit suicide, sadness, fear)

Box 67.14 Du-17 – summary of functions

- Extinguishes interior Wind (epilepsy, lockjaw)
- Benefits the eyes (blurred vision, myopia, eye pain, excessive lacrimation)
- Benefits the Brain (feeling of heaviness of the head, dizziness)
- Calms the Mind and open the Mind's orifices (manic behaviour)

DU-17 NAOHU *BRAIN WINDOW*

Location

On the head, 2.5 *cun* directly above the midpoint of the posterior hairline, 1.5 *cun* above Du-16 Fengfu, in the depression superior to the exterior occipital protuberance.

Nature

Meeting point of Governing Vessel and Bladder channels.

Actions

Extinguishes interior Wind.
Benefits the eyes.
Benefits the Brain.
Calms the Mind and open the Mind's orifices.

Indications

Epilepsy, lockjaw.
Blurred vision, myopia, eye pain, excessive lacrimation.
Feeling of heaviness of the head, dizziness.
Manic behaviour.

Comments

This point is used mostly to subdue interior Wind affecting the brain. It is therefore indicated for epilepsy, Wind-stroke and severe giddiness.

Box 67.14 summarizes the functions of Du-17.

> **Box 67.15 Du-19 – summary of functions**
> - Calms the Mind and opens the Mind's orifices (manic behaviour, anxiety, mental restlessness, insomnia)

DU-19 HOUDING *POSTERIOR VERTEX*

Location
On the head, 5.5 *cun* directly above the midpoint of the posterior hairline, 3 *cun* above Du-17 Naohu.

Nature
None.

Actions
Calms the Mind and opens the Mind's orifices.

Indications
Manic behaviour, anxiety, mental restlessness, insomnia.

Comments
Du-19 has a powerful calming effect on the Mind and is very often used in severe anxiety, especially in combination with Ren-15 Jiuwei.

Box 67.15 summarizes the functions of Du-19.

DU-20 BAIHUI *HUNDRED MEETINGS*

Location
On the head, 5 *cun* directly above the midpoint of the anterior hairline.

Nature
Meeting point of Governing Vessel with Bladder, Gall Bladder, Triple Burner and Liver channels.
Point of the Sea of Marrow.

Actions
Extinguishes interior Wind.
Subdues Liver-Yang.
Raises Yang.
Benefits the Brain and the sense organs.
Lifts the Mind.
Promotes resuscitation.

Indications
Wind-stroke, hemiplegia, opisthotonos, loss of consciousness, epilepsy.
Headache, dizziness, tinnitus, blurred vision.
Prolapse of Internal Organs (stomach, uterus, bladder), prolapse of anus.
Dizziness, brain noise, tinnitus, poor memory, nasal obstruction, nasal discharge, nosebleed, blurred vision.
Depression.
Loss of consciousness.

Comments
Du-20 is at the vertex of the head, the place of maximum potential of energy and also the convergence area of Yang channels. For this reason, it has a dual function as it can either expel Excess Yang from the head or promote the rising of Yang to the head.

Du-20's action in extinguishing interior Wind and subduing Liver-Yang is related to its first function. For this reason, this is an important point for headaches from Liver-Yang rising or Liver-Wind.

Du-20 is a meeting point of many Yang channels, which carry clear Yang to the head: it therefore has a powerful effect in stimulating the ascending of Yang. When used with direct moxa, it stimulates the ascending of clear Qi to the head, and is therefore used for prolapse of the Internal Organs, such as stomach, uterus, bladder, anus or vagina. It is especially indicated for prolapse of anus, which lies on the Governing Vessel's pathway. Du-20 is effective not only in actual prolapses but also for incontinence of urine, very frequent urination and generally sinking of Qi with a feeling of bearing down in the lower abdomen.

When using this point with moxa to raise the Yang, caution must be exercised to make sure that there are no Heat symptoms at all. Also, this point should not be stimulated with moxa if the person suffers from high blood pressure.

This point's lifting action on Yang has a mental effect in that it promotes the rise of clear Yang to the Brain and the Mind. In my experience, Du-20 has a powerful effect in lifting depression and clearing of the mind.

Finally, it promotes resuscitation when the person is unconscious, especially combined with Du-26 Renzhong and P-6 Neiguan.

Box 67.16 summarizes the functions of Du-20.

Box 67.16 Du-20 – summary of functions

- Extinguishes interior Wind (Wind-stroke, hemiplegia, opisthotonos, loss of consciousness, epilepsy)
- Subdues Liver-Yang (headache, dizziness, tinnitus, blurred vision)
- Raises Yang (prolapse of Internal Organs (stomach, uterus, bladder), prolapse of anus)
- Benefits the Brain and the sense organs (dizziness, brain noise, tinnitus, poor memory, nasal obstruction, nasal discharge, nosebleed, blurred vision)
- Lifts the Mind (depression)
- Promotes resuscitation (loss of consciousness)

Box 67.17 Du-23 – summary of functions

- Opens the nose (nasal congestion, nasal discharge, loss of sense of smell, nasal polyps, sneezing, nosebleed)
- Benefits the eyes (blurred vision, pain in the eyes, myopia)

DU-23 SHANGXING *UPPER STAR*

Location

On the head, 1 *cun* directly above the midpoint of the anterior hairline.

Nature

One of Sun Si Miao's Ghost points.

Actions

Opens the nose.
Brightens the eyes.

Indications

Nasal congestion, nasal discharge, loss of sense of smell, nasal polyps, sneezing, nosebleed.
Blurred vision, pain in the eyes, myopia.

Comments

Du-23 is mostly used for chronic nose disorders such as allergic rhinitis or sinusitis, to open the nose and resolve Dampness from the nose and sinuses.

Box 67.17 summarizes the functions of Du-17.

DU-24 SHENTING *MIND COURTYARD*

Location

On the head, on the midline, 0.5 *cun* directly above the midpoint of the anterior hairline.

Box 67.18 Du-24 – summary of functions

- Calms and lifts the Mind, opens the Mind's orifices (manic depression, depression, anxiety, poor memory, insomnia)
- Extinguishes internal Wind (opisthotonos, epilepsy, dizziness, vertigo)
- Benefits the nose (clear nasal discharge (allergic rhinitis), nasal congestion, nosebleed)
- Brightens the eyes (lacrimation, blurred vision)

Nature

Meeting point of Governing Vessel and Stomach channels.

Actions

Calms and lifts the Mind, opens the Mind's orifices.
Extinguishes internal Wind.
Benefits the nose.
Brightens the eyes.

Indications

Manic depression, depression, anxiety, poor memory, insomnia.
Opisthotonos, epilepsy, dizziness, vertigo.
Clear nasal discharge (allergic rhinitis), nasal congestion, nosebleed.
Lacrimation, blurred vision.

Comments

The most important aspect of Du-24's energetic action is its downward movement: it makes Qi descend and subdues rebellious Yang. This is a very important and powerful point to calm the Mind. It is frequently combined with G.B.-13 Benshen for severe anxiety and fears.

An important feature of this point that makes it particularly useful is that it can both calm and lift the Mind: therefore it used not only for anxiety and insomnia but also for depression and sadness. It is also used in psychiatric practice for schizophrenia and split thoughts.[3]

The name of this point refers to its strong influence on the Mind and Spirit. The courtyard was traditionally considered to be a very important part of the house as it was the place from which visitors took their first impressions; it is the entrance. Thus, this point could be said to be the 'entrance' to the Mind and Spirit and its being a courtyard highlights its importance.

Box 67.18 summarizes the functions of Du-24.

DU-26 RENZHONG
MIDDLE OF PERSON

Location
On the face, at the junction of the superior third and middle third of the philtrum.

Nature
Meeting point of the Governing Vessel, Large Intestine and Stomach channels.
One of Sun Si Miao's Ghost points.

Actions
Promotes resuscitation and extinguishes interior Wind.
Opens the nose.
Calms the Mind and opens the Mind's orifices.
Benefits the lumbar spine.
Regulates the Water Passages of the Upper Burner.

Indications
Loss of consciousness, coma, Wind-stroke, lockjaw, deviation of eye and mouth, epilepsy.
Nosebleed, clear nasal discharge, loss of sense of smell.
Manic depression.
Stiffness and pain of the lumbar spine in the midline, inability to bend forward.
Oedema of the upper part of the body.

Comments
Du-26 is used to promote resuscitation when the person is unconscious. Like Du-23, it opens the nose passages.

An empirical use of this point is as a distal point for acute sprain of the lower back, but only when the pain is on the spine itself. In these cases it is usually reduced while the patient is standing and gently bending backwards and forwards.

Du-26 regulates the Water Passages of the Upper Burner and can therefore resolve oedema of the face and hands. Its alternative name, *Shuigou* 'Water Ditch', is related to this function.

Box 67.19 summarizes the functions of Du-26.

Fig. 67.3 illustrates the target areas of the Governing Vessel points.

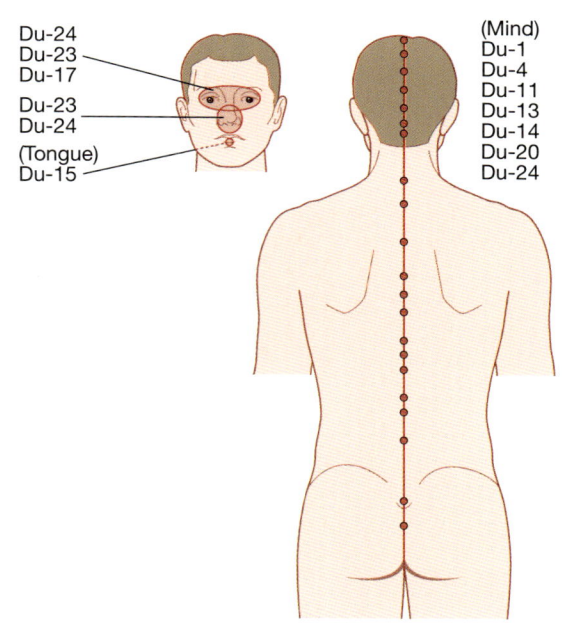

Figure 67.3 Target areas of Governing Vessel points

Box 67.19 Du-26 – summary of functions

- Promotes resuscitation and extinguishes interior Wind (loss of consciousness, coma, Wind-stroke, lockjaw, deviation of eye and mouth, epilepsy)
- Opens the nose (nosebleed, clear nasal discharge, loss of sense of smell)
- Calms the Mind and opens the Mind's orifices (manic depression)
- Benefits the lumbar spine (stiffness and pain of the lumbar spine in the midline, inability to bend forward)
- Regulates the Water Passages of the Upper Burner (oedema of the upper part of the body)

END NOTES
1. The 'Room of Sperm' is not an anatomical, physical structure but it simply indicates the Lower *Dan Tian* in a man where sperm was thought to be made by the Kidneys.
2. Classic of Difficulties, p. 90.
3. Dr Zhang Ming Jiu, personal communication, Nanjing 1982.

SECTION 2   PART 7

Extra Points 68

SISHENCONG *FOUR MIND ALERTNESS*

Location

A group of four points at the vertex, one *cun* from Du-20 Baihui in a cross-formation (Fig. 68.1).

Actions

Extinguishes interior Wind.
Calms the Mind.
Brightens the eyes and benefit the ears.

Indications

Epilepsy, Wind-stroke.
Manic depression, insomnia.
Blurred vision, deafness.

Comments

The actions and functions of these points are similar to those of Du-20 Baihui. These points are mostly used as local points for the treatment of epilepsy.
Box 68.1 summarizes the functions of Shishencong.

Box 68.1 Sishencong – summary of functions

- Extinguishes interior Wind (epilepsy, Wind-stroke)
- Calms the Mind (manic depression, insomnia)
- Brightens the eyes and benefit the ears (blurred vision, deafness)

YINTANG *SEAL HALL*

Location

On the midline of the body in between the eyebrows (Fig. 68.2).

Actions

Extinguishes Wind.
Calms the Mind.
Benefits the nose.

Indications

Epilepsy, vertigo, convulsions.
Anxiety, insomnia, fright.
Nasal congestion and discharge, sneezing.

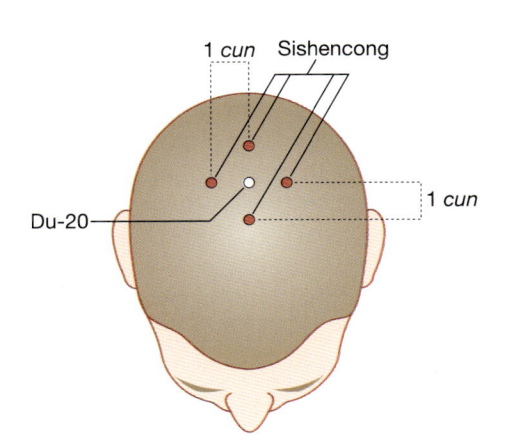

Figure 68.1 Sishencong

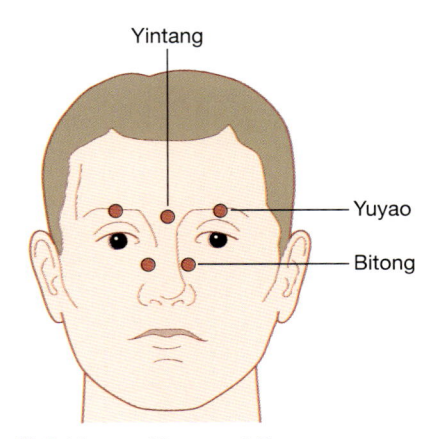

Figure 68.2 Yintang, Yuyao and Bitong

Comments

Yintang point extinguishes interior Wind and it relieves convulsions in children. It is therefore used at the late stages of children's febrile diseases. More commonly in everyday practice, Yintang is used to calm the Mind and to relieve anxiety and insomnia.

Box 68.2 summarizes the functions of Yintang.

> **Box 68.2 Yintang – summary of functions**
>
> - Extinguishes Wind (epilepsy, vertigo, convulsions)
> - Calms the Mind (anxiety, insomnia, fright)
> - Benefits the nose (nasal congestion and discharge, sneezing)

TAIYANG *GREATER YANG*

Location

In a depression 1 *cun* posterior to the midpoint between the lateral end of the eyebrow and the outer canthus (Fig. 68.3).

Actions

Subdues Liver-Yang.
Brightens the eyes.

Indications

One-sided headache on the temple, dizziness, tinnitus.
Blurred vision, redness and swelling of the eye, pain in the eyes.

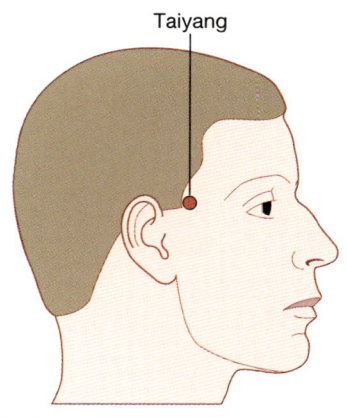

Figure 68.3 Taiyang

Comments

Taiyang is very frequently used as a local point for headaches due to rising of Liver-Yang or Liver-Fire when the headaches occur on the temple.

It can also be used for eye problems due to Heat, either exterior as in Wind-Heat or interior as in Liver-Fire.

Box 68.3 summarizes the functions of Taiyang.

> **Box 68.3 Taiyang – summary of functions**
>
> - Subdues Liver-Yang (one-sided headache on the temple, dizziness, tinnitus)
> - Brightens the eyes (blurred vision, redness and swelling of the eye, pain in the eyes)

YUYAO *FISH SPINE*

Location

In the middle of the eyebrow (see Fig. 68.2).

Actions

Subdues Liver-Yang.
Brightens the eyes.

Indications

Headache behind the eyes, dizziness, blurred vision.
Redness, swelling and pain of the eyes, blurred vision, twitching of eyelids, drooping of eyelid.

Comments

Yuyao is used for eye disorders, such as blurred vision or floaters, particularly deriving from Liver-Blood deficiency.

It is also a useful local point for headaches from Liver-Yang rising when they occur behind one eye. It also treats dull headaches from Liver-Blood deficiency occurring behind both eyes.

Box 68.4 summarizes the functions of Yuyao.

> **Box 68.4 Yuyao – summary of functions**
>
> - Subdues Liver-Yang (headache behind the eyes, dizziness, blurred vision)
> - Brightens the eyes (redness, swelling and pain of the eyes, blurred vision, twitching of eyelids, drooping of eyelid)

BITONG *FREE NOSE PASSAGES*

Location
On the side of the nose, half way between the glabella and the tip of the nose (see Fig. 68.2).

Actions
Opens the nose.

Indications
Sneezing, allergic rhinitis, congested nose, nasal discharge, sinusitis, blocked sinuses, facial pain.

Comments
This is a very useful point to use for allergic rhinitis or sinusitis to open the nasal passages. It also opens the maxillary sinuses. I find this point more effective than L.I.-20 Yingxiang for such problems. L.I.-20 is better at expelling Wind from the face (hence facial paralysis), while Bitong is better at opening the nasal and sinus passages.

I locate the point Bitong slightly higher than what is described in other books, as I was taught by my teachers in Nanjing. The 'Manual of Acupuncture' locates this point at the highest point of the nasolabial groove.[1]

Box 68.5 summarizes the functions of Bitong.

> **Box 68.5 Bitong – summary of functions**
> - Opens the nose (sneezing, allergic rhinitis, congested nose, nasal discharge, sinusitis, blocked sinuses, facial pain)

JINGZHONG *MIDDLE OF PERIODS*

Location
On the lower abdomen, 3 *cun* from the midline, level with Ren-6 Qihai (Fig. 68.4).

Actions
Regulates the Uterus and menstruation.

Indications
Irregular periods, mid-cycle bleeding.

Comments.
Jingzhong is mostly used for irregular periods and mid-cycle bleeding.

Box 68.6 summarizes the functions of Jingzhong.

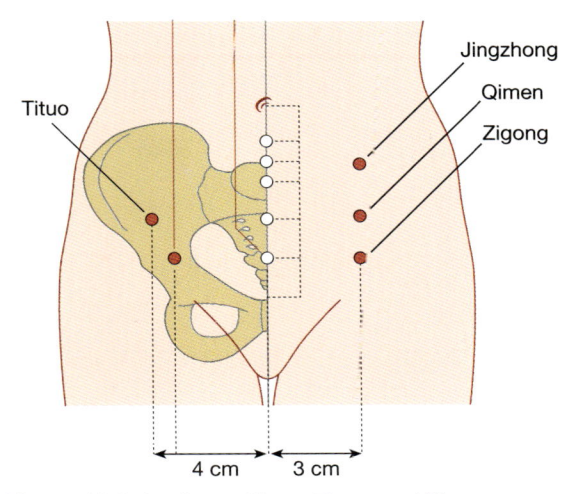

Figure 68.4 Jingzhong, Qimen, Zigong and Tituo

> **Box 68.6 Jingzhong – summary of functions**
> - Regulates the Uterus and menstruation (irregular periods, mid-cycle bleeding)

QIMEN *DOOR OF QI*

Location
On the lower abdomen, 3 *cun* from the midline, level with Ren-4 Guanyuan (see Fig. 68.4).

Actions
Regulates the Uterus and menstruation.

Indications
Infertility, heavy periods.

Comments
Qimen has a special action in infertility and excessive menstrual bleeding.

Box 68.7 summarizes the functions of Qimen.

> **Box 68.7 Qimen – summary of functions**
> - Regulates the Uterus and menstruation (infertility, heavy periods)

ZIGONG PALACE OF CHILD

Location
On the lower abdomen, 3 *cun* lateral to Ren-3 Zhongji (see Fig. 68.4).

Actions
Regulates the Uterus and menstruation.

Indications
Infertility, irregular periods, painful periods, prolapse of uterus, heavy periods.

Comments
Zigong is used to tonify the Kidneys and to regulate menstruation. It is especially indicated for menorrhagia, metrorrhagia and infertility in women. It has a long history of use for infertility.

It is interesting to note that the three extra points on the abdomen, all of which influence menstruation and fertility, are all 3 *cun* from the midline and therefore between the Stomach and Spleen channels: these are Jingzhong (level with Ren-6), Qimen (level with Ren-4) and Zigong (level with Ren-3). It looks almost as if there were another channel between these two channels on the abdomen.

Box 68.8 summarizes the functions of Zigong.

Box 68.8 Zigong – summary of functions

- Regulates the Uterus and menstruation (infertility, irregular periods, painful periods, prolapse of uterus, heavy periods)

TITUO LIFT AND SUPPORT

Location
On the lower abdomen, 4 *cun* lateral to the midline, level with Ren-4 Guanyuan (see Fig. 68.4).

Actions
Raises Qi.
Invigorates Blood.

Indications
Prolapse of uterus.
Painful periods, abdominal pain, abdominal masses, myoma.

Comments
Tituo is an important local point for abdominal pain and abdominal masses from Blood stasis: it affects Blood in the Penetrating Vessel. In modern China, this point is frequently used for myomas ('fibroids').

Box 68.9 summarizes the functions of Tituo.

Box 68.9 Tituo – summary of functions

- Raises Qi (prolapse of uterus)
- Invigorates Blood (painful periods, abdominal pain, abdominal masses, myoma)

DINGCHUAN STOPPING ASTHMA

Location
This point is 0.5 *cun* lateral to Du-14 Dazhui (Fig. 68.5).

Actions
Promotes the descending of Lung-Qi and calms asthma.

Indications
Asthma, wheezing, breathlessness, cough.

Comments
This point is mostly used to calm an acute attack of asthma.

Box 68.10 summarizes the functions of Dingchuan.

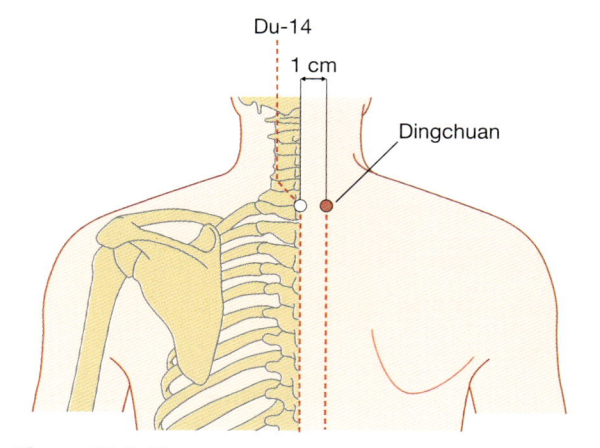

Figure 68.5 Dingchuan

> **Box 68.10 Dingchuan – summary of functions**
> - Promotes the descending of Lung-Qi and calms asthma (asthma, wheezing, breathlessness, cough)

JINGGONG *PALACE OF ESSENCE*

Location
On the back, 0.5 *cun* lateral to the point BL-52 Zhishi (Fig. 68.6).

Actions
Nourishes the Kidney-Essence.

Indications
Infertility.

Comments
Jinggong is used to tonify the Kidney and, specifically, the Kidney-Essence.

Box 68.11 summarizes the functions of Jinggong.

> **Box 68.11 Jinggong – summary of functions**
> - Nourishes the Kidney-Essence (infertility)

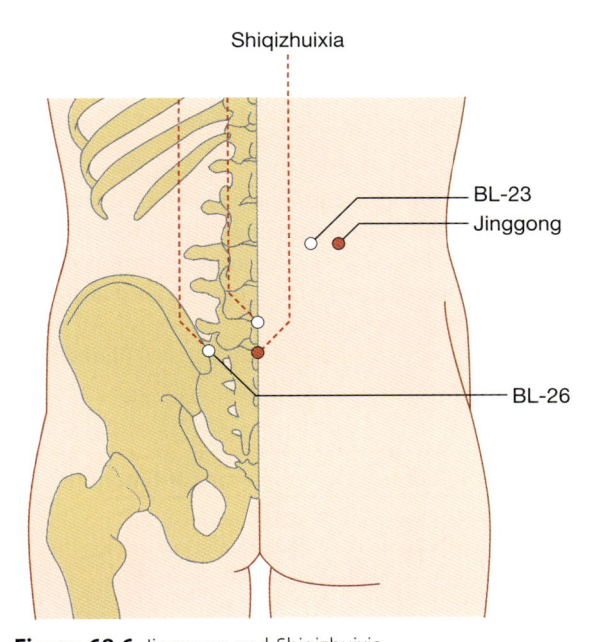

Figure 68.6 Jinggong and Shiqizhuixia

HUATUOJIAJI *HUA TUO BACK FILLING POINTS*

Location
A group of points on both sides of the spine 0.5 *cun* from the midline in correspondence with the intervertebral spaces from the first thoracic to the fifth lumbar vertebra (Fig. 68.7).

Actions
Regulates the Internal Organs.
Benefits the back and spine.

Indications
For diseases of the relevant organs.
Backache.

Comments
These points are named after the famous doctor *Hua Tuo* who lived during the Han dynasty. It is thought that he used these points as Back Transporting points.

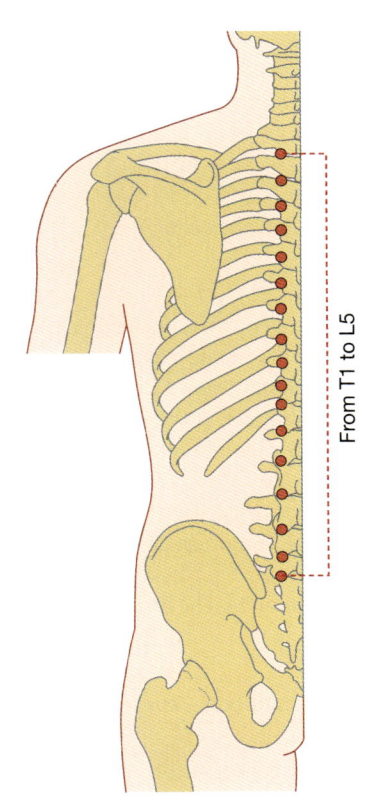

Figure 68.7 Huatuojiaji

The action of these points is similar to that of the corresponding Back Transporting points. However, they are not often used in this way as the Back Transporting points would be more effective.

They are, however, frequently used as local points for backache and are particularly useful to correct deviations of vertebrae.

Box 68.12 summarizes the functions of Huatuojiaji.

Box 68.12 Huatuojiaji – summary of functions

- Regulates the Internal Organs (for diseases of the relevant organs)
- Benefits the back and spine (backache)

SHIQIZHUIXIA *BELOW THE 17TH VERTEBRA*

Location
This point is located on the midline of the back below the tip of the fifth lumbar vertebra (see Fig. 68.6).

Actions
Removes obstructions from the channel.
Benefits the lower back.

Indications
Chronic or acute lower backache.

Comments
This point is excellent as a local point for the treatment of chronic or acute lower backache whether the ache is on the midline or bilateral. It is only used if the ache is quite low down on the sacrum or just above it. I usually combine this point with BL-26 Guanyuanshu.

In my experience, this point is superior to Du-3 Yaoyangguan or Du-4 Mingmen for the treatment of lower backache.

Box 68.13 summarizes the functions of Shiqizhuixia.

Box 68.13 Shiqizhuixia – summary of functions

- Removes obstructions from the channel
- Benefits the lower back (chronic or acute lower backache)

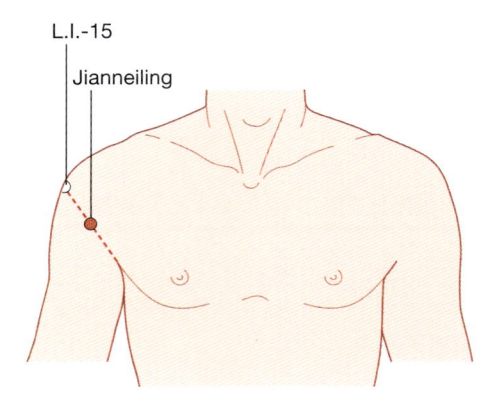

Figure 68.8 Jianneiling

JIANNEILING *INNER SHOULDER MOUND*

Location
Midway between the end of the anterior axillary fold and L.I.-15 Jianyu (Fig. 68.8).

Actions
Removes obstructions from the channel.
Expels Dampness and Cold.

Indications
Stiffness and pain of the shoulder, difficulty in adducting the arm, feeling of heaviness of the arm, numbness.

Comments
This is an extremely useful local point for the treatment of shoulder pain or frozen shoulder. It is selected when the pain radiates towards the anterior aspect of the shoulder (Lung channel). This point is called also Jianqian *Front of the Shoulder*.

Box 68.14 summarizes the functions of Jianneiling.

Box 68.14 Jianneiling – summary of functions

- Removes obstructions from the channel
- Expels Dampness and Cold (stiffness and pain of the shoulder, difficulty in adducting the arm, feeling of heaviness of the arm, numbness)

BAXIE EIGHT PATHOGENIC FACTORS

Location

On the dorsum of the hand, on the webs between the five fingers of both hands. When one hand is made into a fist, three of these points are in the depression between the metacarpal heads proximal to the web margins. The other point is equidistant between the thumb and index metacarpals proximal to the web margins (Fig. 68.9).

Actions

Relaxes the sinews.
Expels Wind-Dampness.

Indications

Numbness, stiffness, redness, swelling, spasm and pain of the fingers, Painful Obstruction Syndrome (*Bi* Syndrome) of the fingers.

Comments

These points are very frequently used for Painful Obstruction Syndrome of the hand and fingers. They eliminate Wind and Damp and relax the tendons.

They also move Blood in the hand and fingers and are therefore used for chronic Atrophy Syndrome of the hands.

Box 68.15 summarizes the functions of Baxie.

> **Box 68.15 Baxie – summary of functions**
>
> - Relaxes the sinews
> - Expels Wind-Dampness (numbness, stiffness, redness, swelling, spasm and pain of the fingers, Painful Obstruction Syndrome (*Bi* Syndrome) of the fingers)

SIFENG FOUR CRACKS

Location

On the palmar surface, in the transverse creases of the proximal interphalangeal joints of the four fingers (excluding the thumb) (Fig. 68.10).

Actions

Resolves Dampness and food retention in children.

Indications

Childhood Nutritional Impairment, Accumulation Disorder in children, food retention, poor digestion, diarrhoea.

Comments

These points are mostly used in young children to promote digestion. The points should be needled and then a yellow fluid extracted from them. However, they are effective also if there is no yellow fluid coming out.

Box 68.16 summarizes the functions of Sifeng.

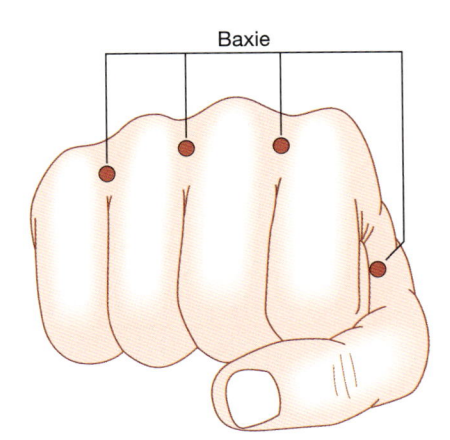

Figure 68.9 Baxie

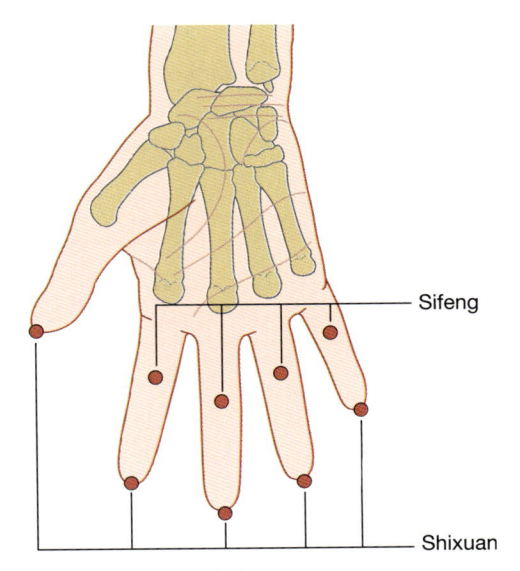

Figure 68.10 Sifeng and Shixuan

> **Box 68.16 Sifeng – summary of functions**
>
> - Resolves Dampness and food retention in children (Childhood Nutritional Impairment, Accumulation Disorder in children, food retention, poor digestion, diarrhoea)

SHIXUAN TEN DECLARATIONS

Location

On the tips of the 10 fingers, about 0.1 *cun* distal to the nails (see Fig. 68.10).

Actions

Clears Heat.
Extinguishes interior Wind.
Opens the orifices.
Promotes resuscitation.

Indications

Febrile disease, Summer-Heat invasion.
Wind-stroke, clonic spasms, epilepsy.
Loss of consciousness.

Comments

These points are used in acute situations when the person is unconscious in cases of Wind-stroke.

Box 68.17 summarizes the functions of Shixuan.

> **Box 68.17 Shixuan – summary of functions**
>
> - Clears Heat (febrile disease, Summer-Heat invasion)
> - Extinguishes interior Wind (Wind-stroke, clonic spasms, epilepsy)
> - Opens the orifices
> - Promotes resuscitation (loss of consciousness)

XIYAN KNEE EYES

Location

Two points in the depressions medial and lateral to the patellar ligaments. The lateral Xiyan is identical to ST-35 Dubi (Fig. 68.11).

Actions

Expels Wind-Damp.
Benefits the knees.

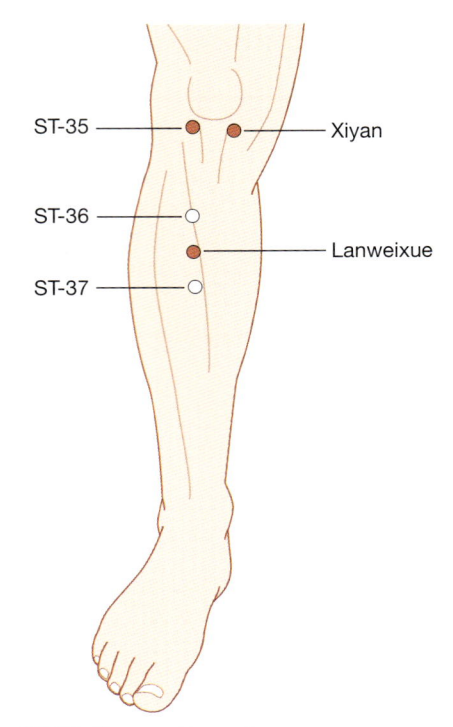

Figure 68.11 Xiyan and Lanweixue

Indications

Swelling and pain of the knee, rigidity of the knee, weakness and numbness of the knee, Painful Obstruction Syndrome (*Bi* Syndrome) of the knee.

Comments

These are important local points for Painful Obstruction Syndrome of the knees, especially when the pain is in the front of the knee or deep inside the joint.

The needle should be inserted obliquely, slightly upwards and medially towards the centre of the joint to a depth of at least 0.25 *cun*.

These points give particularly good results if moxa is burned on the needles.

Box 68.18 summarizes the functions of Xiyan.

> **Box 68.18 Xiyan – summary of functions**
>
> - Expels Wind-Damp
> - Benefits the knees (swelling and pain of the knee, rigidity of the knee, weakness and numbness of the knee, Painful Obstruction Syndrome (*Bi* Syndrome) of the knee)

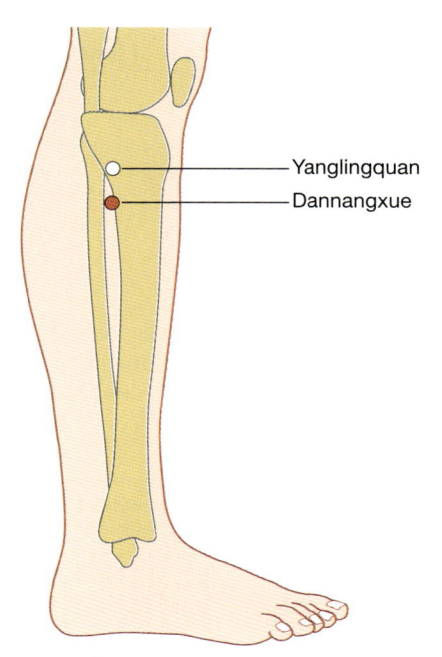

Figure 68.12 Dannangxue

DANNANGXUE *GALL BLADDER POINT*

Location

This point is situated about 1 *cun* below G.B.-34 Yanglingquan. Its location is not fixed as the needle is inserted in the area below G.B.-34 wherever it is tender on pressure (Fig. 68.12).

Actions

Resolves Damp-Heat from the Gall Bladder.

Indications

Jaundice, cholecystitis, cholelithiasis.

Comments

This point is frequently used (if it is tender on pressure) to expel Damp-Heat from the Gall Bladder in cholecystitis or cholelithiasis.

Box 68.19 summarizes the functions of Dannangxue.

Box 68.19 Dannangxue – summary of functions

- Resolves Damp-Heat from the Gall Bladder (jaundice, cholecystitis, cholelithiasis)

LANWEIXUE *APPENDIX POINT*

Location

On the Stomach channel in between ST-36 Zusanli and ST-37 Shangjuxu, on the right leg only. The location of this point is also variable and it is located wherever it is tender on pressure between ST-36 and ST-37 (see Fig. 68.11).

Actions

Stops abdominal pain.
Resolves Damp-Heat.

Indications

Acute and chronic appendicitis.

Comments

This point is used in an acute attack of appendicitis to stop pain. It can also be used in chronic appendicitis.

It is also a useful diagnostic aid in the diagnosis of appendicitis (including the chronic kind) if it is tender on pressure.

Box 68.20 summarizes the functions of Lanweixue.

Box 68.20 Lanweixue – summary of functions

- Stops abdominal pain
- Resolves Damp-Heat (acute and chronic appendicitis)

BAFENG *EIGHT WINDS*

Location

On the dorsum of the foot, on the webs between the five toes, proximal to the margins of the webs (Fig. 68.13).

Actions

Relaxes the sinews.
Expels Wind-Dampness.

Indications

Numbness, stiffness, redness, swelling, spasm and pain of the toes, Painful Obstruction Syndrome (*Bi* Syndrome) of the toes.

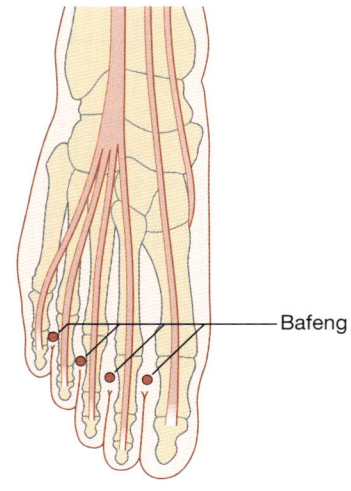

Figure 68.13 Bafeng

Box 68.21 Bafeng – summary of functions

- Relaxes the sinews
- Expels Wind-Dampness (numbness, stiffness, redness, swelling, spasm and pain of the toes, Painful Obstruction Syndrome (*Bi* Syndrome) of the toes)

Comments

These points are used in a similar way to Baxie for Painful Obstruction Syndrome of the feet.

Box 68.21 summarizes the functions of Bafeng.

END NOTE

1. Deadman P, Al-Khafaji M 1998 A Manual of Acupuncture. Journal of Chinese Medicine Publications, Hove, England, p. 568.

PART 8

Principles of Treatment

INTRODUCTION

Part 8 is divided into two chapters:

| Chapter 69 | Principles of treatment |
| Chapter 70 | Principles of the combination of points |

Chapter 69 discusses the importance of formulating a rational plan of treatment in order to be able to respond to clinical situations effectively. For example, this chapter discusses when one should treat the Root (*Ben*) of a condition, when one should concentrate on treating the Manifestation (*Biao*), when to tonify the body's Qi and when to expel pathogenic factors.

Chapter 70 discusses the principles governing the combination of acupuncture points.

PART 8

Principles of Treatment 69

Key contents

The Root and the Manifestation
Treat the Root only
Treat both the Root and the Manifestation
Treat the Manifestation first, and the Root later
Multiple Roots and Manifestations

- Multiple Roots, each giving rise to different Manifestations
- One Root giving rise to different Manifestations
- The Root coincides with the Manifestation

When to tonify Upright Qi, when to expel pathogenic factors
Tonify Upright Qi
Expel pathogenic factors
Tonify Upright Qi and expel pathogenic factors

- First tonify Upright Qi, then expel the pathogenic factors
- First expel the pathogenic factors, then tonify Upright Qi
- Tonify Upright Qi and expel the pathogenic factors simultaneously

Differences between acupuncture and herbal therapy in the application of the treatment principle

After making a diagnosis and identifying the patterns, the next logical step is that of determining the principle of treatment to be adopted. The practitioner of Chinese medicine will need to formulate a rational and coherent plan of action as to what should be treated first, what is primary and what is secondary in the patient's condition, what is the relative importance of the acute or chronic condition and what method of treatment should be used.

Over the centuries, Chinese medical theory has answered these questions and provided a coherent system of principles of treatment. In practice, these principles provide a logical framework according to which a practitioner can evaluate the objectives of his or her treatment. A principle of treatment should always be established before treatment commences. This is achieved by a rigorous analysis of the clinical manifestations and a synthesis of the patient's condition and therapeutic needs at that particular time. The principles of treatment do not necessarily follow logically from the identification of the relevant pattern of disharmony except in a few, simple conditions.

Most of the conditions we see in practice are characterized by multiple patterns and a coexistence of Deficiency and Excess. Thus, although our diagnosis of the patterns involved may be absolutely correct, the success of the treatment depends very much on the adoption of the correct strategy and method of treatment.

For example, although we may correctly diagnose a Spleen deficiency and Dampness, should we concentrate on tonifying the former or eliminating the latter, or should we do both simultaneously? In my experience, the adoption of the correct treatment principle in deciding whether to tonify the body's Qi or eliminate pathogenic factors is absolutely crucial to the success of the treatment.

Clinical note

The adoption of the correct treatment principle in deciding whether to tonify the body's Qi or to eliminate pathogenic factors is absolutely crucial to the success of the treatment

Thus, the therapeutic encounter starts with diagnosis using the tools of observation, interrogation, palpation and hearing/smelling; using these tools, we identify the patterns of disharmony. After that, we need to identify and evaluate carefully the Root and Manifestation, distinguishing between Fullness and Emptiness. It is only after doing this that we can formulate a suitable treatment strategy and method (Fig. 69.1).

A few examples will clarify this:

- A patient with chronic bronchitis presents with an acute attack of Wind-Cold or Wind-Heat (a common cold or influenza, for example). Should we treat the acute attack first and ignore the chronic condition? Or should we treat both at the same time?
- A patient with deficiency of Qi causing great tiredness also has symptoms of Dampness and a thick-sticky tongue coating. Should we concentrate on tonifying Qi or on eliminating Dampness? Or on doing both simultaneously?
- A patient has been having a recurrent temperature and flu-like symptoms for weeks; she is completely exhausted, but her pulse is Full and Wiry. Should we tonify her body's Qi or expel the exterior pathogenic factor still lingering in the Interior?
- An old man has deficiency of Yin with rising of Liver-Yang causing hypertension. We need to reduce Liver-Yang, but as the patient is old and frail, will reducing Liver-Yang weaken his energy?
- An elderly patient suffers from a Kidney deficiency but also from pronounced Blood stasis, Phlegm and Heat. Should we concentrate on tonifying the Kidneys or on invigorating Blood, clearing Heat and resolving Phlegm? Or should be we do both simultaneously? If we choose to invigorate Blood, resolve Phlegm and clear Heat, would that weaken this elderly person?

These are a few examples of complex situations encountered in clinical practice every day, requiring a clear differentiation between what is primary and what is secondary, an assessment of the patient's condition and a clear principle of treatment and plan of action.

The principles of treatment can be discussed from three points of view:

1. The 'Root' ('*Ben*') and the 'Manifestation' ('*Biao*')
2. When to tonify the Upright Qi (*Zheng Qi*) and when to eliminate pathogenic factors
3. The question of when to tonify and when to reduce

Points 2 and 3 will actually be discussed together as they are concerned with the same basic issue so that the discussion will be under the following headings:

- The Root and the Manifestation
  - Treat the Root only
  - Treat both the Root and the Manifestation
  - Treat the Manifestation first, and the Root later
  - Multiple Roots and Manifestations
    - Multiple Roots, each giving rise to different Manifestations
    - One Root giving rise to different Manifestations
    - The Root coincides with the Manifestation
- When to tonify Upright Qi (*Zheng Qi*), when to expel pathogenic factors
  - Tonify Upright Qi
  - Expel pathogenic factors
  - Tonify Upright Qi and expel pathogenic factors
    - First tonify Upright Qi, then expel the pathogenic factors
    - First expel the pathogenic factors, then tonify Upright Qi
    - Tonify Upright Qi and expel the pathogenic factors simultaneously
- Differences between acupuncture and herbal therapy in the application of the treatment principle

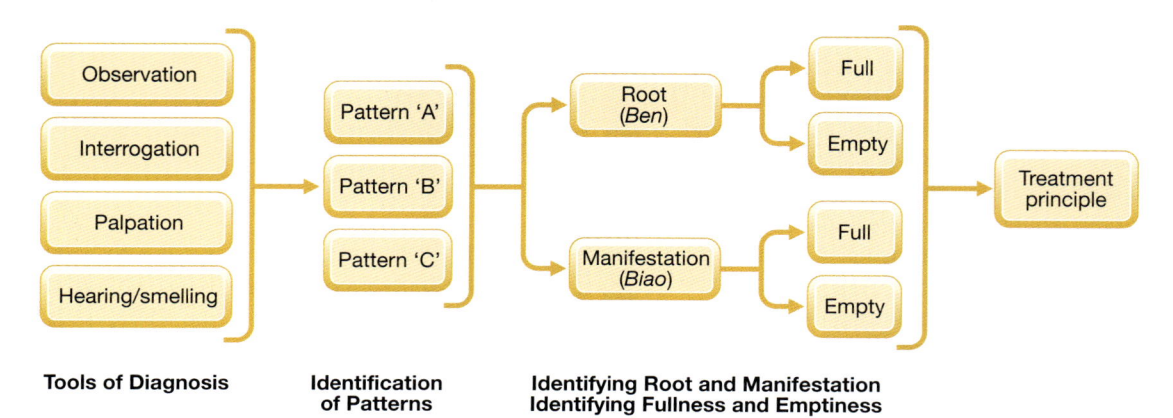

Figure 69.1 The Root (*Ben*) and the Manifestation (*Biao*)

THE ROOT AND THE MANIFESTATION (*BEN* AND *BIAO*)

The Root is called '*Ben*' in Chinese, which literally means 'root', and the Manifestation is called '*Biao*', which literally means 'outward sign' or 'manifestation', i.e. the outward manifestation of some inner, unseen root. The Root and Manifestation can be compared to a tree, its root being the Root and its branches the Manifestation (Fig. 69.2).

Root and Manifestation acquire different meanings in different contexts. These are:

1. From the point of view of Upright Qi (*Zheng Qi*) and pathogenic factors: the Root is the Upright Qi and the Manifestation is the pathogenic factors
2. From the point of view of pathology: the Root is the root of the disease and Manifestation is the clinical manifestations. Example: invasion of external Wind is the Root and its clinical manifestations the Manifestation
3. From the point of view of patterns: the original pattern is the Root and the one originating from it is the Manifestation (e.g. Spleen-Qi deficiency leading to Dampness)
4. From the point of view of onset of the disease: the Root is the initial condition while the Manifestation is the later condition
5. From the point of view of duration of the disease: the Root is a chronic disease while the Manifestation is an acute disease

Thus when treatment of Root or Manifestation is discussed, we need to be clear about the particular standpoint or context being considered. For example, to say that in a certain case the Root needs to be treated first, could mean that the Upright Qi needs to be treated first, or that the root (or cause) of the disease needs treating, or that the chronic conditions should be treated first.

In clinical practice, however, Root and Manifestation are usually considered in the second and third contexts: that is, as root and clinical manifestations of the disease and as original and deriving pattern (Figs 69.3 and 69.4).

Box 69.1 summarizes the Root and Manifestation.

When considering the Root and Manifestation, it is important to understand the connection between the two. They are not separate entities, but two aspects of a contradiction, like Yin and Yang. As their names

---

Box 69.1 Root and Manifestation

Two main meanings:
1. The Root is the root of the condition (e.g. Wind-Cold) and the Manifestation is the clinical manifestations (aversion to cold, fever, Floating pulse, etc.)
2. The Root of the condition is the original pattern (e.g. Spleen-Qi deficiency) and the Manifestation is the deriving pattern (e.g. Dampness)

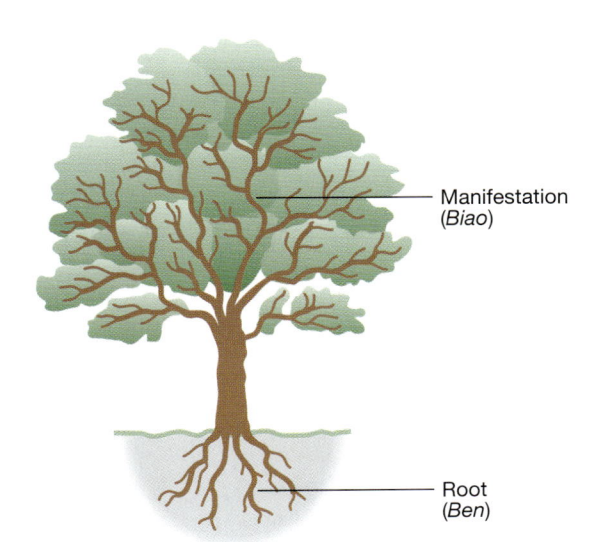

Figure 69.2 Root and Manifestation as a tree

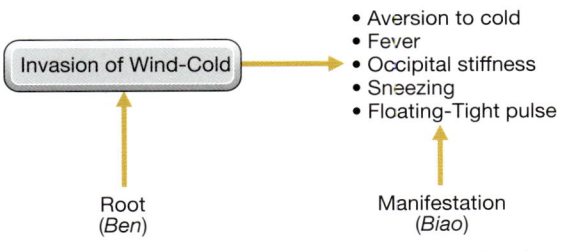

Figure 69.3 Root and Manifestations as root and clinical manifestations of a condition

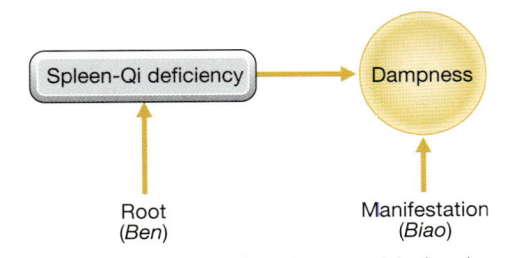

Figure 69.4 Root and Manifestations as original and deriving patterns

suggest, they are related to one another, just as the roots of a tree are connected to its branches, the former under the ground and invisible, the latter above the ground and visible (see Fig. 69.2).

The same relation exists between the root of a disease and its clinical manifestations: they are indissolubly related and they form two aspects of the same entity. There is no separation between the two. For this reason, it is not entirely correct to translate 'Ben' as 'cause' since the relation between the Root and Manifestation is not a causal one. The root is not the 'cause' of the branches, but the two together form the entity of a tree. The art of diagnosis consists precisely in identifying the Root (i.e. the root of symptoms and signs) by looking at the Manifestation (i.e. the clinical manifestations).

For example, if a person has diarrhoea, chilliness, tiredness, poor appetite, abdominal distension, a Weak pulse and a Pale tongue, the complex of these clinical manifestations clearly points to its Root: that is, Spleen-Yang deficiency. In this simple example, therefore, Spleen-Yang deficiency is the Root and all the symptoms and signs are the Manifestation of the disease. It is only when we master the art of pattern identification that we can identify the Root by looking at the pattern woven by the Manifestation, much like a botanist can identify a tree by looking at its leaves.

To give an example of original and deriving pattern as Root and Manifestation, Spleen-Qi deficiency may be the original pattern (Root) and Dampness the deriving pattern (Manifestation). In endometriosis, often a deficiency of Kidney-Yang is the Root while Blood stasis is the Manifestation.

Please note that clinical situations may be very complicated as a Manifestation may, in turn, become a Root. In the example given above, Kidney-Yang deficiency (Root) may give rise to Blood stasis (Manifestation) and this, in turn, may cause Dryness (a Manifestation) (Fig. 69.5).

In some cases, we may actually mistakenly see a Manifestation as a Root. The following brief case history will clarify this.

Case history 69.1

Before reporting the case history I should discuss briefly the pathology of severe metrorrhagia (heavy and irregular menstrual bleeding, called *Beng Lou* in Chinese medicine). There are two basic causes of heavy and irregular menstrual bleeding: either deficient Qi fails to hold Blood, which leaks out, or Heat in the Blood pushes the Blood out of the vessels. In the first case, heavy bleeding will be accompanied by general symptoms and signs of Qi deficiency such as tiredness, pale face, shortness of breath, poor appetite, loose stools, Pale tongue and Empty pulse. When bleeding is due to Blood-Heat there will be general signs of Heat such as a red face, a feeling of heat, thirst, insomnia, a Red tongue and a Rapid-Overflowing pulse.

A 36-year-old woman had been suffering from chronic menorrhagia: the bleeding was so irregular and constant that some months she did not know when her period occurred as she was bleeding every day. She presented with general symptoms of Qi deficiency such as a pale and sallow complexion, tiredness, a weak voice, loose stools and a Weak pulse. I therefore concluded that the bleeding was due to Qi deficiency and treated her by tonifying Qi. This produced no results. I reassessed the diagnosis and discovered that she often felt thirsty, her cheeks were occasionally flushed, her tongue had a slight redness on the sides and her pulse was very slightly Rapid. I therefore concluded that my original diagnosis was wrong and that the bleeding was actually due to Blood-Heat. When I changed my treatment by cooling Blood, this produced immediate results.

If the bleeding was due to Blood-Heat, what are we to make of her Qi deficiency symptoms? What had happened was that the Qi deficiency was actually the result rather than the cause of bleeding. In cases of heavy, prolonged bleeding, the chronic loss of blood induces a deficiency of Blood: as Blood is the mother of Qi, this will eventually induce

Kidney-Yang deficiency → Blood stasis → Dryness

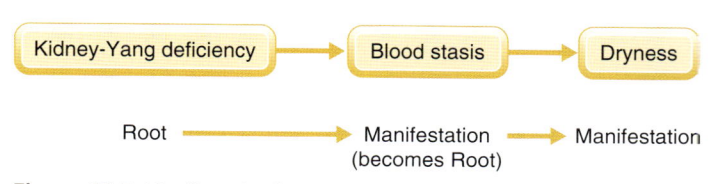

Root → Manifestation (becomes Root) → Manifestation

Figure 69.5 Manifestation becoming secondary Root

a Qi deficiency. In this patient's case, therefore, Qi deficiency was a Manifestation rather than a Root, as follows:

Blood-Heat	**Blood deficiency**	**Qi deficiency**
Root	***Manifestation***	***Manifestation***
	(Bleeding causes Blood deficiency)	(Blood deficiency causes Qi deficiency)

Why do we need to identify the Root? In the course of a disease, the clinical manifestations can be very numerous and complicated and sometimes contradictory. Different clinical manifestations will appear and develop in the course of a long chronic illness; they may combine with superseding acute symptoms, interior conditions may overlap with exterior ones, Deficient conditions may coexist with Excess ones, Cold can coexist with Heat, and so on.

Identification of the Root (which need not be a single one, but could be a multiple one) allows us to understand and unravel the numerous clinical manifestations to see the underlying pattern and decide on the principle of treatment according to the condition of the patient and the character of the diseases.

There is a saying in Chinese medicine 'To treat a disease, find the Root'. This succinctly summarizes the importance of always tracing the clinical manifestations back to their Root in order to treat a disease. This is because, generally speaking, the Root is the primary aspect of the contradiction: that is, it is generally primary in relation to the clinical manifestations. As the Root is primary, treatment of the clinical manifestations is usually carried out by treating the Root.

For example, if a patient complains of acute occipital headache, a slight temperature, a stiff neck, aversion to cold, a runny nose, sneezing and a Floating-Tight pulse, all these clinical manifestations (the Manifestation) obviously point to their root (the Root), which is invasion of the Lung's Defensive Qi portion by exterior Wind-Cold. This pattern was discussed in detail in the chapter on the identification of patterns according to pathogenic factors (ch. 43; see also chs 44 and 45). In this case treatment is aimed at the Root: that is, expelling Cold, releasing the Exterior and restoring the diffusing and descending of Lung-Qi. When this is done, all the clinical manifestations will disappear.

This is a simple example as to how the various clinical manifestations form a pattern, which, when properly identified using the tools of Chinese diagnosis and pattern identification, leads us to recognize the Root and treat it accordingly. In this example, if the practitioner were not skilled in Chinese diagnosis and pattern identification and unable to identify the Root, he or she might set about treating each of the clinical manifestations individually, which would of course be wrong.

Another example: a patient suffers from a low-grade fever in the afternoon, night sweating, a feeling of heat in the palms and soles, a dry mouth at night and has a Red tongue without coating. These are the clinical manifestations that, when properly interpreted, lead us to identify their root: that is, Yin deficiency. To treat all the various clinical manifestations, it is sufficient to treat the Root (i.e. tonify Yin).

Another example: a patient has an unremitting high fever, irritability, thirst, a Rapid pulse, a Red tongue with yellow coating and very cold limbs. In this case there is a contradiction as the patient has a high fever but cold limbs. However, taking all the clinical manifestations into account, we can identify interior Heat as the Root. The correct treatment is therefore to clear interior Heat, in spite of the cold limbs. These are due to interior Heat obstructing the circulation of Yang Qi to the limbs, so that there can be the apparent paradox that the stronger the Heat, the colder the limbs.

Similar examples could be given of original patterns being the Root and deriving patterns being the Manifestation. For example, a deficiency of Spleen-Qi (Root) may give rise to Dampness (Manifestations); a deficiency of Lungs, Spleen and Kidneys (Root) may give rise to Phlegm (Manifestation); a deficiency of Kidney-Yang (Root) may produce Empty-Cold (Manifestation); Qi stagnation (Root) may give rise to Blood stasis (Manifestation); Cold in the Uterus (Root) may cause Blood stasis (Manifestation), etc.

Box 69.2 summarizes original and deriving patterns.

Box 69.2 Original and deriving patterns

Root and Manifestation

Common examples of original and deriving patterns as Root and Manifestation:

Root	*Manifestation*
Spleen-Qi deficiency	Dampness
Lungs, Spleen and Kidney deficiency	Phlegm
Kidney-Yang deficiency	Empty-Cold
Qi stagnation	Blood stasis
Cold in the Uterus	Blood stasis
Liver-Blood deficiency	Liver-Wind

In conclusion, generally speaking, the Root is primary and is treated first. However, under certain circumstances, the Manifestation can become primary and needs to be treated first, even though the ultimate aim is always to treat the Root. The decision to treat the Root or the Manifestation depends on the severity and urgency of the clinical manifestations.

There are three possible courses of action:

1. Treat the Root only
2. Treat both the Root and the Manifestation
3. Treat the Manifestation first, and the Root later

The discussion will be done under four topics:

1. Treat the Root only
2. Treat both the Root and the Manifestation
3. Treat the Manifestation first, and the Root later
4. Multiple Roots and Manifestations
   a) Multiple Roots, each giving rise to different Manifestations
   b) One Root giving rise to different Manifestations
   c) The Root coincides with the Manifestation

Treat the Root only

Generally speaking, treating the Root only is sufficient to clear all clinical manifestations in most cases. The method of treating the Root can be used in both interior or exterior as well as chronic or acute diseases. Examples of this approach have been given above: in case of Spleen-Yang deficiency (the Root) causing the previously mentioned clinical manifestations, treating the Root (i.e. tonifying and warming the Spleen) will be the correct approach, which, in time, should clear all the clinical manifestations.

Similarly, for the clinical manifestations caused by Wind-Cold or those caused by Yin deficiency, in both these cases it will be sufficient to treat the Root (i.e. expel Wind-Cold in the former case, and nourish Yin in the latter) to clear all the clinical manifestations.

Treating only the Root in cases of original and deriving patterns is done only when the clinical manifestations reflect primarily the Root (original pattern) and the clinical manifestations of the Manifestations are few and mild. For example, in case of Spleen-Qi deficiency (Root) giving rise to Dampness (Manifestation), tonifying the Spleen is enough to resolve Dampness only if the symptoms of Dampness are very mild: in most cases, attention should be given to treating the Manifestation as well, i.e. resolving Dampness.

The approach of treating the Root only is applicable in cases when the clinical manifestations are not too severe. If the clinical manifestations are severe or even life-threatening, the approach should be changed, as will be explained below.

Box 69.3 summarizes the approach of treating the Root only.

Treat both the Root and the Manifestation

This approach is widely used in practice. In chronic cases when the clinical manifestations are severe and distressing for the patient, it is necessary to treat both the Root and the Manifestation simultaneously. This approach is also applied when the clinical manifestations themselves are such that they would perpetuate the original problem. For example, in the case of a woman with Qi deficiency leading to excessive menstrual bleeding (Qi not holding Blood), prolonged menstrual bleeding over many years will in itself lead to further deficiency of both Blood and Qi.

To return to the previous example of Spleen-Yang deficiency: if this is causing very severe and debilitating diarrhoea, particularly in an elderly patient, it would be necessary to treat the Root (i.e. tonify and warm the Spleen), but at the same time also take active steps to treat the Manifestation (i.e. stop the diarrhoea). In acupuncture terms this would involve using points which are known to stop diarrhoea (whatever the cause), such as ST-25 Tianshu and ST-37 Shangjuxu. By contrast, if the diarrhoea was not so severe and the patient not old, it would be sufficient to simply treat the chronic deficiency of Spleen-Yang.

In the case of a patient suffering from Spleen-Yang deficiency causing severe oedema, the correct approach would again be to treat both the Root (i.e. tonify and warm the Spleen) and the Manifestation (i.e. eliminate the oedema). In acupuncture terms, this would involve combining the reinforcing method (to tonify the Spleen) with the reducing method (by reducing points

---

Box 69.3 Treating the Root only

In the case of original and deriving patterns, treating the Root only is applicable when the clinical manifestations of the Manifestation are few and mild

to move fluids, such as Ren-9 Shuifen, ST-28 Shuidao and BL-22 Sanjiaoshu).

In the case of a child who has severe whooping cough caused by Phlegm-Heat in the Lungs, it would be necessary again to adopt the method of treating both the Root (by clearing Lung-Heat and resolving Phlegm) and the Manifestation (by stopping the cough). This is the correct approach since the cough is very distressing and debilitating to the child, so it would be wrong to simply treat the Root and wait for the symptoms to improve. This example can be compared and contrasted with a case of a chronic slight dry cough caused by Yin deficiency, in which case the cough is not bad or serious enough to warrant treating the Manifestation.

In the case of original and deriving patterns, treating both the Root and the Manifestation simultaneously is a strategy that is applied very often and it is indeed the most common strategy. For example, if Spleen-Qi deficiency (Root) gives rise to Dampness (Manifestation) one usually tonifies Spleen-Qi and resolves Dampness simultaneously.

However, please note that when we treat both the Root and the Manifestation with herbal medicine, it is not a case of giving 50% of herbs for the Root and 50% for the Manifestation. We still need to make a conscious choice between a formula that treats the Root (e.g. tonify the Spleen) and one that treats the Manifestation (e.g. resolve Dampness).

With herbal medicine, treating both Root and Manifestation means that we choose a formula that treats one or the other and we then modify it. In the example given, formulae that tonify the Spleen are very different from those that resolve Dampness. For example, if we choose to treat the Root, we might use Liu Jun Zi Tang *Six Gentlemen Decoction* that tonifies Spleen-Qi; if we choose to treat the Manifestation, we might use Huo Po Xia Ling Tang *Agastache–Magnolia–Pinellia–Poria Decoction*. In either case, we would then modify the formula by adding herbs that resolve Dampness to the former and herbs that tonify the Spleen to the latter.

With acupuncture, the approach is different because acupuncture works in a different way. Acupuncture points have a broader and more 'neutral' action. The same acupuncture point may tonify the Spleen and resolve Dampness and Ren-12 Zhongwan would be a good example of this.

Box 69.4 summarizes the approach of treating the Root and the Manifestation at the same time.

> **Box 69.4 Treating the Root and the Manifestation simultaneously**
>
> Treating the Root and the Manifestation simultaneously is a strategy that is applied very often whenever the Manifestation produces severe symptoms and signs

> **Box 69.5 Treating the Manifestation first and the Root later**
>
> The strategy of treating the Manifestation first and the Root later is applied when the former is producing severe and distressing symptoms which need to be addressed urgently, often in acute cases

Treat the Manifestation first and the Root later

Under certain circumstances the Root becomes secondary and the Manifestation needs to be treated first, and usually urgently too. This approach is applicable in all cases when the clinical manifestations are very severe or even life-threatening: this is especially common in acute cases.

For example, a patient has a productive cough with profuse watery sputum, breathlessness, chilliness, a thick sticky coating and a Slippery pulse. The clinical manifestations reflect Spleen-Yang deficiency (the Root) causing retention of Phlegm in the Lungs (the Manifestation). In this case, if the clinical manifestations are severe and acute (particularly in an elderly person), the correct approach is to deal with the Manifestation first, by resolving Phlegm and stimulating the descending of Lung-Qi. Later, when the symptoms of Phlegm have subsided, one can treat the Root (i.e. tonify and warm the Spleen).

Another example: a woman suffering from dysmenorrhoea caused by stasis of Blood, itself caused by deficiency of Qi. In this case, the correct approach is to concentrate on treating the Manifestation (i.e. move Blood and stop pain) before or during the period, and treating the Root (i.e. tonify Qi) just after and in between periods.

Box 69.5 summarizes the approach of treating the Manifestation first and the Root later.

Multiple Roots and Manifestations

So far, fairly simple examples have been given when only one Root gives rise to one Manifestation. In reality, however, actual clinical cases are often more complex. There can be more than one Root as well as more than one Manifestation.

There are three possible situations:

1. Multiple Roots, each giving rise to different Manifestations
2. One Root giving rise to different Manifestations
3. The Root coincides with the Manifestation

Multiple Roots, each giving rise to different Manifestations

It is very common to have more than one Root. This is due to the fact that, in the course of one's life, several different causes of disease occurring at different times may overlap. For example, a previous trauma to a joint may predispose someone to subsequent invasion of exterior Cold and Dampness in that joint. Or someone may suffer from a Liver disharmony caused by dietary reasons and later on in life develop Liver-Yang rising from repressed anger. Thus there can be different Roots, each reflected in various different Manifestations.

For example, a patient may have Liver-Fire (the Root) caused by certain emotional problems over a long period of time. Later on, he or she may be exposed to Cold, invading the channels of the shoulder and causing pain and stiffness. In this case there are two separate roots, one being Liver-Fire (caused by emotional problems), the other being exterior Cold invading the shoulder channels (caused by exposure to exterior Cold). It would be wrong then in this case to try and interpret all the clinical manifestations in the light of one Root only, such as Liver-Fire. As for the treatment, when there is more than one Root, each one must be treated.

Of course, there is often an interaction between two separate Roots. In the above example, if a person suffers from Liver-Fire, if he or she suffers an invasion of Wind leading to Painful Obstruction Syndrome (*Bi* Syndrome), he or she will be more likely to develop Damp-Heat in the joints.

Another example: a patient may suffer from Kidney-Yang deficiency (the Root) caused by excessive sexual activity. Later in life he also suffers from stagnation of Liver-Qi (another Root) caused by emotional problems. In this case there are two separate Roots (Kidney-Yang deficiency and Liver-Qi stagnation) from two different causes, and it would be wrong to try and weave all the clinical manifestations into a common pattern.

> **Box 69.6 Multiple Roots**
>
> - Multiple Roots, each giving rise to different Manifestations
> - One Root giving rise to different Manifestations
> - The Root coincides with the Manifestation

Of course the different Roots often do not coexist independently as in the above examples, but may also interact with one another, further complicating the picture. For instance, in the example just given, the stagnant Liver-Qi may invade the Spleen and cause Spleen-Yang deficiency, which would further aggravate the Kidney-Yang deficiency.

One Root giving rise to different Manifestations

One Root can give rise to several different Manifestations. For example, if a patient (particularly a woman) suffers from Spleen-Qi deficiency, this can give rise to oedema (because Spleen-Qi is unable to transport and transform fluids) and also to deficiency of Blood (because the Spleen is unable to make Blood). There will therefore be two Manifestations (the oedema and the deficiency of Blood) arising from the same Root. The treatment in this case is still simply directed at treating the Root.

The Root coincides with the Manifestation

In certain cases the Root and the Manifestation coincide. This can happen only when the clinical manifestations are caused by external physical trauma, such as in an accident. For example, if a person has an accident to the knee, this will cause stagnation of Qi and/or Blood in the knee channels leading to pain. In this case, the stagnation of Qi (the Root) coincides with the knee pain (the Manifestation).

Box 69.6 summarizes manifestations with multiple Roots.

WHEN TO TONIFY UPRIGHT QI, WHEN TO EXPEL PATHOGENIC FACTORS

The question of whether to tonify the body's Qi or to expel pathogenic factors is the second important question to consider when working out a plan of treatment and it is one that is absolutely crucial. We may be very skilled at diagnosis and at identifying the patterns with great clinical acumen, but if the treatment strategy is wrong, all our skill will come to nothing and the patient will not get better and, in some cases, he or she may get worse. The strategic question of whether to tonify the body's Qi or expel pathogenic factors is closely related to the choice of actual method of treatment: that is, whether to tonify (reinforce in acupuncture) or to reduce, so that the two can be discussed together.

The following case history will illustrate this point.

Case history 69.2

A 48-year-old woman had been suffering from asthma for a long time. She had clear symptoms of Spleen-Yang deficiency (tiredness, loose stools, Weak pulse, Pale tongue) and of Kidney-Yang deficiency (backache, frequent pale urination). The deficiency of Yang of the Spleen and Kidneys led to the formation of Damp-Phlegm, which obstructed the Lungs, causing breathlessness, a feeling of oppression of the chest and a cough with expectoration of sticky sputum. The asthma was caused both by the failure of Lung-Qi to descend and of Kidney-Yang to receive Qi.

The patient used two inhalers: *Becotide* (cortisone) and *Ventolin*.

The strategy of treatment adopted was to concentrate on eliminating pathogenic factors (i.e. resolve Phlegm) with herbal treatment and to both tonify the body's Qi (i.e. tonify Spleen- and Kidney-Yang) and resolve Phlegm with acupuncture. I used points such as ST-36, SP-6, KI-7, Ren-12 and BL-23 to tonify Spleen- and Kidney-Yang also with the use of moxa; and points such as LU-5, LU-7 and BL-13 to restore the descending of Lung-Qi.

As for the herbal treatment, I used a *Three Treasures* remedy called *Limpid Sea* (a variation of Er Chen Tang) to resolve Phlegm and another called *Clear Qi* (a variation of Su Zi Jiang Qi Tang) to restore the descending of Lung-Qi. I did not administer any herbal tonics of Spleen- and Kidney-Yang.

I treated her along these lines for several months with excellent results as her asthma improved greatly even after stopping her medication. After about a year, as her asthma and cough had greatly improved and the sputum reduced, I decided that it was time to turn the attention from resolving Phlegm to tonifying the body's Qi (i.e. tonify Spleen- and Kidney-Yang). I therefore asked her to stop taking *Limpid Sea* (which resolves Phlegm) and *Clear Qi* (which restores the descending of Lung-Qi) and prescribed *Strengthen the Root* instead (a variation of You Gui Wan) to tonify Kidney-Yang. In only 1 day she got much worse, her asthma returned and she could hardly breathe. This is a very good example of how the treatment might be 'right' in terms of pattern identification but wrong in terms of strategy and principle of treatment.

In this case, it would have been better not to switch the emphasis of treatment from tonifying the body's Qi to expelling pathogenic factors: the correct strategy would have been to expel pathogenic factor and tonify the body's Qi simultaneously.

'Upright Qi' (*Zheng Qi*) is not a particular type of Qi but simply the sum total of all of the body's Qi, mostly in relation to its capacity to fight pathogenic factors. Upright Qi could therefore also be described as the body's resistance to disease. It is a term which is used only in relation and in contrast to pathogenic factors.

Pathogenic factors (in Chinese called '*Xie*', which means 'evil') indicate any disease factor, whether exterior (such as external Wind, Dampness, Cold, Heat) or interior (such as Phlegm, Fire, interior Wind, interior Cold, stasis of Blood or stagnation of Qi).

An Excess (or Full) condition is characterized by the presence of a pathogenic factor, whether interior or exterior, while the Upright Qi is still relatively intact and fights the pathogenic factor.

A Deficient condition is characterized by weakness of the Upright Qi and the absence of a pathogenic factor.

A mixed Deficient/Excess condition is characterized by weakness of the Upright Qi, but also by the presence of a pathogenic factor. Although there is a pathogenic factor, the Upright Qi is weak and does not react adequately or successfully to the pathogenic factor. This is a very common situation in practice, probably more common than a purely Excess condition (Table 69.1 and Box 69.7).

All the various pathological changes and developments of a disease can be seen as various stages in the struggle between the Upright Qi and pathogenic factors. All the numerous changes, improvements and aggravations are due to fluctuations in the relative strength of the Upright Qi and pathogenic factors.

Table 69.1 Definition of Full and Empty conditions

	Zheng Qi	Pathogenic factor
Full	Zheng Qi intact, fighting pathogenic factor	Pathogenic factor present
Empty	Zheng Qi weak	No pathogenic factor
Full/Empty	Zheng Qi compromised, fighting pathogenic factor weakly	Pathogenic factor present

> **Box 69.7 Full and Empty patterns**
>
> - A Full condition is characterized by the presence of a pathogenic factor, whether interior or exterior, while the Upright Qi is still relatively intact and fights the pathogenic factor
> - An Empty condition is characterized by weakness of the Upright Qi and the absence of a pathogenic factor
> - A mixed Full/Empty condition is characterized by weakness of the Upright Qi, but also by the presence of a pathogenic factor. Although there is a pathogenic factor, the Upright Qi is weak and does not react adequately or successfully to the pathogenic factor

When planning a treatment it is essential to have a clear idea as to the relative strengths of Upright Qi and pathogenic factors, or whether there is a pathogenic factor at all. This is important in order to adopt the correct strategy of treatment. The main question is whether the condition calls for tonification of the Upright Qi, or expulsion of pathogenic factors, or both. If both are required, should they be applied simultaneously or in succession, and if so, which one should be applied first?

In order to answer these questions we can consider three possible approaches:

1. Tonify Upright Qi
2. Expel the pathogenic factors
3. Tonify Upright Qi and expel the pathogenic factors

In this last case there are still three possible courses of action:

1. First tonify Upright Qi, then expel the pathogenic factors
2. First expel the pathogenic factors, then tonify Upright Qi
3. Tonify Upright Qi and expel the pathogenic factors simultaneously

It should be noted that although in many cases the Root (*Ben*) coincides with a deficiency and the Manifestation (*Biao*) with a pathogenic factor, this is by no means always so. The case of a deficiency of Spleen-Qi (Root) leading to Dampness (Manifestations) or that of Liver-Blood deficiency (Root) leading to Liver-Yang rising (Manifestations) are common examples in which the Root is a Deficient pattern and the Manifestation an Excess one.

However, there are many cases when this is not so. An exterior invasion of a pathogenic factor is an obvious example in which the Root (e.g. external Wind) is a Full condition. In the case of Cold invading the Uterus and causing Blood stasis, both the Root (Cold) and the Manifestation (Blood stasis) are Full. Finally, a Full-type Manifestation can itself become a Root. Phlegm is a common example of this as Phlegm itself is a Full-type Manifestation deriving from a Deficient Root (Spleen and Kidney deficiency). After a prolonged time, Phlegm itself can become a cause of further pathology and therefore turn into a Root.

Tonify Upright Qi (*Zheng Qi*)

'Tonifying the Upright Qi' includes any method that strengthens the body condition and increases resistance to disease. This may be achieved with acupuncture, herbal treatment, exercise, diet, *Qi Gong*, meditation or often simply rest. More specifically, from the acupuncture point of view, it implies tonification of Qi, Blood, Yin, Yang, Essence (*Jing*) and Original Qi (*Yuan Qi*), by use of the reinforcing method of needling or moxibustion.

The strategy of tonifying the Upright Qi is applicable when this is weak, or more specifically, in purely Empty patterns: that is, when the Upright Qi is deficient and there are no pathogenic factors. This approach can also be used in mixed Deficiency/Excess patterns but only if the pattern is predominantly Deficient. In such a case tonifying Upright Qi strengthens Qi so that it can eliminate any pathogenic factor that there might be. Hence the saying: 'Support Upright Qi to eliminate pathogenic factors'.

It must be stressed, however, that this approach is applicable only if a mixed Deficient/Excess pattern is predominantly Deficient. If, on the contrary, there is a strong pathogenic factor, tonifying Upright Qi may not only fail to eliminate it, but, actually, in certain cases, even reinforce it and make the condition worse. This is more likely to happen when herbal medicine, rather than acupuncture, is used (see below).

The approach of tonifying Upright Qi is applicable only in interior conditions, as exterior conditions are by definition of the Excess type, being characterized by the presence of an exterior pathogenic factor. Only in very few cases of exterior conditions is it necessary to combine expelling the pathogenic factor with tonifying Upright Qi. This will be discussed later within this chapter.

Examples of purely Deficient patterns, when the approach of tonifying Upright Qi is applicable, are Spleen-Qi deficiency (manifesting with lack of appetite, tiredness, loose stools and an Empty pulse) or Blood deficiency (manifesting with dizziness, blurred vision, poor memory, scanty periods, a Choppy pulse and a Pale tongue).

An example of a mixed Deficiency/Excess pattern, but predominantly Deficient, might be that of Stomach and/or Spleen deficiency allowing themselves to be invaded by Liver-Qi (manifesting with tiredness, no appetite, loose stools, an Empty pulse, a slight dull epigastric pain and slight nausea). The last two symptoms are due to stagnant Liver-Qi invading the Stomach. In this case, however, it is not that Liver-Qi invades the Stomach, but rather that Stomach-Qi is weak and allows itself to be invaded by Liver-Qi. This is borne out by the prevalence of Deficiency symptoms and signs. In this case, the correct course of action is to tonify the Stomach, so that when this is strengthened, Liver-Qi will not be able to invade it.

In mixed Full–Empty conditions in which the Emptiness predominates and therefore tonification of the Upright Qi is called for, the pulse is an important factor in the determination of the correct treatment principle. In fact, the strength of the pulse is an important factor in deciding the relative importance of the Deficiency or the Excess. For example, in the example given above of deficient Stomach and Spleen being invaded by stagnant Liver-Qi, an Empty or Weak pulse indicates that the Deficiency predominates; if the pulse were Wiry and Full, it would indicate that the Excess (i.e. Liver-Qi stagnation) predominates.

> **Box 69.8 Tonify Upright Qi**
>
> The strategy of tonifying the Upright Qi is applicable when this is weak, or more specifically, in purely Empty patterns, i.e. when the Upright Qi is deficient and there are no pathogenic factors

Box 69.8 summarizes the approach of tonifying Upright Qi.

Expel the pathogenic factors

'Expelling pathogenic factors' includes any method that eliminates pathogenic factors, whether exterior or interior. This might be acupuncture, herbal treatment, massage or cupping.

From acupuncture's point of view, it involves eliminating the pathogenic factors by using the reducing method, bleeding or cupping.

This approach is applicable only in purely Excess patterns characterized by the presence of an exterior or interior pathogenic factor. Expelling the pathogenic factor will remove any obstruction caused by it and will indirectly contribute to strengthening Upright Qi (because it can circulate unhampered by the obstruction of the pathogenic factors). Hence the saying: 'Eliminate the pathogenic factors to strengthen Upright Qi'. In my experience, this is very true in practice as I have seen over and over again how expelling pathogenic factors improves a person's Qi and, contrary to what one might think, gives patients more energy.

> **Clinical note**
>
> Expelling pathogenic factors often produces an increase in a patient's energy as his or her Qi flows unencumbered by obstructions

It is important to note that the decision to expel a pathogenic factor by using a reducing method must be based purely on the Excess character of the pattern and not on subjective feelings about the patient. We should not '*translate subjective emotional feelings into a desire to tonify or sedate*'.[1] In other words, if the pattern identification is correct and the pattern is definitely of an Excess character, a reducing method is called for, even if the patient might be elderly or apparently weak. If the pattern is of an Excess character and the pathogenic factor is expelled, the patient will feel better and have more energy because the obstruction of the pathogenic factor is removed.

This is especially true in exterior conditions, when it is necessary to use the reducing method to expel the exterior pathogenic factor. Were the reinforcing method used to tonify Qi, the patient would become worse because tonifying Qi in acute exterior conditions tends also to 'tonify' the pathogenic factor, and thus aggravate the situation. For example, if a patient has symptoms of an attack of Wind-Cold (such as an aversion to cold, a runny nose, sneezing, a stiff neck, and a Floating-Tight pulse), this is an Excess condition, even though the person might have suffered from deficiency of Qi or Blood previous to the exterior attack.

This condition is therefore treated by expelling the pathogenic factor, in this case Wind-Cold. We can later attend to the underlying deficiency and tonify Qi and Blood, but only after the pathogenic factor has been expelled completely. Of course, in a few cases, when the patient is extremely weak and debilitated, it might be necessary to combine the reducing method to expel the pathogenic factor, with the reinforcing method to tonify Qi. This is, however, rarely necessary and it will be discussed under the next heading.

Another example of an Excess pattern, in this case interior, which requires treatment by the method of expelling pathogenic factors, is that of Liver-Fire, with symptoms and signs such as thirst, red eyes, a red face, a bitter taste, constipation, dark urine, headaches, irritability, a Red tongue with yellow coating and a Rapid and Wiry pulse.

Please note that the method of expelling pathogenic factors may also be applied in mixed Full–Empty conditions. I would do this when the pathogenic factors are strong and are causing most of the clinical manifestations. In addition, I would do this only in the beginning of the treatment to rid the body of pathogenic factors so that it will be easier to tonify the Upright Qi later.

For example, if we see a patient suffering from chronic fatigue syndrome with a very pronounced Dampness in the digestive system and the muscles and a Spleen deficiency but with most of the clinical manifestations caused by the Dampness, I would start the treatment by giving him or her a herbal prescription to eliminate Dampness. After some weeks of this treatment, I would then also tonify the Spleen.

Box 69.9 summarizes the approach of expelling pathogenic factors.

> **Box 69.9 Expelling pathogenic factors**
>
> The strategy of expelling pathogenic factors is applicable only in purely Excess patterns characterized by the presence of an exterior or interior pathogenic factor

Tonify Upright Qi and expel the pathogenic factors

Tonifying the Upright Qi and expelling pathogenic factors includes three possibilities:

> 1. First tonify Upright Qi, then expel the pathogenic factors
> 2. First expel the pathogenic factors, then tonify Upright Qi
> 3. Tonify Upright Qi and expel the pathogenic factors simultaneously

First tonify Upright Qi, then expel the pathogenic factors

This approach is used when there is a pathogenic factor to be expelled, but the Upright Qi is too weak to use a reducing method, as this would weaken it further. This situation is, however, rather rare and applies only to exterior patterns, when a very weak and possibly elderly person has been attacked by an exterior pathogenic factor and Upright Qi is extremely weak. In this situation it is not possible to expel the pathogenic factor as the reducing method might further weaken Upright Qi. One can therefore first tonify Upright Qi, and then expel the pathogenic factor.

For example, if a very weak elderly person with chronic bronchitis has an attack of Wind-Cold one could tonify Qi first, and then expel Wind-Cold. This approach, however, is seldom necessary and is not widely applied.

It must be noted here that tonifying Upright Qi alone is not sufficient to expel the pathogenic factor.

This approach does not apply to interior conditions, as in these cases one can tonify the body's Qi and expel the pathogenic factor simultaneously.

Box 69.10 summarizes the approach of first tonifying Upright Qi, then expelling the pathogenic factors.

First expel the pathogenic factors, then tonify Upright Qi

This approach is suitable when there is a pathogenic factor and Upright Qi is weak, but eliminating the

> **Box 69.10 First tonify Upright Qi, then expel pathogenic factors**
>
> Tonifying the Upright Qi before expelling pathogenic factors is used in interior and exterior conditions when the patient's Qi is very depleted. It is a rarely used strategy

pathogenic factor is called for due to the urgency or severity of the clinical manifestations. This approach is also used because tonifying Upright Qi alone can in certain cases also stimulate the pathogenic factor.

This strategy is widely used in clinical practice both in exterior and interior conditions. In fact, when there is a pathogenic factor and the body's Qi is weak, this is the standard procedure to adopt, apart from a few rare cases already mentioned. It is important to stress that if the diagnosis and identification of patterns is correct and elimination of pathogenic factors is called for, eliminating pathogenic factors will not 'weaken' the patient.

We can expel the pathogenic factor first using the reducing method (with acupuncture). Once the pathogenic factor is expelled and the Excess-type clinical manifestations have gone, only then can we tonify Upright Qi. This approach is applicable in both exterior and interior conditions, but particularly in exterior ones. When tonifying the Upright Qi, we should pay attention that there is no pathogenic factor left.

Exterior patterns

In exterior patterns this is generally the approach adopted. For example, if a patient previously suffering from deficiency of Qi is attacked by exterior Wind-Heat and has symptoms of fever, headache, slight sweating, aversion to cold, body aches and Floating-Rapid pulse, the correct approach would be to expel Wind-Heat and release the Exterior (by reducing such points as L.I.-4 Hegu, L.I.-11 Quchi or T.B.-5 Waiguan).

When the exterior symptoms have totally gone (no fever, no body aches, no aversion to cold, no Floating pulse), only then can one tonify the Upright Qi. Tonifying the Upright Qi before the Wind-Heat has been expelled can somehow stimulate the Wind-Heat too and lead to a worsening of the condition. For example, the fever might rise.

It is also important to pay attention to this point even when a fairly long time has elapsed after an exterior attack. In certain cases, if the exterior pathogenic factor is not expelled properly, it can penetrate the Interior and lurk there for a long time after the initial attack. To continue with the previous example of attack of Wind-Heat, the person would find it difficult to recover from the attack, experience great tiredness and become prone to strange recurrent sore throats: these would be due to some remaining Heat 'lurking' in the Interior.

In Chinese this is called 'residual pathogenic factor'. In these cases it is important to be able to recognize it and clear the remaining Heat before tonifying the Upright Qi, as normally one would tend to tonify the Upright Qi straight away since the person would complain of great tiredness.

Symptoms and signs of 'residual pathogenic factor' after an exterior attack would be tiredness, a feeling of heat, recurrent sore throats, a Red tongue with a thin yellow coating in the area between the tip and the centre (Lung area) and a slightly Rapid pulse. In this case we could use points to clear interior Heat such as LU-5 Chize, L.I.-11 Quchi or Du-14 Dazhui.

Interior patterns

In interior patterns the strategy of expelling pathogenic factors first and tonifying the Upright Qi later is used whenever the symptoms caused by the pathogenic factors are severe so that they need to be dealt with. A very common example of such a situation is postviral fatigue syndrome.

In this disease, there is always an underlying deficiency but also usually Dampness: it is the Dampness that causes the tiredness, feeling of heaviness, digestive symptoms and muscle ache. In my experience, it is nearly always necessary to start the treatment by resolving Dampness without tonifying the Upright Qi: this approach applies particularly if herbal treatment is given.

Another example: a patient with a chronic Kidney- and Heart-Yang deficiency suffers an acute episode of total retention of urine leading to hypertension and oedema. In this case the pathogenic factor is 'Water overflowing', causing oedema and retention of urine. Since this needs to be dealt with without delay, one must first expel the pathogenic factor, in this case 'Water overflowing', by using a reducing method (on points such as SP-9 Yinlingquan, ST-28 Shuidao, Ren-9 Shuifen, Ren-5 Shimen, BL-39 Weiyang and BL-22 Sanjiaoshu) as the Lower Burner is in an Excess condition. After the oedema is resolved and the

> **Box 69.11 First expel the pathogenic factors, then tonify Upright Qi**
>
> Expelling pathogenic factors first before tonifying the Upright Qi is used when the clinical manifestations of pathogenic factors are pronounced and causing painful and/or distressing symptoms. It is a widely used strategy in interior and exterior conditions

> **Box 69.12 Tonify Upright Qi and expel the pathogenic factors simultaneously**
>
> The strategy of tonifying the Upright Qi and expelling pathogenic factors simultaneously is used when the Upright Qi is deficient and pathogenic factors are evident but not so much as to require expelling before tonifying the Upright Qi

urinary function restored, one can tonify Kidney- and Heart-Yang.

Another example: a patient with a chronic condition of Liver-Blood deficiency has an acute episode of Liver-Wind causing a temporary spasm of a cerebral vessel and a small stroke, with temporary giddiness, numbness, paralysis of mouth and slurred speech. In this case, it is essential to eliminate the pathogenic factor first (i.e. the Liver-Wind) by using the reducing method (on points such as LIV-3 Taichong). Only when Liver-Wind has been extinguished and the symptoms of it are gone can we tonify Liver-Blood.

The strategy of expelling pathogenic factors before tonifying the Upright Qi is not only applicable in acute and urgent cases such as those mentioned above but also in chronic cases where the symptoms do not have a character of urgency but are, nevertheless, distressing and painful.

For example, a patient may suffer from a chronic deficiency of Liver- and Kidney-Yin leading to the rising of Liver-Yang. This would cause severe headaches as well as dizziness, irritability, and so on. Although the symptoms are not acute or urgent, the headaches may, nevertheless, be extremely painful and distressing. It is therefore necessary to subdue Liver-Yang first, and then tonify Liver- and Kidney-Yin.

In conclusion, in interior patterns the strategy of expelling pathogenic factors first and tonifying the Upright Qi later is very widely used. In particular, I prefer to use this strategy in cases of Dampness, Phlegm and Blood stasis.

Box 69.11 summarizes the approach of first expelling the pathogenic factors, then tonifying Upright Qi.

Tonify the Upright Qi and expel the pathogenic factors simultaneously

This is a widely used approach in cases when there is a pathogenic factor and the Upright Qi is relatively weak, but not so weak as to need to be tonified first (as in the first case above).

This approach can be used only in interior conditions, as in exterior conditions it is usually necessary to expel the pathogenic factor first and then tonify the Upright Qi.

Thus, this strategy is used in cases of mixed Deficiency/Excess interior patterns. Many examples could be given. If there is a condition of Liver-Yin deficiency with rising of Liver-Yang, one can simultaneously tonify Liver-Yin and subdue Liver-Yang. In case of Spleen-Qi deficiency leading to the formation of Dampness, one can tonify Spleen-Qi and resolve Dampness at the same time.

From the acupuncture point of view, this involves using the reinforcing method on some points and the reducing method on others. In the two above examples, one could tonify KI-3 Taixi, SP-6 Sanyinjiao and LIV-8 Ququan to nourish Liver-Yin and reduce LIV-3 Taichong and G.B.-43 Xiaxi to subdue Liver-Yang. In case of Spleen deficiency with Dampness, one could tonify BL-20 Pishu and ST-36 Zusanli to tonify Spleen-Qi and reduce SP-9 Yinlingquan and SP-6 Sanyinjiao to eliminate Dampness.

Box 69.12 summarizes the approach of tonifying Upright Qi and expelling the pathogenic factors simultaneously.

DIFFERENCES BETWEEN ACUPUNCTURE AND HERBAL THERAPY IN THE APPLICATION OF THE TREATMENT PRINCIPLE

We have so far discussed the treatment principle and methods without differentiating between acupuncture and herbal therapy. However, there are important differences in the way acupuncture and herbal therapy work, especially in the way they tonify the Upright Qi and expel pathogenic factors.

Herbal therapy works by ingesting herbs which have a direct, internal influence on the body's physiology and pathology. For examples, herbs that drain Dampness via urination (such as Fu Ling *Poria*) are actual diuretics. Herbal medicines are plant drugs that have specific characteristics: that is, a determinate flavour or taste and 'temperature' or nature.

The five tastes are sour, bitter, sweet, pungent and salty and the nature of the herbs can be hot, warm, cold or cool. The combination of a taste and nature produces specific effects on the body's physiology. For example, pungent cold herbs will clear Heat, expelling it outwards, bitter cold herbs drain Fire with a downward movement, sweet cold herbs nourish Yin, sweet warm herbs tonify Qi and Yang, etc.

Table 69.2 compares the five tastes of herbs.

The nature and taste of the herbs has to be carefully balanced and adapted to the patient's condition, bearing in mind also possible side-effects. For example, although bitter cold herbs are called for to expel Damp-Heat, we should bear in mind that the continued administration of bitter cold herbs may injure the Spleen. Similarly, pungent herbs are called for to move Qi and Blood, but their continued administration may eventually injure Qi and Yin.

Conversely, in order to tonify the Upright Qi, we need to use sweet herbs (cool to nourish Yin and warm to tonify Qi and Yang): the prolonged use of sweet herbs may tend to give rise to some Dampness. For this reason, tonic prescriptions often include one or two herbs with a pungent taste to move Qi.

By contrast, acupuncture works in a completely different way as no substances are ingested. To tonify the Upright Qi, acupuncture stimulates the Qi of the Internal Organs to work better and therefore produce Qi and Blood; to expel pathogenic factors, acupuncture works mainly by moving Qi of various organs.

For example, in order to resolve Phlegm, acupuncture relies on the stimulation of Qi of the Lungs, Spleen, Kidneys and Triple Burner so that fluids are transformed, transported and excreted. In contrast, herbal medicine resolves Phlegm by the ingestion of herbs that have a drying nature and physically dry up Phlegm (and for this reason, their prolonged use may tend to injure Yin).

Therefore, when tonifying the Upright Qi, acupuncture does not tend to cause Dampness in the way that herbal tonics may do; when expelling pathogenic factors, acupuncture does not damage Blood or Yin in the way that certain herbs may do.

To sum up, when tonifying the Upright Qi and expelling pathogenic factors, herbal medicine may have certain side-effects that acupuncture generally does not have.

With particular regard to the alternative treatment strategies of tonifying the Upright Qi versus expelling pathogenic factors, herbal therapy needs to be carefully evaluated. Many of the potential pitfalls mentioned above apply to herbal therapy more than acupuncture.

For example, the choice as to whether we should tonify the Upright Qi or expel pathogenic factors acquires particular importance when herbal medicine is used. In fact, if we wrongly tonify the Upright Qi, we wrongly use sweet herbs which may tend to create Dampness and even 'tonify' the pathogenic factors; if we wrongly expel pathogenic factors, we wrongly use bitter, pungent or salty herbs which may injure the Spleen or damage Yin or Blood.

This problem does not arise so much with acupuncture as, even when we use the reinforcing method to tonify the Upright Qi, the very insertion of a needle in a channel produces a movement of Qi and Blood so that there is no danger that such tonification may give rise to Dampness. Conversely, when we use acupuncture to expel pathogenic factors, there is no danger of injuring Blood, Yin or the Spleen.

Also, acupuncture tends to be more self-balancing and 'neutral' than herbal medicine and therefore the potential for side-effects is much less. Moreover, many acupuncture points would simultaneously tonify Qi and expel pathogenic factors. For example, the point Ren-12 Zhongwan tonifies the Spleen and Stomach but it also resolves Dampness.

Table 69.2 The five tastes of herbs

Taste	Effect	Side-effect
Sour	Astringent	Make Phlegm worse
Bitter	Clear, drain, dry	Injure Spleen, injure Yin
Sweet	Tonify	Create Dampness
Pungent	Move, disperse	Injure Yin
Salty	Purge, soften	Injure fluids

Case history 69.3 – Man, age 44

Clinical manifestations
This man had been suffering from headaches for a long time, on either temple. The ache was intense and of a stabbing character; there was occasionally vomiting, numbness of the right arm and thirst. He also suffered from tinnitus of the left ear for 3 years with a low-pitched sound. His sleep was not good as he often woke up and was unable to fall asleep again.
Pulse: Wiry, especially on the left side.
Tongue: body colour normal, sides slightly pale.

Diagnosis
Liver-Blood deficiency with Liver-Yang rising.

Explanation
The symptoms of Liver-Blood deficiency are numbness of the right arm, Pale tongue-sides and insomnia. The symptoms of Liver-Yang rising are intense temporal headache, vomiting, tinnitus and a Wiry pulse.

Treatment principle
This is a Deficient, interior pattern. Deficiency of Liver-Blood is the Root as it is the primary aspect of the condition, and Liver-Yang rising is the Manifestation.

In this case we need to tonify Upright Qi (i.e. nourish Liver-Blood) and to expel the pathogenic factor (i.e. subdue Liver-Yang). Here we treat the Root and the Manifestation simultaneously as the symptoms are severe and distressing. Had the patient had more symptoms of Liver-Blood deficiency and only slight occasional headaches, treating only the Root (i.e. nourishing Liver-Blood) might have been sufficient.

Case history 69.4 – Woman, age 35

Clinical manifestations
Prior to the initial consultation this patient had had a very heavy cold with a congested chest, an occipital headache and alternating feelings of heat and cold. When she came for the consultation she complained of a feeling of exhaustion, alternating feelings of heat and cold, slight depression, a slight hypochondrial pain and loose stools.
Pulse: Wiry.
Tongue: body colour normal, thin white coating in the Lung area.

Diagnosis
This was originally an attack of exterior Wind-Cold at the Lesser Yang stage; now it is still at the Lesser Yang stage, but combined with the Greater Yin stage (see ch. 44).

Explanation
The symptoms of the Lesser Yang pattern are alternating feeling of heat and cold, hypochondrial pain, slight depression and a Wiry pulse. The symptoms of the Greater Yin pattern are exhaustion and loose stools.

Although this patient was seen 3 weeks after the onset, the pattern was still partially at the Lesser Yang stage, and the pulse was all important in the diagnosis. Since this was Wiry and Full, it indicated that the pattern was still primarily of an Excess character, even though the patient felt very tired, which is a Deficiency symptom.

Treatment principle
Since the pattern is still primarily of an Excess nature and is characterized by the presence of a pathogenic factor (Wind-Cold turned into Heat at the Lesser Yang stage), the correct approach is to concentrate on expelling the pathogenic factor, even though the patient feels tired. When the pathogenic factor has been expelled, one can tonify the Upright Qi, in this case Spleen-Qi.

This was the plan of treatment adopted and in the first treatment T.B.-5 Waiguan, T.B.-6 Zhigou and Du-14 Dazhui were needled with reducing method, to clear Heat and regulate the Lesser Yang. Reducing these points produced a nearly immediate and dramatic improvement including the return of her energy. After reducing similar points again in the second treatment and the disappearance of the Lesser Yang symptoms (hypochondrial pain and Wiry pulse), attention was diverted to tonifying the body's Qi, reinforcing LU-9 Taiyuan, SP-6 Sanyinjiao, ST-36 Zusanli and P-6 Neiguan.

This is an example of the principle of expelling a pathogenic factor first and tonifying the Upright Qi later. From the point of view of Root and Manifestation, the Root is represented by the Heat which is half in the Interior and half in the Exterior (Lesser Yang stage), producing the various clinical manifestations. In this case, only the Root was treated, clearing all the clinical manifestations.

Case history 69.5 – Woman, age 38

Clinical manifestations
This woman had suffered from hypochondrial pain on the right side and a feeling of a 'lump' in the right abdominal region for a long time. In addition, she also suffered from diarrhoea if she ate too many cold and raw foods. For the last year she sweated slightly at night. Her urination was frequent and pale, she felt very cold all the time and the menstrual blood had clots but was not dark.
Pulse: Deep-Weak-Minute.
Tongue: Pale on the sides, Bluish-Purple on the root and centre.

Diagnosis
Long-standing Liver-Blood deficiency giving rise to slight Yin deficiency (just starting) and causing stasis of Blood.

There is also a Kidney-Yang deficiency causing interior Cold and stasis of Blood in the Lower Burner.

Explanation
This is a complicated situation. There are two Roots, each of them giving rise to two Manifestations.

The first Root is the chronic deficiency of Liver-Blood as manifested in the pale sides of the tongue. This gives rise to a slight deficiency of Yin (night sweating) and also to stasis of Blood (feeling of a lump in the abdomen, clots in the menstrual blood and Purple colour of the tongue on the root and centre).

The second Root is Kidney-Yang deficiency (feeling cold, diarrhoea from cold and raw foods, frequent pale urination and Deep-Minute pulse), causing interior Cold and stasis of Blood in the Lower Burner (tongue body Purple). In this case, therefore, the stasis of Blood can be attributed both to the chronic deficiency of Liver-Blood and to the obstruction from interior Cold. For this reason, the tongue is Bluish-Purple. The bluish colour indicates Cold while the Purple colour indicates stasis.

As for the relative strength of Upright Qi and pathogenic factors, this is an interior condition characterized by extreme weakness of the Upright Qi (deficiency of Liver-Blood and Kidney-Yang) and by the presence of pathogenic factors, which are the stasis of Blood and the interior Cold. It is therefore a mixed Deficiency/Excess condition. The Deficiency patterns are the Liver-Blood and Kidney-Yang deficiency; the Excess factors are the interior Cold and the stasis of Blood.

Treatment principle
As the symptoms of the Manifestation (Blood stasis and Cold) are not pronounced, in this case treatment must be aimed primarily at tonifying the body's Qi, hence concentrating on treating the Root; however, the Manifestation can be treated simultaneously. Treating the Root (i.e. tonifying the Upright Qi) can be achieved by tonifying LIV-8 Ququan, SP-6 Sanyinjiao, BL-18 Ganshu and BL-17 Geshu to tonify Liver-Blood and KI-3 Taixi and BL-23 Shenshu to tonify Kidney-Yang.

The clinical manifestations of the Manifestation can be treated simultaneously to relieve the symptoms caused by the stasis of Blood with such points as P-6 Neiguan and SP-10 Xuehai to move Blood.

Case history 69.6 – Woman, age 24

Clinical manifestations
This patient had an exterior condition overlapping a chronic interior one, and only came for treatment after the exterior condition had set in and penetrated to the Interior.

As this is a complicated case, I shall give the clinical manifestations in three groups: the underlying chronic condition; the acute, exterior attack; and the sequelae of such an attack (when she came for treatment).
1. *Chronic condition*: propensity to catching colds, giddiness, Deep-Fine Pulse, both Rear positions very Weak.
   Tongue: Pale-Purple, dry.
2. *Acute, exterior attack*: temperature of 101°F (38.5°C), feeling of heaviness, body aches, headache, 'buzzing in ears', giddiness.
3. *Sequelae*: constant temperature of 99.5°F (37.5°C), lack of balance and coordination, tinnitus, nystagmus, extreme tiredness, poor sleep, lethargy, feeling of heaviness of the legs, numbness of limbs, occipital headache. In particular, the lack of balance and coordination was very pronounced and led Western doctors to suspect a neurological lesion.

Diagnosis and explanation
1. *Chronic condition*: severe Kidney-Yang deficiency. In this case the tongue is dry from deficient

Yang-Qi unable to transport fluids to it. It is also Purple as the deficiency of Kidney-Yang has caused interior Cold, which, in turn, causes stasis of Blood.
2. *Acute, exterior attack*: this was an attack of exterior Wind-Damp-Heat.
3. *Sequelae*: these are caused by the exterior pathogenic factors penetrating in the Interior. The Heat and Dampness have become interior and caused the constant low-grade temperature. Once in the Interior, they disturb the circulation of Qi and Blood and, overlapping with the pre-existing condition of Kidney-Yang deficiency, they cause the rising of Liver-Wind (nystagmus, lack of balance and coordination). These are caused by interior Wind arising from the deficiency of Blood and Kidney-Yang. In addition, Damp-Heat is steaming in the Interior, causing the constant low-grade temperature, numbness, extreme tiredness, feeling of heaviness and lethargy.

Treatment principle
The patient only came at the sequelae stage, when the condition was an interior one. It was characterized by an extreme deficiency of Upright Qi and by the presence of formerly exterior pathogenic factors, now become interior (Damp-Heat).

In addition, the exterior attack had also given rise to another interior pathogenic factor: that is, Liver-Wind. This is a good example of a situation when the Manifestation becomes primary. The Root is represented by the chronic condition of Kidney-Yang deficiency, which must eventually be treated as it also predisposes to Liver-Wind. However, the Manifestation in this case assumes primary importance as it causes symptoms which require urgent treatment. The Manifestation in this case is represented partly by the Damp-Heat and partly by Liver-Wind. Both these, particularly the Liver-Wind, need to be treated without delay.

Treatment in this case was aimed at treating the Manifestation first, and expelling the pathogenic factors first, and later tonifying the Upright Qi. The treatment was aimed at clearing interior Heat, resolving Dampness, extinguishing Wind and pacifying the Liver. Various groups of points were used at different times to achieve these aims. L.I.-11 Quchi and Du-14 Dazhui were used to clear interior Heat. Points on the Governing Vessel (*Du Mai*) are particularly important to clear latent interior Heat resulting from invasion of previously exterior Heat. Points such as SP-9 Yinlingquan, SP-6 Sanyinjiao, Ren-9 Shuifen and BL-22 Sanjiaoshu were used to resolve Dampness; LIV-3 Taichong, G.B.-20 Fengchi and Du-16 Fengfu were used to subdue Liver-Wind. Only after the symptoms of Damp-Heat and Liver-Wind had gone, was the treatment aimed at tonifying Kidney-Yang by tonifying and warming (with moxa) BL-23 Shenshu, Ren-4 Guanyuan and KI-7 Fuliu.

Case history 69.7 – Woman, age 72

Clinical manifestations
This patient had been suffering from chronic bronchitis and emphysema for a very long time. She caught colds easily, was breathless and coughed up a lot of sticky yellow sputum.
Pulse: Slippery, both Front positions Weak.
Tongue: Red, sticky yellow coating.

During the course of treatment she caught a heavy cold and had the following symptoms: aversion to cold, a headache, cough, runny nose, sneezing, breathlessness and a Floating pulse.

Diagnosis
Retention of Phlegm-Heat in the Lungs and Spleen-Qi deficiency. During the acute exterior attack: invasion of Lung's Defensive Qi portion by exterior Wind-Cold.

Explanation
This condition is chronic and, as often happens in chronic conditions, there is interior Heat. There is also Phlegm, which is caused by deficient Spleen-Qi being unable to transform fluids, which accumulate into Phlegm.

The Spleen-Qi deficiency is the Root and the retention of Phlegm in the Lungs is the Manifestation.

The Upright Qi is weak and there is a pathogenic factor in the form of Phlegm-Heat; hence the condition is a mixed Deficient/Excess one.

The acute attack of Wind-Cold represents another Root, causing the various clinical manifestations.

Treatment principle
Treatment must primarily be aimed at the Root (i.e. tonifying Spleen-Qi) because as long as the Spleen is weak, new Phlegm will always be formed. However, the clinical manifestations are in this case severe and

distressing and also need treatment. So in this case both the Root and the Manifestation need to be treated simultaneously and the treatment must combine tonifying the Upright Qi (in this case Spleen-Qi) with resolving the pathogenic factor (in this case Phlegm-Heat).

During the acute attack of common cold, the treatment principle is entirely different. In this case, treatment of the acute condition takes precedence over the chronic one as this patient has emphysema and chronic bronchitis, and therefore an exterior attack of Wind-Cold can have very serious consequences if not treated promptly. The Wind-Cold attack, for instance, could very easily turn into pneumonia, considering the tendency to lung trouble and the retention of Phlegm-Heat in the Lungs.

During the acute attack of Wind-Cold, the primary aim of treatment is to expel the pathogenic factor first and tonify the Upright Qi later. Points used to expel Wind-Cold were LU-7 Lieque and BL-12 Fengmen with cupping.

Learning outcomes

In this chapter you will have learned:
- The absolute importance of adopting the correct treatment principle to successfully treat disease
- The different meanings of Root (*Ben*) and Manifestation (*Biao*) in different contexts
- How the Root and Manifestation relate to each other – their essential unity
- How a Manifestation can become a Root of further Manifestations
- The importance of tracing clinical manifestations back to their Root in order to treat
- When to use the approach of treating the Root only (when clinical manifestations of the Manifestation are few and mild)
- When to treat the Root and Manifestation simultaneously (if the Manifestation is producing severe symptoms)
- When to treat the Manifestation first and the Root later (when symptoms of the Manifestation are distressing, often in acute cases)
- How multiple Roots can develop through life, giving rise to different Manifestations
- How one Root can give rise to different manifestations
- How the Root can coincide with its Manifestation (from external physical trauma)
- The importance of knowing when to tonify Qi or expel pathogenic factors, which depends on clearly understanding the relative strengths of the Upright Qi and any pathogenic factors
- When to use the strategy of tonifying the Upright Qi only (if the condition is predominantly Deficient)
- When to expel pathogenic factors only (in purely Excess patterns)
- When to tonify the Upright Qi and expel pathogenic factors simultaneously (or one before the other)
- The importance of being aware of residual pathogenic factors, which may need to be expelled before tonifying the Upright Qi
- The difference between herbal treatment and acupuncture, particularly in the way they tonify the Upright Qi and expel pathogenic factors

Self-assessment questions

1. What are the two main meanings of the terms Root and Manifestation?
2. Under which conditions would you treat the Root of a disease only?
3. Why would you treat both Root and Manifestation together in the case of a woman with Qi deficiency leading to excessive menstrual bleeding?
4. Under what circumstances would you treat the Manifestation first and the Root later?
5. Identify the Root and Manifestation in a case of trauma causing pain from stagnation of Qi and Blood in the shoulder.
6. Does the Root always coincide with deficiency, and the Manifestation with a pathogenic factor?
7. Give an example of Root from Fullness and Manifestation with Emptiness.
8. Give three ways of tonifying the Upright Qi, other than acupuncture.
9. Would you consider just tonifying the Upright Qi to treat an exterior condition?
10. A patient seems weak and sickly. All other clinical manifestations point towards their condition being Excess. Would you tonify or reduce?
11. Would you tonify the Upright Qi and expel the pathogenic factor simultaneously in a case of an invasion of Wind-Heat?

See p. 1266 for answers

END NOTE

1. 1982 Report on Dr T Kaptchuk Seminar, Journal of Oriental Medicine (Australia), 1:18.

PART 8

Principles of Combination of Points | 70

After identifying the patterns and formulating a plan of treatment, the next step for an acupuncturist is that of the selection of points to use. There are two different considerations:

- The selection of points according to their action
- The combination of points according to channel dynamics

In other words, in order to give an effective acupuncture treatment, it is not enough to select the points according to their individual characteristics and energetic action. We must also be able to combine points harmoniously according to their action within the channel system.

Acupuncture works via the channels, not just via isolated points, so that each point should be considered not only for its individual action but also for its place within the channel system. Even if we master the action of each individual point, this is still not enough to give an effective acupuncture treatment, as each point must be seen not in isolation but within the dynamics of the channel system so as to attain a harmonious combination of points.

For example, one might treat Spleen-Qi deficiency and Liver-Qi stagnation by tonifying BL-20 Pishu and BL-21 Weishu and reducing BL-18 Ganshu and BL-19 Danshu. Although technically correct from the point of view of energetic action of the individual points, it would be an unbalanced point prescription as all the points selected are on the back.

To give another example, one might treat Liver and Kidney Yin deficiency by tonifying KI-3 Taixi, LIV-3 Taichong, SP-6 Sanyinjiao and KI-6 Zhaohai. Again, this would be correct according to the functions of the individual points, but also rather unbalanced as all the points are on the distal part of the legs.

Let us then look at the principles regulating the combination of points according to the channel system dynamics.

The balance of the point combination is essential to the success of an acupuncture treatment. Indeed, a balanced point combination is as important to the therapeutic result as the needling technique. The latter is of course very important to the success of an acupuncture treatment but the harmonious combination of points is often overlooked: they are both important because they reflect two different viewpoints. In a way, the stress placed on needling technique is based on a point-centred view of acupuncture, while the stress placed on the combination of points is based on a channel-centred view of acupuncture. Both of these points of view are important and both need to be taken into account.

The stress placed on needling technique is based on a point-centred view of acupuncture, while the stress placed on the combination of points is based on a channel-centred view of acupuncture

Although the needling technique is indeed very important, we should not place too much stress on it: in fact, when the point combination is harmonious, we bring into play the circulation of Qi in the channel system so that Qi is moved effectively, somewhat reducing the need for vigorous needling manipulation.

For example, ST-40 Fenglong is said to resolve Phlegm and, in case of a severe Phlegm pattern, we should needle this point with a reducing method: the more Full the condition, the stronger the reducing technique required. However, resolving Phlegm with acupuncture involves a lot more than simply reducing ST-40. In particular, it involves regulating the Qi Mechanism by harmonizing the ascending/descending and entering/exiting of Qi: acupuncture can resolve Phlegm only by regulating Qi.

By combining ST-40 with other points according to the principles outlined below, the movement of Qi is encouraged by the 'communication' among the points rather than just by the stimulation of one point. The combination of points also regulates the ascending/descending and entering/exiting of Qi. For example, in order to resolve Phlegm, ST-40 could be combined with LU-7 Lieque, Ren-12 Zhongwan, Ren-9 Shuifen, BL-22 Sanjiaoshu and KI-7 Fuliu. Apart from the fact that the other points also contribute to resolving Phlegm, such a combination balances Yin with Yang points as well as points on the arms with points on the legs.

The discussion on the principles governing the balance of points will be under the following topics:

- Balancing distal and local points
- Balancing upper and lower parts of the body
- Balancing left and right
- Balancing Yin and Yang
- Balancing front and back

Before proceeding with the discussion on point balancing, we should review briefly the circulation of Qi in the channel system.[1]

The head is the highest part of the body not only anatomically but also energetically according to the flow of Qi in the 12 channels. It is, in fact, the area of maximum potential of energy in the circulation of Qi in the channels. Qi circulates in the channels because there is a difference of potential between the chest and the head.

'Potential energy' is a stored energy: an object can store energy as the result of its position. For example, the heavy ram of a pile driver is storing energy when it is held at an elevated position. Similarly, a drawn bow is able to store energy as the result of its position. Potential energy is the stored energy of position possessed by an object.

Gravitational potential energy is the energy stored in an object as the result of its vertical position (i.e. height). The energy is stored as the result of the gravitational attraction of the Earth for the object. The gravitational potential energy of the heavy ram of a pile driver is an example of gravitational potential energy (Fig. 70.1).

The Qi at the top of the head possesses a 'gravitational potential energy' as a result of its position at the top of the body. In the circulation of Qi in the channel system, the top of the head has the maximum and the

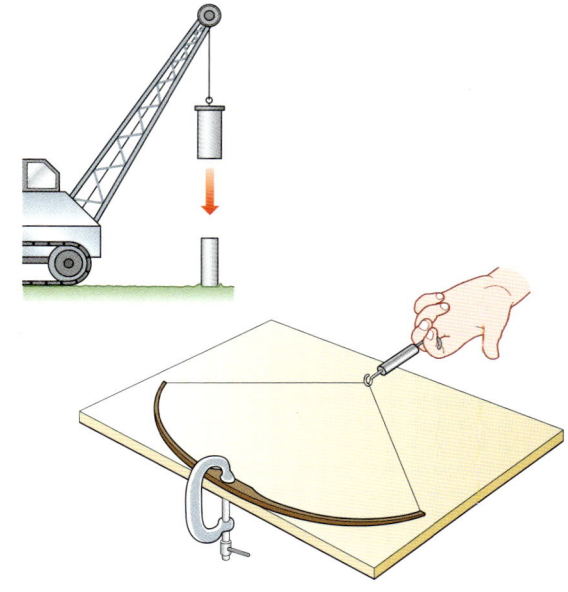

Figure 70.1 Potential energy

chest/abdomen the minimum potential. Qi circulates precisely because of the difference in potential between the head and the chest.

If we consider the first four channels, for example, we see that Qi starts at the chest area in the Lung channel: this is the area of minimum potential of energy. In order to understand this we can visualize a certain amount of water at the bottom of a hill, where its potential of producing energy is minimal or nil. If we slowly carry this water up the hill, gradually its potential of producing energy will increase, as we know. When the water reaches the top of the hill, its potential of producing energy (e.g. hydroelectric energy) will be maximum. The bottom of the hill corresponds to the chest, half-way up the hill corresponds to the hands (or feet) and the top of the hill corresponds to the head (Fig. 70.2).

Thus, from the Lung channel in the chest, Qi starts to move upwards towards the head. At the fingertips, Qi changes polarity, i.e. it flows from the Yin Lung channel to the Yang Large Intestine channel, but it is still flowing towards the head and its potential is increasing. When it reaches the head the potential is at its maximum and it then starts decreasing as it flows towards the feet. At the feet, Qi changes polarity, i.e. it flows from the Yang Stomach channel to the Yin Spleen channel, but its potential is still decreasing as it flows

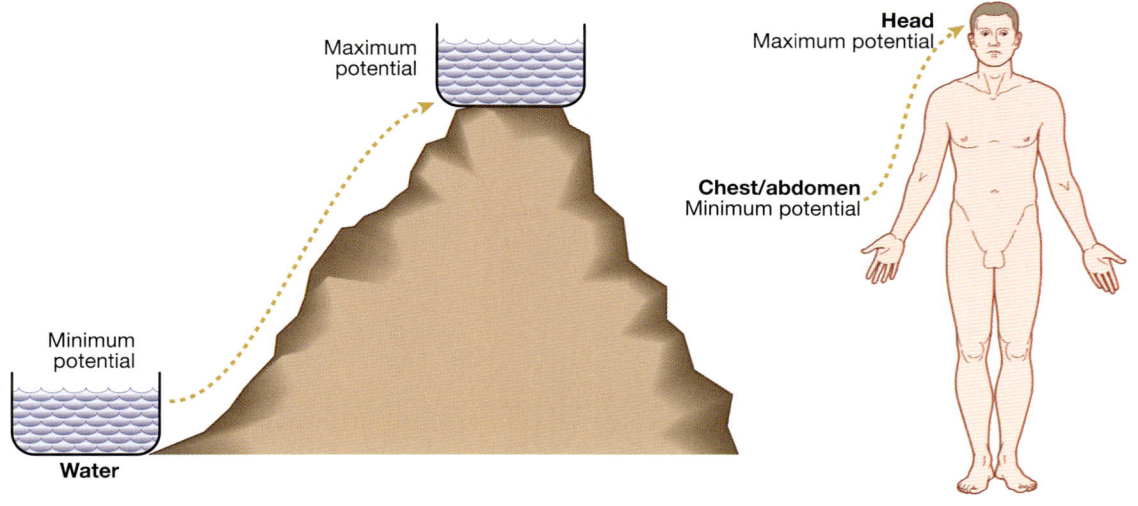

Figure 70.2 Potential energy in Qi circulation

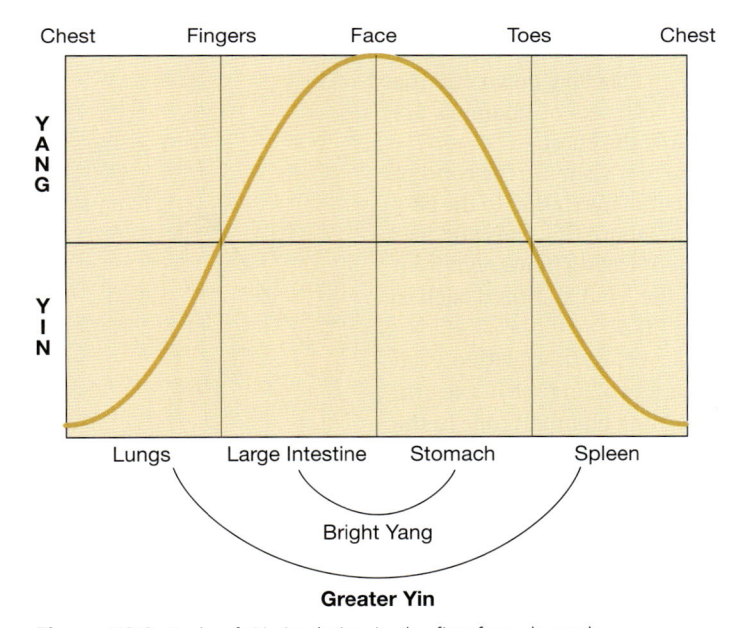

Figure 70.3 Cycle of Qi circulation in the first four channels

towards the chest area. When it reaches the chest the potential is minimum (the water has reached the bottom of the hill again). The Qi from the Spleen channel then connects internally with the Heart channel and a new four-channel cycle starts in exactly the same way. The cycle of Qi in the first four channels can be seen in Figure 70.3. Figure 70.4 shows the circulation of Qi in the 12 channels.

Please note that, in order to visualize this circulation of Qi in relation to the changing gravitational potential energy, it is best to visualize the body without arms and legs. This is because although the three Yin channels of the arm flow down the arm and the three Yang channels of the arm flow up the arm, they are both actually flowing *up* towards the head. Similarly, for the Yang and Yin channels of the legs: that is, although

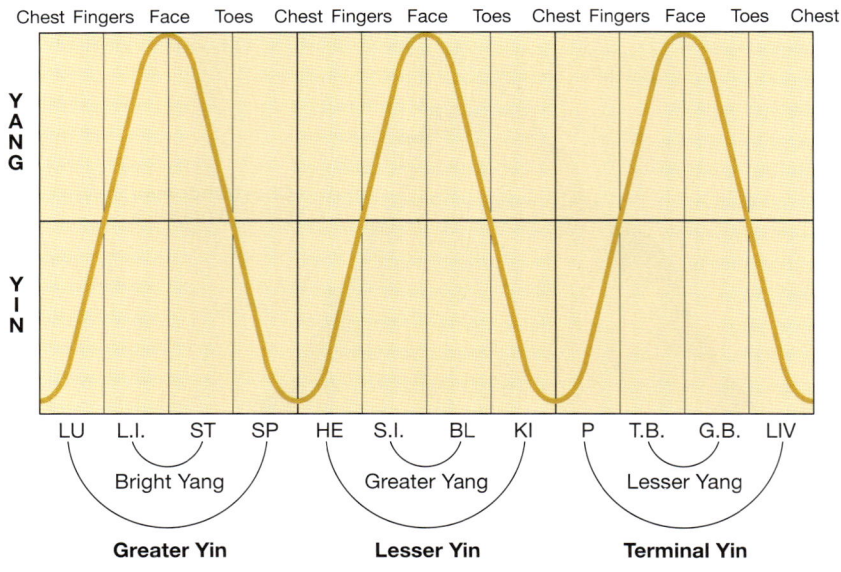

Figure 70.4 Cycle of Qi circulation in the 12 channels

the three Yang channels of the leg flow down and the three Yin channel flow up, both sets of channels are actually flowing *down* towards the chest.

In other words, in order to best visualize the concept of gravitational energy potential in relation to the flow of Qi in the body, it is best to ignore the arms and legs and visualize the movement of Qi as a movement from the chest (via the arms) to the head and then back to the chest (via the legs) (Fig. 70.5).

If we look at Figure 70.4, we see that, within each set of four channels, there are two Yin (one in the arm and one in the leg) and two Yang channels (one in the arm and one in the leg). These channels form pairs of connected channels of same polarity (both Yang or both Yin), same level of energy (see below) and opposite location, i.e, one in the arm, the other in the leg as follows:

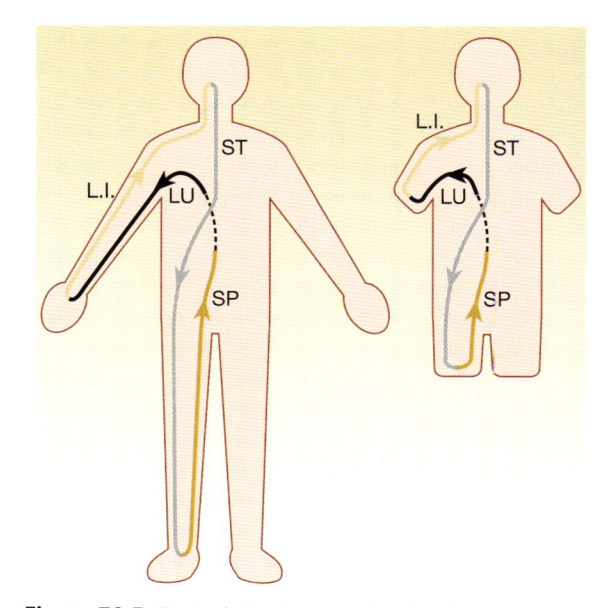

Figure 70.5 Qi circulation between head and chest

In fact, the above names refer to the amount of Yang or Yin energy in the daily cycle as follows:

	Arm	*Leg*
Greater Yang	Small Intestine	Bladder
Lesser Yang	Triple Burner	Gall Bladder
Bright Yang	Large Intestine	Stomach
Greater Yin	Lung	Spleen
Lesser Yin	Heart	Kidneys
Terminal Yin	Pericardium	Liver

- Greater Yang and Greater Yin: maximum Yang and Yin, respectively
- Lesser Yang and Lesser Yin: minimum Yang and Y n, respectively
- Bright Yang and Terminal Yin: average Yang and Yin, respectively

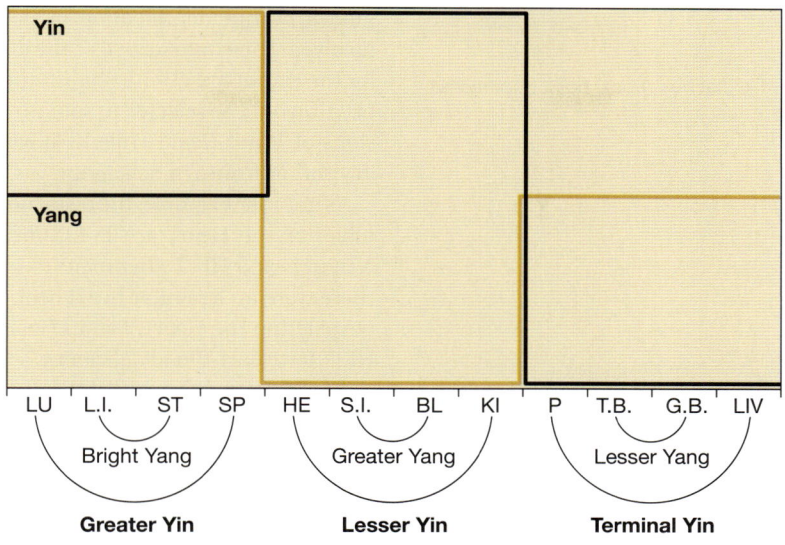

Figure 70.6 Ebb and flow of Yin and Yang in the daily cycle of the 12 channels

If we look at Figure 70.4, we see that in the early morning, Yin is at its maximum (Greater Yin) and Yang at its average level (Bright Yang); in the middle of the day Yang is at its maximum (Greater Yang) and Yin at its minimum (Lesser Yin); and in the evening/night Yang is at its lowest level (Lesser Yang) while Yin is at its average level (Terminal Yin) (Fig. 70.6).

BALANCING DISTAL AND LOCAL POINTS

'Local' points are those situated in close proximity of the area where the clinical manifestations occur: for example, in ear problems with pain and discharge, the points around the ears are local points.

'Distal' points are those that affect a certain area although they are situated away from the area where the clinical manifestations occur: in the above example of ear problems, distal points would be those on the arm.

Generally speaking, local and distal points are situated on the same channel, the former in the area of the clinical manifestations, the latter at the other end of the channel. In the above example, if the channel involved were the Triple Burner channel, T.B.-21 Ermen is a local point and T.B.-5 Waiguan a distal point.

However, distal points are not necessarily only those of the channel involved. In the above example of ear problems due to the Triple Burner channel, L.I.-4 Hegu would also act as a distal point. Furthermore, although I have mentioned T.B.-5 Waiguan as a distal point, any point on the Triple Burner below the elbow would also act as a distal point.

In theory, any point situated at a distance from where the problem lies could be defined as a 'distal' point. For example, if the problem is in the gums along the Stomach channel, ST-4 Dicang, ST-5 Daying and ST-6 Jiache are local points and ST-44 Neiting (located on the foot) the distal point (Fig. 70.7). However, with very few exceptions, this relationship generally works only in one way: that is, while ST-44 is a distal point for problems of the gums, points around the gums (ST-4, ST-5, ST-6) are *not* distal points for foot problems.

Therefore, with only a few exceptions, 'distal' points are the points situated on the arms and legs, and specifically those below the elbows and knees. As mentioned in chapter 50, the points below the elbows and knees are particularly dynamic points which affect distal parts of the body. Obviously, in the case of articular problems below the elbows and knees, local and distal points coincide: for example, in a wrist problem along the Small Intestine channel, S.I.-5 (normally a distal point) acts also as a local point.

We can therefore say that, with few exceptions, distal points are those on the limbs below the elbows and knees while local points are those on the trunk and head. The combination of local and distal points is the most widely used technique of balancing of points.

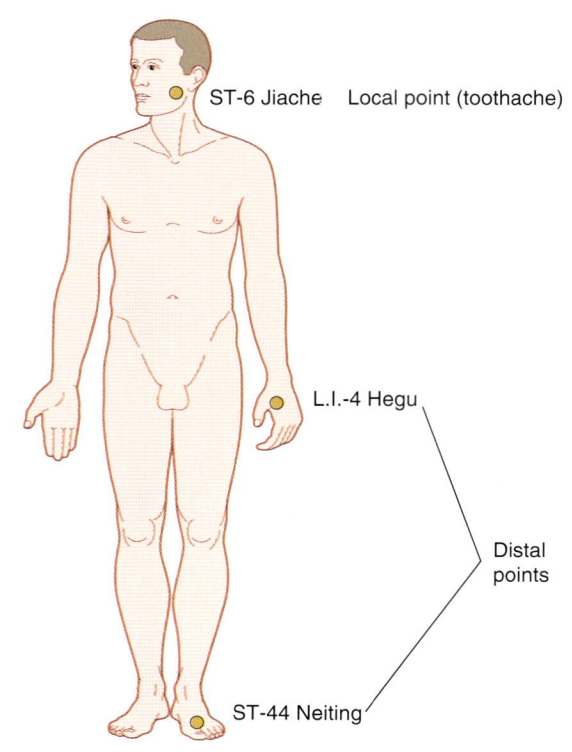

Figure 70.7 Local and distal points

In acute cases, the distal points have the effect of removing obstructions from the channel and expelling pathogenic factors and they are therefore usually needled with reducing method. The local points have the function of supporting the eliminating action of the distal points and focusing it on the desired area: they are usually needled with even method.

For example, in treating an acute sprain of the lower back with bilateral pain on the lower back, one might choose BL-40 Weizhong as a distal point (needled with reducing method) and BL-26 Guanyuanshu as a local point (needled with even method). Sometimes distal points are needled before inserting the local ones. The example of ST-38 Tiaokou for acute sprain of the shoulder has already been given above.

In chronic cases, distal and local points simply reinforce each other's function. Table 70.1 lists the main distal and local points according to areas. This table lists points from different channels and the choice of which point to use has to be guided by other factors, chiefly a proper identification of the channel involved.

As mentioned above, the points in the table are from different channels and their choice has to be further guided by the identification of patterns and channel involved. For example, two of the distal points indicated for the throat are LU-11 Shaoshang and KI-6 Zhaohai: LU-11 would be selected in sore throat from acute invasions of Wind-Heat, while KI-6 would be chosen for a dry throat from Yin deficiency.

As another example, the distal points indicated in the table for the Heart are P-4 Ximen, P-5 Jianshi, P-6 Neiguan and HE-7 Shenmen: P-4 would be chosen if there were an irregular heart beat, P-5 if Phlegm were obstructing the Heart, P-6 in Heart-Qi deficiency, and HE-7 for Heart-Blood deficiency.

As mentioned above, distal points are not only those on the channel involved: for example, in an eye problem deriving from the Bladder channel, distal points would be those on the other extremity of the Bladder channel on the foot. However, L.I.-4 Hegu would also be an effective distal point because it is a point that is used as a distal point for all problems of the face.

In particular, when distal points are selected, the close connection between channels of the same polarity, for example Greater Yang (Small Intestine and Bladder), Lesser Yang (Triple Burner and Gall Bladder), Bright Yang (Large Intestine and Stomach), Greater Yin (Lung and Spleen), Lesser Yin (Heart and Kidneys) and Terminal Yin (Pericardium and Liver) should be borne in mind. These channel pairs unite corresponding arm and leg channels of the same polarity and same 'potential' as described at the beginning of this chapter.

This pairing means that distal points of paired channels may affect the same areas. For example, in ear problems stemming from the Triple Burner channel, the applicable distal points are points on this channel below the elbow, especially T.B.-5 Waiguan and T.B.-2 Yemen. However, due to the close connection between the Triple Burner and Gall Bladder channels within the Lesser Yang pairing, points on the Gall Bladder channel below the knee may also be selected as distal points for ear problems (e.g. G.B.-43 Xiaxi).

Thus, the distal points of paired channels are almost interchangeable: for example, T.B.-2 Yemen and G.B.-43 for ear problems, L.I.-4 Hegu and ST-44 Neiting for gum problems, etc. However, it is interesting to note that such connection and interchangeability is closer for the Yang than it is for the Yin channels. The reason for this is that while the Yang channels connect directly and superficially on the head/face, the Yin channels connect on the chest/abdomen but only at a

Table 70.1 Distal and local points according to areas

Area/organ	Local points	Distal points
Face	Yintang	L.I.-4 Hegu, ST-44 Neiting
Temples	Taiyang, G.B.-8 Shuaigu	T.B.-3 Zhongzhu, T.B.-5 Waiguan, G.B.-43 Xiaxi
Occiput	G.B.-20 Fengchi, BL-10 Tianshu	S.I.-3 Houxi, BL-65 Shugu
Vertex	Du-20 Baihui	LIV-3 Taichong
Eye	BL-1 Jingming, ST-1 Chengqi, Yuyao	L.I.-4 Hegu, LIV-3 Taichong, HE-5 Tongli, S.I.-6 Yanglao, T.B.-3 Zhongzhu
Nose	Yintang, Yingxiang, Bitong	LU-7 Lieque, L.I.-4 Hegu
Teeth	ST-4 Dicang, ST-6 Jiache, ST-7 Xiaguan	L.I.-4 Hegu (upper), ST-44 Neiting (lower)
Ear	T.B.-17 Yifeng, S.I.-19 Tinggong, G.B.-2 Tinghui, T.B.-21 Ermen	T.B.-2 Yemen, T.B.-3 Zhongzhu, T.B.-5 Waiguan, G.B.-43 Xiaxi
Tongue	Ren-23 Lianquan	P-8 Laogong, HE-5 Tongli, KI-6 Zhaohai
Throat	Ren-22 Tiantu	L.I.-4 Hegu, LU-11 Shaoshang, KI-6 Zhaohai
Lungs	LU-1 Zhongfu, BL-13 Feishu, Ren-17 Shanzhong, Ren-22 Tiantu	LU-7 Lieque, LU-5 Chize
Heart	BL-15 Xinshu, BL-14 Jueyinshu, Ren-14 Juque, Ren-15 Jiuwei	P-6 Neiguan, HE-7 Shenmen, P-5 Jianshi, P-4 Ximen
Stomach	BL-21 Weishu, Ren-12 Zhongwan	P-6 Neiguan, ST-36 Zusanli, SP-4 Gongsun
Liver	BL-18 Ganshu, LIV-14 Qimen	LIV-3 Taichong, G.B.-34 Yanglingquan
Gall Bladder	BL-19 Danshu, G.B.-24 Riyue	G.B.-34 Yanglingquan, Dannangxue
Intestines	BL-25 Dachangshu, ST-25 Tianshu	ST-36 Zusanli, SP-6 Sanyinjiao, ST-37 Shangjuxu, ST-39 Xiajuxu
Bladder	Ren-3 Zhongji, BL-28 Pangguangshu, Ren-2 Qugu, BL-32 Ciliao	SP-6 Sanyinjiao, BL-63 Jinmen
Urethra	Ren-2 Qugu, BL-34 Xialiao	LIV-5 Ligou, BL-63 Jinmen
Anus	Du-1 Changqiang, BL-54 Zhibian, G.B.-30 Huantiao	BL-57 Chengshan, BL-58 Feiyang

deep level (see Figs 70.4 and 70.5): thus, we can look upon the Yang channels (e.g. Greater Yang of Small Intestine and Bladder) almost as a single channel joined directly and superficially on the face. So we could look upon the Large Intestine and Stomach channel, for example, as one channel from this point of view. The same applies to Triple Burner–Gall Bladder and Small Intestine–Bladder.

Thus, in the case of the Yang channels, we have a choice of distal points to use, either on the hands or feet, as the points are quite interchangeable. When there is such a choice, we should bear in mind that the distal points of the legs have a stronger effect than those of the arm. For example, for Stomach-Heat affecting the gums, ST-44 Neiting has a stronger effect that L.I.-4 Hegu.[2]

For the Yin channels, it is somewhat different. The Yin channels all end or start in the chest or abdominal cavity and they do merge into one another, but only internally, whereas the Yang channels merge into each other directly and superficially on the face. Thus, in the case of the Yin channels, we do not have the same free choice of distal points as for the Yang channels. For example, P-6 Neiguan and LIV-3 Taichong have some

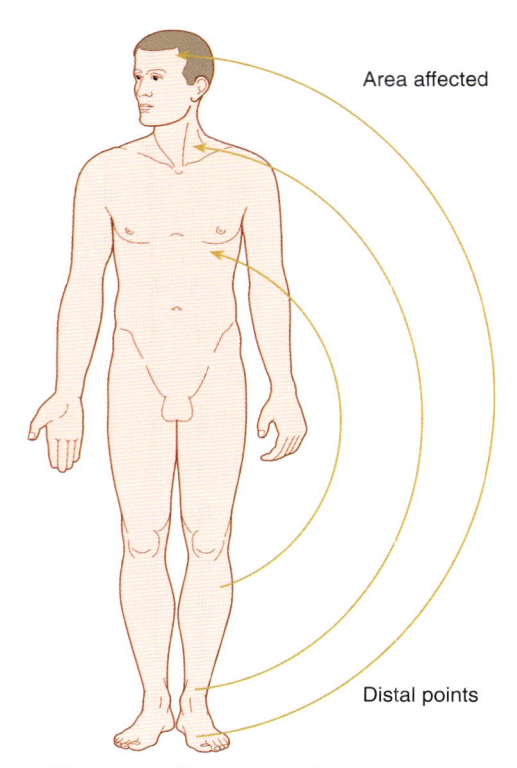

Figure 70.8 Areas affected by distal points

> **Box 70.1 Distal and local points**
>
> - Local points are those in the head and trunk; distal points are the points on the arms and legs below the elbows and knees
> - The arm and leg points of channels of the same polarity and potential (e.g. Greater Yang, Greater Yin, etc.) are almost interchangeable (e.g. L.I.-4 and ST-44)
> - Leg distal points are stronger than arm distal points
> - A distal point may be on a channel different to the channel where the local problem lies (e.g. L.I.-4 for Bladder channel eye problems)

common properties in so far as they both move Liver-Qi, but, besides that, they have quite different actions and there is not really a question of choice between them as a distal point.

Finally, with regard to the local area affected by distal points, there is an important general principle that states 'the farther, the further': that is, the further away a distal point is from a given area, the more it will influence it. For example, it we take a long channel such as the Stomach channel, ST-45 Lidui and ST-44 Neiting will affect the other end of the channel (i.e. the eye and forehead); distal points slightly further up such as ST-41 Jiexi will affect a lower section of the other end of the channel (i.e. the throat). Figure 70.8 illustrates this principle.

Box 70.1 summarizes distal and local points.

Channel problems

In channel problems, the use of local points only might sometimes be sufficient, but it is much more common to balance the local points with distal ones. The distal points actually play an important role in clearing the channel from obstructions (which may be from exterior Cold, Dampness or Wind, or from stagnation of Qi and/or Blood or Phlegm).

When choosing a distal point, we should keep in mind that distal points on the feet are more powerful than those on the hands. If we want to moderate the effect of the treatment because the patient is rather weak or old, we can then choose a distal point on the hands. For example, both L.I.-4 Hegu and ST-44 Neiting have an effect on the face and teeth and both can be used to clear Heat in the Stomach channel affecting the face, and they are somewhat interchangeable. To give another example, both T.B.-5 Waiguan and G.B.-43 Xiaxi affect the temple area and can be used as distal points for the treatment of migraine headaches on the temple.

The main distal points for channel problems according to channels are:

> *Lungs*: LU-7 Lieque
> *Large Intestine*: L.I.-4 Hegu
> *Stomach*: ST-40 Fenglong
> *Spleen*: SP-5 Shangqiu
> *Heart*: HE-5 Tongli
> *Small Intestine*: S.I.-3 Houxi
> *Bladder*: BL-60 Kunlun
> *Kidneys*: KI-4 Dazhong
> *Pericardium*: P-6 Neiguan
> *Triple Burner*: T.B.-5 Waiguan
> *Gall Bladder*: G.B.-41 Zulinqi
> *Liver*: LIV-5 Ligou

It must be stressed that this is a list of the most effective distal points according to my experience. As mentioned above, any point below the elbow and knee may be used as a distal point. Moreover, other practitioners' experience may be different from mine and therefore other distal points may also be as effective.

The choice of distal points must also be made on the basis of the area involved. The main distal points according to areas are:

> *Neck*: G.B.-39 Xuanzhong, S.I.-3 Houxi, T.B.-5 Waiguan, T.B.-8 Sanyangluo, Bl-60 Kunlun *Secondary points*: ST-40 Fenglong and KI-4 Dazhong
> *Shoulder*: T.B.-5 Waiguan, L.I.-4 Hegu, LU-7 Lieque, T.B.-1 Guanchong, L.I.-1 Shangyang, ST-38 Tiaokou, BL-58 Feiyang
> *Elbow*: L.I.-4 Hegu, T.B.-5 Waiguan, L.I.-1 Shangyang
> *Wrist*: ST-36 Zusanli, SP-5 Shangqiu, G.B.-40 Qiuxu
> *Fingers*: no distal points (see above)
> *Lower back*: BL-40 Weizhong, BL-60 Kunlun, BL-59 Fuyang, BL-62 Shenmai, Du-26 Renzhong
> *Sacrum*: BL-40 Weizhong, BL-58 Feiyang
> *Hip*: G.B.-41 Zulinqi, BL-62 Shenmai
> *Knee*: SP-5 Shangqiu, S.I.-5 Yanggu
> *Ankle*: no distal points
> *Toes*: L.I.-4 Hegu

The main local points according to area are:

> *Neck*: BL-10 Tianzhu, G.B.-20 Fengchi
> *Shoulder*: L.I.-15 Jianyu, T.B.-14 Jianliao, Jianneiling (extra point)
> *Elbow*: L.I.-11 Quchi, T.B.-10 Tianjing, S.I.-8 Xiaohai
> *Wrist*: T.B.-4 Yangchi, L.I.-5 Yangxi, S.I.-5 Yanggu, S.I.-4 Wangu, P-7 Daling
> *Fingers*: T.B.-3 Zhongzhu, L.I.-3 Sanjian, Baxie (extra points)
> *Lower back*: BL-23 Shenshu, BL-26 Guanyuanshu, BL-25 Dachangshu, BL-24 Qihaishu, Shiqizhuixia (extra point), Du-3 Yaoyangguan
> *Sacrum*: BL-32 Ciliao, Shiqizhuixia, BL-27 Xiaochangshu, BL-28 Pangguangshu
> *Hip*: G.B.-30 Huantiao, G.B.-29 Juliao
> *Knee*: Xiyan (extra points), ST-36 Zusanli, SP-9 Yinlingquan, LIV-7 Xiguan, LIV-8 Ququan, KI-10 Yingu, G.B.-34 Yanglingquan, BL-40 Weizhong, SP-10 Xuehai
> *Ankle*: SP-5 Shangqiu, G.B.-40 Qiuxu, ST-41 Jiexi, BL-60 Kunlun
> *Toes*: Bafeng (extra points), SP-3 Taibai

Acute cases

In acute cases, the distal point is used first on its own with a reducing method in order to clear the obstruction of the pathogenic factors and open the channel to make it ready for the use of the local points. A few examples will clarify this technique.

In acute sprain of the lower back on the midline, just above the sacrum, one can reduce Du-26 Renzhong first while the patient gently bends forwards and backwards. This helps to clear the obstruction in the channel (the Governing Vessel in this case). After the manipulation of the distal point, the patient lies down and local points are used according to tenderness. These may also be cupped after insertion of the needle (Fig. 70.9). Incidentally, the use of Du-26 Renzhong as a distal point is an example of a distal point located on the head rather than on the limbs below the elbows and knees.

In acute sprain of the shoulder joint affecting the Large Intestine channel one can strongly reduce ST-38 Tiaokou, while the patient gently moves and rotates the arm, perhaps with the help of a third person if possible (Fig. 70.10). After manipulation of the distal point, local points are used according to tenderness and according to the channel involved. If the affected channel is the Small Intestine, BL-58 Feiyang is used as a distal point instead.

In acute sprain of the neck with pronounced rigidity, one can use the point G.B.-39 Xuanzhong with reducing method while the patient moves the head from side to side gently. After withdrawing G.B.-39, local points in the neck are needled (Fig. 70.11).

The arm–leg correspondence of paired channels with the same polarity and potential (e.g. Small Intestine and Bladder, Large Intestine and Stomach, Lungs

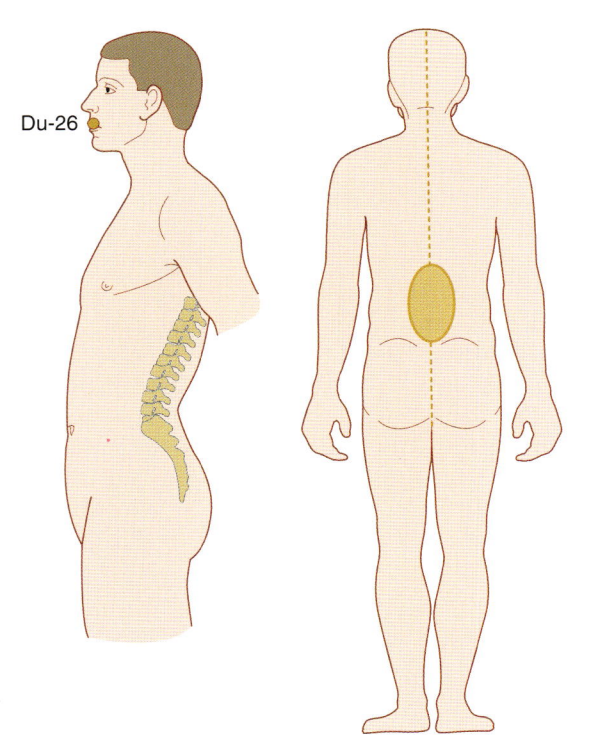

Figure 70.9 Du-26 as distal point for backache

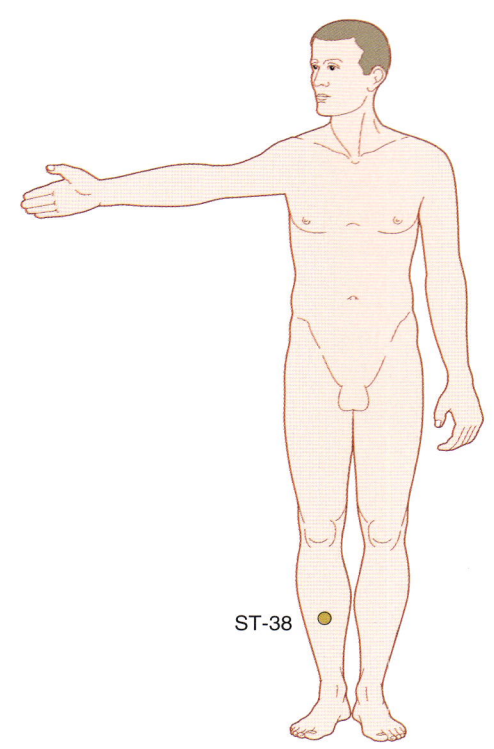

Figure 70.10 ST-38 as distal point for the shoulder

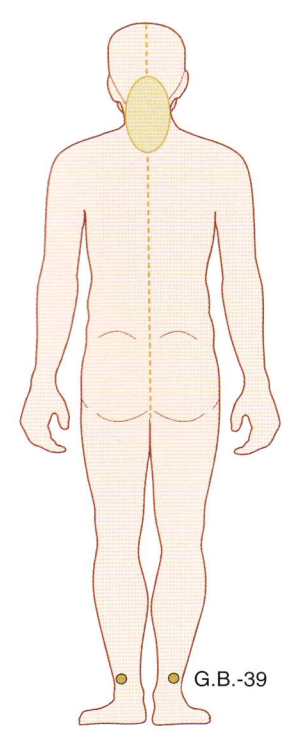

Figure 70.11 G.B.-39 as distal point for the neck

and Spleen, etc.) is used in the treatment of acute sprain of the joints. This is based on the principle of correspondence between shoulder and hip, elbow and knee, wrist and ankle, and on the relationship of leg and arm channels of the same polarity: that is, Lung–Spleen, Heart–Kidney, Pericardium–Liver, Large Intestine–Stomach, Triple Burner–Gall Bladder and Small Intestine–Bladder.

In acute sprain of a joint, one should first of all identify the channel involved and then choose as the distal point a point on the related paired channel of the same polarity and potential on the other limb and often on the opposite side. Some examples will clarify this.

In acute sprain of the wrist one would use a distal point on the feet, choosing the channel on the foot related to the involved channel of the wrist. For example, supposing the main tenderness is on the point T.B.-4 Yangchi, one can choose the leg channel related to the Triple Burner channel with an upper–lower relation (i.e. the Gall Bladder channel). On the Gall Bladder channel one would choose the point with a corresponding location to the wrist point (i.e. on the ankle joint): this would be G.B.-40 Qiuxu.

Supposing the main tender point is LU-7 Lieque, the point used on the foot would have been SP-5 Shangqiu (based on the correspondence between wrist and ankle). If the sprain had been on the elbow and the main tenderness on L.I.-11 Quchi, the point of the foot chosen would have been ST-36 Zusanli (based on the correspondence between elbow and knee). If the tenderness is on L.I.-15 Jianyu in the shoulder, the point on the leg chosen would be ST-31 Biguan (based on the correspondence between shoulder and hip). Figure 70.12 illustrates the correspondence among points of the Bright Yang channels according to this theory, as an example.

As mentioned above, according to this method, these distal points are often used on the opposite side (Fig. 70.13).

Bearing in mind the above correspondences between joints and related leg and arm channels, we can make a table of related distal points to use for each

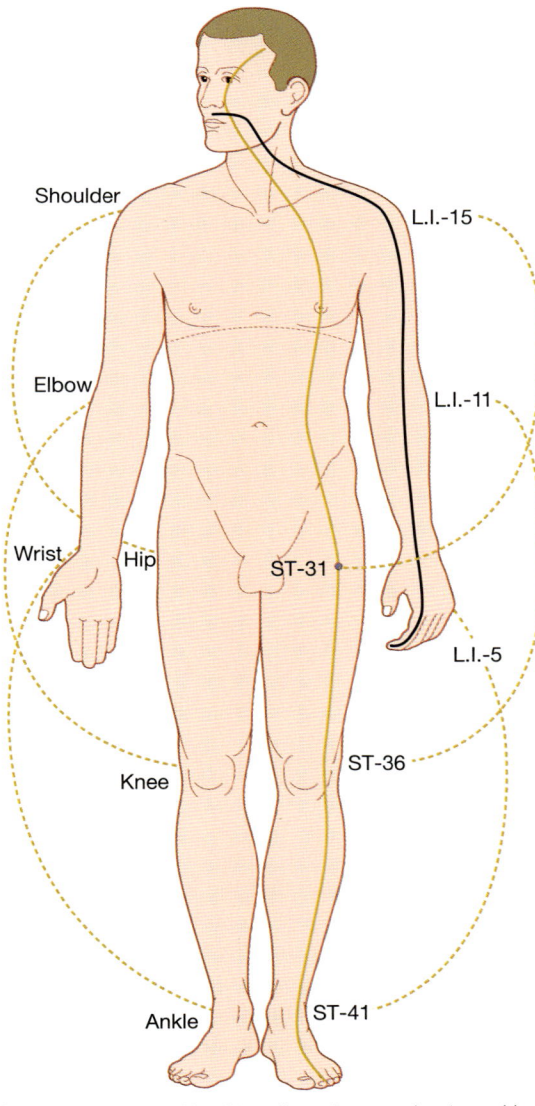

Figure 70.12 Shoulder–hip, elbow–knee and wrist–ankle correspondence in Bright Yang channels

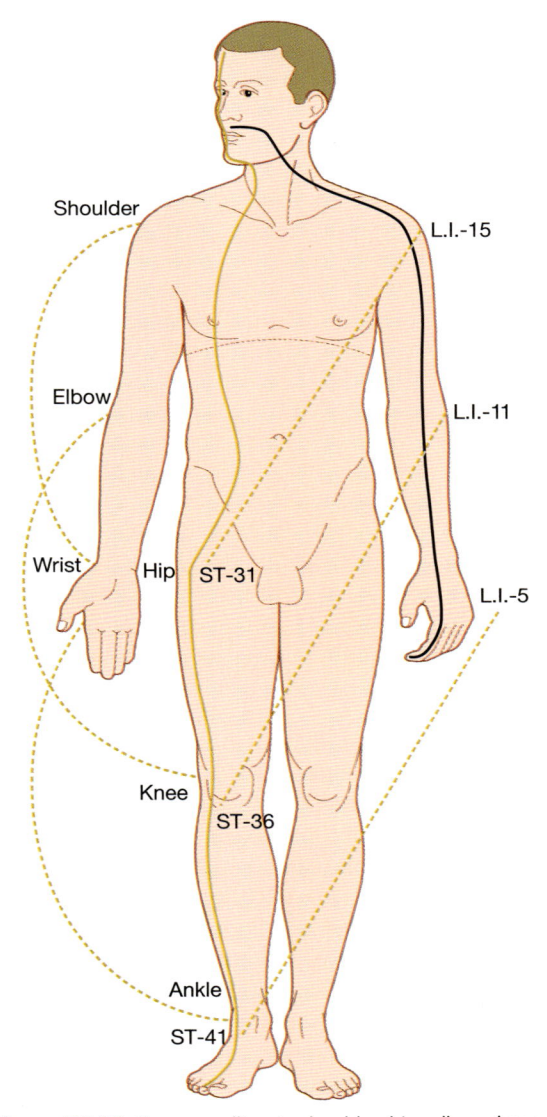

Figure 70.13 Cross-needling in shoulder–hip, elbow–knee and wrist–ankle correspondence in Bright Yang channels

joint according to the two above correspondences (Table 70.2).

Chronic cases

The combination of distal and local points in chronic channel problems is also nearly always used and, in this case, local and distal points reinforce each other's action on the channel.

The main distal and local points are the same as those indicated above.

Organ problems

In interior organ problems, the method of combining distal with local points is always used. One cannot treat the Internal Organs without using distal points, and the local points are often not necessary, except in chronic conditions.

Of course, countless examples could be given of the use of distal points to treat Internal Organ diseases,

Table 70.2 Correspondence of points to joints of the upper and lower part of the body

Joint	Arm	Leg
Shoulder		
Large Intestine	L.I.-15 Jianyu	ST-31 Biguan
Triple Burner	T.B.-14 Jianliao	G.B.-30 Huantiao
Small Intestine	S.I.-10 Naoshu	BL-36 Chengfu
Elbow		
Large Intestine	L.I.-11 Quchi	ST-36 Zusanli
Triple Burner	T.B.-10 Tianjing	G.B.-34 Yanglingquan
Small Intestine	S.I.-8 Xiaohai	BL-40 Weizhong
Wrist		
Large Intestine	L.I.-5 Yangxi	ST-41 Jiexi
Triple Burner	T.B.-4 Yangchi	G.B.-40 Qiuxu
Small Intestine	S.I.-5 Yanggu	BL-60 Kunlun

such as LIV-3 Taichong to treat Liver diseases, ST-36 Zusanli to treat Stomach diseases, and so on.

In chronic conditions of the Internal Organs it is essential to use local points in combination with distal ones. The local points used are mainly the Back Transporting points and Front Collecting points for the relevant Internal Organs. For example, in chronic deficiency of Spleen-Qi, it would be essential to use BL-20 Pishu and/or Ren-12 Zhongwan; in chronic conditions of the Lungs, LU-1 Zhongfu and/or BL-13 Feishu, etc.

When treating chronic headaches some local points on the head are added to the point prescription to treat the Manifestation while the distal points treat the Root. For example, in a chronic case of headaches due to deficiency of Kidney-Yin with rising of Liver-Yang, one can use KI-3 Taixi, SP-6 Sanyinjiao, G.B.-43 Xiaxi and LIV-3 Taichong to treat the Root (i.e. tonify Kidney-Yin and subdue Liver-Yang).

To treat the Manifestation, it would be necessary to add local points according to the channel involved such as G.B.-9 Tianchong and G.B.-6 Xuanli for the Gall Bladder channel or BL-7 Tongtian for the Bladder channel. Assuming the headaches occur always on the left side, I would use KI-3 and SP-6 bilateral, LIV-3 on the right, G.B.-43 on the left (to treat the Gall Bladder channel on the left side) and the local points also on the left side (Fig. 70.14).

The use of local points on the head is important to remove the local stagnation of Qi or Blood in the head which results from chronic headaches, especially if they always occur on the same spot.

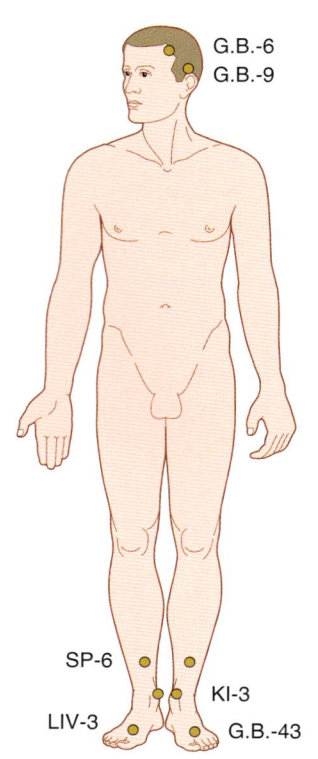

Figure 70.14 Point combination for headaches from Liver-Yang rising and Kidney-Yin deficiency

BALANCING UPPER AND LOWER PARTS OF THE BODY

The channel system forms a closed circuit of energy circulation with a maximum potential of energy on the head, minimum on the chest and average on the hands and feet. In order to maintain the balance between the upper and lower part of the body, it is important to balance the chosen points between these two areas.

After a needle is inserted in a point, it tends to cause a rush of energy towards the top of the body, particularly for the points at the opposite end: that is, the lower part of the body. This movement of Qi is irrespective of the channel's direction of flow. Keeping this in mind, it

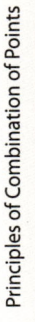

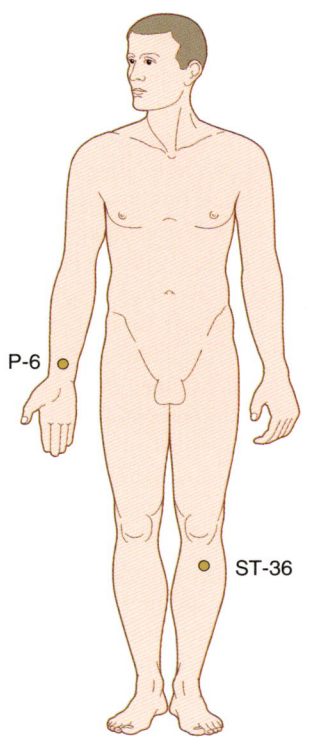

Figure 70.15 Left–right combination of P-6 Neiguan and ST-36 Zusanli

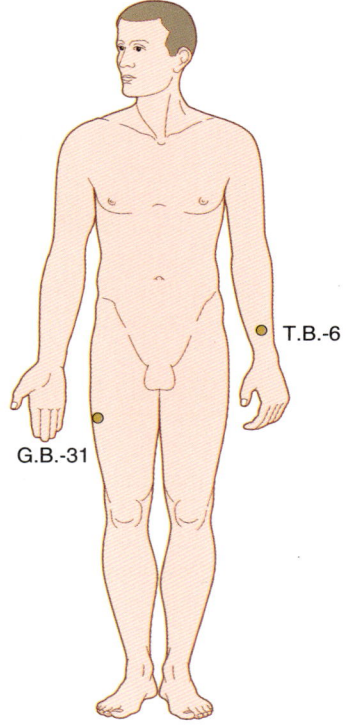

Figure 70.16 Left–right combination of T.B.-6 Zhigou and G.B.-31 Fengshi

is important to balance the points on the upper part of the body with those of the lower part.

An example of point prescription balancing upper and lower part of the body might be L.I.-4 Hegu and LIV-3 Taichong (called the '*Four Gates*'). This combination clears Wind from the head and has a powerful calming effect.

Another example might be the combination of P-6 Neiguan with ST-36 Zusanli. P-6 harmonizes the upper and middle part of the Stomach and subdues rebellious Qi (which causes nausea and vomiting), while ST-36 tonifies Stomach-Qi (Fig. 70.15). The combination of these two points provides a balanced tonification of Stomach and Spleen and can be used in many cases of epigastric problems.

Another example might be the combination of T.B.-6 Zhigou with G.B.-31 Fengshi (Fig. 70.16). These two points clear Wind-Heat from the Blood and can be used for herpes zoster or any skin disease manifesting with a red and itchy rash that changes position rapidly. This combination would be particularly effective if the flanks are affected.

Balancing upper and lower parts of the body achieves a particularly dynamic effect when it is combined with the balancing or Yin–Yang and left–right. For example, this is achieved by using P-6 Neiguan on one side with ST-40 Fenglong on the other.

Of course, there are numerous examples of achieving a balance by using upper and lower points together; such combinations are frequently used. However, this does not mean that one should always balance upper with lower part. In some cases, one might deliberately want to choose an unbalanced point prescription to obtain a specific effect.

For example, if there is an imbalance of energy between the upper and lower part of the body, with a very red face, hypertension, dizziness, anxiety and insomnia caused by a deficiency of Kidney-Yin (Deficiency below) and the rising of Liver-Yang (Excess above), one might choose to needle only KI-1 Yongquan in order to draw the excess Qi on the top downwards.

On the other hand, if a woman suffers from prolapse of the uterus caused by the sinking of Spleen-Qi, one might deliberately use a point on the upper part of the body in order to draw Qi upwards: for example, moxibustion on Du-20 Baihui. In both cases, the channel system dynamics is exploited to draw the energy to the upper or the lower part of the body.

There is another case in which the principle of balancing top with bottom is not applied: this is when a distal point is reduced in acute cases of sprain of the back or a joint. For example, one can strongly reduce the point Du-26 Renzhong for acute sprain of the lower back on the midline over the sacrum.

BALANCING LEFT AND RIGHT

The balancing of points on the left and right sides of the body is something that should be kept in mind when formulating a balanced point combination. There are two aspects to the question of balancing right and left sides when needling. The first is balancing the point combination in terms of left–right when treating a unilateral joint or channel problem; the second is the deliberate use of unilateral points to achieve specific effects.

Balancing left and right when treating a unilateral problem

When treating a unilateral joint or channel problem (e.g. a unilateral neck ache or a unilateral elbow pain) with several points on the affected side attention should be paid to balance left and right by adding one or two points on the opposite side. One can combine this approach with that of balancing Yin and Yang. For example, if we are treating a chronic left shoulder pain along the Large Intestine channel, we might use L.I.-15 Jianyu, L.I.-11 Quchi and L.I.-4 Hegu, all on the left. One way of balancing left and right might be to needle LU-7 Lieque on the right side: this would achieve the effect of balancing left and right and also Yin and Yang.

In some cases, we can balance left and right, Yin and Yang and upper and lower. In the same example of left shoulder pain using L.I.-15 Jianyu, L.I.-11 Quchi and L.I.-4 Hegu all on the left, we might balance these points on the left with LIV-3 Taichong on the right: this achieves a balance of left–right, Yin–Yang and upper–lower. Of course, one would not needle LIV-3 simply to balance the points on the left, but it would be particularly indicated if the patient suffered from a Liver disharmony.

Unilateral needling

Generally speaking, in the majority of cases, bilateral needling is the rule. Such a technique is adopted when a strong effect is needed; however, there are cases when unilateral needling is just as effective.

Points can be needled unilaterally in order to balance the left and right sides. This technique obtains the same therapeutic effect using fewer needles, which is always a bonus, especially for nervous patients, those who are being treated for the first time or those who have a severe deficiency of Qi and Blood. Even in other normal cases, reducing the number of needles used to the minimum without compromising the therapeutic effect is a desirable goal.

Unilateral needling balancing a point on the left with another on the right side can sometimes give even better results than bilateral needling. In particular, if the points balanced between left and right are also at opposite ends (i.e. one on the arm and the other on the leg), the effect is particularly dynamic. It is as if a pressure was applied along the tangent of a circle at opposite ends making it spin (Fig. 70.17). I therefore tend to use unilateral needling to move Qi and Blood and bilateral needling to tonify Qi and nourish Blood or Yin.

> **Clinical note**
>
> I tend to use unilateral (crossed-over) needling to move Qi and Blood and bilateral needling to tonify Qi and nourish Blood and Yin

Figure 70.17 Unilateral needling

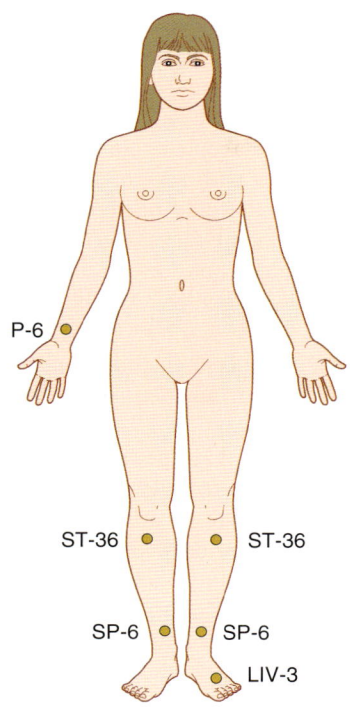

Figure 70.18 Left–right combination of P-6 Neiguan and LIV-3 Taichong with ST-36 Zusanli and SP-6 Sanyinjiao

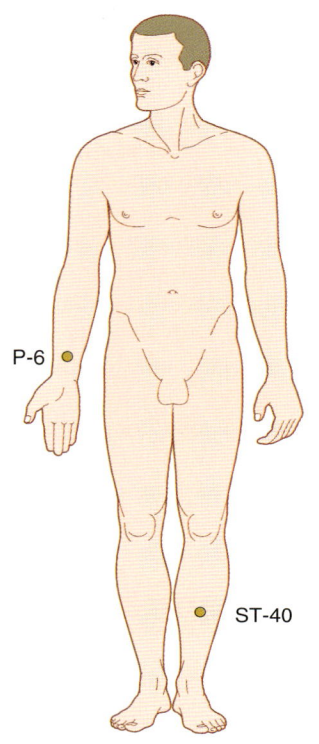

Figure 70.19 Left–right combination of P-6 Neiguan and ST-40 Fenglong

An example of unilateral needling could be the needling of P-6 Neiguan on the right side and LIV-3 Taichong on the left. LIV-3 eliminates stagnation of Liver-Qi or Blood and P-6 moves Blood and calms the Mind. The combination of these two points can therefore eliminate stagnation of Liver-Qi or Blood, particularly if it derives from bottling-up of emotional problems. Very often this situation is also accompanied by a deficiency of Stomach and Spleen, which may arise independently or as a result of invasion of stagnant Liver-Qi to Stomach and Spleen. In such cases, one could combine the needling of P-6 on one side, LIV-3 on the other and ST-36 Zusanli and SP-6 Sanyinjiao bilaterally (Fig. 70.18). The combination of these four points (with six needles instead of eight) can tonify the Stomach and Spleen, calm the Mind and eliminate stagnation of Liver-Qi or Blood.

Another example could be the combination of P-6 Neiguan on one side and ST-40 Fenglong on the other (Fig. 70.19). P-6 harmonizes the Stomach and ST-40 calms the Stomach in Excess patterns: this combination has a good effect in treating Stomach problems of Excess nature. Besides its effect on the Stomach, this particular combination is also used for acute bruising of the ribcage.

Unilateral needling is particularly effective when using two channels of the same polarity, one of the arm the other of the leg: for example, Triple Burner and Gall Bladder (Lesser Yang), Pericardium and Liver (Terminal Yin), and so on. For example, one can use T.B.-5 Waiguan on one side and G.B.-43 Xiaxi on the other for Lesser Yang type of headaches or L.I.-4 Hegu and ST-36 Zusanli for Bright Yang headaches.

The method of using unilateral needling of points on arm and leg channels of the same polarity can be used in the treatment of sprains, as illustrated above, and be combined with the method of using the opposite side (see Figs 70.12 and 70.13). For example, in sprain of the right wrist with tenderness on T.B.-4 Yangchi, one would use G.B.-40 Qiuxu on the left side, so using a point on the related leg channel of the same polarity on the opposite side to the sprained side.

Sometimes unilateral needling is used with the Connecting (*Luo*) points. These are often used on the opposite side to the diseased side, in chronic conditions when the channel is in a deficient state. The use of the Connecting point of the exteriorly–interiorly related channel (either with reducing or even method) will achieve the effect of balancing the left and right side of the channel. For example, if we are treating a chronic pain of the arm along the Large Intestine channel and the channel on the diseased side is in an Empty condition (manifested by dull ache and slight wasting of the muscles), we could use LU-7 Lieque on the healthy side with reducing or even method to balance left and right and shift Qi from the healthy to the diseased side.

The use of the opening and coupled points of the extraordinary vessels is, of course, a good example of the use of unilateral needling and balancing of left and right (ch. 52).

Clinical note

Examples of cross-over unilateral needling:
- P-6 and LIV-3: move Qi, calm the Mind, settle the Ethereal Soul
- P-6 and ST-40: Full patterns of the Stomach, calm the Mind, open the chest
- T.B.-5 and G.B.-43: Lesser Yang headaches
- T.B.-6 and G.B.-41: breast problems
- T.B.-6 and G.B.-31: expel Wind-Heat in skin diseases
- L.I.-4 and ST-36: harmonize the rising and descending of Qi and regulate digestion
- L.I.-4 and ST-44: harmonize the rising and descending of Qi, clear Stomach-Heat
- HE-7 and LIV-3: calm the Mind and settle the Ethereal Soul

BALANCING YIN AND YANG

Balancing the Yin and Yang character of the point used is also important. The nature of the acupuncture points gives us a great choice in the use of points, and we should not think that in order to treat a Yin organ a Yin channel should be used as it is possible to use a Yang channel to treat a Yin organ, or vice versa. For example, ST-36 Zusanli tonifies the Spleen.

This makes it possible to have a wide choice in the balancing of Yin and Yang points.

Generally speaking, it is better to balance Yin and Yang points within one treatment. The excessive use of Yang points may make a person slightly uneasy or edgy, while the excessive use of Yin points may make a person tired. Especially when several points of one polarity are used, it is a good idea to balance them with one or more points of the opposite polarity.

To use the same example as above, if one is treating a shoulder problem with several points on the Large Intestine channel, it would be good to balance them with a single Yin point such as LIV-3 Taichong. This balancing technique could be combined with balancing of left and right and top and bottom. Thus, one might use L.I.-15 Jianyu, L.I.-11 Quchi and L.I.-4 Hegu on the left side and LIV-3 Taichong on the right: that is, balancing Yin and Yang, left and right and top and bottom (Fig. 70.20).

Of course, balancing points should not be chosen just for the sake of balance, but preferably according to a presenting pattern. In other words, it is always better if there is more than one reason for using a certain point.

In balancing Yin and Yang, it is particularly advisable to pay attention to balancing Yang channels with

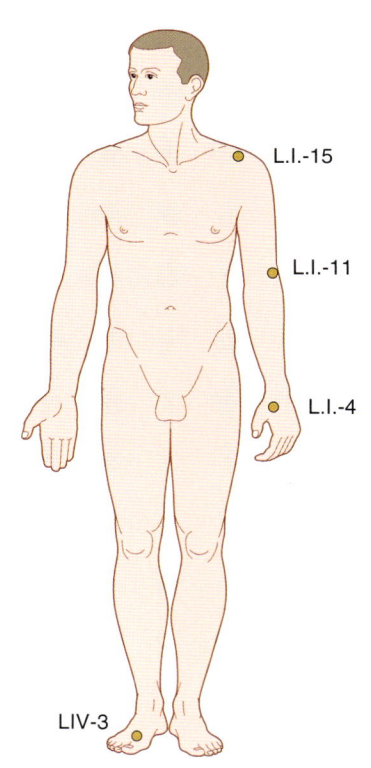

Figure 70.20 Balancing Yin and Yang channels

the Yin channel of the Yin organ across the Overacting cycle of the Five Elements, as follows:

> Gall Bladder–Spleen
> Small Intestine–Lungs
> Stomach–Kidneys
> Large Intestine–Liver
> Bladder–Heart

The example of balancing a series of points on the Large Intestine channels with a point on the Liver channel has been given above. Another example of the balancing of points of Yang channels with points of Yin channels across the Overacting sequence might be the use of SP-6 Sanyinjiao or SP-3 Taibai to balance a series of points on the Gall Bladder channel, such as G.B.-30 Huantiao, G.B.-31 Fengshi and G.B.-34 Yanglingquan treating a sciatica, for example.

The 'Simple Questions' deals with the effects of overaction across the Overacting cycle in chapter 69.[3]

BALANCING FRONT AND BACK

Generally speaking it is not necessary to balance front and back within one treatment. The front points are usually used in acute cases, while the back ones are used in chronic cases. However, this distinction is by no means absolute and both sets of points could be used for acute or chronic cases.

In chronic cases it is often necessary to treat both front and back points. In particular, in very chronic conditions, it is nearly always necessary to use the Back Transporting points at some time during the course of treatment. If treatments are given frequently (i.e. two or three times a week), one can alternate points on the front with those on the back within each treatment: this is a good way to balance the front and back. If treatment is given at more infrequent intervals, points on both the front and back can be used during one treatment. If both back and front points are used in the same treatment, it is better to start with the back points.

Balancing the front and back points can be useful to correct an excessively strong reaction to a treatment. Supposing one has used several back points during one treatment and the patient experiences a fairly strong reaction (whether the treatment was the right one or not), one could correct this by using points on the front in a successive treatment. This method applies to all other categories of balancing mentioned. If a patient experiences a strong reaction, one can analyse the point prescription used and see if it was unbalanced in any way: for example, too many Yin (or Yang) points, too many front (or back) points, too many points on the top (or bottom), too many points on the left (or right) or too many distal (or local) points. If the point prescription appears to be unbalanced, one can balance it appropriately using the opposite type of points.

END NOTES

1. The correlation between Qi circulation in the channel and potential of energy was first formulated by Dr J Lavier in 'Storia, Dottrina e Pratica dell'Agopuntura Cinese', Edizione Mediterranee, Roma, 1966, p. 83.
2. It is an interesting concept that the distal points of the legs (further away from the affected arm) are stronger than those of the arm. This phenomenon could be compared to a lever in physics in which the longer the arm, the easier it is to operate.
3. 1979 The Yellow Emperor's Classic of Internal Medicine – Simple Questions (Huang Ti Nei Jing Su Wen 黄帝内经素问), People's Health Publishing House, Beijing, first published c.100 BC, p. 403–407.

Appendix 1
Prescriptions

AI FU NUAN GONG WAN

Artemisia-Cyperus Warming the Uterus Pill
Ai Ye Folium Artemisiae argyi 9 g
Wu Zhu Yu Fructus Evodiae 4.5 g
Rou Gui Cortex Cinnamomi 4.5 g
Xiang Fu Rhizoma Cyperi 9 g
Dang Gui Radix Angelicae sinensis 9 g
Chuan Xiong Rhizoma Chuanxiong 6 g
Bai Shao Radix Paeoniae alba 6 g
Huang Qi Radix Astragali 6 g
Sheng Di Huang Radix Rehmanniae 9 g
Xu Duan Radix Dipsaci 6 g

AN CHONG TANG

Calming the Penetrating Vessel Decoction
Bai Zhu Rhizoma Atractylodis macrocephalae 9 g
Huang Qi Radix Astragali 9 g
Long Gu Fossilia Ossis mastodi 12 g
Mu Li Concha Ostreae 12 g
Sheng Di Huang Radix Rehmanniae 6 g
Bai Shao Radix Paeoniae alba 6 g
Wu Zei Gu Endoconcha Sepiae 6 g
Qian Cao Gen Radix Rubiae 6 g
Xu Duan Radix Dipsaci 6 g

AN SHEN DING ZHI WAN

Calming the Spirit and Settling the Will-Power Pill
Fu Ling Poria 9 g
Fu Shen Sclerotium Poriae pararadicis 9 g
Ren Shen Radix Ginseng 9 g
Yuan Zhi Radix Polygalae 9 g
Shi Chang Pu Rhizoma Acori tatarinowii 4.5 g
Long Chi Fossilia Dentis mastodi 4.5 g

BA XIAN CHANG SHOU WAN

Eight Immortals Longevity Pill
Mai Men Dong Radix Ophiopogonis 6 g
Wu Wei Zi Fructus Schisandrae 6 g
Shu Di Huang Radix Rehmanniae preparata 24 g
Shan Zhu Yu Fructus Corni 12 g
Shan Yao Rhizoma Dioscoreae 12 g
Ze Xie Rhizoma Alismatis 9 g
Mu Dan Pi Cortex Moutan 9 g
Fu Ling Poria 9 g

BA ZHENG SAN

Eight Rectifications Powder
Mu Tong Caulis Akebiae 3 g
Hua Shi Talcum 12 g
Che Qian Zi Semen Plantaginis 9 g
Qu Mai Herba Dianthi 6 g
Bian Xu Herba Polygoni avicularis 6 g
Shan Zhi Zi Fructus Gardeniae jasminoidis 3 g
Da Huang Radix et Rhizoma Rhei 6 g
Deng Xin Cao Medulla Junci 3 g
Gan Cao Radix Glycyrrhizae 3 g

BAI HE GU JIN TANG

Lilium Consolidating Metal Decoction
Bai He Bulbus Lilii 15 g
Mai Men Dong Radix Ophiopogonis 9 g
Xuan Shen Radix Scrophulariae 9 g
Sheng Di Huang Radix Rehmanniae 9 g
Shu Di Huang Radix Rehmanniae preparata 9 g
Dang Gui Radix Angelicae sinensis 6 g
Bai Shao Radix Paeoniae alba 9 g
Jie Geng Radix Platycodi 6 g
Chuan Bei Mu Bulbus Fritillariae cirrhosae 6 g
Gan Cao Radix Glycyrrhizae 3 g

BAI HU TANG

White Tiger Decoction
Shi Gao Gypsum fibrosum 30 g
Zhi Mu Rhizoma Anemarrhenae 9 g
Zhi Gan Cao Radix Glycyrrhizae preparata 3 g
Geng Mi Semen Oryzae sativae 9 g

BAI TOU WENG TANG

Pulsatilla Decoction
Bai Tou Weng *Radix Pulsatillae* 6 g
Huang Lian *Rhizoma Coptidis* 9 g
Huang Bo *Cortex Phellodendri* 9 g
Qin Pi *Cortex Fraxini* 9 g

BAN XIA HOU PO TANG

Pinellia-Magnolia Decoction
Ban Xia *Rhizoma Pinelliae preparatum* 9–12 g
Hou Po *Cortex Magnoliae officinalis* 9 g
Fu Ling *Poria* 12 g
Zi Su Ye *Folium Perillae* 6 g
Sheng Jiang *Rhizoma Zingiberis recens* 15 g
BAN XIA TANG (from "Spiritual Axis")
Pinellia Decoction
Ban Xia *Rhizoma Pinelliae preparatum* 10 g
Shu Mi Husked sorghum 10 g

BAN XIA TANG (FROM "THOUSAND GOLDEN DUCATS PRESCRIPTIONS")

Pinellia Decoction
Ban Xia *Rhizoma Pinelliae preparatum* 10 g
Rou Gui *Cortex Cinnamomi* 3 g
Gan Jiang *Rhizoma Zingiberis* 3 g
Gan Cao *Radix Glycyrrhizae* 3 g
Ren Shen *Radix Ginseng* 6 g
Xi Xin *Herba Asari* 1.5 g
Fu Zi *Radix Aconiti lateralis preparata* 3 g
Chuan Jiao *Pericarpium Zanthoxyli* 3 g

BAN XIA TANG (FROM "SECRET PRESCRIPTIONS OF A FRONTIER OFFICIAL")

Pinellia Decoction
Ban Xia *Rhizoma Pinelliae preparatum* 10 g
Sheng Jiang *Rhizoma Zingiberis recens* 6 g
Jie Geng *Radix Platycodi* 3 g
Wu Zhu Yu *Fructus Evodiae* 3 g
Qian Hu *Radix Peucedani* 6 g
Bie Jia *Carapax Trionycis* 6 g
Zhi Shi *Fructus Aurantii immaturus* 6 g
Ren Shen *Radix Ginseng* 6 g
Bing Lang *Semen Arecae* 14 nuts

BAO HE WAN

Preserving and Harmonizing Pill
Shan Zha *Fructus Crataegi* 9 g
Shen Qu *Massa Medicata Fermentata* 9 g
Lai Fu Zi *Semen Raphani* 6 g
Chen Pi *Pericarpium Citri reticulatae* 6 g
Ban Xia *Rhizoma Pinelliae preparatum* 9 g
Fu Ling *Poria* 9 g
Lian Qiao *Fructus Forsythiae* 3 g

BAO YIN JIAN

Protecting Yin Decoction
Sheng Di Huang *Radix Rehmanniae* 24 g
Shu Di Huang *Radix Rehmanniae preparata* 15 g
Bai Shao *Radix Paeoniae alba* 12 g
Shan Yao *Rhizoma Dioscoreae* 12 g
Huang Qin *Radix Scutellariae* 9 g
Huang Bo *Cortex Phellodendri* 9 g
Xu Duan *Radix Dipsaci* 6 g
Gan Cao *Radix Glycyrrhizae* 3 g

BAO YUAN TANG

Preserving the Source Decoction
Huang Qi *Radix Astragali* 6 g
Ren Shen *Radix Ginseng* 6 g
Zhi Gan Cao *Radix Glycyrrhizae preparata* 3 g
Rou Gui *Cortex Cinnamomi* 1.5 g

BEI MU GUA LOU SAN

Fritillaria-Trichosanthes Powder
Zhe Bei Mu *Bulbus Fritillariae thunbergii* 4.5 g
Gua Lou *Fructus Trichosanthis* 3 g
Tian Hua Fen *Radix Trichosanthis* 2.4 g
Fu Ling *Poria* 2.4 g
Chen Pi *Pericarpium Citri reticulatae* 2.4 g
Jie Geng *Radix Platycodi* 2.4 g

BU FEI TANG

Tonifying the Lungs Decoction
Ren Shen *Radix Ginseng* 9 g
Huang Qi *Radix Astragali* 24 g
Shu Di Huang *Radix Rehmanniae preparata* 24 g

Wu Wei Zi Fructus Schisandrae 6 g
Zi Wan Radix Asteris 9 g
Sang Bai Pi Cortex Mori 12 g

BU GAN TANG

Tonifying the Liver Decoction
Dang Gui Radix Angelicae sinensis 9 g
Chuan Xiong Rhizoma Chuanxiong 6 g
Bai Shao Radix Paeoniae alba 9 g
Shu Di Huang Radix Rehmanniae preparata 15 g
Suan Zao Ren Semen Ziziphi spinosae 6 g
Mu Gua Fructus Chaenomelis 6 g
Zhi Gan Cao Radix Glycyrrhizae preparata 3 g

BU SHEN AN TAI YIN

Tonifying the Kidneys and Calming the Foetus Decoction
Dang Shen Radix Codonopsis 6 g
Huang Qi Radix Astragali 6 g
Dang Gui Radix Angelicae sinensis 6 g
Bai Zhu Rhizoma Atractylodis macrocephalae 6 g
Fu Shen Sclerotium Poriae pararadicis 6 g
Tu Si Zi Semen Cuscutae 6 g
Shan Zhu Yu Fructus Corni 4.5 g
Suan Zao Ren Semen Ziziphi spinosae 3 g
Shen Qu Massa Medicata Fermentata 6 g
Sheng Jiang Rhizoma Zingiberis recens 3 slices
Da Zao Fructus Jujubae 3 dates

BU SHEN GU CHONG WAN

Tonifying the Kidneys and Consolidating the Penetrating Vessel Pill
Tu Si Zi Semen Cuscutae 6 g
Xu Duan Radix Dipsaci 6 g
Ba Ji Tian Radix Morindae officinalis 6 g
Du Zhong Cortex Eucommiae 6 g
Lu Jiao Shuang Cornu Cervi degelatinatum 6 g
Dang Gui Radix Angelicae sinensis 6 g
Shu Di Huang Radix Rehmanniae preparata 9 g
Gou Qi Zi Fructus Lycii 9 g
E Jiao Colla Corii asini 6 g
Dang Shen Radix Codonopsis 6 g
Bai Zhu Rhizoma Atractylodis macrocephalae 9 g
Da Zao Fructus Jujubae 3 dates
Sha Ren Fructus Amomi 3 g

BU SHEN YANG XUE TANG

Tonifying the Kidneys and Nourishing Blood Decoction
Yin Yang Huo Herba Epimedii 6 g
Xian Mao Rhizoma Curculiginis 6 g
Zi He Che Placenta hominis 6 g
Nu Zhen Zi Fructus Ligustri lucidi 6 g
Dang Gui Radix Angelicae sinensis 6 g
Bai Shao Radix Paeoniae alba 9 g
Dang Shen Radix Codonopsis 6 g
Gou Qi Zi Fructus Lycii 6 g
Tu Si Zi Semen Cuscutae 6 g
Xiang Fu Rhizoma Cyperi 3 g

BU ZHONG YI QI TANG

Tonifying the Centre and Benefiting Qi Decoction
Huang Qi Radix Astragali 12 g
Ren Shen Radix Ginseng 9 g
Bai Zhu Rhizoma Atractylodis macrocephalae 9 g
Dang Gui Radix Angelicae sinensis 6 g
Chen Pi Pericarpium Citri reticulatae 6 g
Sheng Ma Rhizoma Cimicifugae 3 g
Chai Hu Radix Bupleuri 3 g

CANG FU DAO TAN WAN

Atractylodes-Cyperus Conducting Phlegm Pill
Cang Zhu Rhizoma Atractylodis 9 g
Xiang Fu Rhizoma Cyperi 9 g
Zhi Ke Fructus Aurantii 9 g
Fu Ling Poria 9 g
Chen Pi Pericarpium Citri reticulatae 6 g
Dan Nan Xing Rhizoma Arisaematis preparatum 4.5 g
Gan Cao Radix Glycyrrhizae 3 g
Sheng Jiang Rhizoma Zingiberis recens 3 slices
Shen Qu Massa Medicata Fermentata 6 g

CHAI HU SHU GAN TANG

Bupleurum Soothing the Liver Decoction
Chai Hu Radix Bupleuri 6 g
Bai Shao Radix Paeoniae alba 4.5 g
Zhi Ke Fructus Aurantii 4.5 g
Zhi Gan Cao Radix Glycyrrhizae preparata 1.5 g
Chen Pi Pericarpium Citri reticulatae 6 g
Xiang Fu Rhizoma Cyperi 4.5 g
Chuan Xiong Rhizoma Chuanxiong 4.5 g

CHANG TAI BAI ZHU SAN

Long [Life] Foetus Atractylodes Powder
Bai Zhu Rhizoma Atractylodis macrocephalae 6 g
Chuan Xiong Rhizoma Chuanxiong 3 g
Chuan Jiao Pericarpium Zanthoxyli 3 g
Sheng Di Huang Radix Rehmanniae 6 g
E Jiao Colla Corii asini 6 g
Mu Li Concha Ostreae 9 g
Fu Ling Poria 6 g

CHEN XIANG JIANG QI TANG

Aquilaria Descending Qi Decoction
Chen Xiang Lignum Aquilariae resinatum 9 g
Xiang Fu Rhizoma Cyperi 6 g
Sha Ren Fructus Amomi 3 g
Gan Cao Radix Glycyrrhizae 3 g

DA BU YIN WAN

Great Tonifying Yin Pill
Zhi Mu Rhizoma Anemarrhenae 120 g
Huang Bo Cortex Phellodendri 120 g
Shu Di Huang Radix Rehmanniae preparata 180 g
Gui Ban Plastrum Testudinis 180 g
Pig's bone-marrow 120 g

DA BU YUAN JIAN

Great Tonifying the Original [Qi] Decoction
Ren Shen Radix Ginseng 3 g
Shan Yao Rhizoma Dioscoreae 6 g
Shu Di Huang Radix Rehmanniae preparata 9 g
Du Zhong Cortex Eucommiae 6 g
Dang Gui Radix Angelicae sinensis 6 g
Shan Zhu Yu Fructus Corni 3 g
Gou Qi Zi Fructus Lycii 6 g
Zhi Gan Cao Radix Glycyrrhizae preparata 3 g

DA DING FENG ZHU

Big Stopping Wind Pearl
Ji Zi Huang Egg yolk 2 yolks
E Jiao Colla Corii asini 9 g
Bai Shao Radix Paeoniae alba 18 g
Zhi Gan Cao Radix Glycyrrhizae preparata 12 g
Wu Wei Zi Fructus Schisandrae 6 g
Sheng Di Huang Radix Rehmanniae 18 g
Mai Men Dong Radix Ophiopogonis 18 g

Huo Ma Ren Semen Cannabis 6 g
Gui Ban Plastrum Testudinis 12 g
Bie Jia Carapax Trionycis 12 g
Mu Li Concha Ostreae 12 g

DAN SHEN YIN

Salvia Decoction
Dan Shen Radix Salviae miltiorrhizae 30 g
Tan Xiang Lignum Santali albi 4.5 g
Sha Ren Fructus Amomi 4.5 g

DAN ZHI XIAO YAO SAN

Moutan-Gardenia Free and Easy Wanderer Powder
Dang Gui Radix Angelicae sinensis 3 g
Bai Shao Radix Paeoniae alba 3 g
Fu Ling Poria 3 g
Bai Zhu Rhizoma Atractylodis macrocephalae 3 g
Chai Hu Radix Bupleuri 3 g
Bo He Herba Menthae haplocalycis 3 g
Mu Dan Pi Cortex Moutan 1.5 g
Shan Zhi Zi Fructus Gardeniae jasminoidis 1.5 g
Zhi Gan Cao Radix Glycyrrhizae preparata 1.5 g

DANG GUI JI XUE TENG TANG

Angelica-Ji Xue Teng Decoction
Dang Gui Radix Angelicae sinensis 15 g
Shu Di Huang Radix Rehmanniae preparata 15 g
Long Yan Rou Arillus Longan 6 g
Bai Shao Radix Paeoniae alba 9 g
Dan Shen Radix Salviae miltiorrhizae 9 g
Ji Xue Teng Caulis Spatholobi 15 g

DANG GUI JIAN ZHONG TANG

Angelica Strengthening the Centre Decoction
Dang Gui Radix Angelicae sinensis 9 g
Yi Tang Maltosum 30 g
Bai Shao Radix Paeoniae alba 18 g
Gui Zhi Ramulus Cinnamomi 9 g
Sheng Jiang Rhizoma Zingiberis recens 10 g
Zhi Gan Cao Radix Glycyrrhizae preparata 6 g
Da Zao Fructus Jujubae 12 dates

DANG GUI LONG HUI TANG

Angelica-Gentiana-Aloe Decoction
Dang Gui Radix Angelicae sinensis 6 g
Long Dan Cao Radix Gentianae 6 g

Lu Hui Herba Aloes 6 g
Shan Zhi Zi Fructus Gardeniae jasminoidis 4.5 g
Huang Lian Rhizoma Coptidis 3 g
Huang Bo Cortex Phellodendri 6 g
Huang Qin Radix Scutellariae 6 g
Da Huang Radix et Rhizoma Rhei 6 g
Mu Xiang Radix Aucklandiae 3 g

DANG GUI GUI ZHI TANG

Angelica-Ramulus Cinnamomi Decoction
Dang Gui Radix Angelicae sinensis 9 g
Gui Zhi Ramulus Cinnamomi 1g
Bai Shao Radix Paeoniae alba 3 g
Ban Xia Rhizoma Pinelliae preparatum 6 g
Zhi Gan Cao Radix Glycyrrhizae preparata 0.6 g
Pao Jiang Rhizoma Zingiberis officinalis recens (fried) 2 slices
Da Zao Fructus Jujubae 3 dates

DANG GUI SHAO YAO SAN

Angelica-Paeonia Powder
Dang Gui Radix Angelicae sinensis 3 g
Bai Shao Radix Paeoniae alba 15 g
Fu Ling Poria 4 g
Bai Zhu Rhizoma Atractylodis macrocephalae 4 g
Ze Xie Rhizoma Alismatis 8 g
Chuan Xiong Rhizoma Chuanxiong 8 g
Zhi Gan Cao Radix Glycyrrhizae preparata 3 g

DANG GUI SI NI TANG

Angelica Four Rebellious Decoction
Dang Gui Radix Angelicae sinensis 12 g
Bai Shao Radix Paeoniae alba 9 g
Gui Zhi Ramulus Cinnamomi 9 g
Xi Xin Herba Asari 1.5 g
Zhi Gan Cao Radix Glycyrrhizae preparata 5 g
Da Zao Fructus Jujubae 8 pieces
Mu Tong Caulis Akebiae 3 g

DAO CHI SAN

Conducting Redness Powder
Sheng Di Huang Radix Rehmanniae 15 g
Mu Tong Caulis Akebiae 3 g
Zhu Ye Folium Phyllostachys nigrae 3 g
Gan Cao Radix Glycyrrhizae 3 g

DAO CHI QING XIN TANG

Conducting Redness and Clearing the Heart Decoction
Sheng Di Huang Radix Rehmanniae 6 g
Mu Tong Caulis Akebiae 3 g
Mai Men Dong Radix Ophiopogonis 6 g
Fu Shen Sclerotium Poriae pararadicis 6 g
Mu Dan Pi Cortex Moutan 6 g
Lian Zi Xin Plumula Nelumbinis nuciferae 6 g
Hua Shi Talcum 6 g
Gan Cao Radix Glycyrrhizae 3 g
Hu Po Succinum 3 g
Zhu Ye Folium Phyllostachys nigrae 6 g

DI SHENG TANG

Supporting the Sage Decoction
Chi Shao Radix Paeoniae rubra 6 g
Ban Xia Rhizoma Pinelliae preparatum 6 g
Ze Lan Herba Lycopi 6 g
Ren Shen Radix Ginseng 6 g
Sheng Jiang Rhizoma Zingiberis recens 3 slices
Chen Pi Pericarpium Citri reticulatae 3 g
Gan Cao Radix Glycyrrhizae 3 g

DI TAN TANG

Scouring Phlegm Decoction
Ban Xia Rhizoma Pinelliae preparatum 6.6 g
Chen Pi Pericarpium Citri reticulatae 6 g
Fu Ling Poria 6 g
Zhi Shi Fructus Aurantii immaturus 6 g
Zhu Ru Caulis Bambusae in Taeniam 2.1g
Dan Nan Xing Rhizoma Arisaematis preparatum 6.6 g
Shi Chang Pu Rhizoma Acori tatarinowii 3 g
Ren Shen Radix Ginseng 3 g
Gan Cao Radix Glycyrrhizae 1.5 g

DING XIANG SHI DI TANG

Caryophyllum-Diospyros Decoction
Ding Xiang Flos Caryophylli 6 g
Shi Di Calyx Khaki 6 g
Ren Shen Radix Ginseng 3 g
Sheng Jiang Rhizoma Zingiberis recens 6 g

DUO MING SAN

Seizing Life Powder
Mo Yao *Myrrha* 6 g
Xue Jie *Resina Daemonoropis* 6 g

E JIAO JI ZI HUANG TANG

Gelatinum Corii Asini-Egg Yolk Decoction
E Jiao *Colla Corii asini* 6 g
Ji Zi Huang Egg yolk, 2 yolks
Sheng Di Huang *Radix Rehmanniae* 12 g
Bai Shao *Radix Paeoniae alba* 9 g
Zhi Gan Cao *Radix Glycyrrhizae preparata* 1.5 g
Gou Teng *Ramulus Uncariae cum Uncis* 6 g
Shi Jue Ming *Concha Haliotidis* 15 g
Mu Li *Concha Ostreae* 12 g
Fu Shen *Sclerotium Poriae pararadicis* 12 g
Luo Shi Teng *Caulis Trachelospermi jasminoides* 9 g

ER CHEN TANG

Two Old Decoction
Ban Xia *Rhizoma Pinelliae preparatum* 15 g
Chen Pi *Pericarpium Citri reticulatae* 15 g
Fu Ling *Poria* 9 g
Zhi Gan Cao *Radix Glycyrrhizae preparata* 3 g

FO SHOU SAN

Buddha's Hand Powder
Dang Gui *Radix Angelicae sinensis* 6 g
Chuan Xiong *Rhizoma Chuanxiong* 4 g

FU TU DAN

Poria-Cuscuta Pill
Tu Si Zi *Semen Cuscutae* 150 g
Wu Wei Zi *Fructus Schisandrae* 210 g
Shan Yao *Rhizoma Dioscoreae* 60 g
Lian Zi *Semen Nelumbinis* 60 g
Fu Ling *Poria* 90 g

GAN JIANG LING ZHU TANG

Glycyrrhiza-Zingiber-Poria-Atractylodes Decoction
Gan Cao *Radix Glycyrrhizae* 6 g
Gan Jiang *Rhizoma Zingiberis* 12 g
Fu Ling *Poria* 12 g
Bai Zhu *Rhizoma Atractylodis macrocephalae* 6 g

GE GEN QIN LIAN TANG

Pueraria-Scutellaria-Coptis Decoction
Ge Gen *Radix Puerariae* 9 g
Huang Qin *Radix Scutellariae* 9 g
Huang Lian *Rhizoma Coptidis* 4.5 g
Gan Cao *Radix Glycyrrhizae* 3 g

GE XIA ZHU YU TANG

Eliminating Stasis below the Diaphragm Decoction
Dang Gui *Radix Angelicae sinensis* 9 g
Chuan Xiong *Rhizoma Chuanxiong* 3 g
Chi Shao *Radix Paeoniae rubra* 6 g
Hong Hua *Flos Carthami* 9 g
Tao Ren *Semen Persicae* 9 g
Wu Ling Zhi *Faeces Trogopterori* 9 g
Yan Hu Suo *Rhizoma Corydalis* 3 g
Xiang Fu *Rhizoma Cyperi* 3 g
Zhi Ke *Fructus Aurantii* 5 g
Wu Yao *Radix Linderae* 6 g
Mu Dan Pi *Cortex Moutan* 6 g
Gan Cao *Radix Glycyrrhizae* 9 g

GU CHONG TANG

Consolidating the Penetrating Vessel Decoction
Bai Zhu (chao) *Rhizoma Atractylodis macrocephalae* (fried) 30 g
Huang Qi *Radix Astragali* 18 g
Shan Zhu Yu *Fructus Corni* 24 g
Bai Shao *Radix Paeoniae alba* 12 g
Long Gu (duan) *Fossilia Ossis mastodi* (calcined) 24 g
Mu Li (duan) *Concha Ostreae* (calcined) 24 g
Hai Piao Xiao *Endoconcha Sepiae* 12 g
Zong Lu Tan *Fibra Stipulae Trachycarpi* (charred) 6 g
Wu Bei Zi *Galla Rhois chinensis* 1.5 g
Qian Cao Gen *Radix Rubiae* 9 g

GU TAI JIAN

Consolidating the Foetus Decoction
Huang Qin *Radix Scutellariae* 6 g
Chen Pi *Pericarpium Citri reticulatae* 3 g
Bai Zhu *Rhizoma Atractylodis macrocephalae* 9 g
Dang Gui *Radix Angelicae sinensis* 6 g
Bai Shao *Radix Paeoniae alba* 9 g
E Jiao *Colla Corii asini* 6 g
Sha Ren *Fructus Amomi* 3 g

GUI PI TANG

Tonifying the Spleen Decoction
Ren Shen Radix Ginseng 6 g (or **Dang Shen** Radix Codonopsis 12 g)
Huang Qi Radix Astragali 15 g
Bai Zhu Rhizoma Atractylodis macrocephalae 12 g
Dang Gui Radix Angelicae sinensis 6 g
Fu Shen Sclerotium Poriae pararadicis 9 g
Suan Zao Ren Semen Ziziphi spinosae 9 g
Long Yan Rou Arillus Longan 12 g
Yuan Zhi Radix Polygalae 9 g
Mu Xiang Radix Aucklandiae 3 g
Zhi Gan Cao Radix Glycyrrhizae preparata 4 g
Sheng Jiang Rhizoma Zingiberis recens 3 slices
Hong Zao Fructus Jujubae 5 dates

GUI SHEN WAN

Restoring the Kidneys Pill
Tu Si Zi Semen Cuscutae 6 g
Du Zhong Cortex Eucommiae 4 g
Gou Qi Zi Fructus Lycii 6 g
Shan Zhu Yu Fructus Corni 4 g
Dang Gui Radix Angelicae sinensis 6 g
Shu Di Huang Radix Rehmanniae preparata 6 g
Shan Yao Rhizoma Dioscoreae 6 g
Fu Ling Poria 6 g

GUI ZHI TANG

Ramulus Cinnamomi Decoction
Gui Zhi Ramulus Cinnamomi 9 g
Bai Shao Radix Paeoniae alba 9 g
Sheng Jiang Rhizoma Zingiberis recens 9 g
Da Zao Fructus Jujubae 12 dates
Zhi Gan Cao Radix Glycyrrhizae preparata 6 g

GUI ZHI FU LING WAN

Ramulus Cinnamomi-Poria Pill
Gui Zhi Ramulus Cinnamomi 9 g
Fu Ling Poria 9 g
Chi Shao Radix Paeoniae rubra 9 g
Mu Dan Pi Cortex Moutan 9 g
Tao Ren Semen Persicae 9 g

GUN TAN WAN

Vapourizing Phlegm Pill
Duan Meng Shi Lapis Micae seu Chloriti (calcined) 30 g
Da Huang Radix et Rhizoma Rhei 240 g
Huang Qin Radix Scutellariae 240 g
Chen Xiang Lignum Aquilariae resinatum 15 g

HAO QIN QING DAN TANG

Artemisia-Scutellaria Clearing the Gall-Bladder Decoction
Qing Hao Herba Artemisiae annuae 4.5 g
Huang Qin Radix Scutellariae 4.5 g
Zhu Ru Caulis Bambusae in Taeniam 9 g
Zhi Shi Fructus Aurantii immaturus 4.5 g
Chen Pi Pericarpium Citri reticulatae 4.5 g
Ban Xia Rhizoma Pinelliae preparatum 4.5 g
Chi Fu Ling Poria rubrae 9 g
Bi Yu San Jasper powder:
　Hua Shi Talcum
　Gan Cao Radix Glycyrrhizae
　Qing Dai Indigo pulverata Levis

HEI SHEN SAN

Black [Bean] Spirit Powder
Hei Da Dou Semen Glycines 6 g
Shu Di Huang Radix Rehmanniae preparata 6 g
Dang Gui Radix Angelicae sinensis 6 g
Rou Gui Cortex Cinnamoni 3 g
Bao Jiang Rhizoma Zingiberis officinalis recens (fried) 3 slices
Gan Cao Radix Glycyrrhizae 3 g
Bai Shao Radix Paeoniae alba 6 g
Pu Huang Pollen Typhae 6 g

HUA CHONG WAN

Dissolving Parasites Pill
He Shi Fructus Carpesii abrotanoidis 1500 g
Bing Lang Semen Arecae 1500 g
Ku Lian Gen Pi Cortex Meliae radicis 1500 g
Qian Dan Minium 1500 g
Ming Fan Alumen 375 g

HUA GAN JIAN

Transforming the Liver Decoction
Qing Pi Pericarpium Citri reticulatae viride 6 g
Chen Pi Pericarpium Citri reticulatae 6 g
Bai Shao Radix Paeoniae alba 6 g
Mu Dan Pi Cortex Moutan 4.5 g
Shan Zhi Zi Fructus Gardeniae jasminoidis 4.5 g
Ze Xie Rhizoma Alismatis 4.5 g
Chuan Bei Mu Bulbus Fritillariae cirrhosae 6 g

HUANG LIAN E JIAO TANG

Coptis-Colla Asini Decoction
Huang Lian *Rhizoma Coptidis* 12 g
Huang Qin *Radix Scutellariae* 6 g
E Jiao *Colla Corii asini* 9 g
Bai Shao *Radix Paeoniae alba* 6 g
Ji Zi Huang egg yolk 2 yolks

HUANG QI JIAN ZHONG TANG

Astragalus Strengthening the Centre Decoction
Huang Qi Radix Astragali 9 g
Yi Tang Maltosum 18 g
Gui Zhi Ramulus Cinnamomi 9 g
Bai Shao Radix Paeoniae alba 18 g
Zhi Gan Cao Radix Glycyrrhizae preparata 6 g
Sheng Jiang Rhizoma Zingiberis recens 9 g
Da Zao Fructus Jujubae 12 dates

HUO XIANG ZHENG QI SAN

Agastache Upright Qi Powder
Huo Xiang Herba Pogostemonis 12 g
Hou Po Cortex Magnoliae officinalis 9 g
Chen Pi Pericarpium Citri reticulatae 9 g
Zi Su Ye Folium Perillae 6 g
Bai Zhi Radix Angelicae dahuricae 6 g
Ban Xia Rhizoma Pinelliae preparatum 9 g
Da Fu Pi Pericarpium Arecae 9 g
Bai Zhu Rhizoma Atractylodis macrocephalae 12 g
Fu Ling Poria 9 g
Jie Geng Radix Platycodi 9 g
Zhi Gan Cao Radix Glycyrrhizae preparata 3 g

JIAN LING TANG

Constructing Roof Tiles Decoction
Shan Yao Rhizoma Dioscoreae 30 g
Huai Niu Xi Radix Achyranthis bidentatae 30 g
Dai Zhe Shi Haematitum 24 g
Long Gu Fossilia Ossis mastodi 18 g
Mu Li Concha Ostreae 18 g
Sheng Di Huang Radix Rehmanniae 18 g
Bai Shao Radix Paeoniae alba 12 g
Bai Zi Ren Semen Platycladi 12 g

JIE DU HUO XUE TANG

Expelling Poison Invigorating Blood Decoction
Lian Qiao Fructus Forsythiae 6 g
Ge Gen Radix Puerariae 6 g
Chai Hu Radix Bupleuri 4.5 g
Gan Cao Radix Glycyrrhizae 6 g
Sheng Di Huang Radix Rehmanniae 6 g
Chi Shao Radix Paeoniae rubra 4.5 g
Dang Gui Radix Angelicae sinensis 6 g
Hong Hua Flos Carthami 3 g
Tao Ren Semen Persicae 4.5 g
Zhi Ke Fructus Aurantii 6 g
Bai Shao Radix Paeoniae alba 6 g

JIN GUI SHEN QI WAN

Golden Chest Kidney-Qi Pill
Fu Zi Radix Aconiti lateralis preparata 3 g
Gui Zhi Ramulus Cinnamomi 3 g
Shu Di Huang Radix Rehmanniae preparata 24 g
Shan Zhu Yu Fructus Corni 12 g
Shan Yao Rhizoma Dioscoreae 12 g
Ze Xie Rhizoma Alismatis 9 g
Mu Dan Pi Cortex Moutan 9 g
Fu Ling Poria 9 g

JIN SUO GU JING WAN

Metal Lock Consolidating the Essence Pill
Sha Yuan Ji Li Semen Astragali complanati 60 g
Qian Shi Semen Euryales 60 g
Lian Xu Stamen Nelumbinis nuciferae 60 g
Long Gu Fossilia Ossis mastodi 30 g
Mu Li Concha Ostreae 30 g
Lian Zi Semen Nelumbinis 120 g

JING FANG SI WU TANG

Schizonepeta-Ledebouriella Four Substances Decoction
Jing Jie Herba Schizonepetae 4.5 g
Fang Feng Radix Saposhnikoviae 6 g

Shu Di Huang Radix Rehmanniae preparata 6 g
Dang Gui Radix Angelicae sinensis 6 g
Chuan Xiong Rhizoma Chuanxiong 4.5 g
Bai Shao Radix Paeoniae alba 6 g
Zi Su Ye Folium Perillae 3 g

JU PI ZHU RU TANG

Citrus-Bambusa Decoction
Chen Pi Pericarpium Citri reticulatae 9 g
Zhu Ru Caulis Bambusae in Taeniam 9 g
Ren Shen Radix Ginseng 3 g
Sheng Jiang Rhizoma Zingiberis recens 18 g
Gan Cao Radix Glycyrrhizae 6 g
Da Zao Fructus Jujubae 5 dates

LI YIN JIAN

Regulating Yin Decoction
Shu Di Huang Radix Rehmanniae preparata 9 g
Dang Gui Radix Angelicae sinensis 9 g
Zhi Gan Cao Radix Glycyrrhizae preparata 3 g
Bao Jiang Rhizoma Zingiberis preparatum (fried) 3 slices

LI ZHONG TANG

Regulating the Centre Decoction
Gan Jiang Rhizoma Zingiberis 9 g
Ren Shen Radix Ginseng 9 g
Bai Zhu Rhizoma Atractylodis macrocephalae 9 g
Zhi Gan Cao Radix Glycyrrhizae preparata 3 g

LI ZHONG WAN

Regulating the Centre Pill
Gan Jiang Rhizoma Zingiberis 9 g
Ren Shen Radix Ginseng 9 g
Bai Zhu Rhizoma Atractylodis macrocephalae 9 g
Zhi Gan Cao Radix Glycyrrhizae preparata 3 g

LI ZHONG AN HUI TANG

Regulate the Middle and Calming Roundworms Decoction
Ren Shen Radix Ginseng 2.1g
Bai Zhu Rhizoma Atractylodis macrocephalae 3 g
Fu Ling Poria 3 g
Chuan Jiao Pericarpium Zanthoxyli 0.9 g
Wu Mei Fructus Mume 0.9 g
Gan Jiang Rhizoma Zingiberis 1.5 g

LIAN PO YIN

Coptis-Magnolia Decoction
Huang Lian Rhizoma Coptidis 3 g
Hou Po Cortex Magnoliae officinalis 6 g
Shan Zhi Zi Fructus Gardeniae jasminoidis 9 g
Dan Dou Chi Semen Sojae praeparatum 9 g
Shi Chang Pu Rhizoma Acori tatarinowii 3 g
Ban Xia Rhizoma Pinelliae preparatum 3 g
Lu Gen Rhizoma Phragmitis communis 15 g

LIANG DI TANG

Two "Di" Decoction
Sheng Di Huang Radix Rehmanniae 18 g
Di Gu Pi Cortex Lycii 9 g
Xuan Shen Radix Scrophulariae 12 g
Mai Men Dong Radix Ophiopogonis 9 g
Bai Shao Radix Paeoniae alba 12 g
E Jiao Colla Corii asini 9 g

LIANG FU WAN

Alpinia-Cyperus Pill
Gao Liang Jiang Rhizoma Alpiniae officinari 6 g
Xiang Fu Rhizoma Cyperi 6 g

LIANG GE SAN

Cooling the Diaphragm Powder
Da Huang Radix et Rhizoma Rhei 600 g
Mang Xiao Sulfas Natrii 600 g
Gan Cao Radix Glycyrrhizae 600 g
Huang Qin Radix Scutellariae 300 g
Shan Zhi Zi Fructus Gardeniae jasminoidis 300 g
Lian Qiao Fructus Forsythiae 1200 g
Bo He Herba Menthae haplocalycis 300 g

LIANG SHOU TANG

Two Receiving Decoction
Bai Zhu Rhizoma Atractylodis macrocephalae 9 g
Ren Shen Radix Ginseng 9 g
Chuan Xiong Rhizoma Chuanxiong 6 g
Shu Di Huang Radix Rehmanniae preparata 9 g
Shan Yao Rhizoma Dioscoreae 6 g
Shan Zhu Yu Fructus Corni 4.5 g
Qian Shi Semen Euryales 6 g
Bian Dou Semen Lablab album 6 g
Ba Ji Tian Radix Morindae officinalis 6 g

Du Zhong Cortex Eucommiae 6 g
Bai Guo Semen Ginkgo 6 g

LING GAN WU WEI JIANG XIN TANG

Poria-Glycyrrhiza-Schisandra-Zingiberis-Asarum Decoction
Fu Ling Poria 12 g
Gan Cao Radix Glycyrrhizae 9 g
Gan Jiang Rhizoma Zingiberis 9 g
Xi Xin Herba Asari 9 g
Wu Wei Zi Fructus Schisandrae 6 g

LING GUI ZHU GAN TANG

Poria-Ramulus Cinnamomi-Atractylodis-Glycyrrhiza Decoction
Fu Ling Poria 12 g
Gui Zhi Ramulus Cinnamomi 9 g
Bai Zhu Rhizoma Atractylodis macrocephalae 6 g
Zhi Gan Cao Radix Glycyrrhizae preparata 3 g

LING JIAO GOU TENG TANG

Cornu Antelopis-Uncaria Decoction
Ling Yang Jiao Cornu Saigae tataricae 4.5 g
Gou Teng Ramulus Uncariae cum Uncis 9 g
Sang Ye Folium Mori 6 g
Ju Hua Flos Chrysanthemi 9 g
Bai Shao Radix Paeoniae alba 9 g
Sheng Di Huang Radix Rehmanniae 15 g
Fu Shen Sclerotium Poriae pararadicis 9 g
Chuan Bei Mu Bulbus Fritillariae cirrhosae 12 g
Zhu Ru Caulis Bambusae in Taeniam 15 g
Gan Cao Radix Glycyrrhizae 2.5 g

LIU JUN ZI TANG

Six Gentlemen Decoction
Ren Shen Radix Ginseng 3 g
Bai Zhu Rhizoma Atractylodis macrocephalae 4.5 g
Fu Ling Poria 3 g
Zhi Gan Cao Radix Glycyrrhizae preparata 3 g
Chen Pi Pericarpium Citri reticulatae 3 g
Ban Xia Rhizoma Pinelliae preparatum 4.5 g

LIU WEI DI HUANG WAN

Six-Ingredient Rehmannia Pill
Shu Di Huang Radix Rehmanniae preparata 24 g
Shan Zhu Yu Fructus Corni 12 g
Shan Yao Rhizoma Dioscoreae 12 g
Ze Xie Rhizoma Alismatis 9 g
Mu Dan Pi Cortex Moutan 9 g
Fu Ling Poria 9 g

LONG DAN XIE GAN TANG

Gentiana Draining the Liver Decoction
Long Dan Cao Radix Gentianae 6 g
Huang Qin Radix Scutellariae 9 g
Shan Zhi Zi Fructus Gardeniae jasminoidis 9 g
Ze Xie Rhizoma Alismatis 9 g
Mu Tong Caulis Akebiae 9 g
Che Qian Zi Semen Plantaginis 9 g
Sheng Di Huang Radix Rehmanniae 12 g
Dang Gui Radix Angelicae sinensis 9 g
Chai Hu Radix Bupleuri 9 g
Gan Cao Radix Glycyrrhizae 3 g

LU JIAO TU SI ZI WAN

Cornus Cervi-Cuscuta Pill
Lu Jiao Shuang Cornu Cervi degelat natum 9 g
Tu Si Zi Semen Cuscutae 9 g
Mu Li Concha Ostreae 12 g
Bai Zhu Rhizoma Atractylodis macrocephalae 6 g
Du Zhong Cortex Eucommiae 6 g
Lian Xu Semen Nelumbinis nuciferae 6 g
Bai Guo Semen Ginkgo 6 g
Qian Shi Semen Euryales 6 g

MA HUANG TANG

Ephedra Decoction
Ma Huang Herba Ephedrae 9 g
Gui Zhi Ramulus Cinnamomi 6 g
Xing Ren Semen Armeniacae 9 g
Zhi Gan Cao Radix Glycyrrhizae preparata 3 g

MA XING SHI GAN TANG

Ephedra-Prunus-Gypsum-Glycyrrhiza Decoction
Ma Huang Herba Ephedrae 12 g
Shi Gao Gypsum fibrosum 48 g
Xing Ren Semen Armeniacae 18 g
Zhi Gan Cao Radix Glycyrrhizae preparata 6 g

MA ZI REN WAN

Cannabis Pill
Huo Ma Ren Semen Cannabis 9 g
Da Huang Radix et Rhizoma Rhei 6 g
Xing Ren Semen Armeniacae 4.5 g
Zhi Shi Fructus Aurantii immaturus 6 g
Hou Po Cortex Magnoliae officinalis 4.5 g
Bai Shao Radix Paeoniae alba 4.5 g

MU XIANG LIU QI YIN

Aucklandia Flowing Qi Decoction
Mu Xiang Radix Aucklandiae 6 g
Ban Xia Rhizoma Pinelliae preparatum 6 g
Chen Pi Pericarpium Citri reticulatae 3 g
Hou Po Cortex Magnoliae officinalis 4.5 g
Qing Pi Pericarpium Citri reticulatae viride 3 g
Gan Cao Radix Glycyrrhizae 3 g
Xiang Fu Rhizoma Cyperi 6 g
Zi Su Ye Folium Perillae 3 g
Ren Shen Radix Ginseng 6 g
Fu Ling Poria 6 g
Mu Gua Fructus Chaenomelis 3 g
Shi Chang Pu Rhizoma Acori tatarinowii 3 g
Bai Zhu Rhizoma Atractylodis macrocephalae 4.5 g
Bai Zhi Radix Angelicae dahuricae 3 g
Mai Men Dong Radix Ophiopogonis 6 g
Cao Guo Fructus Tsaoko 3 g
Rou Gui Cortex Cinnamomi 1.5 g
E Zhu Rhizoma Curcumae 3 g
Da Fu Pi Pericarpium Arecae 3 g
Ding Xiang Flos Caryophylli 3 g
Bing Lang Semen Arecae 3 g
Huo Xiang Herba Pogostemonis 3 g
Mu Tong Caulis Akebiae 1.5 g

NEI BU WAN

Inner Tonification Pill
Lu Rong Cornu Cervi pantotrichum 3 g
Tu Si Zi Semen Cuscutae 6 g
Rou Cong Rong Herba Cistanches 6 g
Sha Yuan Zi Semen Astragali complanati 6 g
Huang Qi Radix Astragali 6 g
Sang Piao Xiao Ootheca Mantidis 6 g
Rou Gui Cortex Cinnamomi 2 g
Fu Zi Radix Aconiti lateralis preparata 2g
Bai Ji Li Fructus Tribuli 3 g
Zi Wan Radix Asteris 3 g

NUAN GAN JIAN

Warming the Liver Decoction
Dang Gui Radix Angelicae sinensis 6 g
Gou Qi Zi Fructus Lycii 9 g
Xiao Hui Xiang Fructus Foeniculi 6 g
Rou Gui Cortex Cinnamomi 3 g
Wu Yao Radix Linderae 6 g
Chen Xiang Lignum Aquilariae resinatum 3 g
Fu Ling Poria 6 g
Sheng Jiang Rhizoma Zingiberis recens 3 slices

PING WEI SAN

Balancing the Stomach Powder
Cang Zhu Rhizoma Atractylodis 12 g
Hou Po Cortex Magnoliae officinalis 9 g
Chen Pi Pericarpium Citri reticulatae 9 g
Zhi Gan Cao Radix Glycyrrhizae preparata 3 g

QI GONG WAN

Arousing the Uterus Pill
Ban Xia Rhizoma Pinelliae preparatum 6 g
Cang Zhu Rhizoma Atractylodis 6 g
Chen Pi Pericarpium Citri reticulatae 3 g
Fu Ling Poria 6 g
Xiang Fu Rhizoma Cyperi 6 g
Shen Qu Massa Medicata Fermentata 6 g
Chuan Xiong Rhizoma Chuanxiong 4.5 g

QI JU DI HUANG WAN

Lycium-Chrysanthemum-Rehmannia Pill
Gou Qi Zi *Fructus Lycii* 12 g
Ju Hua *Flos Chrysanthemi* 9 g
Shu Di Huang *Radix Rehmanniae preparata* 24 g
Shan Zhu Yu *Fructus Corni* 12 g
Shan Yao *Rhizoma Dioscoreae* 12 g
Ze Xie *Rhizoma Alismatis* 9 g
Mu Dan Pi *Cortex Moutan* 9 g
Fu Ling *Poria* 9 g

QING GAN YIN JING TANG

Clearing the Liver and Guiding the Period Decoction
Dang Gui Radix Angelicae sinensis 6 g
Bai Shao Radix Paeoniae alba 6 g
Sheng Di Huang Radix Rehmanniae 6 g
Gan Cao Radix Glycyrrhizae 3 g
Shan Zhi Zi Fructus Gardeniae jasminoidis 6 g
Huang Qin Radix Scutellariae 4 g
Chuan Lian Zi Fructus Toosendan 3 g
Qian Cao Gen Radix Rubiae 6 g
Bai Mao Gen Rhizoma Imperatae 6 g
Chuan Niu Xi Radix Cyathulae 3 g
Mu Dan Pi Cortex Moutan 6 g

QING HAI WAN

Clearing the Sea Pill
Shu Di Huang Radix Rehmanniae preparata 9 g
Bai Zhu Rhizoma Atractylodis macrocephalae 6 g
Bai Shao Radix Paeoniae alba 6 g
Xuan Shen Radix Scrophulariae 6 g
Sang Ye Folium Mori 3 g
Shan Zhu Yu Fructus Corni 6 g
Shan Yao Rhizoma Dioscoreae 6 g
Mu Dan Pi Cortex Moutan 6 g
Di Gu Pi Cortex Lycii 6 g
Bei Sha Shen Radix Glehniae 6 g
Shi Hu Herba Dendrobii 6 g
Mai Men Dong Radix Ophiopogonis 6 g
Wu Wei Zi Fructus Schisandrae 4.5 g
Long Gu Fossilia Ossis mastodi 9 g

QING JING SAN

Clearing the Menses Powder
Mu Dan Pi Cortex Moutan 6 g
Bai Shao Radix Paeoniae alba 6 g
Shu Di Huang Radix Rehmanniae preparata 6 g
Di Gu Pi Cortex Lycii 15 g
Qing Hao Herba Artemisiae annuae 6 g
Fu Ling Poria 3 g
Huang Bo Cortex Phellodendri 1.5 g

QING LUO YIN

Clearing the Connecting Channels Decoction
Xian Jin Yin Hua Flos Lonicerae japonicae recens 6 g
Xian Bian Dou Hua Flos Dolichoris Lablab recens 6 g
Xi Gua Shuang Mirabilitum Preparata Citrulli 6 g
Si Gua Pi Pericarpium Luffae acutangulae 6 g
Xian He Ye Folium Nelumbinis nuciferae recens 6 g
Xian Zhu Ye Herba Lophateri gracilis recens 6 g

QING QI HUA TAN TANG

Clearing Qi and Resolving Phlegm Decoction
Dan Nan Xing Rhizoma Arisaematis preparatum 6 g
Ban Xia Rhizoma Pinelliae preparatum 6 g
Gua Lou Ren Semen Trichosanthis 6 g
Huang Qin Radix Scutellariae 4.5 g
Chen Pi Pericarpium Citri reticulatae 3 g
Xing Ren Semen armeniacae 4.5 g
Zhi Shi Fructus aurantii immaturus 4.5 g
Fu Ling Poria 6 g

QING RE AN TAI YIN

Clearing Heat and Calming the Foetus Decoction
Huang Lian Rhizoma Coptidis 3 g
Huang Qin Radix Scutellariae 6 g
Ce Bai Ye Cacumen Platycladi 6 g
Chun Gen Bai Pi Cortex Ailanthi 6 g
E Jiao Colla Corii asini 6 g
Shan Yao Rhizoma Dioscoreae 6 g

QING RE GU JING TANG

Clearing Heat and Consolidating the Menses Decoction
Huang Qin Radix Scutellariae 4.5 g
Shan Zhi Zi Fructus Gardeniae jasminoidis (charred) 6 g
Sheng Di Huang Radix Rehmanniae 9 g
Di Gu Pi Cortex Lycii 6 g
Di Yu Radix Sanguisorbae 6 g
E Jiao Colla Corii asini 6 g
Ou Jie Nodus Nelumbinis Rhizomatis 6 g
Zong Lu Zi Fructus Trachycarpi 4.5 g
Gui Ban Plastrum Testudinis (toasted) 12 g
Mu Li Concha Ostreae 12 g
Gan Cao Radix Glycyrrhizae 3 g

QING RE TIAO XUE TANG

Clearing Heat and Regulating Blood Decoction
Mu Dan Pi Cortex Moutan 6 g
Sheng Di Huang Radix Rehmanniae 9 g
Huang Lian Rhizoma Coptidis 4.5 g
Dang Gui Radix Angelicae sinensis 9 g

Bai Shao Radix Paeoniae alba 9 g
Chuan Xiong Rhizoma Chuanxiong 6 g
Hong Hua Flos Carthami 6 g
Tao Ren Semen Persicae 6 g
E Zhu Rhizoma Curcumae 6 g
Xiang Fu Rhizoma Cyperi 6 g
Yan Hu Suo Rhizoma Corydalis 6 g

QING WEI SAN

Clearing the Stomach Powder
Huang Lian Rhizoma Coptidis 1.8 g
Sheng Ma Rhizoma Cimicifugae 3 g
Mu Dan Pi Cortex Moutan 1.5 g
Sheng Di Huang Radix Rehmanniae 0.9 g
Dang Gui Radix Angelicae sinensis 0.9 g

QING YING TANG

Clearing Nutritive-Qi Decoction
Shui Niu Jiao Cornu Bubali 18 g
Xuan Shen Radix Scrophulariae 9 g
Sheng Di Huang Radix Rehmanniae 15 g
Mai Men Dong Radix Ophiopogonis 9 g
Jin Yin Hua Flos Lonicerae 9 g
Lian Qiao Fructus Forsythiae 6 g
Huang Lian Rhizoma Coptidis 4.5 g
Zhu Ye Folium Phyllostachys nigrae 3 g
Dan Shen Radix Salviae miltiorrhizae 6 g

QING ZAO RUN CHANG TANG

Clearing Dryness and Moisteting the Intestines Decoction
Sheng Di Huang Radix Rehmanniae 9 g
Shu Di Huang Radix Rehmannia preparata 6 g
Dang Gui Radix Angelicae sinensis 6 g
Huo Ma Ren Semen Cannabis 4.5 g
Gua Lou Ren Semen Trichosanthis 6 g
Yu Li Ren Semen Pruni 6 g
Shi Hu Herba Dendrobi 9 g
Zhi Ke Fructus aurantii 3 g
Qing Pi Pericarpium Citri reticulatae viride 3 g
Jin Ju Fructus Fortunaellae margaritae 4.5 g

QU TIAO TANG

Expelling Tapeworms Decoction
Nan Gua Zi Semen Cucurbitae moschatae 60–120 g
Bing Lang Semen Arecae 30–60 g

REN SHEN BU FEI TANG

Ginseng Tonifying the Lungs Decoction
Ren Shen Radix Ginseng 9 g
Huang Qi Radix Astragali 24 g
Shu Di Huang Radix Rehmanniae preparata 24 g
Wu Wei Zi Fructus Schisandrae 6 g
Zi Wan Radix Asteris 6 g
Sang Bai Pi Cortex Mori 6 g

ROU FU BAO YUAN TANG

Cinnamomum-Aconitum Preserving the Source Decoction
Rou Gui Cortex Cinnamomi 1.5 g
Fu Zi Radix Aconiti lateralis preparata 3 g
Huang Qi Radix Astragali 6 g
Ren Shen Radix Ginseng 6 g
Zhi Gan Cao Radix Glycyrrhizae preparata 3 g

SAN JIA FU MAI TANG

Three Carapaces Restoring the Pulse Decoction
Zhi Gan Cao Radix Glycyrrhizae preparata 18 g
Sheng Di Huang Radix Rehmanniae 18 g
Bai Shao Radix Paeoniae alba 18 g
Mai Men Dong Radix Ophiopogonis 15 g
Huo Ma Ren Semen Cannabis 9 g
E Jiao Colla Corii asini 9 g
Mu Li Concha Ostreae 15 g
Bie Jia Carapax Trionycis 24 g
Gui Ban Plastrum Testudinis 30 g

SAN MIAO HONG TENG TANG

Three Wonderful Sargentodoxa Decoction
Cang Zhu Rhizoma Atractylodis
Huang Bo Cortex Phellodendri
Yi Yi Ren Semen Coicis
Hong Teng Caulis Sargentodoxae
Xiao Ji Herba Cephalanoplos
Da Ji Herba seu Radix Cirsii japonici
Xian He Cao Herba Agrimoniae
Yi Mu Cao Herba Leonuri
Xia Ku Cao Spica Prunellae
Xiang Fu Rhizoma Cyperi
Bai Jiang Cao Herba Patriniae

SAN REN TANG

Three Seeds Decoction
Xing Ren Semen Armeniacae
Hua Shi Talcum
Tong Cao Medulla Tetrapanacis
Bai Dou Kou Fructus Amomi rotundus
Zhu Ye Folium Phyllostachys nigrae
Yi Yi Ren Semen Coicis
Ban Xia Rhizoma Pinelliae preparatum

SAN ZI YANG QIN TANG

Three-Seed Nourishing the Ancestors Decoction
Bai Jie Zi Semen Sinapis 6 g
Su Zi Fructus Perillae 6 g
Lai Fu Zi Semen Raphani 6 g

SANG JU YIN

Morus-Chrysanthemum Decoction
Sang Ye Folium Mori 7.5 g
Ju Hua Flos Chrysanthemi 3 g
Lian Qiao Fructus Forsythiae 4.5 g
Bo He Herba Menthae haplocalycis 2.4 g
Jie Geng Radix Platycodi 6 g
Xing Ren Semen Armeniacae 6 g
Lu Gen Rhizoma Phragmitis 6 g
Gan Cao Radix Glycyrrhizae 3 g

SANG PIAO XIAO SAN

Ootheca Mantidis Powder
Sang Piao Xiao Ootheca Mantidis 9 g
Long Gu Fossilia Ossis mastodi 12 g
Ren Shen Radix Ginseng 9 g
Fu Shen Sclerotium Poriae pararadicis 9 g
Yuan Zhi Radix Polygalae 3 g
Shi Chang Pu Rhizoma Acori tatarinowii 6 g
Zhi Gui Ban Plastrum Testudinis (honey-fried) 9 g
Dang Gui Radix Angelicae sinensis 6 g

SANG XING TANG

Morus-Prunus Decoction
Sang Ye Folium Mori 3 g
Shan Zhi Zi Fructus Gardeniae jasminoidis 3 g
Dan Dou Chi Semen Sojae praeparatum 3 g
Xing Ren Semen Armeniacae 4.5 g
Zhe Bei Mu Bulbus Fritillariae thunbergii 3 g
Nan Sha Shen Radix Adenophorae 6 g
Li Pi Fructus Pyri 3 g

SHA SHEN MAI DONG TANG

Glehnia-Ophiopogon Decoction
Sha Shen Radix Adenophorae seu Glehniae 9 g
Mai Men Dong Radix Ophiopogonis 9 g
Yu Zhu Rhizoma Poligonati odorati 5 g
Sang Ye Folium Mori 4.5 g
Tian Hua Fen Radix Trichosanthis 4.5 g
Bian Dou Semen Lablab album 4.5 g
Gan Cao Radix Glycyrrhizae 3 g

SHAO FU ZHU YU TANG

Lower Abdomen Eliminating Stasis Decoction
Xiao Hui Xiang Fructus Foeniculi 6 g
Gan Jiang Rhizoma Zingiberis 2 g
Rou Gui Cortex Cinnamomi 1.5 g
Yan Hu Suo Rhizoma Corydalis 6 g
Mo Yao Myrrha 6 g
Pu Huang Pollen Typhae 6 g
Wu Ling Zhi Faeces Trogopterori 4.5 g
Dang Gui Radix Angelicae sinensis 9 g
Chuan Xiong Radix Chuanxiong 4.5 g
Chi Shao Yao Radix Paeoniae rubra 6 g

SHAO YAO TANG

Paeonia Decoction
Bai Shao Radix Paeoniae alba 30 g
Dang Gui Radix Angelicae sinensis 15 g
Gan Cao Radix Glycyrrhizae 6 g
Mu Xiang Radix Aucklandiae 6 g
Bing Lang Semen Arecae 6 g
Huang Lian Rhizoma Coptidis 15 g
Huang Qin Radix Scutellariae 15 g
Da Huang Radix et Rhizoma Rhei 9 g
Guan Gui Cortex Cinnamomi loureiroi 7.5 g

SHE GAN MA HUANG TANG

Belamcanda-Ephedra Decoction
She Gan Rhizoma Belamcandae 9 g
Ma Huang Herba Ephedrae 12 g
Zi Wan Radix Asteris 9 g
Kuan Dong Hua Flos Tussilaginis farfarae 9 g
Ban Xia Rhizoma Pinelliae preparatum 9 g
Xi Xin Herba Asari 9 g

Wu Wei Zi Fructus Schisandrae 3 g
Sheng Jiang Rhizoma Zingiberis recens 12 g
Da Zao Fructus Jujubae 3 pieces

SHEN FU TANG

Ginseng-Aconitum Decoction
Ren Shen Radix Ginseng 30 g
Fu Zi Radix Aconiti lateralis preparata 15 g

SHEN GE SAN

Ginseng-Gecko Powder
Ren Shen Radix Ginseng 12 g
Ge Jie Gecko 12 g

SHEN LING BAI ZHU SAN

Ginseng-Poria-Atractylodes Powder
Ren Shen Radix Ginseng 1000 g
Bai Zhu Rhizoma Atractylodis macrocephalae 1000 g
Fu Ling Poria 1000 g
Zhi Gan Cao Radix Glycyrrhizae preparata 1000 g
Shan Yao Radix Dioscoreae 1000 g
Bian Dou Semen Lablab album 750 g
Lian Zi Semen Nelumbinis 500 g
Yi Yi Ren Semen Coicis 500 g
Sha Ren Fructus Amomi 500 g
Jie Geng Radix Platycodi 500 g

SHEN QI SI WU TANG

Ginseng-Astragalus-Four Substances Decoction
Ren Shen Radix Ginseng 9 g
Huang Qi Radix Astragali 9 g
Dang Gui Radix Angelicae sinensis 6 g
Bai Shao Radix Paeoniae alba 9 g
Shu Di Huang Radix Rehmanniae preparata 6 g
Chuan Xiong Rhizoma Chuanxiong 6 g

SHENG HUA TANG

Generating and Resolving Decoction
Dang Gui Radix Angelicae sinensis 24 g
Chuan Xiong Rhizoma Chuanxiong 9 g
Tao Ren Semen Persicae 6 g
Pao Jiang Rhizoma Zingiberis officinalis recens (fried) 1.5 g
Zhi Gan Cao Radix Glycyrrhizae preparata 1.5 g

SHENG MAI SAN

Generating the Pulse Powder
Ren Shen Radix Ginseng 1.5 g
Mai Men Dong Radix Ophiopogonis 1.5 g
Wu Wei Zi Fructus Schisandrae 7 seeds

SHENG YANG TANG

Raising the Yang Decoction
Zhi Gan Cao Radix Glycyrrhizae preparata 6 g
Ma Huang Herba Ephedrae 12 g
Fang Feng Radix Saposhnikoviae 12 g
Qiang Huo Rhizoma seu Radix Notopterygii 18 g

SHENG YU TANG

Sage Healing Decoction
Sheng Di Huang Radix Rehmanniae 9 g
Shu Di Huang Radix Rehmanniae preparata 9 g
Chuan Xiong Rhizoma Chuanxiong 9 g
Ren Shen Radix Ginseng 9 g
Dang Gui Radix Angelicae sinensis 1.5 g
Huang Qi Radix Astragali 1.5 g

SHI WEI SAN

Pyrrosia Powder
Shi Wei Folium Pyrrosiae 9 g
Dong Kui Zi Fructus Malvae 6 g
Qu Mai Herba Dianthi 6 g
Hua Shi Talcum 6 g
Che Qian Zi Semen Plantaginis 6 g

SHI XIAO SAN

Breaking into a Smile Powder
Pu Huang Pollen Typhae 6 g
Wu Ling Zhi Faeces Trogopterori 6 g

SHOU TAI WAN

Foetus Longevity Pill
Tu Si Zi Semen Cuscutae 6 g
Sang Ji Sheng Herba Taxilli 6 g
Xu Duan Radix Dipsaci 6 g
E Jiao Colla Corii asini 6 g

SI JUN ZI TANG

Four Gentlemen Decoction
Ren Shen *Radix Ginseng* 9 g
Bai Zhu *Rhizoma Atractylodis macrocephalae* 9 g
Fu Ling *Poria* 9 g
Zhi Gan Cao *Radix Glycyrrhizae preparata* 3 g

SI MO TANG

Four Milled-Herb Decoction
Ren Shen *Radix Ginseng* 3 g
Bing Lang *Semen Arecae* 9 g
Chen Xiang *Lignum Aquilariae resinatum* 3 g
Wu Yao *Radix Linderae* 9 g

SI NI SAN

Four Rebellious Powder
Chai Hu *Radix Bupleuri* 9 g
Zhi Shi *Fructus Aurantii immaturus* 9 g
Bai Shao *Radix Paeoniae alba* 12 g
Zhi Gan Cao *Radix Glycyrrhizae preparata* 6 g

SI NI TANG

Four Rebellions Decoction
Fu Zi *Radix Aconiti lateralis preparata* 6 g
Gan Jiang *Rhizoma Zingiberis* 4.5 g
Zhi Gan Cao *Radix Glycyrrhizae preparata* 6 g

SI WU MA ZI REN WAN

Four Substances Cannabis Pill
Dang Gui *Radix Angelicae sinensis* 6 g
Chuan Xiong *Rhizoma Chuanxiong* 3 g
Shu Di Huang *Radix Rehmanniae preparata* 6 g
Bai Shao *Radix Paeoniae alba* 6 g
Huo Ma Ren *Semen Cannabis* 9 g
Da Huang *Radix et Rhizoma Rhei* 6 g
Xing Ren *Semen Armeniacae* 4.5 g
Zhi Shi *Fructus aurantii immaturus* 6 g
Hou Po *Cortex Magnoliae officinalis* 4.5 g
Bai Shao *Radix Paeoniae alba* 4.5 g

SI WU TANG

Four Substances Decoction
Shu Di Huang *Radix Rehmanniae preparata* 9 g
Bai Shao *Radix Paeoniae alba* 9 g
Dang Gui *Radix Angelicae sinensis* 9 g
Chuan Xiong *Rhizoma Chuanxiong* 3 g

SU ZI JIANG QI TANG

Perilla-Seed Subduing Qi Decoction
Su Zi *Fructus Perillae* 9 g
Ban Xia *Rhizoma Pinelliae preparatum* 9 g
Hou Po *Cortex Magnoliae officinalis* 6 g
Qian Hu *Radix Peucedani* 6 g
Rou Gui *Cortex Cinnamomi cassiae* 3 g
Dang Gui *Radix Angelicae sinensis* 6 g
Sheng Jiang *Rhizoma Zingiberis recens* 2 slices
Su Ye *Folium Perillae* 5 leaves
Zhi Gan Cao *Radix Glycyrrhizae preparata* 6 g
Da Zao *Fructus Jujubae* 1 date

SUO GONG ZHU YU TANG

Contracting the Uterus and Eliminating Stasis Decoction
Dang Gui *Radix Angelicae sinensis* 9 g
Chuan Xiong *Rhizoma Chuanxiong* 6 g
Pu Huang *Pollen Typhae* 6 g
Wu Ling Zhi *Faeces Trogopterori*
Dang Shen *Radix Codonopsis* 6 g
Zhi Ke *Fructus Aurantii* 4.5 g
Yi Mu Cao *Herba Leonuri* 6 g

SUO QUAN WAN

Contracting the Spring Pill
Wu Yao *Radix Linderae* 9 g
Yi Zhi Ren *Fructus Alpiniae oxyphyllae* 9 g

TAO HE CHENG QI TANG

Prunus Conducting Qi Decoction
Tao Ren *Semen Persicae* 50 pieces
Da Huang *Radix et Rhizoma Rhei* 12 g
Gui Zhi *Ramulus Cinnamomi* 6 g
Mang Xiao *Sulfas Natrii* 6 g
Zhi Gan Cao *Radix Glycyrrhizae preparata* 6 g

TAO HONG SI WU TANG

Persica-Carthamus Four Substances Decoction
Shu Di Huang *Radix Rehmanniae preparata* 12 g
Dang Gui *Radix Angelicae sinensis* 10 g
Bai Shao *Radix Paeoniae alba* 12 g

Chuan Xiong Radix Chuanxiong 8 g
Tao Ren Semen Persicae 6 g
Hong Hua Flos Carthami 4 g

TIAN DI JIAN

Heaven and Earth Decoction
Tian Men Dong Radix Asparagi 9 g
Shu Di Huang Radix Rehmanniae preparata 9 g

TIAN MA GOU TENG YIN

Gastrodia-Uncaria Decoction
Tian Ma Rhizoma Gastrodiae 9 g
Gou Teng Ramulus Uncariae cum Uncis 9 g
Shi Jue Ming Concha Haliotidis 6 g
Sang Ji Sheng Herba Taxilli 9 g
Du Zhong Cortex Eucommiae 9 g
Chuan Niu Xi Radix Cyathulae 9 g
Shan Zhi Zi Fructus Gardeniae jasminoidis 6 g
Huang Qin Radix Scutellariae 9 g
Yi Mu Cao Herba Leonori 9 g
Ye Jiao Teng Caulis Polygoni multiflori 9 g
Fu Shen Sclerotium Poriae pararadicis 6 g

TIAN TAI WU YAO SAN

Top-Quality Lindera Powder
Wu Yao Radix Linderae 15 g
Mu Xiang Radix Aucklandiae 15 g
Xiao Hui Xiang Fructus Foeniculi 15 g
Qing Pi Pericarpium Citri reticulatae viride 15 g
Gao Liang Jiang Rhizoma Alpiniae officinari 15 g
Bing Lang Semen Arecae 2 pieces
Jin Ling Zi Fructus Meliae toosendan 10 pieces

TIAN WANG BU XIN DAN

Heavenly Emperor Tonifying the Heart Pill
Sheng Di Huang Radix Rehmanniae 12 g
Xuan Shen Radix Scrophulariae 6 g
Mai Men Dong Radix Ophiopogonis 6 g
Tian Men Dong Radix Asparagi 6 g
Ren Shen Radix Ginseng 6 g
Fu Ling Poria 6 g
Wu Wei Zi Fructus Schisandrae 6 g
Dang Gui Radix Angelicae sinensis 6 g
Dan Shen Radix Salviae miltiorrhizae 6 g
Bai Zi Ren Semen Platycladi 6 g

Suan Zao Ren Semen Ziziphi spinosae 6 g
Yuan Zhi Radix Polygalae 6 g
Jie Geng Radix Platycodi 3 g

TIAO WEI CHENG QI TANG

Regulating the Stomach Conducting Qi Decoction
Da Huang Radix et Rhizoma Rhei 12 g
Mang Xiao Sulfas Natrii 9 g
Zhi Gan Cao Radix Glycyrrhizae preparata 6 g

TIAO ZHENG SAN

Regulating the Upright Powder
Bai Zhu Rhizoma Atractylodis macrocephalae 6 g
Cang Zhu Rhizoma Atractylodis 6 g
Fu Ling Poria 6 g
Chen Pi Pericarpium Citri reticulatae 3 g
Zhe Bei Mu Bulbus Fritillariae Thunbergii 6 g
Yi Yi Ren Semen Coicis 12 g

TONG YOU TANG

Penetrating the Depth Decoction
Zhi Gan Cao Radix Glycyrrhizae preparata 1.5 g
Hong Hua Flos Carthami 1.5 g
Sheng Di Huang Radix Rehmanniae 3 g
Shu Di Huang Radix Rehmannia preparata 3 g
Sheng Ma Rhizoma Cimicifuage 6 g
Tao Ren Semen Persicae 6 g
Dang Gui Radix Angelicae sinensis 6 g
Bing Lang Semen Arecae 3 g

TU SI ZI WAN

Cuscuta Pill
Tu Si Zi Semen Cuscutae 6 g
Lu Rong Cornu Cervi pantotrichum 3 g
Rou Cong Rong Herba Cistanches 6 g
Shan Yao Rhizoma Dioscoreae 3 g
Fu Zi Radix Aconiti lateralis preparata 3 g
Wu Yao Radix Linderae 3 g
Wu Wei Zi Fructus Schisandrae 3 g
Sang Piao Xiao Ootheca Mantidis 3 g
Yi Zhi Ren Fructus Alpiniae oxyphyllae 3 g
Duan Mu Li Concha Ostreae (calcined) 6 g
Ji Nei Jin Endothelium Corneum gigeriae galli 1.5 g

WAN DAI TANG

Ending Vaginal Discharge Decoction
Bai Zhu Rhizoma Atractylodis macrocephalae 30 g (fried)
Shan Yao Rhizoma Dioscoreae 30 g (fried)
Ren Shen Radix Ginseng 6 g
Bai Shao Radix Paeoniae alba 15 g (fried)
Che Qian Zi Semen Plantaginis 6 g (fried)
Cang Zhu Rhizoma Atractylodis 9 g
Gan Cao Radix Glycyrrhizae 3 g
Chen Pi Pericarpium Citri reticulatae 1.5 g
Jing Jie Herba Schizonepetae 1.5 g (charred)
Chai Hu Radix Bupleuri 1.8 g

WEI LING TANG

Stomach "Ling" Decoction
Fu Ling Poria 9 g
Cang Zhu Rhizoma Atractylodis 6 g
Chen Pi Pericarpium Citri reticulatae 3 g
Bai Zhu Rhizoma Atractylodis macrocephalae 6 g
Gui Zhi Ramulus Cinnamomi 6 g
Ze Xie Rhizoma Alismatis 6 g
Zhu Ling Polyporus 6 g
Hou Po Cortex Magnolia officinalis 6 g
Zhi Gan Cao Radix Glycyrrhizae preparata 3 g
Da Zao Fructus Jujubae 3 pieces
Sheng Jiang Rhizoma Zingiberis recens 3 slices

WEN DAN TANG

Warming the Gall-Bladder Decoction
Ban Xia Rhizoma Pinelliae preparatum 6 g
Fu Ling Poria 5 g
Chen Pi Pericarpium Citri reticulatae 9 g
Zhu Ru Caulis Bambusae in **Taeniam** 6 g
Zhi Shi Fructus Aurantii immaturus 6 g
Zhi Gan Cao Radix Glycyrrhizae preparata 3 g
Sheng Jiang Rhizoma Zingiberis recens 5 slices
Da Zao Fructus Jujubae 1 date

WEN JING TANG

Warming the Menses Decoction
Wu Zhu Yu Fructus Evodiae 9 g
Gui Zhi Ramulus Cinnamomi 9 g
Sheng Jiang Rhizoma Zingiberis recens 6 g
Dang Gui Radix Angelicae sinensis 9 g
Chuan Xiong Rhizoma Chuanxiong 4.5 g
Bai Shao Radix Paeoniae alba 9 g
Dang Shen Radix Codonopsis 12 g
Mai Men Dong Radix Ophiopogonis 6 g
E Jiao Colla Corii asini 9 g
Mu Dan Pi Cortex Moutan 4.5 g
Ban Xia Rhizoma Pinelliae preparatum 6 g
Zhi Gan Cao Radix Glycyrrhizae preparata 3 g

WEN SHEN TIAO QI TANG

Warming the Kidneys and Regulating Qi Decoction
Du Zhong Cortex Eucommiae 9 g
Xu Duan Radix Dipsaci 9 g
Sang Ji Sheng Herba Taxilli 15 g
Wu Yao Radix Linderae 6 g
Tu Si Zi Semen Cuscutae 9 g
Ai Ye Folium Artemisiae argyi 9 g
Gou Ji Rhizoma Cibotii 6 g

WU HU TANG

Five Tigers Decoction
Ma Huang Herba Ephedrae 2.1 g
Shi Gao Gypsum fibrosum 4.5 g
Xing Ren Semen Armeniacae 3 g
Gan Cao Radix Glycyrrhizae 1.2 g
Sheng Jiang Rhizoma Zingiberis recens 3 slices
Da Zao Fructus Jujubae 1 date
Xi Cha Fine green tea 2.4 g

WU LING SAN

Five-Ingredient Poria Powder
Ze Xie Rhizoma Alismatis 4 g
Fu Ling Poria 2.3 g
Zhu Ling Polyporus 2.3 g
Bai Zhu Rhizoma Atractylodis macrocephalae 2.3 g
Gui Zhi Ramulus Cinnamomi 1.5 g

WU MEI WAN

Prunus Mume Pill
Wu Mei Fructus Mume 24 g
Chuan Jiao Pericarpium Zanthoxyli 1.5 g
Xi Xin Herba Asari 1.5 g
Huang Lian Rhizoma Coptidis 9 g
Huang Bo Cortex Phellodendri 6 g
Gan Jiang Rhizoma Zingiberis 6 g
Fu Zi Radix Aconiti lateralis preparata 3 g

Gui Zhi *Ramulus Cinnamomi* 3 g
Ren Shen *Radix Ginseng* 6 g
Dang Gui *Radix Angelicae sinensis* 3 g

WU REN WAN

Five-Seed Pill
Tao Ren *Semen Persicae* 9 g
Xing Ren *Semen armeniacae* 9 g
Bai Zi Ren *Semen Platycladi* 6 g
Song Zi Ren *Semen Pini tabulaeformis* 3 g
Yu Li Ren *Semen Pruni* 3 g
Chen Pi *Pericarpium Citri reticulatae* 9 g

WU YAO SAN

Linderia Powder
Wu Yao *Radix Linderae* 6 g
Xiang Fu *Rhizoma Cyperi* 6 g
Su Zi *Fructus Perillae* 4.5 g
Chen Pi *Pericarpium Citri reticulatae* 3 g
Chai Hu *Radix Bupleuri* 6 g
Mu Dan Pi *Cortex Moutan* 6 g
Gui Zhi *Ramulus Cinnamomi* 3 g
Mu Xiang *Radix Aucklandiae* 3 g
Dang Gui *Radix Angelicae sinensis* 6 g
Chuan Xiong *Rhizoma Chuanxiong* 3 g
Bo He *Herba Menthae haplocalycis* 3 g
Gan Cao *Radix Glycyrrhizae* 3 g

WU ZHI SAN

Five Citrus Powder
Bai Zhi *Radix Angelicae dahuricae* 3 g
Chen Pi *Pericarpium Citri reticulatae* 3 g
Hou Po *Cortex Magnolia officinalis* 6 g
Dang Gui *Radix Angelicae sinensis* 6 g
Chuan Xiong *Rhizoma Chuanxiong* 4.5 g
Bai Shao *Radix Paeoniae alba* 6 g
Fu Ling *Poria* 6 g
Jie Geng *Radix Platycodi* 3 g
Cang Zhu *Rhizoma Atractylodis* 6 g
Zhi Ke *Fructus aurantii* 6 g
Ban Xia *Rhizoma Pinelliae preparatum* 6 g
Ma Huang *Herba Ephedrae* 3 g
Gan Jiang *Rhizoma Zingiberis* 3 g
Rou Gui *Cortex Cinnamomi* 3 g
Gan Cao *Radix Glycyrrhizae* 3 g
Sheng Jiang *Rhizoma Zingiberis recens* 3 slices

WU ZHU YU TANG

Evodia Decoctoin
Wu Zhu Yu *Fructus Evodiae* 9 g
Sheng Jiang *Rhizoma Zingiberis recens* 6 g
Ren Shen *Radix Ginseng* 9 g
Da Zao *Fructus Jujubae* 3 dates

XI JIAO DI HUANG TANG

Cornus Rhinoceri Rehmannia Decoction
Shui Niu Jiao *Cornu Bubali* 6 g
Sheng Di Huang *Radix Rehmanniae* 24 g
Chi Shao *Radix Paeoniae rubra* 9 g
Mu Dan Pi *Cortex Moutan* 6 g

XIANG LENG WAN

Aucklandia-Sparganium Pill
Mu Xiang *Radix Aucklandiae* 6 g
Ding Xiang *Flos Caryophylli* 3 g
San Leng *Rhizoma Sparganii* 6 g
Zhi Ke *Fructus Aurantii* 6 g
Qing Pi *Pericarpium Citri reticulatae viride* 3 g
Chuan Lian Zi *Fructus Toosendan* 3 g
Xiao Hui Xiang *Fructus Foeniculi* 6 g
E Zhu *Rhizoma Curcumae* 6 g
Sheng Jiang *Rhizoma Zingiberis recens* 3 slices

XIAO CHAI HU TANG

Small Bupleurum Decoction
Chai Hu *Radix Bupleuri* 24 g
Huang Qin *Radix Scutellariae* 9 g
Ban Xia *Rhizoma Pinelliae preparatum* 24 g
Sheng Jiang *Rhizoma Zingiberis recens* 9 g
Ren Shen *Radix Ginseng* 9 g
Zhi Gan Cao *Radix Glycyrrhizae preparata* 9 g
Da Zao *Fructus Jujubae* 12 pieces

XIAO JIAN ZHONG TANG

Small Strengthening the Centre Decoction
Yi Tang *Maltosum* 18 g
Gui Zhi *Ramulus Cinnamomi* 9 g
Bai Shao *Radix Paeoniae alba* 18 g
Zhi Gan Cao *Radix Glycyrrhizae preparata* 6 g
Sheng Jiang *Rhizoma Zingiberis recens* 9 g
Da Zao *Fructus Jujubae* 12 dates

XIAO QING LONG TANG

Small Green Dragon Decoction
Ma Huang Herba Ephedrae 9 g
Gui Zhi Ramulus Cinnamomi 9 g
Gan Jiang Rhizoma Zingiberis 9 g
Xi Xin Herba Asari 3 g
Wu Wei Zi Fructus Schisandrae 6 g
Bai Shao Radix Paeoniae alba 9 g
Ban Xia Rhizoma Pinelliae preparatum 9 g
Zhi Gan Cao Radix Glycyrrhizae preparata 3 g

XIAO YAO SAN

Free and Easy Wanderer Powder
Bo He Herba Menthae haplocalycis 3 g
Chai Hu Radix Bupleuri 9 g
Dang Gui Radix Angelicae sinensis 9 g
Bai Shao Radix Paeoniae alba 12 g
Bai Zhu Rhizoma Atractylodis macrocephalae 9 g
Fu Ling Poria 15 g
Gan Cao Radix Glycyrrhizae 6 g
Sheng Jiang Rhizoma Zingiberis recens 3 slices

XIE BAI SAN

Draining the White Powder
Sang Bai Pi Cortex Mori 30 g
Di Gu Pi Cortex Lycii 30 g
Zhi Gan Cao Radix Glycyrrhizae preparata 3 g
Geng Mi Semen Oryzae sativae 15 g

XIE XIN TANG

Draining the Heart Decoction
Da Huang Radix et Rhizoma Rhei 6 g
Huang Lian Rhizoma Coptidis 3 g
Huang Qin Radix Scutellariae 3 g

XING SU SAN

Prunus-Perilla Powder
Zi Su Ye Folium Perillae 6 g
Qian Hu Radix Peucedani 6 g
Xing Ren Semen Armeniacae 6 g
Jie Geng Radix Platycodi 6 g
Zhi Ke Fructus Aurantii 6 g
Chen Pi Pericarpium Citri reticulatae 6 g
Fu Ling Poria 6 g
Ban Xia Rhizoma Pinelliae preparatum 6 g
Sheng Jiang Rhizoma Zingiberis recens 6 g
Da Zao Fructus Jujubae 2 dates
Gan Cao Radix Glycyrrhizae 3 g

XUAN FU DAI ZHE TANG

Inula-Haematite Decoction
Xuan Fu Hua Flos Inulae 9 g
Dai Zhe Shi Haematitum 3 g
Ban Xia Rhizoma Pinelliae preparatum 9 g
Sheng Jiang Rhizoma Zingiberis recens 6 g
Ren Shen Radix Ginseng 6 g
Zhi Gan Cao Radix Glycyrrhizae preparata 3 g
Da Zao Fructus Jujubae 12 dates

XUE FU ZHU YU TANG

Blood Mansion Eliminating Stasis Decoction
Dang Gui Radix Angelicae sinensis 9 g
Sheng Di Huang Radix Rehmanniae 9 g
Chi Shao Radix Paeoniae rubra 6 g
Chuan Xiong Rhizoma Chuanxiong 5 g
Tao Ren Semen Persicae 12 g
Hong Hua Flos Carthami 9 g
Chai Hu Radix Bupleuri 3 g
Zhi Ke Fructus Aurantii 6 g
Niu Xi Radix Achyranthis bidentatae 9 g
Jie Geng Radix Platycodi 5 g
Gan Cao Radix Glycyrrhizae 3 g

YAN HU SUO TANG

Corydalis Decoction
Yan Hu Suo Rhizoma Corydalis 45 g
Pu Huang Pollen Typhae 15 g
Chi Shao Radix Paeoniae rubra 15 g
Dang Gui Radix Angelicae sinensis 15 g
Guan Gui Cortex Cinnamomi loureiroi 15 g
Jiang Huang Rhizoma Curcumae longae 90 g
Ru Xiang Olibanum 90 g
Mo Yao Myrrha 90 g
Mu Xiang Radix Aucklandiae 90 g
Zhi Gan Cao Radix Glycyrrhizae preparata 7.5 g

YANG YIN QING FEI TANG

Nourishing Yin and Clearing the Lungs Decoction
Sheng Di Huang Radix Rehmanniae 6 g
Xuan Shen Radix Scrophulariae 4.5 g
Mai Men Dong Radix Ophiopogonis 3.6 g

Bai Shao (chao) *Radix Paeoniae alba* (fried) 2.4 g
Mu Dan Pi *Cortex Moutan* 2.4 g
Chuan Bei Mu *Bulbus Fritillariae cirrhosae* 2.4 g
Bo He *Herba Menthae haplocalycis* 1.5 g
Gan Cao *Radix Glycirrhizae* 1.5 g

YI GAN SAN

Restrain the Liver Powder
Bai Zhu (fried) *Rhizoma Atractylodis macrocephalae* 3 g
Fu Ling *Poria* 3 g
Dang Gui *Radix Angelicae sinensis* 3 g
Chuan Xiong *Radix Chuanxiong* 2.4 g
Gou Teng *Ramulus Uncariae cum Uncis* 3 g
Chai Hu *Radix Bupleuri* 1.5 g
Gan Cao *Radix Glycyrrhizae* 1.5 g

YI GUAN JIAN

One Linking Decoction
Bei Sha Shen *Radix Glehniae* 10 g
Mai Men Dong *Radix Ophiopogonis* 10 g
Dang Gui *Radix Angelicae sinensis* 10 g
Sheng Di Huang *Radix Rehmanniae* 30 g
Gou Qi Zi *Fructus Lycii* 12 g
Chuan Lian Zi *Fructus Toosendan* 5 g

YI JIA JIAN ZHENG QI SAN

First Variation of Upright Qi Powder
Huo Xiang *Herba Pogostemonis* 6 g
Hou Po *Cortex Magnoliae officinalis* 6 g
Xing Ren *Semen Armeniacae* 6 g
Fu Ling Pi *Cutis Poriae* 6 g
Chen Pi *Pericarpium Citri reticulatae* 3 g
Shen Qu *Massa Medicata Fermentata* 4.5 g
Mai Ya *Fructus Hordei germinatus* 4.5 g
Yin Chen Hao *Herba Artemisiae scopariae* 6 g
Da Fu Pi *Pericarpium Arecae* 3 g

YI QI GU CHONG TANG

Benefiting Qi and Consolidating the Penetrating Vessel Decoction
Huang Qi *Radix Astragali* 15 g
Bai Zhu *Rhizoma Atractylodis macrocephalae* 6 g
Dang Shen *Radix Codonopsis* 9 g
Ai Ye *Folium Artemisiae argyi* 4.5 g
Xian He Cao *Herba Agrimoniae* 6 g

Jing Jie *Herba Schizonepetae* 6 g (charred)
Dang Gui *Radix Angelicae sinensis* 6 g
Xu Duan *Radix Dipsaci* 6 g
Sheng Ma *Rhizoma Cimicifugae* 3 g
Gan Cao *Radix Glycyrrhizae* 3 g

YI YIN JIAN

One Yin Decoction
Sheng Di Huang *Radix Rehmanniae* 6 g
Shu Di Huang *Radix Rehmanniae preparata* 9 g
Bai Shao *Radix Paeoniae alba* 6 g
Mai Men Dong *Radix Ophiopogonis* 6 g
Gan Cao *Radix Glycyrrhizae* 3 g
Huai Niu Xi *Radix Achyranthis bidentatae* 4.5 g
Dan Shen *Radix Salviae miltiorrhizae* 6 g

YI WEI TANG

Benefitting the Stomach Decoction
Sha Shen *Radix Adenophorae seu Glehniae* 9 g
Mai Men Dong *Radix Ophiopogonis* 15 g
Sheng Di Huang *Radix Rehmanniae* 15 g
Yu Zhu *Rhizoma Polygonati odorati* 4.5 g
Bing Tang Rock candy 3 g

YIN CHEN HAO TANG

Artemisia Yinchenhao Decoction
Yin Chen Hao *Herba Artemisiae scopariae* 6 g
Shan Zhi Zi *Fructus Gardeniae jasminoidis* 9 g
Da Huang *Radix et Rhizoma Rhei* 6 g

YIN JIA WAN

Lonicera-Amyda Pill
Jin Yin Hua *Flos Lonicerae* 6 g
Bie Jia *Carapax Trionycis* 9 g
Lian Qiao *Fructus Forsythiae* 6 g
Sheng Ma *Rhizoma Cimicifugae* 6 g
Hong Teng *Caulis Sargentodoxae* 6 g
Pu Gong Ying *Herba Taraxaci* 6 g
Da Qing Ye *Folium Isatidis* 6 g
Yin Chen Hao *Herba Artemisiae scopariae* 4.5 g
Hu Po *Succinum* 6 g
Jie Geng *Radix Platycodi* 3 g
Zi Hua Di Ding *Herba Violae*
Pu Huang *Pollen Typhae*
Chun Gen Bai Pi *Cortex Ailanthi*

YIN QIAO SAN

Lonicera-Forsythia Powder
Jin Yin Hua *Flos Lonicerae* 9 g
Lian Qiao *Fructus Forsythiae* 9 g
Jie Geng *Radix Platycodi* 3 g
Niu Bang Zi *Fructus Arctii* 9 g
Bo He *Herba Menthae haplocalycis* 3 g
Dan Dou Chi *Semen Sojae praeparatum* 3 g
Jing Jie *Herba Schizonepetae* 6 g
Zhu Ye *Folium Phyllostachys nigrae* 3 g
Lu Gen *Rhizoma Phragmitis* 15 g
Gan Cao *Radix Glycyrrhizae* 3 g

YOU GUI WAN

Restoring the Right [Kidney] Pill
Fu Zi *Radix Aconiti lateralis preparata* 3 g
Rou Gui *Cortex Cinnamomi* 3 g
Du Zhong *Cortex Eucommiae* 6 g
Shan Zhu Yu *Fructus Corni* 4.5 g
Tu Si Zi *Semen Cuscutae* 6 g
Lu Jiao Jiao *Colla Cornu Cervi* 6 g
Shu Di Huang *Radix Rehmanniae preparata* 12 g
Shan Yao *Rhizoma Dioscoreae* 6 g
Gou Qi Zi *Fructus Lycii* 6 g
Dang Gui *Radix Angelicae sinensis* 4.5

YU YUN TANG

Promoting Pregnancy Decoction
Yin Yang Huo *Herba Epimedii* 6 g
Ba Ji Tian *Radix Morindae officinalis* 9 g
Lu Jiao Jiao *Colla Cornu Cervi* 6 g
Zi He Che *Placenta hominis* 6 g
Shan Zhu Yu *Fructus Corni* 6 g
Dang Shen *Radix Codonopsis* 6 g
Dang Gui *Radix Angelicae sinensis* 9 g
Yi Mu Cao *Herba Leonuri* 4.5 g

YUE JU WAN

Gardenia-Ligusticum Pill
Cang Zhu *Rhizoma Atractylodis* 6 g
Chuan Xiong *Rhizoma Chuanxiong* 6 g
Xiang Fu *Rhizoma Cyperi* 6 g
Shan Zhi Zi *Fructus Gardeniae jasminoidis* 6 g
Shen Qu *Massa Medicata Fermentata* 6 g

ZENG YE TANG

Increasing Fluids Decoction
Xuan Shen *Radix Scrophulariae* 18 g
Mai Men Dong *Radix Ophiopogonis* 12 g
Sheng Di Huang *Radix Rehmanniae* 12 g

ZHEN GAN XI FENG TANG

Pacifying the Liver and Subduing Wind Decoction
Huai Niu Xi *Radix Achyrantis bidentatae* 15 g
Dai Zhe Shi *Haematitum* 15 g
Long Gu *Fossilia Ossis mastodi* 12 g
Mu Li *Concha Ostreae* 12 g
Gui Ban *Plastrum Testudinis* 12 g
Xuan Shen *Radix Scrophulariae* 12 g
Tian Men Dong *Radix Asparagi* 12 g
Bai Shao *Radix Paeoniae alba* 12 g
Yin Chen Hao *Herba Artemisiae scopariae* 6 g
Chuan Lian Zi *Fructus Toosendan* 6 g
Mai Ya *Fructus Hordei germinatus* 6 g
Gan Cao *Radix Glycyrrhizae* 6 g

ZHENG QI TIAN XIANG SAN

Upright Qi Heavenly Fragrance Powder
Wu Yao *Radix Linderae* 6 g
Gan Jiang *Rhizoma Zingiberis* 3 g
Zi Su Ye *Folium Perillae* 6 g
Chen Pi *Pericarpium Citri reticulatae* 4.5 g

ZHI DAI WAN

Stopping Vaginal Discharge Pill
Fu Ling *Poria* 6 g
Zhu Ling *Polyporus* 6 g
Ze Xie *Rhizoma Alismatis* 6 g
Chi Shao *Radix Paeoniae rubra* 6 g
Mu Dan Pi *Cortex Moutan* 6 g
Yin Chen Hao

Appendix 2
Glossary of Chinese Terms

ENGLISH-PINYIN GLOSSARY OF CHINESE TERMS

General

Ancestral muscles	Zong Jin 宗 筋
Area below the xyphoid process	Xin xia 心 下
Central-lower abdominal area	Xiao Fu 小 腹
Centre of the Thorax	Shan Zhong 膻 中
Cun (acupuncture unit of measurement)	Cun 寸
Deep layer of skin	Ge 革
Diffusing [of Lung-Qi]	Xuan Fa 宣 发
Eight Ramparts	Ba Kuo 八 廓
Eye System	Mu Xi 目 系
Fat and Muscles	Fen Rou 分 肉
Fat Tissue	Gao 膏
Field of Elixir	Dan Tian 丹 田
The Five Wheels	Wu Lun 五 轮
Great Connecting channel of the Stomach (manifesting in apical pulse)	Xu Li 虚 里
Hypochondrium	Xie Lei 胁 肋
Identification of patterns	Bian Zheng 辨 证
Image	Xiang 象
Lateral-lower abdominal area	Shao Fu 少 腹
Membranes	Huang 肓
Muscles or flesh	Rou 肉
Pathogenic factor	Xie 邪
Pathogenic factor	Xie Qi 邪 气
Pores (including sebaceous glands)	Xuan Fu 玄 府
Sinews	Jin 筋
Six Climates	Liu Qi 六 气
Six Evils (external pathogenic factors)	Liu Xie 六 邪
Six Excesses (excessive climates)	Liu Yin 六 淫
Spaces and Texture (also space between the skin and muscles)	Cou Li 腠 里
"Streets", "avenues", "crossroads", (symbols for channels of the abdomen controlled by the Penetrating Vessel)	Jie 街
Subcutaneous muscles	Ji 肌
Superficial layer of skin	Fu 肤
Transformation and transportation (of the Spleen)	Yun Hua 运 化
Uterus Channel	Bao Luo 胞 络
Uterus Vessel	Bao Mai 胞 脉

Symptoms and signs

Accumulation (or nodules)	Jie 结
Alopecia	Tou Fa Tuo Luo 头 发 脱 落
Alternation of chills and fever	Han Re Wang Lai 寒 热 往 来
Aversion to cold	Wu Han 恶 寒
(Simultaneous) Aversion to cold and fever	Wu Han Fa Re 恶 寒 发 热
Aversion to food	Yan Shi 厌 食
Aversion to wind	Wu Feng 恶 风
Blood masses	Ji 积
Blood masses	Zheng 癥
Bluish-greenish (colour)	Qing 青
Blurred vision	Mu Hun 目 昏
Blurred vision	Mu Xuan 目 眩
Brain noise	Nao Ming 脑 鸣
Breakdown	Jue 厥
Breathlessness	Chuan 喘
Collapse	Tuo 脱
Contraction of the fingers	Shou Zhi Luan 手 指 挛
Depression	Yu Zheng 郁 症
Deviation of eye and mouth	Kou Yan Wai Xie 口 眼 歪 斜
Difficulty in defecation	Li Ji Hou Zhong 里 急 后 重

English	Chinese
Discharge from the eyes	Yan Chi 眼眵
Distension	Zhang 胀
Dizziness	Tou Yun 头晕
Dizziness	Xuan Yun 眩晕
Drooping head	Tou Qing 头倾
Eczema	Shi Zhen 湿疹
Emission of heat, fever	Fa Re 发热
Empty, Emptiness, Deficiency	Xu 虚
Fear of cold (in exterior invasions of Wind)	Wei Han 畏寒
Feeling of distension	Zhang 胀
Feeling of fullness	Man 满
Feeling of heaviness of the body	Shen Zhong 身重
Feeling of heaviness of the head	Tou Zhong 头重
Feeling of oppression	Men 闷
Feeling of stuffiness	Pi 痞
Five Flaccidities	Wu Ruan 五软
Five-palm heat	Wu Xin Fa Re 五心发热
Fullness	Man 满
Five Retardations	Wu Chi 五迟
Floaters	Mu Hua 目花
Foetus' Qi rebelling upwards	Tai Qi Sharg Ni 胎气上逆
Four Rebellious	Si Ni 四逆
Fright palpitations	Jing Ji 惊悸
Full, Fullness, Excess	Shi 实
Gnawing hunger	Cao Za 嘈杂
Greying of the hair	Tou Fa Bian Bai 头发变白
Heart feeling vexed	Xin Zhong Ao Nong 心中懊
Heaviness	Zhong 重
Hemiplegia	Ban Shen Bu Sui 半身不遂
Numbness and/or tingling	Ma Mu 麻木
Oppression	Men 闷
Panic palpitations	Zheng Chong 怔忡
Papule	Qiu Zhen 丘疹
Phlegm-Fluids (or Phlegm-Fluids in Stomach and Intestines)	Tan Yin 痰饮
Phlegm-Fluids above the diaphragm	Zhi Yin 支饮
Phlegm-Fluids in the hypochondrium	Xuan Yin 玄饮
Phlegm-Fluids in the limbs	Yi Yin 溢饮
Pustule	Nong Pao 脓泡
Qi oedema	Qi Zhong 气肿
Qi masses	Jia 瘕
Qi masses	Ju 聚
Quivering eyeball	Mu Chan 目颤
Rash	Zhen 疹
Rebellious-Qi breathing	Shang Qi 上气
Red points (on the tongue)	Dian 点
Regurgitation of food	Fan Wei 反胃
Reverse period	Ni Jing 逆经
Robbing of Qi (very feeble voice with interrupted speech)	Duo Qi 夺气
Root	Ben 本
Shivers	Han Zhan 汗颤
Shiver sweating	Zhan Han 颤汗
Shortness of breath	Duan Qi 短气
Short retching with low sound	Gan Ou 干呕
Slippery (tongue coating)	Hua 滑
Sticky (tongue coating)	Ni 腻
Stone moth (swollen tonsils)	Shi E 石蛾
Streaming eyes	Liu Lei 流泪
Stuffiness	Pi 痞
Sweating from Breakdown	Jue Han 厥汗
Tidal fever	Hu Re 湖热
Toxic Heat	Re Du 热毒
Tremor of the feet	Zu Chan 足颤
Tremor of the hands	Shou Chan 手颤
Vesicle	Pao 泡
Vesicle	Shui Pao 水泡
Vomiting (with sound)	Ou Tu 呕
Vomiting (without sound)	Tu 吐
Vomiting	Ou Tu 呕吐
Water oedema	Shui Zhong 水肿
Water pox (chicken pox)	Shui Dou 水痘
Weak breathing	Qi Shao 气少
Wheal	FengTuan 风团
Wheezing	Xiao 哮
Wind hidden rash (urticaria)	Feng Yin Zhen 风瘾疹
Wind rash (German measles)	Feng Zhen 风疹

Disease-symptoms

Abdominal masses	Ji Ju 积 聚
Abdominal masses (in women)	Zheng Jia 癥 瘕
Accumulation Disorder (in children)	Ji Dai 积 滞
Atrophy Syndrome	Wei Zheng 痿 症
Bleeding between Periods	Jing Jian Qi Chu Xue 经 间 期 出 血
Blood Painful-Urination Syndrome	Xue Lin 血 淋
Breakdown Syndrome	Jue Zheng 厥 症
Breast lumps	Ru Pi 乳 癖
Chicken pox	Shui Dou 水 痘
Childhood Nutritional Impairment	Gan 疳
Depression Pattern	Yu Zheng 郁 症
Diaphragm Choking	Ye Ge 噎 膈
Dizziness of Pregnancy	Zi Yun 子 晕
Dysentery	Li Ji 痢 疾
Early Periods	Yue Jing Xian Qi 月 经 先 其
Eczema (dermatitis)	Shi Zhen 湿 疹
Epilepsy	Dian Xian 癲 痫
Exhaustion	Xu Lao 虚 劳
Exhaustion	Xu Sun 虚 损
Facial paralysis	Mian Tan 面 瘫
Fatigue Painful-Urination Syndrome	Lao Lin 劳 淋
Five Flaccidities	Wu Ruan 五 软
Five Retardations	Wu Chi 五 迟
Flooding and Trickling	Beng Lou 崩 漏
German measles	Feng Zhen 风 疹
Goitre	Ying 瘿
Heat Painful-Urination Syndrome	Re Lin 热 淋
Heavy Periods	Yue Jing Guo Duo 月 经 过 多
Hernial and Genito-Urinary Disorders	Shan 疝
Irregular Periods	Yue Jing Xian Hou Wu Ding Qi 月 经 先 后 无 定 期
Late Periods	Yue Jing Hou Qi 月 经 后 期
Lung-Exhaustion	Fei Xu Lao 肺 虚 劳
Malaria	Nue Ji 疟 疾
Manic depression	Dian Kuang 癲 狂
Measles	Ma Zhen 麻 疹
Nodules	Tan He 痰 核
No Periods	Bi Jing 闭 经
Oedema of Pregnancy	Zi Zhong 子 肿
Painful Obstruction Syndrome	Bi Zheng 痹 症
Painful-Urination Pregnancy	Zi Lin 子 淋
Painful Urination Syndrome	Lin Zheng 淋 症
Paralysis	Tan Huan 瘫 缓
Pi Masses	Pi Kuai 痞 块
Qi Painful-Urination Syndrome	Qi Lin 气 淋
Scanty Periods	Yue Jing Guo Shao 月 经 过 少
Scrofula	Luo Li 瘰 疬
Sticky Painful-Urination Syndrome	Gao Lin 膏 淋
Stone Painful-Urination Syndrome	Shi Lin 石 淋
Urticaria	Yin Zhen 瘾 疹
Warm disease	Wen Bing 温 病
Warm epidemic pathogenic factor	Wen Yi 温 疫
Wind-stroke	Zhong Feng 中 风

Vital substances

Central Qi	Zhong Qi 中 气
Corporeal Soul	Po 魄
Defensive Qi	Wei Qi 卫 气
Emperor Fire	Jun Huo 君 火
Essence	Jing 精
Ethereal Soul	Hun 魂
Exuberant Fire (pathological)	Zhuang Huo 壮 火
Fire of the Gate of Life	Ming Men Huo 命 门 火
Gate of Life	Ming Men 命 门
Gathering Qi (of the chest)	Zong Qi 宗 气
Heavenly Gui	Tian Gui 天 癸
Intellect	Yi 意
Marrow	Sui 髓
Mind (the Shen of the Heart) or Spirit (the complex of Heart-Shen, Corporeal Soul, Ethereal Soul, Intellect and Will-Power)	Shen 神
Minister Fire	Xiang Huo 相 火
Nutritive Qi	Ying Qi 营 气

Original Qi	Yuan Qi 原 气	Terminal Yin	Jue Yin 厥 阴
Physiological Fire of the body	Shao Huo 少 火	Uterus Channel	Bao Luo 胞 络
		Uterus Vessel	Bao Mai 胞 脉
Post-Natal Qi	Hou Tian Zhi Qi 后 天 之 气	Well point	Jing Xue 井 穴
Pre-Natal Qi	Xian Tian Zhi Qi 先 天 之 气	Yang Linking Vessel	Yang Wei Mai 阳 维 脉
Saliva	Xian 涎	Yang Stepping Vessel	Yang Qiao Mai 阳 蹻 脉
Spittle	Tuo 唾	Yin Linking Vessel	Yin Wei Mai 阴 维 脉
True Qi	Zhen Qi 真 气	Yin Stepping Vessel	Yin Qiao Mai 阴 蹻 脉
Upright Qi	Zheng Qi 正 气		
Will-Power	Zhi 志		

Emotions

Anger	Nu 怒
Fear	Kong 恐
Joy	Xi 喜
Pensiveness	Si 思
Sadness	Bei 悲
Shock	Jing 惊
Worry	You 忧

Pulse positions

Front (pulse position)	Cun 寸
Middle (pulse position)	Guan 关
Rear (pulse position)	Chi 尺

Pulse qualities

Big	Da 大
Choppy	Se 涩
Deep	Chen 沉
Empty	Xu 虚
Fine	Xi 細
Firm	Lao 牢
Floating	Fu 浮
Full	Shi 实
Hasty	Cu 促
Hidden	Fu 伏
Hollow	Kou 芤
Hurried	Ji 急
Irregular or Intermittent	Dai 代
Knotted	Jie 结
Leather	Ge 革
Long	Chang 长
Minute	Wei 微
Moving	Dong 动
Overflowing	Hong 洪
Rapid	Shu 数
Scattered	San 散
Short	Duan 短
Slippery	Hua 滑
Slow	Chi 迟
Slowed-Down	Huan 缓
Soggy	Ru 濡
Soggy	Ruan 软
Tight	Jin 紧
Weak	Ruo 弱
Wiry	Xian 弦

Channels and points

Accumulation point	Xi Xue 郄 穴
Back-Transporting points	(Bei) Shu Xue 背 俞 穴
Bright Yang	Yang Ming 阳 明
Connecting channel	Luo Mai (Xue) 络 脉（穴）
Connecting point	Luo Xue 络 穴
Directing Vessel	Ren Mai 任 脉
Divergent channel	Jing Bie 经 别
Five Transporting points	Wu Shu Xue 五 输 穴
Front-Collecting points	Mu Xue 幕 穴
Gathering point	Hui Xue 会 穴
Girdle Vessel	Dai Mai 带 脉
Governing Vessel	Du Mai 督 脉
Greater Yang	Tai Yang 太 阳
Greater Yin	Tai Yin 太 阴
Lesser Yang	Shao Yang 少 阳
Lesser Yin	Shao Yin 少 阴
Main channel	Jing Mai 经 脉
Minute Connecting channel	Sun Luo 孙 络
Muscle channel	Jing Jin 经 筋
Penetrating Vessel	Chong Mai 冲 脉
River point	Jing Xue 经 穴
Sea point	He Xue 合 穴
Source point	Yuan Xue 原 穴
Space between skin and muscles	Cou Li 腠 里
Spring point	Ying Xue 荥 穴
Stream point	Shu Xue 输 穴
Superficial Connecting channel	Fu Luo 浮 络

Methods of treatment

Benefit the throat	Li Hou 利 喉
Break-up Blood	Po Xue 破 血
Brighten the eyes	Li Mu 利 目

Calm the Foetus	An Tai 安胎
Calm the Liver	Ping Gan 平肝
Circulate Defensive Qi	Liu Wei 疏卫
Clear Heat	Qing (Re) 清热
Clear (Heat)	Xie 泄
Consolidate	Gu 固
Consolidate Collapse	Gu Tuo 固脱
Consolidate the Exterior	Gu Biao 固表
Dispel stasis (of Blood)	Gong Yu 功瘀
Dissipate accumulation or dissipate nodules	San Jie 散结
Drain (method of treatment as opposed to Bu 补, tonify)	Xie 泻
Drain (Fire)	Xie 泻
Eliminate stagnation (of Qi)	Jie Yu 解郁
Eliminate stasis (of Blood)	Hua Yu 化瘀
Eliminate stasis (of Blood)	Qu Yu 去瘀
Expel (external Wind)	Qu (Feng) 去风
Expel Cold	San Han 散寒
Extinguish Wind (internal)	Xi Feng 熄风
Harmonize Nutritive and Defensive Qi	Tiao He Ying Wei 调和营卫
Invigorate Blood	Huo Xue 活血
Moderate urgency	Huan Ji 缓急
Move downwards	Xie Xia 泻下
Move Qi	Li Qi 理气
Nourish (Blood)	Yang (Xue) 养血
Open (the chest)	Tong Yang 通畅（胸）
Open the nose	Xuan Tong Bi 宣通鼻窍
Open the orifices	Kai Qiao 开窍
Open the orifices	Tong Qiao 通窍
Pacify (the Liver)	Shu (Gan) 疏肝
Promote healing of tissues	Sheng Xin 生新
Promote resuscitation	Xing Zhi 醒志
Reduce (as a needle technique)	Xie 泻
Regulate the period	Tiao Jing 调经
Regulate the Water passages	Li Shui Dao 理水道
Relax the sinews	Shu Jin 舒筋
Release (the Exterior)	Jie (Biao) 解表
Remove obstructions from the breast's Connecting channels	Tong Ru 通乳络
Remove obstructions from the Connecting channels	Tong Luo 通络
Resolve Dampness	Hua Shi 化湿
Resolve Dampness	Li Shi 利湿
Resolve Phlegm	Hua Tan 化痰
Restore the diffusing of Lung-Qi	Xuan Fei 宣肺
Tonify (or reinforce as a needle technique)	Bu 补
Transform Water	Li Shui 利水
Use pungent herbs to open and bitter ones to make Qi descend	Xin Kai Ku Jiang 辛开苦降
Warm the menses	Wen Jing 温经

Pathogenic factors

Cold	Han 寒
Dampness	Shi 湿
Dryness	Zao 燥
Fire	Huo 火
Heat	Re 热
Pathogenic factor	Xie 邪
Pathogenic factor	Xie Qi 邪气
Phlegm	Tan 痰
Phlegm-Fluids in general and also Phlegm-Fluids in the Stomach	Tan Yin 痰饮
Phlegm-Fluids in the hypochondrium	Xuan Yin 悬饮
Phlegm-Fluids in the limbs	Yi Yin 溢饮
Phlegm-Fluids in the diaphragm	Zhi Yin 支饮
Summer-Heat	Shu 暑
Toxic Heat	Re Du 热毒
Warm epidemic pathogenic factor	Wen Yi 温疫
Wind-Cold	Feng Han 风寒
Wind-Heat	Feng Re 风热

PINYIN-ENGLISH GLOSSARY OF CHINESE TERMS

General

Ba Kuo 八廓	The Eight Ramparts
Bao Luo 胞络	Uterus Channel
Bao Mai 胞脉	Uterus Vessel
Bian Zheng 辨证	Identification of patterns
Cou Li 腠里	Spaces and Texture (also space between the skin and muscles)

Cun 寸	Cun (acupuncture unit of measurement)	Dian 点	Red points (on the tongue)
Dan Tian 丹田	Field of Elixir	Duan Qi 短气	Shortness of breath
Fen Rou 分肉	Fat and Muscles	Duo Qi 夺气	Robbing of Qi (very feeble voice with interrupted speech)
Fu 肤	Superficial layer of skin	E Xin 恶心	Nausea
Gao 膏	Fat Tissue	Fa Re 发热	Emission of heat, fever
Ge 革	Deep layer of skin	Fan Wei 反胃	Regurgitation of food
Huang 肓	Membranes	Fan Zao 烦燥	Mental restlessness
Ji 肌	Subcutaneous muscles	FengTuan 风团	Wheal
Jie 街	"Streets", "avenues", "crossroads", symbols for channels of the abdomen controlled by the Penetrating Vessel	Feng Yin Zhen 风瘾疹	Wind hidden rash (urticaria)
		Feng Zhen 风疹	Wind rash (German measles)
		Fu 腐	Mouldy
Jin 筋	Sinews	Gan Ou 干呕	Short retching with low sound
Liu Qi 六气	6 Climates	Han Re Wang Lai 寒热往来	Alternation of chills and fever
Liu Xie 六邪	6 Evils (external pathogenic factors)		
		Han Zhan 汗颤	Shivers
Liu Yin 六淫	6 Excesses (excessive climates)	Hu Re 湖热	Tidal fever
Mu Xi 目系	Eye System	Hua 滑	Slippery (tongue coating)
Rou 肉	Muscles or flesh	Ji 积	Blood masses
Shan Zhong 膻中	Centre of the Thorax	Jia 瘕	Qi masses
Shao Fu 少腹	Lateral-lower abdominal area	Jiao Qi 脚气	Leg Qi
Wu Lun 五轮	The Five Wheels	Jie 结	Accumulation (or nodules)
Xie Lei 胁肋	Hypochondrium	Jing Ji 惊悸	Fright palpitations
Xiang 象	Image	Ju 聚	Qi masses
Xiao Fu 小腹	Central-lower abdominal area	Jue 厥	Breakdown
Xie 邪	Pathogenic factor	Jue Han 厥汗	Sweating from Breakdown
Xie Qi 邪气	Pathogenic factor	Kou Chuang 口疮	Mouth ulcers
Xin xia 心下	Area below the xyphoid process	Kou Yan Wai Xie 口眼歪斜	Deviation of eye and mouth
Xu Li 虚里	Great Connecting channel of the Stomach (manifesting in apical pulse)		
		Li Ji 里急	Internal urgency (or tension of lining)
Xuan Fa 宣发	Diffusing [of Lung-Qi]	Li Ji Hou Zhong 里急后重	Difficulty in defecation
Xuan Fu 玄府	Pores (including sebaceous glands)		
Yun Hua 运化	Transformation and transportation (of the Spleen)	Liu Lei 流泪	Streaming eyes
		Ma Mu 麻木	Numbness and/or tingling
Zong Jin 宗筋	Ancestral muscles	Ma Zhen 麻疹	Hemp rash (measles)
		Man 满	Feeling of fullness

Symptoms and signs

Ban 斑	Macule (in tongue diagnosis, red spots)	Men 闷	Feeling of oppression
		Mu Chan 目颤	Quivering eyeball
Ban Shen Bu Sui 半身不遂	Hemiplegia	Mu Hua 目花	Floaters
		Mu Hun 目昏	Blurred vision
Ben 本	Root	Mu Xuan 目眩	Blurred vision
Bi Yuan 鼻渊	"Nose pool" (sinusitis)	Nao Ming 脑鸣	Brain noise
Biao 标	Manifestation	Ni 腻	Sticky (tongue coating)
Cao Za 嘈杂	Gnawing hunger	Ni Jing 逆经	Reverse period
Chuan 喘	Breathlessness	Nong Pao 脓泡	Pustule
Dao Han 盗汗	Night-sweating	Ou 呕	Vomiting (with sound)
		Ou Tu 呕吐	Vomiting

Pao 泡		Vesicle
Pi 痞		Feeling of stuffiness
Qi Shao 气少		Weak breathing
Qi Zhong 气肿		Qi oedema
Qing 青		Bluish-greenish (colour)
Qiu Zhen 丘疹		Papule
Re Du 热毒		Toxic Heat
Ru E 乳蛾		Milky moth (swollen tonsils)
Shang Qi 上气		Rebellious-Qi breathing
Shen Zhong 身重		Feeling of heaviness of the body
Shi 实		Full, Fullness, Excess
Shi E 石蛾		Stone moth (swollen tonsils)
Shi Zhen 湿疹		Eczema
Shou Chan 手颤		Tremor of the hands
Shou Zhi Luan 手指挛		Contraction of the fingers
Shui Dou 水痘		Water pox (chicken pox)
Shui Pao 水泡		Vesicle
Shui Zhong 水肿		Water oedema
Si Ni 四逆		Four Rebellious
Tai Qi Shang Ni 胎气上逆		Foetus' Qi rebelling upwards
Tan He 痰核		Nodules
Tan Yin 痰饮		Phlegm-Fluids (or Phlegm-Fluids in Stomach and Intestines)
Tou Zhong 头重		Feeling of heaviness of the head
Tou Fa Bian Bai 头发变白		Greying of the hair
Tou Fa Tuo Luo 头发脱落		Alopecia
Tou Qing 头倾		Drooping head
Tou Yun 头晕		Dizziness
Tu 吐		Vomiting (without sound)
Tuo 脱		Collapse
Wei Han 畏寒		Fear of cold (in exterior invasions of Wind)
Wu Chi 五迟		Five Retardations
Wu Feng 恶风		Aversion to wind
Wu Han 恶寒		Aversion to cold
Wu Han Fa Re 恶寒发热		(Simultaneous) Aversion to cold and fever
Wu Ruan 五软		Five Flaccidities
Wu Xin Fa Re 五心发热		5-palm heat
Xiao 哮		Wheezing
Xin Fan 心烦		Mental restlessness
Xin Zhong Ao Nong 心中懊		Heart feeling vexed
Xu 虚		Empty, Emptiness, Deficiency
Xuan Yin 玄饮		Phlegm-Fluids in the hypochondrium
Xuan Yun 眩晕		Dizziness
Yan Chi 眼眵		Discharge from the eyes
Yan Shi 厌食		Aversion to food
Yi Yin 溢饮		Phlegm-Fluids in the limbs
Yu Zheng 郁症		Depression
Yue 哕		Long retching with loud sound
Zhan Han 颤汗		Shiver sweating
Zhang 胀		Feeling of distension
Zhen 疹		Rash
Zheng 癥		Blood masses
Zheng Chong 怔忡		Panic palpitations
Zhi Yin 支饮		Phlegm-Fluids above the diaphragm
Zu Chan 足颤		Tremor of the feet

Disease-symptoms

Ben Tun 奔豚		Running Piglet Syndrome
Beng Lou 崩漏		Flooding and Trickling
Bi Jing 闭经		No Periods
Bi Zheng 痹症		Painful Obstruction Syndrome
Dian Kuang 癫狂		Manic depression
Dian Xian 癫痫		Epilepsy
Fei Xu Lao 肺虚劳		Lung-Exhaustion
Feng Zhen 风疹		German measles
Gan 疳		Childhood Nutritional Impairment
Gao Lin 膏淋		Sticky Painful-Urination Syndrome
Ji Dai 积滞		Accumulation Disorder (in children)
Ji Ju 积聚		Abdominal masses
Jing Jian Qi Chu Xue 经间期出血		Bleeding between Periods
Jue Zheng 厥症		Breakdown Syndrome
Lao Lin 劳淋		Fatigue Painful-Urination Syndrome
Li Ji 痢疾		Dysentery
Lin Zheng 淋症		Painful Urination Syndrome
Luo Li 瘰疬		Scrofula
Ma Zhen 麻疹		Measles
Mian Tan 面瘫		Facial paralysis
Nue Ji 疟疾		Malaria
Pi Kuai 痞块		Pi Masses
Qi Lin 气淋		Qi Painful-Urination Syndrome
Re Lin 热淋		Heat Painful Urination Syndrome
Ru Pi 乳癖		Breast lumps
Shan 疝		Hernial and Genito-Urinary Disorders

Shi Lin 石淋	Stone Painful-Urination Syndrome	Sui 髓	Marrow
Shi Zhen 湿疹	Eczema (dermatitis)	Tian Gui 天癸	Heavenly Gui
Shui Dou 水痘	Chicken pox	Tuo 唾	Spittle
Tan He 痰核	Nodules	Wei Qi 卫气	Defensive Qi
Tan Huan 瘫缓	Paralysis	Xian 涎	Saliva
Wei Zheng 痿症	Atrophy Syndrome	Xian Tian Zhi Qi 先天之气	Pre-Natal Qi
Wen Bing 溫病	Warm disease		
Wen Yi 溫疫	Warm epidemic pathogenic factor	Xiang Huo 相火	Minister Fire
Wu Chi 五迟	Five Retardations	Yi 意	Intellect
Wu Ruan 五软	Five Flaccidities	Ying Qi 营气	Nutritive Qi
Xu Lao 虛劳	Exhaustion	Yuan Qi 原气	Original Qi
Xu Sun 虛损	Exhaustion	Zhen Qi 真气	True Qi
Xue Lin 血淋	Blood Painful-Urination Syndrome	Zheng Qi 正气	Upright Qi
Ye Ge 噎膈	Diaphragm Choking	Zhi 志	Will-Power
Yin Zhen 癮疹	Urticaria	Zhong Qi 中气	Central Qi
Ying 瘿	Goitre	Zhuang Huo 壮火	Exuberant Fire (pathological)
Yu Zheng 郁症	Depression Pattern	Zong Qi 宗气	Gathering Qi (of the chest)
Yue Jing Guo Duo 月经过多	Heavy Periods		
Yue Jing Guo Shao 月经过少	Scanty Periods		

Emotions

Bei 悲	Sadness
Jing 惊	Shock
Kong 恐	Fear
Nu 怒	Anger
Si 思	Pensiveness
Xi 喜	Joy
You 忧	Worry

Yue Jing Hou Qi 月经后期	Late Periods
Yue Jing Xian Hou Wu Ding Qi 月经先后无定期	Irregular Periods
Yue Jing Xian Qi 月经先其	Early Periods
Zheng Jia 癥瘕	Abdominal masses (in women)
Zhong Feng 中风	Wind-stroke
Zi Lin 子淋	Painful-Urination Pregnancy
Zi Yun 子晕	Dizziness of Pregnancy
Zi Zhong 子肿	Oedema of Pregnancy

Channels and points

Bao Luo 胞络	Uterus Channel
Bao Mai 胞脉	Uterus Vessel
Chong Mai 冲脉	Penetrating Vessel
Cou Li 腠里	Space between skin and muscles
Dai Mai 带脉	Girdle Vessel
Du Mai 督脉	Governing Vessel
Fu Luo 浮络	Superficial Connecting channel
He Xue 合穴	Sea point
Hui Xue 会穴	Gathering point
Jing Xue 井穴	Well point
Jing Xue 经穴	River point
Jing Bie 经别	Divergent channel
Jing Jin 经筋	Muscle channel
Jing Mai 经脉	Main channel
Jue Yin 厥阴	Terminal Yin
Luo Mai (Xue) 络脉 (穴)	Connecting channel
Luo Xue 络穴	Connecting point
Mu Xue 募穴	Front-Collecting points

Vital substances

Hou Tian Zhi Qi 后天之气	Post-Natal Qi
Hun 魂	Ethereal Soul
Jing 精	Essence
Jun Huo 君火	Emperor Fire
Ming Men 命门	Gate of Life
Ming Men Huo 命门火	Fire of the Gate of Life
Po 魄	Corporeal Soul
Shao Huo 少火	Physiological Fire of the body
Shen 神	Mind (the Shen of the Heart) or Spirit (the complex of Heart-Shen, Corporeal Soul, Ethereal Soul, Intellect and Will-Power)

Ren Mai 任脉	Directing Vessel	
Shao Yang 少阳	Lesser Yang	
Shao Yin 少阴	Lesser Yin	
Shu Xue 输穴	Stream point	
(Bei) Shu Xue 背俞穴	Back-Transporting points	
Sun Luo 孙络	Minute Connecting channel	
Tai Yang 太阳	Greater Yang	
Tai Yin 太阴	Greater Yin	
Wu Shu Xue 五输穴	Five Transporting points	
Xi Xue 郄穴	Accumulation point	
Yang Ming 阳明	Bright Yang	
Yang Qiao Mai 阳跷脉	Yang Stepping Vessel	
Yang Wei Mai 阳维脉	Yang Linking Vessel	
Yin Qiao Mai 阴跷脉	Yin Stepping Vessel	
Yin Wei Mai 阴维脉	Yin Linking Vessel	
Ying Xue 荣穴	Spring point	
Yuan Xue 原穴	Source point	

Pulse positions

Chi 尺	Rear (pulse position)
Cun 寸	Front (pulse position)
Guan 关	Middle (pulse position)

Pulse qualities

Chang 长	Long
Chen 沉	Deep
Chi 迟	Slow
Cu 促	Hasty
Da 大	Big
Dai 代	Irregular or Intermittent
Dong 动	Moving
Duan 短	Short
Fu 浮	Floating
Fu 伏	Hidden
Ge 革	Leather
Hong 洪	Overflowing
Hua 滑	Slippery
Huan 缓	Slowed-Down
Ji 急	Hurried
Jie 结	Knotted
Jin 紧	Tight
Kou 芤	Hollow
Lao 牢	Firm
Ru 濡	Soggy
Ruan 软	Soggy
Ruo 弱	Weak
San 散	Scattered
Se 涩	Choppy
Shi 实	Full
Shu 数	Rapid
Wei 微	Minute
Xi 细	Fine
Xian 弦	Wiry
Xu 虚	Empty

Methods of treatment

An Tai 安胎	Calm the Foetus
Bu 补	Tonify (or reinforce as a needle technique)
Gong Yu 功瘀	Dispel stasis (of Blood)
Gu 固	Consolidate
Gu Biao 固表	Consolidate the Exterior
Gu Tuo 固脱	Consolidate Collapse
Hua Shi 化湿	Resolve Dampness
Hua Tan 化痰	Resolve Phlegm
Hua Yu 化瘀	Eliminate stasis (of Blood)
Huan Ji 缓急	Moderate urgency
Huo Xue 活血	Invigorate Blood
Jie (Biao) 解表	Release (the Exterior)
Jie Yu 解郁	Eliminate stagnation (of Qi)
Kai Qiao 开窍	Open the orifices
Li Hou 利喉	Benefit the throat
Li Mu 利目	Brighten the eyes
Li Qi 理气	Move Qi
Li Shi 利湿	Resolve Dampness
Li Shui 利水	Transform Water
Li Shui Dao 理水道	Regulate the Water passages
Liu Wei 疏卫	Circulate Defensive Qi
Ping Gan 平肝	Calm the Liver
Po Xue 破血	Break-up Blood
Qing (Re) 清热	Clear Heat
Qu (Feng) 去风	Expel (external Wind)
Qu Yu 去瘀	Eliminate stasis (of Blood)
San Han 散寒	Expel Cold
San Jie 散结	Dissipate accumulation or dissipate nodules
Sheng Xin 生新	Promote healing of tissues
Shu (Gan) 疏肝	Pacify (the Liver)
Shu Jin 舒筋	Relax the sinews
Tiao He Ying Wei 调和营卫	Harmonize Nutritive and Defensive Qi
Tiao Jing 调经	Regulate the period
Tong Luo 通络	Remove obstructions from the Connecting channels
Tong Qiao 通窍	Open the orifices

Tong Ru 通乳络	Remove obstructions from the breast's Connecting channels	
Tong Yang 通畅 (胸)	Open (the chest)	
Wen Jing 温经	Warm the menses	
Xi Feng 熄风	Extinguish Wind (internal)	
Xie 泻	Reduce (as a needle technique)	
Xie 泄	Clear (Heat)	
Xie 泻	Drain (Fire)	
Xie 泻	Drain (method of treatment as opposed to Bu 补, tonify)	
Xie Xia 泻下	Move downwards	
Xin Kai Ku Jiang 辛开苦降	Use pungent herbs to open and bitter ones to make Qi descend	
Xing Zhi 醒志	Promote resuscitation	
Xuan Fei 宣肺	Restore the diffusing of Lung-Qi	
Xuan Tong Bi 宣通鼻窍	Open the nose	
Yang (Xue) 养血	Nourish (Blood)	

Pathogenic factors

Feng Han 风寒	Wind-Cold
Feng Re 风热	Wind-Heat
Han 寒	Cold
Huo 火	Fire
Re 热	Heat
Re Du 热毒	Toxic Heat
Shi 湿	Dampness
Shu 暑	Summer-Heat
Tan 痰	Phlegm
Tan Yin 痰饮	Phlegm-Fluids in general and also Phlegm-Fluids in the Stomach
Wen Yi 温疫	Warm epidemic pathogenic factor
Xie 邪	Pathogenic factor
Xie Qi 邪气	Pathogenic factor
Xuan Yin 悬饮	Phlegm-Fluids in the hypochondrium
Yi Yin 溢饮	Phlegm-Fluids in the limbs
Zao 燥	Dryness
Zhi Yin 支饮	Phlegm-Fluids in the diaphragm

Appendix 3
Chronology of Chinese Dynasties

Xia: 21st to 16th century BC

Shang: 16th to 11th century BC

Zhou: 11th century to 771 BC

Spring and Autumn Period: 770–476 BC

Warring States Period: 475–221 BC

Qin: 221–206 BC

Han: 206 BC–AD 220

Three Kingdoms Period: AD 220–280

Jin: 265–420

Northern and Southern dynasties: 420–581

Sui: 581–618

Tang: 618–907

Five Dynasties: 907–960

Song: 960–1279

Liao: 906–1125

Jin: 1115–1234

Yuan: 1271–1368

Ming: 1368–1644

Qing: 1644–1911

Republic of China: 1912–1949

People's Republic of China: 1949–

Appendix 4
Bibliography

ANCIENT CLASSICS
(LISTED IN CHRONOLOGICAL ORDER)

1. 1979 The Yellow Emperor's Classic of Internal Medicine-Simple Questions (*Huang Di Nei Jing Su Wen* 黄帝内经素问), People's Health Publishing House, Beijing. First published c. 100 BC.
2. Tian Dai Hua 2005 The Yellow Emperor's Classic of Internal Medicine-Simple Questions (*Huang Di Nei Jing Su Wen* 黄帝内经素问), People's Health Publishing House, Beijing. First published c. 100 BC.
3. 1981 Spiritual Axis (*Ling Shu Jing* 灵枢经), People's Health Publishing House, Beijing. First published c. 100 BC.
4. Tian Dai Hua 2005 Spiritual Axis (*Ling Shu Jing* 灵枢经), People's Health Publishing House, Beijing. First published c. 100 BC.
5. Nanjing College of Traditional Chinese Medicine 1979 A Revised Explanation of the Classic of Difficulties (*Nan Jing Jiao Shi* 难经校释), People's Health Publishing House, Beijing. First published c. AD 100.
6. Qin Yue Ren 2004 Classic of Difficulties (*Nan Jing Jiao Shi* 难经校释), Scientific and Technical Documents Publishing House, Beijing. First published c. AD 100.
7. Wu Chang Guo 1985 The Classic of the Central Organ (*Zhong Zang Jing* 中藏经), Jiangsu Scientific Publishing House. The Classic of the Central Organ was written by Hua Tuo c. AD 198.
8. Nanjing College of Traditional Chinese Medicine, Shang Han Lun Research Group 1980 Discussion on Cold-induced Diseases (*Shang Han Lun* 伤寒论), Shanghai Scientific Publishing House, Shanghai. The Shang Han Lun was written by Zhang Zhong Jing and first published c. AD 220.
9. Duan Guang Zhou et al. 1986 A Manual of the Essential Prescriptions of the Golden Chest (*Jin Gui Yao Lue Shou Ce* 金匮要略手册) Science Publishing House. The Essential Prescriptions of the Golden Chest was written by Zhang Zhong Jing and first published c. AD 220.
10. Traditional Chinese Medicine Research Institute 1959 An Explanation of the Essential Prescriptions of the Golden Chest (*Jin Gui Yao Lue Yu Yi* 金匮要略喻译), People's Health Publishing House, Beijing, p. 61. The Essential Prescriptions of the Golden Chest was written by Zhang Zhong Jing and first published c. AD 220.
11. He Ren 1979 A Popular Guide to the Essential Prescriptions of the Golden Chest (*Jin Gui Yao Lue Tong Su Jiang Hua* 金匮要略通俗讲话) Shanghai Science Publishing House, Shanghai. The Essential Prescriptions of the Golden Chest was written by Zhang Zhong Jing and first published c. AD 220.
12. 1981 A New Explanation of the Essential Prescriptions of the Golden Chest (*Jin Gui Yao Lue Fang Xin Jie* 金匮要略方新解), Zhejiang Scientific Publishing House, Zhejiang. The Essential Prescriptions of the Golden Chest was written by Zhang Zhong Jing and first published c. AD 220.
13. He Ren 2005 Essential Prescriptions of the Golden Chest (*Jin Gui Yao Lue* 金匮要略通俗讲话), People's Health Publishing House, Beijing. Shanghai. The Essential Prescriptions of the Golden Chest was written by Zhang Zhong Jing and first published c. AD 220.
14. Fuzhou City People's Hospital 1984 The Pulse Classic (*Mai Jing* 脉经), People's Health Publishing House, Beijing. The Pulse Classic was written by Wang Shu He and first published c. AD 280.
15. Shandong College of Traditional Chinese Medicine 1984 An Explanation of the Pulse Classic (*Mai Jing Jiao Shi* 脉经校释), People's Health Publishing House, Beijing. The Pulse Classic was written by Wang Shu He and first published c. AD 280.
16. Shandong College of Traditional Chinese Medicine 1979 The ABC of Acupuncture (*Zhen Jiu Jia Yi Jing* 针灸甲乙经), People's Health Publishing House, Beijing. The ABC of Acupuncture was written by Huang Fu Mi and first published AD 282.
17. 1981 An Elucidation of the Yellow Emperor's Classic of Internal Medicine (*Huang Di Nei Jing Tai Su* 黄帝内经太素), People's Health Publishing House, Beijing. An Elucidation of the Yellow Emperor's Classic of Internal Medicine was written by Yang Shang Shan and first published AD 581–618.
18. Ding Guang Di 1991 Discussion of the Origin of Symptoms in Diseases (*Zhu Bing Yuan Hou Lun* 诸病源候论), People's Health Publishing House, Beijing. The Discussion of the Origin of Symptoms in Diseases was written by Chao Yuan Fang in AD 610.
19. 1982 Thousand Golden Ducats Prescriptions (*Qian Jin Yao Fang* 千金要方), People's Health Publishing House, Beijing. The Thousand Golden Ducats Prescriptions was written by Sun Si Miao in AD 652.
20. 1976 Discussion on Stomach and Spleen (*Pi Wei Lun* 脾胃论), People's Publishing House, Beijing. The Discussion on Stomach and Spleen was written by Li Dong Yuan and first published in 1249.
21. Yang Jian Bing 2002 A Vernacular Explanation of the Discussion on Stomach and Spleen (*Pi Wei Lun Bai Hua Jie* 脾胃论白话解), San Qin Publishing House, Xian. The Discussion on Stomach and Spleen was written by Li Dong Yuan and first published in 1249.
22. Kang Suo Bin 2002 A New Explanation of the Guide to Acupuncture Channels (*Quan Xin Zhen Jing Zhi Nan* 诠新针经指南), Hebei Science and Technology Publishing House, Hebei, Shijiazhuang. The Guide to Acupuncture Channels was written by Han Dou in 1295.
23. 1988 Original Mirror on Regulating Exhaustion (*Li Xu Yuan Jian* 理虚元鉴), People's Health Publishing House, Beijing. The Original Mirror on Regulation Exhaustion was written by Zhu Qi Shi and first published c. 1520.
24. 1991 Gatherings from Eminent Acupuncturists (*Zhen Jiu Ju Ying* 针灸聚英), Shanghai Science and Technology Publishing House, Shanghai. The Gatherings from Eminent Acupuncturists was written by Gao Wu and first published in 1529.
25. Wang Luo Zhen 1985 A Compilation of the Study of the Eight Extraordinary Vessels (*Qi Jing Ba Mai Kao Jiao Zhu* 奇经八脉考校注), Shanghai Science Publishing House, Shanghai. The Study of the Eight Extraordinary Vessels was written by Li Shi Zhen and first published in 1578.
26. Heilongjiang Province National Medical Research Group 1984 An Explanation of the Great Compendium of Acupuncture (*Zhen Jiu Da Cheng Jiao Shi* 针灸大成校释), People's Health Publishing House, Beijing. The Great Compendium of Acupuncture was written by Yang Ji Zhou and first published in 1601.

27. 1980 The Great Compendium of Acupuncture (*Zhen Jiu Da Cheng* 针灸大成), People's Health Publishing House, Beijing. The Great Compendium of Acupuncture was written by Yang Ji Zhou and first published in 1601.
28. Wu Zhan Ren, Yu Zhi Gao 1987 Correct Seal of Medical Circles (*Yi Lin Zheng Yin* 医林正印), Jiangsu Science Publishing House, Nanjing. The Correct Seal of Medical Circles was written by Ma Zhao Sheng and first published in 1605.
29. 1982 Classic of Categories (*Lei Jing* 类经), People's Health Publishing House, Beijing. The Classic of Categories was written by Zhang Jie Bin (also called Zhang Jing Yue) and first published in 1624.
30. 1986 Complete Book of Jing Yue (*Jing Yue Quan Shu* 京岳全书). Shangai Scientific Publishing House, Shanghai. The Complete Book of Jing Yue was written by Zhang Jing Yue and first published in 1624.
31. Chinese Medicine Research Group of the Zhejiang Province 1985 A Discussion of Epidemic Warm Diseases with Notes and Commentary (*Wen Yi Lun Ping Zhu* 温疫论评注), People's Health Publishing House, Beijing. The Discussion of Epidemic Warm Diseases was written by Wu You Ke in 1642.
32. Shan Chang Hua 1990 An Explanation of the Acupuncture Points (*Jing Xue Jie* 经穴解), People's Health Publishing House, Beijing. An Explanation of the Acupuncture Points was written by Yue Han Zhen and first published in 1654.
33. 1977 Golden Mirror of Medicine (*Yi Zong Jin Jian* 医宗金鉴), People's Health Publishing House, Beijing. The Golden Mirror of Medicine was written by Wu Qian and first published in 1742.
34. Nanjing College of Traditional Chinese Medicine 1978 A Study of Warm Diseases (*Wen Bing Xue* 温病学), Shanghai Science Publishing House, Shanghai. The Study of Warm Diseases was written by Ye Tian Shi in 1746.
35. Wang Zhen Kun 1995 A New Explanation of the Systematic Differentiation of Warm Diseases (*Wen Bing Tiao Bian Xin Jie* 温病条辨新解), Xue Yuan Publishing House, Beijing. The Systematic Differentiation of Warm Diseases was written by Wu Ju Tong in 1798.
36. 1973 Fu Qing Zhu's Gynaecology (*Fu Qing Zhu Nu Ke* 傅青主女科) Shanghai People's Publishing House, Shanghai. Fu Qing Zhu was born in 1607 and died in 1684. Fu Qing Zhu's Gynaecology was first published in 1827.
37. 1979 Discussion on Blood Patterns (*Xue Zheng Lun* 血证论), People's Health Publishing House. The Discussion on Blood Patterns was written by Tang Zong Hai and first published in 1884.
38. Pei Zheng Xue 1979 A Commentary on the Discussion on Blood Patterns (*Xue Zheng Lun Ping Shi* 血证论评释), People's Health Publishing House, Beijing. The Discussion on Blood Patterns was written by Tang Zong Hai and first published in 1884.
39. 1988 Origin of Diseases Dictionary (*Bing Yuan Ci Dian* 病源辞典), Tianjin Ancient Texts Publishing House, Tianjin. The Origin of Diseases Dictionary was written by Wu Ke Qian.

MODERN TEXTS

Publications without an author are listed in chronological order. Those with an author are listed in alphabetical order.
Texts in chronological order:

1. Nanjing College of Traditional Chinese Medicine-Warm Diseases Research Group 1959 Teaching Reference Material on the School of Warm Diseases (*Wen Bing Xue Jiao Xue Can Kao Zi Liao* 温病学教学参考资料), Jiangsu People's Publishing House.
2. Guangdong College of Traditional Chinese Medicine 1964 A Study of Diagnosis in Chinese Medicine (*Zhong Yi Zhen Duan Xue* 中医诊断学), Shanghai Scientific Publishing House, Shanghai.
3. Guangzhou Army Health Department 1974 A New General Outline of Chinese Medicine, (*Xin Bian Zhong Yi Xue Gai Yao* 新编中医学概要), People's Health Publishing House, Beijing.
4. Shanghai College of Traditional Chinese Medicine 1974 A Study of Acupuncture (*Zhen Jiu Xue* 针灸学), People's Health Publishing House, Beijing.
5. 1978 Fundamentals of Chinese Medicine (*Zhong Yi Ji Chu Xue* 中医基础学), Shandong Scientific Publishing House, Jinan.
6. 1979 Patterns and Treatment of Kidney Diseases (*Shen Yu Shen Bing de Zheng Zhi* 肾与肾病的证治), Hebei People's Publishing House, Hebei.
7. Anwei College of Traditional Chinese Medicine 1979 Clinical Manual of Chinese Medicine (*Zhong Yi Lin Chuang Shou Ce* 中医临床手册), Anwei Scientific Publishing House, Anwei.
8. Acupuncture Research Group 1980 A Simple Compilation of Acupuncture (*Zhen Jiu Xue Jian Bian* 针灸学简编), People's Health Publishing House, Beijing.
9. Beijing College of Traditional Chinese Medicine 1980 Practical Chinese Medicine (*Shi Yong Zhong Yi Xue* 实用中医学), Beijing Publishing House, Beijing.
10. 1980 Concise Dictionary of Chinese Medicine (*Jian Ming Zhong Yi Ci Dian* 简明中医辞典), People's Health Publishing House, Beijing.
11. 1981 Differentiation of Diseases and Patterns in Internal Medicine (*Nei Ke Bian Bing Yu Bian Zheng* 内科辨病与辨证), Heilongjiang People's Publishing House.
12. 1981 Syndromes and Treatment of the Internal Organs (*Zang Fu Zheng Zhi* 脏腑证治), Tianjin Scientific Publishing House, Tianjin. Scientific Publishing House, Tianjin.
13. Anwei College of Traditional Chinese Medicine and Shanghai College of Traditional Chinese Medicine 1987 Dictionary of Acupuncture (*Zhen Jiu Xue Ci Dian* 针灸学辞典), Shanghai Scientific Publishing House, Shanghai.
14. All-China Research Group in Chinese Medicine 1995 Great Dictionary of Chinese Medicine (*Zhong Yi Da Ci Dian* 中医大辞典), People's Health Publishing Company, Beijing.

Texts by author:

15. Chen Jin Guang 1992 Complete Textbook of Chinese Patterns in Contemporary Chinese Medicine (*Xian Dai Zhong Yi Lin Zheng Quan Shu* 现代中医临证全书), Beijing Publishing House, Beijing.
16. Chen You Bang 1990 Chinese Acupuncture Therapy (*Zhong Guo Zhen Jiu Zhi Liao Xue* 中国针灸治疗学), China Science Publishing House, Shanghai.
17. Cheng Bao Shu 1988 Great Dictionary of Acupuncture (*Zhen Jiu Da Ci Dian* 针灸大辞典), Beijing Science Publishing House, Beijing.
18. Fang Wen Xian 1989 A Manual of New Treatment of Internal Medicine Diseases in Chinese Medicine (*Zhong Yi Nei Ke Zheng Zhuang Xin Zhi Shou Ce* 中医内科症状新治手册), China Standard Publishing House, Beijing.
19. Fang Wen Xian 1989 Manual of Differentiation and Treatment of Symptoms in Internal Chinese Medicine (*Zhong Yi Nei Ke Zheng Zhuang Zhi Shou Ce* 中医内科症辨治手册), China Standard Publishing House, Beijing.
20. Gu He Dao 1979 History of Chinese Medicine (*Zhong Guo Yi Xue Shi Lue* 中国医学史略), Shanxi People's Publishing House, Taiyuan.
21. Gu Yu Qi 2005 Chinese Medicine Psychology (*Zhong Yi Xin Li Xue* 中医心理学), China Medicine Science and Technology Publishing House, Beijing.
22. Guo Zhen Qiu 1985 Diagnosis in Chinese Medicine (*Zhong Yi Zhen Duan Xue* 中医诊断学), Hunan Science Publishing House, Changsha.
23. Guo Zi Guang 1985 A New Compilation of Difficult Syndromes in Chinese Medicine (*Zhong Yi Qi Zheng Xin Bian* 中医奇证新编), Hunan Science Publishing House, Changsha.
24. Hu Xi Ming 1989 Great Treatise of Secret Formulae in Chinese Medicine (*Zhong Guo Zhong Yi Mi Fang Da Quan* 中国中医秘方大全), Literary Publishing House, Shanghai.
25. Huang Long Xiang 1997 Collected Works of Famous Outstanding Acupuncturists (*Zhen Jiu Ming Zhu Ji Cheng* 针灸名著集成), Hua Xia Publishing House, Beijing.
26. Huang Tai Tang 2001 The Treatment of Difficult Diseases in Chinese Internal Medicine (*Nei Ke Yi Nan Bing Zhong Yi Zhi Liao Xue*

内科医难病中医治疗学), Chinese Herbal Medicine Science Publishing House, Beijing.

27. Ji Jie Yin 1984 Clinical Records of Tai Yi Shen Acupuncture (*Tai Yi Shen Zhen Jiu Lin Zheng Lu* 太乙神针灸临证录), Shanxi Province Scientific Publishing House, Shanxi.
28. Jiao Shun Fa 1987 An Enquiry into Chinese Acupuncture (*Zhong Guo Zhen Jiu Xue Qiu Zhen* 中国针灸求真), Shanxi Science Publishing House.
29. Li Shi Zhen 1985 Clinical Application of Frequently Used Acupuncture Points (*Chang Yong Shu Xue Lin Chuang Fa Hui* 用输穴临床发挥), People's Health Publishing House, Beijing.
30. Li Wen Chuan, He Bao Yi 1987 Practical Acupuncture (*Shi Yong Zhen Jiu Xue* 实用针灸学), People's Health Publishing House, Beijing.
31. Li Zheng Quan 1992 A Practical Study of the Stomach and Spleen in Chinese Medicine (*Shi Yong Zhong Yi Pi Wei Xue* 实用中医脾胃学), Chongqing Publishing House, Chongqing.
32. Liu Guan Jun 1990 Acupuncture Theory and Clinical Patterns (*Zhen Jiu Ming Li Yu Lin Zheng* 针灸明理与临证), People's Health Publishing House, Beijing.
33. Liu Han Yin 1988 Practical Treatise of Acupuncture (*Shi Yong Zhen Jiu Da Quan* 实用针灸大全), Beijing Publishing House, Beijing.
34. Lu Fang 1981 Identification of Diseases and Patterns in Internal Medicine (*Nei Ke Bian Bing Yu Bian Zheng* 内科辨病与辨证), Heilongjiang People's Publishing House, Harbin.
35. Luo Yuan Kai 1986 Gynaecology in Chinese Medicine (*Zhong Yi Fu Ke Xue* 中医妇科学), Shanghai Science and Technology Press, Shanghai.
36. Qin Bo Wei 1991 The Essence of Medical Records of Famous Doctors of the Qing Dynasty (*Qing Dai Ming Yi Yi An Jing Hua* 清代名医医案精华), Shanghai Science and Technology Press, Shanghai.
37. Shan Yu Dang 1984 Selection of Acupuncture Point Combinations from the Discussion on Cold-induced Diseases (*Shang Han Lun Zhen Jiu Pei Xue Xuan Zhu* 伤寒论针灸配穴选注), People's Health Publishing House, Beijing.
38. Shen Quan Yu, Wu Yu Hua and Shen Li Ling 1989 The Treatment of Manic-Depression and Epilepsy (*Dian Kuang Dian Zheng Zhi* 癫狂痫证治), Ancient Chinese Medicine Texts Publishing House, Beijing.
39. Shi Yu Guang 1988 Essential Clinical Experience of Famous Modern Doctors (*Dang Dai Ming Yi Lin Zheng Jing Hua* 当代名医临证精华), Ancient Chinese Medicine Texts Publishing House, Beijing.
40. Shi Yu Guang 1992 Essential Clinical Experience of Famous Modern Doctors – Manic-Depression and Epilepsy (*Dang Dai Ming Yi Lin Zheng Jing Hua* 当代名医临证精华), Ancient Chinese Medicine Texts Publishing House, Beijing.
41. Wang Jin Quan 1987 Discussion on Categories of Syndromes from the Yellow Emperor's Classic of Internal Medicine (*Nei Jing Lei Zheng Lun Zhi* 内经类证论指), Shanxi Science Publishing House, Xian.
42. Wang Ke Qin 1988 Theory of the Mind in Chinese Medicine (*Zhong Yi Shen Zhu Xue Shuo* 中医神主学说), Ancient Chinese Medical Texts Publishing House, Beijing.
43. Wang Li Cao 1997 A Collection of Chinese Acupuncture Prescriptions (*Zhong Guo Zhen Jiu Chu Fang Da Cheng* 中国针灸处方大成), Shanxi Science Publishing House, Taiyuan.
44. Wang Xin Hua 1983 Selected Historical Theories of Chinese Medicine (*Zhong Yi Li Dai Yi Lun Xuan* 中医历代医论选), Jiangsu Scientific Publishing House.
45. Wang Xue Tai 1988 Great Treatise of Chinese Acupuncture (*Zhong Guo Zhen Jiu Da Quan* 中国针灸大全), Henan Science Publishing House.
46. Wang Yong Yan 2004 Chinese Internal Medicine (*Zhong Yi Nei Ke Xue* 中医内科学), People's Health Publishing House, Beijing.
47. Wang Zhi Xian 1987 A Record of the Treatment of 30 Types of Diseases (*San Shi Zhong Bing Zhi Yan Lu* 三十种病治验录), Shanxi Science Publishing House, Taiyuan.
48. Wang Zhong Heng 1995 Collection of Patterns and Treatment of Difficult Diseases in Internal Medicine (*Nei Ke Za Bing Zheng Zhi Ji Jin* 内科杂病证治集锦), Chinese Medicine Ancient Texts Publishing House, Beijing.
49. Xia De Xin 1989 Clinical Manual of Internal Medicine (*Zhong Yi Nei Ke Lin Chuang Shou Ce* 中医内科临床手册), Shanghai Science Publishing House, Shanghai.
50. Xu Ben Ren 1986 Clinical Acupuncture (*Lin Chuang Zhen Jiu Xue* 临床针灸学), Liaoning Scientific Publishing House, Liaoning.
51. Xu Rong Juan 2004 Internal Medicine (*Nei Ke Xue* 内科学), Chinese Herbal Medicine Publishing House, Beijing.
52. Yang Jia San 1988 Great Dictionary of Chinese Acupuncture (*Zhong Guo Zhen Jiu Da Ci Dian* 中国针灸大辞典), Beijing Sports College Publishing House, Beijing.
53. Yang Jia San 1989 A Study of Acupuncture (*Zhen Jiu Xue* 针灸学), Beijing Science Publishing House, Beijing.
54. Ye Ren Gao 2003 Patterns of Internal Chinese Medicine (*Zhong Yi Nei Ke Zheng Hou* 中医内科证候), People's Health Publishing House, Beijing.
55. Yu Zhong Quan 1988 A Practical Study of the Differentiation of Acupuncture Points (*Jing Xue Bian Zheng Yun Yong Xue* 经穴辨证运用学), Sichuan Science Publishing House, Chengdu.
56. Zeng Shi Zu 1992 Dietary Treatment, Massage and Herbal Treatment for Epilepsy and Hysteria (*Zhi Liao Dian Xian, Yi Bing, Xiao Fang, An Mo Shi Liao* 治疗癫痫癔病效方按摩食疗), Shanxi Science and Technology Publishing House, Xian.
57. Zhai Ming Yi 1979 Clinical Chinese Medicine (*Zhong Yi Lin Chuang Ji Chu* 中医临床基础), Henan Publishing House, Henan.
58. Zhang Bo Yu 1986 Chinese Internal Medicine (*Zhong Yi Nei Ke Xue* 中医内科学), Shanghai Science Publishing House, Shanghai.
59. Zhang Fa Rong 1989 Chinese Internal Medicine (*Zhong Yi Nei Ke Xue* 中医内科学), Sichuan Science Publishing House, Chengdu.
60. Zhang Qi Wen 1995 Menstrual Diseases (*Yue Jing Bing Zheng* 月经病证), People's Hygiene Publishing House, Beijing.
61. Zhang Shan Chen 1982 Essential Collection of Acupuncture Points from the ABC of Acupuncture (*Zhen Jiu Jia Yi Jing Shu Xue Zhong Ji* 针灸甲乙经腧穴重辑), Shandong Scientific Publishing House, Shandong. First published AD 282.
62. Zhang Shan You 1980 An Explanation of Passages Concerning Acupuncture from the Yellow Emperor's Classic of Internal Medicine (*Nei Jing Zhen Jiu Lei Fang Yu Shi* 内经针灸类方语释), Shandong Scientific Publishing House, Shandong.
63. Zhang Sheng Xing 1984 A Compilation of Explanations of the Meaning of the Acupuncture Points Names (*Jing Xue Shi Yi Hui Jie* 经穴释义汇解), Shanghai Science Publishing House, Shanghai.
64. Zhang Yuan Kai 1985 Medical Collection of Four Doctors from the Meng He Tradition (*Meng He Si Jia Yi Ji* 孟河四家医集), Jiangsu Province Scientific Publishing House, Nanjing.
65. Zhou Chao Fan 2000 Essential Chinese Medicine Treatment Principles in Successive Dynasties (*Li Dai Zhong Yi Zhi Ze Jing Hua* 历代中医治则精华), Chinese Herbal Medicine Publishing House, Beijing.

JOURNALS

1. Liao Ning Journal of Chinese Medicine (*Liao Ning Zhong Yi* 辽宁中医), Shenyang, Liao Ning.
2. Journal of Chinese Medicine (*Zhong Yi Za Zhi* 中医杂志), China Association of Traditional Chinese Medicine and China Academy of Traditional Chinese Medicine, Beijing.
3. Journal of Nanjing University of Traditional Chinese Medicine (*Nanjing Zhong Yi Yao Da Xue Xue Bao* 南京中医药大学学报), Nanjing University of Traditional Chinese Medicine, Nanjing.

ENGLISH LANGUAGE TEXTS

Listed in alphabetical order.
1. Ames R. T. (editor) 1994 Self as Person in Asian Theory and Practice, State University of New York Press, New York.
2. Ames R. T. and Hall D. 2001 Focusing the Familiar – A Translation and Philosophical Interpretation of the Zhongyong, University of Hawaii Press, Honolulu.
3. Ames R. T. and Rosemont H. 1999 The Analects of Confucius – A Philosophical Translation, Ballantine Books, New York.
4. Ames R. T., Kasulis T. P. and Dissanayake W. 1998 Self as Image in Asian Theory and Practice, State University of New York Press, New York.
5. Ames R. T. and Hall D. L. 2003 Daodejing – "Making This Life Significant" A Philosophical Translation, Ballantine Books, New York.
6. Beaven D. W. and Brooks S. E. 1988 Colour Atlas of the Tongue in Clinical Diagnosis, Wolfe Medical Publications Ltd, London.
7. Beijing, Shanghai and Nanjing College of Traditional Chinese Medicine 1980 Essentials of Chinese Acupuncture, Foreign Languages Press, Beijing.
8. Bensky D. and O'Connor J. 1981 Acupuncture. a Comprehensive Text, Eastland Press, Seattle.
9. Bensky D., Clavey S. and Stöger E. Materia Medica 2004 3rd Edition, Eastland Press, Seattle.
10. Bockover M. (editor) 1991 Rules, Ritual and Responsibility – Essays Dedicated to Herbert Fingarette, Open Court, La Salle, Illinois.
11. Chang C. 1977 The Development of Neo-Confucian Thought, Greenwood Press Publishers, Westport, Connecticut.
12. Chang L. S. and Feng Y. 1998 The Four Political Treatises of the Yellow Emperor, University of Hawai'i Press, Honolulu.
13. Chen Xin Nong 1987 Chinese Acupuncture and Moxibustion, Foreign Languages Press, Beijing.
14. Claremont de Castillejo I 1997 Knowing Woman – A Feminine Psychology, Shambhala, Boston.
15. Clavey S. 2003 Fluid Physiology and Pathology in Traditional Chinese Medicine, Edinburgh.
16. Crabbe J. (editor) 1999 From Soul to Self, Routledge, London.
17. Damasio A. 1994 Descartes' Error – Emotion, Reason and the Human Brain, Penguin Books, London.
18. Damasio A. 1999 The Feeling of What Happens – Body and Emotion in the Making of Consciousness, Harcourt Inc., San Diego.
19. Damasio A. 2003 Looking for Spinoza – Joy, Sorrow and the Feeling Brain, Harcourt Inc., San Diego.
20. Davidson R. and Harrington A. 2002 Visions of Compassion – Western Scientists and Tibetan Buddhists Examine Human Nature, Oxford University Press, Oxford.
21. Deadman P. and Al-Khafaji M. 1998 A Manual of Acupuncture, Journal of Chinese Medicine Publications, Hove, England.
22. Edelman G. M. and Tononi G. 2000 A Universe of Consciousness – How Matter Becomes Imagination, Basic Books, New York.
23. Edelman G. M. 2005 Wider than the Sky – The Phenomenal Gift of Consciousness, Yale University Press, New Haven.
24. Farquhar J. 1994 Knowing Practice – The Clinical Encounter of Chinese Medicine, Westview Press, Boulder, USA.
25. Fingarette H. 1972 Confucius – The Secular as Sacred, Waveland Press, Prospect Heights, Illinois.
26. Fung Yu Lan 1966 A Short History of Chinese Philosophy, Free Press, New York.
27. Gardner D K 2003 Zhu Xi's Reading of the Analects, Columbia University Press, New York.
28. Gernet J 1983 China and the Christian Impact: a Conflict of Cultures, Cambridge University Press.
29. Giles H. 1912 Chinese-English Dictionary, Kelly & Walsh, Shanghai
30. Gluck A. 2007 Damasio's Error and Descartes' Truth, University of Scranton Press, London.
31. Graham A. C. 1986 Yin-Yang and the Nature of Correlative Thinking, Institute of East Asian Philosophies, Singapore
32. Graham A. C. 1999 The Book of Lieh-Tzu – A Classic of Tao, Columbia University Press, New York.
33. Greene B. 2000 The Elegant Universe, Vintage, London
34. Greenfield S. 2000 The Private Life of the Brain, Penguin Books, London.
35. Hall D. L. and Ames R. T. 1998 Thinking from the Han – Self, Truth and Transcendence in Chinese and Western Culture, State University of New York Press, New York.
36. Helms J. M. 1995 Acupuncture Energetics – A Clinical Approach for Physicians, Medical Acupuncture Publishers, California.
37. Holcombe C. 1994 In the Shadow of the Han, University of Hawaii, Honolulu.
38. Huang Siu-chi 1999 Essentials of Neo-Confucianism, Greenwood Press, Westport, Connecticut.
39. James S. 2003 Passion and Action – The Emotions in Seventeenth-Century Philosophy, Clarendon Press, Oxford.
40. Jones D. (editor) 2008 Confucius Now, Open Court, Chicago
41. Jung C. G. 1961 Modern Man in Search of a Soul, Routledge & Kegan Paul, London.
42. Kaptchuk T. 2000 The Web that has no Weaver – Understanding Chinese Medicine, Contemporary Books, Chicago.
43. Kasulis T. P., Ames R. T. and Dissanayke W. 1993 Self as Body in Asian Theory and Practice, State University of New York Press, New York.
44. Kim Yung Sik 2000 The Natural Philosophy of Chu Hsi, American Philosophical Society, Philadelphia.
45. Kovacs J and Unschuld P 1998 Essential Subtleties on the Silver Sea – The *Yin Hai Jing Wei*: a Chinese Classic of Opthalmology, University of California Press, Berkeley.
46. Lange C. G. and James W. 1922 The Emotions, Vol. 1, Williams and Wilkins Company, Baltimore.
47. Lau D. C. and Ames R. T. 1998 Yuan Dao – Tracing Dao to its Source, Ballantine Books, NewYork.
48. Ledoux J. 1996 The Emotional Brain, Simon & Shuster Paperbacks, New York
49. Lewis T., Amini F. and Lannon R. 2000 A General Theory of Love, Random House, New York.
50. Lewis M. and Haviland-Jones J. M. (editors) 2004 Handbook of Emotions, Guildford Press, New York.
51. Liu Bing Quan 1988 Optimum Time for Acupuncture – A Collection of Traditional Chinese Chronotherapeutics, Shandong Science and Technology Press, Jinan.
52. Maciocia G. 2004 The Diagnosis of Chinese Medicine, Churchill Livingstone, Edinburgh
53. Maciocia G. 2005 The Foundations of Chinese Medicine 2nd Edition, Churchill Livingstone, Edinburgh.
54. Maciocia G. 2007 The Practice of Chinese Medicine 2nd Edition, Churchill Livingstone, Edinburgh.
55. Marks J. and Ames R. T. 1995 Emotions in Asian Thought. State University of New York Press, New York.
56. Matsumoto K. and Birch S. 1988 Hara Diagnosis: Reflections on the Sea, Paradigm Publications, Brookline.
57. Needham J. 1977 Science and Civilization in China, Vol. 2, Cambridge University Press, Cambridge.
58. Needham J. and Lu G. D. 1980 Celestial Lancets, Cambridge University Press, Cambridge.
59. Ng On-cho 2001 Cheng-Zhu Confucianism in the Early Qing, State University of New York Press, New York.
60. Ni Yi Tian 1996 Navigating the Channels of Traditional Chinese Medicine, Complementary Medicine Press, San Diego.
61. Nisbett R. E. 2003 The Geography of Thought – How Asians and Westerners Think Differently and Why, The Free Press, New York.
62. Qiu Mao Liang 1993 Chinese Acupuncture and Moxibustion, Churchill Livingstone, Edinburgh.
63. Pert C. 1997 Molecules of Emotion – The Science of Mind-Body Medicine, Scribner, New York.
64. Redfield Jamison K. 1993 Touched with Fire – Manic-depressive Illness and the Artistic Temperament, Free Press, New York.
65. Redfield Jamison K. 1995 An Unquiet Mind, Picador, London.

66. Russell B. 2002 History of Western Philosophy, Routledge, London.
67. Sartre J. P. 2004 Sketch for a Theory of the Emotions, Routledge, London.
68. Searle J. R. 2004 Mind, Oxford University Press, Oxford.
69. Solomon R. C. 1993 The Passions – Emotions and the Meaning of Life, Hackett Publishing Company, Indianapolis.
70. Sorabji R. 2002 Emotion and Peace of Mind – From Stoic Agitation to Christian Temptation, Oxford University Press, Oxford.
71. Tallis F. 2004 Love Sick, Century, London.
72. Taylor C. 2003 Sources of the Self – The Making of the Modern Identity, Cambridge University Press, Cambridge.
73. Trimble M. R. 2007 The Soul in the Brain, John Hopkins University Press, Baltimore.
74. Unschuld P. 1985 Medicine in China – A History of Ideas, University of California Press, Berkeley.
75. Unschuld P. 1986 Nan Ching – The Classic of Difficult Issues, University of California Press, Berkeley.
76. Unschuld P. 2000 Medicine in China – Historical Artefacts and Images, Prestel, Munich.
77. Unschuld P. 2003 "Huang Di Nei Jing Su Wen: Nature, Knowledge, Imagery in an Ancient Chinese Medical Text", University of California Press, Berkeley.
78. Wang Ai He 1999 Cosmology and Political Culture in Early China, Cambridge University Press, Cambridge.
79. Wilhelm R. (translator) 1962 The Secret of the Golden Flower, Harcourt, Brace & World, Inc., New York, N.Y.
80. Wollheim R. 1999 On the Emotions, Yale University Press, New Haven.
81. Scalp-NeedlingTherapy 1975, Medicine and Health Publishing Co., Hong Kong.

TEXTBOOKS OF WESTERN MEDICINE

1. American Psychiatric Association. *Diagnostic and Statistical Manual for Mental Disorders, fourth edition (DSM-IV)*. Washington, DC: American Psychiatric Press, 1994.
2. Baldry P. E. 1994 Acupuncture, Trigger Points and Musculoskeletal Pain, Churchill Livingstone, Edinburgh.
3. Baldry P. E. 2001 Myofascial Pain and Fibromyalgia Syndromes, Churchill Livingstone, Edinburgh.
4. Bowlby J. 1980 Loss Sadness and Depression, The Hogarth Press, London.
5. Burkitt D. 1980 Don't Forget Fibre in Your Diet, Martin Dunitz, London.
6. Everard M. L. Respiratory Syncytial Virus Bronchiolitis and Pneumonia. In: Taussig L., Landau L. editors 1998 Textbook of Paediatric Respiratory Medicine, St Louis, Mosby.
7. Graf P. and Birt A. "Chapter 2 Explicit and Implicit Memory Retrieval: Intentions and Strategies," Implicit Memory and Metacognition, ed. Reder, L (Mahwah, NJ: Lawrence Erlbaum Associates, 1996).
8. Grahame-Smith D., and Aronson J. 1995 Clinical Pharmacology and Drug Therapy, Oxford University Press, Oxford.
9. Haslett C., Chilvers E., Hunter J. and Boon N. 1999 Davidson's Principles and Practice of Medicine, Churchill Livingstone, Edinburgh.
10. Hickling P. and Golding J. 1984 An Outline of Rheumatology, Wright, Bristol.
11. Kay A. B. 1989 Allergy and Asthma, Blackwell Scientific Publications, Oxford.
12. Kumar P. J. and Clark M. L. 1987 Clinical Medicine, Bailliere Tindall, London
13. Kumar P. and Clark M. 2005 Clinical Medicine, Elsevier, London.
14. Lane D. J. 1996 Asthma: the Facts, Oxford University Press, Third Edition, Oxford.
15. Laurence D. R. 1973 Clinical Pharmacology, Churchill Livingstone, Edinburgh.
16. Mygind N. et al. 1990 Rhinitis and Asthma, Munksgaard, Lund Sweden.
17. Robins L. N. and Regier D.A. (editors) 1991 Psychiatric disorders in America: the Epidemiologic Catchment Area Study, New York, The Free Press.
18. Seligman M. E. P. 1975 Helplessness, W.H. Freeman and Company, San Francisco.
19. Shepherd C. 1989 Living with M.E., Cedar, William Heinemann Ltd., London.
20. Smith D. G. 1989 Understanding M.E., Robinson Publishing, London.
21. Souhami R. and Moxham J. 1994 Textbook of Medicine, Churchill Livingstone, Edinburgh.
22. Wallace D. and Wallace J. 2002 All About Fibromyalgia, Oxford University Press, Oxford.

FOREIGN LANGUAGE TEXTS

1. Battaglia F. et al 1957 Enciclopedia Filosofica, Casa Editrice Sansoni, Firenze.
2. Eyssalet J-M. 1990 Le Secret de la Maison des Ancêtres, Guy Trédaniel Editeur, Paris.
3. Granet M. 1973 La Religione dei Cinesi, Adelphi, Milano.
4. Lamanna E. P. 1967 *Storia della Filosofia* (History of Philosophy), Vol 1, Le Monnier, Florence.
5. Middleton E. et al 1991 Treatise of Allergology, Italian Edition, Momento Medico.

Appendix 5
The Classics of Chinese Medicine

The following is a brief description of the classics of Chinese medicine that I mention most frequently. As I mention some of the classics extensively, it might help the reader to see these in their historical context. This is not a comprehensive list of the classics of Chinese medicine (which would have to be much longer) but simply of those which I mention most frequently. For each classic, I also give the reasons why I mention them frequently and what they add to our clinical practice in the 21st century.

THE YELLOW EMPEROR'S CLASSIC OF INTERNAL MEDICINE (BETWEEN 300 AND 100 BC, WARRING STATES PERIOD, QIN AND HAN DYNASTIES)

Huang Di Nei Jing

The authorship and date of the "Yellow Emperor's Classic of Internal Medicine" is the subject of intense conjecture. The best source for a discussion of the authorship and date of this classic is Unschuld's "Huang Di Nei Jing Su Wen: Nature, Knowledge, Imagery in an Ancient Chinese Medical Text".[1]

What is certain is that the Yellow Emperor's Classic of Internal Medicine was written between 300 and 100 BC and that it was changed by many different authors over the centuries. My Chinese teachers in Nanjing thought that this classic could not be older than the times of Zou Yan (c. 350–270 BC) who was the formulator of the main theory of the 5 Elements.

That this classic received the contributions and changes by many different authors is obvious from the variety of subjects treated and most of all, by the apparent lack of coordination among subjects. What is also generally accepted is that the bulk of the text we use nowadays was compiled by Wang Bing during the Tang dynasty (AD 762). The text was subsequently edited three times during the Song dynasty (960–1279).

The "Yellow Emperor's Classic of Internal Medicine" consists of two parts, each in 81 chapters: the "Simple Questions" (*Su Wen*) and the "Spiritual Axis" (*Ling Shu*). Generally speaking, the "Simple Questions" deals more with the general theory of Chinese medicine while the "Spiritual Axis" is mostly about acupuncture.

The importance of the "Yellow Emperor's Classic of Internal Medicine" in the history of Chinese medicine cannot be overemphasized. It is the earliest source of physiology, pathology, diagnosis and treatment in Chinese medicine. Besides medicine, this classic also contains theories of metereology, astrology and calendar. The following is a partial list of the main topics of significance of the "Yellow Emperor's Classic of Internal Medicine":

1. It established a systematic theory of the channels.
2. It deals in depth with the theories of Yin-Yang and the 5 Elements.
3. It discusses the nature and origin of different types of Qi.
4. It describes the physiology and pathology of the Internal Organs.
5. It determines the location of 160 acupuncture points and their names.
6. It describes the various types of needles and their use.
7. It defines the function of the acupuncture points and their contra-indications.
8. It discusses many needling techniques including the reinforcing and reducing methods.
9. It describes the diagnosis, identification of patterns and treatment of many diseases.

From a philosophical point of view, it is clear that the "Yellow Emperor's Classic of Internal Medicine" was influenced by several different philosophical trends which arose during the Warring States Period (475–221 BC). In particular, this classic shows the influence of the Confucian, Daoist, Legalist and Naturalist schools of thought.

The influence of the Naturalist School (called "School of Yin-Yang") is manifested throughout this classic because the theory of Yin-Yang and the 5 Elements pervades the whole book.

The influence of the Daoist school of thought is evident in the frequent discussion of the ways or "nourishing life" (*yang sheng*), i.e. advice on breathing, exercises, diet, and life-style to prolong life and avoid disease.

The influence of the Confucian school is manifested by the conception of the Internal Organs as ministers of a government. The political views of Confucianism are very much reflected in Chinese medicine where the Internal Organs are compared to government officials with the Heart being the Emperor or Monarch. Each internal organ is compared to a Minister and health depends on good "governance" by the Internal Organs.

There are other aspects of the Confucian philosophy that pervade the "Yellow Emperor's Classic of Internal Medicine". One is the view of the lifestyle practices of *yang sheng* ("nourishing life") as a ritual with its rules and duties. The Confucian philosophy was all about ethics and the practices that would ensure harmony in the family, society and the State. Rites (*Li*) were considered to be part of this ethics system and they were considered very important by Confucius. Interestingly, the character *Li* for "rites" has similarities to that for "body" (*Ti*).

禮 Li (rites, ritual)
體 Ti (body)

The left side of the character for *Li* (rites) is the same as what is on the left of *Shen*, i.e. something supernatural, or something also related to sacrificial rites. The right side represents a sacrificial vessel.

The right side of the character for *Ti* (the body) is the same as above, i.e. a sacrificial vessel while the left side represents bones, i.e. the structure of the body.

The implication is that the body is like a rite, and that the rules of *Yang Sheng* are like a ritual with its rules of conduct. Obeying these rules is called *shun* which means "to conform with" while disobeying them is called *ni*, i.e. rebelling, going against the rules. Interestingly these two terms occur frequently in Chinese medicine and in the "Yellow Emperor's Classic of Internal Medicine". *Ni* is the term used for "rebellious" Qi (or counterflow Qi), while *shun* is its opposite, i.e. Qi that flows in the correct direction.

Thus, ill health is not only a medical problem but also an ethical one stemming from not abiding by the rules of behaviour.

Finally, the "Yellow Emperor's Classic of Internal Medicine" bears the imprint also of the Legalist School. The Legalist School was called the School of Law (*Fa Jia*) in ancient China. This school of thought flourished during the Warring States Period and it prevailed during the Qin dynasty (221–206 BC), a brief dynasty started by the first emperor Qin Shi Huang Di who enthusiastically adopted the principles of government advocated by the Legalist School. Qin Shi Huang Di was the emperor who had the terracotta army built.

The state of Qin in Western China was the first to adopt Legalist doctrines. The Qin were so successful that by 221 BC they had conquered the other Chinese states and unified the empire after centuries of war. Legalist ideas on human nature, society and government could not be further from those of Confucius: the Legalists thought that human nature is essentially unruly and order in society can be kept only by strict laws and harsh punishments, not through ethical behaviour as the Confucianists thought.

What is interesting about the Legalist school from the Chinese medicine point of view, is the fact that the Qin dynasty (which adopted Legalist ideas) was the first to unify China. They established irrigation, unified weights, coins, Chinese script, measures and other things such as the gauge of wheel axles throughout China. The first Qin emperor also initiated a huge program of road building and canals digging. Another important innovation of the Qin dynasty was the fostering of trade among various regions of China on a huge scale.

The Qin dynasty therefore provided the first model of a unified state with an emperor, a central government, local officials, thousands of miles of new roads and a state-wide irrigation system. This provided the first three metaphors of Chinese medicine, i.e. the political metaphor in which the Heart is the emperor, the other Internal Organs are the officials; the road metaphor in which the channels are like a system of roads; and the water metaphor in which Qi, Blood and Body Fluids flow in a system of canals, rivers and reservoirs.

One can see an influence of the Legalist school also in the therapeutic approach of the "Yellow Emperor's Classic of Internal Medicine", i.e. just as human nature cannot be relied upon and must be "straightened" with strict laws and harsh punishments, the body's Qi must be regulated by attacking pathogenic factors decisively and by making sure that the "ruler" and officials do their jobs properly.

Indeed, one could see some of the therapeutic interventions of Chinese medicine – burning moxa, using sweating, vomiting and purging, expelling pathogenic factors, etc. are almost like Legalist "punishments"!

THE CLASSIC OF DIFFICULTIES (CA. 100 BC, HAN DYNASTY)

Nan Jing

The Nan Jing was written in approximately 100 BC by Qin Yue Ren who used as a pseudonym the name of an ancient, mythical doctor called Bian Que. However, like the *Nei Jing*, the date of compilation of the *Nan Jing* is a subject of controversy. Its date is put by some authors as late as 600 AD. The best discussion of the origin of the *Nan Jing* is in Unschuld's "Nan Ching – The Classic of Difficult Issues".[2]

The *Nan Jing* is a gem of a book, in its Chinese edition a very thin and small book full of clinical insights. The attraction of the book for me is that, unlike the *Nei Jing*, it clearly seems to have been written by one author because there is quite a logical progression among chapters.

The *Nan Jing* consists of 81 short chapters. The importance of the *Nan Jing* in the history of Chinese medicine cannot be overestimated. For example, the *Nan Jing* was the first text to advocate taking the pulse at the radial artery: previously the pulse was taken in nine different positions of the body on the arms, legs and neck. This classic was also the first to develop the theory of the Original Qi (*Yuan Qi*) and the role of the Triple Burner in relation to it.

The following is a partial list of the reasons of the importance of the *Nan Jing*:

1. It added to the knowledge of the eight extraordinary vessels compared to that of the *Nei Jing*.
2. It developed the theory of the 5 Transporting (*Shu*) points further than what is discussed in the *Nei Jing*.
3. It put forward for the first time the technique of reinforcing and reducing points according to the Mother-Child relationships within the 5-Element theory (e.g. that the Wood point tonifies the Heart channel because it pertains to Wood, the Heart pertains to Fire and Wood is the Mother of Fire).
4. It established the practice of feeling the pulse at the radial artery.
5. It developed the theory of the Original Qi (*Yuan Qi*) and Gate of Life (*Ming Men*).

ESSENTIAL PRESCRIPTIONS OF THE GOLDEN CHEST (AD 220, HAN DYNASTY)

Jin Gui Yao Lue

Written by Zhang Zhong Jing. This is a classic I also quote frequently. In the field of mental-emotional problems, it is the source of three important formulae, i.e. Ban Xia Hou Po Tang *Pinellia-Magnolia Decoction*, Gan Mai Da Zao Tang *Glycyrrhiza-Triticum-Jujuba Decoction* and Bai He Tang *Lilium Decoction*.

THE PULSE CLASSIC (AD 280, THREE KINGDOMS PERIOD)

Mai Jing

Written by Wang Shu He. The Pulse Classic is very important in the development of pulse diagnosis. This classic consolidated and further developed the assignment of the three pulse positions to organs, first done by the *Nan Jing*. The Pulse Classic describes 24 pulse qualities and their clinical significance systematically.

DISCUSSION OF THE ORIGIN OF SYMPTOMS IN DISEASES (AD 610, SUI DYNASTY)

Zhu Bing Yuan Hou Lun

Written by Chao Yuan Fang. This book is one of the first books describing the symptoms, patterns and treatment of diseases systematically. I consult this book when researching the pathology and treatment of a particular condition.

THOUSAND GOLDEN DUCATS PRESCRIPTIONS (AD 652, TANG DYNASTY)

Qian Jin Yao Fang

Written by Sun Si Miao. This book is one of the few to bear a Buddhist influence. Sun Si Miao was an expert on diet and sexuality. He was one of the fist doctors to describe goitre and correctly attribute it to living in mountainous regions (with water deprived of iodine): he correctly prescribed the use of seaweeds to treat this condition.

In my mind, Sun Si Miao is forever linked to the formulation of the prescription Wen Dan Tang *Warming the Gall-Bladder Decoction* which I use extensively in the treatment of mental-emotional conditions.

DISCUSSION ON STOMACH AND SPLEEN (1249, SONG DYNASTY)

Pi Wei Lun

Written by Li Dong Yuan. The Discussion on Stomach and Spleen is a very important classic in the history of Chinese medicine. Li Dong Yuan is the founder of the School of Stomach and Spleen which attributes a central importance to the Stomach and Spleen in pathology and treatment.

In my mind, the importance of this classic lies especially in the formulation of the prescription Bu Zhong Yi Qi Tang *Tonifying the Centre and Benefiting Qi Decoction*. This is a very important prescription for many different conditions and, in mental-emotional problems, I use it for depression.

Li Dong Yuan was the first to formulate the theory of "Yin Fire", a condition characterized by Heat above deriving from a deficiency of the Stomach and Spleen and of the Original Qi (*Yuan Qi*). In my opinion, Yin Fire is a common pathology in many modern, Western diseases such as chronic fatigue syndrome.

QI JING BA MAI KAO (1578, MING DYNASTY)

A Study of the Eight Extraordinary Vessels

Written by Li Shi Zhen. The importance of this book cannot be overemphasized: for anyone uses the eight extraordinary vessels, this book is a must. First, this is the first book that describes the pathways of the extraordinary vessels in detail, point by point. It also describes the pathology of rebellious Qi of the Penetrating Vessel (*Chong Mai*) which is so common in practice.

I have consulted and quoted this book extensively when writing the Channels of Acupuncture.

A STUDY OF THE PULSE BY THE PIN HU LAKE MASTER (1578, MING DYNASTY)

Pin Hu Mai Xue

Written by Li Shi Zhen. This is another must to understand pulse diagnosis. Li Shi Zhen gives the best description of the pulse qualities and their clinical significance.

COMPENDIUM OF ACUPUNCTURE (1601, MING DYNASTY)

Zhen Jiu Da Cheng

Written by Yang Ji Zhou. This book is a must for acupuncturists. It occupies a fundamental place in the acupuncture literature for several reasons:

1. It summarized the acupuncture experience of previous centuries.
2. It describes many different needling techniques many of which are used today.
3. It dealt with internal medicine, gynaecology and pediatrics.
4. It has many case histories with point prescriptions.
5. It uses the identification of patterns with point prescriptions.
6. It introduced massage therapy for children.

I have used this book extensively when writing the Channels of Acupuncture.

CLASSIC OF CATEGORIES (1624, MING DYNASTY)

Lei Jing

Written by Zhang Jing Yue (also called Zhang Jie Bin). This is a very important book in the history of Chinese medicine. Its importance lies in its discussion of theories from the *Nei Jing* arranged according to topics. It therefore joints together scattered passages from the *Nei Jing* according to topics and diseases.

JING YUE QUAN SHU (1624, MING DYNASTY)

Complete Book of Jing Yue

Written by Zhang Jing Yue (also called Zhang Jie Bin). This book discusses the diagnosis, pathology and treatment of many different conditions. Zhang Jing Yue formulated the prescriptions Zuo Gui Wan *Restoring the Left [Kidney] Pill* and You Gui Wan *Restoring the Right [Kidney] Pill* which tonify Kidney-Yin and Kidney-Yang respectively. I personally use these two formulae to tonify the Kidneys much more often than Liu Wei Di Huang Wan *Six Ingredients Rehmannia Pill* and Jin Gui Shen Qi Wan. *Golden Chest Kidney-Qi Pill*.

AN EXPLANATION OF THE ACUPUNCTURE POINTS (1654, QING DYNASTY)

Jing Xue Jie

Written by Yue Han Zhen. This is not a famous classic but it is a gem of a book that I use extensively to consult the actions and functions of acupuncture points. The book explains the meaning of the points names and it discusses the actions and functions of points according to channel affected, which is very useful. I find the book also interesting because it gives the action of the points (e.g. Spleen-12 moves Qi) which many people think it is a modern adaptation of Chinese acupuncture.

YI ZONG JIN JIAN (1742, QING DYNASTY)

Golden Mirror of Medicine

Written by Wu Qian. This book discusses the diagnosis, pathology and treatment of many different diseases in the field of internal medicine, gynaecology and pediatrics. It is a mine of information and a book that I consult frequently when writing my books.

DISCUSSION ON BLOOD PATTERNS (1884, QING DYNASTY)

Xue Zheng Lun

Written by Tang Zong Hai. This is an important book for the treatment of bleeding disorders. It formulates the four-pronged approach to the treatment of bleeding.

END NOTES

1. Unschuld P 2003 "Huang Di Nei Jing Su Wen: Nature, Knowledge, Imagery in an Ancient Chinese Medical Text", University of California Press, Berkeley.
2. Unschuld P 1986 Medicine in China – Nan-Ching, University of California Press, Berkeley.

Appendix 6
Self-Assessment Answers

CHAPTER 1

1. Yin represents the shady side of a hill and Yang the sunny side.
2. As we face South (in the Northern hemisphere) the sun rises (Yang movement) on our left and it sets (Yin movement) on our right.
3. Heaven is above and is Yang: it is imagined like a round vault. Earth is below and can be parcelled out in fields.
4. Summer and spring pertain to Yang and winter and autumn pertain to Yin.
5. The water of the lake is Yin: the heat of the sun (Yang) transforms the Yin (water) into a more dispersed, subtle form (Yang), i.e. vapour.
6. Yin decreases.
7. Yang is in apparent excess.
8. Liver-Blood and Liver-Qi are an example of the Yin–Yang opposition of Structure–Function. Liver-Blood is the 'structure' of the Liver (Yin) and the free flow of Liver-Qi is its function (Yang). The two are interdependent.
9. Hot–cold, dry–wet, rapid–slow, restless–quiet, excitement–inhibition.
10. Excess of Yang is Full-Heat, Excess of Yin is Full-Cold, Deficiency of Yang is Empty-Cold, Deficiency of Yin is Empty-Heat.

CHAPTER 2

1. Water, Fire, Wood, Metal, Earth, i.e. 1(6), 2(7), 3(8), 4(9) and 5(10).
2. Five basic processes of Nature, five qualities of natural phenomena, five phases of a cycle, five inherent capabilities of change of phenomena.
3. Water at the bottom, Fire at the top, Wood on the left, Metal on the right and Earth in the centre.
4. *The Liver is the Mother of the Heart*: the Liver stores Blood and Heart-Blood houses the Mind. *The Spleen is the Mother of the Lungs*: the Spleen provides Food-Qi to the Lungs where it interacts with air to form True Qi. *The Lungs are the Mother of the Kidneys*: Lung-Qi descends to meet the Kidneys, the Kidneys 'grasp' Qi.
5. *The Liver controls the Stomach and Spleen*: the free flow of Liver-Qi helps the Stomach to ripen and rot food and the Spleen to transform and transport. *The Heart controls the Lungs*: the Heart governs Blood, the Lungs govern Qi, Qi and Blood mutually assist and nourish each other. *The Spleen controls the Kidneys*: the Spleen's transforming and transporting helps the Kidney's excretion of fluids.
6. *Water as the foundation*: the Kidneys store the Essence and are the source of all Yin and Yang energies of the body. *Earth in the Centre*: the Stomach and Spleen are the origin of Post-Natal Qi and occupy a central position in physiology. *Vertical axis of Heart and Kidneys*: Heart and Kidneys must communicate with each, with Fire going down and Water going up.
7. *The Liver over-acts on Stomach and Spleen*: rebellious Liver-Qi may invade the Stomach, causing its Qi to go up (instead of down), and the Spleen, causing its Qi to descend (instead of ascending). *The Spleen over-acts on the Kidneys*: if the Spleen does not transform and transport fluids, these will accumulate and obstruct the Kidneys.

The Kidneys over-act on the Heart: Empty-Heat arising from Kidney-Yin deficiency rises up to harass the Heart.
8. *Wood*: shouting, sour, anger. *Fire*: laugh, bitter, joy. *Earth*: singing, sweet, pensiveness. *Metal*: crying, pungent, sadness. *Water*: groaning, salty, fear.
9. Eating too much salt may lead to hardening of the arteries. The salty taste pertains to the Kidneys; an excessive consumption of this taste may over-act on the Heart. The Heart controls the blood vessels and these are affected by the excessive salt consumption.

CHAPTER 3

1. One part portrays uncooked rice and another the steam deriving from its cooking. It refers to the dual nature of Qi: that is, it is substantial (like rice) but it can be transformed into more subtle forms of energy (like vapour).
2. It determines growth, reproduction and development; it is the basis for Kidney-Qi; it produces Marrow; it is the basis for constitutional strength.
3. Essence, Qi and Mind (*Jing, Qi, Shen*). They represent three different states of aggregation of Qi, from Essence being the densest to Mind being the most rarefied and non-substantial. This highlights the close relationship existing in Chinese medicine between body and mind: the state of the Essence and Qi influences the Mind and vice versa.
4. It is the Motive Force of all physiological processes; it is the basis of Kidney-Qi; it facilitates the transformation of Qi; it facilitates the transformation of Blood; it comes out at the Source points.
5. From the Stomach and Spleen.
6. It is formed from Food-Qi combining with air in the Lungs.
7. It is formed from Gathering Qi under the transforming action of Original Qi.
8. Nutritive Qi: refined, circulates in the channels, nourishes. Defensive Qi: coarse, circulates outside the channels, protects and warms.
9. It is the complex movements of Qi all over the body, including ascending, descending, entering and exiting.
10. Heart-Qi descends, Lung-Qi primarily descends, Liver-Qi flows in all directions.
11. It is formed from Food-Qi in the Heart under the influence of Original Qi and Essence.
12. The Heart governs Blood, the Liver stores Blood, the Spleen makes Blood.
13. Qi is the commander or Blood, Blood is the mother of Qi. Qi moves Blood, Blood nourishes Qi.
14. The Spleen transforms and transports fluids, the Lungs make fluids descend, the Kidneys transform and excrete fluids.
15. Blood and Body Fluids (including sweat) have a relationship of mutual interchange; therefore depleting one might deplete the other.
16. A red tip of the tongue indicates Heart-Heat. As all emotions affect the Heart (as well as their relevant organ) because the Heart houses the Mind which 'feels' the emotions, the tip of the tongue becomes easily red when the person is affected by any emotion.

CHAPTER 4

1. The Triple Burner makes the Original Qi separate and differentiate into its different forms in different places around the body, thus allowing the Original Qi to facilitate the transformation of Qi in different parts of the body.
2. The right Kidney is identified with the Fire of the Gate of Life and the left is the Kidney proper.
3. 'The transformation of Qi relies on <u>warmth</u> as transformation is a Yang process.'
4. In the Upper Burner Qi goes up and exits (under control of the Lungs); in the Middle Burner Qi goes up and down and in and out (under the control of Stomach and Spleen); in the Lower Burner, Qi mostly descends and exits (under the control of the Kidneys, Bladder and Intestines).
5. 'Heaven (<u>Yang</u>) is Above and it <u>descends</u> but <u>descending</u> is a Yin *movement*. Earth (<u>Yin</u>) is Below and it <u>ascends</u> but <u>ascending</u> is a Yang *movement*.'
6. Lung-Qi, Heart-Qi, Kidney-Qi, Stomach-Qi, Bladder-Qi, Large- and Small Intestine-Qi all descend.
7. Greater Yang (Small Intestine), Lesser Yang (Triple Burner) and Bright Yang (Large Intestine).
8. The space between the skin and the muscles is part of the Triple Burner cavities, and the movement of Qi in and out of this space relies on the entering and exiting of Lung-Qi.
9. The Triple Burner, the Liver and whichever channels traverse the joint in question.
10. The Membranes wrap and anchor the organs, muscles and bones, and connect the organs to each other.
11. 'The Ethereal Soul is sometimes defined as the '<u>coming</u> and <u>going</u> of the Mind'.'
12. The Stomach and Spleen are central physiologically as they are the source of Qi and Blood and therefore all the organs rely on them for nourishment. Anatomically they are central as they are in the Middle Burner, at the crossroads of many processes and movements of Qi.
13. The Liver is in the Lower Burner (and on the left energetically) and sends Qi up; the Lungs are in the Upper Burner (and on the right energetically) and send Qi downwards.
14. Qi stagnation.
15. Because the failure of the Lung-Qi to descend affects the Liver and the rising of Liver-Yang.

CHAPTER 5

1. Blood.
2. Blood.
3. Sinews. The Liver.
4. Nose.
5. Lungs.
6. Ethereal and Corporeal souls.
7. Dampness.
8. Liver.
9. Spittle.
10. Scorched.

CHAPTER 6

1. The Heart influences the circulation of Blood throughout the body; the Heart is also the place where Food-Qi is transformed into Blood.
2. The Heart influences the state of the blood vessels.
3. A hard blood vessel may indicate Heart-Blood stasis.
4. A dull-pale complexion indicates Heart-Blood deficiency.
5. Mental activity (including emotions), consciousness, memory, thinking, sleep.
6. Primarily Heart-Blood.
7. A Heart pathology which may be either a deficiency or Heart-Fire.
8. Because the Heart houses the Mind, which is the only one of the five spiritual aspects that recognizes and feels the emotions.
9. A deficiency of Heart-Yang would cause spontaneous daytime sweating.

CHAPTER 7

1. Sending Blood to the sinews and muscles during exercise and storing Blood in relation to menstruation.
2. During exercise, the Blood of the Liver goes to sinews and muscles; during rest, it goes back to the Liver where it helps to restore energy.
3. The Liver stores Blood and is closely connected to the Uterus. When Liver-Blood is abundant, menstruation is normal; if Liver-Blood is scanty, the periods are scanty; if Liver-Blood is stagnant, the periods are painful; if Liver-Blood has Heat, the periods are heavy.
4. In relation to the emotional state, in relation to digestion and in relation to the flow of bile.
5. The smooth flow of Liver-Qi ensures that Spleen-Qi ascends and Stomach-Qi descends, thus helping the transformation and transportation function of the Spleen and the rotting and ripening function of the Stomach. If Liver-Qi is stagnant, Spleen-Qi fails to ascend, causing loose stools, and Stomach-Qi fails to descend, causing hiccup, nausea, vomiting.
6. The smooth flow of Liver-Qi is very important for the emotional state. If Liver-Qi flows smoothly, the person is happy and relaxed; if Liver-Qi stagnates, the person is moody, irritable or depressed; if Liver-Qi rebels upwards (Liver-Yang rising), the person is prone to outbursts of anger.
7. Anger causes Liver-Qi to rise excessively (called Liver-Yang rising); this may cause headaches.
8. Muscle cramps.
9. Blurred vision or floaters.
10. The Ethereal Soul is responsible for life dreams, projects, aims, sense of direction, ideas, inspiration and creativity. It is the 'coming and going of the Mind (*Shen*)' and gives the Mind the above attributes.
11. The Ethereal Soul gives the Mind the 'coming and going', i.e. searching, ideas, inspiration, creativity, exploring; the Mind must control (keep in check) the 'coming and going' of the Ethereal Soul and must integrate the material deriving from the Ethereal Soul. If the Ethereal Soul does not 'come and go' enough (either because it is weak or because the Mind overcontrols it), the person is depressed; if the Ethereal Soul 'comes and goes' too much (either because it is overactive or because the Mind does not control it enough), the person is manic.

CHAPTER 8

1. The Lungs inhale air, which is considered a type of Qi in Chinese medicine. The Lungs govern Qi also by playing a role in the formation of Qi by inhaling air, which, after mixing with the Food-Qi of the Spleen, forms Gathering Qi. Gathering Qi forms True Qi under the influence of Original Qi.
2. The Lungs govern Qi; Qi is the commander of Blood and Blood is the mother of Qi. Nutritive Qi and Blood flow side by side in both channels and blood vessels. Blood relies on the propelling action of Qi to flow in the blood vessels. It is for these reasons that the Lungs influence the blood vessels.
3. The Lungs diffuse Qi and body fluids to the space between the skin and muscles. Qi is present in the space between skin and muscles in the form of Defensive Qi, which protects the body from invasions of external pathogenic factors. The Lungs also diffuse body fluids to the space between skin and muscles where they form sweat and moisten that space. This also contributes to the protection from external pathogenic factors.
4. The Lungs descend Qi to the Kidneys, which respond by holding Qi: the coordination between Lungs and Kidneys harmonizes respiration.

The Lungs also descend body fluids to the Kidneys, which evaporate them and send the resulting 'steam' up to the Lungs to keep them moist. Furthermore, the Lungs descend fluids to the Bladder from where they are excreted as urine.

5. The diffusing function of the Lungs ensures the correct entering and exiting of Qi, especially in the Upper Burner and in the space between skin and muscles. The descending of Lung-Qi ensures that Qi descends from the Upper towards the Lower Burner and, by so doing, it is a vital part of the ascending–descending of Qi.
6. The Lungs are like a Prime Minister (with the Heart being the Emperor) in charge of the administration of the country. Just as the Prime Minister in ancient China would be in charge of administration of every aspect of social life, the Lungs regulate all physiological activities. They do so in three main ways: by governing Qi, by being in charge of respiration and by controlling all channels and blood vessels. The combination of these three activities means that the Lungs, through Qi, breathing and every channel and blood vessel, have an influence on all physiological activities (as Qi is the basis of all transportation and transformation).
7. The diffusing of Qi and fluids towards the space between skin and muscles regulates the fluids of the Upper Burner and regulates sweat. For this reason the Upper Burner is compared to a 'mist'. The descending of Qi and fluids to the Lower Burner (Kidneys and Bladder) ensures that fluids move from the Upper to the Lower Burner and also that they are excreted properly through the Bladder.
8. The Lungs house the Corporeal Soul. This is described as the 'entering and exiting' of the Essence. By this is meant that, through the Corporeal Soul, the Essence 'enters and exits': this indicates that the Essence plays a role in all physical processes. In particular, following the Corporeal Soul (and therefore the Lungs), the Essence goes to the space between the skin and muscles where it plays a role in the protection from exterior pathogenic factors.
9. The Lungs diffuse Qi and fluids to the skin and to the space between the skin and muscles. When Qi is properly regulated and the Lungs diffuse Defensive Qi to this space, the person has a good resistance to pathogenic factors. If the Lungs fail to diffuse Qi to this space (because of Lung-Qi deficiency), the space is said to be too 'open' and that makes the person prone to invasions of external pathogenic factors. When the Lungs diffuse fluids to the space between skin and muscles, sweating is properly regulated. When the diffusing of fluids in this space by the Lungs is impaired (through Lung-Qi deficiency), the person may sweat excessively.

CHAPTER 9

1. The Spleen's function of transformation and transportation is essential in the making of Qi and Blood. The Spleen provides the first transformation of food essences, which, through a process of transformation, make Food-Qi (*Gu Qi*). Food-Qi goes to the Lungs to mix with air and form Gathering Qi, and to the Heart to make Blood. The Spleen's function of transportation is essential for the correct movement of food essences and Food-Qi.
2. After the fluids ingested reach the Stomach, the Spleen transforms them into a clear and a turbid part; it then transports the clear part upwards to the Lungs and the impure part downwards to the Intestines.
3. To the Lungs (to form Gathering Qi) and to the Heart (to form Blood).
4. Spleen-Qi ascends and Stomach-Qi descends. This coordination of ascending and descending of Qi in the Middle Burner is essential for the transformation and transportation of food essences, Qi and fluids upwards and downwards.
5. Firstly, the Spleen controls Blood in the sense that it holds the blood in the blood vessels; secondly, the Spleen controls Blood in the sense that Food-Qi is the basis for the formation of Blood.
6. Spleen-Qi ascends towards the head: this is the ascending of clear Qi or clear Yang, which brightens the sense orifices. A feeling muzziness and heaviness of the head may be due either to deficient Spleen-Qi not ascending to the head, or to retention of Dampness in the head, itself due to the failure of Spleen-Qi to ascend.
7. Spleen-Qi nourishes the muscles by bringing Qi and food essences to them. A deficiency of Spleen-Qi in this area is a very frequent cause of a feeling of tiredness.
8. Spleen-Qi raises the internal organs: a deficiency of this function may therefore cause a prolapse of an organ.
9. The Intellect (*Yi*) controls memory, focusing, concentration and ideas. It is responsible not so much for memory of past events, but memory as the capacity for storing data in the course of one's work or schoolwork.
10. Pensiveness consists in thinking too much, brooding, dwelling on the past, even to the point of obsessive thinking. Pensiveness 'knots' Spleen-Qi, i.e. it causes it to stagnate.

CHAPTER 10

1. The oil in the lamp represents Kidney-Yin and the flame represents Kidney-Yang. If the oil decreases, the flame will also decrease; if the oil increases too much, it may smother the flame.
2. Because they are fundamentally one and interdependent: deficiency of one necessarily implies deficiency of the other.
3. Growth, reproduction, development, sexual maturation, 7- and 8-year cycles, conception, pregnancy, menopause, ageing.
4. The decline of Kidney-Essence in menopausal women means that the Essence does not nourish the Marrow and bones so that they become brittle, leading to osteoporosis.
5. The Kidneys are the 'gate' that controls urination; the Kidneys influence the Lower Burner's excretion of fluids; Kidney-Yang influences the Intestines' capacity for transforming and separating fluids; the Kidneys receive fluids from the Lungs and send vaporized fluids back up to the Lungs; Kidney-Yang provides heat to the Spleen for the transformation and transportation of fluids.
6. If the Kidneys do not receive and hold Qi down, it will escape upwards causing breathlessness and asthma.
7. Urinary incontinence, spermatorrhoea or diarrhoea (leaking from urethra, spermatic duct or anus).
8. The Kidneys control the Gate of Life or Minister Fire, which provides heat for all our bodily functions. When Spleen-Yang and Kidney-Yang are depleted, producing symptoms of tiredness, exhaustion and oedema, it is necessary to tonify the Minister Fire of the Kidneys.
9. Putrid, black, salty, cold, groan.
10. Interior Dryness can come from Stomach deficiency, from profuse loss of fluids (as in sweating or diarrhoea) or from smoking. Internal Dryness would injure Kidney Yin.

CHAPTER 11

1. The Pericardium functions as an external covering of the Heart by protecting the Heart from attacks by exterior pathogenic factors. (It is believed that if the Heart is attacked by a pathogenic factor, the Mind-Spirit will be affected, which may be fatal. If a pathogenic factor does attack the Heart, it will first attack the Pericardium: for this reason, the Heart has no Stream-transporting point.)
2. According to the theory of the Internal Organs, the two primary functions of the Pericardium are similar to those of the Heart: to govern Blood and house the Mind-Spirit.
3. Points on the Pericardium channel can invigorate Blood or cool Blood.
4. Points on the Pericardium channel can stimulate or calm the Mind-Spirit. For example P-6 Neiguan stimulates the mood to relieve depression, while P-7 Daling calms the Mind to relieve anxiety.
5. The Pericardium channel influences the area at the centre of the thorax.
6. In terms of channel relationships, the Pericardium channel has an interior–exterior relationship with the Triple Burner channel, the Pericardium being Yin and the Triple Burner Yang.

7. The Minister Fire arises from in between the Kidneys where the Fire of the Gate of Life resides. The Minister Fire communicates upwards with the Liver, Triple Burner and Pericardium. From the channel perspective, the Pericardium is interiorly–exteriorly related to the Triple Burner; from the Five-Element perspective, the Pericardium and Triple Burner are called 'Minister Fire' as they are like Ministers assisting the Emperor, i.e. the Heart. Therefore the 'Minister Fire' that arises from the Fire of the Gate of Life is different from the 'Minister Fire' in the context of the Five Elements.

CHAPTER 12

Heart and Lungs
1. The Heart governs Blood and the Lungs govern Qi; the relationship between the Heart and Lungs is essentially the relationship between Qi and Blood.
2. Qi and Blood are mutually dependent, as Qi is the commander of Blood and Blood is the mother of Qi. Blood needs the power of Qi in order to circulate in the blood vessels. Blood also needs the warmth of Qi to circulate, while Qi needs the 'immersion', or liquid quality, of Blood as a vehicle to circulate.
3. If Lung-Qi is deficient, it can lead to stagnation of Qi of the Heart, which, in turn may cause Heart-Blood stasis.
4. Excessive Heart-Fire dries up the Lung fluids, causing a dry cough, dry nose and thirst.
5. It is common for both Heart- and Lung-Qi to be deficient at the same time as they are both situated in the chest and both are influenced by Gathering Qi.
6. Gathering Qi collects in the chest, influencing both Heart and Lung function and the circulation of both Qi and Blood. If Gathering Qi is weak, the Qi and Blood of the Lung and Heart will be diminished, leading to symptoms such as a weak voice and cold hands.
7. Sadness depletes both Heart and Lung Qi.

Heart and Liver
1. The Heart governs Blood while the Liver stores Blood and regulates blood volume: these two activities must be coordinated and harmonized.
2. Liver-Blood deficiency can cause Heart-Blood deficiency as not enough Blood is stored by the Liver to nourish the Heart, causing palpitations and insomnia. In Five-Element terms, this would be described as the 'Mother not nourishing the Child'.
3. Deficient Heart-Blood may disrupt the Liver's ability to regulate the Blood, giving rise to symptoms such as dizziness and excessive dreaming. In Five-Element terms, this would be described as the 'Child draining the Mother'.
4. The Heart houses the Mind (*Shen*) and the Liver houses the Ethereal Soul (*Hun*). The Ethereal Soul represents the 'coming and going' of the Mind, giving what might be described as 'movement' to the Mind, in the sense of inspiration, vision and a sense of direction.
5. The Heart houses the Mind (*Shen*), influencing the mood and spirits of a person, while the Liver is responsible for the smooth flow of Qi. This smooth flow of Qi ensures that the person's emotions are experienced in a balanced fashion: they are not repressed, and expressed appropriately rather than inappropriately.

Heart and Kidneys
1. The Heart belongs to Fire, the Kidneys to Water. Fire is Yang in nature and corresponds to movement; Water is Yin in nature and corresponds to stillness. It is important that the Heart and Kidneys are in balance as they represent the two polarities of Yin and Yang:
   i. from a Five-Element perspective, Fire and Water control each other. Fire dries up Water and Water douses Fire
   ii. from an organ perspective, Fire and Water interact and mutually support each other. Just as Lung-Qi in the Upper Burner descends to be grasped by Kidney-Qi in the Lower Burner, Heart-Qi of the Upper Burner descends to be grasped by Kidney-Qi. While Heart-Qi descends to the Kidneys, Kidney-Qi ascends to the Heart. More specifically, Heart-Yang descends to warm Kidney-Yin; Kidney-Yin ascends to nourish and cool Heart-Yang. This is known as the 'mutual support of Fire and Water', or the 'mutual support of Heart and Kidneys'.
2. If Kidney-Yang is deficient, the Kidneys are unable to perform their function of transforming fluids, which can overflow upwards, causing the pattern 'Water insulting the Heart'.
3. If Kidney-Yin is deficient, it cannot rise to nourish Heart-Yin. This leads to the development of Empty-Heat within the Heart, manifesting in symptoms such as palpitations, mental restlessness, insomnia, malar flush and night sweats.
4. The Heart houses the Mind, while the Kidneys store the Essence. Mind and Essence have a common root as Essence is the fundamental substance from which the Mind is derived. Essence, Qi and Mind are three different states of condensation of Qi, the Essence being densest, Qi more rarefied, and Mind the most subtle and immaterial.
5. If a person's Essence is weak, this will be reflected in the state of the Mind: the person will lack vitality, self-confidence and will-power.
6. If the Mind is perturbed by emotional problems, the Mind will be unable to direct the Essence, manifesting in a lack of motivation and a sense of permanent fatigue.
7. The spiritual aspect of the Kidney organ is known as the *Zhi*, or Will-power.
8. If Kidney-Essence is weak, the Will-power will be consequently diminished. This will affect the Mind in a negative fashion: the person will be depressed and lacking in vitality, will-power and determination.
9. The menstrual cycle is a flow of Kidney-Yin and Kidney-Yang as the Kidneys are the origin of *Tian Gui*, which is the basis for menstrual blood. During the first half of the menstrual cycle, Yin grows to reach its maximum at ovulation. At ovulation, Yin begins to decrease and Yang to increase, reaching a maximum just before the onset of the period. This ebb and flow of Yin and Yang is determined by Kidney-Yin and Kidney-Yang. Ovulation marks a change from Yin to Yang (Yin has reached its maximum), while the onset of the period marks a change from Yang to Yin.
10. (i) While the Kidneys provide the material basis (*Tian Gui*) for the ebb and flow of Yin and Yang, the Heart provides the impetus for the transformation of Yin to Yang and vice versa. (ii) Heart-Qi and Heart-Blood descend during the period to promote the downward flow of blood during the period and the discharge of the eggs during ovulation.

Liver and Lungs
1. The relationship between the Liver and Lungs reflects the relationship between Qi and Blood. The Lungs govern Qi, and the Liver stores and regulates Blood: Qi and Blood rely on each other to perform their respective functions.
2. The Liver relies on Lung-Qi to regulate Blood because Lung-Qi drives Blood within the blood vessels (Qi being the commander of Blood).
3. Liver-Blood provides the moisture and nourishment necessary for Lung-Qi to circulate properly (Blood being the mother of Qi).
4. Lung-Qi descends, while Liver-Qi ascends. Although Liver-Qi flows in all directions, in this context it ascends to coordinate the movement of Qi with the Lungs. It should be remembered that this is the normal physiological ascending movement and not the pathological ascending movement of Liver-Yang rising. The descending of Lung-Qi is dependent on the ascending of Liver-Qi and vice versa.
5. If Lung-Qi is deficient and fails to descend, it can affect the Liver function of the smooth flow of Qi, preventing Liver-Qi from rising and making it stagnate. In such cases, a person will experience listlessness (from deficiency of Qi), depression (from stagnation of Liver-Qi), cough and pain in the hypochondrial region. This situation corresponds to 'Wood insulting Metal'.

Liver and Spleen

1. Liver-Qi: (i) ensures the smooth flow of Qi around the body; (ii) ensures the smooth flow of bile, which aids digestion.
2. The normal direction of Spleen-Qi is upwards.
3. Stagnant Liver-Qi disrupts the upward flow of Spleen-Qi. This manifests as abdominal distension, pain in the hypochondrial region and loose stools. According to the theory of the Five Elements, this situation corresponds to 'Wood overacting on Earth'.
4. If Spleen-Qi is deficient, its function of transformation and transportation of food and fluids will be impaired. Food and fluids will not be digested properly and will be retained in the Middle Burner, often also with the formation of Dampness. This in turn may impair the circulation of Liver-Qi and impair the smooth flow of Qi in the Middle Burner, causing abdominal distension, pain in the hypochondrial region and irritability. According to the theory of the Five Elements, this situation corresponds to 'Earth insulting Wood'.
5. The Spleen makes Blood; the Liver stores Blood.

Liver and Kidneys

1. Liver-Blood nourishes and replenishes Kidney-Essence, and Essence in turn contributes in the making of Blood as Essence produces Bone Marrow, which makes Blood. The Kidneys also contribute to the making of Blood through the action of Original Qi: Original Qi facilitates the transformation of Food-Qi into Blood in the Heart.
2. Kidney-Yin nourishes Liver-Yin and Liver-Blood. In Five-Element terms this situation is known as 'Water nourishes Wood'.
3. Without the nourishment of Liver-Blood, Kidney-Essence may become weak, leading to symptoms such as deafness, tinnitus and nocturnal emissions.
4. If Kidney-Yin is deficient, Liver-Yin (and therefore Liver-Blood) will also become deficient, as Kidney-Yin is the basis of Liver-Yin. Deficiency of Liver-Yin may lead to the rising of Liver-Yang, with symptoms such as blurred vision, tinnitus, dizziness, headaches and irritability.
5. The Liver stores Blood and is responsible for supplying the Uterus with Blood. The Kidneys are the origin of *Tian Gui*, which is the substance from which menstrual blood derives. Therefore healthy functioning of the Liver and Kidney organs is paramount to ensure a healthy and regular menstrual cycle.
6. The Liver and Kidney channels are closely linked to the Directing and Penetrating Vessels (*Ren Mai* and *Chong Mai*).

Spleen and Lungs

1. The Spleen extracts refined Essence from food and sends it up to the Lungs where it is combined with air to form Gathering Qi.
2. Lung-Qi descends. The Spleen relies on the descending movement of Lung-Qi to aid its role of transformation and transportation of Body Fluids. If the Spleen cannot transform and transport fluids, oedema may occur.
3. If Spleen-Qi is deficient, Food-Qi will be deficient and the production of Qi, especially the Qi of the Lungs, will be impaired. Symptoms such as shortness of breath, fatigue and a weak voice may occur. This situation may be described in Five-Element terms as 'Earth not producing Metal'.
4. If Spleen-Qi is deficient, fluids will not be transformed, leading to the formation of Phlegm. Phlegm usually settles in the Lungs, impairing Lung function. It is said that 'The Spleen is the origin of Phlegm and the Lungs store it'.

Spleen and Kidneys

1. Post-Heaven Qi continually replenishes Pre-Heaven Qi with the Qi derived from food. Pre-Heaven Qi assists in the production of Post-Heaven Qi by providing the heat necessary for digestion and transformation (via the Fire of the Gate of Life).
2. If Spleen-Qi is deficient, not enough Qi will be produced to replenish Kidney-Essence, leading to a weakness of Kidney-Essence. This may cause fatigue, low backache, lack of appetite, tinnitus and dizziness.
3. If Kidney-Yang is deficient, the Fire of the Gate of Life cannot warm and aid the Spleen in its function of transformation and transportation of food and fluids, resulting in symptoms such as loose stools, diarrhoea and a feeling of chilliness. Dampness may accumulate and oedema may occur. In Five-Element terms this situation may be described as 'Fire not producing Earth'.
4. Kidney-Yang provides the heat necessary for the Spleen to transform and transport fluids. As it transports and transforms fluids, Spleen-Qi aids the Kidneys in their role of the transformation and excretion of fluids. If Spleen-Qi cannot transform and transport fluids, these may accumulate, forming Dampness. The formation of Dampness impairs the Kidney's function of governing Water; in turn, this further worsens the condition of Dampness.

Lungs and Kidneys

1. The Lungs send Qi and fluids down to the Kidneys. The Kidneys respond by holding the Qi down, evaporating some of the fluids, and sending the resulting vapour back up to the Lungs to keep them moist.
2. Gathering Qi and Original Qi assist each other. Gathering Qi of the chest flows downwards to aid the Kidneys, and Original Qi of the Kidneys flows upwards to aid respiration.
3. If Lung-Qi is deficient, it cannot send fluids downwards and the Lungs cannot communicate with the Kidneys and Bladder, causing incontinence or retention of urine.
4. If Kidney-Yang is deficient and cannot transform and excrete the fluids in the Lower Burner, they may accumulate and form oedema. This may impair the Lung descending and dispersing function, causing symptoms such as shortness of breath or cough.
5. A deficiency of Kidney-Yin results in deficiency of fluids of the Lower Burner. Fluids fail to rise to moisten the Lungs, resulting in a deficiency of Lung-Yin. Symptoms resulting from a deficiency of Kidney- and Lung-Yin include a dry throat at night, a dry cough, night sweating and a feeling of heat in the palms and soles of the feet.

Spleen and Heart

1. The Spleen makes Blood (because it provides Food-Essence, which is the basis for Blood), while the Heart governs Blood.
2. If Spleen-Qi is deficient and cannot make enough Blood, this may lead to a deficiency of Heart-Blood, with symptoms such as dizziness, palpitations, poor memory and insomnia.

CHAPTER 13

1. Poor appetite, belching, nausea, vomiting all indicate weak Stomach 'receiving'.
2. The role of the Stomach in the transformation of food makes it (along with the Spleen) the origin of all Qi and Blood produced after birth. Because of this, 'Stomach-Qi' has become synonymous with a good prognosis and life itself.
3. A thin, white coat with root.
4. Tiredness and weakness of the muscles of the limbs.
5. If Stomach-Qi fails to descend, food will stagnate in the Stomach, causing sensations of fullness and distension, sour regurgitation, belching, hiccups, nausea and vomiting.
6. The Kidneys transform fluids in the Lower Burner. If this Kidney function is impaired, fluids will stagnate in the Lower Burner and overflow upwards to the Stomach, impairing the digestion. A long-standing deficiency of fluids in the Stomach (Stomach-Yin) will nearly always cause a deficiency of Kidney-Yin.
7. Stomach-Fire or Stomach Phlegm-Fire.
8. The rotting and ripening of the Stomach coordinates closely with the Spleen's transformation and transportation of food essences. The Spleen's transportation of Food-Qi to the whole body depends on Stomach-Qi. The Stomach's function as origin of fluids relies on the Spleen transforming Body Fluids.

CHAPTER 14

1. The 'clean' part is transported by the Spleen to all parts of the body to nourish the tissues. The 'dirty' part is transmitted to the Large Intestine and Bladder for excretion.
2. They are transmitted to the Large Intestine, partly for reabsorption, partly for excretion in stools.
3. Scanty, dark urination.
4. The Small Intestine influences judgement, mental clarity, and gives us the ability to clearly distinguish the relevant issues before we make a decision. The Gall Bladder gives us the courage to make the decision.
5. Because the Small Intestine and Heart are interiorly–exteriorly related. The Heart-Fire is transmitted to the Small Intestine, which interferes with the separation of fluids and causes Blood to extravasate, resulting in blood in the urine.

CHAPTER 15

1. Abdominal distension, constipation.
2. The Large Intestine reabsorbs the appropriate amount of fluids, ensuring that the bowels are neither too dry nor too wet.
3. L.I.-4 Hegu.
4. If Lung-Qi is deficient and does not descend, the Qi of the Large Intestine may be unable to descend, causing constipation. If, on the other hand, there is constipation, stagnation in the Large Intestine may impair the descending of Lung-Qi, resulting in breathlessness.

CHAPTER 16

1. It is the only Yang organ that does not deal with food, drink and their waste products, and that does not communicate with the exterior directly (via the mouth, rectum or urethra). Because it stores a refined substance, bile, the Gall Bladder more closely resembles a Yin organ.
2. The Gall Bladder stores and excretes bile into the Intestines to aid digestion. It also transmits the Minister Fire of the Kidneys to warm the Spleen and Intestines to aid digestion. Gall Bladder-Qi is part of the free flow of Liver-Qi, which promotes the smooth flow of bile into the intestines. Gall Bladder-Qi also helps the ascending and free flow of Liver-Qi, which, in relation to transformation in the Stomach and Spleen, helps Stomach-Qi to descend and Spleen-Qi to ascend.
3. The Liver nourishes the sinews with its Blood, whereas the Gall Bladder provides Qi to the sinews to ensure proper movement and agility.
4. A deficient Gall Bladder causes indecision, timidity and the tendency to be discouraged at the slightest adversity.
5. Gall Bladder-Qi helps the ascending and free flow of Liver-Qi on a mental level, stimulating the movement of the Ethereal Soul, which in turns gives movement to the Mind, resulting in inspiration, planning, ideas, initiative and creativity.
6. Once all issues have been clarified, the Gall Bladder gives the courage to act.

CHAPTER 17

1. From Kidney-Yang and the Fire of the Gate of Life.
2. Abundant, clear urination.
3. Heart-Qi descends towards the Small Intestine and Bladder, assisting in the excretion of urine. The Bladder Divergent channel flows through the Heart. Heart disharmonies can be transmitted to the Bladder via the Small Intestine, resulting in urinary symptoms.
4. Lung-Qi descends to the Kidneys and Bladder to promote transformation and excretion of urine.
5. The Kidney and Bladder are interiorly–exteriorly related. Kidney-Yang provides Qi and heat for fluid transformation in the Bladder, whilst the Bladder transforms and excretes the Kidneys' 'dirty' fluids.

CHAPTER 18

1. (i) Middle Burner transmits Original Qi to Spleen to transform and transport food essence; (ii) Lower Burner ensures Original Qi warms Kidneys to transform fluids; (iii) Upper Burner facilitates transformation of Gathering Qi into True Qi; (iv) Upper Burner facilitates transformation of Food-Qi into Blood in the Heart.
2. 'The Nutritive Qi originates from the Middle Burner; the Defensive Qi originates from the Lower Burner.'
3. Chapter 8 of the 'Simple Questions' states 'The Triple Burner is the official in charge of ditches'; the metaphor is one of irrigation.
4. Upper Burner: sweat; Middle Burner: Stomach fluids; Lower Burner: urine.
5. The Upper Burner lets out Defensive Qi (directing it to the Lungs); the Middle Burner lets out Nutritive Qi (directing it to all the organs); the Lower Burner lets out waste fluids (directing them to the Bladder).
6. Original Qi provides the heat necessary for transformation of food. The Triple Burner acts as an intermediary to transmit this heat to the Spleen.
7. a) 'The Upper Burner is like a mist'; b) 'The Middle Burner is like a maceration chamber'; c) 'The Lower Burner is like a drainage ditch'.
8. Upper Burner: Gathering Qi (*Zong Qi*); Middle Burner: Nutritive Qi (*Ying Qi*); Lower Burner: Original Qi (*Yuan Qi*).
9. The Triple Burner controls the entering and exiting of Qi and fluids in the joint cavities, which contributes to lubricating the synovial membranes.
10. The Triple Burner acts as a 'hinge' on a psychic level, providing a balance between the outgoing movement of relating to others, and the inward movement towards oneself.

CHAPTER 19

1. Because whilst they are hollow like the other Yang organs, they store Yin essence rather than excreting.
2. If Kidney-Essence is weak the Directing and Penetrating Vessels will be empty, the Uterus will be inadequately supplied with Blood and Essence, resulting in amenorrhoea.
3. Menstrual blood (*Tian Gui*) is a precious fluid deriving directly from the Kidney-Essence, different in origin and nature from normal Blood in the body. The Kidney is also the mother of the Liver (in a Five-Element sense), which provides Blood to the Uterus, and is closely connected to the Directing and Penetrating Vessels, which regulate Qi and Blood in the Uterus.
4. (i) Heart-Qi and -Blood descend to the Uterus to promote discharge of menstrual blood during a period and discharge eggs at ovulation; (ii) Heart-Qi and -Blood descend to bring about the transformation of Yang to Yin with the onset of the period and of Yin to Yang with ovulation; (iii) Heart-Blood nourishes the Uterus; (iv) Heart-Yang descends to meet Kidney-Essence to form menstrual blood (*Tian Gui*).
5. The Liver has the function of storing and regulating Blood and ensuring the smooth flow of Qi. If Liver-Qi becomes stagnant, it may cause Liver-Blood stasis, which affects the Uterus, causing pain and dark, clotted blood.
6. The Kidneys and the Heart: Kidney-Essence produces Marrow, which fills the Brain and spinal cord. Heart-Blood is responsible for nourishing the Brain.
7. Decline of Kidney-Essence in the elderly causes a deficiency of Marrow, which fails to nourish the bones, causing osteoporosis.
8. Because they are hollow and 'house' the Blood (and are also related to the Kidneys via the Kidneys' role of assisting the production of Blood).
9. Shortness of breath and dislike of speaking.
10. Du-20 Baihui and Du-16 Fengfu.

CHAPTER 20

1. Anger makes Qi rise.
2. Fear makes Qi descend.
3. All emotions affect the Heart, which, due to its function of housing the Mind and consciousness, is the only organ which can recognize and feel emotional stress. Emotions from other internal organs can therefore indirectly cause Heart-Heat, which causes a red tongue tip.
4. The emotions cause stagnation of Qi. When Qi is 'compressed' for any length of time, it will lead to Heat and then Fire.
5. Any of the following: headache, dizziness, tinnitus, stiff neck, blotches on the neck, red face.
6. Any of the following: palpitations, insomnia, restlessness, talking a lot, red tongue tip.
7. 'Sadness dissolves Qi, and affects the Heart and the Lungs.'
8. Their worrying has knotted their Qi, primarily affecting the Spleen.
9. Fear depletes Kidney-Yin, which leads to Empty-Heat in the Heart, resulting in symptoms of palpitations, insomnia, etc.
10. Shock is reflected in the 'moving' pulse: short, rapid, slippery, shaped like a bean, and seeming to vibrate as it pulses.

CHAPTER 21

1. If the weather is particularly excessive, even a person with strong Defensive Qi would be relatively weaker, and an external invasion may occur. This may also happen if the weather changes rapidly.
2. The Lungs and autumn.
3. The Four Levels are Defensive Qi (*Wei*), Qi, Nutritive Qi (*Ying*) and Blood (*Xue*). The Defensive Qi level is on the Exterior, the rest are on the Interior.
4. Because they have a tendency to Heat, the invading Wind is likely to combine with this to manifest a pattern of Wind-Heat, despite it being the middle of winter.
5. Wind-Cold is said to penetrate via the skin and Wind-Heat via nose and mouth.
6. An exterior pattern is defined by the location of the pathogenic factor, being in the space between the skin and the muscles and the channels (the 'Exterior' of the body).
7. Aversion to cold from an exterior invasion arises suddenly and is not relieved by covering oneself. The cold feeling from Yang deficiency is chronic and is relieved by covering oneself.
8. By palpating the patient's forehead and back of hands, which would feel hot to the touch.
9. Three of the following: aversion to cold, fever, sore throat, sneezing, runny nose, occipital stiffness, Floating pulse.
10. Cold invading the Stomach, Cold invading the Intestines, Cold invading the Uterus

CHAPTER 22

1. A poor constitution can be caused by: parents in poor health; parents who are too old; conception when drunk; consumption by pregnant mother of alcohol, drugs or cigarettes; medicinal drugs during pregnancy; shock to the mother during pregnancy.
2. Very small ears with short ear lobes can indicate a poor constitution.
3. Overwork causes Yin deficiency, particularly Kidney-Yin deficiency (and even Kidney-Essence deficiency if extreme).
4. Lack of exercise will cause the Qi to stagnate and can lead to Dampness.
5. Excessive sexual desire might be caused by Kidney-Yin deficiency with Empty-Heat or Full-Heat of the Liver and/or Heart. Lack of sexual desire can be caused by Kidney-Yang deficiency.
6. Eating a lot of salads and fruit weakens the Spleen, which then fails to transform and transport food and fluids properly, leading to weight gain.
7. Beta-blockers tend to make the pulse slow and deep.
8. Long-term use of cannabis seems to cause Kidney deficiency and weaken the *Zhi*, as well as adversely affecting the Heart-Blood.

CHAPTER 23

1. The face, the ear, the tongue and the second metacarpal bone.
2. The complexion, the eyes, the state of mind and the breathing.
3. Any three of the following: red complexion, wide teeth, pointed, small head, well-developed shoulder muscles, curly or not much hair, small hands and feet, walking briskly.
4. Two small transverse cracks in the Lung area on the tongue, and a pulse that runs from the Front position up towards the base of the thumb medially.
5. Chronic Blood or Yin deficiency.
6. Kidney-Yin deficiency with Empty-Heat.
7. Liver-Blood deficiency with internal Wind.
8. A complexion with 'lustre' (bright, glowing and with shine) has 'spirit'. A complexion with 'moisture' (skin firm and moist) is said to have 'Stomach-Qi'.
9. Damp-Heat with a prevalence of Heat is likely to show as a bright orange-yellow colour, whereas if Dampness is prevalent the colour would be a smoky, dull-yellow.
10. The Spleen.
11. Heat in the Stomach and Spleen.
12. 'Water oedema' (*shui zhong*) is due to Yang deficiency and the skin pits and changes colour on pressure. 'Qi oedema' (*Qi zhong*) is due to either Qi stagnation or Dampness and the skin does not pit or change colour on pressure.
13. Liver-Wind and Phlegm, which affect the channels and sinews.
14. The Stomach.
15. Blood stasis.
16. Empty-Heat of the Stomach.
17. Full-Heat or Yin deficiency.
18. The presence of a pathogenic factor.
19. A very wet tongue shows that deficient Yang-Qi is unable to transform and transport fluids, which accumulate as Dampness.
20. It indicates a deficiency condition, that the channel is starved of Qi and Blood.

CHAPTER 24

1. Pain; food and taste; stools and urine; thirst and drink; energy levels; head, face and body; chest and abdomen; limbs; sleep; sweating; ears and eyes; feeling of cold, feeling of heat and fever; emotional symptoms; sexual symptoms; women's symptoms; children's symptoms.
2. Because when the traditional 10 questions were formulated, febrile diseases were very common in China and would have formed the major part of a doctor's practice.
3. All pain from a Full condition is seen to be caused by obstruction to the circulation of Qi in the channels.
4. Blood stasis causes severe, boring or stabbing pain with a fixed location.
5. That it is a Full condition.
6. Liver-Fire.
7. An Empty Pattern.
8. Spleen-Qi deficiency.
9. Kidney-Qi deficiency.
10. A Cold pattern (usually of Stomach or Spleen).
11. Liver-Qi stagnation.
12. Liver-Blood deficiency.
13. Damp-Heat in the Stomach channel.
14. Heat or Empty-Heat of the Stomach.
15. Internal Wind and Phlegm.
16. Dampness or Liver-Qi stagnation.
17. Yang deficiency (ameliorated by heat), Heart-Blood deficiency (with palpitations and dizziness), Liver-Qi stagnation.

18. Yin deficiency (of Heart, Liver or Kidneys).
19. The Lungs or the Heart.
20. Kidney deficiency.
21. Any three of the following: intense feeling of cold and shivers; body feels cold and relatively hard to touch; pain; full pulse; sudden onset.
22. 'Fever' literally means 'emission of heat', and therefore it means that the patient's body feels objectively hot on palpation.
23. Heart-Yin deficiency.
24. The Kidneys or the Heart.
25. Blood deficiency.

CHAPTER 25

1. *Superficial level*: Qi and Yang organs; Exterior diseases; Heart and Lungs.
   Middle level: Blood; Stomach and Spleen diseases; Stomach and Spleen.
   Deep level: Yin and Yin organs; Interior diseases; Liver and Kidneys.
2. Lifting (upwards): to check the strength of the pulse at the superficial level.
   Pressing (downwards): to check the strength of the pulse at the middle and deep level
   Pushing (lateral–medial): to check the pulse for qualities.
   Rolling (proximal–distal): to check the length of the pulse (or for children under 1)
3. The pulse of the labourer would most likely be considerably stronger.
4. That both the deep level and the rear positions can be felt clearly, and thus the Kidneys are strong.
5. (a) Feel the pulse as a whole; (b) feel whether the pulse has spirit, Stomach Qi and root; (c) feel the three levels and the three positions; (d) feel the strength of the pulse; (e) feel the overall quality of the pulse; (f) feel the quality of individual pulse positions.
6. An invasion of Wind-Cold.
7. Qi and Yang deficiency.
8. Slow and Weak: Empty-Cold (Yang deficiency); Slow and Full: Full-Cold.
9. 68 beats per minute.
10. Rapid and Floating-Empty.
11. Phlegm, Dampness, retention of food or pregnancy.
12. Blood deficiency or Dampness with severe Qi deficiency.
13. Liver disharmony, Pain or Phlegm.
14. A Knotted pulse is slow and stops at irregular intervals, and indicates Cold and Heart-Yang deficiency.
15. *Depth*: Floating – Deep – Hidden – Firm – Leather.
    Rate: Slow – Rapid – Slowed-down – Hurried – Moving.
    Strength: Empty – Full – Weak – Scattered.
    Size: Big – Overflowing – Fine – Minute.
    Length: Long – Short – Moving.
    Shape: Slippery – Choppy – Wiry – Tight – Moving – Hollow – Firm.
    Rhythm: Knotted – Hasty – Intermittent.
16. Spleen- and Stomach-Yang deficiency.
17. The coldness is particularly in the fingers and toes.
18. The area just below the xiphoid process reflects the state of the Upper Burner Qi.
19. Heart-Blood stasis.
20. A deficiency of Original Qi.

CHAPTER 26

1. A Cold pattern or Lung-Qi deficiency.
2. An Empty condition.
3. Liver-Qi invading the Stomach.
4. Qi stagnation of the Liver or the Lungs.
5. Damp-Heat.
6. The organs of the digestive system, particularly the Stomach or Large Intestine.
7. Damp-Heat in the Large Intestine.

CHAPTER 27

1. Invasion of Cold in the Stomach, invasion of Cold in the Intestines, invasion of Cold in the Uterus.
2. Any three of the following: Qi stagnation, Blood stasis, internal Wind, internal Dampness, internal Cold, Phlegm, Heat, Fire.
3. It requires the presence of a pathogenic factor together with intact Upright Qi.
4. Full pain would be severe and intense. Empty pain is milder and tends to be an ache rather than a pain.
5. A mixed Full/Empty condition requires the presence of a pathogenic factor, while the Upright Qi is deficient.
6. This is a Full/Empty condition. Because the Upright Qi is deficient, the clinical manifestations will be relatively mild.
7. Because the Upright Qi is not strong enough to deal with the pathogenic factor, in this case transforming the Dampness. Moreover, Dampness is notoriously 'heavy' and 'sticky' and therefore difficult to get rid of.
8. Heat will dry the Body Fluids and injure Yin.

CHAPTER 28

1. Excess of Yang = Full-Heat; Deficiency of Yang = Empty-Cold; Excess of Yin = Full-Cold; Deficiency of Yin = Empty-Heat.
2. 'Full-Cold tends to weaken Yang Qi; this leads to Yang deficiency, which, in turn, will lead to Empty-Cold.'
3. (i) An external Yang pathogenic factor. (ii) Internally generated Heat. (iii) Heat from transformation of other pathogenic factors.
4. Any three of the following: dietary factors (cold foods); excessive physical work; overwork; Full-Cold.
5. Overwork
6. Dryness (dry mouth, dry eyes, dry skin, etc.).
7. In Excess of Yang, clear Heat. In Deficiency of Yang, tonify Yang. In Excess of Yin, expel Cold. In Deficiency of Yin, nourish Yin.

CHAPTER 29

1. 'The key words in the pathology of the Qi Mechanism are not 'Deficiency' or 'Excess' but rather 'derangement', 'disruption' and 'obstruction' of Qi.'
2. Emotions and diet.
3. Stomach-Qi should descend. If it rebels upwards it can cause hiccups, nausea, vomiting and belching.
4. The 'coming and going' of the Ethereal Soul (housed in the Liver) gives the Mind the capacity for relationships, for projecting outwards, and for having ideas, plans, inspiration, etc.
   If Liver-Qi fails to ascend, there is often depression and a lack of direction.
5. The person's arm will feel stiff below the elbow and soft and flabby above.
6. The ascending of Qi brings the clear Yang upwards to 'brighten' the orifices and enable the functioning of the sense organs.
7. The space between the skin and muscles would become too 'open'. Defensive Qi would not circulate well, the pores would be too open and the body would be prone to invasion by pathogenic factors.
8. The Triple Burner regulates the transformation, transportation and excretion of fluids. Correct entering/exiting of Qi in and out of the Triple Burner cavities is therefore essential for a proper fluid metabolism.
9. Excessive entering of the Corporeal Soul may cause impotence, while excessive exiting may cause excessive sexual desire.
10. Excessive exiting of Qi would cause stagnation in the Membranes, causing abdominal distension and pain.

CHAPTER 30

1. The Exterior is the space between skin and muscles (where Defensive Qi and sweat are located) and the channels. An exterior pattern refers to the location of the disease (in the Exterior).
2. Aversion to cold and fever.
3. Thirst (Hot) or its absence (Cold) and a Tight (Cold) or Rapid (Hot) Pulse.
4. Three factors: sweating (Empty) or its absence (Full); pulse (Slow in Empty and Tight in Full); severity of body aches (severe in Full, less so in Empty).
5. Aversion to cold would change to an aversion to heat.
6. Any three of: thirst, a feeling of heat, some mental restlessness, red face, dry stools, scanty dark urine, a Rapid-Full pulse, and a Red tongue with yellow coating.
7. Full-Heat causes severe mental restlessness, agitation, anxiety and insomnia with agitated sleep. Empty-Heat causes a vague mental restlessness that is worse in the evening, anxiety with fidgeting, and waking up frequently during the night.
8. Any of the following: feeling cold, cold limbs, no thirst, pale face, abdominal pain aggravated on pressure, desire to drink warm liquids, loose stools, clear abundant urination, Deep-Full-Tight pulse and a Pale tongue with thick white coating.
9. Spleen-Yang deficiency. This is an example of Empty-Cold.
10. These symptoms are an example of Heat above and Cold below.
11. A *Full* condition is characterized by the presence of a pathogenic factor (interior or exterior) and by the fact that the body's Qi is relatively intact. An *Empty* condition is characterized by weakness of the body's Qi and the absence of a pathogenic factor.
12. Any three of the following: a weak voice, dull lingering pain, a very pale face, slight sweating, listlessness, curling up in bed and quiet disposition are signs of an Empty condition.
13. Any three of the following: a dull-pale face, pale lips, blurred vision, dry hair, tiredness, poor memory, numbness or tingling, insomnia, scanty periods or amenorrhoea, a Fine or Choppy pulse and a Pale-Thin tongue.

CHAPTER 31

1. Qi deficiency, Qi sinking, Qi stagnation and rebellious Qi.
2. Feeling of distension, distending pain that moves from place to place, mental depression, irritability, gloomy feeling, frequent mood swings, frequent sighing.
3. Heart-Blood deficiency.
4. The Liver.
5. Skin diseases with itching, heat and redness.
6. Excessive consumption of drying foods (such as baked foods) or irregular eating.
7. A Swollen tongue body, a sticky tongue coating and a Slippery or Wiry pulse.
8. Numbness.
9. The Lungs, the Stomach or the Heart.
10. A feeling of swelling in the throat, difficulty in swallowing, a feeling of oppression of chest and diaphragm, irritability, moodiness, depression, Wiry pulse.

CHAPTER 32

1. The Heart governs Blood, controls the blood vessels, manifests in the complexion, houses the Mind, opens into the tongue and controls sweat.
2. Prolonged sadness and grief cause deficiency of Qi and if prolonged may lead to stagnation of Qi, which then turns into Heat in the Heart.
3. Normally the pulse would be Empty. In severe cases it might feel slightly Overflowing and Empty.
4. The feeling of stuffiness in the chest is due to Heart-Yang not moving Qi in the chest and leading to stagnation of Qi in the chest. This is important as it can lead to Heart-Blood stasis, which is involved in angina pectoris and coronary heart disease.
5. Because Defensive Qi is lost with the sweating, which means a further loss of Yang. Also, losing fluids from sweating leads to Blood deficiency, which will further weaken the Heart.
6. Long-term sadness will disturb the Mind, which will depress the function of the Heart. Since the Heart governs Blood, this will lead to Heart-Blood deficiency.
7. Palpitations from Heart-Qi deficiency occur more in daytime, those from Heart-Blood deficiency more in the afternoon/evening.
8. Normally the pulse is Floating-Empty, or Rapid-Fine if Empty-Heat is present. The pulse is often weak on both Rear positions due to a weakness of Kidney-Yin, and can be Overflowing on both Front positions if Empty-Heat is flaring up.
9. Red with a yellow coating, with a red and swollen tip. Possibly a Heart-crack.
10. The Spleen, unable to transform and transport fluids, is responsible for the formation of Phlegm.
11. It is commonly seen following an attack of Wind-Stroke, with the Phlegm misting the Mind causing coma and aphasia.
12. The tongue would be slightly Pale-Purple on the sides in the chest area.
13. Chest pain, which can vary from a mild pricking sensation to an intense stabbing pain.

CHAPTER 33

1. The Pericardium is the centre of the thorax where it influences both the Heart and Lungs and therefore the Gathering Qi (*Zong Qi*). The Pericardium channel is the propulsive agent for the Qi and Blood of both Heart and Lungs.
2. Because when the Heat penetrates the Nutritive Qi level, it injures the Yin.
3. Pericardium pathology in the mental–emotional sphere would be characterized by problems relating to others, the 'movement' towards others in social, intimate and familial interactions.
4. Blood deficiency of the Pericardium.
5. It is due to the influence of the Pericardium on the Lungs.
6. Spleen deficiency would lead to the formation of Phlegm. Fire, by condensing Body Fluids, would contribute to the build-up of Phlegm.
7. Either the whole tongue body would be purple, or purple just in the chest area on the sides.

CHAPTER 34

1. The Liver stores Blood, ensures the smooth flow of Qi, controls the sinews, manifests in the nails, opens into the eyes, controls tears, houses the Ethereal Soul, is affected by anger.
2. Rapid changes (skin conditions); up and down fluctuation (energy levels, mood); irritability; pain; eye problems; distension; gynaecological problems.
3. A feeling of distension and a Wiry pulse.
4. The tongue might have red sides.
5. Rebellious Liver-Qi, with symptoms of belching, irritability and a Wiry pulse (on the Liver and Stomach positions).
6. LIV-14 Qimen.
7. Dark, clotted menstrual blood and pain.
8. The Fire dries up Body Fluids, causing dryness in the intestines.
9. A feeling of fullness of and heaviness and a sticky-yellow tongue coating.
10. You would look at the nails, which may be withered and brittle from lack of nourishment.
11. Liver-Yin deficiency.
12. Subdue Liver-Yang and nourish Yin or Blood.
13. Tremor, tic, numbness/tingling, dizziness, convulsions and paralysis.

14. Ren-10 Xiawan and Ren-13 Shangwan.
15. Liver- and Heart-Blood deficiency.

CHAPTER 35

1. Governing Qi and respiration.
2. Because they are the most susceptible to invasion by exterior pathogenic factors.
3. Artificial dryness from centrally heated environments can cause Lung Dryness.
4. Cold, raw, greasy and dairy foods would encourage the production of Phlegm.
5. The pulse is often Weak on both Front positions.
6. Poor posture (stooping over a desk for long hours) or excessive use of the voice (teachers).
7. Aversion to cold, sneezing, fever and a Floating pulse.
8. Aversion to cold is due to the obstruction of the Defensive Qi by Wind in the space between the skin and the muscles, so that it is unable to warm the muscles.
9. The Lung-Defensive Qi portion is obstructed by exterior Wind-Cold, so that the Lungs are unable to direct fluids downwards, causing facial oedema.
10. Diet (hot foods) and smoking.
11. Phlegm in the throat and a Swollen tongue.
12. (i) Damp-Phlegm in the Lungs: profuse white sticky sputum; (ii) Cold-Phlegm in the Lungs: white, watery sputum; (iii) Phlegm-Heat in the Lungs: sticky yellow or green sputum; (iv) Dry-Phlegm in the Lungs: scanty sputum, difficult to expectorate; (v) Phlegm-Fluids obstructing the Lungs: white, watery, foamy sputum.
13. Emotional problems such as sadness, grief and worry.

CHAPTER 36

1. During puberty, during each period and after childbirth.
2. Excessive consumption of cold and raw foods, eating at irregular times, excessive eating, eating too little or eating a protein-deficient diet.
3. The Spleen transports Food-Qi to the four limbs and throughout the body. If Spleen-Qi is deficient, the limbs and body will be deprived of nourishment and feel weak and tired.
4. Because of the impairment in the Spleen's transformation and transportation of fluids.
5. Diet: inadequate consumption of Blood-forming foods (meat and grains).
6. Cold-Dampness invading the Spleen.
7. Spleen-Qi deficiency and Heat (often in the Stomach).
8. Palpitations, insomnia, tiredness, loose stools and scanty periods.
9. If the Spleen is deficient and fails in its function of transformation and transportation, fluids accumulate into Dampness. Dampness obstructs the flow of Qi in the Middle Burner. After a long period of time, the obstruction of Dampness gives rise to Heat.

CHAPTER 37

1. 'Kidney-Yin is the root of the Liver, Heart and Lungs. Kidney-Yang is the root of the Spleen, the Lungs and the Heart.'
2. The age and health of the parents at conception.
3. Although fear makes Qi descend, if it is long-standing it makes Qi rise, causing dry mouth, malar flush, mental restlessness and insomnia.
4. Overwork: working long hours without adequate rest for many years under stressful conditions.
5. Because the declining Kidney-Essence and the Fire of the Gate of Life are unable to nourish the sexual organs.
6. Chronic illness, excessive sexual activity, excessive physical work and diet.
7. Deficient Kidney-Yin fails to produce enough Marrow to fill the brain, resulting in dizziness and vertigo.
8. Night sweating is due to deficient Yin being unable to hold Defensive Qi in the body, so that precious Yin nutritive essences are lost with the sweat.
9. Dribbling after urination, chronic vaginal discharge and backache.
10. The asthma is characterized by difficult inhalation (difficult exhalation comes more from a Lung imbalance).
11. Weak knees, falling hair and weak sexual activity.
12. Palpitations and cold hands.
13. Insomnia with falling asleep easily but waking several times in the night and in the early hours of the morning.
14. It is due to deficient Liver-Blood failing to nourish the Uterus and deficient Kidney-Essence unable to promote conception.
15. Floating-Empty and Rapid or Deep-Weak on both Rear positions and relatively Overflowing on both Front positions.

CHAPTER 38

1. The main Stomach function is the 'rotting and ripening' of food.
2. Because of its central position in the Middle Burner, at the centre of all the Qi pathways of the other organs.
3. The Stomach, with the Spleen, is the Root of Post-Heaven Qi, which means it is the source of all the Qi produced by the body after birth. If the Stomach is not functioning properly, not enough Qi will be produced, and a person will experience tiredness.
4. The tongue should have a coating with a root. A pulse with Stomach-Qi should be gentle and relatively soft.
5. Generally the Stomach prefers foods which are moist and not too dry.
6. Because of the natural flow of Qi around different organs during the day; it is important not to eat at a time when Stomach-Qi is inactive.
7. Tiredness, particularly in the mornings (7–9 a.m.).
8. Because of the relationship between the Stomach and Large Intestine (Bright Yang).
9. It would have an absence of coating in the centre, or else have a rootless coating.
10. Irregular eating habits and emotional strain (anger, frustration, resentment).
11. Full-Heat obstructs the Stomach and prevents descent of Stomach-Qi, which rebels upwards.
12. If the Cold is not expelled it will injure the Yang of the Stomach. The symptoms will change over time to those of Empty-Cold and Yang deficiency.
13. These symptoms are due to Damp-Heat in the Stomach channel on the face.
14. The retention of Food in the Stomach blocks the Middle Burner and prevents Heart-Qi from descending, which disturbs the Mind, causing insomnia.
15. Because Blood stasis can potentially cause serious diseases, e.g. cancer, stroke, etc.

CHAPTER 39

1. 'The Small Intestine transforms food in coordination with the Spleen, whilst it transforms fluids in coordination with the Bladder and Kidney-Yang.'
2. Mental clarity, discrimination and the capacity for sound judgement.
3. Heart-Fire blazing.
4. They would dislike pressure on the abdomen as this would aggravate the obstruction from the stagnation of Qi.
5. Excessive consumption of cold and raw foods.
6. A Cold condition of the Spleen and Intestines favours infestation by worms.
7. Borborygmi.

CHAPTER 40

1. Controlling passage and conduction, and transforming stools and reabsorbing fluids.
2. Exposure over a prolonged period of time, inadequate clothing in cold/damp weather and sitting on cold/damp ground.
3. Sadness (depletes Lung- and Large Intestine-Qi), worry (depletes Lung-Qi causing stagnation in Large Intestine) and anger (stagnates Qi).
4. Retention of Dampness in the Large Intestine prevents its function of absorbing fluids and excreting stools, hence fluids are not absorbed and diarrhoea results.
5. 'Heat in the Large Intestine is an Excess pattern with Full-Heat and Dryness.'
6. Heat obstructing the Large Intestine is an acute pattern which appears during febrile diseases, and is always characterized by fever.
7. The pain is severe and cramping in quality as the Cold contracts and causes cramps and spasms.
8. Qi stagnation is characterized by distension, so in this case abdominal distension.
9. Stomach-Yin deficiency.
10. Large Intestine Cold is characterized by Empty-Cold and is a chronic condition. Cold invading the Large Intestine is an acute condition characterized by Full-Cold.
11. Qi deficiency (Spleen, Stomach and Large Intestine) and Qi sinking (Spleen).

CHAPTER 41

1. On the Liver ensuring the smooth flow of Qi.
2. External Dampness and excessive consumption of greasy-fatty and dairy foods.
3. A thick sticky yellow coating, either bilateral in two strips or unilateral.
4. Cholelithiasis or stones in the Gall Bladder.
5. This is something of a trick question, as there is no actual aetiology as such; rather, this pattern describes a certain character of the person rather than a set of clinical manifestations.

CHAPTER 42

1. The Bladder receives the 'dirty' part of fluids after separation from the Small Intestine.
2. Exposure to damp weather, sitting on damp surfaces or living in a damp place.
3. Because the invading Dampness will combine with Heat in a person of a Yang constitution. Given time, Damp-Cold often turns into Damp-Heat in any case.
4. Thick sticky yellow coating on the root with red spots.
5. Dampness obstructs the water passages of the Lower Burner and interferes with the Bladder function of Qi transformation.
6. Kidney-Yang deficiency.

CHAPTER 44

1. The 'Discussion of Cold-Induced Diseases' (*Shang Han Lun*) by Zhang Zhong Jing in the third century AD.
2. Aversion to cold, headache and stiff neck and a Floating pulse.
3. External Wind obstructs the Great Yang channels (Small Intestine and Bladder) which run through this area.
4. Because this pattern is characterized by deficiency of Nutritive Qi, which fails to hold sweat in the space between the skin and muscles.
5. Floating-Tight.
6. It is caused by the pathogenic factor impairing the Bladder's function of Qi transformation.
7. As the pathogenic factor affects the functioning of the Bladder and is at the Blood level.
8. Big thirst, sweating, fever and pulse.
9. The pulse in the channel pattern is Overflowing-Rapid or Big-Rapid. The pulse in the organ pattern is Deep-Full-Slippery-Rapid, which reflects the deeper location of the Fire.
10. Alternating shivers and fever.
11. Spleen-Yang deficiency.
12. Pale Wet tongue with white coating. Deep-Weak-Slow pulse.
13. Heat above (thirst, feeling of energy rising, pain and heat sensation of heart region, hunger) and Cold below (no desire to eat, cold limbs, vomiting).

CHAPTER 45

1. In the 18th century (1746).
2. Three of the following: they all manifest with fever; the pathogenic factor enters through the nose and mouth; they are infectious; the pathological developments are rapid; the pathogenic factor of Warm Diseases has a strong tendency to injure Yin.
3. That pathogenic factors can enter through the nose and mouth and are infectious.
4. Three of the following signs and symptoms (of Full Interior Heat): fever, thirst, feeling of heat, mental restlessness, Red tongue with thick yellow coating and a Rapid-Full pulse.
5. Fever at night, and a Deep-Red tongue without coating.
6. Macules.
7. A spot under the skin which cannot be felt on palpation.
8. Because the Wind obstructs the Defensive Qi in the space between the skin and muscles so that it cannot warm the body.
9. External Wind, Dampness and interior Heat.
10. That they are thirsty but do not really desire to drink much.
11. The Heat impairs the descending of Lung-Qi.
12. Drain Fire (from the Stomach and Intestines).
13. The Lesser Yang pattern of the Six Stages.
14. Because sweat comes from the space between the skin and muscles, whereas the Dampness is in the Interior.
15. Red without coating (as the Heat has injured the Yin).
16. Fever at night, bleeding, internal Wind.
17. Kidney deficiency.
18. Lesser Yang type (Qi level), Bright Yang type (Qi level), and Lesser Yin type (Blood level).

CHAPTER 46

1. The patterns of the Middle Burner are essentially the same as some of those of the Qi level and those of the Lower Burner are essentially the same as some of those of the Blood level. The patterns of the Upper Burner occur at three depths: Defensive Qi, Qi and Nutritive Qi levels.
2. At the Qi level.
3. Three of the following: high fever at night, a burning sensation of the epigastrium, cold limbs, delirium and aphasia.
4. Yes.
5. Deep-Red tongue without coating, Floating-Empty and Rapid pulse.
6. Nourish Yin, extinguish Wind, stop convulsions.

CHAPTER 47

1. The channels pertain to the Exterior (the superficial energetic layers of the body), the organs pertain to the Interior (the deep energetic layer of the body).
2. Exterior invasion, overuse of a part of the body, injury and Internal Organ disharmony.
3. Qi and Blood gather at the joints. Joints are places where Qi enters and exits, and goes from Interior to Exterior (or vice versa). They are also places where pathogenic factors easily settle.

4. In Full conditions there may be a red colour, indicating Heat, or a bluish colour, indicating Cold. In Empty conditions, there may be a pale streak along the course of the channel.
5. Hot palms.
6. Sensation of cold in the teeth.
7. Weakness of the leg muscles.
8. Kidney channel.
9. Triple Burner channel.
10. Itching in the genital region, impotence, swelling and pain in testicle, abnormal erection, contraction of scrotum or vagina, persistent erection.

CHAPTER 49

1. Deficient Gall Bladder.
2. Phlegm in the chest, cough and tiredness caused by a deficient Spleen, leading to the formation of Phlegm, which obstructs the Lungs.
3. Water not generating Wood.
4. In the Earth Element (the face colour usually shows the origin of the disharmony).
5. Kidney and Heart not harmonized, or Kidney and Heart-Yin deficiency with Empty-Heat.

CHAPTER 50

1. The Gall Bladder channel (where it is the fourth).
2. It is superficial, unstable, has an outward centrifugal movement and is easily influenced and changed.
3. Defensive Qi.
4. The Well points.
5. The Stream points.
6. ST-37 for the Large Intestine; ST-39 for the Small Intestine; BL-39 for the Triple Burner.
7. 'The Sea points of the Yang channels are often used to treat skin diseases.'
8. When giving preventative seasonal treatment.
9. 'If a channel is deficient we can choose the point on that channel corresponding to the 'Mother' Element in order to tonify it.'
10. Dampness: Earth points. Wind: Wood points.

CHAPTER 51

1. The Yin organs.
2. Original Qi (*Yuan Qi*).
3. (i) The Connecting (*Luo*) channel itself which is the pathway of Qi departing from each connecting point. (ii) The area of the body that lies between the main channel and the skin.
4. Stagnation of Qi and Blood.
5. BL-47 Hunmen.
6. Ren-3 Zhongji.
7. LIV-13 Zhangmen (Yin organs) and Ren-12 Zhongwan (Yang organs).
8. The Sea of Marrow. Du-20 Baihui (upper), Du-16 Fengfu (lower).
9. On the neck (apart from LU-3 Tianfu and P-1 Tianchi).
10. Bladder, Stomach, Triple Burner and Gall Bladder.

CHAPTER 52

1. Two of the following: (i) they do not belong to the main channel system; (ii) they do not have exterior–interior relationships; (iii) they add something to the channel system.
2. The overflow Qi from the vessels irrigates the space between skin and muscles. Because all the extraordinary vessels derive from the Kidneys; this explains the Kidneys' role in resistance to pathogenic factors.
3. 'The extraordinary vessels integrate the Six Extraordinary Yang Organs with the Internal Organs.'
4. The eyes.
5. The Yin and Yang Stepping Vessels.
6. The Kidney channel.
7. The two Linking Vessels link the Yin and Yang channels and harmonize Interior–Exterior and Nutritive Qi–Defensive Qi.
8. It divides the body into two halves and harmonizes Above and Below.
9. The Penetrating Vessel.
10. LU-7 Lieque and KI-6 Zhaohai *in this order*.

CHAPTER 53

1. It originates between the two kidneys, flows down to the perineum at Ren-1 Huiyin, goes to Du-1 Changqiang and flows along the spine, over the head, down to the upper lip.
2. 'The Governing vessel is called the "Sea of Yang channels" as it exerts an influence on all the Yang channels and it can be used to strengthen the Yang of the body.'
3. The Directing Vessel (to nourish Yin).
4. The Penetrating Vessel is described as the 'Sea of the five Yin and six Yang Organs'[5], the 'Sea of the 12 Channels'[6] and the 'Sea of Blood'.
5. All the points of the Penetrating Vessel on the lower abdomen (ST-30 Qichong and the Kidney lower-abdominal points) affect the Kidneys and the Uterus.
6. It originates from between the Kidneys, it is responsible for the 7-year cycles of women and for the transformation of Kidney-Essence into menstrual blood, controls all Blood Connecting channels and flows through the Uterus.
7. Rebellious Qi of the Penetrating Vessel.
8. ST-30 Qichong.
9. 'The Directing Vessel corresponds to Qi, the Penetrating Vessel to Blood.'
10. The Kidney Divergent channel (at the level of BL-23).
11. KI-6 Zhaohai.
12. 'In cases of insomnia, the Yin Stepping Vessel is tonified and the Yang Stepping Vessel drained.'
13. Through its function of absorbing excess of Yang in the head, which can cause mania, agitation, insomnia, etc.
14. Two of the following: nourish Blood and Yin; mental–emotional problems; headaches.
15. The sides of the body.

CHAPTER 69

1. (i) Root is the root of the condition and Manifestation is the clinical manifestations; (ii) Root is the original pattern and Manifestation is the deriving pattern.
2. When the clinical manifestations reflect primarily the Root and they are few and mild.
3. Because the longer she continues to bleed, the more it will perpetuate the Root problem of Qi deficiency.
4. In all cases where clinical manifestations are acute, severe or life-threatening.
5. In this case the Root (stagnation of Qi and Blood) and the Manifestation (pain) coincide.
6. Often, but not always. For instance with Cold invading the Uterus causing Blood stasis (both Root and Manifestation are Full).
7. Blood stasis leading to Dryness; Heat leading to Yin deficiency.
8. Herbal treatment, exercise, diet, *Qi Gong*, meditation, and rest.
9. No. Exterior conditions are by definition of the Excess type, characterized by the presence of a pathogenic factor.
10. If the pattern you have identified from the clinical manifestations is of an Excess nature you should reduce, despite subjective feelings about the patient.
11. No. In exterior conditions the pathogenic factor needs to be expelled before tonifying the Upright Qi.

Index

Page numbers followed by 'f' indicate figures, 't' indicate tables, and 'b' indicate boxes.

A

Abdomen
  palpating, 394, 394b
  Yang and Yin Linking Vessels and, combined pathology of, 936
Abdominal branch, of Penetrating Vessel, 906
Abdominal distension
  Blood deficiency causing, 1003
  Qi stagnation in Large Intestine and, 695b
Abdominal pain, 353, 353b
  Girdle Vessel and, 920
  Yin Stepping Vessel and, 924
Accumulation *(Xi)* points, 858–859, 859b
Acupuncture
  for Bladder deficient and Cold, 719
  for Blood deficiency of Pericardium, 520
  for Blood rebelling upwards after childbirth, 815
  for Blood stasis
    in Directing and Penetrating Vessels, 811
    of Pericardium, 527–528
    in Stomach, 671–672
  for Cold
    in Directing and Penetrating Vessels, 811
    invading Large Intestine, 695, 698–699
    invading Stomach, 665
  for Cold-Phlegm in Lungs, 588–589
  for Damp-Cold in Bladder, 717–718
  for Damp-Heat
    in Bladder, 716
    in Directing and Penetrating Vessels, 812–813
    in Gall Bladder, 707
    in Large Intestine, 690
    in Spleen, 789
    in Stomach, 668
  for Damp-Phlegm in Lungs, 587
  for Dampness
    in Directing and Penetrating Vessels, 811
    in Gall Bladder, 705
    and Phlegm in Uterus, 814
  differences between herbal therapy and, 1184–1189
    case history, 1186b–1189b
  in Directing Vessel, 808
  for Dry Large Intestine, 697–698
  for Dry-Phlegm in Lungs, 592
  for empty Directing and Penetrating Vessels, 810
  for Empty-Heat, in Directing and Penetrating Vessels, 812
  in Fetus Cold, 815
  in Fetus Heat, 815
  for food retention in Stomach, 670
  for Full-Cold in Directing and Penetrating Vessels, 813
  for Full-Heat
    in Directing and Penetrating Vessels, 812
    in Small Intestine, 679
  for Gall Bladder deficiency, 709
  in Girdle Vessel, 815
  in Governing Vessel, 807
  for Heart-Blood deficiency, 497–498
  for Heart-Blood stasis, 512
  for Heart-Fire blazing, 501–502
  for Heart-Qi deficiency, 492–493
  for Heart-Qi stagnation, 508
  for Heart-Vessel obstructed, 510
  for Heart-Yang collapse, 496
  for Heart-Yang deficiency, 494
  for Heart-Yin deficiency, 499
  for Heat
    in Large Intestine, 691–692, 694
    in Pericardium, 517
  for invasion of Wind-Cold with prevalence of Wind, 755
  for Liver-Blood deficiency, 550
    and Heart-Blood deficiency, 567
  for Liver-Blood stasis, 541–542
  for Liver-Fire
    blazing, 544
    insulting Lungs, 564–565
  for Liver-Qi stagnation, 534
    turning into Heat, 536
  for Liver-Yang rising, 554–555
  for Liver-Yin deficiency, 552
  in Lower Burner, 790
  for Lung- and Heart-Qi deficiency, 594–595
  for Lung Dryness, 578
  for Lung-Heat, 585
  for Lung-Qi deficiency, 575
  for Lung-Yin deficiency, 577
  in Middle Burner, 789
  Nutritive Qi and, 517
  and Original Qi, 52
  in Penetrating Vessel, 810
  for Pericardium-Fire, 522
  for Phlegm-Fire
    harassing Heart, 504
    harassing Pericardium, 524
  for Phlegm-Fluid in Lungs, 593
  for Phlegm-Heat in Lungs, 590
  for Phlegm misting Mind, 506
  for Qi stagnation
    in Large Intestine, 696
    in Pericardium, 526
  for rebellious Liver-Qi, 538
    invading Spleen, 561–562
    invading Stomach, 563
  for Small Intestine deficient and Cold, 684–685
  for Small Intestine-Qi pain, 681
  for Small Intestine-Qi tied, 682
  for stagnant Cold in Uterus, 814
  for stagnant Heat in Directing and Penetrating Vessels, 813
  for stagnation of Cold in Liver channel, 547
  for Stomach- and Spleen-Qi deficiency, 673
  for Stomach- and Spleen-Yin deficiency, 674
  for Stomach deficient and Cold, 658
  for Stomach-Heat, 663–664
  for Stomach-Qi deficiency, 656
  for Stomach-Qi rebelling upwards, 666–667
  for Stomach-Qi stagnation, 661–662
  for Stomach-Yin deficiency, 660
  for unstable Directing and Penetrating Vessels, 810
  in Upper Burner, 788
  in Uterus deficient and Cold, 813
  for Wind-Cold invasion of Lungs, 580–581
  for Wind-Heat invasion of Lungs, 582
  for Wind-Water invasion of Lungs, 583
  wrong treatment with, 293
  in Yang Linking Vessel, 819
  in Yang Stepping Vessel, 817
  in Yin Linking Vessel, 817
  in Yin Stepping Vessel, 816
  Yin-Yang imbalance and, 423b
Acupuncture points, 826
  nature of, 1206
Acute cases, distal and local points, 1196
Acute Dampness, 741–742, 742b
Acute febrile diseases, 1084
Adult life, cause of disease, 249–250
Affections, 72
Age
  Kidney-Essence and, 624
  sexual activity and, 286
Amenorrhoea, ST-29 Guilai *Return* and, 982–983
'An Explanation of the Acupuncture Points', 999, 1003

'Ancestral muscles,' Penetrating Vessel and, 913–914, 913f
Anger, 259–260, 259f–260f, 260b
    Heart and, 491
    irritability and, 365, 365b
    Large Intestine and, 688
    Liver and, 125, 125f, 531, 531b
    Stomach and, 259
Animals, correspondences of the Five Elements, 26t
Antibiotics, 293, 293f–294f
    Stomach-Yin deficiency and, 659
Anus area, distal and local points, 1197t
Anxiety
    full and empty causes of, 364f
    patterns in, 364b
    symptoms of, 363–364, 365b
Apical (heart) beat, palpating, 392–393, 392b, 392f
Artificial 'climates,' as causes of disease, 272, 272b
Artificial 'dryness,' Lung Dryness and, 578
Asthma, LU-6 and, 953
Atrophy of limbs, 354
Atrophy (Wei) syndrome
    ST-31 Biguan Thigh Gate and, 984
    Yin Stepping Vessel and, 924
Attack of Cold, 755, 756b
Attack of Wind, 754–755, 755f
Aversion to Cold, 274–276, 275b, 275f, 360, 453–454
    Defensive-Qi level, 770
    Greater Yang stage, 753–754, 754f
    Wind-Heat and, 730
Aversion to Wind, 275

B

Babies, index finger diagnosis in, 323–324, 323f
Back
    and front of body, Yin-Yang, 9
    Governing Vessel strengthens, 893–894
Back Transporting (Shu) points, 37b, 853–857, 854b, 854f, 855t, 857b
    palpation, 394
    sense organs and, 99b
Backache, 352
    Du-26 as distal point for, 1199f
    Governing Vessel and Heart point combination for, 1011, 1011f
    Yang Stepping Vessel and, 927
Bacteria, and viruses, 269, 270b
Bafeng Eight Winds, 1167–1168, 1168b, 1168f
Bailao, 1032–1033
Balancing
    distal and local points, 1195–1202, 1196f, 1197t, 1198b
    front and back, 1207
    function
        of extraordinary vessels, 872–874, 873f, 874b
        of Liver, 126–127
    left and right sides of body, 1204–1206
    upper and lower body, 1202–1204, 1202t
    Yin-Yang, 1206–1207
Baxie Eight Pathogenic Factors, 1165, 1165b, 1165f
Beishu, 1032
Belching, diagnosis by, 398–399

Bile
    Gall Bladder stores and excretes, 209–210, 210b–211b
    smooth flow of Liver-Qi and, 122, 122b
Biliary ascariasis, ST-2 Sibai Four Whites and, 975
Bitong Free Nose Passage, 1159f, 1161, 1161b
Bitter taste, 114
BL-1 Jingming Eye Brightness, 1027–1028, 1029b
BL-2 Zanzhu (Cuanzhu) Gathered Bamboo, 1029, 1029b
BL-5 Wuchu Five Places, 1029, 1029b
BL-7 Tongtian Penetrating Heaven, 1029–1030, 1030b
BL-9 Yuzhen Jade Pillow, 1030, 1030b
BL-10 Tianzhu Heaven Pillar, 1030–1031, 1031b
BL-11 Dazhu Big Shuttle, 1031–1033, 1033b
BL-12 Fengmen Wind Door, 1033, 1033b
BL-13 Feishu Lung Back Transporting Point, 1034, 1034b, 1049f
BL-14 Jueyinshu Terminal Yin Back Transporting Point, 1035, 1035b
BL-15 Xinshu Heart Back Transporting Point, 1035, 1036b
BL-16 Dushu Governing Vessel Back Transporting Point, 1036, 1036b
BL-17 Geshu Diaphragm Back Transporting Point, 1036–1037, 1037b
BL-18 Ganshu Liver Back Transporting Point, 1037–1038, 1038b
BL-19 Danshu Gall Bladder Back Transporting Point, 1038, 1038b
BL-20 Pishu Spleen Back Transporting Point, 1039, 1039b, 1043b
BL-21 Weishu Stomach Back Transporting Point, 1039–1040, 1040b
BL-22 Sanjiaoshu Triple Burner Back Transporting Point, 1040–1041, 1041b, 1041f
BL-23 Shenshu Kidney Back Transporting Point, 1041–1042
BL-24 Qihaishu Sea of Qi Back Transporting Point, 1043, 1043b
BL-25 Dachangshu Large Intestine Back Transporting Point, 1043–1044, 1044b
BL-26 Guanyuanshu Origin Gate Back Transporting Point, 1044, 1044b
BL-27 Xiaochangshu Small Intestine Back Transporting Point, 1044–1045, 1045b
BL-28 Pangguanshu Bladder Back Transporting Point, 1045, 1045b
BL-30 Baihuanshu White Ring Transporting Point, 1045–1046, 1046b
BL-32 Ciliao Second Crevice, 1046
BL-36 Chengfu Receiving Support, 1046, 1047b
BL-37 Yinmen Huge Gate, 1047, 1047b
BL-39 Weiyang Supporting Yang, 1047, 1047b
BL-40 Weizhong Supporting Middle, 1047–1048, 1048b
BL-42 Pohu Door of the Corporeal Soul, 1048–1049, 1049b
BL-43 Gaohuangshu Transporting Point of Gaohuang, 1049–1050, 1050b
BL-44 Shentang Mind Hall, 1050, 1050b
BL-47 Hunmen Door of the Ethereal Soul, 1050–1051, 1051b
BL-49 Yishe Intellect Abode, 1051, 1051b

BL-51 Huangmen Door of Gaohuang, 1052, 1052b
BL-52 Zhishi Room of Will-Power, 1052–1053, 1054b
BL-53 Baohuang Bladder Vitals, 1053–1054, 1054b
BL-54 Zhibian Lowermost Edge, 1054, 1055b
BL-57 Chengshan Supporting Mountain, 1055, 1055b
BL-58 Feiyang Flying Up, 1055–1056, 1056b
BL-59 Fuyang Instep Yang, 1056, 1056b
BL-60 Kunlun kunlun (Mountains), 1056–1057, 1057b
BL-62 Shenmai Ninth Channel, 1057–1058, 1058b
BL-63 Jinmen Golden Door, 1058, 1058b
BL-64 Jinggu Capital Bone, 1058–1059, 1059b
BL-65 Shugu Binding Bone, 1059, 1059b
BL-66 Tonggu Passing Valley, 1059, 1060b
BL-67 Zhiyin Reaching Yin, 1060, 1060b
Black colour
    face, 316, 316b
    of Kidneys, 165
Bladder
    aspects of, 216–217
    and Body fluids, 68
    Damp-Cold in, 716–718
        acupuncture for, 717–718
        aetiology of, 717
        clinical manifestations of, 716–717, 717b, 717f
        pathological precursors of pattern in, 717, 718f
        pathology of, 717
        treatment for, 717–718
    Damp-Heat in, 714–716, 715f, 716b, 718b
        acupuncture for, 716
        aetiology of, 714
        case history for, 716b
        clinical manifestations of, 714, 714b
        emotional strain and, 714
        exterior pathogenic factors and, 714, 714b
        herbal formula for, 716, 718
        pathological developments from pattern, 715
        pathological precursors of pattern, 715, 715f
        pathology of, 715
        treatment for, 715–716
    Dampness in, 741
    deficient and Cold, 718–720, 720b
        acupuncture for, 719
        aetiology of, 718
        clinical manifestations of, 718, 718b, 719f
        excessive physical exercise and, 718
        excessive sexual activity and, 718
        exterior pathogenic factors and, 718
        herbal formula for, 719–720
        pathological developments from pattern, 719
        pathological precursors of pattern in, 718, 719f
        pathology of, 718
        treatment for, 719–720
    distal and local points, 1197t
    functions of, 215–217, 215b
    HE-5 Tongli Inner Communication and, 1009, 1009f
    invasion of external Dampness in, 740

line, spiritual aspects and, 112b
LU-5 and, 953
pathology of ascending/descending of Qi and, 429
relationship between Small Intestine and, 215, 215f, 216b
removes Water by Qi transformation, 215–216, 216b
and REN-3 Zhongji *Middle Pole*, 1131
and REN-4 Guanyuan *Gate of the Original Qi*, 1133
Bladder channel, 1027–1061
connecting pathway of, 1027, 1028f
main pathway of, 1027, 1027f
patterns, 800
points, 1028b
target areas of, 1060f
Bladder patterns, 713–721, 714b
Empty, 718–721
Full, 714–718
general aetiology of, 713–714, 714b
emotional strain and, 713
excess sexual activity and, 713–714
excessive physical exercise and, 714
exterior pathogenic factors of, 713
Qi transformation and, 713
Bleeding
from Fire, 747
gums, 351, 351b
'Bloating.' *see* Distension.
Blood, 61–66, 63b
and Body fluids, 69–70, 70f
Directing Vessel and, 898
and Essence, 66
Fire damage and, 747
and Food-Qi, 52, 52f
functions of, 63, 63b
and Heart, 63, 63f, 107–108, 108b
Heat in, 66, 66b, 475, 475f, 476b
and Kidneys, 65
L.I.-11 and, 967
and Liver, 63f–64f, 64, 118–120
and Lungs, 64–65
Marrow and, 242
pathology of, 66, 66b
pattern identification, 471–476
and Qi, 65–66, 65f, 175–176
and Body fluids, pattern identification, 448, 469–481, 469b
circulation, 243
generates, 65
holding, 65
movement, 65
nourishment, 65–66
Original Qi, 51
Yin-Yang, 11
rebelling upwards after childbirth, 815
in relation with internal organs, 63–65
and REN-4 Guanyuan *Gate of the Original Qi*, 1132
source of, 61–63, 62f
SP-6 Sanyinjiao *Three Yin Meeting* and, 1001
and Spleen, 63f, 64
Spleen not controlling, 605–606, 605b–606b, 605f–606f
volume regulation, 118–119
Yin Linking Vessel and, 932
Blood accumulation, Greater Yang stage, 756–757, 757b

Blood Connecting channels, SP-21 Dabao *General Control* and, 1005
Blood deficiency, 66, 473, 473b, 473f
causing abdominal distension, 1003
Heart, 496–498, 496f–497f, 497b–498b, 565–567, 567b, 612–614, 612b, 612f–613f, 614b
case history in, 498b
of Pericardium, 518–520, 518b, 519f, 520b
Spleen, 606–607, 606b, 607f–608f, 608b, 612–614, 612b, 612f–613f, 614b, 616–617, 616b–617b, 616f–617f
see also Liver-Blood deficiency
Blood level (*Xue*), 768, 768t–769t, 776–778
Lesser Yin type, Latent Heat, 781, 781t
Blood loss, 476, 476b
Heart-Blood deficiency, 496
Heart-Qi deficiency, 492
Kidney-Essence deficiency, 634
Kidney-Yin deficiency, 627
Liver and, 532
Liver-Blood deficiency and, 548
Blood stasis, 66, 66b, 405–406, 406b, 406f, 473–475, 474b–475b
causes of, 474f
Cold and, 732–733, 733b
and Dampness in Directing and Penetrating Vessels, 811–812
Heart, 474, 510–512, 511f–512f, 512b
case history in, 512b
Intestines, 474
Liver, 474, 538–542, 539f, 540b–542b, 541f, 568f
case history of, 542b
Lungs, 474
as pathogenic factors, 726
in Penetrating and Directing Vessels, 811
Penetrating Vessel and, 911, 911b
of Pericardium, 526–528, 526b, 527f, 528b
Phlegm and, 409, 409f
and stagnation of Qi, 474, 474t
Stomach, 474, 670–672, 670b–672b, 670f–671f
Uterus, 474–475
Blood vessels, 243
extraordinary vessels, 871
functions of, 243b
Heart and, 108–109, 108b
LU-9 and, 957
Lungs and, 131, 131b
Blue face colour, 316, 316b
Blue tongue, 327
Bluish-purple tongue, 326, 327f
Blurred vision, 359
Bodily secretions, odour of, 399–400
Body, 352b
cavities, Triple Burner as, 226–229, 227f–229f, 229b
Defensive-Qi portion of, Summer-Heat and, 737
diagnosis by observation, 307–311, 311b
Five-Element types of, 307–311
movements and demeanour, 313, 313b
sides, Yang Linking Vessel and, 935
signs, 311, 312f, 313b
symptoms, 349–352
three divisions of, Triple Burner as, 224–226, 225f, 226b
see also Balancing; Constitution

Body and Mind interaction, 254, 254f–255f, 255b
Body fluids (*Jin-Ye*), 66–70
and Bladder, 68
and Blood, 69–70, 70f
deficiency of, 476–477, 476b–477b, 477f
descending of, 132, 132b–133b, 132f
diffusing of, 131–132, 131f, 132b
and Kidneys, 67–68
loss of, 627
and Lungs, 67, 131–132
pathology of, 70, 70b
pattern identification, 476–481
and Qi, 69, 69f, 131–132, 131f, 132b
and Blood, pattern identification, 448, 469–481, 469b
relations with internal organs, 67–68
retention of. *see* Oedema
and Small Intestine, 68
source of, 66–67, 67f
and Spleen, 67, 68f
and Stomach, 68
and Triple Burner, 68
types of, 69, 69b
see also Fluids; Water
Body hair, Lungs manifest in, 137, 137b, 138f
Body odour, 399
Body structures, Yin-Yang and, 9–11, 9f, 9t
'Bone diseases', 1032
Bone Painful Obstruction Syndrome, G.B.-39 and, 1115
Bones, 242–243, 243b
entering-exiting of Qi in, 83, 83b
extraordinary vessels, 871
Kidneys controlling, 158–160, 160b
Marrow and, 242
Borborygmi, diagnosis by, 398
Brain, 240–241, 240f
extraordinary vessels, 871
functions of, 241b
Governing Vessel nourishes, 894
Kidney-Essence and, 159b–160b, 159f
Kidneys filling up, 158–160, 160b
Marrow and, 242
Mind in, 112
see also Sea of Marrow
Breast
female, Penetrating Vessel and, 911–912, 912f
lumps, 393b–394b
palpating, 393–394
problems, ST-18 Rugen *Breast Root* and, 978
Breath odour, 399–400, 400b
Breathing, 139
diagnosis by, 398
equalizing, 382
Bright Yang
channels
cross-needling in shoulder-hip, elbow-knee and wrist-ankle correspondence in, 1201f
shoulder-hip, elbow-knee and wrist-ankle correspondence in, 1201f
Heat in, 789, 789b
Latent Heat, 779

patterns
  channel, 757–758, 757f, 758b
  channel and organ, differences between, 759t
  organ, 758–759, 758f, 759b
  stage, 757–759

C

Cannabis, 294
Catarrh, chronic, in children, 371
Causes of disease, 248, 248f
  external, 267–278, 267b
  internal, 251–266, 251b–252b
  miscellaneous, 279–295, 279b
  of pain, 344b
Central Qi (Zhong Qi), 56, 56b
'Centre of the thorax,' Pericardium as, 524–528
Centripetal forces, of Gui, 1034
Channel(s)
  Bladder, 1027–1061
    connecting pathway of, 1027, 1028f
    main pathway of, 1027, 1027f
    points, 1028b
  Dampness in, 738
    chronic, 742
  diagnosis by observation of, 331–332, 332b
  ebb and flow of Yin and Yang in, 1195f
  invasion of acute, external Dampness in, 741
  invasion of Cold in, 734
  invasion of Wind in, 731
  Lungs and, 131, 131b
  non-substantial Phlegm, 478–479
  pathology of ascending/descending of Qi in, 429–431, 430f
  pathology of entering/exiting of Qi in, 432–433, 432f, 432t, 433f
  pathology/patterns
    Bright Yang, 757–758, 757f, 758b
    Greater Yang stage, 754–755
    identification of, 794–805, 795b
    Latent Heat bright Yang type, 779
    multiple, simultaneous, 885
  Pericardium as, 170–171, 170f
  problems, 1198–1201
    HE-4 Lingdao Spirit Path and, 1009
  Transporting points, 829
  vs. organs, 795–797, 796f
  in pulse diagnosis, 378f, 379
  Yang, and DU-20 Baihui Hundred Meetings, 1155
  see also specific channels
Chest, 352–353, 352f
  pain, 353
    LU-1 and, 950
  palpating, 392–394, 393b
Childbirth, 370
  Blood rebelling upwards after, 815
  Kidney-Essence deficiency, 634
  Kidney-Qi not firm, 630
Childhood, cause of disease, 249
Children's symptoms, 370–372, 371b
Chinese and Western medicine, emotions in, 251–253, 252f–253f
Chinese herbs, overdosage of, 627–628
Chinese medical theory, 205
Chinese medicine
  Five Elements in, 26–41
  general theory of, 2

nature of 'symptoms' in, 337
vs. Western medicine, in exterior pathogenic factor, 269
Choppy (Se) pulse, 385, 385b
Chronic cases
  balancing front and back, 1207
  distal and local points, 1196
    channel, 1201
    organ, 1202
Chronic conditions, complicated, 885
Chronic constipation, SP-15 Daheng Big Horizontal Stroke and, 1005
Chronic Dampness, 741, 742b
Chronic diseases
  Back Transporting (Shu) points, 853
  and Spleen-Qi deficiency, 599
Chronic illness
  Kidney, 624–625, 627, 632, 636
  Stomach-Qi deficiency and, 655
'Classic of Difficulties'
  pulse position in, 376t, 377f
  source (Yuan) points, 847, 847f, 848f
  Transporting (Shu) points, 834–835, 835b, 841t
Clear discharge, Cold and, 733–734
Clear Qi, 1179b
Climate(s)
  application in clinical practice, 30
  correspondences of the Five Elements, 26t
  in diagnosis, Five Elements, 37, 37b
  as external cause of disease, 267b–269b, 268–269, 268f
  and Spleen-Qi deficiency, 599
  see also External pathogenic factors; specific factors
Climatic factors, as patterns of disharmony, 271–272, 272b, 272f
Cocaine, 294
Cognition, 71
Cold, 457–459, 732–736, 751
  attack of, 755, 756b
  characteristics of, 734b
  Directing and Penetrating Vessels deficient and, 811
  exterior, 454, 454b
  external, 733f, 735b, 735f
  feeling, 359–360, 360b
  Fetus, 815
  and Heat
    alternating, 361
    combined, 460–461
    extraordinary channels, 886
    mutual consuming of Yin-Yang, 16b
    Yin-Yang imbalance, 12
  internal, 733f, 735–736
  and Kidney, 165
  in Large Intestine, 687, 694–695, 694b–695b, 694f–695f, 698–699, 698b–699b, 698f–699f
  L.I.-1 and, 962
  LU-7 and, 954
  Lungs and, 141
  pain, 344
  seasons and, 725
  and Small Intestine, 684–685, 684b–685b, 684f
  sores, 351

stagnation
  in Liver channel, 546–547, 547f, 548b
  in Uterus, 814
  Stomach and, 654, 657–658, 657f–658f, 658b, 664b–665b, 664f–665f
  symptoms and signs of invasion of, 276
  transformation, Lesser Yin stage, 761, 761f, 762b
  Uterus deficient and, 813–814
  Wind and, 729
  see also Aversion to Cold; Cold-Dampness; Cold-Phlegm; Wind-Cold
Cold-Dampness, invading Spleen, 608–610, 608f–609f, 609b–610b
Cold feet, 355, 391b
Cold foods, 291, 653
Cold hands, 355, 355b, 391b
Cold-Phlegm, 480
  in Lungs, 587–589, 587f–588f, 588b–589b
Collapse
  of Large Intestine, 699–701, 699b–700b, 700f
  of Yang, 778, 778b
  of Yin, 778, 778b
Collecting (Mu) points, front, 854–855, 855t, 857–858, 858b
Colour(s)
  application in clinical practice, 30
  correspondences of the Five Elements, 26t
  in diagnosis
    Five Elements, 34–35, 35b
    menstrual blood, 369
    urine, 347
  of ears, 319
  of eyes, 317, 317f
  of face, 313–316
  of Liver, 125
  of Lungs, 141
  of mouth, 319
  of nose, 318
  of skin, 324
  Spleen, 151
  of tongue-body, 325–327
  of tongue coating, 330
Command points, 864–865
Complexion
  Heart manifests in, 109, 109b
  lustre and moisture, 314, 314b
  normal attributes of, 314–315, 315b
  organs and, 114, 125
Conception, 47
  weak constitution and, 280
Conduction, Large Intestine controls passage and, 205, 206b
Connecting channels, 848
  Bladder, 800
  diagnosis by observation of, 331, 332b
  Gall Bladder, 802
  of Governing Vessel, 893
  Heart, 799
  Kidneys, 801
  Large Intestine, 798
  Liver, 803–805
  Lungs, 797
  Pericardium, 802
  Small Intestine, 800
  and source (Yuan) points, 848, 849f
  Spleen, 799

1270

Stomach, 798–799
Triple Burner, 802
Connecting *(Luo)* points, 848–853, 853*b*
Consciousness, 71, 241
Constipation, 346, 346*b*
  Lung-Qi and, 955
Constitution, 283*b*
  assessment of, 282–283
  Essence as basis of strength, 49
  hereditary, 280, 280*f*
  importance in health and disease, 279
  Kidneys, hereditary weakness, 623, 632, 634, 636
  Lung-Qi deficiency and, 574, 574*f*
  prenatal, 281
  Stomach-Yin deficiency and, 659
  weak, 279–283
Constitutional traits, observation of, 304–306, 307*b*
Contraction
  Cold and, 733
  of limbs, 322, 322*b*
Controlling sequence, Five Elements, 24, 24*f*, 27–28, 27*f*
Convulsions, 127, 727
Corporeal Soul *(Po)*, 101, 111, 1034, 1048
  entering-exiting of Qi, 81
  Lungs house, 138–140, 139*f*, 140*b*
Cosmological sequence, Five Elements, 23, 28–30, 29*b*, 29*f*
Cough, diagnosis by, 398
Cracked tongue, 329, 329*f*–330*f*
Cyclical movement, Yin-Yang as phases, 5–6, 5*f*–6*f*, 5*t*

D

Damp(ness), 151, 151*b*, 545, 545*b*, 598*b*, 737–743, 739*b*
  and Blood stasis, in Directing and Penetrating Vessels, 811–812
  in channels, 738
  characteristics of, 737
  classification of, 740*f*
  climatic, 737
  dirty, 738
  external, 739–741, 741*b*
  external Summer-Heat with, 741
  in Gall Bladder, 704–706, 704*b*, 704*f*
    acupuncture for, 705
    aetiology of, 704
    clinical manifestations of, 704
    diet and, 704
    external pathogenic factors and, 704
    pathological developments from pattern, 705
    pathological precursors of pattern of, 705, 705*f*
    pathology of, 704–705, 705*f*
    treatment for, 705–706
  heavy, 738
  internal, 739, 741–742, 742*b*
  in internal organs, 738
  in Large Intestine, 687
  L.I.-11 and, 967
  with Liver-Qi stagnation, 617–620, 618*b*–619*b*, 618*f*–619*f*
  in Lower Burner, 918–919
  in Lungs, 572–573
  manifestations of, 738*b*, 739*f*

and Phlegm, differences between, 743
Qi and, 416*f*
  External Wind and, 417*f*
qualities of, 738*b*
seasons and, 725
skin and, 738
SP-3 Taibai *Supreme White* and, 997
SP-6 Sanyinjiao *Three Yin Meeting* and, 1000
Spleen loathes, 152
sticky, 738–739
Summer-Heat and, 737
symptoms and signs of, 997
  invasion, 276–277
in Uterus, 814
Damp-Cold, in Bladder, 716–718
  acupuncture for, 717–718
  aetiology of, 717
  clinical manifestations of, 716–717, 717*b*, 717*f*
  pathological precursors of pattern in, 717, 718*f*
  pathology of, 717
  treatment for, 717–718
Damp-Heat, 772, 772*b*
  in Bladder, 714–716, 715*f*, 716*b*, 718*b*
    acupuncture for, 716
    aetiology of, 714
    case history for, 716*b*
    clinical manifestations of, 714, 714*b*
    emotional strain and, 714
    exterior pathogenic factors and, 714, 714*b*
    herbal formula for, 716, 718
    pathological developments from pattern, 715
    pathological precursors of pattern, 715, 715*f*
    pathology of, 715
    REN-3 Zhongji *Middle Pole*, 1131
    treatment for, 715–716
  in Directing and Penetrating Vessels, 812–813
  expelling, 1185
  in Gall Bladder, 706–707, 706*b*–708*b*, 706*f*–707*f*
  and Liver, 710–712, 710*b*–711*b*, 710*f*–711*f*
  in Large Intestine, 688–690, 688*b*–690*b*, 689*f*–690*f*
    case history of, 690*b*
    L.I.-11 and, 967
  in Liver, 544–546, 544*b*, 545*f*–546*f*, 546*b*
  in Small Intestine, 988
  in Spleen, 610–612, 610*b*–612*b*, 610*f*–611*f*, 789, 790*b*
  in Stomach, 667–668, 667*b*–668*b*, 667*f*–668*f*
  and Spleen, 775, 775*b*
Damp-Phlegm, 479
  in Lungs, 585–587, 585*b*, 585*f*–586*f*, 587*b*
Dannangxue *Gall Bladder Point*, 1167, 1167*b*, 1167*f*
Dashu, 1032
Deafness, 358
  S.I.-19 Tinggong *Listening Palace* and, 1026
Decision-making, Gall Bladder controls, 210–211, 212*f*
Deep *(Chen)* pulse, 384, 384*b*
Deep-red tongue, 326

Defensive Qi *(Wei Qi)*, 55, 55*b*, 1028
  circadian rhythm and, Yin and Yang Stepping Vessels and, 930, 931*f*
  extraordinary vessels and, 870–871, 870*f*, 871*b*, 930
  Four Levels, 767, 770–773
  function, 58
  Kidney-Yin deficiency, 628
  Lung-Qi and, 136–137, 428, 428*b*, 428*f*
  'Lung's Defensive Qi portion', 453
  and Nutritive Qi, 11, 55–56, 56*b*, 56*f*, 755
  Triple Burner and, 221, 223, 229
  Wind-Cold invasion of Lungs and, 579–580
  Yang and Yin Linking Vessels and, combined pathology of, 936
Deficiency/excess conditions, extraordinary channels, 886
Density of matter, Yin-Yang as states of, 6–7, 7*t*
Depression, 362–363, 364*b*
  SP-1 Yinbai *Hidden White* and, 996
Descending branch, of Penetrating Vessel *(Chong Mai)*, 906–907
Development, Essence, 48–49
Deviated tongue, 329
Diagnosis, 298–299
  by hearing and smelling, 397–400, 397*b*
  by interrogation, 335–372, 335*b*
  by observation, 301–333, 301*b*
  by palpation, 373–396, 373*b*
Diaphragm, Phlegm-Fluids above, 480–481, 480*f*
Diarrhoea, 346–347, 346*b*
Diet, 290–292, 292*b*
  Blood deficiency and, 496, 548, 565, 612
  Gall Bladder and, 703
    Damp-Heat in, 706
    Dampness in, 704
  and Liver, Damp-Heat in, 710
  Heart and, 496, 500, 502, 508, 565, 612
  Kidney-Yang deficiency and, 625, 636
  Large Intestine and, 688
    Damp-Heat, 688
    Dry, 697
    Qi stagnation, 695
  Liver and, 531, 535, 537, 543, 545, 548, 553, 560, 565
  Lungs and, 573, 578, 586, 588–589, 591, 593, 614
  Mind and, 505
  Pericardium and, 520, 522
  Small Intestine and, 677
    Full-Heat, 679
    Small Intestine-Qi pain, 680
  Spleen and, 560, 598, 612, 614
  Spleen-Qi deficiency and, 599
  Stomach and, 653–654
    and Cold, 657
    Damp-Heat in, 667
    Heat, 663
    Qi deficiency, 655
    Qi rebelling upwards, 666
    Qi stagnation, 660
    Yin deficiency, 659
  see also Eating; Food
Digestion
  Kidneys warming the Stomach and Spleen to aid, 164
  smooth flow of Liver-Qi and, 121, 121*f*–122*f*, 122*b*

Digestive symptoms, in children, 370
Dingchuan *Stopping Asthma*, 1162, 1162f, 1163b
Directing Vessel *(Ren Mai)*, 808, 808f, 877b, 877f, 897–901, 897f, 1129–1145, 1129b
　activates Triple Burner, 898–899
　case history of, 901b–902b
　classical indications of, 900–901, 901b
　clinical applications of, 898–900, 900b
　connecting channel pathway, 1129, 1129f
　controls fat tissue and membranes, 899, 899b
　descending of Lung-Qi and Kidneys' receiving of Qi and, 898
　epigastric points in, 980
　and Governing Vessel, 876–878, 883–884, 892, 900
　herbs/herbal therapy for, 808, 901
　LU-7 and, 955
　main channel pathway, 1129, 1129f
　moves Qi in Lower Burner and Uterus, 898
　nourishes Yin, 898
　pathway of, 897, 897b
　and Penetrating Vessel, 876–877
　　combined patterns, 810
　　comparison and differentiation of, 914, 914f–915f
　points, 897
　　combination of, 900
　　target areas, 1145f
　regulates Uterus and Blood, 898
　transformation, transportation and excretion of fluids and, 898
　Uterus and, 236–237, 236f, 237b
Directions
　application in clinical practice, 30
　correspondences of the Five Elements, 26t
Dirty Dampness, 738
Disease, causes of
　external, 267–278, 267b
　internal, 251–266, 251b–252b
　miscellaneous, 279–295, 279b
Disharmony, 455
　and climatic factors, 271–272, 272b, 272f
　in Liver, internal Wind and, 732
　in observation of constitutional traits, 304
Distal point
　areas affected by, 1198f
　balancing, 1195–1202, 1196f
　　according to area, 1197t
　choice of, 1199
　Du-26 as, for backache, 1199f
　G.B.-39 as, for neck, 1200f
　pairing, 1196
　ST-38 as, for shoulder, 1200f
Distension
　abdominal, 695b
　epigastric, 660b
　Liver-Qi stagnation and, 532, 532b, 532f
　Qi stagnation and, 405, 471
Distinct face colour, 316, 316f
Dizziness, 350, 350b
　ST-8 Touwei *Head Corner* and, 977
Domestic animals, correspondences of the Five Elements, 26t
Dreams
　and Bladder, 216
　and Gall Bladder, 213
　and Heart, 115

　and Kidney, 165
　and Large Intestine, 206
　and Liver, 126
　and Lungs, 141
　and Small Intestine, 202
　and Spleen, 151–153
　and Stomach, 198, 198b
　and Triple Burner, 230
Drugs
　medicinal, 293, 294f
　recreational, 294
　Stomach-Yin deficiency and, 659
Dry(ness), 743–745
　clinical manifestations of, 743
　exterior, 577–578
　external, 744
　internal, 744f
　internal causes of, 744b
　and Kidneys, 166
　and Large Intestine, 697, 697b–698b, 697f
　and Lungs, 141, 572
　seasons and, 725
　and Spleen, 152–153
　symptoms and signs of invasion of, 277
　and Wetness, 12
Dry eyes, 359
Dry-Heat, 772–773, 773b
Dry-Phlegm, in Lungs, 591–592, 591b–592b, 591f–592f
Dry skin, in diagnosis by observation, 324
Drying Fire, 747
DU-1 Changqiang *Long Strength*, 1148, 1148b
DU-2 Yaoshu *Transporting Point of Lower Back*, 1148, 1148b
DU-3 Yaoyangguan *Lumbar Yang Gate*, 1148–1149, 1149b
DU-4 Mingmen *Gate of Life*, 1149–1150, 1150b
DU-8 Jinsuo *Tendon Spasm*, 1150, 1150b
DU-9 Zhiyang *Reaching Yang*, 1151, 1151b
DU-11 Shendao *Mind Way*, 1151, 1151b
DU-12 Shenzhu *Body Pillar*, 1151–1152, 1152b
DU-13 Taodao *Kiln Way*, 1152, 1152b
DU-14 Dazhui *Big Vertebra*, 1152–1153, 1153b
DU-15 Yamen *Door to Dumbness*, 1153, 1153b
DU-16 Fengfu *Wind Palace*, 1154, 1154b
DU-17 Naohu *Brain Window*, 1154, 1154b
DU-19 Houding *Posterior Vertex*, 1155, 1155b
DU-20 Baihui *Hundred Meetings*, 1155, 1156b
DU-23 Shangxing *Upper Star*, 1156, 1156b
DU-24 Shenting *Mind Courtyard*, 1156, 1156b
DU-26 Renzhong *Middle of Person*, 1157, 1157b
Dysmenorrhoea, ST-29 Guilai *Return* and, 982–983

E

Earache, in children, 370–371
Ear(s), 358, 358b
　diagnosis by observation, 319, 319b
　distal and local points, 1197t
　Kidney channels and Triple Burner channels in, 1088
　Kidneys open into, 161, 161b
　microsystem in diagnosis, 302, 304f
　problems, Yang Linking Vessel and, 935–936
　symptoms, 358–359
　see also Hearing

Earth
　body type, 307–308, 309b, 309f
　insulting Wood, 823
　not generating Metal, 822
　overacting on Water, 822
　role in seasonal cycle, 30
'Earth mechanism', 1002
Eating
　conditions of, 292, 654, 654b
　insufficient, 291
　see also Diet; Food
Ecstasy, 294
Eight Extraordinary Vessels, 867–887, 867b–868b, 889–939, 889b–890b
　clinical use of, 880–887, 884b, 886b
　functions of, 868–874, 874b
　pattern identification according to, 794, 807–819
　and six extraordinary Yang organs, 871–872
　use of, 885–887
Eight Principles, pattern identification of, 448, 451–467, 451b, 453b
Ejaculation, recommended frequency of, 286t
Elbow problems, S.I.-7 Zhizheng *Branch to Heart Channel* and, 1020
Elements. *see* Five Elements.
Emotion(s)
　application in clinical practice, 31
　as cause of disease, 253–254, 254b
　correspondences of the Five Elements, 26t
　in diagnosis, Five Elements, 36, 36b
　effects on body, 257–258, 258f, 259b
　internal organs and, 99–100, 99f–100f, 100b
　Liver and, 531
　Liver-Qi and, smooth flow of, 120–121
　Lungs and, 573
　Mind *(Shen)* and, 177, 177f
　positive counterpart of, 255
　Qi mechanism and, 427
　questions, 341
　symptoms, 361–366
Emotional frame, at meal times, 654
Emotional problems
　LU-7 and, 955
　Lung- and Heart-Qi deficiency and, 594
Emotional stress/strain
　Bladder patterns and, 713
　Blood deficiency and, 496, 518, 548, 565, 612
　Blood stasis, 510
　Damp-Heat and
　　in Bladder, 714
　　in Gall Bladder, 706
　　in Gall Bladder and Liver, 710
　Gall Bladder and, 703
　Heart, 498, 500, 502, 507
　Heart-Blood, 496, 510, 612
　Heart-Blood deficiency and, 565
　Heart-Vessel, 508
　Kidney, 623
　and Large Intestine, 687–688
　　Damp-Heat, 688–689
　　Qi stagnation, 696
　Liver and, 532–533, 535, 537, 543, 553, 560
　Liver-Blood deficiency and, 548, 565
　Lungs and, 574, 576, 590
　Pericardium and, 518, 520, 522, 525

Qi stagnation and, 405
on Small Intestine, 677–678
  Full-Heat, 679
  Small Intestine-Qi pain, 680
Spleen and, 560, 598, 612
and Spleen-Qi deficiency, 599
Stomach and, 654, 654b
  Damp-Heat in, 667
  Heat, 663
  Qi rebelling upwards, 660b
  Qi stagnation, 660, 660b
see also Fear; Mental-emotional problems; Pensiveness; Worry
Emptiness, of Girdle Vessel, 920, 920b
Empty Blood, 463, 464b
  case history in, 463b
Empty-Cold, 359, 408, 459, 459f, 460b, 736
  case history in, 460b
  clinical manifestations of, 360b
  Full-Cold and, 459t, 732, 733f, 736t
  main clinical manifestations of, 736
  origin of, 736f
Empty conditions/patterns, 411–412, 412b, 461–464
  of Bladder, 718–721
  depression, 362
  Directing and Penetrating Vessels, 810
  of Gall Bladder, 708–709
  Heart, 491
  of Liver, 548–552
  of Lungs, 573–578
  pain, 343
  Small Intestine, 684–685
see also Full/Empty conditions/patterns
Empty Fire, vs. full-Fire, 749, 749b, 749t
Empty-Heat, 456–457, 457b–458b, 457f, 638–640, 638b, 638f–639f, 640b, 644
  case history in, 457b
  in Directing and Penetrating Vessels, 812
  from Kidneys, 1065
  manifestations of, 639f
  nourishing Yin and clearing, 808
  Stomach-Yin deficiency and, 658
  Yin deficiency and, 422–423
Empty Qi, 462–463, 463b
  case history in, 463b
Empty symptoms, of Connecting channels, 851, 852t
Empty-Wind agitating interior, 777–778, 778b
Empty (Xu) pulse, 384, 385b
Empty Yang, 463, 463b
  case history in, 463b
Empty Yin, 464, 464b
  case history in, 464b–465b
Energetic actions, of points, Transporting points, 832–833
Energetic dynamics, of extraordinary vessels, 874–880, 874t–875t, 875f–876f, 878b
Energetic influence, of Connecting points, 851–853, 853b
Energy levels, 348–349, 348b
  questions on, 342
see also Tiredness
Enuresis, LU-5 and, 953
Epigastric distension, 660b
Epigastric fullness, ST-19 Burong Full and, 979
Epigastrium, 353
  discomfort in, in Stomach deficient and Cold, 657b

Essence (Jing), 46–50
  as basis of Kidney-Qi, 49, 49f
  common root of Mind and, 178, 179f
  and Kidney, 623
  pathology of entering/exiting of Qi in, 435–436, 436b
  Post-Heaven, 48, 157, 158f
  Pre-Heaven, 47–48, 47f, 157, 158f
  relationship with Blood, 66
  storage in Kidneys, 48–50
  types of, 46b
Essence-Qi-Mind (Jing-Qi-Shen), 30
Ethereal Soul (Hun), 100, 111, 1053
  in depression, 362–363
  entering-exiting of Qi and, 83–84, 84f
  Liver and, 111
  Liver-Blood deficiency and, 549, 566
  Liver houses, 124–125, 124f
  Liver-Qi and, smooth flow of, 120–121
  and Mind (Shen), 120–121, 177, 355f
  relationship between Gall Bladder and, 212f
  and REN-4 Guanyuan Gate of the Original Qi, 1132
  in sleep disturbance, 355
Excitement-inhibition, 12
Exercise, lack of, 285
Expelling pathogenic factors, 1181–1182, 1181b–1182b
  tonifying Upright Qi and, 1182–1184
    expelling pathogenic factors first then tonifying Upright Qi, 1182–1184, 1183b
    simultaneously tonifying Upright Qi and expelling pathogenic factors, 1184, 1184b
    tonifying Upright Qi first then expelling pathogenic factors, 1182, 1184b
'Explanation of the Acupuncture Points', 1049, 1053
Exterior, of body
  case history in, 455b
  definition of, 453
Exterior Cold, 454, 454b
  Heat in, 460
Exterior dryness, 577–578
Exterior-interior
  of body, Yin-Yang, 10
  patterns, 453–455
Exterior pathogenic factors, 267, 344
  Bladder deficient and Cold, 718
  Bladder patterns and, 713
  clinical manifestations of, 272–274, 273f, 274b
  consequences of invasion of, 277–278, 277b
  Damp-Heat in Bladder and, 714, 714b
  Heart, 490
  Large Intestine, 687
    Dry, 697
  in Lungs, 572–574, 572b, 579, 586, 588, 590
  penetration of, 272f–273f
  of Pericardium, 490, 515–517, 516b, 516f
  Spleen, 598
  Stomach, 654–655, 657
  symptoms and signs of, 276–277
  in Western and Chinese medicine, 269
Exterior patterns, 453
  clinical manifestations of, 453–455, 454b
  Empty, 454, 454b, 729
  Full, 454, 454b

Heat, 454, 454b
  Cold in, 460
  in tonifying Upright Qi and expelling pathogenic factors, 1183
Exterior Wind, Governing Vessel expels, 895–896
External causes of disease, 267–278, 267b
  vs. internal causes, 254, 254f
External Cold, 733f, 734, 735b, 735f
External Damp-Heat, invasion of, at Defensive Qi level, 741
External Dampness, 739–741, 741b
External Dryness, 744
External Heat, 498
External pathogenic factors, 403–404, 404b, 404f
  and Damp-Heat in Gall Bladder, 706
  and Liver, 710
  Gall Bladder and, 703–704
    Dampness in, 704
  Liver, 530–531, 530b–531b
see also Climate(s); Pathogenic factors; specific factors
External Wind, 727–731
  invasions of, 729f, 732b
Extraordinary vessels. see Eight Extraordinary Vessels; specific vessels
Extraordinary Yang organs, 234–245, 235b
Eye(s), 358–359, 359b
  area, distal and local points, 1197t
  diagnosis by observation of, 317–318, 317f–318f, 318b
  extraordinary vessels and, 930, 930f
  L.I.-1 and, 962
  Liver-Blood moistens, 119–120, 119f
  Liver opens into, 123, 123b
  symptoms, 358–359
  and Wood (and Liver), 31
  Yang Stepping Vessel and, 927
Eye problems
  ST-1 Chengqi Containing Tears and, 974
  ST-2 Sibai Four Whites and, 975
Eye system, 863f, 864b
  extraordinary vessels and, 929, 929f
  points, 863–864, 863f–864f, 864b

F

Face, 350–351
  areas, 316–317
    distal and local points, 1197t
  colour, 313–316
  feeling of Heat in, 350
  L.I.-4 and, 963
  LU-7 and, 955
  microsystem in diagnosis, 302, 302f–303f
  pain, 350–351, 350b
  paralysis of
    G.B.-14 and, 1105
    ST-3 Juliao Great Crevice and, 975
    ST-4 Dicang Earth Granary and, 975
    ST-6 Jiache Jaw Chariot and, 976
    ST-7 Xiaguan Lower Gate and, 976
  Wind and, 728, 731, 731b
  symptoms, 349–352
see also Complexion
Fat tissue (Gao)
  Directing Vessel controls, 899
  entering/exiting of Qi in, 83
  pathology of, 437–438, 437b

Fear, 264–265, 264f, 265b
    of cold, 275
    symptoms of, 363–364, 365b
Feelings, 72
Feet
    cold, 391b
    palpation of, 390–391
    Qi circulation to, Penetrating Vessel and, 913
Fetus, 239
    Cold, 815
    Heat, 814–815
Fever, 359–361
    aversion to Cold and, 275–276, 275f, 276b
    intermittent, Yang Linking Vessel and, 935
    simultaneous aversion, 361
    Stomach-Yin deficiency and, 659
    Wind invasion and, 728–729
Fine (Xi) pulse, 386, 386b
Finger(s)
    diagnosis of, in babies, 323–324, 323f
    Pericardium and Triple Burner channel connection in, 1088, 1088f
Fire, 411, 411b, 543f, 745–750
    aetiology of, 746f
    body type, 307, 308b, 308f
    drying, 747
    Full vs. Empty, 749, 749b, 749t
    general clinical manifestations of, 747–748
    and Heart, 31
    and Heat, 410
        differences between, 746–747
    insulting Water, 823
    Kidneys as origin of, 157f
    main characteristics of, 747b
    nature of, 746
    not generating Earth, 822
    organs affected by, 748, 748f
    overacting on Metal, 822
    as pathogenic factor, 747
    pathological, 745f
    physiological, 745f
    related to tongue, 31
    seasons and, 726
    symptoms and signs of invasion of, 277
    and Water, mutual assistance of, 11–12, 178
Fire of the Gate of Life (Ming Men), 77f, 78b
    and Essence, 77, 77f
    functions of, 164b–165b
    and Gathering Qi, 77, 77f
    Kidney-Qi not firm, 630
    for Qi transformation, 76–78, 78b
    storage in Kidney, 156
Firm (Lao) pulse, 387, 387b
Five Command points, 864–865, 864b
Five Elements, 19–41, 19b
    in acupuncture treatment, 38–39
    as basic qualities, 22, 22b
    body types, 307–311
    in Chinese medicine, 26–41
    correspondences, 25, 25f–26f, 26t, 311, 311b
    in diagnosis, 34–37
    in herbal and diet therapy, 39–41, 40f
    historical development of, 20
    interrelationships, 23–25
    as movements, 22, 22b, 22f
    in nature, 20–25
    nature of, 20b
    odours, 399b

in pathology, 31–34
pattern identification according to, 794, 821–823, 821b
in physiology, 26–31
    system correspondences in, 30–31
sounds and smells, 398f
as stages of seasonal cycle, 22–23, 23b, 23f
and Transporting (Shu) points, 838–839, 841b
treatment according to
    Five Transporting points, 39, 39f
    various sequences, 38–39, 38f
'Five-palm Heat', 457
Five Transporting points (Shu points), 829–843, 829b, 834b
Flaccid tongue, 328
Flaccidity of limbs, 321–322, 322b, 354
Floating face colour, 316, 316b
Floating (Fu) pulse, 383–384, 384f
    Greater Yang stage, 753–754, 754f
Fluids, 69
    excretion of, Triple Burner and, 222–223, 222b–223b, 222f
    origin, Stomach, 197, 197b
    reabsorption by Large Intestine, 206, 206b
    and REN-9 Shuifen Water Separation, 1138
    separation, Small Intestine, 202, 202b, 202f
    thirst and drink, 347, 348b
    transformation/transportation
        and excretion, Directing Vessel and, 898
        Spleen, 144–145, 145b, 146f
Food, 345b
    modern changes in, 290–291
    nature of, 653, 653b
    Pre-Heaven Essence, 48
    retention of, 344, 668–672, 669b–670b, 669f
    'rotting and ripening' of, 194, 194b, 198, 224–226
    Sea of Food, 872
    and taste, 345, 345b
    types and energetic effect of, 291–292
Food essences, transportation of, 144–145, 194–195, 195b–196b, 195f, 243
Food-Qi (Gu Qi), 52–53, 53b
    and Blood, 52, 52f
    and Gathering Qi, 52f, 53–54
    and Spleen, 143, 182
        transformation/transportation, 144–145
Forgetfulness, LU-3 and, 951
Four crevices, 1046
'Four Flowers', 1037
'Four Gates', 964
Four Levels
    pattern identification according to, 724, 765–785, 765b, 767f, 779b
    Six Stages and Three Burners, relationship between, 781–785, 782f–784f
    theory of, 270, 270b, 271f
Four Seas, 243–245, 244b
    and extraordinary vessels, 872, 873b
    points of, 244b, 859–860, 860b
    symptoms of, 244b
Front and back of body
    balancing, 1207
    Yin-Yang, 9
Front-collecting (Mu) points, 854–855, 855t, 857–858, 858b

Frontal headaches, ST-8 Touwei Head Corner and, 977
Full-Cold, 359, 408, 457–459, 458f, 459b, 735–736
    case history in, 459b
    clinical manifestations of, 359b, 735
    in Directing and Penetrating Vessels, 813
    and Empty-Cold, 459t, 732, 733f, 736t
Full conditions/patterns, 411, 412b, 412f, 461–462, 462b
    of Bladder, 714–718
    of Gall Bladder, 704–707
    of Large Intestine, 688–696
    of Liver, 532–547
    of Lungs
        exterior, 579–584
        interior, 584–593
        pain, 343
    of Small Intestine, 678–683
    of Spleen, 608–612
    of Stomach, 660–672
        ST-19 Burong Full and, 979
        ST-20 Chengman Supporting Fullness and, 979
Full/empty conditions/patterns, 412–415, 413b, 461–464, 461b
    of Liver, 552–559
    mixed, 462, 462b
    pathogenic factors and, interactions of, 403, 415–417
        no pathogenic factor-deficient Upright Qi, 413, 413b
        no pathogenic factor-normal Upright Qi, 413, 413b
        strong pathogenic factor-deficient Upright Qi, 414, 414b
        strong pathogenic factor-strong Upright Qi and, 413–414, 414b
        weak pathogenic factor-deficient Upright Qi, 415, 415b
        weak pathogenic factor-strong Upright Qi, 414–415, 415b
Full-Fire, vs. empty Fire, 749, 749b, 749t
Full-Heat, 455–456, 455f–456f, 456b
    case history in, 456b
    in Directing and Penetrating Vessels, 812
    and Empty-Heat, 458t
    in Small Intestine, 678–680, 678b, 679f, 680b
    taste and, 345
Full (Shi) pulse, 385, 385b
Full symptoms, of Connecting channels, 851, 852t
Fullness
    feeling of, 979
    of Girdle Vessel, 920, 920b

G

Gall Bladder, 243
    area, distal and local points, 1197t
    aspects of, 211–213
    controls decisiveness, 210–211, 211b
    controls sinews, 211
    Damp-Heat in, 706–707, 706b–708b, 706f–707f
    Dampness in, 704–706, 704b, 704f–705f, 706b, 742
    deficient, 706f, 708–709, 708b–709b, 708f–709f

and DU-9 Zhiyang *Reaching Yang*, 1151
extraordinary vessels, 871
as extraordinary Yang organ, 243
functions of, 209–213, 209b
Heat in, 774–775, 775b
herbal formula for, 709
invasion of external Dampness in, 741
relationship between Ethereal Soul and, 212f
relationship between Heart and, 211f
and Small Intestine, 203, 203f
storage and excretion of bile by, 209–210, 210f
see also under Liver
Gall Bladder channel, 1099–1118
  connecting channel pathway, 1099, 1100f
  main channel pathway, 1099, 1099f
  patterns, 802–803
  points, overview of, 1100b
  target areas in, 1118f
Gall Bladder patterns, 703–712, 704b
  combined, 710–712
  Empty, 708–709
  Full, 704–707
  general aetiology of, 703–704, 704b
    diet in, 703
    emotional strain and, 703
    external pathogenic factors and, 703–704
Gall Bladder Point Dannangxue, 1167, 1167b, 1167f
Gall Bladder-Qi, ascending of, 210f, 212
Gall Bladder Qi deficiency, HE-7 Shenmen *Mind Door* and, 1011
Gall Bladder stones, non-substantial Phlegm, 479
'Gaohuang', 1073
Gate of life *(Ming Men)*, 163f
  Kidney control of, 162–164, 163f
Gate of Stomach, Kidneys as, 166, 197
Gathering *(Hui)* points, 859, 859b
Gathering Qi *(Zong Qi)*, 53–54, 54b, 133, 133f
  chest palpation, 392–393
  Fire of the Gate of Life and, 77, 77f
  and Food-Qi, 52–53, 52f
  and Lungs, 53, 183–184
  Pericardium and, 518, 518f
  Sea of Qi and, 53–54, 245
  Triple Burner and, 221, 229
G.B.-1 Tongziliao *Pupil Crevice*, 1100, 1100b
G.B.-2 Tinghui *Hearing Convergence*, 1100–1101, 1101b
G.B.-4 Hanyan *Jaw Serenity*, 1101, 1101b
G.B.-5 Xuanlu *Hanging Skull*, 1101, 1101b
G.B.-6 Xuanli *Deviation from Hanging Skull*, 1101–1102, 1102b
G.B.-8 Shuaigu *Leading Valley*, 1102, 1102b
G.B.-9 Tianchong *Penetrating Heaven*, 1102–1103, 1103b
G.B.-11 Touqiaoyin (head) *Yin Orifices*, 1103, 1103b
G.B.-12 Wangu *Whole Bone*, 1103–1104, 1104b
G.B.-13 Benshen *Mind Root*, 1104, 1105b
G.B.-14 Yangbai *Yang White*, 1105, 1105b
G.B.-15 Linqi *Falling Tears*, 1105, 1106b
G.B.-17 Zhengying *Top Convergence*, 1106, 1106b
G.B.-18 Chengling *Spirit Receiver*, 1106, 1106b
G.B.-19 Naokong *Brain Cavity*, 1106–1107, 1107b

G.B.-20 Fengchi *Wind Pool*, 1107–1108, 1108b, 1108f
G.B.-21 Jianjing *Shoulder Well*, 1108–1109, 1109b
G.B.-22 Yuanye *Axilla Abyss*, 1109, 1109b
G.B.-24 Riyue *Sun and Moon*, 1109, 1109b
G.B.-25 Jingmen *Capital Door*, 1110, 1110b
G.B.-26 Daimai *Girdle Vessel*, 1110, 1110b
G.B.-29 Juliao *Squatting Crevice*, 1110–1111, 1111b
G.B.-30 Huantiao *Jumping Circle*, 1111, 1111b
G.B.-31 Fengshi *Wind Market*, 1112, 1112b
G.B.-33 Xiyangguan *Knee Yang Gate*, 1112, 1112b
G.B.-34 Yanglingquan *Yang Hill Spring*, 1112–1113, 1113b, 1117t
G.B.-35 Yangjiao *Yang Crossing*, 1113, 1113b
G.B.-36 Waiqiu *Outer Mound*, 1113–1114, 1114b
G.B.-37 Guangming *Brightness*, 1114, 1114b
G.B.-38 Yangfu *Yang Aid*, 1114, 1114b
G.B.-39 Xuanzhong *Hanging Bell*, 1115, 1115b
G.B.-40 Qiuxu *Mound Ruins*, 1115–1116, 1116b, 1117t
G.B.-41 Zulinqi (foot) *Falling Tears*, 1116, 1116b
G.B.-43 Xiaxi *Stream Insertion*, 1116–1117, 1117b, 1117t
G.B.-44 Zuqiaoyin (foot) *Yin Orifice*, 1117, 1117b, 1117t
Gender, and pulse, 382–383
Generating sequence, Five Elements, 24, 24f, 27–28, 27f–28f, 32–34, 34f
  patterns, 821–822
Ghost points, 862–863, 862t
Girdle Vessel *(Dai Mai)*, 815–816, 816f, 878–880, 878b, 879f–880f, 918–922, 918f, 1110
  abdominal pain and, 920
  affects Qi of Stomach channel in legs, 919, 919f
  case history of, 922b
  classical indications of, 920–921, 921b
  clinical applications of, 918–920, 921b
  energetic sphere of, 919f
  in gynaecology, 920
  harmonizes Liver and Gall Bladder, 918
  herbs/herbal therapy for, 815–816, 921–922
  hips and, 920
  pathway of, 918, 918b
  points of, 918, 918b
  regulates circulation of Qi in legs, 919
  resolves Dampness in Lower Burner, 918–919
Goitre, ascending and descending of Qi and, 951
Gong Sun, 999
Governing Vessel *(Du Mai)*, 807–808, 808f, 877b, 877f, 892–897, 1073, 1147–1157, 1147b
  back and, 893–894
  classical indications of, 896, 896b
  clinical applications of, 893–896, 896b
  connecting channel pathway of, 1147, 1147f
  and Directing Vessel, 876–878, 883–884, 892, 900
  expels exterior Wind, 895–896

extinguishes interior Wind, 896
herbs/herbal therapy for, 807–808, 896–897
main channel pathway of, 1147, 1147f
Mind and, 894–895, 894f
nourishes brain and Marrow, 894, 894f
opening and coupled points, 882–883, 882f
opening point of, 1017, 1018f
pathway of, 892–893, 892f, 893b
points of, 892
  combination of, 900
REN-1 Huiyin *Meeting of Yin*, 1130
target areas of, 1157f
tonifies Kidney-Yang, 893, 895b
Grains, correspondences of the Five Elements, 26t
Gravitational potential energy, 1192
  concept of, 1194, 1194t
Greasy foods, 292
Great connecting channel of Spleen, 799, 996f, 1005
'Great Dictionary of Chinese Acupuncture', 1003–1004
Greater Yang channels, 1031
Greater Yang stage, 753–754, 754b, 754f, 755t
Greater Yin *(Tai Yin)* stage, 760–761, 760f, 761b
Green face colour, 315–316, 316b
Greenish complexion, 125
Grief, 366
  and Heart, 490–491, 491b
  and Lungs, 140, 140b, 140f, 573, 573b, 573f
  see also Sadness
Groaning, 165
Growth
  Essence, 48–49
  Kidneys governing, 157–158, 158b
  Liver influences, 126
'Guan', 1082–1083
'Guest-host', 954
Gui Zhi Tang, 1032
Gums
  bleeding, 351, 351b
  diagnosis by observation, 319, 319b
Gynaecology
  Girdle Vessel and, 920
  see also Directing Vessel *(Ren Mai);* Penetrating Vessel *(Chong Mai)*

H

Haemorrhage, differentiation of causes of, 476t
Hair
  body, Lungs manifest in, 137, 137b, 138f
  diagnosis by, 313
  Kidneys manifesting in, 161, 161b
Hands
  cold, 391b
  diagnosis areas, 391f
  dorsum and palms, comparison, 391
  organ positions in, 392f
  palpation of, 391–392
Hard-soft swellings/masses, 12
Hasty *(Cu)* pulse, 388, 388b
HE-1 Jiquan *Supreme Spring*, 1007–1008, 1008b
HE-3 Shaohai *Lesser-Yin Sea*, 1008, 1008b
HE-4 Lingdao *Spirit Path*, 1008–1009, 1009b

HE-5 Tongli *Inner Communication*, 1009, 1009b, 1009f–1010f
HE-6 Yinxi *Yin Crevice*, 1010, 1010b
HE-7 Shenmen *Mind Door*, 1010–1011, 1011f–1012f, 1012b
  comparison between P-7 Daling and, 1084t
HE-8 Shaofu *Lesser-Yin Mansion*, 1012, 1012b
HE-9 Shaochong *Lesser-Yin Penetrating*, 1013, 1013b
Head
  branch, of Penetrating Vessel (Chong Mai), 906
  diagnosis, 349–350
  and face, diagnosis of, 313–317
  LU-7 and, 955
  symptoms, 349
  Yang and Yin Linking Vessels and, combined pathology of, 936
  Yang Stepping Vessel and, 926–927
Head-body, Yin-Yang, 9–10
Headache, 349–350, 349b
  Greater Yang stage, 753
  in Liver-Yang rising, 552
  soon after orgasm, 368
  Yin Linking Vessel and, 933
Hearing, diagnosis by, 397–399
Heart, 107, 107b
  apical beat, palpating, 392–393
  area, distal and local points, 1197t
  and Blood, 63, 63f
  Blood deficiency, 496–498, 496f–497f, 497b–498b
  Blood stasis and, 474, 510–512, 511f–512f, 512b
    case history in, 512b
  dreams and, 115
  and DU-9 Zhiyang *Reaching Yang*, 1151
  emotions and, 257, 257f, 257f, 490–491, 491b, 491f
    anger, 259–260
    fear, 265
    joy, 112–113, 261, 490
    pensiveness, 264
    shock, 265
  and Emperor-Fire, 31
  external, 498
  functions of, 107–114
  and Gathering Qi, 53
  HE-5 Tongli *Inner Communication* and, 1009, 1009f
  and joy, 112–113, 261, 490
  and Kidneys, 29, 60–61, 61f, 177–179, 180b
    not harmonized, 642–644, 642b, 642f–643f, 644b
  and Liver, 176–177, 177b, 177f
  and Lungs, 28, 133, 134f, 175–176, 175f, 176b
  P-4 action for, 1081
  pathology of ascending/descending of Qi and, 428, 428b, 428f
  Penetrating Vessel and, 912
  Phlegm, non-substantial, 479
  Phlegm-Fire harassing, 502–504, 503b, 503f–504f, 505b
    case history in, 504b–505b
  Phlegm obstructing, 1081

relationships, 114
  between Bladder, Small Intestine and, 216f
  between Gall Bladder and, 211f
  between Pericardium, Liver, Uterus and, 1083f
  role of, in sexual arousal, 368f
  sayings, 115
  and Small Intestine, 202–204, 203b, 203f
  and Spleen, 28, 184–187, 184f, 185b
  sweat and, 102
  tongue related to, 31
  Uterus and, 237, 237b, 237f–238f, 239b
Heart-Blood deficiency, 612–614, 612b, 612f–613f, 614b
  Liver-Blood deficiency and, 565–567, 565b–567b, 565f–567f
Heart channel, 1007–1014
  anti-itching effect of, 1011
  antispasmodic effect of, 1011
  connecting channel pathway of, 1007, 1007f
  main channel pathway of, 1007, 1007f
  patterns, 799
  points of, 1007, 1007b
    comparison, 1013t
  target areas, 1014f
Heart crack, 108, 108f
Heart deficiency, 1081
Heart Empty-Heat, HE-1 Jiquan *Supreme Spring* and, 1008
Heart-Fire, 203–204, 748, 1084
  blazing, 500–502, 500f–501f, 501b–502b
    case history in, 502b
  HE-3 Shaohai *Lesser-Yin Sea* and, 1008
  Small Intestine and, 679, 679f
Heart patterns, 489–513, 489b
  aetiology (general) of, 490–491, 490b
  combined, 513
  deficiency-excess, 510–512
  empty, 491
  excess, 500–510
Heart-Qi
  deficiency, 491–493, 492f, 493b
    Lung-Qi deficiency and, 594–596, 594b–595b, 594f–595f
  HE-5 Tongli *Inner Communication* and, 1009
  stagnation, 506–508, 507f–508f, 508b
Heart-Vessel obstructed, 508–510, 509b–510b, 509f
Heart-Yang
  collapse, 494–496, 495f, 496b
  deficiency, 493–494, 493f–494f, 494b, 736
Heart-Yin
  deficiency, 498–500, 498f–499f, 500b
    case history in, 500b
  HE-1 Jiquan *Supreme Spring* and, 1008
  HE-6 Yinxi *Yin Crevice* and, 1010
Heat, 410, 410b
  in Blood, 475, 475f, 476b
  in Bright Yang, 789, 789f
  Cold and
    mutual consuming of, Yin-Yang, 16b
    Yin-Yang imbalance, 12
  and DU-9 Zhiyang *Reaching Yang*, 1151
  and DU-13 Taodao *Kiln Way*, 1152
  exterior, 454, 454b
  extreme, generating wind, 556, 556b

feeling of, 359–361, 360b
  in diseases of exterior origin, 361, 361b
  exterior conditions, 360–361
  in skin, 390
Fetus, 814–815
and Fire, 411
  differences between, 746–747
Heart loathes, 114–115
in Kidneys, 790, 790b
in Large Intestine, 691–692, 691b–692b, 691f
latent, 779–781, 779f–780f, 781t
L.I.-11 and, 967
Liver-Qi stagnation turning into, 535–536, 535b, 536f, 537b
in Lungs, 584–585, 584b–585b, 584f–585f, 773, 773b, 788, 788b
in Nutritive Qi level, 767–768, 775–776, 776b
obstructing Large Intestine, 692–694, 692b, 692f–693f, 694b
pain, 344
in Pericardium, 516–517, 516b–517b, 517f, 776, 776b, 788–789, 789b
stagnant, in Directing and Penetrating Vessels, 813
in Stomach, 663, 773–774, 774b
toxic, 749–750, 750b
transformation, Lesser Yin stage, 761–762, 762b, 762f
victorious agitates Blood, 776–777, 777b
victorious stirring Wind, 777, 777b
Yin and empty Heat, 416f
Heat above-Cold below, 460
Heaven and Earth, Yin-Yang of, 5–6
Heavenly Star points, of Ma Dan Yang, 862
Heaviness, of limbs, 355
Heavy Dampness, 738
Herbal formula
  for Heart-Blood deficiency, 498
  for Heart-Blood stasis, 512
  for Heart-Fire blazing, 502
  for Heart-Qi deficiency, 493
  for Heart-Qi stagnation, 508
  for Heart-Vessel obstructed, 510
  for Heart-Yang collapse, 496
  for Heart-Yang deficiency, 494
  for Heart-Yin deficiency, 499
  for Large Intestine
    Cold, 695, 699
    collapse of, 699–701
    Damp-Heat, 690, 690b
    Dry, 698
    Heat, 692
    obstructing Heat, 694
    Qi stagnation, 696
  for Liver-Blood stasis, 542
  for Liver-Qi stagnation, 534–535
  Middle Burner, 789–790
  for Phlegm-Fire harassing Heart, 504
  for Phlegm misting Mind, 506
  for rebellious Liver-Qi, 538
  Six Stages, 755
  for Small Intestine
    Cold, 685
    Full-Heat, 680
    Small Intestine-Qi pain, 681
    Small Intestine-Qi tied, 682
    worm infestation, 683

for stagnation of Cold in Liver channel, 547
for Stomach
    Blood stasis, 672
    and Cold, 658, 665
    Damp-Heat, 668
    food retention, 670
    Heat, 664
    Qi deficiency, 656
    Qi stagnation, 662
    rebellious Qi, 667
    Stomach- and Spleen-Qi deficiency, 673
    Stomach- and Spleen-Yin deficiency, 674–675
    Yin deficiency, 660
    Upper Burner, 788
Herbal medicine, wrong treatment with, 293
Herbal therapy
    differences between acupuncture and, 1184–1189
        case history, 1186b–1189b
    Directing Vessel and, 901
    Girdle Vessel and, 921–922
    Governing Vessel and, 896–897
    Penetrating Vessel and, 915–916
    Yang Linking Vessel and, 936
    Yang Stepping Vessel and, 928
    Yin Linking Vessel and, 934
    Yin Stepping Vessel and, 925
Herbs
    Directing Vessel, 808
    Girdle Vessel, 815–816
    Governing Vessel, 807–808
    Penetrating Vessel, 810
    taste of, 1185, 1185t
    Yang Stepping Vessel, 817
    Yin Stepping Vessel, 816–817
Hereditary constitution, 280, 280f
Hernial and genitourinary disorders, LIV-1 and, 1120
Hiccup, diagnosis by, 398
Hidden (Fu) pulse, 388, 388b
Hips
    Girdle Vessel and, 920
    Yang Stepping Vessel and, 927
Historical perspective
    exterior pathogenic factors, 270–271, 271b
    Five Elements, 20
    Heart and Mind, 112
    pulse diagnosis, 375
    Six Stages, 751
    Yin-Yang, 4, 4f
Holding function, of Qi, 58
Hollow (Kou) pulse, 387, 387b
Hookworms, 683
Hot, 455–457
    and Cold, combined, 460–461
Hot-Cold, 455–459
Hot foods, 292, 653
'Huangshu', 1073
Huatuojiaji Hua Tuo back Filling Points, 1163–1164, 1163f, 1164b
Hurried (Ji) pulse, 388–389, 388b
Hypochondrium, 353
    Phlegm-Fluids in, 480
Hypogastrium, 353

I

Ideas, 72
Illness, condition of, 358

Immunizations, in children, 371–372
Impotence, 367, 367b
Index finger, in babies, diagnosis of, 323–324, 323f
Individual part, and whole, correspondence between, 302–303, 303b
Influenza, LU-7 and, 954
'Injury from Cold' (Shang Han), 752, 752f
Insight, 71
Insomnia, 355–356, 356b
    SP-6 Sanyinjiao Three Yin Meeting and, 1001
Insulting sequence, Five Elements, 24–25, 25f, 32, 33f–34f
    patterns, 823
Integrating function, of extraordinary vessels, 872–874, 873f, 874b
Intellect (Yi), 100–101, 111, 997
    Spleen houses, 149–150, 150b
Intelligence, 72, 241
Interdependence of Yin-Yang, 7, 13–14
Interior conditions, 359–360
Interior Full-Cold, 458–459
Interior patterns, 455, 455f
    in tonifying Upright Qi and expelling pathogenic factors, 1183–1184
Interior Wind, Governing Vessel extinguishes, 896
Intermittent (Dai) pulse, 388, 388b
Internal branch, of Penetrating Vessel (Chong Mai), 905–906
Internal causes of disease, 251–266, 251b–252b
Internal Cold, 408, 408b, 733f, 735–736
    origin of, 736f
Internal conditions, Upright Qi and, 414–416
Internal Dampness, 407, 407b, 739, 741–742, 742b
Internal diseases, Qi mechanism and, 426
Internal Dryness, 744–745
    origin of, 744f
Internal Full-Heat, 456
Internal organs
    chronic Dampness in, 741–742
    climates and, 101, 101b
    colours and, 102, 103b
    correspondences, 97, 97b
    Dampness in, 738
    emotions and, 99–100, 99f, 100b, 254b, 255–256, 255f, 256b–257b
    external manifestations of, 101, 101b
    fluids and, 101–102, 102b
    functions of, 97–105, 97b
    interrelationships of, 94, 98
    invasion of external Dampness in, 740–741
    odours and, 102, 102b
    pathology of ascending/descending of Qi in, 427–429
    relationship between Minister Fire and, 172f
    and the sense organs, 98–99, 99b
    sounds and, 103, 103b
    and spiritual aspects, 100–101, 100b–101b
    tastes and, 103, 103b
    theory of, 94
    tissues and, 98, 98b
    vital substances and, 98, 98b
    Yang (Fu), 103–105, 104b
    Yin (Zang), 103–105, 104b
Internal pathogenic factors, 404–411, 404f

Internal Wind, 406–407, 407b, 727–728, 732, 732b, 1064
Interrogation
    aspects of, 337b
    diagnosis by, 335–372, 335b
    identification of patterns and, 339–340
    nature of diagnosis by, 337
    procedure for, 339, 339f
    questions in, 338, 338f, 342–372, 342b
    traditional, 340–341
    for Western patients, 341–342
Interstitial cystitis, 720–721
Intertransformation of Yin-Yang, 16–17
Intestinal gas odour, 400
Intestines
    area, distal and local points, 1197t
    Blood stasis symptoms and signs, 474
    Dampness in, 742
    Dry-Heat, 774, 774b
    Fire in, 748
    invasion of Cold and, 734
    invasion of external Dampness in, 740
    Phlegm-Fluids in, 480
Irritability, 365, 365b
Itching, Wind and, 728
Itchy skin, in diagnosis by observation, 324

J

Jianneiling Inner Shoulder Mound, 1164, 1164b, 1164f
Jinggong Palace of Essence, 1163, 1163b, 1163f
Jingzhong Middle of Periods, 1161, 1161b, 1161f
Joints
    entering-exiting of Qi in, 82–83, 82f
    invasion of Cold in, 734
    invasion of Wind in, 731
    non-substantial Phlegm, 479
    pain, 354, 354f
    painful obstruction (Bi) syndrome in, 321
    pathology of entering/exiting of Qi in, 434–435, 435b
    SP-5 Shangqiu Metal Mound and, 1000
    swelling of, 321, 321b
Joy, 261, 261b, 261f
    and Heart, 112–113, 261, 490

K

KI-1 Yongquan Bubbling Spring, 1063–1064, 1064b
KI-2 Rangu Blazing Valley, 1064–1065, 1065b
KI-3 Taixi Greater Stream, 1065, 1066b
KI-4 Dazhong Big Bell, 1066, 1066b
KI-5 Shuiquan Water Spring, 1066–1067, 1067b
KI-6 Zhaohai Shining Sea, 1067, 1067b
KI-7 Fuliu Returning Current, 1068, 1068b
KI-8 Jiaoxin Meeting the Spleen Channel, 1068–1069, 1069b
KI-9 Zhubin Guest House, 1069, 1069b
KI-10 Yingu Yin Valley, 1069–1070, 1070b
KI-11 Henggu Pubic Bone, 1070, 1070b
KI-12 Dahe Big Glory, 1070–1071, 1071b
KI-13 Qixue Qi Hole, 1071–1072, 1072b
KI-14 Siman Four Fullnesses, 1072, 1072b
KI-16 Huangshu Transporting Point of 'Huang,', 1073, 1074b
    relationship between BL-17 and, 1073f

1277

KI-17 Shangqu *Bent Metal*, 1073–1074, 1074*b*
KI-21 Youmen *Door of Darkness*, 1074, 1074*b*
KI-23 Shenfeng *Mind Seal*, 1075, 1075*b*
KI-24 Lingxu *Spirit Burial-Ground*, 1075, 1075*b*
KI-25 Shencang *Mind Storage*, 1075–1076, 1076*b*
KI-27 Shufut *Transporting Point Mansion*, 1076, 1076*b*
Kidney(s), 155–167, 155*b*
　and Blood, 65
　and Body fluids, 67–68, 477
　Cold in, 165, 734
　Dampness in, 742
　Empty-Heat from, 1065
　fear and, 265
　Fire of the Gate of Life and, 77
　functions of, 157–164
　and Heart, 28–29, 177–179, 180*b*
　　not harmonized, 642–644, 642*b*, 642*f*–643*f*, 644*b*
　Heat in, 790, 790*b*
　and Liver, 28, 181–182, 182*b*, 182*f*
　and Lungs, 183–184, 184*b*, 184*f*, 632
　and Qi
　　failing to receive, 631–633, 632*b*–633*b*, 632*f*–633*f*
　　pathology of ascending/descending of, 429, 429*b*, 429*f*
　relationships, 165, 165*b*
　　with Bladder, 216–217
　and REN-3 Zhongji *Middle Pole*, 1131
　and REN-4 Guanyuan *Gate of the Original Qi*, 1132
　as Root of Pre-Heaven Qi, 166
　sayings, 165–166, 166*b*
　shock and, 265
　and Spleen, 183, 183*b*, 183*f*
　and *Tian Gui*, 157*f*
　Uterus and, 237, 237*f*–238*f*, 239*b*
Kidney channel, 1063–1077
　connecting pathway of, 1063, 1064*f*
　main pathway of, 1063, 1063*f*
　patterns, 800–801
　points of, 1063*b*
　　target areas, 1076*f*
　Triple Burner channels and, in ears, 1088
Kidney-Dryness, 745, 745*b*
Kidney-Essence, 49, 241, 242*b*, 1042
　deficiency, 633–635, 633*f*–635*f*, 634*b*–635*b*
　and extraordinary vessels, 869–870, 870*b*
　functions of, 50*b*, 158, 158*b*
　REN-1 Huiyin *Meeting of Yin*, 1130
　sexual life and, 285, 286*f*
Kidney patterns, 621–649, 621*b*, 623*b*, 648*b*–649*b*
　aetiology (general), 623–624, 624*b*
　combined, 640–649
Kidney-Qi
　basis of
　　Essence as, 49, 49*f*
　　Original Qi, 51
　Directing Vessel promotes receiving of, 898
　direction of, 60, 60*f*
　not firm, 629–631, 629*b*, 630*f*–631*f*, 631*b*
Kidney stones, non-substantial Phlegm, 479

Kidney-Yang, 1068
　deficiency, 621*t*–622*t*, 622*b*, 622*f*, 625–627, 625*b*, 625*f*–626*f*, 627*b*, 736, 1178
　　precursors of, 626*f*
　　and Spleen-Yang deficiency, 646–649, 646*b*, 647*f*, 648*b*
　　Water overflowing, 635–637, 636*b*–637*b*, 636*f*–637*f*
　and DU-4 Mingmen *Gate of Life*, 1149–1150
　Governing Vessel tonifies, 893, 895*b*
　Kidney-Yin and, 155*f*–156*f*, 156, 156*b*, 158*f*
Kidney-Yin, 457, 1042, 1068
　deficiency, 621*t*–622*t*, 622*b*, 622*f*, 627–629, 627*b*–629*b*, 627*f*–628*f*
　　Empty-Heat blazing, 638–640, 638*b*, 638*f*–639*f*, 640*b*
　　and Liver-Yin deficiency, 557, 558*b*, 640–642, 640*b*, 640*f*–641*f*, 642*f*
　　and Lung-Yin deficiency, 644–646, 644*b*, 644*f*–645*f*, 646*b*
　　point combination for headaches from, 1202*f*
　　Stomach-Yin deficiency and, 659*b*
Knees, weak, 355
Knotted (*Jie*) pulse, 388, 388*b*

L
Lactation
　S.I.-1 Shaoze *Lesser Marsh* and, 1016
　ST-18 Rugen *Breast Root* and, 978
Lanweixue *Appendix Point*, 1166*f*, 1167, 1167*b*
Large Intestine
　aspects of, 206–207
　　mental, 206, 206*b*
　Cold in, 687, 694–695, 694*b*–695*b*, 694*f*–695*f*, 698*b*–699*b*, 698*f*–699*f*
　collapse of, 699–701, 699*b*–700*b*, 700*f*
　controls passage and conduction, 205, 206*b*
　Damp-Heat in, 688–690, 688*b*–690*b*, 689*f*–690*f*
　Dry, 477, 697, 697*b*–698*b*, 697*f*
　functions of, 205–207, 205*b*
　Heat in, 691–692, 691*b*–692*b*, 691*f*
　　obstructing, 692–694, 692*b*, 692*f*–693*f*, 694*b*
　Lung-Qi and, 955
　pathology of ascending/descending of Qi and, 429
　Qi stagnation in, 695–696, 695*b*–696*b*, 696*f*
　relationship between Lungs and, 206–207, 206*f*
Large Intestine channel, 961–971
　connecting pathway of, 961, 961*f*
　main pathway of, 961, 961*f*
　patterns, 798
　points of, 961*b*
　　target areas of, 971*f*
Large Intestine patterns, 687–701, 687*b*
　aetiology (general) of, 687–688, 688*b*
　Empty, 697–701
　Full, 688–696
Latent Heat, 779–781, 779*f*–780*f*, 781*t*
Lateral abdominal pain, ST-27 Daju *Big Greatness* and, 981
Laughing, 114
Leather (*Ge*) pulse, 387, 387*b*

Left-right combination
　of P-6 Neiguan and LIV-3 Taichong with ST-36 Zusanli and SP-6 Sanyinjiao, 1205*f*
　P-6 Neiguan and ST-36 Zusanli, 1203*f*
　P-6 Neiguan and ST-40 Fenglong, 1205*f*
　of T.B.-6 Zhigou and G.B.-31 Fengshi, 1203*f*
Left side
　Liver arises from, 127
　and right side, balancing, 1204–1206
Leg problems, ST-32 Futu *Crouching Rabbit* and, 984
Legs, Girdle Vessel and, 919
Lesser Yang stage, 759–760, 760*b*, 760*f*
Lesser Yang type, Latent Heat, 779
Lesser Yin stage, 761–762, 761*f*–762*f*, 762*b*
Lesser Yin type, Latent Heat, 781
Lethargy, 356, 357*b*
Leucorrhoea, 370
L.I.-1 Shangyang *Metal Yang*, 962, 962*b*
L.I.-2 Erjian *Second Interval*, 962–963, 963*b*
L.I.-3 Sanjian *Third Interval*, 963, 963*b*
L.I.-4 Hegu *Enclosed Valley*, 963–964, 964*b*
L.I.-5 Yangxi *Yang Stream*, 964–965, 965*b*
L.I.-6 Pianli *Lateral Passage*, 965, 965*b*
L.I.-7 Wenliu *Warm Gathering*, 965–966, 966*b*
L.I.-10 Shousanli *Arm Three Miles*, 966, 967*b*
L.I.-11 Quchi *Pool on Bend*, 967, 967*b*
L.I.-12 Zhouliao *Elbow Crevice*, 968, 968*b*
L.I.-14 Binao *Upper Arm*, 968, 968*b*
L.I.-15 Jianyu *Shoulder Bone*, 968–969, 969*b*
L.I.-16 Jugu *Great Bone*, 969, 969*b*
L.I.-17 Tianding *Heaven's Tripod*, 969, 969*b*
L.I.-18 Futu *Support the Protuberance*, 969–970, 970*b*
L.I.-20 Yingxiang *Welcome Fragrance*, 970, 970*b*
Libido, lack of, 625
　in men, 367
　in women, 367*b*, 368
Life cycles, and extraordinary vessels, 871, 871*b*
Life habits
　Lung-Qi deficiency, and Spleen-Qi deficiency, 614–615
　Lung-Yin deficiency and, 576
　Lungs and, 574
　Phlegm-Heat and, 589
Lifestyle, Lungs and, 573
Limbs
　anterior-medial surface of, 10
　diagnosis by observation, 321–324
　numbness/tingling of, 354
　palpating, 390–392
　Phlegm-Fluids in, 480
　posterior-lateral surface of, 10
　Spleen controls, 148, 148*b*, 152
　symptoms, 353–355
　tremor of, 354
　weakness of, 354
Limpid Sea, 1179*b*
Lips
　diagnosis by observation, 319, 319*b*
　Spleen manifests in, 149, 149*b*
Liquids (*Ye*), 69
LIV-1 Dadun *Big Mound*, 1120, 1120*b*
LIV-2 Xingjian *Temporary In-Between*, 1120–1121, 1121*b*
　and LIV-3 Taichong, 1122*t*

LIV-3 Taichong *Bigger Penetrating*, 1121–1122, 1122*b*
  and LIV-2 Xingjian, 1122*t*
LIV-4 Zhongfeng *Middle Seal*, 1123, 1123*b*
LIV-5 Ligou *Gourd Ditch*, 1123, 1123*b*
LIV-6 Zhongdu *Middle Capital*, 1124, 1124*b*
LIV-7 Xiguan *Knee Gate*, 1124, 1124*b*
LIV-8 Ququan *Spring on Bend*, 1124–1125, 1125*b*
LIV-13 Zhangmen *Completion Gate*, 181*b*, 859, 1125, 1125*b*
LIV-14 Qimen *Cyclic Gate*, 181*b*, 1125–1126, 1126*b*
Liver, 117–128, 117*b*
  area, distal and local points, 1197*t*
  and Blood, 63*f*–64*f*, 64, 118–120, 118*b*–119*b*, 118*f*
  Blood stasis and, 474, 538–542, 539*f*, 540*b*–542*b*, 541*f*, 568, 568*f*
  combined patterns of, 559–570
  Damp-Heat in, 544–546, 544*b*, 545*f*–546*f*, 546*b*
  Dampness in, 742
  and DU-9 Zhiyang *Reaching Yang*, 1151
  empty-Wind, 791–792, 791*b*
  Ethereal Soul and, 111
  External Wind and, 728
  eyes and, 31
  functions of, 118–125
  Gall Bladder and
    Damp-Heat in, 710–712, 710*b*–711*b*, 710*f*–711*f*
    Girdle Vessel harmonizes, 918
  and Heart, 27, 176–177, 177*b*, 177*f*
  houses Ethereal Soul *(Hun)*, 124–125, 124*f*
  and Kidneys, 181–182, 182*b*, 182*f*
  and Lungs, 179–181, 180*b*–181*b*, 563–565
  pathology, 'feel' for, 530*b*
  pathology of ascending/descending of Qi and, 428–429, 428*f*
  and Qi, direction, 59, 59*f*–60*f*
  relationships, 125–126, 125*b*
    with Gall Bladder, 213
    between Pericardium, Heart, Uterus and, 1083*f*
  sayings, 126–127
  and Spleen, 28, 181, 181*b*, 181*f*
  and Stomach, 28
  tears and, 101–102
  Triple Burner and, 222*b*
  Uterus and, 238, 238*f*, 239*b*
  Wind and, 727
  see also Triple Burner
Liver-Blood deficiency, 176*b*, 548–550, 548*b*–550*b*, 548*f*, 550*f*, 616–617, 616*b*–617*b*, 616*f*–617*f*
  case history of, 550*b*
  generating wind, 559, 559*b*
  Heart-Blood deficiency and, 565–567, 565*b*–567*b*, 565*f*–567*f*
  Liver-Qi stagnation and, 568, 568*f*
  Liver-Yang rising and, 558, 558*b*, 568, 569*f*
  and Spleen-Blood deficiency, 616–617, 616*b*–617*b*, 616*f*–617*f*
Liver channel, 1119–1127
  Cold stagnation in, 546–547, 547*f*, 548*b*
  connecting channel pathway in, 1119, 1119*f*
  External Wind and, 731, 731*b*

main channel pathway in, 1119, 1119*f*
patterns, 803–805
  Pericardium patterns and, 515
points of, 1119*b*
target areas of, 1126*f*
Liver-Fire, 748
  blazing, 542–544, 542*b*, 543*f*–544*f*, 544*b*
    Liver-Yang rising and, 746–747
  generating wind, 558–559, 559*b*
  insulting Lungs, 563–565, 564*f*, 565*b*
  Liver-Qi stagnation and, 569–570, 569*f*
  vs. Liver-Yang rising, 554*t*
Liver-Heat stirs Wind, 790, 791*b*
Liver patterns, 529–570, 529*b*
  aetiology of, general, 530–532, 532*b*
  combined, 559–570
  Empty, 548–552
  Full, 532–547
  Full/Empty, 552–559
Liver-Qi, 529, 1113
  BL-2 and, 1029
  and Gall Bladder, 210
  rebellious, 536–538, 537*b*–538*b*, 537*f*–538*f*, 569, 569*f*
    invading Spleen, 560–562, 560*b*–562*b*, 560*f*–561*f*
    invading Stomach, 562–563, 562*f*–563*f*, 563*b*
Liver-Qi stagnation, 532–535, 532*b*–535*b*, 532*f*, 534*f*
  case history of, 535*b*
  Liver-Yang rising, 568, 568*f*
  Spleen obstruction by Dampness with, 617–620, 618*b*–619*b*, 618*f*–619*f*
  turning into Heat, 535–536, 535*b*, 536*f*, 537*b*
  vs. rebellious Liver-Qi, 539*t*
Liver-Wind, agitating within, 555–559, 556*b*, 556*f*
Liver-Yang
  Gall Bladder deficiency and, 708, 709*f*
  G.B.-13 and, 1104
Liver-Yang rising, 429, 429*b*, 552–555, 552*b*–555*b*, 554*f*
  case history of, 555*b*
  combined patterns of, 568, 568*f*
  generating wind, 557–558
  Liver-Fire blazing upwards and, 746–747
  Liver-Qi stagnation and, 568, 568*f*
  Lungs, Liver-Fire insulting, 553*f*
  in pain, 344
  point combination for headaches from, 1202*f*
  Qi mechanism and, 426
  rebellious Liver-Qi and, 569, 569*f*
Liver-Yin deficiency, 550–552, 551*b*–552*b*, 551*f*–552*f*
  and Kidney-Yin deficiency, 640–642, 640*b*, 640*f*–641*f*, 642*b*
  Liver-Yang rising deriving from, 557, 557*b*
Local point, balancing, 1195–1202, 1196*f*
  according to area, 1197*t*
  main, 1199
Lochia, odour, 400
Long *(Chang)* pulse, 385, 385*b*
Long tongue, 329
Lower body, and upper body, balancing, 1202–1204, 1202*t*

Lower Burner, 88, 88*f*
  Body fluid excretion and, 223
  Dampness in, 918–919
    KI-7, 1068
  Directing Vessel and, 898
  dreams and, 230
  fluid transformation, 216
  Girdle Vessel and, 918–919
  like a ditch, 225*f*, 226, 226*b*
  patterns, 790–792
  Qi of, 226*b*
  and REN-7 Yinjiao *Yin Crossing*, 1135
  and Stomach function, 197
Lower Sea points, 395, 835
LSD, 294
LU-1 Zhongfu *Central Palace*, 949–950, 950*b*
LU-2 Yunmen *Cloud Door*, 950–951, 951*b*
LU-3 Tianfu *Heavenly Palace*, 951–952, 952*b*, 952*f*
LU-5 Chize *Foot Marsh*, 952–953, 953*b*
LU-6 Kongzui *Convergence Hole*, 953, 954*b*
LU-7 Lieque *Branching Cleft*, 954–956, 954*f*, 956*b*
LU-8 Jingqu *River [Point] Ditch*, 956, 956*b*
LU-9 Taiyuan *Supreme Abyss*, 956–957, 957*b*
LU-10 Yuji *Fish Border*, 957–958, 958*b*
LU-11 Shaoshang *Lesser Metal*, 958
Lumps, hard-soft, 12
Lung(s), 129–142, 129*b*
  area, distal and local points, 1197*t*
  and Blood, 64–65
  Blood stasis symptoms and signs, 474
  and Body fluids, 67, 477
  Damp-Phlegm in, 585–587, 585*b*, 585*f*–586*f*, 587*b*
  Defensive-Qi portion of
    invasion of Cold in, 734
    Wind invasion in, 728–731
  as delicate organ, 141–142
  diffusing and descending of, 131–132, 133*b*, 134*f*
  Fire in, 748
  functions of, 130–140, 571
  and Gathering Qi, 53, 133, 133*f*, 183–184
  governs 100 vessels, 141
  and Heart, 175–176, 175*f*, 176*b*
  Heat in, 788, 788*b*
  and Kidneys, 28, 183–184, 184*b*, 184*f*, 632
  and Liver, 28, 179–181, 180*f*, 181*b*
  Liver-Fire insulting, 563–565, 564*f*, 565*b*
  LU-1 tonifies, 950
  pathology, 'feel' for, 571*b*
  Phlegm-Fluids obstructing, 592–593, 592*b*–593*b*, 592*f*–593*f*
  Phlegm in
    obstructing, 1080
    substantial, 478
  and Qi
    direction, 59, 59*f*–60*f*
    pathology of ascending/descending of, 428, 428*b*, 428*f*
  relationships, 140–141
    between Large Intestine and, 206–207, 206*f*
  sadness and, 261–262
  sayings, 141–142
  and Spleen, 182–183, 182*f*, 183*b*
  Triple Burner and, 222*b*
  and True Qi *(Zhen Qi)*, 54

Wind and, 572, 579–581, 579b, 579f–580f, 581b, 727
worry and, 263
Lung channel, 949–959
  connecting pathway of, 949, 949f
  main pathway of, 949, 949f
  patterns, 797
  Pericardium patterns and, 515
  points of, 949b
    target areas of, 959f
Lung-Defensive Qi, L.I.-1 and, 962
Lung-Dryness, 577–578, 577b–578b, 578f, 745, 745b
Lung-Heat, 584–585, 584b–585b, 584f–585f, 773, 773b
Lung patterns, 571–596, 571b
  aetiology of, general, 572–573, 573b
  combined, 594–596
  Empty, 573–578
  Full
    exterior, 579–584
    interior, 584–593
Lung-Qi
  deficiency, 573–575, 574b–575b, 574f–575f, 736
    and Spleen-Qi deficiency, 614–616, 614b, 614f–615f, 616b
  descending of, 898
  Directing Vessel and, 898
  direction of, 180
  and DU-12 Shenzhu *Body Pillar*, 1152
  Heart-Qi deficiency and, 594–596, 594b–595b, 594f–595f
  Large Intestine and, 955
  L.I.-4 and, 964
  and Liver-Blood, 180
  and Liver-Qi, 180–181
  and REN-17 Shanzhong (or Tanzhong) *Middle of chest*, 1143
  and REN-22 Tiantu *Heaven Projection*, 1144
  stimulation of, 184b
Lung-Yin deficiency, 576–577, 576b–577b, 576f–577f
  and Kidney-Yin deficiency, 644–646, 644b, 644f–645f, 646b
'Lung's Defensive Qi portion', 453
Luo channels, 1083
Lustre
  of complexion, 314
  of eyes, 317

M

Macules, 769
'Magnificent Six', 1037
Main channel patterns
  Bladder, 800, 801f
  Gall Bladder, 802, 803f
  Heart, 799, 800f
  Kidneys, 800, 801f
  Large Intestine, 798, 798f
  Liver, 803, 803f
  Lungs, 797, 797f
  Pericardium, 801–802, 802f
  Spleen, 799, 799f
  Stomach, 798, 798f
  Triple Burner, 802, 802f

Malnutrition, 291
Manifestation (*Biao*), 1172f, 1173–1178, 1173b, 1175t
  becoming secondary root, 1177b
  one root giving rise to different, 1178
  treating first before root, 1177, 1177b
  see also Root (*Ben*), and manifestation (*Biao*)
Marrow, 241–242
  and Blood, 62
  extraordinary vessels, 871
  functions of, 242, 242b
  Governing Vessel nourishes, 894
  Kidney-Essence and, 49, 159f, 160b
  Kidneys producing, 158–160, 160b
  Sea of Marrow, 241, 244b, 860
Medicinal drugs, 293, 293f
Membranes (*Huang*)
  Directing Vessel controls, 899, 899b
  entering-exiting of Qi in, 83
  pathology of entering/exiting of Qi in, 436–437, 437b
  Penetrating Vessel and, 911
  Qi movement and, Triple Burner and, 227–228
Memory, 71, 150, 240–241
  Spleen influence on, 150b, 150f
Men
  sexual activity, 623, 624f
  sexual symptoms, 367
  Uterus in, 240
Menstrual blood (*Tian Gui*), 64, 64b, 148, 237, 287, 287f
Menstrual cycle, 236–237, 368–369
  Heart and Kidneys in, 178–179, 179f
  phases of, 239, 239f
Menstrual disorders, and REN-5 Shimen *Stone Door*, 1134
Menstruation, 108, 182f, 239, 368–370
  extraordinary vessels, 871
  Heart and, 237
  Liver-Blood regulates, 119, 119b
  and REN-3 Zhongji *Middle Pole*, 1131
  and REN-4 Guanyuan *Gate of the Original Qi*, 1132
  and REN-7 Yinjiao *Yin Crossing*, 1135
Mental aspect
  of Bladder, 216
  of Gall Bladder, 211–213
  of Small Intestine, 202
  of Stomach, 197–198
  of Triple Burner, 229–230, 230b, 230f
Mental-emotional problems, 886
  Yang Stepping Vessel and, 927
  Yin Linking Vessel and, 933, 933b
  see also Fear; Pensiveness; Worry
Mental overwork, 284
Mental restlessness, 499
  SP-1 Yinbai *Hidden White* and, 996
Metacarpal bone, microsystem of, in diagnosis, 304f
Metal
  body type, 308–309, 310b, 310f
  insulting Fire, 823
  not generating Water, 822
  overacting on Wood, 822
Microsystems, in diagnosis, 302–303, 304f–305f

Middle Burner, 87–88, 120–121
  crossing of Qi in, 85, 85b
  and fluids, 222–223
  and Food Qi, 52
  like a maceration chamber, 225–226, 225f
  patterns, 789
  and Qi, 221, 223, 226b
    Liver, 120–121
    Spleen, 150
  and Stomach function, 194, 196
  see also Triple Burner
Mind (*Shen*), 70–73, 100
  and emotions, 177, 177f
  entering-exiting of Qi in, 83–84
  and Essence, common root of, 178, 179f
  and Ethereal Soul, 84f
  Fire and, 747
  functions of, 71b
  Governing Vessel strengthens, 894–895, 894f, 895b
  Heart houses, 109–112, 109b–110b, 110f, 164
  L.I.-5 and, 965
  L.I.-7 and, 966
  obstruction of, 951–952
  pathology of entering/exiting of Qi in, 436, 436b, 436f
  Pericardium and, 518–524
  Phlegm misting, 505–506, 505f–506f, 506b
  and REN-4 Guanyuan *Gate of the Original Qi*, 1132
  and REN-14 Juque *Great Palace*, 1141
  and REN-15 Jiuwei *Dove Tail*, 1142–1143
  S.I.-3 Houxi *Back Stream* effect in, 1017–1018
  S.I.-5 Yanggu *Yang Valley* and, 1019
  sleep disturbance, 355, 355f
  see also Essence-Qi-Mind (*Jing-Qi-Shen*); Mental aspect; Spirit; Three treasures
Mind-spirit, Pericardium and, 171, 171b
Minister Fire
  and Gall Bladder, 209–210
  Pericardium and, 171–172, 172b, 172f
  relationship between internal organs and, 172f
  in sexual activity, 368
  sexual arousal and, 288
  Triple Burner and, 228–229, 231
  see also Fire of the Gate of Life (*Ming Men*)
Minute Connecting channels, 999, 999f
Minute (*Wei*) pulse, 386, 386b
Misting
  Heart, 479
  Mind, 505–506, 505f–506f, 506b
Mixed deficient/excess condition, 1179
Mixed full-empty conditions, 462, 462b
Moist face colour, 316, 316b
Moisture
  complexion, 314, 314b
  and texture of skin, 390, 390b
  of tongue, 331, 331b
Mother-child relationship
  Five Elements, 838
  Gall Bladder and Heart, 211
Motive force, Original Qi, 51
Mouth
  diagnosis by observation, 319, 319b
  Spleen opens into, 148–149, 149b
  ulcers, 351, 351b

Movement(s)
  body, 313, 313b
  of Ethereal Soul, 363, 363b, 363f
  Five Elements as, 22, 22b, 22f
  Qi. see Qi mechanism/movement
Moving (Dong) pulse, 388, 388b
Moxibustion, and REN-6 Qihai Sea of Qi, 1134–1135
Muscle channel, Gall Bladder and, 929–930
Muscle channel patterns
  Bladder, 800
  Gall Bladder, 803
  Heart, 799
  Kidney, 801
  Large Intestine, 798
  Liver, 803–805
  Lungs, 797
  Pericardium, 802
  Small Intestine, 800, 800f
  Spleen, 799
  Stomach, 799
  Triple Burner, 802
Muscles
  acne in limbs, 354
  'ancestral muscles,' Penetrating Vessel and, 913–914, 913f
  invasion of Cold and, 734
  Spleen controls, 148, 148f
Mutual consuming of Yin-Yang, 7–8, 8f, 14–16, 14f

N

Nails
  diagnosis by observation, 323
  Liver manifests in, 123
Nasal mucus, 102
  Lungs control, 138, 139b
Nasal obstruction, LU-7 and, 954
'Naturalist School', 4
Nausea, HE-4 Lingdao Spirit Path and, 1009
Neck
  G.B.-39 as distal point for, 1200f
  stiffness, Greater Yang stage, 753, 754f
'Nei Guan', 1082–1083
Neurological problems, extraordinary vessels, 886
Night sweating, 628
Non-substantial Phlegm, 479b
Nose
  area, distal and local points, 1197t
  diagnosis by observation, 318, 318b
  Lungs open into, 137–138, 138b
  problems, L.I.-20 and, 970
  runny, 351
  see also Smell(s)
Numbers, and Five Elements, 24f, 26t
Numbness/tingling, 352
  of limbs, 354, 354b
  Wind and, 727
Nutritive Qi (Ying Qi), 54, 54b
  and Defensive Qi, 11, 55–56, 56b, 56f, 755
  Heat, 767–768, 775–776
    in Pericardium, 517, 776, 776b, 788–789, 789b
  Lesser Yin type, Latent Heat, 781
  in Middle Burner, 221, 223
  Yang and Yin Linking Vessels and, combined pathology of, 936
  Yin-Yang, 11

O

Observation, diagnosis by, 301–333
Occipital points, of eye system, 863, 864f
Occiput area, distal and local points, 1197t
Occupation, and pulse, 383, 383b
Odours. see Smell(s).
Oedema, 477–478, 477f, 478b
  Kidney-Yang deficiency, 635
  of limbs, 321, 321b
Old age, Kidney-Essence and, 624
Opening and closing, Kidneys control, 165–166
Opposition of Yin-Yang, 11–13, 11b, 11t
Organ(s)
  assignment to pulse position, 375–376
  and Body fluids, 67–68
  emotions and, 254b, 255–256, 255f, 256b–257b
  entering/exiting of Qi in, pathology of, 433–434, 435t
  function-structure of, Yin-Yang, 10–11, 10f, 13–14
  involved in urination, 217f
  Kidneys as source of physiological Fire for all, 164
  'lifting' of, by Spleen-Qi ascending, 147, 147b, 149f
  pathology/patterns
    affecting different channels, 885–886
    Bright Yang, 758–759, 758f, 759b
    Greater Yang stage, 756–757, 757f
    Latent Heat, Bright Yang type, 779
  Pericardium as, 169–170, 170b
  problems, distal and local points, 1201–1202
  and REN-15 Jiuwei Dove Tail, 1142–1143
  spiritual aspects of, 110–112, 111b–112b
  vs. channel, 795–797, 796f
  in pulse diagnosis, 378f, 379
  Yang, six extraordinary, 871–872, 872b, 872f
Orgasm, in women, 368
Orifices
  and extraordinary vessels, 872, 873b
  lower, Kidneys control, 162, 162b
  pathology of ascending/descending of Qi in, 431, 431f–432f, 431t
  pathology of entering/exiting of Qi in, 435, 435b, 435t
Original Qi (Yuan Qi), 50–52
  and DU-4 Mingmen Gate of Life, 1150
  and Fire of the Gate of Life, 77f
  functions of, 52b
  and Gathering Qi, 53, 183–184
  and Kidney-Qi, 630
  mobilized by Triple Burner, 219–220, 220b, 220f, 224, 224b
  motive force for Qi transformation, 75–76, 76b, 76f
  and REN-3 Zhongji Middle Pole, 1131
  and REN-4 Guanyuan Gate of the Original Qi, 1132
  and REN-5 Shimen Stone Door, 1134
  root of, 164
  and Triple Burner, 76, 76f, 1090–1091
Original Yang, 50–51
  and REN-7 Yinjiao Yin Crossing, 1136
Original Yin, 50–51
  and REN-7 Yinjiao Yin Crossing, 1136

Over-acting sequence, Five Elements, 24, 24f, 32, 32f, 34f
  patterns, 822
Overdosage, of Chinese herbs, 627–628
Overeating, 291
  Stomach and, 653
Overflowing (Hong) pulse, 385–386, 386b
Overthinking, 365, 366b
Overwork, 283–284, 284b, 624
  Heart-Yin deficiency and, 498
  Kidney-Yin deficiency and, 627
  Lung- and Heart-Qi deficiency and, 594
  see also Physical work, excessive

P

P-1 Tianchi Heavenly Pool, 1079–1080, 1080b
P-3 Quze Marsh on Bend, 1080, 1080b
P-4 Ximen Cleft Door, 1081, 1081b
P-5 Jianshi Intermediary, 1081–1082, 1082b
P-6 Neiguan Inner Gate, 1082–1083, 1083b
P-7 Daling Great Hill, 1083–1084, 1084b
  comparison of HE-7 Shenmen and, 1084t
P-8 Laogong Labour Palace, 1084, 1085b
P-9 Zhongchong Centre Rush, 1085, 1085b
Pain, 343–344
  epigastrium, 353
  eye, 358–359
  facial, 350–351, 350b
  factors affecting, 343t
  hypogastrium, 353
  location of, 344t
  Small Intestine-Qi, 680–681, 680b–681b, 680f–681f
  SP-6 Sanyinjiao Three Yin Meeting and, 1001
  urination, 347
  in whole body, 351
  see also Abdominal pain
Painful obstruction syndrome (Bi), 109, 455, 1048
  Cold and, 734
  Damp, 741
  of foot, 990
  of hip, SP-12 Chongmen Penetrating Door and, 1004
  of joints, 321
  of knee, 985
  L.I.-3 and, 963
  L.I.-15 and, 969
  LU-5 and, 953
  S.I.-4 Wangu Wrist Bone and, 1018–1019
  S.I.-8 Xiaohai Small Intestine Sea and, 1020
  S.I.-9 Jianzhen Upright Shoulder and, 1021
  S.I.-10 Naoshu Humerus Transporting Point and, 1021
  ST-34 Liangqiu Beam Mound and, 985
  T.B.-5 and, 1091
  T.B.-8 and, 1094
  Wind and, 727, 731
Pale tongue, 325, 325b, 325f
Palpation, diagnosis by, 373–396, 373b
'Palpitations', 492
Pancreas, 144
Papules, 769
Paralysis
  of limbs, 322, 322b
  Wind and, 727–728, 731, 731b
Parasites, 292–293
  see also Worm infestation
Parotitis (mumps), toxic Heat in, 1025

Pathogenic factors, 1179
  evolution of, 415b
  expelling, 1181–1182, 1181b–1182b
  and Five Elements, 839, 840t, 841b
  full/empty conditions, interactions of, 403
  identification of patterns and, 724–750
    case history for, 742b
  internal, 404–411, 404f
  nature of, 403–411
  no pathogenic factor-deficient Upright Qi, 413, 413b
  no pathogenic factor-normal Upright Qi, 413, 413b
  Phlegm and, 410
  residual, 1183
  strong pathogenic factor-deficient Upright Qi, 414, 414b
  strong pathogenic factor-strong Upright Qi and, 413–414, 414b
  Upright Qi and, 412–413, 413f, 413t, 415–417, 416b, 416f
  weak pathogenic factor-deficient Upright Qi, 415, 415b
  weak pathogenic factor-strong Upright Qi, 414–415, 415b
  see also External pathogenic factors
Pathological colours, 315–316
Pathology, 402
  Blood, 66, 66b
  of exterior pathogenic factors, 272–274, 272f–273f, 274b
  of Full and Empty conditions, 403–417, 403b
  of pain, 343–344
  of Qi mechanism, 425–438, 425b–426b
  of Yin-Yang imbalance, 419–424, 419b
Pattern identification
  according to 12 channels, 794–805, 795b
  according to Eight Extraordinary Vessels, 794, 807–819
  according to Eight Principles, 448, 451–467, 451b
  according to Five Elements, 794, 821–823, 821b
  according to Qi-Blood-Body fluids, 448, 469–481, 469b
  Four Levels, 724, 765–785, 765b
  by interrogation, 337
  Six Stages, 724, 751–764, 751b
  Three Burners, 724, 787–792, 787b
Penetrating Vessel (Chong Mai), 809–810, 809f, 876–878, 877b, 877f, 902–916, 903f, 998
  'ancestral muscles' and, 913–914, 913f
  Blood stasis and, 911, 911b
  branches of, 902, 905–907
  case history of, 916b–917b
  classical indications of, 915, 916b
  clinical applications of, 905–914, 915b
  female breast and, 911–912, 912f
  Heart and, 912
  herbs/herbal therapy for, 810, 915–916
  membranes and, 911
  pathway of, 902–905, 905b
  points of, 902, 905b
  Qi circulation to feet and, 913
  rebellious Qi of, 909–911, 909f–910f, 910b
  and REN-1 Huiyin Meeting of Yin, 1130

and REN-4 Guanyuan Gate of the Original Qi, 1132–1133
  as Sea of Blood, 244, 907–908, 908b, 1070
  ST-30 Qichong Penetrating Qi and, 983
  Stomach and, 912–913
  Uterus and, 236–237, 236f, 237b
  various names of, 907–908
Pensiveness, 264, 264b, 264f
  Spleen affected by, 150, 150b–151b, 598
Pericardium, 96, 169–173, 169b
  Blood deficiency of, 518–520, 518b, 519f, 520b
  Blood stasis of, 526–528, 526b, 527f, 528b
  as 'centre of the thorax', 524–528
  as channel, 170–171, 170f
  connections, 169f
  external pathogenic factors and, 490
  Fire, 520–522, 520b, 521f, 522b
  Heart and, 228–229, 229f, 515
  Heat in, 516–517, 516b–517b, 517f, 776, 776b, 788–789, 789b
  as 'house' of Mind, 518–524
  invasion of exterior pathogenic factors in, 515–517, 516b, 516f
  and Mind-spirit, 171, 171b
  and Minister Fire, 171–172, 172b, 172f
  names for, 169
  as organ, 169–170, 170b
  pathology of, 'feel' for, 516b
  patterns, 515–528, 515b
  Qi stagnation in, 524–526, 525b–526b, 525f–526f
  relationship between Heart, Liver, Uterus and, 1083f
  T.B.-6 and, 1093
  Triple Burner and, 228–232, 229f
  and Uterus, 172–173
Pericardium channel, 1079–1086
  connecting pathway of, 1079, 1079f
  main pathway of, 1079, 1079f
  patterns, 801–802
  points, 1079b, 1082
    target areas of, 1085f
  and Triple Burner channel, connection at the fingertips, 1088, 1088f
Periorbital points, of eye system, 863, 863f
Pharynx, diagnosis by observation, 320, 320b
Phlegm, 408–410, 408b, 479b, 481b
  case history for, 480b
  changing, 409
  chronic retention of, in Lungs, 997–998
  and Dampness, differences between, 743
  essential manifestations of, 408b
  joint pain, 344
  LU-1 and, 950
  lumps and, 409
  misting Mind, 505–506, 505f–506f, 506b
  and origin of many diseases, 410
  and pathogenic factors, 410
  pattern identification, 478–481
  Qi mechanism and, 409
  ST-40 Fenglong Abundant Bulge and, 988–989
  stasis and, 409, 409f
  Stomach and Spleen, damage to, 410
  types of, 479–481, 479t
  as Yin pathogenic factor, 408–409

Phlegm-Fire
  harassing Heart, 502–504, 503b, 503f–504f, 505b
    case history in, 504b–505b
  harassing Pericardium, 522–524, 522b, 523f, 524b
Phlegm-fluids, 480–481
  obstructing Lungs, 592–593, 592b–593b, 592f–593f
Phlegm-Heat, 479, 662
  in Lungs, 589–591, 589b, 589f–590f, 591b
Physical exercise, excessive
  Bladder deficient and Cold, 718
  Liver-Blood deficiency and, 548
Physical work, excessive, 284–285, 284b–285b
  Blood deficiency and, 565
  Heart-Vessel obstructed, 508
  Kidney patterns, 625, 630, 632, 636
  Phlegm-Fluids obstructing Lungs and, 593
  Spleen- and Heart-Blood deficiency, 612
  see also Overwork
Physiological activities, Lungs regulate, 132–134, 134b
Pinworms, 683
Planets, correspondences of the Five Elements, 26t
Planning, Liver controls, 126
'Plum stone in the throat', 533
'Plum-stone syndrome', 480
Point(s)
  categories, 828
    functions of specific, 845–865, 845b
  combination of, 1191–1207
    balancing distal and local points, 1195–1202, 1198b
    regulating principles, 1191
  combinations, 12 Heavenly Star points, 862
  extra, 1159–1168
  extraordinary vessels, 880–881, 881b
    opening, vs. points on, 881–884
    see also specific vessels
  palpating, 394–395
  on vessel, 883–884
  see also Acupuncture; specific points
Poisons, 292–293
Post-Heaven Essence, 48
Post-Heaven Qi, 283
  Spleen, 152
Postviral fatigue syndrome, 414, 1183
Potential energy, 1192, 1192f
  in Qi circulation, 1193f
Pre-Heaven Essence, 47–48, 47f, 279
  and DU-4 Mingmen Gate of Life, 1149
Pre-Heaven Qi, 623
Pregnancy, 239, 370
  weak constitution and, 280
Premature ejaculation, 367, 367b
Prenatal constitution, 281
Prenatal period, cause of disease in, 249
Principles of treatment, 1170
  Yin-Yang imbalance and, 423–424, 423b
Protecting function, of Qi, 58
Puberty, 48
Pulse
  in assessment of constitution, 282, 282f
  clinical significance of, 379, 380t
  correspondence of, 376f
  extraordinary channels, 883, 883f
  factors to take into account, 382–383

floating, Greater Yang stage, 753–754, 754f
LU-9 and, 957
method for taking, 380–382, 382b–383b
   arranging the fingers, 380
   levelling the arm, 380, 381f
   moving the fingers, 382
   placing the fingers, 380
   regulating the fingers, 380–382
   time, 380
   using the fingers, 382
nine regions of, 375t
normal, 383, 383b
positions, assignment to organs, 375–376
qualities, 383–389, 389t
reconciliation of contradictions, 376–379
and Stomach-Qi, 195
Stomach-Qi and, 652
'Pulse classic,' pulse position in, 376t
Pulse diagnosis, 134b, 374–389
   and interrogation, 340
   three levels, 379–380
'Pulse Study of Bin-Hu Lake,' pulse position in, 376t
Pungent taste, 141
Purple tongue, 326–327, 327b
Putrid smell, 165

Q

Qi, 50–61
   ascending of, Spleen controls, 145–147, 147b
   and Blood, 65–66, 65f
   Blood-Body fluids
      pattern identification, 448, 469–481
      see also under Blood; Body fluids
   and Body fluids, 69, 69f
   circulation
      in channels, 1193f–1194f
      between head and chest, 1194f
      potential energy in, 1193f
      see also Qi mechanism/movement
   concept of
      in medicine, 45–73
      in philosophy, 43–45, 44f–45f
   Dampness and, 416f
      External Wind and, 417f
   deficiency, 61, 470, 470b, 475
      haemorrhage and Blood deficiency and, 416f
      see also specific organs/types
   descending, Stomach controls, 196–197, 196b–197b
   diffusing of, Lungs control, 131–132
   emotions and, 256, 256f
   forms of, 50
   functions of, 57–58, 57b, 57f
   improper direction of, 427
   Kidney failing to receive, 631–633, 632b–633b, 632f–633f
   Liver ensures smooth flow of, 120–122, 120b–121b, 120f
   Lungs govern, 130–131, 130b–131b, 130f
   original. *see* Original Qi *(Yuan Qi)*
   and overwork, 283–284, 284f
   pathology of, 61, 61b
   pattern identification, 470–471
   raising of, Spleen controls, 149
   rebellious. *see* Rebellious Qi

and REN-17 Shanzhong (or Tanzhong) *Middle of Chest*, 1143
reservoirs, extraordinary vessels as, 868–869, 869b, 869f, 882–883, 883f
respiration and, 130–131, 130b, 130f
sinking. *see* Qi sinking
stagnation. *see* Qi stagnation
transformation. *see* Qi transformations
'types' of, 46, 46f
   see also specific organs/types
worry knots, 263
Qi Ji, 1002
Qi level *(Qi)*, 767, 768t, 773–775
Qi mechanism/movement, 58–61, 58f, 59b, 78–84, 79f, 86b, 86f
   ascending-descending, 79–80, 90b
      pathology of, 426–431
   derangement of, 426
   entering-exiting, 80–84, 80f–81f
      channels in, 80–81
      pathology of, 432–438
      Triple Burner and, 226–227, 229
   Heart and Kidneys as root, 86, 86f–87f
   Liver and Lungs as outer wheel, 85, 85f–86f
   pathology of, 425–438, 425b–426b
      Phlegm and, 409
   Stomach and Spleen as central axis, 84–85, 84f–85f
Qi oedema, 321
Qi-Phlegm, 480
Qi reception
   Kidney control, 160–161, 161b, 161f
   Kidney function of, 164
Qi sinking, 61, 470, 471b
   Spleen, 603–604, 603b–605b, 603f–604f, 699
Qi stagnation, 61, 405, 405b, 456, 471, 471b
   and Blood stasis, 66, 66b, 474, 474t
   Heart, 506–508, 507f–508f, 508b
   in Large Intestine, 695–696, 695b–696b, 696f
   in Pericardium, 524–526, 525b–526b, 525f–526f
   use of Connecting points to treat, 852–853
Qi transformations, 75–92, 75b
   Bladder removes Water by, 215–216, 216b
   dynamics of, 78–86, 87b
   Fire of the Gate of Life as warmth for, 76–78, 78b
   Original Qi as motive force for, 75–76, 76b, 76f
   pathology of, 89–91
      Heart, 90–91
      Kidneys, 90–91
      Liver, 89–90, 89f–90f
      Lungs, 89–90, 89f–90f
      Spleen, 89
      Stomach, 89
   physiology of, 78–86, 87b
   REN-3 Zhongji *Middle Pole*, 1131
   role, Original Qi, 51
   Triple Burner and, 87–88, 88b–89b, 88f
Qijie, 983
Qimen *Door of Qi*, 1161, 1161b, 1161f
Quivering tongue, 329

R

Raising function, of Qi, 58
Rancid smell, 125

Rapid *(Shu)* pulse, 384, 384b
Rapidity-slowness, Yin-Yang, 12
Rates, normal, 384t
Rebellious Qi, 61, 471, 472f–473f, 810, 1071
   Four Seas and, 244
   KI-14 for, 1072
   Penetrating Vessel and, 909–911, 909f–910f, 910b
   types of, 472t
   see also Liver-Qi, rebellious
Receiving functions
   of Small Intestine, 201, 201b–202b, 201f
   of Stomach, 193–194, 194b
Recreational drugs, 294
Rectus abdominis, Penetrating Vessel and, 913
Red colour
   of eye, 317
   of face, 315, 315b
Red complexion, 114
Red tongue, 325–326, 326b, 326f
   Wind-Heat and, 730
Reddish-purple tongue, 326, 327f
Redness-paleness, Yin-Yang, 12
Regulating function, of extraordinary vessels, 872–874, 873f, 874b
REN-1 Huiyin *Meeting of Yin*, 1129–1130, 1130b
REN-2 Qugu *Curved Bone*, 1130–1131, 1131b
REN-3 Zhongji *Middle Pole*, 1131, 1131b, 1133t
REN-4 Guanyuan *Gate of the Original Qi*, 178b, 900, 1042, 1068, 1132–1133, 1133b, 1133t, 1135t
REN-5 Shimen *Stone Door*, 1133–1134
REN-6 Qihai *Sea of Qi*, 1134–1135, 1135b, 1135t
REN-7 Yinjiao *Yin Crossing*, 1135–1136, 1136b
REN-8 Shenque *Spirit Palace*, 1136–1138, 1137f, 1138b
REN-9 Shuifen *Water Separation*, 1138, 1138b, 1139f
REN-10 Xiawan *Lower Epigastrium*, 1138–1139, 1139b
REN-11 Jianli *Building Mile*, 1139, 1139b
REN-12 Zhongwan *Middle of Epigastrium*, 1139–1140, 1140b, 1140f
REN-13 Shangwan *Upper Epigastrium*, 1140–1141, 1141b
REN-14 Juque *Great Palace*, 1141, 1142b, 1142f
REN-15 Jiuwei *Dove Tail*, 1142–1143, 1143b
Ren-17 Shanzhong, 53–54, 54f, 176b, 859
REN-17 Shanzhong (or Tanzhong) *Middle of Chest*, 1143, 1143b
REN-22 Tiantu *Heaven Projection*, 1144, 1144b
REN-23 Lianquan *Corner Spring*, 1144, 1144b
REN-24 Chengjiang *Saliva Receiver*, 1144–1145, 1145b
Reproduction
   Essence, 48–49
   Kidneys governing, 157–158, 158b
   see also Childbirth; Conception
'Residual pathogenic factor', 1183
Resolute organ, Liver as, 126
Respiration, 130–131, 130b–131b, 130f
Respiratory symptoms, in children, 370–371
Restless-quiet, Yin-Yang, 12
Retention of food, 344, 668–672, 669f, 670b

Rigidity
  of limbs, 322, 322b
  from Wind, 727
Rising, Liver influences, 126
River *(Jing)* point, 833, 833b, 835–837, 841t
Root, normal pulse, 383
Root *(Ben)*, 1172f, 1173–1178, 1173b, 1175t, 1177b
  identification of, 1175
  and manifestation *(Biao)*, 1172f, 1173–1178, 1173b, 1175t
    multiple, 1177–1178, 1178b
    as original and deriving patterns, 1173f, 1175b
    as root and clinical manifestations of condition, 1173f
    treating root only, 1176, 1176b–1177b
    treatment of both, 1176–1177
    as tree, 1173f
  multiple, giving rise to different manifestations, 1178
  one, giving rise to different manifestations, 1178
  secondary, manifestation becoming, 1174f
  treating manifestation before, 1177
Root of Original Qi *(Yuan Qi)*, 164
'Root of Post-Heaven Qi', 147, 194
Rotten smell, 102, 140–141
'Rotting and ripening' of food, 194, 194b, 198, 224–226
Roundworms, 683
Running piglet syndrome, 1071
Runny nose, 351
  LU-7 and, 954

S
Sadness, 176, 176b, 261–262, 262b–263b, 262f, 366, 366b
  and Heart, 490–491, 491b
  and Large Intestine, 687–688
  and Liver, 531
  LU-3 and, 951
  and Lungs, 140, 140b, 140f, 573, 573b, 573f
Saliva, 102
  Spleen controls, 149, 149b
Salty taste, 165
Sayings
  Heart, 115
  Kidneys, 165–166, 166b
  Liver, 126–127
  Lungs, 141–142
  Spleen, 151–153
Scattered face colour, 316, 316b
Scattered *(San)* pulse, 387, 388b
Scattering, of Summer-Heat, 737
Sciatica, Yang Stepping Vessel and, 927, 927b
Scorched smell, 102, 114
Sea *(He)* point, 833, 833b, 835–838, 841t
Sea of Blood, 244, 244b, 860
  BL-11 and, 1032
  Penetrating Vessel as, 244, 907–908, 908b
Sea of Food, 244b, 245, 860, 983
Sea of Marrow, 241, 244, 244b, 860
Sea of Qi, 244b, 245, 860, 977
  and Gathering Qi, 53–54, 245
Sea of the 12 channels, Penetrating Vessel as, 908, 908b

Sea of the five Yin and six Yang organs, Penetrating Vessel as, 908, 909b
'Sea of the Yin channels', 897
'Sea of Yang channels', 893
Seasons
  application in clinical practice, 30
  correspondences of the Five Elements, 26t
    and pulse, 382
  Summer-Heat as pathogenic factor, 725, 736
  Transporting *(Shu)* points, 838, 838b
Sense organs/orifices
  application in clinical practice, 30
  correspondences of the Five Elements, 26t
  Five Elements in diagnosis, 37, 37b
  pathology of ascending/descending of Qi in, 431, 431f–432f, 431t
  see also specific sense organs/orifices
Senses, 72, 241
  see also specific senses
Sexual activity
  beneficial effects of, 289–290, 290f
  excessive, 285–290, 286b, 286t, 290b
    Bladder deficient and Cold, 718
    Bladder patterns and, 713–714
    and Kidney, 623–625, 627, 630, 636
    Kidney-Essence, 634
  insufficient, as cause of disease, 288–289, 289b
Sexual desire, 289, 289b
Sexual disease, in women, 288, 288f
Sexual frustration, 289
Sexual life, questions about, 342
Sexual symptoms, 366–368
  men, 367
  questions, 366
  women, 367–368
  see also Sexual activity, excessive
Sexuality, differences between men's and women's, 287–288
Shan Zhong, 518
'Shang', 1074
Shiqizhuixia *Below the 17th Vertebra*, 1163f, 1164, 1164b
Shivers, 275
Shixuan *Ten Declarations*, 1165f, 1166, 1166b
Shock, 265–266, 265b, 265f
Short *(Duan)* pulse, 385, 385b
Short tongue, 329
Shoulder
  joint, empirical distal point for pain and stiffness of, 988
  pain, LU-1 and, 950
  ST-38 as distal point for, 1200f
Shoulder problems
  S.I.-9 Jianzhen *Upright Shoulder* and, 1021
  S.I.-12 Bingfeng *Watching Wind* and, 1022
  S.I.-13 Quyuan *Bent Wall* and, 1023
  S.I.-14 Jianwaishu *Transporting Point of the Outside of the Shoulder* and, 1023
Shouting, 126
'Shu', 1073
'Shuttle', 1032
S.I.-1 Shaoze *Lesser Marsh*, 1016, 1016b
S.I.-2 Qiangu *Front Valley*, 1016, 1017b
S.I.-3 Houxi *Back Stream*, 1017–1018, 1018b, 1018f
S.I.-4 Wangu *Wrist Bone*, 1018–1019, 1019b
S.I.-5 Yanggu *Yang Valley*, 1019, 1019b

S.I.-6 Yanglao *Nourishing the Elderly*, 1019, 1020b
S.I.-7 Zhizheng *Branch to Heart Channel*, 1020, 1020b
S.I.-8 Xiaohai *Small Intestine Sea*, 1020, 1021b
S.I.-9 Jianzhen *Upright Shoulder*, 1021, 1021b
S.I.-10 Naoshu *Humerus Transporting Point*, 1021, 1021b
S.I.-11 Tianzong *Heavenly Attribution*, 1021–1022, 1022b
S.I.-12 Bingfeng *Watching Wind*, 1022, 1022b
S.I.-13 Quyuan *Bent Wall*, 1022–1023, 1023b
S.I.-14 Jianwaishu *Transporting Point of the Outside of the Shoulder*, 1023, 1023b
S.I.-15 Jianzhongshu *Transporting Point of the Centre of the Shoulder*, 1023–1024, 1024b, 1024f
S.I.-16 Tianchuang *Heavenly Window*, 1024, 1024b
S.I.-17 Tianrong *Heavenly Appearance*, 1024–1025, 1025b
S.I.-18 Quanliao *Zygoma Crevice*, 1025, 1025b
S.I.-19 Tinggong *Listening Palace*, 1025–1026, 1026b
Sifeng *Four Cracks*, 1165, 1165f, 1166b
Sighing, diagnosis by, 398
Sinews
  of arm, LU-5 and, 953
  Gall Bladder controls, 211, 211b
  invasion of Cold and, 734
  Liver-Blood moistens, 119–120, 119f
  Liver controls, 122–123, 122b–123b
  SP-5 Shangqiu *Metal Mound* and, 1000
Singing, 151
Sinking Qi. *see* Qi sinking.
Sishencong *Four Mind Alertness*, 1159, 1159b, 1159f
Six extraordinary Yang organs, 234–245, 235b
Six Stages
  pattern identification according to, 724, 751–764, 751b, 753f
  theory of, 270, 270b
Skin
  chronic Dampness in, 742
  Connecting points, 853
  Dampness in, 738
  diagnosis by observation, 324, 324b
  Lungs, control of, 135–136, 136b–137b, 136f–137f
  non-substantial Phlegm, 478
  palpating, 389–390
  rashes and Warm disease, 769–770, 769f–770f, 769t
  Wind and, 728, 731, 731b
  see also Space between skin and muscles (*Cou Li* space)
Sleep, 71
  in children, 371
  symptoms, 355–356
  Yin Stepping Vessel and, 923–924, 924f
Slippery *(Hua)* pulse, 385, 385b
Slow *(Chi)* pulse, 384, 384b
Slowed-down *(Huan)* pulse, 386, 386b
Small Intestine
  aspects of, 201
  and Body fluids, 68
  connections with organs, 678f
  and fluids, 202, 202b, 202f, 215
  Full-Heat in, 678–680, 679f, 680b

functions of, 201–204, 201*b*
HE-5 Tongli *Inner Communication* and, 1009, 1009*f*
pathology of ascending/descending of Qi and, 429
relationship between Bladder and, 215, 215*f*–216*f*, 216*b*
worm infestation in, 683, 683*b*, 683*f*
Small Intestine channel, 1015–1026
 connecting channel pathway of, 1015*f*
 main channel pathway of, 1015, 1015*f*
 patterns, 800
 points of, 1015, 1015*b*
 target areas, 1026*f*
Small Intestine patterns, 677–685, 677*b*
 aetiology (general) of, 677–678, 678*b*
 Empty, 684–685
 Full, 678–683, 678*b*, 679*f*
Small Intestine-Qi
 pain, 680–681, 680*b*–681*b*, 680*f*–681*f*
 tied, 681–682, 681*f*–682*f*, 682*b*
Smell(s)
 in diagnosis, 399–400
 Five Elements and, 36, 36*b*
 of Heart, 114
 of Kidneys, 165
 of Liver, 125
 of Lungs, 140–141
 sense of, loss of, LU-7 and, 954
 of Spleen, 151
Smoking, 573, 576, 589
Sneezing, LU-7 and, 954
Soggy *(Ru)* pulse, 387, 387*b*
Sore throat, LU-11 and, 958
Sound(s)
 application in clinical practice, 31
 correspondences of the Five Elements, 26*t*
 diagnosis by, Five Elements, 35, 35*b*
 five-elements, 398*f*
 Heart, 114
 internal organs and, 103, 103*b*
 Kidney, 165
 Liver, 126
 Lungs, 141
 Spleen, 151
Sour taste, 125
Source *(Yuan)* points, 52*b*, 845–847
 and Connecting channels, 848, 849*f*
 Connecting points in, conjunction with, 850–851, 851*b*
 and Original Qi, 51–52, 51*f*
SP-1 Yinbai *Hidden White*, 995–996, 996*b*
SP-2 Dadu *Big Capital*, 996–997, 997*b*
SP-3 Taibai *Supreme White*, 997–998, 998*b*
SP-4 Gongsun *Minute Connecting Channels*, 998–999, 999*b*, 999*f*
SP-5 Shangqiu *Metal Mound*, 999–1000, 1000*b*
SP-6 Sanyinjiao *Three Yin Meeting*, 1000–1001, 1001*b*
SP-8 Diji *Earth Pivot*, 1001–1002, 1002*b*
SP-9 Yinlingquan *Yin Mound Spring*, 1002, 1002*b*
SP-10 Xuehai *Sea of Blood*, 1003–1004, 1003*f*, 1004*b*
SP-12 Chongmen *Penetrating Door*, 1004, 1004*b*
SP-15 Daheng *Big Horizontal Stroke*, 1004–1005, 1005*b*

SP-21 Dabao *General Control*, 1005, 1005*b*
Space between skin and muscles *(Cou Li* space)
 entering-exiting of Qi in, 81–82, 81*f*, 82*b*
 pathology of, 433, 434*b*, 434*f*
 Lungs control, 135–136, 136*b*–137*b*, 136*f*–137*f*
Spasticity, of limbs, 323, 323*b*
Speech
 Heart controls, 115
 see also Sound(s)
Sperm, 287, 287*f*
 production of, 240
Spinal branch, of Penetrating Vessel *(Chong Mai)*, 906
Spinal cord, Kidney-Essence and, 159*f*
Spine, SP-3 Taibai *Supreme White* and, 998
Spirit
 diagnosis by observation, 306–307, 307*b*
 normal pulse, 383
 Yin organs, 110, 111*f*
'Spiritual axis'
 Connecting *(Luo)* points, 851, 851*b*
 source *(Yuan)* points, 845–847, 846*f*, 847*b*
 Transporting *(Shu)* points, 835–837, 836*b*, 841*t*
Spittle, 102
 Kidneys control, 161, 162*b*
Spleen, 143–153, 143*b*
 and Blood, 63*f*, 64
 and Body fluids, 67, 68*f*
 Cold-Dampness invading, 608–610, 608*f*–609*f*, 609*b*–610*b*
 controls Blood, 147–148, 147*b*–148*b*, 147*f*
 damage to, Phlegm and, 410
 Damp-Heat in, 610–612, 610*b*–612*b*, 610*f*–611*f*, 789, 790*b*
 Dampness in, 741
 functions of, 144–150
 great connecting channel of, 799, 996*f*, 1005
 and Heart, 184–187, 184*f*, 185*b*
 insufficient eating and, 291
 intellect *(Yi)* and, 111
 and Kidneys, 28, 183, 183*b*, 183*f*
 and Liver, 181, 181*b*, 181*f*
 LU-1 tonifies, 950
 and Lungs, 28, 182–183, 182*f*, 183*b*
 not controlling Blood, 605–606, 605*b*–606*b*, 605*f*–606*f*
 origin of birth and development, 152
 pathology of ascending/descending of Qi and, 427, 427*b*, 427*f*
 raises clear (Yang) upwards, 152, 152*f*
 rebellious Liver-Qi invading, 560–562, 560*b*–562*b*, 560*f*–561*f*
 relationships, 151
 sayings, 151–153
 and Stomach, 60, 61*f*
  centre role, 29
  as support for Heart, 30
 transformation and transportation of, 145*f*, 146*b*
  fluids, 145, 146*f*
  food Essences and Qi, 144–145
 Uterus and, 238, 238*f*, 239*b*
 worry and, 263
 see also Stomach, and Spleen

Spleen-Blood deficiency, 606–607, 606*b*, 607*f*–608*f*, 608*b*, 612–614, 612*b*, 612*f*–613*f*, 614*b*, 616–617, 616*b*–617*b*, 616*f*–617*f*
Spleen channel, 995–1006
 connecting channel pathway of, 995, 996*f*
 main channel pathway of, 995, 995*f*
 patterns, 799
 points of, 995, 995*b*
 target areas, 1006*f*
Spleen patterns, 597–620, 597*b*, 620*b*
 aetiology (general), 598, 598*b*
 combined, 612–620
 Empty, 599–607
 Full, 608–612
Spleen-Qi
 ascending, 146–147, 146*f*
 deficiency, 145*b*, 148*b*, 599–601, 599*b*–601*b*, 599*f*–601*f*, 606*b*, 606*f*
 and Lung-Qi deficiency, 614–616, 614*b*, 614*f*–615*f*, 616*b*
 pathology of, 615*f*
 Stomach-Qi deficiency and, 657*b*, 672–673, 672*b*–673*b*, 672*f*–673*f*
 variations of, 600*f*
 and Food-Qi, 52
 and REN-12 Zhongwan *Middle of Epigastrium*, 1140
 sinking, 603–604, 603*b*–605*b*, 603*f*–604*f*, 699
Spleen-Yang deficiency, 602, 602*b*–603*b*, 602*f*–603*f*, 736, 1176
 and Kidney-Yang deficiency, 646–649, 646*b*, 647*f*, 648*b*
Spleen-Yin
 deficiency, Stomach-Yin deficiency and, 673–675, 673*b*–675*b*, 674*f*–675*f*
 and REN-12 Zhongwan *Middle of Epigastrium*, 1140
Spring *(Ying)* point, 832–834, 833*b*, 836–838, 841*t*
Sputum odour, 400
ST-1 Chengqi *Containing Tears*, 974, 974*b*
ST-2 Sibai *Four Whites*, 974–975, 975*b*
ST-3 Juliao *Great Crevice*, 975, 975*b*
ST-4 Dicang *Earth Granary*, 975, 976*b*
ST-6 Jiache *Jaw Chariot*, 976, 976*b*
ST-7 Xiaguan *Lower Gate*, 976, 977*b*
ST-8 Touwei *Head Corner*, 977, 977*b*
ST-9 Renying *Person's Welcome*, 977, 978*b*
ST-12 Quepen *Empty Basin*, 978, 978*b*
ST-18 Rugen *Breast Root*, 978, 979*b*
ST-19 Burong *Full*, 979, 979*b*
ST-20 Chengman *Supporting Fullness*, 979, 979*b*
ST-21 Liangmen *Beam Door*, 979–980, 980*b*
ST-22 Guanmen *Pass Gate*, 980, 980*b*
ST-25 Tianshu *Heavenly Pivot*, 980–981, 981*b*
ST-27 Daju *Big Greatness*, 981, 982*b*
ST-28 Shuidao *Water Passages*, 982, 982*b*
ST-29 Guilai *Return*, 982–983, 983*b*
ST-30 Qichong *Penetrating Qi*, 983, 984*b*
ST-31 Biguan *Thigh Gate*, 984, 984*b*
ST-32 Futu *Crouching Rabbit*, 984, 984*b*
ST-34 Liangqiu *Beam Mound*, 985, 985*b*
ST-35 Dubi *Calf Nose*, 985, 985*b*
ST-36 Zusanli *Three Miles of the Foot*, 985–987, 987*b*

ST-37 Shangjuxu *Upper Great Emptiness*, 987, 987b
ST-38 Tiaokou *Narrow Opening*, 987–988, 988b
ST-39 Xiajuxu *Lower Great Emptiness*, 988, 988b
ST-40 Fenglong *Abundant Bulge*, 988–989, 989b, 989f
ST-41 Jiexi *Dispersing Stream*, 989–990, 990b
ST-42 Chongyang *Penetrating Yang*, 990, 990b
ST-43 Xiangu *Sinking Valley*, 990–991, 991b
ST-44 Neiting *Inner Courtyard*, 991, 991b
ST-45 Lidui *Sick Mouth*, 991–992, 992b
Stage of development, correspondences of the Five Elements, 26t
Stagnation
  Cold, 546–547, 547f, 548b, 814
  Heat, in Directing and Penetrating Vessels, 813
  of Qi, pain and, 344
Stasis of Blood, pain and, 344
Sticky Dampness, 738–739
Stiff neck, Greater Yang stage, 753, 754f
Stiff tongue, 328, 329f
Stomach
  anger and, 259
  area, distal and local points, 1197t
  aspects of, 193
  Blood stasis, 474, 670–672, 670b–672b, 670f–671f
  and Body fluids, 68, 477
  Cold and, 654, 657–658, 657f–658f, 658b, 664–665, 664b–665b, 664f–665f
  damage to, Phlegm and, 410
  Damp-Heat in, 667–668, 667b–668b, 667f–668f
  Dampness in, 741
  functions of, 193–199, 193b
  gate of Kidney, 166
  invasion of Cold and, 734
  invasion of external Dampness in, 740
  pathology of ascending/descending of Qi and, 427–428, 427f, 428b
  Penetrating Vessel and, 912–913
  Phlegm-Fluids in, 480
  rebellious Liver-Qi invading, 562–563, 562f–563f, 563b
  retention of food in, 668–672, 669f, 670b
  'rotting and ripening' of food, 194, 194b, 198
  as Sea of Food, 244
  and Spleen, 60, 61f, 197b–198b, 198–199, 198f
    central role, 29, 56
  Damp-Heat in, 775, 775b
  Essence-Qi-Mind, 50
  as 'Root of Post-Heaven Qi', 194
  as 'Root of the Post-Heaven Essence', 48
  smooth flow of Liver-Qi, 120
  as support for Heart, 30
  transformation of fluids, 152
  Uterus and, 238–239, 238f, 239b
Stomach channel, 973–993
  connecting channel pathway of, 973, 974f
  in legs, Girdle Vessel affects Qi of, 919, 919f
  main channel pathway of, 973, 973f
  patterns, 798–799
  points of, 973, 973b
    target areas, 992f

Stomach-Dryness, 744, 744b
Stomach-Fire, 663, 663b, 748
  Phlegm-Fire, 198
Stomach-Heat, 662–664, 662b, 662f–663f, 664b, 773–774, 774b, 990
  case history, 664b
Stomach patterns, 651–675, 651b–652b
  aetiology of, 653–655, 655b
  combined, 672–675
  Empty, 654
  Full, 660–672
Stomach problems, ST-21 Liangmen *Beam Door* and, 980
Stomach-Qi, 146, 194, 196f, 198, 1082
  deficiency of, 655–657, 655b, 655f, 657b
    aetiology of, 655
    clinical manifestations of, 655
    pathology of, 655–656, 656f
    treatment of, 656–657
  and pulse diagnosis, 383
  rebelling upwards, 666–667, 666f, 667b
  and REN-10 Xiawan *Lower Epigastrium*, 1138
  and REN-12 Zhongwan *Middle of Epigastrium*, 1140
  and REN-13 Shangwan *Upper Epigastrium*, 1140–1141
  stagnation of, 660–662, 661f, 662b
Stomach-Yin
  deficiency of, 658–660, 658b–660b, 659f–660f
  and Spleen-Yin deficiency, 673–675, 673b–675b, 674f–675f
  and REN-12 Zhongwan *Middle of Epigastrium*, 1140
Stools, 345–347
  constipation, 346, 346b
  diarrhoea, 346–347, 346b
  Large Intestine transforms, 206
  odour, 400
Stream (*Shu*) point, 833–834, 833b, 836–838, 841t
'Streets of Qi', 983
Strength and skill, Kidneys controlling, 166
Strong prenatal constitution, 281, 281f
Substantial *vs* non-substantial
  Phlegm, 478–481
  Yin-Yang, 12
Sugar, 292
Summer-Heat, 736–737, 771–772, 772b
  characteristics of, 737b
  clinical manifestations of, 737
  Dampness and, 737, 741
  interior Heat of, 737
  as pathogenic factor, 725, 737
  scattering of, 737
  symptoms and signs of invasion of, 276
  top of body and, 737
Sun Si Miao's ghost points, REN-1 Huiyin *Meeting of Yin*, 1130
Supraclavicular fossa
  Stomach channel and, 973
  superficial pathway of channel from, 1015
Sweat/sweating, 357
  causes of, 357b
  in full and empty conditions, 357
  Heart and, 102, 113–114, 113f
  night, 628
  odour, 400

quality of, 358
slight, 755
symptoms, 357–358
Upper Burner and, 222–223
Sweet foods, 292
Sweet taste, 151
Swelling, of skin, in diagnosis by observation, 324
Swollen tongue, 327–328, 328f

T
Taiyang *Greater Yang*, 1160, 1160b, 1160f
Tapeworms, 683
Taste(s)
  application in clinical practice, 30
  correspondences of the Five Elements, 26t
  Five Elements in diagnosis, 36, 37b
  and Heart, 114
  of herbs, 1185, 1185t
  internal organs and, 103, 103b
  and Kidney, 165
  and Liver, 125
  and Lungs, 141
  sense of, 148–149
  and Spleen, 151
T.B.-1 Guanchong *Penetrating the Gate*, 1088, 1089b
T.B.-2 Yemen *Fluid Door*, 1089, 1089b
T.B.-3 Zhongzhu *Middle Islet*, 1089–1090, 1090b
T.B.-4 Yangchi *Yang Pond*, 1090–1091, 1091b
T.B.-5 Waiguan *Outer Gate*, 1091–1092, 1092b, 1117t
T.B.-6 Zhigou *Branching Ditch*, 1092–1093, 1093b, 1117t
T.B.-7 Huizong, 858
T.B.-7 Huizong *Converging Channels*, 1093, 1093b
T.B.-8 Sanyangluo *Connecting Three Yang*, 1093–1094, 1094b
T.B.-10 Tianjing *Heavenly Well*, 1094, 1094b
T.B.-13 Naohui *Shoulder Convergence*, 1094–1095, 1095b
T.B.-14 Jianliao *Shoulder Crevice*, 1095, 1095b
T.B.-15 Tianliao *Heavenly Crevice*, 1095, 1095b
T.B.-16 Tianyou *Window of Heaven*, 1096, 1096b
T.B.-17 Yifeng *Wind Screen*, 1096, 1097b
T.B.-21 Ermen *Ear Door*, 1096–1097, 1097b
T.B.-23 Sizhukong *Silk Bamboo Hole*, 1097, 1097b
Tears, Liver controls, 124
Teeth, diagnosis by observation, 319, 319b
Temperature, of skin, 389–390, 390b
Temples area, distal and local points, 1197t
Temporal points, of eye system, 863, 863f
Tendinitis, L.I.-12 and, 968
Tendinomuscular problems, Connecting points, 851–852
Terminal Yin (*Jue Yin*) stage, 762–764, 763b, 763f
Terminology, problems in interrogation, 338–339
Texture, of skin, 390, 390b
Thenar eminence, diagnosis by observation, 323, 323b
Thin face colour, 316, 316b
Thin tongue, 327
Thinking, 71, 241

Thirst, in diagnosis, 347, 348b
Three Burners
　pattern identification according to, 724, 787–792, 787b
　theory of, 271
　see also Triple Burner
Three treasures, 253, 253f
　Essence as basis of, 50, 50t
　for Stomach
　　Blood stasis, 672
　　Damp-Heat, 668
　　Qi deficiency, 657
　　Stomach- and Spleen-Qi deficiency, 673
　　Yin deficiency, 660
Throat
　area, distal and local points, 1197t
　diagnosis by observation, 320
　problems, L.I.-18 and, 970
Thyroid Phlegm swellings, S.I.-7 Zhizheng Branch to Heart Channel and, 1020
Tight (Jin) pulse, 386, 386b
Time, of meals, 653–654, 654b
Tingling. see Numbness/tingling.
Tinnitus, 358
　S.I.-19 Tinggong Listening Palace and, 1026
Tiredness, 651b
　after ejaculation, 367
　in the morning, 655b
Tissues
　application in clinical practice, 30
　correspondences of the Five Elements, 26t
　in diagnosis, Five Elements, 37, 37b
Tituo Lift and Support, 1161f, 1162, 1162b
Tongue
　area, distal and local points, 1197t
　in assessment of constitution, 282, 282f
　drug effects on, 293, 293f–294f
　Heart opens into, 113, 113b
　Stomach-Qi and, 652, 652f
Tongue coating, 195f–196f, 330–331, 330f, 331b
　Stomach-Qi and, 194–195
Tongue diagnosis
　and interrogation, 340
　microsystem, 302
　by observation, 324–331, 324f–325f, 325b
Tongue shape, 327–330, 327b
Tonification and drainage points, 838, 838t
Tonifying Upright Qi (Zheng Qi), 1180–1181, 1181b
　and expelling pathogenic factors, 1182–1184
　　expelling pathogenic factors first then tonifying Upright Qi, 1182–1184, 1183b
　　simultaneously tonifying Upright Qi and expelling pathogenic factors, 1184, 1184b
　　tonifying Upright Qi first then expelling pathogenic factors, 1182, 1184b
Tonsillitis, toxic Heat in, 1025
Tonsils
　diagnosis by observation, 320, 320b
　swollen, LU-11 and, 958
Toothmarked tongue, 330
Toxic Heat, 749–750, 750b
Transformation
　and conservation, Yin-Yang, 12–13, 13t
　of fluids, 898
　　Triple Burner and, 1090

interaction between Yin and Yang and, 420–421, 421b, 421f
Large Intestine, 206
role, Qi, 57
Transforming functions, of Small Intestine, 201, 201b–202b, 201f
Transportation
　of fluids, 898
　of food essences, 194–195, 195b–196b, 195f, 243
　function of Qi, 57–58
　of Qi, control by Triple Burner, 221–222, 221f, 222b
Transporting points (Shu points), 829–843, 829b, 833t, 834b, 841t
　channels and, 829
　energetic actions of, 832–833
　from the classics, 834–839
　see also Back Transporting (Shu) points
Trauma, 292, 292b
Treatment principles, 1171–1189, 1171b
　application of, differences between acupuncture and herbal therapy in, 1184–1189
　case history, 1186b–1189b
　case history of, 1174b–1175b
Tremor of limbs, 323, 323b, 354
Triple Burner, 135, 219–232, 219b
　aspects of, 229–232
　and Body fluids, 68
　cavities, 82, 82f
　　pathology of entering/exiting of Qi and, 433, 434b
　Directing Vessel activates, 898–899
　four views of, 223–229
　functions of, 219–223, 220b
　Original Qi as conduit of, 51
　Original Qi mobilization by, 219–220, 220b, 220f
　and pulse diagnosis, 378
　Qi transportation and penetration and, 221–222, 221f, 222b
　transformation of Qi and, 87–88, 88b–89b, 88f
　see also Three Burners
Triple Burner channel, 1087–1097
　connecting channel pathway in, 1087, 1087f
　main channel pathway in, 1087, 1087f
　patterns, 802
　points, overview of, 1087b
　target areas of, 1097f
True cold-false heat, 461, 461t
True heat-false cold, 461, 461t
True Qi (Zhen Qi), 54–56, 54b, 54f
12 Heavenly Star points, of Ma Dan Yang, 862

U
Ulcers
　mouth, 351, 351b
　with swelling, Fire and, 747–748
Undereating, Stomach and, 653
Unilateral needling, in balancing left and right sides of the body, 1204–1206, 1204b, 1204f, 1206b
Unilateral problem, balancing left and right when treating, 1204
Unstable Directing and Penetrating Vessels, 810

Upper body, and lower body, balancing, 1202–1204, 1202t
Upper Burner, 87, 135, 146
　like a mist, 225, 225f, 226b
　patterns, 787–789
　Qi, 221, 223–224, 226b
　sweat and, 222–223
Upper Sea points, 835
Upright Qi (Zheng Qi), 56, 57b, 986
　deficient
　　no pathogenic factor and, 413, 413b
　　strong pathogenic factor and, 414, 414b
　　weak pathogenic factor and, 415, 415b
　pathogenic factors and, 412–413, 413f, 413t, 415–417, 416b, 416f, 1178–1184
　　case history of, 1179b
　　full-empty conditions in, 1180b, 1180t, 1181
　　strong, weak pathogenic factor and, 414–415, 415b
　tonifying, 1180–1181, 1181b
　　and expelling pathogenic factors, 1182–1184
Urethra area, distal and local points, 1197t
Urinary function, SP-6 Sanyinjiao Three Yin Meeting and, 1000–1001
Urinary retention, LU-7 and, 955
Urination, frequent, LU-5 and, 953
Urine
　diagnosis, 347, 347b
　excretion of, 226
　odour, 400
　production of, 215
Uterus, 235–240, 235f–236f
　Blood stasis symptoms and signs, 474–475
　Dampness in, 742
　　and Phlegm, 814
　deficient and Cold, 813–814
　Directing Vessel and, 236–237, 236f, 237b, 898
　extraordinary vessels, 871
　functions of, 240b
　invasion of Cold and, 734
　invasion of external Dampness in, 740
　Kidneys warming, 164
　in men, 240
　Penetrating Vessel and, 236–237, 236f, 237b
　Pericardium and, 172–173, 1082
　relationship between Pericardium, Heart, Liver and, 1083f
　and REN-3 Zhongji Middle Pole, 1131
　and REN-4 Guanyuan Gate of the Original Qi, 1132
　and REN-7 Yinjiao Yin Crossing, 1135
　and Spleen, 238, 238f, 239b
　stagnant Cold in, 814
　Triple Burner's transformation and penetration of Qi and, 1092–1093
Uterus channel, 237

V
Vagina, Governing Vessel and, 893
Vaginal discharge
　colour of, 125
　odour, 400
Vegetarianism, 291
Vertex area, distal and local points, 1197t
Vesicles, 769

1287

Viruses, and bacteria, 269, 270b
Vital substances, 43–74, 43b
   internal organs and, 98, 98b
Voice
   diagnosis by, 397–398, 398b
   excessive use of, 574, 576
   Lungs govern, 141
   see also Sound(s)
Vomiting, 345b
   diagnosis by, 398
   and food, 345

W

Waist
   structures above and below, 10
   Yang and Yin Linking Vessels and, combined pathology of, 936
Warm diseases, 268, 270, 765
   Four Levels, 766–768
   nature of, 766
   and skin rashes, 769–770, 769f–770f, 769t
   and Wind-Heat, 766, 766b
'Warm epidemic pathogenic factors', 268
Warming function, of Qi, 58
Water
   accumulation, Greater Yang stage, 756, 756b
   body type, 309, 310f, 311b
   and Fire
     mutual assistance of, 178
     in sexual activity, 289–290
   as foundation, 29
   insulting Earth, 823
   Kidneys as origin of, 157f
   Kidneys control, 160b
   Kidneys govern, 160
   not generating Wood, 822
   overacting on Fire, 822
   overflowing, Kidney-Yang deficiency, 635–637, 636b–637b, 636f–637f
   removal of, by Bladder, 215–216, 216b
   see also Body fluids (Jin-Ye); Fluids
Water oedema, 321
'Water overflowing', 1183–1184
Water passages
   L.I.-6 and, 965
   Lungs and Kidneys, 184
   Lungs regulate, 134–135, 135b, 135f
   Triple Burner and, 222–223, 223b
Weak constitution, 279–283
   causes of, 280, 280f, 281b
   see also Constitution
Weak-floating (Ru) pulse, 387, 387b
Weak knees, 355
Weak prenatal constitution, 281–282, 282f
Weak (Ruo) pulse, 387, 387b
Weeping, 141
   LU-3 and, 951
   LU-7 and, 955
Well (Jing) point, 832, 832b, 834, 836, 841t
Western medicine, vs. Chinese medicine, in exterior pathogenic factor, 269
Western patients, diagnostic questions for, 341–342
White colour
   of eye, 317
   of face, 315, 315b
Whole body microsystems, in diagnosis, 302–303, 305f

Whooping cough, LU-5 and, 953
Will-power (Zhi), 101, 111, 150, 178
   Kidney control, 162b
   Kidney house, 162
Wind, 727–732
   attack of, 754–755, 755b
   bacteria and viruses in relation to, 269, 270b
   Chinese characters for, 270f
   clinical manifestations of, 727
   Cold and, 729
   convulsions and, 727
   and DU-16 Fengfu Wind Palace, 1154
   external, 728–731, 895–896
   Fire and, 747
   Heat victorious stirring, 777, 777b
   internal, 732, 732b, 896
   itching and, 728
   L.I.-1 and, 962
   Liver and, 125, 127, 727–728
   Liver-Heat stirs, 790, 791b
   Lungs and, 572, 579–581, 579b, 579f–580f, 581b, 727
   movement of manifestations and, 727
   numbness/tingling and, 727
   paralysis and, 727, 731b
   rapid changes and, 727
   rapid onset of, 727
   relationships of, 725
   skin and, 728
   symptoms and signs of invasion of, 276
   top part of the body and, 727
   tremors and, 727
   see also Climate(s)
Wind-Cold, 730, 730b
Wind-Cold invasion
   Cold prevalent, 755, 756b
   of Lungs, 572, 579–581, 579b, 579f–580f, 581b
   Wind prevalent, 754–755, 755b
Wind-Dampness, 730, 730b
Wind-Dryness, 730, 730b
Wind-Heat, 455, 730, 730b, 770–771, 771b, 771t
   and DU-14 Dazhui Big Vertebra, 1153
   invasion of Lungs, 581–582, 581b–582b, 581f–582f
   in Lung's Defensive-Qi portion, 787–788, 788b
   T.B.-5 and, 1091
   T.B.-6 and, 1093
   and Warm diseases, 766, 766b
Wind-Phlegm, 480
Wind-stroke
   HE-1 Jiquan Supreme Spring and, 1008
   HE-9 Shaochong Lesser-Yin Penetrating and, 1013
Wind-Water, 731
   invasion of Lungs, 582–584, 582b, 583f, 584b
Window of Heaven points, 860–861, 861b, 861f
Wiry (Xian) pulse, 386, 386b
Wisdom, 72
Women
   breast palpation, 393
   Directing Vessel and, 898
   Governing Vessel and, 892–893
   Liver-Blood deficiency in, 549, 568
     Heart-Blood deficiency and, 566

   Liver-Qi stagnation in, 533–534, 534b, 568
   sexual activity, 623, 624f
   sexual disease in, 288
   sexual symptoms, 367–368, 368b
   symptoms, 368–370, 369b
   vegetarianism in, 291
   Yin Linking Vessel and, 932
Wood, 21
   body type, 307, 308b, 308f
   eyes and, 31
   insulting Metal, 823
   not generating Fire, 821–822
   overacting on Earth, 822
   system correspondences related to, 30
   Triple Burner and, 229, 230f
Worm infestation, 293, 683, 683b, 683f
Worry, 263, 263b, 263f, 365, 366b
   and Heart, 491
   and Large Intestine, 688
   and Liver, 531
   and Lungs, 140, 140b, 140f, 573
   and Spleen, 598
   see also Pensiveness
Wrong treatment, 293

X

Xiphoid process
   area below, 393b
   palpating, 393, 393f
Xiyan Knee Eyes, 1166, 1166b, 1166f

Y

Yang
   Cold injures, 732
   collapse of, 465–467, 778, 778b
   consumption of, 15, 15f
   deficiency of, 419, 420f, 421, 422b, 477
   excess of, 15, 15f, 419, 421, 421b
   three types of, 421
   'original', 50–51
   and REN-4 Guanyuan Gate of the Original Qi, 1132
Yang Linking Vessel (Yang Wei Mai), 818–819, 877–878, 878b, 934–936, 934f
   body sides and, 935
   case history of, 936b
   classical indications of, 936, 936b
   clinical applications of, 935–936, 936b
   ear problems and, 935–936
   herbs/herbal therapy for, 819, 936
   intermittent fevers and, 935
   pathway of, 935, 935b
   points of, 934, 935b
   Yin Linking Vessel and, combined pathology of, 936–938, 937b
Yang organs, 10, 94, 103–105, 104b, 190
   correspondences of the Five Elements, 26t
   extraordinary vessels, 871
   positions for, 376b
   six extraordinary, 234–245, 235b
   Triple Burner as, 223–224, 223f, 224b
Yang-Qi, 58
Yang Stepping Vessel (Yang Qiao Mai), 817, 817f, 877, 877b, 883, 884f, 925–928, 926f, 1056–1057
   absorbs excess Yang from head, 926–927
   in backache and sciatica, 927, 927b
   case history of, 928b
   classical indications of, 928, 928b

clinical applications of, 926–927, 927b
eyes and, 927
herbs/herbal therapy for, 817, 928
hip and, 927
L.I.-16 and, 969
mental problems and, 927
pathway of, 925–926, 926b
points of, 925, 926b
Yin Stepping Vessel and, combined pathology of, 929–931, 931b
Yellow colour
of face, 315, 315b
of skin, 324
of Spleen, 151
'Yellow Emperor's Classic', 170
Yin
collapse of, 465, 778, 778b
consumption of, 15–16, 15f
deficiency of, 419, 422–423, 423b
Directing Vessel nourishes, 898
excess of, 15, 15f, 419, 420f, 422, 422b
types of, 422, 422f
Fire damage and, 747
L.I.-4 and, 964
'original', 50–51
and overwork, 283–284, 284f
Summer-Heat injures, 737
Yin Linking Vessel nourishes, 932
Yin channels, Connecting (Lou) points of, 998
Yin Linking Vessel *(Yin Wei Mai)*, 817–818, 818f, 877–878, 878b, 931–934, 932f
case history of, 934b
classical indications of, 933, 933b
clinical applications of, 932–933, 933b
headaches and, 933
herbal therapy and, 934
mental-emotional problems and, 933, 933b
nourishes Blood and Yin, 932
pathway of, 932, 932b
points of, 931, 932b
Yang Linking Vessel and, combined pathology of, 936–938, 937b
Yin organs, 10, 94, 96, 103–105, 104b
correspondences of the Five Elements, 26t
emotions and, 255
interrelationships, 175–187, 175b
Yin Stepping Vessel *(Yin Qiao Mai)*, 816–817, 816f, 877, 877b, 922–925, 923f, 1065, 1067, 1069
abdominal pain and, 924
atrophy *(Wei)* syndrome and, 924
case history of, 925b
classical indications of, 924–925, 925b
clinical applications of, 923–924, 924b
herbs/herbal therapy for, 816–817, 925
pathway of, 922–923, 923b
points of, 922, 923b
sleep and, 923–924, 924f
Yang Stepping Vessel and, combined pathology of, 929–931, 931b
Yin-Yang, 3–17, 3b
application to medicine, 9–11
ascending-descending of Qi and, 79–80, 80f
balance of, 15f
balancing channels, 1206f
and body structures, 9–11, 9f, 9t
case history in, 465b–466b
concept of, 3
correspondences of the Five Elements, 26t
in daily cycle, 5, 6f
ebb and flow of, in channels, 1195f
in Eight Principles, 465–467
function-structure of organs, 10–11, 10f, 13–14
historical development of, 4, 4f
imbalance of, 419–420, 420b
acupuncture treatment method and, 423b
Heat-Cold patterns and, 420, 420b, 420f
pathology of, 419–424, 419b
principles of treatment for, 423–424, 423b
interactions between, transformation and, 420–421, 421b, 421f
interdependence of, 7, 13–14
intertransformation of, 8, 16–17
mutual consuming of, 7–8, 8f, 14–16, 14f
nature of concept, 4–8, 4f–5f
opposition of, 11–13, 11b, 11t
principles of, 11–17
relationship of, 7–8
in seasonal cycle, 6, 6f
symbol of, 6, 7f
transformation/change-conservation/storage/sustainment in, 12–13, 13t
Yintang *Seal Hall*, 1159–1160, 1159f, 1160b
Yuyao *Fish Spine*, 1159f, 1160, 1160b

Z

Zigong *Palace of Child*, 1161f, 1162, 1162b

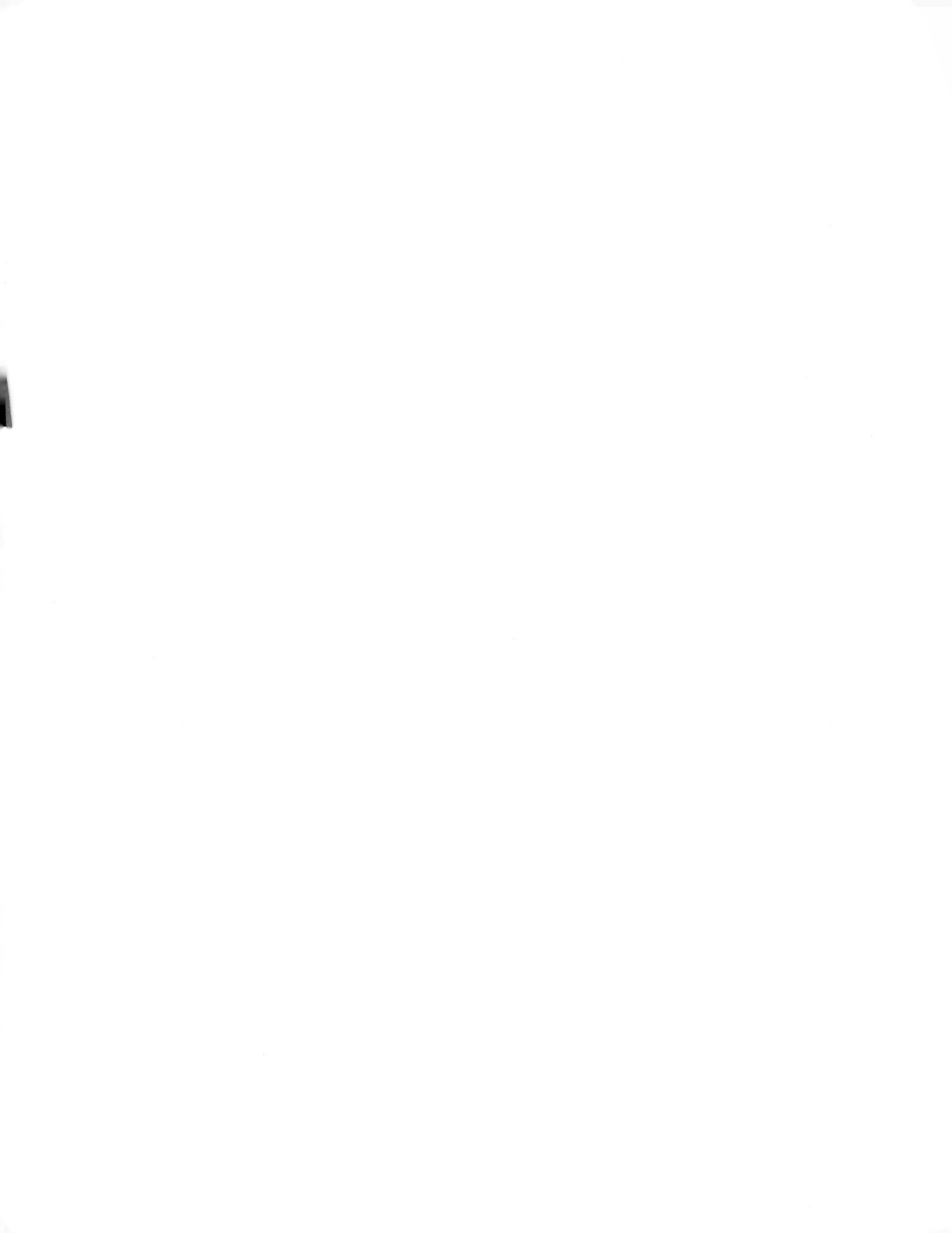

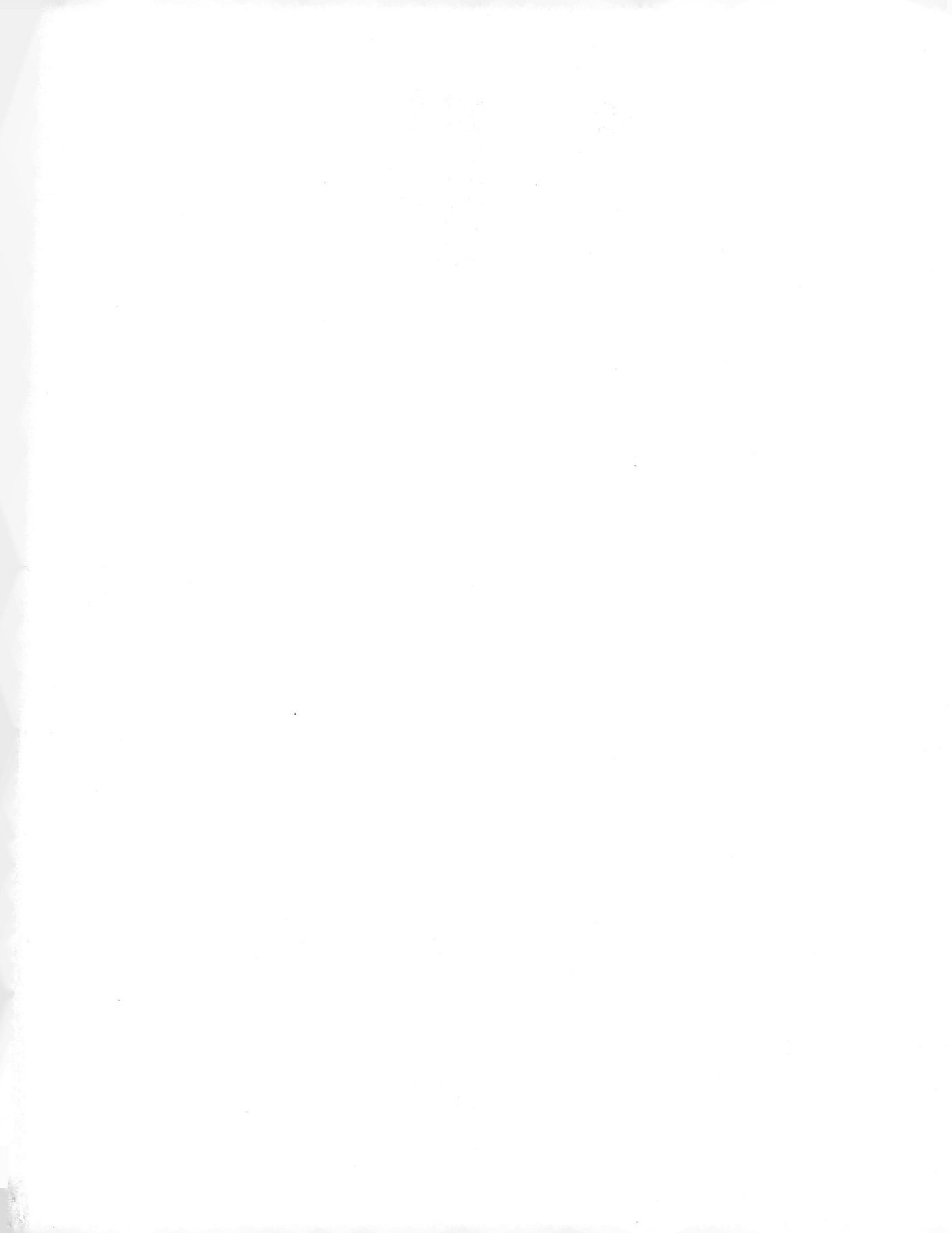